D1401169

I

Pathology: Implications for the Physical Therapist

Pathology: Implications for the Physical Therapist

Catherine Cavallaro Goodman, M.B.A., P.T.

School of Pharmacy and Allied Health Sciences
Physical Therapy Department
University of Montana
Missoula, Montana

William G. Boissonnault, M.S., P.T.

Rehabilitation Team Supervisor: Orthopedics
University of Wisconsin Hospital/Clinics
Associate Lecturer
University of Wisconsin–Madison Physical Therapy Program
Madison, Wisconsin

Assistant Professor, University of St. Augustine Center of Health Sciences
St. Augustine, Florida

Clinical Assistant Professor, Department of Rehabilitation Sciences
University of Tennessee–Memphis College of Allied Health Sciences
Memphis, Tennessee

Adjunct Faculty, Massachusetts General Hospital
Institute of Health Professions
Boston, Massachusetts

Instructor, Krannert Graduate School of Physical Therapy
University of Indianapolis
Indianapolis, Indiana

W.B. SAUNDERS COMPANY
A Division of Harcourt Brace & Company
Philadelphia London Toronto Montreal Sydney Tokyo

W.B. SAUNDERS COMPANY
A Division of Harcourt Brace & Company

The Curtis Center
Independence Square West
Philadelphia, Pennsylvania 19106

Library of Congress Cataloging-in-Publication Data

Goodman, Catherine Cavallaro.
Pathology : implications for the physical therapist / Catherine Cavallaro Goodman, William G. Boissonnault.—1st ed.

p. cm.

ISBN 0–7216–5636–6

1. Pathology. 2. Musculoskeletal system—Pathophysiology. 3. Nervous system—Pathophysiology. 4. Physical therapy. I. Boissonnault, William G. II. Title.

[DNLM: 1. Pathology. 2. Physical Therapy. QZ 140 G653p 1998]

RB111.G66 1998 149′.97—dc21

DNLM/DLC 97–7701

PATHOLOGY: IMPLICATIONS FOR THE PHYSICAL THERAPIST ISBN 0–7216–5636–6

Printed in the United States of America.

Last digit is the print number: 9 8 7 6 5 4 3 2 1

To Margaret M. Biblis, formerly senior editor, health-related professions, W.B. Saunders, in recognition of all you have done for the physical therapy profession through the many fine publications you have engineered.

C.C.G.

To the next generation: Joshua, Jacob, Eliya, Becky, Brandee, and Paul.

W.G.B.

Medical Consultant

Michael B. Koopmeiners, M.D.

Associate Professor, Institute of Physical Therapy
St. Augustine, Florida

Family Practice Physician
Health Partners Maplewood Clinic
Maplewood, Minnesota

Special Consultants

Kenda S. Fuller, P.T., N.C.S.

Certified Specialist in Neurologic Physical Therapy
Clinical Coordinator of Outpatient Physical Therapy
Rehabilitation Medicine
Clinical Instructor, Physical Therapy Program
University of Colorado Health Sciences Center
Denver, Colorado

Teresa E. Kelly Snyder, M.N., R.N., C.S.

Clinical Specialist in Medical-Surgical Nursing
Associate Professor of Nursing
Montana State University
Bozeman, Montana

contributors

Sharon M. Konecne, M.H.S., P.T.
Master of Health Care Systems
Oncology Physical Therapist
Lutheran Medical Center
Wheat Ridge, Colorado

Jim Miedaner, M.S., P.T.
Associate Director, Physical Therapy Department
University of Wisconsin Hospital and Clinics
Madison, Wisconsin

Terry Randall, M.S., P.T., O.C.S., A.T., C.
Captain, Army Medical Specialist Corps
Assistant Chief, Physical Therapy
Reynolds Army Hospital
Ft. Sill, Oklahoma

Marcia B. Smith, P.T., Ph.D.
Assistant Professor
Rehabilitation Medicine
Physical Therapy Program
University of Colorado Health Sciences Center
Denver, Colorado

Pam Unger, P.T.
Community General Hospital
Center for Wound Management
Reading, Pennsylvania

reviewers

Kay Biediger, M.S., P.T.
Director of Rehabilitation Services
St. Patrick Hospital
Missoula, Montana

Barbara Butler, M.S., P.T.
Surgical Chest Clinical Specialist
University of Michigan Medical Center
Ann Arbor, Michigan

Sharon McHugh Funk, P.T.
University of Colorado Health Sciences Center
Mountain States Regional Hemophilia Center
Denver, Colorado

Christine M. Fry, M.S., A.T., C.
Athletic Treatment Center
University of Montana
Missoula, Montana

Rose Heeg, S.P.T.
University of Montana
Missoula, Montana

Ellen Hillegass, M.M.Sc., P.T., C.C.S.
Georgia State University
Department of Physical Therapy
College of Health Sciences
Atlanta, Georgia

Elizabeth G. Hockey, M.Ed., P.T.
Department of Rehabilitation Services
University Hospitals of Cleveland
Cleveland, Ohio

Leonard N. Matheson, Ph.D., C.V.E.
Director, ERIC Human Performance Laboratory
Assistant Research Professor
Program in Occupational Therapy
Washington University School of Medicine
St. Louis, Missouri

Jeffrey L. Newman, P.T.
Chief, Physical Therapy
Veterans Affairs Medical Center
Minneapolis, Minnesota

Donna S. Oldfield, P.T.
Gulf State Hemophilia Diagnostic and Treatment Center
University of Texas–Houston
Houston, Texas

Catherine G. Page, Ph.D.
Director of Physical Therapy Program
Nova Southeastern University
North Miami Beach, Florida

Michael Schmitt, P.T.
St. Joseph's Hospital of Atlanta
Atlanta, Georgia

Lana Sineath, P.T., R.N.
Medical University of South Carolina (MUSC)
Medical Center, 3 SW Hospital
Charleston, South Carolina

Joanne Watchie, M.A., P.T., C.C.S.
University of Southern California University Hospital
Mount Saint Mary's
Los Angeles, California

Mitchel A. Woltersdorf, Ph.D., P.T.
Wesley Rehabilitation Hospital
College Hill Psychiatric Group
Wichita, Kansas

Vicky Wyder, P.T.
Chief Physical Therapist
Somerset Medical Center
Somerville, New Jersey

foreword

The role of all health-care providers has experienced tremendous change over the last 20 years. It was once said about Henry Ford, "It will take us 100 years to figure out whether you hurt us or helped us, but you sure didn't leave us like you found us." A similar statement can be made concerning changes in medicine.

While all change is loss and all loss must be grieved, change also presents some significant opportunities. To take full advantage of these opportunities and to solidify the therapist's role as a collaborative practitioner, a sound knowledge of clinical pathology is important. It is rare that providers address a medical condition that does not have some potential overlap into other areas of the person's life. As a physician, I cannot treat asthma without addressing the significant impact of breathing difficulties on the patient's day-to-day functioning. There are similar examples in a therapy setting, such as considering the presence of lupus (systemic lupus erythematosus) in a person with a recent total hip replacement or understanding vascular disease as it relates to the treatment of a patient with leg pain.

The text provides information for the therapist to better appreciate the significant overlaps between neuromusculoskeletal conditions and other medical pathologic conditions. In particular, the therapist must evaluate how comorbidities and prescribed medical treatment can affect clinical decision making. The emphasis on clinical application is a unique feature of this textbook. Too frequently, pathology is presented in such a way that it fails to emphasize the clinical importance to the therapist. This text demonstrates that pathology can be clinically relevant.

It is my personal hope that this text will increase effective communication between therapists and physicians. This can be achieved by providing a common understanding and language for communication between the therapist and physician. In this process, physicians can enhance their knowledge of the therapist's role in treating neuromusculoskeletal pathology. Collaborative practice and optimum patient outcome require strong working relationships between all members of the health-care delivery team.

As the primary medical consultant to this project, it is difficult to express my opinion of this text without the potential of seeming pretentious. The contributing authors did the hard work. Their eagerness to produce an excellent product, willingness to do the extensive research, and openness to feedback have resulted in this final product, an excellent resource for the therapist.

I have been privileged to know and to work with many wonderful therapists during my medical career. Recognizing my inadequacies and taking advantage of learning opportunities that were available by discussing mutual cases with therapists has been one of the better professional decisions I have made during my career. Participating in the completion of this text has been an enjoyable learning experience for me. My contact with the authors of this text reinforces the respect I have for their profession and the care they render our mutual patients. It has been an honor to write this foreword.

Michael B. Koopmeiners, M.D.

preface

The ever-evolving health-care delivery system presents physical and occupational therapists with multiple challenges and responsibilities. Limitations imposed by prospective reimbursement systems have resulted in hospital admissions only in the case of serious illness, earlier discharge from the acute care setting, and limited outpatient visits. These factors have resulted in therapists evaluating and treating clients who are critically ill or who have significant health problems, necessitating changes in therapy approaches and techniques.

In addition, nearly two thirds of hospitalized clients who present with an acute episode of a chronic health problem are age 65 years or older. A multitude of co-morbidities, such as diabetes mellitus, hypertension, and atherosclerotic cardiovascular disease, can exist in this population as well as in clients seen in outpatient settings.

The therapist must recognize when medical complications require precautions or even possibly represent a contraindication to certain techniques or to therapy altogether. A thorough understanding of the pathologic processes and of the medical diagnostic and treatment procedures is vital to develop a rehabilitation program that is safe and effective.

The purpose of this textbook is to provide information designed to facilitate the students' and clinicians' understanding of how pathologic processes can affect their practice. Toward that end, whenever possible or appropriate we have provided a feature, *Special Implications for the Therapist*, specifically for the therapist to consider prior to establishing a treatment plan. The information in these sections quickly outlines any special considerations necessary for each pathologic condition presented.

The text is organized into four major sections. The introductory section presents a broad overview of pathologic concepts, taking into consideration biopsychosocial aspects of health, aging, illness, and disease. Many conditions affect multiple body organs and systems, including the neuromusculoskeletal system. We thought it would be helpful for the student to step back and view pathologic conditions from an overall perspective, rather than just focus on the individual body parts affected. For this reason, we included the chapter Problems Affecting Multiple Systems (Chapter 4) before turning the focus toward individual disease entities.

Section 2 deals with pathology of the individual organs and body systems. Diseases of these anatomic structures constitute what is traditionally referred to as clinical medicine. Section 3 covers pathology of the musculoskeletal system; the neurologic system is discussed separately in Section 4.

Each disease process is discussed from the perspective of a traditional medical model (e.g., definition, incidence, etiology, pathogenesis, clinical manifestations) with a clinical emphasis (e.g., medical diagnosis and treatment, special implications for the therapist). Whenever possible, other considerations, such as nutrition, medication, psychosocial status, and emotional response to the illness and/or treatment, are included.

For example, pharmacology is the medical treatment of choice for many conditions; the therapist must recognize when drug therapy may have a direct impact on proposed exercise or another therapy program. Drug interactions or drug effects may mimic symptoms of pathology or, conversely, mask symptoms of underlying pathology. The therapist is often the first to observe any of these effects and must be able to recognize the need for further medical investigation.

Finally, a chapter is included with a clinical focus on laboratory test results. These test results reflect the components of the medical management discussed throughout the text that are particularly pertinent to the therapist. As with the specific results of pathologic processes, a therapist must know when test results indicate a need for necessary precautions or a contraindication to therapy.

All in all, clinical pathology as it relates to practice has been our focus. We have made every attempt to look toward the future of therapy practice and to provide the reader with as much clinically oriented information as possible. We welcome any input you may like to offer in making this a text for clinicians in any health-care setting.

Catherine Cavallaro Goodman
William G. Boissonnault

acknowledgments

Though we may receive credit for this project, we are eager to recognize the contributions of many family members, friends, and professionals, both in our immediate circles and across the country in what is affectionately referred to as "the family of physical therapists." In particular, we would like to especially mention the following:

All of the members of our families for their patience, understanding, cooperation, and support . . . for providing extra childcare and extra meals, guarding office doors, listening to us vent, and anything else they would add to this list.

All of the physical therapists, physicians, pathologists, and researchers who released their findings and manuscripts to us prior to publication.

The many authors and publishers who have allowed us to publish some of their tables and figures to help present the information in a quick-reference format for both students and clinicians.

To Elaine Wilder, M.A., P.T., Margaret Herning, Ph.D., P.T., and Rosemary Norris, M.S., P.T., School of Allied Health Professions, Department of Physical Therapy, St. Louis University Health Sciences Center, St. Louis, for their patient and valiant efforts to provide us with information about pathology across the lifespan.

All those who made it possible to use their photographs, especially Jeffrey P. Callen, M.D., Pam Unger, Kurt Dasse, Johnson and Johnson Interventional Systems, and Carol Lynn Daly (Thomas Jefferson University, Philadelphia).

The physicians of our communities for sharing books, materials, and counsel, especially Rae Johnston, Peggy Schlesinger, Stephen Speckart, and Judy Visscher in Missoula, Montana, and Carol Foster in Denver.

Many organizations, such as the National Hemophilia Foundation, American Heart Association, Alliance for Aging, APTA Aquatic Section (Ann Charness, President), American Society for the Advancement of Lymphedema Management, Centers for Disease Control and Prevention, National Multiple Sclerosis Society, National Stroke Association, and The National Institutes of Health, for assistance in finding data and references.

The staff of St. Patrick Hospital, Missoula, Montana, especially the medical library staff, Marianne Farr and Kathy Murphy; Kay Biediger, Director of Rehabilitation Services, and the physical therapy staff; and Vicki Tomascak, B.S., B.A., M.T.-A.S.C.P., C.I.C. certified, infection control coordinator.

Lynn Palmer, for her patience and persistence related to the preparation of certain parts of the manuscript.

The physical therapy students of Krannert Graduate School of Physical Therapy, University of Indianapolis, for information presented in their professional papers, especially Jane Ford and Marilyn Mason.

The Director of Rehabilitation Services, Patricia Sanders-Hall, and the physical therapy staff at the University of Colorado Hospital, Denver, and the students and faculty of the University of Colorado Health Sciences Center Physical Therapy Program for review and comments regarding the text.

M. (Peg) Waltner, developmental editor, who did a fabulous job of organizing the various sections of the manuscript.

All of the staff at W.B. Saunders who contributed their skills and efforts toward this project.

To these people and to the many others who remain unnamed but not forgotten, we say thank you. Your support and encouragement have made this text possible.

Catherine Cavallaro Goodman
William G. Boissonnault
Kenda S. Fuller
Michael B. Koopmeiners

contents

section 1

Introduction

SECTION 1

chapter 1

Introduction to Concepts of Pathology

Catherine C. Goodman

THE PATHOGENESIS OF DISEASE

Pathology is defined as the branch of medicine that investigates disease, especially structural and functional changes in body tissues and organs that cause or are caused by disease (O'Toole, 1992). *Clinical pathology* in medicine refers to pathology applied to the solution of clinical problems, especially the use of laboratory methods in clinical diagnosis. *Pathogenesis* is the development of unhealthy conditions or disease, more specifically the cellular events and reactions and other pathologic mechanisms that occur in the development of disease.

In this text, we examine the pathogenesis of each disease or condition, that is the progression of each pathologic condition on the cellular level as well as its clinical presentation, when signs and symptoms are manifested. For the therapist, clinical pathology has a different meaning as we explore the effects of pathologic processes (i.e., disease) on the individual's functional abilities and limitations. The relationship between impairment and functional limitation is the key focus in therapy.

Using this revised definition of clinical pathology, we ask, *How does this particular disease or condition affect this person's functional abilities and functional outcome? What precautions should be taken when someone with this condition is exercising? Should vital signs be monitored during therapy for this disease? How will that information affect the treatment plan?*

We must evaluate each individual client on the basis of the clinical presentation in conjunction with the underlying pathology. For example, the person with osteoporosis may require joint mobilization, but this technique must be modified for the presence of osteoporosis. Or the individual with cardiac valvular disease may need a different exercise program than that prescribed for a healthy athlete. Or the adult with musculoskeletal symptoms of thoracic spine pain, muscle spasm, and loss of thoracic motion who has a primary medical diagnosis (e.g., posterior penetrating ulcer) will be unaffected by therapy techniques.

This text explores the advances in medicine that have resulted in a population with greater longevity but also with a more complex pathologic picture. Orthopedic and neurologic conditions no longer present as singular phenomena; they frequently occur in a person with other medical pathology. We must be cognizant of the impact of other conditions and diseases on the individual's neuromusculoskeletal system and take the necessary steps to provide safe *and* effective treatment.

CONCEPTS OF HEALTH AND ILLNESS

(Ignatavicius and Bayne, 1991)

Health

Many people and organizations have attempted to define the concept of health but no universally accepted definition has been adopted. A dictionary definition describes health in terms of an individual's ability to function normally in society. Some definitions characterize health as a disease-free state or condition. The World Health Organization (WHO) (1947) has defined health as a state of complete physical, mental, and social well-being, and not merely as the absence of disease or infirmity. All of these definitions present health as an "either/or" circumstance—an individual is either healthy or ill.

Health may be viewed as a continuum on which wellness—at one end—is the optimal level of function, and illness—at the opposite end—may be so unfavorable as to result in death. Health is a dynamic process that varies with changes in interactions between an individual and the internal and external environments. This type of definition recognizes health as an individual's level of wellness. Health reflects a person's biologic, psychological, spiritual, and sociologic state. The *biologic* or physical state, refers to the overall structure of the individual's body tissues and organs as well as to the biochemical interactions and functions within the body. The *psychological* state includes the individual's mood, emotions, and personality. The *spiritual* aspect of health addresses the individual's religious needs, which may be affected by illness or injury. The *sociologic* or social state, refers to the interaction between the individual and the social environment. A high level of wellness or holistic health is achieved when the biopsychosocial needs of a person are met.

Illness

Definition

Illness is often defined as sickness or deviation from a healthy state, and the term has a broader meaning than *disease*. Disease refers to a biologic or psychological alteration that results in a malfunction of a body organ or system. Disease is usually the term that is used to describe a biomedical condition that is substantiated by objective data, such as elevated temperature or presence of infection (as demonstrated by positive blood cultures). Illness is the perception and response of the person to not being well. Illness includes disturbances in normal human biologic function as well as personal, interpersonal, and cultural reactions to disease. Disease can occur in an individual without the person's being aware of illness and without others perceiving illness. However, a person can feel very ill even though no obvious pathologic processes can be identified (Coe, 1970).

Acute Illness

Acute illness usually refers to an illness or disease that has a relatively rapid onset and short duration. The condition frequently responds to a specific treatment and is usually self-limiting, although exceptions to this definition are numerous, such as viral infections, which need no pharmacologic treatment, or acute lymphocytic leukemia, which frequently results in death. If no complications occur, most acute illnesses end in a full recovery, and the individual returns to the previous level of functioning. *Subacute* refers to a condition or illness that is somewhat acute (i.e., between acute and chronic). Chronic conditions sometimes flare up and may be referred to as subacute.

Acute illnesses usually follow a specific sequence, or stages of illness, from onset through recovery. The first stage involves the experience of physical symptoms (e.g., pain, shortness of breath, fever), cognitive awareness (i.e., the symptoms are interpreted to have meaning), and an emotional response, usually one of denial, fear, or anxiety.

Subsequent stages of an acute illness may include assumption of a "sick" role as the person recognizes the problem as being sufficient to require contact with a health care professional. If the illness is confirmed, the individual continues in the sick role; if it is not confirmed, a return to normalcy may occur or the person may continue to seek health care to identify the illness. A stage of dependency[1] occurs when the person receives and accepts a diagnosis and treatment plan. Depending on the severity of the illness, the individual may give up independence and control and assume a more dependent sick role. During this stage, sick people often become more passive and concerned about themselves. Most people move to the final stage of recovery or rehabilitation. During this stage, the individual gives up the sick role and resumes more normal activities and responsibilities. Individuals with long-term or chronic illnesses may require a longer period of time to adjust to new lifestyles.

Chronic Illness

Chronic illness describes illnesses that include one or more of the following characteristics: permanent impairment or disability, residual physical or cognitive disability, or the need for special rehabilitation and/or long-term medical management. Chronic illnesses and conditions may fluctuate in intensity as acute exacerbations occur that cause physiologic instability and necessitate additional medical management. A person who has exacerbations of chronic illness may progress through the stages of illness described in the previous section.

Psychological Aspects *(Berman and Blumenfield, 1992)*

The most important factor influencing psychological reactions to illness is the premorbid (before illness) psychological profile of the affected person. For example, a person with a dependent-type personality may become very dependent, perhaps seeking unusually great amounts of advice or reassurance from the health care specialist or expecting attention beyond that required for the degree of illness present. A narcissistic (self-centered) person may be particularly concerned about the need to take medication or the loss of the ability to work. The stoic person (indifferent to or unaffected by pain) may have difficulty admitting to being sick at all.

Other factors that affect a person's psychological reaction include the extent of the illness and the particular symptoms that develop. Extremely mild disease may have little effect, whereas completely unexpected and debilitating illness may be very distressing. A common reaction to any illness is fear related to the loss of control over one's own body. Denial is an unconscious defense mechanism that allows a person to avoid painful reality as long as possible. Denial can be a natural part of the process of dealing with illness, which culminates in acceptance.

Noncompliance with treatment may have a psychological basis (e.g., denial—"*There is nothing wrong with me, therefore I do not need medical treatment*"), but it may also occur as a result of previous experience. For example, noncompliance with prescribed corticosteroid therapy may be based on aversion to side effects experienced during use of this drug during previous disease flare. With chronic autoimmune diseases (e.g., connective tissue diseases), denial may continue for years as a coping mechanism for the individual who continues to decline in physical functional capacity.

It is important to recognize that psychological or psychiatric symptoms, such as impairment of memory, personality changes (e.g., paranoia), loss of impulse control, or mood disorders (e.g., persistent depression or elation) can have a functional or organic basis. Functional symptoms occur without significant physical dysfunction of brain cells, whereas organic symptoms can be caused by abnormal physiologic changes in brain tissue. An example of a functional symptom is depression that is considered to be the psychological consequence of a general medical condition (e.g., myocardial infarction).

Organic symptoms occur as a direct physiologic consequence of a medical condition, such as multiple sclerosis, stroke, or hypothyroidism. For example, a person with systemic lupus erythematosus (SLE) may experience symptoms of organic mental disorders secondary to SLE-mediated vasculitis, called *lupus cerebritis*, or a person with endstage liver disease may develop hepatic encephalopathy when toxic substances in the blood, such as ammonia, reach the brain. Onset of corticosteroid-induced psychological symptoms is another example of an organic basis for symptomatology. In this instance, symptoms may be rapid or delayed, are frequently dose-related, and subside as the corticosteroids are tapered.

Disability Classifications *(Fuller and Huber, 1995; Jette, 1986)*

According to the Centers for Disease Control and Prevention, during the 1991 to 1992 year, about 48.9 million persons (19% of the total U.S. population) had a disability (MMWR, 1994). Among this population, 3.8 million persons (approximately 8%) were younger than 17 years.

Physical Disability

The WHO (1990) has developed an International Classification of Impairments, Disabilities, and Handicaps (ICIDH) to

[1] This type of dependency in the psychologically and emotionally balanced person represents the awareness, acceptance, and reliance on diagnosis and care beyond self-help. This definition of dependency differs from dependency associated with dependent personality disorder, in which the affected person lacks self-confidence or the ability to function independently, and allows others to assume responsibility for his or her care.

provide a conceptual framework for standardization of data and monitoring of chronic and disabling conditions. The ICIDH clarifies the concepts common to rehabilitation and further defines impairments, disability, and handicap.

Impairment is any loss or abnormality of psychological, physiologic, or anatomic structure or function (e.g., range-of-motion limitations, decreased strength or muscle performance, edema, lack of sensation). Impairments can be temporary or permanent and are considered to occur at the organ level. Another example is proprioceptive loss in an extremity resulting in decreased sensory input to the central nervous system.

Disability is any restriction or lack of ability to perform an activity in a normal manner or within the normal range. A person's disability status or activity restriction describes how the impairment affects activities at work or home or participation in sports. The disability resulting from an impairment in proprioception might be excessive weight shift away from the affected extremity. The person may be at greater risk of falling. Not all disease leads to impairment, and not all impairment leads to disability. For example, diabetes can result in impairment (e.g., diminished circulation), but not all persons with diabetes sustain a disability (e.g., vision loss or amputation) (Clifton, 1995).

Handicap is a disadvantage for an impaired or disabled individual that limits or prevents the fulfillment of normal life roles. An example of a handicap would be the inability to be independently mobile in the community due to lack of stability required in the diverse environmental situations encountered there.

A second system often used by health care professionals to classify the impact of disease or trauma is the Nagi health status model (Nagi, 1969). The Nagi model differs from the ICIDH in the use of the terms *functional limitation* and *disability* (Table 1–1). Nagi proposed that functional limitations were the result of impairments and consisted of an individual's inability to perform the tasks and roles that constitute usual activities for that individual. According to the Nagi model, disability is defined as the patterns of behavior that emerge over long periods of time when functional limitations cannot be overcome to create "normal" task performance or role fulfillment.

Cognitive Disability (*Woltersdorf, 1992*)

Problems such as depression and cognitive impairments often are undiagnosed (Clopton and McMahon, 1992), and although therapists cannot diagnose these impairments, recognizing the deficits is important. There are five types of cognitive deficit associated with specific areas of brain damage and linked to possible causes that may be barriers to successful treatment (Table 1–2).

Executive functions may be described as cortical functions involved in formulating goals and in planning, initiating, monitoring, and maintaining behavior (Lezak, 1983). *Behavior* is defined here in its broadest terms to include not only overt motor behavior but also affective and social behavior. A person with executive function deficits typically appears inert or apathetic. Clinically, these patients typically have a right hemisphere lesion and apraxia, unilateral neglect, or both. When frontal lobe damage occurs, the effects of impaired executive functions may be attributed to depression. Although the two may occur simultaneously, depression is usually characterized by a lack of energy, whereas impaired executive functions are demonstrated by a lack of involvement.

Complex problem-solving may be described as the effective handling of new information. Impaired problem-solving results in concrete thinking, inability to distinguish the relevant from the irrelevant, erroneous application of rules, and difficulty generalizing from one situation to another. For example, when a client learns how to accomplish wheelchair transfers and then generalizes that information to various settings (bed to chair, chair to toilet, chair to car, in hospital, at home) he or she is using new information in complex problem-solving.

Information processing involves the speed with which information travels from one part of the brain to another and the amount of information assimilated at that speed (Lezak, 1983). Whereas complex problem-solving has to do with the orchestration of information, information processing involves the efficient transfer of information. As a result of genetic, environmental, and educational factors, some people are more proficient processors than others. As a result of trauma, some people may lose processing ability and speed. Noise levels, external sensory stimulation (e.g., presence of other people and other activities), presentation of more than one kind of information at a time (e.g., providing a written home program then discussing the time of the next appointment) are examples of distractions to persons with reduced information-processing abilities.

Memory deficits occur when there is a failure to store or retrieve information. Before it can be determined that the person is experiencing a memory lapse, it must be established that the material was learned in the first place. Memory problems typically are acquired rather than developmental. Depression may masquerade as memory loss, but the depressed person is usually less attentive or interactive with the environment and therefore registers (or learns) less. For example, a client may appear to be suffering from a memory dysfunction when, in fact, the decreased attention span is a result of depression that has reduced learning.

Learning disability occurs in a person with normal or near-normal intelligence as difficulty acquiring information in specific domains, such as spelling, arithmetic, reading, and visual-spatial relationships. Therapists most commonly encounter learning disabilities manifested as noncompliance with written treatment programs, repeated tardiness or absence for treatment sessions, and an overly anxious approach to the

TABLE 1-1 Disability Classifications

ICIDH Model	Nagi Model
Disease	Disease
Impairment	Impairment
Disability	Functional limitations
Handicap	Disability

ICIDH, International Classification of Impairments, Disabilities, and Handicaps.
Data from Fuller K, Huber L: Improving postural control through integration of sensory inputs and visual biofeedback. Top Stroke Rehabil 1:32–47, 1995.

TABLE 1-2 Types of Cognitive Deficits

Type	Lesion	Etiology	Therapist Strategies
Decreased executive functions	Right hemisphere lesion; frontal lobe damage	Car accidents; whiplash injuries; exposure to organic solvents; AIDS/HIV complications; Korsakoff's disease; Parkinson's disease; craniotomy	More active role in maintaining treatment program, educating family and client's employer, teaching self-monitoring skills; include pacing in treatment regimen; use home trainers; closely monitor all clinic activities; teach time management techniques; include client in group activities; do not take socially inappropriate behavior personally
Poor complex problem-solving	Diffuse and/or global cortical damage	Exposure to occupational toxins; postsurgical anoxia; stroke; hydrocephalus; small-vessel disease associated with hypertension	Fragment treatment program into small pieces and reassemble pieces into coherent whole when each has been well-learned; turn the new into the familiar through repetition; reduce complexity of treatment components, avoid abstract visual aids and abstract verbal explanations
Slowed information processing	Diffuse cortical or subcortical system damage; reticular activating system of the brainstem	Alcohol abuse; drug abuse; exposure to toxins; developmental delays; traumatic brain injury	Slow the rate of presentation; remove environmental distractors; do not speak loudly as though client were hearing impaired; simply present one type of information at a time, making sure the client understands you before you move on
Memory deficits	Temporal lobe damage	Alcohol abuse; temporal lobe injuries; seizures; traumatic brain injury; exposure to toxins; age-related deterioration	Make certain that no learning or emotional disorder is involved; use external aids and multichannel approaches to improve retention of information; determine which aid or approach works best for each individual
Learning disabilities	Unclear	Unknown; possibly traumatic birth, genetic predisposition; early acquired brain damage; metabolic abnormalities	Avoid written material unless it is appropriate to the person's reading level; use nonverbal modes of communication

Adapted from Woltersdorf MA: Beyond the sensorimotor strip. Clin Manage 12:63–69, 1992.

physical symptoms that have brought the client to the therapist in the first place.

Special Implications for the Therapist **1-1**

COGNITIVE DISABILITY

Although therapists cannot diagnose cognitive deficits, the therapist's evaluation and clinical observations may help identify cognitive deficits that might interfere with treatment. Appropriate referral is always recommended when problems beyond our expertise are suspected. Specific rehabilitation and training strategies for persons with cognitive disabilities are available (Woltersdorf, 1992).

Theories of Health and Illness *(Black, 1993)*

Many theories exist as to the cause of illnesses. In the latter part of the 19th century, Pasteur's *germ theory* promoted our understanding of infectious disease. Pasteur proposed that a specific microorganism was capable of causing an infectious disease. The germ theory cannot explain all diseases, and other more complex theories have been postulated.

The *biomedical model* explains disease as a result of malfunctioning organs or cells. Within this model, conditions can be classified as diseases if they have a recognized cause and if there is a consistently identifiable group of signs and symptoms. The biomedical model focuses on cause-and-effect relationships but does not take into account psychosocial components of disease, such as varying reactions to a disease due to age, lifestyle, personality, and compliance with therapy.

In the past, the high death rate from epidemics of infectious diseases meant that many people did not live long enough for chronic illnesses to develop, especially those that occur with aging. With the development of penicillin in 1928, and with the subsequent development of other antibiotics, people in the 20th century have had reduced mortality from infectious disease. Heart disease and cancer have become the center of focus. However, many diseases previously under control (e.g., tuberculosis) are resurging with increasing resistance to one or more antibiotics (Tomasz, 1994). Resistant infections kill 19,000 US hospital patients and contribute to the deaths of 58,000 every year (CDC, 1994).

Homeostatic or *multicausal theories* have been proposed to take into account the many additional factors associated with health and the development of illness (Fig. 1–1). Many of these variables are discussed further in Chapter 3. Homeostasis is the body's ability to maintain its internal environment in a constant state of equilibrium despite external influences that promote imbalance. The body's ability to maintain temperature, blood pressure, and levels of fluid and electrolytes, serum glucose, blood oxygen, and carbon dioxide within a given range are examples of homeostasis.

The *general adaptation syndrome* describes a response to stress that, regardless of diagnosis, has common symptoms, such as appetite loss, weight loss, myalgias, and fatigue. The entire body responds to stress in an attempt to maintain or adapt through the autonomic and central nervous systems. If the demand or stress continues, the adaptive capacity of the body can be exceeded, and disease may result. This theory suggests that stress causes disease by placing excessive demands on the body, which in turn produces high levels of adaptive hormones, such as glucocorticoids (which reduce inflammation) and mineralocorticoid hormones (which regulate electrolyte and water metabolism). These hormones lower the body's resistance to disease and cause organ damage.

Psychosocial theories of disease attempt to integrate physiologic, psychological, and social factors to explain disease. An individual's degree of resistance to microbes depends largely on how well he or she is coping. Resistance to infectious disease, allergies, and possibly cancer depends on a well-functioning immune system. People who cope poorly with stress have significantly impaired immune responses, as manifested by a diminished activity level in natural killer cells. These are a special type of leukocyte that destroys viruses and cancer cells without having previously encountered them. Biopsychosocial concepts as they relate to health are discussed more fully in Chapter 2.

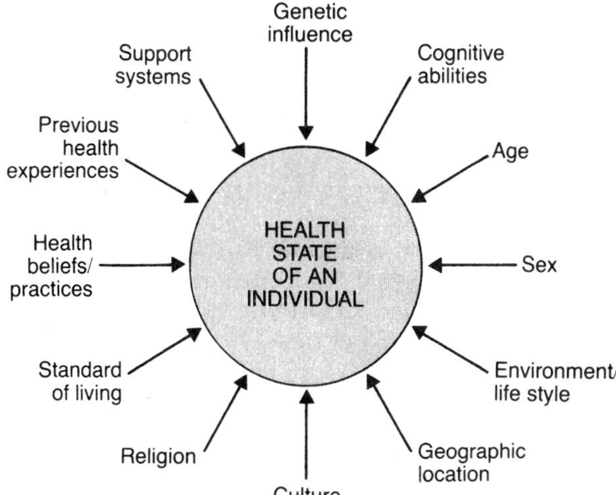

Figure 1–1. Multiple variables influence the health and illness of an individual. *(From Ignatavicius DD, Bayne MV: Medical-Surgical Nursing. Philadelphia, WB Saunders, 1991, p 8.)*

Genetic Aspects of Disease *(Black, 1993)*

In addition to research on the biopsychosocial aspects of diseases, there has been a great deal of recent research into the genetic aspects of diseases. Recent technology has enabled researchers to identify the actual gene that encodes a particular disorder. It may be possible in the near future to treat altered gene structure (called gene therapy) to attempt to eliminate certain disease processes. More specifically, gene therapy is the process in which specific malfunctioning cells are targeted and repaired or replaced with corrected genes. It is hoped that the altered cells will yield daughter cells with healthy genes; these offspring cells will help eliminate the diseased cells. Research is ongoing into such cures for cystic fibrosis, brain cancer, Duchenne's muscular dystrophy, hypercholesterolemia, diabetes, hemophilia, Parkinson's disease, and adenosine deaminase enzyme (ADA) deficiency. The laboratory studies and recent advances in the collection of immune cells now makes clinical trials of gene therapy feasible.

HEALTH PROMOTION AND DISEASE PREVENTION

Health Promotion

Health promotion as a concept and as an active process is built on the principles of self-responsibility, nutritional awareness, stress reduction and management, and physical fitness. Health promotion is not limited to any particular age group but rather extends throughout the life span from before birth (e.g., prenatal care) through old age. Health promotion programs that encompass the entire life span are applicable to persons of both sexes and all socioeconomic and cultural backgrounds, to those who have no health problems, and to those with chronic illnesses and disabilities. Many types of health promotion programs are in existence, such as health screening, wellness, safety, stress management, or support groups for specific diseases (Brunner and Suddarth, 1988).

Disease Prevention

It has been recognized that preventing disease is more cost-effective than treating disease, and this has therefore been addressed by greater numbers of health care professionals. Preventive medicine as a branch of medicine is categorized as primary, secondary, or tertiary.

Primary prevention is geared toward removing or reducing disease risk factors, for example, by maintaining adequate levels of calcium intake and regular exercise as a means of preventing osteoporosis and subsequent bone fractures, or by giving up or not starting smoking to reduce multiple causes of morbidity. Use of seatbelts, helmets by motorcyclists and bicyclists, and immunizations are other examples of primary prevention strategies.

Secondary prevention techniques are designed to promote early detection of disease and to employ preventive measures to avoid further complications. Examples of secondary prevention include skin tests for tuberculosis or screening procedures such as mammography, colonoscopy, or routine cervical Papanicolaou smear.

Tertiary prevention measures are aimed at limiting the

impact of established disease (e.g., radiation or chemotherapy to control localized cancer) (Schroeder and McPhee, 1994). Tertiary prevention involves rehabilitation and may end when no further healing is expected. The goal of tertiary prevention is to return the person to the highest possible level of functioning and to prevent severe disabilities (Ignatavicius and Bayne, 1991).

References

Berman HM, Blumenfield MM: Psychiatric symptoms in systemic lupus erythematosus. J Musculoskel Med 9:81–94, 1992.

Black JM: Theories of health and illness. *In* Black JM, Matassarin-Jacobs E, (eds): Luckmann and Sorensen's Medical-Surgical Nursing, ed 4. Philadelphia, WB Saunders, 1993, pp 43–58.

Brunner LS, Suddarth DS: Textbook of Medical-Surgical Nursing, ed 6. Philadelphia, JB Lippincott, 1988.

Clopton N, McMahon T: Patient compliance. Clin Management 12:59–65, 1992.

Clifton DW: "Tolerated treatment well" may no longer be tolerated. PT Magazine 3:24–27, 1995.

Coe R: Sociology of Medicine. New York, McGraw-Hill, 1970.

Cohen M (Centers for Disease Control and Prevention spokesman): Personal communication, 1994.

Disabilities among children aged ≤ 17 years—United States, 1991–1992. MMWR 44:609–613, 1995.

Fuller K, Huber L: Improving postural control through integration of sensory inputs and visual biofeedback. Top Stroke Rehab 1:32–47, 1995.

Ignatavicius DD, Bayne MV: Medical-Surgical Nursing. Philadelphia, WB Saunders, 1991.

Jette AM: Functional disability and rehabilitation of the aged. Top Geriatr Rehab 1:1–7, 1986.

Lezak, M: Neuropsychological Assessment. New York, Oxford University Press, 1983.

Nagi SZ: Disability and Rehabilitation. Columbus, Ohio State University Press, 1969.

O'Toole M (ed): Miller-Keane Encyclopedia and Dictionary of Medicine, Nursing, and Allied Health, ed 5. Philadelphia, WB Saunders, 1992.

Prevalence of disabilities and associated health conditions—United States, 1991–1992. MMWR 43:730–731, 737–739, 1994.

Schroeder SA, McPhee SJ: General approach to the patient; health maintenance and disease prevention; and common symptoms. *In* Tierney LM, McPhee SJ, Papadakis MA (eds): Current Medical Diagnosis and Treatment, ed 33. Norwalk, Conn, Appleton & Lange, 1994, pp 1–15.

Tomasz A: American Association for the Advancement of Science, annual meeting, San Francisco, February 1994.

Woltersdorf MA: Beyond the sensorimotor strip. Clin Management 12:63–69, 1992.

World Health Organization: Constitution of the World Health Organization: Chronicle of the World Health Organization. Geneva, Switzerland, 1947, p 1.

World Health Organization: International classification of impairments, disabilities, and handicaps: A manual of classification relating to the consequences of disease. Geneva, Switzerland, 1990.

SECTION 1

chapter 2

Biopsychosocial Concepts Related to Health Care

Catherine C. Goodman

OVERVIEW

During the last two decades basic scientists and clinicians have started to consider the complex biopsychosocial phenomena associated with disease, illness, and injury. Multidisciplinary team and managed care approaches to such conditions now address the needs of the client in terms of the psychological impact, social needs, and comprehensive biologic picture that goes beyond medication and surgical intervention as the primary forms of medical treatment. During the 1980s, the medical model was influenced by a movement toward what was then called *holistic health*, the notion that the physical, mental, social, and spiritual aspects of a person's life must be viewed as an integrated whole. Since that time it has become well established that social support plays a key role in promoting health, decreasing susceptibility to disease, and facilitating recovery from illness or injury. Client care must be focused on emotional and social needs as well as physical needs (see Fig. 1–1).

Now that technology has provided opportunities for research on the body's response to disease at the cellular and tissue level, a new concept has developed called *psychoneuroimmunology*. This study of behavioral-neural-endocrine-immune system interactions has provided a basis for exploring the idea that behavior can alter immune function and vice versa, that is, that immunologic changes account for some behaviors (Ader et al., 1991). The interactions between these systems may also provide the means whereby psychosocial factors and emotional states influence the development and progression of infectious, autoimmune, and neoplastic diseases. The association between stressful life experiences and changes in immune function do not establish a causal link between stress, immune function, and disease as this chain of events has not yet been definitively established. However, major links between these systems have been identified and a new understanding of interactive biologic signaling has begun.

Psychoneuroimmunology is just beginning to identify the reciprocal relations between neural and immune function, endocrine and immune function, and behavior and immune function. Researchers are beginning to develop the means to explore these relations and their clinical and therapeutic implications (Ader et al., 1995; see also Chapter 5).

PERSONAL HEALTH CARE AND PREVENTIVE MEDICINE

Variations in Client Populations

Geographic Variations (*Rubin and Farber, 1994*)

The geographic and political climates of countries play a role in determining how people live and the health problems that commonly develop. For example, in the United States obesity, alcoholism, sedentary lifestyle, and tobacco use have contributed significantly to the most common causes of morbidity and mortality (Table 2–1, Fig. 2–1).

A half century ago a few physicians cultivated an interest in diseases that seemed to have strict geographic boundaries. As a result, a discipline called *geographic pathology* developed. Geographic pathology was concerned with diseases endemic (present in a community at all times) to certain areas of the world, most often parasitic and infectious diseases that seemed unique to individual geographic regions.

With the discovery that chemical agents are mediators of a variety of tissue changes, and with the recognition that many of these causative agents are environmental contaminants, a component called *occupational disease* was added. Disease caused by contaminants was included to constitute the field of *environmental pathology*. For further discussion, see Chapter 3.

Race

Race or ethnic background predisposes people to certain diseases and chronic conditions. Data indicate that some conditions are more prevalent in certain races; for example, nonwhite people (black, Native Americans, and Asians) are three times more likely to die of hypertension than white people of the same age group.[1] In the past, six causes of death were identified that together accounted for more than 80% of mortality in nonwhite people, including cancer, cardiovascular disease and stroke, chemical dependency, diabetes, homicides and accidents, and infant mortality (NCHS, 1985). Other conditions that are peculiar to ethnic or racial groups include Tay-Sachs disease (Jewish people of northeastern European origin are most susceptible), cystic fibrosis (inci-

[1] This likely reflects an actual increased incidence among nonwhites but may also reflect poor treatment received by this group. Ethnic differences in hypertensive responses (and other conditions) are being investigated (Sherwood et al., 1995).

TABLE 2–1 The Five Leading Causes of Death in the United States and Associated Modifiable Risk Factors

Cause of Death	Risk Factors
1. Heart disease	Tobacco use Elevated serum cholesterol High blood pressure Obesity Diabetes mellitus Sedentary lifestyle
2. Malignant neoplasms	Tobacco use Improper diet Alcohol Occupational and environmental exposures
3. Cerebrovascular disease	High blood pressure Tobacco use Elevated serum cholesterol
4. Chronic obstructive pulmonary disease	Tobacco use Occupational and environmental exposures
5. Accidental injuries	Seat belt nonuse Cycle helmet nonuse Alcohol and other substance abuse Reckless driving Occupational hazards Guns in the home Stress and fatigue

* According to the World Health Organization, infection and parasitic diseases are the leading causes of death worldwide, although heart disease, stroke, and cancer now kill almost as many people. Smoking remains the world's largest single preventable cause of illness and death (J Commun Dis 28:215–219, 1996).

Adapted from National Center for Health Statistics/U.S. Department of Health and Human Services: Health United States: 1994. DHHS Publication No. (PHS) 95-1232, 1995 and DHHS Publication No. (PHS) 95-1120, 5-0920, March 1995.

dence highest in whites, rare in Asians), and sickle cell disease (affects blacks, especially Africans).

Minorities are also less likely to have access to health care services and especially in obtaining specialty care. Problems with language differences arise with as many as one fourth of the minority population who do not speak English as a first language requiring an interpreter (often unavailable) when seeking health care (Davis, 1994).

Race, culture, and ethnicity are important factors in an individual's response to pain and disease. It is important to remember that people of any culture may deal with pain and disability differently than expected. The therapist's own cultural influences on pain assessment and treatment must be considered as well. The results of classic studies on cultural and ethnic influences on pain are summarized in Table 2–2. Research in the area of aging and ethnic or racial background is needed; most research excludes minorities.

Age and Gender

Age and gender play important roles in the development of most diseases. Age often represents the accumulated effects of genetic and environmental factors over time. Today life expectancy is 78.5 years for women and 71.8 years for men.[2] In 1900, people over 65 years old constituted 4% of the US population. By 1988, that proportion was up to 12.4% (DHHS, 1990) and it is predicted that by 2025 one third of all Americans will be 65 years old or older (White House Conference on Aging, 1994). The most rapid population increase over the next decade will be among those over 85 years of age (DHHS, 1990). Additionally, almost 80% of babies born today will live to see their 65th birthday. This aging trend of the US population will be reflected in the kinds of clients and problems therapists will treat in the coming decades.

Gender differences may represent either environmental or genetic factors. Diseases with rates of occurrence that differ between men and women may reflect lifestyle or environmental differences or anatomic and hormonal differences (Williams, 1994). It is now understood that there are major gender differences in such things as risk factors, response to medications, response to surgical procedures, and response to treatment. For example, 1 year after a heart attack, nearly one half of men but only one third of women survive; osteoporosis affects up to 60% of women over the age of 45 and 90% over the age of 75; and the human immunodeficiency virus (HIV) has become the number one killer of women of reproductive age in many major cities (Blumenthal, 1995b). As of the 1990s medical research subjects are no longer only males; results of research on male subjects will no longer be extrapolated to treating and preventing diseases in women[3]. New studies evaluating differences between the sexes regarding a variety of factors are currently underway (Warner et al., 1995; Howard et al., 1995; Burker et al., 1994).

Gender expectations play a role in response to health issues in most cultures in the United States. Males are expected to show less expression of pain than females. In most cultures, men will be less expressive in describing pain. In some cultures, male children are held in higher esteem than female children and are more likely to receive necessary care and follow-up prescribed. Additionally, researchers are now examining whether people are more vulnerable to environmental and biologic challenges during periods of critical biochemical change than in times of relative quiescence. For example, are social, biologic, or psychological changes that affect health magnified during puberty, pregnancy, and menopause, compared with other periods in a woman's life cycle? (Rodin, 1994).

There are few differences between men and women in response to exercise so few adjustments need to be made when prescribing exercise for the female as opposed to the male. Aging has a more important role in the endurance capacity of women, which may be attributed more to physical inactivity than to gender. It is important to match the intensity of the exercise to the capacity of the individual. When

[2] Whites and blacks have similar life expectancies at age 65 years; there is a higher death rate among younger blacks.

[3] Recently, a new position within the Department of Health and Human Services was developed (Deputy Assistant Secretary for Women's Health) to make women's health a top priority in the United States. Future research studies will emphasize gender differences in the causes, treatment, and prevention of diseases.

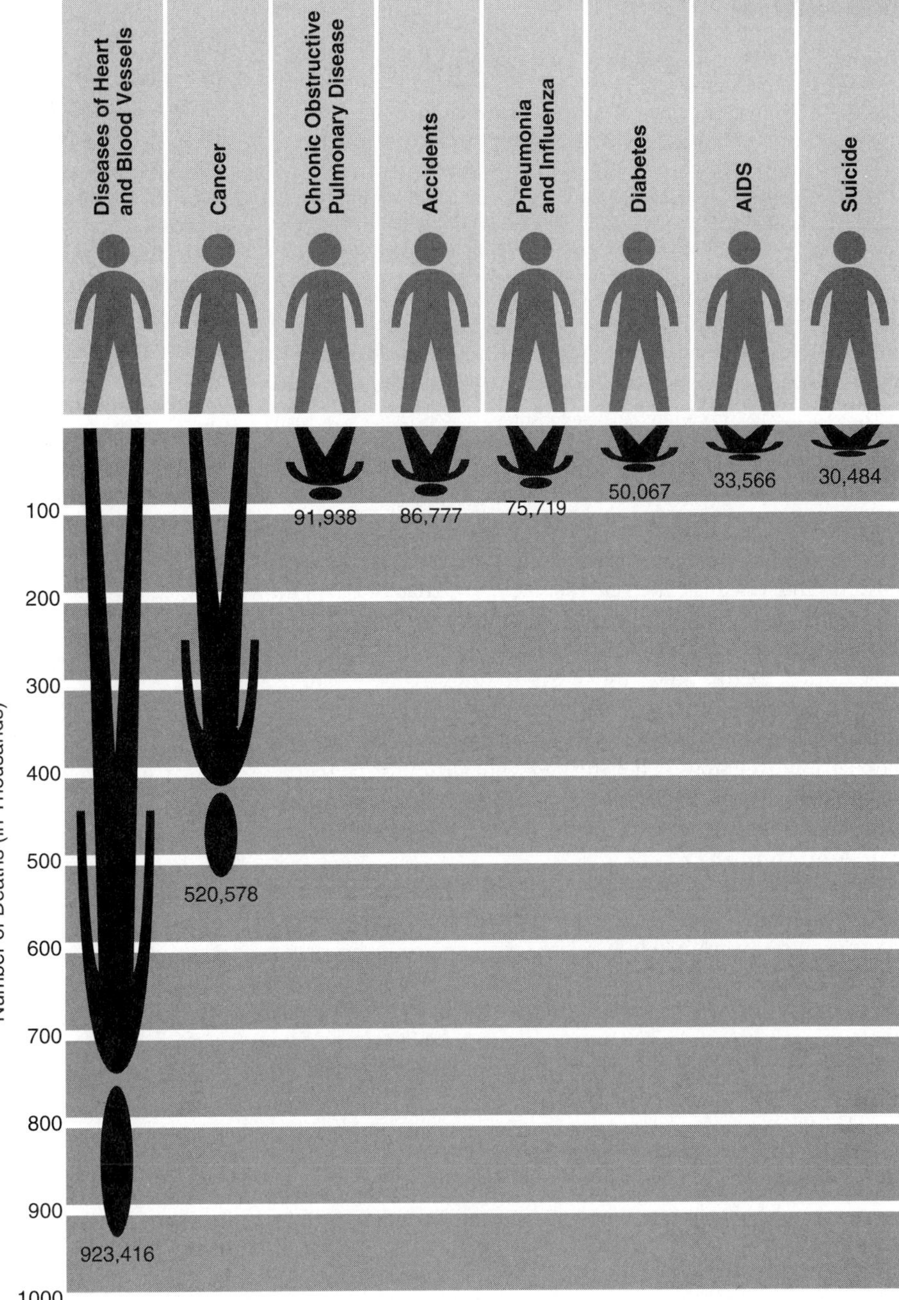

Figure **2–1.** Deaths from the leading causes, United States, 1992 (final mortality statistics). The total for Diseases of Heart and Blood Vessels represents the combined total for the categories Heart Diseases and Cerebrovascular Disease in Table 2–1. (*Data from Kochanek KD, Hudson BL: Advance Report of Final Mortality Statistics, 1992. Monthly Vital Statistics Report 43(6):1–73, March 22, 1995, and American Heart Association: Death from the Leading Causes: Still Number One. Publication No. 04–9550, Dallas, American Heart Association 1994.*)

training heart rate has not been determined through prescreening exercise testing, an exercise protocol should progress in slow stepwise increments (Wilmore, 1993).

Variations in Lifestyle

More than half of deaths from the leading causes in the United States (see Table 2–1) result from behavioral and lifestyle factors such as diet, exercise, smoking, and substance abuse. More than any other intervention, changing behavior and lifestyle could help prevent death, enhance the quality of life, and reduce the escalating costs of treating chronic illnesses (Blumenthal, 1995a). Deaths from heart disease in the United States have been reduced by 52% over the last two decades as a result of changes in diet and lifestyle. It is predicted that before the turn of the century cancer will replace heart disease as the number one cause of mortality in the United States (NCHS, 1995).

Variations in lifestyle influencing clients' perceptions of health care may occur as a result of cultural, religious, or socioeconomic factors. Although clinical manifestations of a disease or condition are essentially the same across cultures, how a person (or family member) responds or interprets the

TABLE 2-2 CULTURAL RESPONSES TO PAIN

English	Stoic reaction to pain; high tolerance for pain; refuse pain intervention
Irish	Denial of pain; expression of pain limited and minimized; unwilling to accept treatment to relieve pain
Italian	Suffer loudly and want everyone to know about the pain; react out of proportion to the painful stimuli present; enjoy the sympathy and secondary gains associated with painful condition
Jewish	Suffer loudly and involve family closely with the suffering; want great detail about the cause of pain; often react out of proportion to the painful stimuli

Adapted from Zborowski M: People in Pain. San Francisco, Jossey-Bass, 1969.

experience can vary. This phenomenon of response based on cultural influence is called *cultural relativity*, that is, behavior must be judged first in relation to the context of the culture in which it occurs (Wong, 1993).

Cultural factors may also prevent illness. For example, people belonging to religious faiths that proscribe (forbid) drinking or smoking have lower cancer rates than the general population. Religious beliefs related to health must be recognized and respected. Detailed summaries of religious beliefs that may affect health care are available (Wong, 1993; Keegan, 1993).

The most adverse influence on health is socioeconomic status, with a higher percentage of low–socioeconomic class persons suffering from health-related problems than any other group. Lack of health insurance coverage may result in delayed or postponed diagnosis and treatment of health problems. Differences in attitudes toward health have been found to be greater between social classes than between races or ethnic groups.

The homeless have become one of the fastest growing populations in need of health care in the United States. Traditionally, the homeless consisted primarily of older, single men, often alcoholics, but now this group includes families and children who are runaways or adolescent throwaways. An estimated 100,000 children in the United States are homeless and more than half are under 5 years of age (Shulsinger, 1991).

Other risk factors in lifestyle affecting health status and health care include personal habits such as rest and sleep; diet, including calcium, fat, and fiber intake; level of activity and exercise; stress and coping ability; substance abuse; high-risk sexual activity; travel; and environmental or occupational status. Most of these factors are discussed in greater detail elsewhere in this book.

Special Implications for the Therapist **2-1**

ADAPTING TREATMENT TO THE INDIVIDUAL

In any setting, it is important for therapists to be aware of their own attitudes and values regarding lifestyle choices; responses to pain, illness, and disability; and health practices. It may be beneficial to adapt the individual treatment program to ethnic practices and beliefs. Health care education may be most effective if provided without trying to change the individual's or family's longstanding beliefs. Knowing what is needed to effectively rehabilitate an individual does not assure success unless provided within a cultural and socioeconomic framework acceptable to the individual or family.

In the past, studies examining personal factors to treatment failure have focused primarily on the client, not on the practitioner (Dunbar-Jacob, 1993). Taking a closer look at ourselves and understanding certain psychological concepts, for example; transference, countertransference,* direction of care (toward the client or therapist?) can help the health professional become more effective, efficient, and consistent in the delivery of health care (Woltersdorf, 1994,1995).

* *Transference* is defined as the unconscious transfer of emotions and beliefs about significant others (such as parents) onto an unsuspecting party, usually an authority figure (such as a health care provider). *Countertransference* is the authority figure's reciprocal transfer of emotions and beliefs that do not belong to the client (Gorkin, 1987).

Substance Abuse

Substance abuse is defined as the excessive use of mood-affecting chemicals (Box 2–1) that are a potential or real threat to either physical or mental health (Kneisl, 1993). Substance abuse has become increasingly prevalent in American society among persons of every social, economic, professional, and educational status. The reasons for this phenomenon are multifactorial including personality characteristics, genetic influences, peer pressure, parental and cultural influences, nonadaptive coping skills, and as a means of self-treatment in posttraumatic stress disorder, a syndrome with symptoms resulting from past trauma outside normal human experience (Cottler, 1992; Clark et al., 1994). Alcoholism is the most common drug abuse problem in the United States affecting more than 15 million Americans, including the aging population.

Substance abuse may take the form of both addiction and habituation leading to psychological craving or dependence,

BOX **2-1**
Mood-Affecting Chemicals*

- Tobacco
- Alcohol (wine, beer, liquor)
- Caffeine-containing substances:
  - Coffee
  - Black tea
  - Some carbonated beverages
  - Medications, including many over-the-counter medications
  - Chocolate
- Prescription drugs
- Illicit drugs (e.g., hallucinogens, cocaine, marijuana)
- Over-the-counter medications

* These are listed in order of societal impact.

physiologic dependence accompanied by withdrawal symptoms[4] when use is discontinued, and tolerance[5]. The addiction may lead to a lifestyle (e.g., prostitution, theft, violent crime) that puts the person at considerable risk for illness, disease, and injury. Substance abuse is estimated to be a factor in half of all highway fatality accidents.

Varying center-based statistics show that 25% to 50% of all people with spinal cord injury (SCI) have substance abuse problems compared with an estimated 10% of the general population. The statistics for alcohol and drug use at the time of injury are as high as 68% to 80% (Johnson, 1995). Among a sample of people admitted to one center, nearly half of all people who sustained an SCI were intoxicated when injured; although many newly admitted clients with SCI reduce or eliminate alcohol use during their hospitalization, 56% resume drinking after 1 year (Schmidt, 1995).

Aging and Substance Abuse *(Reichel, 1995)*. Alcohol is by far the most serious drug problem among the elderly or aging population. Many older persons view alcohol problems in a moral context associated with feelings of shame and weakness which prevents them from seeking help. An elderly person is at greater risk for difficulties with alcohol than a young person for several reasons. Both total body water and lean body mass are reduced as one ages. Even though ethanol metabolism is not decreased in the elderly (unless there is some underlying condition), blood alcohol levels are less diluted and thus higher in the older person than in the younger person when both are given equivalent amounts determined by body surface area. Thus, the same person as he or she ages can achieve higher blood alcohol levels with no increase in the amount ingested, all other factors remaining constant (Hartford and Damorajski, 1982). Illness, malnutrition, the administration of other hepatotoxic drugs, or drugs that require breakdown in the liver may all increase an elderly person's sensitivity to alcohol.

Many over-the-counter liquid cold remedies, as well as mouthwashes and cough syrups, contain alcohol which the aging person may consume as a substitute for drinking. Signs and symptoms of alcohol abuse may occur, but the person denies alcohol intake. Further questioning may be necessary to uncover these hidden problems with alcohol.

The older person is even more vulnerable to the detrimental effects of alcohol on cognitive function than the younger person. These effects on cognitive function occur even with light social drinking and are similar to those associated with aging. Alcohol can mimic or exacerbate cognitive changes linked both with normal aging and Alzheimer's disease (Atkinson and Kofoed, 1984).

Sleep disorders are common among older people leading to the use of alcohol and other sedative or hypnotic drugs as chemical management for insomnia. Alcohol does act to decrease sleep latency (the time between falling asleep and the first rapid-eye-movement or REM period), which increases with age, but it also tends to further reduce REM and stages 3 and 4 of non-REM sleep, which is already decreased in the elderly. The net result is a virtual elimination of the restful and restorative portions of the sleep cycle. This can be further complicated by alcohol withdrawal occurring during sleep with the accompanying sympathetic discharge and arousal (Hartford and Damorajski, 1982).

Abuse of sedative-hypnotics, taken either for sleep or anxiety, is a common form of drug abuse among the elderly (Salzman, 1984). Complications of these drugs may be related to the development of toxic levels from the long half-lives of these compounds along with their slow metabolic breakdown in the elderly. Slowed response, hypersomnia, and increasing confusion are sometimes thought to relate to aging when actually they are symptoms of toxic drug levels. Withdrawal symptoms may occur when the medication is abruptly discontinued as a result of hospitalization or other change in life circumstances. Symptoms can be severe and may include tachycardia, hyperthermia, hypertension, altered mental states, seizures, and opisthotonos (severe spasm of the body backward into extension) (Miller et al., 1985). Frequently the withdrawal is not recognized or diagnosed immediately.

Pathogenesis and Clinical Manifestations. People who use and abuse illicit drugs, any substances mentioned in Box 2–1, or any combination of these substances have special health care needs. Specific effects and adverse reactions depend on the drug type such as caffeine, cannabis (e.g., marijuana and hashish), CNS stimulants (e.g., amphetamines, cocaine), CNS depressants (e.g., alcohol, sedatives, tranquilizers), narcotics (e.g., opium, morphine, codeine, heroin), and tobacco (Table 2–3).

Stimulants such as caffeine, cocaine, and amphetamines affect the cardiovascular system and stimulate the sympathetic nervous system to increase production of adrenaline, causing the effects listed in Table 2–3. Caffeine in toxic amounts (more than 250 mg/day or 3 cups of caffeinated coffee) may also produce additional symptoms (see Table 2–3). Death can occur as a result of interaction between depressants such as alcohol combined with certain medications. The many respiratory diseases directly attributable to tobacco are discussed in Chapter 12. Additionally, cigarettes have been linked to fatal breast cancer (Calle et al., 1994).

Illicit drug use or abuse may damage neurotransmitter receptor sites; the subsequent imbalance produces symptoms that may mimic other psychiatric illnesses such as agitated depression or amphetamine (speed)-induced seizures or paranoia. Repeated stimulation of the brain, called *kindling*, increases susceptibility to focal brain activity with minimal stimulation until the individual experiences spontaneous effects without the use of chemicals (Brophy, 1994). The effects of kindling may be manifested as mood swings, panic, psychosis, and occasionally seizures. Behavioral effects are also noted such as poor work performance, job loss, pathologic lying, truancy, paranoia and aggression, violence, marital problems, or erratic behavior. Nonspecific signs such as red eyes, fatigue, signs of upper respiratory infection (especially cough), heart palpitations, avoidance of eye contact, confusion, or evidence of trauma may be present.

---

[4] Withdrawal is the pattern of physical responses that appears when regular drug use is discontinued. When a physically dependent person abruptly stops consumption, signs and symptoms of withdrawal occur. Most withdrawal reactions produce an effect opposite to that of the ingested substance (e.g., a depressant causes hyperactivity during withdrawal) (Kneisl, 1993).

[5] The central nervous system (CNS) adapts to the continued presence of a substance by compensating for its effect in a process referred to as "tolerance." As a result, the person has to take increased quantities of the substance to obtain the same effect or to feel "normal." This phenomenon leads to physical dependence and pathologic organ changes (Kneisl, 1993).

TABLE 2-3 SPECIFIC EFFECTS AND ADVERSE REACTIONS TO SUBSTANCES

CAFFEINE	CANNABIS	DEPRESSANTS	NARCOTICS	STIMULANTS	TOBACCO
Nervousness Irritability Agitation Sensory disturbances Tachypnea Urinary frequency Sleep disturbances Fatigue Muscle tension Headaches Intestinal disorders Enhances pain perception Heart palpitation Vasoconstriction	Short-term memory loss Sedation Tachycardia Euphoria Increased appetite Relaxed inhibitions Fatigue Paranoia Psychosis Ataxia, tremor Paresthesias	Vasodilation Fatigue Depression Altered pain perception Slurred speech Altered behavior Slow, shallow breathing Clammy skin Coma (overdose)	Euphoria Drowsiness Respiratory depression	Increased alertness Excitation Euphoria Increased pulse rate Increased blood pressure Insomnia Loss of appetite Agitation, increased body temperature, hallucinations, convulsions, death (overdose)	Increased heart rate Vasoconstriction Decreased O_2 to heart Increased risk of thrombosis Loss of appetite Poor wound healing

Medical Management. Substance abuse of any kind requires an overall treatment program including counseling, education, behavior modification, and for some substances, pharmacologic help. In the rehabilitation of SCI and traumatic brain-injured (TBI) clients, pain may be undertreated causing some clients to turn to other, sometimes illicit, drugs to self-medicate. Timely, effective treatment for pain control is the goal in treatment before substance abuse becomes a problem.

Special Implications for the Therapist **2-2**

SUBSTANCE ABUSE

Substance abuse can impair or slow the rehabilitation process, especially delaying wound healing. The client using any substances discussed in this section should be encouraged to reduce (eliminate if possible) intake of these chemicals during the rehabilitation process.* Not only will the healing process accelerate but levels of perceived pain can be reduced when these substances are eliminated.

As part of the assessment process, therapists can screen for the presence of chemical substances by asking about the use of prescribed drugs, over-the-counter drugs and self-prescribed drugs such as nicotine, caffeine, alcohol, or street drugs. It may be helpful to assess the behavioral impact of substance abuse by asking, "Are you concerned about your chemical use? Has anyone around you raised concern about your chemical use?" An appropriate final question may be "Are there any drugs or substances you take (use) that you haven't told me about yet?" Specific interviewing techniques are provided in more appropriate sources (Coulehan and Block, 1992; Goodman and Snyder, 1995; Boissonnault and Koopmeiners, 1994). The National Council on Alcoholism and Drug Dependence has also published a self-test for assessing the signs of alcoholism (NCADD, 1990).

If the client reports the use of substances, the therapist may want to ask whether the person has discussed this with his or her physician or other health care personnel. Encourage the client to seek medical attention or inform the individual that you plan to discuss this as a medical problem with the physician. You can take the approach that this situation is no different from a case of undiagnosed or untreated angina. The client's health is impaired by the use and abuse of substances and therapy will not be effective as long as the person is under the influence of chemicals.

With the SCI and TBI population, the therapist must be alert to any suspicious signs or symptoms of substance abuse (see Clinical Manifestations). Medical professionals should also be observant for excessive sleeping and unusual symptoms such as muscular inflammation and myopathies, which can occur with the use of street drugs.

Tobacco

Heavy smoking is commonly associated with chronic alcohol abuse (Matsuo et al., 1987), and both addictions have a negative influence on bone formation, probably the result of defective osteoblastosis (de Vernejoul et al., 1983). Women who smoke are at significantly higher risk of developing osteoporosis late in life and subsequent bone fractures compared with nonsmokers (Slemenda, 1994; Hopper and Seeman, 1994). See also Special Implications for the Therapist: Osteoporosis, Chapter 20. The effects of tobacco use (see Table 2–3) have a direct impact on the client's ability to exercise and must be considered when starting a treatment or exercise program. In addition to the overall effects of nicotine, inhaled nicotine has additional pulmonary effects. The combination of smoking and coffee ingestion raises the blood pressure of hypertensive clients about 15/33 mm Hg for as long as 2 hours (Freestone and Ramsay, 1982), requiring careful monitoring of vital signs during exercise.

The detrimental effects of cigarette smoking on wound healing and peripheral circulation are well documented (Sherwin and Gastwirth, 1990; Kyro et al., 1993; Silverstein, 1992; Jones and Triplett, 1992). The relationship between smoking and pain has also been documented; study results demonstrated that pain in the extremities was related more clearly to smoking than the pain in the neck or back. A link between smoking and back pain in occupations requiring physical exertion was also established (Boshuizen et al., 1993). Whenever possible, clients who smoke should be encouraged to stop smoking or at least reduce tobacco use prior to surgery and when recovering from wounds or injuries resulting from trauma or disease. The National Cancer Institute (800-4-CANCER) provides educational materials for health professionals that contain practical steps toward stopping smoking.

Cigarette smoking is a risk factor for diabetes, complicating vascular disease (Mitchell et al., 1990; Moss et al., 1992). Smoking may especially exacerbate circulatory problems leading to foot amputation in people with diabetes (Calhoun et al., 1994). This population generally has a lower oxygen supply to the lower extremities because they are subject to advanced atherosclerosis. Since good oxygen supply is required for wound healing in soft tissue, it is imperative that people with a history of diabetes and smoking, now presenting with pressure ulcers or other foot complications, receive adequate arterial blood supply to the lower extremities. See further discussion in Chapters 9 and 10.

Depressants *(Kneisl, 1993)*

Alcohol, barbiturates, and similarly acting sedatives, hypnotics, and antianxiety agents are CNS depressants. Approximately 30% of hospitalized people (including the elderly) are alcohol abusers and many traumatic injuries occur as a result of excessive alcohol consumption. Alcohol affects many body systems (Fig. 2–2) but the effects on the neurologic and musculoskeletal systems are of particular interest to therapists.

Alcoholic polyneuropathy is a degenerative process involving mutliple nerves and occurs as a result of nutritional deficiencies associated with chronic alcoholism. It occurs most frequently between ages 40 and 70 and develops slowly over a long period of time. Some people with neuropathies are asymptomatic but neurologic assessment usually reveals varying degrees of motor, reflex, and sensory loss, which typically occur in the feet before the hands, moving distal to proximal. Sensory disturbances usually appear first and are described as tingling, pricking, burning, or numbing sensations. Safety precautions are very important for people with diminished sensation. See also Table 10–22: Guidelines for Skin Care. Calf muscles may be tender to the touch and diminished sensation and weak muscles may result in a wide-stance gait.

Alcohol ingestion may damage skeletal muscle, resulting in subclinical, acute, or chronic alcoholic myopathy. The pathologic process is the same as in alcoholic cardiomyopathy (see Chapter 10). *Acute alcoholic myopathy* is a syndrome of muscle pain, tenderness, and edema occurring after acute excesses of alcohol ingestion. The proximal muscles of the extremities, the pelvic and shoulder girdles, and the muscles of the thoracic cage are most commonly affected. Symptoms may subside in 1 to 3 weeks with cessation of alcohol use but may recur with repeated alcohol ingestion. Treatment consists of a well-balanced diet with supplemental vitamins and abstinence from alcohol. *Chronic alcoholic myopathy* is characterized by muscle weakness and wasting involving the same muscle groups described in acute alcoholic myopathy. Onset is slow and insidious with no history of pain or tenderness. Treatment is the same as for acute alcoholic myopathy.

Prolonged use of excessive alcohol contributes to three known skeletal complications: a syndrome of nontraumatic hip osteonecrosis (Matsuo et al., 1987), deficient bone metabolism leading to osteomalacia and osteoporosis (Shapira, 1990), and an increased incidence of fractures and other injuries secondary to trauma and falls (Nilsson, 1970; Kristensson et al., 1980). Impaired coordination due to high blood alcohol levels is a contributing factor to falls.

Saturday night palsy, an injury to the radial nerve in the spiral groove, may occur during deep sleep in intoxicated persons. Prolonged compression of the radial nerve results in paralysis of the extensor muscles of the wrist and fingers (O'Toole, 1992). The nerve may be injured at or above the elbow; its purely motor posterior interosseous branch, supplying the extensors of the wrist and fingers, may be involved immediately below the elbow, but then there is sparing of the extensor carpi radialis longus, so that the wrist can still be extended. The triceps muscle is spared because of its more proximal nerve supply (Aminoff, 1994). See also Chapter 34.

Stimulants

The use of chemical stimulants such as caffeine, cocaine, and amphetamines has a direct effect on the CNS and may enhance a person's perception of pain. Pain can be relieved by reducing the daily intake of these chemicals but care must be taken to avoid the caffeine withdrawal syndrome (e.g., symptoms of headache, lethargy, fatigue, muscle pain, and stiffness) (Couturier et al., 1992; Hughes et al., 1991). The negative effects of caffeine on TBI are also problematic for the therapist having to work with the agitation often present in this group.

Caffeine also increases urinary excretion of calcium leading to osteoporosis. According to at least one study (Barrett-Connor et al., 1994), lifetime caffeinated coffee intake equivalent to 2 cups per day is associated with decreased bone density in older women who do not drink milk on a daily basis. People taking stimulants such as cocaine and amphetamines are easily provoked into aggressive, violent behavior. A calm approach is essential and realistic goals for client behavior and rehabilitation are important.

Cannabis

The effects of cannabis derivatives usually last a few hours and with repeated use, less of the drug is needed

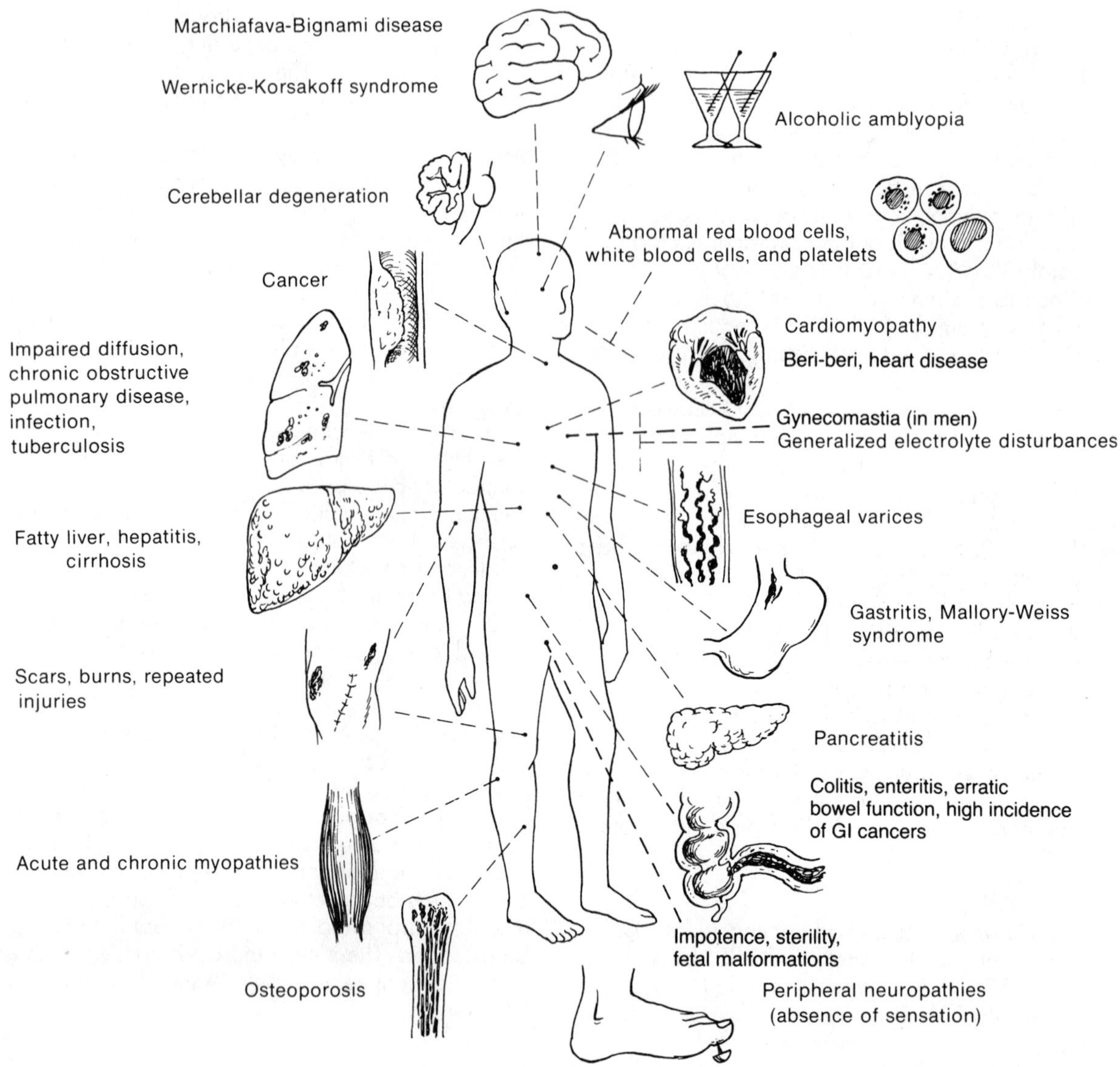

Figure **2–2.** Clinical problems resulting from alcohol abuse. Not all of the conditions pictured in this figure are discussed in this text. *(From Kneisl CR: Nursing care of clients with substance abuse.* In *Black JM, Matassarin-Jacobs E (eds): Luckmann and Sorensen's Medical-Surgical Nursing ed 4. Philadelphia, WB Saunders, 1993, p 2207.)*

to produce the same effects. The agent persists in the body as an active metabolite as long as 8 days after use, so less of the drug is needed to produce the same effects during this time (Jaffe, 1980). As with any substance, clients are encouraged to eliminate the use of cannabis derivatives during the rehabilitation process. Relapse or worsening of symptoms in persons with a history of psychological disorders occurs with the use of cannabis (Hutchinson, 1992).

* Primary intervention or care for the chemically dependent person is essential. However, the realistic picture is more often one of a person who has a pattern of substance abuse and either denies the problem or admits "failure" in the past. For example, failure is most commonly admitted by people who smoke or chew tobacco and have repeatedly tried to quit.

Eating Disorders

Anorexia Nervosa

Anorexia nervosa (AN) is a refusal to eat. It is characterized by severe weight loss in the absence of obvious physical cause and attributed to emotions such as anxiety, irritation, anger, and fear. This condition is characterized by distorted thinking, including a fear of becoming obese despite progressive weight loss, accompanied by the perception that the body is fat when it is underweight. The person may use laxatives, diuretics, exercise and self-induced vomiting to achieve additional weight loss. The effects of starvation have psychological, emotional, and physical sequelae, and medical complications that may lead to death.

Anorexia nervosa occurs predominantly in adolescent and young adult females from middle and upper class families,

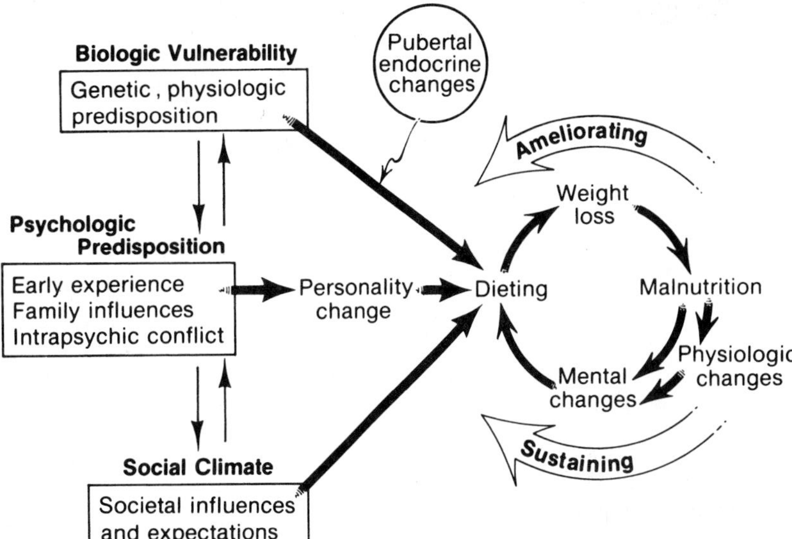

Figure **2–3.** Biopsychosocial model for anorexia nervosa. See text discussion. (*From Lucas AR: Toward an understanding of anorexia nervosa as a disease. Mayo Clin Proc 56:254, 1981.*)

often at or near the onset of menstruation (menarche). There is an increased incidence of AN among sports participants, especially sports that emphasize leanness such as gymnastics, wrestling, diving, figure skating and distance running, and in ballet dancers. AN occurs in men in approximately 5% to 10% of cases; it is suspected that this figure is a low estimate as it is likely that more males suffer from AN than come to health professionals' attention.

Although attributed to psychological and emotional factors (e.g., the need for control is a common variable; fear of growing up; fear of sexuality; rejection of self), the cause of AN is unknown. During the past several decades, single-factor causal theories have been replaced by the view that anorexia nervosa is a multifactorial biopsychosocial disorder (Fig. 2–3). Specific early experiences and family influences may create intrapsychic conflicts that determine the psychological predisposition. The challenges and conflicts of pubertal endocrine changes (biologic factors) may initiate the disorder. Social factors, such as the American cultural obsession with thinness, reinforce the pursuit of thinness. The cumulative effect leads to dieting and other means of weight loss. This in turn results in malnutrition and "starvation neurosis." The vicious circle of psychological dysfunction fostering further dieting and psychological denial becomes established and may lead to death (Lucas, 1981; Bo-Linn, 1993; Garner, 1993).

Clinical Manifestations. Besides the obvious lack of appetite and refusal to eat with weight loss, other signs and symptoms may occur, such as cessation of menstrual cycle (amenorrhea), muscle and fat atrophy giving the person a skeleton-like appearance, postural hypotension, edema, bradycardia, hypothermia and cold intolerance, constipation, anemia, and sleep disturbance.

Physical manifestations may include dry skin, brittle nails, and lanugo (the fine hair sometimes seen on the body of the newborn infant) owing to loss of body fat and secondary to hypothermia. When AN is accompanied by self-induced vomiting, further complications include electrolyte imbalance, dental caries (the acid content of vomitus erodes tooth enamel), esophagitis, starvation-induced cardiac failure, and possible death. Mitral valve prolapse (MVP) may occur secondary to starvation-induced decrease in left ventricular volume (see Special Implications for the Therapist related to MVP, Chapter 10). Behavioral symptoms are listed in Table 2–4.

Bone density is decreased in anorexic (and bulimic; see next section) women, possibly the result of estrogen deficiency, low intake of nutrients, low body weight, early onset and long duration of amenorrhea, low calcium intake, reduced physical activity, and hypercortisolism (Salisbury and Mitchell, 1992; Foster, 1994).

Medical Management. Diagnostic criteria may be taken from the American Psychiatric Association's *Diagnostic and Statistical Manual of Mental Disorders* (DSM-IV, 1994).[6] (Box 2–2). There is no universally accepted treatment for anorexia nervosa. Treatment is difficult and lengthy and may include behavior therapy, demand feeding, behavioral contracts, psychotherapy, family therapy, modifying food habits, and correction of nutritional status, which may require hospitalization. Estrogen hormone replacement is now considered an important part of medical treatment for women with anorexia who have experienced prolonged absence of menses (Mickley, 1992). As mentioned, starvation-induced cardiac failure and death is possible.

Special Implications for the Therapist **2–3**

ANOREXIA NERVOSA

Rehabilitation may be required for the person with AN to regain muscle mass lost as a result of low calorie

[6] The term "mental disorder" unfortunately implies a distinction between "mental" and "physical" when in fact there is much "physical" in "mental" disorders and much "mental" in "physical" disorders. The problem raised by the term "mental disorders" has been much clearer than its solution and the term persists for lack of an appropriate substitute (DSM-IV, 1994).

TABLE 2-4 COMMON BEHAVIORAL SYMPTOMS OF EATING DISORDERS

SYMPTOMS	ANOREXIA NERVOSA*	BULIMIA NERVOSA*	BINGE EATING DISORDER
Excessive weight loss in relatively short period of time	+	−	−
Continuation of dieting although bone-thin	+	−	−
Dissatisfaction with appearance; belief that body is fat, even though severely underweight	+	−	−
Unusual interest in food and development of strange eating rituals	+	+	−
Eating in secret	+	+	+
Obsession with exercise	+	+	−
Serious depression	+	+	+
Binging—consumption of large amounts of food	−	+	+
Vomiting or use of drugs to stimulate vomiting, bowel movements, and urination	−	+	−
Binging but no noticeable weight gain	−	+	−
Disappearance into bathroom for long periods of time to induce vomiting	−	+	−
Abuse of drugs or alcohol	−	+	+

* Some individuals suffer from anorexia and bulimia and have symptoms of both disorders.
Adapted from Hoffman L: Eating Disorders. National Institutes of Health, NIH Publication No. 93-3477, Bethesda, Md, January 1993.

diets, malnutrition, binging, and purging. It is important for the therapist to be aware of some of the physical side effects of previously diagnosed AN. Vital sign instability can be severe, including orthostatic hypotension, irregular and decreased pulse, and bradycardia and hypothermia, which can result in cardiac arrest. Heart rate must be monitored and maintained within safe limits during exercise. Poor nutritional status and dehydration also contribute to poor wound healing.

Posture is often poor because of the loss of upper body muscle mass. Exercise tolerance may be low and endurance reduced significantly as a result of malnutrition. Clients may be resistive to exercise or may engage in excessive exercise to "vent" or "work off" their feelings. Consulting with other members of the health care team such as psychologists and psychiatrists can help in providing a behavioral approach to physical therapy and especially to an exercise program (Box 2–3).

The health care provider must also remain aware of the possibility of undiagnosed anorexia nervosa (or bulimia; see next section) in any population group, but especially preadolescents, adolescents, and young adults. A musculoskeletal problem can be an indication of an eating disorder. Overuse injuries such as shin splints, tendinitis, stress fractures, or hip or back pain can occur from excessive exercise; the individual may continue to exercise despite fatigue, weakness, and pain. Early detection and prompt referral to an appropriate center with expertise in treating this illness is essential (Edwards, 1993).

Bulimia Nervosa

Bulimia nervosa, also known as compulsive eating, is characterized by episodic binge eating (consuming large amounts of food at one time) followed by purging behavior such as self-induced vomiting, fasting, laxative and diuretic abuse, and excessive exercising. Risk factors are the same as for anorexia nervosa and the bulimic person has a preoccupying pathologic fear of becoming overweight despite the fact that she or he is usually within normal weight standards. There is an awareness that the eating pattern is abnormal and self-recrimination is frequent. In contrast to persons with anorexia nervosa who restrict food as a means of gaining control over problems, people with bulimia react to distress by the binge-purge cycle.

Approximately 50% of persons with bulimia are also an-

BOX 2–2
Diagnostic Criteria for Anorexia Nervosa

A. Refusal to maintain body weight at or above a minimal normal weight for age and height or failure to make expected weight gain during period of growth, leading to body weight 15% below that expected.

B. Intense fear of gaining weight or becoming fat, even though underweight.

C. Disturbance in the way in which one's body weight, size, or shape is experienced, e.g., the person claims to "feel fat" even when emaciated and believes that one area of the body is "too fat" even when obviously underweight; undue influence of body weight or shape on self-evaluation, or denial of the seriousness of the current low body weight.

D. In females, absence of at least three consecutive menstrual cycles when otherwise expected to occur (primary or secondary amenorrhea). A woman is considered to have amenorrhea if her periods occur only following hormone (e.g., estrogen) administration.

Adapted from American Psychiatric Association: Diagnostic and Statistical Manual of Mental Disorders, ed 4 [DSM-IV]. Washington, DC, Author, 1994.

BOX **2–3**

Behavioral Goals and Guidelines for Eating Disorders

- Obtain an accurate exercise history.
- Determine the person's target heart rate and teach how and why it is important to monitor heart rate during exercise.
- Develop a well-rounded program of exercise including stretching exercises, breathing techniques, light weights for upper extremity toning, aerobic exercise, and cooldown.
- Convey to the person that the treatment or exercise plan is to help and protect the person's overall health status and is not meant to control the person.
- Instruct each person how to determine the appropriate frequency, intensity, and duration of each component of exercise. Monitor daily and weekly amounts of exercise using a chart or written record and use this tool to help the person develop a consistent and appropriate level of exercise.
- Encourage the client whenever possible to make decisions about the treatment plan; this will help provide a sense of control and increase self-confidence.
- Draw the person out as to his or her attitude toward exercise and consistently encourage recognition of exercise as part of the overall health plan, not just a means of losing weight.
- Exercise is only one tool for stress relief; encourage each individual to develop alternative ways of expressing feelings.
- Modifying thought patterns and changing behavior is a slow process. Encouragement and support are essential. Reinforce even small steps and successes.
- Watch for signs of dissociation (e.g., glazed look or faraway expression) and assist the person to remain aware of the effect of exercise on the physical body; paying attention to the physical discomfort will help prevent working through fatigue, striving for the "runner's high," overexercising, and overuse injuries.
- Avoid making value judgments about the client's body or physical condition. When the client makes comment such as, "I lost/gained a pound this week" or "I cannot believe how fat my arms are," do not react or judge by saying, "You are not supposed to be weighing yourself" or "You are not fat at all!" Seek professional guidance to handle such situations.

orexic, forming a condition called *bulimarexia*. This is characterized by periods of starving to lose weight, alternating with periods of binging and purging. There may be periods of normal eating but the pattern of fasting or binging will resume at some point in time.

The exact cause of bulimia nervosa is unknown. Several theories include a primary neurologic dysfunction; an electrical disorder, similar to epilepsy; disturbance in the appetite and satiety center of the hypothalamus; and a learned behavior for dealing with stress and unpleasant feelings. A vicious circle of depression, overeating to feel better, vomiting and purging to maintain normal weight, and subsequent depression perpetuates this disorder.

Clinical Manifestations. The effects of bulimia nervosa are similar to self-induced vomiting in anorexia nervosa: erosion of the tooth enamel and subsequent dental decay, irritation of the throat and esophagus, fluid and electrolyte imbalances, and rectal bleeding associated with laxative abuse. Binge eating results in abdominal distention and pain until relieved by vomiting or laxative use. Other symptoms may include mood changes, secretiveness, impulsive behaviors, sleep difficulties, and obsession with food and exercise (see Table 2–4).

Medical Management. The DSM-IV provides diagnostic criteria for this condition. Treatment is also similar to the intervention recommended for anorexia, including psychotherapy, family therapy, and self-help groups. Pharmacotherapy may include fluoxetine hydrochloride (Prozac) and a monoamine oxidase inhibitor (tranylcypromine sulfate) to decrease the urge to binge.

Special Implications for the Therapist **2–4**

BULIMIA NERVOSA

Bulimia contributes to problems associated with fluid depletion as well as temperature regulation. For people who use vomiting to purge and abuse laxatives or diuretics, significant dehydration and potassium loss are quite frequent. The immediate outcome of such behavior is usually muscle cramping (including irregular heartbeat as the heart muscle cramps), fatigue, and low blood pressure on standing (Shafe and Parsons, 1992). In such situations, the therapist should delay treatment until electrolyte levels are within normal limits and encourage fluid intake and reduced activity level. In the more extreme condition, incoordination, confusion, and disorientation may be observed requiring medical attention.

Most deadly among the forms of purging is the abuse of ipecac, an emetic (a syrup that induces vomiting) used to treat poison victims. Many people who try it once find it so unpleasant that they avoid further use, but repeated use can cause toxic levels in the body producing myopathy with arm or leg weakness, or affecting the heart and causing sudden death (Mickley, 1992).

See also Special Implications for the Therapist: Anorexia Nervosa.

Obesity

Definition. *Obesity* is medically defined as weight greater than 20% of desirable weight for adults of a given sex, body structure, and height. This definition may be somewhat misleading as obesity by dictionary definition is an excessive accumulation of fat in the body. A person's body weight may be in excess of the normal range according to a height and weight chart, but if there is not excess body fat, that person is not considered obese. A more precise definition has been suggested (O'Toole, 1992): *overweight* describes someone who weighs 10% more than his or her optimum weight; *obese* persons weigh 15% more, and *grossly obese* persons weigh 20% or more above the optimum weight for height and body type. See also Diagnosis, this section, for other forms of measurement of body fat or obesity.

There are two types of obesity: exogenous, resulting from excessive caloric intake, and endogenous, resulting from inherent metabolic problems (Ravussin and Swinburg, 1992). Fewer than 1% of obese people have an identifiable secondary cause of obesity such as hypothyroidism and Cushing's disease (Baron, 1994). Child-onset obesity can be caused by a greater than normal number of fat cells (hyperplasia) or a greater than normal size of fat cells (hypertrophy).

Etiology. Genetic factors appear to play an important, although as yet unknown, role in obesity. After a 40-year search, scientists have found a gene for obesity in mice that may have a counterpart in humans. Several new studies (Zhang et al., 1994; Considine et al., 1995) support a growing consensus that several genes are involved in the body's mechanisms for controlling weight, but how this contributes to obesity still remains unknown.

Non–insulin-dependent diabetes mellitus (NIDDM or type II) is often associated with obesity. Excessive food intake stimulates hyperinsulinemia. Through a negative-feedback mechanism, excessive insulin levels decrease the number of insulin receptor sites on adipose cells. The decrease in insulin receptor sites decreases the amount of glucose that can enter the cells. This promotes high blood levels of glucose. The excess glucose is stored as glycogen in the liver or as triglycerides in adipose cells, thereby enhancing hypertrophy and hyperplasia of fat cells in the already obese person. Weight reduction does reverse this process (Huether and McCance, 1994).

Other causes of obesity may include depression, smoking cessation, endocrine and metabolic disturbances (uncommon and may actually occur secondary to the obesity), polycystic ovary syndrome, low set-point (obese people have a lower point at which appetite is stimulated by the ventromedial hypothalamus), delayed puberty, and failure of aging people to adjust food intake to lowered metabolism and diminished activity. "Yo-yo dieting," or weight cycling with fluctuations of body weight produced by repeated cycles of weight loss and gain, appears to contribute to the inability to lose weight on a long-term basis (Brownell and Rodin, 1994). Low socioeconomic status is also associated with obesity.

Pathogenesis. The pathogenesis of obesity is not understood. There are several theories to explain the physiology of obesity. The most obvious cause of obesity is an excessive intake of calories in proportion to the expenditure of calories. Inactivity and a high fat, low carbohydrate diet with excess intake of refined sugar are contributing factors to excess adipose and weight gain.

The Na^+, K^+-ATPase (adenosine triphosphatase) pump is believed to play a major role in the development of obesity. This enzyme pump transports sodium out of the cell and potassium into the cell at the expense of cellular energy in the form of adenosine triphosphate. Obese people have fewer ATPase pumps than the nonobese, leading to less energy release and obesity.

The *fat cell* or *adipose cell theory* postulates that some people have an excessive number of fat cells (adipocytes) and the size of the fat cells is increased. The *lipoprotein lipase (LPL) theory* suggests that LPL (the enzyme that helps fat to be deposited in adipocytes) is elevated in obese persons and weight reduction stimulates even more production of LPL, causing fat cells to return to their hypertrophic size.

Clinical Manifestations. The outward signs and symptoms of obesity are readily observable (excess body fat), but the effects and complications of obesity are less easily identified at onset. Obesity is associated with significant increases in both morbidity and mortality and is associated with three leading causes of death: cardiovascular disease, cancer,[7] and diabetes mellitus.

More specifically, shortness of breath, atherosclerosis and high blood pressure, increased susceptibility to infectious diseases, and psychological disturbances such as irritability, loneliness, depression, and tension can be linked to obesity. Other complications may include nephrotic syndrome and renal vein thrombosis, other thromboembolic disorders, digestive tract diseases such as gallstones and reflux esophagitis, obstructive sleep apnea and subsequent pulmonary compromise with decreased gas exchange, vital capacity, and expiratory volume.

Medical Management

Diagnosis. In most cases, physical examination is sufficient to detect excess body fat and also provides an assessment of the degree and distribution of body fat, overall nutritional status, and signs of secondary causes of obesity. Using calipers (the pinch test) to measure subcutaneous fat is one way to determine the presence of obesity. A fold of skin and subcutaneous fat from various body locations (e.g., midbiceps, midtriceps, and subscapular or inguinal areas) greater than 1 in. indicates excessive body fat. This measurement is taken into consideration along with body type and height.

Other procedures include electrical devices using light rays to measure the change in body composition as people progress through a weight loss program and relative weight (measured body weight divided by the desirable weight × 100) and body mass index (BMI) (measured body weight in kilograms divided by height in meters squared; Table 2–5) (Baron, 1994).

Treatment. A multidisciplinary approach with emphasis on weight loss maintenance should include balanced low fat diets, behavior modification, exercise, and social support. Medications for obesity are widely available over the counter and by a prescription. The use of pharmacologic agents to inhibit appetite and increase metabolic rate is highly controversial and provides, at best, only a short-term benefit.

[7] Obesity is a risk factor for breast, cervical, endometrial, and liver cancer in women and for prostate, colon, and rectal cancer in men (American Cancer Society, 1986; Boeck et al., 1993).

TABLE 2-5 Body Mass Index (BMI) to Determine Obesity Classification

Classification	BMI (kg/m^2)*
Underweight	<20
Normal	20–25
Overweight	25–30
Obese	30–40
Severely obese	>40

* To calculate your BMI using pounds and inches, multiply your weight in pounds by 700 and divide the product by your height in inches squared. For example, if you weigh 155 lbs, multiply 155 × 700 = 108,500. Now calculate your height in inches squared; for example, if you are 5 ft 8 in. or 68 in. tall, your height squared is 68^2 = 4624; 108,500 divided by 4624 = 23.4 is considered within the normal classification.

Surgical treatment may be considered for some obese persons if serious attempts to lose weight have failed and complications of obesity are life-threatening. There are several surgical procedures designed to reduce the ability of the body to ingest or absorb nutrients (e.g., jaw wiring, stomach stapling [gastroplasty], and gastric bypass). The once common intestinal bypass surgery has been abandoned because of unacceptable long-term complications. The failure rate for the still used gastric bypass is close to 50% (Baron, 1994).

Prognosis. Little progress has been made in the successful treatment of obesity, especially when therapy is confined to dietary measures alone (Kayman et al., 1990). The death rate increases in proportion to the degree of obesity and in the presence of complications. For example, among the cardiovascular problems associated with obesity, hypertension in combination with obesity increases the risk for development of cerebrovascular disease, specifically cerebral thrombosis (Heyden, 1971). Following weight loss in the obese, there is usually a decrease in blood pressure, as well as in the work of the heart (MacMahon et al., 1986).

Patterns of fat distribution are important in determining the risk factor of obesity (Ostlund, 1990). Visceral fat within the abdominal cavity is more hazardous to health than subcutaneous fat around the abdomen. Upper body obesity around the waist and flank is a greater health hazard than lower body obesity marked by fat in the thighs and buttocks. People who are obese with high waist-to-hip ratios (greater than 1.0 in men, 0.8 in women) have a significantly greater risk of diabetes mellitus, stroke, coronary artery disease, and early death than equally obese people with lower ratios (Baron, 1994).

Although the connection between obesity (BMI greater than 30) and coronary heart disease is well established, it remains unknown whether there is a similar link for mild overweight. A recent study has shown that even people (specifically women in this study) whose BMI at midlife (30 to 55 years of age) was between 23 and 24.9 had a 50% higher risk of heart attack compared with those whose BMI was under 20. Women whose BMI was greater than 29 had a 3.6 times greater risk of heart attack compared with the leanest group (Willett et al., 1995).

Weight loss alters conditions associated with obesity. Elevated blood pressure may be reduced with regression of left ventricular hypertrophy, total and high-density lipoprotein cholesterol are favorably changed, and glucose tolerance improves in those with NIDDM. The addition of exercise to a comprehensive program of caloric reduction and behavior modification can improve results (Elliot and Goldberg, 1994). Regular exercise can maximize body composition change and increase the probability of maintaining a weight loss (King, 1989a).

Special Implications for the Therapist **2-5**

OBESITY

Problems associated with obesity commonly seen in a therapy program include back pain, skin breakdown, and cardiopulmonary compromise. Obesity is a known risk factor in the development of NIDDM often accompanied by diabetic neuropathy, foot ulcerations, and neuropathic fractures.

Since obesity is often associated with an increased prevalence of cardiovascular risk factors, graded exercise testing may be indicated prior to prescribing an exercise program. Even morbidly obese people can be evaluated on the treadmill with some modification in the testing protocol such as beginning with slow walking without treadmill elevation, followed by gradual increases in speed to achieve maximal exertion (Foss et al., 1976; Elliot and Goldberg, 1994).

Prescribing exercise for obese persons follows the principles used with healthy people (Box 2–4), including modifications for mechanical limitations,

BOX **2-4**
Strategies to Facilitate Successful Exercise Programs

- Ask the client if he or she is currently exercising regularly (or was prior to illness or injury). Provide a brief description of benefits that the person could achieve from such a program.
- Allow the person to respond to the recommendation for an exercise program. Encourage the person to verbalize any thoughts or reactions to your suggestions.
- Determine whether the person believes that an exercise program will benefit him or her personally. Help the individual to set personal goals for exercise.
- Elicit from the client a statement accepting an exercise program.
- If resistance to the idea of an exercise program is encountered, give the person an opportunity to list potential barriers to exercise. Ask the person to develop a list of "facilitators," i.e., ways to overcome potential barriers.
- Whenever possible provide a written (preferably just pictures because of the potential of undisclosed illiteracy) of the proposed exercise program. Review progress and reward attempts, successes, and progression of the exercise program.
- Make it fun to foster long-term adherence.

Adapted from Butler RM, Rogers FJ: Exercise in healthy individuals. *In* Goldberg L, Elliot DL (eds): Exercise for Prevention and Treatment of Illness. Philadelphia, FA Davis, 1994, p 21.

awareness of potential hazards of exercise (Box 2–5), and awareness of the greater heat intolerance of the obese (Bar-Or et al., 1969). Some equipment modifications may be necessary if the client is too large to use a stationary bicycle or exceeds the manufacturer's recommended weight capacity. For example, a stationary bike can be pedaled by the client while seated in a chair behind the bike.

There is a higher incidence of exercise-related injury among the obese (Goodman and Kenrick, 1975; Pollock, 1977) requiring extra caution in the first few weeks. Recommendations include adequate warmup and stretching, and progressive increases in intensity, frequency, and duration. Severe obesity contributes to back pain and back injury and affects foot mechanics, which can lead to foot and ankle problems. Selection of appropriate footwear with possible orthotic devices that provide heel support or compensatory foot pronation is recommended to make exercise safer and more comfortable (Buskirk, 1993; Messier et al., 1994).

Aerobic exercise with a frequency of four times a week to produce significant weight loss is recommended because it provides the greatest caloric expenditure per minute of training (Pollock et al., 1969; Pollock, 1972). However, compliance and caloric expenditure are the early goals toward achieving a habit of regular exercise rather than an immediate increase in aerobic endurance. The influence of body weight on exertion and lower-extremity trauma may support an initial program of stationary cycling. Aquatic exercise programs can be an important part of reducing strain on joints by providing non–weight bearing exercise for the obese person (Cirullo, 1994; Huey, 1994; Buskirk, 1993).

Resistive exercises and weightlifting can be structured to produce aerobic gains by using a circuit style with low resistance, multiple repetitions, and short rests between sets. For most individuals, caloric expenditure with traditional strength-training techniques is not as great as with circuit lifting or aerobic conditioning, but strength training does use calories and can increase lean body mass (Kuehl et al., 1990; Geissler et al., 1989).

Behavior modification focusing on routine daily activities requiring no special equipment and involving only simple lifestyle changes may be the only type of physical activity that is continued for any length of time. For example, less reliance on vehicular transportation, parking a distance from the destination, avoiding elevators and using stairs, delivering messages within the work structure rather than telephoning, and walking 10 minutes during lunch are useful and easily accommodated suggestions for increasing energy expenditure (Buskirk, 1993).

For the therapist, working with the obese person poses a definite risk to good health. Using proper body mechanics, careful planning for transfers, and obtaining adequate help are essential during any hands-on therapy*.

BOX **2–5**
Potential Hazards of Exercise for the Obese Person

Precipitation of angina pectoris or myocardial infarction
Excessive rise in blood pressure
Aggravation of degenerative arthritis and other joint problems
Ligamentous injuries
Injury from falling
Excessive sweating
Skin disorders, chafing
Hypohydration and reduced circulating blood volume
Heat stroke or heat exhaustion

From Skinner JS: Exercise Testing and Exercise Prescription for Special Cases: Theoretical Basis and Clinical Application, ed 2. Philadelphia, Lea & Febiger, 1993, p 205.

* A useful book written by the National Back Pain Association (1994) with advice to prevent lifting injuries, *The Guide to the Handling of Patients,* can be obtained from IMPACC-USA, 1 Washington St. Greenville, ME 04441; see also Main, K.: *A Manual of Handling People: A Health and Safety Guide for Caregivers.* Helios Therapy Resources, 1955 West Grant Rd., #230-A, Tucson, AZ 85745 (800-759-9920, Dept. A).

Domestic Violence

Domestic violence or domestic abuse has reached epidemic proportions in the United States. Each year a reported 3 to 4 million women are battered, as well as a smaller unknown number of men, including the elderly. There is no clear profile of the type of person who may be in an abusive relationship; pregnant women and women with disabilities are as much at risk as the able-bodied person. Domestic violence occurs across all races and socioeconomic groups. Clinical manifestations of domestic violence are many and varied (Box 2–6). Behavioral symptoms may include hyperventilation, sleep disturbances, mood and appetite disorders, interpersonal distrust, social isolation, decreased libido, depression, substance abuse, and suicidal ideation or attempts.

BOX **2–6**
Clinical Manifestations of Domestic Violence

Injuries (e.g., contusions, lacerations, fractures)
Headaches
Low back pain
Breast or chest pain
Chronic pain disorder
Somatoform pain disorder
Abdominal pain
Gastrointestinal symptoms
Irritable bowel syndrome
Dysphagia (from choking)
Head or face trauma
- Hearing loss
- Ocular motor dysfunction
- Vestibular dysfunction
- Recurrent sinus infections
- Temporomandibular joint pain–dysfunction
- Deviated septum (broken nose)

Sexual assault
- Anuresis (retention of urine)
- Dyspareunia (difficult or painful coitus)
- Recurrent genitourinary infections
- Temporomandibular joint pain–dysfunction

Reports of elder abuse vary from 200,000 to nearly 2 million. The exact incidence is unknown. Complaints include cold food; lack of privacy; physical, sexual, and verbal abuse; and poor care. A significant number of the homebound elderly are also victims of "passive judgment," arising from a lack of knowledge, time, or ability to cope with the problems of a dependent elder.

Signs of passive neglect can be difficult to detect and the elderly are often reluctant to report mistreatment, fearing nursing home placement. Behavioral warning signs of abuse may include depression, poor hygiene, confusion, hostility, unresponsiveness, longing for death, frequent physician visits or changes, and multiple visits to the emergency department. Physical manifestations may include fractures, bruises, malnutrition, and pressure ulcers.

Special Implications for the Therapist **2-6**

DOMESTIC VIOLENCE

Frequently, domestic violence remains undetected and goes unreported. The therapist is able to develop a trusting relationship with clients and may become the first professional to identify the problem. During the therapy interview, the question, "Were you or have you been assaulted or hit?" can elicit the underlying cause for the injury or presenting symptoms.* It may be necessary to ask this question later after the therapist has developed rapport with the client. Questions should be asked with sensitivity and compassion but also directly and specifically. For example, if an injury seems questionable or the client presentation is suspicious of abuse, the therapist may ask, "Were you hit, kicked, or pushed? Is there anything else about your situation you would like to tell me?" A series of questions can be used as an abuse assessment screening (McFarlane and Parker, 1992).

A majority of the elderly are cared for at home by family members who are at least 50 years old and unprepared physically, emotionally, or financially for the added responsibility. Neglect is often not intentional or willful but rather the result of lack of information or misjudgment. Spouses may also physically abuse their partner. The home health therapist is often in the best position to evaluate or screen for potential mistreatment. Questions asked by the therapist in any setting or comments made by the client may reveal the need for further evaluation by the physician, social worker, or visiting nurse.

The health care professional should be familiar with community services available for the battered person whose safety is at risk. Local hospitals may have a consultant or domestic violence task force available to provide assistance once the problem has been identified. Telephone numbers for local shelters or hot lines should be posted.

---

* *Assault* is defined as a physical or verbal attack. Many people who have been physically struck, pushed, or kicked do not consider the action an assault, especially if inflicted by someone they know. Therefore it may be necessary to use some other word besides "assaulted."

Variations in Exercise and Health

Poor eating habits and a sedentary lifestyle are major risk factors for disease. Hypercholesterolemia, obesity, and muscular atrophy are only a few of the potential results of inactivity leading to atherosclerosis, constipation, hypertension, cardiorespiratory disorders, and some cancers. Regular physical activity can play an important role in the promotion and maintenance of health. The beneficial effect of physical activity and exercise on the immune system, the body's response to illness and injury, and psychological well-being have been widely accepted. In addition to the traditionally recognized benefits such as improved range of motion, strength, and endurance, exercise also enhances the immune system, and improves mobility and function. Health care providers should take a proactive role toward exercise (Butler and Rogers, 1994).

Collectively, research results suggest that regular exercise improve one's sense of well-being, defined as a sense of body shape and appearance, health, fitness, safety, and security (Pierce et al., 1993; Plante and Rodin, 1990; Steptoe and Cox, 1988). Moderate-intensity exercise such as walking at least 2 to 3 hours a week seems to provide as much benefit as higher levels of exertion. The effect of training intensity as well as the breadth of emotional benefit from physical activity has not been determined (Benight and Taylor, 1994).

The importance of exercise in the prevention and rehabilitation of individual diseases is documented throughout this book. Even though the benefits of exercise are becoming widely known, most Americans remain sedentary. It is estimated that less than 10% of sedentary adults will begin an exercise program in a given year, and long-term adherence remains poor among those who do attempt to exercise regularly. About 50% of persons will discontinue exercise during the first year (Oldridge, 1982; Dishman et al., 1985). Gender does not appear to be a significant predictor of exercise compliance (Emery et al., 1992).

Exercise may be contraindicated in some conditions; orthopedic problems are a common reason for noncompliance with an exercise program. Other barriers reported include increased demands at work or home, travel requirements, scheduling conflicts, and illnesses (Durbeck, 1972). The elderly face additional problems of deconditioning or loss of balance and stability as a result of disease or illness. The most successful exercise programs take into consideration the person's functional capacity, medical status, and personal interests. Some helpful strategies for facilitating an exercise program (whether for a specific body part or as an overall fitness program) are listed in Box 2–4.

The need for individual exercise prescription, principles of exercise training, and components of exercise (e.g., frequency, intensity, duration) in relation to diseases and chronic conditions are of particular interest to the therapist. Whenever possible, specific information related to these aspects of exercise are included in Special Implications for the Therapist. The reader is referred to more basic texts for the underlying rationale related to exercise and disease (Skinner, 1993; Goldberg and Elliot, 1994; ACSM, 1991).

Psychological Risks of Exercise *(Benight and Taylor, 1994)*

There are few psychological problems associated with exercising but some people become obsessed, even fanatical, about exercise. Any interruption in their exercise routine or schedule causes anger, irritability, and depression. There is no doubt that some people become addicted to exercise and that certain clinical problems (e.g., anorexia nervosa, obsessive-compulsive personality disorder) are associated with excessive exercise.

Special Implications for the Therapist **2–7**

THE "ADDICTED" EXERCISER

The therapist should be alert to the occasional client who becomes "addicted" to exercise. Clinical characteristics of such a person may include training to the exclusion of other important activities, dysphoria (depression accompanied by anxiety; disquiet) or panic when the exercise schedule is disrupted, exercising against medical advice, exercising more than once a day, and exercising to decrease or maintain an excessively low body weight (see also Anorexia Nervosa) (Hauck and Blumenthal, 1992). On the whole, the challenge of achieving adherence to a regular exercise program far outweighs concern about the occasional person who becomes obsessed with habitual exercise (see Box 2–4).

STRESS, COPING, AND ADAPTATION

Stress

Definition and Overview. *Stress* is a collective term used to describe the many social (e.g., change in job, residence, or marital status), psychological (e.g., anxiety, fear of the unknown), and physiologic (e.g., blood loss, anesthesia, pain, immobility, infection) factors that cause neurochemical changes within the body. Holmes and Rahe (1967) first developed and researched the notion that life changes (either personal or work-related) as a source of stress can eventually lead to disease. Table 2–6 summarizes their findings on major life change events. The body's response to any stress, whether caused by events perceived as positive or negative, is to mobilize its defenses to maintain homeostasis (Box 2–7). The success of the stress response in maintaining homeostatic balance is determined by the person's age, sex, physical condition, and the duration of the stress.

TABLE 2–6 Top-Rated Social Stressors

Event	Life Change Units*
Death of spouse	100
Divorce	73
Separation from mate	65
Confinement in an institution	63
Death of a close family member	63
Major personal injury or illness	53
Marriage	50
Being fired	47
Reconciliation with mate	45
Retirement from work	45
Major change in family member's health or behavior	44
Pregnancy	40
Sexual difficulties	39
Gaining a new family member	39
Major business readjustment	39
Major change in financial status	38
Death of a close friend	37
Changing to a different line of work	36
Major changes in arguments with partner	35
Heavy debt	31
Foreclosure on a mortgage or loan	30
Major change in responsibilities at work	29
Son or daughter leaving home	29
Trouble with in-laws	29
Outstanding personal achievement	28
Partner beginning or ceasing to work outside the home	26
Beginning or ceasing formal schooling	26
Change in living conditions	25

* The amount of life stress that a person has experienced in a given period of time (e.g., 1 year) is measured by the total number of life change units (LCUs). These units are obtained by adding the values shown in the right-hand column associated with events that the person has experienced during the target time period. People who encounter more than 150 LCUs/year will experience a decline in health the following year; a score between 150 and 300 LCUs carries a 50% chance of major illness; a score greater than 300 LCUs will increase the chance of major illness by 70%.

Modified from Holmes TH, Rahe RH: The Social Adjustment Rating Scale. J Psychosom Res 11:213–218, 1967.

Risk Factors. Personality traits, rotating shift work (regularly changing work hours), work environment (e.g., exposure to noise, excessive or extreme temperatures, chemicals, vibration, or extremes of lighting or glare), safety hazards, social factors, and recent life changes (e.g., death of a child or spouse, marital separation or divorce, pregnancy or birth, a move, change in job or retirement) are a few of the known risk factors linked to stress. Although many factors causing stress have been studied, the ability to predict a stress response in any given individual remains poor.

Pathogenesis (Seward, 1990). Research supports a strong correlation between stress response and the manifestation of various disorders (Box 2–8) but a direct link has not been established. How stress produces disease is frequently debated and the exact pathophysiologic mechanism remains unknown. One theory holds that certain kinds of stress are consistently likely to produce given physiologic responses, and, consequently, specific pathologic states.

BOX **2–7**

Physiologic Adaptation Response to Stress

- Increased heart rate
- Contraction of the spleen
- Release of glucose
- Redirection of blood supply
- Changes in respiratory system
- Decrease in blood clotting time
- Dilation of pupils

From Ignatavicius DD, Bayne MV: Surgical Nursing. Philadelphia, WB Saunders, 1991, pp 87–88.

BOX **2-8**
Stress-Related Conditions and Diseases

Allergic and hypersensitivity diseases
Anorexia nervosa
Asthma
Bulimia
Cancer
Cerebrovascular accident
Connective tissue disease
Crohn's disease (regional enteritis)
Emphysema
Gastrointestinal ulcers
Headache
Hypertension
Infections
Irritable bowel syndrome
Myocardial infarction
Obesity
Peripheral vascular disease
Sexual dysfunction
Tuberculosis
Ulcerative colitis

At one time it was thought that a direct link could be established between stress events and illness or between personality type and illness. At that time, it was not uncommon to hear professionals speak of a colitis, ulcer, or stroke personality. However, none of these theories have held up under investigation. At this time, only personality (angry, hostile type A behavior) has been *directly* linked with (heart) disease. See discussion, Chapter 10.

From Ignatavicius DD, Bayne MV: Surgical Nursing. Philadelphia, WB Saunders, 1991, p 89.

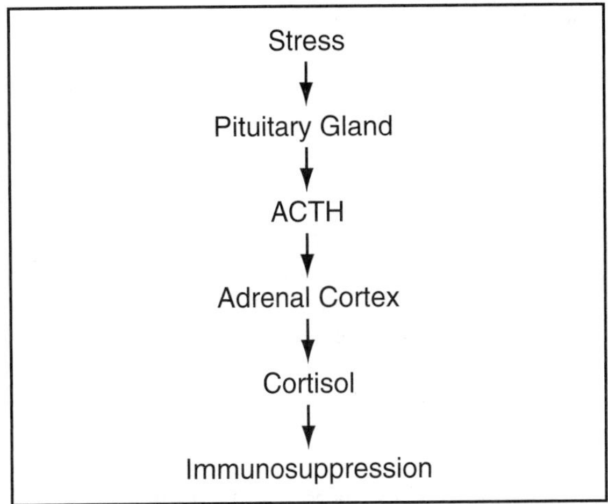

Figure **2-4.** The stress response algorithm. *(From Bancroft B: Immunology simplified. Semin Perioperative Nurs 3:70–78, 1994.)*

Another viewpoint is that stress is "nonspecific" and that personal factors such as conditioning and heredity determine which organ system, if any, will be affected by a variety of stressors. A given individual may have a specific susceptible organ that will be the target of a variety of stresses; thus, some people are gastrointestinal reactors; others are cardiac or muscle tension reactors. Familial patterns may account for the hereditary factor determining which organ system is affected. Low back pain, abdominal pain, and migraine headaches affecting adults often also occurred in the parents. Finally, stress may be viewed as a nonspecific force that exacerbates existing disease states.

The stress response has been associated with a variety of physiologic changes that may be postulated as mediators in the development of disease. The hypothalamic-pituitary axis, the autonomic nervous system, and the catecholamine response are often cited as stress-sensitive systems. These and other neurologic and endocrine systems may be important factors in the chain of events leading to cardiovascular, gastrointestinal, endocrine, and other stress-related disorders.

Recently there has been a surge of information on how the stress response systems interact in combination with a proposed neuroendocrine-neuroimmune stress response to affect autoimmunoregulation. Findings that link immune and neuroendocrine function may provide explanations of how the emotional state or response to stress can modify a person's capacity to cope with infection or cancer and influence the course of autoimmune disease (Reichlin, 1993). For example (Fig. 2-4), ongoing stress causes adrenocorticotropic hormone releasing factor (ACTH-RF) to be released from the hypothalamus, causing ACTH to be released from the pituitary gland. Stress hormones (e.g., cortisol) are then released from the adrenal glands, causing immunosuppression, that is, decreased numbers of lymphocytes (white blood cells) and antibodies, thus increasing vulnerability to infectious diseases, including viral-induced cancers (Ader et al., 1995; Fricchione and Stefano, 1994; see also Chapter 5).

Stress can play a key role in psychogenic pain, that is, pain believed to be caused by emotional factors rather than the result of physiologic dysfunction. Although psychogenic pain begins without a physical basis, repeated severe stress most likely alters the complex physiology of pain transmission, modulation, and perception. When the psychogenic effects of stress, anxiety, fear, and anger produce painful alterations in physiology, this is referred to as *psychophysiologic pain* (Matassarin-Jacobs, 1993). For example, stress can produce chronic excessive muscle contraction with resultant ischemia, and pain with eventual functional impairment.

On the other hand, there is evidence to suggest that psychological distress does not cause conditions such as headaches. Rather, chronic headaches can trigger stress, depression, and other psychological disorders. According to one study (Tramuta, 1994), when headaches with an underlying medical diagnosis were treated, the likelihood of psychiatric disorder also lessened.

Clinical Manifestations. Therapists frequently treat people with neuromusculoskeletal dysfunction, especially head, neck, and back pain without an identified point of injury or cause. Stress, reaction to stress, and posttraumatic stress disorder are common causes of physical manifestations treated by the therapist. Muscle tension and pain, restlessness, irritability, fatigue, increased startle reaction, breath holding, hyperventilation, tachycardia, palpitations, and sleep disturbances are some of the more common symptoms reported to the therapist. Frequently, clients self-medicate using chemical (alcohol, nicotine, drugs) or food substances; the alert therapist may help assist the client by facilitating treatment for this aspect of the person's stress response.

Psychological Aspects *(Brophy, 1994).* Psychological (psychiatric) disorders may result from disturbance of one or more interrelated factors including biologic function, coping mechanisms, learned behavior, and social and environmental conditions. Psychological disorders of biologic origin may be secondary to identifiable physical illness, acquired through trauma such as head injury, the side effects of medication, or caused by biochemical disturbances in the brain. Other commonly observed psychological disorders in a therapy practice are discussed here, including anxiety disorders, psychophysiologic or psychosomatic disorders, chronic pain disorders, and mood disorders (especially depression).

Special Implications for the Therapist **2-8**

STRESS

The therapist may be called upon to assist the client in reducing the physical impact of stress on the body as well as providing a means of physical or emotional control. *Progressive muscle relaxation* (*PMR*), breathing exercises, exercise, and biofeedback are the primary tools used in therapy to teach the client effective stress-reducing techniques (Thompson et al., 1993).

Since stress commonly causes muscle tension producing somatic symptoms such as headaches and neck and back pain, control of muscle tension appears to help reduce the physical effects of such tension as well. PMR involves the alternate tensing and relaxing of all major muscle groups, usually in sequential steps. It is easy to teach and inexpensive.

Breathing exercises can be helpful in restoring normal respiration by providing moments of deep breathing because the person in a stressful situation tends to breathe shallowly or even unconsciously holds his or her breath. Teaching diaphragmatic breathing skills and suggesting ways clients can remember to check their breathing (e.g., whenever the telephone rings, setting their watches to beep on the hour, at every stop sign when in an automobile) can aid in reducing the chest and upper body muscle tension that accompanies altered breathing patterns.

Exercise is only one of the behavioral and psychological therapies recommended for the treatment of selected clients, such as those with coronary disease. Exercise training, type A behavior* modification, psychological counseling, smoking cessation, and dietary modification are also considered important in the overall holistic treatment approach to many people. For example, aerobic exercise has been found to consistently attenuate (weaken or reduce) the psychophysiologic responses to stress, particularly in type A personalities (Blumenthal and Wei, 1993). Type A "beliefs" may predispose individuals to health problems through impaired interactions with their interpersonal environment (Watkins et al., 1992), as will mechanisms that increase cardiovascular and neuroendocrine responses (Fredrikson and Blumenthal, 1992). In this particular population, aerobic training blunts their cardiovascular and adrenal response to stress.

Although physical exercise may be considered a stressor itself, there are significant differences in the way the body responds to exercise vs. the way the body responds to a mental stressor. A key difference is between the diastolic and systolic blood pressure responses. Exercise results in a rise in the systolic pressure and possibly a small increase in diastolic pressure, whereas mental stress produces a significant increase in both diastolic and systolic blood pressures. Blood vessels dilate during physical exercise to increase the blood supply to the muscles. During this vasodilation the diastolic blood pressure tends to stabilize or increase mildly, whereas during mental stress, although the muscles may isometrically contract (muscle tension), there is no substantial movement of the body by the muscles and no metabolic reason for vasodilation to occur. Decreased vagal activity may contribute to the exaggerated diastolic blood pressure reactivity to mental stress (Jiang et al., 1993).

Biofeedback can be an effective means of training persons to reverse the subtle changes in blood pressure, muscle tension, and heart rate that accompany a stress-induced somatic response. Biofeedback involves using electronic instrumentation to signal selected somatic changes. Surface electrodes are sensitive to small changes in the electrical activity of the muscles signaling to the client by way of sound or sight the need to practice physiologic quieting techniques (e.g., visualization, imagery, deep breathing).

* A behavior pattern associated with the development of coronary heart disease, characterized by excessive competitiveness and aggression and a fast-paced lifestyle. Persons exhibiting type A behavior are constantly struggling to accomplish ill-defined or broadly encompassing goals in the shortest time possible. This type of behavior has been shown to be as significant as other risk factors in the development of coronary artery disease and myocardial infarction when accompanied by hostility associated with anger (Mittleman et al., 1994). The opposite type of behavior, exhibited by persons who are relaxed, unhurried, and less aggressive, is called type B (O'Toole, 1992; Friedman and Rosenman, 1981).

Anxiety Disorders

Anxiety is defined as a generalized emotional state of fear and apprehension that is usually associated with a heightened state of physiologic arousal such as elevation in heart rate and sweat gland activity. The most common anxiety disorders encountered in the therapy practice include adjustment disorder with anxious mood, general anxiety disorder, posttraumatic stress disorder (PTSD), panic disorder, and obsessive-compulsive disorder (OCD). Frequently, somatic symptoms referable to the autonomic nervous system or to a specific organ system (e.g., chest pain, dyspnea, palpitations, paresthesias) occur. Anxiety can become self-generating because the symptoms reinforce the reaction, causing a spiral effect. Stimulants such as caffeine, cocaine or other stimulant drugs, or medications containing caffeine, or stimulants used in treating asthma can also trigger anxiety disorders and contribute to this spiral effect (Hendrix, 1993).

The *adjustment disorder* is usually a temporary phenomenon in response to a stressor such as a traumatic injury (e.g., SCI, cerebrovascular accident, total body burns), change in family system due to debility of the wage earner, or a known organic condition such as a pulmonary embolus with a life-threatening status. During the adjustment phase, the person gathers resources to maintain self-worth, acceptance, and ability to cope. For some people, the adjustment stage becomes more of a maladjustment stage, in which case the person remains unable to come to terms with fear, disbelief, anger, guilt, or depression and remains hampered by the disease's real or perceived impairment (Sanford and Petajan, 1988). When viewed by the client as an unpredictable, variable, and disabling condition, chronic illnesses such as obstructive pulmonary disease (COPD) or multiple sclerosis are often associated with such an adjustment disorder.

General anxiety disorders are marked by a focus on physical or emotional pain; the person either notices pain more or interprets pain as being more significant than a nonanxious person would. Disability, pain behavior such as limping and grimacing, and medication-seeking may develop. Symptoms may present as physical, behavioral, cognitive, or psychological (Table 2–7).

Posttraumatic stress disorder (DSM-IV, 1994) is the development of characteristic symptoms following exposure to an extreme traumatic stressor involving direct personal experience of an event that involves actual or threatened death or serious injury, or other threat to one's physical integrity; or witnessing an event that involves death, injury, or threat to someone else. The person's response to the event involves intense fear, helplessness, or horror (or in children, disorganized or agitated behavior).

Traumatic events that are experienced may include military combat, violent personal assault (sexual assault, physical attack, robbery, mugging), being kidnapped or taken hostage, terrorist attack, torture, incarceration as a prisoner of war or in a concentration camp, natural or manmade disasters, a severe automobile accident, or being diagnosed with a life-threatening illness. For children, sexually traumatic events may include developmentally inappropriate sexual experiences without threatened or actual violence or injury.

PTSD can occur at any age, including childhood. Symptoms usually begin within the first 3 months after the trauma, although there may be a delay of months, or even years, before symptoms appear. The person with PTSD experiences persistent symptoms of anxiety or increased arousal that were not present before the trauma. These symptoms may include difficulty falling or staying asleep, hypervigilance and exaggerated startle response, or difficulty concentrating on or completing tasks. Children may also exhibit various physical symptoms such as headaches and stomachaches. There may be other associated conditions such as panic disorder, agoraphobia, obsessive-compulsive disorder, social phobia, specific phobia, major depressive disorder, somatization disorder, and substance abuse disorders.

Panic disorder is characterized by periods of sudden, unprovoked, intense anxiety with associated physical symptoms lasting a few minutes to less than 2 hours. Initial panic attacks may develop during a period of extreme stress, or following surgery, a serious accident, illness, or childbirth. The premenstrual period is one of heightened vulnerability. Panic disorder may be due to an inherently unstable autonomic nervous system, coupled with cognitive distress (Papp et al., 1993). Worrisome signs and symptoms such as marked dyspnea, tachycardia, palpitations, headaches, dizziness, paresthesias (nose, cheeks, lips, fingers, toes), choking, smothering feelings, nausea, and bloating are associated with feelings of alarm and a sense of impending doom. Recurrent sleep panic attacks (not nightmares) occur in about 30% of panic disorders. Residual sore muscles are a consistent finding following the panic attack; the person with sleep panic attacks awakens feeling fatigued, stiff, and sore.

Obsessive-compulsive disorder (OCD) is characterized by obsessions (constantly recurring thoughts such as fear of exposure to germs) and compulsions (repetitive actions such as washing the hands hundreds of times a day). The motivating force behind such behaviors was thought to be the need to maintain control but the fact that some people with OCD respond well to specific medications suggests the disorder may have a neurobiologic basis (Hendrix, 1991). Most clients do not mention the symptoms or the disorder (if diagnosed) and must be asked about their presence and effect on the person's life and rehabilitation. A person is not considered to have OCD unless the obsessive and compulsive behaviors are extreme enough to interfere with daily activities.

People with OCD should not be confused with a much

TABLE 2–7 SYMPTOMS OF ANXIETY

PHYSICAL	BEHAVIORAL	COGNITIVE	PSYCHOLOGICAL
Increased sighing respirations	Hyperalertness	Fear of losing one's mind	Phobias
Increased blood pressure	Irritability	Fear of losing control	Obsessive-compulsive behaviors
Tachycardia	Uncertainty		
Shortness of breath	Apprehensiveness		
Dizziness	Difficulty with memory or concentration		
Lump in throat	Sleep disturbance		
Muscle tension			
Dry mouth			
Diarrhea			
Nausea			
Clammy hands			
Sweating			
Pacing			
Chest pain*			

* Chest pain associated with anxiety accounts for more than half of all emergency room admissions for chest pain. The pain is substernal, a dull ache which does not radiate, and is not aggravated by respiratory movements, but *is* associated with hyperventilation and claustrophobia.

larger group of individuals who are sometimes called "compulsive" because they hold themselves to a high standard of performance in their work and even in their recreational (or rehabilitation) activities (Hendrix, 1991). Compulsive exercising sometimes accompanied by bulimia or other eating disorders can interfere with the rehabilitation process. Major depression is present in two thirds of cases of OCD.

Special Implications for the Therapist **2-9**

ANXIETY DISORDERS

Although panic disorder clients may fear exercise, panic attacks during exercise are rare. If a client experiences a panic attack during therapy, reassurance and distraction frequently work well to help the person move through the episode. Hyperventilation may be an accompanying symptom requiring intervention. A paper bag is used for rebreathing in such instances.

Recognizing signs and symptoms of previously undiagnosed anxiety disorders can provide the client with beneficial treatment once referred to a physician. Medications can provide significant relief from the symptoms of anxiety disorders in more than half of all cases. Combining physical therapy with behavioral therapy can often accelerate both the physical and psychological rehabilitation process.

Uncontrolled and controlled studies on the effects of exercise on anxiety provide support for regular physical activity as a treatment for anxiety disorders (Moses, 1989; King, 1989b; Cameron and Hudson, 1986). The exact mechanism whereby exercise reduces symptoms of anxiety has not been determined. Hypotheses include the following: (1) exercise creates cognitive distraction from stressful stimuli; (2) exercise promotes a sense of personal empowerment and control; (3) exercise provides social reinforcement and support; (4) exercise improves physiologic responses to stressful conditions resulting in lower overall sympathetic reactivity under stress; and (5) exercise provides quicker sympathetic recovery after exposure to stress (Benight and Taylor, 1994).

The therapist must remain alert to the possibility of suicide or alcohol abuse sometimes combined with dependence on sedatives. Suspicion of either should be reported to the case manager, counselor, or physician. See also the discussion of suicide in Special Implications for the Therapist 2–13: Coping and Adapting. Clients with obsessive-compulsive tendencies must be given specific guidelines for any home program prescribed. Specific limits for numbers of repetitions must be provided, including the strict admonishment to avoid "checking" their pain or loss of motion "to see if it is any better yet."

Psychophysiologic Disorders

Psychophysiologic disorders, also referred to as psychosomatic disorders, are any disorders in which the physical symptoms may be caused or exacerbated by psychological factors. Common examples include migraine headaches, low back pain, gastric ulcer, or irritable bowel syndrome. Previously it was believed that psychological factors caused these conditions. More recently the existing lack of certainty about the actual role of psychological factors in causing these conditions has led researchers to suggest that psychological factors are more likely to be contributory to physical conditions.

Psychophysiologic disorders are generally characterized by subjective complaints that exceed objective findings, symptom development in the presence of psychosocial stresses, and physical symptoms involving one or more organ systems. This category includes *somatoform disorder*, *psychogenic pain disorder*, and *factitious disorder*.

Somatoform Disorder

Somatoform disorder is the presence of physical symptoms that suggest a medical condition causing significant impairment in social, occupational, or other areas of functioning. The physical symptoms associated with somatoform disorders are not intentional or under voluntary control, which differentiates it from factitious disorder and malingering.

Persons who are unable to cope with emotional problems or conflicts may develop physical symptoms as a means of coping, because it may be easier to accept physical symptoms as a cause of unhappiness or conflict than to admit to an underlying emotional or psychological cause. The disorder is characterized by vague, multiple, recurring physical complaints that have no biologic or physiologic cause. This disorder was previously included in the group of psychologic conditions called hysterical neurosis (conversion type).

Frequently, the term somatoform disorder is used interchangeably with somatization disorder, but in fact somatoform disorder includes six distinct conditions, namely somatization disorder, undifferentiated somatoform disorder, conversion disorder, pain disorder, hypochondriasis, and body dysmorphic disorder.

Specific symptoms of *somatization disorder* (Briquet's syndrome) (Box 2–9) may include double or blurred vision, food sensitivity, abdominal pain or bloating, bowel problems, vomiting, fainting, headaches, chest pain, nonexertional dyspnea, painful menstruation, or sexual indifference. These symptoms are often presented in a dramatic and exaggerated way, but the person is vague about the exact nature of the symptoms. Depression and anxiety are often key components of this disorder. The person will consult with multiple physicians and receive a variety of treatment approaches, often including multiple surgeries, with apparent unsuccessful outcome.

Undifferentiated somatoform disorder is characterized by unexplained physical complaints lasting at least 6 months that are below the threshold for a diagnosis of somatization disorder. The most frequent complaints are chronic fatigue, loss of appetite, or gastrointestinal or genitourinary symptoms that cannot be fully explained by any known general medical condition. Physical symptoms or impairment are beyond what would be expected from the history, physical examination, or laboratory findings.

Hypochondriasis is marked by a preoccupation with one's health and exaggeration of normal sensations and minor complaints into a serious illness. Hypochondriasis is focused on a single illness, unlike somatization, which is accompanied by multiple complaints. With hypochondriasis, symptoms are amplified and the client is hyperresponsive to the treatment administered, especially in the therapy setting. No amount

BOX **2–9**
Diagnostic Criteria for Somatization Disorder

A. A history of many physical complaints beginning before age 30 years that occur over a period of several years and result in treatment being sought or significant impairment in social, occupational, or other important areas of functioning.

B. Each of the following criteria must have been met, with individual symptoms* occurring at any time during the course of the disturbance:

1. *Four pain symptoms:* a history of pain related to at least four different sites or functions (e.g., head, abdomen, back, joints, extremities, chest, rectum, during menstruation, during sexual intercourse, or during urination)
2. *Two gastrointestinal symptoms:* a history of at least two gastrointestinal symptoms other than pain (e.g., nausea, bloating, vomiting other than during pregnancy, diarrhea, or intolerance of several different foods)
3. *One sexual symptom:* a history of at least one sexual or reproductive symptom other than pain (e.g., sexual indifference, erectile or ejaculatory dysfunction, irregular menses, excessive menstrual bleeding, vomiting throughout pregnancy)
4. *One pseudoneurologic symptom:* a history of at least one symptom or deficit suggesting a neurologic condition not limited to pain (conversion symptoms such as impaired coordination or balance, paralysis or localized weakness, difficulty swallowing or lump in throat, aphonia, urinary retention, hallucinations, loss of touch or pain sensation, double vision, blindness, deafness, seizures; dissociative symptoms such as amnesia; or loss of consciousness other than fainting)

C. Either (1) or (2):

1. After appropriate investigation, each of the symptoms in criterion B cannot be fully explained by a known general medical condition or the direct effects of a substance (e.g., a drug of abuse, a medication)
2. When there is a related general medical condition, the physical complaints or resulting social or occupational impairment are in excess of what would be expected from the history, physical examination, or laboratory findings

D. The symptoms are not intentionally produced or feigned (as in factitious disorder or malingering).

* Symptoms are listed in the approximate order of their reported frequency.
Adapted from American Psychiatric Association: Diagnostic and Statistical Manual of Mental Disorders, ed 4. [DSM-IV]. Washington, DC, Author, 1994.

of reassurance can convince the person that he or she is healthy; hypochondriasis is often common in panic disorders.

Somatoform pain disorder is another type of somatization disorder frequently encountered in the therapy setting. Pain disorder is characterized by pain as the predominant focus of clinical attention, but psychological factors have an important role in the onset, severity, exacerbation, or maintenance of this disorder (DSM-IV, 1994). This condition may be viewed as (1) pain disorder associated with psychological factors; (2) pain disorder associated with a general medical condition; and (3) pain disorder associated with both psychological factors and a medical condition. There are both acute and chronic forms of somatoform pain disorder. Chronic pain associated with a known medical condition (e.g., neoplasm, diabetic polyneuropathy, postoperative pain) is discussed in the next section, Chronic Pain Disorders.

Body dysmorphic disorder is a particular type of somatization disorder frequently encountered in people who have undergone amputation, extensive surgery, or had burns with significant scarring and those with weight control problems (Woltersdorf, 1995). There is a preoccupation with the imagined or exaggerated defect in personal appearance.

Conversion is a psychodynamic phenomenon rather than a behavioral response to illness or injury and is quite rare in the chronically disabled population. Conversion is defined as a transformation of an emotion into a physical manifestation. The person is unable to verbally express an emotion (considered threatening or unacceptable) and expresses a physical symptom instead. Conversion symptoms are peripheral and anesthetic, most commonly presenting as paralysis of the limbs or loss of vision without physical explanation or findings.

Psychophysiologic symptoms associated with conversion occur when anxiety activates the autonomic nervous system (an unconscious, unintentional process), resulting in tachycardia, hyperventilation, and vasoconstriction. Other symptoms may include hysterical pain response[8] and symptoms related to voluntary motor or sensory functioning, referred to as pseudoneurologic. Motor symptoms or deficits include localized weakness or paralysis, impaired coordination or balance, aphonia (loss of voice), difficulty swallowing or a sensation of a lump in the throat, and urinary retention. Sensory changes include loss of touch or pain sensation, double vision, blindness, deafness, and hallucinations. Seizure or convulsions may also occur. No cause or disease can explain the distribution of such symptoms; the physician must carefully differentiate conversion symptoms from physical disorders with unusual presentations such as multiple sclerosis.

Psychogenic Pain Disorder

Psychogenic pain is often ill-defined, and its anatomic distribution depends more on the person's concepts of disease and dysfunction than on the actual course of the clinical disease. The client presents with multiple unrelated symptoms, and the fluctuations in the course of symptoms are determined more by crises in the person's psychosocial life than by physical changes.

Factitious Disorder

Factitious disorder is characterized by somatic symptom production that is intentional or self-induced for the purpose of

[8] Excessive pain without organic cause.

gaining attention by deceiving health care personnel or for personal gain (DSM-IV, 1994). A parent may fabricate an illness in a child so that treatment can be given to satisfy a somatoform disorder in the parent. The person's motivation is often unclear; frequently the client is already involved in some way with the health care profession (e.g., works in a physician's office). Adolescents often feign illness or injury to receive attention they feel they lack at home.

Symptoms that are intentionally produced do not count toward a diagnosis of somatoform disorder, but factitious or malingering symptoms are often mixed with other nonintentional symptoms, resulting in a diagnosis of somatoform disorder and a factitious disorder or malingering. In factitious disorder, the motivation is to assume the sick role and to obtain medical evaluation and treatment, whereas in malingering, more external incentives are apparent, such as financial compensation, avoidance of duty, evasion of criminal prosecution, or obtaining drugs.

Factitious disorder is characterized by signs and symptoms that are predominantly psychological or physical. When an individual presents with a medical condition in an attempt to get admitted to (or to stay in) a hospital, the disorder is referred to as *Munchausen's syndrome*. The symptoms are determined by the person's medical knowledge, sophistication, and imagination.

Medical Management

Diagnosis (DSM-IV, 1994). With all psychophysiologic disorders, the physician must rule out general medical conditions that are characterized by vague, multiple, and confusing somatic symptoms, such as hyperparathyroidism, acute intermittent porphyria, multiple sclerosis, or systemic lupus erythematosus. The onset of multiple physical symptoms late in life is almost always due to a general medical condition.

Several criteria must be met before a somatoform disorder can be established (see Box 2–9; Table 2–8). For all psychophysiologic disorders (somatoform disorders, psychogenic pain disorder, factitious disorder), there is remarkable absence of findings in laboratory test results to support the subjective report of symptoms. Likewise, the physical examination is remarkable for the absence of objective findings to fully explain the many subjective symptoms.

Prognosis. The course of psychophysiologic disorders varies with each type of disorder. Within the somatoform disorders, somatization disorder and undifferentiated somatoform disorder are chronic and unpredictable and rarely remit. Conversion is often of short duration and hospitalized individuals have remission within 2 weeks in most cases. A good prognosis for conversion is associated with acute onset, presence of clearly identifiable stress at the time of onset, a short interval between onset and the initiation of treatment, above average intelligence, and symptoms of paralysis, aphonia, and blindness. Poor prognostic indicators include symptoms of tremors and seizures. Pain disorder resolves relatively quickly when associated with an acute episode, but there is a wide range of variability in the course of chronic pain (see also Chronic Pain Disorders). Hypochondriasis is usually chronic but can remit completely, especially in the absence of a personality disorder and the absence of a secondary gain. Body dysmorphic disorder often has a continuous course once it is diagnosed. Symptoms are almost always present, although the intensity may vary over time. The course of psychogenic pain disorder or factitious disorder may be limited to one or more brief episodes, but it is more often of a chronic nature with a lifelong pattern of hospitalization.

Special Implications for the Therapist **2–10**

PSYCHOPHYSIOLOGIC DISORDERS

The health care professional who can communicate a willingness to consider all aspects of illness, whether physiologic or psychological, can foster a trusting relationship with the client. Such an attitude promotes client self-disclosure and a reliance on confidentiality. As with all psychologically based illnesses, the therapist is encouraged to practice in cooperation with the other team members, especially when behavioral or psychological approaches are the basis of medical treatment.

TABLE 2–8 Somatoform Disorders

Disorder	Presentation	Criteria
Somatization disorder (Briquet's syndrome)	Multiple focal symptom focus	Begins before age 30, extends over a period of years, characterized by a combination of pain, gastrointestinal, sexual, or pseudoneurologic symptoms
Undifferentiated somatoform disorder	Diffuse symptom focus	Unexplained physical complaints that are below the threshold for the diagnosis of somatization disorder; complaints must be present for at least 6 mo
Hypochondriasis	Single symptom focus	Preoccupation with the fear of having, or the idea that one has, a serious disease based on the person's misinterpretation of body symptoms
Somatoform pain disorder	Pain is the predominant focus	Pain the prime complaint with psychological factors having an important role in the onset, worsening, or maintenance of the disorder
Body dysmorphic disorder	Body part distortion	Preoccupation with an imagined or exaggerated defect in physical appearance
Conversion disorder	Motor/sensory symptoms	Involves unexplained symptoms affecting voluntary motor or sensory functions that mimic a general medical or neurologic condition; psychological factors are associated with the presentation of the symptoms

Adapted from Woltersdorf MA: Hidden disorders: Psychological barriers to treatment success. Phys Ther 3:58–66, 1995.

Somatoform Disorders *(Woltersdorf, 1995)*

Somatoform disorders can account for 80% of all physician visits and make up a large portion of clients in a therapy setting. Personality disorders, though rare in the general population, are common in the medical arena (Sweet and Reynolds, 1992). Somatoform clients are often described as "whiners" and can present with a bewildering array of symptoms, all of which are highly resistant to improvement through therapy or other medical or psychological treatment.

The essential markers for the somatoform disorders are the absence or inadequacy of physical findings, insatiable complaints, excessive social and occupational consequences, preoccupation with problems, and lack of obvious secondary or material gain. This is not to say that adopting the sometimes enjoyable sick role has no gain associated with it, but not material or monetary gain. However, somatoform disorders can coexist with a concurrent physical illness, emphasizing the need for ongoing evaluation.

These persons frequently seek treatment from several physicians concurrently, which may lead to complicated and sometimes hazardous combinations of treatment (polypharmacy). Frequent use of medications may lead to side effects and substance-related disorders. The therapist is encouraged to maintain close communication with the physician if either of these situations is suspected or discovered.

Working with individuals who have somatoform disorders places the therapist at risk for personal and professional burnout. To preserve one's sanity and maintain a professional perspective, persons with somatoform disorders must be identified. Most people with somatoform disorders are not helped by any kind of physical or occupational therapy. A brief summary of the somatoform disorders and possible clinical strategies are provided in Table 2–9. The reader is referred to articles on these topics written specifically for the health care professional for more specific details (see Woltersdorf, 1992, 1994, 1995; DSM-IV, 1994).

Chronic Pain Disorders

Definition and Overview. Chronic pain has been recognized as pain which persists past the normal time of healing (Bonica, 1953).[9] This may be less than 1 month, or more often, more than 6 months. The International Association for the Study of Pain has settled on 3 months as the dividing line between acute and chronic pain (Merskey, 1986). Chronic pain appears to be frequently associated with depressive disorders, whereas acute pain appears to be more commonly associated with anxiety disorders. The associated mental disorders may precede the pain disorder (and possibly predispose the individual to it), co-occur with it, or result from it (DSM-IV, 1994).

The Subcommittee on Taxonomy of the International Association for the Study of Pain has proposed a five-axis system for categorizing chronic pain (Table 2–10) according to (1) anatomic region; (2) organ system; (3) temporal characteristics of pain and pattern of occurrence; (4) person's statement of intensity and time since onset of pain; and (4) etiology. This five-axis system focuses primarily on the physical manifestations of pain but provides for comments on the psychological factors on both the second axis where the involvement of a mental disorder can be coded and on the fifth axis where possible etiologies include "psychophysiologic" and "psychological."

Incidence. Chronic pain disorders can occur at any age and are relatively common. For example, it is estimated that in any given year, 10% to 15% of adults in the United States have some form of work disability due to back pain alone. Females appear to experience certain chronic pain conditions such as headaches and musculoskeletal pain more often than do males (DSM-IV, 1994).

Etiology. Among the most common general medical conditions associated with chronic pain are various *musculoskeletal conditions* (e.g., disk herniation, osteoporosis, osteoarthritis or rheumatoid arthritis, myofascial syndromes), *neuropathies* (e.g., diabetic neuropathies, postherpetic neuralgia), and *malignancies* (e.g., metastatic lesions in bone, tumor infiltration of nerves) (DSM-IV, 1994). The most common chronic pain conditions encountered by the therapist are listed in Box 2–10. Chronic pain may be a form of self-defense as a result of domestic violence or abuse. See also Somatoform Disorders and Domestic Violence in this chapter.

Chronic postoperative pain occurs in a small percentage of people after the following procedures: thoracotomy with pain caused by tumor recurrence or invasion of the chest wall, mastectomy with pain from interruption of the intercostobrachial nerve (branches from the brachial plexus to the thoracic region), surgical amputation followed by phantom limb pain, and chemotherapy when associated with neuropathies producing painful dysesthesias (abnormal sensations) of the feet and hands.

Physiologic, Psychological, and Behavioral Response *(Ludwig-Beymer and Huether, 1993).* Physiologic responses to chronic pain depend on the persistent (e.g., low back pain) or intermittent (e.g., migraine headache) nature of the pain. Intermittent pain produces a physiologic response similar to that of acute pain, whereas persistent pain allows for physiologic adaptation (e.g., normal heart rate, blood pressure, and respiratory rate).

Chronic pain produces significant behavioral and psychological changes. A constellation of life changes that produce altered behavior in the individual and that persist even after the cause of the pain has been eradicated make up the *chronic pain syndrome* (Zohn and Mennell, 1988). Painful symptoms out of proportion to the injury or which are not consistent with the objective findings may be a red flag indicative of systemic disease or a psychogenic pain disorder. This can be differentiated from a chronic pain syndrome in that the syndrome is characterized by multiple complaints, excessive preoccupation with pain or physical symptoms, and frequently, excessive drug use. The person exhibiting symptoms of a chronic pain syndrome may isolate himself or herself

[9] In order to prevent confusion the reader should keep in mind that chronic pain disorders cn be psychologically based (somatoform pain disorder), a result of a general medical condition, or a mixture of both. The American Psychiatric Association's *Diagnostic and Statistical Manual of Mental Disorders* (DSM-IV, 1994) classifies conditions with a psychological basis. The International Association for the Study of Pain has also developed diagnostic criteria specific to pain disorders.

TABLE 2–9 Clinical Strategies for Somatoform Disorders

Disorder	Problem	Solution
Personality disorders	Rigid, inflexible, interpersonal style that has no correlation to the current personal relationship or needs of the setting of the moment	*Do:* focus on the physical needs of the client, remind self that you are not there to satisfy all the needs of the client, remain professional, document objectively any troublesome exchanges. *Don't:* try to be their friend, ever take any client's response personally, allow emotions to creep into your documentation.
Somatization disorder	Bewildering array of physical complaints that exceed findings	*Do:* keep accurate records of all physical findings, assess regularly, mention their progress frequently, focus on what you can change (stiffness) and avoid what you can't (nausea), praise their strengths. *Don't:* tell them it's in their head even though you're right, don't confront the obvious contradictions.
Undifferentiated somatoform disorder	Diffuse, ambiguous complaints	*Do:* assess for physical findings only. *Don't:* become more than a therapist for them; refer appropriately.
Hypochondriasis	Intense, single-symptom focus	Same as somatization disorder.
Somatoform pain disorder	Pain, pain, pain	*Do:* remember pain cannot be measured directly, focus on the indirect effects of pain, have a multidisciplinary approach, demand regular improvement and set criteria early in treatment for what improvement looks like. *Don't:* get angry at them, confront their inconsistencies; document objectively and unemotionally.
Body dysmorphic disorder	Excessive concerns about appearances	*Do:* focus on their strengths, stay upbeat, downplay any undue attention to the actual area of disfigurement. *Don't:* have them talk about their feelings about the body part in question, tell them they're being unreasonable, say you know how they feel.
Conversion disorder	Motor/sensory inconsistencies	Same as somatization disorder.

Modified from Woltersdorf MA: Hidden disorders: Psychological barriers to treatment success. PT Magazine 3(12):58–66, 1995.

socially from other people and be fatigued, tense, fearful, and depressed. There are chronic pain cases in which a diagnosis is finally made (e.g. spinal stenosis or thyroiditis) and the treatment is specific, not one of pain management alone.

Persons with chronic pain often are depressed, have sleep disturbances, and may become preoccupied with the pain. People with chronic pain often attempt to maintain their former lifestyle in order to appear as normal as possible, even denying pain and engaging in activities that exacerbate their painful symptoms. They may not report the full extent of their pain for fear of being labeled a complainer or hypochondriac. The need to hide the pain conflicts with the need to have someone understand the pain. The result is emotional and psychological conflicts. See Coping and Adapting later in this chapter.

Symptom Magnification Syndrome. *Sympton magnification syndrome (SMS)* is defined as "a self-destructive, socially reinforced *behavioral response* pattern consisting of reports or displays of symptoms which function to control the life of the sufferer" (Matheson, 1986, 1987). At the present time, SMS is not listed in the DSM-IV. It is likely that in the future SMS will be categorized as a somatoform disorder, possibly a variant of somatoform pain disorder of a chronic nature.

The term was first coined by Leonard N. Matheson in 1977 to describe persons whose symptoms have reinforced their self-destructive behavior, that is, the symptoms have become the predominant force in the client's function, rather than the physiologic phenomenon of the injury determining outcome (unless physiologic changes occur leading to deconditioning). Conscious symptom magnification is referred to as "malingering," whereas unconscious symptom magnification is labelled "illness behavior" or somatoform disorder.

SMS can fall into several categories and the reader is referred to Matheson (1991) for an in-depth understanding of this syndrome. Three signs indicating that a client may be exhibiting symptom magnification are the following:

1. Ineffective strategy for balancing symptoms against activities.
2. Client acts as if the future cannot be controlled because of the presence of symptoms; limitation is blamed on symptoms: "My [back] pain won't let me. . . "
3. Client may exaggerate limitations beyond those that are reasonable in relation to the injury; client applies minimal effort on maximum performance tasks and overreacts to loading during objective examination.

Medical Management

Diagnosis. In conjunction with the proposed five-axis system for categorizing chronic pain (see Table 2–10), the physician may use the diagnostic criteria outlined in DSM-IV (Box 2–11).

Prognosis. There is a wide range of variability in the course of chronic pain. In most cases, symptoms persist for many years, but function can improve when the individual partici-

TABLE 2-10 Classification of Chronic Pain

Axis I: Regions
Head, face, and mouth
Cervical region
Upper shoulder and upper limbs
Thoracic region
Abdominal region
Low back: lumbar spine, sacrum, and coccyx
Lower limbs
Pelvic region
Anal, perineal, and genital region
More than 3 major sites

Axis II: Systems
Nervous system (central, peripheral, and autonomic) and special senses; physical disturbance or dysfunction
Nervous system (psychological and social)*
Respiratory and cardiovascular systems
Musculoskeletal system and connective tissue
Cutaneous and subcutaneous and associated glands (breast, apocrine, etc.)
Gastrointestinal system
Genitourinary system
Other organs or viscera (e.g., thyroid, lymphatic, hemapoietic)
More than one system

Axis III: Temporal Characteristics of Pain: Pattern of Occurrence
Not recorded, not applicable, or not known
Single episode, limited duration (e.g., ruptured aneurysm, sprained ankle)
Continuous or nearly continuous, nonfluctuating (e.g., low back pain, some cases)
Continuous or nearly continuous, fluctuating severity (e.g., ruptured intervertebral disk)
Recurring irregularly (e.g., headache, mixed type)
Recurring regularly (e.g., premenstrual pain)
Paroxysmal (e.g., tic douloureux)
Sustained with superimposed paroxysms
Other combinations
None of the above

Axis IV: Person's Statement of Intensity: Time Since Onset of Pain†
Not recorded, not applicable, or not known

Mild:	≤1 mo
	1–6 mo
	>6 mo
Medium:	≤1 mo
	1–6 mo
	>6 mo
Severe:	≤1 mo
	1–6 mo
	<6 mo

Axis V: Etiology
Genetic or congenital disorders (e.g., congenital dislocation)
Trauma, operation, burns
Infective, parasitic
Inflammatory (no known infective agent), immune reactions
Neoplasm
Toxic, metabolic (e.g., alcoholic neuropathy, anoxia, vascular, nutritional, endocrine), radiation
Degenerative, mechanical‡
Dysfunctional (including psychophysiologic)§
Unknown or other
Psychological origin (e.g., conversion hysteria, depressive hallucination)

* To be coded for psychiatric illness without any relevant lesion.
† Determine the time at which pain is recognized retrospectively as having started even though the pain may occur intermittently. Grade for intensity in relation to the level of the current pain problem.
‡ For example, a lumbar puncture headache would be mechanical.
§ For example, migraine headache, tension headache, or irritable bowel syndrome; syndromes where a pathophysiologic alteration is recognized are also included. Emotional causes may or may not be present.
Adapted from Merskey H (ed): Classification of chronic pain: Scheme for coding chronic pain diagnoses. Pain (suppl 3):S10–S11, 1986.

pates in regularly scheduled activities such as volunteer or paid work.

Special Implications for the Therapist **2-11**

CHRONIC PAIN DISORDERS

It is counterproductive to speculate about whether the client's pain is "real." It is real to the person, and acceptance of the pain as part of the clinical picture places the therapist in alliance with the client toward mutually acceptable goals. Focusing on improving functional outcomes rather than on reducing the pain should be the underlying direction in therapy.

Chronic anxiety and depression may produce heightened irritability, overreaction to stimuli, and a heightened awareness of the symptoms. The person may become preoccupied with the details of anatomic function and how each movement or external event affects the symptoms. This self-focus must be redirected toward improving function and differs from the overdramatization of the discomfort that is sometimes helpful in alleviating the problem in certain cultures (see Table 2–2). The cornerstone of a unified approach to chronic pain syndrome is a comprehensive behavioral program. Whenever possible, the therapist should reinforce the behavioral approaches used by the other

BOX 2–10
Chronic Pain Conditions

Arthritis
Persistent neck/back pain
Neuralgias
Peripheral neuropathies
Peripheral vascular disease
Causalgia
Reflex sympathetic dystrophy
Hyperesthesia
Myofascial pain syndrome
Fibromyalgia syndrome
Phantom limb pain
Cancer
Postoperative pain
Spinal stenosis

Adapted from Ludwig-Beymer P, Huether SE: Pain, temperature regulation, sleep, and sensory function. *In* Black JM, Matassarin-Jacobs E (eds): Luckmann and Sorensen's Medical-Surgical Nursing, ed 4. Philadelphia, WB Saunders, 1993, p 446.

members of the team. Some general guidelines are outlined in Box 2–12.

Persons whose pain is associated with severe depression and those whose pain is related to a terminal illness, most notably cancer, appear to be at increased risk for suicide. See discussion of suicide in Special Implications for the Therapist 2–9: Anxiety Disorders, 2–12: Depression, and 2–13: Coping and Adapting. Persons with recurrent acute or chronic pain are sometimes convinced that there is a health professional somewhere who has the "cure" for the pain. Pain may lead to inactivity and social isolation, which in turn can lead to additional psychological problems (e.g., depression) and a reduction in physical endurance that results in fatigue and additional pain (DSM-IV, 1994).

BOX 2–11
Diagnostic Criteria for Pain Disorder

A. Pain in one or more anatomic sites is the predominant focus of the clinical presentation and is of sufficient severity to warrant clinical attention.
B. The pain causes clinically significant distress or impairment in social, occupational, or other important areas of functioning.
C. Psychological factors are judged to have an important role in the onset, severity, exacerbation, or maintenance of the pain.
D. The symptom or deficit is not intentionally produced or feigned (as in factitious disorder or malingering).
E. The pain is not better accounted for by a mood, anxiety, or psychotic disorder and does not meet criteria for dyspareunia.

Adapted from American Psychiatric Association: Diagnostic and Statistical Manual of Mental Disorders [DSM-IV]. Washington, DC, Author, 1994, p 461.

BOX 2–12
Behavioral Goals and Guidelines for Chronic Pain Syndrome

- Identify and eliminate pain reinforcers.
- Decrease drug use.
- Use positive reinforcers that shift the focus from pain.
- Concentrate on abilities, not disabilities.
- Avoid the concept of cure: concentrate on control of pain and improved function.
- Avoid discussion of pain except as arranged by the team (e.g., only during monthly reevaluation, only with a designated team member).
- Use a home program to focus on function and functional outcome (e.g., self-help tasks within capabilities).
- The client should keep a log of accomplishments so that progress can be measured and remembered.
- Measure success by what the individual client can accomplish, not based on others' success.
- Take one day at a time. Direct energy toward solving today's problems rather than focusing on the future.
- Avoid negative reinforcers such as sympathy and attention to symptoms (especially pain).
- Encourage tolerance to increasing activity levels.
- Gradual progress is better than quick results with increased symptoms.
- Teach the client how and when to ask for and accept help when necessary. Do not offer help or yield to the demands of someone who does not need help.

Adapted from Brophy JJ: Psychiatric disorders. *In* Tierney LM, McPhee SJ, Papadakis MA (eds): Current Medical Diagnosis and Treatment. Norwalk, Conn, Appleton & Lange, 1994, pp 855–911.

Symptom Magnification

It is important for health care providers to recognize that we often contribute to symptom magnification syndrome by focusing on the relief of symptoms, especially pain, as the goal of therapy. Reducing pain is an acceptable goal for some clients, but for those who experience pain after their injuries have healed, the focus should be restoration, or at least, improvement of function. Instead of asking if the client's symptoms are "better," "same," or "worse," it may be more appropriate to inquire as to functional outcomes, for example, what can the client accomplish at home that she or he was unable to attempt at the beginning of treatment, last week, or even yesterday? Materials and courses on symptom magnification and functional capacity evaluations are available.

Mood Disorders

Depression

Definition and Overview. *Depression* in psychiatric terms is a morbid sadness, dejection, or a sense of melancholy, distinguished from grief, which is a normal response to a personal loss (DSM-IV, 1994; O'Toole, 1992). Mild, sporadic depression is a relatively common phenomenon experienced by almost everyone at some time, referred to as the "common cold of emotions." Depression is the most commonly seen mood disorder within a therapy practice, often associated with other physical illnesses (Table 2–11).

Depression is a normal response to (not a cause of) pain which may influence the client's ability to cope with pain. While anxiety is more apparent in acute pain episodes, depression occurs more often in clients with chronic pain (Sternbach, 1974). When the pain is relieved, the depression usually disappears (Matassarin-Jacobs, 1993).

Mood disorders can be classified into three broad types: major depressive disorder, organic mood disorder, and bipolar illness (manic depression). The most common type of depression observed is *major depressive disorder*, formerly referred to as endogenous or reactive depression.[10] Major depressive disorder can occur as a single isolated episode lasting weeks to months, or intermittently throughout a person's life. This type of depression may be seen as an adjustment disorder with depressive mood and occurs as a result of external circumstances (e.g., environmental stress, loss, or trauma). Profound depression may be an illness itself, considered as an affective or anxiety disorder, or it may be symptomatic of another psychiatric disorder such as schizophrenia (O'Toole, 1992).

Organic mood disorder is also biologically based; structural changes in the brain associated with disease (e.g., multiple sclerosis) or brain trauma (e.g., left-sided cerebrovascular accident, traumatic brain injury) can cause depressive reactions, either on a short-term or recurring basis (see Table 2–11). Anticonvulsant medications such as valproic acid (Depakote) and carbamazapine (Tegretol) are often effective, especially in the traumatic brain-injured (TBI) population.

Bipolar disorder or *manic depressive disorder* is characterized by cyclical mood swings that often include intense outbursts of high energy and activity, elevated mood, a decreased need for sleep, and a flight of ideas (mania) followed by extreme depression (Table 2–12); each may last from days to months. The cause is a biochemical dysfunction; evidence that a gene,

TABLE 2–11 Physical Illnesses Commonly Associated with Depression

Central Nervous System
Parkinson's disease
Cerebral arteriosclerosis
Stroke
Alzheimer's disease
Temporal lobe epilepsy
Postconcussion injury
Multiple sclerosis
Miscellaneous focal lesions

Endocrine, Metabolic
Hyperthyroidism
Hypothyroidism
Addison's disease
Cushing's disease
Hypoglycemia
Hyperglycemia
Hyperparathyroidism
Hyponatremia
Diabetes mellitus

Viral
Acquired immunodeficiency syndrome
Hepatitis
Pneumonia
Influenza

Nutritional
Folic acid deficiency
Vitamin B_6 deficiency
Vitamin B_{12} deficiency

Cancer
Pancreatic
Bronchogenic
Renal
Ovarian

Miscellaneous
Systemic lupus erythematosus
Pancreatitis
Sarcoidosis
Syphilis
Porphyria
Myocardial infarction

From Tollefson GD: Recognition and treatment of major depression. Am Fam Physician 42(suppl 5):S59–S69, 1990.

TABLE 2–12 Clinical Manifestations of Bipolar Disorder

Mania	Depression
Excessive "high" or euphoric feelings	Persistent sad, anxious, or empty mood
Sustained period of behavior different from usual	Feelings of hopelessness or pessimism
Increased energy, activity, restlessness, racing thoughts, and rapid talking	Feelings of guilt, worthlessness, or helplessness
Decreased need for sleep	Loss of interest or pleasure in ordinary activities, including sex
Unrealistic beliefs in one's abilities and powers	Decreased energy, feeling fatigued, or being "slowed down"
Extreme irritability and distractibility	Difficulty concentrating, remembering, making decisions
Uncharacteristically poor judgment	Restlessness or irritability
Increased sexual drive	Sleep disturbances
Abuse of drugs, particularly cocaine, alcohol, and sleeping medications	Loss of appetite and weight, or weight gain
Obnoxious, provocative, or intrusive behavior	Chronic pain or other persistent bodily symptoms that are not caused by physical disease
Denial that anything is wrong	Thoughts of death or suicide; suicide attempts

Adapted from Bipolar Disorder: Manic-Depressive Illness. National Institute of Mental Health Publication No. (ADM) 89-1609, Rockville, Md, 1989.

[10] These older terms have been discarded because many reactive depressions, contrary to previous thinking, require drug therapy and intensive intervention (Crump, 1993).

possibly on chromosome 18 or 21, promotes this type of depression has been found (Detera-Wadleigh et al., 1994; Berrettini et al., 1994). Treatment is typically pharmacologic.

Incidence (DSM-IV, 1994). Major depressive disorder is the most common adult psychiatric disorder beginning at any age with an average onset in the mid-20s. In the United States, over 2.5 million men and 5.0 million women meet the criteria for major depression over a 6-month period (Robins, 1984) and it appears to be occurring at earlier ages for those born in the last decade. In prepubertal children, boys and girls are equally affected. Rates in men and women are highest in the 25- to 44-year-old age group, whereas rates are lower for both men and women over age 65 years.

Etiology and Risk Factors. Predisposing factors for the development of depression may be genetic, familial, or psychosocial, or the depression may occur in association with medical illness or surgical procedures. Other conditions associated with depression include chronic illnesses such as rheumatoid arthritis, multiple sclerosis, chronic heart disease, or hypothyroidism. Up to 20% to 25% of individuals with certain general medical conditions (e.g., diabetes, myocardial infarction, carcinomas, stroke) will develop major depressive disorder during the course of their disease (DSM-IV, 1994) (see Table 2–11).

Depression may occur as a result of medications (especially sedatives, hypnotics, cardiac drugs, antihypertensives, steroids) (Table 2–13), alcohol or drug abuse (especially cocaine dependence), or exposure to heavy metals or toxins (e.g., gasoline, paint, organophosphate insecticides, nerve gas, carbon monoxide, carbon dioxide); this type of depression may be labeled substance-induced mood disorder[11]. Other causes of depression among the general population include prenatal and postpartum depression occurring in approximately 20% of all pregnancies and seasonal affective disorder (SAD), a dysfunction of circadian rhythms that occurs more commonly in the winter as a result of decreased exposure to sunlight.

TABLE 2–13 Drugs Commonly Associated with Depression

Psychoactive Agents
Amphetamines
Cocaine
Benzodiazepines
Barbiturates
Neuroleptics

Antihypertensive Drugs
β-Blockers, especially propranolol (Inderal)
α_2-Adrenergic antagonists
Reserpine (Serpalan, Serpasil)
Methyldopa (Aldomet, Amodopa)
Hydralazine (Alazine, Apresoline)

Analgesics
Salicylates
Propoxyphene (Darvon, component of Dolene)
Pentazocine (Talwin)
Morphine
Meperidine (Demerol)

Cardiovascular Drugs
Digitalis
Digoxin (Lanoxin)
Procainamide (Pronestyl)
Disopyramide (Norpace)

Anticonvulsants
Phenytoin (Dilantin)
Phenobarbital

Hormonal Agents
Corticosteroids
Oral contraceptives

Miscellaneous
Histamine H_2 receptor antagonists, especially cimetidine (Tagamet)
Metoclopramide (Reglan)
Levodopa (Dopar, Larodopa)
Nonsteroidal anti-inflammatory drugs
Antineoplastic agents
Disulfiram (Antabuse)

Adapted from Tollefson GD: Recognition and treatment of major depression. Am Fam Physician 42(suppl 5):S59–S69, 1990.

Pathogenesis. Several theories of pathogenesis based on etiologic factors have been examined by researchers. These include biochemical mechanisms, neuroendocrine mechanisms, sleep abnormalities, genetics, and psychosocial factors. Recent study of the *biochemical basis* of depression has centered on two primary neurotransmitters: norepinephrine and serotonin (Richelson, 1991). As demonstrated in animal models, antidepressant drugs decrease the sensitivity of postsynaptic β-adrenergic and 5-hydroxytryptamine receptors by blocking the reuptake of the neurotransmitters into nerve endings. This change occurs 1 to 3 weeks after treatment, correlating with the delay seen clinically in the effectiveness of antidepressants. Researchers have found changes in dopaminergic activity, acetylcholine, vasopressin, and endorphins associated with mood disorders, particularly depression.

Neuroendocrine abnormalities, such as in the limbic-hypothalamic-pituitary-adrenal axis, have been implicated in the cause of depression, prompting a search for a reliable serum abnormality that could be used as a "depression test." Some examples of possible abnormalities include oversecretion of cortisol and suppressed nocturnal secretion of melatonin and decreased prolactin production in response to tryptophan administration. There is also a known association between hormonal variations such as low testosterone levels in men and basal levels of follicle-stimulating hormone (FSH) and luteinizing hormone (LH) in women and some depressions.

Sleep abnormalities are consistently associated with depression, including decreased rapid-eye-movement (REM) latency (the time between falling asleep and the first REM period), longer first REM period, less continuous sleep, and early-morning awakenings. Animal studies have shown that many antidepressants can "reset the internal clock." Whether these sleep abnormalities represent causes or effects of depression remains unknown.

Genetic-based pathogenesis is suspected for bipolar depression based on a clear familial pattern and chromosomal link-

[11] The DSM-IV (1994) categorizes this type of depression separately from the three broad types outlined at the beginning of this section.

TABLE 2–14 Side Effects of Tricyclic Antidepressants

Type	Mild Effects	Severe and Toxic Effects
Anticholinergic	Dry mouth Blurred vision Constipation Urinary hesitancy Central anticholinergic*	Dental decay Peritonitis Parotitis (inflammation of parotid gland) Acute glaucoma Falls and fractures (secondary to sedation or hypotension)
Neurologic	Sedation Disturbed sleep, nightmares Transient increase in anxiety Lower seizure threshold Fine tremor‡ Disturbed balance Analgesia	Seizures Choreoathetoid movements† Ataxia, coma, respiratory depression
Cardiovascular	Prolonged conduction time (quinidine-like effect) Postural hypotension‡ Increased heart rate	Heart block† Ventricular dysrhythmias† Asystole† Hypotension
Endocrine, metabolic	Weight gain, craving for sweet foods Fluctuation in blood glucose levels Decreased libido and impaired erection and ejaculation Gynecomastia Fluid retention	
Hematologic		Blood dyscrasias
Dermatologic	Skin rash Photosensitivity	
Gastrointestinal	Nausea, epigastric distress, diarrhea, vomiting	Hepatitis (rare)

* Central anticholinergic syndrome occurs because acetylcholine stores are depleted in the aging brain and adding an anticholinergic drug will make existing symptoms worse. Symptoms may include disorientation, confusion, hallucinations, delusions, decreased sweating, tachycardia, increased temperature, mydriasis (dilation of the pupil of the eye).
† Occurs with overdose.
‡ Frequent and troublesome in elderly people.
Adapted from Williams GO: Management of depression in the elderly. Prim Care 16:451–474, 1989.

age studies. There is evidence that the key gene involved in the transmission of bipolar disease is X-linked. There may also be a familial pattern in the development of major depressive disorder as this type of depression occurs up to three times more often in first-degree biologic relatives of persons with this disorder.

Psychosocial factors, such as life events and perceived stress, are clearly associated with depression, but it is difficult to establish whether they cause depression or merely determine when a susceptible person will experience depression. Episodes of major depressive disorder often follow a severe psychosocial stressor, such as the death of a loved one or divorce. Psychosocial events as stressors may play a more significant role in the precipitation of the first or second episodes of major depressive disorder, but play less of a role in the onset of subsequent episodes. Hospitalized clients are particularly susceptible to feelings of depression and a sense of loss and despair.

Clinical Manifestations. Depressed mood and loss of interest in usually pleasurable activities are the hallmarks of depression (see Table 2–12). Over 95% of depressed persons report decreased energy, even for minor daily tasks. The inability to accomplish new or challenging activities often results in occupational or school dysfunction; 90% report having problems with concentration and memory. Difficulty concentrating and marked forgetfulness is particularly common in depressed elderly people and is called *pseudodementia* (Crump, 1993).

Persons with mood disorders, particularly depressive disorders, may present with somatic complaints, most commonly headache, gastrointestinal disturbances, or unexplained pain (Box 2–13) (see also earlier discussion under Somatoform Disorders). Other mental disorders frequently co-occur with major depressive disorder such as anxiety, substance-related disorders, panic disorder, obsessive-compulsive disorder, anorexia nervosa, bulimia nervosa, and borderline personality disorder.

Almost 80% of depressed persons report problems with sleep, including early-morning and frequent nocturnal awakenings. Among the elderly, depression is often the cause of sleep disturbances but depression may be the first symptom of systemic illness. Often depression by itself or linked with

BOX **2–13**
Somatic Symptoms Associated with Depression*

Weakness
Headaches
Excess perspiration
Dizziness
Dry mouth
Rapid breathing
Blurred vision
Constipation
Tinnitus
Dry skin
Delayed ejaculation
Flushing
Slurred speech
Premature ejaculation
Chest pain
Excessive salivation
Amenorrhea
Impotence
Lack of orgasms
Loss of libido
Excessive libido
Polymenorrhea
Difficulty with urination

* Refers to nonmedicated persons. Listed in order of decreasing prevalence.
Adapted from Mathew RJ, Weinman ML, Mirabi M: Physical symptoms of depression. Br J Psychiatry 139:293–296, 1981.

acute confusion, falling, incontinence, or syncope signify underlying disease requiring medical referral.

Medical Management

Diagnosis. Primary care physicians detect only 33% to 50% of depressed outpatients (Wells, 1989). Over 50% of persons with depression present with somatic complaints or "masked" depression (Lesse, 1983). The application criteria based on the DSM-IV (1994) remain problematic with as many as 50% of persons with depressive symptoms being unclassified using these diagnostic criteria (Barrett, 1988).

The diagnosis of manic episodes associated with bipolar disorder is difficult, especially without knowledge of the baseline behavior of the person in question. The behavior of the person during a manic episode is described in Table 2–12. Driven behaviors such as late-night telephone calls, impulsive sexual liaisons, pathologic gambling, and excessively flamboyant dress and behavior are also characteristic.

Depression associated with underlying diseases may be identified by a comprehensive history, physical examination, and basic laboratory studies, including a complete blood count, erythrocyte sedimentation rate, chemistry panel, and thyroid function tests.

Treatment. Depression can be treated effectively with one of several antidepressant drugs, and, depending on its cause and severity, cognitive-behavioral therapies (Hendrix, 1993). Bipolar disorders are treated with lithium carbonate. The physician will use the history, laboratory findings, and physical examination to determine whether the depression is a mood disorder due to a general medical condition (i.e., the direct physiologic consequence of a medical condition such as multiple sclerosis, stroke, or hypothyroidism) or if the depression is considered to be the psychological consequence of having the general medical condition (e.g., myocardial infarct). There may be no etiologic relationship between the depression and the medical condition. The medical management of general medical conditions with accompanying major depressive disorder is more complex, with a less favorable prognosis than just the medical condition alone.

Prognosis. Depression is a chronic relapsing disorder associated with high mortality and the severity of the initial depressive episode appears to predict persistence. Chronic general medical conditions are also a risk factor for more persistent episodes. Up to 15% of persons diagnosed with this disorder die by suicide. Epidemiologic evidence also suggests that there is a fourfold increase in death rates in persons with major depressive disorder who are over age 55 years. Persons with this condition admitted to nursing homes may have a markedly increased likelihood of death in the first year.

Special Implications for the Therapist **2–12**

DEPRESSION

Depression occurs in over 50% of people with Parkinson's disease and strokes. In these, as well as in other clients, the therapist may detect early signs of depression such as pessimistic statements about the illness and its prognosis (poor in the individual's mind) and passive noncompliance during therapy with minimal or no compliance in following a home program or in following (performing) postoperative or rehabilitative exercises. When depression is noted, it should be included as a problem in the care plan; the team can then develop strategies to help the person.

The client with mood disorders may cry easily and often for no apparent reason. Such a situation can be handled by offering reassurance and redirecting the person's attention toward the treatment or other more positive topics. Using the acronym PLISSIT* may help provide the therapist with some direction early on in treatment: *P*ermission: Acknowledge the presence of the depression and give the person permission to feel depressed. *L*imited *i*nformation: "Of course you are feeling down. You broke your hip, it hurts, and you cannot get around." Again, this acknowledges and validates the person's experience. *S*pecific *s*uggestions: For example, knowing that depression often causes the person to avoid social contact and to seek isolation which then contributes to the depression, encourage the person to make telephone contact with at least one person every day or listen to upbeat music every morning and every evening or make arrangements to exercise with someone else (even if only for 10 minutes once a week: it is a start!). *I*ntensive *t*herapy: The client is referred to appropriate specific therapy from other trained professionals (Annon, 1976).

Depression may also lead to anger observed as outbursts of hostility, attempts to sabotage treatment efforts, or blame for the injury placed on the work site or employer. Sometimes the client sees the therapist as an extension of the employer and carries over anger into the rehabilitation process. The therapist can persist in asking questions and actively listening without communicating judgment when the client expresses despair, anger, or negative feelings. The therapist can offer encouragement by pointing out improvements in symptoms or function. See also Special Implications for the Therapist 2–13: Coping and Adapting.

Although the physician must differentiate between pseudodementia of depression and dementia in the aging, the therapist's observations may be helpful toward this end. For example, characteristically, a person with dementia who does not know the answer to a question becomes tangential, changing the subject or resorting to confabulation. In contrast, a person with depression gives up easily and responds by saying, "I don't know." With some encouragement and extra time, the depressed person often makes an appropriate response, but the person with dementia moves further from the topic with each comment. People with depression commonly have global memory loss, whereas dementia results in loss of recent memory but retention of detail for remote memory (Crump, 1993). It is possible for dementia and depression to coexist.

Additionally, a recent study has reported that depression is a risk factor for osteoporosis, especially among the aging population. Hyperadrenocorticism (Cushing's syndrome; see discussion in Chapter 9), well known to be associated with depression, is the most reasonable pathophysiologic mechanism to explain the findings of this study. Treatment for persons who are experiencing major depression may provide the additional benefit of fracture prevention (Schweiger et al., 1994).

Suicide and Depression

Treatment of depression (whether pharmacologic or psychotherapy) does not change or alleviate symptoms immediately; most drugs used to treat depression require 3 to 4 weeks before a true mood-elevating effect is perceived. The physical symptoms of sleep and appetite disturbances, fatigue, and agitation are the first to improve with medication. Cognitive symptoms such as low self-esteem, guilt, uncertainty, pessimism, and suicidal thoughts resolve more slowly (HWHW, 1995).

Although some severely depressed people lack the energy necessary to complete an impulsive act such as suicide, close observation is required during the early weeks of pharmacologic treatment. As energy is restored, but before a stable elevation of mood is achieved, the individual is at increased risk for suicide. See further discussion of suicide in this chapter (Special Implications for the Therapist 2–9: Anxiety Disorders; and 2–13: Coping and Adapting). Encourage the client to continue taking the prescribed medications and to contact his or her physician before discontinuing or tapering dosage.

Side effects of antidepressant medications are common and may affect multiple systems. The therapist should be alert to any mention of these and encourage the affected person to discuss these symptoms with the prescribing physician. The therapist may be able to offer some practical suggestions such as an over-the-counter artificial saliva spray for dry mouth; an education and prevention and management program for orthostatic hypotension (see under Postural hypotension, Chapter 10); or reduced caffeine intake for persons experiencing tremor.

Exercise and Depression

Exercise has a known benefit in clinical depression although any discussion of how exercise might alleviate depression is speculative because the biologic cause of depression is not well understood. In some cases, exercise can alleviate depression immediately, independent of achieving fitness, although there is some evidence that exercise must be continued to remain effective (Benight and Taylor, 1994). Exertion appears to increase the levels of various neurotransmitters (e.g., dopamine and serotonin) in the same direction as do antidepressants (Brown and Van Huss, 1973; Brown, 1979). Exercise also appears to increase levels of β-endorphins, which are believed to be low in depressed persons (Berk, 1981).

For the client taking tricyclic antidepressants (TCAs), heart rate during peak exercise should be monitored (see Appendix B) because the anticholinergic effect of these medications significantly increases heart rate. These drugs may cause a number of other side effects as a result of increased norepinephrine levels such as dry mouth, blurred vision, urinary retention, constipation, palpitations, and orthostatic hypotension (Table 2–14). The last can be the source of dizziness and fainting, increasing the risk of falls and accidents, especially in the elderly. Elderly people taking TCAs are at greater risk for heat stroke, especially in the summer. These people are not able to adjust easily to ambient air temperatures which may affect their exercise program or pool therapy.

Other medications such as fluoxetine (Prozac), bupropion (Wellbutrin), and monoamine oxidase inhibitors (MAOIs) such as phenelzine (Nardil) may cause headaches and insomnia. Since some of these medications' side effects are dose-related, the therapist should encourage the client to report any symptoms to the prescribing physician.

* Although PLISSIT was developed as a model for sexual health interventions (Annon, 1976), this same concept can be applied to depression.

Coping and Adapting

People react to a stressful event using coping mechanisms, also called *relief behaviors*. Behavioral or cognitive coping mechanisms are used to resolve, reduce, or replace the level of stress, depression, and anxiety. When the stress is resolved, accepted, or changed, adaptation occurs implying that a sense of equilibrium is restored to the person disordered by stress (Ignatavicius and Bayne, 1991).

The body also has coping mechanisms, referred to as the *generalized adaptation response* to stressors with multiple physiologic events (Fig. 2–5). The first stage is the alarm stage or "fight-or-flight response" when the autonomic nervous system activates the body's involuntary responses such as hormone secretions, metabolism, and fluid regulation. Once the body recognizes continued threat, physiologic forces are mobilized

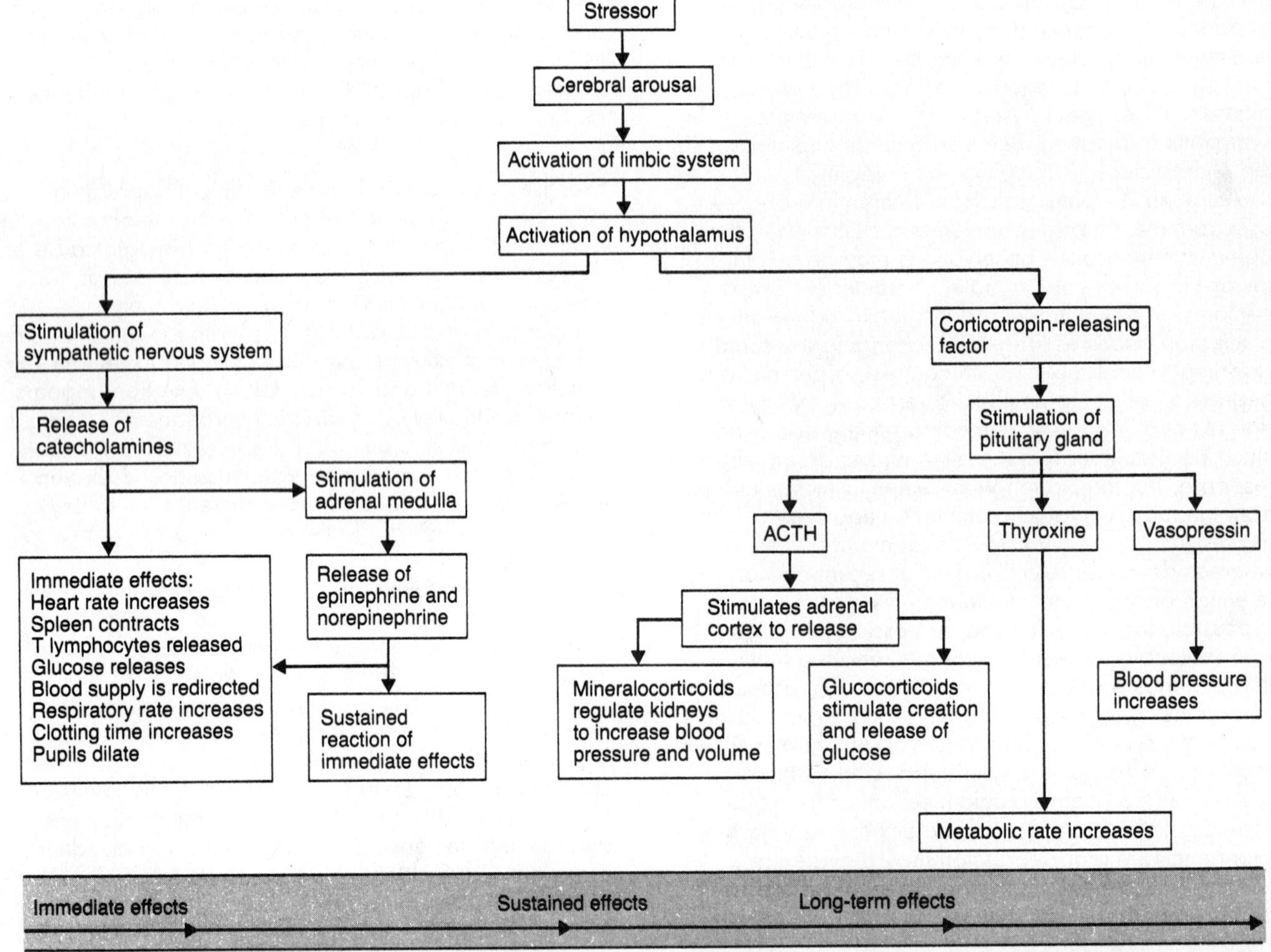

Figure 2–5. The general adaptation syndrome. See text discussion. *(From Ignatavicius DD, Bayne MV: Medical-Surgical Nursing. Philadelphia, WB Saunders, 1991, p 88.)*

to maintain an increased resistance to stressors and return to a state of homeostasis. Chronic resistance eventually causes damage to the involved systems as the body enters a stage of exhaustion, possibly resulting in diseases of adaptation or stress-related diseases (see Boxes 2–7 and 2–8).

The process of coping with chronic pain, trauma, or illness is ongoing. Each change in the downward course of the illness requires new and painful acceptance of the disease and its limitations. Behavioral or cognitive coping may be adaptive (e.g., talking or reading about the problem, prayer or seeking God) or maladaptive, such as denial and distancing or the use of alcohol or drugs. When a person is unable to mobilize the necessary resources to manage stress, death from disease may result or suicide may be the final step to conflict resolution.

Special Implications for the Therapist **2–13**

COPING AND ADAPTING

Clients frequently present with somatic symptoms with an underlying psychosocial basis (see Psychophysiologic Disorders). It is not easy for people to make necessary changes (or they would have done so long ago) and denial often obscures the picture. Patience is a vital tool for the therapist working with clients who are having difficulty adjusting to the stress of illness and disability or the client who has a psychological disorder. Relaxation, breathing, and exercise techniques are helpful in reducing the reaction to stressful events. The health care provider also assists the client in recognizing physical responses to stress and teaches how to use these techniques early in the stressful situation or event.

The therapist may need to develop personal coping mechanisms when working with clients who have chronic illnesses or psychological disturbances. Preexisting character issues or the presence of psychological problems in a client (e.g., anxiety, panic disorder, depression) can create obstacles to rehabilitation or prevent progress. Recognizing problems that are psychologically based vs. conditions that are the direct result of organic dysfunction such as disease or traumatic injury will assist the therapist in coping with clients who are hostile, ungrateful, adversarial, noncompliant, or negative. As part of the treatment team, a psychiatrist, psychologist, or counselor can assist other members of the health care team to better understand individual clients, thereby reducing the therapist's stress and maximizing the client's recovery. Knowing what to say when a client becomes provocative, insulting, or angry is an important coping mechanism for the therapist. See also Special Implications for the Therapist 2–10: Psychophysiologic Disorders, this chapter.

Other basic techniques for coping with anxious, depressed, angry, or otherwise psychologically compromised clients may include reassurance and education, cognitive restructuring, and operant conditioning. Reassurance can be provided by letting the person know that his or her experience is normal and by providing education about the condition and outlining the steps to recovery. Cognitive restructuring guides the client to focus on active coping behaviors and improving function instead of focusing on physical symptoms and pain. Reinforcing positive active behaviors and ignoring pain-related behaviors is called operant conditioning (see Box 2–12).

All suicidal thoughts and acts must be taken seriously and responded to appropriately. Observe for changes in client mood, such as calmness or tranquillity in a formerly hostile, angry, or depressed client. Such a behavior change may be a prelude to a suicidal event. Comments such as, "I won't be seeing you again," or "Next time you see me, I'll be riding in a hearse" may be a form of suicidal communication. People who are suicidal may also be manipulative; therefore, therapy staff needs to be aware of and manage their own feelings while empathizing with the client's point of view (Thompson et al., 1993). When in doubt, report concerns to the appropriate resource (e.g., physician or counselor when one is involved).

References

ACSM (American College of Sports Medicine): Guidelines for Graded Exercise Testing and Exercise Prescription, ed 4. Philadelphia, Lea & Febiger, 1991.

Ader R, Felten DL, Cohen N (eds): Psychoneuroimmunology, ed 2. San Diego, Academic Press, 1991.

Ader R, Cohen N, Felten D: Psychoneuroimmunology: Interactions between the nervous system and the immune system. Lancet 345:99–103, 1995.

American Cancer Society. Cancer Facts. New York, Author, 1986.

Aminoff MJ: Nervous system. *In* Tierney LM, McPhee SJ, Papadakis MA: Current Medical Diagnosis and Treatment, ed 33. Norwalk, Conn, Appleton & Lange, 1994, pp 798–854.

Annon JS: The PLISSIT model: A proposed conceptual scheme for the behavioral treatment of sexual problems. J Sex Educ Ther 2:1–15, 1976.

Atkinson RM, Kofoed LL: Alcohol and drug abuse in old age. *In* Walsh CC (ed): Geriatric Medicine, vol 2: Fundamentals of Geriatric Care. New York, Springer-Verlag, 1984.

Baron RB: Nutrition. *In* Tierney, LM, McPhee SJ, Papadakis MA: Current Medical Diagnosis and Treatment, ed 33. Norwalk, Conn, Appleton & Lange, 1994, pp 1025–1052.

Bar-Or O, Lundegren HM, Buskirk ER: Heat tolerance of exercising obese and lean women. J Appl Physiol 26:403–409, 1969.

Barrett JE: The prevalence of psychiatric disorders in a primary care practice. Arch Gen Psychiatry 45:1100–1116, 1988.

Barrett-Connor E, Change JC, Edelstein SL: Coffee-associated osteoporosis offset by daily milk consumption. JAMA 271:280–283, 1994.

Benight CC, Taylor CB: Exercise, emotions, and Type A behavior. *In* Goldberg L, Elliot DL (eds): Exercise for Prevention and Treatment of Illness. Philadelphia, FA Davis, 1994, pp 319–332.

Berk L: Beta-endorphin response to exercise in athletes and nonathletes (abstract). Med Sci Sports Exerc 13:134, 1981.

Berrettini WH, Ferraro TN, Goldin LR, et al: Chromosome 18 DNA markers and manic-depressive illness: Evidence for a susceptibility gene. Proc Natl Acad Sci U S A 91:5918–5921, 1994.

Blumenthal JA, Wei J: Psychobehavioral treatment in cardiac rehabilitation. Cardiol Clin 11:323–331, 1993.

Blumenthal SJ: Healthy Women 2000 Forum. *In* The 10 Steps to Good Health, April 25, 1995. Washington, DC, 1995a.

Blumenthal SJ: Women's Health: An International Perspective. World Conference of Physical Therapists '95, June 25–30. Washington, DC, 1995b.

Boeck MA, Chen C, Cunningham-Rundles S: Altered immune function in a morbidity obese pediatric population. Ann N Y Acad Sci 699:253–256, 1993.

Boissonnault WG, Koopmeiners MB: Medical history profile: Orthopaedic physical therapy outpatients. J Orthop Sports Phys Med 20:2–10, 1994.

Bo-Linn G: Obesity, anorexia nervosa, bulimia and other eating disorders. *In* Sleisenger, MH, Fordtran JS (eds): Gastrointestinal Disease, ed 5. Philadelphia, WB Saunders, 1993, pp 2109–2136.

Bonica JJ: The Management of Pain. Philadelphia, Lea & Febiger, 1953.

Boshuizen HC, Verbeek JH, Broersen JPJ, et al: Do smokers get more back pain? Spine 18:35–40, 1993.

Brophy JJ: Psychiatric disorders. *In* Tierney LM, McPhee SJ, Papadakis MA (eds): Current Medical Diagnosis and Treatment. Norwalk, Conn, Appleton & Lange, 1994, pp 855–911.

Brown B: Chronic response to rat brain norepinephrine and serotonin levels of endurance training. J Appl Psychol 46:19–23, 1979.

Brown B, Van Huss W: Exercise and brain catecholamines. J Appl Physiol 34:664–669, 1973.

Brownell KD, Rodin J: Medical, metabolic, and psychological effects of weight cycling. Arch Intern Med 154:1325–1330, 1994.

Burker EJ, Fredrikson M, Rifai N, et al: Serum lipids, neuroendocrine, and cardiovascular responses to stress in men and women with mild hypertension. Behav Med 19:155–161, 1994.

Buskirk ER: Obesity. *In* Skinner JS: Exercise Testing and Exercise Prescription for Special Cases: Theoretical Basis and Clinical Application, ed 2. Philadelphia, Lea & Febiger, 1993, pp 185–210.

Butler RM, Rogers FJ: Exercise in healthy individuals. *In* Goldberg L, Elliot DL (eds): Exercise for Prevention and Treatment of Illness. Philadelphia, FA Davis, 1994, pp 3–23.

Calhoun J, Anger DM, Stafford D, et al: An outcome and transcutaneous oxygen study on smoking in diabetics with lower extremity ulcers and surgery. Presented at the American Orthopaedic Foot and Ankle Society Annual Meeting, Coeur d'Alene, Idaho, June 30–July 3, 1994.

Calle EE, Miracle-McMahill HL, Thun MJ, Heath CW: Cigarette smoking and risk of fatal breast cancer. Am J Epidemiol 139:1001–1007, 1994.

Cameron O, Hudson C: Influence of exercise on anxiety level in patients with anxiety disorders. Psychosom Med 27:720–723, 1986.

Cirullo J (ed): Aquatic Physical Therapy. Orthopedic Physical Therapy Clinics (OPTC). Philadelphia, WB Saunders, 1994.

Clark LA, Watson D, Mineka S: Temperament, personality, and mood and anxiety disorders reviewed. J Abnorm Psychol 103:103–116, 1994.

Considine RV, Considine EL, Williams CJ, et al: Evidence against either a premature stop codon or the absence of obese gene mRNA in human obesity. J Clin Invest 95:2986–2988, 1995.

Cottler LB: Posttraumatic stress disorder among substance users from the general population. Am J Psychiatry 149:664, 1992.

Coulehan JL, Block MR: The Medical Interview. Philadelphia, FA Davis, 1992.

Couturier EGM, Hering R, Steiner TJ: Weekend attacks in migraine patients: Caused by caffeine withdrawal? Cephalalgia 12:99–100, 1992.

Crump WJ: Depression Monograph 171, Series III. Kansas City, Mo, American Academy of Family Physicians (AAFP), 1993.

Davis K: The Commonwealth Fund Minority Health Survey. New York, Louis Harris & Associates, 1994.

Detera-Wadleigh SD, Hsieh WT, Berrettini WH, et al: Genetic linkage mapping for a susceptibility locus to bipolar illness: Chromosomes 2, 3, 4, 7, 9, 10p, 11p, 22, and Xpter. Am J Med Genet 54:206–218, 1994.

de Vernejoul MC, Bielakoff J, Herve M, et al: Evidence for defective osteoblastic function. A role of alcohol and tobacco consumption in osteoporosis in middle-aged men. Clin Orthop 179:107–115, 1983.

DHHS (Department of Health and Human Services): Health People 2000, Publication No. 91-50212, Washington, DC, Author, 1990.

Dishman RK, Sallis JF, Orentstein DR: The determinants of physical activity and exercise. Public Health Rep 100:158–171, 1985.

Diagnostic and Statistical Manual of Mental Disorders, ed 4 [DSM-IV]. Washington, DC, American Psychiatric Association, 1994.

Dunbar-Jacob J: Contributions to patient adherence: Is it time to share the blame? Health Psychol 12:91–93, 1993.

Durbeck DC: The National Aeronautics and Space Administration–US Public Health Service Health Evaluation and Enhancement Program: Summary of results. Am J Cardiol 30:784–790, 1972.

Edwards KI: Obesity, anorexia, and bulimia. Med Clin North Am 77:899–909, 1993.

Elliot DL, Goldberg L: Exercise and obesity. *In* Goldberg L, Elliot DL (eds): Exercise for Prevention and Treatment of Illness. Philadelphia, FA Davis, 1994, pp 211–221.

Emery CF, Hauck ER, Blumenthal JA: Exercise adherence or maintenance among older adults: 1-year follow-up study. Psychol Aging 7:466–470, 1992.

Foss ML, Lampman RM, Schteingart D: Physical training program for rehabilitating extremely obese patients. Arch Phys Med Rehabil 57:425–429, 1976.

Foster DW: Anorexia nervosa and bulimia. *In* Isselbacher KJ, Braunwald E, Wilson JD, et al (eds): Harrison's Principles of Internal Medicine, ed 13. New York, McGraw-Hill, 1994, pp 452–454.

Fredrikson M, Blumenthal JA: Serum lipids, neuroendocrine, and cardiovascular responses to stress in healthy Type A men. Biol Psychol 34:45–58, 1992.

Freestone S, Ramsay LE: Effect of coffee and cigarette smoking on the blood pressure of untreated and diuretic-treated hypertensive patients. Am J Med 73:348–353, 1982.

Fricchione GL, Stefano GB: The stress response and autoimmunoregulation. Adv Neuroimmunol 4:13–27, 1994.

Friedman M, Rosenman RH: Type A Behavior and Heart. New York, Fawcett Crest, 1981.

Garner DM: Pathogenesis of anorexia nervosa. Lancet 341:1631–1635, 1993.

Geissler CA, Miller DS, Shah M: The daily metabolic rate of the post-obese and the lean. Am J Clin Nutr 45:914–920, 1989.

Goldberg L, Elliot DL (eds): Exercise for Prevention and Treatment of Illness. Philadelphia, FA Davis, 1994.

Goodman CC, Snyder TE: Differential Diagnosis in Physical Therapy, ed 2. Philadelphia, WB Saunders, 1995.

Goodman CE, Kenrick MM: Physical fitness in relation to obesity. Obes Bar Med 4:12, 1975.

Gorkin M: The Uses of Counter-Transference. Northvale, NJ, Jason Aronson, 1987.

Hartford JR, Damorajski T: Alcoholism in the geriatric population. J Am Geriatr Soc 30:18, 1982.

Hauck ER, Blumenthal JA: Obsessive and compulsive traits in athletes. Sports Med 14:215–227, 1992.

Hendrix ML: Obsessive Compulsive Disorder. Washington, DC, National Institutes of Health, 1991.

Hendrix ML: Understanding Panic Disorder. Washington DC, National Institutes of Health, 1993.

Heyden S: Weight and weight history in relation to cerebrovascular and ischemic heart disease. Arch Intern Med 128:956, 1971.

Holmes TH, Rahe RH: The Social Adjustment Rating Scale. J Psychosom Res 11:213–218, 1967.

Hopper JL, Seeman E: The bone density of female twins discordant for tobacco use. N Engl J Med 330:387–392, 1994.

Howard BV, Hannah JS, Heiser CC, et al: Effects of sex and ethnicity on responses to a low-fat diet: A study of African Americans and whites. Am J Clin Nutr 62:488S–492S, 1995.

Huether SE, McCance KL: Alterations of digestive function. *In* McCance KL, Huether SE (eds): Pathophysiology: The Biologic Basis for Disease in Adults and Children, ed 2. St Louis, Mosby–Year Book, 1994, pp 1320–1375.

Huey L: Water healing your hips. Swim 10:17–20, 1994.

Hughes JR, Higgins ST, Bickel WK, et al: Caffeine self-administration, withdrawal, and adverse effects among coffee drinkers. Arch Gen Psychiatry 48:611–617, 1991.

Hutchinson S: The nursing process with psychoactive substance use disorder. *In* Wilson, HS, Kneisl CR (eds): Psychiatric Nursing, ed 4. Redwood City, Calif, Addison-Wesley, 1992.

HWHW (Harvard Women's Health Watch): Depression. Cambridge, Mass, Author, (2):2, 1995.

Ignatavicius DD, Bayne MV: Surgical Nursing. Philadelphia, WB Saunders, 1991.

Jaffe J: Addictions: Issues and Answers. New York, Harper & Row, 1980.

Jiang W, Hayano J, Coleman ER, et al: Am J Cardiol 72:551–554, 1993.

Johnson K: Personal communication, August, 1995.

Jones JK, Triplett RG: The relationship of cigarette smoking to impaired intraoral wound healing: A review of evidence and implications for patient care. J Oral Maxillofac Surg 50:237–239, 1992.

Kayman S, Burold W, Stern JS: Maintenance and relapse after weight loss in women: Behavioral aspects. Am J Clin Nutr 52:800–807, 1990.

Keegan L: Spirituality. *In* Black JM, Matassarin-Jacobs E (eds): Luckmann and Sorensen's Medical-Surgical Nursing, ed 4. Philadelphia, WB Saunders, 1993, pp 89–102.

King AC: Diet vs. exercise in weight maintenance. Arch Intern Med 149:2741–2746, 1989a.

King AC: The influence of regular aerobic exercise on psychological health: A randomized, controlled trial of healthy middle-aged adults. Health Psychol 8:305–324, 1989b.

Kneisl CR: Nursing care of clients with substance abuse. *In* Black JM, Matassarin-Jacobs E (eds): Luckmann and Sorensen's Medical-Surgical Nursing, ed 4. Philadelphia, WB Saunders, 1993, pp 2199–2216.

Kristensson H, Lunden A, Nilsson BE: Fracture incidence and diagnostic roentgen in alcoholics. Acta Orthop Scand 51:205–207, 1980.

Kuehl K, Elliot DL, Goldberg L: Predicting caloric expenditure during multistation resistance exercise. J Appl Sport Sci 4:63–67, 1990.

Kyro A, Usenius JP, Aarnio M, et al: Are smokers a risk group for delayed healing of tibial shaft fractures? Ann Chir Gynaecol 82:254–262, 1993.

Lesse S: The masked depression syndrome—Results of a seventeen-year clinical study. Am J Psychother 37:456–475, 1983.

Lucas AR: Toward an understanding of anorexia nervosa as a disease. Mayo Clin Proc 56:254–261, 1981.

Ludwig-Beymer P, Huether SE: Pain, temperature regulation, sleep, and sensory function. *In* Black JM, Matassarin-Jacobs E (eds): Luckmann and Sorensen's Medical-Surgical Nursing, ed 4. Philadelphia, WB Saunders, 1993, pp 437–476.

MacMahon SW, Wilcken DEL, MacDonald GJ: The effect of weight reduction on left ventricular mass: A randomized controlled trial in young overweight hypertensive patients. N Engl J Med 314:334–379, 1986.

Matassarin-Jacobs E: Pain assessment and intervention. *In* Black JM, Matassarin-Jacobs E (eds): Luckmann and Sorensen's Medical-Surgical Nursing, ed 4. Philadelphia, WB Saunders, 1993, pp 311–358.

Matheson LN: Symptom magnification casebook. Anaheim, Calif, Employment and Rehabilitation Institute of California, 1987.

Matheson LN: Symptom magnification syndrome structured interview: Rationale and procedure. J Occup Rehabil 1:43–56, 1991.

Matheson LN: Work capacity evaluation: Systematic approach to industrial rehabilitation. Anaheim, Calif, Employment and Rehabilitation Institute of California, 1986.

Matsuo KM, Mirohata T, Sugioka Y: Influence of alcohol intake, cigarette smoking and occupational status on idiopathic osteonecrosis of the femoral head. Clin Orthop 234:115–123, 1987.

McFarlane J, Parker B: Assessing for abuse during pregnancy: Severity and frequency of injuries and associated entry into prenatal care. JAMA 267:3176–3179, 1992.

Merskey H (ed): Classification of chronic pain: Descriptions of chronic pain syndromes and definitions of pain terms. Pain (suppl 3), S5, 1986.

Messier SP, Davies, AB, Moore DT, et al: Severe obesity: Effects on foot mechanics during walking. Foot Ankle Int 15:29–34, 1994.

Mickley DW: Medical dangers of anorexia nervosa and bulimia nervosa. *In* Lemberg R (ed): Controlling Eating Disorders with Facts, Advice, and Resources. Phoenix, Oryx Press, 1992, pp 37–40.

Miller F, Whitcup S, Sacks M, et al: Unrecognized drug dependence and withdrawal in the elderly. Drug Alcohol Depend 15:177, 1985.

Mitchell BC, Hawthorne VM, Vinik AI: Cigarette smoking and neuropathy in diabetic patients. Diabetes Care 13:434–437, 1990.

Mittleman MA, Maclure M, Sherwood JB, et al: Triggering of myocardial infarction onset by episodes of anger (abstract). Circulation 89:936, 1994.

Moses J: The effects of exercise training on mental well-being in the normal population: A controlled trial. J Psychosom Res 33:47–61, 1989.

Moss SE, Klein R, Klein BE: The prevalence and incidence of lower

extremity amputation in a diabetic population. Arch Intern Med 152:610–616, 1992.
NCADD (National Council on Alcoholism and Drug Dependence): What Are the Signs of Alcoholism? New York, Author, 1990.
NCHS (National Center for Health Statistics): Vital statistics of the United States 1980, Vol 11. Mortality, Part B, US Department of Health and Human Services Publication No. (PHS) 85-01102, Washington, DC, US Government Printing Office, 1985.
NCHS (National Center for Health Statistics), Vital Statistics Report, Washington, DC, US Government Printing Office, Vol 43, No 6, Supplement March 22, 1995.
NIDA (National Institute on Drug Abuse): Statistics 1994, Rockville, Md, 1995.
Nilsson BE: Conditions contributing to fractures of the femoral neck. Acta Chir Scand 136:383–384, 1970.
Oldridge NB: Compliance and exercise in primary and secondary prevention of coronary heart disease: A review. Prev Med 11:56–70, 1982.
Ostlund RE: The ratio of waist to hips circumference, plasma insulin level, and glucose intolerance as independent predictors of the HDL_2 cholesterol level in older adults. N Engl J Med 322:229–234, 1990.
O'Toole M (ed): Miller-Keane Encyclopedia and Dictionary of Medicine, Nursing, and Allied Health, ed 5. Philadelphia, WB Saunders, 1992.
Papp LA, Klein DF, Gorman JM: Carbon dioxide hypersensitivity, hyperventilation, and panic disorder. Am J Psychiatry 150:1149–1157, 1993.
Pierce TW, Madden DJ Siegel WC, et al: Effects of aerobic exercise on cognitive and psychosocial functioning in patients with mild hypertension. Health Psychol 12:286–291, 1993.
Plante T, Rodin J: Physical fitness and enhanced psychological health. Curr Psychol 9:3–24, 1990.
Pollock ML: Effects of frequency and duration of training on attrition and incidence of injury. Med Sci Sports Exerc 9:31, 1977.
Pollock ML: Effects of training two days per week at different intensities on middle-aged men. Med Sci Sports Exerc 4:192–197, 1972.
Pollock ML, Cureton TK, Greninger L: Effects of frequency of training on working capacity, cardiovascular function, and body composition of adult men. Med Sci Sports Exerc 1:70–74, 1969.
Ravussin E, Swinburg GA: Pathophysiology of obesity. Lancet 340:404–408, 1992.
Reichel W: Care of the Elderly: Clinical Aspects of Aging, ed 4. Baltimore, Williams & Wilkins, 1995.
Reichlin S: Neuroendocrine-immune interactions. N Engl J Med 329:1246–1253, 1993.
Richelson E: Biological basis of depression and therapeutic relevance [erratum appears in J Clin Psychiatry 52:353, 1991]. J Clin Psychiatry 52(Suppl 6):4–10, 1991.
Robins LN: Lifetime prevalence of specific psychiatric disorders in three sites. Arch Gen Psychiatry 41:949–958, 1984.
Rodin J: Unpublished data reported in The Pennsylvania Gazette, University of Pennsylvania, Philadelphia, March 1994, pp 19–26.
Rubin E, Farber JL: Environmental and Nutritional Pathology. *In* Rubin E, Farber JL (eds): Pathology, ed 2. Philadelphia, JB Lippincott, 1994, pp 289–336.
Salisbury JJ, Mitchell JE: Bone mineral density and anorexia nervosa in women. Am J Psychiatry 149:415–416, 1992.
Salzman C: Clinical Geriatric Psychopharmacology. New York, McGraw-Hill, 1984.
Sanford ME, Petajan JH: Multiple Sclerosis and Your Emotions. New York, National Multiple Sclerosis Society, 1988.
Schmidt M: Personal communication, August, 1995.
Schweiger U, Deuschle M, Körner A, et al: Low lumbar bone mineral density in patients with major depression. Am J Psychiatry 151:1691–1693, 1994.
Seward JP: Occupational stress. *In* LaDou J (ed): Occupational Medicine. Norwalk, Conn, Appleton & Lange, 1990, pp 467–481.
Shafe MC, Parsons JM: Eating disorders: A holistic approach to treatment. *In* Lemberg R (ed): Controlling Eating Disorders with Facts, Advice, and Resources. Phoenix, Oryx Press, 1992, pp 138–144.
Shapira D: Alcohol abuse and osteoporosis. Semin Arthritis Rheum 19:371–376, 1990.
Sherwin MA, Gastwirth CM: Detrimental effects of cigarette smoking on lower extremity wound healing. J Foot Surg 29:84–87, 1990.
Sherwood A, May CW, Siegel WC, et al: Ethnic differences in hemodynamic responses to stress in hypertensive men and women. Am J Hypertens 8:552–557, 1995.
Shulsinger E: Needs of sheltered homeless children. J Pediatr Health Care 4:136–140, 1991.
Silverstein P: Smoking and wound healing. Am J Med 93(1A):22S–24S, 1992.
Skinner JS (ed): Exercise Testing and Exercise Prescription for Special Cases, ed 2. Philadelphia, Lea & Febiger, 1993.
Slemenda CW: Cigarettes and the skeleton. N Engl J Med 330:430–431, 1994.
Steptoe A, Cox S: Acute effects of aerobic exercise on mood. Health Psychol 7:329–340, 1988.
Sternbach RA: Pain Patients: Traits and Treatment. New York, Academic Press, 1974.
Sweet J, Reynolds C: Handbook of Clinical Psychology in Medical Settings. New York, Plenum Press, 1992.
Thompson JM, McFarland GK, Hirsch JE, et al: Mosby's Clinical Nursing, ed 3. St Louis, Mosby–Year Book, 1993.
Tramuta G: Psychological Disorders Associated with Chronic Headaches. Germantown, Pa, Comprehensive Headache Center, 1994.
Warner JG, Jr, Brubaker PH, Zhu Y, et al: Long-term (5 year) changes in HDL cholesterol in cardiac rehabilitation patients. Do sex differences exist? Circulation 92:773–777, 1995.
Watkins PL, Ward CH, Southard DR, et al: The Type A belief system: Relationships to hostility, social support, and life stress. Behav Med 18:27–32, 1992.
Wells KB: Detection of depressive disorder for patients receiving prepaid or fee-for-service care. Results from the Medical Outcomes Study. JAMA 262:3298–3302, 1989.
White House Conference on Aging: Demographics associated with aging. Washington DC, Author, 1994.
Willett WC, Manson JE, Stampfer MJ, et al: Weight, weight change, and coronary heart disease in women: Risk within the 'normal' weight range. JAMA 273:461–465, 1995.
Williams RR: Genes and environmental interaction: Familial diseases. *In* McCance KL, Huether SE (eds): Pathophysiology: The Biologic Basis for Disease in Adults and Children, ed 2. St Louis, Mosby–Year Book, 1994, pp 166–201.
Wilmore JH: Importance of differences between men and women for exercise testing and exercise prescription. *In* Skinner JS (ed): Exercise Testing and Exercise Prescription for Special Cases, ed 2. Philadelphia, Lea & Febiger, 1993, pp 41–56.
Woltersdorf MA: Beyond the sensorimotor strip. Clin Manage 12:63–69, 1992.
Woltersdorf MA: Hidden disorders: Psychological barriers to treatment success. PT Magazine 3(12):58–66, 1995.
Woltersdorf MA: Transference: Whistling in the dark. PT Magazine 2(1):60–65, 1994.
Wong DL: Whaley & Wong's Essentials of Pediatric Nursing, ed 4. St Louis, Mosby–Year Book, 1993.
Zhang Y, Proenca R, Maffei M, et al: Positional cloning of the mouse obese gene and its human homologue. Nature 372:425–432, 1994.
Zohn DA, Mennell J: Musculoskeletal Pain: Diagnosis and Physical Treatment, ed 2. Boston, Little, Brown, 1988.

SECTION 1

chapter 3

Environmental and Occupational Medicine

Catherine C. Goodman

ENVIRONMENTAL MEDICINE[1] *(Gochfeld, 1995c)*

Environmental medicine[1] and a newly emerging branch of medicine called clinical ecology study the results of interaction between humans and the environment. Many diseases (e.g., contact dermatitis, obstructive lung disease, nephropathy, neuropathy, various cancers) occur when the body is exposed to some agent or stressor in the environment. Usually the focus of environmental medicine is on chemical and physical hazards in the environment.

The *environment* is defined as all agents outside the body, including infectious organisms, toxins, and food. Intrinsic factors include the genetic makeup of the host as well as the individual's underlying state of health and history of past illnesses. Disease results from an interplay of the environment and these intrinsic factors when the host defenses are overcome. *Occupational medicine* is a specialty involving the health of workers and workplaces and can be considered a special form of environmental medicine.

Industrial, occupational, and environmental illnesses, injuries, and diseases widely affect the population. Hazardous waste sites, nuclear energy leaks, contaminated drinking water, low-level exposures to untested chemical compounds, repeated exposure to electromagnetic waves and second-hand smoke are examples of problems the American public will continue to face.

Whether at home, in the workplace, or in the community at large, chemical, physical, biologic, psychosocial, and traumatic hazards exist. *Chemical agents* are responsible for the majority of environmental toxic reactions; *physical agents* include radiation, vibration, temperature, and noise; *biologic agents* include bacteria and viruses, allergens, and fungi (molds); *psychosocial factors* (see Chapter 2) are an important consideration for environmental medicine; and *macro-* and *microtrauma*, include mechanical factors such as cumulative or repetitive trauma (e.g., carpal tunnel syndrome), as well as trauma induced by recreational activities or accidents outside the workplace.[2]

Multiple agencies exist for the investigation and regulation of environmental health care. The National Institute for Occupational Safety and Health (NIOSH) is the federal research agency that conducts studies to develop safety and health standards. It does not have legal authority to adopt or enforce regulations. The Occupational Safety and Health Administration (OSHA) is the primary regulatory agency that determines which of the standards proposed by NIOSH will be adopted and enforced.[3] Its standards are law throughout the United States, and its compliance officers can inspect the workplace at any time to determine the status of health and safety (LaDou, 1990). There are many other government and private agencies and organizations concerned with these regulatory issues.

Ergonomics *(Khalil et al., 1994)*

Derived from the Greek *ergon* work, and *nomos*, law, ergonomics is the study of work and of the relationship between humans and their working and physical environment. This relationship includes other people, equipment, environmental conditions, and tasks. Humans have limitations arising from factors such as gender differences, race (e.g., differences in size, weight, and body proportions), aging, physical fitness, diet, stress, as well as pain and injury. Our abilities (and limitations) combined with the necessary acquired skills, determine how well we perform our daily tasks. Ergonomics helps people recognize their abilities and limitations for safe and effective performance within the environment.

Work environments are often designed without adequate consideration for the people who will use them. Inadequate workplace design can contribute to stress, injury, pain, job-related disabilities, and subsequently, lost productivity. If products are designed without considering the human factor, health and safety hazards can occur.

Ergonomics is an interdisciplinary field of study that integrates engineering, medicine, and physical and behavioral management sciences and addresses issues arising from the interaction of humans in an increasingly technological society. As a field of study, ergonomics deals with job design, work performance, health and safety, stress, posture, body mechanics, biomechanics, anthropometry (measurement of body size, weight, and proportions), manual material handling, equipment design, quality control, environment, workers' education and training, and employment testing.

[1] Environmental medicine as a broad term encompasses industrial and occupational medicine as well as environmentally induced illnesses and conditions and is used throughout this chapter to refer to all three branches of study.

[2] It should be noted that in comparison to all the possible hazards listed above, morbidity and mortality from the voluntary intake of tobacco smoke, alcohol, and illicit psychoactive drugs far exceed effects from all other environmental hazards combined (Rubin and Farber, 1994a).

[3] Congress has now prohibited OSHA from formulating any further new safety regulations, including completion of a draft entitled *OSHA Ergonomics Program Guidelines 3123* which would help therapists establish their role in work injury management. The move reflected both a general antiregulatory mood in Congress and a specific effort to cut US Department of Health and Human Services appropriations for OSHA (PT Magazine, 1995).

Ergonomic Certification

Board certification in professional ergonomics (BCPE) credentials engineering ergonomists through a certification examination. The BCPE recognizes ergonomics primarily from the standpoint of engineering and design, defining *ergonomics* as "a body of knowledge about human abilities, limitations, and other characteristics that are relevant to design. The practice of ergonomics is the application of this knowledge to the design of tools, machines, systems, tasks, jobs, and work environments for safe, comfortable effective human use." Most often BCPE-certified ergonomists have engineering and industrial psychology backgrounds and begin working toward improved industrial productivity first before targeting improved safety.

This approach differs from the rehabilitation ergonomics common in the rehabilitation field. Concentrating on improved safety focuses on physiologic improvement which in turn increases productivity. The Ergonomic Research and Rehabilitation Society (ERRS), an organization representing health ergonomists, describes rehabilitation ergonomists as "health care professionals who utilize knowledge of the relationship between pathology and work, to match the demands of the job to the capacity of the worker." In other words, rehabilitation ergonomists work with people who do not fit the normal standards but require modification to safely and productively perform their job or task. Another organization, the National Interdisciplinary Committee on Health Ergonomics, is currently developing its own set of standards to create certification for the health or rehabilitation ergonomist.

Incidence *(LaDou, 1990)*

The rapid proliferation of new industrial materials, new production methods, and new commercial products in the 20th century (particularly since World War II) has progressed with little known until recently about their effects on the environment and on human health. Only about 10,000 of the estimated 60,000 chemicals used commercially today have been tested for toxicity in animals. While toxicity testing lags far behind the rate of new developments, the incidence of work- and environment-related illness in humans increases.

Each year in the United States, over 2 million people suffer permanent or temporary disability from various causes, including occupational illness and occupational injury. Although the number of people with disabilities resulting from occupational illness is not known, it has been estimated that there are at least 390,000 new cases of disabling occupational illness and as many as 100,000 deaths from occupational diseases each year.

It is likely that because of the difficulty of diagnosis and the likelihood that occupational illness claims will be disputed by employers, these figures are gross underestimates of the true incidence of environmentally induced illnesses. The National Academy of Sciences estimates that 15% of the population experiences some degree of chemical sensitivity, and chemical-related injury and illness are dramatically on the rise. The Social Security Administration recognized chemical sensitivity as an environmental illness and disability in 1988.

Etiology

Specific sources of environmental exposure are listed in Box 3–1. Construction and architectural modifications introduced in the 1970s as a result of the worldwide energy crisis have resulted in better insulated and tighter buildings with reduced ventilation. The indoor air pollution, which has developed in tight, energy-efficient homes and buildings with poor ventilation and reduced air-exchange rates, is called the *sick building syndrome* or *building-related illness*.

BOX 3–1
Environmental Exposure Sources

- Indoor air pollution (includes mold and mildew)
- Outdoor air pollution
- Asbestos exposure in buildings
- Manmade mineral fibers
- Fire and pyrolysis products*
- Water pollution
- Food
- Soil
- Physical agents
  - Ionizing radiation
  - Radon
  - Nonionizing radiation
  - Electromagnetic fields
  - Vibration
  - Heat stress
  - High-altitude and aerospace medicine
  - Chemical agents
  - Biologic agents
  - Heavy metals
- Waste
  - Solid waste
  - Hazardous waste
  - Incinerator waste

* Pyrolysis (incomplete combustion) of wood releases many compounds that are highly toxic and can react with other organics to produce new toxic and irritant chemicals. Incomplete combustion and firefighting water also may produce highly acidic aerosols. Many toxic products are released by smoldering or partially controlled fires (Gochfeld, 1995b).

Data from Brooks SM, Gochfeld M, Herzstein J et al: Environmental Medicine. St Louis, Mosby–Year Book, 1995.

Other sources of *indoor air pollution* include tobacco smoke (see Environmental Tobacco Smoke, Chapter 12); fireplaces; space heaters; stoves; pilot lights; gas ranges; mothballs; cleaning fluids; glues; photocopiers; formaldehyde in foam, glues, plywood, particle board, carpet backing, and fabrics; and infectious and allergic agents such as dust mites, cockroaches, bacteria, fungi, viruses, and pollen. Many investigations of workplace environments have clearly documented the role of occupational air pollutants in causing health complaints and disease (Fernandez-Caldas et al., 1995; Gold, 1992).

Outdoor air pollution has long been associated with clinically significant adverse health effects. Although exposure to air pollution is classified separately as indoor and outdoor, the concept of total personal exposure, whether exposure occurs in the home, office, outdoors at home or at work, in a car, movie theater, and so on, is relevant to every individual. People considered especially susceptible to air pollution include cigarette smokers, the elderly, infants, and young children, and persons with chronic obstructive pulmonary disease (COPD) or coronary heart disease (CHD). The consequences

TABLE 3–1 CONSEQUENCES OF AIR POLLUTION IN SUSCEPTIBLE PERSONS

POPULATION	PATHOGENESIS	CONSEQUENCES
Persons with asthma	Increased airway responsiveness	Increased risk of exacerbation of respiratory symptoms
Cigarette smokers	Impaired defense clearance, lung injury	Increased damage through synergism (combined effect)
Elderly	Impaired respiratory defenses, reduced functional reserve	Increased risk of respiratory infection, increased risk of clinically significant effects on function
Infants	Immature defense mechanisms of the lung	Increased risk of respiratory infection
Persons with CHD	Impaired myocardial oxygenation	Increased risk of myocardial ischemia
Persons with COPD	Reduced level of lung function	Increased risk of clinically significant effects on function

CHD, coronary heart disease; COPD, chronic obstructive lung disease.
Modified from Utell MJ, Samet JM: Air pollution in the outdoor environment. *In* Brooks SM, Gochfeld M, Herzstein J, et al: Environmental Medicine. St Louis, Mosby–Year Book, 1995, p 466.

of air pollution on these populations are listed in Table 3–1 (Utell and Samet, 1995).

Carbon monoxide (CO), an odorless, tasteless, and colorless gas, is a common environmental pollutant from automobile exhaust emissions, fires, and in some areas, home heating systems. It does not produce lung injury, but does have an effect on tissue oxygenation. CO combines 240 times more quickly with hemoglobin than does oxygen, so when carbon dioxide is bound to hemoglobin, its oxygen-carrying capacity is decreased. In the presence of CO, oxygen is not released normally by the blood, resulting in tissue hypoxia. Exposure to CO causes impaired visual acuity, headache, nausea, fatigue, behavioral change, ataxia, and hypoxic damage to the heart or brain. A characteristic cherry-red (lips) cyanosis due to the bright red color of carboxyhemoglobin (COHb) may occur if the COHb concentration is above 40%.

Other air pollutants include smog, a combination of smoke and fog that develops when car exhaust fumes containing nitrous oxides and hydrocarbons are photochemically oxidized.[4] Nitrogen dioxide and ozone are toxic byproducts of this reaction. Ozone is also produced in the welding process when oxygen is ionized. Both of these byproducts are toxic to the respiratory tract, damaging ciliated endothelial cells lining bronchioles and impairing the mucociliary clearance mechanism. Those persons who are very young, very old, heavy smokers, or who have preexisting lung disease are at increased risk in the presence of these toxins (Pearlstein, 1987).

Asbestos continues to be a significant occupational hazard. Abatement workers employed to remove asbestos in buildings wear protective clothing to decrease exposure but still are considered at risk. Long latency (exposure occurring 30 or more years ago continues to affect former workers) and long-term low-level exposure to the presence of indoor asbestos remain risk factors (Landrigan and Kazemi, 1991). See Chapter 12 for a discussion of asbestosis.

Manmade vitreous fibers containing mineral wool, glass wool or fiber, and ceramic fiber have replaced asbestos in the workplace. The nonoccupational exposure to manmade minerals does not put consumers at substantial risk; health issues related to these materials mainly occur among workers with long duration of exposure. Clinical consequences are similar to those of asbestos, including pulmonary fibrosis, bronchogenic carcinoma, mesothelioma, and possibly other types of cancers (Brooks, 1995).

Two million people are treated annually for *burns*, including civilians and firefighters. Death can occur as a result of smoke inhalation and myocardial infarction. Musculoskeletal injuries associated with fires and firefighting account for 35% of the nonfatal injuries (Washburn et al., 1980).

Water pollution in the form of contamination of drinking water by toxic chemicals has become widely recognized as a public health issue since the late 1970s. Increased monitoring since then has shown that many pesticides and industrial chemicals can be detected in drinking water. Studies are being carried out to assess cancer risks associated with water pollution (Brown and Jackson, 1995).

Food is one of the major environmental agents to which we are exposed. In many documented cases, reversible and irreversible human and ecological damage has occurred as a result of pollution-induced food contamination. As scientific and epidemiologic information accumulates, our society is questioning to what degree these technologies and byproducts contribute to the steadily rising incidence of certain cancers, autoimmune and other chronic diseases, birth defects, and other health problems for which the cause is not well understood. Pesticide residues in food, hormone residues, food irradiation (a method of preservation and protection from microbial contamination), and food additives and preservatives are major consumer concerns (Lechowich, 1992; Shank and Carson, 1992). At present, there are no conclusive studies to substantiate these concerns but research is ongoing in this area.

Contaminated soil is often the main source of chemical exposure for humans, and there is an active interchange of chemicals between soil and water, air, and food. Direct contact and ingestion of soil are important exposure pathways and inhalation of volatile compounds or dust must also be considered. The movement of contaminants through soil is

[4] Ozone and nitrogen, the components of smog, result from the action of sunlight on the products of vehicular internal combustion engines. Automobiles and trucks emit unburnt hydrocarbons and nitrogen dioxide. Ultraviolet irradiation of these compounds leads to complex chemical reactions that produce ozone, various nitrates, and other organic and inorganic compounds constituting smog (Rubin and Farber, 1994b).

very complex, some moving rapidly and others slowly, eventually reaching and contaminating surface or ground water, on which people rely for drinking and other purposes (Gochfeld, 1995d).

Physical agents (see Box 3–1) are the source of much environmental damage. *Ionizing radiation* is the form of radiant energy capable of disrupting the atoms and molecules in the tissues through which it passes. Because all living material is composed of atoms joined into molecules, it is vulnerable to ionization by high-energy radiation. These disruptions produce ions and free radicals (unstable oxygen molecules)[5] which in turn can cause further biochemical damage, including somatic effects such as cell death, and genetic effects, including reproductive effects and cancer. Radiation-induced changes can cause genetic mutations and structural rearrangements in chromosomes that can be transmitted from generation to generation (Burger, 1995).

Nonionizing radiation is the result of electromagnetic waves entering the body and acting on neutral atoms or molecules with sufficient force to remove electrons, creating an ion. Sources of nonionizing radiation are light (ultraviolet, visible, and infrared), radiofrequency and microwave, and electromagnetic fields, particularly from electrical power and appliances. Exposure to this type of radiation commonly occurs as a result of the use of a wide variety of industrial and electronic devices (e.g., microwave ovens, scanning lasers in stores, high-intensity lamps, video display terminals (Sheedy, 1995; Scullica et al., 1995), cellular phones, scanning radar).

A wide range of adverse health effects have been attributed to ionizing radiation, including visual (Kosnik, 1995; Muhlbach et al., 1995), thermal, behavioral, central nervous system (CNS), and auditory effects; effects on the blood-brain barrier; and immunologic, endocrinologic (including effects on biorhythm), hematologic, developmental, and cardiovascular effects (Burger and Gochfeld, 1995). See also Tables 5–9 and 5–10.

Radon, a product of the breakdown of radium, poses an environmental risk because of its carcinogenic (especially lung cancer) properties. Exposure is predominantly naturally occurring rather than generated by human polluters and is present in poorly ventilated homes in the form of an odorless gas. Other sources include radioactive waste and underground mines; exposure to tobacco smoke multiplies the risk of concurrent exposure to radon (Schoenberg, 1990; Klotz, 1995).

Vibration is divided into two types: whole-body vibration (WBV) and hand-arm vibration (HAV). Truck and bus drivers, heavy equipment operators, miners, and others are at increased risk for WBV. Major clinical concerns of WBV exposure are chronic back pain and degenerative disk diseases, and circulatory and digestive system disorders (Wilder et al., 1982; Hulshof and van Zanten, 1987). Vibration-induced white finger disease is the most common example of an occupational injury caused by vibration of the hands. This condition occurs secondary to use of hand tools such as power saws, grinders, sanders, pneumatic drills, jackhammers, and other equipment used in construction, foundry work, machining and mining (Cohen, 1990a).

Heat stress exceeding human tolerance can result in heat disorders (e.g., stroke, exhaustion, cramps, dehydration, prickly heat) and heat illnesses (e.g., chronic heat exhaustion, reduced heat tolerance, anhidrotic heat exhaustion), some of which are fatal. In a therapy setting, the groups of people most likely to experience heat stress include the elderly during temperature extremes, industrial workers, outdoor sports participants, agricultural workers, pregnant women, and people taking mood-altering drugs (i.e., they lose touch with their environment), as well as antidepressants such as tricyclic antidepressants which affect the body's ability to respond to temperature changes.

High-altitude environment (8000 to 14,000 feet) is characterized by atmosphere with decreasing partial pressure of oxygen and decreasing temperature. Hypoxia (reduced availability of oxygen to the body) appears to be the underlying cause of most of the physiologic changes of elevated altitude. Acute altitude sickness includes acute mountain sickness, high-altitude pulmonary edema, and high-altitude cerebral edema. These three probably represent a continuum of disease, but each have different symptom complexes, pathogenesis, and slightly different treatment. Persons with cardiopulmonary and other diseases (e.g., sickle cell disease) are at increased risk for worsening of the medical disorder and possibly at increased risk for acute altitude illnesses with ascent to high altitudes (Bullock, 1995). Aviation and aerospace illnesses are rarely encountered by the therapist and are beyond the scope of this book.

Chemical agents (e.g., organic and inorganic) and *biologic agents* (e.g., viruses, bacteria, allergens) can lower the body's resistance making a person more susceptible to infectious diseases. Chemical agents are numerous and can be classified by use (e.g., agricultural chemicals, automotive products, pharmaceutical agents, cleaning agents, paints, dyes, explosives, and so on), by their mechanism of action (e.g., enzyme disruption, metabolic poison, irritants, free radical formation), and by their target organ(s) (e.g., neurotoxins, hepatotoxins, cardiotoxins and so on). Although there are many toxic effects, they can be broken down into three main categories: local acute effects, systemic effects, and idiosyncratic (unpredictable) effects (Gochfeld, 1995a). Biologic agents are discussed in Chapters 6 and 8.

Heavy metals, such as lead, arsenic, and mercury, actually fall under the chemical agents category but are mentioned separately here because of their prevalence and uniqueness as environmental toxins. The ingestion of *lead* paints found in older residential neighborhoods is a continuing problem among the pediatric population; adults are often exposed to lead in the manufacture of brass, batteries, bullets, solder, and glass. Lead is stored in the body predominantly in bone, but may adversely affect many organ systems, including the central nervous, gastrointestinal, hemopoietic, reproductive, and renal systems (Bauer and Watson, 1994). The implications of lead poisoning are discussed later in this chapter.

Arsenic is used in the manufacture of glass, pesticides, and wood preservatives and has been found to contaminate water, beer, and seafood. Arsenic binds to tissue proteins and is

[5] Free radicals, also known as "reactive oxygen species," have now been implicated in more than 50 medical conditions, including various forms of cancer, heart disease, premature aging, cataracts, and the acquired immunodeficiency syndrome (AIDS). The balance of radical and nonradical reactive oxygen can be upset by many factors such as cigarette smoke, air pollution, anticancer drugs (e.g., doxorubicin [Adriamycin]), ultraviolent light, pesticides and other chemicals, uncontrolled diabetes, radiation, emotional stress, and asbestos and related fibers (Cooper, 1994). When any of these factors rob normal oxygen atoms of electrons, free radicals occur. The free radicals attempt to replace their missing electrons by scavenging the body and taking electrons from healthy cells, generating more free radicals.

concentrated in the liver, skin, kidney, nervous system, and bone (the last to a lesser extent than lead). The symptoms of acute inorganic arsenic poisoning may include severe burning of the mouth and throat, abdominal pain, nausea, vomiting, diarrhea, hypotension, and muscle spasms. In severe cases, cardiomyopathy, jaundice, renal impairment, red cell hemolysis, ventricular arrhythmias, coma, seizures, and intestinal hemorrhage are seen. Chronic arsenic poisoning is characterized by an irregular dusky pigmentation and hyperkeratosis of the skin that looks like "raindrops on a dusty road." Painful dysesthesia in the hands and feet, bone marrow depression, transverse white striae of the nails, altered mentation, and occasionally garlic-odor perspiration may occur. Cancer of the skin and lungs has been associated with arsenic poisoning (Bauer and Watson, 1994).

Mercury is used in electrical products and dental amalgams and as a fungicide. Although inorganic mercury is poorly absorbed from the gastrointestinal tract, mercury vapor is well absorbed through the lungs, and organic mercury compounds are well absorbed from the gut. Inorganic mercury poisoning causes irritation of the mouth and pharynx and is accompanied by vomiting, dehydration, abdominal cramps, and bloody diarrhea. Death can occur from acute renal failure. Chronic exposure to inorganic mercury may cause additional symptoms of gingivitis, speech defects, tremor, and chronic personality disorder called the Mad Hatter syndrome characterized by unusual shyness, labile affect, and decline in intellect. Organic mercury poison affects the nervous system resulting in dysarthria, ataxia, paresthesias, and constricted visual fields. Organic mercury can cross the placenta causing fatal mental retardation, cerebral palsy, and seizures (Bauer and Watson, 1994).

The effects of exposure to solid, hazardous, and incinerator *waste* are not likely to be encountered directly in a therapy practice. Information from current studies on the latent effects of waste exposure and epidemiologic studies are limited at this time.

Risk Factors

Environmental pathogenesis requires an understanding of *latency*, the concept that a disease agent may initiate a series of internal reactions that do not manifest as overt disease for many years or even decades as the body strives to maintain a state of optimal health or homeostasis. Many factors such as route of exposure (e.g., inhalation, ingestion, absorption through the skin), magnitude or concentration (dose) of exposure, duration (e.g., minutes, hours, days, lifetime), frequency (e.g., seasonal, daily, weekly, monthly), play into the development of progressive and overt disease. Likewise, personal factors that vary from one person to another may affect pathogenesis and must be considered. These include age, sex, race, nutritional status, personal habits and lifestyle, genetic makeup and host susceptibility, and the strength of individual defense mechanisms. The host-agent-environment interactions are immensely complex and poorly understood at this time.

Risk factors for musculoskeletal occupational injury have been identified by OSHA. If workers are exposed to one or more of these factors (Box 3–2) during their shift, this signals increased risk requiring preventive intervention.

BOX 3–2
Risk Factors for Musculoskeletal Injury

1. Performance of the same motions or motion pattern every few seconds for more than 2 hours at a time
2. Fixed or awkward work postures for more than a total of 2 hours (e.g., overhead work, twisted or bent back, bent wrist, kneeling, stooping, or squatting)
3. Use of vibrating or impact tools or equipment for more than a total of 2 hours
4. Unassisted manual lifting, lowering, or carrying of anything weighing more than 25 lbs more than once during the work shift
5. Piece rate or machine-paced work for more than 4 hours at a time

Data from Occupational Safety and Health Administration (OSHA): Draft Proposed Ergonomic Protection Standard. Washington, DC, Author, March 13, 1995.

Pathogenesis

Once a hazardous substance is released into the environment, it may be transported and transformed in a variety of complex ways (Koren, 1991). For example, a chemical may be modified by the environment before entering the body; be transformed by chemical or biochemical processes; or undergo vaporization, diffusion, dilution, or concentration by physical or biologic processes. Plants and animals may accumulate small doses of a chemical agent and bioconcentrate them to the degree that they become hazardous when consumed by humans.

All cells respond to a variety of different adverse environmental stimuli with a cellular defense response now commonly referred to as the "stress response." Molecules released by the cells in response to stress are called "stress proteins." Increased levels of these proteins after a cellular injury from a toxic chemical seem to act as molecular chaperones that facilitate the synthesis and assembly of new reparative proteins (Welch, 1993). Cells that produce high levels of stress proteins seem better able to survive ischemic damage; stress proteins may be influential in certain immunologic responses and may also be a requirement for cells to recover from a metabolic insult.[6]

Some persons, once sensitized to chemicals, develop increasingly severe reactions to more and more chemicals at smaller and smaller concentrations. The allergic response that occurs does not appear to be a typical response, perhaps suggesting immune system modulation. One theory, supported by animal studies (Miller, 1992), suggests that some chemicals damage the limbic system, the part of the brain most vulnerable to the environment through the olfactory nerve. The limbic system is crucial to emotional responses, laying down new memories, and involuntary nervous system

[6] This finding may lead to further research investigating the role of pharmacology in raising the levels of stress proteins to provide additional protection to injured tissues and organs. Such a therapeutic approach could have other applications outside environmental medicine such as to reduce tissue damage from surgery-induced ischemia or to help protect isolated organs used for transplantation, which often suffer from ischemia and reperfusion injury. Immunologists have also discovered a possible connection between stress proteins and autoimmune disease (Welch, 1993).

functions. Damage could scramble signals to mood, memory, digestive, respiratory and other critical body functions (Miller, 1992).

Clinical Manifestations

An environmental illness may manifest in a variety of ways. The illness may present as a newly developed clinical syndrome or an aggravation or change in a preexisting condition (Cullen et al., 1995). The Environmental Protection Agency (EPA, 1993) identifies seven categories of human health effects from hazardous exposures: (1) carcinogenicity, that is, can cause cancer; (2) heritable genetic and chromosomal mutations, that is, can cause mutations in genes and chromosomes that will be passed on to the next generation, such as by ionizing radiation; (3) developmental toxicity, that is, can cause birth defects or miscarriages; (4) reproductive toxicity, that is, can damage the ability of men and women to reproduce; (5) acute toxicity, that is, can cause death from even short-term exposure to the lungs, through the mouth, or the skin; (6) chronic toxicity, that is, can cause long-term damage other than cancer, such as liver, kidney, or lung damage; and (7) neurotoxicity, that is, can harm the nervous system by affecting the brain, spinal cord, or nerves.

Local toxicities from exposure to environmental agents can occur such as ocular damage, mucous membrane complaints (eye, nose, and throat irritation), chemical burns to skin, noise-induced hearing loss, and vestibular disorders. Systemic toxicities can involve any organ system (Table 3–2). The clinical syndrome may mimic a wide range of psychiatric, metabolic, nutritional, inflammatory, and degenerative diseases. Of particular interest to the therapist may be the effects on the nervous system. Neurologic symptoms are common presenting symptoms in people seen by occupational and environmental health professionals. Cognitive difficulties, headaches, fatigue, dizziness, and limb paresthesias are frequently experienced but these are nonspecific and seldom point to a single disease or cause.

Neurotoxicity *(So, 1995)*

Many toxins manifest as a nonspecific syndrome of distal sensorimotor impairment that is indistinguishable from the neuropathy due to common systemic diseases (e.g., diabetes mellitus, vitamin B_{12} deficiency, alcoholism, uremia). Toxins such as lead have a striking predilection for motor fibers and usually produce minimal sensory symptoms.

Neurologic symptoms that appear immediately after acute exposure are usually due to the physiologic effects of the specific (usually chemical) agent. These symptoms subside with cessation of exposure and elimination of the compound from the body. By contrast, delayed neurologic disorders are generally a result of pathologic alterations of the nervous system. Symptoms appear in a subacute manner over days or weeks after short-term exposure. In the case of long-term exposure, symptoms may appear insidiously and progress over many weeks or months. Recovery can be expected after cessation of exposure, but the recovery is slow and depends on the extent of neuronal damage, the half-life of the chemical (i.e., continued exposure until the drug is out of the system), and the adverse effects of chelates used in the chemotherapy of metal poisoning.

Neurotoxicants do not cause focal (asymmetrical) neuro-

TABLE 3–2 Systemic Manifestations of Toxicity

Optic	Optic nephropathy, optic neuritis, optic atrophy
Cardiovascular	Cardiac arrhythmia Coronary artery disease Hypertension Myocardial injury Nonatheromatous ischemic heart disease Peripheral arterial occlusive disease
Respiratory system	Airway inflammation and hyperreactivity Bronchitis Asthma Hypersensitivity pneumonitis Pneumoconiosis Interstitial fibrosis Asbestosis Silicosis Granuloma formation Diffuse alveolar damage
Gastrointestinal (GI) tract	Cancer
Liver	Acute or subacute hepatocellular injury Cirrhosis Angiosarcoma Carcinoma Hepatitis
Kidney and urinary tract	Acute renal disease Chronic renal failure Tubulointerstitial nephritis Nephrotic syndrome Rapidly progressive glomerulonephritis
Central nervous system	Sensorimotor polyneuropathies (mild to severe weakness) Muscular fasciculations and weakness Reduced or absent reflexes Cranial neuropathy Prominent autonomic dysfunction Encephalopathy Cerebellar ataxia
Hematopoietic system	Aplastic anemia Hemolytic anemia Myelodysplastic syndromes Multiple myeloma Toxic thrombocytopenia Porphyria
Immune system	Allergic disease Allergic rhinitis Bronchial asthma GI allergy (food) Atopic dermatitis Urticaria Anaphylaxis Autoimmune diseases Neoplasia
Reproductive system	Menstrual disorders Altered fertility or infertility Spontaneous abortion or stillbirth Birth defects, low birth weight Cancer Reduced libido or impotence Altered or reduced sperm production Premature menopause

logic syndrome. Neurotoxins reach the nervous system by the systemic route and cause neurologic symptoms and deficits in a difuse and symmetrical manner resulting in a clinical syndrome referred to as polyneuropathy. Any significant asymmetry in the presentation, such as weakness or numbness affecting one limb or one side of the body, is not likely to be attributed to neurotoxicity. Multiple neurologic syndromes are possible from a single toxin. Although the effects of neurotoxins are symmetrical, neurons from different parts of the nervous system react differently to the agent.

Toxic polyneuropathy affects the distal limbs first, reflecting the greater vulnerability of the longest nerve axons. Sensory disturbances are usually reported as a tingling or burning sensation distributed in a stocking-and-glove pattern (see Fig. 34–5). The toes and the feet are affected first; hand symptoms are seldom present during the early stage. Involvement of the motor nerve fibers, if present, manifests first as atrophy and weakness of the intrinsic foot and hand muscles, bilaterally. More severe cases may present with footdrop or wristdrop, reflecting degeneration of motor axons to the lower leg and forearm muscles.

Neuropathic pain is commonly encountered in people with peripheral neuropathies regardless of the cause. In other words, pain patterns associated with chemically induced peripheral neuropathies do not differ significantly from the clinical picture of pain associated with neuropathy of other causes. Often this pain bears little relationship to the severity of neuropathy and may intensify during a period of recovery or it may remit paradoxically as the neuropathy progresses, often with further loss of sensation. Pain is not a reliable indicator of neurologic progression or recovery.

Medical Management

Clinical assessment may include assessing the details of exposure and correlating them with the medical condition. Various testing procedures may be developed on the basis of the historical informaton provided by the client. The clinical presentation, environmental history, and results of laboratory tests assist the physician in demonstrating a correlation between exposure and the clinical manifestations. Nerve conduction velocity (NCV) studies and electromyography (EMG) are the primary tools for the laboratory evaluation of neuromuscular disorders. A toxic polyneuropathy is characterized by a diffuse and relatively symmetrical pattern of NCV abnormalities.

Removal from exposure is essential in the treatment of exposure-linked toxicity. This may be accomplished through the protective use of appropriate clothing, mask, gloves, and so on. Specific treatment protocols depend on the agent involved (e.g., pesticide poisoning requires symptom-specific therapy such as intravenous anticonvulsants to halt a seizure; antihistamines are used for allergic reactions), the particular organ system involved, and the presenting pathologic condition.

Special Implications for the Therapist 3–1

ENVIRONMENTAL HAZARDS

Given the context of industrial, occupational, and environmental medicine and the single overriding factor of latency, health care professionals must view each client's health status holistically, as a composite of the individual's total life experience. Whenever symptoms present in the absence of a clearly identifiable history or cause, the client's past medical history must be carefully reviewed. Any information elicited by the therapist but unknown to the physician must be documented and reported.

Air Pollution

Clinical studies of people and heart disease have been carried out to evaluate the effects of carbon monoxide exposure on exercise capacity. During exercise, persons with coronary artery disease experience a decreased time to occurrence of myocardial ischemia when exposed to CO compared to healthy subjects (Alfred, 1989; Kleinman, 1989; Sheps, 1987). Additionally, as the CO binds to hemoglobin to form carboxyhemoglobin the reduced capacity of the blood to deliver oxygen to the tissues results in increased frequency of arrhythmias (Sheps, 1990). Health care providers can reasonably advise clients to stay indoors during pollution episodes. Vigorous exercise outdoors, which increases the dose of pollution delivered to the respiratory tract, also should be avoided at such times (Utell and Samet, 1995).

Respiratory protective equipment has been developed for use in the workplace to minimize exposure to toxic gases and airborne particles. Many of these devices, particularly those likely to be most effective, add to the work of breathing and are not well tolerated by persons with respiratory disease. Under most circumstances, health care providers should not suggest respiratory protection as a method for reducing the risks of air pollution. Similarly, air cleaners have not been shown to have health benefits (Utell and Samet, 1995).

Burns *(Gochfeld, 1995b)*

Aside from the acute injurious effects of fire, clinicians must be alert to the pathophysiologic changes associated with exposure to heat and smoke and to the chronic sequelae, both physical and psychological (Table 3–3). In addition to the management of burns and trauma, it is necessary to evaluate clients for all acute systemic effects of exposure to smoke, heat, or toxic substances; recognize toxic effects that may be obscured by more serious traumatic effects; be alert for delayed consequences; and recognize acute and chronic exposure and health effects due to toxic chemicals in smoke, especially among firefighters.

Carbon monoxide is always present at fires. The main symptoms of CO poisoning are dizziness, headache, nausea, weakness, and tachypnea, followed at higher amounts by loss of consciousness, coma, convulsions, and death.

Carbon Monoxide

Subacute and long-term exposure to CO may accelerate atherosclerosis and increases the risk of arrhythmias even as much as 2 weeks after exposure. Acute myonecrosis (death of individual muscle fibers) has been associated with CO poisoning (Herman, 1988). The incidence of CO poisoning in homes with faulty furnaces has become an increasing problem, especially

TABLE 3-3 Types of Fire-Related Acute and Chronic Injury

Acute	Chronic
Burns (superficial, deep, internal)	Chronic cardiovascular disease
Dermal reactions to toxicants	Chronic respiratory disease
Eye irritation and burns	Noise-induced hearing loss
Smoke inhalation	Posttraumatic stress disorder
Cardiovascular strain	Elevated risk of cancer
Musculoskeletal trauma	
Heat stress	
Neuropsychiatric effects	
Renal damage	

Data from New Jersey State Department of Health: Firefighting in New Jersey: Hazards and methods of control. Trenton, Author, 1982; and International Association of Fire Fighters: 1982 Annual Death and Injury Survey. Washington, DC, Author, 1983.

in the Midwest. Inexpensive CO monitoring devices have helped to identify many previously undetected cases of high levels of CO in private homes.

Lead

The brain is the target of lead toxicity in children but adults usually present with manifestations of peripheral neuropathy. Typically, the radial and peroneal nerves are affected resulting in wristdrop and footdrop, respectively. Lead anemia and lead nephropathy may also occur. See also Neurotoxicity.

Heat Stress

Muscle cramps and distal extremity edema, dehydration, and electrolyte imbalance are the most commonly observed phenomena associated with heat stress in a therapy practice. The implications surrounding these adverse effects are discussed fully in Chapter 4.

High Altitude

The underlying cause of changes in exercise capacity associated with high altitude is not completely understood. The primary effect of altitude on exercise capacity is through effects on the cardiovascular system, with decrease in maximum oxygen consumption (VO_{2max}) and decrease in maximum heart rate. With continued exposure to increased altitude, exercise capacity dose seem to improve, but never reaches that attained at sea level (Bullock, 1995; Grover et al., 1986). Persons with congestive heart failure or coronary artery disease are more likely to be symptomatic at high altitudes. Those persons with either of these conditions are likely to experience reduced exercise capacity (Hultgren, 1992; Morgan, 1990).

Neurotoxicity *(So, 1995)*

Litigation and other potential sources of secondary gains frequently complicate environmental or occupational exposures that result in neurologic disorders. Psychological factors may have profound effects on the client's perception of neurologic symptoms, even in those persons with genuine organic disease. Emotional issues must be recognized and addressed throughout the rehabilitation process.

Coasting is the phenomenon of continuing clinical progression of neurologic deficits after removal of the offending toxin. Weakness or sensory deficits of these neuropathies often worsen for as long as 4 to 5 months after cessation of exposure, reflecting the delayed neuronal death or degeneration induced by the toxin.

Neurologic recovery is facilitated by the plasticity of the nervous system (i.e., its ability to adapt to injury). Peripheral sensory and motor nerve fibers have a remarkable capacity to regenerate after removal of the neurotoxin. Although the neurons in the CNS lack the ability to multiply, surviving neurons may eventually take over the function of degenerated neurons and partially restore neurologic function. Physical therapy is beneficial during the recovery time to facilitate this process. When given sufficient time (18 to 24 months), partial clinical improvement is demonstrable in the majority of cases.

OCCUPATIONAL INJURIES AND DISEASES

Occupational Injuries

Overall workplace injuries in private industry, estimated at 10 million annually in 1987 (Pollack and Keimig, 1987), had declined to 6.5 million in 1995 (Bureau of Labor Statistics, 1997) but these may be grossly underreported, especially if no loss of work time occurs. The most common occupational injuries involve the musculoskeletal system with over 1 million workers sustaining back injuries each year.

The number of low back injuries in the workplace has been decreasing, but the incidence of upper extremity injuries now accounts for nearly two thirds of workplace disorders. The US Department of Labor has cited carpal tunnel syndrome and other cumulative trauma disorders (Table 3–4) as the cause of two thirds of all industrial workplace disorders,

TABLE 3-4 Work-Related Conditions of the Hand and Arm

Cumulative Trauma Disorders	Repetitive Strain Injury
Carpal tunnel syndrome	Carpal tunnel syndrome
de Quervain's disease	Cervical radiculopathy
Epicondylitis	Thoracic outlet syndrome
Ganglionic cysts	Pronator syndrome
Neuritis in the fingers	Cubital tunnel syndrome
Tenosynovitis of the finger extensor tendons	Distal ulnar neuropathy
Tenosynovitis and peritendinitis crepitans of the radial styloid housing the abductor pollicis longus and extensor pollicis brevis	

Adapted from LaDou J (ed): Occupational Medicine. Norwalk, Conn, Appleton & Lange, 1990, p 47.

affecting more than 5 million Americans (Ellis, 1995). Other commonly sustained workplace injuries include eye injuries, fractures, amputations, and lacerations severe enough to require medical treatment.

The incidence of carpal tunnel syndrome alone has continued to rise annually by 7% to 10% from the early 1990s to the present. In addition to workers who spend hours at the computer, carpal tunnel syndrome has been reported in meat packers, assembly line workers, jackhammer operators, athletes, and homemakers.[7] The major causes of occupational deaths are work-related motor vehicle accidents, falls, trauma, and electric shock.

More recently, there has been an increase to almost epidemic proportions in the incidence of a form of repetitive strain injury (RSI) (see Table 3–5) which occurs primarily among keyboard operators. The use of the term "strain" may be a misnomer as the symptoms occur in response to static muscle overload or maintenance of constrained postures rather than repetitive or dynamic muscle load.

The clinical features of this syndrome vary and may include chronic neck pain and arm and hand pain associated with weak grip and tight proximal muscles. There may be dysesthesia and variable hand and forearm swelling. These symptoms lead to inability to perform previous work tasks or leisure activities that require repetitive movement or maintained positions. Physical, ergonomic, environmental, and psychological factors are all attributed to the development of this condition. The higher incidence of RSI in women is more likely to be related to their predominance in occupations at risk for RSI rather than to their physical or psychological makeup (Hazleman, 1994).

Therapists often play a significant role in the prevention (e.g., job site analysis and workstation redesign) and rehabilitation of occupational injuries. Work hardening is a fairly recent innovation in rehabilitation specifically geared toward reemployment. Unlike conventional programs, it does not focus on such goals as symptom reduction or increased physical capacity. Through graded work simulations conducted in a realistic industrial or office setting, injured persons rebuild physical and psychological fitness to work (Matheson, 1993).

Occupational Pulmonary Diseases

Many acute and chronic pulmonary diseases are directly related to inhalation of noxious substances encountered in the workplace. Disorders caused by chemical agents are classified as (1) pneumoconioses, (2) hypersensitivity pneumonitis, (3) obstructive airway disorders, (4) toxic lung injury, (5) lung cancer, and (6) pleural diseases (Stauffer, 1994).

Asbestos and other silicates such as kaolin, mica, and vermiculite can cause *pneumoconiosis*. Asbestos-induced diseases cause lung inflammation and fibrosis as a result of activation of alveolar macrophages. Coal worker's pneumonoconiosis is another parenchymal lung disease caused by inhalation of coal dust. *Hypersensitivity pneumonitis* has many other names (e.g., extrinsic allergic alveolitis, farmer's lung, detergent worker's lung) and is characterized by a granulomatous inflammatory reaction in the pulmonary alveolar and interstitial spaces. Occupational asthma (*airway obstruction*) follows workplace exposure to inhaled gases, dusts, fumes, or vapors. Silicosis is a parenchymal *toxic lung disease* caused by inhalation of crystalline silica, a component of rock and sand. Workers at risk include miners, tunnelers, quarry workers, stonecutters, sandblasters, foundry workers, glass blowers, and ceramic workers. These conditions are discussed more fully in Chapter 12.

Occupational Cancer *(Fischman et al., 1990)*

It is estimated that 30% to 40% of the population in the industrialized world will develop malignant disease during their lifetime. Various studies have attributed 70% to 80% of cancer cases in humans to environmental causes. Alteration or mutation in the genetic material (DNA) may occur as a result of exposure to carcinogenic chemicals or radiation. Both experimental animal models of cancer and the study of human cancers with known causes have revealed the existence of a significant interval between first exposure to the responsible agent and the first manifestation of a tumor. This time period is referred to as the induction period, latency period, or induction-latency period.

For humans, the length of the induction-latency period varies from a minimum of 4 to 6 years for radiation-induced leukemias to 40 or more years for some cases of asbestos-induced mesotheliomas. For most tumors, the interval ranges from 12 to 25 years; such a long time period may easily obscure the relationship between a remote exposure and a newly discovered tumor. Individual cancers are discussed in organ-specific chapters; see also Chapter 7.

Acute Radiation Syndrome

Acute radiation syndrome is caused by brief but heavy exposure of all or part of the body to ionizing radiation. The radiation disrupts chemical bonds, which causes molecular excitation and free radical formation. Highly reactive free radicals react with other essential molecules such as nucleic acids and enzymes and this in turn disrupts cellular function. The clinical presentation and severity of illness are determined by the dosage, body distribution, and duration of exposure. Tissues with the most rapid cellular turnover are the most radiosensitive and include reproductive, hematopoietic, and gastrointestinal tissues (Cohen, 1990b). For further discussion, see Radiation Injuries, Chapter 4.

Occupational Infections

Occupational infections are diseases caused by work-associated exposure to microbial agents, including bacteria, viruses, fungi, and protozoa. What distinguishes an infection as occupational is that some aspect of the work involves contact with a biologically active organism. Occupational infection can occur following contact with infected persons, as in the case of health care workers; with infected animal or human tissue, secretions, or excretions, as in laboratory workers; with asymptomatic or unknown contagious humans, as happens during business travel; or with infected animals, as in agriculture (e.g., brucellosis) (Cohen, 1990b). Tuberculosis, hepatitis B, and AIDS are the most likely occupational infections encountered in a therapy practice. See further discussion of these elsewhere in this book.

---

[7] Carpal tunnel syndrome is also correlated to medical conditions such as thyroid problems, arthritis, liver disease, multiple myeloma, and diabetes, as well as to other musculoskeletal disorders such as thoracic outlet syndrome and cervical spine disorders. See also Compression/Entrapment Syndromes, Chapter 34.

Occupational Skin Disorders *(Nethercott, 1990)*

Work-related dermatoses account for 20% of all cases of occupational disease in the United States and contact dermatitis (acute, chronic or allergic) is the most common of those skin disorders. Dermatoses are more prevalent in some states such as California and Florida; contact dermatitis from plants is common among agricultural workers. Other agents include irritating chemicals such as solvents, cutting oils, detergents, alkalis, and acids.

Other types of occupational skin disorders include contact urticaria, psoriasis, vitiligo (areas of depigmentation), chloracne (Fig. 3–1), actinic skin damage known as "farmer's skin" or "sailor's skin," cutaneous malignancy, and cutaneous infections. For further discussion of specific skin disorders, see Chapter 8.

Latex Rubber Allergy

In the health care industry, dentists, surgeons, nurses, and therapists have been increasingly affected by sensitivity to rubber gloves (Fig. 3–2). As many as 12% of health care providers have developed latex hypersensitivity reactions compared with less than 1% in the general population (Gritter, 1995). The recent epidemic of latex allergy may be attributed to the increased use of natural rubber latex gloves in response to universal precautions required for human immunodeficiency virus. The increased demand for gloves may have temporarily changed manufacturing procedures, resulting in a poor-quality, highly allergenic product (Sussman and Beezhold, 1995).

This occupational sensitivity to rubber (latex proteins and in some cases, the associated cornstarch glove powder) has resulted in mild to severe allergic contact dermatitis. Symptoms range from mild contact dermatitis, hives, and rhinitis to bronchospasm and severe anaphylactic reactions. The affected person may experience shortness of breath, facial flushing, wheezing, urticaria (hives), or skin rash, which can spread from the hands, up the arms, to the face, and swelling of the lips, eyes, ears, and larynx (laryngeal edema can prevent the person from speaking).

Once sensitized, some health care workers are at risk for severe systemic allergic reactions which can be fatal in a small number of cases (Scarbeck, 1993). Several potential sources of powder-free, natural hypoallergenic latex[8] may be tolerated by latex-sensitive persons (Carey et al., 1995) but no single replacement glove has been found for all people affected. Cotton liners or barrier creams can be effective treatments. A latex-free environment, described as one in which there is no latex glove use by any personnel and no direct client contact with latex devices (catheters, condoms, adhesives, tourniquets, and anesthetic equipment), may be required for complete recovery (AAAI, 1993). Nonlatex gloves (vinyl or synthetic latex such as neoprene) have equal barrier protection compared with latex gloves but the vinyl appears to tear more easily and is therefore substantially more permeable (Korniewicz et al., 1990; DeGroot-Kosolcharoen and Jones, 1989).

Latex-induced rhinitis has also been reported as a new form of occupational rhinitis and occupational asthma secondary to airborne latex allergens in operating rooms, intensive care units, and dental suites. The elimination of wearing latex gloves has not been successful as latex allergens are airborne (Moneret-Vautrin et al., 1994).

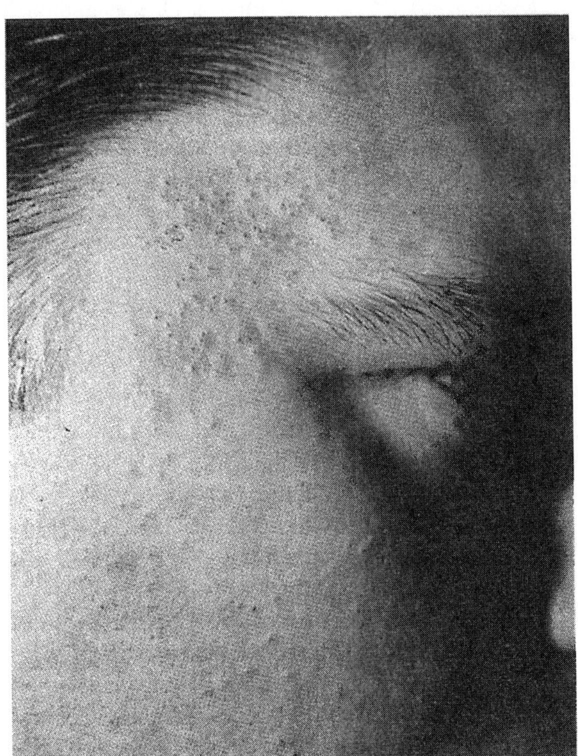

Figure 3–1. Chloracne. (*From Raffle PAB, Adams PH: Hunter's Diseases of Occupations, ed 8. London, Edward Arnold, 1994, p 708.*)

Special Implications for the Therapist **3–2**

LATEX RUBBER ALLERGY

Should anyone in the rehabilitation or therapy department develop symptoms in association with the use of latex gloves, emergency medical care may be required. In a hospital setting, a physician can be paged immediately; other locations may require an emergency medical team (911 or ambulance service). Check with the facility for incident report requirements. For the health care worker with a known sensitivity, a medical-alert bracelet should be worn and the individual should have autoinjectable epinephrine (EpiPen) for use if another reaction occurs. Further episodes may be avoided using nonlatex medical products (see previous discussion).

Military-related Diseases

Seven diseases (asthma, laryngitis, chronic bronchitis, emphysema, and three eye ailments) have been identified by the Department of Veterans Affairs for compensation as a result of exposure to toxic chemicals during World War II (PT Bull, 1993a). Survivors of the Vietnam War who have been exposed to the defoliant Agent Orange are at risk for

[8] Nonallergenic natural rubber latex is not currently available.

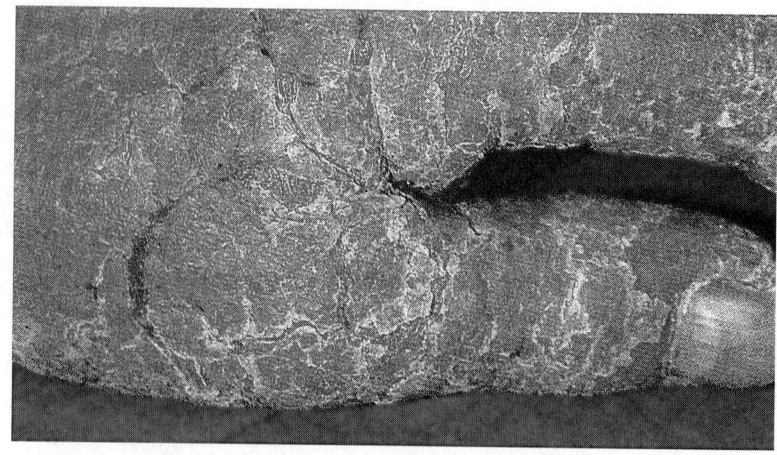

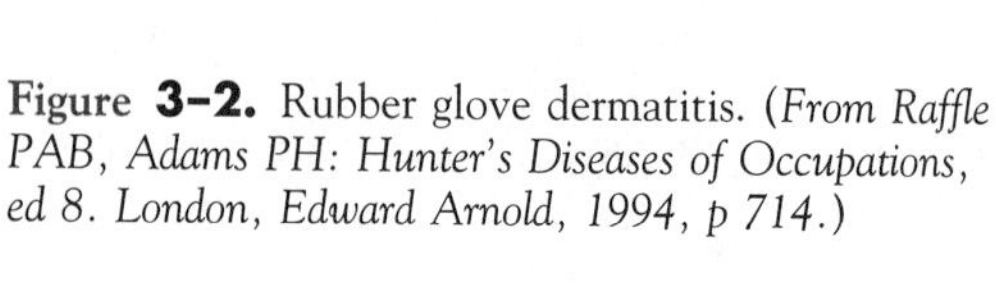

Figure 3–2. Rubber glove dermatitis. (*From Raffle PAB, Adams PH: Hunter's Diseases of Occupations, ed 8. London, Edward Arnold, 1994, p 714.*)

the development of soft tissue sarcoma, non-Hodgkin's lymphoma, Hodgkin's disease, and a skin-blistering disease, chloracne (Dalager et al., 1991; PT Bull, 1993b; Uzych, 1991). More recently a group of symptoms presented by participants in the Gulf War have been identified.

The Gulf War Syndrome

Whether or not there is an actual "Gulf War syndrome" (GWS) remains a hotly debated topic. According to the Centers for Disease Control and Prevention (CDC), Americans who served in the Persian Gulf War are significantly more likely than others to suffer from more than a dozen disorders known generically as Gulf War syndrome. The CDC does not term this phenomenon the GWS, but reports that people who went to the Persian Gulf are experiencing problems (referred to as Persian Gulf illness or PGI) that those who did not go are not experiencing. On the other hand, the Department of Defense does not support the existence of this illness, reporting only that the results of medical examinations of 10,000 veterans and family members affected revealed multiple illnesses with overlapping symptoms (Joseph, 1995).

Incidence, Etiology, and Clinical Manifestations

Of the 700,000 troops dispatched to the Persian Gulf between August 1990 and June 1991, as of January 1997, more than 84,000 veterans have filed with the federal registry reports of symptoms that include (in order of frequency) fatigue, skin rash, headache, muscle and joint pain, memory loss, shortness of breath, sleep disturbances, diarrhea and other gastrointestinal symptoms, and depression. CDC data show that the GWS affects 27% of veterans compared to 2% of nonveterans. Fatigue has been reported to affect 54% of Gulf War veterans compared with 16% of non–Gulf War veterans.

No known cause has been proved[9] but possible causes include chemical or biologic weapons used on allied forces, insecticides, Kuwaiti oil well fires, parasites, or pills protecting against nerve gas, and inoculations against petrochemical exposure administered by the military that had unexpected side effects or reacted with one another to create adverse symptoms. In 1993, the Birmingham, Alabama VA Center was designated as a national pilot center to study the possible neurologic effects of exposure to environmental agents in the Persian Gulf. Other designated environmental hazards research centers are located in Boston; East Orange, NJ; and Portland, Oregon. Currently, more than 30 studies are underway to examine the various explanations for this phenomenon.

[9] The U.S. Department of Defense recently announced that a greater number of PGW veterans than originally estimated were potentially exposed to nerve agents from the demolition of Iraqi chemical weapons in 1991. For more information, contact the VA Persian Gulf Information Helpline at 800-PGW-VETS. First-hand incidents can be reported to the Gulf War Incident-Reporting Hotline at 800-472-6719.

Medical Management

No specific treatment beyond symptomatic measures exists for the Gulf War Illnesses. One program at the Walter Reed Army Medical Center in Washington, D.C. is approaching PGI using a chronic pain–work hardening protocol toward improved function and increased tolerance for work and activity. The long-term prognosis is unknown, but according to an as yet unpublished Pentagon study, only a small percentage of those persons affected by PGI are seriously ill. Eighty-one percent of those participating in the survey have missed no work in the previous 3 months and only 7% missed a week or more in that period.

References

AAAI (American Academy of Allergy and Immunology): Committee report. J Allergy Clin Immunol 92:16–18, 1993.

Alfred EN: Short-term effects of carbon monoxide exposure on the exercise performance of subjects with coronary artery disease. N Engl J Med 321:1426, 1989.

Bauer RL, Watson WA: Clinical toxicology. *In* Stein JH (ed): Internal Medicine, ed 4. St Louis, Mosby–Year Book, 1994, pp 2789–2799.

Brooks SM: Man-made mineral fibers. *In* Brooks SM, Gochfeld M, Herzstein J, et al: Environmental Medicine. St Louis, Mosby–Year Book, 1995, pp 455–461.

Brown JP, Jackson RJ: Water pollution. *In* Brooks SM, Gochfeld M, Herzstein J, et al: Environmental Medicine. St Louis, Mosby–Year Book, 1995, pp 479–487.

Bullock L: High-altitude and aerospace medicine. *In* Brooks SM, Gochfeld M, Herzstein J, et al: Environmental Medicine. St Louis, Mosby–Year Book, 1995, pp 576–591.

Bureau of Labor Statistics: Workplace Injuries and Illnesses in 1995. US Department of Labor News Release No. 97-76. Washington, DC, 1997.

Burger J: Ionizing radiation. *In* Brooks SM, Gochfeld M, Herzstein J, et al: Environmental Medicine. St Louis, Mosby–Year Book, 1995, pp 524–533.

Burger J, Gochfeld M: Nonionizing radiation. *In* Brooks SM, Gochfeld M,

Herzstein J, et al: Environmental Medicine. St Louis, Mosby–Year Book, 1995, pp 542–553.
Carey AB, Cornish K, Schrank P: Cross-reactivity of alternate plant sources of latex in subjects with systemic IgE-mediated sensitivity to *Hevea brasiliensis* latex. Ann Allergy Asthma Immunol 74:317–320, 1995.
Cohen R: Injuries due to physical hazards. *In* LaDou J (ed): Occupational Medicine. Norwalk, Conn, Appleton & Lange, 1990a, pp 106–131.
Cohen R: Occupational infections. *In* LaDou J (ed): Occupational Medicine. Norwalk, Conn, Appleton & Lange, 1990b, 170–181.
Cooper KH: Antioxidant Revolution. Nashville, Thomas Nelson, 1994.
Cullen MR, Rosenstock L, Brooks SM: Clinical approach and establishing a diagnosis of an environmental medical disorder. *In* Brooks SM, Gochfeld M, Herzstein J, et al: Environmental Medicine. St Louis, Mosby–Year Book, 1995, pp 217–231.
Dalager, NA, Kang HK, Burt VL, Weatherbee L: Non-Hodgkin's lymphoma among Vietnam veterans. J Occup Environ Med 33:774–779, 1991.
DeGroot-Kosolcharoen J, Jones JM: Permeability of latex and vinyl gloves to water and blood. Am J Infect Control 17:196–201, 1989.
Ellis J: Incidence of carpal tunnel syndrome is rising. PT Bull 10:6–9, October 6, 1995.
EPA (Environmental Protection Agency): Categories of released chemicals reported to the toxic release inventory, 1993.
Fernandez-Caldas E, Fox RW, Richards IS, et al: Indoor air pollution. *In* Brooks SM, Gochfeld M, Herzstein J, et al: Environmental Medicine. St Louis, Mosby–Year Book, 1995, pp 419–437.
Fischman ML, Cadman EC, Desmond S: Occupational cancer. *In* LaDou J (ed): Occupational Medicine. Norwalk, Conn, Appleton & Lange, 1990, pp 182–208.
Gochfeld M: Chemical agents. *In* Brooks SM, Gochfeld M, Herzstein J, et al: Environmental Medicine. St Louis, Mosby–Year Book, 1995a, pp 592–614.
Gochfeld M: Fire and pyrolysis products. *In* Brooks SM, Gochfeld M, Herzstein J, et al: Environmental Medicine. St Louis, Mosby–Year Book, 1995b, pp 470–478.
Gochfeld M: Overview of environmental medicine. *In* Brooks SM, Gochfeld M, Herzstein J, et al: Environmental Medicine. St Louis, Mosby–Year Book, 1995c, pp 3–8.
Gochfeld M: Soil: Sources, dynamics, and routes of exposure. *In* Brooks SM, Gochfeld M, Herzstein J, et al: Environmental Medicine. St Louis, Mosby–Year Book, 1995d, pp 515–523.
Gold DR: Indoor air pollution. Clin Chest Med 13:215–229, 1992.
Gritter M: Latex hypersensitivity. Nursing95 25(5):33, 1995.
Grover RF, Weil JV, Reeves JT: Cardiovascular adaptation to exercise at high altitude. Exerc Sport Sci Rev 14:269, 1986.
Hazleman BL: Repeated movements and repeated trauma. *In* Raffle PAB, Adams PH, Baxter PJ (eds): Hunter's Diseases of Occupations, ed 8. London, Edward Arnold, 1994, pp 515–529.
Herman GD: Myonecrosis in carbon monoxide poisoning. Vet Hum Toxicol 20:28, 1988.
Hulshof C, van Zanten B: Whole-body vibration and low-back pain: A review of epidemiologic studies. Int Arch Occup Environ Health 59:205, 1987.
Hultgren HN: High-altitude medical problems. *In* Rubenstein E, Federman DD (eds): Scientific American Medicine. New York, Scientific American, 1992.
Joseph S: No unique illness afflicts Gulf veterans. News release. Washington D.C., August 2, 1995.
Khalil TM, Abdel-Moty E, Steele-Rosomoff R, Rosomoff HL: The role of ergonomics in the prevention and treatment of myofascial pain. *In* Rachlin ES: Myofascial pain and fibromyalgia: Trigger point management. St Louis, Mosby–Year Book, 1994, pp 487–523.
Kleinman MT: Effects of short-term exposure to carbon monoxide in subjects with coronary artery disease. Arch Environ Health 44:361, 1989.
Klotz JB: Radon. *In* Brooks SM, Gochfeld M, Herzstein J, et al: Environmental Medicine. St Louis, Mosby–Year Book, 1995, pp 534–541.
Koren H: Environment and humans. *In* Koren H (ed): Handbook of Environmental Health and Safety: Principles and Practices. Chelsea, Mich, Lewis, 1991.
Korniewicz DM, Laughton BE, Cyr WH, et al: Leakage of virus through used vinyl and latex examination gloves. J Clin Microbiol 28:787–789, 1990.
Kosnik W: Effects of a laser-induced temporary scotoma on target acquisition performance. Hum Factors 37:356–370, 1995.
LaDou J (ed): Occupational Medicine. Norwalk, Conn, Appleton & Lange, 1990.
Landrigan PJ, Kazemi H: The third wave of asbestos disease: Exposure to asbestos in the workplace. Ann N Y Acad Sci 643:1, 1991.
Lechowich RV: Current concerns in food safety. *In* Finley JW, Robinson SF, Armstrong DJ (eds): Food Safety Assessment. Washington, DC, American Chemical Society, 1992.
Matheson LN: Work hardening for patients with back pain. J Musculoskel Med 10:53–63, 1993.
Miller CS, Bell IR, Schwartz, GE: An olfactory-limbic model of multiple chemical sensibility syndrome: Possible relationship to kindling and affective spectrum disorders. Soc Bio Psychiatry 32:218–242, 1992.
Moneret-Vautrin DA, Kohler DJC, Stringini R, et al: Occupational rhinitis and asthma to latex. Rhinology 32:198–202, 1994.
Morgan BJ: The patient with coronary heart disease at altitude: Observations during acute exposure to 3100 meters. J Wilderness Med 1:147, 1990.
Muhlbach L, Bocker M, Prussog A: Telepresence in videocommunications: A study on stereoscopy and individual eye contact. Hum Factors 37:290–295, 1995.
Nethercott JR: Occupational skin disorders. *In* LaDou J (ed): Occupational Medicine. Norwalk, Conn, Appleton & Lange, 1990, pp 209–220.
Pearlstein MF: Occupational lung disease. *In* Frownfelter DL: Chest Physical Therapy and Pulmonary Rehabilitation, ed 2. Chicago, Mosby–Year Book, 1987, pp 128–144.
Pollack ES, Keimig DG (eds): National Research Council, Panel on Occupational Safety and Health Statistics: Counting Injuries and Illnesses in the Workplace: Proposals for a Better System. Washington, DC, National Academy Press, 1987.
PT Bull: VA may see more ailments caused by toxins. January 20, 1993a.
PT Bull: Two diseases added to list attributed to Agent Orange. August 11, 1993b.
PT Magazine: OSHA update from the editors. 3(11):65, 1995.
Rubin E, Farber JL: Environmental and nutritional pathology. *In* Rubin E, Farber JL (eds): Pathology, ed 2. Philadelphia, JB Lippincott, 1994a, pp 289–335.
Rubin E, Farber JL: The respiratory system. *In* Rubin E, Farber JL (eds): Pathology, ed 2. Philadelphia, JB Lippincott, 1994b, pp 556–617.
Scarbeck K: Latex: Is it safe? Acad Gen Dentistry 21:2–6, 1993.
Schoenberg JB: Case-control study of residential radon and lung cancer among New Jersey women. Cancer Res 50:6520, 1990.
Scullica L, Rechichi C, De Moja CA: Protective filters in the prevention of asthenopia at a video display terminal. Percept Mot Skills 80:299–303, 1995.
Shank FR, Carson KL: What is safe food? *In* Finley JW, Robinson SF, Armstrong DJ (eds): Food Safety Assessment. Washington, DC, American Chemical Society, 1992.
Sheedy JE: Focus on computer-generated eye problems. Occup Health Saf 64:46–60, 1995.
Sheps DS: Lack of effect of low levels of carboxyhemoglobin on cardiovascular function in patients with ischemic heart disease. Arch Environ Health 42:108, 1987.
Sheps DS: Production of arrhythmias by elevated carboxyhemoglobin in patients with coronary artery disease. Ann Intern Med 113:343, 1990.
So YT: Nervous system. *In* Brooks SM, Gochfeld M, Herzstein J, et al: Environmental Medicine. St Louis, Mosby–Year Book, 1995, pp 318–325.
Stauffer JL: Pulmonary diseases. *In* Tierney LM, McPhee SJ, Papadakis MA (eds): Current Medical Diagnosis and Treatment, ed 33. Norwalk, Conn, Appleton & Lange, 1994, pp 207–279.
Sussman GL, Beezhold DH: Allergy to latex rubber. Ann Intern Med 122:43–46, 1995.
Utell MJ, Samet JM: Air pollution in the outdoor environment. *In* Brooks SM, Gochfeld M, Herzstein J, et al: Environmental Medicine. St Louis, Mosby–Year Book, 1995, pp 462–469.
Uzych L: Agent Orange, the Vietnam war, and lasting health effects. Environ Health Perspect 95:211, 1991.
Washburn AE, Harlow DW, Horn S: United States firefighter deaths in the line of duty during 1979: Natl Fire Protection Assoc Fire Command 47:30, 1980.
Welch W: How cells respond to stress. Sci Am 268(5):56–64, 1993.
Wilder, DG, Woodworth BB, Frymoyer JW: Vibration and the human spine. Spine 7:243, 1982.

SECTION 1

chapter 4

Problems Affecting Multiple Systems

Catherine C. Goodman and
Teresa E. Kelly Snyder

TERMINOLOGY ASSOCIATED WITH FLUID AND ELECTROLYTE IMBALANCE

(O'Toole, 1992)

Acidemia Abnormal acidity of the blood; decreased pH of the blood.

Acidosis Pathologic condition resulting from accumulation of acid or depletion of the alkaline reserve (bicarbonate content) in the blood and body tissues; characterized by an increase in hydrogen ion concentration (decrease in pH); the opposite of alkalosis.

Alkalemia Abnormal alkalinity or increased pH of the blood.

Alkalosis Pathologic condition resulting from accumulation of base or from loss of acid without comparable loss of base in the body fluids; characterized by decrease in hydrogen ion concentration (increase in pH); the opposite of acidosis.

Dehydration Removal or loss of water from the body or a tissue; water deficit; severe dehydration may lead to acidosis, accumulation of waste products in the body (uremia), and fatal shock.

Diuretic An agent that promotes increased urine excretion.

Electrolyte A substance that develops an electrical charge when dissolved in water (e.g., sodium, potassium, calcium, chloride, and bicarbonate); the terms *serum electrolytes* and *plasma electrolytes* are used interchangeably, even though serum is the portion of plasma left after clotting factors and blood cells have been removed.

Extracellular fluid Fluid outside the cells.

Fluid volume deficit (FVD) The result of water and electrolyte loss usually due to loss of body fluids (e.g., losses of gastrointestinal secretions, excessive urine output, increased metabolism as a result of fever, or severe perspiration, especially in the absence of fluid replacement).

Hypercalcemia Excess of calcium in the blood.

Hyperkalemia Above-normal serum potassium concentration.

Hypernatremia Greater than normal serum sodium level (>145 mEq/L) indicative of water loss exceeding sodium loss.

Hypocalcemia Diminished calcium in the blood.

Hypokalemia Below normal potassium concentration in the blood.

Hyponatremia Below normal serum sodium level (<135 mEq/L); salt depletion.

Hypovolemia Abnormally decreased volume of circulating fluid (plasma) in the body.

Interstitial fluid The extracellular fluid bathing most tissues, excluding the fluid within the lymph and blood vessels.

Intracellular fluid Fluid within a cell or cells.

Intravascular fluid Fluid within the blood vessels.

Membrane potential The electrical tension or pressure that exists on two sides of a membrane or across a cell wall.

Osmolality The measure of dissolved particles per unit of solution; serum osmolality is the measure of the number of dissolved particles per unit of water in serum; a measurement of the hydration status within the cells.

SIADH Syndrome of inappropriate antidiuretic hormone secretion; in conditions causing SIADH, either too much antidiuretic hormone (ADH) is released or the renal response to ADH is intensified.

Serum Blood serum; the clear, liquid portion of the plasma that remains after the blood cells have been separated out.

Many conditions and diseases seen in the rehabilitation setting (Box 4–1) can affect multiple organs or systems. In particular, such conditions can affect acid-base and/or fluid and electrolyte balance. Additionally, a single disease or pathologic condition can predispose a person to associated secondary illnesses. For example, specific types of pneumonia can be associated with seizures, alcoholism, diabetes mellitus, sickle cell disease, and chronic lung and renal disease. The consequences of immunodeficiency, such as occurs with acquired immunodeficiency syndrome (AIDS), predisposes the person to many kinds of opportunistic infections. Although medical conditions encountered in the clinic or home health-care setting are discussed individually in the appropriate chapter, it is important for the health-care provider to understand the systemic as well as the local effects of such disorders.

The scope of this test does not allow for an in-depth discussion of each condition or disease and its related multiple

BOX **4-1**
Conditions that Affect Multiple Systems

- Autoimmune disorders
- Burns
- Cancer
- Cystic fibrosis
- Connective tissue diseases
  - Rheumatoid arthritis
  - Progressive systemic sclerosis (scleroderma)
  - Polymyositis
  - Sjögren's syndrome
  - Systemic lupus erythematosus
  - Polyarteritis nodosa
- Diabetes
- Environmental and occupational diseases
- Genetic diseases
- Malnutrition or other nutritional imbalance
- Metabolic disorders
- Multiple organ dysfunction syndrome (MODS)
- Sarcoidosis
- Shock
- Trauma
- Tuberculosis
- Vasculitis

systemic effects. This chapter provides a brief listing of the systemic effects of commonly encountered pathologic conditions and a basic presentation of acid-base and fluid and electrolyte imbalances.

SYSTEMIC EFFECTS OF PATHOLOGY

(Harruff, 1994)

Systemic Effects of Acute Inflammation

Acute inflammation can be described as the initial response of tissue to injury, particularly bacterial infections and necrosis, involving vascular and cellular responses. Local signs of inflammation (e.g., redness, warmth, swelling, pain, and loss of function) are commonly observed in the therapy setting. Local inflammation can lead to abscesses, when excessive suppuration (formation of pus) occurs; chronic inflammation; and the formation of adhesions. Systemic effects of acute inflammation include fever, tachycardia, and a hypermetabolic state. These effects produce characteristic changes in the blood, such as elevated serum protein levels (C-reactive protein, serum amyloid A, complement, and coagulation factors) and an elevated white blood count (leukocytosis).

Systemic Effects of Chronic Inflammation

Chronic inflammation is the result of persistent injury, repeated episodes of acute inflammation, infection, cell-mediated immune responses, and foreign body reactions. It is the tissue response to injury that is characterized by accumulation of lymphocytes, plasma cells, and macrophages (mononuclear inflammatory cells) and production of fibrous connective tissue (fibrosis).[1] The associated fibrosis causes progressive tissue damage and loss of function. Systemic effects of chronic inflammation may include low-grade fever, malaise, weight loss, anemia, fatigue, leukocytosis, and lymphocytosis (caused by viral infection). Inflammatory activity can be detected by the erythrocyte sedimentation rate (ESR). In general, as the disease improves, the ESR decreases.

Systemic Factors Influencing Healing

In addition to local factors that affect healing (e.g., infection, blood supply, extent of necrosis, presence of foreign bodies, protection from further trauma or movement), a variety of systemic factors influence healing as well. Systemic factors may include general nutritional status (especially protein and vitamin C); psychological well-being; presence of cardiovascular disease, cancer, hematologic disorders (e.g., neutropenia) systemic infections, and diabetes mellitus; and whether the person is undergoing corticosteroid or immunosuppressive therapy.

Healing in specific organs varies according to the underlying cause and site of the injury. For example, myocardial infarctions heal exclusively by scarring, and the heart is permanently weakened. A cerebrovascular accident (CVA or stroke) may cause permanent disability, and healing occurs by the formation of nervous tissue (e.g., astrocytes, oligodendrocytes, and microglia) rather than by collagenous scar formation; this process is called *gliosis*.

In other organs, effective tissue regeneration depends primarily on the site of injury. Necrosis of only parenchymal (functional visceral) cells with retention of the existing stroma (framework or structural tissue) may permit regeneration and restoration of normal anatomy, whereas necrosis that involves the mesenchymal framework (connective tissue including blood and blood vessels) usually results in scar formation (e.g., as in hepatic cirrhosis).

Consequences of Immunodeficiency

Immunodeficiency diseases are caused by congenital (primary) or acquired (secondary) failure of one or more functions of the immune system, predisposing the affected individual to infections that a noncompromised immune system could easily resist. The therapist is more likely to encounter individuals with acquired (rather than congenital) immunodeficiency from nonspecific causes, such as occur with viral and other infections, malnutrition, alcoholism, aging, autoimmune diseases, diabetes mellitus, cancer, chronic diseases, steroid therapy, cancer chemotherapy and radiation therapy.

Predisposition to opportunistic infections, resulting in clinical manifestations of those infections, is the primary consequence of immunodeficiency. Selective B-cell deficiencies predispose an individual to bacterial infections. T-cell deficiencies predispose to viral and fungal infections. Combined deficiencies (including AIDS) are particularly severe because they predispose to many kinds of viral, bacterial, and fungal infections.

Systemic Effects of Neoplasm *(Hobson and Webster, 1987)*

Malignant tumors, by their destructive nature and uncontrolled growth patterns, produce many local and systemic effects. Locally, the rapid growth of the tumor encroaches on healthy tissue, causing destruction, necrosis, ulceration, and hemorrhage. Pain may or may not occur, depending on how

[1] Fibroblasts and small blood vessels, along with collagen fibers synthesized by fibroblasts, constitute fibrosis. Grossly, fibrotic tissue is light gray and has a dense, firm texture that causes contraction of the normal tissue (Harruff, 1994).

close tumor cells, swelling, or hemorrhage occurs to the nerve cells. This process also occurs locally at metastatic sites. Pain may occur as a late symptom as a result of infiltration, compression, or destruction of nerve tissue. Secondary infections frequently occur as a result of the host's decreased immunity and can lead to death.

The person with a malignant neoplasm frequently presents with systemic symptoms such as gradual or rapid weight loss, muscular weakness, anorexia, anemia, and coagulation disorders (granulocyte and platelet abnormalities). Continued spread of the cancer may lead to gastrointestinal, pulmonary, or vascular obstruction. Other vital organs may be affected; in the brain increased intracranial pressure by tumor cells can cause partial paralysis and eventual coma. Hemorrhage caused by direct invasion or necrosis in any body part leads to further anemia or even death if the necrosis is severe.

Advanced cancers produce cachexia (wasting) as a result of tissue destruction and the body's nutrients being used by the malignant cells for further growth. Multiple mechanisms may be involved in this process, including release of tumor necrosis factor (also called cachectin). Paraneoplastic syndromes (see Chapter 7) are produced by hormonal mechanisms rather than by direct tumor invasion. For example, hypercalcemia can be caused in cases of lung cancer by the secretion of a peptide with parathyroid hormone, and polycythemia can be caused by the secretion of erythropoietin by renal cell carcinoma. Neuromuscular disorders such as Eaton-Lambert syndrome, polymyositis/dermatomyositis, and hypertrophic pulmonary osteoarthropathy are other examples of paraneoplastic syndromes that can occur as a systemic effect of neoplasm (see Tables 7–6 and 7–7).

ADVERSE DRUG REACTIONS *(Harruff, 1994; Berkow and Fletcher, 1992)*

Definition and Overview. Adverse drug reactions (ADRs) are defined as harmful effects produced by medications or prescription drugs. The term usually excludes nontherapeutic overdosage, such as accidental exposure or attempted suicide. Side effects are usually defined as predictable pharmacologic effects that occur within therapeutic dose ranges and are undesirable in the given therapeutic situation. Overdosage toxicity is the predictable toxic effect that occurs with dosages in excess of the therapeutic range for a particular person.

ADRs are classified as *mild* (no antidote, therapy, or prolongation of hospitalization necessary); *moderate* (change in drug therapy required), although not necessarily a cessation of therapy; may prolong hospitalization or require special treatment); *severe* (potentially life-threatening, requires discontinuation of the drug and specific treatment of the adverse reaction); and *lethal* (directly or indirectly leads to the death of the person).

Incidence, Risk Factors, and Etiology. Although it is recognized that ADRs are not uncommon, the exact incidence among ambulatory or outpatient clients remains undetermined. Specific studies have been conducted to determine the rate of ADR-related admissions to hospitals or the rate of ADRs associated with immunizations (Bates et al., 1993; Duclos et al., 1993; Prevots et al., 1994). Up to 5% of hospitalized clients experience an ADR, but this figure is considered conservative (Larson, 1993); 2% to 12% of those may be fatal reactions. Risk factors include age, gender, race (occurring most frequently in elderly white women), concomitant alcohol consumption, new drugs, number of drugs, dosage, duration of treatment, noncompliance (e.g., unintentional repeated dosage), and presence of underlying conditions (e.g., hepatic or renal insufficiency) (Abrams et al., 1995).

Halothane (anesthesia)-induced hepatic necrosis and anaphylactic reaction to penicillin are among the most common fatal reactions. The drugs most commonly associated with ADRs in the elderly can be categorized according to the site of care (Table 4–1). The risk of fatal reaction is increased in elderly persons taking multiple drugs.

ADRs may be dose-related (predictable drug injury) or non–dose-related (unpredictable or idiosyncratic drug injury). The causes and pathophysiologic mechanisms by which these two types of ADRs occur are listed in Table 4–2. Cardiac or pulmonary toxicity may occur as a result of the irradiation and immunosuppressive drugs given to prepare recipients for organ transplantation or for any type of cancer. Some of the

TABLE 4-1 Relationship Between Adverse Drug Reactions (ADRs) and Site of Care for the Elderly

Most common causes of hospital-acquired ADRs	Most common causes of nursing home–acquired ADRs
Digoxin	Tranquilizers (phenothiazines)
Aminoglycoside antibiotic	Sedative-hypnotics
Anticoagulants (heparin and warfarin)	Warfarin (Coumadin)
	Antacids
Insulin overdose	Oral hypoglycemics
Steroid-induced GI bleeding	Digoxin
Aspirin	Aspirin

From Abrams WR, Berkow R (eds): The Merck Manual of Geriatrics. Rahway, NJ, Merck & Co, 1990, p 192.

TABLE 4-2 Causes of Adverse Drug Reactions

Dose-Related Effects	Non–Dose-Related Effects
Drug toxicity (overdose)	Immunologic reactions
Variations in pharmaceutical preparations	Immediate hypersensitivity or anaphylaxis
Genetic variations in drug metabolism	Cytotoxic reactions
Preexisting liver disease	Immune complex reactions
Renal failure	Delayed hypersensitivity
Heart failure	Idiosyncratic reactions (individual susceptibility; nonimmunologic)
Thyroid disease	
Drug interactions	
Antineoplastic drugs (bone marrow and immune system suppression)	

Adapted from Harruff RC: Pathology Facts. Philadelphia, JB Lippincott, 1994, p 47.

more common specific target organs and effects are listed in Table 4–3.

Clinical Manifestations. Rashes, fever, and jaundice are common signs of drug overdosage toxicity. Elderly people may develop ADRs that are clearly different from those seen in younger persons (Box 4–2). Early symptoms of salicylate intoxication include tinnitus, deafness, disequilibrium, drowsiness, and a moderate delirium (Andreoli et al., 1993). Digitalis toxicity is a life-threatening condition that may present with systemic or cardiac manifestations (see Table 10–9). (See also Chemotherapy later in this chapter.)

Medical Management. Differentiating an ADR from underlying disease requires a thorough history, especially when a symptom appears 1 to 2 months after a medication regimen has been started. Monitoring blood cell counts and levels of liver enzymes, electrolytes, blood urea nitrogen (BUN), and creatinine is indicated for certain drugs. Digoxin and other cardiotropic drugs cause arrhythmias that require electrocardiographic (ECG) monitoring. With dose-related ADRs, dose modification is usually all that is required, whereas with non–dose-related ADRs, the drug therapy is usually stopped and re-exposure avoided.

Special Implications for the Therapist **4–1**

EXERCISE AND DRUGS

Exercise can produce dramatic changes in the way drugs are absorbed, distributed, localized, transformed, and excreted in the body (pharmacokinetics). The magnitude of these changes is dependent on the characteristics of each drug (e.g., route of administration, chemical properties) as well as exercise-related factors (e.g., exercise intensity, mode, and duration). A single exercise session can cause sudden changes in pharmacokinetics that may have an immediate impact on people who exercise during therapy. Exercise training can also produce changes in pharmacokinetics, but these tend to occur over a longer period and to cause a slower and fairly predictable change in a person's response to certain medications. A detailed description of the effects of exercise, physical agents, and manual techniques on drug bioavailability is available (Ciccone, 1995; Dossing, 1985).

For the most part, drugs administered locally by transdermal techniques or by subcutaneous or intramuscular injection are potentially absorbed more with increased systemic bioavailability in the presence of exercise, local heat, or massage of the administration site. In addition, allergic and potentially fatal anaphylactic drug reactions are mediated by exercise. The therapist should always consider the possibility that anyone in therapy taking drugs may have an altered response to those drugs as a result of interventions used in therapy (Ciccone, 1995).

Nonsteroidal Anti-inflammatory Drugs

Nonsteroidal anti-inflammatory drugs (NSAIDs, pronounced *en'-seds*) are a heterogeneous group of drugs that are useful in the symptomatic treatment of inflammation; some appear to be most useful as analgesics. NSAIDs are commonly used postoperatively for discomfort, for painful musculoskeletal conditions, especially among the elderly population and in the treatment of inflammatory rheumatic diseases. These medications may consist of over-the-counter preparations such as acetylsalicylic acid (ASA or aspirin), other salicylates and ibuprofen (e.g., Advil, Motrin, Nuprin, Medipren, Rufen), or prescription drugs (Table 4–4).

The incidence of significant adverse reactions to NSAIDs is low. However, the widespread use of NSAIDs results in a substantial number of people being affected. The more commonly occurring side effects of NSAIDs are stomach upset and stomach pain, possibly leading to ulceration. Most susceptible individuals are persons age 65 years or older, especially those with a history of ulcer disease. Side effects are generally dose-related, but other risk factors include taking NSAIDs longer than 3 months, taking high-dose or multiple NSAIDs, and receiving corticosteroid therapy at the same time (Lichtenstein et al., 1995).

NSAIDs are associated with a wide spectrum of potential clinical toxicities, which occur most often in the gastrointestinal tract, central nervous system, hematopoietic system, kidneys, skin, and liver (Table 4–5). NSAIDs limit the capacity of the kidneys to respond to ischemic stress and decrease renal blood flow and clearance. This results in an accelerated tendency for damage in persons with preexisting renal disease (Perneger et al., 1994). Slow-acting antirheumatic drugs, such as gold and penicillamine, are well known for renal toxic effects, which resolve completely once the drug has been discontinued (Moots and Bacon, 1994).

NSAIDs are all potent platelet inhibitors. Aspirin is the most powerful agent, because its effects on platelets are irreversible; a single dose of aspirin impairs clot formation for 5 to 7 days, and two aspirin can double bleeding time. All NSAIDs, to varying degrees, can cause sodium retention and edema is susceptible persons (Schlegel and Paulus, 1986). NSAIDs may also attenuate (weaken or lessen) the antihypertensive effects of diuretics, β-blockers, angiotensin-converting enzyme inhibitors, and other antagonists.[2]

Special Implications for the Therapist **4–2**

NONSTEROIDAL ANTI-INFLAMMATORY DRUGS (NSAIDs)

The therapist is advised to observe for any side effects or adverse reactions to NSAIDs, especially among elderly clients; those taking high doses of NSAIDs for long periods (e.g., for rheumatoid arthritis); those with peptic ulcer, renal or hepatic disease, congestive heart failure, or hypertension; and those treated with anticoagulants. NSAIDs have antiplatelet effects that can increase the anticoagulant effects of drugs such as warfarin (Coumadin). Easy bruising and bleeding under the skin may be early signs of hemorrhage.

[2] One study (Houston et al., 1995) has shown verapamil, a calcium-channel blocker, to be unaffected by concomitant administration of ibuprofen or naproxen. Verapamil may therefore offer some advantage in maintaining control of blood pressure in persons who regularly take NSAIDs.

TABLE 4-3 EFFECTS OF ADVERSE DRUG REACTIONS

HEART

Cardiomyopathy
- Adriamycin

Myocardial infarction
- Oral contraceptives

LUNG

Alveolitis and interstitial fibrosis
- Nitrofurantoin
- Busulfan
- Bleomycin

Asthma
- Aspirin
- Propranolol

Pneumonia
- Steroids
- Immunosuppressive therapy

GASTROINTESTINAL TRACT

Gingival hyperplasia
- Phenytoin (Dilantin)

Gastritis and peptic ulcer
- Steroids
- Aspirin
- Other NSAIDs

Pseudomembranous colitis
- Broad-spectrum antibiotics

LIVER

Fatty change
- Tetracycline
- Aspirin (pediatrics: Reye's syndrome)

Cholestatic jaundice
- Phenothiazines
- Sex steroids

Hepatitis
- Halothane
- Isoniazid

Massive necrosis
- Halothane
- Acetaminophen (overdose)

Adenoma
- Oral contraceptives

FETAL INJURY

Phocomelia
- Thalidomide

Vaginal carcinoma
- Diethylstilbestrol

Discoloration of teeth
- Tetracycline

Multiple congenital anomalies
- Antineoplastic agents
- Phenytoin
- Sodium warfarin

KIDNEYS

Acute interstitial nephritis
- Methicillin
- Other antibiotics
- Contrast dye for imaging studies

Acute tubular necrosis
- Gentamicin
- Amphotericin B

Chronic interstitial nephritis and papillary necrosis
- Phenacetin
- Acetaminophen
- Aspirin

ENDOCRINE SYSTEM

Adrenocortical atrophy
- Steroids

SKELETAL SYSTEM

Osteoporosis
- Steroids

CENTRAL NERVOUS SYSTEM

Intracranial hemorrhage
- Warfarin; heparin

Cerebral infarction
- Oral contraceptives

Pseudodementia
- Benzodiazepines
- Narcotics

BLOOD AND BONE MARROW

Anemias
- Penicillins
- Cephalosporins
- Methyldopa
- Antimalarial drugs
- Sulfonamides
- Nitrofurantoin
- Methotrexate
- Phenytoin
- Antineoplastic agents

Thrombocytopenia
- Quinidine

SKIN

Urticaria
- Penicillins
- Contrast dye for imaging studies

Erythema nodosum
- Sulfonamides
- Oral contraceptives

EARS, NOSE, THROAT (ENT)

Deafness
- Aminoglycosides

EYES

Asthma induced by β-blockers used for glaucoma

Adapted from Harruff RC: Pathology Facts. Philadelphia, JB Lippincott, 1994, pp 47–48.

BOX 4–2
Common Signs and Symptoms of Adverse Drug Reactions in the Elderly

Restlessness
Falls
Depression
Confusion
Loss of memory
Constipation
Incontinence
Extrapyramidal syndromes (e.g., parkinsonism, tardive dyskinesia)

From Abrams WB, Berkow R (eds): The Merck Manual of Geriatrics. Rahway, NJ, Merck & Co, 1990, p 191.

Ulcer presentation without pain occurs more frequently in elderly people and in those taking NSAIDs. Frequently, people who take prescription NSAIDs also take Advil or aspirin (Boissonnault and Koopmeiners, 1994). Combining these medications increases the risk for development of peptic ulcer disease (Agrawal, 1991). Any client with gastrointestinal symptoms should report these to the physician. Musculoskeletal symptoms may recur after discontinuing NSAIDs, owing to the masking effects of anti-inflammatory agents and the fact that they do not prevent tissue injury and have no major effect on the underlying disease process (Schumacher et al., 1993; Moncur and Williams, 1995). Once the drug is discontinued, painful musculoskeletal symptoms caused by underlying ulcer disease may return.

The influence of NSAIDs on blood pressure in normotensive and hypertensive persons remains questionable, although NSAIDs have a potential to interact with antihypertensive agents. Anyone with coronary artery disease who is taking NSAIDs may also be at slight risk for myocardial ischemia as a result of increased myocardial oxygen demand (e.g., exercise or fever) (Yost and Morgan, 1994). It is important to check blood pressure the first few weeks of therapy and to periodically check thereafter to identify any adverse blood pressure response to the combination of NSAIDs, antihypertensive agents, and increased activity (Gurwitz et al., 1994; Radack and Deck, 1987).

TABLE 4–4 Nonsteroidal Anti-inflammatory Drugs (NSAIDs)*

Generic Name	Brand Name
Diclofenac sodium	Voltaren
Diflunisal	Dolobid
Etodolac	Lodine
Fenoprofen calcium	Nalfon
Flurbiprofen	Ansaid
Ibuprofen	Motrin, Advil, Nuprin, Rufen
Indomethacin	Indocin
Ketoprofen	Orudis
Ketorolac tromethamine	Toradol
Meclofenamate sodium	Meclomen
Mefenamic acid	Ponstel
Nabumetone	Relafen
Naproxen	Naprosyn, Anaprox
Phenylbutazone	Butazolidin
Piroxicam	Feldene
Sulindac	Clinoril
Tolmetin sodium	Tolectin

* The listing of these drugs does not imply endorsement.
Adapted from Babb RR: Gastrointestinal complications of nonsteroidal anti-inflammatory drugs. West J Med 157:444–447, 1992.

TABLE 4–5 Possible Systemic Effects of NSAIDs

Site	Symptom
Gastrointestinal	Indigestion Gastroesophageal reflux Exacerbate peptic ulcers GI hemorrhage and perforation
Hepatic	Cholecystic hepatitis Transaminase elevation
Renal	Interstitial nephritis (rare) Acute renal failure Nephrotic syndrome
Hematologic	Thrombocytopenia Neutropenia Hemolytic anemia Red cell aplasia Prolonged bleeding time
Cardiovascular	Blunt action of cardiovascular drugs (e.g., diuretics, ACE inhibitors, β-blockers) Possible influence on blood pressure Increase fluid retention Isolated lower extremity edema
Cutaneous	Skin reactions and rashes Photosensitivity Urticaria (hives)
Respiratory	Bronchospasm Pneumonitis
Central nervous system	Headache Dizziness Personality change Aseptic meningitis Tinnitus Confusion (elderly treated with indomethacin, naproxen, ibuprofen)

Adapted from Moncur C, Williams HJ: Rheumatoid arthritis: Status of drug therapies. Physical Therapy 75:511–525, 1995.

Immunosuppressants

Immunosuppressants work by decreasing bone marrow production of white blood cells (WBCs) or by selectively inhibiting components of the immune response. Most immunosup-

TABLE 4–6 Major Immunosuppressant Drugs

Drugs	Indications for Use
Corticosteroids (see Box 4–4)	Variety of inflammatory conditions Tissue and organ transplantation Autoimmune diseases
Cyclosporine, tacrolimus (FK-506)	Organ transplantation
Alkylating agent Cyclophosphamide	Lymphoma, leukemia Autoimmune diseases
Antimetabolite Azathioprine (Imuran)	Renal transplantation Pemphigus (skin disease) Neoplasm

Adapted from Long BC, Wright ER: Persons with problems of the immune system. *In* Phipps WJ, Long BC, Woods NF, et al (eds): Medical Surgical Nursing: Concepts and Clinical Practice, ed 4. St. Louis, Mosby–Year Book, 1991, p 2202.

pressants (Table 4–6) are used for organ transplants to prevent rejection, with autoimmune diseases, or for neoplasms. Usually, intensive immunosuppression is required only during the first few weeks after organ transplantation or during rejection crises. Subsequently, the immune system accommodates to the graft and can be maintained with relatively small doses of immunosuppressive drugs, with fewer adverse effects.

Immunosuppression may lead to CNS complications either directly (e.g., cyclosporine-induced CNS lesions)[3] or indirectly (e.g., increased susceptibility to infectious agents, many of which, such as fungi and viruses, involve the CNS). Neurologic effects associated with immunosuppression are listed in Box 4–3. This phenomenon may be reversible on withdrawal of the drug (Singh et al., 1994). Temporary peripheral neuropathy and paresthesias may result in varying combinations and degrees of weakness in the intrinsic muscles of the hands and feet; wristdrop or footdrop may result.

Cyclophosphamide, methotrexate, and azathioprine may be used in the management of severe, active rheumatoid arthritis (RA). The dosage used to treat RA is much lower than the dose used to treat cancer. Likewise, the side effects are fewer than those associated with doses to treat cancer. In cases of inflammatory conditions resistant to corticosteroids, immunosuppressive agents such as cyclophosphamide, chlorambucil, and azathioprine may be used.

The most serious adverse reactions to immunosuppressants are renal failure (e.g., albuminuria, hematuria, proteinuria) and hepatotoxicity. There is a substantial risk of secondary infection, because all immunologic reactions are suppressed; overwhelming infection is the leading cause of death in transplant recipients. Other risks of immunosuppression include reactivation of latent herpes viruses (cytomegalovirus, herpes simplex virus, varicella-zoster virus). The most common side effects are mouth sores (oral *Candida* infection), gum hyperplasia, tremors, and headache (Skidmore-Roth, 1995).

BOX 4–3
CNS Effects of Immunosuppression

Confusion
Psychosis
Cortical blindness
Quadriplegia
Tremors
Seizures
Coma

Special Implications for the Therapist **4–3**

IMMUNOSUPPRESSANTS

Careful handwashing is essential before contact with any client who is immunosuppressed. If the therapist has a known infectious or contagious condition, he or she should *not* work with the immunosuppressed client (see Table 6–6). Both client and therapist can wear a mask in the presence of an upper respiratory infection.

Peripheral neuropathies and subsequent functional impairment can be addressed by the therapist while the client waits for resolution of these side effects. Upper extremity splinting (e.g., cock-up splint for the hand) may be appropriate, or an ankle-foot orthosis to prevent falls and assist in continued and safe ambulation may be provided (Hamburgh, 1992). (See also discussion Cancer and Exercise in Chapter 7.)

Corticosteroids

Naturally occurring corticosteroids are hormones produced by the adrenal cortex; synthetic equivalents can be prescribed as medication. All hormones, whether produced by the adrenal cortex or produced elsewhere, are steroid-based, with similar chemical structures but quite different physiologic effects. Generally they are divided into *glucocorticoids* (cortisol, or hydrocortisone, cortisone, and corticosterone), which mainly affect carbohydrate and protein metabolism and the immune system; *mineralocorticoids* (aldosterone, desoxycorticosterone, corticosterone), which regulate electrolyte and water metabolism; and *androgens* (androsterone and testosterone), which cause masculinization. See Box 4–4 for a list of commonly prescribed synthetic corticosteroids.

Glucocorticoids are used to decrease inflammation in a broad range of local or systemic conditions (Box 4–5), for immunosuppression (see previous section, Immunosuppressants), and as an essential replacement steroid for adrenal insufficiency. Some products may be given for allergy, adrenal insufficiency (e.g., Addison's disease), or cerebral edema. Mineralocorticoids are given for adrenal insufficiency or adrenogenital syndrome. Therapists most often see people who have received prolonged, systemic corticosteroid therapy in the treatment of cancer; organ, tissue, and bone marrow trans-

[3] The pathogenetic mechanism of cyclosporine toxicity is not yet understood. One possible explanation is that cyclosporine enhances platelet aggregation associated with systemic thromboembolic complications (Choudhury et al., 1985; Thomson et al., 1985). Other theories include the role of hypomagnesemia or low serum cholesterol level (low-density lipoprotein functions as a cyclosporine carrier in the plasma). Low cholesterol levels may lead to an increased concentration of cyclosporine within the lipoprotein particles, thereby facilitating the transmembrane transport of cyclosporine through the blood-brain barrier and affecting the CNS (Gurecki et al., 1985).

BOX **4–4**
Commonly Prescribed Corticosteroids

Betamethasone
Cortisone
Desoxycorticosterone
Dexamethasone
Fludrocortisone
Fluprednisolone
Hydrocortisone
Methylprednisolone
Paramethasone
Prednisolone
Prednisone
Triamcinolone

plants; collagen diseases (e.g., systemic lupus erythematosus, scleroderma); rheumatic diseases; and respiratory diseases (e.g., asthma) (Grant, 1994).

Anabolic androgenic steroids (anabolic steroids), synthetic derivatives of the hormone testosterone, are most commonly used to develop secondary male characteristics (androgenic function) and to build muscle tissue (anabolic function). Studies show a high estimated prevalence of anabolic steroid use among adolescent athletes, especially in football, track and field, swimming, and basketball (Buckley, 1988; Potteiger and Stilger, 1994). The use of this type of steroid is illegal and potentially unsafe, unless given under the direction of a licensed physician; most of these drugs cannot even be prescribed legally.

BOX **4–5**
Therapeutic Use of Corticosteroids

Adrenal insufficiency
Alcoholic hepatitis
Allergic disorders
Asthma (oral agents)
Autoimmune disorders
- Rheumatic fever
- Systemic lupus erythematosus

Blood dyscrasia
- Idiopathic thrombocytopenic purpura
- Aplastic anemia
- Acquired hemolytic anemia

Cancer chemotherapy
Chronic obstructive disease (oral agents)
Chronic active hepatitis
Giant cell arteritis
Gout
Hypopituitarism
Immunosuppression
Inflammatory bowel disease
- Regional enteritis (Crohn's disease)
- Ulcerative colitis

Myocarditis
Neoplastic diseases (Hodgkin's disease, lymphoma, acute leukemia)
Nephritis
Pericarditis
Pruritus
Psoriasis
Rheumatic diseases (e.g., rheumatoid arthritis, ankylosing spondylitis)
Sarcoidosis
Shock (e.g., acute adrenal insufficiency)
Systemic lupus erythematosus
Topical dermatologic therapy (skin disorders)

Adverse Effects of Corticosteroids[4]

Corticosteroids are much superior to NSAIDs as effective anti-inflammatory agents, but long-term use to sustain the benefits of these drugs is accompanied by an increased risk of side effects and adrenal suppression (George and Kirwan, 1990). Additionally, their long-term use as an anti-inflammatory agent is not warranted, because steroids neither cure nor alter the natural course of disease. Long-term use of corticosteroids is necessary for adrenal insufficiency.

The *most common* adverse effects of corticosteroids include change in behavior (e.g., insomnia, euphoria), gastrointestinal irritation, metabolic reactions (e.g., hypokalemia, hyperglycemia), and sodium and fluid retention with edema formation (Table 4–7); most adverse reactions are dose-related. The *most serious* side effects of steroid use are the masking of inflammation, gastrointestinal tract ulceration, and development of diabetes mellitus.

Severe adrenal insufficiency may follow sudden withdrawal of the medication. During or after steroid withdrawal, especially in the presence of infection or other types of stress, the person may experience vomiting, orthostatic hypotension, hypoglycemia, restlessness, anorexia, malaise, and fatigue. These symptoms should be reported to the physician. In the rehabilitation setting, it is important to know the effects of corticosteroids on skin and connective tissue, the musculoskeletal system, the gastrointestinal system, the liver, and the cardiovascular system.

Effects on the skin and connective tissue include excessive hair growth (hirsutism), thinning of the subcutaneous tissue accompanied by splitting of elastic fibers with resultant red or purple striae (stretch marks), and ecchymoses (bruising). Glucocorticoids alter the response of connective tissue to injury by inhibiting collagen synthesis, which is why these agents are used to suppress manifestations of the collagen diseases. Clients who are taking steroids experience delayed wound healing with decreased wound strength, inhibited tissue contraction for wound closure, and impeded epithelization. Fortunately, vitamin A has been shown to reverse the healing impairments caused by steroids (Goodman, 1990).

Effects of hydrocortisone in physiologic quantities on the musculoskeletal system include smooth muscular contraction, but in large doses it causes muscle weakness and atrophy due to inhibition of protein synthesis. Specifically, because of the glucocorticoid receptor sites that exist in skeletal muscle, muscle is one of the target organs for corticosteroids. The resulting decreased oxidative metabolism, enhanced glucose synthesis, and inhibited protein synthesis lead to muscle wasting. The glucocorticoid action reduces the uptake of amino acids by skeletal muscle and inhibits amino acid incorporation

[4] Generally, glucocorticoids cause fluid imbalances and mineralocorticoids cause electrolyte imbalances. However, mineral corticosteroids are used minimally (e.g., for adrenal insufficiency or adrenogenital syndrome). Most adverse effects seen by the clinical therapist will be related to glucocorticosteroids. Adverse effects of anabolic steroids primarily occur in an athletic or sports training setting.

TABLE 4-7 Possible Adverse Effects of Prolonged Systemic Corticosteroids

Site	Symptom
Metabolic	Obesity, increased glucose/protein metabolism Electrolyte and fluid imbalance Fluid retention/edema Potassium loss (hypokalemia) Calcium loss (hypocalcemia) Corticosteroid withdrawal syndrome Growth retardation (children) Hyperuricemia (cyclosporine-induced)
Endocrine	Diabetes (new-onset) Hirsutism (hair growth) Cushing's syndrome (hypercortisolism)
Cardiovascular	Accelerated atherosclerosis Increased blood pressure
Immune system	Increased risk of opportunistic infections Bone marrow suppression, malignancy
Musculoskeletal	Myopathy Osteoporosis Osteonecrosis, avascular necrosis of femoral head Tendon rupture
Gastrointestinal	Peptic ulcer disease Pancreatitis
Central nervous system	Change in behavior (insomnia, euphoria) Psychosis, depression Benign intracranial hypertension
Ophthalmologic	Cataracts, glaucoma
Dermatologic	Acne Striae ("stretch marks") Alopecia (baldness or hair loss) Bruising, hematomas Skin atrophy, delayed wound healing

Adapted from Moncur C, Williams HJ: Rheumatoid arthritis: Status of drug therapies. Physical Therapy 75:511–525, 1995.

into proteins. The overall effect is a negative nitrogen balance, resulting in increased protein wasting, weight loss, muscle atrophy, and myopathy (Mandel, 1982; Price and Wilson, 1992).

Corticosteroid-induced myopathies are characterized by loss of muscle substance and focal myositis. Four functional classifications of muscle weakness, referred to as steroid myopathy, can occur in persons with corticosteroid-induced myopathy (Table 4–8). Recovery from corticosteroid-induced myopathy can occur with dose reduction; improvement in strength may occur within 2 to 3 weeks. Complete resolution may take from 1 to 4 months to 1 to 2 years, depending on the underlying diagnosis prior to treatment with corticosteroids (e.g., organ transplantation requiring lifetime administration of corticosteroids) (Grant, 1994).

Use of corticosteroids for longer than 6 months results in osteoporosis from altered resorption of calcium (hypocalcemia), inhibition of osteoblast collagen synthesis, elevation

TABLE 4-8 Functional Classifications of Corticosteroid-Induced Myopathy

Level	Function
Advanced	Person has difficulty climbing stairs
High	Person cannot rise from a chair
Intermediate	Person cannot walk without assistance
Low	Person cannot elevate extremities or move in bed

Adapted from Askari A, Vignos PJ, Moskoweitz RW: Steroid myopathy in connective tissue disease. Am J Med 61:485–492, 1976.

of parathormone levels that amplify osteoclastic bone resorption, and enhanced renal excretion of calcium (Parrillo and Fauci, 1979; Weiss, 1989). Users of anabolic steroids may experience an increased susceptibility to tendon strains and injuries (especially biceps and patellar tendons), because muscle size and strength increase at a rate far greater than tendon and connective tissue strength. Adolescent steroid use may lead to accelerated maturation and premature epiphyseal closure (Potteiger and Stilger, 1994). Long-term exposure to corticosteroids increases the risk of avascular necrosis, which often requires orthopedic intervention (e.g., total hip replacement) (Prosnitz et al., 1981).

Effects on the gastrointestinal tract, liver, and cardiovascular system include peptic ulcer (especially in people with RA), decreased clotting function leading to subsequent bruising and hematomas, and hypertension, hypervolemia, edema, and congestive heart failure, respectively (Berkow and Fletcher, 1992). Any person receiving corticosteroids should also be taking a gastrointestinal protective drug (e.g., Pepcid).

Special Implications for the Therapists **4-4**

CORTICOSTEROIDS

Inflammation and Infection

In the rehabilitation setting, large doses of steroids are administered early in the treatment of traumatic brain-injured (TBI) and spinal cord–injured (SCI) clients to control cerebral or spinal cord edema. Suppression of the inflammatory reaction in persons who are given large doses of steroids may be so complete as to mask the clinical signs and symptoms of major diseases, perforation of a peptic ulcer, or spread of infection. In the orthopedic population, local symptoms of pain or discomfort are also masked, so the therapist must exercise caution during evaluation or treatment to avoid exacerbating the underlying inflammatory process.

Increased susceptibility to the infections associated with impaired cellular immunity and the decreased rate of recovery from infection associated with corticosteroid use requires careful infection control. Special care should be taken to avoid exposing immunosuppressed clients to infection, and everyone in contact with that person should follow strict handwashing policies (see Infectious Diseases, Chapter 6). Some facilities recommend that persons with a WBC count of $<1,000$ mm^3 or a neutrophil count of <500 mm^3 wear a protective mask. (See Table 7–3.) Therapists should ensure that anyone who is immunosuppressed is provided with equipment that has been disinfected according to universal precautions (see Appendix A).

Depending on the therapy treatment prescribed, the therapist may schedule the client according to the timing of the medication dosage. For example, with a chronic condition such as adhesive capsulitis, the goal may be to increase joint accessory motion, which requires more vigorous joint mobilization techniques. Masking local painful symptoms may help the client to remain relaxed during mobilization procedures. When pain can be predicted (i.e., pain is brought on by therapy treatment), the drug's peak effect should be timed to coincide with the painful event. For nonopioids, such as corticosteroids (including NSAIDs), the peak effect occurs approximately 2 hours after oral administration. However, in a condition such as shoulder impingement syndrome, teaching the client proper positioning and functional movement to avoid painful impingement may require treatment without the maximal benefit of medication. The therapy session could be scheduled for a time just before the next scheduled dosage. If back pain occurs in a person who is receiving corticosteroids, diagnostic measures should be undertaken to rule out osteoporosis or compression fracture.

Intra-articular Injections (Moncur and Williams, 1995)

Occasionally, intra-articular injections of corticosteroids are necessary to control acute inflammation in a joint that is otherwise uncontrollable. Such injections can provide prolonged relief and improve the client's mobility and function. The rationale for use in the joint is to suppress the synovitis, because no evidence currently indicates that intra-articular injections retard the progression of erosive disease. Intra-articular injections must be carefully selected, and no single joint should have more than 3 or 4 injections before other procedures are pursued (Paulus and Bulpitt, 1993).

Most steroid injections are accompanied by an anesthetizing agent, such as lidocaine or bupivacaine, which usually provides immediate pain relief, although the anti-inflammatory may require 2 to 3 days to take effect. During this time, the client should be advised to continue using proper supportive positioning and to avoid movements that would otherwise aggravate the previous symptoms. There remains some controversy as to whether the person can bear weight on the joint for several days after the injection; a less conservative approach permits nonstrenuous activity (Chatham et al., 1989; Neustadt, 1985). Vigorous exercise may speed resorption of the steroid from the joint and reduce the intended effect. Intra-articular injection of corticosteroid may also result in pigment changes that are most noticeable among dark-skinned people.

Exercise and Steroids

The harmful side effects of glucocorticoid steroids can be delayed or reduced in their severity by regular aerobic exercise and proper nutrition (Hickson and Marone, 1993; Kavanagh et al., 1988; Schols, 1993). Unfortunately, these clients are often too sick to engage in exercise at all, much less at a level of intensity that would reverse myopathy. Whenever possible, the therapist can help to emphasize the importance of exercise, especially activities that produce significant stress on the weight-bearing joints (e.g., walking; jogging is not usually recommended), to decrease the calcium loss from long bones that is attributable to prolonged steroid use. It is essential to consult with the client's oncologist before initiating aerobic exercise, especially in clients who have received high-dose chemotherapy or radiation to the thoracic region, as cardiac and pulmonary toxicity can occur. (See also Radiation Injuries and Chemotherapy.)

Strength training or stair exercise is one way to maintain the large muscle groups of the legs, which are most affected by the muscle-wasting properties of corticosteroids (Painter, 1993). The treatment plan should also include closed-chained exercises to prevent shearing forces across joint lines and to allow for normal joint loading (Sawyer et al., 1990), prevention of vertebral compression fractures, and education about proper body mechanics during functional activities (Grant, 1994).

Client education about the importance of proper footwear and choice of exercise surfaces is important for the individual receiving long-term corticosteroid therapy. For the person at risk of avascular necrosis of the femoral head, exercising the surrounding joint musculature in a non–weight-bearing position may be required.

Monitoring Vital Signs

Long-term use of corticosteroids may result in electrolyte imbalances (e.g., hypokalemia, metabolic alkalosis, sodium and fluid retention, edema, hypertension), which necessitates monitoring of vital signs during aerobic activity, because of the demand placed on the cardiovascular system in conjunction with these adverse effects (Grant, 1994). (See Guidelines for Activity and Exercise, Appendix B.)

Laboratory Values

The therapist can monitor protein wasting by checking certain laboratory values. An elevation in the percentage of blood creatinine (normal value, 0.6 to 1.2 mg/dL) accompanied by serum enzymes within normal limits (e.g., creatine phosphokinase [CPK], aldose, and serum glutamic oxaloacetic transaminase [SGOT]) may indicate protein wasting. Rising creatinine levels may indicate muscle wasting from an increase in corticosteroid dosage or from exercise levels that are beyond the client's physiologic capabilities (Grant, 1994).

Steroids, Nutrition, and Stress

Persons taking steroids may be advised to increase their dietary intake of potassium, to counteract the loss of potassium in the urine, or to take antacids, to decrease gastric irritation. Protein intake is recommended for muscle growth to offset steroid-induced catabolism. Corticosteroids stimulate gluconeogenesis and interfere with the action of insulin in peripheral cells, which may result in diabetes mellitus or may aggravate existing conditions in diabetes. Regular blood glucose monitoring is recommended to detect steroid-induced diabetes mellitus. Some facilities establish exercise protocols based on blood glucose levels. For example, at the Johns Hopkins Hospital, Baltimore, exercise is not recommended for persons with blood glucose levels >250 mg/dL (Grant, 1994).

Clients taking replacement glucocorticoids (e.g., for Addison's disease) may need to increase the required dosage during stressful situations (e.g., emotional stress, dental extractions, minor surgery, upper respiratory infections). Temporary mineralocorticoid dosage increases may also be indicated if the client receiving replacement mineralocorticoid experiences profuse diaphoresis for any reason (strenuous physical exertion, heat spells, fever) (Loriaux, 1993). Either of these situations requires physician evaluation.

Psychological Considerations

Corticosteroid use can result in a range of mood changes from irritability, euphoria, and nervousness to more serious depression and psychosis (Grant, 1994; Price and Wilson, 1992). The intensity of changes in mood may depend on the dosage administered, the sensitivity of the individual, and the underlying personality. When intense changes are observed, the physician should be notified so that an adjustment in dosage can be made.

Chronic corticosteroid use may alter a person's body image because of changes in adipose tissue distribution, thinning of skin, and development of stretch marks. The classic characteristics of a "cushingoid" appearance may develop, including a moon-shaped face, enlargement of the supraclavicular and cervicodorsal fat pads ("buffalo hump"), and truncal obesity (see Figs. 9–5 to 9–7). Some people may be extremely self-conscious about these cosmetic changes and others may be emotionally devastated by them; caution is required in discussing assessment findings with the client.

The therapist needs to be aware of the affected individual's coping abilities (Snyder, 1992). Treatment intervention can include educating the individual about traditional stress-management techniques. Therapists can facilitate psychosocial support by contacting social work and clinical nurse specialists to integrate programs such as survivorship support groups and image consultants.

Anabolic Steroids (Potteiger and Stilger, 1994)

Therapists working with athletes, especially adolescent athletes, may observe signs and symptoms of (illegal) anabolic steroid use, including rapid weight gain (10 to 15 lb in 3 weeks); elevated blood pressure and associated edema; acne on the face, upper back, and chest; alterations in body composition, with marked muscular hypertrophy; and disproportionate development of the upper torso along with stretch marks around the back and chest. After prolonged anabolic steroid use, jaundice may develop.

Other signs of steroid use include needle marks in the large muscle groups, development of male pattern baldness, gynecomastia (breast enlargement), and frequent hematoma or bruising. Among females secondary male characteristics may develop, such as a deeper voice, breast atrophy, and abnormal facial and body hair. Irreversible sterility can occur (females being affected more than males), and menstrual irregularities may develop in women.

Changes in personality may occur; the athlete may become more aggressive or experience mood swings and psychological delusions (e.g., believe he or she is indestructible). "Roid rages," characterized by sudden outbursts of uncontrolled emotion, may be observed. The therapist who suspects an athlete may be using anabolic steroids should report findings to the physician. The therapist may consider approaching that person to discuss the situation. Testing for elevated blood pressure may provide an opportunity for evaluation of anabolic steroid use. Information as to the long-term adverse effects of anabolic steroids should be provided as part of the education process for all athletes. The therapist or trainer can provide healthy and safe strength training, stressing the importance of nutrition and proper weight-training techniques.

Radiation Injuries

Definition and Overview. Radiation therapy, or radiotherapy, is the treatment of disease (usually cancer) by delivery of radiation to a particular area of the body. Radiation reactions and injuries are the harmful effects (acute, delayed, or chronic) to body tissues of exposure to ionizing radiation.

Ionizing radiation interacts with nuclear DNA directly or indirectly, to stop cellular reproductive capacity. Radiation therapy may be delivered by isotopes implanted in the tumor or a body cavity, by external-beam sources delivered in the form of electromagnetic waves (e.g., x-rays or γ-rays), or as streams of particles (e.g., electrons). X-rays generated by linear accelerators and γ-rays generated by radioactive isotopes (e.g., cobalt 60, radium 226, cesium 137) are used for the treatment of visceral tumors, as they penetrate to great depths before reaching full intensity and thereby spare the skin from toxic effects. Electron beam irradiation is most useful in the treatment of superficial tumors, as energy is deposited at the skin and quickly dissipates, sparing the deeper tissues from toxic effects (Andreoli et al., 1993).

Etiology and Risk Factors. Localized radiation therapy for acne, enlarged thymus, or tumors (e.g., skin cancer or leukemia) accounts for most instances of radiation injury. Whole-body irradiation occurs with nuclear reactor accidents or nuclear explosions; it is also administered prior to bone marrow transplantation. Other risk factors include environmental exposure (e.g., to radon, which causes lung cancer); atomic bomb survivors were found to have breast cancer, leukemia, and thyroid cancer; and radium dial painters were found to have breast and oral cancer.

Congenital anomalies after intrauterine exposure (especially if it occurs during early pregnancy) may include microcephaly, growth and mental retardation, hydrocephalus, spina bifida, blindness, cleft palate, and club foot.

Clinical Manifestations. Immediate and delayed effects of radiation (the latter caused by excessive doses) listed in Table

4–9 vary with radiation site, dose, and time (Abrams and Berkow, 1992; O'Toole, 1992). In general, most side effects will not begin before a week to 10 days after the first treatment. Side effects vary from individual to individual, but they typically continue throughout the course of treatment and for several weeks after the last treatment.

When the radiation field includes sites of active bone marrow (e.g., sternum, iliac crests, long bones), hematopoiesis is altered, and myelosuppression can occur (McDonald, 1992). Radiation therapy to the breast and axillary areas after lumpectomy or mastectomy or to the long bones for the treatment of metastatic lesions may result in fibrosis and atrophy of the soft tissues, which in turn result in decreased range of motion and edema (Hamburgh, 1992). Many women have developed brachial plexus injury, often resulting in severe pain and loss of use of the arm, after radiotherapy for breast cancer (Sikora, 1994). Radiation of the pelvic cavity often causes dense pelvic adhesions that can cause painful motion restrictions.

Radiation Syndromes

Although the side effects of radiation just described are common, an acute radiation sickness syndrome occasionally develops (Table 4–10). This condition is a systemic reaction that occurs most often when the therapy is given in a large dosage to large areas over the abdomen; it occurs less often when radiotherapy is given over the thorax, and rarely when it is given over the extremities. Thoracic radiation may result in pericarditis and pneumonitis, which can progress to pulmonary fibrosis weeks, or even months, after radiation treatments have ended. Radiation esophagitis can cause difficulty swallowing and severe pain with eating and swallowing.

TABLE 4–9 IMMEDIATE AND DELAYED EFFECTS OF IONIZING RADIATION*

IMMEDIATE	DELAYED (CHRONIC) EFFECT
Anorexia, nausea, vomiting, diarrhea	Skin scarring
Urinary dysfunction	Telangiectasis (vascular lesion)
Skin toxic effects	Cataract
Erythema	Myelopathy (spinal cord dysfunction)
Epilation or hair loss at roots	Cerebral injury
Destruction of fingernails	Obliterative endarteritis
Epidermolysis (loose skin)	Pericarditis
Xerostomia (dry mouth)	Hypothyroidism
Stomatitis (inflammation of mouth mucosa)	Pulmonary fibrosis
	Hepatitis
	Intestinal stenosis
	Nephritis
	Skin cancer (squamous cell)
	Amenorrhea
	Decreased fertility (both sexes)
	Decreased libido (females only)
	Brachial plexus injury (breast cancer)

* The health-care professional must remember that some of the delayed effects of radiation, such as cerebral injury, pericarditis, pulmonary fibrosis, hepatitis, intestinal stenosis, other GI disturbances, and nephritis, may be signs of recurring cancer. The physician should be notified by the affected individual of any new symptoms, change in symptoms, or increase in symptoms.

TABLE 4–10 ACUTE RADIATION SICKNESS SYNDROMES

Hematopoietic syndrome	Anorexia, nausea, vomiting, diarrhea (limited) Thrombocytopenia Hemorrhage Fatal infection
Gastrointestinal syndrome	Nausea, vomiting, profuse diarrhea (dehydration) Hypovolemic shock, sepsis
Cerebral syndrome (fatal)	Convulsions, coma Cerebral edema Rapid death

Adapted from Harruff, RC: Pathology Facts. Philadelphia, JB Lippincott, 1994, p 50.

Radiation Enterocolitis

Radiation therapy is used frequently for cancer of the bladder, prostate, rectum, colon, and female genital organs. The symptoms of radiation enteritis are the same as those of chronic intestinal obstruction (e.g., dysphagia; abdominal pain, distention, and spasm; reflexive vomiting [associated with pain]; constipation; constitutional symptoms; dehydration). Radiation colitis is manifested by bleeding and diarrhea.

Radiation Lung Disease *(Roberts et al., 1993; Stauffer, 1994)*

The lung is a radiosensitive organ that can be affected by external beam radiation therapy. The pulmonary response is determined by the volume of lung radiated, the dose and rate of therapy, and enhancing factors, such as concurrent chemotherapy, previous radiation therapy in the same area, and simultaneous withdrawal of corticosteroid therapy.

Symptomatic radiation lung injury occurs in about 10% of clients treated with megavoltage therapy for carcinoma of the breast, 5% to 15% of clients treated for carcinoma of the lung, and 5% to 35% of clients treated for lymphoma.

There are two phases of pulmonary response to radiation: an acute phase (radiation pneumonitis) and a chronic phase (radiation fibrosis). *Radiation pneumonitis* usually occurs 2 to 3 months (range, 1 to 6 months) after completion of radiotherapy, and it is characterized by insidious onset of dyspnea, persistent dry cough, chest fullness or pain, weakness, and fever. In severe disease, respiratory distress and cyanosis occur that are characteristic of adult respiratory distress syndrome (ARDS).

Pulmonary function studies reveal reduced lung volumes, reduced lung compliance, hypoxemia, reduced diffusing capacity, and reduced maximum voluntary ventilation. Treatment is symptomatic and consists of administration of aspirin and cough suppressants and bed rest. Acute respiratory failure is treated appropriately when present. Although there is no proof that corticosteroids are effective in radiation pneumonitis, prednisone is prescribed immediately, with early tapering of dosage. Radiation pneumonitis usually resolves in 2 to 3 weeks, and death from ARDS is unusual.

Pulmonary radiation fibrosis occurs in nearly all clients who receive a full course of radiation therapy for cancer of the lung or breast. Pulmonary fibrosis occurs approximately 6 to 12 months after resolution of radiation pneumonitis, although radiation fibrosis can develop without radiation pneumonitis. Most people are asymptomatic, but progressive dyspnea may develop slowly. No specific therapy is necessary, and corticosteroids have no value.

Cutaneous Effects of Radiation

Although all body systems can be affected by radiation, the skin is the system at greatest risk for injury, including open, weeping wounds and alterations in the mucosal integrity.[5] Cellular breakdown in the epidermis results in an inflammatory process similar to a sunburn. *First-degree* reactions resemble a sunburn and can destroy hair roots, causing the hair to fall out. *Second-degree* reactions, also called dry desquamation, produce bright red erythema. Sweat glands and hair follicles are damaged and the hair falls out, which may be irreversible. *Third-degree* reactions, also called moist desquamation, are characterized by a dark purple color and possible formation of blisters and ulcers. If the area is exposed to air, scabbing can occur over the exposed area. *Fourth-degree* reactions (rare) occur as a result of radiation overdose and are characterized by tissue necrosis.

Effects of Radiation on the Nervous System

Injury of the nervous system can also occur as a complication of excessive radiation dosage to tissue. Both acute and subacute transient symptoms may develop early, but progressive, permanent, and often disabling nervous system damage may not be evident for months to years after radiation therapy. Acute encephalopathy consisting of headache, nausea and vomiting, somnolence (sleepiness), and progressive neurologic signs may develop after the first or second dose of radiation. This condition becomes less severe as the radiation therapy continues, after treatment with corticosteroid hormones. Early-delayed encephalopathy occurs in the first 2 to 4 months after therapy. Early-delayed radiation myelopathy (functional disturbance or pathologic change in the spinal cord) follows radiation therapy to the neck or upper thorax and is characterized by Lhermitte's sign (an electric shock-like sensation radiating down the back and into the legs on flexion of the neck). This syndrome resolves spontaneously. Late-delayed radiation damage to the nervous system may appear months to years after treatment, including brachial neuropathy after radiation for breast or lung cancer and Brown-Séquard syndrome (weakness and proprioceptive sensory loss on one side of the body and loss of pain and temperature sensation on the other side leading to eventual paraplegia) after radiation for extraspinal tumors (e.g., Hodgkin's disease).

Medical Management. Treatment of systemic reactions is symptomatic and supportive. No truly effective antinausea drug is available, although some medications are used as needed. When radiation dosage levels are sufficient to cause damage to gastrointestinal mucosa, bone marrow, and other vital tissues, blood and platelet transfusions, antibiotics, fluid and electrolyte maintenance, and other supportive medical measures may be used.

Prognosis depends on the dose, the rate at which it was received, and its distribution within the body. Serial hematologic and bone marrow studies may be used to accurately determine the prognosis. Death occurs within hours to days in the presence of the cerebral syndrome, within days with gastrointestinal syndrome, and within weeks with hematopoietic syndrome.

[5] This is also true for the gastrointestinal and genitourinary mucosa.

Special Implications for the Therapist **4-5**

RADIATION

Radiation Hazard for Health-Care Professionals

People who receive external radiation do not give off radiation to persons who come in contact with them. Internal implants can present some hazards to others as long as the implant is in place. Pregnant staff members should avoid all contact with the internally radiated client.

When administering direct care, staff members should plan interventions so that each task can be accomplished as quickly as possible. Distance provides some protection; therefore, it is advisable to use positions that place the staff person as far away from the radioactive implant as possible. For example, if the implant is in the pelvis, the caregiver might stand at the head or foot, rather than at the side, of the bed.

The use of protective lead aprons or portable shields may be recommended according to the hospital protocol. Each staff member is encouraged to know and follow the recommended policies and procedures for the given institution (O'Toole, 1992). A film badge worn on the outside of any protective devices or clothing worn by caregivers records the cumulative dose of radiation received and is used to monitor exposure over a period of time.

Some sources of radiation (e.g., iodine 131, phosphorus 32) are excreted in body fluids (e.g., urine, sweat, tears, saliva) for several days after it has been administered to the client. These clients are placed in strict radioactive isolation during hospitalization and treatment. All articles used by the client, such as toothpicks, tissues, and bed linens, are considered as a possible radiation hazard. Disposal of all such items should follow hospital protocol.

Postradiation Therapy

For the client who is in the process of receiving external radiation therapy, handwashing before treating the client is essential to protect him or her from infection. Skin care precautions include the following: avoid topical use of alcohol or other drying agents, lotions, gels, oils, or salves; do not wash away markings for target area; avoid positions in which the client is lying on the target area; avoid exposure to direct sunlight, heat lamps, or other sources of heat, including thermal modalities.

Radiation to the low back may cause nausea, vomiting, or diarrhea because the lower digestive tract is exposed to the radiation (National Cancer Institute,

1991). Radiation of the pelvic cavity often causes dense pelvic adhesions that can cause painful motion restrictions. The therapist's role in the postradiation treatment of these clients is to increase range of motion and provide stretching exercises. Early, aggressive intervention by the therapist is essential to prevent or minimize restrictive scarring.

Some effects of radiation on the nervous system can develop as late as a year after treatment. Anyone presenting with neurologic signs or symptoms of unknown cause must be questioned about past medical history and the possibility of prior radiation treatment.

Postradiation Infection

Signs and symptoms of infection are often absent because the immunosuppressed person cannot mount an adequate inflammatory response. Fever may be the first and only sign of infection. Swelling, redness, and pus are absent in infected tissue. The therapist must observe very carefully for any sign of infection, anemia, or bleeding and other signs of thrombocytopenia (see Chapter 11).

Chemotherapy

Systemic chemotherapy plays a major role in the management of the 60% of malignancies that are not curable by regional modalities. As with radiation therapy, chemotherapy acts by interfering with cell division by chemically interacting with DNA. Myelosuppression (inhibits bone marrow production of blood cells and platelets) as a result of specific chemotherapeutic agents or drug combinations is the primary factor that predisposes the individual to infection. With increased dosages or more frequent administration of drugs, more profound and prolonged myelosuppression is occurring (Wujcik, 1993).

The patterns of toxicity of some commonly used cytotoxic drugs are outlined in Table 4–11. Certain agents cause breaks in the integrity of the oral and gastrointestinal mucosa, which provide openings for normal flora (bacteria normally present in the gut) to invade the bloodstream. This loss of mucosal integrity from chemotherapy or radiation therapy predisposes the gastrointestinal tract to invasion by bacteria, fungi, or viruses (Wujcik, 1993). Persons who have received anthracycline antibiotics (i.e., doxorubicin) as part of a chemotherapeutic regimen may develop cardiac toxic effects (e.g., arrhythmias, conduction disturbances).

Fluid and electrolyte imbalances associated with the use of chemotherapy are discussed later in this chapter. Cardiac arrhythmias may be the first sign that a chemotherapeutic agent is becoming cardiotoxic. Delayed-onset cardiac toxic effects as a result of chemotherapeutic agents may appear as a chronic cardiomyopathy. Other cardiac problems that may develop include acute or chronic pericarditis, conduction disturbances, accelerated and radiation-induced coronary artery disease, and valvular dysfunction. The development of accelerated atherosclerosis associated with cardiac radiation can lead to coronary ischemia and myocardial infarction.

TABLE 4–11 Major Toxicities of Commonly Used Cancer Chemotherapeutic Agents

Short-Term Effect	Long-Term Effect
Nausea, vomiting	Leukemia
Alopecia (hair loss)	Cardiomyopathy
Myelosuppression	Pulmonary fibrosis
Hypersensitivity	Hemolytic-uremic syndrome
Tissue necrosis	Peripheral neuropathy
Stomatitis	Premature menopause, sterility
Renal failure	
Hemorrhagic cystitis	
Ileus	

Andreoli TE, Bennett JC, Carpenter CCJ, et al: Cecil Essentials of Medicine, ed 3. Philadelphia, WB Saunders, 1993, p 427.

Special Implications for the Therapist **4-6**

CHEMOTHERAPY

The period following chemically induced remission is critical for each client who is now highly susceptible to spontaneous hemorrhage and infection. The usual precautions for thrombocytopenia (see Chapter 11) and infection control must be adhered to strictly. The importance of strict handwashing technique with an antiseptic solution cannot be overemphasized. The therapist should be alert to any sign of infection and report any potential site of infection, such as mucosal ulceration or skin abrasion or tear (even a hangnail). Check skin for petechiae, ecchymoses, chemical cellulitis, and secondary infection.

Follow precautions as outlined for anemia (see Anemia: Chapter 11). Concepts regarding exercise following cancer treatment and the use of physical agents (thermal and mechanical modalities) are presented in Chapter 7; see also Table 7–10.

Neuropathy can occur as a result of the neurotoxic effects of chemotherapy. For the client on bedrest, prevention of pressure ulcers through client and family education and positioning with appropriate protection (e.g., footboard to prevent footdrop, protective coverings, such as sheepskin and eggshell foam) are also important. For the mobile client, safety standards must be followed during ambulation because of weakness and numbness of the extremities.

Bone marrow suppression is a common and serious side effect of many chemotherapeutic agents (and can be a side effect of radiation therapy in some instances). It is extremely important to monitor the hematology values in clients receiving these treatment modalities. Before any type of vigorous exercise or rehabilitative treatment is initiated, laboratory values should be monitored (see Table 7–3).

Drug-induced mood changes ranging from feeling of well-being and euphoria to depression and irritability may occur; depression and irritability may also be associated with the cancer. Knowing these and other potential side effects of medications used in the treatment of cancer can help the therapist better understand client reactions during rehabilitation or therapy treatment.

SPECIFIC DISORDERS AFFECTING MULTIPLE SYSTEMS

Vasculitic Syndromes *(Hunder, 1993)*

Vasculitis is a term that applies to a diverse group of diseases characterized by inflammation in blood vessel walls. The primary forms of vasculitis encountered in a therapy practice include giant cell (temporal) arteritis, polyarteritis nodosa, hypersensitivity vasculitis, Kawasaki disease, and thromboangiitis obliterans. These are discussed in greater detail in Chapter 10. Because the pathogenesis of most forms of vasculitis remains poorly understood and cases of vasculitis show great variability, it may not be possible to apply a specific disease label to such cases. Such instances of vasculitis may be diagnosed as *systemic vasculitis*.

Blood vessels of different sizes in various parts of the body may be affected by vasculitis, causing a wide spectrum of clinical manifestations. The inflammation often causes narrowing or occlusion of the vessel lumen and produces ischemia of the tissues that are supplied by the involved vessels. The inflammation may weaken the vessel wall, resulting in aneurysm or rupture. Major symptoms of small blood vessel vasculitis are skin lesions that may be accompanied by fever, malaise, and myalgia. Conditions characterized by this type of small-vessel involvement include temporal arteritis, Sjögren's syndrome, connective tissue disorders, chronic active hepatitis, ulcerative colitis, malignancies, biliary cirrhosis, and infections such as bacterial endocarditis.

Vasculitis may occur either as a primary disease or as a secondary manifestation of other illnesses, such as rheumatoid arthritis (RA), childhood dermatomyositis, systemic lupus erythematosus, mixed connective tissue disease, and systemic sclerosis. The next section contains a more detailed description of rheumatoid vasculitis; the other conditions are discussed elsewhere in the text.

TABLE 4-12 Extra-Articular Manifestations of Rheumatoid Arthritis

Cardiac
- Conduction defects (usually asymptomatic)
- Pericarditis

Hematologic
- Anemia of chronic disease
- Felty's syndrome (splenomegaly and neutropenia)

Neurologic
- Compression neuropathies
- Polyneuropathy

Nodulosis (subcutaneous nodules)

Ocular
- Episcleritis (inflammation of the superficial sclera and conjunctiva)
- Scleritis (inflammation of the sclera)
- Sicca syndrome (dry eyes)

Pulmonary
- Effusions
- Interstitial fibrosis
- Nodules
- Pleurisy

Vasculitis
- Mononeuritis multiplex
- Nailfold infarctions
- Digital gangrene
- Skin changes (ulcers, purpura, bullae)
- Peripheral neuropathy

Adapted from Eggert JR, Messner RP: Rheumatoid arthritis: Early clinical picture and diagnosis. J Musculoskel Med 12:19–30, 1995.

Rheumatoid Arthritis *(Moots and Bacon, 1994)*

Considering the multiple systemic processes that occur in RA, the condition might be more appropriately termed *rheumatoid disease*. Although RA is best known as a disease affecting synovial tissue, extra-articular rheumatoid nodules can appear at almost any body site, including the pleura, pericardium, and parenchyma of any organ. Serositis (inflammation of the serous membrane) can also involve the heart and lungs (Table 4–12).

Certain autoimmune disorders appear to be associated with RA, most notably fibrosing alveolitis and Sjögren's syndrome. The chronic immune stimulation that occurs in people with RA can give rise to amyloidosis, Felty's syndrome (splenic disease), or lymphadenopathy. Other extra-articular conditions that can occur with RA include anemia, osteopenia, and cardiac or renal involvement; the extra-articular features of RA are more common in men.

Rheumatoid vasculitis is the least frequent extra-articular manifestation of RA, but because the vasculitic lesions can cause infarction or dysfunction in major organs (including the brain), vasculitis is associated with considerable morbidity and mortality. Vasculitis usually develops when joint disease is relatively quiet; early onset in the course of RA is associated with a poor prognosis. (See also pulmonary manifestations of RA in Collagen Vascular Disease, Chapter 10.)

Clinical features of systemic rheumatoid vasculitis are diverse, because any size blood vessel may be involved anywhere in the body (Scott et al., 1981). Skin ulcers and unexplained weight loss are clues to vasculitis. The most frequent findings are cutaneous lesions, such as nail-edge infarctions (Fig. 4–1), rashes, and skin ulcers. Skin ulcers usually develop suddenly as deep, punched-out lesions at sites that are unusual for venous ulceration, such as the dorsum of the foot or the upper calf. Peripheral neuropathies (mononeuritis multiplex) present with sensory symptoms of paresthesia or numbness and motor impairment (e.g., weakness in the muscles supplied by the affected nerve). Systemic manifestations of rheumatoid vasculitis may include unexplained weight loss, anorexia, and malaise. Malaise may be related to the widespread release of cytokines (substances released by lymphocytes with various immunologic functions) and may be accompanied by fatigue, low-grade fever, and night sweats. Individuals with severe RA who experience any of these symptoms should be referred to the physician for further evaluation.

Anemia in the presence of RA is usually proportional to the disease severity, and it resolves as RA is brought under control. Iron deficiency is often caused by gastrointestinal bleeding as a result of therapy with NSAIDs or inadequate food intake, especially in persons with systemic illness. The anemia is treated by controlling the underlying RA and the therapist should follow special precautions related to anemia

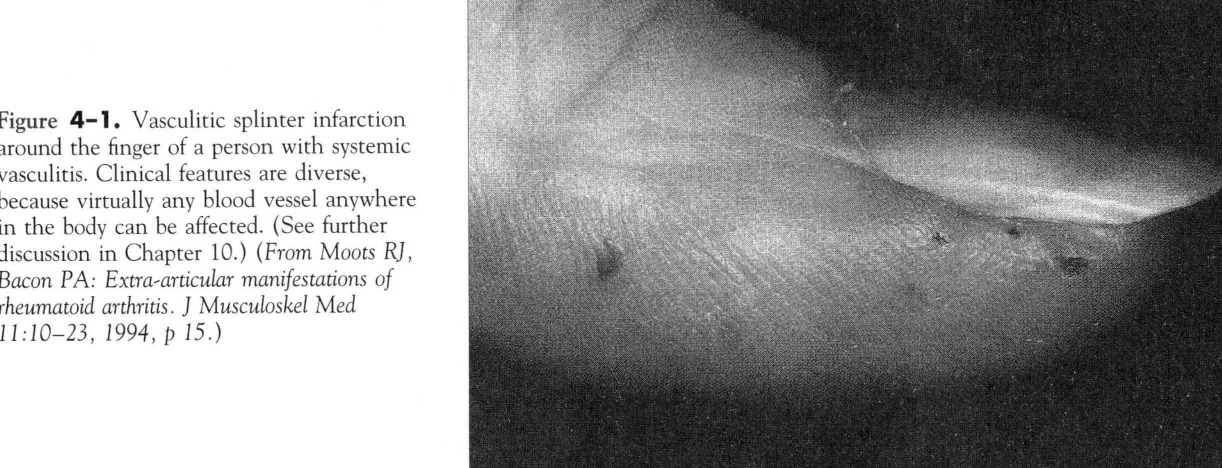

Figure 4-1. Vasculitic splinter infarction around the finger of a person with systemic vasculitis. Clinical features are diverse, because virtually any blood vessel anywhere in the body can be affected. (See further discussion in Chapter 10.) (*From Moots RJ, Bacon PA: Extra-articular manifestations of rheumatoid arthritis. J Musculoskel Med 11:10–23, 1994, p 15.*)

until the disease is under control (see Special Implications: Anemia, Chapter 11).

Osteopenia may result from general immobility, but it may also be an inherent part of RA (Reid et al., 1986). Initially, areas around the joints are affected. With longstanding disease, osteoporosis may become generalized and can lead to fractures following minimal stress. Management with corticosteroids increases the incidence of osteoporosis and related complications.

Systemic Lupus Erythematosus

Lupus erythematosus is a chronic inflammatory disorder of the connective tissues that appears in two forms: discoid lupus erythematosus (DLE), which affects only the skin, and systemic lupus erythematosus (SLE), which affects multiple organ systems as well as the skin and can be fatal. SLE may involve every organ system, but cardiovascular, renal, or neurologic complications are prevalent. Like RA, SLE is characterized by recurring remissions and exacerbations, which are especially common during the spring and summer. SLE affects women eight times as often as men, increasing to 15 times as often during childbearing years (Norris et al., 1995). (For further discussion of DLE see Chapter 8; see Chapter 5 for a complete discussion of SLE.)

Systemic Sclerosis

Systemic sclerosis, also known as progressive systemic sclerosis (PSS), scleroderma, and the CREST (*c*alcinosis, *r*aynaud's phenomenon, *e*sophageal dysmotility, *s*clerodactyly, and *t*elangiectasia) syndrome is a diffuse connective tissue disease characterized by fibrotic, degenerative, and occasionally inflammatory changes throughout the body. Most commonly affected sites include the skin, blood vessels, synovial membranes, skeletal muscles, and internal organs, especially the esophagus, gastrointestinal tract, thyroid, heart, lungs, and kidneys. It affects women more than men, especially between ages 30 and 50 years. Approximately 30% of people with PSS die within 5 years of onset (Norris et al., 1995). (See Integumentary System, Chapter 8, for complete discussion of this condition. See also Systemic Sclerosis Lung Disease, Chapter 12.)

Tuberculosis

Tuberculosis (TB) is an acute or chronic infection caused by *Mycobacterium tuberculosis*. Although the primary infection site is the lungs, mycobacteria commonly exist in other parts of the body; this is referred to as *extrapulmonary tuberculosis*. The extrapulmonary sites may include the renal system, skeletal system (osteomyelitis; vertebral TB is known as Pott's disease), gastrointestinal tract, meninges (tuberculous meningitis), and genitals. Extrapulmonary tuberculosis occurs with greatly increased frequency in persons with human immunodeficiency virus (HIV) infection. (Pulmonary tuberculosis is discussed in depth in Chapter 12. Tuberculous spondylitis [Pott's disease] is discussed in Chapter 21.)

Sarcoidosis

Sarcoidosis is a multisystem disorder characterized by the formation of granulomas, a formation of inflammatory cells (e.g., mononuclear inflammatory cells or macrophages), usually surrounded by a rim of lymphocytes. These granulomas may develop in the lungs, liver, bones or eyes (see Table 12–11) and may be accompanied by skin lesions (see Fig. 12–13). In the United States, sarcoidosis occurs predominantly among blacks, affecting twice as many women as men. Acute sarcoidosis usually resolves within 2 years. Chronic, progressive sarcoidosis, which is uncommon, is associated with pulmonary fibrosis and progressive pulmonary disability (Norris et al., 1995). (See Chapter 12 for a complete discussion of this condition.)

Multiple Organ Dysfunction Syndrome

(Haak et al., 1994)

Overview. Care of critically ill people has progressed significantly during the last 50 years. Significant advances have been made in the care of shock, acute renal failure, acute brain injury, and acute respiratory failure, and more people are surviving these conditions. However, despite these advances, progressive deterioration of organ function occurs in people who are critically ill or injured. People frequently die of complications of disease, rather than from the disease itself. Multiple organ dysfunction syndrome (MODS) is often the final complication of a critical illness; it accounts for most deaths in noncoronary intensive care units (Beal and Cerra, 1994).

Definition, Etiology, and Risk Factors. MODS, formerly called multiple organ failure syndrome (MOFS), is the progressive failure of two or more organ systems after a very severe illness or injury. Although sepsis and septic shock are the most common causes, infection is not necessary to its development. MODS also can be triggered by persistent inflammatory processes, necrosis, severe trauma, pulmonary contusion, major surgery, multiple blood transfusions, burns, circulatory shock, acute pancreatitis, acute renal failure, and adult respiratory distress syndrome (ARDS).

Systemic inflammatory response syndrome (SIRS), formerly called *sepsis syndrome*, characterizes the clinical manifestations of hypermetabolism (e.g., increased temperature, heart rate, and respirations) present in many clients with MODS. Because it is a response to tissue insult or injury, SIRS is present in most individuals admitted to a critical care unit (CCU).

After an initial insult or injury, other factors can increase a person's chances of developing MODS/SIRS, including inadequate or delayed resuscitation, age over 65 years, alcoholism, diabetes, surgical complications (e.g., infection, hematoma formation), bowel infarction, or the previous existence of organ dysfunction (e.g., renal insufficiency) (Beal and Cerra, 1994).

Pathogenesis. The physiologic changes in MODS/SIRS are complex and incompletely understood at this time. In response to illness or traumatic injury, the neuroendocrine system activates stress hormones (e.g., cortisol, epinephrine, norepinephrine, endorphins) to be released into the circulation, whereas the sympathetic nervous system is stimulated to compensate for complications such as fluid loss and hypotension. Because of the initial insult and subsequent release of mediators, three major plasma enzyme cascades are activated with the overall effect of massive uncontrolled systemic immune and inflammatory responses. This hyperinflammation and hypercoagulation perpetuates edema formation, cardiovascular instability, endothelial damage, and clotting abnormalities. At the same time, initial oxygen consumption demand increases, because the oxygen requirements at the cellular level increase. Flow and oxygen consumption are mismatched because of a decrease in oxygen delivery to the cells caused by maldistribution of blood flow, myocardial depression, and a hypermetabolic state. Tissue hypoxia with cellular acidosis and impaired cellular function result in multiple organ dysfunction characteristic of MODS.

Clinical Manifestations. A clinical pattern in the development of MODS has been well established. After the precipitating event, low-grade fever, tachycardia, dyspnea, SIRS, and altered mental status develop. The lung is the first organ to fail, resulting in ARDS (see Chapter 12). Between 7 and 10 days, the hypermetabolic state intensifies, gastrointestinal bacteremia is common, and signs of liver and kidney failure develop. During days 14 to 21, renal and liver failures progress to a severe status and the gastrointestinal and immune systems fail, with eventual cardiovascular collapse. Ischemia and inflammation are responsible for the central nervous system manifestations.

Protein metabolism is also affected, and amino acids derived from skeletal muscle, connective tissue, and intestinal viscera become an important energy source. The result is a significant loss of lean body mass, a condition termed *autocannibalism* (Cerra et al., 1980).

Medical Management. Prevention and early detection and supportive therapy are essential for MODS, as no specific medical treatment exists for this condition. A way to halt the process, once it has begun, has not yet been discovered. Pharmacologic treatment may include antibiotics to treat infection, inotropic agents (e.g., dopamine, dobutamine) to counteract myocardial depression, and supplemental oxygen and ventilation to keep oxygen saturation levels at or above 90%. Fluid replacement and nutritional support are also provided. The recent development of monoclonal antibodies to modulate or inhibit the immune and inflammatory responses may lead to more specific pharmacologic treatment.

MODS is the major cause of death (usually occurring between days 21 and 28) following septic, traumatic, and burn injuries (Bone, 1991; Lekander and Cerra, 1990). If the affected individual's condition has not improved by the end of the third week, survival is unlikely. The mortality rate of MODS is 60% to 90% and approaches 100% if 3 or more organs are involved, sepsis is present, and the individual is older than 65 years (Bone, 1991; Huddleston, 1992).

Special Implications for the Therapist **4-7**

MULTIPLE ORGAN DYSFUNCTION SYNDROME

Only the critical care or burn unit therapist will encounter the client with MODS/SIRS. The hypermetabolism associated with this condition is accompanied by protein catabolism, primarily of skeletal muscle and visceral organs. Lean body mass can be significantly depleted in 7 to 10 days (Lekander and Cerra, 1990), necessitating skin precautions and skin care.

FLUID AND ELECTROLYTE IMBALANCES[6]

(Metheny, 1992; O'Toole, 1992)

Observing clinical manifestations of fluid or electrolyte imbalances may be an important aspect of client care, especially in the acute care and home health-care settings. Identifying clients at risk for such imbalances is the first step toward early detection. Although the causes of fluid and electrolyte

[6] This is a brief presentation of the normal homeostatic processes of fluid and electrolyte balance. The interactions of these systems and how they maintain fluid and electrolyte balance and acid-base regulation are beyond the scope of this text. For a more in-depth study of these and other concepts presented in this text, the reader is referred to Guyton AC, Hall JE: *Textbook of Medical Physiology*, ed 9. Philadelphia, WB Saunders, 1996; Sirica AE (ed): *Cellular and Molecular Pathogenesis*. Philadelphia, Lippincott-Raven, 1995; or other similar texts. Because of the many terms associated with this topic, a list of terminology is provided at the beginning of this chapter.

BOX 4–6
Factors Affecting Fluid and Electrolyte Balance in Elderly Adults

- Acute illness (fever, diarrhea, vomiting)
- Bowel cleansing for gastrointestinal diagnostic testing
- Change in mental status
- Constipation
- Decreased thirst mechanism
- Difficulty swallowing
- Excessive sodium intake
  - Diet
  - Sodium bicarbonate antacids (e.g., alka-seltzer)
  - Water supply or water softener
  - Decreased taste sensation (increased salt intake)
- Excessive calcium intake
  - Alkaline antacids
- Immobility
- Laxatives (habitual use for constipation)
- Medications
  - Antiparkinsonian drugs
  - Diuretics
  - Propranolol
- Tamoxifen (breast cancer therapy)
- Sodium-restricted diet
- Urinary incontinence (voluntary fluid restriction)

imbalance are many and varied, generally, any disease process or injury, medication, medical treatment, dietary restrictions, and imbalance of fluid intake with fluid output can disrupt fluid and electrolyte balance. The most common causes in a therapy practice include burns, surgery, diabetes mellitus, malignancy, acute alcoholism, socioeconomic status, and factors affecting the elderly (Box 4–6).

Aging and Fluid and Electrolyte Balance

The volume and distribution of body fluids composed of water, electrolytes, and non-electrolytes vary with age, sex, and amount of adipose tissue. Throughout life, a slow decline occurs in the volume of body fluids; body water decreases with increased body fat, because fat is free of water; therefore, obesity decreases the relative amount of water in the body.

Fluid Imbalances

Overview. Approximately 45% to 60% of the adult human body is composed of water, which contains the electrolytes that are essential to human life (see Electrolytes). This life-sustaining fluid is found within various body compartments, including the intracellular (within cells), interstitial (space between cells), intravascular (within blood vessels), and transcellular compartments.[7] The fluid in the interstitial and intravascular compartments comprises approximately one-third the total body fluid, called the *extracellular fluid* (ECF). Fluid found inside the cells accounts for the remaining two-thirds of total body fluid, called the *intracellular fluid* (ICF).

The cell membrane is water permeable with equal concentrations of dissolved particles on each side of the membrane maintaining equal volumes of ECF and ICF and preventing passive shifts of water. Passive shifts occur only if an inequality occurs on either side of the membrane in the concentration of solutes that cannot permeate the membrane. Water can also move with sodium ion movement.

Five types of fluid imbalances may occur: (1) ECF volume deficit (ECFVD); (2) ECF volume excess (ECFVE); (3) ECF volume shift; (4) ICF volume excess (ICFVE); and (5) ICF volume deficit (ICFVD).[8] The material in this section is presented on the bases of three broad categories: fluid deficit, fluid excess, and fluid shift.

Etiology and Pathogenesis. Maintaining constant internal conditions (homeostasis) requires the proper balance between the volume and distribution of ECF and ICF to provide nutrition to the cells, allow excretion of waste products, and promote production of energy and other cell functions. Maintenance of this balance depends on the differences in the concentrations of ICF and ECF fluids, the permeability of the membranes, and the effect of the electrolytes in the fluids.

A fluid imbalance occurs when either gains or losses of body fluids and electrolytes cause fluid deficit or a fluid excess. Sodium is the major ion that influences water retention and water loss. A deficit of body fluids occurs with either an excessive loss of body water or an inadequate compensatory intake. The result is an insufficient fluid volume to meet the needs of the cells. It is manifested by dehydration (Box 4–7), hypovolemia (such as blood or plasma loss), or both. Severe fluid volume deficit can cause vascular collapse and shock.

An *excess* of water occurs when there is an overabundance of water in the interstitial fluid spaces or body cavities (edema) or within the blood vessels (hypervolemia). A *fluid shift* occurs when vascular fluid moves to interstitial or intracellular spaces or interstitial or intracellular fluid moves to vascular fluid space. Fluid that shifts into the interstitial space (i.e., fluid that is not in the vascular compartment) and remains there is referred to as *third-space fluid*. Third-space fluid is commonly seen in a therapy practice as a result of altered capillary permeability secondary to tissue injury or inflammation, but the most common cause is liver disease. Decreased serum protein (albumin) associated with liver disease and/or states of malnutrition result in third-space fluid.

Other areas called potential spaces can fill with fluid in the presence of inflammation or fluid imbalances. Examples of potential spaces include the peritoneal cavity fluid (e.g., ascites) and the pleural cavity (e.g., pleural effusion).

Clinical Manifestations. *Fluid volume deficit* (FVD) is most often accompanied by symptoms related to a decrease in cardiac output, such as decreased blood pressure, increased pulse, and orthostatic hypotension. FVD can occur from loss of blood (whether obvious hemorrhage or occult gastrointestinal bleeding); loss of plasma (burns, peritonitis); or loss of

[7] Fluid in the transcellular compartment is present in the body but is separated from body tissues by a layer of epithelial cells. This fluid includes digestive juices, water, and solutes in the renal tubules and bladder, intraocular fluid, joint-space fluid, and cerebrospinal fluid (Lehman, 1991).

[8] A simpler approach to this subject is to view fluid shifts in terms of intravascular or extravascular movement. Movement from the vascular space to the extravascular areas, and vice versa, takes place easily and is the first mechanism of extracellular movement. *Increased intravascular fluid* results in congestive heart failure, increased pulse, and increased respiration. *Decreased intravascular fluid* results in decreased blood pressure, increased pulse, and increased respirations. However, *increased extravascular fluid* may cause edema, ascites, or pleural effusion. *Decreased extravascular fluid* results in decreased skin turgor and fatigue.

BOX 4-7
Clinical Manifestations of Dehydration

Absent perspiration, tearing, and salivation
Body temperature (subnormal or elevated)
Confusion
Disorientation; comatose; convulsions
Dizziness when standing
Dry, brittle hair
Dry mucous membranes
Headache
Incoordination
Irritability
Lethargy
Postural hypotension
Rapid pulse
Rapid respirations
Skin changes
  Color: gray
  Temperature: cold
  Turgor: poor
  Feel: Dry, clammy, thickened, doughy
Sunken eyeballs
Sunken fontanel (children)

body fluids (diarrhea, vomiting, diaphoresis, lack of fluid intake), resulting in dehydration. Hypernatremia occurs if the body fluid loss is a loss of body water without solute components (e.g., diabetes insipidus). Most often, however, body fluid losses contain both body water and its solute components. The affected individual experiences symptoms of thirst, weakness, dizziness, decreased urine output, fever, weight loss, and altered levels of consciousness (i.e., confusion, coma). Significant decreases in systolic blood pressure (<70 mm Hg) result in symptoms of shock and require immediate medical treatment and possibly life-sustaining emergency management.

Fluid volume excess (FVE) is primarily characterized by weight gain and edema of the extremities. With intravascular FVE, other clinical manifestations include dyspnea, engorged neck and hand veins, and a bounding pulse. In the early stages, if the fluid is in the third space (interstitial fluid between cells), the person may not exhibit any of these symptoms.

Fluid shift from the vascular to the extravascular (interstitial) spaces (e.g., burns, peritonitis) is manifested by signs and symptoms similar to fluid volume deficit and shock, including skin pallor, cold extremities, weak and rapid pulse, hypotension, oliguria, and decreased levels of consciousness. When the fluid returns to the blood vessels, the clinical manifestations are similar to those of fluid overload such as bounding pulse, engorgement of peripheral and jugular veins,[9] and an increased blood pressure.

Medical Management. The extracellular fluid (ECF) is the only fluid compartment that can be readily monitored; clinically, the status of intracellular fluid (ICF) is inferred from analysis of plasma and the condition of the person. A fluid balance record is kept on any individual who is susceptible or already experiencing a disturbance in the balance of body fluids. In addition, medical evaluation of clinical signs and laboratory tests are helpful in the assessment of a person's hydration status. Laboratory tests may include serum osmolality, sodium, hematocrit, and blood urea nitrogen (BUN) measurements (see Laboratory Values, Chapter 35).

Serum osmolality measures the concentration of particles in the plasma portion of the blood. Osmolality increases with dehydration and decreases with overhydration. Serum sodium is an index of water deficit or excess; an elevated level of sodium in the blood (hypernatremia) would indicate that the loss of water from the body has exceeded the loss of sodium such as occurs in the administration of osmotic diuretics, uncontrolled diabetes insipidus, and extensive burns. Hematocrit increases with dehydration and decreases with excess fluid. BUN serves as an index of kidney excretory function; BUN increases with dehydration and decreases with overhydration (see Table 35–11).

Treatment is directed to the underlying cause; in the case of fluid volume deficit, the aim is to improve hydration status. This may be accomplished through replacement of fluids and/or electrolytes by oral, nasogastric, or intravenous means, including tube feeding or parenteral hyperalimentation, which is administered via a venous catheter, usually inserted into the superior vena cava.

Special Implications for the Therapist **4-8**

FLUID IMBALANCES

Monitoring Fluid Balance

Fluid balance is so critical to physical well-being and cardiopulmonary sufficiency that fluid input and output records are frequently maintained at bedside. The therapist may be involved in maintaining these records, which also include fluid volume lost in wound drainage, gastrointestinal output, and fluids aspirated from any body cavity. Body weight may increase by several pounds before edema is apparent. The dependent areas manifest the first signs of fluid excess. Individuals on bed rest show sacral swelling; people who can sit on the edge of the bed or in a chair for prolonged periods tend to show swelling of the feet and hands (Dean, 1996).

Water and fluids should be offered frequently to the elderly and to clients with debilitating diseases to prevent body fluid loss and hypernatremia. However, increasing fluid intake in clients with congestive heart failure or severe renal disease is usually contraindicated. Caffeinated fluids and alcohol can increase water loss, thereby increasing the serum sodium level; these beverages should be avoided to prevent fluid loss due to this diuretic effect (Kee, 1993). Water is the preferred fluid for hydration except in athletic or marathon race situations, which require replacement of electrolytes.

Dehydration

Dehydration (water deficit) degrades endurance exercise performance, and physical work capacity is diminished even at marginal levels of dehydration

[9] The jugular pulse is not normally visible. If the jugular pulse is noted 2 cm above the sternal angle when the individual sits at a 45-degree angle, it may be a sign of fluid overload.

(defined clinically as a 1% loss of body weight through fluid loss). Alterations in VO_{2max} occur with a 2% or more deficit in body water loss. Greater body water deficits are associated with progressively larger reductions in physical work capacity. Dehydration results in larger reductions in physical work capacity in a hot environment (e.g., aquatic or outdoor setting) as compared to a thermally neutral environment. Prolonged exercise that places large demands on aerobic metabolism is more likely to be adversely affected by dehydration than is short-term exercise (Pandolf, 1993).

Core body temperature increases predictably as the percentage of dehydration increases. The heart rate increases about 6 beats/minute for each 1% increase in dehydration (Adolph, 1947).* Individuals exercising in the heat (including aquatic exercise) should be encouraged to drink water in excess of normal desired amounts. When exercise is expected to cause an increase of more than 2% in dehydration, target heart rate modifications are necessary (Pandolf, 1993).

Severe losses of water and solutes can lead to hypovolemic shock. It is important for the therapist to be aware of possible fluid losses or water shifts in any client who is already compromised by advanced age or by the presence of an ileostomy or tracheostomy that results in a continuous loss of fluid. Because the response to fluid loss is highly individual, it is important to recognize the early clinical symptoms of fluid loss (see Box 4–7) and to carefully monitor clients who are at risk (e.g., observe for symptoms, monitor vital signs). People at risk for profound and potentially fatal fluid volume deficit, as in severe and extensive burns, should be assessed frequently and regularly for mental acuity and orientation to person, place, and time.

Skin Care

Careful handling of edematous tissue is essential to maintaining the integrity of the skin, which is stretched beyond its normal limits and has a limited blood supply. Turning and repositioning the client must be done gently to avoid friction. A break in or abrasion of edematous skin can readily develop into a pressure ulcer. Client education may be necessary in the proper application and use of anti-embolism stockings, lower-extremity elevation, and the need for regular exercise. Clients should be cautioned to avoid crossing the legs, putting pillows under the knees, or otherwise creating pressure against the blood vessels (O'Toole, 1992).

* This is not true for elderly people who may have limited rate changes with increased activity. Cardiac medications such as digoxin also prevent the heart rate from responding to increased activity. Heart transplant recipients also have a unique situation as the heart has been denervated (see Special Implications for the Therapist: Heart Transplantation, Chapter 10). Elderly individuals with hypovolemia cannot compensate with an increased heart rate as younger people can, so shock is more difficult to treat.

Electrolyte Imbalances

Overview. Electrolytes are chemical substances that separate into electrically charged particles, called *ions*, in solution. This process allows the ions in the body fluids to conduct an electrical charge necessary for metabolic activities and essential to the normal function of all cells. The electrolytes that consist of positively charged ions, or *cations*, are sodium (Na^+), potassium (K^+), calcium (Ca^+), and magnesium (Mg^{2+}), and those that consist of negatively charged ions, or *anions*, are chloride (Cl^+), bicarbonate (HCO_3^-), and phosphate (PO_4^{3-}).

Concentration gradients of sodium and potassium across the cell membrane produce the membrane potential and provide the means by which electrochemical impulses are transmitted in nerve and muscle fibers. *Sodium* affects the osmolality of blood and therefore influences blood volume and pressure and the retention or loss of interstitial fluid. Sodium imbalance affects the osmolality of the extracellular fluid and is often associated with fluid volume imbalances. Adequate *potassium* is necessary to maintain function of the sodium-potassium pump, which is essential for the normal muscle contraction-relaxation sequence. Imbalances in potassium affect muscular activities, notably those of the heart, intestines, and respiratory tract, and neural stimulation of the skeletal muscles.

Calcium influences the permeability of cell membranes and thereby regulates neuromuscular activity. Calcium plays a role in the electrical excitation of cardiac cells and in the mechanical contraction of the myocardial and vascular smooth muscle cells. An imbalance in calcium concentrations affects the bones, kidneys, and gastrointestinal tract.

Magnesium enhances neuromuscular integration and stimulates parathyroid hormone (PTH) secretion, thus regulating intracellular fluid calcium levels. Magnesium assists in regulating skeletal muscle activity through this influence on calcium utilization by depressing acetylcholine release at synaptic junctions. Magnesium imbalances cause irritability of the nervous system affecting the musculoskeletal and cardiac systems.

Etiology and Pathogenesis. An electrolyte imbalance exists when the serum concentration of an electrolyte is either too high or too low. Stability of the electrolyte balance depends on adequate intake of water and the electrolytes and on homeostatic mechanisms within the body that regulate the absorption, distribution, and excretion of water and its dissolved particles. Bodily fluid loss associated with weight loss, excessive perspiration, or chronic vomiting and diarrhea are the most common causes of electrolyte imbalance. Many other conditions can interfere with these processes and result in an imbalance (Table 4–13).

Oxygen deprivation is accompanied by electrolyte disturbances, particularly loss of potassium, calcium, and magnesium from cells. Myocardial cells deprived of necessary oxygen and nutrients lose contractility, thereby diminishing the pumping ability of the heart. Diuretics also can produce mild to severe electrolyte imbalance. These factors explain the careful observation of specific electrolyte levels in the cardiac client.

Clinical Manifestations. In a therapy practice, paresthesias, muscle weakness, muscle wasting, muscle tetany, and bone pain are the most likely symptoms first observed with electrolyte imbalances. (See Common Causes of Fluid and Electrolyte Imbalances: Clinical Manifestations; see also Table 4–14.)

Medical Management. Potassium, calcium, and, to a lesser extent, magnesium imbalances are reflected on ECG (Fig.

TABLE 4-13 CAUSES OF ELECTROLYTE IMBALANCES

	RISK FACTORS FOR IMBALANCE
POTASSIUM	
Hypokalemia	Dietary deficiency (rare) Intestinal or urinary losses as a result of diarrhea or vomiting (anorexia, dehydration), drainage from fistulas, overuse of gastric suction Trauma (injury, burns, surgery): damaged cells release potassium, are excreted in urine Chronic renal disease Medications such as potassium-wasting diuretics, steroids, sodium-containing antibiotics Acid-base imbalances Hyperglycemia Cushing's syndrome, primary aldosteronism, excessive ingestion of licorice, severe magnesium deficiency
Hyperkalemia	Conditions that alter kidney function or decrease its ability to excrete potassium Intestinal obstruction that prevents elimination of potassium in the feces Addison's disease Chronic heparin therapy, lead poisoning, insulin deficit Trauma: crush injuries, burns
SODIUM	
Hyponatremia	Inadequate sodium intake (low-sodium diets) Excessive intake or retention of water (kidney failure and heart failure) Excessive water loss and electrolytes (vomiting, excessive perspiration, tap-water enemas, suctioning, use of diuretics) Loss of bile (high in sodium) as a result of fistulas, drainage, gastrointestinal surgery, and suction Trauma (loss of sodium through burn wounds, wound drainage from surgery) IV fluids that do not contain electrolytes Adrenal gland insufficiency (Addison's disease) or hyperaldosteronism Cirrhosis of the liver with ascites Syndrome of inappropriate antidiuretic hormone secretion (SIADH): brain tumor, cerebrovascular accident, pulmonary disease, neoplasm with ADH production, medications
Hypernatremia	Decreased water intake (comatose, mentally confused, or debilitated client) Water loss (excessive sweating, diarrhea, failure of kidney to reabsorb water from urine) ADH deficiency (diabetes insipidus) Excess adrenocortical hormones (Cushing's syndrome) IV administration of high-protein, hyperosmotic tube feedings and diuretics
CALCIUM	
Hypocalcemia	Inadequate dietary intake of calcium and vitamin Impaired absorption of calcium from intestinal tract (severe diarrhea, overuse of laxative, and enemas containing phosphates; phosphorus tends to be more readily absorbed from the intestinal tract than calcium and suppresses calcium retention in the body) Hypoparathyroidism (injury, disease, surgery) Severe infections or burns Overcorrection of acidosis Pancreatic insufficiency Renal failure Hypomagnesemia
Hypercalcemia	Hyperparathyroidism, hyperthyroidism, adrenal insufficiency Tumors (bone, lung, stomach, and kidney) Multiple fractures Excess intake of calcium (excessive antacids), excess intake of vitamin D, milk alkali syndrome Osteoporosis, immobility, multiple myeloma Thiazide diuretics Sarcoidosis
MAGNESIUM	
Hypomagnesemia	Decreased magnesium intake or absorption (chronic malnutrition, chronic diarrhea, bowel resection with ileostomy or colostomy, chronic alcoholism, prolonged gastric suction, acute pancreatitis, biliary or intestinal fistula, diuretic therapy)

TABLE 4–13 CAUSES OF ELECTROLYTE IMBALANCES *(Continued)*

	RISK FACTORS FOR IMBALANCE
MAGNESIUM	
	Excessive loss of magnesium (diabetic ketoacidosis, severe dehydration, hyperaldosteronism and hypoparathyroidism, diuretic therapy)
Hypermagnesemia	Chronic renal and adrenal insufficiency Overuse of antacids and laxatives containing magnesium Severe dehydration (resulting oliguria can cause magnesium retention) Overcorrection of hypomagnesemia Near-drowning (aspiration of sea water)

Adapted from Norris J (ed): Professional Guide to Diseases, ed 5. Springhouse, Pa, Springhouse Corporation, 1995.

4–2). Values for sodium or chloride can be measured in plasma. A sweat test for sodium and chloride levels can be done if cystic fibrosis is suspected. Elevated values in the presence of a family history or clinical findings of cystic fibrosis are diagnostic. Intracellular levels of electrolytes cannot be measured; therefore, all values for electrolytes are expressed as serum values. Serum values for electrolytes are given as milliequivalents per liter (mEq/L) or milligrams per deciliter (mg/dL) (see Table 35–8). As with fluid imbalances, the underlying cause of electrolyte imbalances must be determined and corrected.

Special Implications for the Therapist **4–9**

ELECTROLYTE IMBALANCES

Encourage adherence to a sodium-restricted diet prescribed for clients. The use of over-the-counter medications for people on a sodium-restricted diet should be approved by the physician. Encourage activity altered by rest periods. Lying down favors diuresis of edematous fluid (Schrier, 1986). Monitor for worsening of the underlying cause of fluid or electrolyte imbalance and report significant findings to the nurse or physician. If dyspnea and orthopnea are present, teach the client to use a semi-Fowler position (head elevated 18 to 20 in. from horizontal with knees flexed) to promote lung expansion. Frequent position changes are important in the presence of edema; edematous tissue is more prone to skin breakdown than is normal tissue.

Elderly persons have frequent problems with hypokalemia most often associated with the use of diuretics. Assessment for signs and symptoms of electrolyte imbalance must be ongoing, and changes need to be reported immediately. Decreased potassium levels can result in fatigue, muscle cramping, and cardiac dysrhythmias, usually manifested by an irregular pulse rate or complaints of dizziness and/or palpitations. Fatigue and muscle cramping increase the chance of musculoskeletal injury. Observing for accompanying signs and symptoms of fluid and electrolyte imbalances will help promote safe and effective exercise for anyone with the potential for these disorders.

With appropriate medical therapy, cardiac, muscular, and neurologic manifestations associated with electrolyte imbalances can be corrected. Delayed medical treatment may result in irreversible damage or death.

Common Causes of Fluid and Electrolyte Imbalances

The exact mechanisms of fluid and electrolyte imbalances are outside the scope of this text. A brief description of the common causes encountered in a therapy practice is included here.

Pathogenesis. *Burns*, *surgery*, and *trauma* may result in a fluid volume shift from the vascular spaces to the interstitial spaces. Tissue injury causes the release of histamine and bradykinin, which increases capillary permeability, allowing fluid, protein, and other solutes to shift into the interstitial spaces. In the case of burns, the fluid shifts out of the vessels into the injured tissue spaces as well as into the normal (unburned) tissue. This causes severe swelling of these tissues and a significant loss of fluid volume from the vascular space, which results in hypovolemia. Severe hypovolemia can result in shock, vascular collapse, and death. In the case of major tissue damage, potassium is also released from the damaged tissue cells and can enter the vascular fluids, causing hyperkalemia (Kee, 1993).

In an attempt to treat shock, large quantities of fluid are administered intravenously to maintain blood pressure, cardiac output, and renal function. After 24 to 72 hours, capillary permeability is usually restored and fluid begins to leave the tissue spaces and shift back into the vascular space. If renal function is not adequate, the accumulation of fluid used for treatment and fluid returning from the tissue spaces into the vascular space can cause fluid volume overload. Fluid overload can then cause congestive heart failure.

Diabetes mellitus may result in a condition called *diabetic ketoacidosis*, as a result of overproduction of ketone bodies and the accompanying metabolic acidosis that occurs (see discussion, Chapter 9). As the pH of the blood decreases (acidosis), the accumulating hydrogen moves from the extracellular fluid to the intracellular fluid. Movement of hydrogen into the cells promotes the movement of potassium out of the cells and into the extracellular fluid. As the potassium

TABLE 4–14 Clinical Features of Various Electrolyte Imbalances

System Dysfunction		
Potassium Imbalance		
	Hypokalemia	**Hyperkalemia**
Cardiovascular	Dizziness, hypotension, arrhythmias, ECG changes (flattened T waves, elevated U waves, depressed ST segment), cardiac arrest (with serum potassium levels <2.5 mEq/L)	Tachycardia and later bradycardia, ECG changes (tented and elevated T waves, widened QRS, prolonged PR interval, flattened or absent P waves, depressed ST segment), cardiac arrest (with levels >7.0 mEq/L)
Gastrointestinal	Nausea and vomiting, anorexia, diarrhea, abdominal distention, paralytic ileus or decreased peristalsis	Nausea, diarrhea, abdominal cramps
Musculoskeletal	Muscle weakness and fatigue, leg cramps	Muscle weakness, flaccid paralysis
Genitourinary	Polyuria	Oliguria, anuria
CNS	Malaise, irritability, confusion, mental depression, speech changes, decreased reflexes, respiratory paralysis	Hyperreflexia progressing to weakness, numbness, tingling, and flaccid paralysis
Acid-base balance	Metabolic alkalosis	Metabolic acidosis
Calcium Imbalance		
	Hypocalcemia	**Hypercalcemia**
CNS	Anxiety, irritability, twitching around mouth, laryngospasm, convulsions, Chvostek's sign, Trousseau's sign	Drowsiness, lethargy, headaches, depression or apathy, irritability, confusion
Musculoskeletal	Paresthesia (tingling and numbness of the fingers), tetany or painful tonic muscle spasms, facial spasms, abdominal cramps, muscle cramps, spasmodic contractions	Weakness, muscle flaccidity, bone pain, pathologic fractures
Cardiovascular	Arrhythmias, hypotension	Signs of heart block, cardiac arrest in systole, hypertension
Gastrointestinal	Increased GI motility, diarrhea	Anorexia, nausea, vomiting, constipation, dehydration, polydipsia
Other	Blood-clotting abnormalities	Renal polyuria, flank pain, and, eventually, azotemia
Sodium Imbalance		
	Hyponatremia	**Hypernatremia**
CNS	Anxiety, headaches, muscle twitching and weakness, convulsions	Fever, agitation, restlessness, convulsions
Cardiovascular	Hypotension; tachycardia; with severe deficit, vasomotor collapse, thready pulse	Hypertension, tachycardia, pitting edema, excessive weight gain
Gastrointestinal	Nausea, vomiting, abdominal cramps	Rough, dry tongue; intense thirst
Genitourinary	Oliguria or anuria	Oliguria
Respiratory	Cyanosis with severe deficiency	Dyspnea, respiratory arrest, and death (from dramatic rise in osmotic pressure)
Cutaneous	Cold clammy skin, decreased skin turgor	Flushed skin; dry, sticky mucous membranes
Magnesium Imbalance		
	Hypomagnesemia	**Hypermagnesemia**
Neuromuscular	Hyperirritability, tetany, leg and foot cramps, Chvostek's sign (facial muscle spasms induced by tapping the branches of the facial nerve)	Diminished reflexes, muscle weakness, flaccid paralysis, respiratory muscle paralysis that may cause respiratory embarrassment
CNS	Confusion, delusions, hallucinations, convulsions	Drowsiness, flushing, lethargy, confusion, diminished sensorium
Cardiovascular	Arrhythmias, vasomotor changes (vasodilation and hypotension), occasionally, hypertension	Bradycardia, weak pulse, hypotension, heart block, cardiac arrest (common with serum levels of 25 mEq/L)

From Norris J (ed): Professional Guide to Diseases, ed 5. Springhouse, Pa, Springhouse Corporation, 1995, pp 890–900.

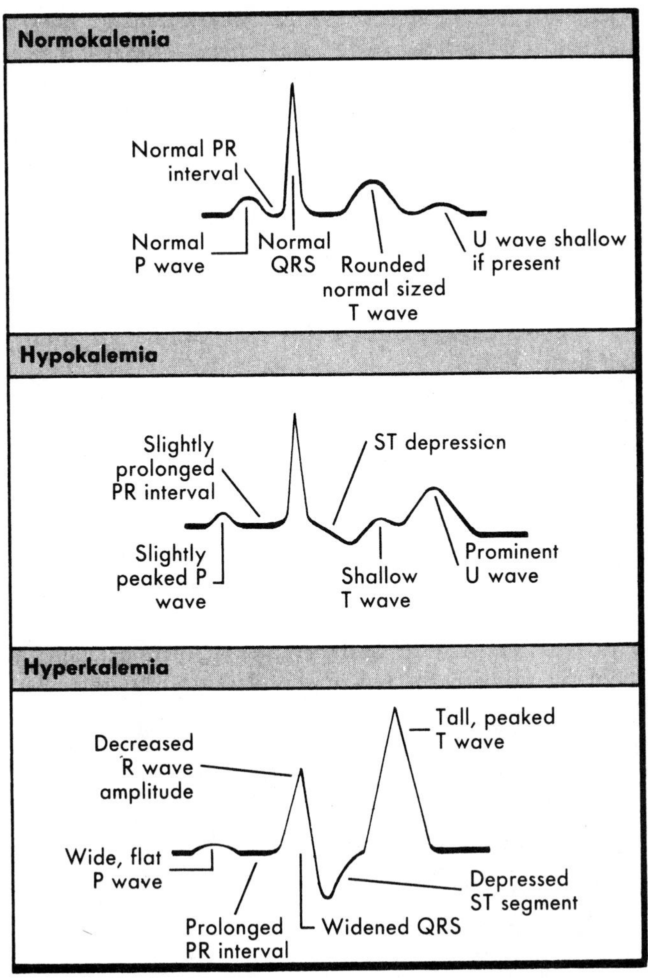

Figure **4–2.** ECG changes with potassium (K^+) changes. (*From McCance KL, Huether SE: Pathophysiology: The Biologic Basis for Disease in Adults and Children, ed 2. St Louis, Mosby-Year Book, 1994, p 105.*)

enters the vascular space, the plasma potassium levels increase. However, since severe diuresis is also occurring, the accumulated potassium is quickly excreted in the urine. As a result, severe potassium losses occur (hypokalemia), which unless treated immediately, cause life-threatening cardiac dysrhythmias.

Malignant tumors can produce "remote effects" as a result of impaired hormonal regulation of body water and electrolytes. Production of these hormones is not regulated by normal suppression feedback loops; consequently, the ectopic hormone[10] continues to be released by the tumor, often causing life-threatening electrolyte imbalances. The generally accepted theory that accounts for the production of ectopic hormones is faulty genetic regulation by the malignant tumor itself (Metheny, 1992). One example of this phenomenon is the ectopic production of antidiuretic hormone (ADH) by lung carcinomas resulting in severe water retention.

Tumor-induced imbalances can affect the central nervous system and cause neurologic syndromes referred to as *paraneoplastic syndromes* (see complete discussion, Chapter 7). The neurologic syndromes are generally produced by cancer stimulation of antibody production (Odell, 1993). For example, cancer cells produce antibodies that impair presynaptic calcium-channel activity, which hinders the release of acetylcholine. In the Lambert-Eaton myasthenic syndrome (LEMS), autoantibodies directed against the presynaptic calcium channels at the neuromuscular junction cause impaired release of acetylcholine from the presynaptic nerve terminals, resulting in muscle weakness (Henson and Posner, 1993; Odell, 1993).

A more local effect of malignancy occurs when metastases to the skeletal system produce hypercalcemia from the osteolysis of bone. The treatment of malignancies also can create fluid and electrolyte imbalances such as occurs with hormonal treatment for breast cancer (tamoxifen); hyponatremia and hypokalemia may also result from nausea and vomiting caused by chemotherapy, and hyponatremia from water intoxication may occur in association with the use of certain chemotherapeutic drugs (e.g., vincristine and cyclophosphamide).

Clinical Manifestations. The effects of a fluid or electrolyte imbalance are not isolated to a particular organ or system (Box 4–8). Symptoms most commonly observed by the therapist may include skin changes, neuromuscular irritability (muscle fatigue, twitching, cramping, or tetany), CNS involvement, edema, and changes in vital signs, especially tachycardia and postural (orthostatic) hypotension (see Box 10–10 for causes of orthostatic hypotension).

Skin changes include changes in skin turgor and alterations in skin temperature. In a healthy individual, pinched skin will immediately fall back to its normal position when released, a measure of skin turgor. In a person with fluid volume deficit (FVD) such as dehydration, the skin flattens more slowly

BOX **4–8**
Clinical Manifestations of Fluid/Electrolyte Imbalance*

- Skin changes
  - Poor skin turgor
  - Changes in skin temperature
- Neuromuscular irritability
  - Muscle fatigue
  - Muscle twitching
  - Muscle cramping
  - Tetany
- CNS involvement
  - Changes in deep tendon reflexes
  - Convulsions
  - Depression
  - Memory impairment
  - Delusions
  - Hallucinations
- Edema
- Changes in vital signs
  - Tachycardia
  - Postural hypotension
  - Altered respirations

* Only signs and symptoms most likely to be seen in a therapy practice are included here.

[10] Hormone that arises at or is produced at an abnormal site or in a tissue where it is not normally found.

after the pinch is released, and may even remain elevated for several seconds (Fig. 4–3). Tissue turgor can vary with age, nutritional state, race, and complexion and must be accompanied by other signs of FVD to be considered meaningful. Skin turgor may be more difficult to assess in the elderly owing to reduced skin elasticity compared to that of younger clients. Skin temperature may become warm and flushed as a result of vasodilation (e.g., in metabolic acidosis) or pale and cool due to peripheral vasoconstriction compensating for hypovolemia.

Neuromuscular irritability can occur as a result of imbalances in calcium, magnesium, potassium, and sodium. (See Chapter 20 for discussion of osteoporosis associated with calcium loss.) Specific signs of neuromuscular involvement associated with these imbalances occur because of increased neural excitability, specifically increased acetylcholine action at the nerve ending, resulting in lowering of the threshold of the muscle membrane (Schrier, 1986). Tetany (continuous muscle spasm) is the most characteristic manifestation of hypocalcemia. The affected person may report a sensation of tingling around the mouth (circumoral paresthesia) and in the hands and feet as well as spasms of the muscles of the extremities and face. Less overt signs (latent tetany) can be elicited through Trousseau's sign (Fig. 4–4), Chvostek's sign (Fig. 4–5), and changes in deep tendon reflexes (DTRs) (Table 4–15). Many other factors can produce abnormalities in DTRs requiring the therapist to evaluate altered DTRs in light of other clinical signs and client history.

Nervous system involvement may occur in the peripheral system (hyperkalemia) or the central nervous system (hypocalcemia). Central nervous system manifestations of hypocalcemia may include convulsions, irritability, depression, mem-

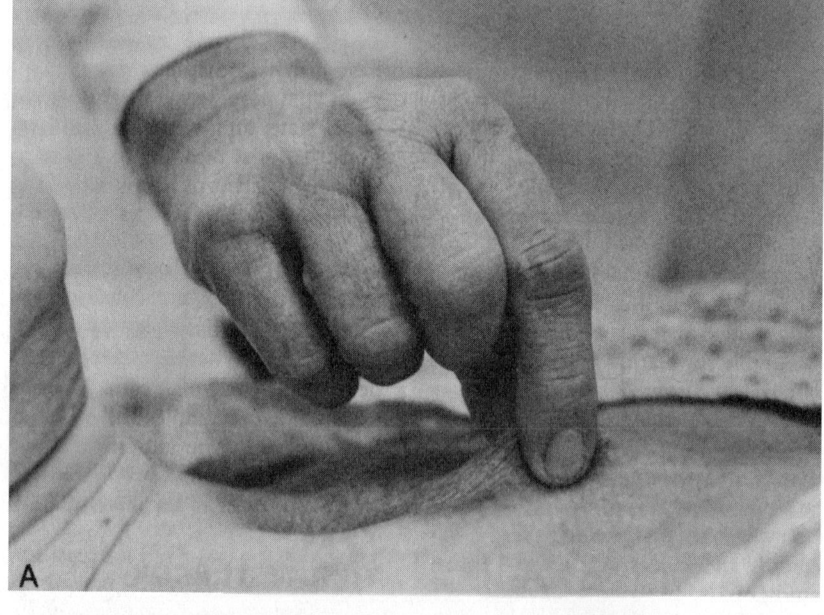

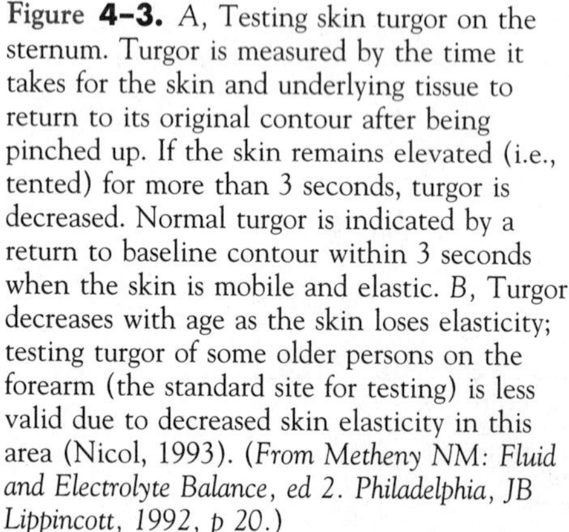

Figure 4–3. *A*, Testing skin turgor on the sternum. Turgor is measured by the time it takes for the skin and underlying tissue to return to its original contour after being pinched up. If the skin remains elevated (i.e., tented) for more than 3 seconds, turgor is decreased. Normal turgor is indicated by a return to baseline contour within 3 seconds when the skin is mobile and elastic. *B*, Turgor decreases with age as the skin loses elasticity; testing turgor of some older persons on the forearm (the standard site for testing) is less valid due to decreased skin elasticity in this area (Nicol, 1993). (*From Metheny NM: Fluid and Electrolyte Balance, ed 2. Philadelphia, JB Lippincott, 1992, p 20.*)

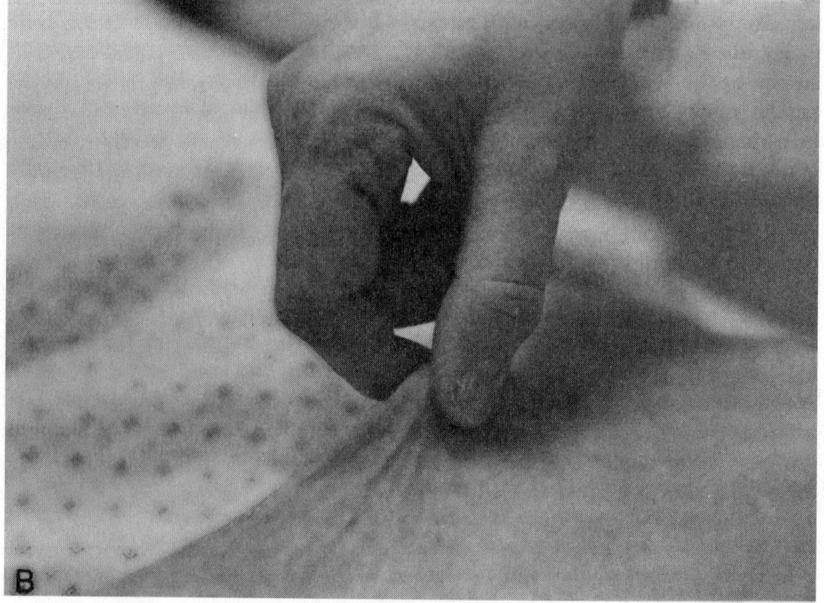

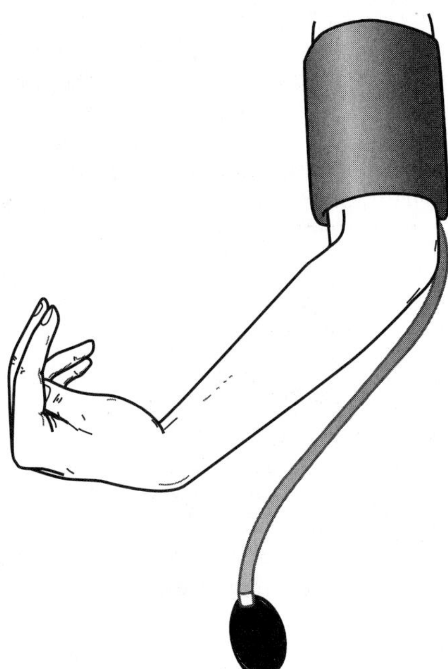

Figure **4–4.** Carpopedal attitude of the hand, a form of latent tetany associated with hypocalcemia, is called *Trousseau's sign*. This can be tested for by inflating a blood pressure cuff on the upper arm to a level between diastolic and systolic blood pressure and maintaining this inflation for 3 minutes. A positive test results in the carpal spasm shown here.

ory impairment, delusions, and hallucinations. In chronic hypocalcemia, the skin may be dry and scaling, the nails become brittle, and the hair is dry and falls out easily.

Hypokalemia seen in a therapy practice can be associated with diuretic therapy; excessive sweating, vomiting, or diarrhea; diabetic acidosis; trauma; or burns. It is also accompanied by muscular weakness that can progress to flaccid quadriparesis (Valtier et al., 1989). The weakness is initially most prominent in the legs, especially the quadriceps; it extends to the arms, with involvement of the respiratory muscles soon after (Metheny, 1992). Finally, a condition called *rhabdomyolysis* (disintegration of striated muscle fibers with excretion of myoglobin in the urine) can occur with potassium or phosphorus depletion.

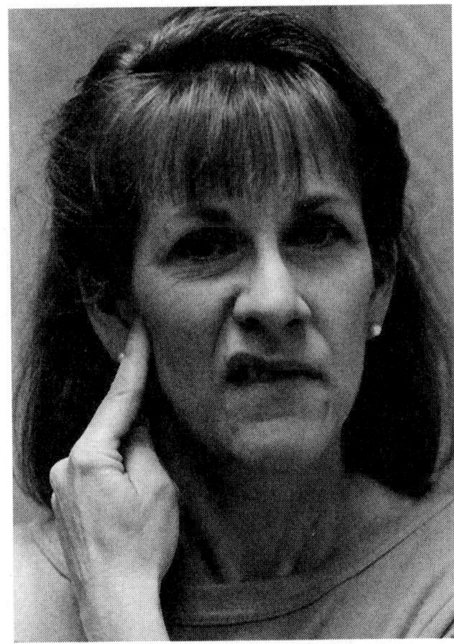

Figure **4–5.** To check for *Chvostek's sign*, tap the facial nerve above the mandibular angle, adjacent to the ear lobe. A facial muscle spasm that causes the person's upper lip to twitch, as shown, confirms tetany.

TABLE 4–15 CHANGES IN DEEP TENDON REFLEXES (DTR) ASSOCIATED WITH FLUID/ ELECTROLYTE IMBALANCE

Increased (Hyperactive)	Decreased (Hypoactive)
Hypocalcemia	Hypercalcemia
Hypomagnesemia	Hypermagnesemia
Hypernatremia	Hyponatremia
Hyperkalemia	Hypokalemia
Alkalosis	Acidosis

Edema, defined as an excessive accumulation of interstitial fluid (fluid that bathes the cells), may be either localized or generalized. Generalized edema may be characterized by shortness of breath, ankle swelling that subsides after lying down, nocturia, and orthopnea. Other manifestations of generalized edema may include decreased urinary output; weight gain; bounding or arrhythmic pulse; labored, shallow, and increased respiratory rate; distended neck veins at 45 degrees elevation of the head; changes in venous and arterial blood pressure; and abnormal laboratory findings (e.g., electrolytes, serum creatinine, blood urea nitrogen, hemoglobin, and hematocrit). Pulmonary edema results from excessive shifting of fluid from the vascular space into the pulmonary interstitium and air spaces. When edema forms as a result of salt retention, the clinical picture is usually one of "pitting" edema (Fig. 4–6).

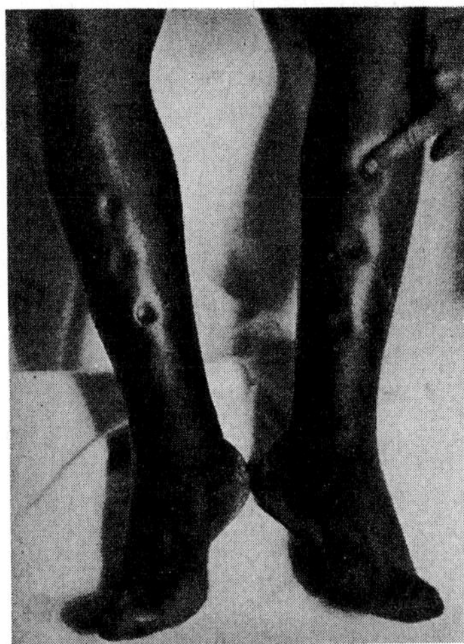

Figure **4–6.** Severe, bilateral, dependent, pitting edema occurs with some systemic diseases, such as congestive heart failure and hepatic cirrhosis. (*From Delp MH, Manning RT: Major's Physical Diagnosis: An Introduction to the Clinical Process, ed 9. Philadelphia, WB Saunders, 1981, p 327.*)

Vital sign changes, including pulse, respirations, and blood pressure, may signal early development of fluid volume changes. Decreased blood pressure and tachycardia are usually the first signs of the decreased vascular volume associated with FVD as the heart pumps faster to compensate for the decreased plasma volume. Irregular pulse rates and dysrhythmias may also be associated with magnesium, potassium, or calcium imbalances.

Deep, rapid respirations may be a compensatory mechanism for metabolic acidosis or a primary disorder causing respiratory alkalosis. Slow, shallow respirations may be a compensatory mechanism for metabolic alkalosis or a primary disorder causing respiratory acidosis. Weakness or paralysis of respiratory muscles can occur in severe hypokalemia or hyperkalemia and in severe magnesium excess.

Orthostatic hypotension is another sign of volume depletion (hypovolemia). Moving from a supine to standing position causes an abrupt drop in venous return, which is normally compensated for by sympathetically mediated cardiovascular adjustments. For example, in the healthy individual, increased peripheral resistance and increased heart rate maintain cardiac return. Blood pressure is unaffected or characterized by a small decrease in systolic pressure, and the diastolic pressure may actually rise a few millimeters of mercury. In contrast, for the person with FVD, systolic pressure may fall 20 mm Hg or more, accompanied by an increase in the pulse rate greater than 15 beats/minute (Kokko and Tannen, 1990). The decreased volume results in compensatory increases in pulse rate as the heart attempts to increase output in the face of decreased stroke volume. As fluid volume depletion worsens, blood pressure becomes low in all positions due to loss of compensatory mechanisms and autonomic insufficiency. Conditions such as diabetes, associated with autonomic neuropathy, can also produce orthostatic blood pressure and pulse changes. (See also Orthostatic Hypotension, Chapter 10.)

Special Implications for the Therapist **4-10**

ASSESSMENT OF FLUID AND ELECTROLYTE IMBALANCE

Assessment of fluid and electrolyte balance is based on both subjective and objective findings (Table 4–16). At the bedside or in the home health-care setting, the therapist must be alert to complaints of headache, thirst, and nausea and changes in dyspnea, skin turgor, and muscle strength. More objective assessment of fluid and electrolyte balance is based on fluid intake, output, and body weight. (See also Special Implications 4–8 and 4–9: Fluid Imbalances and Electrolyte Imbalances.)

ACID-BASE IMBALANCES *(Hansen, 1993)*

Normal function of body cells depends on regulation of hydrogen ion concentration (H^+) so that H^+ levels remain within very narrow limits. Acid-base imbalances occur when these limits are exceeded and are recognized clinically as abnormalities of serum pH (i.e., the measure of acidity or alkalinity of blood). Normal serum pH is 7.35 to 7.45 (slightly alkaline). Cell function is seriously impaired when pH falls to 7.2 or lower or rises to 7.55 or higher (see Laboratory Values, Chapter 35).

Three physiologic systems act interdependently to maintain normal serum pH: immediate buffering of excess acid or base by the *blood buffer systems*, excretion of acid by the *lungs* (occurs within hours), and excretion of acid or reclamation of base by the *kidneys* (occurs within days). The four general classes of acid-base imbalance are respiratory acidosis, respiratory alkalosis, metabolic acidosis, and metabolic alkalosis. Table 4–17 summarizes these four imbalances (see also Table 35–9).

Acidosis refers to any pathologic process causing a relative excess of acid in the body. This can occur as a result of accumulation of acid or depletion of the alkaline reserve (bicarbonate content, HCO_3^-) in the blood and body tissues. *Acidemia* refers to excess acid in the blood and does not necessarily confirm an underlying pathologic process. The same distinction may be made between the terms *alkalosis* and *alkalemia;* alkalosis indicates a primary condition resulting in excess base in the body. Although efforts have been made to standardize acid-base terminology, these terms are often used interchangeably.

Incidence. The incidence of acid-base imbalances in hospital settings is high. One study (Palange, 1990) reported an overall incidence of acid-base imbalances of 56%, with

TABLE 4-16 ASSESSMENT OF FLUID AND ELECTROLYTE IMBALANCE

Area	Fluid Excess/Electrolyte Imbalance	Fluid Loss/Electrolyte Imbalance
Head and neck	Distended neck veins, facial edema	Thirst, dry mucous membranes
Extremities	Dependent edema, "pitting," discomfort from weight of bed covers	Muscle weakness, tingling, tetany
Skin	Warm, moist, taut, cool feeling when edematous	Dry, decreased turgor
Respiration	Dyspnea, orthopnea, productive cough, moist breath sounds	Changes in rate and depth of breathing
Circulation	Hypertension, jugular pulse visible at 45° sitting angle, atrial arrhythmias	Pulse rate irregularities, arrhythmia, postural hypotension, tachycardia
Abdomen	Increased girth, fluid wave	Abdominal cramps

Adapted from Phipps WJ, Long BC, Woods NF, et al (eds): Medical Surgical Nursing: Concepts and Clinical Practice, ed 4. St. Louis, Mosby–Year Book, 1991, p 561.

TABLE 4–17 OVERVIEW OF ACID-BASE IMBALANCES

MECHANISM	ETIOLOGY	CLINICAL MANIFESTATIONS	TREATMENT
Respiratory Acidosis			
Hypoventilation	COPD Neuromuscular disease Guillain-Barré Myasthenia gravis Respiratory center depression Drugs Barbiturates Sedatives Narcotics Anesthetics CNS lesions Tumor Stroke Inadequate mechanical ventilation	Restlessness, disorientation, confusion, sleepiness, coma, headache, dyspnea, cyanosis, decreased deep tendon reflexes, hyperkalemia, pH <7.35, Pa_{CO_2} >45 mm Hg	Treat underlying cause; support ventilation; correct electrolyte imbalance
Excess CO_2 production	Hypermetabolism Sepsis Burns Total parenteral nutrition Enteral feeding (gastrostomy)		
Respiratory Alkalosis			
Hyperventilation	Hypoxemia Emphysema Pneumonia ARDS Impaired lung expansion Pulmonary fibrosis Ascites Scoliosis Pregnancy* Congestive heart failure Pulmonary embolism Stimulation of respiratory center Bacterial toxins (sepsis) Ammonia (hepatic failure) Salicylates (aspirin overdose) CNS trauma CNS tumor Excessive exercise Extreme stress Severe pain	Tachypnea, dizziness, difficulty concentrating, numbness and tingling, blurred vision, diaphoresis, dry mouth, muscle cramps, carpopedal spasms, muscle twitching and weakness, arrhythmias, pH >7.45, Pa_{CO_2} <35 mm Hg, hypokalemia, hypocalcemia (see Table 4–14)	Treat underlying cause; increase CO_2 retention (rebreathing, sedation)
Metabolic Acidosis			
Acid excess	Renal failure Diabetic or alcoholic ketoacidosis Lactic acidosis Ingested toxins Aspirin Antifreeze Severe diarrhea	Hyperventilation (compensatory), muscular twitching, weakness, malaise, nausea, vomiting, diarrhea, headache, hyperkalemia, pH <7.35, HCO_3^- <22 mm Hg, Pa_{CO_2} normal or slightly decreased, coma (death)	Treat underlying cause, correct electrolyte imbalance sodium bicarbonate ($NaCO_3$)
Base deficit	Renal failure		
Metabolic Alkalosis			
Fixed acid loss (with base excess)	Hypokalemia Diuresis Steroids Vomiting Nasogastric suctioning	Hypoventilation (compensatory); dysrhythmias, nausea, prolonged vomiting, diarrhea, confusion, irritability, agitation, restlessness, muscle twitching, cramping, weakness, Trousseau's sign, paresthesias, convulsions, coma, hypokalemia, hypocalcemia, pH >7.45, Pa_{CO_2} normal or slightly increased	Treat underlying cause; administer potassium chloride
Excessive HCO_3^- intake	Peptic ulcer Milk-alkali syndrome Excessive intake of antacids Overcorrection of acidosis Massive blood transfusion		

Table continued on following page

TABLE 4–17 Overview of Acid-Base Imbalances (Continued)

Mechanism	Etiology	Clinical Manifestations	Treatment
Metabolic Alkalosis			
Excessive HCO_3^- resorption	Hyperaldosteronism Cushing's disease Licorice intoxication (rare)		

COPD, chronic obstructive pulmonary disease; ARDS, adult respiratory distress syndrome.
* In the third trimester of pregnancy, the hormone progesterone also stimulates respiration.
Adapted from Hansen MJ: Acid-Base Imbalances. *In* Black JM, Matassarin-Jacobs E (eds.): Luckmann and Sorensen's Medical-Surgical Nursing, ed 4. Philadelphia, WB Saunders, 1993, pp 303–304.

respiratory alkalosis being the most common imbalance, followed by respiratory acidosis, metabolic alkalosis, and metabolic acidosis. Ten percent of the population studied had more than one acid-base imbalance at the same time.

Clinical Manifestations. A guide to the clinical presentation of acid-base imbalances is shown in Table 4–18. Besides the major distinguishing characteristics of acid-base imbalance described in this chapter, potassium excess (hyperkalemia) is associated with both respiratory and metabolic acidosis, and neuromuscular hyperexcitability is associated with both respiratory and metabolic alkalosis (Dean, 1996).

Medical Management

Diagnosis. The blood test used most often to measure the effectiveness of ventilation and oxygen transport is oxygen saturation. However, this test only provides information about the levels of arterial oxygen and does not provide information about carbon dioxide level or pH. A more comprehensive procedure is the arterial blood gas test (ABG). (See Laboratory Values, Table 35–21.) This measurement is important in the diagnosis and treatment of ventilation, oxygen transport, and acid-base problems. The test measures the amount of dissolved oxygen and carbon dioxide in arterial blood and indicates acid-bases status by measurement of the arterial blood pH. The pH is inversely proportional to the hydrogen ion concentration in the blood. Therefore, as the hydrogen ion concentration increases (acidosis), the pH decreases; as the hydrogen ion concentration decreases (alkalosis), the pH increases.

The pCO_2 is a measure of the partial pressure of carbon dioxide in the blood. pCO_2 is termed the respiratory component in acid-base measurement, because the carbon dioxide level is primarily controlled by the lungs. As the carbon dioxide level increases, the pH decreases (respiratory acidosis); as the carbon dioxide level decreases, the pH increases (respiratory alkalosis) (Pagana and Pagana, 1995).

TABLE 4–18 Signs and Symptoms of Common Acid-Base Disturbances

Respiratory Acidosis	Metabolic Acidosis
Hypercapnia	Bicarbonate deficit
Hypoventilation	Hyperventilation
Headache	Headache
Visual disturbances	Mental dullness
Confusion	Deep respirations
Drowsiness	Stupor
Coma	Coma
Hyperkalemia	Hyperkalemia
Ventricular fibrillation	Cardiac arrhythmias
Depressed deep tendon reflexes	
Respiratory Alkalosis	**Metabolic Alkalosis**
Hypocapnia	Bicarbonate excess
Lightheadedness	Depressed respirations
Numbness/tingling of digits	Numbness/tingling of digits
Tetany	Muscle twitching, tetany
Convulsions	Convulsions
Hypokalemia	Hypokalemia
Cardiac arrhythmias	Cardiac arrhythmias

Adapted from Dean E: Monitoring systems in the intensive care unit. *In* Frownfelter D, Dean E: Principles and Practice of Cardiopulmonary Physical Therapy, ed 3. Chicago, Mosby–Year Book, 1996, p. 236.

Treatment. Treatment in acid-base imbalances is directed toward the underlying cause as well as toward correction of any coexisting electrolyte imbalance. For example, respiratory infections contributing to ventilatory failure are managed with appropriate antibiotic therapy. Use of pharmaceutical agents that depress the respiratory control center is minimized. Dialysis may be indicated in renal failure or overdose of toxins. Respiratory support may be required via hydration, pulmonary hygiene, oxygen therapy, and possibly, continuous mechanical ventilation.

Respiratory Acidosis *(O'Toole, 1992)*

Respiratory acidosis is nearly always due to hypoventilation and subsequent retention of carbon dioxide. In a therapy setting, respiratory acidosis is most commonly observed in the population with chronic obstructive pulmonary disease (COPD), whenever the diaphragm is impaired (e.g., Guillain-Barrè syndrome, myasthenia gravis, chest wall deformities), secondary to burns, and as a result of lesions of the CNS (e.g., tumor, stroke, muscular dystrophy).

The respiratory system has an important role in maintaining acid-base equilibrium. In response to an increase in the hydrogen ion concentration in body fluids, the respiratory rate increases, causing more carbon dioxide (CO_2) to be released from the lung. Anything that impairs this CO_2 exhalation causes the CO_2 to accumulate in the blood, where it unites with water to form carbonic acid (H_2CO_3), decreasing the blood pH.

Respiratory acidosis can be acute, due to a sudden failure in ventilation, or chronic, as with long-term pulmonary disease (e.g., COPD). In the *acute* episode, the blood buffer systems cannot compensate to restore the acid-base balance because normal blood circulation and tissue perfusion are impaired. The lungs and kidneys are little help because the lungs are malfunctioning and the kidneys require more time to compensate than the acute condition permits. *Chronic* respiratory acidosis results from gradual and irreversible loss of ventilatory function. Although there is increased retention of CO_2, the kidneys have time to compensate by retaining bicarbonate and thereby maintaining a pH within tolerable limits. However, if even a minor respiratory infection develops, the person is subjected to a rapidly developing state of acute acidosis, because the lungs cannot remove more than a minimal amount of CO_2.

Clinical Manifestations. Acute respiratory acidosis produces CNS disturbances that reflect changes in the pH of cerebrospinal fluid (CSF) rather than increased CO_2 levels in cerebral circulation. Effects range from restlessness, confusion, and apprehension to somnolence (sleepiness), with a fine or flapping tremor (see Asterixis, Chapter 14), or coma. The person may report headaches and shortness of breath with retraction and use of accessory muscles. On examination, deep tendon reflexes may be depressed. This disorder may also cause cardiovascular abnormalities, such as tachycardia, hypertension, atrial and ventricular arrhythmias, and, in severe acidosis, hypotension with vasodilation (bounding pulses and warm periphery) (Norris et al., 1995).

Respiratory Alkalosis

Respiratory alkalosis, the opposite of respiratory acidosis, occurs as a result of an accumulation of base or loss of acid without compensation, most commonly when the lungs excrete excessive amounts of carbon dioxide (hyperventilation). Conditions associated with respiratory alkalosis fall into two categories: *pulmonary*, caused by hypoxemia in early-stage pulmonary problems (e.g., pulmonary edema, pulmonary embolism, pneumonia, and acute asthma), and by overuse of a mechanical ventilator, and *nonpulmonary*, which includes anxiety, hysteria, pain, hypoxia, fever, high environmental temperature, pregnancy, poisoning, early cerebral vascular accident (CVA), and central nervous system disease (see Table 4–17) (O'Toole, 1992).

Clinical Manifestations. The cardinal sign of respiratory alkalosis is deep, rapid breathing, possibly exceeding 40 breaths/minute (much like the Kussmaul's respirations that characterize diabetic acidosis) (see Table 4–18). Such hyperventilation usually leads to CNS and neuromuscular disturbances, such as dizziness or light-headedness (due to below-normal CO_2 levels that decrease cerebral blood flow), inability to concentrate, tingling and numbness of the extremities and around the mouth, blurred vision, diaphoresis, dry mouth, muscle cramps, carpopedal (wrist and foot) spasms, twitching (possibly progressing to tetany), and muscle weakness. Severe respiratory alkalosis may cause cardiac arrhythmias, convulsions, and syncope (Norris et al., 1995).

Metabolic Acidosis

Metabolic acidosis is an accumulation of acids or a deficit of bases, usually resulting from an accumulation in the blood of acids (e.g., ketone bodies and lactic acid, or, in the presence of renal impairment, phosphoric or sulfuric acids). This type of acidosis can occur with an acid gain (e.g., diabetic ketoacidosis, lactic acidosis, poisoning, renal failure) or bicarbonate loss (e.g., diarrhea; see Table 13–2). Specific etiologies are listed in Table 4–17. *Ketoacidosis* occurs when insufficient insulin for the proper use of glucose results in increased breakdown of fat. This accelerated fat breakdown produces ketones and other acids. While the body attempts to neutralize these increased acids, the plasma bicarbonate (HCO_3^-) is used up. In the case of *renal failure*, the failing kidney cannot rid the body of excess acids and cannot produce the necessary bicarbonate to buffer the acid load that is accumulating in the body. *Lactic acidosis* occurs as excess lactic acid is produced during strenuous exercise or when oxygen is insufficient for proper use of carbohydrate, glucose, and water. *Severe diarrhea* depletes the body of highly alkaline intestinal and pancreatic secretions (Lehman, 1995).

Clinical Manifestations. The symptoms of metabolic acidosis can include muscular twitching, weakness, malaise, nausea, vomiting, diarrhea, and headache (see Table 4–18). Compensatory hyperventilation may occur as a result of stimulation of the hypothalamus. As the acid level goes up, these symptoms progress to stupor, unconsciousness, coma, and death. The breath may have a fruity odor in the presence of acetone associated with ketoacidosis.

Metabolic Alkalosis

Metabolic alkalosis occurs when there is either an abnormal loss of acid or excess accumulation of bicarbonate. This condition is associated with hypokalemia (potassium deficiency) commonly seen in hospitalized clients secondary to taking certain medications (e.g., diuretics, steroids). Postoperative loss of acids through vomiting or gastric suctioning may also result in metabolic alkalosis. In the outpatient setting, excessive use of antacids and milk (milk alkali syndrome) may occur in people with peptic ulcers associated with NSAIDs. Other causes are listed in Table 4–17.

Clinical Manifestations. Signs and symptoms occur as the body attempts to correct the acid-base imbalance, primarily through hypoventilation. Respirations are shallow and slow as the lungs attempt to compensate by building up carbonic acid stores. Clinical manifestations may be mild at first, with muscle weakness, irritability, confusion, and muscle twitching (see Table 4–18). If untreated, the condition progresses and the person may become comatose, with possible convulsive seizures and respiratory paralysis.

Aging and Acid-Base Regulation *(Hansen, 1993)*

The normal aging process results in decreased ventilatory capacity as well as loss of alveolar surface area for gas exchange; thus, the elderly are prone to respiratory acidosis due to hypoventilation and to respiratory alkalosis due to hypoxemia. Elderly persons are frequently taking multiple medications for hypertension or cardiovascular disease; these drugs may contribute to hypokalemia (potassium deficiency) and metabolic alkalosis. Respiratory compensation in these conditions can be compromised owing to the structural and functional changes mentioned. Decreased cardiac output in the aging person diminishes renal perfusion and glomerular filtration. Aldosterone is less effective in the elderly, as is ammonia buffering. These changes limit renal compensation for respiratory imbalances and place the individual at higher risk for metabolic imbalance.

Special Implications for the Therapist **4-11**

ACID-BASE IMBALANCES

The therapist must observe clients at risk for acid-base imbalance for any early symptoms. This is especially true for persons with known pulmonary, cardiovascular, or renal disease; clients in a hypermetabolic state, such as occurs in fever, sepsis, or burns; clients receiving total parenteral nutrition or enteral tube feedings that are high in carbohydrate; mechanically ventilated clients; clients with insulin-dependent diabetes; elderly clients, whose age-related decreases in respiratory and renal function may limit their ability to compensate for acid-base disturbances; and clients with vomiting, diarrhea (see Table 13–2), or enteric drainage (Hansen, 1993). Specific reference values in acid-base disorders are listed in Tables 4–17 and 35–9.

Client and family education in the prevention of acute episodes of metabolic acidosis, particularly diabetic ketoacidosis, is essential. A fruity breath odor from rising acid levels (acetone) may be detected by the therapist treating someone who has uncontrolled diabetes. The therapist should not be hesitant to ask the client about this breath odor, as immediate medical intervention is required for diabetic ketoacidosis. Always monitor the vital signs of a person with diabetes. A rising pulse rate and a drop in blood pressure occur in the presence of metabolic acidosis.

Safety measures to avoid injury during involuntary muscular contractions are the same as for convulsions or epileptic seizures. Vigorous restraint can cause orthopedic injuries as the muscles contract strongly against resistance. Placing padding to protect the person is a key to prevention of injury.

Measures that facilitate breathing are essential to client care during respiratory acidosis. Frequent turning, coughing, and deep breathing exercises to encourage oxygen-carbon dioxide exchange are beneficial. Postural drainage, unless contraindicated by the client's condition, may be effective in promoting adequate ventilation (O'Toole, 1992).

In the case of respiratory hyperventilation, rebreathing carbon dioxide in a paper sack is helpful, as is encouraging the individual to hold the breath. Oxygen may be given to reduce respiratory effort and the resultant blowing off of CO_2 in the person who has anoxia caused by pulmonary infection or congestive heart failure. Individuals with COPD may retain CO_2; the use of oxygen is contraindicated in these clients, as it can further depress the respiratory drive, causing death.

Any client receiving diuretic therapy must be monitored for signs of potassium depletion (e.g., postural hypotension, muscle weakness, and fatigue; see Table 4–14) and alkalosis (see Tables 4–17 and 4–18). Decreased respiratory rate may be an indication of compensation by the lungs, but this assessment must be made by the physician. Signs of neural irritability, such as Trousseau's sign (see Fig. 4–4) may be seen when taking blood pressure measurements, and they are helpful in detecting early stages of tetany due to calcium deficiency.

References

Abrams WB, Beer MH, Berkow R (eds): The Merck Manual of Geriatrics, ed 2. Rahway, NJ, Merck & Co, 1995.

Adolph EF: Physiology of Man in the Desert. New York, Interscience Publishers, 1947.

Agrawal N: Risk factors for gastrointestinal ulcers caused by non-steroidal anti-inflammatory drugs (NSAIDs). J Fam Pract 32:619–624, 1991.

Andreoli TE, Bennett JC, Carpenter CC, et al: Cecil Essentials of Medicine, ed 3. Philadelphia, WB Saunders, 1993.

Bates DW, Leape LL, Petrycki S: Incidence and preventability of adverse drug events in hospitalized adults. J Gen Intern Med 8:289–294, 1993.

Beal AL, Cerra FB: Multiple organ failure syndrome in the 1990s: Systemic inflammatory response and organ dysfunction. JAMA 271:226–233, 1994.

Berkow R, Fletcher AJ (eds): The Merck Manual of Diagnosis and Therapy, ed 16. Rahway, NJ, Merck Sharp & Dohme Research Laboratory, 1992.

Boissonnault WG, Koopmeiners MB: Medical history profile: Orthopaedic physical therapy outpatients. J Orthop Sports Phys Ther 20:2–10, 1994.

Bone RC: The pathogenesis of sepsis. Ann Intern Med 115:457–459, 1991.

Buckley WE: Estimated prevalence of anabolic steroid use among male high school seniors. JAMA 260:3441–3445, 1988.

Cerra FB, Siegel JH, Coleman B, et al: Septic autocannibalism: A failure of exogenous nutritional support. Ann Surg 192:570–580, 1980.

Chatham WW, Williams GV, Moreland LW, et al: Intra-articular injections: Should you rest joints? Arthritis Rheum 32(suppl 1):R45, 1989.

Choudhury N, Neild GH, Brown A, et al: Thromboembolic complications in cyclosporin-treated kidney allograft recipients. Lancet 1:606, 1985.

Ciccone CD: Introduction: Pharmacology. Physical Therapy 75:342–351, 1995.

Dean E: Monitoring systems in the intensive care unit. *In* Frownfelter DL, Dean E: Principles and Practice of Cardiopulmonary Physical Therapy, ed 3. St. Louis, Mosby–Year Book, 1996, pp 229–247.

Dossing M: Effect of acute and chronic exercise on hepatic drug metabolism. Clin Pharmacokinet 10:426–431, 1985.

Duclos P, Pless R, Koch J, Hardy M: Adverse events temporally associated with immunizing agents. Can Fam Physician 39:1907–1913, 1993.

George E, Kirwan JR: Corticosteroid therapy in rheumatoid arthritis. Baillieres Clin Rheumatol 4:621–647, 1990.

Goodman T: Skin ulcers. AORN J 52:24–37, 1990.

Grant J: Corticosteroid side effects: Implications for PT. PT Magazine 2:56–60, 1994.

Gurecki J, Warty V, Sanghvi A: The transport of cyclosporine in association with plasma lipoproteins in heart and liver transplant patients. Transplant Proc 17:1997–2002, 1985.

Gurwitz JH, Avorn J, Bohn RL, et al: Initiation of antihypertensive treatment during nonsteroidal anti-inflammatory drug therapy. JAMA 272:781–786, 1994.

Haak SW, Richardson SJ, Davey SS: Alterations of cardiovascular function. *In* McCance KL, Huether SE (eds): Pathophysiology: The Biologic Basis for Disease in Adults and Children, ed 2. St Louis, Mosby-Year Book, 1994, pp 1000–1084.

Hamburgh RR: Principles of cancer treatment. Clin Manage 12:37–41, 1992.
Hansen MJ: Acid-base imbalances. *In* Black JM, Matassarin-Jacobs E (eds): Luckmann and Sorensen's Medical-Surgical Nursing, ed 4. Philadelphia, WB Saunders, 1993, pp 297–310.
Harruff RC: Pathology Facts. Philadelphia, JB Lippincott, 1994.
Henson JW, Posner JB: Neurological complications. *In* Holland JF, Frei E, Bast RC (eds): Cancer Medicine, ed 3, vol 2. Philadelphia, Lea & Febiger, 1993, pp 2268–2286.
Hickson RC, Marone JR: Exercise and inhibition of glucocorticoid-induced muscle atrophy. Exerc Sport Sci Rev 21:135–167, 1993.
Hobson L, Webster C: Oncology. *In* Frownfelter DL: Chest Physical Therapy and Pulmonary Rehabilitation, ed 2. Chicago, Year Book Medical Publishers, 1987, pp 608–633.
Houston MC, Weir M, Gray J, et al: The effects of nonsteroidal antiinflammatory drugs on blood pressures of patients with hypertension controlled by verapamil. Arch Intern Med 155:1049–1054, 1995.
Huddleston VB: Multisystem organ failure: Background and etiology. *In* Huddleston, VB (ed): Multisystem Organ Failure. St Louis, Mosby–Year Book, 1992, pp 3–15.
Hunder GG: Vasculitic syndromes: An update on diagnosis and management. J Musculoskel Med 10:50–60, 1993.
Kavanagh T, Yacoub MH, Mertens DJ, et al: Cardiorespiratory responses to exercise training after orthotopic cardiac transplantation. Circulation 77:162–171, 1988.
Kee J: Fluid and electrolyte balance. *In* Black JM, Matassarin-Jacobs E (eds): Luckmann and Sorensen's Medical-Surgical Nursing, ed 4. Philadelphia, WB Saunders, 1993, pp 259–296.
Kokko J, Tannen R: Fluids and Electrolytes, ed 2. Philadelphia, WB Saunders, 1990.
Larson EB: Adverse drug effects: The harder we look, the more we find. J Gen Intern Med 289–294, 1993.
Lehman MK: Acid-base imbalance. *In* Phipps W, Long B, Woods N, Cassmeyer V (eds): Medical-Surgical Nursing: Concepts and Clinical Practice, ed 5. St Louis, Mosby–Year Book, 1995, pp 569–575.
Lekander BJ, Cerra FB: The syndrome of multiple organ failure. Crit Care Nurs Clin North Am 2:331–342, 1990.
Lichtenstein DR, Syngal S, Wolfe MM: Nonsteroidal antiinflammatory drugs and the gastrointestinal tract: The double-edged sword. Arthritis Rheum 38:5–18, 1995.
Loriaux TC: Nursing care of clients with adrenal, pituitary, and gonadal disorders. *In* Black JM, Matassarin-Jacobs E (eds): Luckmann and Sorensen's Medical-Surgical Nursing, ed 4. Philadelphia, WB Saunders, 1993, pp 1837–1862.
Mandel S: Steroid myopathy: Insidious cause of muscle weakness. Postgrad Med J 72:207–214, 1982.
McDonald A: Altered protective mechanisms. *In* Hassey Dow K, Hilderley LJ: Nursing Care in Radiation Oncology. Philadelphia, WB Saunders, 1992, pp 96–125.
Metheny NM: Fluid and Electrolyte Balance: Nursing Considerations, ed 2. Philadelphia, JB Lippincott, 1992.
Moncur C, Williams HJ: Rheumatoid arthritis: Status of drug therapies. Physical Therapy 75:61–75, 1995.
Moots RJ, Bacon PA: Extra-articular manifestations of rheumatoid arthritis. J Muculoskel Med 11:10–23, 1994.
Mulberg AC, Linz C, Tucker L, et al: Identification of NSAID-induced gastroduodenal injury in children with juvenile rheumatoid arthritis. J Pediatr 122:647–649, 1995.
National Cancer Institute: Multiple Myeloma. Bethesda, Md, US Department of Health and Human Services, December, 1991.
Neustadt DH: Intra-articular therapy in rheumatoid synovitis of the knee: Effects of post injection rest regimen. Clin Rheumatol Pract 3:65–68, 1985.
Norris J, McMahon E, Fandek N, et al: Professional Guide to Diseases, ed 5. Springhouse, Pa, Springhouse Corporation, 1995.
Odell WD: Ectopic hormones and humoral syndromes of cancer. *In* Holland JF, Frei E, Bast RC (eds): Cancer Medicine, ed 3, vol 1. Philadelphia, Lea & Febiger, 1993, pp 896–904.
Ostrov BE: Variability complicates systemic-onset juvenile rheumatoid arthritis. J Musculoskel Med 12:26–36, 1995.
O'Toole M (ed): Encyclopedia and Dictionary of Medicine, Nursing, and Allied Health, ed 5. Philadelphia, WB Saunders, 1992.
Pagana KD, Pagana TJ: Mosby's Diagnostic and Laboratory Test Reference, ed 2. St Louis, Mosby–Year Book, 1995.
Painter P: End-stage renal disease. *In* Skinner JS (ed): Exercise Testing and Exercise Prescription, ed 2. Philadelphia, Lea & Febiger, 1993, pp 351–362.
Palange P: Incidence of acid-base and electrolyte disturbances in a general hospital: A study of 110 consecutive admissions. Recenti Prog Med 8:788–791, 1990.
Pandolf KB: Importance of environmental factors for exercise testing and exercise prescription. *In* Skinner JS: Exercise Testing and Exercise Prescription, ed 2. Philadelphia, Lea & Febiger, 1993, pp 87–109.
Parrillo JE, Fauci AS: Mechanisms of glucocorticoid actions on immune processes. Ann Rev Pharmacol Toxicol 19:179–210, 1979.
Paulus HE, Bulpitt KJ: Nonsteroidal antiinflammatory agents and corticosteroids. *In* Schumacher HR, Klippel JH, Koopman WJ (eds): Primer on the Rheumatic Diseases, ed 10. Atlanta, Ga, Arthritis Foundation, 1993, pp 298–303.
Perneger TV, Whelton PK, Klag MJ: Risk of kidney failure associated with the use of acetaminophen, aspirin, and other NSAIDs. N Engl J Med 331:1675–1679, 1994.
Potteiger JA, Stilger VG: Anabolic steroid use in the adolescent athelete. J Athletic Training 29:60–63, 1994.
Prevots DR, Sutter RW, Strebel PM, et al: Completeness of reporting for paralytic poliomyelitis, United States, 1980 through 1991: Implications for estimating the risk of vaccine-associated disease. Arch Pediatr Adolesc Med 148:479–485, 1994.
Price SA, Wilson L: Pathophysiology: Clinical Concepts of Disease Processes. St Louis, Mosby–Year Book, 1992.
Prosnitz LR, Lawson JP, Friedlander GE, et al: Avascular necrosis of bone in Hodgkin's disease patients treated with combined modality therapy. Cancer 47:2793–2797, 1981.
Radack K, Deck C: Do nonsteroidal antiinflammatory drugs interfere with blood pressure control in hypertensive patients? Gen Intern Med 2:108–112, 1987.
Reid DM, Nicoll JJ, Smith MA, et al: Corticosteroids and bone mass in asthma: Comparison with rheumatoid arthritis and polymyalgia rheumatica. BMJ 293:1463–1466, 1986.
Roberts CM, Foulcher E, Zunders JJ, et al: Radiation pneumonitis: A possible lymphocyte-mediated hypersensitivity reaction. Ann Intern Med 118:696–700, 1993.
Sawyer M, Peterson JA, Einhorn A: Closed chain exercises: What it is and what you should know about it. Randall Wellness Newsletter 2:4–6, 1990.
Schlegel SI, Paulus HE: Nonsteroidal antiinflammatory drugs: Use in rheumatic disease, side effects and interactions. Bull Rheum Dis 36:1–8, 1986.
Schols AMWJ: The effects of nutritional support and anabolic steroids on physiologic function in patients with COPD. Am Rev Respir Dis 147:1151, 1993.
Schrier R: Renal and electrolyte disorders, ed 3. Boston, Little, Brown, 1986.
Schumacher HR, Klippel JH, Koopman WJ (eds): Primer on the Rheumatic Diseases, ed 10. Atlanta, Ga, Arthritis Foundation, 1993.
Scott DI, Bacon PA, Tribe CR: Systemic rheumatoid vasculitis: A clinical and laboratory study of 50 cases. Medicine 60:288–297, 1981.
Sikora K: Enraged about radiotherapy. BMJ 308:188–189, 1994.
Singh N, Yu VL, Gayowski T: Central nervous system lesions in adult liver transplant recipients: Clinical review with implications for management. Medicine 73:110–118, 1994.
Skidmore-Roth L: Mosby's 1995 Nursing Drug Reference. St Louis, Mosby-Year Book, 1995.
Snyder R: Coping: You and your patient with cancer. Clin Manage 12:64–69, 1992.
Stauffer JL: Pulmonary diseases. *In* Tierney LM, McPhee SJ, Papadakis MA (eds). Current Medical Diagnosis and Treatment, ed 33. Norwalk, Conn, Appleton & Lange, 1994, pp 207–279.
Thomson AW, Webster LM, Aldridge RD, et al: Cyclosporin and leukocyte procoagulant activity. Lancet 2:1396, 1985.
Valtier B, Mion G, Pham L, et al: Severe hypokalemic paralysis from an unusual cause mimicks the Guillain-Barré syndrome. Intensive Care Med 15:534, 1989.
Wallace CA, Levinson JE: Outcome and treatment for the 1990s. Rheum Dis Clin North Am 17:891–905, 1991.
Weiss MM: Corticosteroids in rheumatoid arthritis. Semin Arthritis Rheum 19:9–21, 1989.
Wujcik D: Infection control in oncology patients. Nursing Clin North Am 28:639–647, 1993.
Yost JH, Morgan GJ: Cardiovascular effects of NSAIDs. J Musculoskel Med 11:22–34, 1994.

section 2

Clinical Medicine

SECTION 2

chapter 5

The Immune System

Catherine C. Goodman and
Teresa E. Kelly Snyder

TERMINOLOGY ASSOCIATED WITH IMMUNOLOGY

Agglutination Clumping antigens together in the presence of specific antibodies to inactivate the antigens.

Anaphylaxis An unusual or exaggerated allergic reaction to foreign protein or other substances such as drugs; venom of bees, hornets, and wasps; pollens; mold; and animal dander.

Antigen Any foreign substance in the body that does not have the characteristic cell surface markers of the individual and is capable of eliciting an immune response; proteins, large polysaccharides, and large lipoprotein complexes that stimulate an immune response are antigens.

Arachidonic acid An unsaturated fatty acid, it is converted into a wide array of inflammatory substances, most notably prostaglandins (PGs) and leukotrienes (LTs); these substances in turn mobilize part of the body defenses that repair tissue and fight infection.

B cell Cells derived from hematopoietic stem cells that mature in the bone marrow (or lymphoid organs other than the thymus); they are responsible for the production of immunoglobulins; also called B lymphocytes, B cells secrete antibodies and are responsible for humoral-mediated immunity.

B lymphocyte See B cell.

Chemotaxis The movement of white blood cells (WBCs) toward the site of the damaged tissue.

Complement A complex of 20 distinct serum proteins which produce a specific effect, in this case, immune cytolysis, that is, dissolution of cells by antibodies.

Cytokines Self-regulating proteins released by macrophages and involved in triggering the immune response; there are five classes of cytokines: colony-stimulating factor (CSF), interferon (IFN), interleukin (IL), tumor necrosis factor (TNF), and transforming growth factor (TGF).

Emigration The process by which WBCs leave the blood vessel and enter the damaged area.

Hapten A molecule, that is not antigenic alone but when bound with larger molecules (carriers), becomes antigenic or immunogenic.

Immunocompetence The ability to mount an immune response.

Immunocompromise A state in which the individual is at an increased risk for infection as a result of an ineffective host state; the individual who is immunosuppressed often is also immunocompromised.

Immunoglobulins Antibodies or γ-globulins of which there are five classes: IgM, IgG, IgA, IgD, and IgE.

Immunosuppression An artificial reduction of immune response that involves the suppression of the production of antibodies or sensitization of lymphocytes, for example, giving drugs that prevent transplant rejection.

Interleukins Interleukins are a large group of cytokines sometimes called lymphokines when produced by the T lymphocytes or monokines when produced by mononuclear phagocytes; interleukins have a variety of effects, but most direct other cells to divide and differentiate.

Interferons Interferons are a family of related proteins called cytokines that are produced by either virally infected body cells or activated T cells for the purpose of amplifying the immune response; they are classified into three major groups: α, β, and γ.

Leukotrienes Made from arachidonic acid, leukotrienes perform a variety of functions; they are many times more inflammatory than histamine or prostaglandin compounds responsible for symptoms associated with allergy; initially helpful because they signal the WBCs to accumulate in an infected area, leukotrienes also produce asthma and hypersensitivity reactions, stimulate suppressor T cells and inhibit helper T cells.

Lymphocytes Any of the mononuclear, nonphagocytic, leukocytes found in the blood, lymph, and lymphoid tissues; they are divided into two classes of immune cells: B lymphocytes and T lymphocytes responsible for humoral and cellular immunity, respectively.

Lymphokines Lymphokines are protein mediators released by sensitized lymphocytes on contact with antigen; believed to play a role in macrophage activation; referred to as cytokines when released by macrophages.

Lymphopenia A reduction in the number of lymphocytes in the circulating blood.

Monoclonal antibodies Antibodies made in the laboratory to specific antigens, for example, to tumor antigens (lymphoma), to cytokines (TNF), to markers on certain T cells (killer T cells) such as OKT3.

Natural killer (NK) cells Cytotoxic T cells responsible for directly attacking and killing target invader cells with which they come into contact; sometimes the NK cells attack and kill the body's normal cells.

Neuroimmunoendocrinology The study of neuroendocrine influences on immune function.

Neuroimmunomodulation The influence of the nervous system on the immune response.

Opportunistic infection Infection caused by microbes that cannot be defeated by a weakened immune system; examples include tuberculosis, candidiasis, *Pneumocystis carinii* pneumonia, cytomegalovirus.

Opportunistic tumors Tumors that may develop when the immune system is suppressed: examples are Kaposi's sarcoma, non-Hodgkin's lymphoma, lymphoma.

Phagocytosis The process by which microbes or particles are engulfed, killed, degraded, and ingested.

Psychoneuroimmunology The study of the effects of psychological status on immune function.

Serotonin A hormone and inhibitory central nervous system neurotransmitter; it has many physiologic properties, including inhibition of gastric secretion, stimulation of smooth muscle, and production of vasoconstriction.

Substance P A peptide composed of 11 amino acids present in nerve cells scattered throughout the body and in special endocrine cells in the gut; it seems to be an excitatory sensory neurotransmitter involving pain, touch, and temperature.

T cell WBC that is processed in the thymus and then produces lymphokines; responsible in part for carrying out the immune response; also called T lymphocyte.

T lymphocyte See T cell.

Tumor necrosis factor (TNF, cachectin) A lymphokine that has many systemic functions; one is to modulate metabolism of fat cells; systemic TNF release may be the final common pathway for the clinical manifestation of shock; use of monoclonal antibodies to inhibit systemic TNF release is currently being investigated; TNF is produced in response to cancer but it is just too much and needs an inhibiting factor (an antibody against TNF).

Immunology is the study of the physiologic mechanisms that allow the body to recognize materials as foreign and to neutralize or eliminate them.[1] There are two nonspecific (or innate immunity) lines of defense against pathogens. The first is the skin and its mucosal barriers and the second is a nonspecific inflammatory response to all forms of cellular injury or death. The primary role of the immune system as a more specific line of defense (acquired immunity) is to recognize and destroy foreign substances such as bacteria, viruses, fungi, and parasites and to prevent the proliferation of mutant cells, such as those involved in malignant transformation.

When the immune system is working properly, it protects the organism from infection and disease; when it is not, the failure of the immune system can result in localized or systemic infection or disease. In fact, the significance of a healthy immune system is apparent in states or diseases characterized by immunodeficiency, as occurs in human immunodeficiency virus (HIV) infection or in persons on immunosuppressive medication. Without an effective immune system, an individual is at risk for the development of overwhelming infection, malignant disease, or both.

Not all immune system responses are helpful, as in the case of organ or tissue transplant rejection. Additionally, excessive or inappropriate activity of the immune system can result in hypersensitivity states, immune complex disease, or autoimmune disease.

The Major Histocompatibility Complex

Since the basis of immunity depends on the immune cells' ability to distinguish self from nonself, all cells of the body contain specific cell surface markers or molecules that are as unique to that person as a fingerprint. The immune system recognizes these cell markers and tolerates them as self, in other words, produces self-tolerance. These cell markers are present on the surface of all body cells and are known as the major histocompatibility complex (MHC) proteins. They were originally discovered on leukocytes and are commonly called human leukocytic antigens (HLAs). There are five specific HLAs within the MHC markers (HLA-A, HLA-B, HLA-C, referred to as class I antigens and HLA-D and HLA-DR, referred to as class II antigens)[2]. The cell markers are essential for immune function. They not only determine which antigens an individual responds to and how strongly, but also allow immune system cells to recognize and communicate with one another.

HLA antigens are inherited and can predispose or increase an individual's susceptibility to certain diseases (usually autoimmune) (see Table 35–17). Such diseases encompass many that affect the joints, endocrine glands, and skin, including rheumatoid arthritis, Graves' disease, psoriasis, and many others. Not all persons with a certain HLA pattern will develop the disease, but they have a greater probability for its development than the general population.

Antigens

Any foreign substance in the body that does not have the characteristic cell surface markers of that individual and is capable of eliciting an immune response is referred to as an antigen. Bacteria, viruses, parasites, foreign tissue cells, and even large protein molecules are recognized as antigens or called "antigenic." On encountering an antigen, the immune system recognizes it as nonself, and the appropriate immune response is mounted against the antigen. A single bacterium contains hundreds of antigenic sites, and therefore has multiple sites capable of stimulating an immune response.

The subunits of an antigen that elicit an immune response are called epitopes. These molecules protrude from the surface of an antigen and actually combine with an antibody (Fig.

[1] For more specific information regarding types of immunity and the structure and function of the immune system, the reader is referred to Bancroft (1994) and Janusek (1993).

[2] Class I antigens are found on nucleated cells and platelets; class II antigens are found on monocytes, macrophages, B cells, activated T cells, vascular endothelial cells, Langerhans' (skin) cells, and dendritic (nerve) cells. There is a third class of antigens (class III) including certain complement proteins (C2, C4, and factor B).

5–1). Each antigen may display hundreds of epitopes. The more epitopes there are, the greater the antigenicity of a substance and the greater the immune response. Antibodies produced in response to an antigen are protein molecules structured in such a way that they only interact with the antigen that induced their synthesis, much as a key is made to fit a lock.

Types of Immunity *(Janusek, 1993)*

Two types of immunity are recognized: innate and acquired immunity. *Innate immunity* acts as the body's first line of defense to prevent the entry of pathogens. Most organisms enter the body by penetrating the epithelial surface of the respiratory, gastrointestinal, or genitourinary tract. These portals of entry are protected by many physical and biochemical defenses such as skin barrier, acid secretions producing unfavorable pH, lysosomes that destroy cell walls of bacteria, phagocytes that engulf and destroy foreign particles, and natural killer (NK) cells which attack and destroy virus-infected cells and tumor cells.

Acquired immunity is characterized by specificity and memory. This type of immunity results when a pathogen gains entry to the body, and the body produces a specific response to the invader. Acquired immunity has a memory so that when the same organism is encountered again, the body can respond even more rapidly to it. These immune responses can occur as a result of active or passive immunity (Table 5–1). Active immunity includes natural immunity and artificial immunity which is intended or deliberate. Active acquired immunity refers to protection acquired by introduction (either artificially by vaccination or naturally from environmental exposure) of an antigen into a responsive host. This type of immunity is expected to last a lifetime but there are occasional exceptions.

Passive acquired immunity occurs when antibodies or sensitized lymphocytes produced by one person are transferred to another. Preformed antibodies made in a laboratory or made by someone else is another form of passive immunity. For example, the transplacental transfer of antibodies from mother to fetus, the transfer of antibodies to an infant through breast milk or receiving immune serum globulin (γ-globulin) provides immediate protection but does not result in the formation of memory cells and therefore provides only temporary immunity. This type of immunity (passive acquired) lasts only until the antibodies are degraded, which may be only a few weeks to months.

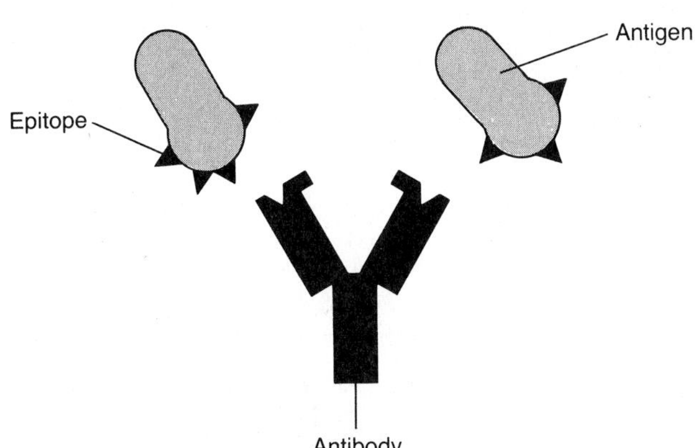

Figure 5–1. Epitopes protrude from the surface of an antigen and combine with the appropriate receptor of an antibody, much as a key fits a lock. (*From Black JM, Matassarin-Jacobs E (eds): Luckmann and Sorensen's Medical-Surgical Nursing, ed 4. Philadelphia, WB Saunders, 1993, p 530.*)

TABLE 5–1 TYPES OF ACQUIRED IMMUNITY

TYPE OF IMMUNITY*	HOW ACQUIRED	LENGTH OF RESISTANCE
Natural		
Active	Natural contact and infection with the antigen	May be temporary or permanent
Passive	Natural contact with antibody transplacentally or through colostrum and breast milk	Temporary
Artificial		
Active	Inoculation of antigen	May be temporary or permanent
Passive	Inoculation of antibody or antitoxin	Temporary

* Active immunity occurs when a person produces his or her own antibodies to the infecting organism; passive immunity occurs when the antibody is formed in another host and is transferred to an individual.
Adapted from Thompson JM, McFarland GK, Hirsch JE, Tucker SM: Mosby's Clinical Nursing, ed 3. St Louis, Mosby–Year Book, 1993, p 1035.

Cells of the Immune System

Throughout the body, there are multiple portals of entry for disease-causing microbes to penetrate. In order to rapidly respond to any pathogen or foreign microorganism, cells, tissues, and organs constituting the immune system are widely distributed throughout the body. In this way, the immune cells remain mobile, able to circulate, moving in and out of tissues searching for pathogens, cellular debris, virus-infected cells, and tumor cells (i.e., immune surveillance). For a discussion of lymphoid organs, see Chapter 11; see also Figure 11–1.

Leukocytes

The immune system contains an immense arsenal of white blood cells (WBCs) or leukocytes aimed at protecting the body against foreign invasion. Infection stimulates WBC production in hemapoietic tissue (site of blood cell formation, e.g., bone marrow, spleen) and leads to an increase in the number of circulating WBCs (leukocytosis). A reduction in the total number of circulating WBCs (leukopenia) occurs in conditions marked by bone marrow suppression, increased peripheral destruction of WBCs (e.g., splenomegaly), or increased "use" of WBCs in the case of overwhelming sepsis. Five types of leukocytes are recognized: the neutrophil, eosinophil, basophil,[3] monocyte, and lymphocyte. Each of these cell types has a specific phagocytic function in the immune system (see Disorders of Leukocytes, Chapter 11). Neutrophils, eosinophils, basophils, and monocytes are classified as cells that function in nonspecific or innate immunity.

[3] Because of their granular appearance, neutrophils, eosinophils, and basophils are collectively referred to as granulocytes. Granulocytes are short-lived (2 to 3 days) compared with monocytes and macrophages, which may live for months or years.

Neutrophils

Neutrophils, the most numerous of these WBCs, derive from bone marrow and increase dramatically in number in response to infection and inflammation. Neutrophils not only kill invading organisms but may also damage host tissues. In the process of phagocytosis, bacteria or debris is engulfed, then digested by enzymes contained within the neutrophils. Neutrophils die after phagocytosis; the accumulation of dead neutrophils contributes to the formation of pus.

Eosinophils

Eosinophils, also derived from bone marrow, multiply in both allergic disorders and parasitic infestations. The exact phagocytic function of eosinophils is not clearly understood. Their products may diminish the inflammatory response in allergic disorders.

Basophils

Basophils circulate in peripheral blood and function similarly to mast cells in allergic disorders. This type of leukocyte has cell surface receptors for the antibody IgE. When cross-linked by an IgE-antigen complex, basophils release vasoactive mediators characteristic of the allergic response.

Monocytes and Macrophages

Monocytes circulate in the blood but when they migrate to tissues, they mature into macrophages, which means "large eaters." The engulfment of a pathogen by a macrophage is an essential first step leading to a specific immune response (Fig. 5–2). After phagocytes digest the pathogens, antigenic material appears on their surface to identify them more specifically as foreign invaders. In this process, phagocytes (primarily macrophages) serve as antigen-presenting cells (APCs) to introduce the pathogen to lymphocytes.

The macrophage or APC processes the pathogen and presents a small part of it (the epitope; see Fig. 5–1) to a specific cell of the immune system known as the helper/inducer lymphocyte, or T4 lymphocyte (also referred to as CD4 lymphocyte[4]). To prompt the T4 lymphocyte to recognize the processed pathogen, the macrophage releases interleukin-1 (IL-1),[5] a chemical messenger with many roles. In this way, the macrophage processes the antigen and then signals the lymphocytes to stimulate the specific immune response. Macrophages also participate in the defense against tumor cells and secrete numerous molecules called monokines that assist in the immune and inflammatory response. Stimulation of macrophages can boost the immune response.

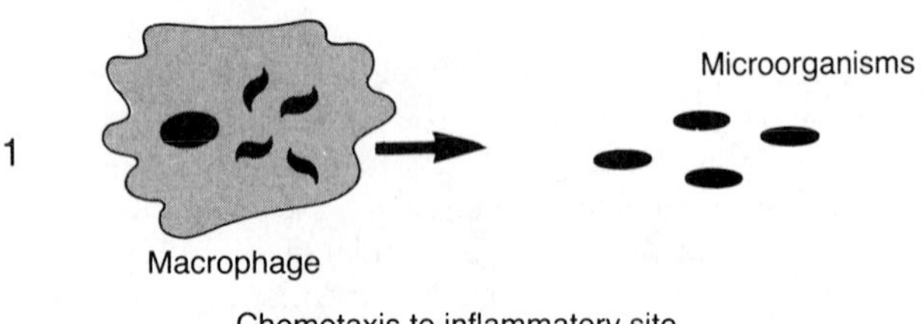

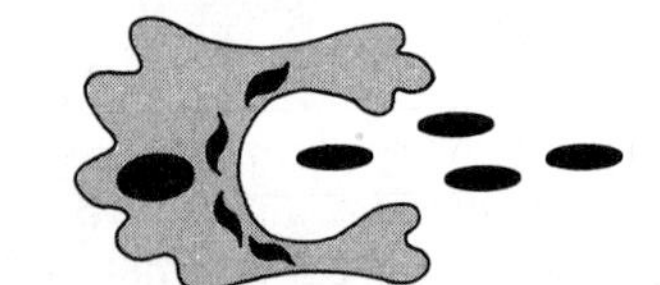

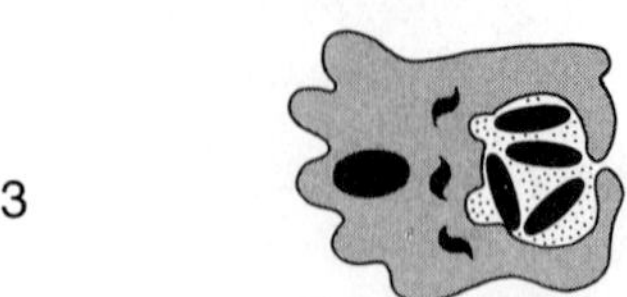

Figure **5–2.** (*1*) Macrophages migrate to an inflammatory site by chemotaxis. (*2*) Macrophages engulf the microorganisms by extending pseudopodia around them. A phagosome or phagocytic vacuole forms around the microorganisms. (*3*) Lysosomes attach to the phagosome and release their enzymes, which destroy the microorganisms. (*From Black JM, Matassarin-Jacobs E (eds): Luckmann and Sorensen's Medical-Surgical Nursing, ed 4. Philadelphia, WB Saunders, 1993, p 533.*)

Lymphocytes *(Wilder, 1996)*

Lymphocytes originate from stem cells in the bone marrow and differentiate or mature into either B or T cells (Fig. 5–3). Both T and B lymphocytes continuously recirculate between blood, lymph, and lymph nodes. The B cell is thought to mature and become immunocompetent in the bone marrow. The surface of B lymphocytes is coated with immunoglobulin or antibody. When stimulated by an antigen, B cells further differentiate into plasma cells or memory cells, which secrete antibodies into the bloodstream. The activation of B cells and the production of antibodies is the component of the immune system called humoral immunity, and it is particularly useful in fighting bacterial infections (see Humoral Immune Response, this chapter).

The T cell differentiates in the thymus gland (see Fig. 11–1) where it learns to discriminate self from nonself. After interaction with a specific antigen, the activated lymphocyte will produce numerous additional lymphocytes called sensitized T cells. This T-cell subpopulation has three primary functions. The most numerous of the T cells, *helper T cells* constituting 75% of all T cells, assist the B cells to mature and produce antibody by secreting protein mediators called lymphokines.[6] Lymphokines enhance the production of antibodies by the B cells following initial response to antigens and also activate macrophages to more effectively promote phagocytosis of invaders. The human immunodeficiency virus (HIV) destroys or inactivates these helper T cells and leaves

[4] Microscopically, T lymphocytes appear identical, but they can be distinguished by means of distinctive molecules called cluster designations (CDs) located on their cell surface. For example, all mature T cells carry markers known as T2, T3, T5, and T7 (or CD2, CD3, CD5, and CD7). T4 (CD4) are the "helper" T cells and T8 (CD8) are cytotoxic T cells. Another group of T lymphocytes are identified as "natural killer" (NK) cells for their ability to kill certain tumor cells and virus-infected cells without prior sensitization or activation.

[5] Interleukins are one type of cytokine, a protein released by macrophages to trigger the immune response. See Cytokines, later in this section. Some of the multiple functions of IL-1 include increasing the temperature set-point in the hypothalamus; increasing serotonin in the brainstem and duodenum causing sleep and nausea, respectively; stimulating the production of prostaglandins, leading to a decrease in the pain threshold, resulting in myalgias and arthralgias; increasing the synthesis of collagenases, resulting in the destruction of cartilage; and most important, kicking the T4 cells into action.

[6] There are many different lymphokines identified, including, but not limited to, chemotactic factor, macrophage-activating factor, interleukin-1, interleukin-2, interferon, T cell replacement factor, and transfer factor.

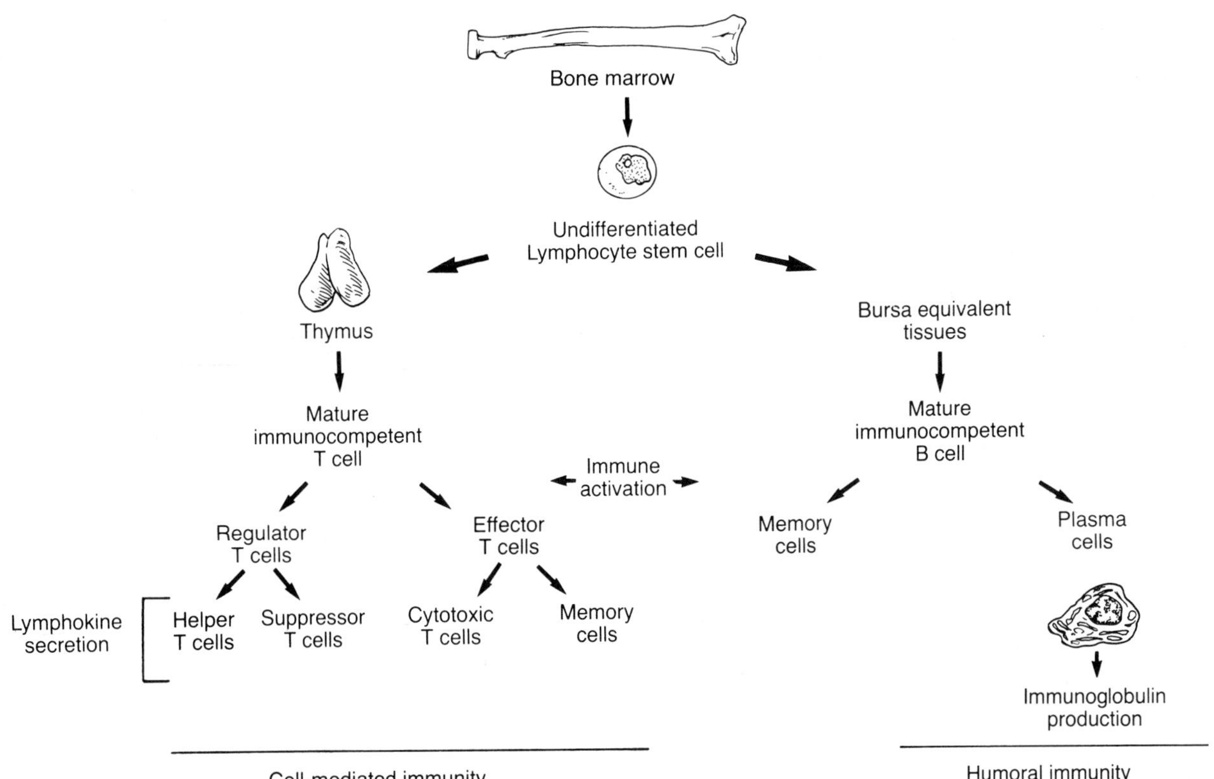

Figure **5-3.** The pathway of lymphocyte maturation. Undifferentiated lymphocyte stem cells are derived from the bone marrow. Those stem cells that are processed in the thymus differentiate into mature immunocompetent T cells, whereas those that are processed in bone marrow become mature immunocompetent B cells. Activation of either T or B cells by antigens leads to proliferation of immune cells that mediate either cell-mediated immunity or humoral immunity. (*From Black JM, Matassarin-Jacobs E (eds): Luckmann and Sorensen's Medical-Surgical Nursing, ed 4. Philadelphia, WB Saunders, 1993, p 533.*)

the body at risk for infectious agents such as cytomegalovirus (CMV).

Cytotoxic T cells, also called *natural killer cells,* directly attack and kill target invader cells with which they come into contact, and sometimes kill the body's normal cells. *Suppressor T cells* suppress both helper and cytotoxic T cell functions, thereby reducing the immune response, an important function when the body's immune system attacks its own normal tissue. This recognition and response is known as immune tolerance (Guyton, 1992). The loss of immune tolerance can result in autoimmune disease in young and old.

T lymphocytes contribute to the immune response in two major ways. They are capable of turning the entire immune system "on" and just as capable of turning the entire immune system "off" through the actions of the helper/inducer T4 lymphocytes (the "on" cells) and the cytotoxic/suppressor T8 lymphocytes (the "off" cells).[7] The production and activation of T cells is the component of the immune response called cell-mediated immunity and is primarily responsible for fighting invading pathogens such as viruses, fungi, bacteria, and so on (see Cell-Mediated Immune Response, this chapter).

Cytokines *(Norris, 1995)*

Cytokines are self-regulating proteins released by macrophages. Cytokines are involved in communication between cells and in triggering the immune response, inducing acute inflammatory events, and in modulating the transition from acute to (or persistence of) chronic inflammation (Burger and Dayer, 1995).[8] Cytokines are categorized as (1) colony-stimulating factor (CSF); (2) interferon (IFN); (3) interleukins (IL); (4) tumor necrosis factor (TNF); and (5) transforming growth factor (TGF).

Colony-stimulating factors function primarily as hematopoietic growth factors, guiding the division and differentiation of bone marrow stem cells. They also influence the functioning of mature lymphocytes, monocytes, macrophages, and neutrophils. CSFs are now synthesized and administered pharmaceutically to stimulate WBC production (e.g., filgrastim [Neupogen]) or to stimulate red blood cell production (e.g., epoetin alfa; human albumin [Epogen, EPO]).

Interferons are proteins secreted by various leukocytes that act early to limit the spread of viral infections by protecting noninfected cells. They also inhibit tumor growth. Their primary function is to determine how well tissue cells interact with cytotoxic cells and lymphocytes. *Interleukins* are a large

[7] Autoimmune diseases are possible examples wherein suppressor T8 cells (CD8) are not functioning properly and do not get "turned off."

[8] The mechanisms of cytokine regulation are currently being discovered and described and hold promise for therapeutic potential against inflammatory processes and sepsis. The complex network of signaling pathways (signaling cascade) of cytokines that contribute to modulation of TNF and interleukin bioactivity are just beginning to be unraveled by researchers (Stewart and Marsden, 1995). As more knowledge is gained about the cytokine network in human diseases, additional avenues for treatment through inhibition of cytokine effects are certain to be developed (Arend, 1995).

group of cytokines sometimes called lymphokines when produced by the T lymphocytes or monokines when produced by mononuclear phagocytes. Interleukins have a variety of effects, but most interleukins direct other cells to divide and differentiate.

Tumor necrosis factors are believed to play an important role in mediating inflammation and cytotoxic reactions (along with interleukins). TNFs produce necrosis of tumor cells by eliminating the blood supply to these growths.[9] Small amounts of TNF are beneficial in promoting wound healing and preventing tumors but large amounts are accompanied by symptoms of fever, weight loss, and tissue damage that can cause more problems than the benefits provided.[10] *Transforming growth factor* demonstrates both inflammatory and anti-inflammatory effects. It is believed to be partially responsible for tissue fibrosis associated with many diseases. It demonstrates immunosuppressive effects on T cells, B cells, and NK cells.

The Complement System

The complement system consists of 20 serum proteins which are key components in the inflammatory response. When activated, these proteins interact in a cascade-like process to assist immune cells by coating microorganisms so they can be more easily phagocytosed, and to participate in bacterial lysis. In some cases the invading organisms are eliminated from the body. Sometimes the inflammation produced by the complement cascade (immune response) walls off the microorganism by forming, for example, a cyst or tubercle that protects the rest of the body from infection (Benhaim and Hunt, 1992). This system promotes inflammation but causes some damage to normal tissue around the foreign tissue, and in some cases, the process can be injurious to the host (Bullock, 1992).

Complement activation takes place through one of two pathways. In the classic pathway, binding of the antigen and immunoglobulin (IgM or IgG) forms antigen-antibody complement complexes that activate the first complement component, C1. This, in turn, activates C4, C2, and C3. The second pathway to complement activation occurs when inflammation or coagulation takes place.

THE IMMUNE RESPONSE *(Table 5–2)*

The immune response primarily involves the interaction of lymphocytes (T and B cells), macrophages, and their products with antigens. These cells may be circulating or may be localized in the tissues and organs of the immune system, the thymus, lymph nodes, spleen, and tonsils (see Fig. 11–1).

TABLE 5–2 Unique Characteristics of the Immune System

Self or nonself recognition	Recognizes host cells as nonantigenic and responds only to foreign agents as antigens; in autoimmune disease, there is a breakdown in this distinction, and the immune system attacks host cells as if they were antigens
Antibody production	Produces specific antibodies that target specific antigens for destruction; produces new antibodies in response to new antigens
Memory	Remembers antigens that have invaded the body in the past, allowing a quicker response to subsequent invasion by the same antigen
Self-regulation	Monitors its own performance, turning on when antigens invade and turning off when infection is eradicated, preventing destruction of healthy tissue

Adapted from Thompson JM, McFarland GK, Hirsch JE, Tucker SM: Mosby's Clinical Nursing, ed 3. St Louis, Mosby–Year Book, 1993.

The thymus participates in the maturation of T lymphocytes (cell-mediated immunity) where the cells are "instructed" to differentiate self from nonself. In contrast, B lymphocytes (humoral immunity) mature in the bone marrow. The key mechanisms of the B lymphocytes is their production of immunoglobulin (antibodies) and the subsequent activation of the complement cascade. The lymph nodes, spleen, liver, and intestinal lymphoid tissue help remove and destroy circulating antigens in the blood and lymph (Norris, 1995).

Antigen presentation and IL-1 release by macrophages prompt the T4 lymphocyte to activate the specific immune response. An array of responses is possible including (1) B lymphocyte activation to produce a specific antibody to the pathogen; (2) activation of cytotoxic T lymphocytes and NK cells to directly attack cells that have been transformed by a virus or a malignant process; (3) activation of macrophages and neutrophils to stimulate an increased release of WBCs from the bone marrow; and (4) activation of the suppressor T8 lymphocyte to eventually slow down the immune response so that host damage does not occur (Bancroft, 1994).

Types of Immune Responses *(Bancroft, 1994)*

The two types of immune responses that occur are *cell-mediated immunity* and *humoral immunity*. Although these two responses are often discussed separately, they are two arms of the immune system and work together; failure in one can alter the effectiveness of the other. These two types of responses overlap and interact considerably but the distinction is useful in understanding how the immune system is activated.

Cell-Mediated Immune Response

Cell-mediated immunity is the arm of the immune system that is responsible on a day-to-day basis for the recognition and removal of bacteria, viruses, fungi, parasites, tumors, and foreign tissue. Cellular immune responses are primarily directed by T lymphocytes which represent 70% to 80% of the blood lymphocytes. T cells are thought to originate from stem

[9] Researchers are testing the effectiveness of TNF as a form of cancer treatment by collecting lymphocytes from a tumor, injecting TNF, and then reinfusing these cells back into the affected person in an attempt to increase the TNF's ability to more effectively target and attack the person's tumor cells.

[10] It has been recently discovered that the drug thalidomide inhibits the production of TNF but does not block it completely. Thalidomide was once banned because it caused severe birth defects when taken as a sedative by pregnant women in their first trimester. Researchers have discovered new uses for this drug as a cure for graft-vs.-host disease in bone marrow transplant recipients, to stop drastic weight loss in people with tuberculosis or acquired immunodeficiency syndrome (AIDS), and as an inhibitor of tumor growth (Weinroth et al., 1995; Bron, 1994). The drug is not available for clinical use as yet but clinical trials in the National Institutes of Health are currently underway.

cells in the bone marrow, but mature in the thymus gland (thus the designation *T* for *t*hymus). The T cells develop distinctive receptors on their cell surfaces and proliferate rapidly in the thymus. These cells then leave the thymus and exist mainly in lymph nodes and in part of the white pulp of the spleen, or they may enter the blood circulation and extravascular areas waiting to encounter antigens (Bullock, 1992).

T lymphocytes interact directly with their targets, attacking body cells that have been invaded by pathogens. This direct attack is referred to as cell-mediated immunity and is responsible for the rejection of transplanted tissue, delayed hypersensitivity reactions (e.g., contact dermatitis), and some autoimmune diseases. Cell-mediated immunity is the basis for many skin tests (e.g., tuberculin test, allergy testing). Cellular immunity cannot be transferred passively to another person.

Clinical conditions that compromise the cell-mediated T lymphocyte function include HIV infection and AIDS with a progressive reduction in T4 lymphocytes over the duration of the illness (Jones et al., 1991). The elderly show reduced numbers of circulating lymphocytes (Neiderman and Fein, 1986), and malnourished people show defects in most tests of T cell function (Meakins and Nohr, 1983). Other conditions known to affect T cell number or responsiveness include stress, malignancy, general anesthesia, thermal injury, surgery, diabetes, and immunosuppressive drugs (including corticosteroids).

Humoral Immune Response

The B lymphocytes are responsible for the arm of the immune system referred to as humoral immunity (also called immunoglobulin-related immunity), named after "humors," the ancients' name for body fluids. These cells also originate in the bone marrow and mature in the bone marrow or in some other part of the immune system.

When B lymphocytes recognize a specific foreign substance or antigen, they change into protein-synthesizing cells known as plasma cells and memory B cells (see Fig. 5–3). The plasma cell produces and secretes into body fluids a specific antibody to that antigen. Memory cells produced in connection with humoral immunity circulate between the blood, lymphoid system, and tissues for about a year or even longer. They are responsible for the more rapid and sustained immune response that occurs with repeated exposure to the same antigen.

The B lymphocyte–plasma cell interaction is capable of producing five types of antibodies or immunoglobulins (Ig) in response to specific antigens. Because of these antibodies the humoral immune response may be referred to as the antibody immune response. The five types of antibodies are IgG, IgM, IgA, IgD, and IgE; major functions of immunoglobulins are listed in Box 5–1.

IgM predominates in the primary or initial immune response and is the largest immunoglobulin; because of its size it is found almost exclusively in the intravascular compartment. IgG is the major antibacterial and antiviral antibody and is the predominant immunoglobulin in blood; it is responsible for the protection of the newborn during the first 6 months of life and is the only immunoglobulin to cross the placenta. It is the major immunoglobulin synthesized during the secondary immune response (after IgM initially responds to foreign pathogens) conferring long-term or permanent immunity. *IgA* defends external body surfaces and is the predominant immunoglobulin on mucous membrane surfaces and is found in secretions such as saliva, breast milk, urine, seminal fluid, tears, nasal fluids, and respiratory, gastrointestinal, and genitourinary secretions. *IgD* is the predominant antibody found on the surface of B lymphocytes and serves mainly as an antigen receptor and may function in controlling lymphocyte activation or suppression. *IgE* is a primary factor in eliminating parasitic infections such as roundworms and is therefore significant in the immune responses of people in developing countries where adequate nutrition, hygiene, and primary medical care are lacking. IgE also functions during allergic reactions by lysing the mast cells and releasing histamine in association with allergies, anaphylaxis, extrinsic asthma, and urticaria (hives). This response of IgE is a normal reaction but becomes excessive in people with allergies.

BOX 5–1
Major Functions of Immunoglobulins

- Immunoglobulins directly attack antigens, destroying or neutralizing them through the processes of agglutination, precipitating the toxins out of solution, neutralizing antigenic substances, and lysing the organism's cell wall
- Immunoglobulins activate the complement system
- Immunoglobulins activate anaphylaxis by releasing histamine in tissue and blood
- Immunoglobulins stimulate antibody-mediated hypersensitivity

From Thompson JM, McFarland GK, Hirsch JE, Tucker SM: Mosby's Clinical Nursing, ed 3. St Louis, Mosby–Year Book, 1993, p 1034.

The type of antibody produced depends on genetic variability, the specific antigenic stimulus, and whether it is a first or subsequent exposure to that antigen. The humoral immune response is more rapid than the cell-mediated response and is more frequently a factor in resistance to acute bacterial infections. Humoral immunity can be transmitted to another person, either by inoculation or by maternal transfer via placenta or breast milk (Thompson et al., 1993). This transfer is called passive immunity.

Aging and the Immune System *(Brink and Reichel, 1995; Rote, 1994a)*

Aging is accompanied by immune dysregulation as immune function declines with increasing age. There is involution (shriveling) of the thymus, the central lymphoid organ for T cell development.[11] By age 45 to 50 years thymus size is only 5% to 15% of its maximum size (which is reached at sexual maturity). As a result of thymic atrophy, the level of thymic hormone production and the capacity of the thymus to mediate T cell differentiation decreases. No thymic hormone is detected by age 60.

Numbers of circulating T cells do not decrease with age, but T cell function may deteriorate. In addition to diminished

[11] The thymus gland is essential to the differentiation of bone marrow lymphocytes into thymic or T lymphocytes, needed for both humoral and cellular immunity (Fretwell, 1993).

T cell function, specific antibody responses to antigenic challenge diminish by 50% to 80% and there is also increased antibody production against self-antigens (autoantibodies). Aging is associated with the accumulation of mutations in regulatory genes, leading to the loss of coordinated control of cell growth and function. For example, immunologic system cells such as T and B lymphocytes are regulated by specific hormones such as IL-1, IL-2, TNF, and interferon, all of which control proliferation and differentiation in lymphocytes in response to antigenic exposure. How mutations in regulatory genes interfere with hormones such as these to alter the immune response is discussed further in Chapter 7.

Cell-mediated immunity is similarly impaired, apparently by the same mechanisms, as fewer cells are available to mediate the reaction. The diminished cell-mediated immunity can result in the reactivation of dormant infections such as herpes zoster and tuberculosis (Ben-Yehuda and Weksler, 1992). Age-related increase in autoimmune activity is both a cellular and a humoral phenomenon and limited studies suggest that reduced humoral and cellular immunocompetence, reduced suppressor cell activity, and increased autoantibody activity are all associated with reduced survival (Fretwell, 1993).

TABLE 5–3 Factors Affecting Immunity

Aging
Sex and hormonal influences
Nutrition/malnutrition
Environmental pollution
Exposure to toxic chemicals
Trauma
Presence of concurrent illnesses and diseases
Malignancy
Diabetes mellitus
Chronic renal failure
HIV infection
Iatrogenic
Urinary catheters
Nasogastric tubes
Endotracheal tubes
Chest tubes
Intracranial pressure monitor
External fixation devices
Implanted prostheses
Immunosuppressive drugs
General anesthesia
Sexual practices

FACTORS AFFECTING IMMUNITY

(Rote, 1994a)

In addition to the effects of aging, other factors can affect the immune system. These factors may include nutrition, environmental pollution and exposure to chemicals that influence the host defense, prior or ongoing trauma or illnesses, medications, splenectomy (removal of the spleen), influences of the endocrine and neurochemical systems, stress and psychological well-being, as well as socioeconomic status (Fretwell, 1993). These factors, as well as clinical conditions that contribute to an immunocompromised state,[12] are listed in Table 5–3. Some factors such as the iatrogenically introduced interventions listed and sexual practices do not alter the immune system directly but increase a person's exposure to pathogens.

Nutritional status can have a profound effect on immune function. Severe deficits in calorie or protein intake or vitamins such as vitamin A or vitamin E can lead to deficiencies in T cell function and numbers. Deficient zinc intake can profoundly depress both T and B cell function. Zinc is required as a cofactor for at least 70 different enzymes, some of which are found in lymphocytes and are necessary for their function. Secondary zinc deficiencies may be associated with malabsorption syndrome, chronic renal disease, chronic diarrhea, or burns or severe psoriasis (loss of zinc through the skin). Dietary changes may alter aspects of immunity, although research in this area is limited (McMurray et al., 1990; Richter et al., 1991). Additionally, morbid obesity may alter the immune system by creating a vulnerability to certain diseases, including cancer (Boeck et al., 1993).

Some *medications* (e.g., cancer chemotherapeutic agents) profoundly suppress blood cell formation in the bone marrow. Other drugs (e.g., analgesics, antithyroid medications, anticonvulsants, antihistamines, antimicrobial agents, and tranquilizers) induce immunologic responses that destroy mature granulocytes. Many drugs also affect B and T cell function, especially against antigens that require the interaction of helper T cells and B cells for antibody production. These complications have been observed since the advent of potent immunosuppressive (e.g., corticosteroids) and chemotherapeutic drugs as treatment of persons with autoimmune diseases, transplants, or cancer. Depression of B and T cell formation is manifested as a progressive increase in infections with opportunistic microorganisms (e.g., *P. carinii*, cytomegalovirus, and *Candida albicans* and other fungi).

Surgery and *anesthesia* can also suppress both T and B cell function for up to 1 month postoperatively (Lynch and Kirov, 1986). Because of the invasive nature of any surgical procedure, and because defects in immunity have been described in most major illnesses, it is logical to assume that the majority of hospitalized surgical clients are immunocompromised to some degree. Surgery to remove the spleen results in a depressed humoral response against encapsulated bacteria, especially *Streptococcus pneumoniae*, *Haemophilus influenzae*, *Staphylococcus aureus*, the group A streptococci, and *Neisseria meningitidis* (see Specific Infectious Diseases, Chapter 6).

Burns cause increased susceptibility to severe bacterial infections as a result of decreased neutrophil function, decreased complement levels, decreased cell-mediated immunity, and decreased primary humoral responses. Blood serum from clients with burns also contains nonspecific immunosuppressive factors that will suppress all immune responses, regardless of the antigen involved.

The relationship between *stress*, *psychological well-being*, and *socioeconomic status* and susceptibility to disease through depressed immune function has recently become an area of intense research interest. In the past, there were anecdotal

[12] The terms *immunosuppression* and *immunocompromise* are frequently used interchangeably to refer to an individual whose immune system function is decreased. However, the two terms are not synonymous. See Terminology Associated with Immunology for definitions.

reports of increased incidence of infection and malignancy associated with periods of both intense and relatively minor stress (see Table 2–7). In the new and expanding world of psychoneuroimmunology, almost any stress seems capable of altering immune function (Eichner and Calabrese, 1994). The role of stress in the development of pathology is discussed in Chapter 2. Likewise, the role of environmental pollution and exposure to chemicals on susceptibility to immune system dysfunction and development of disease is discussed in Chapter 3.

INTERACTIONS BETWEEN THE IMMUNE AND CENTRAL NERVOUS SYSTEMS

(Ader et al., 1991, 1995; Reichlin, 1993)

The role of the nervous and endocrine systems in homeostasis has now been shown to include interaction with the immune system.[13] Two pathways link the brain and the immune system: the autonomic nervous system and neuroendocrine outflow via the pituitary. Immune responses alter neural and endocrine functions, and in turn, neural and endocrine activity modify immunologic function.[14]

Many regulatory peptides and their receptors previously thought to be limited to the brain or to the immune system are now known to be expressed by both. Findings that link immune and neuroendocrine function may help explain how emotional state or response to stress can modify a person's capacity to cope with infection or cancer and influence the course of autoimmune disease. Whether emotional factors can influence the course of autoimmune disease, cancer, and infection in humans is a subject of intense research that has not been clearly elucidated as yet.

The CNS can be involved in immune reactions arising from within the brain or in response to peripheral immune stimuli. Activated immunocompetent cells such as monocytes, lymphocytes, and macrophages can cross the blood-brain barrier and take up residence in the brain, where they secrete their full repertoire of cytokines and other inflammatory mediators such as leukotrienes and prostaglandins. All aspects of immune and complement cascades can occur in the brain.

A number of cytokines called neurocytokines (e.g., IL-1, -2, -4, and -6, neuroleukin, and TNF-α) are formed by glia (the supporting structure of nervous tissue) (Benveniste, 1992; Gurney et al., 1986). The activation of cytokines in the CNS occurs in response to local tissue injury and can lead to profound changes in neural functions, ranging from mild behavioral disturbances to anorexia, drowsiness, sleep disturbances, coma, dementia, and the destruction of neurons (Benveniste, 1992; Dinarello and Wolff, 1993). The activation of cytokines in neural tissue by injury or toxins has a positive benefit as well by stimulating the production of nerve growth factor (Friedman et al., 1990).

Based on studies utilizing animal models, researchers suggest that immunocompetence can be regulated by the brain. Much of this neuroimmunomodulation takes place through the hypothalamic-pituitary system but also through the sympathetic nervous system, the latter by the release of catecholamines at autonomic nerve endings and from the adrenal medulla. The principal immunoregulatory organs (lymph nodes, thymus, spleen, and intestinal Peyer's patches) are abundantly supplied by autonomic nerve fibers (Felten et al., 1985). Sensory neurons contain a variety of neurotransmitters and neuropeptides that can influence lymphocyte function but it remains unknown whether these secretions have a systemic effect.

IMMUNOLOGY AND EXERCISE *(Eichner and Calabrese, 1994)*

Much research interest today centers on the exercise-associated changes in numbers or function of lymphocytes and granulocytes, and in levels of immunoglobulins and the implications for interactions with viral infections, especially HIV infection (see also HIV and Exercise, this chapter). In general, these immune changes are mixed, mild, and brief. Clinical studies are not consistently conclusive and eliminating cofactors, especially the impact of psychological stress, is difficult (Eichner, 1993).

Brisk exercise (even brief, heavy exertion, such as maximal bicycle ergometry for 30 or 60 seconds) increases the WBC count in proportion to the effort (Gray et al., 1992; Nieman et al., 1992). This exercise-induced increase in WBCs (including lymphocytes and NK cells) is largely the result of the mechanical effects of an increased cardiac output and the physiologic effects of a surge in serum epinephrine concentration.

Further studies on the effect of exercise and the function of NK cells, levels of serum immunoglobulins, and levels of polymorphonuclear neutrophils (PMNs) are underway (Eichner, 1993; Field et al., 1991; Nieman et al., 1990). Most researchers agree that the number of NK cells and the function or activity of these cells in the blood increases during exercise. This phenomenon, referred to as *NK enhancement*, is temporary and seems to be the result of a surge in epinephrine levels as well as from cytokines released during exercise (Sprenger et al., 1992). NK enhancement by exercise occurs in everyone regardless of sex, age, or level of fitness training; however, once a person is accustomed to a given exercise level, the NK enhancement falls off, suggesting it is a response not to exercise per se but to physiologic stress (Eichner, 1993).

Little is known about the effect of exercise on serum immunoglobulins and results of research have had little clinical relevance. Studies of salivary immunoglobulins, proteins that are key in defense against microorganisms in the nose and throat, have shown mixed results. More research is needed for a definitive understanding of this aspect of exercise.

Exercise triggers a rise in blood levels of PMNs (McCarthy and Dale, 1988). The exercise-evoked increase in the PMN count is greater if the exercise has an eccentric component, such as downhill running. If the exercise goes beyond 30 minutes, there tends to be a second, or delayed, rise in PMNs over the next 2 to 4 hours, while the exerciser is at rest. This delayed rise in PMNs is probably the result of cortisol which spurs release of PMNs from the bone marrow and hinders

---

[13] The study of immune responses involving the central nervous system (CNS) has been called neuroimmunology. Newer terms include neuroimmunomodulation, psychoneuroimmunology, and neuroimmunoendocrinology (see Terminology Associated with Immunology, this chapter, for definitions).

[14] The immune system has the capacity not only to sense the presence of foreign molecules but also to communicate this to the brain and neuroendocrine system. This interaction is termed "bidirectional communication" between the immune and neuroendocrine systems (Blalock, 1989).

the exit of PMNs from the bloodstream (McCarthy and Dale, 1988).

After brief, gentle exercise, the PMN count soon returns to baseline, but after prolonged, strenuous exercise, this return to normal may take 24 hours or longer (Eichner, 1993). One study suggests that a bout of vigorous exercise may increase resistance to infection by priming the killing capacity of PMNs, but prolonged periods of intensive training may do the opposite (Smith et al., 1990).

Other immune factors may play a role in exercise and immunologic function. It has been established that strenuous exercise can damage enough tissue to evoke the *acute phase response* in humans (Cannon and Kluger, 1983; Weight et al., 1991). This complex cascade of reactions can modulate immune defense by activating complement and spurring the release of TNF, interferons, interleukins, and other cytokines. Much more research is needed before we can understand the clinical applications of this exercise-induced acute phase response.

Special Implications for the Therapist **5–1**

IMMUNOLOGY AND EXERCISE

For anyone (especially competitive athletes) wondering whether or not to exercise in the presence of an acute viral or bacterial infection (e.g., when manifesting constitutional symptoms), do a "neck check." If the symptoms are located "above the neck," such as a stuffy or runny nose, sneezing, or a scratchy throat, exercise should be performed cautiously through the scheduled workout at half speed. If, after 10 minutes, the symptoms are alleviated, the workout can be finished with the usual amount of frequency, intensity, and duration. If, instead, the symptoms are worse and the head is pounding or throbbing with every footstep, the exercise program should be stopped and the person should rest. If there is a fever or there are symptoms "below the neck," such as aching muscles, a hacking cough, diarrhea, or vomiting, exercise should not be initiated (Eichner, 1992). See also specific exercise guidelines for the HIV-infected person, this chapter.

IMMUNODEFICIENCY DISEASES

In immunodeficiency, the immune response is absent or depressed as a result of a primary or secondary disorder. Primary immunodeficiency reflects a defect involving T cells, B cells, or lymphoid tissues. Secondary immunodeficiency results from an underlying disease or factor that depresses or blocks the immune response.

Primary Immunodeficiency

Primary immunodeficiency disorders are congenital. These disorders are associated with failure of organ development necessary for lymphocyte maturation resulting in dysfunctions of B cells, T cells, phagocytosis, antibody, or the complement system. Other causes of primary immunodeficiency may include a specific enzyme deficiency or an undefined failure of lymphocyte maturation (Harruff, 1994). Table 5–4 summarizes these conditions. No further discussion of these conditions is included in this book because these congenital conditions are rarely encountered by the therapist.

Secondary Immunodeficiency

Secondary immunodeficiency disorders such as leukemia or Hodgkin's disease follow and result from an earlier disease or event. Multiple, diverse, and nonspecific defects in the immune defenses occur in viral and other infections, and in malnutrition, alcoholism, aging, autoimmune disease, diabetes mellitus, cancer, chronic disease, steroid therapy, cancer chemotherapy, and radiation. More specific causes such as AIDS also contribute to secondary immunodeficiency (Norris, 1995).

Iatrogenic Immunodeficiency

Immunodeficiency induced by immunosuppressive drugs, radiation therapy, or splenectomy is referred to as *iatrogenic* immunodeficiency. Immunosuppressive drugs fall into several categories including cytotoxic drugs, corticosteroids, cyclosporin, and antilymphocyte serum or antithymocyte globulin (ATG). *Cytotoxic drugs* kill immunocompetent cells while they are replicating but since most cytotoxic drugs are not selective, all rapidly dividing cells are affected. Not only are lymphocytes as well as phagocytes eliminated but these drugs interfere with lymphocyte synthesis and release of immunoglobulins and lymphokines.

Other effects of this nonselectivity of cytotoxic drugs are discussed in Chapter 4 and may include bone marrow suppression with neutropenia, anemia, and cytopenia; gonadal suppression with sterility; alopecia; hemorrhagic cystitis; and vomiting, nausea, and stomatitis. The risk of lymphoproliferative malignancy is also increased (see Tables 4–11 and 7–9).

Corticosteroids are used to treat immune-mediated disorders because of their potent anti-inflammatory and immunosuppressive effects. Corticosteroids stabilize the vascular membrane, blocking tissue infiltration by neutrophils and monocytes, thus inhibiting inflammation. They also "kidnap" T cells in the bone marrow, causing lymphopenia. Corticosteroids also appear to inhibit immunoglobulin synthesis and to interfere with the binding of the immunoglobulin to antigen.

Cyclosporin, a relatively new immunosuppressive drug, selectively suppresses the proliferation and development of helper T cells, resulting in depressed cell-mediated immunity. This drug is used primarily to prevent rejection of organ transplants but is also being investigated for use in several other disorders. *Antilymphocyte serum* or *antithymocyte globulin* is an anti–T cell antibody that reduces T cell number and function, thereby suppressing cell-mediated immunity. It has been used effectively to prevent cell-mediated rejection of tissue grafts or transplants. See further discussion under Adverse Drug Reactions: Immunosuppressants, in Chapter 4.

Radiation therapy is cytotoxic to most lymphocytes, inducing profound lymphopenia, resulting in immunosuppression. Irradiation of all major lymph node areas, a procedure known as total nodal irradiation (TNI), is used to treat disorders such as Hodgkin's lymphoma. It is being investigated for its effectiveness in severe rheumatoid arthritis, lupus nephritis, and prevention of kidney transplant rejection. *Splenectomy*

TABLE 5-4 Immunodeficiency Disorders

Primary Immunodeficiency Disorders	Secondary Immunodeficiency Diseases	Acquired Immunodeficiency Syndrome (AIDS)
Immunodeficiency disorders associated with B cells or antibody X-linked infantile agammaglobulinemia Transient hypogammaglobulinemia Common variable hypogammaglobulinemia (e.g., autoimmune diseases such as hemolytic anemia and systemic lupus erythematosus) Selective immunoglobulin disorders (e.g., IgA deficiency) Immunodeficiency disorders associated with T cells and cell-mediated immunity Congenital thymic aplasia (e.g., DiGeorge syndrome) Severe combined immunodeficiency disease (SCID) Heterogeneous group of immune disorders in which stem cells fail to differentiate into T or B cells (high susceptibility to any type of microbial infection) Phagocytic dysfunctions Deficiency of antibodies, complement components, or lymphokines, or defects in phagocytic cell metabolic pathways (e.g., Chédiak-Higashi syndrome and chronic granulomatous diseases) Diseases caused by abnormalities in complement system May result in recurrent bacterial infections and increased susceptibility to autoimmune diseases	Diseases in which the immune dysfunction is secondary to other diseases Loss of T or B cells from leukemia or other malignant disorders Tumor invasion of bone marrow Sequelae from surgery, trauma, anesthesia, burns; result of chronic diseases such as diabetes, renal failure, cirrhosis Treatment of cancer Chemotherapeutic agents Radiation therapy Bone marrow transplant Organ transplantation or graft-vs.-host disease Other factors Age Stress Malnutrition Radiation exposure	Human immunodeficiency virus–related diseases Reduction of CD4+ helper lymphocyte cells and functional impairment

Modified from Benjamini E, Leskowitz S: Immunology: A short course, ed 2. New York, Wiley-Liss, 1991; and Lewis SM, Collier IC: Medical-Surgical Nursing: Assessment and Management of Clinical Problems. St Louis, Mosby–Year Book, 1992.

increases a person's susceptibility to infection, especially with pyogenic bacteria such as *S. pneumoniae*. This risk of infection is even greater when the person is very young or has an underlying reticuloendothelial disorder. These persons should be observed carefully for any signs of infection (see Table 6–1).

Consequences of Immunodeficiency *(Schaffer et al., 1996)*

Persons who are immunocompromised from any of the immunodeficiency disorders (see Table 5–4) are at increased risk of developing infection because their impaired immune system does not provide adequate protection against invading microorganisms. Normal mechanical defense mechanisms may be affected (respiratory, gastrointestinal systems). Body flora that are normally harmless (such as *Candida*) may become pathogenic and a source of infection.

Additional risk factors for people who are already immunocompromised include poor physiologic and psychological health status, old age, coexistence of other diseases or conditions, invasive procedures (e.g., surgery, invasive lines), and treatments (e.g., chemotherapy, radiation therapy, bone marrow transplantation). The weakened immune system can cause the person to become susceptible to common everyday infectious agents, such as influenza viruses and *S. aureus*, as well as the more exotic organisms, such as *Histoplasma capsulatum* and *Toxoplasma gondii*.

Special Implications for the Therapist **5-2**

INFECTION CONTROL IN IMMUNODEFICIENCY DISORDERS

Although infection control strategies such as handwashing, standard precautions, and disinfection are important for all people treated in the health care system, they are especially critical for individuals whose immune systems are altered by primary immunodeficiency disorders, secondary immunodeficiency disorders, and HIV infection.

It is important that health care providers stop and

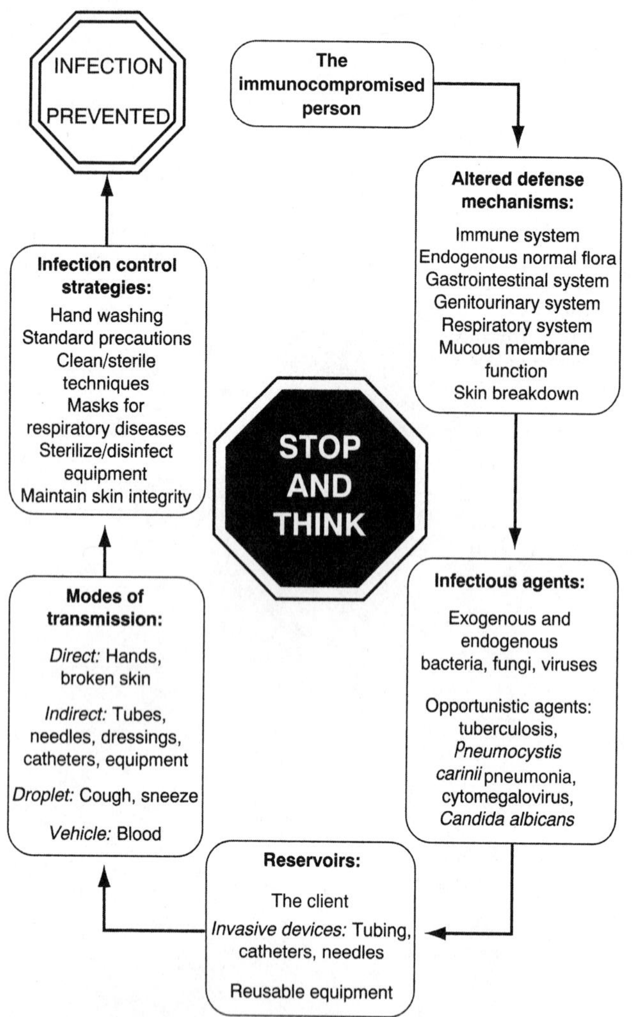

Figure **5-4.** Factors affecting the immunocompromised person, leading to the selection of the correct infection control strategies to prevent infectious complications. (*From Schaffer SD, Garzon LS, Heroux DL, et al: Pocket Guide to Infection Prevention and Safe Practice. St Louis, Mosby–Year Book, 1996, p 222.*)

think about altered defense mechanisms infectious agents, reservoirs, modes of transmission, and infection control strategies to prevent infection in this population (Schaffer et al., 1996) (Fig. 5–4; see also Chapter 7).

Acquired Immunodeficiency Syndrome (AIDS)

Overview and Definition *(Norris, 1995)*. Currently one of the most widely publicized diseases, AIDS was first recognized in homosexual men in 1981. The natural history of AIDS begins with infection by the HIV retrovirus[15] which is detectable only by laboratory tests, and ends with the severely immunocompromised, terminal stage of this disease. Great variation exists among individuals as to the amount of time that passes between acute HIV infection, the appearance of symptoms, the diagnosis of AIDS, and death.

AIDS is characterized by progressive destruction of cell-mediated (T cell) immunity as well as changes in humoral immunity and even elements of autoimmunity because of the central role of the CD4+ T lymphocyte in immune reactions (see Monocytes and Macrophages earlier in this chapter for a discussion of CD4+ cells). The resultant immunodeficiency leaves the affected person susceptible to opportunistic infections, including unusual cancers, and other abnormalities that characterize this syndrome.

The Centers for Disease Control and Prevention (CDC) revised the definition of AIDS in 1992 to include those who are infected with HIV type 1 (HIV-1) and who have a CD4 count below 200/μL (the normal CD4 lymphocyte count is 600 to 1200/μL) or 14% of the total lymphocyte count, even if the person has no other signs or symptoms of infection. The AIDS definition was further expanded in 1993 to include diseases affecting women (e.g., cervical cancer) and persons with tuberculosis or depressed immune systems.

Incidence. At the end of 1993, the CDC estimated that at least 1 million Americans were carrying the HIV virus, most of them asymptomatic, while reports of 355, 953[16] cases of AIDS among adults and adolescents in the United States and its territories (Guam, Puerto Rico, and the Pacific and Virgin Islands) have been reported. Of these known AIDS cases, slightly more than half were white Americans, and the rest were blacks, Latinos, Asians, and Native Americans. Despite being the number one cause of death in American men aged 25 to 44 and the fourth leading cause of death in women in the same age group, the rate at which AIDS is spreading has leveled off and the number of new cases reported annually is declining (Selik et al., 1995).

Estimates of babies born with the HIV virus annually range from 1630 to 1760 but numbers appear to be dropping since 1991, possibly attributable to a decline in fertility among women of childbearing age who are infected with HIV, more abortions, or a stable state of infection among affected women (CDC, 1995).

Etiology and Risk Factors. The primary cause is the retrovirus (HIV) type 1. Transmission of HIV occurs by exchange of body fluids (notably blood and semen) and is associated with high-risk behaviors. Most commonly affected groups include sexually active homosexual and bisexual men, intravenous (IV) drug users who share contaminated equipment, recipients of contaminated blood or blood products (a risk now diminished by routine testing of all blood products), people with hemophilia who received blood products prior to 1985, heterosexual partners of persons in the former groups, and newborns of HIV-infected women (via the placenta from mother to fetus, by cervical or blood contact at delivery, and in breast milk). Additionally, a recent report indicated there is a substantial prevalence of HIV infection among heterosexual

[15] A retrovirus contains reverse transcriptase, an enzyme required for successful infection by the virus. Before viral replication can occur in the host cell, this enzyme must copy all the genetic information of the virus from viral RNA to viral DNA. Once the viral genome is transcribed, it can be integrated into the host's DNA and duplicated many times. This extra step formerly gave these viruses the term "slow" viral infections and previously explained why some people infected with HIV may live many years without signs or symptoms of infection.

[16] These numbers represent only the cases actually reported by physicians; it is likely that many people with AIDS go unreported for various reasons.

alcoholics attributed to unsafe sex practices rather than to IV drug use (Avins et al., 1994).

HIV is not transmitted by fomites (e.g., coffee cups, drinking fountains, telephone receivers), or by casual household or social contact. The average time between exposure to the virus and diagnosis (latency period) of AIDS is 8 to 10 years, but incubation time can vary on either side of those numbers.

Pathogenesis. HIV is a retrovirus that predominantly infects human T4 (helper) lymphocytes, the major regulators of the immune response, and destroys or inactivates them. HIV is unique in that despite the body's immune responses following initial infection, some HIV invariably escapes. Recently researchers have discovered large amounts of HIV "hiding" in the immune cells lining the surface of adenoids (Frankel et al., 1996). This discovery is important because it supports the idea that there is a significant amount of viral reproduction in a person with a latent infection. This information alters the formally held view that HIV–1 is a slow or covert process when in fact the virus's growth continues in the period between infection and the onset of AIDS. It is theorized that the use of a preventive vaccine could stop hidden viral production.

Once HIV enters the body, cells containing the CD4 antigen (including macrophages and T4 cells) serve as receptors for the HIV retrovirus, allowing direct passage of the infection into target cells previously identified (e.g., gastrointestinal tract, uterine cervical cells, and neuroglial cells). After invading a cell, a virus particle called a *virion* injects the core proteins and the two strands of viral RNA into the cell.[17] This replication of the HIV virus can cause cell death, or it may remain latent (dormant and concealed[18]). Seroconversion (becoming HIV positive) takes place during the first 3 to 6 weeks of this replication process, but after a few months, very little virus is found in the blood; only HIV antibodies remain in the serum.

During the period of clinical latency, the virus continues to kill the CD4 cells in the lymph nodes.[19] Once all of these cells are depleted, the virus once again enters the blood and clinically apparent disease occurs (Fig. 5–5). HIV infection leads to profound pathology, either directly by destruction of CD4+ cells, other immune cells, or neuroglial cells; or indirectly, through the secondary effects of CD4+ T cell dysfunction and resultant immunosuppression. The decline in CD4 cells results in progressive loss of immune system function and the development of a wide variety of clinical signs and symptoms (Pantaleo et al., 1993). A decrease in the CD4 count to less than 200 is associated with the development of opportunistic infections (Lane, 1992).

This infectious process may take one of three forms: (1) immunodeficiency with opportunistic infections and unusual malignancies; (2) autoimmunity such as rheumatoid arthritis, lymphoid interstitial pneumonitis, hypergammaglobulinemia, and production of autoimmune antibodies; and (3) neurologic dysfunction including AIDS dementia complex, HIV encephalopathy, and peripheral neuropathies.

The rapid convergence of information from diverse areas of AIDS research makes it impossible to present the most up-to-date information. Scientists are reporting new discoveries daily about the pathogenesis of HIV disease. For example, researchers are studying how different strains of HIV use recently discovered cell surface molecules, in addition to the well-known CD4 molecule, to bind to and enter target cells. Another consideration is how different strains of HIV have a preference for certain cells; strains that infect macrophages and T cells are the main ones found early in the disease. Later, strains appear that replicate efficiently in T cells but not in macrophages. Finally, mutations in the human genes for HIV co-receptors may help explain why some people do not become infected despite repeated exposure and why some who are infected may have different rates of disease progression (Fauci, 1997).

Clinical Manifestations. HIV infection manifests itself in many different ways (Table 5–5). During the latent stage the person demonstrates laboratory evidence of seroconversion (HIV positive) but remains asymptomatic. Some individuals develop an acute, self-limiting infectious mononucleosis-like illness or a more subtle viral-like syndrome followed by a period of clinical latency that may last a decade or more. During that latent period, the infected person is clinically healthy and capable of normal daily activities, normal work habits, and unrestricted level and duration of exercise (Eichner and Calabrese, 1994).

As the infection progresses and the immune system becomes increasingly more compromised, a variety of symptoms may develop including persistent generalized adenopathy; nonspecific symptoms such as weight loss, fatigue, night sweats, and fevers; neurologic symptoms resulting from HIV encephalopathy; or an opportunistic infection (e.g., *Pneumocystis carinii* pneumonia [PCP], cytomegalovirus, toxoplasmosis) or malignancy (e.g., lymphoma, Kaposi's sarcoma).

CMV is associated with HIV retinitis, which can cause blindness and peripheral neuropathy; PCP produces pulmonary symptoms such as dyspnea on exertion, nonproductive cough, and weight loss, and toxoplasmosis is a parasitic disease that affects the CNS. In addition to the symptoms that may occur with opportunistic diseases, treatment with multiple medications can cause adverse side effects, sometimes creating a confusing clinical picture.

The CNS appears to be more frequently attacked by HIV than the peripheral nervous system. HIV or AIDS encephalopathy, also referred to as AIDS dementia complex (ADC), is a primary infection of the brain by HIV. Symptoms range from subtle alterations in memory to obvious confusion and disorientation. Behavioral disturbances include apathy, lethargy, and social withdrawal. Early motor deficits may include

[17] All human cells contain DNA and RNA, known collectively as nucleic acids. The DNA is located in the cell nucleus, and the RNA is located in the cytoplasm of the cell. Viruses contain only one of the nucleic acids and are categorized as belonging to the DNA group (e.g., herpes and mononucleosis) or the RNA group (e.g., measles and mumps). HIV is classified as a lentivirus, a subclass of retroviruses that contain RNA. When the RNA virus intitiates replication in the living host cell, it must convert its RNA genetic information into a DNA template in order to replicate (Minerbo, 1992).

[18] Eventually the viruses in latently infected cells are reactivated and infectious virions are produced and released. By the time this happens, the immune system has been compromised and is ineffective and unable to mount a specific immune response to these virions. The immune system dysfunction is even more exaggerated if the host has become further immunocompromised by opportunistic diseases.

[19] The regulation of HIV expression by modules secreted by immune cells is even more complex than previously realized. The initially expanded clones that can kill HIV-infected cells are found in the bloodstream rather than in the lymph nodes, where the virus is replicating. The gene (*vpr*) within HIV that stops production of the CD4 T lymphocytes has now been identified. Current research focus is on understanding how the *vpr* gene prevents these disease-fighting cells from dividing. New drugs to block the gene's actions and allow immune cells to continue multiplying and fighting HIV would be the next step (Jowett et al., 1995; Levy et al., 1995).

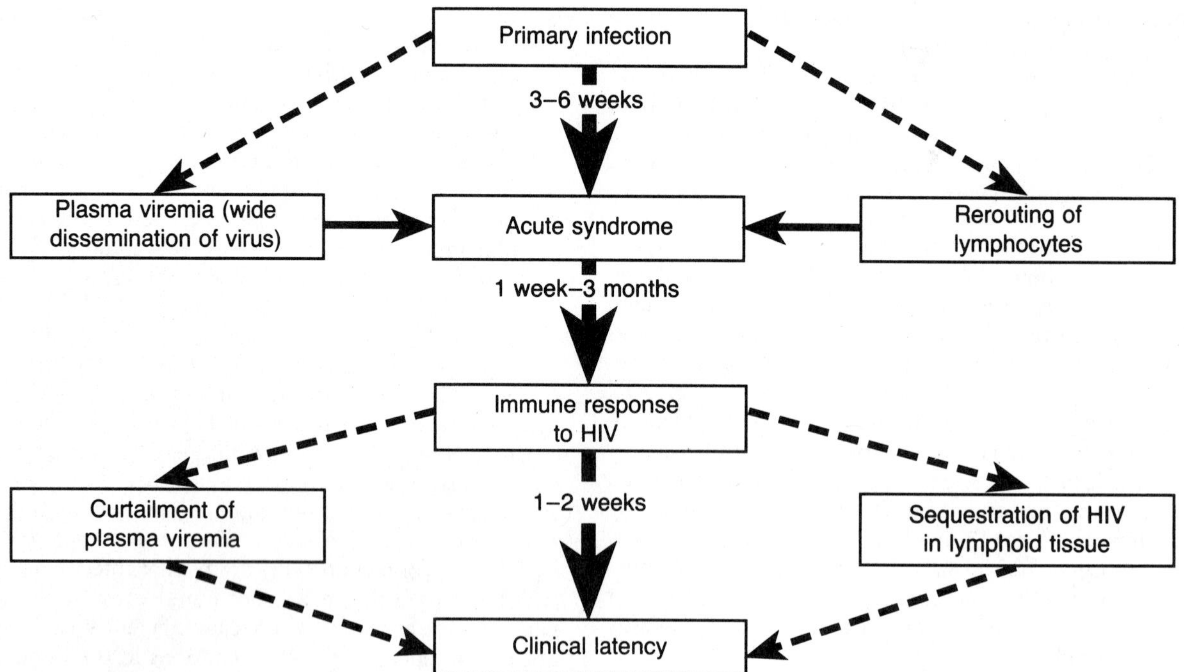

Figure **5–5.** The progression of HIV infection from primary infection through acute HIV syndrome to the stage of clinical latency. (*From Graziosi C, Pantaleo G, Demarest JF, et al: Model of HIV progression: HIV-1 Infection in the lymphoid organs. AIDS 7 (suppl 2):S53–58, 1993.*)

ataxia; leg weakness with gait disturbances; tremor, and loss of fine motor coordination. In the most advanced stages of the disease, severe dementia, mutism, incontinence, and paraplegia may occur. A detailed summary of nervous system disorders associated with HIV (including treatment) is available (Obbens and Galantino, 1992).

AIDS is associated with neuromusculoskeletal diseases such as osteomyelitis, bacterial myositis, non-Hodgkin's lymphoma, and infectious arthritis (Steinbach et al., 1993). Peripheral neuropathy, drug-induced myopathy, and musculoskeletal pain syndromes associated with the wasting process in AIDS may occur secondary to weight loss and malnutrition (e.g., mineral and vitamin deficiencies, especially vitamin B deficiency).[20] As the HIV epidemic affects more women, increasing cases of pelvic inflammatory disease (PID) are being reported (Irwin et al., 1994). Pain is a common symptom in all these conditions.

The pain of peripheral neuropathy is characterized by burning, tingling, hypersensitivity, proprioceptive losses, and in severe cases, secondary motor deficits. Symptoms are usually reported in the hands and feet, but other parts of the body may be affected such as the face or trunk. Polymyositis involves bilaterally symmetrical proximal muscle weakness and arthritis may precede or accompany seroconversion. The arthritis tends to be severe and does not necessarily respond to conventional medications (Steinbach et al., 1993).

HIV-associated myopathy presents with a progressive painless weakness in the proximal limb muscles. The weakness is symmetrical and often involves the muscles of the face and neck. This type of myopathy may occur in HIV-infected clients at every stage of illness (Simpson and Bender, 1988). Muscle biopsies have shown necrosis of muscle fibers with and without inflammatory infiltrates. No evidence has been found of direct HIV infection of the muscle, and the underlying cause has not been determined. The fact that these clients improve on corticosteroids or plasmapheresis may point to an underlying autoimmune defect. Drug-induced myopathy is discussed in Chapter 4.

Medical Management

Diagnosis. In order to establish uniformity in reporting AIDS cases, the CDC has established diagnostic criteria for the confirmation of AIDS. The most commonly performed test is the ELISA (enzyme-linked immunosorbent assay) test, an antibody test to indicate HIV infection indirectly by revealing HIV antibodies (indicating exposure to the virus). However, antibody testing is not always reliable because the body takes a variable amount of time to produce a detectable level of antibodies. This "window" may vary from a few weeks to as long as 35 months in one documented case. Consequently, a person infected with HIV could test negative for HIV antibodies. Antibody tests are also unreliable in neonates because transferred maternal antibodies persist for 6 to 10 months (Norris, 1995). The Western blot test is a more expensive test that may be used when there is a concern about false-positive tests because it is more specific, that is, in identifying individuals with *negative* test results.

The current CDC AIDS surveillance definition requires direct testing including antigen tests (p24 antigen), HIV cultures, nucleic acid probes of peripheral blood lymphocytes,

[20] Studies have shown a clear relationship between vitamin B_{12} deficiency and dysfunction of the central and peripheral nervous systems. Some of the clinical abnormalities of the nervous system seen in people infected with HIV-1 are similar to those that have been described in persons with vitamin B_{12} deficiency. The theory that vitamin replacement therapy should be a treatment approach in treating nervous system deficits in AIDS clients has not yet been proved effective (Robertson et al., 1993).

TABLE 5-5 Symptomatic Classification of HIV Infections

Group I: Acute Infection	Group II: Asymptomatic Infection	Group III: Persistent Generalized Lymphadenopathy	Group IV: Other Diseases
After initial infection brief febrile illness; generalized rash and mononucleosis-like symptoms	Period of asymptomatic infection; normal function; infection can pass to others; may last years undetected	Painless enlargement of lymph nodes usually at 2+ extrainguinal sites	May occur with or without lymph node swelling; 5 subgroups A–E: *Group A:* Constitutional diseases, formerly AIDS-related complex (ARC) or wasting syndrome *Group B:* Neurologic disease including dementia, myelopathy and peripheral neuropathy *Group C:* Secondary infectious diseases such as *Pneumocystis carinii* pneumonia (PCP), toxoplasmosis, cytomegalovirus (CMV), tuberculosis, oral hairy leukoplakia, multidermatomal herpes zoster, oral candidiasis, and others *Group D:* Secondary cancers, including Kaposi's sarcoma, non-Hodgkin's lymphoma, primary lymphoma *Group E:* Other conditions not included in groups A–D

Adapted from Galantino ML: Clinical Assessment and Treatment of HIV: Rehabilitation of a Chronic Illness. Thorofare, NJ, Slack, 1992.

and the polymerase chain reaction (PCR). Additional laboratory confirmation of HIV infection is required; a CD4+ T lymphocyte count of fewer than 200/μL is also considered diagnostic. T lymphocyte counts monitor the progression of HIV.

Treatment. No cure has been found for AIDS. Several different groups are using different strategies to explore various types of vaccines. Until a vaccine is available, the goal of treatment has been to stop HIV from replicating. Treatment approaches have been centered around the use of a combination of anti-HIV drugs (e.g., nucleoside analogues, proteinase inhibitors, reverse-transcriptase inhibitors) to stop HIV from replicating by targeting the reverse transcriptase enzyme (Lipsky, 1996). Viral-load testing is now available that allows a physician to measure the amount of HIV in a person's bloodstream to guide treatment.

In some studies, use of the protease inhibitors, a class of drugs that can stop virus replication with other AIDS drugs, has shown that virus levels can fall to undetectable levels. It remains to be seen if the immune system can recover completely after persistent decrease of viral load to low levels and whether successful treatment can bring lymphocyte activation back to normal. Treatment with these new drug "cocktails" are apparently most effective for people who have been infected only a short time and who still have healthy immune systems. Despite treatment advances, the virus becomes resistant to all of the protease inhibitors and is changing almost as fast as the drugs being developed to fight it. The subtypes of HIV-1 have been identified and labeled HIV-A, -B, -C, -D, -E, -F, and -G.

Other treatment interventions being investigated include the use of interferon-α, and gene therapy and immune reconstitution or restoration. If, as suspected, there are multiple variants of HIV in a single host and the virus is capable of mutating easily, treatment approaches geared toward enhancing host resistance and restoring or building the immune system will be more successful than trying to kill the virus[21] (Bridges and Sarver, 1995).

There is no known curative treatment for AIDS dementia complex (ADC). Palliative and supportive treatment help maintain nutritional status and relieve pain and other distressing physical and psychological symptoms while maintaining as much function as possible. Many pathogens in AIDS respond to anti-infective drugs but recur when the treatment ends. Many clients need anti-infective medications for life or until the drug is no longer tolerated or effective (Norris, 1995).

Prognosis. The development of combination therapies is extending the lives of AIDS clients, keeping many healthy enough to avoid hospitalization. Promising new drug treatment has been so effective for people infected only a short time that some researchers question whether a cure may have been found for this particular group of individuals. For those people long infected with HIV the prognosis remains poor, with secondary infections remaining the leading cause of death in AIDS. However, persons with AIDS are living longer with lower CD4 levels because prophylaxis and treatment of *P. carinii* pneumonia saves many who would have died sooner in the earlier days of the AIDS epidemic (Osmond et al., 1994).

[21] This same principle of using drugs to boost the immune system, called biotherapy, immunotherapy, or immunologic therapy, is also being applied in the use of genetically engineered IL-2 to treat tumors of the kidney and skin (Rosenberg et al., 1994).

Special Implications for the Therapist **5-3**

ACQUIRED IMMUNODEFICIENCY SYNDROME (AIDS)

Prevention of Transmission

Health care workers may be concerned about potential contact with AIDS clients in the workplace. Health care considerations are primarily directed at preventing the transmission of the virus when caring for someone with AIDS. Recommendations for preventing the spread of the virus consist of the use of universal precautions (see Appendix A: Summary of Universal Precautions). Specific recommendations for health care professionals working with AIDS and HIV-positive clients are included in Box 5–2. Everyone with AIDS is immunodeficient and every precaution must be taken to prevent infection for that person.

An HIV-infected person does not need a private room unless there is a communicable disease that requires respiratory isolation (e.g., tuberculosis). Hepatitis would require universal precautions but not isolation. The virus is not transmitted through casual nonintimate contact or social encounters such as eating in restaurants or using public transportation or public bathroom facilities because the virus does not live long or replicate outside the body.

Direct contact of cuts, scratches, abrasions, or mucosal surfaces with material or secretions containing live contaminated virus (e.g., blood, semen, saliva, tears, urine, cerebrospinal fluid, amniotic fluid, solid tissue, and vaginal secretions) is required for transmission of the virus. For the health care worker this means possible transmission may occur through parenteral (i.e., subcutaneous, intramuscular, or IV) inoculation, through needle sticks, broken glass, or spillage of infected material onto the worker's abraded skin or mucous membranes. Neither ingestion nor inhalation has been shown to be a mode of transmission (Cohen, 1990).

Health care workers at potential risk of contact with HIV-infected body fluids include blood bank technologists, dialysis technicians, emergency department personnel, morticians, dentists, medical technicians, surgeons, and laboratory workers. Therapists are not considered at risk unless working in one of these capacities or performing wound care or debridement with an infected client.

Few studies have evaluated the risk of transmission of blood-borne pathogens during sports or athletic activity. However, the risk of transmission of HIV has been evaluated by both the National Football League and the National Collegiate Athletic Association. Both groups conservatively estimate that the risk of HIV transmission on the playing field is well below one per 1 million games (Brown and Drotman, 1993; Dick and Worthman, 1994).

Guidelines for Infected Health Care Workers

Any health care worker with HIV or the most virulent form of hepatitis B should not perform "exposure-prone" procedures in which blood contact might occur. Permission and guidance from special review committees is required before an infected health care worker can perform such procedures. For the therapist, this would primarily exclude wound care including debridement and dressing changes. According to guidelines drafted by the CDC, at a minimum the potential client must be informed of the worker's HIV (or hepatitis B) status if the therapist is to engage in high-risk activity such as debridement or other wound care (CDC, 1989).

HIV and Exercise *(Eichner and Calabrese, 1994; McGrew, 1995)*

Unlike other infections, HIV directly affects the immune system. If exercise has clinically significant effects on immune responsiveness, there is potential to alter the natural history of HIV infection in a beneficial manner through the use of exercise. A growing number of studies are now addressing the issue of the relationship between exercise and HIV infection. The results are summarized here.

Exercise is considered safe for HIV-infected persons and may provide pain relief, reduction of stress, reduction of muscle atrophy, and improved function, as well as enhanced immune function (the latter by increasing the number of CD4 cells) (LaPerrierre et al., 1988, 1990, 1991). Exercise training in the form of moderate aerobic exercise (defined differently with different studies) may attenuate some of the psychological and immunologic sequelae of an acute stressor for both the asymptomatic HIV-infected person as well as for the persons with advanced infection (Ironson et al., 1992; Schlenzig et al., 1989).

Exercise programs to increase strength and body mass are particularly relevant to HIV because wasting is one of the most devastating aspects of this infection. In contrast to people suffering from simple starvation who lose adipose tissue but initially retain lean body mass, people with HIV infection lose lean body mass as well. Exercise training, including strength training, may have the potential to (possibly only temporarily) reverse the wasting effects. The limits of strength training and the

BOX **5-2**

Universal AIDS/HIV Precautions for Health Care Workers (HCWs)

- Use protective barriers (gloves, eye shields, gowns) when handling blood, body fluids, and infectious fluids
- Wash hands, skin, and mucous membranes immediately and thoroughly if contaminated by blood or other body fluids
- Prevent needle or scalpel sticks
- Ventilation devices are available for resuscitation
- Any HCW with open wounds or skin lesions should not treat clients or handle equipment until the lesion(s) heals
- Pregnant HCWs should take extra precautions. See Appendix A, Summary of Universal Precautions

Adapted from CDC (Centers for Disease Control and Prevention): Guidelines for prevention of HIV and hepatitis B virus transmission to health care and public safety workers. MMWR 38:S1–6, 1989.

resultant benefits in strength and body mass have not been determined yet.

The effects of exercise demands on an HIV-infected, high-level athlete in competition on levels of psychological stress and immune function remain unclear. There are potential adverse effects of the stresses of competition such as increased upper respiratory infections in marathon runners (Nieman et al., 1990). Exercise recommendations for HIV-infected athletes are summarized in Box 5–3.

HIV and Rehabilitative Therapy

From a rehabilitation point of view, HIV is considered a chronic illness on a continuum (i.e., from being asymptomatic to exhibiting mild to severe symptoms) rather than as a terminal illness. In addition to physical fitness and strength training, therapists must look at activities of daily living and work simplification. Home programs must be simple and easily incorporated into activities of daily living. Often AIDS clients are overwhelmed by the disease process, the complicated treatment, the multiple health care appointments, and scheduling to manage all of these tasks. Adding an exercise program may result in frustration and noncompliance unless the person can see a clear benefit and way to manage yet another aspect of the treatment program.

For the client with neurologic involvement (e.g., related to toxoplasmosis or AIDS encephalitis), rehabilitative therapy can help the person to regain lost function and recover some skills. These clients seem to respond well to stroke or head-injured treatment programs. PNF (proprioceptive neuromuscular facilitation) and Bobath techniques may be more beneficial for the lower-level functioning clients (Keller, 1994). The therapist must be prepared for seizures which may occur as a result of nervous system involvement, sometimes for the first time during a therapy session.

The presence of peripheral neuropathies may signal nutritional deficiencies requiring nutritional counseling. This is especially true for the client who has the wasting syndrome that often accompanies HIV infection and AIDS. The body may begin to draw from its own stores of fat, affecting the myelin sheaths of nerves which are protected by fat. Without proper nutrition, therapy involving balance training, extremity strengthening and stretching, and motor skills may be limited in benefit.

For individuals with painful myopathy in the large muscle groups, progressive resistance training with weights or Theraband to strengthen specific muscles may be beneficial. Muscle spasms accompanying myopathy may respond well to gentle but consistent stretching exercises. Postexercise soreness is common in the AIDS group experiencing muscle pain. A longer rest period between exercises may be necessary.

Improper body mechanics and poor postural alignment may occur in the person who has developed muscle weakness and fatigue following progression of the disease process, malnutrition, or the wasting syndrome. Again, postural awareness, stretching and strengthening of specific muscles, and attention to nutrition may be part of the treatment plan.

Muscle and joint mobilization techniques as well as breathing exercises are essential for the person who has been immobilized for any length of time as a result of respiratory or other disease involvement. The rib cage is one area where normal respiratory and accessory movements are essential for adequate lung ventilation, energy conservation, correct posture, and balance reactions.

For the client with malignancy, guidelines for the treatment of the oncologic client are discussed in Chapter 7. See also Kaposi's Sarcoma, Chapter 8.

BOX **5-3**

Exercise Recommendations for HIV-Infected Athletes*

- Before initiating any exercise program, the athlete must have a complete physical examination
- A graded exercise test may be a necessary part of the evaluation to determine how much exercise the person can tolerate and what baseline of exercise should be established to start
- Exercise is a safe and beneficial activity for the HIV-infected person
- For healthy, asymptomatic HIV-infected persons, unrestricted exercise activity and competition are acceptable; overtraining should be avoided
- For persons with more advanced HIV infection, who are experiencing mild to moderate symptoms, athletic competition is not considered advisable given the stress of competition and its effect on the immune system; training may continue without competition
- Symptomatic persons should avoid exhaustive exercise but may be able to continue exercise training under close supervision
- Exercise training programs may need to be modified to include mild exercise and energy conservation techniques for anyone during the acute stage of an opportunistic infection
- For the noncompetitive person, exercise should begin while healthy with strategies to help maintain an exercise program throughout the course of the illness
- HIV-infected persons, through the use of exercise, can play an important role in the management of their illness, while improving quality of life
- Exercise has the potential to offer subtle and effective behavioral therapeutic benefits regardless of ethnicity, exposure category, or gender

* General principles included here apply to all HIV-infected persons, including those who are not athletes or competitive in athletics or sports.

Modified from Calabrese LH, LaPerrierre A: Human immunodeficiency virus infection, exercise, and athletics. Sports Med 15:6, 1993.

Chronic Fatigue and Immune Dysfunction Syndrome

Overview. Chronic fatigue and immune dysfunction syndrome (CFIDS), chronic fatigue syndrome (CFS), chronic Epstein-Barr virus (CEBV), myalgic encephalomyelitis, neuromyasthenia, and the "yuppie flu" all denote a recently publicized but not new illness (Strauss, 1991; Norris, 1995). The name chronic fatigue syndrome (CFS) indicates that this illness is not a single disease but the result of a combination of factors.

Incidence and Risk Factors. The number of reported cases of CFS depends on the case definition used. The CDC has initiated a physician-based surveillance team in four cities to determine the prevalence, incidence, course, and impact of this illness. The incidence among the general population appears to be between 5 and 11 per 100,000 (Gunn et al., 1993). Medical skepticism as to the existence of CFS may account for the broad range of percentages reported (Jason et al., 1995). Some researchers suggest an increasing trend based on increasing prevalence rates (Minowa and Jiamo, 1996).

More than 80% of persons with CFS are women, and most are middle-class and white, with an average age at onset of 30 years. These data indicate that factors of race, sex, and socioeconomic status can predispose a person to this syndrome, but the reason for this remains unknown.

Etiology. Most people relate the onset of their illness to a particular infection, one that they might have had before (e.g., respiratory or gastrointestinal illness, flulike disease, bronchitis, sore throat, cold) without long-lasting consequences. The exact cause of CFS is unknown but researchers suspect it may be found in human herpesvirus 6 or other herpesviruses, enteroviruses, or retroviruses. Rising levels of antibodies to Epstein-Barr virus (EBV), another herpesvirus, was once thought to be the cause of CFS but is now considered a result of this disease.

CFS may be associated with a reaction to viral illness that is complicated by a dysfunctional immune response and by other factors that may include the age, sex, genetic predisposition, or neuropsychological makeup of the individual; prior illness (especially acute infection); stress; or environment. Another possible but still unproven theory is that severe allergies can trigger this syndrome; some people believe this disorder should be called the "total allergy syndrome."

Pathogenesis. More remains unknown about CFS than is currently known. Research findings of immunologic dysfunction and neuroendocrine changes suggest the possible dysregulation of interactions between the nervous system and the immune system (Farrar et al., 1995). It is clear that certain components of the immune system behave abnormally. IL-2 and interferon-γ produced in the presence of infectious processes or malignancy may not be made in normal amounts in people with CFS. There is a slight increase in WBCs that usually accumulate during an infectious process, and NK cells are slightly decreased. This small reduction in NK cell activity is identical to findings in persons diagnosed with clinical depression (Strauss, 1991). The connection between depression, the immune system, and CFS remains unclear.

Clinical Manifestations. The foremost characteristic symptom of CFS is prolonged (lasting more than 6 months), often overwhelming fatigue that is commonly associated with a varying complex of other symptoms. These symptoms result in at least 50% reduction in activity. To aid the identification of this disease, the CDC has developed a "working case definition" to group symptoms and classify severity (Table 5–6). Other common symptoms are depression, memory loss, and an inability to concentrate. The pattern of symptoms (frequency and duration) varies from individual to individual. Some persons are ill all the time, whereas others are well except for a single fatigue episode every several weeks. There appears to be no way to accurately predict exacerbations and remissions.

Medical Management

Diagnosis, Treatment, and Prognosis. No single test confirms the presence of CFS; physicians must rely on the client's history and the CDC criteria (see Table 5–6). Even so, the CDC criteria are a working concept that may not include all forms of this disease and are based on symptoms that can result from other diseases (e.g., systemic lupus erythematosus, cancer, Lyme disease, arthritis). Diagnosis is often difficult and uncertain. The presence of antibodies to EBV does not necessarily mean the person has CFS although some people with CFS do, in fact, have high levels of EBV antibodies. Others with the syndrome have normal or no antibodies to the virus.

Likewise, no treatment is known to cure CFS. Experimental treatments include antiviral acyclovir and selected immunomodulating agents such as IV γ-globulin, ampligen, transfer factor, and others. Symptomatic treatment may include monoamine oxidase inhibitor antidepressants (MAOIs) or tricyclic antidepressants (e.g., doxepin, amitriptyline, sertraline [zoloft]), histamine H_2 receptor-blocking agents (cimetidine), and antianxiety agents (alprazolam). In some persons, avoidance of environmental irritants and certain foods may help to relieve symptoms.

Only 5% to 10% of persons with CFS recover completely from this illness; many are left feeling extremely weak, tired, and depressed long after the main symptoms of the infection have resolved.

Special Implications for the Therapist **5-4**

CHRONIC FATIGUE SYNDROME *(Sistu, 1995)*

The client with CFS is treated following guidelines and protocols for autoimmune disorders such as fibromyalgia (see also Fibromyalgia, this chapter). Pacing, energy conservation (see Box 7–1), physiologic quieting, stress management, and balancing life activities are extremely helpful in preventing worsening of fatigue and maintaining an even flow of energy from day to day. Support groups may be beneficial in providing emotional and psychological support as well as helping the individual to keep up with latest research results and progress in medical treatment.

Although abnormal lung function or low concentration of oxygen with accompanying dyspnea or shortness of breath is not a clinical feature of this disease, anyone who is severely deconditioned and then tries to do even light exercise may experience dyspnea. Always assess for conditioning before initiating even a simple exercise program with anyone who has had CFS longer than 6 months.

Assessment of vital signs may demonstrate very large fluctuations in pulse rate and blood pressure which are

TABLE 5-6 CRITERIA FOR DIAGNOSING CHRONIC FATIGUE SYNDROME*

MAJOR CRITERIA	SYMPTOM CRITERIA	PHYSICAL CRITERIA
1. New onset of persistent or relapsing debilitating fatigue in a person without a history of similar symptoms; fatigue does not resolve with bed rest and is severe enough to reduce or impair average daily activity by 50% for 6 mo 2. Exclusion of other disorders after evaluation through history, physical examination, and laboratory findings	1. The main symptom complex develops over a few hours or days 2. Profound or prolonged fatigue, especially after exercise levels that would have been easily tolerated before 3. Low-grade fever 4. Sore throat 5. Painful lymph nodes 6. Muscle weakness 7. Muscle discomfort or myalgia 8. Sleep disturbances (insomnia or hypersomnia) 9. Headaches of a new type, severity, or pattern 10. Migratory arthralgias without joint swelling or redness 11. Photophobia, forgetfulness, irritability, confusion, depression, transient visual scotomata, difficulty thinking, and inability to concentrate	Three criteria must be recorded on at least two occasions, at least 1 mo apart 1. Low-grade fever 2. Nonexudative pharyngitis 3. Palpable or tender nodes

* To meet the Centers for Disease Control and Prevention (CDC) case definition, a person must fulfill the 2 major criteria, and either 8 of the 11 symptom criteria, or 6 of the 11 symptom criteria and 2 of the 3 physical criteria.

not consistent with the person's position or movement. Whereas the blood pressure and pulse rate normally show a slight increase as a physiologic response to a change in position from sitting to standing, orthostatic hypotension is marked in the CFS population. Vital signs may stay the same or even decrease, resulting in dizziness, lightheadedness, or loss of balance. The symptoms may result in decreased self-confidence in the ability to pursue activities.

The therapist must evaluate for altered breathing patterns, components of poor posture, and inefficient movement patterns contributing to pain. Addressing these areas is an important part of the rehabilitation process. Stretching, strengthening, and cardiovascular training are essential aspects of therapy. Like persons with fibromyalgia, those diagnosed with CFS must progress slowly and avoid overexertion since they frequently do not have the internal mechanism to alert them to stop an activity.

HYPERSENSITIVITY DISORDERS

An exaggerated or inappropriate immune response may lead to various hypersensitivity disorders. Such disorders are classified as type I, II, III, or IV, although some overlap exists (Table 5–7). Overreaction to a substance, or hypersensitivity, is often referred to as an allergic response and although the term "allergy" is widely used, the term "hypersensitivity" is more appropriate. Hypersensitivity designates an increased immune response to the presence of an antigen (referred to as an allergen) that results in tissue destruction. There are two general categories of hypersensitivity reactions: immediate and delayed, based on the rapidity of the immune response.

Type I Hypersensitivity (Immediate Hypersensitivity, Allergic Disorders, Anaphylaxis)

Type I hypersensitivity reactions include hay fever, allergic rhinitis, urticaria, extrinsic asthma, and anaphylactic shock. In this type of immediate hypersensitivity response, IgE, instead of IgG, is produced in response to a pathogen (allergen). IgE resides on mast cells in connective tissue, especially the upper respiratory tract, gastrointestinal tract, and dermis. When IgE meets the pathogen again, an immediate response occurs with histamine release along with other inflammatory mediators (e.g., chemotactic factors, prostaglandins, and leukotrienes) that enhance and prolong the response initiated by histamine.

If this response becomes systemic, widespread release of histamine results in systemic vasodilation, bronchospasm, and increased mucous secretion, and edema referred to as anaphylaxis. Classic associated signs and symptoms are wheezing, hypotension, swelling, urticaria, and rhinorrhea (clear runny nose often accompanied by sneezing). Anaphylaxis is a life-threatening emergency; bee stings remain the number one cause of anaphylaxis. Other triggers include penicillin, foods, animal dander, children, semen, and latex.

Type II Hypersensitivity (Cytotoxic Reactions to Self-Antigens)

When the body's own tissue is recognized as foreign or nonself, activation of complement occurs with subsequent agglutination (clumping together) and phagocytosis of the identified pathogens. This means the cellular membrane of normal tissues (e.g., red blood cells, leukocytes, and platelets) is disrupted and ultimately destroyed. Self-antigen disorders include blood transfusion reactions, hemolytic disease of the newborn, autoimmune hemolytic anemia, and myasthenia gravis.

TABLE 5-7 Clinical Manifestations of Hypersensitivity Disorders

Type I	Type II	Type III	Type IV
Varies according to the allergies present Classic symptoms Wheezing Hypotension Swelling Urticaria Rhinorrhea Anaphylaxis	General: malaise, weakness Dermal: hives, erythema Respiratory: sneezing, rhinorrhea, dyspnea Upper airway: hoarseness, stridor; tongue and pharyngeal edema Lower airway: dyspnea, bronchospasm, asthma (air trapping), chest tightness, wheezing Gastrointestinal: increased peristalsis, vomiting, dysphagia, nausea, abdominal cramps, diarrhea Cardiovascular: tachycardia, palpitations, hypotension, cardiac arrest CNS: Anxiety, seizures	Headache Back (flank) pain Chest pain similar to angina Nausea and vomiting Tachycardia Hypotension Hematuria Urticaria	Fever Arthralgias Lymphadenopathy Urticaria Anemia

A second type of hypersensitivity response occurs when there is a cross-reaction from exogenous pathogens with endogenous body tissues as occurs in rheumatic fever. For example, group A hemolytic streptococci (the exogenous pathogen) are attacked by the immune system but the body also misinterprets the mitral valve (endogenous body tissue) as a foreign microorganism (i.e., as streptococcus) and attacks normal, healthy tissue in the same way it attempts to destroy the true pathogenic microorganisms. Another example of this type of cross-reaction is an exogenous virus causing the immune system to attack the peripheral nervous system as nonself, as occurs in Guillain-Barré syndrome.

Type III Hypersensitivity (Immune Complex Disease)

Normally, excessive circulating antigen-antibody complexes called immune complexes are effectively cleared by the reticuloendothelial system. When circulating immune complexes (antigen-antibody complexes) successfully deposit in tissue around small blood vessels, they activate the complement cascade and cause acute inflammation and local tissue injury. The subsequent vasculitis most commonly affects the skin; the joints, causing synovitis, as in rheumatoid arthritis; the kidneys, causing nephritis; the pleura, causing pleuritis; and the pericardium, causing pericarditis.

Systemic lupus erythematosus (SLE) is the classic picture of vasculitis occurring in various organ systems. The antigen is the individual's own nucleus of cells; antinuclear antibodies (ANAs) are made which in turn complex with the antigen and are deposited in the skin, joints, and kidneys causing acute immune injury. Other examples of this hypersensitivity reaction occur in association with infections such as hepatitis B and bacterial endocarditis; malignancies; or following drug or serum therapy.

Type IV Hypersensitivity (Cell-Mediated Immunity)

Type IV is a delayed hypersensitivity response such as the reaction that occurs in contact dermatitis after sensitization to an allergen (commonly a cosmetic, adhesive, topical medication, or plant toxin such as poison ivy), latex sensitivity, or the response to a tuberculin skin test present 48 to 72 hours after the skin test. In this type of reaction, the antigen is processed by macrophages and presented to T cells. The sensitized T cells then release lymphokines, which recruit other lymphocytes, monocytes, macrophages, and PMNs. Graft-vs.-host disease (GVHD) and transplant rejection are also examples of type IV reactions.

Special Implications for the Therapist 5-5

HYPERSENSITIVITY DISORDERS

Immediate action is required for any client experiencing a type I hypersensitivity reaction or anaphylaxis. When a severe reaction occurs, the health care professional must call for emergency assistance.

Type IV reactions may occur in response to lanolin added to lotions, ultrasound gels, or other preparations used in massage or soft tissue mobilization, requiring careful observation of all people for delayed skin reactions to any of these substances. With the first exposure, no reaction necessarily occurs but antigens are formed and on subsequent exposures, hypersensitivity reactions are triggered. Anyone with known hypersensitivity should have a small area of skin tested before use of large amounts of topical agents in the therapy setting. Careful observation throughout treatment is recommended.

AUTOIMMUNE DISEASES

Definition and Overview. Autoimmune diseases fall into a category of conditions in which the cause involves immune mechanisms directed against self-antigens. More specifically, the body fails to distinguish self from nonself, causing the immune system to direct immune responses against normal (self) tissue and become self-destructive. Autoimmune disease can be viewed as a spectrum of disorders. Some diseases in this category are systemic; others involve a single organ (Table 5–8) (O'Toole, 1992).

At one end of the continuum are organ-specific diseases, in which there is localized tissue damage resulting from the presence of specific autoantibodies. An example is Hashimoto's disease of the thyroid, characterized by a specific lesion in the thyroid gland with production of antibodies with absolute specificity for certain thyroid constituents.

TABLE 5-8 AUTOIMMUNE DISORDERS

ORGAN-SPECIFIC	SYSTEMIC
Addison's disease	Amyloidosis
Chronic active hepatitis	Ankylosing spondylitis
Diabetes mellitus	Mixed connective tissue disease
Giant cell arteritis	Myasthenia gravis
Hemolytic anemia	Polymyalgia rheumatica
Idiopathic thrombocytopenic purpura	Progressive systemic sclerosis (scleroderma)
Polymyositis/dermatomyositis	Psoriasis (psoriatic arthritis)
Postviral encephalomyelitis	Reiter's syndrome
Primary biliary cirrhosis	Rheumatoid arthritis
Thyroiditis	Sarcoidosis
Graves' disease	Sjögren's syndrome
Hashimoto's disease	Systemic lupus erythematosus
Ulcerative colitis	

In the middle of the continuum are disorders in which the lesion tends to be localized in one organ, but the antibodies are not organ-specific. An example is primary biliary cirrhosis, in which there is inflammatory cell infiltration of the small bile ductule, but the serum antibodies are not specific to liver cells.

At the other end of the spectrum are non–organ-specific diseases, in which lesions and antibodies are widespread throughout the body and not limited to one target organ. SLE is an example of this type of autoimmune disease. Identification of ANAs that attack the nucleic acids (DNA and RNA) and other components of the body's own tissues established SLE as an autoimmune disease.

In this book, with the few exceptions included in this chapter (e.g., fibromyalgia, CFS, SLE), autoimmune disorders are discussed individually in the most appropriate chapter. For example, Reiter's syndrome, rheumatoid arthritis, and Sjögren's syndrome are discussed in Chapter 23. Polymyositis, dermatomyositis, and progressive systemic sclerosis are discussed in Chapter 8. Giant cell arteritis is discussed in Chapter 10, sarcoidosis in Chapter 12, and so on.

Etiology and Risk Factors. Although the autoimmune disorders are regarded as acquired diseases, their causes often cannot be determined. Autoimmunity is believed to result from a combination of factors, including genetic, hormonal (women are affected more often than men by autoimmune diseases), and environmental influences (e.g., exposure to chemicals, other toxins, or sunlight; drugs that may destroy suppressor T cells). In most autoimmune disorders, there is a known or suspected genetic susceptibility and certain HLA types show increased risk, such as ankylosing spondylitis with HLA-B27 (see Table 35–17).

Other factors implicated in the development of immunologic abnormalities resulting in autoimmune disorders include viruses, stress, cross-reactive antibodies, and most recently, there have been case reports of various autoimmune diseases occurring in women who have had silicone gel breast implants. This organ-specific autoimmune disease has been associated with musculoskeletal problems (see discussion in Chapter 6).

Pathogenesis. There are many hypotheses to explain autoimmune diseases, including escape of a normally sequestered antigen; production of antibodies against microorganisms that cross-react with normal tissue components; modification of cell surface antigens or defective recognition of antigens; depression of suppressor T cell activity; inappropriate helper T cell activity; and polyclonal B cell stimulation (Harruff, 1994). Whatever the underlying pathogenesis, autoimmune disorders involve disruption of the immunoregulatory mechanism, causing normal cell-mediated and humoral immune responses to turn self-destructive, resulting in tissue damage.

Some known pathophysiologic mechanisms include hypersensitivity reactions that mediate autoimmune diseases. Examples of these are the cytolytic and cytotoxic reactions that produce autoimmune hemolytic anemia, Graves' disease, Hashimoto's disease, myasthenia gravis, and insulin-dependent diabetes mellitus (IDDM). Immune complex hypersensitivity causes much of the tissue damage in systemic autoimmune diseases, such as SLE, rheumatoid arthritis, and progressive systemic sclerosis. See discussions of these conditions in this and other chapters.

Many autoimmune diseases are associated with characteristic autoantibodies. In other words, the body begins to manufacture antibodies directed against the body's own cellular components or specific organs. These antibodies are known as autoantibodies, in this case producing autoimmune diseases. For example, SLE is associated with anti-DNA and anti-Sm antigen; Sjögren's syndrome is associated with antiribonucleoproteins (SS-A and SS-B); progressive systemic sclerosis is associated with anticentromere and anti-Scl-70 (DNA topoisomerase); psoriasis and psoriatic arthritis are associated with HLA-B13; and mixed connective tissue disease is associated with antiribonucleoprotein without anti-DNA.

Antibodies specific to hormone receptors on the surface of cells have been found and determined to be partially responsible for some conditions. Examples include myasthenia gravis, in which anti–acetylcholine receptor antibodies are involved; Graves' disease, in which antibodies against components of thyroid cell membranes, including the receptors for thyroid-stimulating hormone (TSH), are responsible; and certain cases of insulin-resistant diabetes mellitus, in which the antibodies affect insulin receptors on cells. Other diseases involving autoimmune mechanisms include rheumatic fever, rheumatoid arthritis, autoimmune hemolytic anemia, idiopathic thrombocytopenic purpura, and postviral encephalomyelitis.

Clinical Manifestations. Autoimmune disorders share certain clinical features and differentiation among them is often difficult because of this. Common findings include synovitis, pleuritis, myocarditis, endocarditis, pericarditis, peritonitis, vasculitis, myositis, skin rash, alterations of connective tissues, and nephritis (Hellman, 1994). Constitutional symptoms such as fatigue, malaise, myalgias, and arthralgias are also common.

Medical Management

Diagnosis. Laboratory tests may reveal thrombocytopenia, leukopenia, immunoglobulin excesses or deficiencies, ANAs, rheumatoid factor, cryoglobulins, false-positive serologic tests, elevated muscle enzymes, and alterations in serum complement. Coombs' test will be positive when hemolytic anemia is present. Some of the laboratory alterations that occur in autoimmune diseases (e.g., false-positive serologic tests, rheumatoid factor) occur in asymptomatic persons. These changes may also be demonstrated in certain asymptomatic relatives of people with connective tissue diseases, in older persons, in persons taking certain medications, and in persons with chronic infectious diseases (Hellman, 1994).

Treatment. Treatment of autoimmune diseases varies with the specific disease. Treatment must maintain a delicate balance between adequate suppression of the autoimmune reaction to avoid continued damage to the body tissues, and maintenance of sufficient functioning of the immune mechanism to protect the person against foreign invaders. In general, autoimmune diseases are treated by the administration of corticosteroids to produce an anti-inflammatory effect and salicylates to provide symptomatic relief.

Systemic Lupus Erythematosus

Definition and Overview. Lupus erythematosus, sometimes referred to as lupus, is a chronic inflammatory autoimmune disorder that appears in several forms, including *discoid lupus erythematosus (DLE)*, which affects only the skin (see Chapter 8), and *systemic lupus erythematosus*, which affects the entire organism (systemic) (Norris, 1995; Pisetsky, 1993; Von Feldt, 1995).

The clinical picture of SLE presents on a continuum with different combinations of organ system involvement. The most common of these presentations are latent lupus, drug-induced lupus, antiphospholipid antibody syndrome, and late-stage lupus. *Latent lupus* describes a constellation of features suggestive of SLE, but does not qualify as classic SLE (Box 5–4). Many persons with latent lupus persist with their clinical presentation of signs and symptoms over many years without ever developing classic SLE.

Drug-induced lupus may be diagnosed in persons without prior history suggestive of SLE in whom the clinical and serologic manifestations of SLE develop while the person is taking a drug. The symptoms cease when the drug is stopped, with gradual resolution of serologic abnormalities. *Antiphospholipid antibody syndrome* describes the association between arterial and venous thrombosis, recurrent fetal loss, and immune thrombocytopenia with a variety of antibodies directed against cellular phospholipid (lipids in cell membranes containing phosphorus) components. This syndrome may be part of the clinical manifestations seen in SLE or it may occur as a primary form without other clinical features of lupus (Love and Santaro, 1990).

Late-state lupus is defined as chronic disease duration of greater than 5 years. In such cases, morbidity and mortality are affected by long-term complications of SLE that result either from the disease itself or as a consequence of its therapy. These late complications may include endstage renal disease, atherosclerosis, pulmonary emboli, and avascular necrosis. In late-stage lupus, when there is no longer any evidence of active disease, and the client is on low-dose or no corticosteroids, cognitive disabilities are a frequent manifestation (Gladman and Urowitz, 1993).

BOX **5–4**

American Rheumatism Association Diagnostic Criteria for Systemic Lupus Erythematosus (SLE)

Abnormal titer of antinuclear antibodies
Butterfly (malar) rash
Discoid rash
Hemolytic anemia, leukopenia, lymphopenia, or thrombocytopenia
Neurologic disorder: seizures or psychoses
Nonerosive arthritis (of two or more peripheral joints)
Oral or nasopharyngeal ulcerations
Photosensitivity
Pleuritis or pericarditis
Positive LE cell preparation, anti-DNA, or anti-Sm test or chronic false-positive serologic test for syphilis
Renal disorder: profuse proteinuria (>0.5 g/day) or excessive cellular casts in urine

A person is considered to have SLE if 4 or more of these 11 criteria are present, serially or simultaneously, during any interval of observation.

Incidence. SLE is primarily a disease of young women. Disease onset may occur from infancy to advanced age but its peak incidence occurs between the ages of 15 and 40; women are affected 10 to 15 times more often than men. The female-to-male ratio is less dramatic (2 : 1) in SLE with onset in childhood or older age. The dramatic age and sex relationship in SLE has led researchers to investigate the importance of the hormonal influence in the pathogenesis. SLE occurs worldwide but is most prevalent among blacks and some Asian and Native American groups; at least 1.4 million Americans have been diagnosed with SLE.

Risk Factors. SLE shows a strong familial link with a much higher frequency among first-degree relatives. Genetically determined immune abnormalities may be triggered by both exogenous and endogenous factors. While the predisposition to disease is hereditary, it is likely to involve different sets of genes in different individuals. As the human genome becomes more extensively mapped, a susceptibility gene may be found, although it remains possible that the differences in disease course among ethnic groups relates solely to their environment and other social factors (Liang et al., 1991).

Other factors predisposing to SLE may include physical or mental stress, which can provoke neuroendocrine changes affecting immune cell function; streptococcal or viral infections; exposure to sunlight or ultraviolet light, which can cause inflammation and tissue damage; immunization; pregnancy[22]; and abnormal estrogen metabolism.[23] SLE may also be triggered or aggravated by treatment with certain drugs (e.g., hydralazine, anticonvulsants, penicillins, sulfa drugs, and oral contraceptives) which could modify cellular responsiveness as well as the immunogenicity of self-antigens.

[22] Whether pregnancy induces lupus flares has not been established; existing data suggest both that it does and that it does not. More studies are needed to further determine the effects of pregnancy on this condition (Boumpas et al., 1995a).

[23] There is a higher incidence of SLE exacerbation among women taking even low-dose estrogen contraceptives. Since there is also an increased risk of thrombosis in young women with SLE, estrogen-containing contraceptives are avoided or used with the lowest effective dose of estrogen. There is no evidence that postmenopausal estrogen replacement therapy is associated with SLE flares and since women in this age range are at increased risk for coronary artery disease and osteoporosis, estrogen replacement therapy can be taken. For all women with SLE who have been treated with cyclophosphamide, there is an increased risk of gynecologic malignancy (Petri, 1994).

Etiology and Pathogenesis. The cause of SLE remains unknown but evidence points to interrelated immunologic, environmental, hormonal, and genetic factors. Whether SLE represents a single pathologic entity with variable expression or a group of related conditions remains unknown. Immune dysregulation in the form of autoimmunity is thought to be the prime causative mechanism.

The central immunologic disturbance in SLE is autoantibody production. The body produces antibodies (e.g., ANAs[24]) against its own cells. Deposition of the formed antigen-antibody complexes at various tissue sites can suppress the body's normal immunity, and damage tissues. In fact, one significant feature of SLE is the ability to produce antibodies against many different tissue components, such as red blood cells, neutrophils, platelets, lymphocytes, or almost any organ or tissue in the body. This wide range of antigenic targets has resulted in SLE being classified as a disease of generalized autoimmunity. Given the clinical diversity of SLE, the disease may be mediated by more than one autoantibody system and several immunopathogenic mechanisms.

Specific pathologic findings are organ-dependent; for example, repeat biopsies of the kidney show inflammation, cellular proliferation, basement membrane abnormalities, and immune complex deposition comprised of IgM, IgG, and IgA. Skin lesions demonstrate inflammation and degeneration at the dermal-epidermal junction with the basal layer being the primary site of injury. Other organ systems affected by SLE are usually studied only at autopsy. Although these tissues may show nonspecific inflammation or vessel abnormalities, pathologic findings are sometimes minimal, suggesting a mechanism other than inflammation as the cause of organ damage or dysfunction.

Clinical Manifestations

Musculoskeletal

Arthralgias and arthritis constitute the most common presenting manifestations of SLE but the onset of SLE may be acute or insidious and produce no characteristic clinical pattern. Other early symptoms may include fever, weight loss, malaise, and fatigue. Acute arthritis can involve any joint but typically affects the small joints of the hands, wrists, and knees. It may be migratory or chronic; most cases are symmetrical but asymmetrical polyarthritis is not uncommon. Unlike rheumatoid arthritis, the arthritis of SLE is not usually erosive or destructive of bone, and symptoms are not usually severe enough to cause joint deformities, but pain can cause temporary functional impairment. When deformities do occur these are most often ulnar deviation, swan-neck deformity, or fixed subluxations of the fingers. Tenosynovitis and tendon ruptures may occur.

Cutaneous and Membranous Lesions

The skin rash occurs most commonly in areas exposed to sunlight (ultraviolet rays). The classic butterfly rash over the nose and cheeks is common (see Fig. 8–16). Discoid lesions associated with DLE are raised, red, scaling plaques with follicular plugging and central atrophy (see Fig. 8–15). This raised edging and sunken center gives tham a coin-like appearance (see Chapter 8).

Vasculitis (inflammation of cutaneous blood vessels) involving small and medium-sized vessels may cause other skin lesions including infarctive lesions of the digits (see Fig. 4–1), splinter hemorrhages, necrotic leg ulcers, or digital gangrene (Arnold et al., 1990). Raynaud's phenomenon occurs in about 20% of persons. Diffuse or patchy alopecia (hair loss) may be temporary with hair regrowth once the disease is under control. However, permanent hair loss can occur from the extensive scarring of discoid lesions. Painless ulcers of the mucous membranes are common involving the mouth, vagina, and nasal septum.

Cardiopulmonary System

Signs of cardiopulmonary abnormalities may develop such as pleuritis, pericarditis, and dyspnea. Myocarditis, endocarditis, tachycardia, and pneumonitis (acute or chronic) may also occur. Pulmonary hypertension and congestive heart failure are less common and usually secondary to a combination of factors. See also discussion of collagen-vascular disease in Chapter 10.

Central Nervous System

CNS involvement, sometimes referred to as "neuropsychiatric manifestations" may produce headaches, irritability, and depression (most commonly), but emotional instability, psychosis, seizures, cerebrovascular accidents, cranial neuropathy, peripheral neuropathy, and organic brain syndrome can also occur (Futrell and Millikan, 1994). Return to the previous level of intellectual function may follow remission of the neuropsychiatric flare, or permanent cognitive impairment may occur. Progressive cognitive impairment, sometimes subtle and sometimes obvious, may develop even in the absence of clinically diagnosed episodes of neuropsychiatric disease (Ginzler, 1992). Persons with SLE may or may not have other signs of lupus when they experience neurologic symptoms.

Other Systems

Pathologic changes may also occur in the kidneys where the glomerulus is the usual site of destruction; other renal effects may include hematuria and proteinuria, progressing to kidney failure. Anemia from decreased erythrocytes is a common finding with associated amenorrhea (cessation of menstrual flow) among women. Sometimes the spleen, and cervical, axillary, and inguinal nodes are enlarged; hepatitis may develop. Nausea, vomiting, diarrhea, and abdominal pain may occur with gastrointestinal involvement.

All symptoms mentioned in this section can occur at the onset or at any time during the course of lupus. The frequency of lupus manifestations at onset and at any time during the course of lupus are shown in Table 5–9. Nearly all persons with SLE experience fluctuations in disease activity with exacerbations and remissions.

Medical Management

Diagnosis. Diagnosis of SLE is difficult because SLE often mimics other diseases and the symptoms are often vague, varying greatly from individual to individual. The American Rheumatism Association has issued a list of criteria for classifying SLE to be used primarily for consistency in epidemio-

[24] High titers of antibodies to ribonucleoprotein are common in SLE but are also present in people with mixed connective tissue disease (overlap connective tissue disease).

TABLE 5-9 Frequency of Lupus Manifestations at Onset and at Any Time During the Course of Lupus

Manifestations	Frequency (%) Onset	Any Time
Arthralgia	77	85
Constitutional	73	84
Skin	57	81
Arthritis	56	63
Renal	44	77
Raynaud's syndrome	33	58
Lymphadenopathy	25	32
CNS	24	54
Pleurisy	23	37
Gastrointestinal	22	47
Pericarditis	20	29
Mucous membranes	18	54
Vasculitis	10	37
Lung	9	17
Myositis	7	5
Nephrotic syndrome	5	11
Azotemia (nitrogen compounds in blood)	3	8
Thrombophlebitis	2	8
Myocarditis	1	4
Pancreatitis	1	4

Adapted from Gladman DD, Urowitz MB: Systemic lupus erythematosus: Clinical manifestations. *In* Schumacher HR (ed): Primer on the Rheumatic Diseases, ed 10. Atlanta, Arthritis Foundation, 1993, pp 106–111.

logic surveys. Usually, four or more of these signs are present at some time during the course of the disease (see Box 5–4).

In addition to the routine history and physical examination, laboratory findings are an important part of the diagnosis of SLE and subsequent monitoring of clinical disease activity. Three studies are particularly helpful: C-reactive protein (CRP) and erythrocyte sedimentation rate (ESR) as general indicators of inflammation; platelet count, urinalysis, and serum creatinine levels for persons with specific target organ involvement; and serologic markers of clinical SLE activity such as levels of antibodies to double-stranded DNA (anti-ssDNA). Numerous studies have confirmed the close association of this last measure (levels of these antibodies) with SLE activity generally, and in particular with the presence and activity of lupus nephritis (Ballou, 1993).

Serial measurement of antibodies such as the antibody to ribosomal P protein (anti-P antibody levels), lymphocytotoxic antibodies, or antiphospholipid antibodies may identify the presence of neuropsychiatric lupus (Ginzler, 1992). Computed tomography (CT) or magnetic resonance imaging (MRI) scans of the head are usually ordered for all persons experiencing new episodes of focal neurologic deficits, seizures, altered consciousness, or psychosis.

Treatment. The objectives of medical treatment are to reverse the autoimmune and inflammatory processes and to prevent exacerbations and complications. Mild symptoms can be managed with nonsteroidal anti-inflammatory drugs to relieve muscle and joint pain while reducing tissue inflammation. Antimalarial agents are useful against the dermatologic, arthritic, and renal symptoms of this disease. Immunosuppressive drugs weaken the body cells that produce the immune and inflammatory responses and are used only with active disease, especially with severe kidney involvement. Corticosteroids and cytotoxic drugs are given in more severe disease that has not responded to these other types of drug therapy.

Prognosis. The prognosis improves with early detection and treatment but remains poor for people who develop cardiovascular, renal, or neurologic complications, or severe bacterial infections. Persons with SLE have an increased prevalence of valvular and atherosclerotic heart disease, apparently because of factors related to the disease itself and to drug therapy (Boumpas et al., 1995a). Symptomatic large vessel occlusive disease in SLE occurring several years after the diagnosis of SLE is associated with a relatively poor short-term outcome (Mitsias and Levine, 1994).

Recent studies have documented a substantial improvement in survival in SLE; 5-year and 10-year survival rates of 90% or more have been reported (Boumpas et al., 1995b).

Special Implications for the Therapists **5-6**

SYSTEMIC LUPUS ERYTHEMATOSUS

Like fibromyalgia, physical and occupational therapy can be important components of the overall treatment plan. Recurrence of disease can be managed with carefully controlled and sometimes restricted activities. After an exacerbation, gradual resumption of activities must be balanced by maximum rest periods, usually 8 to 10 hours of sleep a night and several rest periods during the day. Most of the principles and reference materials outlined in the following section, Fibromyalgia, also apply to SLE. Management of joint involvement follows protocols for rheumatoid arthritis (see Special Implications for the Therapist 23–3: Rheumatoid Arthritis). Clients with skin lesions should be examined thoroughly at each visit. The therapist can be instrumental in teaching and assisting with skin care and prevention of skin breakdown.

Septic arthritis or osteonecrosis may develop as a complication of SLE or its treatment. Septic arthritis is uncommon in SLE but it should be suspected when one joint is inflamed out of proportion to the others. Persons with SLE may develop a drug-related myopathy secondary to corticosteroids or as a complication of antimalarials (see discussion of corticosteroid myopathy, Chapter 4).

High-dose oral corticosteroid treatment remains the major predisposing cause of avascular necrosis in SLE and other autoimmune disorders. The most common site is the femoral head of the hip; less commonly, the femoral condyle of the knee is affected. While the condition may be bilateral, it most often presents with an insidious onset of unilateral hip or knee pain that is worse with ambulating but often present at rest. Symptoms are progressive over weeks to months (Weinstein, 1994).

Anyone taking corticosteroids or immunosuppressants must be monitored carefully for signs of infection, especially persons at heightened risk of infection such as those with renal failure, cardiac valvular abnormalities, or ulcerative skin lesions. See specific side effects and Special Implications: Corticosteroids, Chapter 4. It is important for the client to contact the physician if a fever or any other new symptoms develop.

Observe carefully for any sign of renal involvement such as weight gain, edema, or hypertension. Take seizure precautions if there are signs of neurologic involvement. If Raynaud's phenomenon is present, teach the client to warm and protect the hands and feet. See also Special Implications for the Therapist 10–17: Peripheral Vascular Disease—Raynaud's Phenomenon, Chapter 10.

Fibromyalgia *(Hulme, 1995)*

Definition and Overview. Fibromyalgia or fibromyalgia syndrome, formerly mislabeled or misdiagnosed as fibrocytis, fibromyositis, nonarticular arthritis, myofascial pain, chronic fatigue syndrome, or systemic lupus erythematosus, is a chronic muscle pain syndrome with no known cause and no known cure. It is commonly associated with many other conditions but the link between these disorders is poorly understood.

Fibrositis means inflammation of the fibrous connective tissue and although muscle biopsy studies have failed to demonstrate an inflammatory process, the term *fibrositis* has persisted. Myalgia means muscle pain so fibromyalgia would literally mean pain as opposed to inflammation of the soft tissue. *Fibromyalgia* is becoming the more accepted term. It is considered a syndrome and not a disease and has now been defined by the American College of Rheumatology as pain that is widespread in at least 11 of 18 tender points (see further under Clinical Manifestations and under Diagnosis).

Fibromyalgia has been differentiated from myofascial pain (see Myofascial Pain Syndrome, Chapter 23) in that fibromyalgia is considered a systemic problem with widespread multiple tender points as one of the key symptoms. Myofascial pain is a localized condition specific to a muscle and may involve as few as one or as many as several areas with characteristic trigger points that are painful and refer pain to other areas when pressure is applied.

It has been proposed that fibromyalgia and CFS are two names for the same syndrome, but at present, CFS is thought to differ by the greater degree of fatigue, whereas persons with fibromyalgia tend to experience more pain. In contrast to CFS, fibromyalgia is associated with a variety of initiating or perpetuating factors such as psychologically distressing events, primary sleep disorders, inflammatory rheumatic arthritis, and acute febrile illness. Fibromyalgia and CFS have similar disordered sleep physiology and evidence suggests a reciprocal relationship of the immune and sleep-wake systems. Interference with either system has effects on the other and will be accompanied by the symptoms of CFS (Moldofsky, 1993).

Incidence. Fibromyalgia occurs in 5% to 8% of the US population, affecting at least 6 million Americans and possibly as many as 10 to 12 million (Bennett, 1995). It has now surpassed rheumatoid arthritis as the most common musculoskeletal disorder in the United States (Wolfe et al., 1995a,b). Women are affected more often than men (75% to 80% are women),[25] generally between the ages of 14 and 68 years, although it has been reported in children as young as 6 and adults as old as 85 years.

Risk Factors. Risk factors or triggering events for the onset of fibromyalgia may include prolonged anxiety and emotional stress, trauma (e.g., motor vehicle accident, work injury, surgery), rapid steroid withdrawal, hyperthyroidism, and viral and nonviral infections. Fibromyalgia may also develop with no obvious precipitating events or illnesses. It is more prevalent in minimally to moderately physically fit persons and is not usually found in highly trained athletes; there is a strong correlation between fibromyalgia and anxiety or depression (it remains unclear whether these factors are contributory or a result of this condition).

Etiology. Research is now ongoing to determine the cause of fibromyalgia; most likely the initiation of this condition is multifactorial (Fig. 5–6). Debate continues over whether fibromyalgia is even an organic disease and if so, whether it is caused by abnormal biochemical, metabolic, or immunologic pathology (Hunder et al., 1993). Possible etiologic theories include diet; viral origin; sleep disorder; occupational, seasonal, or environmental influences (Moldofsky, 1994; Waylonis and Perkins, 1994; Waylonis et al., 1994), psychological dysfunction (Yunus, 1994); and a familial or hereditary link (Table 5–10).

Research in the 1990s has demonstrated that fibromyalgia is transmitted as an autosomal dominant trait (Waylonis and Heck, 1992). This heredity factor is thought to be characterized by neurohormonal imbalances (i.e., dysfunction of the body's network of neurotransmitters and hormones causing problems with the body's central pain control mechanisms) that may be triggered by viral infection, traumatic event, or stress (Goldenberg, 1990).

The basis of most viral theories was the discovery that people with cancer temporarily develop fibromyalgia (or CFS) while they receive treatment with IL-2 and interferon-α. These two cytokines are produced by the immune system when the body is fighting an infection. Overproduction of interleukins (the IL-1 β inhibitory theory) has been documented to cause musculoskeletal pain, fatigue, memory problems, and other symptoms of fibromyalgia and CFS that may explain the cause and pathology of both these conditions (Wallace, 1989).

Pathogenesis. Both central and peripheral mechanisms may operate in the pathophysiology of impaired muscle function and pain in fibromyalgia (Bennett and Jacobsen, 1994). The activity of the skeletal muscles, as well as the heart, stomach, intestines, blood vessels, and sweat glands, during daily stress tends to be excessive in fibromyalgia. These organs overactivate resulting in the heart beating faster, the stomach secreting excessive digestive juices and contracting erratically, the smooth muscles of the intestines and bowel

[25] A recent study (Wolfe et al., 1995a) using measures of pain threshold has provided information to suggest that pain threshold is lower in women. A decreased pain threshold correlates with all of the symptoms of fibromyalgia, even in those people who do not meet the criteria for the syndrome. Decreased pain threshold is an intrinsically important aspect of distress associated with fibromyalgia and will be the focus of continuing research efforts to understand and effectively treat this condition.

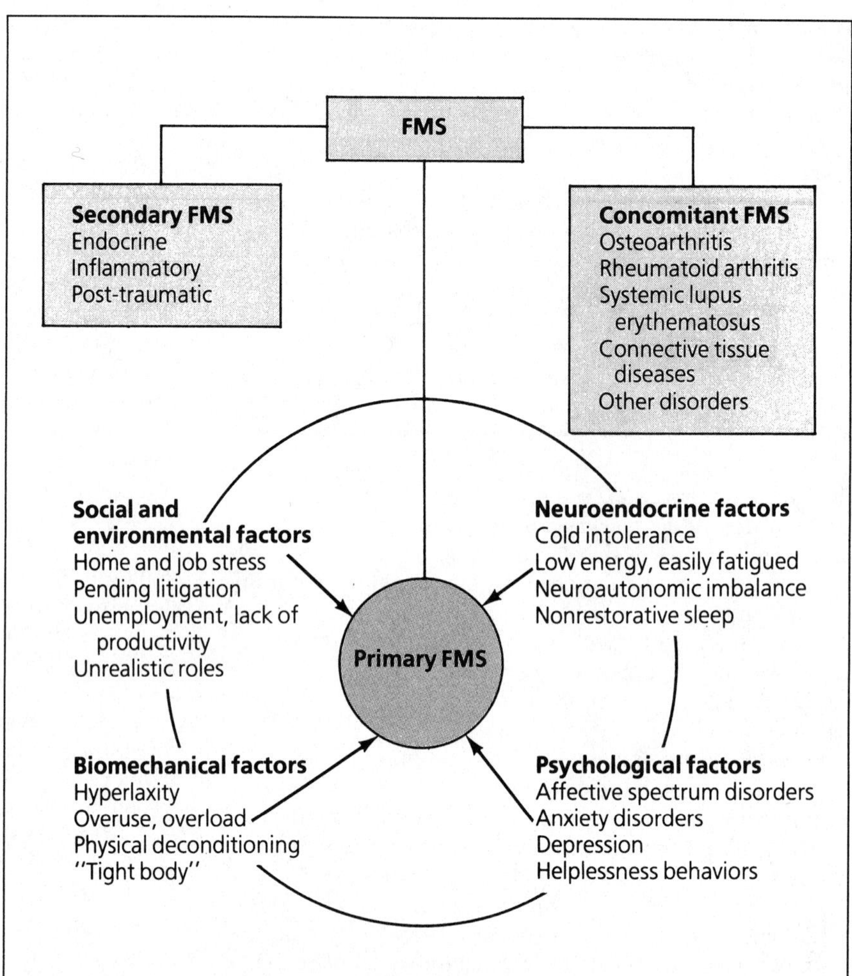

Figure **5-6.** A model of how multiple factors contribute to the development of fibromyalgia syndrome (FMS). The terms primary and secondary fibromyalgia are no longer used in a clinical setting but are important in defining subjects in research protocols. Previously, primary fibromyalgia was the term used to describe fibromyalgia without an apparent underlying cause, whereas secondary fibromyalgia denoted an association with an underlying cause or disease such as rheumatoid arthritis, Lyme disease, or sleep apnea (Freundlich, B., and Leventhal, L., 1993). (*Adapted from Masi T: Aspects of the epidemiology and criteria of myofascial pain and fibromyalgia: Concepts of illness in populations as applied to dysfunctional syndromes. J Musculo Pain 1:113–136, 1993; and Masi AT: Management of fibromyalgia syndrome: A person-centered approach. J Musculo Med 11(8):29, 1994.*)

TABLE 5-10 Theories of the Cause of Fibromyalgia

	Muscle Injury (Bennett, 1989)	Nonrefreshing Sleep (Moldofsky, 1989)	Psychophysiology (Blumer and Heilbronn, 1982)
Preconditioners	Enhanced predisposition to muscle microtrauma	Neurohormonal, other contributors	Masked depression, unbearable guilt and anguish
Stressors	Too much/too little physical activity	Factors altering sleep physiology (e.g., presence of alpha-delta sleep*)	Pain-prone personality, "solid citizen," self-sacrificing, egomanic tendencies
Tissue effects	Muscle microtrauma, local sarcomere injury	Increased pain transmission (substance P), decreased pain tolerance	Central pain perception
Symptoms	Myalgia, fatigue	Myalgia, fatigue, sleep disturbance	Continuous pain, anhedonia, misery, insomnia, fatigue
Physical findings	Deconditioned	Deconditioned	Anergic, detached, passive
Psychological reactions	Anxiety, fatigue	Heightened sensitivities	Hypochondriacal preoccupations, denial
Behavioral pattern	Inactivity, avoidance	Complaining	Passive-dependent suffering, invalid role

* Nonrestorative sleep in which high-frequency brain waves of wakefulness intrude into low-frequency brain waves of deep sleep.
Modified from Masi AT, Yunis MB: Fibromyalgia—Which is the best treatment? A personalized, comprehensive, ambulatory, patient-involved management programme. Baillieres Clin Rheumatol 4:333–370, 1991.

contracting abnormally, breathing becoming rapid and shallow, and blood vessels constricting, decreasing blood flow to body parts.

These and other autonomic nervous system responses may occur in response to a relatively mild life stressor and linger even after cognitive memory of the event is gone.[26] Substance P, a neurotransmitter for pain,[27] may play a role in the transmission of nociceptive information. Elevated levels of substance P have been found in the cerebrospinal fluid of fibromyalgia clients, resulting in an exaggerated response to normal stimuli and an amplified effect on pain (Vaeroy, 1988; Russell et al., 1994).

The role of other pain-inhibiting neurotransmitters, such as serotonin, γ-aminobutyric acid (GABA), enkephalins, epinephrine, and norepinephrine has been studied. While substance P is elevated, decreased levels of all of these neurotransmitters in the cerebrospinal fluid have been observed (Yunus et al., 1992; Russell et al., 1992). Serotonin, a CNS neurotransmitter that is made from tryptophan (an essential amino acid obtained from diet), is necessary for restorative sleep and appears to play a role in pain control, immune system function, vascular constriction and dilation, and even emotions that may contribute to such feelings as depression or anxiety. Several studies have found the concentration of serotonin end products (metabolites) to be lower than normal in clients with fibromyalgia, supporting the hypothesis of aberrant pain perception resulting from a deficiency of serotonin (Russell, 1989; Russell and Vaeroy, 1990; Russell et al., 1992).

Sleep disturbances may contribute to fibromyalgia symptoms; researchers are investigating alterations of the neuroimmunoendocrine systems that accompany disordered sleep physiology, resulting in the nonrestorative sleep, pain, fatigue, and cognitive and mood symptoms that persons with fibromyalgia and CFS experience (Moldofsky, 1995). Persons affected do not enter restorative sleep (phase IV sleep) called rapid eye movement (REM sleep). Deficiency of non-REM sleep also contributes to sleep disturbance by reducing the amount of time the muscles enter a state of resting muscle tone. Eighty percent of the body's growth hormone is secreted by the pituitary gland (under hypothalamic control) during deep sleep, and it is crucial for normal muscle metabolism and tissue repair (Bennett et al., 1992). These types of sleep disturbances are not unique to fibromyalgia but have been observed in many people with rheumatoid arthritis, osteoarthritis, and other painful rheumatic diseases (Moldofsky, 1989).

Clinical Manifestations. Fibromyalgia is characterized by muscle pain as the major symptom, often described as aching or burning, "a migraine headache of the muscles." There is diffuse pain or tender points present on both sides of the body in many muscle groups including the neck, back, arms, legs, jaw, feet, and hands (Fig. 5–7). Sleep disturbances result in fatigue and exhaustion, even after a night's sleep. Symptoms of traumatically induced fibromyalgia are the same as those of spontaneous fibromyalgia (Waylonis and Perkins, 1994).

Other symptoms or associated problems occur with a high frequency (Table 5–11). Symptoms are often exacerbated by stress; physical activity ("overloading it") including overstretching; damp or chilly weather; heat exposure or humidity; sudden change in barometric pressure; trauma; or another illness. Those persons with fibromyalgia who are aerobically fit manifest fewer symptoms than those who remain physically deconditioned and aerobically unfit. Biofeedback specialists have shown that blood circulation to the affected areas is often significantly decreased while at rest and a noticeable decrease in circulation occurs with changes in barometric pressure. During exercise, when circulation should normally increase to muscles and brain, in fibromyalgia, just the opposite happens and circulation is decreased significantly (Hulme, 1995).

The diaphragm is significantly affected in fibromyalgia to the point that it ceases to function as the major breathing muscle and accessory muscles of the neck and upper chest take over. This overwork results in tender points or tightness of the neck and chest muscles. In general, the level of muscular activity in fibromyalgia is high, even when the body is sitting or reclining. During daily activities such as cleaning, cooking, typing, and even socializing, the muscles used for these activities are at a higher level of activity than the muscles of a normal person doing the same tasks. When the activity is over, and the person with fibromyalgia is "resting," those same muscles continue to repeat the activity over and over at a lower intensity so that no outward movement is apparent.

Medical Management

Diagnosis. There is no definitive test currently available to determine the presence of fibromyalgia. The American College of Rheumatology has published the most current diagnostic criteria for classification (see Fig. 5–7). Subjective assessment of tender points can be elicited by the use of an instrument called a dolorimeter, which distributes pressure equally over a discrete point. With a dolorimeter, the pressure required to produce pain in a given area can be recorded (Freundlich and Leventhal, 1993).

Often the diagnosis is determined as a process of elimination by ruling out other conditions (Box 5–5) based on clinical presentation and past medical history. In addition to the presence of tender points (see Fig. 5–7), skin fold tenderness, increased reactive skin hyperemia, and low tissue compliance (in the trapezius and paraspinal regions) provide further diagnostic information (Granges and Littlejohn, 1993). Laboratory tests and radiologic studies give essentially normal results.

Treatment. Approaches to helping clients with fibromyalgia must be holistic and multidisciplinary including education and support, stress management and lifestyle training (including coping strategies, applying work simplification and ergonomic principles, and psychotherapy), medications (including analgesics and antidepressants), local modalities and techniques for muscle pain, and conditioning and aerobic exercise (Nichols and Glenn, 1994). Cognitive behavioral

[26] People who do not have fibromyalgia experience these changes but the autonomic responses occur in smaller amplitude and for a shorter period of time before returning to normal levels. In fibromyalgia, the nervous system's ability to modulate and return to normal is fragile and lacks the subtle ability to respond quickly; responses are more exaggerated and the return to normal takes more time (Yunus, 1992; Hulme, 1995).

[27] The inhibitory system acts to lessen or filter out some of the painful signals transmitted to the brain. These pain stimuli are usually transmitted by substance P. Increased activity of substance P may explain an abnormally decreased pain threshold in fibromyalgia (Yunus, 1992).

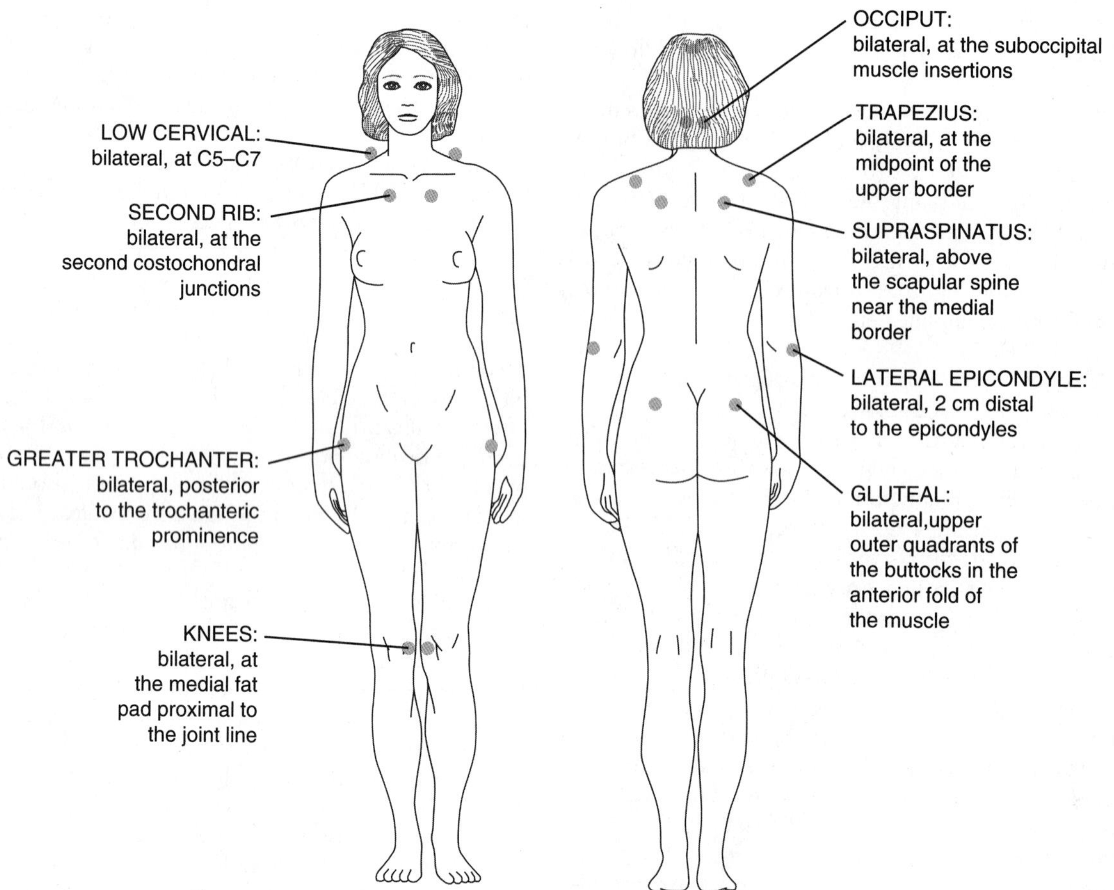

Figure **5-7.** Anatomic locations of tender points associated with fibromyalgia, according to the American College of Rheumatology 1990 classification of fibromyalgia. Digital palpation should be performed with an approximate force of 4 kg (approximately the pressure needed to indent a tennis ball). For a tender point to be considered positive, the subject must state that the palpation was "painful." A reply of "tender" is not considered painful and is not positive.

therapy aimed at altering sensory, affective, cognitive, and behavioral aspects of chronic pain (e.g., pain severity, emotional distress, depression, anxiety, pain behavior) have been shown to be effective over a long period of time, even when the disease process cannot be controlled and symptoms worsen (White and Nielson, 1995).

Prognosis. Many people with mild symptoms are managed without a specialist and have an expected good long-term outcome (Nies, 1995), but most people experience persistent symptoms of fibromyalgia for many years or a lifetime. Symptoms usually remain unchanged or increase with concomitant decrease in function (Ledingham et al., 1993; Hendriksson, 1994; Onchi et al., 1990). The major factor determining the long-term outcome in fibromyalgia is the severity of typical symptoms and the degree of disability at the time of diagnosis.

Special Implications for the Therapist **5-7**

FIBROMYALGIA

Rehabilitative therapy is an important component in managing fibromyalgia. Therapy is helpful first in directing individuals to reach goals of lessening pain and fatigue, and eliminating sleep disturbance. It is essential to combine self-care and management strategies, including an exercise program* to reach the goals of optimal function and fitness while maintaining decreased pain and fatigue, and increasing endurance for daily activities. A cardiopulmonary fitness component should be included at whatever level the individual presents with at the time of assessment.

Aquatic therapy† is an ideal way to begin conditioning with low-level progressive exercises, gradually increasing strength and endurance while improving overall cardiovascular fitness. As with all exercise programs with this population (whether aquatic or other therapy), persons with fibromyalgia fatigue quickly and may have a low tolerance for exertion, requiring short exercise sessions (according to individual tolerance using the rate of perceived exertion; see Chapter 10), possibly even only 5 to 8 minutes at first. The client is encouraged to increase exercise duration in small daily increments, sometimes only by seconds or minutes. Reaching a goal of 30 minutes of daily exercise may take weeks to months;

TABLE 5-11 Clinical Manifestations of Fibromyalgia

Sign or Symptom	Incidence (%)*
Visual problems (e.g., blurring, double vision, bouncing images)	95
Mental and physical fatigue	85
Sleep disturbance/morning fatigue	80
Morning stiffness (persists >30 min)	75
Global anxiety	72
Cognitive (memory) problems (e.g., decreased attention span, impaired short-term memory, decreased concentration)	71
Irritable bowel syndrome	70
Ulcerative colitis	50–60
Headaches	70
Hypersensitivity to noise, odors, heat, or cold	50–60
Mitral valve prolapse	50
Paresthesias	50
Swollen feeling	50
Hypoglycemia (e.g., weakness, irritability, disorientation)	45–50
Pelvic pain	43
Raynaud's phenomenon	38
Sicca syndrome (dry eyes/mouth)	33
Respiratory dysfunction (e.g., dyspnea, erratic breathing patterns during exertion)	33
Auditory problems	31
Temporomandibular dysfunction	25
Irritable bladder syndrome/female urethral syndrome	12
Hyperactive autonomic responses	Unknown
Allergies	Unknown
Restless leg syndrome, nocturnal myoclonus	Unknown
Lack of libido	Unknown

* These figures were compiled from a variety of sources but represent a fairly accurate clinical perspective.

Modified from Hulme J: Fibromyalgia: A handbook for self-care and treatment. Missoula, Mont, Phoenix, 1995, pp 5–8.

some individuals are only able to tolerate one to three daily exercise cycles, each lasting only 5 to 10 minutes.

Persons with fibromyalgia are also more vulnerable to overuse syndromes than people with normal muscle histology, requiring a slower, longer rehabilitation process. This may not be activity-induced as once thought, but rather may occur as a result of sarcolemmal abnormality (Jubrias et al., 1994). At present, until more is known and understood about this phenomenon, an aerobic exercise routine should become a part of the client's life before individual muscle group strengthening is started.

Several studies have supported the hypothesis that a cardiovascular fitness program improves pain ratings and psychological profiles of persons with fibromyalgia, as well as increasing β-endorphin, adrenocorticotropic hormone (ACTH), and cortisol levels in response to exercise at aerobic levels (i.e., 60% of maximal oxygen consumption) (Nichols and Glenn, 1994; McCain et al., 1988).

BOX 5-5
Differential Diagnosis of Fibromyalgia

Hypothyroidism
Polymyalgia rheumatica/giant cell arteritis
Rheumatoid arthritis
Polymyositis/dermatomyositis
Systemic lupus erythematosus
Myofascial pain syndrome
Metabolic myopathy (e.g., alcohol)
Neurosis (depression/anxiety)
Metastatic cancer
Chronic fatigue syndrome
Temporomandibular joint dysfunction
Disk disease

Adapted from Harvey CK, et al: Fibromyalgia. Part 1. Review of the literature. J Am Podiatr Med Assoc 83:413, 1993.

Strategies for work modification and applying ergonomic techniques to increase efficiency and decrease pain are important treatment modalities (Hulme, 1995). A chronic pain program may be appropriate (see Chronic Pain, Chapter 2). The reader is referred to more specific literature for treatment regimens and therapy protocols for this condition‡ (Hulme, 1995; Backstrom, 1992; Rachlin, 1994; Jacobsen et al., 1993).

* Sometimes the person's condition is so acute that exercise is not tolerated immediately. This is often the reason for using modalities in the early stage of therapy. Exercise too soon and too much can set the person back considerably but at the same time the therapist must keep in mind the long-term goal to increase strength and improve aerobic fitness.

† Ideal pool temperature is between 84° and 90°F (compared with 82° to 84°F for the general population and 90° to 94°F for persons with arthritic conditions) (Kuhne, 1995).

‡ Other resources include the Fibromyalgia Network Newsletter, P.O. Box 31750, Tucson, AZ 85751 and the American Fibromyalgia Syndrome Association, P.O. Box 9699, Bakersfield, CA 93389.

ISOIMMUNE DISEASE

Organ and Tissue Transplantation

With recent advances in technology and immunology, organ and tissue transplantation is becoming commonplace. In fact, transplantation of almost any tissue is feasible but the clinical use of transplantation to remedy disease is still limited for many organ systems because of the rejection reaction. Transplant rejection, an isoimmune phenomenon, occurs in response to transplantation because the body usually recognizes the donor tissue as nonself and attempts to destroy the tissue shortly after transplantation.

There are several different types of transplants. *Syngeneic* transplants are between genetically identical members of the same species (identical twins); these are also called *isografts*. *Allograft* (or homograft) transplants are between individuals of the same species (e.g., human to human). Two randomly chosen individuals are almost certainly antigenically different to some degree. Transplants between them are rejected in approximately 2 weeks without the extensive use of immunosuppressive drugs. *Autologous* transplants are within the same individual (e.g., skin graft from leg to hand). *Xenogeneic* (heterograft) transplants are between individuals of different species (e.g., pig to human).

Histocompatibility

In all cases of graft rejection, the cause is incompatibility of cell surface antigens. The rejection of foreign or transplanted tissue occurs because the recipient's immune system recognizes that the surface HLA proteins of the donor's tissue are different from the recipient's. For this reason, HLA matching of donor and recipient greatly enhances the probability of graft acceptance (Rote, 1994b). Certain antigens are more important than others for a successful transplant, including ABO and Rh antigens present on red blood cells and histocompatibility antigens, most importantly the HLA. As expected, there is a better chance of graft acceptance with syngeneic or autologous transplants because the cell surface antigens are identical.

The process of determining histocompatibility, that is, finding compatible donors and recipients, is called tissue typing. Prior to transplantation, testing in the laboratory is carried out to determine whether antibodies incompatible with the donor have been formed by the recipient (a positive crossmatch). If the crossmatch is positive, the transplant will fail; a negative test result is necessary for a successful transplant.

Graft Rejection

Transplant failure is primarily due to histoincompatibility and lack of effective immunosuppressive drugs to prevent rejection. Pretransplant serologic testing is done to avoid transmitting infectious agents (e.g., CMV, hepatitis virus) from donor to recipient. In order to minimize rejection and improve chances of survival, blood types and tissue types are matched as closely as possible between donor and recipient.

In the case of organs such as the lungs, as well as the kidney, heart, liver, and pancreas, a generous blood supply is essential to survival in the recipient's body. As blood is drained from the transplanted organ into the host's general circulation, the body recognizes the transplanted tissue cells as foreign invaders (antigens) and immediately sets up an immune response by producing antibodies. These antibodies are capable of inhibiting metabolism of the cells within the transplanted organ and eventually actively cause their destruction (O'Toole, 1992).

There are three types of transplant rejection—the hyperacute rejection, the acute or late acute rejection, and the chronic rejection—depending on the amount of time that passes between transplantation and rejection. In the *hyperacute rejection* (rare with antibody screening and tissue typing), there is an immediate rejection after transplantation when the recipient has preformed antibodies to donor tissue. This reaction necessitates prompt surgical removal of the transplanted tissue.

The *acute* or *late acute rejection* can appear days or years after the transplantation. This type of rejection involves a combination of cellular and humoral reactions. Clinically, there is sudden onset of organ-related symptoms, which may be associated with fever and graft tenderness. Graft rejection must be differentiated from immunosuppressive toxicity. In the case of acute rejection, if detected in its early stages, this condition can be reversed with immunosuppressive therapy.

Months to years may pass before the *chronic rejection* occurs. This type of rejection develops as a function of the cell-mediated system and is characterized by slow, progressive organ failure. Chronic rejection may be the end result of repeated episodes of cellular rejection, either asymptomatic or clinically apparent. This advanced state of damage is not responsive to therapy (Rubin and Farber, 1994).

Graft-vs.-Host Disease

The discussion of graft rejection describes reactions in a transplant recipient with an intact immune system. In recent years, bone marrow transplantation to bone marrow–depleted or immunodeficient persons has resulted in the complication of graft-vs.-host disease. GVHD occurs when immunocompetent T lymphocytes in the grafted material recognize foreign antigens in the recipient, initiating a type IV hypersensitivity reaction against the recipient's tissues. GVHD may be acute, occurring in the first 1 to 2 months after transplantation, or chronic, developing at least 2 to 3 months after transplantation.

GVHD occurs most commonly after bone marrow and fetal thymus transplantation (obtained from stillborn infants for children with thymic aplasia and consequent lack of normal development of the lymphoid system). It does not occur in autologous bone marrow transplantation or peripheral blood stem cell transplantation but may occur in an allograft or syngeneic transplant, even with a perfect HLA match, because of unidentified and therefore unmatched antigens. Pretransplant immunologic and genetic manipulation using hematopoietic stem cells has minimized GVHD in clients receiving high-dose chemotherapy (Jagannath et al., 1993).

Signs and symptoms of GVHD are fever, exfoliative dermatitis, hepatitis, diarrhea or abdominal pain, ileus, vomiting, and weight loss. GVHD is also characterized by hardening of organ tissues and drying of mucous membranes, especially in the gastrointestinal mucosa, the liver, and the skin, resembling scleroderma (Rote, 1994a). A generalized polyneuropathy coincident with the occurrence of GVHD has been reported (Amato et al., 1993). The neuropathy affected proximal and distal muscles and demonstrated hyporeflexia or areflexia. Electrophysiologic studies did not meet strict criteria for demyelination. The signs of neuropathy improved after immunosuppressive treatment or simultaneous with the resolution of GVHD.

Untreated GVHD is often fatal. Treatment with immunosuppressive therapy including prednisone, cyclosporin, thalidomide, or a combination of these agents has improved the long-term outlook for persons with chronic GVHD (Sullivan et al., 1988; Vogelsang et al., 1992).

Immunosuppression

The fact that a primary role of the immune system is to distinguish between self and nonself presents a major problem facing the candidate for transplantation: the immunologic response of the client to the donor's tissues. In the person with an intact immune system (immunocompetence), the client's immune system recognizes the transplanted tissue or organ as foreign (nonself) and produces antibodies and sensitized lymphocytes against it.

The ultimate objective of immunosuppressive therapy is to block transplant recipient reactivity to the donor's organ while sparing other responses. Since these drugs suppress all immunologic reactions, overwhelming infection is the leading cause of death in transplant recipients. However, increased understanding of rejection mechanisms has made it possible to suppress specific elements of the immune response using monoclonal antibodies in experimental models[28] (Cosimi, 1995). Transferring this information for use in human models with more selective immunosuppressive agents may improve future transplantation success.

[28] Clinical trials with monoclonal antibodies that react with antigens present only on activated T cells (sparing T cells not participating in the rejection reaction) are now in progress.

References

Ader R, Cohen N, Felten D: Psychoneuroimmunology: Interactions between the nervous system and the immune system. Lancet 345:99–103, 1995.

Ader R, Felten DL, Cohen N (eds): Psychoneuroimmunology, ed 2. San Diego, Academic Press, 1991.

Amato AA, Barohn RJ, Sahenk Z, et al: Polyneuropathy complicating bone marrow and solid organ transplantation. Neurology 43:1513–1518, 1993.

Arend WP: Inhibiting the effects of cytokines in human diseases. Adv Intern Med 40:365–394, 1995.

Arnold HL, Odom RB, James WD (eds): Andrews' Diseases of the Skin: Clinical Dermatology, ed 8. Philadelphia, WB Saunders, 1990.

Avins AL, Woods WJ, Lindan CP, et al: HIV infection and risk behaviors among heterosexuals in alcohol treatment programs. JAMA 271:515–518, 1994.

Backstrom G: When Muscle Pain Won't Go Away. Dallas, Taylor, 1992.

Ballou SP: Concurrent laboratory tests best to monitor SLE activity. J Musculoskel Med 10(10):11–12, 1993.

Bancroft B: Immunology simplified. Semin Perioperative Nurs 3:70–78, 1994.

Benhaim R, Hunt TK: Natural resistance to infection: Leukocyte functions. J Burn Care Rehabil 13:289, 1992.

Bennett R, Clark SR, Campbell SM, Burckhardt CS: Low levels of somatomedin-C in patients with FMS: A possible link between sleep and muscle pain. Arthritis Rheum 35:1113–1116, 1992.

Bennett RM: Beyond fibromyalgia: Ideas on etiology and treatment. J Rheumatol 16(suppl 19):185–191, 1989.

Bennett RM: Fibromyalgia: The commonest cause of widespread pain. Compr Ther 21:269–275, 1995.

Bennett RM, Jacobsen S: Muscle function and origin of pain in fibromyalgia. Baillieres Clin Rheumatol 8:721–746, 1994.

Benveniste EN: Cytokines: Influence on glial cell gene expression and function. *In* Blalock JE (ed): Neuroimmunoendocrinology, ed 2. Basel, Karger, 1992, pp 84–105.

Ben-Yehuda A, Weksler M: Host resistance and the immune system. Clin Geriatr Med 8:701–711, 1992.

Blalock JE: A molecular basis for bidirectional communication between the immune and neuroendocrine systems. Physiol Rev 69:1–32, 1989.

Blumer D, Heilbronn M: Chronic pain as a variant of depressive disease: The pain-prone disorder. J Nerv Ment Dis 170:381–406, 1982.

Boeck MA, Chen C, Cunningham-Rundles S: Altered immune function in a morbidly obese pediatric population. Ann NY Acad Sci 699:253–256, 1993.

Boumpas DT, Austin HA, Fessler BJ, et al: Systemic lupus erythematosus: Emerging concepts. Part 1. Ann Intern Med 122:940–950, 1995a.

Boumpas DT, Fessler BJ, Austin HA, et al: Systemic lupus erythematosus: Emerging concepts. Part 2. Ann Intern Med 123:42–53, 1995b.

Bridges SH, Sarver N: Gene therapy and immune restoration for HIV disease. Lancet 345:427–432, 1995.

Brink JJ, Reichel W: Cell biology and physiology of aging. *In* Reichel W (ed): Care of the Elderly: Clinical Aspects of Aging, ed 4. Baltimore, Williams & Wilkins, 1995, pp 472–475.

Bron D: Graft-versus-host-disease. Curr Opin Oncol 6:358–364, 1994.

Brown L, Drotman P: What is the risk of HIV infection in athletic competition. Presented at Ninth International Conference on AIDS, Berlin, June 6–11, 1993.

Bullock B: Normal immunologic response. *In* Bullock B, Rosendahl P: Pathophysiology: Adaptations and Alterations in Function, ed 3. Philadelphia, JB Lippincott, 1992, pp 296–311.

Burger D, Dayer JM: Inhibitory cytokines and cytokine inhibitors. Neurology 45 (suppl 6):S39–43, 1995.

Cannon JG, Kluger MJ: Endogenous pyrogen activity in human plasma after exercise. Science 220:617, 1983.

CDC (Centers for Disease Control and Prevention): Guidelines for prevention of HIV and hepatitis B virus transmission to health care and public safety workers. MMWR 38:S1–6, 1989.

CDC (Centers for Disease Control and Prevention): National notifiable diseases reporting—United States, 1994. JAMA 273:194, 1995.

Cohen R: Occupational infections. *In* LaDou J (ed): Occupational Medicine. Norwalk, Conn, Appleton & Lange, 1990, pp 170–181.

Cosimi AG: Future of monoclonal antibodies in solid organ transplantation. Dig Dis Sci 40:65–72, 1995.

Dick R, Worthman F: Frequency of bleeding and risk of HIV transmission in intercollegiate athletics. Med Sci Sports Exer 5(suppl):S13, 1994.

Dinarello CA, Wolff SM: The role of interleukin-1 in disease. N Engl J Med 328:106–113, 1993.

Eichner ER: Infection, immunity, and exercise: What to tell patients? Physician Sportsmed 21(1):125–135, 1993.

Eichner ER: Neck check. Runner's World 27(1):16, 1992.

Eichner ER, Calabrese LH: Immunology and exercise. Med Clin North Am 78:377–388, 1994.

Farrar DJ, Locke SE, Kantrowitz FG: Chronic fatigue syndome: Etiology and pathogenesis. Behav Med 21:5–16, 1995.

Fauci A: Host factors in the pathogenesis of HIV disease. Presented at the Fourth Annual Conference on Retroviruses and Opportunistic Infections, Washington, DC, Jan 22–26, 1997.

Felten DL, Felten SY, Carlson SL: Noradrenergic and peptidergic innervation of lymphoid tissue. J Immunol 135 (suppl):755s–765s, 1985.

Field CJ, Goureon R, Marliss EB: Circulating mononuclear cell numbers and function during intense exercise and recovery. J Appl Physiol 71:1089, 1991.

Frankel SS, Wenig BM, Burke AP, et al: Replication of HIV-1 in dendritic cell–derived syncytia at the mucosal surface of the adenoid. Science 272:115–117, 1996.

Fretwell MD: Aging changes in structure and function. *In* Carnevali DL, Patrick M (eds): Nursing Management for the Elderly, ed 3. Philadelphia, JB Lippincott, 1993, pp 113–140.

Freundlich B, Leventhal L: The fibromyalgia syndrome. *In* Schumacher HR (ed): Primer on the Rheumatic Diseases, ed 10. Atlanta, Arthritis Foundation, 1993, pp 247–249.

Friedman WJ, Larkfors L, Ayer-LeLievre C, et al: Regulation of beta-nerve growth factor expression by inflammatory mediators in hippocampal cultures. J Neurosci Res 27:374–382, 1990.

Futrell N, Millikan C: When lupus involves the central nervous system. J Musculoskel Med 11(5):53–62, 1994.

Ginzler E: Cognitive dysfunction associated with SLE. J Musculoskel Med 9(3):17–18, 1992.

Gladman DD, Urowitz MB: Systemic lupus erythematosus: Clinical manifestations. *In* Schumacher HR (ed): Primer on the Rheumatic Diseases, ed 10. Atlanta, Arthritis Foundation, 1993, pp 106–111.

Goldenberg DL: Fibromyalgia and chronic fatigue syndrome: Are they the same? J Musculoskel Med 7(5): 1990.

Granges G, Littlejohn GO: A comparative study of clinical signs in fibromyalgia/fibrositis syndrome, healthy and exercising subjects. J Rheumatol 20:344–351, 1993.

Gray AB, Smart YC, Telford RD, et al: Anaerobic exercise causes transient changes in leukocyte subsets and IL-2R expression. Med Sci Sports Exerc 24:1332, 1992.

Gunn WJ, Connell DB, Randall B: Epidemiology of chronic fatigue syndrome: The Centers for Disease Control Study. Ciba Found Symp 173:83–101, 1993.

Gurney ME, Heinrich SP, Lee MR, et al: Molecular cloning and expression of neuroleukin, a neurotrophic factor for spinal and sensory neurons. Science 234:566–574, 1986.

Guyton AC: Human Physiology and Mechanisms of Disease, ed 5. Philadelphia, WB Saunders, 1992.

Harruff HC: Pathology Facts. Philadelphia, JB Lippincott, 1994.

Hellman DB: Arthritis and musculoskeletal disorders. *In* Tierney LM, McPhee SJ, Papadakis MA (eds): Current Medical Diagnosis and Treatment, ed 34. Norwalk, Conn, Appleton & Lange, 1994, pp 664–710.

Hendriksson CM: Long-term effects of fibromyalgia on everyday life. A study of 56 patients. Scand J Rheumatol 23:36–41, 1994.

Hulme J: Fibromyalgia: A Handbook For Self-care and Treatment. Missoula, Mont, Phoenix, 1995.

Hunder GG, Kaye RL, Williams RD: Rheumatology symposium: OA, osteoporosis, fibromyalgia. J Musculoskel Med 10(9):16–34, 1993.

Ironson G, Simoneau J, Antoni MH, et al: Distress, denial, and low compliance predict disease progression in HIV-1 seropositive gay men. *In* Proceedings of American Psychosomatic Society, New York, 1992.

Irwin KL, Rice RJ, Sperling RS, et al: Potential for bias in studies of the influence of human immunodeficiency virus infection on the recognition, incidence, clinical course, and microbiology of pelvic inflammatory disease. Obstet Gynecol 84:463–469, 1994.

Jacobsen S, Danneskiold-Samsoe B, Lund B: Musculoskeletal Pain, Myofascial Pain Syndrome, and the Fibromyalgia Syndrome. Binghamton, NY, Haworth Medical Press, 1993.

Jagannath S, Barlogie B, Tricot G: Hematopoietic stem cell transplantation. Hosp Pract 28(8):79–86, 1993.

Janusek L: Structure and function of the immune system. *In* Black JM, Matassarin-Jacobs E: Luckmann and Sorensen's Medical-Surgical Nursing, ed 4. Philadelphia, WB Saunders, 1993, pp 529–547.

Jason LA, Taylor R, Wagner L, et al: Estimating rates of chronic fatigue syndrome from a community-based sample: A pilot study. Am J Community Psychol 23:557–558, 1995.

Jones D, Adinolfi A, Gallis HA (eds): Overview of HIV Infection in Care of the Patients with HIV Infection. Research Triangle, NC, Glaxo, 1991, pp 5–65.

Jowett JB, Planelles V, Poon B, et al: The human immunodeficiency virus type 1 *vpr* gene arrests infected T cells in the G2 + M phase of the cell cycle. J Virol 69:6304–6313, 1995.

Jubrias SA, Bennett RM, Klug GA: Increased incidence of a resonance in the phosphodiester region of 31P nuclear magnetic resonance spectra in the skeletal muscle of fibromyalgia patients. Arthritis Rheum 37:801–807, 1994.

Keller P: Physical therapy management of patients with HIV-positive/AIDS. Adv Phys Therapists 5:6–7, 17, 1994.

Kuhne L: Improving functional mobility for fibromyalgia patients with aquatic exercise. Presented at Aquatic Therapy Rehabilitation Institute Conference, Las Vegas, August 1995.

Lane HC: Immunoregulation, immune defects, and clinical strategies. Mt Sinai J Med 59:244–252, 1992.

LaPerrierre A, Antoni MH, Klimas N, et al: Psychoimmunology and stress management in HIV-1 infection. *In* Gorman J, Kretzner RM (eds): Psychoimmunology Update. Washington, DC, American Psychiatric Press, 1991.

LaPerrierre A, Antoni MH, Schneiderman N, et al: Exercise intervention attenuates serologic status for HIV-1. Biofeedback Self Regul 15:229, 1990.

LaPerrierre A, O'Hearn P, Ironson G, et al: Exercise and immune function in healthy HIV antibody negative and positive gay males. *In* Proceedings of the Ninth Annual Scientific Sessions of the Society of Social Behavioral Medicine. Boston, 1988, p 28.

Ledingham J, Doherty S, Doherty M: Primary fibromyalgia syndrome—An outcome study. Br J Rheumatol 32:139–142, 1993.

Levy DN, Refaeli Y, Weiner DB: The *vpr* regulatory gene of HIV. Curr Top Microbiol Immunol 193:209–236, 1995.

Liang MH, Partridge AJ, Daltroy LH, et al: Strategies for reducing excess morbidity and mortality in blacks with systemic lupus erythematosus. Arthritis Rheum 34:1187–1196, 1991.

Lipsky JJ: Antiretroviral drugs for AIDS. Lancet 348:800–803, 1996.

Love PE, Santaro SA: Antiphospholipid antibodies: Anticardiolipin and the lupus anticoagulant in systemic lupus erythematosus (SLE) and non-SLE disorders. Ann Intern Med 112:682–698, 1990.

Lynch FA, Kirov SM: Changes in blood lymphocyte populations following surgery. J Clin Lab Immunol 20:75, 1986.

McCain G, Bell D, Mai F, Halliday P: A controlled study of the effects of a supervised cardiovascular fitness training program on the manifestations of primary fibromyalgia. Arthritis Rheum 31:1135–1141, 1988.

McCarthy DA, Dale MM: The leukocytosis of exercise: A review and model. Sports Med 6:333–363, 1988.

McGrew CA: HIV, hepatitis B, and the athlete: What precautions are needed? J Musculoskel Med 12(3):14–20, 1995.

McMurray RW, Bradsher RW, Steele RW, et al: Effect of prolonged modified fast in obese persons on in vitro markers of immunity: Lymphocyte function and serum effects on normal neutrophils. Am J Med Sci 299:379, 1990.

Meakins JL, Nohr CW: Assessment of immunology responsiveness. *In* Kirkpatrick JR (ed): Nutrition and Metabolism in the Surgical Patient. Mt Kisco, NY, Futura, 1983, pp 107–119.

Minerbo GM: Immunologic aspects in HIV. *In* Galantino ML (ed): Clinical Assessment and Treatment of HIV. Thorofare, NJ, Slack, 1992, pp 17–24.

Minowa M, Jiamo M: Descriptive epidemiology of chronic fatigue syndrome based on a nationwide survey. J Epidemiol 6:75–80, 1996.

Mitsias P, Levine SR: Large cerebral vessel occlusive disease in systemic lupus erythematosus. Neurology 44(3 pt 1):385–393, 1994.

Moldofsky H: Chronobiological influences on fibromyalgia syndrome: Theoretical and therapeutic implications. Baillieres Clin Rheumatol 8:801–810, 1994.

Moldofsky H: Fibromyalgia, sleep disorder and chronic fatigue syndrome. Ciba Found Symp 173:262–271, 1993.

Moldofsky H: Nonrestorative sleep and symptoms after a febrile illness in patients with FMS and CFS. J Rheumatol 16(suppl 19):150–153, 1989.

Moldofsky H: Sleep and fibrositis syndrome. Rheum Dis Clin North Am 15:91–103, 1989.

Moldofsky H: Sleep, neuroimmune and neuroendocrine functions in fibromyalgia and chronic fatigue syndrome. Adv Neuroimmunol 5:39–56, 1995.

Neiderman MS, Fein AM: Pneumonia in the elderly. Geriatr Clin North Am 2:247–254, 1986.

Nichols DS, Glenn TM: Effects of aerobic exercise on pain perception, affect, and level of disability in individuals with fibromyalgia. Phys Ther 74:327–332, 1994.

Nieman DC, Henson DR, Johnson R, et al: Effects of brief, heavy exertion on circulating lymphocyte subpopulations and proliferative response. Med Sci Sports Exerc 24:1339, 1992.

Nieman DC, Johanssen IM, Lee JW, et al: Infectious episodes in runners before and after the Los Angeles Marathon. J Sports Med Phys Fitness 30:316, 1990.

Nies KM: Disability, symptom severity predict outcome in fibromyalgia. J Musculoskel Med 12(10):11–12, 1995.

Norris J (ed): Professional Guide to Diseases, ed 5. Springhouse, PA, Springhouse, 1995.

Obbens E, Galantino ML: Rehabilitation perspectives for neurologic complications of HIV. *In* Galantino ML (ed): Clinical Assessment and Treatment of HIV. Thorofare, NJ, Slack, 1992, pp 87–99.

Onchi DR, Dill ER, Katz RS: How often do fibromyalgia patients improve? Pro Ann Sci Meet Am Coll Rheumatol 33:S136, 1990.

Osmond D, Charlebois E, Lang W, et al: Changes in AIDS survival time, 1983–1993. JAMA 271:1083–1087, 1994.

O'Toole M: Miller-Keane Encyclopedia and Dictionary of Medicine, Nursing, and Allied Health, ed 5. Philadelphia, WB Saunders, 1992.

Pantaleo G, Graziosi G, Fauci A: The immunopathogenesis of human immunodeficiency virus infection. N Engl J Med 328:327, 1993.

Petri M: Is estrogen therapy safe in women with lupus? J Musculoskel Med 11(12):11, 1994.

Pisetsky DS: Systemic lupus erythematosus: Epidemiology, pathology, and pathogenesis. *In* Schumacher HR (ed): Primer on the Rheumatic Diseases, ed 10. Atlanta, Arthritis Foundation, 1993, pp 100–105.

Rachlin ES (ed): Diagnosis and Comprehensive Management of Myofascial Pain. St Louis, Mosby–Year Book, 1994.

Reichlin S: Neuroendocrine-immune interactions. N Engl J Med 329:1246–1253, 21, 1993.

Richter EA, Kiens B, Raben A, et al: Immune parameters in male athletes after a lacto-ovo vegetarian diet and a mixed Western diet. Med Sci Sports Exerc 23:517, 1991.

Robertson KR, Stern RA, Hall CD, et al: Vitamin B_{12} deficiency and nervous system disease in HIV infection. Arch Neurol 50:807–811, 1993.

Rosenberg SA, Yang JC, Topalian SL, et al: Treatment of 283

consecutive patients with metastatic melanoma or renal cell cancer using high-dose bolus interleukin-2. JAMA 271:907–913, 1994.
Rote NS: Alterations in immunity and inflammation. *In* McCance KL, Huether S: Pathophysiology: The Biologic Basis for Disease in Adults and Children, ed 2. St Louis, Mosby–Year Book, 1994a, pp 268–298.
Rote N: Immunity. *In* McCance KL, Huether S: Pathophysiology: The Biologic Basis for Disease in Adults and Children, ed 2. St Louis, Mosby–Year Book, 1994b, pp 205–233.
Rubin E, Farber JL: Pathology, ed 2. Philadelphia, JB Lippincott, 1994.
Russell I: Neurohormonal aspects of fibromyalgia syndrome. Rheum Dis North Am 15:149–168, 1989.
Russell IJ, Michalek JE, Vipraio GA, et al: Platelet 3H-imipramine uptake receptor density and serum serotonin levels in patients with fibromyalgia/fibrositis syndrome. J Rheumatol 19:104–109, 1992.
Russell IJ, Orr MD, Littman B, et al: Elevated cerebrospinal fluid levels of substance P in patients with the fibromyalgia syndrome. Arthritis Rheum 37:1593–1601, 1994.
Russell I, Vaeroy H: Cerebrospinal fluid (CSF) biogenic amines in fibromyalgia syndrome. ACR Sci Abstracts S55, 1990.
Schaffer SD, Garzon LS, Heroux DL, et al: Pocket Guide to Infection Prevention and Safe Practice. St Louis, Mosby–Year Book, 1996.
Schlenzig C, Jager H, Rieder H, et al: Supervised physical exercise leads to psychological and immunological improvement in pre-AIDS patients. *In* Proceedings of the Fifth International Conference on AIDS, Montreal, 1989, p 337.
Selik RM, Chu SY, Ward JW: Trends in infectious diseases and cancers among persons dying of HIV infection in the United States from 1987 to 1992. Centers for Disease Control and Prevention (CDC). Ann Intern Med 123:933–936, 1995.
Simpson DM, Bender AN: Human immunodeficiency virus-associated myopathy. Ann Neurol 24:79, 1988.
Sisto SA: Chronic fatigue syndrome. Presented at the World Confederation of Physical Therapy, Washington, DC, June 1995.
Smith JA, Telford RD, Mason IB, et al: Exercise, training, and neutrophil microbicidal activity. Int J Sports Med 11:179, 1990.
Sprenger H, Jacobs C, Nain M, et al: Enhanced release of cytokines, interleukin-2 receptors, and neopterin after long distance running. Clin Immunol Immunopathol 63:188, 1992.
Steinbach LS, Tehranzadeh J, Fleckenstein J, et al: Human immunodeficiency virus infection: Musculoskeletal manifestations. Radiology 186:833–838, 1993.
Stewart RJ, Marsden PA: Biologic control of the tumor necrosis factor and interleukin-1 signaling cascade. Am J Kidney Dis 25:954–966, 1995.
Strauss S: Chronic fatigue syndrome. National Institutes of Health (NIH) Publication No. 91-3059, Bethesda, MD, December 1991.
Sullivan KM, Witherspoon RP, Storb R, et al: Alternating-day cyclosporin and prednisone for treatment of high-risk chronic graft-versus-host disease. Blood 72:555–561, 1988.
Thompson JM, McFarland GK, Hirsch JE, Tucker SM: Mosby's Clinical Nursing, ed 3. St. Louis, Mosby–Year Book, 1993.
Vaeroy H: Elevated CSF levels of substance P and high incidence of Raynaud phenomenon in patients with fibromyalgia. Pain 32:21–26, 1988.
Vogelsang GB, Farmer ER, Hess AD, et al: Thalidomide for the treatment of graft-versus-host disease. N Engl J Med 326:1055–1058, 1992.
Von Feldt JM: Systemic lupus erythematosus. Recognizing its various presentations. Postgrad Med 97:799–886, 1995.
Wallace D: Cytokine and immune regulation in FMS. Arthritis and Rheum 32:1334–1335, 1989.
Waylonis GW, Heck W: Fibromyalgia syndrome. New associations. Am J Phys Med Rehabil 71:343–348, 1992.
Waylonis GW, Perkins RH: Post-traumatic fibromyalgia. A long-term follow-up. Am J Phys Med Rehabil 73:403–412, 1994.
Waylonis GW, Ronan PG, Gordon C: A profile of fibromyalgia in occupational environments. Am J Phys Med Rehabil 73:112–115, 1994.
Weight LM, Alexander D, Jacobs P: Strenuous exercise: Analagous to the acute-phase response? Clin Sci 81:677, 1991.
Weinroth SE, Parenti DM, Simon GL: Wasting syndrome in AIDS: Pathophysiologic mechanisms and therapeutic approaches. Infect Agents Dis 4:76–94, 1995.
Weinstein A: Corticosteroids linked to avascular necrosis in SLE patients. J Musculoskel Med 11(4):16, 1994.
White KP, Nielson WR: Cognitive behavioral treatment of fibromyalgia syndrome: A followup assessment. J Rheumatol 22:717–721, 1995.
Wilder E: Unpublished material.
Wolfe F, Ross K, Anderson J, et al: Aspects of fibromyalgia in the general population: Sex, pain threshold, and fibromyalgia symptoms. J Rheumatol 22:151–156, 1995a.
Wolfe F, Ross K, Anderson J, et al: The prevalence and characteristics of fibromyalgia in the general population. Arthritis Rheum 38:19–28, 1995b.
Yunus MB: Psychological aspects of fibromyalgia syndrome: A component of the dysfunctional spectrum syndrome. Baillieres Clin Rheumatol 8:811–837, 1994.
Yunus MB: Towards a model of pathophysiology of fibromyalgia. Aberrant central pain mechanisms with peripheral modulation. J Rheumatol 19:846–850, 1992.
Yunus MB, Dailey JW, Aldag JC, et al: Plasma tryptophan and other amino acids in primary fibromyalgia: A controlled study. J Rheumatol 19:90–94, 1992.

SECTION 2

chapter 6

Infectious Disease

Catherine C. Goodman

Although humans are continually exposed to a vast array of microorganisms in the environment, only a small proportion of those microbes are capable of interacting with the human host in such a way that infection and disease result. With the steady advances being made in medicine, people are living longer, but infection is still a frequent cause of hospital admission and remains an important cause of death, especially in the aging population.

From 1950 until 1980 the management of communicable infectious diseases was well under control; morbidity and mortality from infectious diseases such as yellow fever, cholera, typhus, malaria, typhoid fever, and plague were no longer serious threats in the United States. The widespread availability and use of sulfa drugs and antibiotics successfully treated tuberculosis, syphilis, gonorrhea, bacterial meningitis, scarlet fever, and rheumatic fever, as well as nosocomial (hospital- or nursing home–acquired) infections (Grimes, 1993). Organized efforts to immunize all children lowered the incidence of vaccine-preventable diseases such as measles, mumps, rubella, diphtheria, tetanus, and poliomyelitis. Research was directed toward preventing and managing chronic disease.

Unfortunately, this period of reduced morbidity and mortality secondary to infectious disease did not last, and in the 1980s new infectious agents appeared. *Legionella*, human immunodeficiency virus (HIV), antibiotic-resistant organisms, and a resurgence of tuberculosis are examples of infectious processes that have returned the focus to the prevention and treatment of infectious diseases. Infectious diseases are spreading more rapidly throughout the world than in the past, facilitated by a combination of environmental disruption and increasing human mobility (Bright, 1995).

While a number of new infectious diseases have appeared in recent years, there has also been a worldwide resurgence of longstanding diseases once thought to be well controlled. Epidemics of destructive organisms have accelerated; one third of the world's population now carries *Mycobacterium tuberculosis*. Organisms travel on the shoes of tourists, in the ballast of cargo ships, and in the blood of humans. When natural systems are weakened by ecological stresses (e.g., pollution, habitat destruction, weather disasters, climate change, famine), they become more vulnerable to damage or destruction by invading organisms, which can result in the spread of infection. Opportunistic organisms take advantage of the weakened defenses (Platt, 1995).

All health care professionals must maintain a vigilant attitude to preventing infectious disease. This requires an understanding of the infectious process, the chain of transmission, and selected aspects of control. In this chapter, a basic understanding of these concepts is provided along with a discussion of a few infectious diseases. Other pertinent infectious diseases are presented in appropriate chapters according to the primary clinical pathology (e.g., pneumonia in Chapter 12, bacterial meningitis in Chapter 25, Sjögren's syndrome in Chapter 23).

SIGNS AND SYMPTOMS OF INFECTIOUS DISEASES *(Thompson et al., 1993)*

Clinical manifestations of infectious disease are many and varied depending upon the etiologic agent (e.g., viruses, bacteria; see Types of Organisms, this chapter) and the system affected (e.g., respiratory, central nervous system [CNS], gastrointestinal, genitourinary). Systemic symptoms of infectious disease can include fever and chills, sweating, malaise, and nausea and vomiting. There may be changes in blood composition, such as an increased number of leukocytes or a change in the types of leukocytes. The elderly may experience a change in mentation (e.g., confusion, memory loss, difficulty concentrating). When observing any person for early signs of infection, the therapist will most likely see one or only a few symptoms listed (Table 6–1).

A change in body temperature is a characteristic systemic symptom of infectious disease (Box 6–1), but fever may accompany noninfectious causes such as inflammatory, neoplastic, and immunologically mediated diseases. *Fever*, a sustained temperature above normal, can be caused by abnormalities of the hypothalamus, brain tumors, dehydration, or toxic substances affecting the temperature-regulating center of the hypothalamus. Certain protein substances and toxins can cause the set-point of the hypothalamic "thermostat" to rise. This results in activation of the hypothalamus to conserve heat and increase heat production. Substances that cause these effects are called pyrogens.

In infectious disease the endotoxins of some bacteria and the extracts of normal leukocytes (interleukin) are pyrogenic. They act to raise the thermostat in the hypothalamus, thus raising the body temperature. Fever patterns may differ depending on the specific infectious disease present and occur clinically on a continuum from fever associated with an acute illness lasting 7 to 10 days, to sepsis and ongoing infection lasting longer than 10 days, to fever of unknown origin (FUO) associated with a possible infectious origin lasting at least 3 weeks. Other causes of FUO include neoplasm (lymphoma and leukemia are the most common), autoimmune disorders such as Still's disease, systemic lupus erythematosus, and polyarteritis nodosa; and miscellaneous diseases including temporal arteritis, sarcoidosis, alcoholic hepatitis, and drug-induced fever, among others.

A general rule, the 102°F rule, divides conditions into two groups: those that do not cause temperature elevations exceeding 102°F (39°C) and those that regularly exceed

TABLE 6–1 Signs and Symptoms of Infectious Disease

Fever, chills, malaise (most common early symptoms)

Enlarged lymph nodes

Integument
- Purulent drainage from open wound or skin lesion
- Skin rash, red streaks
- Bleeding from gums or into joints; joint effusion or erythema

Cardiovascular
- Petechial lesions
- Tachycardia (see also Aneurysm, Thrombophlebitis, Chapter 10)
- Hypotension
- Change in pulse rate (may increase or decrease depending on the type of infection)

Central nervous system
- Altered level of consciousness, confusion, convulsions
- Headache
- Photophobia
- Memory loss
- Stiff neck, myalgia

Gastrointestinal
- Nausea
- Vomiting
- Diarrhea

Genitourinary
- Dysuria or flank pain
- Hematuria
- Oliguria
- Urgency, frequency

Upper respiratory
- Cough
- Hoarseness
- Sore throat
- Nasal drainage
- Sputum production

102°F. Table 6–2 reflects hospital data, whereas the outpatient population is more likely to experience fever accompanied by generalized arthralgias and myalgias associated with a self-limiting illness, or fever with localized symptom(s) such as a sore throat, cough, or right lower quadrant pain, as occurs with bacterial infection. Temperature elevation to 104°F (40°C) may cause delirium and convulsions, particularly in children. An extremely high fever may damage cells irreversibly.

BOX 6–1
Common Causes of Fever in the Hospitalized Person

Atelectasis
Pneumonia
Catheter-related infection
Surgical wound infection
Urinary tract infection
Drugs
Pulmonary emboli
Infected pressure ulcers

From Andreoli TE, Bennett JC, Carpenter CCJ, et al (eds): Cecil Essentials of Medicine, ed 3. Philadelphia, WB Saunders, 1993, p 691.

TABLE 6–2 Most Common Causes of Prolonged Fever*

Conditions in Which Fever Generally Does Not Exceed 102°F	Conditions in Which Fever Regularly Exceeds 102°F
Catheter-associated bacteriuria	Malignant hyperthermia (secondary to anesthesia)
Atelectasis	Transfusion reactions
Phlebitis	Urosepsis
Pulmonary emboli	Intravenous (IV) line sepsis
Dehydration	Prosthetic valve endocarditis
Pancreatitis	Intra-abdominal or pelvic peritonitis or abscess
Myocardial infarction	*Clostridium difficile* colitis
Uncomplicated wound infections	Procedure-related bacteremia
Any malignancy	Nosocomial pneumonia
Cytomegalovirus	Drug fever
Hepatitis	HIV infection
Infectious mononucleosis (Epstein-Barr virus)	Heat stroke
Subacute bacterial endocarditis	Acute bacterial endocarditis
Tuberculosis	Tuberculosis (usually disseminated or extrapulmonary)
	Lymphoma
	Metastasizing carcinoma to liver or central nervous system

* The evaluation of fever magnitude with the 102°F rule is most often done in the acute care setting. This is a general guideline that must be taken into consideration with other presenting factors (Cunha, 1989).
From Cunha BA: Clinical implications of fever. Postgrad Med 85:192, 1989.

Some people with serious infection do not initially develop fever but instead become *tachypneic, confused,* or develop *hypotension.* Most often, this situation occurs in the elderly, hospitalized client with a nosocomial infection or in the immunocompromised person.

Inflammation and its *exudates* may remain localized, may permeate the tissue, or may spread throughout the body via the blood or lymph. Infection can develop, as is the case with an *abscess,* a localized infection and inflammation with purulent exudate. Leukocytes form a wall around the organisms. The abscess deepens as more leukocytes are drawn into the area, more organisms are killed, and more necrotic tissue is dissolved. The exudate may eventually be autolyzed and resorbed by the body, in which case the inflammation and infection are resolved. Rupture of the abscess and drainage into other tissues can spread the infection to other areas of the body.

For example, infectious abdominal disorders (e.g., Crohn's disease, diverticulitis, appendicitis), as well as tuberculosis of the spine, pelvic inflammatory disease, vertebral osteomyelitis, septic arthritis of the sacroiliac joint, and tumor of the thigh, can result in abscess formation in the space between the posterior peritoneum and the psoas and iliac fascia (Maull and Sachatello, 1974; Oliff and Chuang, 1978). A psoas abscess is usually confined within the psoas fascia, but occasionally, because of anatomic relations, infection extends to the buttock, hip, or upper thigh. Such an abscess causes true musculoskeletal symptoms of back pain, or pain referred to the hip or knee, and limited range of hip motion, but from an underlying systemic cause. Flexion deformity of the hip may develop from reflex spasm, and extension of the thigh is very painful; hip abduction and adduction evoke minimal discomfort. An unexplained limp may be the initial symptom and this will be an important clinical clue when taking a history (see Figs. 13–10 and 13–11). Only days to weeks later does lower abdominal pain develop, and the person becomes acutely ill with a high fever.

Rash with fever can result from a local infectious process caused by any microbe that has successfully penetrated the stratum corneum (see Fig. 8–1) and multiplied locally. Skin rashes may also occur with infection elsewhere in the body unrelated to local skin disease (e.g., scarlet fever caused by streptococci; also called scarlatina). The most common types of localized skin lesions associated with infectious disease are maculopapular eruptions (e.g., classic childhood viral illnesses such as measles, rubella, roseola, fifth disease), nodular lesions (e.g., streptococcus, *Pseudomonas*), diffuse erythema (e.g., scarlet fever, toxic shock syndrome), vesiculobullous eruptions (e.g., varicella, herpes zoster), and petechial purpuric eruptions (e.g., Epstein-Barr virus, cytomegalovirus [CMV]). Specific types of skin lesions are discussed in Chapter 8.

Red streaks radiating from an infection site (referred to in lay terms as "blood poisoning") in the direction of a regional lymph node may be associated with lymphangitis secondary to an infection such as cellulitis. Lymphangitis, an acute inflammation of the subcutaneous lymphatic channels, usually occurs as a result of hemolytic streptococci or staphylococci (or both) entering the lymphatic channels from an abrasion or local trauma, wound, or infection (see Chapter 8). The red streak may be obvious or it may be faint and easily overlooked, especially in dark-skinned people. The nodes most frequently affected are the submandibular, cervical, inguinal, and axillary nodes, in that order. Involved nodes are usually tender and enlarged (greater than 3 cm).

Inflamed lymph nodes can be associated with other infectious diseases and may be palpated by the therapist, especially in cervical, axillary, or inguinal areas when there are presenting musculoskeletal symptoms in those areas. For example, intraoral infection may cause an inflamed cervical node leading to spasm of the sternocleidomastoid muscle causing neck pain. Palpation may appear to aggravate a primary spasm as if originating in the muscle, when in fact a lymph node under the muscle is the source of the symptom. In acute infections, nodes are tender asymmetrically, enlarged, and matted together. The overlying skin may be erythematous (red) and warm. Unilaterally warm, tender, enlarged, and fluctuant lymph nodes sometimes associated with elevated body temperature may be caused by pyogenic infections and may require medical referral.

Supraclavicular and inguinal nodes are also common metastatic sites for cancer. Nodes involved with metastatic cancer are usually hard and fixed to the underlying tissue. Changes in size (greater than 1 cm), shape (matted together), and consistency (rubbery or firm) of lymph nodes in more than one area that persist for more than 4 weeks, or the presence of painless, enlarged lymph nodes, should be reported to the physician.

Joint effusion, usually of one joint (monarticular), associated with infectious arthritis can occur as a result of bacterial, mycobacterial, fungal, or viral etiologic agents. Streptococcal bacteremia from any cause can result in suppurative arthritis (inflammatory with pus formation). Bone and joint infections are discussed more completely in Chapter 21.

AGING AND INFECTIOUS DISEASES

(Reichel, 1995)

Although most types of infections are seen in the aging, many infections are indigenous (occur naturally) to this group. The aging person can have more serious infections with little or no fever because of an impaired thermoregulatory system[1] or secondary to the masking effects of drugs such as aspirin, other anti-inflammatory drugs, and corticosteroids. If the febrile response is absent in an elderly person with a serious infection, it is a grave sign. A review of the elderly with fever of unknown origin found that 36% had infections such as endocarditis, intra-abdominal abscess, and tuberculosis (Esposito and Gleckman, 1978).

Early recognition of infection in the elderly is difficult because people underreport symptoms, the presentation is often vague or atypical, and symptoms are difficult to assess. The elderly person may be unable to describe the present illness, past history, or list the medications being taken. A complete physical examination may be difficult because of the person's uncooperativeness, cognitive impairment, neurologic deficits, or contracted limbs. Pain may be poorly localized or absent, as in appendicitis, or it may be confused with preexisting conditions, as in septic arthritis or degenerative joint disease (DJD). A change in mental state with confusion or lethargy may be the earliest sign of acute infection.

Aging is a state of immune dysregulation. There is involution (shriveling) of the thymus and altered T cell–mediated immunity, but also increased antibody production to self-antigens. Diminished cell-mediated immunity results in the reactivation of dormant infections such as herpes zoster and tuberculosis. Influenza deaths after age 65 are increased, and the antibody response to influenza vaccine is decreased (Ben-Yehuda and Weksler, 1992).

The aging process at the tissue and cellular level may lead to increased susceptibility to infection because of atrophic skin, achlorhydria (absence of hydrochloric acid in gastric juice), and decreased cough and gag reflexes, as well as decreased bronchiolar elasticity and mucociliary activity (Rossman, 1986). The most important determining factors of how well aging people can handle infections are related to their underlying mental and physical disability, nutritional status, and the presence of chronic disease such as renal and cardiac impairment or peripheral vascular insufficiency. Environmental factors also play a role in preventing infections. In many aging people physical or psychological impairment and decline may result in indifference to personal hygiene and loss of manual dexterity, body mobility, or vision. Likewise aging spouse caregivers of aging people are significantly more likely

[1] Fever in older people may not be high enough to cause concern because the basal body temperature is low. Temperatures should be taken in the evening and a lower threshold for infection should be used (e.g., oral temperature of 99° or 100°F with a change in function) (Castle et al., 1991).

to have communicable upper respiratory tract infections than are others (Kiecolt-Glaser et al., 1991).

INFECTIOUS DISEASES

Overview and Definitions. Infection is a process in which an organism establishes a parasitic relationship with its host. This invasion and multiplication of microorganisms produce signs and symptoms as well as an immune response. Such reproduction injures the host by causing cellular damage from microorganism-producing toxins or intracellular multiplication, or by competing with the host's metabolism. The host's immune response may compound the tissue damage; such damage may be localized (e.g., as in infected pressure ulcers) or systemic (Norris, 1995).

The development of an infection begins with transmission of an infectious organism (agent, pathogen, pathogenic agent) and depends on a complex interaction of the pathogen, an environment conducive to transmission of the organism, and the susceptibility of the human host. Even after successful transmission of a pathogen, the host may experience more than one possible outcome. The pathogen may merely contaminate the body surface and be destroyed by first-line defenses such as intact skin or mucous membranes that prevent further invasion.

Alternatively, successful invasion and replication of the pathogen, a process called *colonization*, may result in a laboratory-verified condition referred to as *subclinical*, *silent*, or *asymptomatic*, causing no signs and symptoms or immune response. The person with a subclinical condition or colonization may be a carrier and transmit infection to others, but is not susceptible and does not have a clinical infection.

The period of time when the pathogen enters the host to the appearance of clinical symptoms is called the *incubation period*. This period may last from a few days to several months, depending on the causative organism and type of disease. Disease symptoms herald the end of the incubation period. A *latent infection* occurs after a microorganism has replicated but remains dormant or inactive in the host, sometimes for years (e.g., tuberculosis). The host may harbor a pathogen in sufficient quantities to be shed at any time after latency and toward the end of the incubation period. This time period when an organism can be shed is called the *period of communicability*.

From this concept of communicability, communicable diseases can be defined as any disease whereby the causative agent may pass or be carried from one person to another directly or indirectly. It usually precedes symptoms and continues through part or all of clinical disease, sometimes extending to convalescence, but it is important to note that an asymptomatic host can still transmit a pathogen. The communicable period, like the incubation period and mode of transmission, varies with different pathogens and different diseases (Grimes, 1993).

Types of Organisms *(Norris, 1995)*

There is a great variety of microorganisms responsible for infectious diseases, including viruses, mycoplasmata, bacteria, rickettsiae, chlamydiae, protozoa, and fungi (yeasts and molds). All microorganisms can be distinguished by certain intrinsic properties such as shape, size, structure, chemical composition, antigenic makeup, growth requirements, ability to produce toxins, and ability to remain alive (viability) under adverse conditions such as drying, sunlight, or heat. These properties provide the basis for identification and classification of the organisms. Knowledge of the properties permits diagnosis of a specific pathogen in specimens of body fluids, secretions, or exudates. All these properties are important to consider when looking for ways to interfere with the mechanisms of transmission.

Viruses are subcellular organisms made up only of an RNA or a DNA nucleus covered with proteins. They are the smallest known organism, visible only through an electron microscope. Viruses are completely dependent on host cells and cannot replicate unless they invade a host cell and stimulate it to participate in the formation of additional virus particles. The estimated 400 viruses that infect humans are classified according to their size, shape (spherical, rod-shaped, or cubic) or means of transmission (respiratory, fecal, oral, or sexual). Viruses are not susceptible to antibiotics and cannot be destroyed by pharmacologic means. However, antiviral medications can mitigate (moderate) the course of the viral illness. For example, acyclovir, an antiviral medication used for herpesvirus interferes with DNA synthesis causing decreased viral replication and decreasing the time of lesional healing (Skidmore-Roth, 1995).

Mycoplasmata (includes the pleuropneumonia-like organisms (PPLOs) are bacteria that can be separated into 15 different species that have a membrane but lack cell walls. For this reason, antibiotics that are active against bacterial cell walls have no effect on mycoplasmata. At present, mycoplasmata remain sensitive to antibiotics.

Bacteria are single-celled microorganisms with well-defined cell walls that can grow independently on artificial media without the need for other cells. Bacteria can be classified according to shape. Spherical bacterial cells are called *cocci*; rod-shaped bacteria, *bacilli*; and spiral-shaped bacteria, *spirilla* or *spirochetes*. Bacteria can also be classified according to their response to staining (gram-positive, gram-negative, or acid-fast), motility (motile or nonmotile), tendency to capsulation (encapsulated or nonencapsulated) and capacity to form spores (sporulating or nonsporulating).

Rickettsiae are primarily animal pathogens that generally produce disease in humans through the bite of an insect vector such as a tick, flea, louse, or mite and are relatively uncommon in the United States. They are small gram-negative, bacteroid organisms that frequently cause life-threatening infections. Like viruses, these microorganisms require a host for replication. Three categories of the family Rickettsiaceae are *Rickettsia*, *Coxiella*, and *Rochalimaea*. Chlamydiae are smaller than rickettsiae and bacteria but larger than viruses. They too depend on host cells for replication, but unlike viruses they always contain both DNA and RNA and are susceptible to antibiotics.

Protozoa have a single cell unit or a group of nondifferentiated cells, loosely held together and not forming tissues. They have cell membranes rather than cell walls, and their nuclei are surrounded by nuclear membranes. Larger parasites include roundworms and flatworms. *Fungi* are unicellular to filamentous organisms possessing hyphae (filamentous outgrowths) surrounded by cell walls and containing nuclei. Fungi show relatively little cellular specialization and occur as yeast (single-cell oval-shaped organisms) or molds (organisms with branching filaments). Depending on the environment, some fungi may occur in both forms. Fungal diseases in humans are called *mycoses*.

The Chain of Transmission *(Grimes, 1993)*

Infection begins with transmission of a pathogen to the host. Successful transmission depends upon a pathogenic agent, a reservoir, a portal of exit from the reservoir, a mode (mechanism) of transmission, a portal of entry into the host, and a susceptible host. This sequence of events is called the chain of transmission (Table 6–3).

Pathogens

Humans coexist with many microorganisms in complex, mutually beneficial relationships. Even so, many organisms are parasitic, maintaining themselves at the expense of their host. Some parasites arouse a pathologic response in the host and are called *pathogens* or pathogenic agents. As such, pathogens are ineffective parasites because they stimulate a disease response, which may harm the host and eventually kill the pathogen.

The mode of action of a pathogen refers to how the organism produces a pathologic process. Great variation exists among the various pathogens. Some intracellular pathogens, like viruses, invade cells and interfere with cellular metabolism, growth, and replication, whereas others invade and cause hyperplasia, necrosis, and cell death. Some viruses, like CMV, and varicella-zoster virus, create a persistent latent infection.

TABLE 6–3 Chain of Transmission of Infectious Disease

Transmission Chain	Factors
Pathogen or agent	Viruses, mycoplasmata, bacteria, rickettsiae, chlamydiae, protozoa, fungi
Reservoir	Humans (clinical cases, subclinical cases, and carriers)
	Animal, arthropod, plant, soil, food, organic substance
Portal of exit	Genitourinary tract, gastrointestinal tract, respiratory tract, oral cavity, open lesion, blood, vaginal secretions, semen, tears, excretions (urine, feces)
Transmission	Direct: person to person (fecal-oral, sexual, bites, contact with discharge from an ulcer, open sore, or respiratory mucous droplet)
	Indirect: through a vehicle (animate: animal or vector such as mosquito or tick bite; inanimate: food, water, soil, milk, air, intravenous therapy, or catheters)
Modes of entry	Ingestion, inhalation, percutaneous injection, transplacental entry, mucous membranes
Susceptible host	Specific immune reactions
	Nonspecific body defenses
	Host characteristics: age, sex, ethnic group, heredity, behaviors
	Environmental and general health status

Adapted from Thompson JM, McFarland GK, Hirsch JE, Tucker SM: Mosby's Clinical Nursing, ed 3. St Louis, Mosby–Year Book, 1993.

The human immunodeficiency virus (HIV) causes immunosuppression by destroying helper T lymphocytes. Some pathogens, such as the tetanus bacillus, produce a toxin that interferes with intercellular responses. Others, such as group A β-hemolytic streptococci, stimulate a pathologic immune response in the host. Larger parasites, such as roundworms, cause anemia as well as interfere with the function of the gastrointestinal system.

The likelihood of a pathogen producing infectious disease and the type of disease are influenced by the characteristics of the organism. These characteristics include infectivity, pathogenicity, virulence, toxigenicity, and antigenicity. Infectivity, the pathogen's ability to invade and replicate in the host, is facilitated by enzymes produced by the organism. These enzymes dissolve host connective tissue or protect the pathogen from host defenses. Infectivity is high in a disease like measles because it takes very few viruses to establish infection. Infectivity is low in tuberculosis because many bacilli remain dormant and the disease remains quiescent after the initial hypersensitivity to the tuberculin microorganism.

Pathogenicity, the ability of the organism to induce disease, depends on the organism's speed of reproduction in the host, the extent of tissue damage, and the strength of any toxin released by the pathogen. For example, the rabies virus is highly pathogenic; infection with it always results in disease, whereas the poliovirus has a low pathogenicity and only produces disease when multiple conditions are favorable.

Virulence refers to the potency of the pathogen in producing severe disease and is measured by the case-fatality rate (i.e., the number of people who die of the disease divided by the number of people who have the disease). Some pathogens, such as HIV, are highly virulent and some pathogens have changed their virulence over time. *Toxigenicity*, the amount and destructive potential of released toxin, is closely related to virulence. Some bacteria, such as diphtheria and tetanus, secrete water-soluble antigenic exotoxins that are quickly disseminated in the blood, causing potentially severe systemic and neurologic manifestations. Other microorganisms, such as *Shigella*, affecting the intestinal tract and causing dysentery, contain endotoxins in their cell lining that cause local inflammation and destruction of cells.

Antigenicity is the ability of the pathogen to stimulate an immune response in the host and varies greatly among organisms depending on the site of invasion and dissemination in the body. Generally, organisms that invade and localize in tissue initially stimulate a cellular (T cell) response. Organisms that disseminate quickly stimulate a humoral or antibody response. Some organisms, such as the influenza virus, have the potential to alter their antigenic characteristics. This virus is capable of extensive gene rearrangements resulting in significant changes in surface antigen structure. This ability allows new strains to evade host antibody responses directed at earlier strains.

Reservoir

A *reservoir* is an environment in which an organism can live and multiply such as an animal, plant, soil, food, or other organic substance or combination of substances. The reservoir provides the essentials for survival of the organism at specific stages in its life cycle. Some parasites have more than one reservoir such as the yellow fever virus, which can maintain life in humans and other animals. Some parasites require more than one reservoir at different growth stages and still others, such as most sexually transmitted organisms, require only a human reservoir.

Human and animal reservoirs can be symptomatic or asymptomatic carriers of the pathogen. A carrier maintains an environment that promotes growth, multiplication, and shedding of the parasite without exhibiting signs of disease. Hepatitis is a common example of this in humans.

Portal of Exit

The portal of exit is the place from which the parasite leaves the reservoir. Generally, this is the site of growth of the organism and corresponds to the system of entry into the next host. For example, the portal of exit for gastrointestinal parasites is usually the feces, and the portal of entry into a new host is the mouth. There are always exceptions, as is the case with hookworm eggs which are shed in the feces but enter through the skin of a person walking barefoot in soil containing hatched eggs.

Common portals of exit include secretions and fluids (e.g., respiratory secretions, blood, vaginal secretions, semen, tears), excretions such as urine and feces, open lesions, and exudates such as pus from an open wound or ulcer. Some organisms such as HIV have more than one portal of exit. Knowledge of the portal of exit is essential for preventing transmission of a pathogen.

Mode of Transmission

Most infectious diseases are transmitted in one of four ways. *Contact transmission* occurs when the host comes into direct contact (sexual contact, biting, touching, kissing, or direct projection of respiratory mucous droplets) or indirect contact with the source (e.g., contaminated inanimate objects[2] or close-range spread of respiratory droplets). *Airborne transmission* results from the inhalation of contaminated droplets. Airborne transmission requires that the pathogen survive in the air until it is inhaled. *Enteric (oral-fecal) transmission* requires the host to ingest infecting organisms found in feces, often through fecally contaminated food or water. *Vector-borne transmission* is the indirect transmission that occurs when an intermediate carrier (vector), such as a flea or a mosquito, transfers an organism. Living vectors can carry the pathogen internally as a biologic vector or externally by mechanical means (e.g., water, soil, food, milk, biologic products, air). Inanimate objects (fomites) include items such as needles, countertops, eating utensils, and urinary catheters.

Nosocomial infections are infections acquired in a hospital or other institution. This type of infection is usually transmitted by direct contact. Less frequently, transmission occurs by inhalation or by contact with contaminated equipment and solutions. Despite hospital programs of infection control that include surveillance, prevention, and education, about 5% to 7% of hospitals patients contract a nosocomial infection. These infections continue to be a difficult problem because hospital patients today are older and more debilitated than in the past. Additionally, nosocomial infections are more virulent and more resistant to treatment. The increased use of invasive and surgical procedures, immunosuppressants, antibiotics, and the lack of handwashing predisposes people to such infections and superinfections. At the same time, the growing number of personnel that come into contact with the client makes the risk of exposure greater (Norris, 1995).

Portal of Entry

A pathogen may enter a new host by ingestion, by inhalation, by bites, through contact with mucous membranes, percutaneously, or transplacentally. Infectious diseases vary as to the number of organisms and the duration of exposure required to start the infectious process in a new host.

Host Susceptibility

Each person has his or her own susceptibility to infectious disease and this susceptibility can vary throughout time. A susceptible host has personal characteristics and behaviors that increase the probability of an infectious disease developing. Biologic and personal characteristics such as age, sex, ethnicity, and heredity influence this probability. General health and nutritional status, hormonal balance, and the presence of concurrent disease also play a role. Likewise, living conditions and personal behaviors, such as drug use, diet, hygiene, and sexual practices, influence the risk of exposure to pathogens and resistance once exposed.

The aged in hospitals and long-term care facilities are already susceptible hosts, especially if poorly nourished. Immunosuppressive agents and corticosteroids decrease the body's ability to resist infection. Inadequate or absent handwashing or other breaches of aseptic technique result in spread of microorganisms from health care workers to clients and between individuals receiving health care. Contamination of the surfaces of equipment can cause infections. Incorrect isolation procedures such as leaving doors to isolation rooms open or not using masks increase the risk of nosocomial infections.

The presence of underlying medical disorders (e.g., malignancy, diabetes, renal failure, acquired immunodeficiency syndrome [AIDS], and cirrhosis) decrease T cell– and B cell–mediated immune function. Breaches of body integrity such as nasogastric and chest tubes, intubation, urinary catheters, and intravenous (IV) devices impair the body's defense mechanisms, decreasing the ability of the integumentary, gastrointestinal, genitourinary, and respiratory systems to resist invasion by microorganisms (Weber and Rutala, 1993).

Lines of Defense

Susceptibility is also influenced by the presence of anatomic and physiologic defenses, sometimes called lines of defense (Thompson et al., 1993). The *first-line defenses* are external such as intact skin and mucous membranes, oil and perspiration on skin, cilia in respiratory passages, gag and coughing reflexes, peristalsis in the gastrointestinal tract, and the flushing action of tears, saliva, and mucus. These first-line defenses act to bar invasion of pathogens and remove them before they have an opportunity to invade. The chemical composition of body secretions such as tears and sweat, together with the pH of saliva, vaginal secretions, urine, and digestive juices, further prevents or inhibits growth of organisms. Compromise

[2] Inanimate objects can include items such as the telephone, sphygmomanometer, bedside rails, tray tables, countertops, etc. that come into direct contact with the infected person, thus emphasizing the need for thorough handwashing at all times.

in any of these natural defenses increases host susceptibility to pathogen invasion.

Another important first-line defense is the normal flora of microorganisms that inhabit the skin and mucous membranes in the oral cavity, gastrointestinal tract, and vagina. These organisms occur naturally and usually coexist with their host in a mutually beneficial relationship. Through a mechanism called microbial antagonism they control the replication of potential pathogens. The importance of this mechanism is evident when it is disturbed, as happens when extensive antibiotic therapy destroys normal flora in the oral or vaginal cavity resulting in *Candida albicans*, an overgrowth of yeast.

Some normal flora can become pathogenic under specific conditions, such as immunosuppression or displacement of the pathogen to another area of the body. Displacement of normal flora is a common cause of nosocomial infections. This can occur when *Escherichia coli* (*E. coli*) ordinarily normal flora in the gastrointestinal tract, invades the urinary tract. Invasive procedures increase the risk of displacing these organisms.

The *second-line defense*, the inflammatory process, and the *third-line defense*, the immune response, share several physiologic components. These include the lymphatic system, leukocytes, and a multitude of chemicals, proteins, and enzymes that facilitate the internal defenses. Once a microorganism penetrates the first line of defense and invades cells, the inflammatory response is initiated. Inflammation is a local reaction to cell injury of any type whether from physical, chemical, or thermal damage, or microbial invasion. As a response to microbial injury, inflammation is aimed at preventing further invasion by walling off, destroying, or neutralizing the invading organism.

The early inflammatory response is protective, but it can continue for sustained periods of time in some infections, leading to granuloma formation. The production of new leukocytes may be stimulated for weeks or months and is reflected in an elevated white blood cell (WBC) count. However, sustained inflammation can become chronic and result in destruction of healthy tissues. Extensive necrosis from persistent inflammation can increase tissue susceptibility to the infectious agent or provide an ideal setting for invasion by other pathogens.

The first and second lines of defense are nonspecific, that is, they operate against all infectious agents in the same way. In contrast, the immune system responds in a specific manner to individual pathogens, as long as the organism has antigenic characteristics. Generally, antigens are either proteins, large polysaccharides, or large lipoprotein complexes that stimulate an immune response. Not all microorganisms are antigenic, but some are bound by complement or other host-produced substances to form an antigen that elicits an immune response. An immune response is triggered after foreign materials have been cleared from an area of inflammation. For specific details regarding cell-mediated vs. humoral immune responses, see Chapter 5.

Control of Transmission

Much can be done to prevent transmission of infectious diseases, including correction of environmental factors; improved nutrition, living conditions, and sanitation; comprehensive immunizations (including the required immunization of travelers to or emigrants from endemic areas); and drug prophylaxis. Breaking the transmission chain at any of these links can help control transmission of infectious diseases. The link most amenable to control varies with the characteristics of the organism, its reservoirs, the type of pathologic response it produces, and the available technology for control. The general goal is to break the chain at the most cost-effective point or points. That is the point at which the greatest number of people can be protected with available technology and the least amount of resources.

Immunization, by decreasing host susceptibility, can now control many diseases, including diphtheria, tetanus, pertussis, measles, rubella, some forms of meningitis, poliomyelitis, hepatitis A and B, pneumococcal pneumonia, influenza (certain strains),[3] rabies, and tetanus. Through immunization, smallpox (variola) is believed to have been successfully eradicated worldwide.

Vaccines, which contain live but attenuated (weakened) or killed microbes, induce active immunity against bacterial and viral diseases by stimulating antibody formation.[4] These molecules lock onto specific proteins made by a virus or bacterium—often those proteins lodged in the microbe's outer coat. Once antibodies attach to an invading microbe, other immune defenses are evoked to destroy it. Immune globulins contain previously formed antibodies from hyperimmunized donors or pooled plasma and provide temporary passive immunity. Passive immunization is generally used when active immunization is life-threatening or when complete protection requires both active and passive immunization (e.g., immunoglobulins used for hepatitis B or for tetanus) (see Table 5–1).

Prophylactic antibiotic therapy may prevent certain diseases but the risk of superinfection and the emergence of drug-resistant strains makes this impractical. Prophylactic antibiotics are usually reserved for people at high risk of exposure to dangerous infections. Antibiotic-resistant bacteria are on the rise in part because antibiotics have been misused and overused.[5] Crowded conditions (e.g., daycare centers, hospitals, military barracks, and prisons) and prior antibiotic therapy are the principal factors predisposing to colonization and disease (McCracken, 1995; Barnes et al., 1995).

Some bacteria, such as enterococci, which cause wound and blood infections, have developed mutant strains that do not respond to any antibiotic therapy. Enterococcal infections

---

[3] Each year the Centers for Disease Control and Prevention (CDC) issues updated information on the vaccine and antiviral agents available for controlling influenza during the current influenza season.

[4] There may be side effects to immunization such as orchitis (inflammation of a testis) following mumps vaccination in adults (Kuczyk et al., 1994) or reactive arthritis after influenza vaccination (Biasi et al., 1994) and after hepatitis B vaccination (Biasi et al., 1993). Animal studies have shown that progressive autoimmune rheumatoid arthritis and ankylosing spondylitis can occur in genetically susceptible mice following certain immunogens (Buzas et al., 1995; Brennan et al., 1995), but the incidence of significant adverse effects of immunization among humans remains very small (Malleson et al., 1993; Chalmers et al., 1994). The potential increase in susceptibility to influenza and death from respiratory illness in high-risk people (e.g., those with rheumatoid arthritis, the elderly, and chronically ill or immunosuppressed) suggests that the influenza and pneumococcal vaccines should include these groups in standard immunization programs (Fiebach and Beckett, 1994; Chalmers et al., 1994).

[5] This is only a small part of the total picture regarding this issue. Other components of this problem include the extensive use of antibiotics in animals later consumed or whose products are consumed (e.g., milk products) and the fact that a number of pharmaceutical companies have focused their research in noninfectious areas of study because it seemed there were enough antibiotics available. Development of new drugs to treat drug-resistant bacteria is at least 5 to 7 years away and drug companies are not pursuing these new drugs at this time (Cohen, 1994).

are primarily limited to hospitals but the genes for resistance are carried on the bacterial structures (plasmids) which can easily be shared by bacteria of different species. Thus, the resistance could move to pneumococcus and to staphylococcus, other bacteria that cause pneumonia and wound and blood infections, respectively (Sanches et al., 1995). At present, certain strains of pneumococcus are resistant to only one antibiotic so that other antibiotics remain effective against these pneumococci. If those strains become resistant to other (currently effective) antibiotics, there may be no treatment at all (Tomasz, 1995). Before 1980, only a few cases of pneumococcus were resistant to penicillin but within a year, strains resistant to penicillin were reported everywhere and are now common throughout the world.

Improved nutrition, *living conditions*, and *sanitation* through the use of disinfection, sterilization, and anti-infective drugs can inactivate pathogens such as *Staphylococcus aureus*.[6] Transmission to a new portal of entry can be prevented by environmental disinfection; use of barrier precautions (gloves, masks, condoms); proper handling of food; and protection from vectors. Decreasing host susceptibility can be achieved through personal hygiene and avoidance of high-risk behaviors (unsafe sex practices, IV drug use, recapping needles); and effective handwashing. Maintaining the first line of defense is an important consideration for the client whose health status has already been compromised by disease or diagnostic and treatment procedures. Some ways to accomplish this include preoperative and postprocedure assistance to encourage deep breathing, coughing, ambulation, skin care, and maintaining adequate hydration, fluid and electrolyte balance, and proper nutrition to strengthen resistance.

Correction of environmental factors, particularly water treatment, food and milk safety programs, and control of animals, vectors, rodents, sewage, and solid wastes, can best eradicate nonhuman environments (reservoirs) and thus control pathogens. Other prevention methods in this category include proper handling and disposal of secretions, excretions, and exudates; isolation of infected clients; and quarantine of contacts. Specific isolation precautions, based on knowledge of the transmission chain for individual infections, have been recommended by the CDC. The precautions were designed to prevent transmission of pathogens among hospitalized people, health care personnel, and visitors (see Table 6–4). Specific recommendations have been made for individual diseases.

Special Implications for the Therapist **6–1**

CONTROL OF TRANSMISSION

The CDC has set up guidelines for the care of all clients regarding precautions against the transmission of infectious disease (see Appendix A: Summary of Universal Precautions). These should be used with all clients regardless of their disease status. All blood and body fluids are potentially infectious and should be handled as such.

All clients receiving therapy (and thus in contact with health care workers) may be asymptomatic hosts during the period of communicability. The careful use of precautionary measures severely limits the transmission of any disease. In addition, each hospital has isolation precautions organized according to categories of disease to prevent the spread of infectious disease to others. Every health care professional must be familiar with these procedures and follow them carefully. Transmission prevention guidelines and accompanying basic isolation procedures are provided in Table 6–4.

Health care professionals should be concerned about improving their resistance and decreasing their susceptibility to infectious diseases. Maintaining an adequate immunization status is one approach. Every health care worker should be adequately immunized against hepatitis B, measles, mumps, rubella, polio, tetanus, diphtheria, and varicella. The 1991 CDC recommendations for immunization of health care workers are given in Table 6–5.

Nosocomial Infections

Therapists can help prevent nosocomial infections (Table 6–6) by following universal precautions (see Appendix A) and by:

- Following strict infection-control procedures. Make sure to identify each client's individual isolation precautions and procedures. When in doubt, ask the nursing staff regarding the status of the person in question.
- Strictly follow necessary isolation techniques.
- Observe *all* clients for signs of infection (see Table 6–1), especially those persons at high risk. Notify nursing or medical staff of these observations.
- Always follow proper handwashing technique, and encourage other staff members to do so as well. Take time to wash your hands after each and every client.
- Stay away from susceptible, high-risk clients when you have an obvious infection. Make arrangements for some other therapist to treat that client until the contagious period has passed. If in doubt, consult a physician.
- Take special precautions with vulnerable clients, that is, those with Foley catheters, mechanical ventilators, or IV lines, and those recuperating from surgery. Specific tips for preventing infection in these situations are listed in Box 6–2.

Hydrotherapy Protocol

In the past, routine cultures of hydrotherapy equipment were performed to identify and supposedly eliminate colonization of infectious bacteria. In this way, the spread of infection was prevented from equipment to client and from client to client, especially in the acute care setting. Now, under the outcomes based management philosophy, infection control is cost-driven so that the outcome is managed as long as the outcome is what was predicted and intended or improving. For example, in the case of preventing the spread of

[6] This is important since one strain of staphylococcus (methicillin-resistant *S. aureus*, MRSA) is resistant to most antibiotics. Over the past 10 years, MRSA and other resistant strains of *S. aureus* have become the most common causes of hospital and community-acquired infections. MRSA usually develops when multiple antibiotics are used in the treatment of infection and in people who are elderly, debilitated, having surgery or multiple invasive procedures, or being treated in critical care units (Grimes, 1993).

TABLE 6-4 Transmission Prevention Guidelines

To prevent the transmission of infectious diseases in hospitals and other clinical settings, the Centers for Disease Control and Prevention has published a *category-specific* isolation system, which describes six of its seven categories of isolation precautions according to major modes of transmission. The seventh category, *universal precautions*, has been expanded to cover all clients—not just those with known or suspected blood-borne diseases. Because of the special concern about the risk of transmitting human immunodeficiency virus, this category is covered separately.

Type of Isolation and Diseases Requiring Isolation	Private Room	Mask	Gown	Gloves	Special Handling
Strict isolation Prevents transmission of contagious or virulent infections by air or contact. Special ventilation is required *Diseases:* pharyngeal diphtheria, viral hemorrhagic fevers, pneumonic plague, smallpox, varicella-zoster virus (localized in immunocompromised person or disseminated)	X With door closed	X	X	X	X
Contact isolation Prevents transmission of epidemiologically important infections that do not require strict isolation. Health care workers should wear masks, gowns, and gloves for direct or close contact, depending on the infection *Diseases in any age group:* group A streptococcal endometritis; impetigo; pediculosis; *Staphylococcus aureus* or *Streptococcus pneumoniae* infection; rabies; rubella; scabies; staphylococcal scalded skin syndrome; major skin, wound, or burn infection (draining and not adequately covered by dressing); vaccinia; primary disseminated herpes simplex; cutaneous diphtheria; infection or colonization with bacteria that resist antibiotic therapy *Diseases in infants and young children:* acute respiratory infections, influenza, infectious pharyngitis, viral pneumonia, group A streptococcal infection *Diseases in neonates:* gonococcal conjunctivitis, staphylococcal furunculosis, neonatal disseminated herpes simplex	X	O	S	S	X
Respiratory isolation Prevents transmission of infections spread primarily through the air by droplets *Diseases:* *Haemophilus influenzae* epiglottitis, erythema infectiosum, measles, *H. influenzae* or meningococcal pneumonia, meningococcemia, mumps, pertussis	X With door closed	X	—	—	X
Acid-fast bacillus isolation Prevents clients with active pulmonary or laryngeal tuberculosis from transmitting acid-fast bacillus to other clients. Client requires special ventilation. *Disease:* tuberculosis	X With door closed	X*	S	—	X
Enteric precautions Prevent transmission of infection through direct or indirect contact with feces *Diseases:* amebic dysentery; cholera; coxsackievirus disease; acute diarrhea with suspected infection; echovirus disease; encephalitis unless known not to be caused by enteroviruses; *Clostridium difficile* or enterocolitis caused by *Staphylococcus;* enteroviral infection; gastroenteritis caused by *Campylobacter* spp., *Cryptosporidium* spp., *Dientamoeba fragilis, Escherichia coli, Giardia lamblia, Salmonella* spp., *Shigella* spp., *Vibrio parahaemolyticus*, viruses, or *Yersinia enterocolitica;* hand-foot-and-mouth disease; hepatitis A; herpangina, necrotizing enterocolitis; pleurodynia; poliomyelitis; typhoid fever; viral pericarditis, viral myocarditis, and viral meningitis unless known not to be caused by enteroviruses	D	—	S	S	X
Drainage and secretion precautions Prevent transmission of infection from direct or indirect contact with purulent material or drainage *Diseases:* conjunctivitis; minor or limited abscess; minor or limited burn, skin wound, or pressure ulcer infection; herpes zoster (shingles)	—	—	S	S	X

X, always necessary; S, necessary if soiling of hands or clothing is likely; O, necessary for close contact or if client is coughing and does not reliably cover mouth; D, desirable but optional; necessary only if client has poor hygiene.
* Mask must be particulate respirator.
Modified from Norris J (ed): Professional Guide to Diseases, ed 5. Springhouse, Pa, Springhouse, 1995, pp 149–150.

TABLE 6-5 The 1991 CDC Recommendations for Immunization of Health Care Workers (HCWs)

Disease	Recommendation
Hepatitis A	Not routinely recommended for HCWs; recommended for neonatal ICU workers without serologic evidence of previous HAV infection
Hepatitis B	Three-dose series of hepatitis B vaccine for pre-exposure protection
Influenza	Recommended for HCWs who care for persons with chronic illness or clients >65 yr, and for workers who have chronic illness such as chronic obstructive pulmonary disease or cardiac disease; administer annually prior to influenza season (mid-October to mid-November)
Pneumococcus	Recommended for employees > 65 yr or with underlying cardiac, pulmonary, liver, renal, or immunocompromising disease; booster required every 6 to 10 yr
Poliomyelitis	Primary series of oral poliovirus vaccine in childhood is sufficient but should be complete; not recommended during pregnancy
Tetanus, diphtheria	Booster dose of tetanus-diphtheria toxoids, adult type (Td) every 10 years after primary series; tetanus toxoid may be repeated in 5 years if a dirty wound is sustained
Measles	College entrants and HCWs who do not have evidence of immunity to measles (physician-diagnosed measles or laboratory evidence of immunity) should have documentation of 2 doses of measles vaccine received on or after their first birthday; vaccine can be given as MMR*
Mumps	A single dose of live mumps vaccine received on or after the first birthday is sufficient; vaccine can be given as MMR*
Rubella	A single dose of live attenuated rubella vaccine received on or after the first birthday is sufficient; vaccine can be given as MMR*
Varicella-zoster	Two doses of vaccine 4–8 wk apart† for people who have not developed immunity; pregnancy testing is required prior to administration to a menstruating female

* There is no evidence suggesting an increased risk from live measles, mumps, and rubella (MMR) vaccine to persons already immune to these diseases as a result of previous vaccination or natural disease.

† Report by Center for Biologics Evaluation and Research, Food and Drug Administration. National Immunization Program, CDC. MMWR 44:264, 1995. The recommendations of the Advisory Committee on Immunization Practices (ACIP) on the use of varicella vaccine will be published.

From CDC (Centers for Disease Control and Prevention): Update on adult immunization: Recommendations of the Immunization Practices Advisory Committee (ACIP). MMWR 40:RR-12, 1991.

infection through hydrotherapy equipment, good disinfection and cleaning procedures are practiced and monitored closely. This plan is both cost-effective and is accompanied by a high degree of safety. Routine environmental cultures are not cost-effective and therefore are not performed. Many organisms are present normally, and even if present, if no one is infected, these pathogens are not considered a functional problem. Under outcomes based management, when an infectious problem develops, the cause is traced back to the source and eliminated at that point.

Home Health Care

Preventing spread of an infectious disease to the family, the home health therapist, and perhaps the community is a primary concern when preparing the client for return home. The therapist should work closely with the home health nurse and seek guidance if unsure how to handle a specific situation. A list of helpful hints for home health care includes the following (Grimes, 1993):

- Handwashing is the best protection against transmission of infectious diseases, and it is essential after providing direct care and when gloves are removed.
- Staff should leave extraneous clothing and equipment outside the client's area and take in only items that are needed.
- Equipment needed on a regular basis, such as the blood pressure cuff and stethoscope,* should be in the room at the beginning of home health care. When it is no longer needed, equipment should be bagged or covered and taken to the appropriate area for decontamination and reprocessing. Disposable equipment should be contained, labeled, and discarded.
- The therapist should be adequately supplied with gloves, masks, gowns, and disposable plastic aprons. Some plastic bags of different sizes should be carried for your own use as well as to demonstrate to the client's family how to handle soiled linens and trash.
- Paper towels are useful when working in the client's area. Use them as a clean surface during care and to wipe your hands.
- Before going into the client's area, plan what to do and gather the items needed.
- It is important to remember that isolation or precautions can have a negative effect on the family. Help the family to feel comfortable with the techniques needed for isolation. Encourage them to visit with the client and not just be with him or her during care.
- Should the client have a feces-borne infectious disease such as hepatitis A or salmonellosis, it is important to show the family how to bag and launder soiled linens. It is equally important to demonstrate

TABLE 6-6 Summary of Important Recommendations and Work Restrictions for Personnel with Infectious Diseases

Disease	Relieve from Direct Client Contact	Partial Work Restriction	Duration
Conjunctivitis	Yes	Report to the employee health service; employee will be sent home	Until discharge ceases
Cytomegalovirus	No		
Diarrhea			
Acute stage (diarrhea with other symptoms)	Yes		Until symptoms resolve and salmonella is ruled out
Convalescent stage (salmonella [nontyphoid])	No	Should not care for high-risk clients	Until stool is free of organism on two consecutive cultures not less than 24 hr apart
Other enteric pathogens	No		
Enteroviral infections	No	Should not care for infants	Until symptoms resolve
Group A streptococcal disease	Yes		Until 24 hr after adequate treatment is started
Hepatitis, viral			
Hepatitis A	Yes		Until 7 days after onset of jaundice or other symptoms
Hepatitis B	Possibly	Requires individual determination by hospital or facility for workers performing exposure-prone procedures (e.g., wound or burn care)	
Hepatitis C–E	No	None	
Herpes simplex			
Genital	No		
Hands (herpetic whitlow)	Yes	Note: not known whether gloves prevent transmission	Until lesions heal
Orofacial	No	Personnel should not care for infants or high-risk clients	Until lesions heal
HIV	Possibly	Recommendation: †Any health care worker with a known positive antibody can notify the facility, but this is not a requirement; once the worker is identified as HIV positive, hospital or facility will make individual determination. Employees infected with HIV in areas of high multidrug-resistant (MDR) tuberculosis prevalence should be advised against working with high-risk populations (e.g., AIDS and pulmonary cases) (Diekema and Doebbeling, 1995).	
Measles			
Active	Yes		Until 7 days after rash appears
Postexposure (susceptible personnel)	Yes		From 5–21 days after exposure or 7th day after rash appears
Mumps*			
Active	Yes		Until 9 days after onset of parotitis (from 5–26 days after exposure or 9 days after onset of symptoms)
Postexposure	Yes		
Pertussis			
Active	Yes		From beginning of catarrhal stage through 3rd wk after onset of paroxysms, or until 7 days after start of effective therapy

TABLE 6–6 Summary of Important Recommendations and Work Restrictions for Personnel with Infectious Diseases *(Continued)*

Disease	Relieve from Direct Client Contact	Partial Work Restriction	Duration
Postexposure (asymptomatic personnel)	No		
Postexposure (symptomatic personnel)	Yes		Same as active pertussis
Rubella			
Active	Yes		Until 5 days after rash appears
Postexposure (susceptible personnel)	Yes		From 7–21 days after exposure or 5 days after rash appears
Scabies	Yes		Until treated
Staphylococcus aureus (skin lesions)	Yes		Until lesions have resolved
Upper respiratory infections (includes respiratory syncytial virus, RSV)	Yes	Personnel with upper respiratory infections should not care for infants, children, or high-risk clients	Until acute symptoms resolve
Varicella (chickenpox)			
Active	Yes		Until all lesions dry and crust
Postexposure	Yes		From 10–21 days after exposure or, if varicella occurs, until all lesions dry and crust
Zoster (shingles)			
Active	No	Appropriate barrier desirable; personnel should not take care of high-risk clients	Until lesions dry and crust
Postexposure	Yes		From 10–21 days after exposure or, if varicella occurs, until all lesions dry and crust

* At present there are no determinations, only recommendations, regarding potentially transmissible diseases such as hepatitis B or HIV in health-care workers. Whereas the transmission risk of HBV is well documented, transmission of HIV from health-care worker to client is extremely unlikely; if HIV-positive employees follow usual infection control guidelines, the risk of HIV transmission during routine client care is negligible (Diekema and Doebbeling, 1995). Our understanding of these diseases is changing so rapidly that any determination is often outdated before policies can be published. The Centers for Disease Control and Prevention Hospital Infection Control Practices Advisory Council (HICPAC) will publish Personnel Guidelines for Health Care by the end of 1997.

† Mumps vaccine may be offered to susceptible personnel. When given after exposure, mumps vaccine may not provide protection. However, if exposure did not result in infection, immunizing exposed personnel should protect against subsequent infection. Neither mumps immunoglobulin nor immune serum globulin (ISG) is of established value in postexposure prophylaxis. Transmission of mumps among personnel and clients has not been a major problem in hospitals in the United States, probably owing to multiple factors, including high levels of natural and vaccine-induced immunity.

Modified with permission from Immunological Disorders: Manual of Infection Control. Houston, Author, 1986.

how to bag and dispose of soiled paper products such as linen savers, which cannot be flushed down the toilet. Remind the family to wash their hands afterward and do so yourself.

- If the client has hepatitis A or salmonellosis, the family as well as the client should be reminded not to handle raw food served to others, such as lettuce or tomatoes, until the physician determines the client is past the infectious stage.
- In treating clients with blood-borne illnesses, if the client accidently sustains a cut, any spilled blood should be cleaned off with household bleach and water. Razors and toothbrushes should not be shared.
- The therapist should practice self-protection at all times. Use good handwashing technique† and when in doubt, ask for assistance from other, more knowledgeable health care staff.

*Stethoscopes are often contaminated with staphylococci and therefore a potential vector of infection. Such contamination poses a risk to people with open wounds, such as burns. This contamination is greatly reduced by frequent cleaning with alcohol or nonionic detergent; cleaning with antiseptic soap is only 75% effective in reducing the bacterial count (Jones et al., 1995).

†For specifics about handwashing procedures and other infection control guidelines (including managing significant health care worker exposures), see Schaffer et al. (1996).

Diagnosis of Infectious Diseases *(Andreoli et al., 1993)*

Five basic laboratory techniques can be used in the diagnosis of infectious diseases: (1) direct visualization of the organism;

BOX **6-2**
Tips for Preventing Infection

Chest Tube

Prevent chest tube from kinking by carefully coiling the tubing on top of the bed and securing it to the bed linen, leaving room for the person to turn.

Tracheostomy

Contact with secretions occurs with a tracheostomy; follow standard precautions. When there is direct contact and potential splash secondary to expelled secretions, gown, mask, protective facewear, and gloves are needed.

Urinary Catheter

Follow universal precautions for handwashing techniques.

Do not allow the drainage bag spigot to come in contact with a contaminated surface.

When the drainage tubing becomes disconnected, do not touch the ends of the tubing or catheter. Contact the nursing staff for reconnecting.

Before turning, moving, or transferring a catheterized person, locate the proximal end of the tubing and either clamp it to the person's gown or hold it to allow necessary slack during movement. This will help prevent the catheter from accidentally and traumatically being pulled out.

Whenever possible, avoid raising the drainage bag above the level of the person's bladder.

If it becomes necessary to raise the bag during transfers, clamp the tubing but avoid prolonged clamping or kinking of the tubing (except during bladder conditioning).

Avoid allowing large loops of tubing to dangle from the bedside, wheelchair, or walker.

Drain all urine from tubing into the bag before the person exercises or ambulates.

Intravenous (IV) Devices

If you have exudative lesions or weeping dermatitis, refrain from all direct contact with IV or invasive equipment until the condition resolves.

Notify the nursing staff of any suspicious observations, for example, if the IV device is not dripping at a steady rate (either none at all or flowing very fast); if the IV bag is empty; if blood is flowing from insertion of the IV catheter tip into the person's body out into the IV line.

Nasogastric and Feeding Tubes

Care must be taken to avoid excessive movement or pulling and tugging of these tubes.

Wash your hands before and after touching the entry point of the tube into the body.

Adapted from Potter P, Perry A: Fundamentals of Nursing: Concepts, Processes, and Practice. St Louis, Mosby–Year Book, 1993.

(2) detection of microbial antigen; (3) a search for "clues" produced by the host immune response to specific microorganisms; (4) detection of specific microbial nucleotide sequences; and (5) isolation of the organism in culture. Each technique has its use and each has associated advantages and disadvantages.

In many infectious diseases, pathogenic organisms can be directly visualized by microscopic examination of readily available tissue fluids, such as sputum, urine, pus, and pleural, peritoneal, or cerebrospinal fluid. Detection of specific antigens establishes the presence of some diseases such as meningitis, hepatitis B, and some respiratory and genitourinary tract infections. Histopathologic examination of biopsied or excised tissue often reveals patterns of the host inflammatory response that can provide clues to narrow down the diagnostic possibilities. Some viral infections, such as skin or respiratory infections caused by herpesviruses, or pneumonia due to cytomegalovirus produce characteristic changes in host cells visible on cytologic examination. Recent techniques to amplify microbial DNA or RNA sequences for detection have been used to diagnose some infections and are expected to be developed enough to diagnose numerous other infectious diseases. Finally, isolation of a single microbe from an infected site is generally considered evidence that the infection is caused by this organism.

SPECIFIC INFECTIOUS DISEASES

Most infections are confined to specific organ systems. In this book, many of the important infectious disease entities are discussed in the specific chapter dealing with the affected anatomic area. Only the most commonly encountered infectious problems not covered elsewhere are included in this chapter.

Bacterial Infections

Staphylococcal Infections

Overview and Risk Factors. *Staphylococcus aureus* is one of the most common bacterial pathogens normally residing on the skin and is easily inoculated into deeper tissues where it causes suppurative (pus formation) infections (Rubin and Farber, 1994). It is the most common cause of suppurative infections affecting all ages and involving the skin, joints, and bones. It is a leading cause of infective endocarditis. *S. aureus* spreads by direct contact with colonized surfaces or persons. Most people (both children and adults) are intermittently colonized with *S. aureus*, carrying the organism on the skin, in the nares, or on clothing. The organism also survives on inanimate surfaces for long periods of time. Predisposing factors are multiple and varied depending upon the type of disease outcome (Table 6–7).

Burns and surgical wounds often become infected with *S. aureus* from the person's own nasal passages or from medical personnel. Newborns and elderly, malnourished, diabetic, and obese persons all have increased susceptibility. *S. aureus* is the causative organism in half of all cases of septic arthritis, mostly in people 50 to 70 years old. Rheumatoid arthritis and corticosteroid therapy are common predisposing conditions.

Pathogenesis. *S. aureus* cannot invade through intact skin or mucous membranes; infection usually begins with traumatic inoculation of the organism. Once inside the body, the organism is a virulent pathogen, secreting at least five different membrane-damaging enzymes and toxins that harm host

TABLE 6-7 Staphylococcal Infections

Type	Predisposing Factors
Bacteremia	Infected surgical wounds Abscesses Infected intravenous or intra-arterial catheter sites; catheter tips Infected vascular grafts or prostheses Infected pressure ulcers Osteomyelitis Parenteral drug abuse Source unknown (primary bacteremia) Cellulitis Burns Immunosuppression Debilitating diseases (e.g., diabetes, renal failure) Infective endocarditis Cancer (leukemia) or neutropenia after chemotherapy or radiation
Pneumonia	Immunodeficiency (especially elderly and children <2 yr) Chronic lung disease and cystic fibrosis Malignancy Antibiotics that kill normal respiratory flora but spare *Staphylococcus aureus* Viral respiratory infections, especially influenza Blood-borne bacteria spread to the lungs from primary sites of infections (e.g., heart valves, abscesses, pulmonary emboli) Recent bronchial or endotracheal suctioning or intubation
Enterocolitis	Broad-spectrum antibiotics as prophylaxis for bowel surgery or treatment of hepatic coma Elderly; newborn infants (associated with staphylococcal skin lesions)
Osteomyelitis	Hematogenous organisms (blood-borne) Skin trauma Infection spreading from adjacent joint or other infected tissues *Staphylococcus aureus* bacteremia Orthopedic surgery or trauma Cardiothoracic surgery Usually occurs in growing bones, especially femur and tibia of children <12 yr Male sex
Food poisoning	Contaminated food
Skin infections	Decreased resistance Burns or pressure ulcers Decreased blood flow Skin contamination from nasal discharge Foreign bodies Underlying skin diseases, such as eczema and acne Common in persons with poor hygiene living in crowded quarters

Adapted from Norris J (ed): Professional Guide to Diseases, ed 5. Springhouse, Pa, Springhouse, 1995, pp. 154–156.

tissues and are capable of destroying erythrocytes, leukocytes, platelets, fibrinoblasts and other cells.

Many S. *aureus* infections begin as localized infections of the skin and skin appendages and then invade beyond the initial site, spreading by the bloodstream or lymphatic system to almost any location in the body. The bones, joints, and heart valves are the most common sites of metastatic S. *aureus* infections.

Clinical Manifestations. When S. *aureus* is inoculated into a previously sterile site, infection usually produces suppuration and abscess formation. The abscesses range in size from microscopic to lesions several centimeters in diameter and they are filled with pus and bacteria. The clinical manifestations vary enormously according to the site and type of infection and may include furuncles (boils), paronychia (staphylococcal infection of the nail bed), felons (staphylococcal infections on the palmar side of the fingertips), carbuncles (clusters of infected boils), osteomyelitis, infections of burns or surgical wounds, respiratory tract infections, bacterial arthritis, septicemia, bacterial endocarditis, toxic shock syndrome, and food poisoning. Fever and chills, as well as symptoms associated with the affected area, may accompany staphylococcal infection of any body part.

Acute staphylococcus *osteomyelitis*, usually in the bones of the legs, most commonly affects boys between 3 and 10 years of age, most of whom have a history of infection or trauma. Osteomyelitis presenting in the vertebrae affects adults older than 50 years of age, often following staphylococcal infections of the skin or urinary tract, following prostatic surgery, or after pinning of a fracture. Clinical manifestations include abrupt onset of fever, usually 101°F (38.3°C) or lower, shaking chills, pain and swelling over the infected area, restlessness, and headache (see discussion of osteomyelitis in Chapter 21).

Staphylococcus–associated *skin infections* include cellulitis (see cellulitis, Chapter 8), boil-like lesions (furuncles and carbuncles), and small macules or skin blebs that may develop into pus-filled vesicles. Associated symptoms may include mild or spiking fever and malaise.

Medical Management

Diagnosis, Treatment, and Prognosis. Culture of the organism from pus or drainage is usually diagnostic; antibiotic sensitivity testing is important. Isolation of the organism in blood cultures confirms endocarditis in the presence of a new murmur or positive echocardiogram. Treatment may include drainage of any abscesses, administration of antibiotics, and supportive therapy for the specific type and site. Prognosis is good with treatment, although antibiotic resistance is common. Untreated skin infections can become systemic and cause infective endocarditis and visceral abscesses or osteomyelitis; staphylococcal sepsis is potentially lethal.

Special Implications for the Therapist **6-2**

STAPHYLOCOCCAL INFECTIONS

Some organisms such as *S. aureus* (and streptococci) are considered resident organisms because they are not easily removed by scrubbing and often can be cultured from the health care worker's skin. Many health care workers carry *S. aureus* without sequelae but are able to shed organisms into nonintact skin areas of susceptible hosts, causing infections.

For the most part, good handwashing with plain soap is adequate in the therapy setting. Antimicrobial soaps that contain chemicals to kill transient and some resident organisms may be recommended. The choice of using an antimicrobial soap or plain soap is usually based on the need to reduce and maintain minimal counts of resident organisms and to mechanically remove transient organisms (e.g., *Pseudomonas, E. coli,* salmonellae, *Shigella*) (Larson, 1991).

Streptococcal Infections

Group A Streptococci

Streptococcus pyogenes, the prototype of group A streptococci, is one of the most frequent bacterial pathogens of humans of any age (Rubin and Farber, 1994). It causes many diseases of diverse organ systems (Table 6–8) ranging from skin infections, to acute self-limited pharyngitis, to major-illnesses such as rheumatic fever (see Chapter 10). The diseases caused by *S. pyogenes* may be considered in two categories: suppurative (formation of pus) and nonsuppurative. Suppurative diseases occur at sites where the bacteria invade and cause tissue necrosis, usually inciting an acute inflammatory response. Suppurative *S. pyogenes* infections include pharyngitis, scarlet fever, impetigo (pyoderma), streptococcal gangrene, necrotizing fasciitis, cellulitis, myositis, pneumonia (rarely), and puerperal sepsis (following abortion). By contrast, nonsuppurative diseases (e.g., rheumatic fever, acute poststreptococcal glomerulonephritis) occur at sites remote from the site of bacterial invasion.

Signs and symptoms of group A streptococcus depend on the location but typically include fever, chills, sore throat and enlarged lymph nodes with pharyngitis; red "honey-crusted" lesions with impetigo; diffuse inflammation of the skin and subcutaneous tissues with swelling and redness with erysipelas ("skin strep"), a type of skin cellulitis; and a new heart murmur with endocarditis.

Streptococcal Pharyngitis. Streptococcal pharyngitis, commonly known as "strep throat" accounts for 95% of all cases of bacterial pharyngitis. Occurring most commonly from October to April in children aged 5 to 10 years, there has been a recent increase among adults aged 30 to 50 years. This organism frequently colonizes throats of persons with no symptoms; up to 20% of schoolchildren may be carriers (pets may also be carriers).

After a 1- to 5-day incubation period, a temperature of 101° to 104°F (38.3° to 40°C), sore throat with severe pain on swallowing, beefy red pharynx, tonsillar exudate, edematous tonsils and uvula, swollen glands along the jaw line, generalized malaise and weakness, anorexia, and occasional abdominal discomfort may develop. Up to 40% of affected children may have symptoms too mild for diagnosis.

Complications may include otitis media or sinusitis; rarely, bacteremic spread may cause arthritis, endocarditis, meningitis, osteomyelitis, or liver abscess; and poststreptococcal sequelae include acute rheumatic fever or acute glomerulonephritis. Diagnosis is usually by throat culture and treatment is pharmacologic with supportive measures for symptoms.

Scarlet Fever. Scarlet fever usually follows streptococcal pharyngitis, may also follow wound infections or puerperal sepsis. It is caused by a streptococcal strain that releases an erythrogenic toxin and is most common in children 2 to 10 years old. It is spread by inhalation or direct contact and presents as a streptococcal sore throat, fever, strawberry tongue (white-coated tongue with prominent red papillae), and fine erythematous rash that blanches on pressure and resembles sunburn with goose bumps. The rash first appears on the upper chest, then spreads to the neck, abdomen, legs, and arms, sparing the soles and palms. The cheeks may be flushed, with pallor around the mouth. Rarely, complications may include high fever, arthritis, and jaundice.

Impetigo. Impetigo, or streptococcal pyoderma, occurs most commonly in children aged 2 to 5, especially in hot, humid weather. Predisposing factors include close contact in schools, overcrowded living quarters, poor skin hygiene, and minor skin trauma. Small macules appear and rapidly develop into vesicles that become pustular and encrusted causing pain, surrounding erythema, and itching. Scratching spreads infection and may develop into adenitis (glandular inflammation) or cellulitis. Lesions frequently affect the face, heal slowly, and leave depigmented areas.

Streptococcal Gangrene. Group A β-hemolytic streptococcal infections have shown remarkable virulence in recent years, resulting in severe local tissue destruction as occurs in streptococcal gangrene. This is a rare form of gangrene, due to group A (or C or G) streptococci,[7] which usually develops at a site of trauma on an extremity or from an intraoral abscess or dental source affecting the face, head, and neck (Jackson and Sproat, 1995). It may also occur in the absence of an obvious portal of entry. Predisposing factors include surgery, wounds, skin ulcers, intramuscular administration of drugs such as nonsteroidal anti-inflammatory agents (NSAIDs) (Rowan and North, 1995; Pillans and O'Connor, 1995), diabetes mellitus, chronic alcoholism and peripheral vascular disease.

TABLE 6–8 STREPTOCOCCAL INFECTIONS

Streptococcus pyogenes (group A streptococci)
- Streptococcal pharyngitis
- Rheumatic fever
- Scarlet fever (scarlatina)
- Erysipelas
- Impetigo (streptococcal pyoderma)
- Streptococcal gangrene (necrotizing fasciitis)
- Streptococcal cellulitis
- Streptococcal myositis

Streptococcus agalactiae (group B streptococci)
- Neonatal streptococcal infections
- Adult group B streptococcal infection

Streptococcus pneumoniae (group D streptococci)
- Pneumococcal pneumonia
- Otitis media
- Meningitis
- Endocarditis

[7] Other pathogens for this disease include *S. aureus* (Henrich et al., 1995), *Staphylococcus epidermidis* (Leibowitz and Ramakrishnan, 1995), a case where a nonvirulent organism becomes pathogenic as a result of age alone, and *Streptococcus pneumoniae* (Choudhri et al., 1995).

This condition mimics gas gangrene because it develops within 72 hours of onset with the affected person showing a red-streaked, painful skin lesion with dusky red surrounding tissue. Bullae containing yellowish to red-black fluid develop and rupture; the lesion evolves into a sharply demarcated area covered by a necrotic eschar and surrounded by an erythematous border. The involved area resembles a third-degree burn. Extensive necrotic sloughs can result because of deep penetration of the infection along fascial planes (Swartz, 1995).

Other symptoms may include fever, tachycardia, lethargy, prostration, disorientation, hypotension, jaundice, hypovolemia, and severe pain followed by anesthesia due to nerve destruction. Complications may include bacteremia (bacteria in the blood), metastatic abscesses, and death; and secondary thrombophlebitis when the lower extremities are involved.

Streptococci can usually be cultured from the early bullous lesions and frequently from the blood. Treatment is immediate with wide, deep surgical debridement of all necrotic tissue accompanied by high-dose IV antibiotics. If surgical therapy is not an option, the prevention of secondary complications such as infection becomes the goal of treatment until the necrotic process stops and healing begins. In such situations, a moist environment is a recommended choice for topical therapy (Piczon et al., 1995).

Necrotizing Fasciitis *(Swartz, 1995)*. Necrotizing fasciitis, an invasive infection of fascia, is usually caused by multiple pathogens. In the pediatric population,[8] varicella (chickenpox) is an important risk factor for necrotizing fasciitis (varicella gangrenosa) caused by more virulent strains of group A β-hemolytic streptococci (Wilson et al., 1995). In the newborn, necrotizing fasciitis can be a serious complication of omphalitis (inflammation of the umbilical cord).

Other predisposing risk factors include trauma (laceration, abrasion, burn, insect bite); ischemia; surgery (e.g., hemorrhoidectomy, vasectomy); anatomic sites regularly exposed to fecal or oral contamination, such as wounds associated with intestinal surgery; pressure and diabetic ulcers; human bites; infected pilonidal (containing hair) cysts; alcoholism; and parenteral drug abuse (Schecter et al. 1982).

This condition is characterized by infectious thrombosis of vessels passing between the skin and deep circulation, producing skin necrosis superficially resembling ischemic vascular or clostridial gangrene. The affected area is initially erythematous, swollen, without sharp margins, hot, shiny, exquisitely tender, and painful. The process progresses rapidly over several days, with sequential skin color changes from red-purple to patches of blue-gray. Within 3 to 5 days of onset, skin breakdown with bullae containing thick pink or purple fluid and cutaneous gangrene resembling a thermal burn occurs. By this time, the involved area is no longer tender but has become anesthetic secondary to the thrombosis of small blood vessels and destruction of superficial nerves located in the necrotic subcutaneous tissues.

Necrotizing fasciitis can affect any part of the body but is most common on the extremities, particularly the legs. Necrotizing fasciitis from intestinal sources may extend along the psoas muscle to affect the lower extremities, groin, or abdominal wall.

Streptococcal Cellulitis. Streptococcal cellulitis, an acute spreading inflammation of the skin and subcutaneous tissues, usually results from infection of burns or wounds. Recurrent episodes of cellulitis may occur in extremities in which lymphatic drainage has been impaired (e.g., postaxillary node dissection). Lymphangitis may accompany cellulitis or may occur after clinically minor or unapparent skin infection. Lymphangitis is readily recognized by the presence of red, tender, linear streaks directed toward enlarged, tender regional lymph nodes. It is accompanied by systemic symptoms such as chills, fever, malaise, and headache. See also Cellulitis, Chapter 8, and Lymphangitis, Chapter 10.

Myositis. Streptococcal myositis[9] is a rare but potentially life-threatening entity characterized by severe pain and inflammation in the affected muscle (Adams et al., 1986). There is usually marked systemic toxicity. Therapy includes aggressive surgical debridement and IV penicillin. Mortality in reported cases has been high (Bisno, 1995). See also Streptococcal Gangrene, this chapter.

Puerperal Sepsis. Puerperal sepsis follows abortion or delivery when streptococci colonizing the woman or transmitted from medical personel invade the endometrium and surrounding structures, lymphatics, and bloodstream. The resulting endometritis and septicemia may be complicated by pelvic cellulitis, septic pelvic thrombophlebitis, peritonitis, or pelvic abscess. This disease was associated with high mortality in the preantibiotic era. See also Chapter 17.

Group B Streptococci

Group B streptococcal infection (*Streptococcus agalactiae*) is the leading cause of neonatal pneumonia, meningitis, and sepsis. The organism is also an infrequent cause of pyogenic infections in adults. Several thousand neonatal infections with group B streptococci occur in the United States each year, and about 10% of the infected infants die. Group B streptococci are part of the normal vaginal flora and are found in 30% of women. Most newborns born to colonized women acquire the organism as they pass through the birth canal, but less than 1% of these infants develop group B streptococcal infections.

Symptoms of infection in the newborn are not specific, but group B streptococcal infection typically presents as lethargy, poor feeding, and respiratory distress. In the first few days of life, fever may not be present, but if infection occurs several weeks after birth, fever is prominent.

Streptococcus pneumoniae *(Group D Streptococci; Pneumococcal Pneumonia; Pneumococcus)*

Pneumonia and other infections, such as sepsis, otitis media, and meningitis, can be caused by *S. pneumoniae*. This is the most common cause of community-acquired pneumonia,

[8] Isolated cases of this condition caused by chickenpox in adults have been reported (Gonzalez-Ruiz et al., 1995).

[9] This condition can also be caused by bacteria, mycobacteria, fungi, viruses, and protozoan forms. Gas gangrene (discussed in the following section) is a type of myositis, as is psoas abscess associated with enteric infection and pyomyositis, an accumulation of pus in the skeletal muscles, usually caused by *S. aureus*.

accounting for 70% of all cases of bacterial pneumonia. Pneumococcal pneumonia often follows influenza or viral respiratory infection and is frequently seen in clients with chronic diseases, immunosuppression, and in alcohol abusers. Other risk factors include cigarette smoking, aspiration of oral contents, splenectomy, and neurologic impairment.

Clinical manifestations include acute onset of fever, chills, pleuritis with pleuritic chest pain, and dyspnea with productive cough or purulent sputum that may be blood-tinged. Other complications may include empyema, bacteremia, sepsis, meningitis, and septic arthritis. Septic arthritis can occur in a natural or prosthetic joint (Ryczak et al., 1987) or as a complication of rheumatoid arthritis (Morley et al., 1987); underlying chronic joint disease may delay diagnosis. Pneumococcal (septic) arthritis secondary to this pathogen is relatively uncommon and occurs principally in the elderly. The clinical symptoms are similar to other forms of hematogenous pyogenic joint infections. Adjacent osteomyelitis involving the vertebral bones may be detected on radiologic examination (Gelfand and Cleveland, 1992; Musher, 1995).

Diagnosis is made by recognition of abrupt onset of symptoms typical of pneumonia, defining chest film, and laboratory examination of sputum (culture). Immunization is available, recommended for susceptible people (e.g., elderly and asplenic people), and effective against at least 23 strains of the pneumococcal organism. A single dose is usually protective for a lifetime (Cronin, 1993). Prognosis is usually good with treatment, resistance to penicillin occurs but is still uncommon, and the mortality rate is higher (5% to 20%) in those with significant underlying diseases.

Medical Management

Diagnosis, Treatment, and Prognosis. Clinical diagnosis of streptococcal infections is based on recognition of spreading skin infections and other defining clinical presentation. Laboratory diagnosis isolates the organism from the infected region (or blood as in endocarditis). Treatment is with antibiotic therapy (usually penicillin) and prevents long-term sequelae in heart and kidneys. Prognosis is usually good with therapy; toxic shock syndrome associated with streptococcus has a high mortality.

Gas Gangrene (Clostridial Myonecrosis)

Definition and Overview. *Gangrene* is the death of body tissue usually associated with loss of vascular (nutritive, arterial circulation) supply, and followed by bacterial invasion and putrefaction. The three major types of gangrene are dry, moist, and gas gangrene. Dry and moist gangrene result from loss of blood circulation due to various causes; gas gangrene occurs in wounds infected by anaerobic bacteria, leading to gas production and tissue breakdown. This is a rare but severe, painful condition usually following trauma or surgery in which muscles and subcutaneous tissues become filled with gas and an exudate. The disease spreads rapidly to adjacent tissues and can be fatal within hours of onset.

Pathogenesis. Fortunately, the anaerobic conditions necessary to foster clostridial growth are uncommon in human tissues and produced only in the presence of extensive devitalized tissue, as occurs with severe trauma, wartime injuries, and septic abortions. Contributing factors include hypoxia from injury to blood vessels near the wound site, pressure dressings, tourniquets, local injection of vasoconstrictors, foreign bodies, damaged tissues from earlier injury, and concurrent microbial infections. Gas gangrene is most often found in deep wounds, especially those in which tissue necrosis further reduces oxygen supply. Such necrosis releases both carbon dioxide and hydrogen subcutaneously, producing interstitial gas bubbles. Gas gangrene (clostridial myonecrosis) is rare when wounds are promptly and thoroughly cleaned and debrided of traumatized tissue.

Clinical Manifestations. The incubation period for gas gangrene is usually 2 to 4 days after injury. Sudden, severe pain occurring at the site of the wound which is tender and edematous are early signs and symptoms of gas gangrene. The skin darkens because of hemorrhage and cutaneous necrosis. The lesion develops a thick discharge which has a foul odor and may contain gas bubbles. Crepitation may be felt on palpation of the skin from the gas bubbles in muscles and subcutaneous tissue. True gas gangrene produces myositis and anaerobic cellulitis, affecting only soft tissue. The skin over the wound may rupture, revealing dark-red or black necrotic muscle accompanied by a foul-smelling watery or frothy discharge. Associated symptoms may include sweating, low-grade fever, and disproportionate tachycardia followed by hemolytic anemia, hypotension, and renal failure.

Medical Management

Diagnosis, Treatment, and Prognosis. Prevention is the key to avoiding gas gangrene before treatment is required. To prevent gangrene in an open wound, the wound should be kept as clean as possible. Special wound care is particularly important in persons with diabetes mellitus, malnutrition, and immunodeficiency.

Diagnosis based on history and clinical presentation is confirmed by anaerobic cultures of wound drainage and radiographs showing gas in the tissues. Once diagnosed, treatment involves opening the wound widely to admit air and permit drainage. Large, multiple incisions are made through the skin and fascia, sutures and any gangrenous material are removed, and the wound is irrigated. Anti-infective agents are administered but if massive gangrene develops, amputation may be necessary. With prompt treatment, 80% of persons with gas gangrene of the extremities survive; prognosis is poorer for gas gangrene in other sites such as the abdominal wall, uterus, or bowel.

Special Implications for the Therapist **6-3**

GAS GANGRENE

Careful observation may result in early diagnosis. With any postoperative or posttraumatic injury, look for signs of ischemia such as cool skin, pallor or cyanosis, sudden, severe pain, sudden edema, and loss of pulses in the involved limb. Record carefully and immediately report these findings to the medical staff. Throughout this illness, adequate fluid replacement is essential; assess pulmonary and cardiac functions often (Norris, 1995).

Special care to prevent skin breakdown is important and meticulous wound care following surgery is imperative. To prevent gas gangrene, routinely take precautions to render all wound sites unsuitable for growth of clostridia by attempting to keep granulation tissue viable; adequate debridement is imperative to reduce anaerobic growth conditions. Notify the physician immediately of any devitalized tissue. Position the client to facilitate drainage.

Psychological support is critical as these clients can remain alert until death, knowing that death is imminent and unavoidable. The therapist must be prepared for the foul odor from the wound and prepare the client emotionally for the large wound after surgical excision. Wound care requires sterile procedures to prevent spread of bacteria; dispose of drainage material and dressings in double plastic bags for incineration. No special cleaning measures are required after the client is discharged.

Pseudomonas (*Rubin and Farber, 1994*)

Overview. *Pseudomonas aeruginosa* is a major opportunistic pathogen and one of the most frequent hospital- or nursing home–acquired (nosocomial) pathogens. The organism infrequently colonizes humans, but it can cause disease, particularly in the hospital environment, where it is associated with pneumonia, wound infections, urinary tract disease, and sepsis in debilitated persons. Burns, urinary catheterization, cystic fibrosis, chronic lung diseases, neutropenia associated with chemotherapy, and diabetes all predispose to infections with *P. aeruginosa*. This bacterium produces the pigments cyanin and fluorescein that give the color to the "blue pus" seen in some suppurative infections. It thrives on moist environmental surfaces, making swimming pools, Hubbard tanks, and whirlpools, as well as respiratory therapy equipment and liquid soap dispensers, prime targets for growth. This organism is among the most antibiotic-resistant bacteria.

Pathogenesis. *P. aeruginosa* consists of an array of proteins which allow it to attach to, invade, and destroy host tissues, while avoiding host inflammatory and immune defenses. Injury to epithelial cells uncovers surface molecules that serve as binding sites for the pili of *P. aeruginosa*. Many strains of this pathogen produce a proteoglycan that surrounds the bacteria, protecting them from mucociliary action, complement, and phagocytes. The organism releases extracellular enzymes which facilitate tissue invasion and are partially responsible for the necrotizing lesions associated with *Pseudomonas* infections. This pathogen can also invade blood vessel walls and produce systemic pathologic effects through endotoxin and several systemically active exotoxins.

Clinical Manifestations. Signs and symptoms of *Pseudomonas* infection vary with the site of infection and the state of host defenses (Pollack, 1995). If the host has the capacity to respond to the invading bacteria with neutrophils, an acute inflammatory response will result. The *Pseudomonas* organism often invades small arteries and veins, producing vascular thrombosis and hemorrhagic necrosis, particularly in the lungs and skin. Blood vessel invasion predisposes to bacteremia, dissemination (spread), and sepsis (toxins in the blood). Vascular invasion often leads to the rapid development of multiple metastatic nodular lesions in the lungs. Disseminated infections are marked by the development of typical skin lesions called ecthyma gangrenosum. These bullous or pustular eruptions represent sites where the organism has disseminated to the skin, invaded blood vessels, and produced localized hemorrhagic infarctions.

This bacterium can cause infective endocarditis on native heart valves in IV drug users and on prosthetic heart valves; pneumonia in persons with chronic lung disease, congestive heart failure, and malignancies, especially those involving the hematopoietic system and in those who are neutropenic as a result of chemotherapy; CNS infections such as meningitis and brain abscess; and ear, eye, urinary tract, gastrointestinal, skin and soft tissue, and bone and joint infections.

Central Nervous System Infections

Pseudomonas infections of the CNS result from extension from a contiguous structure such as ear, mastoid, or paranasal sinus; direct inoculation into the subarachnoid space or brain by means of head trauma, surgery, or invasive diagnostic procedures (e.g., lumbar punctures, spinal anesthesia, intraventricular shunts); and bacteremic spread from a distant site of infection such as the urinary tract, lung, or endocardium.

The clinical manifestations of *Pseudomonas* meningitis are like those of other forms of bacterial meningitis (see Chapter 25) and include fever, headache, and confusion. The onset of disease may be acute and occur suddenly or may be more gradual and insidious in the absence of systemic signs and symptoms, as in those whose meningitis is related to neurosurgery, extension from a contiguous site of chronic infection, or in persons who are immunosuppressed or have cancer.

Skin and Soft Tissue Infections

Pseudomonas disease of the skin and mucous membranes can result from primary or metastatic foci of infections. Primary skin and soft tissue infections may be either localized or diffuse. Common predisposing factors are a breakdown in the integument, especially resulting from burns, trauma, pressure ulcers, whirlpool use, and chemotherapy-induced neutropenia. Wound infections may have a characteristic fruity odor (sweet, grapelike odor) with a blue-green exudate that forms a crust on wounds. *Pseudomonas* bacteria may produce distinctive skin lesions known as ecthyma gangrenosum characterized by hemorrhage, necrosis, and surrounding erythema. Associated symptoms may include headache, dizziness, earache, sore throat, swollen breasts, sore eyes, sore nose, and abdominal cramps. Fever is uncommon and remains low grade when it occurs.

Pseudomonas burn wound sepsis is a dreaded complication of extensive thermal injuries and is characterized by multifocal black or dark-brown discoloration of the burn eschar; degeneration of the underlying granulation tissue with rapid eschar separation and hemorrhage into subcutaneous tissue; edema or hemorrhagic necrosis of previously healthy tissue adjacent to infected burn sites; and erythematous nodular lesions in unburned skin. Systemic manifestations may include fever or hypothermia, disorientation, hypotension, oliguria, ileus, and leukopenia.

Bone and Joint Infections

Pseudomonas infections of the bones and joints result from hematogenous spread from other primary sites or extension from other sites of infection. Contiguous infections are usually related to penetrating trauma, surgery, or overlying soft tissue infections. *Pseudomonas* osteochondritis can follow puncture wounds of the foot; the sternoclavicular and sacroiliac joints, vertebrae, and symphysis pubis are affected in IV drug users; osteomyelitis occurs in conjunction with vascular insufficiency of the lower extremities in persons with diabetes mellitus; diseased large synovial joints are infected in persons with underlying rheumatoid disease; and infections of the long bones follow open fractures and internal fixation procedures.

Pseudomonas osteochondritis following a puncture wound involves the cartilage of the small joints and the bones of the foot. Typically the person experiences early improvement in pain and swelling following a puncture wound only to have the symptoms recur or worsen several days later. The average duration of symptoms prior to diagnosis is several weeks, and fever and other systemic signs are usually absent. There may be an area of superficial cellulitis on the plantar surface of the foot, or merely tenderness to deep palpation.

Bloodborne *Pseudomonas* appears to have a predilection for the fibrocartilaginous joints of the axial skeleton involving joint space, cartilage, synovium, and contiguous bone. Vertebral osteomyelitis caused by *P. aeruginosa* is occasionally associated with complicated urinary tract infections and genitourinary surgery or instrumentation. This disease occurs most often in elderly people and involves the lumbosacral spine. Physical signs include local tenderness and decreased range of motion in the spine; fever and other systemic symptoms are relatively uncommon. There may be mild neurologic deficits present.

Medical Management

Diagnosis, Treatment, and Prognosis. Diagnosis requires isolation of the *Pseudomonas* organism in blood, spinal fluid, urine, exudate, or sputum culture. Antibiotic therapy is initiated immediately; local *Pseudomonas* infections or septicemia secondary to wound infection requires acetic acid irrigations, topical drug therapy, and debridement or drainage of the infected wound.

P. aeruginosa infections are among the most aggressive human bacterial infections, often progressing rapidly to sepsis, especially in persons with poor immunologic resistance (e.g., premature infants, the elderly, and persons with debilitating disease, burns, or wounds). In local *Pseudomonas* infections, treatment is usually successful and complications are rare. Immediate medical intervention is necessary; septicemic *Pseudomonas* infections are associated with a high mortality. Medical management is directed according to the site of infection and may include antibiotics, surgery, pulmonary therapy, respiratory assistance if necessary, and other supportive measures dictated by the presence of septic shock and other complications.

Special Implications for the Therapist **6-4**

PSEUDOMONAS INFECTIONS

Pseudomonas is a transient organism that is able to survive less than 24 hours on the skin and is easily removed by washing or scrubbing. These organisms use the hands as a short-lived mode of transmission while looking for a susceptible host or reservoir where they can survive. Such transient organisms readily cause infection once they enter a susceptible host. For this reason, person-to-person transmission of *Pseudomonas* via the hands of hospital staff is often assumed but difficult to prove. These types of organisms can be removed by mechanical friction and soap-and-water washing and become the focus of handwashing to prevent further spread (Schaffer et al., 1996; Larson, 1991).

Anyone who is immunocompromised should be protected from exposure to this infection. Wound care requires strict sterile technique.

Viral Infections *(Norris, 1995)*

Cytomegalovirus

Overview and Incidence. Cytomegalovirus or cytomegalic inclusion disease (CID) is a commonly occurring DNA herpes virus group. CMV may occur congenitally, peri- or postnatally, or disseminated in immunocompromised persons and increases in frequency with age. One percent of newborns are infected and four out of five adults over age 35 have been infected with CMV, usually during childhood or early adulthood, and are seropositive. Multiple sites may be affected, including the brain (in utero infection), salivary glands, kidneys, liver, lung, pancreas, thyroid, adrenals, and gastrointestinal tract (Harruff, 1994).

Etiology and Risk Factors. CMV is transmitted by human contact such as through the placenta, urine, breast milk, feces, blood, sexually (semen, vaginal and cervical secretions), through blood transfusions, and transplanted organs (organ recipients have the greatest risk). CMV is extremely common in AIDS.

Pathogenesis and Clinical Manifestations. CMV probably spreads through the body through lymphocytes or mononuclear cells to the lungs (CMV pneumonitis), liver (CMV hepatitis), gastrointestinal tract (CMV gastroenteritis), eyes (CMV retinitis), and CNS where it produces inflammatory reactions. Lesions include diffuse interstitial pneumonitis leading to respiratory distress syndrome; hepatitis, adrenalitis, and intestinal ulcerations; and calcifications around ventricles in neonatal CNS infections.

In normal adults, the infection is usually asymptomatic and runs a self-limiting course. In immunosuppressed persons, transplant recipients, or neonates, there may be fever, splenomegaly, hepatitis, pneumonitis or other pulmonary involvement, or multisystem involvement. In persons with AIDS, infection with CMV can cause the various clinical illnesses listed, but the most common manifestation is chorioretinitis. Early symptoms include mild visual impairment and deficits of peripheral vision; blindness can occur. Peripheral neuropathies and distal sensory axonal neuropathies occurring in the later phases of HIV infection are commonly caused by CMV (Eidelberg et al., 1986; Snider et al., 1988).

Medical Management

Diagnosis, Treatment, and Prognosis. Diagnosis is made by isolating the virus in cultures of urine, saliva, throat, or cervix; serum antibody titers may indicate prior infection that has been reactivated. Treatment is toward relief of symptoms and preventing complications. In the immunosuppressed person pharmacologic treatment with ganciclovir or foscarnet has been proved effective (acyclovir is ineffective). The prognosis for persons with transplanted organs or who are immunocompromised is poor as they may have fatal disseminated infections with respiratory failure (Harruff, 1994).

Special Implications for the Therapist **6–5**

CYTOMEGALOVIRUS

Pregnant women and immunosuppressed persons should avoid exposure to confirmed or suspected CMV infection. Clients with CMV infection should be encouraged to wash their hands thoroughly and frequently to prevent spreading it. It is especially important to impress this on young children. As difficult as it may be, the child should not be allowed to kiss others; parents and others should also avoid kissing the affected child. Health care professionals must observe universal precautions when handling body secretions.

Infectious Mononucleosis *(Norris, 1995)*

Overview. Infectious mononucleosis is an acute infectious disease caused by the Epstein-Barr virus (EBV), a member of the herpesvirus group. It primarily affects young adults and children, although in children it is usually so mild that its presence often goes unnoticed.

Incidence, Etiology, and Risk Factors. Infection with EBV is fairly common in the United States and both sexes are affected equally. Incidence varies seasonally among college students but not among the general population. The reservoir of EBV is limited to humans and probably spreads by the oral-pharyngeal route, since about 80% of people carry EBV in the throat during the acute infection and for an indefinite period afterward. For this reason, it is sometimes called the "kissing disease." It can also be transmitted by blood transfusion and has been reported after cardiac surgery as the "post-pump perfusion" syndrome.

Pathogenesis and Clinical Manifestations. EBV causes lymphoid proliferation in the blood, lymph nodes, and spleen. Characteristically, the virus produces fever, sore throat, headache, and painful cervical lymphadenopathy, as well as hepatic dysfunction, and increased lymphocytes and monocytes. The incubation period is about 10 days in children and from 30 to 50 days in adults.

Temperature fluctuations occur throughout the day, peaking in the evening (101° to 102°F [38.3° to 38.9°C.]). A maculopapular rash closely resembling the rash of rubella occurs in 10% to 15% of those affected. Hepatomegaly may develop and the spleen may enlarge to two to three times its normal size causing left upper quadrant pain with possible referral to the left shoulder and left upper trapezius region. Both the peripheral and central nervous systems can be involved.

Overall major complications are rare but may include splenic rupture, aseptic meningitis, encephalitis, hemolytic anemia, idiopathic thrombocytopenia, and Guillain-Barré syndrome. Symptoms subside about 6 to 10 days after onset of the disease but may persist for weeks.

Medical Management

Diagnosis, Treatment, and Prognosis. The symptoms of EBV infection mimic those of other infectious diseases such as hepatitis, rubella, and toxoplasmosis. Diagnosis is based on three criteria: physical assessment, laboratory tests, and a positive heterophil[10] (Monospot) test. Rising levels of antibodies to EBV were once thought to be the cause of chronic fatigue syndrome but are now considered a result of chronic fatigue syndrome (CFS) (see Chronic Fatigue and Immune Dysfunction Syndrome, Chapter 5). The prognosis is excellent with rest and supportive care but there is no lifetime immunity against this virus; the virus can live indefinitely in B lymphocytes. No other specific intervention alters or shortens the disease process.

Special Implications for the Therapist **6–6**

INFECTIOUS MONONUCLEOSIS

Infectious mononucleosis is probably contagious before symptoms develop until the fever subsides and the oral and pharyngeal lesions disappear. Although infectious mononucleosis appears to be only mildly contagious, adherence to universal precautions, especially good handwashing and avoiding shared dishware or food items with other people, is essential in preventing the health care professional from contracting this condition.

The person with infectious mononucleosis should be cautioned against engaging in excessive activity, especially contact sports, which could result in splenic rupture or lowered resistance to infection. Usually this guideline is appropriate for a period of at least 1 month. Any sign of splenic rupture (abdominal or upper quadrant pain; Kehr's sign, or sudden left shoulder pain; shock) requires immediate medical evaluation. Any soft tissue mobilization or myofascial techniques necessary in the left upper quadrant (especially up and under the rib cage) must take into consideration the enlarged spleen; indirect techniques away from the spleen are indicated.

MISCELLANEOUS INFECTIOUS DISEASES

Infections in Drug Addicts *(Jacobs, 1994)*

The abuse of parenterally administered narcotic drugs has increased enormously in recent years. There are now an estimated 300,000 or more narcotic addicts in the United States, mostly in or near large urban centers. Consequently, health care workers in urban and suburban populations may encounter many problems related to drug abuse, including infections.

Common infections that occur with greater frequency in drug users include (1) skin infections associated with poor hygiene and multiple needle punctures, commonly caused by *S. aureus;* (2) hepatitis, which is nearly universal among habitual drug users and is transmissible both by the parenteral and by the fecal-oral route; (3) aspiration pneumonia and its

[10] Heterophil antibodies (agglutinins for sheep red blood cells) in serum drawn during the acute illness and at 3- to 4-week intervals rise to four times normal.

complications (lung abscess, empyema, brain abscess) resulting from altered consciousness associated with drug abuse; (4) pulmonary septic emboli originating from venous thrombi or endocarditis; (5) sexually transmitted diseases, which are not directly related to drug abuse but occur with greater frequency in population groups that are also involved in drug abuse; (6) higher incidence of AIDS among IV drug abusers and their sexual contacts as well as the offspring of infected women; and (7) infective endocarditis.

Osteomyelitis involving vertebral bodies, sternoclavicular joints, and other sites are found in drug abusers usually from hematogenous distribution of injected organisms or septic venous thrombi. Pain and fever precede radiographic changes by several weeks.

Infections with Prostheses and Implants[11] *(Brause, 1995)*

Overview. Over the past two decades joint replacement surgery has become commonplace which is largely attributed to the success of these procedures in restoring function to people with disabling arthritis. People receiving total joint replacements number in the hundreds of thousands each year worldwide, and virtually millions of people have indwelling prosthetic joints. Likewise, during the past 25 years, many new instrumentation systems for internal fixation of the spine have been developed (Heggeness et al., 1993).

Other types of prostheses or implants susceptible to infection include breast implants, dental implants, cardiac implants, other orthopedic devices and hardware, shunts, and even contact lenses (external to epithelial surfaces that can give rise to serious sight-threatening infections).

Incidence. The successful development of synthetic materials and the introduction of artificial devices into nearly all body systems has been accompanied by the adaptation of microorganisms to the opportunities these devices provide for eluding defenses and invading the host. One percent to 5% of indwelling prostheses become infected (Dickinson and Bisno, 1993). Additionally, as the number of people undergoing cardiac valve replacement has grown, valve reoperations have become increasingly frequent.

On the other hand, bioprostheses, implanted in large numbers in the 1970s and early 1980s, have now gone into the second decade of life since implantation, a time when biodegradation becomes more frequent. Multiple reoperations carry a higher risk of infection (Antunes, 1992). Likewise, as the population ages, an increasing number of total hip, knee, shoulder, elbow, wrist, and finger arthroplasties are coming up for revision. Data concerning arthroplasty loosening associated with infection in this age group are minimal at this time (Ballard et al., 1995). One study of failed implant arthroplasty of the wrist reported a low incidence of only 11% (2 of 19) failed wrist arthroplasties attributed to infection (Ferlic et al., 1992).

Risk Factors. Certain groups have been identified as predisposed toward infection of their prosthetic joints, including those with prior surgery at the site of the prosthesis, rheumatoid arthritis, corticosteroid therapy, diabetes mellitus, poor nutritional status, obesity, and extremely advanced age (Gristina and Kolkin, 1983; Brause, 1986). One case of skin breakdown with sequential infection of silicone metacarpophalangeal joint arthroplasty was attributed to excessive and improper use of the hand (Golz et al., 1992). Risk factors for infection of spinal instrumentation may include IV drug use, paraplegia with neurogenic bladder, and pyelonephritis secondary to renal calculi (Heggeness et al., 1993).

Any factor or event that delays wound healing increases the risk of infection. In the early postimplantation period the fascial layers have not yet healed, and the deep, periprosthesis tissue is not protected by the usual physical barriers. Any superficial infection that develops, such as ischemic necrosis, an infected wound hematoma, wound infection, or suture abscess, can become a preceding event for joint replacement sepsis.

Etiology and Pathogenesis. Prosthetic joints and other implants become infected by two different pathogenic routes: the locally introduced route and the hematogenous route. The locally introduced form of infection accounts for 60% of all prosthetic joint infections and occurs as a result of wound sepsis next to the prosthesis or operative contamination (seeding at the time of the operation). Generally, these infections are caused by a single pathogen, but polymicrobial sepsis can occur.

Staphylococcus (coagulase-negative organisms such as *S. epidermidis*) is the most common etiologic agent, but old *S. aureus* and *Mycobacterium tuberculosis* infections can recur postoperatively. Latent quiescent osteomyelitis can also be reactivated by the disruption of tissue associated with implantation surgery. For example, skin breakdown over prominent hardware with subsequent percutaneous seeding of the implant often occurs in persons who have major neurologic deficits and anesthetic skin (Heggeness et al., 1993).

Any bacterium can induce infection of a total joint replacement by the hematogenous route, which accounts for 20% to 40% of prosthetic joint infections. Hematogenous spread may occur from dentogingival infections, pyogenic skin processes, and genitourinary or gastrointestinal tract infections or procedures.

Prostheses that are cemented into place with polymethyl methacrylate develop infection at the bone-cement interface, whereas cementless prostheses may develop sepsis in the bone contiguous with the metallic alloy. As foreign bodies these prostheses contribute to local sepsis by decreasing the quantity of bacteria necessary to establish infection and by permitting pathogens to persist on their avascular surface, sequestered from circulating immunologic defenses (leukocytes, antibodies, and complement) as well as from systemic antibiotics (Brause, 1986; Petty et al., 1985). Before the development of cementless prostheses,[12] the cement used appeared to predispose toward infection by inhibiting phagocytic, lymphocytic, and complement function.

Clinical Manifestations. Prosthetic joint sepsis produces the cardinal symptoms of inflammation with a wide variability of severity. Most people present with a long course characterized by a progressive increase in joint pain and occasionally

[11] There are four major pathologic processes that may arise in response to any biomedical implant. In addition to infection, there may be inflammation, thrombosis, and neoplasia (Kossovsky and Papasian, 1992; Kossovsky and Freiman, 1994).

[12] These devices have textured surfaces to provide fixation by the growth of adjacent bone into the porous interface of the prosthesis. The performance and durability of this new form of arthroplasty remains uncertain (Brause, 1995).

the formation of cutaneous draining sinuses but without fever, soft tissue swelling, or systemic toxicity. Others present with an acute illness with high fever, severe joint pain, local swelling, and erythema.

The pattern and clinical presentation is determined largely by three factors: the virulence of the infecting pathogen, the nature of the host tissue in which the microorganism grows, and the route of infection. *S. aureus* and β-hemolytic streptococci are particularly virulent pathogens in this situation and usually produce a fulminant (occurring suddenly with great intensity) infection, occasionally with septic shock. Coagulase-negative staphylococci are avirulent but tenacious pathogens consistently associated with a more indolent (slow) course of events.

Characteristics of the involved tissue can influence the type of clinical presentation on the basis of their support of microbial growth. For example, wound hematomas, seromas, and hemarthroses; fresh operative wounds; ischemic wounds; and tissues in diabetic and steroid-treated persons all enhance the ability of bacteria to multiply rapidly.

The hematogenous route of spread theoretically seeds the bone-cement interface. When a blood-borne infection arises in a prosthetic joint several months or years after implantation surgery, the fully healed connective tissue often is capable of restricting the septic process to a relatively small focus at the bone-cement interface. Joint pain is the principal symptom of deep tissue infection irrespective of mode of presentation and suggests either acute inflammation of the periarticular tissue or loosening of the prosthesis due to subacute erosion of bone at the bone-cement interface.

Medical Management

Diagnosis. Clinical manifestations of joint pain, swelling, erythema, and warmth all reflect an underlying inflammatory process in the surrounding tissues but are not specific for infection. When a painful prosthesis is accompanied by fever or purulent drainage from overlying cutaneous sinuses, infection is investigated further. The physician must differentiate infection from aseptic and mechanical problems (e.g., hemarthrosis, gout, mechanical loosening, or dislocation) which are more common causes of inflammatory and painful symptoms in this population. Constant joint pain is suggestive of infection, whereas mechanical loosening commonly causes pain only with motion or with weight bearing (Gristina and Kolkin, 1983).

Radiologic abnormalities may be helpful but generally require 3 to 6 months to demonstrate changes. When both the distal and proximal components of a prosthetic joint demonstrate pathology on radiography, sepsis is more likely than is simple mechanical loosening. However, such radiographic changes are not specific for infection and may also be seen with aseptic processes. Radioisotope scans demonstrate increased uptake in areas of bone with enhanced blood supply or increased metabolic activity (a normal finding during the first 6 months post implantation). Positive scans after 6 months following implantation are abnormal but do not differentiate among inflammation, possible loosening, and infection.

The specific diagnosis of joint replacement infection is dependent upon isolation of the pathogen by aspiration of joint fluid or by culture of tissue obtained at arthrotomy (O'Neill and Harris, 1984). Recently ultrasound-guided (ultrasonography) aspiration in suspected sepsis of arthroplasty has been developed to facilitate this process (Foldes et al., 1995).

Treatment. Prosthesis removal accompanied by extensive and meticulous surgical debridement of surrounding tissue is usually necessary to treat deep infections, especially infections involving the interface between prosthesis and bone (Rasul et al., 1991). Often these procedures produce large skeletal defects, shorten the extremity, and result in severe functional impairment. Bactericidal antibiotic therapy follows surgery for 6 weeks before reimplantation is performed. An alternative treatment protocol for less virulent pathogens involves a one-stage surgical procedure called an exchange operation in which joint and cement extraction are immediately followed by reimplantation of a new prosthesis using cement impregnated with an antibiotic (Duncan and Masri, 1995).

Sometimes surgical intervention is not possible owing to a medical or surgical condition or refusal on the part of the affected client. In such cases, lifelong oral antibiotic treatment may be required to suppress the infection and retain function of the joint. Serial radiographs are needed to monitor for progressive bone resorption at the bone-cement interface. In such cases, the localized septic process may still extend into adjacent tissue compartments or become a systemic infection or the person may develop side effects of chronic antibiotic administration.

Prognosis. Infection associated with prostheses and implants can produce significant morbidity and occasionally death. Early recognition and prompt therapy for infection in any location is critical to reducing the risk of seeding the joint implant hematogenously. Situations likely to cause bacteremia should be avoided (Brause, 1995).

Special Implications for the Therapist **6-7**

INFECTIONS WITH PROTHESES AND IMPLANTS

Many cases of infection after instrumentation or prosthetic implantation occur months to years after the surgery. In most cases, a distant cause of infection can be identified but usually there is no preceding breakdown of the overlying skin to help identify the presence of underlying infection (Heggeness et al., 1993).

Anyone with implants of any kind with onset of increasing musculoskeletal symptoms (especially in the area of the surgery) must be screened for the possibility of infection. The therapist may not be aware of existing hardware and must include questions in the interview to elicit this information. A recent history of infection from dental caries, pulmonary or upper respiratory tract, gastrointestinal tract, or genitourinary tract in such a person requires medical evaluation. Any spontaneous drainage from previous scars or sites of surgery may be a sign of infection and must also be evaluated by a physician.

Breast Implantation

Silicone breast implants (SBIs) are medical devices implanted subcutaneously or subpectorally for cosmetic breast augmentation or reconstruction. With silicone breast implants, thrombosis is not a clinical concern and infection is relatively rare (Freedman and Jackson, 1989). Recently, breast implants have been implicated in a variety of illnesses, the most controversial of which are symptoms of connective tissue diseases or immune-related disorders (Box 6–3). However, evidence to support an autoimmune response to silicone breast implants has not been conclusively proved and to date the largest studies have found no association between the implants and connective tissue diseases or signs and symptoms of these diseases (Sanchez-Guerro et al., 1995; Gabriel et al., 1994, 1995).

The consensus is that the reported cases of connective tissue diseases or immune-related disorders in women with breast implants do not exceed the number of cases normally expected in women (Robertson, 1993). In the meantime, silicone breast implant litigation escalated in the early 1990s so that despite the Food and Drug Administration's (FDA) statement that there is no medical evidence that silicone causes autoimmune disease, silicone gel implants were removed from the market in 1992* (Shiffman, 1994).

Most women with silicone gel–filled breast implants do not experience serious problems but some women experience symptoms otherwise associated with connective tissue and immune-related disorders. Such symptoms may include joint pain and swelling; skin tightness, redness, or swelling; swollen glands or lymph nodes; unusual and unexplained fatigue; swollen hands and feet; and unusual hair loss. The term *human adjuvant disease* is sometimes used to describe the musculoskeletal symptoms accompanying breast implantation.

The most common complication of SBIs is capsule contracture or contracture of the fibrous tissue surrounding the prosthesis, possibly associated with subclinical infection (*S. epidermidis*) (Virden et al., 1992). Other complications may include gel bleed, implant rupture, calcifications around the implant, and possibly interference with mammography in the diagnosis of breast cancer (Shiffman, 1994). Chest pain mimicking a heart attack can occur in women with SBIs. This same phenomenon has been documented in fibromyalgia. Whether or not this symptom occurs only in women with SBI associated with fibromyalgia remains unknown (Thorson, 1994).

Any woman (with or without breast implants) experiencing breast pain or discomfort, changes in size or shape of the breast, color changes in the breast area, discharge from or unusual sensation around the nipple, or unexplained symptoms possibly related to breast tissue should see a medical doctor.

* Silicone implants are still used in FDA clinical trials for women needing reconstructive surgery but no date has been set for when silicone gel implants will again be approved for general use. To report a problem with an implant, write to The Problem Reporting Program, 12601 Twinbrook Parkway, Rockville, MD 20852. For other information on breast implants, write FDA, Breast Implant Information, HFE-88, 5600 Fishers Lane, Rockville, MD 20857; or call (301) 443-3170 (Segal, 1992).

BOX 6–3

Connective Tissue Diseases Most Often Occurring with Silicone Gel Breast Implants*

Fibromyalgia or fibromyalgia-like syndrome (FMS)†
Chronic fatigue syndrome
Scleroderma
Inflammatory arthritis
Sjögren's syndrome
Polymyositis
Rheumatoid arthritis
Undifferentiated connective tissue disease
Raynaud's phenomenon
Systemic lupus erythematosus

* Presented in descending order of frequency.
† Research findings at the 1993 American College of Rheumatology meeting identified fibromyalgia or fibromyalgia-like syndrome as the most common diagnosis in women with silicone breast implants. The frequency of this disorder varied among studies but ranged from 25% to 50%. The second most commonly overlooked diagnosis was chronic fatigue syndrome (CFS) (Thorson, 1994); neither fibromyalgia nor CFS is mentioned in Bridges and Vasey (1993).
Adapted from Bridges AJ, Vasey FB: Silicone breast implants: History, safety, and potential complications. Arch Intern Med 153:2638–2644, 1993.

Lyme Disease *(Norris, 1995)*

Definition and Overview. Lyme disease is an infectious multisystemic disorder caused by a spiral-shaped form of bacteria, *Borrelia burgdorferi*. It is carried by a deer tick (*Ixodes dammini*)[13] and was first recognized (but did not originate) in 1975 when a group of children in Lyme, Connecticut developed an unusual type of arthritis. It often begins in the summer and is now recognized to occur primarily in three parts of the United States: in the Northeast (from Massachusetts to Maryland), in the Midwest (Wisconsin and Minnesota), and in the West (California and Oregon). Although it is endemic to these areas, cases have been reported from 43 states and 20 other countries, including Germany, Switzerland, France, and Australia.

Incidence. Lyme disease has been heralded as the fastest-growing infectious disease in this country after AIDS. In 1992, 5100 cases of Lyme disease had been reported to the CDC; in 1993, 8000 cases were reported, and in 1994, more than 13,000 cases were reported, making this infectious disease more common than measles or meningitis. Both sexes appear to be almost equally affected (CDC, 1995).

Pathogenesis. Lyme disease occurs when a tick injects spirochete-laden saliva into the bloodstream or deposits fecal matter on the skin. After incubating for 3 to 32 days, the spirochetes migrate out to the skin, causing characteristic skin lesions (see Clinical Manifestations). Then the bacteria disseminate to other skin sites or organs via the bloodstream or lymphatic system. The spirochetes' life cycle is not completely understood; it remains unclear whether they survive for years in areas that receive minimal blood supply (e.g., tendons or the synovium in joints) or perhaps just trigger an inflammatory response in the host and then die. The absence of detect-

[13] In addition to deer, these ticks are found on birds and rodents; they are about the size of the period at the end of a sentence. Not all of these ticks carry the bacteria.

able *B. burgdorferi* DNA in the synovial fluid of most people with chronic Lyme arthritis indicates that persistent joint infection is not the causative mechanism (Rahn, 1994).

There are several different strains of the bacterium, each with its own distinct set of proteins, and bacteria within an individual strain may change the shape of their proteins over time so that antibodies can no longer identify and lock onto them. This may account for why people who have been infected once can acquire the infection again (NIH, 1992).

Clinical Manifestations. Lyme disease typically has three stages. After a week or two of flulike symptoms, which may be accompanied by a rash, symptoms usually disappear with other symptoms developing much later. The initial presentation of Lyme disease is a classic skin lesion that resembles a raised, red circle with a clear center called erythema migrans (EM) or bull's-eye rash, often at the site of the tick bite (Fig. 6–1). The red macule or papule that develops may be about the size of a dime and feel hot and itchy and can grow to over 50 cm in diameter. Within a few days, as the infection spreads, more lesions may erupt, and a migratory, ringlike rash, conjunctivitis, or diffuse urticaria (hives) occurs. In 3 to 4 weeks, these lesions are replaced by small red blotches, which persist for several more weeks.

Malaise and fatigue are constant, but other intermittent flulike symptoms may occur, including headache, fever, chills, achiness, and regional lymphadenopathy. Less commonly, meningeal irritation, mild encephalopathy, migrating musculoskeletal pain,[14] and hepatitis may develop. A persistent sore throat and dry cough may appear several days before EM.

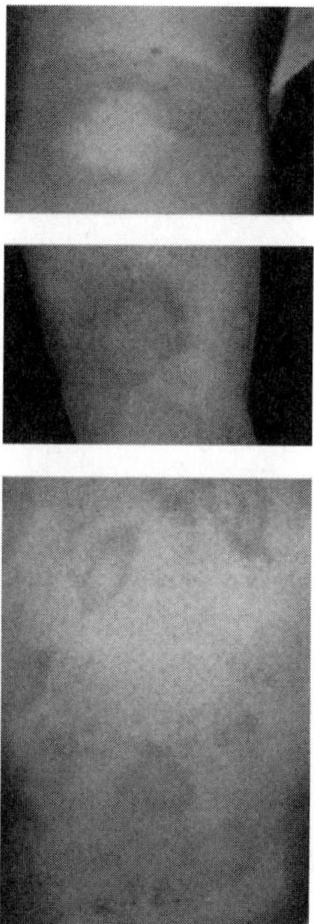

Figure **6–1.** Examples of erythema migrans associated with Lyme disease. Other types of rashes can also occur. (*From National Institutes of Health (NIH): Lyme Disease: The facts, the challenge. NIH Publication No. 92-3193. US Department of Health and Human Services, Bethesda, Md, 1992, p 6.*)

TABLE 6–9 NEUROPSYCHIATRIC MANIFESTATIONS OF LYME DISEASE

NEUROLOGIC MANIFESTATIONS	PSYCHIATRIC MANIFESTATIONS
Cranial neuritis	Anorexia nervosa
Encephalitis	Bipolar disorder
Encephalomyelitis	Dementia
Encephalopathy	Impaired memory
Meningitis	Conceptual and learning ability
Radiculoneuropathies	Attention and verbal fluency
	Major depression
	Obsessive-compulsive disorder
	Panic attacks
	Paranoia
	Schizophrenia

From Fallon BA, Nields JA: Lyme disease: A neuropsychiatric illness. Am J Psychiatry 151:1571–1583, 1994.

Weeks or months later, stage 2 with neurologic[15] or cardiac abnormalities sometimes develops. Infection with *B. burgdorferi* is responsible for a wide spectrum of neurologic and psychiatric symptoms (Table 6–9). Central or peripheral neurologic involvement develops in 40% of persons with Lyme disease. Psychiatric symptoms initially believed to be functional in persons with Lyme borreliosis are now proved to be consequences of the underlying disease (Fallon and Nields, 1994). Neurologic abnormalities may include fluctuating meningoencephalitis with peripheral and cranial neuropathy that usually resolves after weeks or months. Other neurologic complications may include abnormal skin sensations and sensitivities, insomnia or sleep disturbances, memory loss, difficulty with concentration, and hearing loss.

Cardiac abnormalities such as brief, fluctuating atrioventricular heart block may occur. The affected person may experience irregular, rapid, or slowed heart beat; chest pain; fainting; dizziness; and shortness of breath. Fewer than 1 out of 10 people with Lyme disease develop heart problems. These symptoms occur several weeks after infection and rarely last more than a few days or weeks.

Stage 3 begins weeks to years later and occurs in more than half of the persons affected who have not received early treatment. It is primarily characterized by rheumatoid arthritis with marked swelling, especially in the large joints (most often the knee) (Fig. 6–2). Recurrent attacks may precede chronic arthritis with severe cartilage and bone erosion; chronic arthritis develops in about 10% to 20% of untreated persons.

[14] Migratory musculoskeletal pain in joints, bursae, tendons, muscle, or bone may occur in one or a few locations at a time, frequently lasting only hours or days in a given location. Weeks to months later, after the development of a marked cellular and humoral response to the spirochete, untreated persons often have intermittent or chronic monarticular (one joint) or oligoarticular (affecting only a few joints) arthritis. The large joints, particularly the knees, are most commonly affected (Steere, 1995).

[15] Recent studies indicate that the bacteria may invade the brain and spinal cord early in the disease.

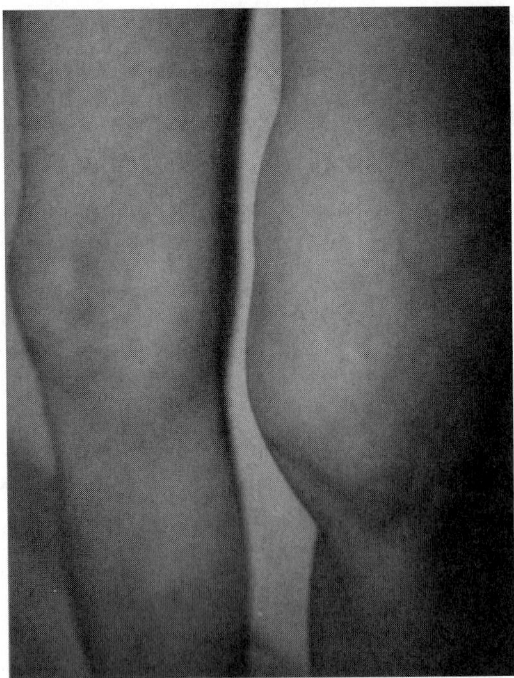

Figure **6–2.** Swollen knee of a youth with Lyme arthritis. (*From National Institutes of Health (NIH): Lyme Disease: The facts, the challenge. NIH Publication No. 92-3193. US Department of Health and Human Services, Bethesda, Md, 1992, p 12.*)

BOX **6–4**
Prevention of Lyme Disease

These precautions are provided for people living in tick-infested areas:

Avoid tick-infested areas, especially in May, June, and July (check with local health departments or park services for the seasonal and geographic distribution in your area).

Walk along cleared or paved surfaces rather than through tall grass or wooded areas.

Wear long-sleeved shirts, long pants tucked into socks, and closed shoes (no part of foot exposed).

Wear light-colored clothing to make it easy to detect ticks.

Shower as soon as possible after being outdoors. Ticks take several hours to attach themselves to the skin and can be washed away first.

Wash clothing worn outdoors immediately and use a dryer (heat kills the ticks). If there is no access to laundry facilities, the clothing should not be stored in the bedroom, or if camping, the clothing should not be stored in the same area where people are sleeping.

If bitten by a tick, remove the tick immediately by grasping it as close to the skin as possible with tweezers and tugging gently. Do not twist or turn the tweezers; pull straight away from the skin. A cotton ball soaked in rubbing alcohol or fingernail polish remover and rubbed against the "head" while tugging gently may help loosen the tick more readily.

To lessen the chance of contact with the bacterium, do not crush the tick's body or handle the tick with bare hands. Clean the bite area thoroughly with soap and water, then swab the area with an antiseptic to prevent bacterial infection.

Whenever possible, save the tick in a glass jar for identification should symptoms develop.

If living in an area in which deer ticks are common, keep the weeds and grass around the house mowed.

Use tick and flea collars on pets; brush and examine them carefully after they have been outdoors. People can use insecticides such as permethrin or insect repellents containing diethyltoluamide (DEET).*

* The use of such chemicals may be objectionable to some people because they may cause neurotoxicity in children. Alternative methods are recommended.

Adapted from NIH (National Institutes of Health): Lyme Disease: The facts, the challenge. Publication No. 92-3193, US Department of Health and Human Services, Bethesda, Md, 1992.

Medical Management

Diagnosis. Prevention is the key to avoiding Lyme disease. Two promising vaccines against Lyme disease are undergoing testing in humans at this time.[16] Studies by NIH-supported researchers suggest that a tick must be attached for many hours to transmit the Lyme disease bacterium, so prompt tick removal could prevent the disease (NIH, 1992). Other precautions are advised for people living in tick-infested areas (Box 6–4).

Because of the wide range of symptoms possible with Lyme disease, it is easily misdiagnosed as rheumatoid arthritis, fibromyalgia, chronic fatigue syndrome, meningitis, or multiple sclerosis. Fatigue, mood changes, and neurologic problems are often mistaken for mental illness or chronic fatigue syndrome (Steere, 1995).

Lyme disease can be diagnosed on the basis of geographic location (travel history is important), clinical presentation, and blood tests. Seropositivity may indicate but does not prove infection with *B. burgdorferi*, whereas seronegativity usually rules out the diagnosis; each symptom, especially in the absence of erythema migrans, requires assessment by differential diagnosis; persistence of symptoms does not prove that infection persists (Sigal, 1995).

A new test called *polymerase chain reaction* (*PCR*) uses gene slicing techniques to detect extremely small quantities of the genetic material of the bacterium itself, enabling earlier diagnosis than the previously used antibody tests (Nocton et al., 1994). The PCR has its limitations and it remains unknown whether persisting PCR positivity means ongoing infection or merely persistence of dead organisms (Sigal, 1994). Two other nonserologic tests are currently under investigation, one of which would require only a urine sample (Ziska, 1995).

Treatment. Lyme disease is treated with oral antibiotics; severe cases may require IV antibiotics for several months or longer. Supportive measures are essential for the associated

[16] Although the American Lyme Disease Foundation supports a vaccine that can be used by people living in high-risk areas, not all people should be vaccinated and exposed to the potential side effects of the immunization. Two drug companies (Connaught Laboratories and Smith-Kline) are working on a vaccine that may require annual boosters to provide continuous protection.

constitutional symptoms (e.g., rest for fatigue and for swollen, inflamed joints; analgesics for pain). Treatment of long-term complications varies according to the affected organs. Arthroscopic surgery may be required for joints damaged by the disease.

Prognosis. Early treatment is vital for the prevention of long-term complications, but even so, complications involving the heart, joints, and nervous system occur in about 15% of persons who do undergo early treatment. For most people, Lyme disease is curable with standard antibiotic therapy and the effects of Lyme disease resolve completely within a few weeks or months of treatment. Unfortunately, there is no natural immunity developed from exposure to Lyme disease and anyone can be reinfected. Although Lyme disease is rarely fatal, heart complications may cause life-threatening cardiac arrhythmias, and infection during pregnancy can cause fetal death. The infection can be transferred to the unborn child and can increase the risk of miscarriage or stillbirth (NIH, 1992).

Special Implications for the Therapist **6-8**

LYME DISEASE

Chronic arthritis is the most widely recognized result of untreated Lyme disease in the United States. Unlike other forms of rheumatoid arthritis, Lyme arthritis does not affect the joints bilaterally, though both sides may be affected alternately. The condition has been called chronic because episodes can last months, occurring intermittently over a period of 1 to 3 years (Steere, 1995). Permanent joint damage and cartilage destruction can occur if excessive use occurs during the inflammatory period. Range-of-motion and strengthening exercises are important but must be carried out carefully and without overexertion.

Nervous system abnormalities can develop weeks, months, or even years following an untreated infection. These symptoms often last for weeks or months and may recur. The therapist may treat such a client at any time during the course of symptomatic presentation. For anyone with known Lyme disease, frequent assessment of the person's neurologic function and level of consciousness is important. Any signs of cardiac abnormality or increased intracranial pressure and cranial nerve involvement (e.g., ptosis, strabismus, diplopia) must be reported to the physician immediately. Both upper and lower extremity peripheral nerve problems can occur and are managed as any neuropathy from other causes.

It has been hypothesized that persons who present with symptoms of multiple sclerosis but respond to antibiotics may have been bitten by ticks years ago. However, in theory, if the person had true multiple sclerosis, antibiotics would not have altered the symptoms present as they do with Lyme disease. Along the same lines, the question has been raised whether fibromyalgia is triggered by Lyme disease or does Lyme disease just manifest clinically as indistinguishable from fibromyalgia (Ziska, 1995)? It is possible that fibromyalgia-like symptoms develop as a result of sleep disturbances during the dissemination stage of Lyme disease. Since the cause of fibromyalgia (independent of Lyme disease) is unknown, linking its development to Lyme disease is even more difficult.

For the present, therapists are encouraged to treat adults with long-term manifestations of Lyme disease using the treatment philosophy adopted for autoimmune disorders (see Fibromyalgia; Systemic Lupus Erythematosus, Chapter 5). Conversely, anyone diagnosed as having fibromyalgia should be screened for Lyme disease. The therapist can start this screening process by asking about a history of exposure (i.e., frequency and location of outdoor activities) if the physician has not already posed these questions.

References

Adams EM, Gudmundsson S, Yocum DE, et al: Streptococcal myositis. Arch Intern Med 145:1020–1023, 1986.

Andreoli TE, Bennett JC, Carpenter CCJ, et al (eds): Cecil Essentials of Medicine, ed 3. Philadelphia, WB Saunders, 1993.

Antunes MJ: Reoperations on cardiac valves. J Heart Valve Dis 1(1):15–28, 1992.

Ballard WT, Callaghan JJ, Johnston RC: Revision of total hip arthroplasty in octogenarians. J Bone Joint Surg [Am] 77:585–589, 1995.

Barnes DM, Whittier S, Gilligan PH, et al: Transmission of multidrug resistant serotype 23F *Streptococcus pneumoniae* in group day care. J Infect Dis 171:890–896, 1995.

Ben-Yehuda A, Weksler M: Host resistance and the immune system. Clin Geriatr Med 8:701–711, 1992.

Biasi D, Carletto A, Caramaschi P, et al.: A case of reactive arthritis after influenza vaccination. Clin Rheumatol 13:645, 1994.

Biasi D, De Sandre G, Bambara LM, et al: A new case of reactive arthritis after hepatitis B vaccination. Clin Exp Rheumatol 11:215, 1993.

Bisno AL: *Streptococcus pyogenes*. *In* Mandell GL, Bennett JE, Dolin R (eds): Principles and Practice of Infectious Diseases, ed 4. New York, Churchill Livingstone, 1995, pp 1786–1798.

Brause BD: Infections associated with prosthetic joints. Clin Rheum Dis 12:523–536, 1986.

Brause BD: Infections with prostheses in bones and joints. *In* Mandell GL, Bennet JE, Dolin R. (eds): Principles and Practice of Infectious Diseases, ed 4. New York, Churchill Livingstone, 1995, pp 1051–1055.

Brennan FR, Mikecz K, Buzas EI, et al: Interferon-gamma but not granulocyte/macrophage colony-stimulating factor augments proteoglycan presentation by synovial cells and chondrocytes to an autopathogenic T cell hybridoma. Immunol Lett 45:87–91, 1995.

Bridges AJ, Vascy FB: Silicone breast implants: History, safety, and potential complications. Arch Intern Med 153:2638–2644, 1993.

Bright C: Infectious diseases are spreading worldwide. PT Bull 10(28):6, 1995.

Buzas EI, Brennan FR, Mikecz K, et al: A proteoglycan (aggrecan)-specific T cell hybridoma induces arthritis in BABL/c mice. J Immunol 155:2679–2687, 1995.

Castle SC, Norman DC, Yeh M, et al: Fever response in the elderly. Are the older truly colder? J Am Geriatr Soc 39:853–857, 1991.

CDC (Centers for Disease Control and Prevention): Lyme disease—United States, 1994. MMWR 44:459–462, 1995.

Chalmers A, Scheifele D, Patterson C, et al: Immunization of patients with rheumatoid arthritis against influenza: A study of vaccine safety and immunogenicity. J Rheumatol 21:1203–1206, 1994.

Choudhri SH, Brownstone R, Hashem F, et al: A case of necrotizing fasciitis due to *Streptococcus pneumoniae*. Br J Dermatol 133:128–131, 1995.

Cohen M: Bacteria seen evolving into untreatable forms: Interview with CDC spokesman. PT Bull 9(9):2, 1994.

Cronin SN: Nursing care of clients with lower airway disorders. *In* Black JM, Matassarin-Jacobs E (eds): Luckmann and Sorensen's Medical-Surgical Nursing, ed 4. Philadelphia, WB Saunders, 1993, pp 1021–1088.

Cunha BA: Clinical implications of fever. Postgrad Med 85:188–200, 1989.

Dickinson GM, Bisno AL: Infections associated with prosthetic devices: Clinical considerations. Int J Artif Organs 16:749–754, 1993.

Diekema DJ, Doebbeling BN: Employee health and infection control. Infection Control Hosp Epidemiol 16:292–301, 1995.

Duncan CP, Masri BA: The role of antibiotic-loaded cement in the treatment of an infection after a hip replacement. Instr Course Lect 44:305–313, 1995.

Eidelberg D, Sotrel A, Vogel H, et al: Progressive polyradiculopathy in acquired immune deficiency syndrome. Neurology 36:912, 1986.

Esposito AL, Gleckman RA: Fever of unknown origin in the elderly. J Am Geriatr Soc 26:498–505, 1978.

Fallon BA, Nields JA: Lyme disease: A neuropsychiatric illness. Am J Psychiatry 151:1571–1583, 1994.

Ferlic DC, Jolly SN, Clayton ML: Salvage for failed implant arthroplasty of the wrist. J Hand Surg [Am] 17:917–923, 1992.

Fiebach N, Beckett W: Prevention of respiratory infections in adults. Influenza and pneumococcal vaccines. Arch Intern Med 154:2545–2557, 1994.

Foldes K, Balint P, Balint G, et al: Ultrasound-guided aspiration in suspected sepsis of resection arthroplasty of the hip joint. Clin Rheumatol 14:327–329, 1995.

Freedman AM, Jackson IT: Infections in breast implants. Infect Dis Clin North Am 3:275–287, 1989.

Gabriel SE, O'Fallon WM, Beard CM, et al: Trends in the utilization of silicone breast implants, 1964–1991, and methodology for a population-based study of outcomes. J Clin Epidemiol 48:527–537, 1995.

Gabriel SE, O'Fallon WM, Kurland LT, et al: Risk of connective-tissue diseases and other disorders after breast implant. N Engl J Med 330:1697–1702, 1994.

Gelfand MS, Cleveland KO: Penicillin-resistant pneumococcal vertebral osteomyelitis. Clin Infect Dis 15:746–749, 1992.

Golz R, Kuschner SH, Gellman H: Sequential infection of silicone metacarpophalangeal joint arthroplasties resulting from skin breakdown. J Hand Surg 17:150–152, 1992.

Gonzalez-Ruiz GL, Cohen SL, Hunt CP, et al: Varicella gangrenosa with toxic shock–like syndrome due to group A streptococcus in an adult: Case report. Clin Infect Dis 20:1058–1060, 1995.

Grimes DE: Nursing care of clients with infectious diseases. *In* Black JM, Matassarin-Jacobs E (eds): Luckmann and Sorensen's Medical-Surgical Nursing, ed 4. Philadelphia, WB Saunders, 1993, pp 579–592.

Gristina AG, Kolkin J: Total joint replacement and sepsis. J Bone Joint Surg [Am] 65:128–134, 1983.

Harruff RC: Pathology Facts. Philadelphia, JB Lippincott, 1994.

Heggeness MH, Esses SI, Errico T, et al: Late infection of spinal instrumentation by hematogenous seeding. Spine 18:492–496, 1993.

Henrich DE, Smith TL, Shockley WW: Fatal craniocervical necrotizing fasciitis in an immunocompetent patient: A case report and literature review. Head Neck 17:351–357, 1995.

Jackson BS, Sproat JE: Necrotizing fasciitis of the head and neck with intrathoracic extension. J Otolaryngol 24:60–63, 1995.

Jacobs RA: General problems in infectious diseases. *In* Tierney LM, McPhee SJ, Papadakis MA (eds): Current Medical Diagnosis and Treatment, ed 33. Norwalk, Conn, Appleton & Lange, 1994, pp 1053–1073.

Jones JS, Hoerle D, Riekse R: Stethoscopes: A potential vector of infection? Ann Emerg Med 26:296–299, 1995.

Kiecolt-Glaser JK, Dura JR, Speicher CE, et al: Spousal caregivers of dementia victims: Longitudinal changes in immunity and health. Psychosom Med 53:345–362, 1991.

Kossovsky N, Freiman CJ: Silicone breast implant pathology: Clinical data and immunologic consequences. Arch Pathol Lab Med 118:686–693, 1994.

Kossovsky N, Papasian N: Mammary implants: A clinical review. J Appl Biomater 3:239–242, 1992.

Kuczyk MA, Denil J, Thon WF: Orchitis following mumps vaccination in an adult. Urol Int 53:179–180, 1994.

Larson E: Guideline for use of topical antimicrobial agents. Am J Infect Control 19:59, 1991.

Leibowitz MR, Ramakrishnan KK: Necrotizing fasciitis: The role of *Staphylococcus epidermidis*, immune status, and intravascular coagulation. Austr J Dermatol 36:29–31, 1995.

Malleson PN, Tekano JL, Scheifele DW, et al: Influenza immunization in children with chronic arthritis: A prospective study. J Rheumatol 20:1769–1773, 1993.

Maull KI, Sachatello C: Retroperitoneal iliac fossa abscess. A complication of suppurative iliac lymphadenitis. Am J Surg 127:270, 1974.

McCracken GH Jr: Emergence of resistant *Streptococcus pneumoniae:* A problem in pediatrics. Pediatr Infect Dis J 14:424–428, 1995.

Morley PK, Hull RG, Hall MA: Pneumococcal septic arthritis in rheumatoid arthritis. Ann Rheum Dis 46:482–484, 1987.

Musher DM: *Streptococcus pneumoniae*. *In* Mandell GL, Bennett JE, Dolan R (eds): Principles and Practice of Infectious Diseases, ed 4. New York, Churchill Livingstone, 1995, pp 1811–1826.

NIH (National Institutes of Health): Lyme disease: The facts, the challenge. NIH Publication No. 92-3193, US Department of Health and Human Services, Bethesda, Md, 1992.

Nocton JJ, Dressler F, Rutledge B, et al: Detection of *Borrelia burgdorferi* DNA by polymerase chain reaction in synovial fluid from patients with Lyme disease. N Engl J Med 330:229–283, 1994.

Norris J (ed): Professional Guide to Diseases, ed 5. Springhouse, Pa, Springhouse, 1995.

Oliff M, Chuang VP: Retroperitoneal iliac fossa pyogenic abscess. Radiology 126:647, 1978.

O'Neill DA, Harris WH: Failed total hip replacement: Assessment by plain radiographs, arthrograms, and aspiration of the hip joint. J Bone Joint Surg [Am] 66:540–546, 1984.

Petty W, Spanier S, Shuster JJ, et al: The influence of skeletal implants on incidence of infection. J Bone Joint Surg [Am] 67:1236–1244, 1985.

Piczon OY, Manahan FJ, Udomsak P, et al: Case study: A modified topical treatment regimen for sodium warfarin–induced necrotizing fasciitis. Ostomy Wound Manage 41:48–50, 52, 54, 1995.

Pillans PI, O'Connor N: Tissue necrosis and necrotizing fasciitis after intramuscular administration of diclofenac. Ann Pharmacother 29:264–266, 1995.

Platt A: Infectious diseases are spreading worldwide. PT Bulletin 10:6, 1995.

Pollack M: *Pseudomonas aeruginosa*. *In* Mandell GL, Bennett JE, Dolin R (eds): Principles and Practice of Infectious Diseases, ed 4. New York, Churchill Livingstone, 1995, pp 1980–2003.

Rahn DW: Lyme disease: Where's the bug? (editorial). N Engl J Med 330:282–283, 1994.

Rasul AT, Tsukayama D, Gustilo RB: Effect of time on onset and depth of infection on the outcome of total knee arthroplasty infections. Clin Orthop 273:98–104, 1991.

Reichel W (ed): Care of the Elderly: Clinical Aspects of Aging, ed 4. Baltimore, Williams & Wilkins, 1995.

Robertson CR: Silicone breast implants not proved as cause of musculoskeletal problems. J Musculoskel Med 10(9):13–14, 1993.

Rossman R: Clinical Geriatrics: Decline in Organ Function with Aging, ed 3. Philadelphia, JB Lippincott, 1986.

Rowan JA, North RA: Necrotizing fasciitis in the puerperium. Am J Obstet Gynecol 173:241–242, 1995.

Rubin E, Farber JL: Pathology, ed 2. Philadelphia, JB Lippincott, 1994.

Ryczak M, Sands M, Brown RB, et al: Pneumococcal arthritis in a prosthetic knee. A case report and review of the literature. Clin Orthop 224:224–227, 1987.

Sanches IS, Ramirez M, Troni H, et al: Evidence for the geographic spread of a methicillin-resistant *Staphylococcus aureus* clone between Portugal and Spain. J Clin Microbiol 33:1243–1246, 1995.

Sanchez-Guerro J, Colditz GA, Karlson EW, et al: Silicone breast implants and the risk of connective tissue diseases and symptoms. N Engl J Med 332:1666–1670, 1995.

Schaffer SD, Garzon LS, Herous DL, et al: Infection Prevention and Safe Practice. St Louis, Mosby–Year Book, 1996.

Schecter W, Meyer A, Schecter G, et al: Necrotizing fasciitis of the upper extremity. J Hand Surg 7:15, 1982.

Swartz MN: Cellulitis and subcutaneous tissue infections. *In* Mandell GL, Bennett JE, Dolin R (eds): Principles and Practice of Infectious Diseases, ed 4. New York, Churchill Livingstone, 1995, pp 909–929.

Segal M: Silicon breast implants: Available under tight controls. FDA Consumer Magazine, US Department of Health and Human Services Publication No. (FDA) 93-4253. Rockville, Md, June 1992.

Shiffman MA: Silicone breast implant litigation (p 1). Med Law 13:681–716, 1994.

Sigal, LH: Lyme disease minus the mythology. J Musculoskel Med 12(5):51–58, 1995.
Sigal LH: The polymerase chain reaction assay for *Borrelia burgdorferi* in the diagnosis of Lyme disease (editorial). Ann Intern Med 120:520–521, 1994.
Skidmore-Roth L: Mosby's 1995 Nursing Drug Reference. St. Louis, Mosby–Year Book, 1995.
Snider WD, Sipson DM, Nielsen S, et al: Neurological complications of acquired immune deficiency syndrome: Analysis of 50 patients. Ann Neurol 14:403, 1988.
Steere AC: Musculoskeletal manifestations of Lyme disease. Am J Med 98(suppl 4A):4A–44S, 1995.
Thompson JM, McFarland GK, Hirsch JE, et al: Mosby's Clinical Nursing, ed 3. St Louis, Mosby–Year Book, 1993.
Thorson K (ed): Silicone breast implants: What's the connection? Fibromyalgia Network 24:15, January 1994.
Tomasz A: The pneumococcus at the gates. N Engl J Med 333:514–515, 1995.
Virden CP, Dobke MK, Stein P, et al: Subclinical infection of the silicone breast implant surface as a possible cause of capsular contracture. Aesthetic Plast Surg 16:173–179, 1992.
Weber DJ, Rutala WA: Environmental issues and nosocomial infections. *In* Wenzel RP (ed): Prevention and Control of Nosocomial Infections, ed 2. Baltimore, Williams & Wilkins, 1993.
Wilson GJ, Talkington DF, Gruber W, et al: Group A streptococcal necrotizing fasciitis following varicella in children: Case reports and review. Clin Infect Dis 20:1333–1338, May 1995.
Ziska M: Personal communication, June 1995.

SECTION 2

chapter 7

Oncology

Catherine C. Goodman

Cancer is a term that refers to a large group of diseases characterized by uncontrolled growth and spread of abnormal cells. Other terms used interchangeably for cancer are malignant neoplasm, tumor, malignancy, and carcinoma. Cancer in its various forms is a genetic disease, characterized by deviations of the normal genetic mechanisms that regulate cell growth (Sandberg, 1994). Only oncologic concepts are presented in this chapter; individual cancers are discussed in the chapters devoted to the affected system. See also Chapter 4.

DEFINITIONS *(Goodman and Snyder, 1995)*

Differentiation

Normal tissue contains cells of uniform size, shape, maturity, and nuclear structure. Differentiation is the process by which normal cells undergo physical and structural changes as they develop to form different tissues of the body. Differentiated cells specialize in different physiologic functions. In malignant cells, differentiation is altered and may be lost completely so that the malignant cell may not be recognizable in relationship to its parent cell. When a tumor has completely lost identity with the parent tissue, it is considered to be undifferentiated (anaplastic). In this case, it may become difficult or impossible to identify the malignant cell's tissue of origin. In general, the less differentiated a tumor becomes, the worse the prognosis.

Dysplasia

A variety of other tissue changes can occur in the body. Some of these changes are benign whereas others denote a malignant or premalignant state. Dysplasia is a general category that indicates a disorganization of cells in which an adult cell varies from its normal size, shape, or organization. This is often caused by chronic irritation as is seen with changes in cervical (uterine) epithelium as a result of longstanding irritation of the cervix. Dysplasia may reverse itself or may progress to cancer.

Metaplasia

Metaplasia is the first level of dysplasia (early dysplasia). It is a reversible and benign but abnormal change in which one adult cell changes from one type to another. For example, the most common type of epithelial metaplasia is the change of columnar epithelium of the respiratory tract to squamous epithelium (Deters, 1995). Although metaplasia usually gives rise to an orderly arrangement of cells, it may sometimes produce disorderly cellular patterns (i.e., cells varying in size, shape, and orientation to one another) (Groenwald, 1993a).

Loss of cellular differentiation is called *anaplasia*. Anaplasia is the most advanced form of metaplasia and is a characteristic of malignant cells only.

Hyperplasia

Hyperplasia refers to an increase in the number of cells in tissue, resulting in increased tissue mass. This type of change can be a normal consequence of physiologic alterations (*physiologic hyperplasia*), such as increased breast mass during pregnancy, wound healing, or bone callus formation. *Neoplastic hyperplasia*, however, is the increase in cell mass due to tumor formation and is an abnormal process.

Tumors

Tumors, or neoplasms, are new growths and may be benign or malignant. The mass of tissue constituting the new growth is a neoplasm that enlarges at the expense of its host, sometimes acting as a parasite by competing for nutrients and threatening the survival of the host. A *primary* tumor arises from cells that are normally local to the given structure, whereas a *secondary* tumor arises from cells that have metastasized from another part of the body. For example, a primary neoplasm *of* bone arises from within the bone structure itself, whereas a secondary neoplasm occurs *in* bone as a result of metastasized cancer cells from another (primary) site.

Carcinoma in situ refers to preinvasive epithelial tumors of glandular or squamous cell origin. These tumors have not broken through basement membranes of the squamous cells and occur in the cervix, skin, oral cavity, esophagus, and bronchus. Carcinoma in situ affecting glandular epithelium occurs in the stomach, endometrium, and large bowel. How long the characteristic cell disorganization and atypical changes last before becoming invasive remains unknown.

Classifications of Neoplasm *(Rubin and Farber, 1994; Vincent and Mirand, 1991)*

A *neoplasm* is defined as an abnormal growth of new tissue that serves no useful purpose and may harm the host organism by competing for vital blood supply and nutrients. A neoplasm can be classified on the basis of cell type, tissue of origin, degree of differentiation, anatomic site, or whether it is benign or malignant.

A benign growth is usually considered harmless and does not spread or invade other tissue. Certain benign growths, recognized clinically as tumors, are not truly neoplastic but rather represent overgrowth of normal tissue elements (e.g., vocal cord polyps, skin tags, hyperplastic polyps of the colon). However, benign growths can become large enough to impair normal body functions as in the case of benign central nervous system (CNS) tumors which can cause disability and even death.

Malignant tumors usually carry the same name as the benign tumor except the suffix *carcinoma* is applied to epithelial cancers and *sarcoma* refers to those of mesenchymal origin. For example, a malignant tumor of the stomach is a gastric adenocarcinoma and an invasive tumor of the skin is a squamous cell carcinoma. The name of the tumor may identify the tissue type of origin, as in adenocarcinoma, squamous cell carcinoma, osteogenic sarcoma, or bronchogenic carcinoma.

When tumors (benign or malignant) are classified by cell type, they are named according to the tissue from which they arise (Table 7–1). The five major classifications of normal body tissue are epithelial, connective and muscle, nerve, lymphoid, and hematopoietic tissue. Not all tissue types fit into one of these five categories, requiring a miscellaneous category (not included in Table 7–1) for other tissues such as the tissues of the reproductive glands, placenta, and thymus.

Epithelium covers all external body surfaces and lines all internal spaces and cavities. The skin, mucous membranes, gastrointestinal tract, and lining of the bladder are examples of epithelial tissue. The functions of epithelial tissues are to protect, excrete, and absorb. Cancer originating in any of these epithelial tissues is called a carcinoma. Tumors derived from epithelial and glandular tissues are called adenocarcinoma.

Connective tissue consists of elastic, fibrous, and collagenous tissues, such as bone, cartilage, and fat. Cancers originating in connective tissue and muscle are called sarcomas. *Nerve tissue* includes the brain, spinal cord, and nerves, and consists of neurons, nerve fibers, dendrites, and a supporting tissue composed of glial cells. Tumors arising in nerve tissue are named for the type of cell involved. For example, tumors arising from astrocytes, a type of glial cell thought to form the blood-brain barrier, are called astrocytomas. Tumors arising in nerve tissue are often benign, but because of their critical location are more likely to be harmful than benign tumors in other sites.

Malignancy originating in *lymphoid tissues*, such as lymph nodes, the spleen, and the intestinal lining, are referred to as lymphomas. Cancers of the hemopoietic tissues are called leukemias.

Staging and Grading *(Beahrs et al., 1992)*

Staging is the process of describing the extent of disease at the time of diagnosis in order to aid treatment planning, predict clinical outcome (prognosis), and compare different treatment approaches. The practice of dividing cancer cases into groups according to stages arose from the fact that survival rates were higher for cases in which the disease was localized than for those in which the disease had extended beyond the site of origin. The stage of disease at the time of diagnosis may reflect not only the rate of growth and extension of the neoplasm but also the type of tumor and the tumor-host relationship.

In one classification scheme called the *TNM classification*, developed by the American Joint Committee on Cancer (AJCC), tumors are staged according to three basic compo-

TABLE 7–1 CLASSIFICATION OF NEOPLASMS BY CELL TYPE OF ORIGIN

TISSUE OF ORIGIN	BENIGN	MALIGNANT
Epithelial tissue		
Surface epithelium (skin) and mucous membrane	Papilloma	Carcinoma
Epithelial lining of glands or ducts	Adenoma	Adenocarcinoma
Pigmented cells (melanocytes of basal layer)	Nevus (mole)	Malignant melanoma
Connective tissue and muscle		
Fibrous tissue	Fibroma	Fibrosarcoma
Adipose	Lipoma	Liposarcoma
Cartilage	Chondroma	Chondrosarcoma
Bone	Osteoma	Osteosarcoma
Blood vessels	Hemangioma	Hemangiosarcoma
Smooth muscle	Leiomyoma	Leiomyosarcoma
Striated muscle	Rhabdomyoma	Rhabdomyosarcoma
Nerve tissue		
Nerve cells	Neuroma	
Glia		Glioma or neuroglioma
Ganglion cells	Ganglioneuroma	Neuroblastoma
Nerve sheaths	Neurilemoma	Neurilemic sarcoma
Meninges	Meningioma	Meningeal sarcoma
Retina		Retinoblastoma
Lymphoid tissue		
Lymph nodes		Lymphoma/lymphosarcoma
Spleen		Lymphoma/lymphosarcoma
Intestinal lining		Lymphoma/lymphosarcoma
Hematopoietic tissue		
Bone marrow		Leukemias, Ewing's sarcoma
Plasma cells		Multiple myeloma

nents (Table 7–2): (1) primary tumor (T); (2) regional lymph nodes (N); and (3) metastasis (M). Numbers are used with each component to denote extent of involvement; for example, T0 indicates undetectable, and T1, T2, T3, and T4 indicate a progressive increase in size or involvement (O'Toole, 1992).

Grading, another way to define a tumor, classifies the degree of malignancy and differentiation and estimates tumor growth. For example, a low-grade tumor typically has cells more closely resembling normal cells, whereas a high-grade tumor has poorly differentiated cells.

CANCER AND AGING

Age is the single most significant risk factor for cancer, and the incidence of most cancers rises exponentially throughout human life. Cancer is the second most common cause of mortality in the elderly, currently causing about 25% of deaths in persons aged 65 years and older. Cancer incidence and mortality rates increase with age until the 84th year when they plateau and may even decline slightly. In the oldest group of persons (i.e., those older than 84 years) cancer is responsible for a smaller proportion of deaths than in younger groups (Brody and Persky, 1990).

Older people may be more susceptible to cancer simply because they have been exposed to carcinogens longer than younger people. The effects of age on immune function and host defense are difficult to determine but may have a link to the increasing incidence of cancer with age. See Aging and the Immune System: Chapter 5.

Studies on how often mutations in cancer-causing genes occur in the elderly are being reported. Aging cells, when copying their genetic material, may begin to err, giving rise to mutations, and the aging immune system may not recognize these mutations as foreign, thus allowing them to proliferate and form a malignant tumor. Researchers report finding that mutations linked with lymphoma and leukemia accumulate with age. For example, people past their 60th birthday face 40 times the risk of non-Hodgkin's lymphoma as those younger than 20 years, and the risk for stomach, colon, lung, breast, and other cancers increases as well (Liu et al., 1994; Arnheim and Cortopassi, 1992).

Cancers that exhibit the most consistent increases in rate with age are leukemia, cancers of the digestive system, and cervical, breast, prostate, and skin cancers. For example, the incidence of myelodysplastic syndrome (MDS, a group of hematopoietic stem cell disorders leading to leukemia) appears to be increasing in the aging population. With MDS, there is a definite increase occurring within each 10-year age group above 50 (Sandberg, 1994).

An increase in cervical cancer associated with age is observed in women age 65 years and older (ACS, 1989). The incidence of breast cancer rises with age and does not level off until age 85 or above, whereas colorectal cancer increases in incidence throughout old age and continues to rise beyond age 85. Nonmelanoma skin cancers are the most common malignancies found in older people. The incidence of both basal and squamous cell carcinomas increases with age. When identified at an early stage, both melanoma and nonmelanoma skin cancers are treatable (Murphy and Coletta, 1995).

TABLE 7-2 TNM STAGING SYSTEM

T: PRIMARY TUMOR	
T_X	Primary tumor cannot be assessed
T_0	No evidence of primary tumor
T_{is}	Carcinoma in situ (confined to site of origin)
T_1, T_2, T_3	Progressive increase in tumor size and involvement locally
N: REGIONAL LYMPH NODES	
N_X	Nodes cannot be assessed
N_0	No metastasis to regional lymph nodes
N_1, N_2, N_3	Increasing degrees of involvement of regional lymph nodes
Note: Extension of primary tumor directly into lymph nodes is considered metastasis to lymph nodes. Metastasis to a lymph node beyond the regional ones is considered distant metastasis.	
M: DISTANT METASTASIS	
M_X	Presence of distant metastasis cannot be assessed
M_0	No distant metastasis
M_1	Presence of distant metastasis

Adapted from O'Toole M (ed): Miller-Keane Encyclopedia and Dictionary of Medicine, Nursing and Allied Health, ed 5. Philadelphia, WB Saunders, 1992.

CANCER AND EXERCISE *(Thompson, 1994)*

Exercise as a Cancer Prevention Strategy

Physical activity is defined as bodily movement caused by skeletal muscle contraction that results in quantifiable energy expenditure. Both epidemiologic and laboratory data indicate that the level of physical activity in which an individual engages may affect cancer risk. Exercise is distinguished from other types of physical activity by the fact that the intensity, duration, and frequency of the activity are specifically designed to improve physical fitness.

Based on available data, a role for exercise in specifically reducing cancer risk has been conjectured and is referred to as the *exercise-cancer hypothesis*. However, the amount of scientific evidence in support of this hypothesis is still quite limited, and there are conflicting reports about the nature of the association.

Some research studies have indicated that both the intensity and duration of exercise affect the development of experimentally induced breast cancer. As exercise intensity increased, the likelihood that such physical activity inhibited carcinogenesis increased. Exercise at lower intensities resulted in either inhibition, no effect, or enhancement of the tumorigenic response depending on the duration of exercise (Thompson, 1994). Another study did not support a protective effect of physical activity during adulthood for breast cancer, but suggested an increased risk among more active women (Dorgan et al., 1994).

Moderate exercise may have an effect on the cytotoxic activity of natural killer (NK) cells. Although the number of NK cells does not change, the cytotoxic activity of resting NK cells is increased (Peters et al., 1994).

Exercise for the Person with Cancer

Generalized weakness associated with cancer treatment can be more debilitating than the disease itself. Whenever possible, exercise, including strength and cardiovascular training, is an essential component for many people with cancer. Improving strength and endurance aids in countering the effects of the disease and the effects of medical interventions. Not all people with cancer are able to participate in aerobic exercise. People who ambulate less than 50% of the time or who are confined to bed and those who fatigue with mild exertion may not be candidates for aerobic exercise (Winningham, 1991). Range of motion and gentle resistive work until tolerance for activity improves are still important (Miller, 1992).

Medical screening should be conducted with *all* clients before their participation in an exercise program (ACSM, 1991). This type of screening is especially important for people with cancer who receive various levels of treatment that can affect the physiologic response to exercise. A detailed medical history is essential and should include conditions not related to cancer, such as hypertension, diabetes, coronary artery disease, preexisting orthopedic conditions, and so on. The person's current physical condition and condition prior to disease onset and age are also important variables (Winningham et al., 1986).

The therapist must understand the stages of the disease and know the type and timing of the radiation and chemotherapy. The body's physiologic response to these agents may affect tolerance for exercise and alter the normal training response (Miller, 1992).

Bone marrow suppression is a common and serious side effect of many chemotherapeutic agents and can be a side effect of radiation therapy in some instances. Therefore, it is extremely important to monitor the hematologic values in clients receiving these treatment modalities. The therapist must review these values before any type of vigorous exercise or activity is initiated. A helpful guideline to indicate when aerobic exercise is contraindicated in chemotherapy clients is given in Table 7–3.

Monitoring physiologic responses (e.g., vital signs) to exercise is important in the immunosuppressed population. Watch closely for early signs (dyspnea, pallor, sweating, fatigue) of cardiopulmonary complications of cancer treatment. The activity level of someone with anemia also may require adjustment. This client may have elevated pulse and respiratory rates because of hypoxia, with increased cardiac output resulting from the body's effort to maintain an adequate oxygen supply. The therapist should always monitor pulse rate, breathing frequency, blood pressure, and signs and symptoms such as pallor and sweating throughout the treatment session. The affected person may become easily fatigued with minimal exertion; interval exercise or a bedside exercise program should be performed during frequent but short sessions throughout the day and may be the only treatment possible in this circumstance (Hamburgh, 1992). See also Special Implications for the Therapist: Anemia, Chapter 11.

Exercise intensity determined by training heart rate may be difficult to use as some people have inappropriate heart responses to exercise and large physiologic changes on a day-to-day basis from disease and treatment, including changes in medications. Exercise intensity can be guided by heart rate ranges based on oxygen consumption or metabolic equivalent (MET) levels (see Myocardial Infarction: Monitoring Vital Signs, Chapter 10) along with monitoring of blood pressure, heart rate (for rhythm changes), and Borg's ratings of perceived exertion scale (see Table 10–14) (Pfalzer, 1987).

Compromised skeletal integrity may prevent weight-bearing activities. Non–weight-bearing aerobic activities, which may be utilized for people with bone and joint disease, include cycling, rowing, and swimming (the last for those who are not immunosuppressed). People with severe muscle weakness may tolerate cycling better than ambulation (Pfalzer, 1987).

Energy-conservation techniques and work simplification (Box 7–1) may be necessary for the person with chronic fatigue and for those whose functional status is declining. Therapeutic exercise should be scheduled during periods when the person has the highest level of energy. Interval exercise may be preferred at first, with work-rest intervals beginning at the person's level of tolerance. This may be no more than 1 minute of exercise activity followed by 1 minute of rest, then 1 minute of exercise, and so on. As the person's endurance level increases, the duration of work may be increased and the interval of rest decreased.

TABLE 7-3 WINNINGHAM CONTRAINDICATIONS TO AEROBIC EXERCISE IN CHEMOTHERAPY CLIENTS

Platelet count	<50,000/μL
Hemoglobin	<10 g/dL
White blood cell count	<3000/μL
Absolute granulocytes	<2500/μL

Data from Winningham ML, MacVicar MG, Burke CA: Exercise for cancer patients: Guidelines and precautions. Physician Sportsmed 14:125–134, 1986.

INCIDENCE

The American Cancer Society (ACS) publishes annual cancer statistics and estimates cancer trends. Data are based on statistics obtained from approximately 500,000 people diagnosed and treated in the previous year at almost 1000 hospitals. These cases represent approximately half of all US cases, allowing individual hospitals to compare their results with regional and national outcomes (Murphy, 1994).

The National Cancer Institute (NCI) established the Surveillance, Epidemiology, and End Results (SEER) Program in 1973 as a way to report population-based data of site-specific incidences of cancer, mortality, and survival rates. This report is based on 12% of the US population, including six large cities.

The incidence of reported cases of cancer has been increasing steadily since 1900. Approximately 1 million new cases of cancer will be diagnosed this year. One in 4 people will be diagnosed with some form of cancer; 1 in 3 will survive 5 years or more after diagnosis and treatment. Cancer claims more than 500,000 lives annually and disrupts many thousands more.

Currently, cancer is the second leading cause of death in the United States, exceeded only by heart disease. There are at least three reasons for this apparent increase: (1) improved diagnostic methods; (2) computerization of statistical gathering and analysis allowing for more accurate reporting; and

BOX 7–1
Tips for Energy Conservation

Energy conservation is an organized procedure for finding ways to reduce the amount of effort and energy needed to accomplish a given task. By reducing the amount of energy needed to accomplish a task, more energy is available.

Applying principles of energy conservation requires self-examination and assessment of habits and priorities. Making these types of changes requires patience but can result in continued activity over a longer period of time:

Schedule the most strenuous activities during the periods of highest energy.

Before starting any activity, analyze the task and answer the following questions:
- Is the task necessary?
- Can it be eliminated or combined?
- Am I doing this out of habit?
- Can it be simplified by combining or eliminating steps?
- Can a larger job be divided up into smaller tasks?
- Are there any assistive devices or tools that could make the task easier?
- Can this be done by someone else?

Alternate more strenuous tasks with easier ones.

Plan frequent rest periods, sit down, or take naps as needed.

Cluster activities so that it is not necessary to make frequent trips or walk long distances at home, school, or work.

Avoid or keep to a minimum the climbing of stairs.

Keep certain tasks such as housekeeping to a minimum.

Sit down to perform activities of daily living (e.g., toothbrushing, hair combing) or household tasks, including meal preparation.

Avoid sitting on low or soft furniture which requires more energy expenditure to get up again.

Adapted from Hamburgh RR: Principles of cancer treatment. Clin Manage 12:37–41, 1992.

(3) longer life span placing older adults at greater risk for many cancers.

ETIOLOGY

The cause of cancer varies and causative agents are generally subdivided into two categories: those of endogenous (genetic) origin and those of exogenous (environmental or external) origin. It is likely that most cancers develop as a result of multiple environmental, viral, and genetic agents working together to disrupt the immune system. Certain cancers show a familial pattern giving people a hereditary predisposition to cancer. The most common cancers showing a familial pattern include breast, ovarian, and colon cancers. Research efforts have been directed at finding genes associated with various cancers that could identify high-risk individuals for screening and early detection.

The ACS estimates that 80% of all cancers are caused by one or more of nearly 500 different cancer-causing agents (e.g., viruses, chemical agents, physical agents, drugs, alcohol, hormones) (Garfinkel, 1995). Etiologic agents capable of initiating the malignant transformation of a cell (i.e., carcinogenesis) are called *carcinogens*. The study of *viruses* as carcinogens is one of the most rapidly advancing areas in cancer research today. Researchers now have evidence that viruses play a role in the pathogenesis of cervical carcinomas, some hepatomas, Burkitt's lymphoma, nasopharyngeal carcinomas, adult T cell leukemias, and indirectly, many Kaposi's sarcomas (Weinberg, 1994). Viruses such as the human immunodeficiency virus (HIV), the causative agent of acquired immunodeficiency syndrome (AIDS), weakens cell-mediated immunity, resulting in malignancies.

Chemical agents (e.g., tar, soot, asphalt, dyes, hydrocarbons, oils, nickel, arsenics) and *physical agents* (e.g., radiation, asbestos) may cause cancer after close and prolonged contact. Most persons affected by chemical agents are workers in industries. Radiation exposure is usually from natural sources,[1] especially ultraviolet radiation from the sun which can cause changes in DNA structure that lead to malignant transformation. Basal and squamous cell carcinoma and malignant melanoma are all linked to ultraviolet exposure. See further discussion of chemical and physical agents in Chapter 3.

Some *drugs*, such as cancer chemotherapeutic agents, are in themselves carcinogenic. Cytotoxic drugs, including steroids, decrease antibody production and destroy circulating lymphocytes. Cancer clients treated with chemotherapy are at risk for future development of leukemia and other cancers. Cancer itself is immunosuppressive; advanced cancer exhausts the immune response (Norris, 1995).

Excessive *alcohol* consumption is associated with cancer of the mouth, pharynx, larynx, and esophagus. It can also indirectly contribute to liver cancer (i.e., alcohol causes liver cirrhosis, which is associated with cancer).

Hormones have been linked to tumor development and growth but the exact relationship between hormonal secretion and action and tumor formation remains undetermined. One of the most controversial topics in this area is the role of estrogen in producing cancer, especially breast and endometrial cancers. Other types of cancer occurring in target or hormone-responsive tissues include ovary and prostate cancers.

RISK FACTORS

In addition to the carcinogens described earlier under Etiology, there are also predisposing factors that influence the host's susceptibility to various etiologic agents. Factors that influence cancer incidence and deaths are listed in Box 7–2. Risk factors for selected cancer sites are listed in Table 7–4. Men and women are susceptible to prostate and cervical cancer, respectively. Lung cancer is now the leading cancer-causing death in both sexes. Cigarette smoking is responsible for about 90% of lung cancer deaths (Fig. 7–1).

Race

Black Americans are diagnosed with cancer and die from it more often than any other racial group in the United States. At present this increased incidence is attributed to prevent-

[1] Notable exceptions include past history of radiation treatment for acne, thymus, or thyroid conditions.

BOX 7–2
Cancer Risk Factors

Personal behaviors
- Tobacco use
- Diet
- Alcohol use
- Sexual and reproductive behavior

Age
Gender
Race
Geographic location
Occupation (see Chapter 3)
Socioeconomic status (see Chapter 2)
Heredity
Presence of precancerous lesions
Stress

able risk factors such as the absence of early screening, delayed diagnosis, and smoking and diet. The number of black American men who smoke is decreasing but the incidence of lung cancer and other smoking-related disease remains high, possibly because black men tend to smoke cigarettes with a higher tar and nicotine content (NCI, 1992).

The number of black American women (aged 45 to 54 years) who have died from lung cancer has increased 30% over the last two decades. Second to breast cancer, lung cancer is the leading cause of cancer death among black American women and the number of black American women of all ages who have died from breast cancer has risen nearly 20% over the last 25 years. Colorectal cancer has increased in both black American men and women; black women are twice as likely to develop cervical cancer and nearly three times as likely to die from it than other women; black American men have the world's highest rate of prostate cancer (NCI, 1992).

Geographic Location

The incidence of different types of cancer varies geographically. Colon cancer is more prevalent in urban than in rural areas, but in rural areas, especially among farmers, skin cancer is more common. The greater susceptibility of certain geographic areas within the United States is probably related to exposure to different carcinogens (Matassarin-Jacobs and Petardi, 1993).

Precancerous Lesions

Precancerous and some benign tumors may undergo transformation later into cancerous lesions and tumors. Common precancerous lesions include pigmented moles, burn scars, senile keratosis, leukoplakia, and benign adenomas or polyps of the colon or stomach. All such lesions need to be examined periodically for signs of changes.

Stress

Recent research suggests a strong link between stress and cancer. Chronic physical or emotional stress can cause hormonal or immunologic changes, or both, which, in turn, can facilitate the growth and proliferation of cancer cells. See Stress, Chapter 2.

TABLE 7–4 Risk Factors for Selected Cancer Sites

Cancer Site	High-Risk Factors
Lung	Heavy smoker (all types) over age 50 yr Smoked a pack a day for 20 yr Started smoking at age 15 yr or earlier Smoker working with or near asbestos Secondary cigarette smoke High levels of indoor radon Occupational and environmental industrial pollutants
Breast	History of previous breast cancer, or benign breast disease Family history of breast cancer (see Chapter 17) Diet high in fat Nulliparous or first child after age 30 yr Early menarche or late menopause
Colon-rectum	History of rectal polyps or colonic adenomatosis Family history of rectal polyps Ulcerative colitis or Crohn's disease Low fiber, high fat diet Obesity, sedentary lifestyle Increasing age
Uterus-endometrium	History of menstrual irregularity Late menopause (after age 55 yr) Nulliparity Infertility through anovulation Diabetes, high blood pressure, obesity Age 50–64 yr
Skin	Excessive exposure to sun History of severe sunburn before age 18 yr Fair complexion, burn easily Presence of congenital moles or history of dysplastic nevi or cutaneous melanoma Family history of melanoma
Oral region	Heavy smoker, tobacco chewer, drinker Poor oral hygiene Long-term exposure to sun (lip) Poorly fitting dentures
Ovary	History of ovarian cancer among close relatives History of breast cancer History of pelvic radiation Nulliparity or delayed age at first pregnancy Age 50–59 yr
Prostate	Increasing age Black adult male Occupations related to the use of cadmium
Stomach	Family history of stomach cancer Diet heavy in smoked, pickled, or salted foods

Adapted from Cohen RF, Frank-Stromborg M: Cancer risk and assessment. *In* Groenwald SL, Frogge MH, Goodman M (eds): Cancer Nursing: Principles and Practices. Boston, Jones & Bartlett, 1990.

Estimated New Cancer Cases*
10 Leading Sites by Sex, United States, 1997

Male	%	%	Female
Melanoma of Skin	3%	3%	Melanoma of Skin
Oral Cavity & Pharynx	3%	30%	Breast
Lung & Bronchus	13%	13%	Lung & Bronchus
Stomach	2%	2%	Pancreas
Colon & Rectum	8%	11%	Colon & Rectum
Kidney & Renal Pelvis	2%	4%	Ovary
Prostate	43%	2%	Cervix Uteri
Urinary Bladder	5%	6%	Corpus & Uterus, NOS
Leukemia	2%	3%	Urinary Bladder
Non-Hodgkin's Lymphoma	4%	4%	Non-Hodgkin's Lymphoma
All Other Sites	16%	21%	All Other Sites

*Excludes basal and squamous cell skin cancer and carcinoma in situ except bladder.

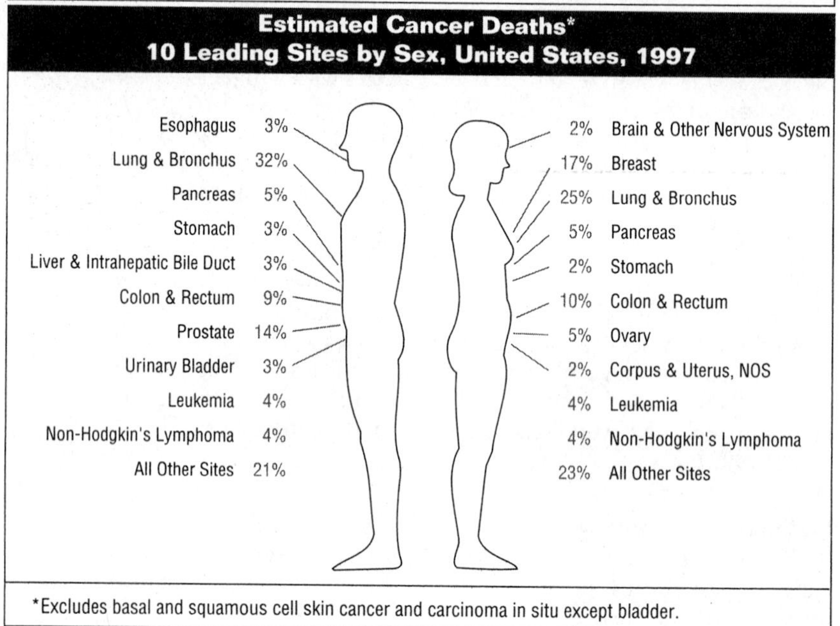

Figure **7–1.** Estimated new cancer cases (*top*) and cancer deaths (*bottom*), 1997, United States (percent distribution of sites by sex). (*From Parker SL, Tong T, Bolden S, et al: Cancer Statistics, 1997. CA Cancer J Clin 47:5–27, 1997.*)

Personal Behavior

Personal behaviors such as tobacco use, diet, alcohol use, and sexual and reproductive behavior are cited as risk factors for the development of cancer. Both epidemiologic and experimental data support the conclusion that *tobacco* (including smokeless tobacco) is carcinogenic and remains the most important cause of cancer. Cigarette smoking is related to nearly 90% of all lung cancers and accumulating evidence suggests that cigarette smoking increases the incidence of cancer of the bladder, pancreas, and to a lesser extent, the kidney, larynx, oral cavity, and esophagus (Henderson et al., 1991).

Diet and its role in the causation of cancer remain unclear. The intake of cured, pickled, smoked, salted, preserved, and unrefrigerated food has been conclusively linked to stomach cancer and it is suspected that there is a correlation between the amount of fat in the diet and the incidence of breast, prostatic, ovarian, and colon cancer in this country (Carroll, 1991; Kelsey and Gammon, 1991; Weisburger and Wynder, 1991). There is a similar correlation between excessive meat consumption and colon cancer (Willet, 1989). The role of fruits and vegetables and their antioxidant qualities in reducing cancer of various sites has been proved (Block et al., 1992), but it remains unclear whether a specific nutrient or some other biologically active substance reduces the risk of cancer.

Alcohol consumption has been linked to increased incidence rates of cancer of the mouth, pharynx, larynx, esophagus, and liver in smokers (ACS, 1992). Alcohol interacts with smoke, increasing the risk of malignant tumors, possibly by acting as a solvent for the carcinogenic smoke products and increasing the absorption of carcinogens (Brennan et al., 1995). Alcohol consumption has been consistently linked to breast and colorectal cancer (Henderson et al., 1991; Kelsey and Gammon, 1991).

Sexual and *reproductive* behaviors are linked to the risk of developing various cancers. For example, the risk of developing cervical cancer is related to age of first sexual intercourse (increased incidence with earlier intercourse) and to the number of sexual partners (increased incidence with increasing number of sexual partners) (ACS, 1992). Pregnancy and childbearing seem to be protective against cancers of the endometrium, ovary, and breast. Other risk factors for breast cancer are discussed in Chapter 17.

PATHOGENESIS *(Mitelman, 1994)*

Early in the study of cancer the concept that neoplasia originates in a single cell by acquired genetic change (see earlier discussions under Etiology and Risk Factors) was proposed and remains today the view of cancer pathogenesis most supported by experimental evidence. This hypothesis, called the *somatic mutation theory*, was first substantiated when investigations of tumors confirmed that tumor cells are characterized by chromosomal abnormalities, numerical as well as structural.[2] The discovery that chromosomal aberration is one of the basic mechanisms of tumor cell proliferation laid the foundation of modern cancer cytogenetics (study of chromosomes in cancer).

At first the question arose: are acquired chromosomal abnormalities the cause of the neoplastic changes in cells or merely the result of the neoplastic state? Chromosomal banding techniques developed in the 1970s have allowed precise identification of chromosomal changes. This information, along with molecular genetic techniques developed during the 1980s, has enabled researchers to investigate this question by examining tumor cells at the level of individual genes.

From these studies two functionally different classes of cancer-relevant genes have been detected: (1) the dominant oncogenes and (2) the recessive tumor suppressor genes. Both gene classes have been detected at just those chromosomal sites that are visibly involved in cancer-associated rearrangements. To date, over 100 genes have been found to be structurally or functionally altered following neoplasia-associated chromosomal abnormalities.

Exactly how these chromosomal changes contribute to the malignant process remains unclear. Chromosomal rearrangements may lead to oncogene activation either by a regulatory change causing increased production of normal oncogene-encoded peptides or by creating a deranged oncogene template that codes for an abnormal protein product. Another proposed mechanism suggests that chromosomal changes inactivate a tumor suppressor gene through chromosomal deletion. Loss of tumor suppressor genes is suspected because chromosomal regions found to be consistently missing in tumor cells have been observed in carcinomas of the lung, breast, bladder, and kidney.

Although much remains to be learned about the cascade of genetic changes for every kind of cancer, continued increasing understanding may suggest a means for interrupting the genetic events leading to cancer and for diagnosing the early stages of tumorigenesis (Sandberg, 1994).

Current Theory of Oncogenesis *(Fearon, 1995)*

The study of viruses in tumors has led researchers to discover small segments of genetic DNA called *oncogenes*. Oncogenes, also called *proto-oncogenes*, have the ability to transform normal cells into malignant cells, independently or incorporated with a virus. Oncogenes are thought to be the abnormal counterparts of *proto-oncogenes*, which aid in regulating biologic functions, such as cell division, in normal cells. Oncogenes may be activated by carcinogens, at which point they alter the regulation of growth in the cell. Oncogenes force a cell to grow even when its surroundings contain none of the cues that normally provoke growth (Weinberg, 1994). Oncogenes are hyperactivated versions of normal cellular growth-promoting genes. By releasing strong, unrelenting growth-stimulating signals into a cell, oncogenes can drive cell growth ceaselessly.

Researchers have also discovered a group of regulatory genes, called *antioncogenes*, now called tumor suppressor genes, that have the opposite effect of oncogenes. When activated, tumor suppressor genes can regulate growth and inhibit carcinogenesis (Vincent and Mirand, 1991). Tumor suppressor genes are the "brakes" to the "stuck accelerator" of the activated oncogene. When defects in the oncogene occur simultaneously with inactivation of growth-suppressing genes, aggressive cell proliferation takes place with the creation of certain types of tumor cells.

Tumor Biochemistry and Pathogenesis *(Weinberg, 1994)*

Carcinogenesis is the process by which a normal cell undergoes malignant transformation. Usually it is a multistep process, involving progressive changes following genetic damage to or alteration of cellular DNA through the development of hyperplasia, metaplasia, dysplasia, carcinoma in situ, invasive carcinoma, and metastatic carcinoma in that order (Hinson and Perry, 1993). These discrete stages in tumor development suggest that a single altered gene only suffices to push a cell part of the way down the path to actual malignancy. The process is completed when multiple, successive changes occur in distinct cellular genes, including activation or overexpression of oncogenes and loss or mutation of tumor suppressor genes.

This requirement for multiple changes creates an important protective mechanism against cancer. If a small number of genetic changes sufficed to transform a normal cell into a malignant one, multiple tumors would develop easily. These multiple barriers, along with the normal circuitry inside cells, ensures that only the rare cell will sustain the requisite number of changes for making a cancer cell.

[2] Chromosomal changes can include addition or deletion of entire chromosomes (numerical changes) or translocations, deletions, inversions, and insertions of parts of chromosomes (structural changes). Translocations occur when two or more chromosomes exchange material and are common in leukemias and sarcomas. Deletions or losses of chromosomal material are common in epithelial adenocarcinomas of the large bowel, lung, breast, and prostate. Chromosomal deletions may lead to neoplastic development when a tumor suppressor gene is lost. Chromosomal inversions and insertions are less common but still cause abnormal juxtaposition (side-by-side placement) of genetic material (Sandberg, 1994).

Invasion and Metastases *(Liotta et al., 1993)*

Malignant tumors differ from benign tumors in their ability to *metastasize* or spread from the primary site to other locations in the body. Metastasis occurs when cells break away from the primary tumor, travel through the body via the blood or lymphatic system, and become trapped in the capillaries of organs. From there, they infiltrate the organ tissue and grow into new tumor deposits. Cancer can also spread to adjacent structures and penetrate body cavities by direct extension. For example, ovarian tumors frequently shed cells into the peritoneal cavity, where they grow to cover the surface of abdominal organs.

Patterns of metastasis differ from cancer to cancer. Although there is no clear explanation of the exact mechanism of metastasis, certain cancers tend to spread to specific organs or sites in the body in a predictable manner. The five most common sites of metastasis are the lymph nodes, liver, lung, bone, and brain.

The spread of cancer may be negatively influenced by a variety of host factors such as the aging or dysfunctional immune system, increasing age, hormonal environment, pregnancy, and stress. Factors that may slow the spread of metastasis include radiation, chemotherapy, anticoagulants, steroids, and other anti-inflammatory agents.

Incidence of Metastasis

Approximately 30% of clients with newly diagnosed cancers have clinically detectable metastases. At least 30% to 40% of the remaining clients who are clinically free of metastases harbor occult (hidden) metastases. Unfortunately, most people have multiple sites of metastatic disease, not all of which present at any one time. The formation of metastatic colonies is a continuous process, commencing early in the growth of the primary tumor and increasing with time.

Even metastases have the potential to metastasize; the presence of large, identifiable metastases in a given organ can be accompanied by a greater number of micrometastases that have been disseminated more recently from the primary tumor or the metastasis. The size variation in metastases and the dispersed anatomic location of metastases can make complete surgical removal of disease impossible, limiting the effective concentration of anticancer drugs that can only be delivered to tumor cells in metastatic colonies.

Mechanism of Metastasis

A complicated series of tumor-host interactions resulting in a metastatic colony is called the *metastatic cascade*. Once a primary tumor is initiated and starts to move by local invasion, blood vessels from surrounding tissue grow into the solid tumor, a process called tumor angiogenesis. Tumor cells invade host blood vessels and are discharged into the venous drainage (Folkman, 1993).

For rapidly growing tumors, millions of tumor cells can be shed into the circulation every day (Liotta et al., 1974, 1993). Only a very small percentage of circulating tumor cells initiate metastatic colonies because most cells released into the bloodstream are quickly eliminated. The greater the number of tumor cells released into the bloodstream, the greater the probability that some cells will survive to form metastases.

Tumors generally lack a well-formed lymphatic network, so communication of tumor cells with lymphatic channels occurs only at the tumor periphery and not within the tumor mass. Lymphatic and hematogenous dissemination occur in parallel (Liotta and Stetler-Stevenson, 1993). Where lymph nodes drain into veins (e.g., lymphatic intersection with the subclavian vein), cancer cells can enter the bloodstream (Groenwald, 1993b).

Clinical Manifestations of Metastasis (Goodman and Snyder, 1995)

Metastatic spread may occur as late as 15 to 20 years after initial diagnosis and treatment, necessitating a thorough past medical history as part of the interview. Metastases to any of four systems are most commonly observed in a therapy practice: (1) the pulmonary system; (2) the hepatic system; (3) the skeletal system; and (4) the CNS system.

Pulmonary System

Pulmonary metastases are the most common of all metastatic tumors because venous drainage of most areas of the body is through the superior and inferior venae cavae into the heart, making the lungs the first organ to filter malignant cells. Parenchymal metastases are asymptomatic until tumor cells have obstructed bronchi resulting in pulmonary symptoms or until tumor cells have expanded and reached the parietal pleura where pain fibers are stimulated.

Pleural pain and dyspnea may be the first two symptoms experienced (Belcher, 1992). Tumor cells traveling from the lung via the pulmonary veins and carotid artery can result in metastases to the CNS. Lung cancer is the most common primary tumor to metastasize to the brain. Any neurologic sign may be the presentation of a silent lung tumor (Gudas, 1987).

Hepatic System

Liver metastases are among the most ominous signs of advanced cancer. The liver filters blood coming in from the gastrointestinal tract, making it a primary metastatic site for tumors of the stomach, colorectum, and pancreas. Symptoms include abdominal pain and tenderness with general malaise and fatigue.

Skeletal System

Bone metastases represent the initial site of metastatic disease in a large proportion of cancer cases and generally indicate a poor prognosis (Belcher, 1992). The primary symptom associated with bone metastases is pain. Although lung, breast, and prostate are the three primary sites responsible for most metastatic bone disease, tumors of the thyroid and kidney, lymphoma, and melanoma can also metastasize to the skeletal system.

In any person with metastasized cancer, bone metastases may be the osteolytic type, marked by areas of decreased bone density, or osteoblastic, appearing as areas of dense scarring and increased bone density. Osteolytic metastases predominate in breast and lung cancer, whereas osteoblastic metastases occur in prostate cancer. The axial skeleton is most commonly involved with spread to the spine, pelvis, ribs, proximal femora, proximal humeri, and skull. Pain is usually deep and worsened by activity, especially weight bearing. Disabling pathologic fractures, especially of the long bones, may occur in up to half of people with osteolytic metastases (Gudas, 1987).

Metastatic involvement of the vertebrae may result in epidural spinal cord compression with resultant quadriplegia or paraplegia and possibly death. The client who presents with spinal cord symptoms caused by metastatic epidural disease and resultant compression may have only transient symptoms with proper medical treatment. Lung and breast cancer are the leading causes of epidural spinal cord compression and this complication is becoming more common as these people are surviving longer (i.e., long enough to develop epidural disease) (Gudas, 1987).

Primary bone tumors, such as osteogenic sarcoma, metastasize initially to the lungs.

Central Nervous System *(Wegman, 1993)*

Many primary tumors may lead to CNS metastases. Lung carcinomas account for approximately half of all metastatic brain lesions. Breast carcinoma, the second leading type of primary tumor involved in brain metastases, accounts for approximately 15% of metastases to the CNS. Metastatic disease in the brain is life-threatening and emotionally debilitating. Metastatic brain tumors can increase intracranial pressure, obstruct the normal flow of cerebrospinal fluid, change mentation, and reduce sensory and motor function.

Primary tumors of the CNS rarely develop metastases outside the CNS despite the highly invasive capacity of these tumors. When metastasis does take place, spread occurs via the cerebrospinal fluid or by direct extension. Spinal cord and nerve root compression cause either insidious or rapid loss of neurologic function. This compression phenomenon occurs in approximately 5% of persons with systemic cancer, most often caused by carcinoma of the lung, breast, prostate, or kidney. Lymphoma and multiple myeloma may also result in spinal cord and nerve root compression. The spinal cord is most often compressed anteriorly by direct growth of a tumor.

Diagnosis of Metastasis

Metastases usually reproduce the cellular structure of the primary growth well enough to enable a pathologist to determine the site of the primary tumor. For example, bone metastases from a carcinoma of the thyroid not only exhibit a microscopic structure similar to the original tumor but may also produce thyroid hormone (Baird, 1991).

CLINICAL MANIFESTATIONS

Local and Systemic Effects

Most cancers in their earliest, most treatable stages are asymptomatic. Later, the rapid growth of the tumor encroaches on healthy tissue, causing destruction, necrosis, ulceration, and hemorrhage and producing many local and systemic effects. Pain may or may not occur depending on how close tumor cells, swelling, or hemorrhage occurs to the nerve cells. This process also occurs locally at metastatic sites. Pain may occur as a late symptom caused by infiltration, compression, or destruction of nerves. Secondary infections frequently occur as a result of the host's decreased immunity and can lead to death.

Systemically, the host frequently presents with a gradual or rapid weight loss, muscular weakness, anorexia, anemia and coagulation disorders (granulocyte and platelet abnormalities; see discussion, Disorders of Hemostasis and Thrombocytopenia, Chapter 11). Anorexia is a common symptom in people with cancer, especially lung carcinoma, hypernephroma, and pancreatic carcinoma. This symptom has been attributed to tumor production of a protein called tumor necrosis factor (TNF), also called cachectin. Fever may be seen with cancer in the absence of infection and is produced either by white blood cells inducing a pyrogen (an agent that causes fever) or by direct tumor production of a pyrogen.

Continued spread of the cancer may lead to gastrointestinal, pulmonary, or vascular obstruction. Other vital organs may be affected such as the brain where increased intracranial pressure by tumor cells can cause partial paralysis and eventual coma. Hemorrhage caused by direct invasion or necrosis in any body part leads to further anemia or death if the necrosis is severe. In addition to the local effects of tumor growth, cancer can produce systemic signs and symptoms that are not direct effects of either the tumor or its metastases. For example, paraneoplastic syndromes are produced by hormonal mechanisms rather than by direct tumor invasion.

Cancer Pain Syndrome

One of the most common symptoms of cancer is the cancer pain syndrome, affecting between 50% and 70% of clients in its early stages and 60% to 90% of clients in its late stages (Johanson, 1991; Brescia et al., 1990). It is estimated that 1.1 million Americans experience cancer-related pain annually (Bonica, 1990). Depression and anxiety may increase the person's perception of pain and often symptoms go unreported or underreported because clients are reluctant to take the pain medication prescribed.[3]

The cause of cancer pain is multifaceted and the characteristics of the pain depend on the tissue structure as well as on the mechanisms involved (Table 7–5). Some pain is caused by pressure on nerves or by the displacement of nerves. Microscopic infiltration of nerves by tumor cells can result in continuous, sharp, stabbing pain generally following the pattern of nerve distribution. Pain may also result from interference with blood supply or from blockage within hollow organs.

A common cause of cancer pain is metastasis of cancer to bone. Lung, breast, prostate, thyroid, and the lymphatics are the primary sites responsible for most metastatic bone disease. Bone metastasis results in increased release of prostaglandins and subsequent bone destruction caused by breakdown and resorption. Bone pain may be mild to intense. Movement, weight bearing, and ambulation exacerbate painful symptoms from bone destruction. Pathologic fractures with resultant muscle spasms can develop; in the case of vertebral involvement, nerve pain may also occur.

Signs and symptoms accompanying mild to moderate superficial pain may include hypertension, tachycardia, and tachypnea (rapid, shallow breathing) as a result of a sympathetic nervous system response. In severe or visceral pain, a parasympathetic nervous system response is more characteristic, with hypotension, bradycardia, nausea, vomiting, tachypnea, weakness, or fainting (Snyder, 1986).

[3] Addiction due to treatment of cancer pain occurs in less than 1% of people who have no prior history of addiction (Cherny and Portenoy, 1994). An unfounded fear of tolerance, addiction, or adverse effects from pain medication may result in underreporting of painful symptoms with subsequent inadequate cancer pain control and unnecessary pain-induced loss of function. Likewise, physicians may hesitate to provide adequate pain medications based on this misconception of client addiction (Jaffe, 1989).

TABLE 7-5 COMMON PATTERNS OF PAIN REFERRAL

PAIN MECHANISM	SITE OF LESION	REFERRAL SITE
Visceral	Diaphragmatic irritation	Shoulder
	Urothelial tract	Inguinal region and genitalia
Somatic	C7, T1 vertebrae	Interscapular
	L1–2 vertebrae	Sacroiliac joint and hip
	Hip joint	Knee
	Pharynx	Ipsilateral ear
Neuropathic	Nerve or plexus	Anywhere in the distribution of a peripheral nerve
	Nerve root	Anywhere in the corresponding dermatome
	Central nervous system	Anywhere in the region of the body innervated by the damaged structure

Modified from Cherny NI, Portenoy RK: The management of cancer pain. CA Cancer J Clin 44:271, 1994.

Spinal cord compression from metastases may present as back pain, leg weakness, and bowel or bladder symptoms. Back pain may precede the development of neurologic signs and symptoms. The presence of jaundice in association with an atypical presentation of back pain may indicate liver metastasis. In a therapy practice, signs of nerve root compression may be the first indication of cancer, in particular of lymphoma, multiple myeloma, or cancer of the lung, breast, prostate, or kidney. Other neurologic or musculoskeletal manifestations of neoplasm are discussed under Paraneoplastic Syndromes.

Pain may also result from iatrogenic causes such as surgery, radiation therapy, or chemotherapy. Immobility and inflammation can lead to pain. Inflammation with its accompanying symptoms of redness, edema, pain, heat, and loss of function may progress to infection, necrosis, and sloughing of tissue. If the inflammatory process alone is present, the pain is characterized by tenderness. Pain may be excruciating in the presence of tissue necrosis and sloughing (Deters, 1995).

Paraneoplastic Syndromes *(Vincent and Mirand, 1991)*

Overview and Definition. In addition to the local effects of tumor growth, cancer can produce systemic signs and symptoms that are not direct effects of either the tumor or its metastases. Neurologic complications are common in cancer. The most frequent neurologic problems are caused directly by three phenomena: (1) tumor metastases to the brain; (2) endocrine, fluid, and electrolyte abnormalities; and (3) paraneoplastic syndromes. The focus in this chapter is on the neurologic manifestations of malignancy caused by paraneoplastic syndromes. See Chapter 4 for a discussion of fluid and electrolyte imbalances and Chapter 26 for a discussion of CNS neoplasms.

When tumors produce signs and symptoms at a site distant from the tumor or its metastasized sites, these "remote effects" of malignancy are collectively referred to as *paraneoplastic syndromes*.

Although malignant cells frequently lose the function, appearance, and properties associated with the normal cells of the tissue of origin, in some cases they can acquire new cellular functions uncharacteristic of the originating tissue. Many of these syndromes involve ectopic hormone production by tumor cells or the secretion of biochemically active substances that cause metabolic abnormalities. For example, tumors in nonendocrine tissues sometimes acquire the ability to produce and secrete hormones which are distributed by the circulation and act on target organs at a site other than the location of the tumor. The most common cancer associated with paraneoplastic syndromes is small cell cancer of the lung, which can produce adrenocorticotropic hormone (ACTH) in amounts sufficient to cause Cushing's syndrome.

Incidence and Etiology. Previously, these syndromes occurred in 10% to 20% of all cancer clients (Croft and Wilkinson, 1965). Paraneoplastic nervous system syndromes are now being identified with increasing frequency because of greater physician awareness and the availability of serodiagnostic tests for some syndromes (Glantz et al., 1994).

The causes of these syndromes are not well understood but four groups of mechanisms have been identified (Rugo, 1994): (1) effects initiated by a variety of vasoactive tumor products such as serotonin, histamine, catecholamines, prostaglandins, and vasoactive peptides, which usually occur in the small bowel and less commonly in the lung or stomach; (2) effects due to the destruction of normal tissues by tumor as occurs when osteolytic skeletal metastases causes hypercalcemia; (3) effects due to unknown mechanisms such as unidentified tumor products or circulating immune complexes stimulated by the tumor (e.g., osteoarthropathy due to bronchogenic carcinoma); and (4) effects caused by autoantibodies (antibodies directed against the host's tissue).

The neurologic syndromes are generally produced by cancer stimulation of antibody production (Dalmau and Posner, 1994; Odell, 1993). Cancer cells produce antibodies that impair presynaptic calcium channel activity hindering the release of the neurotransmitter acetylcholine, resulting in muscle weakness (Henson and Posner, 1993).

Clinical Manifestations. The paraneoplastic syndromes are of considerable clinical importance because they may accompany relatively limited neoplastic growth and provide an early clue to the presence of certain types of cancer. Nonspecific symptoms such as anorexia, malaise, diarrhea, weight loss, and fever may be the first clinical manifestations of a paraneoplastic syndrome. Even these types of nonspecific symptoms occur as a result of the production of specific biochemical products by the tumor itself (Rugo, 1994).

Paraneoplastic syndromes with musculoskeletal manifestations are listed in Table 7–6. Gradual, progressive muscle weakness may develop over a period of weeks to months. The proximal muscles (especially of the pelvic girdle) are most likely to be involved; the weakness does stabilize. Reflexes of the involved extremities are present but diminished.

Muscular and cutaneous disorders associated with malignancy are presented in Table 7–7. Myositis may precede, follow, or arise concurrently with the malignancy and tends to occur most often in older people. Cutaneous paraneoplastic syndromes are a large group of dermatoses that may be associated with an internal malignancy (Cohen, 1994).

TABLE 7-6 PARANEOPLASTIC SYNDROMES: RHEUMATOLOGIC ASSOCIATIONS AND CLINICAL FEATURES

MALIGNANCY	RHEUMATOLOGIC ASSOCIATIONS	CLINICAL FEATURES
Lymphoproliferative disease (leukemia)	Vasculitis	Necrotizing vasculitis
Plasma cell dyscrasia	Cryoglobulinemia	Vasculitis, Raynaud's disease, arthralgia, neurologic symptoms
Hodgkin's disease	Immune complex disease	Nephrotic syndrome
Ovarian cancer	Reflex sympathetic dystrophy	Palmar fasciitis and polyarthritis
Carcinoid syndrome	Scleroderma	Scleroderma-like changes: anterior tibia
Colon cancer	Pyogenic arthritis	Enteric bacteria cultured from joint
Mesenchymal tumors	Osteogenic osteomalacia	Bone pain, stress fractures
Renal cell cancer (and other tumors)	Severe Raynaud's phenomenon	Digital necrosis
Pancreatic cancer	Panniculitis	Subcutaneous nodules, especially males

Adapted from Gilkeson GS, Caldwell DS: Rheumatologic associations with malignancy. J Musculoskel Med 7(1):72, 1990.

There may be rheumatologic symptoms referred to as *carcinoma polyarthritis*. This condition can be differentiated from rheumatoid arthritis by the presence of asymmetrical joint involvement, involvement of primarily the lower extremity, explosive onset, late age of onset, and the presence of malignancy and arthritis together (Gilkeson and Caldwell, 1990).

Neurologic paraneoplastic syndromes are of unknown cause and include subacute cerebellar degeneration, amyotrophic lateral sclerosis, sensory or sensorimotor peripheral neuropathy, Guillain-Barré syndrome, dermatomyositis, polymyositis, myasthenia gravis, and the Lambert-Eaton myasthenic syndrome (LEMS) (Berkow and Fletcher, 1992).

Medical Management

Diagnosis, Treatment, and Prognosis. Serodiagnostic tests are available for some syndromes and characteristic abnormalities in magnetic resonance imaging (MRI) have been identified in association with neurologic paraneoplastic syndromes (Glantz et al., 1994). Biochemical markers in urine provide specific monitoring of the response of bone metastases to treatment. This early diagnosis of paraneoplastic syndromes provides for prevention of tumor progression and subsequent problems such as bone pain, fracture, and hypercalcemia (Walls et al., 1995).

The clinical course of the paraneoplastic syndromes usually parallels the course of the tumor. Therefore, effective medical treatment (rather than rehabilitative therapy) should result in resolution of the presenting neuromuscular symptoms. Some of the cutaneous paraneoplastic syndromes will respond to specific measures, such as systemic corticosteroid therapy, but for the most part, successful resolution requires eradication of the underlying malignancy (Kurzrock and Cohen, 1995).

Likewise, recurrence of the cancer may be first recognized by the return of systemic symptoms associated with the paraneoplastic phenomena. The metabolic or toxic effects of the syndrome (e.g., hypercalcemia, hyponatremia) may constitute a more urgent hazard to life than the underlying cancer.

TABLE 7-7 MUSCULAR AND CUTANEOUS DISORDERS ASSOCIATED WITH MALIGNANCY

MUSCULAR	CUTANEOUS
Amyloidosis	Acanthosis (diffuse thickening)
Amyotrophic lateral sclerosis	Dermatomyositis
Polymyositis	Extramammary Paget's disease
Lambert-Eaton myasthenic syndrome (LEMS)	Nigricans (blackish discoloration; changes in skin pigmentation)
Myasthenia gravis	Pemphigus vulgaris (water blisters)
Metabolic myopathies	Pruritus (itching)
Primary neuropathic diseases	Pyoderma gangrenosum (eruption of skin ulcers)
Type II muscle atrophy	Reactive erythemas (skin redness)

Data from Gilkeson GS, Caldwell DS: Rheumatologic associations with malignancy. J Musculoskel Med 7(1): 70, 1990; and Cohen PR: Cutaneous paraneoplastic syndromes. Am Fam Physician 50:1273–1282, 1994.

Medical Management *(Norris, 1995)*

Diagnosis. Medical history and physical examination are usually followed by more specific diagnostic procedures. Useful tests for the early detection and staging of tumors include radiograph, endoscopy, isotope scan, computed tomography (CT) scan, mammography, MRI, and biopsy. Biopsy of tissue samples is the single most important diagnostic method for the study of tumor. Tissue for biopsy may be taken by curettage (Papanicolaou, or Pap, smear), fluid aspiration (pleural effusion, lumbar puncture or spinal tap), needle aspiration (breast, thyroid), dermal punch (skin or mouth), endoscopy (rectal polyps) or surgical excision (visceral tumors and nodes).

Tumor markers, substances produced and secreted by tumor cells, may be found in the blood serum. The level of tumor marker seems to correlate with the extent of disease. A tumor marker is not diagnostic itself but can signal malignancies. Carcinoembryonic antigen (CEA) is one tumor marker that may indicate malignancy of the large bowel, stomach, pancreas, lungs, breasts, and sometimes sarcomas, leukemias, and lymphomas. CEA blood titers provide a valuable baseline during chemotherapy to evaluate the extent of the tumor spread, regulate drug dosage, determine prognosis after surgery or radiation, and detect tumor recurrence.

Other tumor markers found in the blood (no more specific than CEA) include alphafetoprotein (AFP), a fetal antigen uncommon in adults and suggestive of testicular, ovarian, gastric, pancreatic, liver, or primary lung tumors. Human chorionic gonadotropin (β subunit) may indicate testicular cancer or choriocarcinoma. Prostate-specific antigen (PSA) helps evaluate prostatic cancer.

Treatment *(Norris, 1995)*. Prevention is the first key to the treatment of cancer. Primary prevention may include identification of high-risk individuals and subsequent reduction or elimination of modifiable risk factors (e.g., tobacco use, diet high in unsaturated fats and low in fiber). Screening of the high-risk population is another aspect of primary prevention. Secondary prevention aimed at preventing morbidity and mortality utilizes early detection and prompt treatment. Tertiary prevention focuses on managing symptoms, limiting complications, and preventing disability associated with cancer or its treatment.

Currently, no known specific immunization prevents cancer but research focusing on a cancer vaccine to stimulate an immune response against cancer cells is being investigated in clinical studies. The vaccine specifically evokes the activity of killer T cells to directly target and destroy tumors in all vaccine recipients. A vaccine given on an outpatient basis, would be less dangerous than surgery and less toxic than other cancer treatments, such as chemotherapy and radiation therapy.

Curative vs. Palliative Therapy. Five major therapies are the focus of curative cancer treatment (i.e., with the intent to cure) at this time, including surgery, radiation, chemotherapy, biotherapy (also called immunotherapy), and hormonal therapy.

Palliative (i.e., provides symptomatic relief but does not cure) treatment may include radiation, chemotherapy, physical therapy (e.g., physical agents, exercise, positioning, relaxation techniques, biofeedback, manual therapy), medications, acupuncture, chiropractic care, alternative medicine (e.g., homeopathic and naturopathic treatment), and hospice care. Hospice care attempts to help the person achieve as full a life as possible, with minimal pain, discomfort, and restriction. Many medications, especially morphine, are used for pain control. Emphasis of hospice care is toward emotional and psychological support for the client and the family focusing on death as a natural end to life.

Five Major Treatment Modalities. Each of the five curative therapies mentioned earlier may be used alone or in combination, depending on the type, stage, localization, and responsiveness of the tumor and on limitations imposed by the person's clinical status. *Surgery*, once a mainstay of cancer treatment, is now used most often in combination with other therapies. Surgery may be used curatively, for tumor biopsy and tumor removal, or palliatively to relieve pain, correct obstruction, or alleviate pressure. Surgery can be curative in persons with localized cancer, but 70% of clients have evidence of micrometastases at the time of diagnosis, requiring surgery in combination with other treatment modalities to achieve better response rates (Dietrick-Gallagher and Brasher, 1991). Adjuvant therapy used following surgery may discourage proliferation of any residual cells.

Radiation therapy is used to destroy the dividing cancer cells, while damaging resting normal cells as little as possible. Radiation consists of two types: ionizing radiation and particle radiation. Both types have the cellular DNA as their target; however, particle radiation produces less skin damage. Radiation treatment approaches include external beam radiation and intracavitary and interstitial implants. Radiation may be used preoperatively to shrink a tumor, making it operable, while preventing further spread of the disease during surgery. After the surgical wound heals, postoperative doses prevent residual cancer cells from multiplying or metastasizing.

Normal and malignant cells respond to radiation differently, depending on blood supply, oxygen saturation, previous irradiation, and immune status. Generally, normal cells recover from radiation faster than malignant cells. The success of the treatment and damage to normal tissue also vary with the intensity of the radiation. Although a large single dose of radiation has greater cellular effects than fractions of the same amount delivered sequentially, a protracted schedule allows time for normal tissue to recover in the intervals between individual sublethal doses.

Chemotherapy includes a wide array of chemical agents to destroy cancer cells. It is particularly useful in the treatment of widespread or metastatic disease, whereas radiation is more useful for treatment of localized lesions. Chemotherapy is used in controlling residual disease as well as inducing long remissions and sometimes cures, especially in children with childhood leukemia and adults with Hodgkin's disease or testicular cancer. Several major chemotherapeutic agents are listed in Table 7–8.

Chemotherapeutic drugs can be given orally, subcutaneously, intramuscularly (IM), intravenously (IV), intracavitarily (into a body cavity such as the thoracic, abdominal, or pelvic cavity), intrathecally (through the sheath of a structure such as through the sheath of the spinal cord into the subarachnoid space), and by arterial infusion, depending on the drug and its pharmacologic action and on tumor location. Administration in any form is usually intermittent to allow for bone marrow recovery between doses.

Biotherapy, formerly called immunotherapy, relies on biologic response modifiers (BRMs) to change or modify the

TABLE 7-8 MAJOR CHEMOTHERAPEUTIC AGENTS

AGENT	ACTION
Alkylating agents	Inhibit cell growth and division by reacting with DNA
Nitrosourea	Inhibits cell growth and division by reacting with DNA
Antimetabolites	Prevent cell growth by competing with metabolites in production of nucleic acid
Antitumor antibiotics	Block cell growth by binding with DNA and interfering with DNA-dependent RNA synthesis
Plant alkaloids	Prevent cellular reproduction by disrupting cell mitosis
Steroid hormones	Inhibit the growth of hormone-susceptible tumors by changing their chemical environment

From Norris J (ed): Professional Guide to Diseases, ed 5. Springhouse, Pa, Springhouse, 1995.

TABLE 7–9 Side Effects of Cancer Treatment

Surgery	Radiation	Chemotherapy	Biotherapy	Hormonal Therapy
Disfigurement	Radiation sickness	Gastrointestinal effects	Fever	Nausea
Loss of function	Immunosuppression	Anorexia	Chills	Vomiting
Infection	Decreased platelets	Nausea	Nausea	Hypertension
Increased pain	Decreased white blood cells	Vomiting	Vomiting	Steroid-induced diabetes
Deformity	Infection	Diarrhea	Anorexia	Myopathy (steroid-induced)
	Fatigue	Ulcers	Fatigue	Weight gain
	Fibrosis	Hemorrhage	Fluid retention	Altered mental status
	Burns	Bone marrow suppression	CNS effects	Hot flashes
	Mucositis	Anemia		Sweating
	Diarrhea	Leukopenia		Impotence
	Edema	Thrombocytopenia		Decreased libido
	Hair loss	Skin rashes		
	Delayed wound healing	Neuropathies		
	CNS effects	Hair loss		
	Malignancy	Sterilization		
		Phlebitis		

relationship between the tumor and host by strengthening the host's biologic response to tumor cells. Much of the work related to BRMs is still experimental so the availability of this type of treatment is variable regionally within the United States. The most widely used agents include interferons, which have a direct antitumor effect, and interleukin-2, one type of cytokine, a protein released by macrophages to trigger the immune response (see Chapter 5)(Rosenberg et al., 1994).

Other forms of biotherapy include bone marrow (stem cell) transplantation, monoclonal antibodies, colony-stimulating factors, and hormonal therapy. Bone marrow transplantation (BMT) is used for cancers that are responsive to high doses of chemotherapy or radiation. These high doses kill cancer cells but are also toxic to bone marrow; BMT provides a method for "rescuing" people from bone marrow destruction while allowing higher doses of chemotherapy for a better antitumor result (see Bone Marrow Transplantation, Chapter 11).

Monoclonal antibodies are proteins produced from a single clone of B lymphocytes that can be used alone to produce a massive amount of one specific antibody or bound with radioisotopes and injected into the body to detect cancer by attaching to tumor cells. Research is underway to find a way to use these antibodies as a means of destroying specific cancer cells without disturbing healthy cells (Goldenberg, 1994).

Colony-stimulating factors (CSFs) may be used to support the person with low blood counts related to chemotherapy. CSFs function primarily as hematopoietic growth factors, guiding the division and differentiation of bone marrow stem cells. They also influence the functioning of mature lymphocytes, monocytes, macrophages, and neutrophils.

Hormonal therapy is used for certain types of cancer that have been shown to be affected by specific hormones. For example, the luteinizing-releasing hormone leuprolide is now used to treat prostate cancer. With long-term use, this hormone inhibits testosterone release and tumor growth. Tamoxifen, an antiestrogen hormonal agent, is used in breast cancer to block estrogen receptors in breast tumor cells that require estrogen to thrive.

Local and Systemic Effects of Cancer Treatment. Table 7–9 presents a comparison of the potential side effects associated with the five treatment modalities discussed in this section. See Chapter 4 for discussion of the effects of chemotherapy agents, radiation sickness, CNS effects of immunosuppression, and steroid-induced myopathy.

Pain Control. Pain management and control may depend on the cause of the pain syndrome (see Cancer Pain Syndrome). Treatment approaches may include narcotic[4] and non-narcotic analgesics; chemotherapy or radiation therapy, or both; surgery; nerve blocks; or other more invasive pain control measures such as intraspinal opioids, rhizotomy, or cordotomy.

In 1994 the US Department of Health and Human Services released a clinical practice guideline for clinicians advising medical professionals on the treatment of cancer pain (AHCPR, 1994). Whereas severe cancer pain is treated pharmaceutically, mild to moderate joint and muscle pain can be addressed by the rehabilitation professional. Pain elimination through the use of medication may not be possible without accompanying severe loss of function, an undesirable outcome. Noninvasive physical agents such as cryotherapy, thermotherapy, electrical stimulation, immobilization, exercise, massage, biofeedback, and relaxation techniques may be effective in pain management.

Prognosis. Prognosis is influenced by the type of cancer, the stage and grade of disease at diagnosis, the availability of effective treatment, and the response to treatment. Cancer cells that develop resistance to anticancer drugs can regrow with fatal consequences. Researchers are close to understanding the mechanisms underlying chemotherapeutic failure and

[4] A new method of pain relief called patient-controlled analgesia (PCA) is now being used in many cancer care centers. This system permits the person to self-administer a premeasured dose of analgesic by pressing a button that activates a pump syringe containing the analgesic. Small intermittent doses of the analgesic administered IV maintain blood levels that ensure comfort and minimize the risk of oversedation. Clinical studies report that persons using PCA effectively maintain comfort without oversedation and use less drug than the amount normally given by IM injection (Nolan and Wilson, 1995).

TABLE 7-10 Some Physiologic Effects and Uses of Physical Agents in People with Cancer

	Potential Benefits	General Contraindications and Precautions	Effectiveness
Thermal Agents			
Superficial heating agents such as hot packs, paraffin baths, fluidotherapy, infrared lamps	Increase blood flow to affected area Decrease pain and muscle spasm Increase range of motion Provide mild heat (≤40° C) to trunk and girdle Provide vigorous heat (>40°–45° C) to extremities Increase metabolism Decrease chronic inflammation	Do not use: Over dysvascular tissue (i.e., tissue that has been exposed to radiation therapy) (fibrotic circulatory impairment) With persons who have decreased sensitivity to temperature or pain in affected area In areas of increased bleeding or hemorrhage (e.g., if there has been long-term corticosteroid therapy) Directly over tumor If there is acute injury or inflammation In open wounds (applies especially to paraffin baths and fluidotherapy)	Some studies with animals have been published. Heat and stretch may decrease pain and muscle spasm in abnormal tissue; not proved effective in decreasing deep cancer pain or bone pain.
Deep heat agents such as ultrasound, diathermy, and hydrotherapy	Increase blood flow to affected area Decrease pain and muscle spasm Increase range of motion Provide mild heat (≤40° C) to trunk and girdle Provide vigorous heat (>40°–45° C) to extremities Increase metabolism Decrease chronic inflammation Increase (collagen) tissue extensibility and decrease stiffness Decrease viscosity	Do not use: Over dysvascular tissue (i.e., tissue that has been exposed to radiation therapy) (fibrotic circulatory impairment) With persons who have decreased sensitivity to temperature or pain in affected area In areas of increased bleeding or hemorrhage (e.g., if there has been long-term corticosteroid therapy) Directly over tumor If there is acute injury or inflammation In open wounds When elevation in core body temperature is possible do not use with clients who have cardiopulmonary insufficiency (i.e., clients with acute myocardial infarction, congestive heart failure, hypertension, or severe chronic pulmonary obstructive disease [applies especially to hydrotherapy]) Do not use diathermy with metal implants or pacemakers	Some pretreatment and post-treatment studies with humans and several studies with animals.
Cryotherapy such as cold packs, ice massage, ice towels, cold baths (hydrotherapy), vapocoolant sprays, cold and compression	In acute musculoskeletal trauma: Decrease acute inflammation, edema, pain, bleeding, muscle spasms, muscle spasticity Treat trigger points (myofascial pain) Decrease stiffness Increase relaxation Decrease metabolism Increase viscosity	Do not use: With clients who have sensitivity to or intolerance of cold or who have Raynaud's disease or peripheral vascular disease Over dysvascular tissue (i.e., tissue that has been exposed to radiation therapy) (fibrotic circulatory impairment) If there is transient increase in blood pressure (in hypertension, monitor blood pressure through treatment and discontinue if blood pressure increases) If wound healing is delayed or if nerve is injured (applies especially to irradiation- or chemotherapy-induced nerve injury) May not want to use if client has a psychological aversion to cold	Several studies with humans indicate that vapocoolant spray and stretch combined are effective and that cold and compression combined are effective.

Contrast baths	Decrease pain and stimulate local circulation	See also Hydrotherapy with agitation Do not use: With clients who have peripheral vascular disease, especially small-vessel disease Over dysvascular tissue (i.e., tissue that has been exposed to radiation therapy) (fibrotic circulatory impairment) With persons who have decreased sensitivity to temperature or pain in affected area In areas of increased bleeding or hemorrhage (e.g., if there has been long-term corticosteroid therapy) Directly over tumor If there is acute injury or inflammation When treating a large body surface area, and when elevation or reduction in core body temperature is possible, do not use with clients who have cardiopulmonary insufficiency (i.e., acute myocardial infarction, congestive heart failure, hypertension, severe chronic pulmonary obstructive disease [applies especially to hydrotherapy])	Studies with humans are needed.
Mechanical Agents			
Hydrotherapy with agitation	Stimulates circulation for wound healing Promotes muscle relaxation and pain relief Removes exudates and necrotic tissue Facilitates exercise	Do not use: Over dysvascular tissue (i.e., tissue that has been exposed to radiation therapy) (fibrotic circulatory impairment) With persons who have decreased sensitivity to temperature or pain in affected area In areas of increased bleeding or hemorrhage (e.g., if there has been long-term corticosteroid therapy) Directly over tumor If there is acute injury or inflammation In open wounds If elevation in core body temperature is possible do not use with clients who have cardiopulmonary insufficiency (i.e., acute myocardial infarction, congestive heart failure, hypertension, severe chronic pulmonary obstructive disease [applies especially to hydrotherapy]) Dependent on water temperature: With painful, open lesions, severely traumatized tissue, or recent skin grafts, agitation should be minimized The risk of cross-infection must be controlled (especially in clients with cancer who are immunosuppressed)	Some studies have shown decrease in edema; controversy exists.
Mechanical/external compression (includes use of compression pumps)	Decreases edema (and pain related to edema) Decreases acute inflammation Increases range-of-motion for problems related to edema	Do not use: If client has difficulty tolerating therapy (applies especially to clients with impaired circulation; these individuals must be closely monitored) If client has phlebitis or deep venous thrombosis in area to be compressed The compression pressure setting should never exceed the client's diastolic blood pressure (10 mm Hg $\leq$ the person's normal diastolic blood pressure) Diastolic blood pressure should be measured while the client is in the position of treatment	Several studies with humans have demonstrated efficacy in decreasing edema with cold and compression combined.

Table continued on following page

TABLE 7-10 Some Physiologic Effects and Uses of Physical Agents in People with Cancer *(Continued)*

	Potential Benefits	General Contraindications and Precautions	Effectiveness
Mechanical Agents			
Traction (spinal and peripheral)	Increases motion and mobility in persons who have herniated disks, degenerative joint disease, joint hypomobility, or stiffness	Do not use with clients who have structural disease such as tumor or infection and impaired circulation (i.e., peripheral vascular disease) or when motion and mobility is contraindicated, as with acute sprains, strains, or inflammation, a positive vertebral artery test, or a positive alar ligament test	Although no double-blind studies have been done, a meta-analysis of the literature has indicated effectiveness.
Ultrasound	Softens scar tissue (collagen) Increases extensibility of tissue (tendons) Decreases pain through decreasing muscle spasms and therapy of nerve roots	Do not use: Over growing epiphyses, metal implants, bony prominences, areas of acute hemorrhage, or areas of decreased sensation Over uterus if client could be pregnant With breast implants High frequency affects older pacemakers Cavitation effects may occur on molecular structure with a high dose of radiation	Research on safety of treatment with humans is needed. (If breast implant is inserted beneath pectoralis muscle, e.g., care should be taken in depth of penetration and heating effects of ultrasound.)
Electrical Agents			
Diathermy (see Deep heat agents)		*Do not use with metal implants or pacemakers*	
Neuromuscular electrical stimulation	Decreases muscle spasm Increases relaxation To increase exercise to reduce disuse atrophy, weakness, and pain and to increase blood flow and metabolism Adjunct to healing and therapy for chronic inflammation	Do not use: Over open wound if there has been hemorrhaging If client has spontaneous or pathologic fracture sites With clients who have cardiopulmonary insufficiency in whom increased exercise and metabolism are contraindicated If client has peripheral vascular disease or phlebitis High frequency may affect older pacemakers	Studies with humans and animals have been published that demonstrate effectiveness.
Transcutaneous electrical nerve stimulation (TENS)	Decreases acute pain (i.e., postoperative) and chronic pain	Do not place electrode over open wound High frequency may affect older pacemakers	Studies have shown that TENS may not be effective in controlling deep cancer or bone pain but that it may be helpful in reducing postoperative pain (e.g., post-tumor resection surgery).

Modified from Pfalzer L: Physical agents and the patient with cancer. Clin Manage 12:84–86, 1992.

developing new strategies to circumvent drug resistance (Fisher and Sikic, 1995; Ford, 1995). Generally, the earlier cancers are found, the simpler treatment may be and the greater likelihood of a "cure."

Cancer survival statistics are usually reported as 5-year survival rates. This means that the person who is alive and without evidence of disease for at least 5 years after diagnosis is considered "cured."[5] Although the 5-year determination is arbitrary, in many cancers, this waiting period decreases the probability that the condition will recur or spread. Even without complete remission, cancer can be controlled to provide longer survival time and improved quality of life, but these factors are not reflected in survival rates. Cancer statistics reported usually include a lag time so that rates may not reflect the most recent treatment advances (Wingo et al., 1995).

Survival rates for many cancers have increased from 1960 to the present but not all cancers have been characterized by this increase. For example, while survival rates for Hodgkin's disease, and prostate, testicular, and bladder cancers have increased by at least 25%, the survival rates for cancers of the oral cavity and pharynx, liver, pancreas, esophagus, and colon have decreased or increased less than 5% during the same time period.

A significantly lower survival rate in black Americans for most cancer classifications has been noted (Greenwald and Sandik, 1986). This difference may be due to a variety of factors, including limited access to health care, little or no insurance, lack of a primary health care provider, limited knowledge of the benefits of early diagnosis and treatment, and greater exposure to carcinogens (Matassarin-Jacobs and Petardi, 1993).

Special Implications for the Therapist 7-1
ONCOLOGY/CANCER

Side Effects of Cancer Treatment

The risk of falling is one of the more serious sequelae both of the local effects of cancer and the systemic consequences of cancer treatment. See Adverse Drug Reactions: Radiation Injuries and Chemotherapy, Chapter 4. Weakness, pain, fatigue, orthostatic hypotension, peripheral neuropathy, and diminished flexibility, in various combinations, may result in falls. Anyone with metastasized cancer to the spine or long bones may fracture these bones in a fall (or fall because of pathologic fractures), resulting in serious, long-term disability.

Fall prevention and education are important aspects of the rehabilitation or exercise program. Additionally, the therapist must evaluate each client individually, possibly selecting an assistive device in appropriate cases. A walker with auto-stop wheels in the front may be a safer choice for some people than a standard walker that must be repeatedly lifted during ambulation. A wheelchair may be necessary for someone who experiences dizziness, weakness, fatigue, or signs of disorientation (Hamburgh, 1992).

Physical Agents

The use of physical agents in people who have cancer is summarized in Table 7–10. The reader is encouraged to consult Pfalzer (1992) for references and more specific information about the use of thermal and mechanical agents with this population. Heat modalities should not be used in people undergoing radiation as the thermal effect may enhance the effect of the radiation.

The application of therapeutic ultrasound over tumors is contraindicated, presumably because it is believed that there is an increased risk of metastasis (ter Haar et al., 1988). Studies conducted on mice have shown that a tumor given large doses of ultrasound will spread because of increasing blood supply to the area (Hogan et al., 1982; Lejbkowicz et al., 1993). The concern that electrical and thermal modalities increase blood flow and possibly increase micrometastases in humans has not yet been proved in clinical studies.*

The clinical behavior of the majority of musculoskeletal tumors is such that the symptoms are shared with a wide range of nontumorous orthopedic disorders. Pain, swelling, and local heat accompanying musculoskeletal tumors are also common to inflammatory conditions. In addition, the most likely sites of musculoskeletal tumors are regions frequently involved in sports injuries (Lewis and Reilly, 1987). Occasionally the client does recall some sort of injury at the site of a previously unsuspected tumor and this information further confuses the relationship between trauma and malignancy (Maxwell, 1995).

As a general guideline, some therapists caution that people with cancer should not be treated with electrical or deep-heating thermal physical agents (ultrasound in particular), even at a site distant from the neoplasm, because the effect of ultrasound on micrometastases is not known. Despite this general precaution there are times when tumors are unknowingly sonicated by a therapist, as when tumors of the musculoskeletal system are misdiagnosed (Maxwell, 1995).

Radiation Hazard for the Health Care Worker

Implant radiation therapy requires personal radiation protection for all staff members who come in contact with the client (see Radiation Hazard for Health Care Professionals, Chapter 4).

* For a detailed explanation of the possible physiologic effects of therapeutic ultrasound on tumor angiogenesis, see Maxwell (1995).

CHILDHOOD CANCER *(Ely et al., 1991)*

Incidence and Overview

Each year nearly 10,000 children in the United States are diagnosed with cancer. With recent advances in treatment, 65% of these children will survive 5 years or more, an increase of almost 40% since the early 1960s. Treatment-related deaths have declined as a result of advances in clinical supportive

[5] The terms *survival* and *cure* do not always portray the functional status of a cancer survivor. Many people considered cured are left with physical limitations and movement dysfunctions that interfere with their daily lives.

care (e.g. antibiotic therapy, indwelling venous access lines, blood products, and enteral and parenteral nutrition) that maximize the benefits and minimize the side effects of cancer therapy.

The types of cancers that occur in children vary greatly from those seen in adults. Leukemias and lymphomas (almost half of all childhood cancers involve the blood or blood-forming organs), brain tumors, embryonal tumors, and sarcomas are the most common pediatric malignancies, whereas adenocarcinomas (e.g., lung, breast, colorectal) are more common in adults.

Other differences which must be taken into account when treating the child with cancer include the stage of growth and development, stage of psychosocial and cognitive development, and emotional response to the illness and its treatment. The immaturity of the child's organ systems often has important treatment implications.

Types of Childhood Cancers

Acute lymphoblastic leukemia (ALL), the most common childhood malignancy, accounts for almost one third of all pediatric cancers. White males are affected most often and although the exact cause is unknown, radiation, chromosomal abnormalities, viruses, and congenital immunodeficiencies have all been associated with an increased incidence of leukemia. See also The Leukemias, Chapter 11.

Wilms' tumor, a malignancy that may affect one or both kidneys, occurs in children under the age of 14 years and is slightly more prevalent in females than males. Epidemiologic research suggests an increased incidence in children of men exposed to lead or hydrocarbons. Recently, an association between Wilms' tumor and chromosomal abnormalities has been established, specifically deletion of a suppressor gene located on the short arm of chromosome 11. This chromosomal anomaly is an autosomal dominant trait requiring evaluation of other family members.

Neuroblastoma is the most common extracranial solid tumor in children and the most commonly diagnosed neoplasm during the first year of life. Approximately 500 new cases are diagnosed annually in the United States and the incidence is higher among whites than nonwhites. Neuroblastoma can originate anywhere along the sympathetic nervous system, but more than half the tumors occur in the retroperitoneal area and present as an abdominal mass. Other common sites include the posterior mediastinum, pelvis, and neck. If the bone marrow is involved, bone pain may occur. See discussion of Neuroblastoma in Chapter 26.

Rhabdomyosarcoma is the most common soft tissue sarcoma and the seventh leading cause of cancer in children. This tumor, which is more prevalent in males than females, originates from the same embryonic cells that give rise to striated muscle. The peak incidence is between the age of 2 and 5 years with a second peak occurring between age 15 and 19. The most common tumor sites include the head and neck, genitourinary tract, and extremities. Head and neck tumors can lead to CNS involvement including cranial nerve palsies, meningeal symptoms, and respiratory paralysis. Ninety percent of children with lesions extending into the CNS die.

Other common cancers seen in children are bone cancers, both osteogenic and Ewing's sarcomas (see discussion, Chapter 22), and brain tumors (see Chapter 26).

Late Effects and Prognosis

Survival of children with cancer continues to improve. It is estimated that by the year 2000, 1 in 1000 people between the ages of 20 and 29 will be survivors of childhood cancer. With increasing survival rates, there is a growing concern about the late effects of disease and treatment.

The term *late effects* refers to the damaging effects of surgery, radiation, and chemotherapy on nonmalignant tissues, as well as to the social, emotional, and economic consequences of survival. These effects can appear months to years after treatment and can range in severity from subclinical, to clinical, to life-threatening. Fortunately, not all children experience such effects but those that do often end up in the rehabilitation setting.

Late effects have been identified in almost every organ system. Treatments involving the CNS can cause deficits in intelligence, hearing, and vision. Treatment involving the CNS, head and neck, or gonads can cause endocrine abnormalities such as short stature, hypothyroidism, or delayed secondary sexual development. Surgery and radiation involving the musculoskeletal system have been associated with defects such as kyphosis, scoliosis, and spinal shortening. Finally, the child who has received radiation or chemotherapy has a tenfold greater chance of developing a second malignancy than a child who has never had cancer.

References

ACS (American Cancer Society): Cancer Facts and Figures 1992. New York, American Cancer Society, 1992.

ACS (American Cancer Society): Cancer statistics, 1989. CA Cancer J Clin 30:3–20, 1989.

ACSM (American College of Sports Medicine): Preventive and Rehabilitative Exercise Committee. Guidelines For Exercise Testing and Prescription, ed 4. Philadelphia, Lea & Febiger, 1991.

AHCPR (Agency for Health Care Policy and Research): Management of cancer pain for Adults/Management of cancer pain for children and adolescents. Guideline No. 9, 1994. Available by calling the National Cancer Institute (800) 4-CANCER; or write Cancer Pain Guideline, AHCPR Publications Clearinghouse, P.O. Box 8547, Silver Spring, MD 20907.

Arnheim N, Cortopassi G: Deleterious mitochondrial DNA mutations accumulate in aging human tissues. Mutat Res 275:157–167, 1992.

Baird SB (ed): A Cancer Source Book For Nurses ed 6. Atlanta, American Cancer Society, 1991.

Beahrs OH, Henson DE, Hutter RVP, Kennedy BJ (eds): American Joint Committee on Cancer: Manual For Staging of Cancer ed 4. Philadelphia, JB Lippincott, 1992.

Belcher A: Cancer Nursing. Mosby's Clinical Nursing Series. St Louis, Mosby–Year Book, 1992.

Berkow R, Fletcher AJ (eds): The Merck Manual of Diagnosis and Therapy, ed 16. Rahway, NJ, Merck, 1992.

Block G, Patterson B, Suba, A: Fruit, vegetables, and cancer prevention: A review of the epidemiological evidence. Nutr Cancer 18:1–29, 1992.

Bonica JJ: Cancer pain. *In* Bonica JJ (ed): The Management of Pain ed 2. Philadelphia, Lea & Febiger, 1990, pp 400–460.

Brennan JA, Boyle JO, Koch WM, et al: Association between cigarette smoking and mutation of the p53 gene in squamous-cell carcinoma of the head and neck. N Engl J Med 332:712–717, 1995.

Brescia FJ, Adler D, Gray G, et al: Hospitalized advanced cancer patients: A profile. Pain Symptom Manage 5:221–227, 1990.

Brody JA, Persky VW: Epidemiology and demographics. *In* Abrams WB, Berkow R (eds): The Merck Manual of Geriatrics. Rahway, NJ, Merck, 1990, pp 1115–1127.

Carroll KK: Dietary fats and cancer. Am J Clin Nutr 53:10654–10675, 1991.

Cherny NI, Portenoy RK: The management of cancer pain. CA Cancer J Clin 44(5):262–303, 1994.

Cohen PR: Cutaneous paraneoplastic syndromes. Am Fam Physician 50:1273–1282, 1994.

Croft PB, Wilkinson MW: The incidence of carcinomatous neuropathy in patients with various types of carcinoma. Brain 88:427, 1965.

Dalmau J, Posner JB: Neurologic paraneoplastic antibodies (anti-Yo; anti-Hu; anti-Ri): The case for nomenclature based on antibody and antigen specificity. Neurology 44:2241–2246, 1994.

Deters GE: Cancer. *In* Phipps W, Cassmeyer VL, Sands JK, Lehman MK (eds): Medical-Surgical Nursing: Concepts and Clinical Practice ed 5. St Louis, Mosby–Year Book, 1995, pp 362–442.

Dietrick-Gallagher M, Brasher E: Surgical oncology. *In* Baird SB (ed): A Cancer Source Book for Nurses, ed 6. Atlanta, American Cancer Society, 1991, pp 56–62.

Dorgan JF, Brown C, Barrett M, et al: Physical activity and risk of breast cancer in Framingham Heart Study. Am J Epidemiol 139:662–669, 1994.

Ely T, Giesler D, Moore K: Childhood cancer. *In* Baird SB (ed): A Cancer Source Book for Nurses, ed 6. Atlanta, American Cancer Society, 1991, pp 296–308.

Fearon ER: Oncogenes and tumor suppressor genes. *In* Abeloff MD, Armitage JO, Lichter AS (eds): Clinical Oncology. New York, Churchill Livingstone, 1995, pp 11–40.

Fisher GA, Sikic BI: Clinical studies with modulators of multidrug resistance. Hematol Oncol Clin North Am 9:363–382, 1995.

Folkman J: Tumor angiogenesis. *In* Holland JF, Frei E III, Bast RC Jr, et al (eds): Cancer Medicine, ed 3, vol 1. Philadelphia, Lea & Febiger, 1993, pp 153–170.

Ford JM: Modulators of multidrug resistance. Preclinical studies. Hematol Oncol Clin North Am 9:337–361, 1995.

Garfinkel L: Perspectives on cancer prevention. CA Cancer J Clin 45:5–7, 1995.

Gilkeson GS, Caldwell DS: Rheumatic associations with malignancy. J Musculoskel Med 7:64–79, 1990.

Glantz MJ, Biran H, Myers ME, et al: The radiographic diagnosis and treatment of paraneoplastic central nervous system disease. Cancer 73:168–175, 1994.

Goldenberg DM: New developments in monoclonal antibodies for cancer detection and therapy. CA 44:43–64, 1994.

Goodman CC, Snyder TE: Differential Diagnosis in Physical Therapy, ed 2. Philadelphia, WB Saunders, 1995.

Greenwald P, Sandik EJ (eds): Surveillance in Cancer Control Objectives for the Nation: 1985–2000. NCI Monograph No. 2. Washington DC, United States Government Printing Office, 1986.

Groenwald S: Differences between normal and cancer cells. *In* Groenwald S, Frogge M, Goodman N, Yarbro C (eds): Cancer Nursing: Principles and Practice ed 3. Boston, Jones & Bartlett, 1993a, pp 47–57.

Groenwald S: Invasion and metastasis. *In* Groenwald S, Frogge M, Goodman N, Yarbro C (eds): Cancer Nursing: Principles and Practice, ed 3. Boston, Jones & Bartlett, 1993b, pp 58–69.

Gudas S: The physical therapy challenge in disseminated cancer. APTA Newsletter 5:3, 1987.

Hamburgh, R.R.: Principles of cancer treatment. Clin Manage 12:37–41, 1992.

Henderson BE, Ross RK, Pike MC: Toward the primary prevention of cancer. Cancer Sci 254:1131–1137, 1991.

Henson JW, Posner JB: Neurological complications. *In* Holland JF, Frei E III, Bast RC Jr, et al (eds): Cancer Medicine, ed 3, vol 2. Philadelphia, Lea & Febiger, 1993, pp 2268–2286.

Hinson JA, Perry MC: Small cell lung cancer. CA 43:216–225, 1993.

Hogan RD, Burke KM, Franklin TD: The effect of ultrasound on microvascular haemodynamics in skeletal muscle: Effects during ischaemia. Microvasc Res 23:370–379, 1982.

Jaffe JH: Misinformation: Euphoria and addiction. *In* Hill CS Jr, Fields WS (eds): Drug Treatment of Cancer Pain in a Drug-Oriented Society, New York, Raven Press, 1989, pp 175–180.

Johanson GA: Symptom character and prevalence during cancer patients' last days of life. Am J Hosp Palliative Care 8:6–8, 18, 1991.

Kelsey J, Gammon MD: The epidemiology of breast cancer. CA Cancer J Clin 41:146–165, 1991.

Kurzrock R, Cohen PR: Mucocutaneous paraneoplastic manifestations of hematologic malignancies. Am J Med 99:207–216, 1995.

Lejbkowicz F, Zwiran M, Salzberg S: The response of normal and malignant cells to ultrasound in vitro. Ultrasound Med Biol 19:75–82, 1993.

Lewis MM, Reilly JF: Sports tumors. Am J Sports Med 15:362–365, 1987.

Liotta LA, Kleinerman J, Saidel GM: Quantitative relationships of intravascular tumor cells, tumor vessels, and pulmonary metastases following tumor implantation. Cancer Res 34:997, 1974.

Liotta LA, Stetler-Stevenson WG: Principles of molecular cell biology of cancer: Cancer metastasis. *In* DeVita VT, Hellman S, Rosenberg SA (eds): Cancer: Principles and Practice of Oncology, ed 4. Philadelphia, JB Lippincott, 1993, pp 134–149.

Liotta LA, Stetler-Stevenson WG, Steeg PS: Invasion and metastatis. *In* Holland JF, Frei E III, Bast RC Jr, et al (eds): Cancer Medicine, ed 3, vol. 1. Philadelphia, Lea & Febiger, 1993, pp 138–153.

Liu Y, Hernandez AM, Shibata D, et al: BCL2 translocation frequency rises with age in humans. Proc Natl Acad Sci USA 91:8910–8914, 1994.

Matassarin-Jacobs E, Petardi LA: Basic concepts of neoplastic disorders. *In* Black JM, Matassarin-Jacobs E (eds): Luckmann and Sorensen's Medical-Surgical Nursing, ed 4. Philadelphia, WB Saunders, 1993, pp 473–500.

Maxwell L: Therapeutic ultrasound and tumor metastasis. Physiotherapy 81:272–275, 1995.

Miller LT: Postsurgery breast cancer outpatient program. Clin Manag 12:50–55, 1992.

Mitelman F: Chromosomes, genes, and cancer. CA Cancer J Clin 44:133–135, 1994.

Murphy JB, Coletta EM: Health maintenance and prevention for older persons. *In* Reichel W: Care of the Elderly: Clinical Aspects of Aging, ed 4. Baltimore, Williams & Wilkins, 1995, pp 31–40.

Murphy JP: The national cancer data base: A vital commitment. CA Cancer J Clin 44:69–70, 1994.

NCI (National Cancer Institute): A Guide for Black Americans. NIH Publication No. 93-3412, Bethesda, Md, December 1992.

Nolan MF, Wilson MC: Patient-controlled analgesia: A method for the controlled self-administration of opioid pain medications. Phys Ther 75:374–379, 1995.

Norris J (ed.): Professional Guide to Diseases, ed 5. Springhouse, Pa, Springhouse, 1995.

Odell WD: Ectopic hormones and humoral syndromes of cancer. *In* Holland JF, Frei E III, Bast RC Jr, et al (eds): Cancer Medicine ed 3, vol 1. Philadelphia, Lea & Febiger, 1993, pp 896–904.

O'Toole M (ed): Miller-Keane Encyclopedia and Dictionary of Medicine, Nursing, and Allied Health, ed 5. Philadelphia, WB Saunders, 1992.

Peters C, Lotzerich H, Niemeier B, et al: Influence of a moderate exercise training on natural killer cytotoxicity and personality traits in cancer patients. Anticancer Res 14:1033–1036, 1994.

Pfalzer C: Exercise for patients with disseminated cancer. APTA Newslett 5:5–7, 1987.

Pfalzer L: Physical agents and the patient with cancer. Clin Manage 12:84–86, 1992.

Rosenberg SA, Yang JC, Topalian SL, et al: Treatment of 238 consecutive patients with metastatic melanoma or renal cell cancer using high-dose bolus interleukin 2. JAMA 271:907–913, 1994.

Rubin E, Farber JL: Pathology, ed 2. Philadelphia, JB Lippincott, 1994.

Rugo HS: Cancer. *In* Tierney LM, McPhee SJ, Papadakis MA (eds): Current Medical Diagnosis and Treatment, ed 33. Norwalk, Conn, Appleton & Lange, 1994, pp 61–88.

Sandberg AA: Cancer cytogenetics for clinicians. CA Cancer J Clin 44:136–159. 1994.

Snyder CC: Oncology Nursing. Boston, Little, Brown, 1986.

ter Haar G, Dyson M, Oakley S: Ultrasound in physiotherapy in the United Kingdom: Results of a questionnaire. Physiother Pract 4:69–72, 1988.

Thompson HJ: Effect of exercise intensity and duration on the induction of mammary carcinogenesis. Cancer Res 54(supp 7):1960s–1963s, 1994.

Vincent B, Mirand A: The nature of cancer. *In* Baird SB (ed): A Cancer Source Book For Nurses, ed 6. Atlanta, American Cancer Society, 1991, pp 22–29.

Walls J, Bundred N, Howell A: Hypercalcemia and bone resorption in malignancy. Clin Orthop 312:51–63, 1995.

Wegman J: Central nervous system cancers. *In* Groenwald S, Frogge M, Goodman N, Yarbro C (eds): Cancer Nursing: Principles and Practice, ed 3. Boston, Jones & Bartlett, 1993, pp 959–983.

Weinberg RA: Oncogenes and tumor suppressor genes. CA Cancer J Clin 44:160–170, 1994.

Weisburger JH, Wynder EL: Dietary fat intake and cancer. Hematol Oncol Clin North Am 5:7–23, 1991.

Willet W: The search for the cause of breast and colon cancer. Nature 338:389–394, 1989.

Winningham ML: Walking program for people with cancer. Cancer Nurs 14:270–276, 1991.

Winningham ML, MacVicar MG, Burke CA: Exercise for cancer patients: Guidelines and precautions. Physician Sportsmed 14:121–134, 1986.

Wingo PA, Tong T, Bolden S: Cancer statistics, 1995. CA Cancer J Clin 45:8–30, 1995.

SECTION 2

chapter 8

The Integumentary System

Pamela Unger and
Catherine C. Goodman

TERMINOLOGY ASSOCIATED WITH SKIN DISORDERS

Alopecia Loss of hair; baldness.

Blepharitis Inflammation of the glands and lash follicles along the margin of the eyelids with itching, burning, mucous discharge, crusted eyelids, and loss of eyelashes.

Boil A painful nodule formed in the skin by inflammation of the dermis and subcutaneous tissue, enclosing a central slough or "core"; also called furuncle.

Bulla (pl. bullae) A blister or bleb; a fluid-containing, elevated lesion of the skin.

Carbuncle A group of interconnected boils arising in a cluster of hair follicles.

Comedo (pl. comedones) A plug of keratin and sebum within the dilated opening of a hair follicle frequently containing bacteria; a closed comedo is a whitehead; an open comedo is a blackhead.

Desquamation The shedding of skin in scales or sheets.

Ecchymosis Bruise; localized red or purple discoloration caused by extravasation of blood into dermis and subcutaneous tissues.

Erythema Redness of the skin caused by congestion of the capillaries in the lower layers of the skin; occurs with skin injury, infection, or inflammation.

Excoriation Loss of epidermis, usually from abrasion or scratching.

Fissure A narrow slit in the skin; a crack.

Folliculitis Inflammation of a follicle, one of the tubular cavities of the epidermis enclosing the hairs and from which the hairs grow.

Furuncle See Boil.

Furunculosis Persistent sequential occurrence of boils (furuncles) over a period of weeks or months.

Ichthyosis A group of skin disorders characterized by dryness, roughness, and scaliness of the skin; results in thickening of the skin, sometimes referred to as "alligator skin," "fish skin," "crocodile skin," "porcupine skin."

Induration Hardening.

Keratitis Inflammation of the cornea.

Lichenification Roughened, thick epidermis; accentuated skin markings caused by rubbing or irritation; often involves flexor aspect of extremity. Example: chronic dermatitis.

Maceration Softening of skin from wetting or soaking.

Macule Any change in color in the skin that is flat. Examples: white (vitiligo), brown (café-au-lait spot), purple (petechia).

Nevus (pl. nevi) Mole.

Nodule A deep-seated mass with indistinct borders that elevates the overlying epidermis. Example: tumor. If it moves with the skin on palpation, it is intradermal; if the skin moves over the nodule, it is subcutaneous.

Papule A solid, elevated area less than 1 cm in diameter whose top may be pointed, rounded, or flat. Examples: acne, warts, small lesions of psoriasis; see also Plaque (large papule).

Petechiae Pinpoint, tiny, and sharp circumscribed spots in the superficial layers of the epidermis caused by intradermal or submucous small blood vessel hemorrhage.

Plaque A solid distinct area greater than 1 cm in diameter, usually flat-topped. Example: psoriasis.

Pruritus Itching.

Pustule A vesicle containing a purulent exudate. Examples: acne, folliculitis.

Pyoderma Any purulent (containing or forming pus) skin disease.

Spider angioma A benign tumor made up of dilated blood vessels; a specific form of telangiectasia usually associated with liver disease.

Telangiectasia A vascular lesion formed by dilation of a group of small blood vessels; vascular spider or spider veins; ultraviolet light accelerates the loss of elasticity in the walls of the tiny blood vessels that supply the skin, contributing to their permanent dilation and the formation of telangiectasia.

Urticaria An eruption of itching wheals (hives); a vascular reaction of the skin with the appearance of slightly elevated patches that are redder or paler than the surrounding skin.

Verruca A flesh-colored growth; wart.

Vesicle An elevated lesion less than 1 cm in diameter and containing clear serous fluid. Example: blisters of herpes simplex or herpes zoster.

Wheal A circumscribed area of elevated, flat-topped edema on the body surface. Example: urticaria.

Xeroderma A mild form of ichthyosis; excessive dryness of the skin.

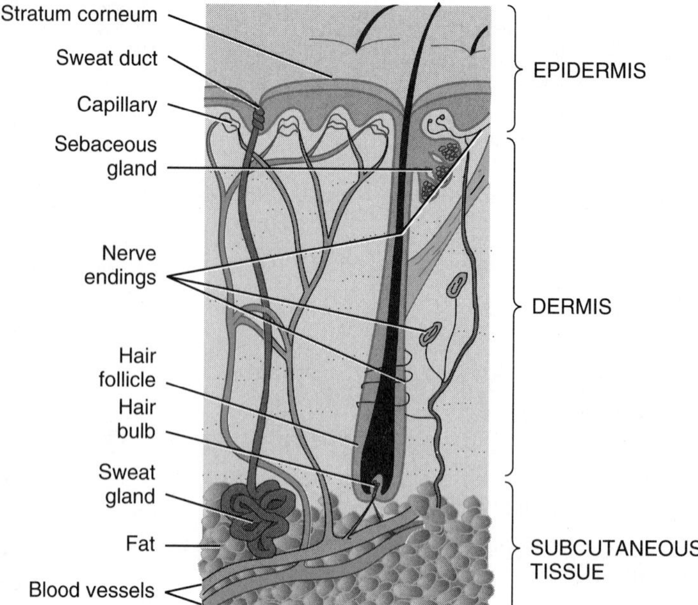

Figure **8–1.** Overall skin structure.

Skin is the largest body organ constituting 15% to 20% of the body weight and consisting of three layers (Fig. 8–1). The structures included in each layer are listed in Table 8–1. The skin differs anatomically and physiologically in different areas of the body but the overall primary function of the skin is to protect the underlying structures from external injury and harmful substances. The skin is primarily an insulator, not an organ of exchange. It has many other different functions including holding the organs together, sensory perception, contributing to fluid balance, controlling temperature, absorbing ultraviolet (UV) radiation, metabolizing vitamin D, and synthesizing epidermal lipids.

TABLE 8–1 Skin Structure

Layer	Structure	Function
Epidermis	Stratum corneum	Protective
	Keratinocytes (squamous cells)	Synthesis of keratin (skin protein)
	Melanocytes	Synthesis of melanin, a pigment
	Langerhans' cells	Antigen presentation; immune response
	Basal cells	Epidermal reproduction
Epidermal appendages	Eccrine unit	Thermoregulation by perspiration
	Apocrine unit (unknown gland)	Production of apocrine sweat; unknown
	Hair follicle	Protection; cavity enclosing hair
	Nails	Protection; mechanical assistance
	Sebaceous glands	Produces sebum (oil to lubricate skin)
Dermis	Collagen, elastin	Skin proteins; skin texture
	Fibroblasts	Collagen synthesis for wound healing
	Macrophages	Phagocytosis of foreign substances; initiates inflammation and repair
	Mast cells	Provides histamine for vasodilation and chemotactic factors for inflammatory responses
	Lymphatic glands	Removal of microbes and excess interstitial fluids; provides lymphatic drainage
	Blood vessels	Provides metabolic skin requirements; thermoregulation
	Nerve fibers	Perception of heat and cold, pain, itching
Subcutaneous tissue	Fat	Energy storage and balance; trauma absorption

Adapted from Nicol NH: Structure and function: Assessment of clients with integumentary disorders. *In* Black JM, Matassarin-Jacobs E (eds): Luckmann and Sorensen's Medical-Surgical Nursing, ed 4. Philadelphia, WB Saunders, 1993, pp 1940–1941.

SKIN LESIONS

Approximately 1 in every 4 people who consult a physician has a skin disorder. Skin lesions can occur as a result of a wide variety of etiologic factors (Box 8–1). Lesions of the skin or disorders with skin manifestations can be classified as *primary* or *secondary* lesions. The primary lesion is the first lesion to appear on the skin and has a visually recognizable structure (e.g., macule, papule, plaque, nodule, tumor, wheal, vesicle, pustule) (see Terminology Associated with Skin Disorders at the beginning of this chapter). When changes occur in the primary lesion, it becomes a secondary lesion (e.g., scale, crust, thickening, erosion, ulcer, scar, excoriation, fissure, atrophy). These changes may result from many factors, including scratching, rubbing, medication, natural disease progression, or processes of healing.

Birthmarks, commonly due to a nevus (pl. nevi), may involve an overgrowth of one or more of any of the normal components of skin such as pigment cells, blood vessels, lymph vessels, and so on. Birthmarks may be classified as pigment cell (e.g., mongolian spot, café au lait spot); vascular (e.g., port-wine stain, strawberry hemangioma); epidermal (e.g., epidermal nevus, nevus sebaceus), or connective tissue (e.g., juvenile elastoma, collagenoma) birthmarks.

Most of these birthmarks do not require treatment. Vascular birthmarks may be removed with laser therapy for cosmetic reasons. The presence of six or more café au lait spots over 5 cm in length require medical investigation as these may be diagnostic of neurofibromatosis or Albright's syndrome. Mongolian spots, blue-black macules, are found over the lumbosacral area in 90% of Native American, black, and Asian infants and can easily be mistaken for a large bruise by the uninformed.

SIGNS AND SYMPTOMS OF SKIN DISEASE

Pruritus (itching) is one of the most common manifestations of skin problems, especially among the chronically ill and the elderly. It can lead to damage if scratching injures the skin's protective barrier, possibly resulting in increased inflammation, infection, and scarring. There are many systemic disorders that may cause pruritus, most commonly diabetes mellitus, drug hypersensitivity, and hyperthyroidism (Box 8–2).

Urticaria, more commonly known as hives, is a vascular reaction of the skin marked by the appearance of smooth, slightly elevated patches (wheals). These are redder or paler than the surrounding skin and are often accompanied by severe itching. These eruptions are usually an allergic response to drugs or infection and rarely last longer than 2 days but may exist in a chronic form, lasting more than 3 weeks and, rarely, months to years.

Rash is a generalized term for an eruption on the skin, most often on the face, trunk, axilla, and groin, and is often accompanied by itching. As such, a rash can present as a continuum anywhere from erythema, to macular lesions, to a raised papular appearance. Rashes typically occur as a secondary response to some primary agent such as exposure to the sun, allergens, irritants, medications, or in association with systemic disease. The most common rashes are diaper rash, drug rash, heat rash, and butterfly rash (a cutaneous reaction across the nose and adjacent areas of the cheeks in the pattern of a butterfly, most often encountered in systemic lupus erythematosus) (see Fig. 8–16).

Xeroderma is a mild form of ichthyosis or excessive dryness of the skin characterized by dry, rough, discolored skin with the formation of scaly desquamation (shedding of the epithelium in small sheets). This problem is accentuated by the use of drying skin cleansers, soaps, disinfectants, solvents, and dry climates.

Other symptoms, such as unusual spots, moles, cysts, fibromas, nodules, swelling, or changes in nail beds, may be observed frequently as more than half of all people have some basic skin problem at some point in their lives (Box 8–3).

BOX **8–1**
Causes of Skin Lesions

- Contact with injurious agents (e.g., chemical toxins)
- Contact with infective organisms
- Reaction to medication
- Physical trauma
- Hereditary factors
- Reaction to allergens
- Systemic origin (e.g., diseases with a cutaneous manifestation)
- Burns (thermal, electrical, chemical, inhalation)
- Neoplasm (chronic ultraviolet B radiation exposure)

BOX **8–2**
Systemic Causes of Pruritus

- Diabetes mellitus
- Drug hypersensitivity
- Hyperthyroidism
- Intestinal parasites
- Iron deficiency anemia
- Kidney disease
- Leukemia
- Liver disease
- Lymphomas
- Polycythemia rubra vera
- Renal disease
- Solid tumor malignancies

BOX **8–3**
Signs and Symptoms of Skin Disorders

- Pruritus
- Urticaria
- Rash
- Xeroderma (dry skin)
- Unusual spots, moles, nodules, cysts
- Edema or swelling
- Changes in appearance of nails
- Changes in skin pigmentation, turgor, texture

Any unusual spot that has appeared recently or changed since its initial appearance should be documented and brought to the physician's attention. On the legs, varicosities and stasis changes from poor venous return may be signaled by changes in skin pigmentation, skin turgor (see Fig. 4–3), and skin texture. Edema of the legs can be a sign of multiple systemic illnesses such as heart, kidney, or liver disease.

AGING AND THE INTEGUMENTARY SYSTEM

The skin undergoes numerous changes that can be seen and felt throughout the life span. The most obvious changes occur first during puberty and again during older adulthood. Hormone changes during puberty stimulate the maturation of hair follicles, sebaceous glands, and apocrine and eccrine units in certain body areas. Mild acne, perspiration and body odor, freckles (promoted by sun exposure), and pigmented nevi (moles) are common occurrences.

During adolescence and adulthood, the use of birth control pills or pregnancy may result in temporary changes in hair growth patterns or hyperpigmentation of the cheeks and forehead known as melasma or "pregnancy mask." Other hormonal abnormalities may result in excessive facial and body hair in women (androgen-related). Hormonal and genetic changes also produce male baldness (alopecia).

The skin exhibits changes that denote the onset of senescence (the process or condition of growing old). These changes may be due to the aging process itself or to the cumulative effects of exposure to sunlight and environmental factors. As aging occurs both structural and functional changes occur in the skin (Table 8–2) resulting clinically in diminished pain perception, increased vulnerability to injury, decreased vascularity, and a weakened inflammatory response.

Visible indications of skin changes associated with aging include gray hair, balding and loss of secondary sexual hair, increased facial hair,[1] lax skin, vascular changes (e.g., decreased elasticity of blood vessel walls; angiomas) (Fig. 8–2), dermal or epidermal degenerative changes, and wrinkling (Kurban and Kurban, 1993). Wrinkling signifies loss of elastin fibers, weakened collagen, and decreased subcutaneous fat and is accelerated by smoking and excessive sun exposure. Many other benign changes may occur including seborrheic keratoses (raised brown or black wartlike growths), lentigines ("liver spots," unrelated to the liver but rather secondary to sun exposure), and skin tags (small flesh-colored papules).

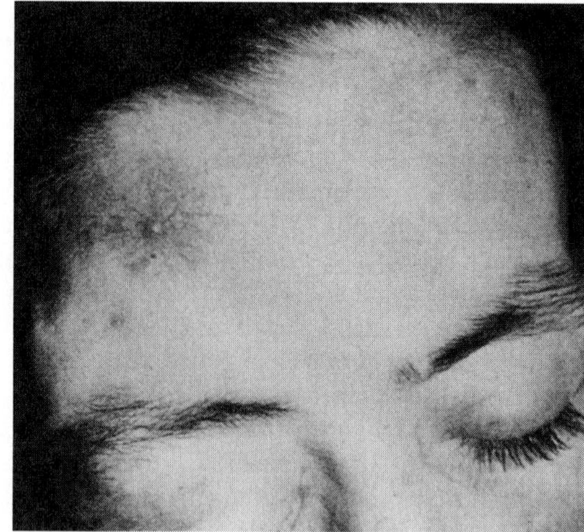

Figure 8–2. Spider angioma (arterial spider, spider telangiectasia, vascular spider) is so called because it consists of a central arteriole, radiating from which are numerous small vessels resembling a spider's legs (ranging from pinhead size to 0.5 cm in diameter). Common sites are the necklace area, the face, forearms, and dorsum of the hand; may be associated with pregnancy, liver disease, or estrogen therapy, or may be normal. *(From Callen JP, Jorizzo J: Dermatological Signs of Internal Disease, ed 2. Philadelphia, WB Saunders, 1995, p 234.)*

TABLE 8–2 Effects of Aging on the Skin

Structural	Functional
Flattening of the dermal-epidermal junction	Altered skin permeability
Changes in basal cells	Decreased inflammatory responsiveness
Decreased number of Langerhans' cells	Decreased immunologic responsiveness
Decreased number of melanocytes	Impaired wound healing
Decreased dermal thickness	Decreased eccrine sweating
Decreased vascularization	Decreased elasticity
Degeneration of elastin fibers	Decreased vitamin D production
Decreased number and altered structure of sweat glands	Impaired sensory perception
Decreased number and distorted structure of specialized nerve endings	
Decreased hair bulb melanocytes	

Adapted from Phillips TJ, Gilchrest BA: Skin changes and disorders. *In* Abrams WB, Berkow R (eds): The Merck Manual of Geriatrics. Rahway, NJ, Merck, 1990, p 1026.

A primary factor in the loss of protective functions of the skin is the diminished barrier function of the stratum corneum (outermost layer of the epidermis; see Fig. 8–1). As this layer becomes thinner, the skin becomes translucent and paper-thin, reacting more readily to minor changes in humidity, temperature, and other irritants. There are fewer melanocytes, with decreased protection against UV radiation. A significant decrease in the number of Langerhans' cells, which remove foreign substances, decreases the skin's immune response with aging. By the time a person reaches 70 years there are only half the number of Langerhans' cells compared to the number in early adulthood. The epidermis is also one of the body's principal suppliers of vitamin D, which is produced when a hormone, 7-dehydrocholesterol, is exposed to sunlight. At age 65, the levels of that hormone are only about 25% of what they were in youth, contributing to vitamin D deficiency and, because vitamin D plays a vital role in building bone, to osteoporosis as well.

[1] For women, excessive facial hair may occur along the upper lip and around the chin. Women may also experience balding after menopause. Men frequently develop increased facial hair in the nares, eyebrows, and helix of the ear.

Special Implications for the Therapist **8-1**

SKIN LESIONS

Any time a client reports signs or symptoms of skin lesions, further evaluation is necessary; documentation and possible medical referral may be required. When examining and documenting the presence of a skin disorder, note the location, size, and any irregularities in skin color, temperature, moisture, ulceration, texture, thickness, mobility, edema, turgor, odor, and tenderness. If more than one lesion is present, note the pattern of distribution: localized or isolated; regional; general; or universal (total), involving the entire skin, hair, and nails. Note whether the lesions are unilateral or bilateral, symmetrical or asymmetrical, and note the arrangement of the lesions (clustered or linear configuration) especially if these occur as a result of contact with clothing, jewelry, or other external object (Norris et al., 1995).

The therapist should remain alert to any skin changes that may indicate the onset or progression of a systemic condition. Certain skin lesions—for example, actinic keratosis, slightly raised, red, scaly papules; sebaceous cysts, enclosed cysts in the dermis—should be examined by a physician because of their premalignant status and infectious potential, respectively. Seborrheic keratosis can be moved with friction and may bleed, causing alarm, but this is not a malignancy; the therapist must avoid contact with the skin in that area.

Care must be taken when using electrical or thermal modalities (heat or cold) with elderly people. Decreased circulation, reduced subcutaneous adipose, and altered metabolism create a situation where initial skin resistance to electricity or poor dissipation of heat or cold can lead to tissue damage. Extra toweling and close supervision are necessary to prevent complications.

COMMONLY OCCURRING SKIN DISORDERS

Atopic Dermatitis

Definition and Incidence. Atopic dermatitis (AD) is a common, chronic relapsing, pruritic type of eczematous disorder. The word "atopic" refers to a group of three associated allergic disorders: asthma, allergic rhinitis (hay fever), and atopic dermatitis. There is usually a personal or family history of allergic disorders present.

Etiology, Risk Factors, and Pathogenesis. The exact cause of atopic dermatitis is unknown. Risk factors include irritants, allergens, physical environment, and emotional stress. The role of food allergy in the etiology of AD remains controversial. Xerosis (abnormal dryness) associated with AD is usually worse during periods of low humidity and over the winter months in northern latitudes.

The underlying biochemical abnormality in xerosis is unknown and the pathologic findings may be a result of the dry skin rather than the cause of the drying effects of this condition. Compared with normal skin, the dry skin of atopic dermatitis has a reduced water-binding capacity, a higher transepidermal water loss, and a decreased water content. Rubbing and scratching of itchy skin are responsible for many of the clinical changes seen in the skin. Hands frequently in and out of water makes the condition worse.

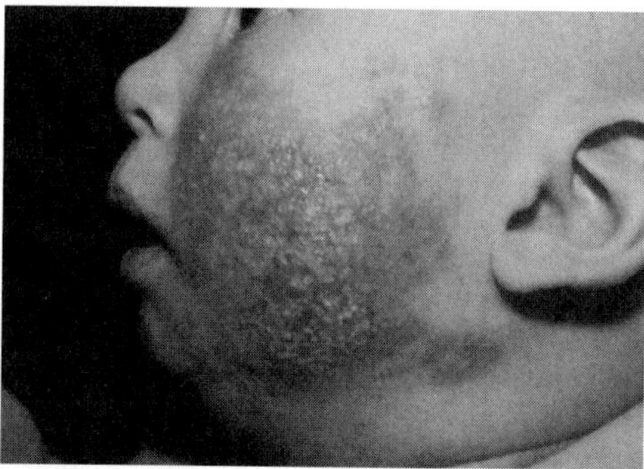

Figure **8-3.** Infantile atopic dermatitis with oozing and crusting lesions. (*From Weston WL, Lane AT: Color Textbook of Pediatric Dermatology. St Louis, Mosby–Year Book, 1991.*)

Clinical Manifestations. Atopic dermatitis begins in many people during infancy in the form of a red, oozing, crusting rash classified as acute dermatitis (Fig. 8–3). As the child grows, the chronic form of dermatitis results in skin that is dry, thickened, and brownish gray in color. The rash tends to become localized to the large folds of the extremities as the person becomes older. It is found mainly on flexor surfaces such as the elbows and knees, neck, sides of the face, eyelids, and the backs of hands and feet. Hand and foot dermatitis can become a significant problem for some people.

Xerosis and pruritus are the major symptoms of atopic dermatitis and cause the greatest morbidity with severely excoriated lesions, infection, and scarring. Viral, bacterial, and fungal secondary skin infections may cause further changes in the skin. *Staphylococcus aureus* is the most common bacterial infection, resulting in extensive crusting with serous weeping, folliculitis (inflammation of hair follicles), pyoderma (pus), and furunculosis (boils).

Medical Management. The goal of medical therapy is to break the inflammatory cycle that causes excess drying, cracking, itching, and scratching. Personal hygiene, moisturizing the skin, avoidance of irritants, topical pharmacology, and sometimes systemic medications (e.g., antibiotics, antihistamines, and rarely, systemic corticosteroids) are treatment techniques currently available. Experimental research using immune response modifiers to treat severe atopic dermatitis is underway.

Special Implications for the Therapist **8-2**

ATOPIC DERMATITIS

The therapist may be instrumental in providing client education that results in proper daily care (hydration and lubrication) of the skin. Daily applications (two or three times daily) of emollients that occlude the skin to prevent evaporation and retain moisture should be recommended. Creams or ointments containing petrolatum or lanolin should be used unless the person is sensitized to lanolin (see Contact Dermatitis) and those that contain urea or lactic acid improve the binding of water in the skin and prevent evaporation.

Understanding the individual disease pattern and identifying exacerbating factors are crucial to effective management of this disorder. It is important to identify and eliminate triggers that cause the atopic dermatitis to flare. Elderly clients should be encouraged to bathe with tepid water using a nondrying, nonperfumed soap or other agent when indicated. Daily bathing should be avoided. Emollients must be applied to the body within 5 minutes after showering or bathing, especially in dry, winter weather, to prevent further skin drying.

Dermatitis must be considered a precaution, if not contraindication, to some treatment modalities used by therapists. The use of water, alcohol, or any topical agents containing alcohol should be avoided. Topical agents, such as ultrasound gel, mobilization creams, and so on, must be used carefully, observing for any skin reaction. A nonreactive response does not guarantee the client will not react when such agents are subsequently applied in future treatment sessions. Caution and careful observation is encouraged.

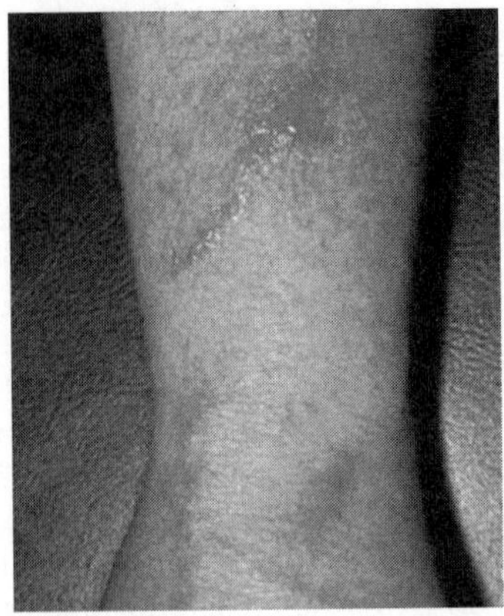

Figure **8-4.** Primary contact dermatitis, a local inflammatory reaction, can occur in response to an irritant in the environment or an allergy. Characteristic location of lesions often give a clue to the cause. Erythema shows first, followed by swelling, wheals, or urticaria, or maculopapular vesicles accompanied by intense pruritus. The example shown here is a result of contact with poison ivy. (*From Hurwitz S: Clinical Pediatric Dermatology: A Textbook of Skin Disorders of Childhood and Adolescence. Philadelphia, WB Saunders, 1981, p 381.*)

Contact Dermatitis

Etiology, Incidence, and Pathogenesis. Contact dermatitis can be an acute or chronic skin inflammation caused by exposure to a chemical, mechanical, physical, or biologic agent. It is one of the most common environmental skin diseases occurring at any age. As people age, they may develop delayed cell-mediated hypersensitivity to a variety of substances that come in contact with the skin.

Common sensitizers include nickel (found in jewelry and many common foods), chromates (used in tanning leathers), wool fats (particularly lanolin found in moisturizers and skin creams), rubber additives (see Latex Rubber Allergy, Chapter 3), topical antibiotics (typically neomycin), and topical anesthetics such as benzocaine or lidocaine (Abrams et al., 1995). Dermatitis of unknown cause is more commonly diagnosed in the elderly population.

A small percentage of the population is allergic to silicone. The therapist is most likely to see this reaction in a sensitized person with an amputation using a silicone-type interface in a prosthetic device (designed to reduce shear, decrease repetitive stress, and absorb shock).

Clinical Manifestations. Intense pruritus (itching), erythema (redness), and edema of the skin occur 1 to 2 days after exposure in previously sensitized persons. Clinical manifestations begin at the site of exposure, but then extend to more distant sites. These conditions may progress to vesiculation, oozing (watery discharges), crusting, and scaling (Fig. 8–4). If these symptoms persist the skin becomes thickened with prominent skin markings and pigmentation changes. The elderly have a less pronounced inflammatory response to standard irritants than do younger persons.

Medical Management

Diagnosis, Treatment, and Prognosis. If contact dermatitis is suspected, the client should be referred to a physician. A detailed history and careful examination are frequently all that are needed to make the diagnosis. It may be necessary to perform patch testing to identify the causative agent.

Primary treatment is removal of the offending agent; treatment of the skin is secondary. The client should be instructed to avoid contact with strong soaps, detergents, solvents, bleaches, and other strong chemicals. The involved skin should be lubricated frequently with emollients. Topical anesthetics or steroids (topical or sometimes systemic), or both, may be prescribed.

Acute lesions usually resolve in 3 weeks; chronic lesions persist until the causative agent has been removed.

Special Implications for the Therapist **8-3**

CONTACT DERMATITIS

The therapy professional should always consider the client's reactions to external substances. This is of particular importance when applying any cream, topical agent, or solution. Various modalities used within the profession may involve causative substances (e.g., whirlpool additives, ultrasound gels, self-sticking electrode pads). The client's skin must always be examined before and after treatment for the appearance of any adverse reactions. The client should be instructed to report any discomfort or unusual findings during or after treatment to the therapist.

The person with contact dermatitis associated with the use of a silicone sleeve or interface with a prosthetic device should be cautioned about the use of soaps that do not include a rinsing agent. Many antibacterial and antiperspirant soaps leave particles on the surface of the skin that act as a barrier on the skin's surface against bacterial invasion. A rash or blister may occur in patchy areas corresponding to pressure points when the friction of the interface drives the soap particles back into the skin (Callaghan, 1996).

The therapist may suggest one of several care plans for this type of contact dermatitis. The use of alcohol-based lubricants or soaps, antifungal or antibacterial soaps without a rinsing agent, and lanolin should be avoided. Soap-free cleansing agents or a soft soap should be used for daily cleansing and a petroleum-based ointment can be applied to the limb before putting on the liner. Water-based ointments should be avoided when using urethane liners because these can cause the normally tacky urethane to adhere to the skin so that when the liner is removed, bits of skin may be pulled off as well. Alcohol-based lubricants or soaps should also be avoided with urethane products as these components act as a solvent on urethane, increasing the stickiness of the urethane (Callaghan, 1996).

Eczema and Dermatitis

Definition and Overview. *Eczema* and *dermatitis* are terms that are often used interchangeably to describe a group of disorders with a characteristic appearance (Nicol, 1993). Eczema or dermatitis is a superficial inflammation of the skin due to irritant exposure, allergic sensitization (delayed hypersensitivity), or genetically determined idiopathic factors. Many types of dermatitis are represented according to these major categories of etiology (e.g., allergic dermatitis, irritant dermatitis, seborrheic dermatitis, nummular eczema, atopic dermatitis, stasis dermatitis).

Eczema or dermatitis has three primary stages; this condition can manifest in any one of the three stages or the three stages may coexist. *Acute dermatitis* is characterized by extensive erosions with serous exudate or by intensely pruritic, erythematous papules and vesicles on a background of erythema. *Subacute dermatitis* is characterized by erythematous, excoriated (scratched or abrased), scaling papules or plaques that are either grouped or scattered over erythematous skin. Often the scaling is so fine and diffuse the skin acquires a silvery sheen. *Chronic dermatitis* is characterized by thickened skin and increased skin marking (called lichenification) secondary to rubbing and scratching; excoriated papules, fibrotic papules, and nodules (prurigo nodularis); and postinflammatory hyper- and hypopigmentation.

Incidence and Etiology. Dermatitis is a common skin disorder in the elderly. It may be caused by hypoproteinemia, venous insufficiency, allergens, irritants, or underlying malignancy such as leukemia or lymphoma. Because the elderly often take multiple medications, dermatitis from drug-drug interaction can occur. The normal aging process with the flattened epidermal-dermal junction and loss of dermis results in skin fragility which contributes to the development of dermatitis.

Stasis Dermatitis

Stasis dermatitis is the development of areas of very dry, thin skin and sometimes shallow ulcers of the lower legs primarily due to venous insufficiency. The client commonly has a history of varicose veins or deep vein thrombosis (see also Venous Diseases, Chapter 10). The process of stasis dermatitis begins with edema of the leg as a result of slowed venous return. As the venous stasis continues, the tissue becomes hypoxic from inadequate blood supply. This poorly nourished tissue begins to necrose. The clinical manifestations include itching, a feeling of heaviness in the legs, brown-stained skin, and open shallow lesions (Fig. 8–5). The lesions are very slow to heal because of a lack of oxygenated blood.

Environmental Dermatoses

It is well documented that exposure to various environmental chemicals and to physical stimuli (Box 8–4) are capable of inducing adverse cutaneous responses. Common environmental skin diseases seen in a therapy practice may include irritant and allergic dermatitis, acne lesions, pigmentary changes (hyperpigmentation, hypopigmentation, or absence of pigment), photosensitivity reactions, scleroderma, infectious disorders, and cutaneous malignancy. Each of these environmentally induced skin conditions is discussed separately in this chapter. See also Chapter 3.

Rosacea *(Goldstein and Odom, 1995)*

Rosacea is a chronic facial disorder of middle-aged and older people. Although this is a form of acne, it is differentiated by age, the presence of a large vascular component (erythema and telangiectasis), and usually the absence of comedones. An acneiform rosacea can occur with papules, pustules, and oily skin. No known cause or factor has been identified to explain the pathogenesis of this disorder. A statistically significant incidence of migraine headaches accompanying rosacea has been reported. Rosacea has often been linked with

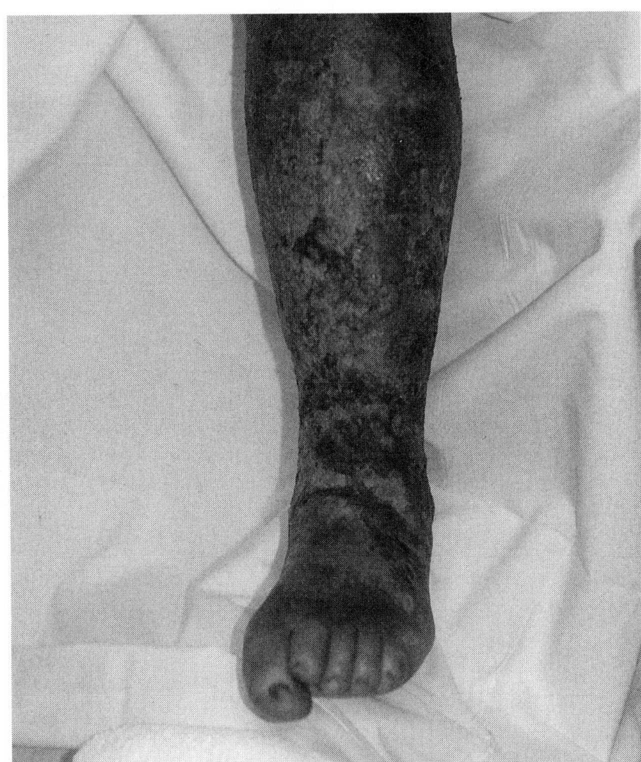

Figure **8–5.** Stasis dermatitis. (*Courtesy of Pam Unger, P.T., Community General Hospital, Center for Wound Management, Reading, Pa, 1995.*)

BOX **8–4**
Environmental Factors That Induce Skin Disease

- Mechanical factors
  - Friction
  - Pressure
  - Vibration
  - Cuts
- Physical factors
  - Heat
  - Cold
  - Humidity
  - Water
  - Sunlight
  - Ultraviolet light
  - Ionizing radiation
- Chemical agents
  - Primary irritants
  - Sensitizers
  - Photoirritants
  - Photosensitizers
- Biologic agents
  - Insect and animal parasites
  - Bacteria
  - Rickettsiae
  - Fungi
  - Viruses
  - Irritant and sensitizing plants and woods

From Brooks SM, Gochfeld M, Herzstein J, et al: Environmental Medicine. St Louis, Mosby–Year Book, 1995.

TABLE **8–3** INFECTIONS OF THE SKIN

TYPE OF INFECTION	TRANSMISSION
Bacterial	
Impetigo contagiosa	Contagious
Pyoderma	Contagious
Folliculitis (pimple, boil)	Contagious; minimal chance of spread
Cellulitis	Contagious*
Viral	
Verrucae (warts)	Contagious; autoinoculable†
Verruca plantaris (plantar wart)	Contagious; autoinoculable
Herpes simplex	
Type 1: cold sore, fever blister	Contagious
Type 2: genital lesion	Contagious
Varicella-zoster virus (herpes zoster; shingles)	Contagious; chickenpox can occur in anyone not previously exposed
Fungal	
Tinea corporis (ringworm)	Person-to-person Animal-to-person Inanimate object-to-person
Tinea capitis (affects scalp)	Person-to-person Animal-to-person
Tinea cruris (jock itch)	Person-to-person
Tinea pedis (athlete's foot)	Transmission to other persons rare despite general opinion to the contrary
Other	
Scabies	Person-to-person; sexually transmitted Inanimate object-to-person
Lice	Same as scabies

* Technically, cellulitis is contagious, but from a practical point of view the chances of this spreading are very low and would require a susceptible host, e.g., an open cut on the therapist's hand coming in contact with blood or pus from client's open wound.
† Capable of spreading infection from one's own body by scratching.
Adapted from Wong D: Whaley and Wong's Essentials of Pediatric Nursing, ed 4. St Louis, Mosby–Year Book, 1993, pp 1030–1032.

gastrointestinal disturbances and a causal relationship between *Helicobacter pylori* (a bacterium that causes gastritis) and rosacea has been established in some cases (Kolibasova et al., 1996).

Clinically, the cheeks, nose, and chin (sometimes the entire face) may have a rosy appearance. The affected person reports burning or stinging with episodes of flushing. Inflammatory papules are prominent and there may be pustules. It is not uncommon to have associated ophthalmic disease, including blepharitis and keratitis.

Medical management aimed at the inflammatory papules, pustules, and surrounding erythema may include topical or systemic therapy. Rosacea tends to be a persistent condition that can be controlled with drugs. Rosacea associated with *H. pylori*–induced gastritis can be effectively treated by addressing the underlying problem. Although therapists do not treat this condition, clients with other diagnoses often present with this condition also. Clients with this condition should see a physician for adequate treatment.

SKIN INFECTIONS

Many of the bacterial, viral, fungal, and other parasitic skin infections encountered by the therapist are not the primary focus of treatment but rather occur in clients who are hospitalized or being treated for some other condition. Many of these skin disorders are contagious (Table 8–3) and require careful handling by all health care professionals to avoid spreading the infection and becoming contaminated themselves. Sources of infection differ depending on the disease and mode of transmission (see also, Chapter 6). Predisposing factors to skin infections include decreased resistance, burns or pressure ulcers, decreased blood flow, contamination from nasal discharge, poor hygiene, and crowded living conditions (Wong, 1993). Only the most common skin infections encountered in the therapy or rehabilitation setting are discussed further in this section.

Bacterial Infections

Normally, the skin harbors a variety of bacterial flora, including the major pathogenic varieties of staphylococci and streptococci. The degree of their pathogenicity depends on the invasiveness and toxigenicity of the specific organisms, the integrity of the skin, the barrier of the host, and the immune and cellular defenses of the host. Organisms usually enter the skin through abrasions or puncture wounds of the hands. Clinical infection develops 3 to 7 days after inoculation. Septicemia can develop if treatment is not provided or if the person is immunocompromised (Shadomy and Utz, 1993).

People at risk for the development of bacterial infections include children and adults who are immunocompromised, as occurs with acquired or inherited immunodeficiency; anyone in a debilitated physical condition; those on immunosuppressive therapy; and those with a generalized malignancy such as leukemia or lymphoma. All of these factors emphasize the importance of careful handwashing and cleanliness to prevent spread of infection before and after caring for infected people and their lesions.

Some conditions (e.g., impetigo) are easily spread by self-inoculation; therefore the affected person must be cautioned to avoid touching the involved area. Follicular lesions should not be squeezed as this will not hasten the resolution of the infection and may increase the risk of making the lesion worse or spreading the infection.

Impetigo

Definition and Overview. Impetigo is a superficial skin infection commonly caused by staphylococci or streptococci. It is most commonly found in infants, young children aged 2 to 5 years, and the elderly. Predisposing factors include close contact in schools, overcrowded living quarters, poor skin hygiene, anemia, malnutrition, and minor skin trauma. It can be spread by direct contact, environmental contamination, or an arthropod vector. Impetigo often occurs as a secondary infection in conditions characterized by a cutaneous barrier broken to microbes, such as eczema or herpes zoster excoriations.

Clinical Manifestations. Small macules (unraised spots) rapidly develop into vesicles (small blisters) which then become pustular (pus-filled). When the vesicle breaks, a thick yellow crust forms from the exudate causing pain, surrounding erythema, regional adenitis (inflammation of gland), cellulitis (inflammation of tissue), and itching. Scratching spreads infection, a process called autoinoculation. Lesions frequently affect the face, heal slowly, and leave depigmented areas. If the infection is extensive, malaise, fever, and lymphadenopathy may also be present.

Medical Management. Single small lesions can often be managed by soaking them for 10 minutes with drying agents (Burrow's solution). Oral antibiotics may be required. Rarely, extensive lesions require systemic antibiotics to reduce the risk of glomerulonephritis and to prevent this contagious condition from spreading. A skin swab may be necessary to determine the contaminating organism.

Cellulitis (Nicol, 1993)

Cellulitis is a suppurative inflammation of the dermis and subcutaneous tissues that spreads widely through tissue spaces. Cellulitis usually occurs in the loose tissue beneath the skin, but may also occur in tissues beneath mucous membranes or around muscle bundles. The skin is erythematous, edematous, tender, and sometimes nodular. Erysipelas, a surface cellulitis of the skin, is characterized by patches of skin that are red with sharply defined borders and that feel hot to the touch. Red streaks extending from the patch indicate that the lymph vessels have been infected. Facial cellulitis involves the face, especially the cheek or periorbital or orbital tissues; the neck may also be affected. Pelvic cellulitis involves the tissues surrounding the uterus and is called parametritis (O'Toole, 1992).

Streptococcus pyogenes or staphylococcus are the usual causes of this infection although other pathogens may be responsible (see also Streptococcal Cellulitis, Chapter 6). Lymphangitis may occur; if cellulitis is untreated (treatment is usually pharmacologic), gangrene, metastatic abscesses, and sepsis can result. Clients at increased risk for cellulitis include the elderly and people with lowered resistance from diabetes, malnutrition, steroid therapy, and the presence of wounds or ulcers. Other predisposing factors include the presence of edema or other cutaneous inflammation or wounds (e.g., tinea, eczema, burns, trauma). There is a tendency for recurrence, especially at sites of lymphatic obstruction. See also Lymphangitis, Chapter 10.

Viral Infections

Viruses are intracellular parasites that produce their effect by using the intracellular substances of the host cells. Viruses are composed only of DNA or RNA, not both, usually enclosed in a protein shell, and are unable to provide for their own metabolic needs or to reproduce themselves. After a virus penetrates a cell of the host organism, it sheds the outer shell and disappears within the cell, where the nucleic acid core stimulates the host cell to form more virus material from its own intracellular substance. In a viral infection the epidermal cells react with inflammation and vesiculation (as in herpes zoster) or by proliferating to form growths (warts).

Herpes Zoster

Definition, Incidence, and Risk Factors. Herpes zoster, or shingles, is a local disease brought about by the reactivation of the same virus that causes a systemic disease called varicella (chickenpox). The initial infection with varicella is common during childhood. Shingles may occur at any age, although peak incidence occurs between ages 50 and 70. The disease is usually brought on by an immunocompromised state as occurs with underlying malignancy or acquired immunodeficiency syndrome (AIDS).

Pathogenesis. Herpes zoster results from reactivation of varicella virus that has been dormant in the cerebral ganglia (extramedullary ganglia of the cranial nerves) or the ganglia of posterior nerve roots from a previous episode of chickenpox. How or why this reactivation occurs is not clearly understood at this time. One explanation is that the virus multiplies as it is reactivated and that it is neutralized by antibodies remaining from the initial infection. If effective antibodies are not present, the virus continues to multiply in the ganglia, destroying the host neuron, and spreading down the sensory nerves to the skin (Norris, 1995).

Clinical Manifestations. The affected person may have some early warning (prodromal symptoms) that the virus has become reactivated especially in repeat incidences. Early symptoms of pain and tingling along the affected spinal or cranial nerve dermatome are usually accompanied by fever, chills, malaise, and gastrointestinal disturbances. One to 3 days later red papules form seen along a dermatome (Fig.

8–6). The lesions most commonly spread unilaterally around the thorax or vertically over the arms or legs (Norris et al., 1995).

Herpes papules rapidly develop into vesicles that vary in size and may be filled with clear fluid or pus. The vesicles are confined to the distribution of the infected nerve root and begin to dry 5 days after eruption with gradual, progressive healing over the next 2 to 4 weeks. Postherpetic neuralgia can occur and increases sharply in occurrence in people over the age of 60. Children are unaffected by postherpetic pain. In the adult, severe neuralgic pain can occur in peripheral areas innervated by the nerves arising in the inflamed root ganglia. The pain may be constant or intermittent and vary from light burning to a deep visceral sensation. The duration of this neuralgic pain can be weeks or months to years. The cause of postherpetic neuralgia is not fully understood. Scarring and degenerative changes involving the nerve trunks, ganglia, and skin may be important factors. The incidence of scarring and hyperpigmentation is much higher in the elderly.

Occasionally, herpes zoster involves the cranial nerves, especially the trigeminal and geniculate ganglia or the oculomotor nerve. Geniculate zoster may cause vesicle formation in the external auditory canal, ipsilateral facial palsy, hearing loss, dizziness, and loss of taste. Trigeminal ganglion involvement causes eye pain, and possibly corneal and scleral damage with loss of vision.

In rare cases, herpes zoster leads to generalized CNS infection, muscle atrophy, motor paralysis (usually transient), acute transverse myelitis, and ascending myelitis. More often, generalized infection causes acute retention of urine and unilateral paralysis of the diaphragm.

Medical Management

Diagnosis. Diagnosis is usually based on clinical examination and recognition of the skin lesions with accompanying systemic signs of infection. Laboratory diagnosis may include culture and histologic examination of skin biopsy. Differentiation of herpes zoster from localized herpes simplex requires staining antibodies from vesicular fluid and identification under fluorescent light.

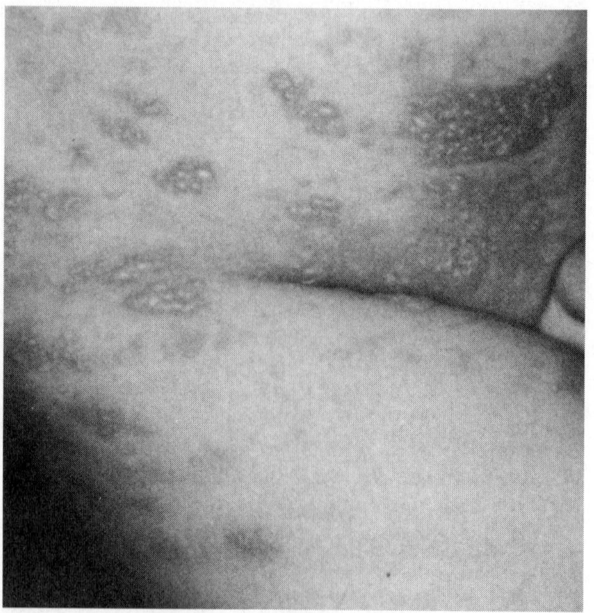

Figure **8–6.** Herpes zoster of the groin. (*From Black JM, Matassarin-Jacobs E (eds): Luckmann and Sorensen's Medical-Surgical Nursing, ed 4. Philadelphia, WB Saunders, 1993, p 1975.*)

Treatment. There is no curative agent for shingles but supportive treatment to relieve itching and neuralgic pain is provided. The use of systemic corticosteroids within the first week of eruption may abort the attack and appears to reduce both the acute symptoms and the risk of postherpetic neuralgia in elderly persons (Abrams et al., 1995). Acyclovir (Zovirax) seems to stop the progression of the rash and prevents visceral complications. A newer oral drug (famciclovir) is comparable to acyclovir in effectiveness but has a longer duration of action and requires less frequent dosage. Hospitalized clients with varicella-zoster should be placed in isolation rooms, and personnel entering the room should wear gowns, gloves, and masks. Eye involvement in zoster requires ophthalmologic evaluation and treatment (Gill and Shandera, 1995).

A live varicella vaccine (Varivax) was approved by the Food and Drug Administration (FDA) for use in persons 12 months of age or older who have not had varicella (Farrington, 1995). Until the varicella vaccine is widely available (and very likely after), the only effective means of preventing or modifying the varicella infection in exposed, susceptible persons remains the varicella-zoster immune globulin (VZIG).[2] This preparation is obtained from pooled plasma donations from individuals with known high titers of antivaricella antibody and recommended for several categories of high-risk exposed susceptible persons. These include the immunocompromised, some healthy persons 25 years or older, pregnant women or women in the health care profession who may be contemplating pregnancy, newborns whose mothers develop varicella between 5 days before and 48 hours after delivery, hospitalized premature infants over 28 weeks of gestational age whose mothers are susceptible, and hospitalized premature infants less mature than 28 weeks regardless of maternal status (Simoes, 1995).

Prognosis. Overall prognosis is good unless the infection spreads to the brain (rare). Most people recover completely, with the possible exception of scarring and, with corneal damage, visual impairment. Occasionally, intractable pain associated with neuralgia may persist for months or years. Those persons who develop postherpetic neuralgia may require further medical intervention.

Special Implications for the Therapist **8–4**

HERPES ZOSTER

Adults with shingles are infectious to persons who have not had chickenpox. For this reason, therapists who have never had chickenpox should receive the vaccination; complications and morbidity associated

[2] At present, the duration of protection from the vaccine remains unknown but it is thought that lifetime protection is NOT provided. Because seroconversion does not take place until 4 to 6 weeks' postvaccination VZIG remains the only immediate treatment for some people.

with adult onset of varicella warrant this precaution. Any female therapist who is pregnant or planning a pregnancy should be tested for immune status if unsure about her previous history of varicella. This is especially important because transmissibility of the virus occurs 2 to 3 days before symptoms occur until all lesions are crusted over. This means anyone receiving treatment by a therapist may be an asymptomatic host during the period of communicability; exposure to self and further transmission to others can occur without the therapist's awareness.

The Centers for Disease Control and Prevention (CDC) has set up guidelines for the care of all clients regarding precautions for the transmission of infectious skin diseases (see Tables 8–3 and 6–6). These Universal precautions (see Appendix A) should be used with all clients regardless of their disease status. All skin lesions are considered potentially infectious and should be handled as such. The careful use of these precautionary measures severely limits the transmission of any disease. In addition, each hospital has isolation precautions organized according to categories of disease to prevent the spread of infectious disease to others. Every health care professional must be familiar with these procedures and follow them carefully. See also Isolation Procedures, Chapter 6, and Table 6–4.

Neither heat nor ultrasound should be used on a person with shingles as these modalities can increase the severity of the person's symptoms. For the person with severe herpetic pain, relaxation techniques may be useful. In the case of unresolved postherpetic neuralgia, the individual may benefit from a program of chronic pain management.

Warts (Verrucae)

Warts are common benign, viral infections of the skin and adjacent mucous membranes caused by human papilloma viruses (HPVs). There are over 50 different varieties of these viruses depending upon their location on the skin. The incidence of warts is highest in children and young adults, but can occur at any age. Transmission is probably through direct contact, but autoinoculation is possible.

Warts may appear singly or as multiple lesions with thick white surfaces containing many pointed projections. Clinical manifestations depend on the type of wart and its location. The most common wart (*verruca vulgaris*) is referred to as such and appears as a rough, elevated, round surface most frequently on the extremities, especially the hands and fingers. *Plantar warts* are slightly elevated or flat, occurring singly or in large clusters referred to as mosaic warts, primarily at pressure points of the feet.

Medical Management *(Arnold et al., 1990)*

Diagnosis. Diagnosis is usually made on the basis of visual examination. Plantar warts can be differentiated from corns and calluses by certain distinguishing features. Plantar warts obliterate natural lines of the skin, may contain red or black capillary dots that are easily discernible if the surface of the wart is shaved down with a scalpel, and are painful on application of pressure. Both plantar warts and corns have a soft, pulpy core surrounded by a thick callous ring; plantar warts and calluses are flush with the skin surface.

Treatment. Some warts respond to simple treatment and some disappear spontaneously. Warts can be chronic or recurrent. There are a multitude of treatment regimens available. The specific choice of treatment method is influenced by the location of the wart(s), the size and number of warts, the presence of secondary infection, the amount of tenderness present on palpation, the age and sex of the client, history of previous treatment, and individual compliance with treatment. Over-the-counter salicylic acid preparations (e.g., Wart-off, Clear Away, Freezone, Wart Remover) applied topically may be used to induce peeling of the skin.

Cryotherapy is performed with either liquid nitrogen or solid carbon dioxide. This procedure is widely used as the cosmetically preferred treatment choice but is painful. The procedure causes epidermal necrosis; the area dries and peels off together with the wart. *Acids* in liquid form or as a paste (salicylic acid and lactic acid) can be painted on warts daily, removed after 24 hours, and reapplied. This treatment choice is not recommended for areas where perspiration is heavy, for areas likely to get wet, or for exposed body parts where patches are cosmetically undesirable. Acid therapy requires a commitment from the client or family to perform it on a daily basis. Electrodesiccation and *curettage* of warts is widely used for common warts and occasionally for plantar warts. High frequency electric current destroys the wart, and is followed by surgical removal of dead tissue at the base with application of an antibiotic ointment and bandage for 48 hours. Atrophic scarring may occur and the recurrence rate is 20% to 40%. The use of mechanical (nonthermal) ultrasound has been advocated by some in the treatment of plantar warts, but this has not been widely accepted by the medical community.

Fungal Infections (Dermatophytoses)

Fungal infections such as ringworm are caused by a group of fungi that invade the stratum corneum, hair, and nails. These are superficial infections that live on, not in, the skin and are confined to the dead keratin layers, unable to survive in the deeper layers. Since the keratin is being shed (desquamated) constantly, the fungus must multiply at a rate that equals the rate of keratin production to maintain itself; otherwise the infection would be shed with the discarded skin cells.

Ringworm (Tinea Corporis)

Dermatophytoses, or fungal infections of the hair, skin, or nails, are designated by the Latin word *tinea,* with further designation related to the affected area of the body (see Table 8–3). Tinea corporis, or ringworm, has no association with worms but rather is marked by the formation of ring-shaped pigmented patches covered with vesicles or scales that often become itchy (Fig. 8–7). Transmission can occur directly through contact with infected lesions or indirectly through contact with contaminated objects such as shoes, towels, or shower stalls.

Diagnosis can be made through laboratory examination of the affected skin. Treatment for any type of ringworm requires maintaining clean, dry skin and the application of antifungal powder or topical agent as prescribed. Treatment with the drug griseofulvin may take weeks to months to complete

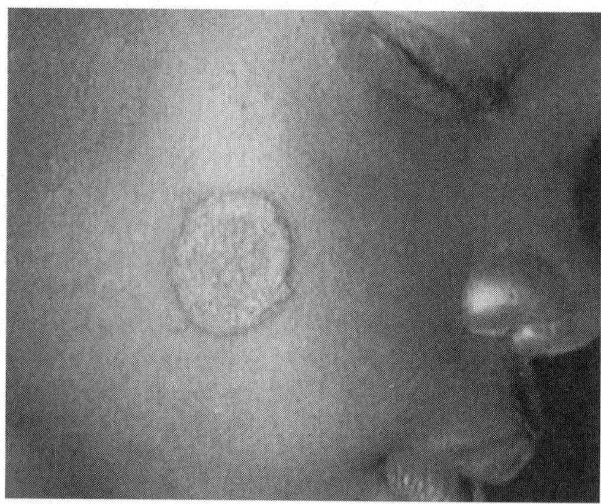

Figure **8–7.** Scales forming multiple circular lesions with clear centers are characteristic of tinea corporis (ringworm). These lesions are hyperpigmented in whites, depigmented in dark-skinned persons, and occur most often on the face, chest, abdomen, and back of arms. (*From Hurwitz S: Clinical Pediatric Dermatology. A Textbook of Skin Disorders of Childhood and Adolescence. Philadelphia, WB Saunders, 1981, p 381.*)

and should be continued throughout the prescribed dosage schedule even if symptoms subside. Possible side effects of this agent include headache, gastrointestinal upset, fatigue, insomnia, and photosensitivity. Prolonged use of this drug requires monitoring of liver function.

Occasionally, an obese client with tinea corporis is referred to therapy for wound care secondary to skin breakdown. Open wet dressings may be applied two to three times daily to areas of moist denuded skin to help decrease inflammation.

Athlete's Foot (Tinea Pedis)

Tinea pedis, or athlete's foot, causes erythema, skin peeling, and pruritus between the toes which may spread from the interdigital spaces to the sole. Severe infection may result in inflammation, with severe itching and pain on walking. Clean, dry socks and adequate footwear (well-ventilated, properly fitting) are important. After washing the feet and drying thoroughly between the toes, antifungal cream or powder (the latter to absorb perspiration and prevent excoriation) can be applied.

Special Implications for the Therapist **8–5**

FUNGAL INFECTIONS

Ringworm

The infectious nature of fungal infections requires specific hygienic measures common to all infectious conditions. Affected persons should not share hair care products (e.g., combs, brushes, headgear), clothes, or other articles that have been in proximity to the infected area. Affected persons must use their own towels and linens. Since the infection can be acquired by animal-to-human transmission (see Table 8–3), all household pets must be examined for the presence of ringworm as well. Other sources of infection include seats with headrests (e.g., theater seats, seats on public transportation, or other public seats that can be shared)(Wong, 1993).

Athlete's Foot

Athlete's foot, often observed by the therapist (see previous description), should be discussed with the client. Although the client may consider this condition a nuisance or a minimal problem that does not require medical attention, it can be an entry point for bacterial infections, especially in the elderly. Keeping athlete's foot under control is an important way to prevent cellulitis, a bacterial infection in the legs, and is especially important in the presence of diabetes (Halpern, 1993).

Other Parasitic Infections

Some parasitic infections of the skin are caused by insect and animal contacts. Contact with insects that puncture the skin for the purpose of sucking blood, injecting venom, or laying their eggs is relatively common. Substances deposited by insects are considered foreign to the host and may create an allergic sensitivity in that individual and produce pruritus, urticaria, or systemic reactions of a greater or lesser degree, depending on the individual's sensitivity.

Scabies (*Abrams et al., 1995*)

Definition. Scabies (mites) is an eruption caused by a mite, *Sarcoptes scabiei*. The female mite burrows into the skin and deposits eggs which hatch into larvae in a few days. Scabies are easily transmitted by skin-to-skin contact, from contact with contaminated objects such as linens, or sexually. Mites can spread rapidly between members of the same household, nursing home, or institution, but the inflammatory response and itching do not occur until approximately 30 to 60 days after initial contact.

Clinical Manifestations. The symptoms include intense pruritus (worse at night), usually excoriated skin, and the burrow, which is a linear ridge with a vesicle at one end. The mite is usually found in the burrow, commonly in the interdigital web spaces, flexor aspects of the wrist (volar surface), the axillae, waistline, on nipples in females, on genitalia in males, and the umbilicus. Intense scratching can lead to severe excoriation and secondary bacterial infection. Itching can become generalized secondary to sensitization.

Medical Management. The mite can be excavated from one end of a burrow with a needle or a scalpel blade and examined under a microscope. In longstanding cases, a mite may not be found. At that point treatment is based on a presumptive diagnosis.

Treatment with a scabicide, usually a lotion or cream containing permethrin or lindane, is applied to the entire body from the neck down. The client must understand that NO area can be missed. After 24 hours, the affected person should bathe. All bed linens and clothes must be laundered in hot water or dry-cleaned. Other household members and those in close contact with the affected person should be treated. A second application of the cream or lotion is applied 7 days later. The same procedure is followed. Itching may persist for 1 to 2 weeks post-treatment until the stratum corneum is replaced, but lesions on the forearms or legs can be occluded with Unna's boots to eliminate the scratch-itch cycle (Fig. 8–8). Widespread bacterial infections require additional treatment with systemic antibiotics.

Special Implications for the Therapist **8–6**

SCABIES

If a hospitalized person has scabies, prevent transmission to self and others by practicing good handwashing technique and by wearing gloves when touching the affected person. Observe wound and skin precautions for 24 hours after treatment of scabies. Gas-autoclave blood pressure cuffs or other equipment used with the affected person before using them on other people. All linens and toweling used must be isolated after use until the person is noninfectious. If treated anywhere outside the hospital room (e.g., on a plinth or treatment mat), the area must be thoroughly disinfected after each session.

Pediculosis (Lousiness)

Pediculosis is an infestation by *Pediculus humanus*, a very common parasite infecting the head, body, and genital area. Transmission is from one person to another, usually on shared personal items such as combs, lockers, clothes, or furniture. Lice are not carried or transmitted by pets. School-age children are easily infected as are people who live in overcrowded surroundings, and those elderly people who have poor personal hygiene, depend on others for care, or live in a nursing home.

Pediculus humanus var. *capitis*, the head louse, is transmitted through personal contact or through shared hairbrushes or shared headwear. Severe itching accompanied by secondary eczematous changes develop and small grayish or white nits (eggs) are usually seen attached to the base of the hairshafts.

Pediculus corporis, the body or clothes louse, produces intense itching which in turn results in severe excoriations from scratching and possible secondary bacterial infections. The lice or nits are generally found in the seams of the affected individual's clothing.

Pediculus pubis or *Phthirus pubis*, the pubis or crab louse, is usually transmitted by sexual contact, but can be transferred on clothing or towels. The lice and nits are usually found at the base of the pubic hairs. Sometimes dark-brown particles (louse excreta) may be seen on underclothes.

Medical Management. Treatment is with the appropriate cleaning solution (e.g., shampoo or soap) specific to the type of louse present. All combs and brushes should be soaked in the cleaning agent and clothing must be boiled, dry-cleaned, or washed in a machine (hot cycle). The seams of the clothing should be pressed with a hot iron. Carpets, car seats, pillows, stuffed animals, rugs, mattresses, upholstered furniture, and similar objects that come in contact with the affected person must be vacuumed or cleaned thoroughly with hot water and the cleaning agent. Any item that cannot be cleaned can be stored in sealed plastic bags for 2 to 3 weeks until all lice have been killed.

Special Implications for the Therapist **8–7**

PEDICULOSIS

The therapist must always be conscious of the personal hygiene of all clients. Anyone can get pediculosis regardless of age, socioeconomic status, or status of personal cleanliness. Wear gloves while carefully inspecting the head of any adult or child who scratches excessively. Look for bite marks, redness, and nits or movement that indicates a louse. If exposed to lice, treatment for the client as well as the therapist may be required depending on the exposure level. Use the same precautions outlined earlier for Scabies.

SKIN CANCER

The American Cancer Society (ACS) estimates that skin cancers are the most prevalent form of cancer, eventually

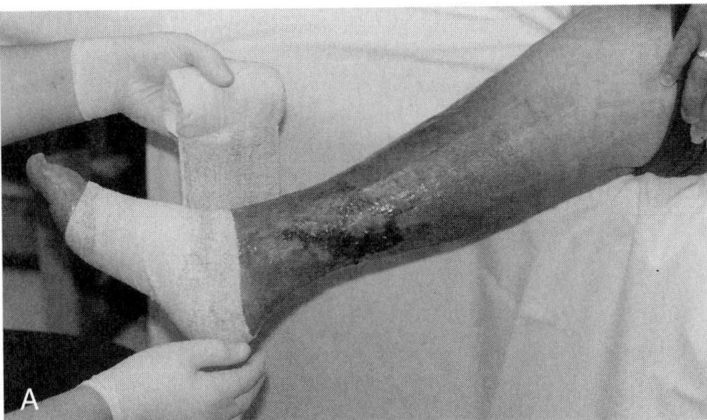

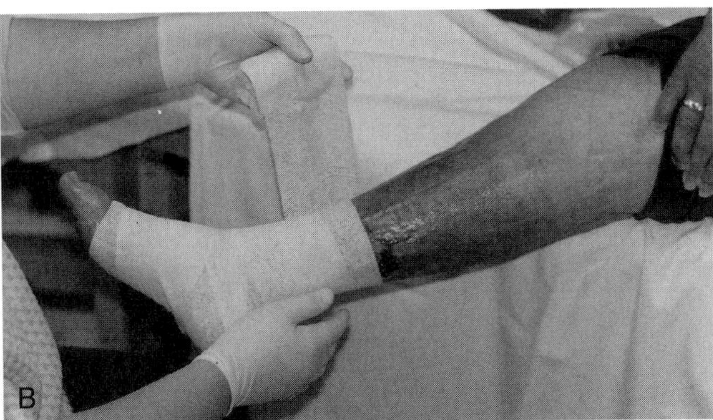

Figure **8–8.** Application of Unna's boot to the forearms or legs can be used with a variety of skin lesions to eliminate the scratch-itch cycle. Unna's boot is a dressing made of gauze impregnated with gelatin, zinc oxide, calamine, and glycerin. The bandage is applied in a spiral fashion and allowed to dry forming a rigid dressing. This dressing can be allowed to stay intact for 7 days. (*Courtesy of Pam Unger, P.T., Community General Hospital, Center for Wound Management, Reading, Pa, 1995.*)

affecting nearly all people older than 65 years of age. Skin cancer is the most rapidly increasing cancer in the United States with up to a million new cases of nonmelanoma skin cancer diagnosed annually in the United States. There is no evidence that this epidemic has peaked (Miller and Weinstock, 1994). Solar radiation (exposure to midrange wavelength ultraviolet B [UVB] radiation) causes most skin cancers and protection from the sun during the first two decades of life significantly reduces the risk of skin cancer (Box 8–5) (Ananthaswamy and Pierceall, 1992; Truhan, 1991). The melanoma rate is rising most rapidly in persons below age 40 and is now the most common cancer in women between the ages of 25 and 29, and second only to breast cancer in the age group from 30 to 34 (Rigel, 1993).

In this section, skin cancer is discussed in three broad categories: benign, premalignant, and malignant. Malignant lesions of the skin are considered as either melanoma or nonmelanoma. Kaposi's sarcoma, which occurs in the skin, is not included in these categories and is discussed separately (Table 8–4).

Benign skin lesions such as seborrheic keratosis, keratoacanthoma, or nevi (moles) do not usually undergo transition to malignant melanoma[3] and do not usually require treatment. Precancerous lesions such as actinic keratosis or Bowen's disease may progress to malignancy and must be carefully evaluated. The most common types of (nonmelanoma) malignant skin cancer are basal call carcinoma and squamous cell carcinoma. These carcinomas occur twice as often in men as in women, and the incidence increases steadily with age. A third type of malignant skin cancer, malignant melanoma, is the most serious skin cancer, resulting in early metastasis and possible death.

BOX **8–5**
Important Trends in Skin Cancer

Incidence
More than 500,000 cases a year with the majority being the highly curable basal or squamous cell cancers; not as common is the most serious malignant melanoma with an estimated 40,300 cases a year.

Mortality
Total estimated deaths in 1997 were 9490, 7300 from malignant melanoma, 2190 from other skin cancers.

Risk factors
Excessive exposure to ultraviolet radiation from the sun; fair complexion; occupational exposure to coal tar, pitch, creosote, arsenic compounds, and radium; skin cancer is negligible in blacks because of heavy skin pigmentation.

Warning signals
Any unusual skin condition, especially a change in the size or color of a mole or other darkly pigmented growth or spot.

Prevention and early detection
Avoidance of sun when ultraviolet light is strongest (e.g., between 10 AM and 3 PM); use sunscreen preparations, especially those containing ingredients such as PABA (para-aminobenzoic acid); basal and squamous cell skin cancers often form a pale, waxlike, pearly nodule, or a red, sharply outlined patch; melanomas are usually dark brown or black; they start as small molelike growths that increase in size, change color, become ulcerated, and bleed easily from a slight injury.

Treatment
There are four methods of treatment: surgery, electrodesiccation (tissue destruction by heat), radiation therapy, and cryosurgery (tissue destruction by freezing); for malignant melanomas, wide and often deep excisions and removal of nearby lymph nodes are required.

Survival
For basal cell and squamous cell cancers, cure is virtually assured with early detection and treatment; malignant melanoma, however, metastasizes quickly; this accounts for a lower 5-year survival rate for white people with this disease.

Modified from Huether SE, Kravitz M: Structure, function, and disorders of the integument. *In* McCance KL, Huether SE (eds): Pathophysiology: The Biologic Basis for Disease in Adults and Children, ed 2. St Louis, Mosby–Year Book, 1994, p 1541.

Benign Tumors

Seborrheic Keratosis

Seborrheic keratosis is a benign proliferation of basal cells occurring most frequently after middle age and presenting as multiple lesions on the chest, back, and face. The lesions often appear following hormonal therapy or inflammatory dermatoses. The areas are waxy, smooth, or raised lesions that vary in color from yellow to flesh tones to dark brown or black. Their size varies from barely palpable to large verrucous (wartlike) plaques. These tumors are usually left untreated unless they itch or cause pain. Otherwise, cryotherapy with liquid nitrogen is an effective treatment.

Nevi (Moles)

Nevi are pigmented or nonpigmented lesions that form from aggregations of melanocytes beginning early in life. Most moles are either brown, black, or flesh-colored and may appear on any part of the skin. They vary in size and thickness, occurring in groups or singly. Nevi seldom undergo transition to malignant melanoma, but as previously mentioned, when malignant melanoma does occur, it often arises from a preexisting mole; the chances of cancerous transformation are increased as a result of constant irritation. Any change in size, color, or texture of a mole; bleeding; or any excessive itching should be reported to a physician.

Precancerous Conditions

There are two common premalignant skin lesions: actinic keratosis and Bowen's disease.

Actinic Keratosis

Actinic (solar) keratosis is a well-defined, crusty, or sandpaper-like patch or bump that appears on chronically sun-exposed areas of the body (e.g., face, ears, lower lip, bald scalp, dorsa of hands and forearms). The base may be light

[3] Although most moles remain benign skin lesions, when malignant melanoma *does* occur, it often arises from a preexisting mole, derived from pigment cells (melanocytes) of the skin.

TABLE 8-4 Types of Skin Cancer

Benign	Premalignant	Nonmelanoma	Melanoma
Seborrheic keratosis	Actinic keratosis	Basal cell carcincoma	Superficial spreading melanoma
Nevi (moles)	Bowen's disease	Squamous cell carcinoma	Nodular melanoma
			Lentigo maligna melanoma
			Acral-lentiginous melanoma

or dark, tan, pink, red, or a combination of these, or it may be the same color as the skin. The scale or crust is horny, dry, and rough; it is often recognized by touch rather than sight. Occasionally it itches or produces a pricking or tender sensation. The skin abnormality or lesion develops slowly to reach a size that is most often from 3 to 6 mm. It may disappear only to reappear later. Often there are several actinic keratoses present at a time. This skin disorder is most common in fair-complexioned, middle-aged men with a history of sun exposure (solar radiation) (Amonette et al., 1993).

Actinic keratosis affects nearly 100% of the elderly white population. There is a small but definite risk of malignant degeneration and subsequent metastatic potential in neglected lesions. It is important that this condition be diagnosed properly as it is often difficult to distinguish a large or hypertrophic actinic keratosis from a squamous cell carcinoma. A biopsy may be indicated.

Not all keratoses need to be removed. The decision about treatment protocol is based on the nature of the lesion and the age and health of the affected person. Treatment may be with 5-fluorouracil (5-FU, Efudex), a topical antimetabolite that inhibits cell division, or masoprocol cream; cryosurgery using liquid nitrogen; or curettage by electrodesiccation (superficial tissue destruction through the use of bursts of electrical current). These clients should be advised to avoid sun exposure and use a high-potency (SPF 15+)[4] sunscreen 30 to 60 minutes before going outside. A recent study has indicated that a low fat diet can reduce the incidence of common precancerous skin lesions such as this one (Black et al., 1995).

Bowen's Disease

Bowen's disease can occur anywhere on the skin (exposed and unexposed areas) or mucous membranes (especially the glans penis in uncircumcised males). It presents as a persistent, brown to reddish-brown, scaly plaque with well-defined margins. Often the person has a history of arsenic exposure in youth. Multiple lesions have been associated with an increased number of internal malignancies and therefore require close follow-up (Abrams et al., 1995; Washington, 1994). Treatment is with surgical excision and topical 5-FU.

Malignant Neoplasms

Basal Cell Carcinoma

Definition and Overview. Basal cell carcinoma is a slow-growing surface epithelial skin tumor originating from undifferentiated basal cells contained in the epidermis. This type of carcinoma rarely metastasizes beyond the skin and does not invade blood or lymph vessels but can cause significant local destruction. Until recently, this tumor rarely appeared before age 40 and was more prevalent in blond, fair-skinned males. More recent research has indicated that in the age group under 30, more women than men develop skin cancer associated with the use of indoor tanning booths with concentrated doses of UV radiation (Dinehart, 1993).[5] It is the most common malignant tumor affecting whites, with a reported 100,000 new cases each year; blacks and Asians are rarely affected.

Etiology and Risk Factors. Prolonged sun exposure is the most common cause of basal cell carcinoma but arsenic ingestion (in drinking water, insecticides), UV radiation exposure, burns, immunosuppression, genetic predisposition, and rarely, the site of vaccinations are other possible causes (Norris et al., 1995). These lesions are seen most frequently in geographic regions with intense sunlight in people with outdoor occupations, and on those areas most exposed, the face and neck. Dark-skinned persons are rarely affected because their basal cells contain the pigment melanin, a protective factor against sun exposure.

Anyone who has had one basal cell carcinoma is at increased risk of developing others. Recurrences of previously treated lesions are possible, usually within the first 2 years after initial treatment.

Pathogenesis. The pathogenesis of basal cell tumors remains uncertain. One theory suggests that these tumors arise as a result of a defect that prevents the cells from being shed by the normal keratinization process. The process of epidermal cell maturation is called keratinization as the cells synthesize a fibrous protein called keratin. Basal cells that lack the normal keratin proteins form basal cell tumors. Another hypothesis is that undifferentiated basal cells become carcinomatous instead of differentiating into sweat glands, sebum, and hair.

Clinical Manifestations. Basal cell carcinoma (Fig. 8–9) typically has a pearly or ivory appearance, rolled edges, and is slightly elevated above the skin surface, with small blood vessels on the surface (telangiectasia) (see Fig. 8–2). The nodule is usually painless and slowly increases in size and may ulcerate centrally. More than 65% of basal cell carcinomas are found on the head and neck. Other locations are the trunk,

[4] SPF 30+ is recommended for people of fair complexion. Sunscreens are not recommended for infants under 6 months of age. Infants should be kept out of the sun or shaded from it. Fabric with a tight weave, such as cotton, is suggested.

[5] About 80% of indoor tanning patrons are women, with an average age of 26 (Dinehart, 1993).

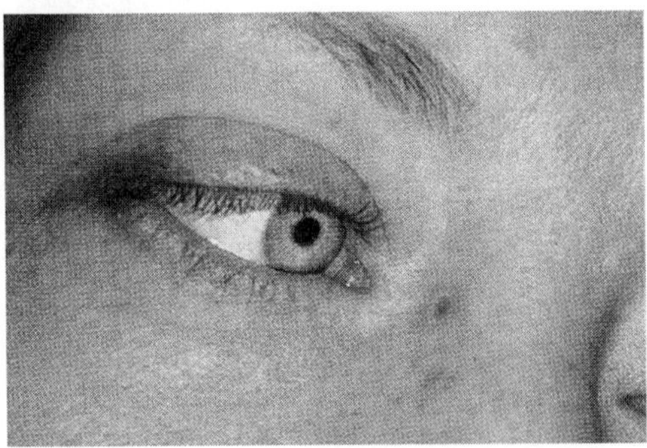

Figure **8-9.** Basal cell carcinoma can appear as a red patch; a shiny pearly or translucent pink, red, or white bump; a crusty, open sore that will not heal; or a scarlike area. There may be a rolled border with an indented center. (*From What You Need To Know About Skin Cancer. New York, Skin Cancer Foundation, 1993.*)

especially the upper back and chest. If these lesions are not detected and treated early, they may invade deep tissues and ulcerate (see Prognosis).

Medical Management

Diagnosis and Treatment. Diagnosis by clinical examination of appearance must be confirmed via biopsy and histologic study. Treatment depends on the size, location, and depth of the lesion and may include curettage and electrodesiccation, chemotherapy, surgical excision, Mohs' chemosurgery (serial application and removal of pathologic tissue using a fixative paste such as zinc chloride), and irradiation. Irradiation is used if the tumor location requires it and in elderly or debilitated people who can not tolerate surgery. Radiation therapy is generally contraindicated in persons less than 50 years of age, because of the risk of recurrence and the development of secondary radiation-induced tumors of the skin (Clark, 1994).

If the tumor is identified and treated early, local excision or even nonexcisional destruction is usually curative. Skin grafting may be required in cases where large areas of tissue have been removed. A new experimental treatment called photodynamic therapy (PDT) is being investigated in the treatment of superficial nonmelanoma skin cancers. This technique requires the administration of a drug that induces photosensitivity, followed in 48 to 72 hours by exposure to light that helps outline the tumor. The tumor cells concentrate this drug so as to allow selective destruction of the cancer cells when exposed to a laser light of 630 nanometers (nm) (Waldow et al., 1987; Clark, 1994). Clinical trials are underway investigating the use of vitamin A analogues called retinoids and the use of immunotherapy with interferon in skin cancer management.

Prognosis. If left untreated, basal cell lesions slowly invade surrounding tissues over months and years, destroying local tissues such as bone and cartilage, especially around the eyes, ears, and nose.

Squamous Cell Carcinoma

Definition and Overview. Squamous cell carcinomas are the second most common skin cancer in whites, usually arising in sun-damaged skin such as the rim of the ear, the face, the lips and mouth, and the dorsa of the hands (Fig. 8–10). It is a tumor of the epidermal keratinocytes and rarely occurs in dark-skinned people.

Squamous cell tumor may be one of two types: in situ (confined to the site of origin) and invasive (infiltrate surrounding tissue). *In situ* squamous cell carcinoma is usually confined to the epidermis but may extend into the dermis. Common premalignant skin lesions associated with in situ carcinomas are actinic keratosis and Bowen's disease (see earlier discussion). *Invasive* squamous cell carcinoma can arise from premalignant lesions of the skin, including sun-damaged skin, actinic dermatitis, scars, whitish discolored areas (leukoplakia), radiation-induced keratosis, tar and oil keratosis, and chronic ulcers and sinuses.

Incidence. As with basal cell carcinoma, fair-skinned people have a higher incidence of squamous cell carcinoma. This particular type of tumor has a peak incidence at 60 years of age and affects men more than women.

Etiology and Risk Factors. Predisposing factors associated with squamous cell carcinoma include overexposure to UV radiation (e.g., outdoor employment or residence in a warm, sunny climate), presence of premalignant lesions such as actinic keratosis or Bowen's disease, radiation therapy, ingestion of herbicides containing arsenic, chronic skin irritation and inflammation, exposure to local carcinogens (tar, oil), and hereditary disease such as xeroderma pigmentosum and albinism. Rarely, squamous cell carcinoma may develop on the site of a smallpox vaccination, psoriasis, or chronic discoid lupus erythematosus.

Pathogenesis. The exact mechanism for the development of squamous cell tumors is unknown. It remains unclear why UV light produces its harmful effects, but possibly it is because of problems in DNA synthesis, DNA repair, or DNA replication.

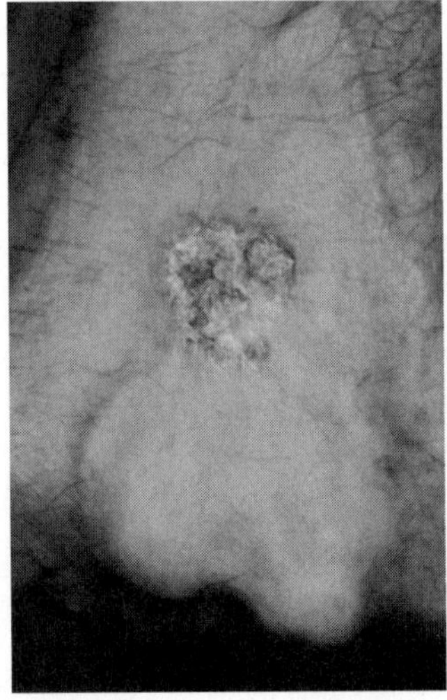

Figure **8-10.** Squamous cell carcinoma can take the form of a persistently scaly red patch that sometimes crusts or bleeds; an open sore that does not heal; or a raised or wartlike growth that may bleed. (*From What You Need To Know About Skin Cancer. New York, Skin Cancer Foundation, 1993.*)

Clinical Manifestations. Squamous cell lesions are more difficult to characterize than basal cell tumors. The squamous cell tumor has poorly defined margins as the edge blends into the surrounding sun-damaged skin. This type of carcinoma can present as an ulcer, a flat red area, a cutaneous horn, an indurated plaque, or a nodule. It may be red to flesh-colored surrounded by scaly tissue. More than 80% of squamous cell carcinomas occur in the head and neck region.

Usually lesions on unexposed skin tend to be more invasive and more likely to metastasize with the exception of lesions on the lower lip and ears. These sites tend to metastasize early, beginning with the process of induration and inflammation of the lesion. Metastasis can occur to the regional lymph nodes, producing characteristic systemic symptoms of pain, malaise, fatigue, weakness, and anorexia.

Medical Management

Diagnosis, Treatment, and Prognosis. An excisional biopsy provides definitive diagnosis and staging (Table 8–5) of squamous cell carcinoma. Other laboratory tests may be appropriate depending on the presence of systemic symptoms. The size, shape, location, and invasiveness of a squamous cell tumor and the condition of the underlying tissue determine the treatment method selected (see under Basal Cell Carcinoma; see also Box 8–5). A deeply invasive tumor may require a combination of techniques. As with all benign, premalignant, or malignant skin lesions, application of strong sunscreening agents containing para-aminobenzoic acid (PABA) is recommended for skin and lips 30 to 60 minutes prior to sun exposure. Wearing protective clothing (hat, tightly woven clothing, long sleeves) is also important.

All the major treatment methods have excellent rates of cure; generally, the prognosis is better with a well-differentiated lesion in an unusual location (Norris et al., 1995).

Malignant Melanoma

Definition and Overview. Malignant melanoma is a neoplasm of the skin originating from melanocytes or cells that synthesize the pigment melanin. The melanomas occur most frequently in the skin but can also be found in the oral cavity, esophagus, anal canal, vagina, meninges, or within the eye. The clinical varieties of cutaneous melanoma are classified into four types (Fig. 8–11):

1. *Superficial spreading melanoma* (SSM) is the most common type of melanoma and accounts for 75% of cutaneous melanomas.[6] SSM can occur on any part of the body, especially in areas of chronic irritation, the legs of females between the knees and ankles, or the upper back in both sexes. SSM is usually diagnosed in people between 20 and 60 years of age. It usually arises in a preexisting mole and presents as a brown or black raised patch with an irregular border and variable pigmentation (red, white, and blue, brown black, black blue). It is usually asymptomatic. With advanced lesions, itching and bleeding may occur.

2. *Nodular melanoma* can be found on any part of the body with no specific site preference. Men between 20 and 60 years of age are affected more often than women. It is often described as a small suddenly appearing but quickly enlarging, uniformly and darkly pigmented papule (may be grayish) accounting for approximately 12% of cutaneous melanomas. This type invades the dermis and metastasizes early.

3. *Lentigo maligna melanoma* (LMM) is a less common type of lesion occurring predominantly on sun-exposed areas, especially the head, neck, and dorsa of hands or under the fingernails in the 50- to 80-year-old age group, accounting for 6% to 10% of cutaneous melanomas. This lesion looks like a large (3 to 6 cm) flat freckle with an irregular border containing varied pigmentation of brown, black, blue black, red, and white found in a single lesion. These lesions enlarge and become progressively irregularly pigmented over time. Approximately one third develop into malignant melanoma and therefore bear careful watching.

4. *Acral-lentiginous melanoma* (ALM) is a relatively uncommon form of melanoma accounting for 5% of all cutaneous melanomas. It is the most common form of melanoma in dark-skinned people (e.g., Africans and Asians). These lesions usually have flat dark-brown portions with raised bumpy areas that are predominantly brown black or blue black. Most common areas include low-pigment sites where hair is absent, such as the palms of the hands, soles of the feet, nail beds of fingers and toes, and mucous membranes (Burstein and Sober, 1993).

Incidence. Malignant melanoma accounts for up to 3% of all cancers, currently affecting 1 in 75 people in the course of a lifetime (Friedman et al., 1991). Epidemiologists, who report that the incidence of melanoma is doubling every 10 to 20 years, call this a "melanoma epidemic" (Bellet et al., 1983; HWHW, 1994). The ACS reported 40,300 new cases of malignant melanoma in 1997 (ACS, 1997), accounting for 7300 deaths, more than from any other skin disorder.

Another study examined the mean number of annual malignant melanoma cases reported to dermatologists in each state and reported an estimated 80,000 new cases, much higher than currently published estimates (Salopek et al., 1995). The peak incidence is between 40 and 60 years, affect-

TABLE 8–5 STAGING OF SQUAMOUS CELL CARCINOMA

Primary tumor (T)	
TX	Primary tumor cannot be assessed
T0	No evidence of primary tumor
Tis	Carcinoma in situ
T1	Tumor ≤2 cm in greatest dimension
T2	Tumor >2 cm but not >5 cm in greatest dimension
T3	Tumor >5 cm in greatest dimension
T4	Tumor invades deep extradermal structures, i.e., cartilage, skeletal muscle or bone
Regional lymph nodes (N)	
NX	Regional lymph nodes cannot be assessed
N0	No regional lymph node metastasis
N1	Regional lymph node metastasis
Distant metastasis (M)	
MX	Presence of distant metastasis cannot be assessed
M0	No distant metastasis
M1	Distant metastasis

Modified from Beahrs OH (ed): American Joint Committee on Cancer (AJCC) Manual for Staging of Cancer, ed 4. Philadelphia, JB Lippincott, 1992.

[6] Percentages of each of the four classifications in this section were obtained from Bouffard et al. (1993).

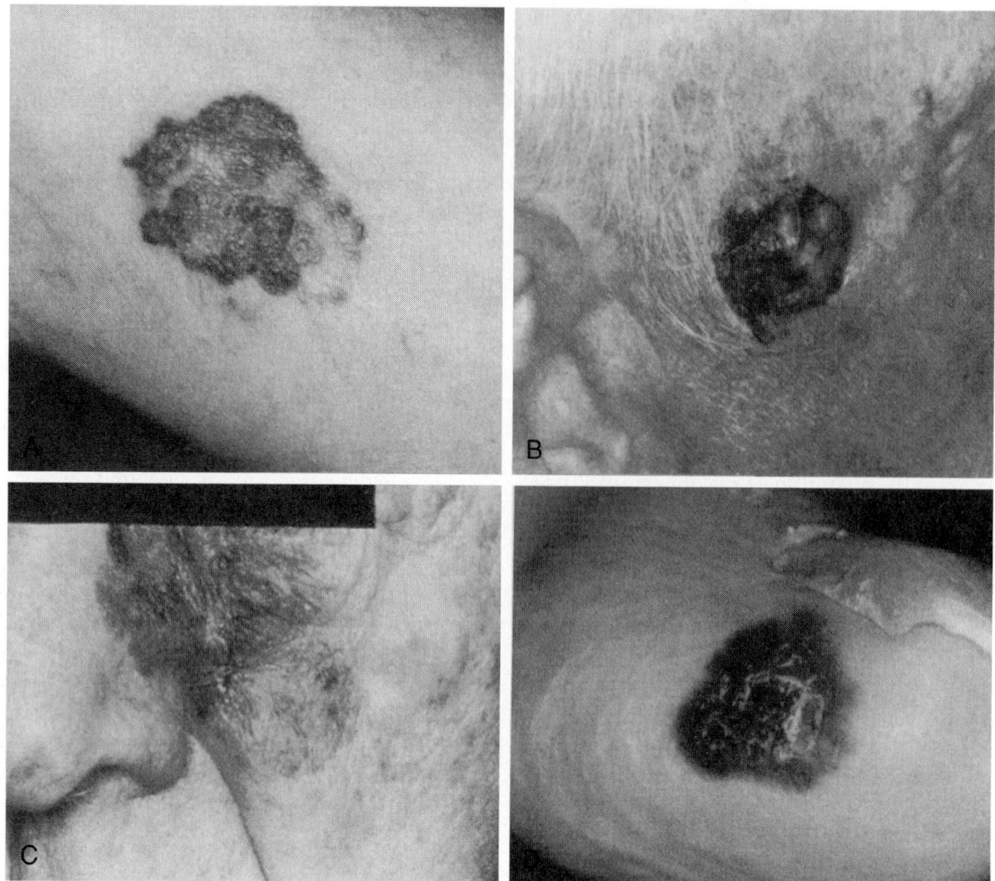

Figure **8-11.** *A*, Superficial spreading melanoma: an irregular margin with multiple colors of black, blue, pale red, and white may be seen. *B*, Nodular lesion of melanoma. *C*, Lentigo maligna: if left alone, progression to lentigo maligna melanoma occurs. *D*, Acral-lentiginous melanoma. (*Courtesy of Dr. Neil A. Fenske, Tampa, Fl.*) (*From Callen JP, Jorizzo J (eds): Dermatological Signs of Internal Disease, ed 2. Philadelphia, WB Saunders, 1995, pp 173–174.*)

ing women more than men but with a greater mortality rate among men (Geller et al., 1992; Vossaert et al., 1992). The incidence is rising in younger age groups but remains rare in children prior to adolescence.

Etiology and Risk Factors. Melanomas appear to be more prevalent among whites of high socioeconomic status (Pion et al., 1995) who take short vacations with intense sun exposure than in people who are at risk of chronic sun exposure. Most people who develop melanoma have blond or red hair, fair skin, and blue eyes; are prone to sunburn; and are of Celtic or Scandinavian ancestry (Box 8–6). Studies have indicated that not only UVB radiation (280 to 320 nm) but UVA (320 to 400 nm) radiation, the type produced by sun lamps, may promote skin cancer. For these reasons, tanning parlors should also be considered a significant risk factor for the development of skin cancer.

Other causative factors implicated in the development of melanoma include genetic predisposition and steroid hormone activity. Melanoma occurs more often within families and among people who have dysplastic nevus syndrome, also known as the atypical mole syndrome (AMS). This is a familial disorder that results in a large number of irregular moles that have an almost 50% chance of developing melanoma during the person's lifetime (Kruger et al., 1992; Marghoob et al., 1994; Schneider et al., 1994). Puberty and pregnancy may enhance growth. Previous history of melanoma places the individual at greater risk of developing a second melanoma.

Pathogenesis. UV radiation continues to be one of the most important causes of malignant melanoma as the sun's UV rays damage the DNA inside the nuclei of the epidermal cells, triggering enzymes to repair the damage. The majority of malignant melanomas appear to be associated with the

BOX **8-6**
Risk Factors for the Development of Malignant Melanoma

- Family history of malignant melanoma
- Presence of blond or red hair
- Presence of marked freckling on the upper back
- History of three or more blistering sunburns prior to age 20 yr
- History of 3 or more years of an outdoor summer job during adolescence
- Presence of actinic keratosis (sharply outlined horny growth)

Modified from Friedman RJ, Rigel DS, Silverman MK, et al: Malignant melanoma in the 1990s. CA Cancer J Clin 41:201–225, 1991.

intensity rather than the duration of sunlight exposure. UV radiation gives rise to a tanning response by introducing lesions in the skin's cellular DNA. The majority of these lesion are excised, disposed of, and successfully corrected by the repair enzymes. DNA repair enzymes may issue the key signal for tanning after UV damage by speeding up production of the UV-absorbing pigment melanin, which erects a dark barrier meant to block sunlight from further destroying DNA. In other words, tanning is the body's attempt to protect against sun damage by UV radiation. The more UV damage to be repaired, the darker the tan (Gilchrest, 1995; Gilchrest et al., 1993).

We differ in our ability to produce repair enzymes which may explain our differences in tanning ability as well as susceptibility to skin cancer. Not all DNA lesions are properly repaired, increasing the risk of skin cancer. Melanomas arise as a result of malignant degeneration of melanocytes located either along the basal layer of the epidermis or in a benign melanocytic nevus (mole or aggregation of melanocytes). These clusters of cells may not be apparent until puberty, when the pigmentation process is initiated by steroid hormones. Malignant growth occurs horizontally along the epidermis (outer layer of skin) before invading the underlying dermis.

Clinical Manifestations. Melanoma can appear anywhere on the body, not just on sun-exposed areas. Common sites are the head and neck in men, the legs in women, and the backs of people exposed to excessive UV radiation. Up to 70% arise from a preexisting nevus. Any change in a skin lesion or nevus (increased size; bleeding; soreness or inflammation; changes in color, pigmentation, or texture) must be examined for melanoma.

Medical Management

Diagnosis. Early recognition of cutaneous melanomas can have a major impact on the surgical cure of this disease. The ACS suggests a monthly self-examination. A skin biopsy with histologic examination can distinguish malignant melanoma from other lesions, determine tumor thickness, and provide staging (Table 8–6; Fig. 8–12). Depending on the depth of the tumor invasion and metastatic spread, other testing procedures may include baseline laboratory studies, a bone scan for metastasis, or computed tomography (CT) scan for metastasis to the chest, abdomen, CNS, and brain.

Treatment. Surgical resection to remove the tumor is necessary when the diagnosis of malignant melanoma has been established. Surgical excision of the primary lesion site may be accompanied by removal of regional lymph nodes (regional lymphadenectomy). Neither cryosurgery with liquid nitrogen nor electrodesiccation are used to treat melanoma, although they are among the acceptable procedures for squamous cell and basal cell tumors.

Deep primary lesions may warrant adjuvant chemotherapy and biotherapy to eliminate or reduce the number of tumor cells, but there is no role at present for chemotherapy or radiation therapy as the initial treatment. Radiation therapy is used for metastatic disease to reduce tumor size and provide palliative relief from painful symptoms; it does not prolong survival time.

Other more investigational techniques may include treatments to boost the immune system such as injecting the tumor with the vaccinia virus, or bacille Calmette-Guérin (BCG), an attenuated strain of the bacterium that is the primary cause of tuberculosis in cattle, which causes tumor regression by stimulating an immune response. There has also been some success with levamisole, an oral immune system stimulant, and with immunotherapy in which the person's own lymphocytes are removed, cultivated in laboratory cultures with the immune-stimulating protein interleukin-2 (IL-2), and returned intravenously (IV) with more IL-2 (HWHW, 1994; Ho, 1995; Barth and Morton, 1995). In addition to immunotherapy to stimulate the immune system, research to treat people with a vaccine made from their own cancer cells is underway.[7] This antimelanoma immunization may be available for high-risk individuals within the next 5 years (Sato et al., 1995; Berd et al., 1993).

Prognosis. The prognosis for all types of melanoma depends primarily on the tumor's depth of invasion, not on the histologic type, that is, the more superficial or "thin" the tumor, the better the prognosis. For example, melanoma lesions less than 0.76 mm deep have an excellent prognosis (5-year survival rate is 90%), whereas deeper lesions (more than 0.76 mm) are at risk for metastasis (5-year survival rate with local metastasis is 55%; 14% when distant metastases are present) (HWHW, 1994). Metastases, usually to the brain, lungs, bones, liver, skin, and CNS are universally fatal, usually within 1 year (Balch et al., 1992).

Prognosis is better for a tumor on an extremity that is drained by one lymphatic network than for one on the head, neck, or trunk, drained by several lymphatic networks. Tumors can recur more than 5 years after primary surgery, requiring close long-term medical follow-up. Education on the effects of UVB exposure can dramatically reduce the incidence of skin cancer.

Special Implications for the Therapist **8–8**

MALIGNANT MELANOMA

During observation and inspection of any client, the therapist should be alert to the potential signs of skin cancer. Therapists should not become overly concerned about small pink spots on the client's skin, as other common skin conditions such as eczema, psoriasis, and seborrheic dermatitis are prevalent in more than half of all people at some time in their lives. Therapists should look for abnormal spots, especially in sun-exposed areas, that are rough in texture, persistently present, and bleed on minimal contact or with minimal friction.*

As discussed in the text, *any* change in a wart or mole (color, size, shape, texture, ulceration, bleeding, itching) should be inspected by a physician. The Skin Cancer Foundation advocates the use of the ABCD method of early detection of melanoma and dysplastic (abnormal in size or shape) moles (Box 8–7). Other signs and symptoms that may be important include

[7] Currently the vaccine must be made from the affected person's own tumor cells, requiring a large tumor to produce the vaccine. Laboratory scientists are working to identify the peptides that trigger the antiimmune response in the vaccine and then synthesizing it to make a more easily reproducible vaccine.

TABLE 8-6 Staging of Malignant Melanoma*

Primary tumor (pT)	
pTX	Primary tumor cannot be assessed
pT0	No evidence of primary tumor
pTis	Melanoma in situ (atypical melanocytic hyperplasia, severe melanocytic dysplasia, not an invasive lesion (Clark's level I)
pT1	Tumor ≤0.75 mm in thickness and invades the papillary dermis (Clark's level II)
pT2	Tumor >0.75 mm but not >1.5 mm in thickness or invades to papillary-reticular dermal interface (Clark's level III)
pT3	Tumor >1.5 mm but not >4 mm in thickness or invades reticular dermis (Clark's level IV)
pT3a	Tumor >1.5 mm but not >3 mm in thickness
pT3b	Tumor >3 mm but not >4 mm in thickness
pT4	Tumor >4 mm in thickness or invades subcutaneous tissue (Clark's level V) or satellite(s) within 2 cm of primary tumor
pT4a	Tumor >4 mm in thickness or invades subcutaneous tissue
pT4b	Satellite(s) within 2 cm of primary tumor
Regional lymph nodes (N)	
NX	Regional lymph nodes cannot be assessed
N0	No regional lymph node metastasis
N1	Metastasis ≤3 cm in greatest dimension in any regional lymph node(s)
N2	Metastasis >3 cm in greatest dimension in any regional lymph node(s) or in-transit metastasis
N2a	Metastasis >3 cm in greatest dimension in any regional lymph node(s)
N2b	In-transit metastasis
N2c	Both (N2a and N2b)
Distant metastasis (M)	
MX	Presence of distant metastasis cannot be assessed
M0	No distant metastasis
M1	Distant metastasis
M1a	Metastasis in skin or subcutaneous tissue or lymph node(s) beyond regional lymph nodes
M1b	Visceral metastasis

* Several systems exist for staging malignant melanoma, including the TNM (tumor, node, metastasis) system, developed by the American Joint Committee on Cancer, and Clark's system, which classifies tumor progression according to skin layer penetration (see Fig. 8–12).
Modified from Beahrs OH (ed): American Joint Committee on Cancer (AJCC) Manual for Staging of Cancer, ed 4. Philadelphia, JB Lippincott, 1992.

irritation and itching; tenderness, soreness, or new moles developing around the mole in question; or a sore that keeps crusting and does not heal within 6 weeks. For any client with a previous history of skin cancer, emphasize the need for continued close follow-up to detect recurrence early. Education on the effects of UV radiation and taking precautions (Box 8–8) can dramatically reduce the incidence of skin cancer.

If surgery included lymphadenectomy, the therapist may be involved in minimizing lymphedema or treating

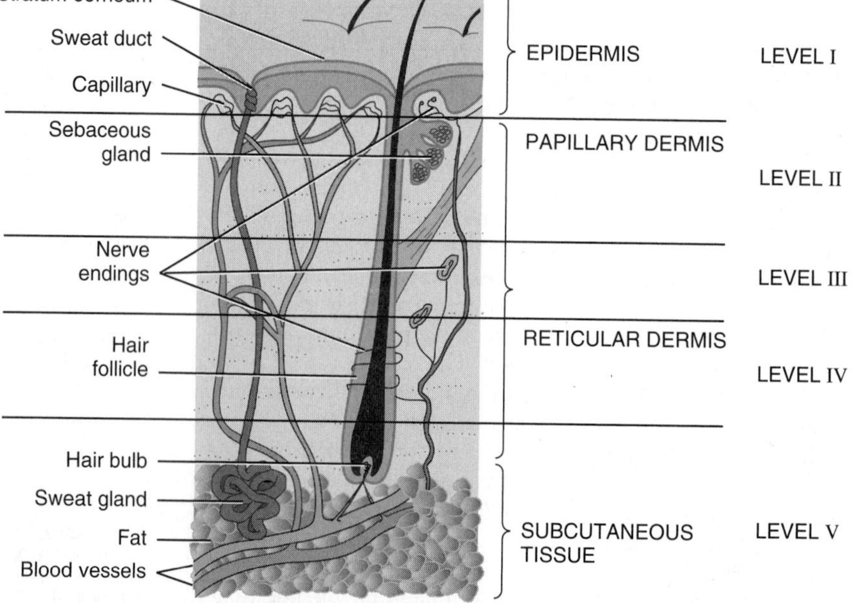

Figure **8–12.** Clark's levels, a system of classifying tumor progression according to skin layer penetration.

BOX **8–7**
ABCD Method of Early Melanoma Detection

A: *asymmetry*: Uneven edges, lopsided in shape, one half unlike the other
B: *border*: Irregularity, irregular edges scalloped or poorly defined edges
C: *color*: Black, shades of brown, red, white, occasionally blue
D: *diameter*: Larger than a pencil eraser

residual lymphedema (see Lymphedema, Chapter 10). Wound care may involve care of a skin graft and the associated donor site; the graft may be as painful as the tumor excision site and just as much at risk for infection. Universal precautions (see Appendix A) are essential for the postoperative as well as immunosuppressed client.

For the dying client, hospice care may include pain control and management. It is important that pain relief not be delayed until after it occurs but rather that a schedule of analgesia to prevent pain or to prevent an increase in pain levels be instituted.

* Keep in mind that seborrheic keratosis commonly bleeds; once diagnosed, this bleeding should not cause undue alarm.

Kaposi's Sarcoma

Definition and Incidence. Kaposi's sarcoma (KS) is a malignancy of angiopoietic tissue that presents as a skin disorder. Until recently, this tumor was most commonly seen in elderly people of central European origin, especially men of Jewish or Italian ancestry (now referred to as *classic* KS). The growth of this tumor is promoted by AIDS-associated immunodeficiency and the incidence has risen dramatically along with the incidence of AIDS (*epidemic* KS) (Safai, 1987). KS may also occur in kidney transplant recipients taking immunosuppressive drugs.

Etiology and Pathogenesis. The endothelial cell is thought to be the cell of origin of KS and genetic or hereditary predisposition may be a factor in the classic form. Immunosuppression allows for opportunistic infection and malignancy in the epidemic type. Among the people who develop AIDS, KS is seen almost exclusively among homosexual men. If a person contracts AIDS as a result of IV drug use or from a transfusion, the chance of developing KS is less than 2%. Recent research has confirmed that epidemic KS is caused by a herpesvirus infection (Roizman, 1995; Cesarman et al., 1995; Moore and Chang, 1995).

BOX **8–8**
Guidelines for Prevention of Skin Cancer

1. Avoid peak hours of sunlight
2. Wear close-woven protective clothing
3. Use a sunscreen of SPF 15 or higher
4. Teach children sun protection
5. Do not work on getting a tan
6. Do not patronize tanning salons
7. Examine your skin regularly
8. If you notice any changes, see your physician promptly

From the Skin Cancer Foundation. Skin Cancer: Preventable and Curable (film). New York, Author, 1990.

Clinical Manifestations. This neoplasm occurs commonly on the lower extremities and the affected areas are red, purple, or dark-blue macules (Fig. 8–13) which slowly enlarge to become nodules or ulcers. Itching and pain in the lesions that impinge on nerves or organs may occur and as the sarcoma progresses causing lymphatic obstruction, the legs become edematous. The lesions may spread by metastasis through the upper body to the face and oral mucosa.

The tumor may be the first manifestation of AIDS and can involve the gastrointestinal tract, lungs, and lymph nodes. Systemic involvement may present with one or more signs and symptoms, including weight loss (10% of body weight), fever of unknown origin that exceeds 100° F (37.8° C) for more than 2 weeks, chills, night sweats, lethargy, anorexia, and diarrhea.

Medical Management. Diagnosis is by skin biopsy that identifies the lesion type and stage. A CT scan may be performed to detect and evaluate possible metastasis. Treatment is not indicated for all people. Indications for excision of local lesions may include painful or obstructive lesions. Systemic lesions are treated with a combination of biotherapy with interferon-α-2b, cytotoxic agents, and radiation. These treatment measures reduce the number of skin lesions but have no effect on advanced disease. General response to treatment is poor, but the 2-year survival rate is better in persons with KS alone than in those with KS and an opportunistic infection. See discussion of AIDS in Chapter 5.

Special Implications for the Therapist **8–9**
KAPOSI'S SARCOMA

The KS skin lesions in the AIDS client are not contagious and the health care provider need have no fear of transmission of KS or HIV through daily contact with the client. Universal precautions must be followed whenever providing care for clients with KS to prevent the spread of infection to the client. Prevention of skin breakdown and wound care are the usual focus of treatment. Clients receiving radiation therapy must keep the irradiated skin dry to avoid possible breakdown and subsequent infection (see Special Implications for the Therapist: Radiation Injuries, Chapter 4).

SKIN DISORDERS ASSOCIATED WITH IMMUNE DYSFUNCTION

Psoriasis

Definition and Incidence. Psoriasis is a chronic, inherited, recurrent inflammatory dermatosis characterized by well-defined erythematous plaques covered with a silvery scale

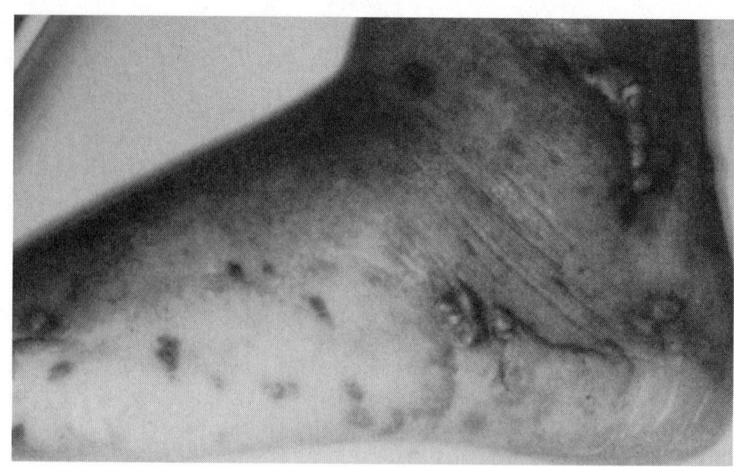

Figure 8–13. Classic Kaposi's sarcoma is present as typical nodular lesions on this ankle and foot. (*From Callen JP, Jorizzo J (eds): Dermatological Signs of Internal Disease, ed 2. Philadelphia, WB Saunders, 1995, p 161.*)

(Fig. 8–14). Psoriasis occurs equally in both sexes and most commonly in young adults (mean age of onset is 27 years of age) but can occur at any age. Although psoriasis can occur in infancy, it is uncommon in children under the age of 6 years. It is uncommon among blacks but affects 1% to 2% of the white population.

Etiology and Risk Factors. The cause of psoriasis is unknown but it appears to be hereditary, that is, the tendency to develop psoriasis is genetically determined. Researchers have discovered a significantly higher than normal incidence of certain human leukocyte antigens (HLAs) in families with psoriasis, suggesting a possible immune disorder. Precipitating factors include trauma, infection (especially β-hemolytic streptococci), pregnancy, and endocrine changes. Cold weather and severe anxiety or emotional stress tend to aggravate psoriasis. Flare-ups are often related to specific systemic and environmental factors, but may be unpredictable.

Pathogenesis. Normally, the life cycle of a skin cell is 28 days: 14 days to move from the basal layer to the stratum corneum and 14 days of normal wear and tear before the cell is sloughed off. In contrast, the turnover time of psoriatic skin is 3 to 4 days. This shortened cycle does not allow time for the cell to mature, resulting in a thick and flaky stratum corneum which in turn produces the cardinal manifestations of psoriasis.

Clinical Manifestations. Psoriasis appears as erythematous papules and plaques covered with silvery scales. The lesions in ordinary cases have a predilection for the scalp, chest, nails, elbows, knees, and buttocks. The occurrence may vary from a solitary lesion to countless patches covering large areas of the body in a symmetrical pattern. Two clearly distinguishing features are the tendency for this condition to recur and to persist. Lesions that develop at the site of a previous injury are known as *Koebner's phenomenon*.

The most common subjective complaint is itching and, occasionally, pain from dry, cracked, encrusted lesions. In approximately 30% of cases, psoriasis spreads to the fingernails, producing small indentations and yellow or brown discoloration. In severe cases, the accumulation of thick, crumbly debris under the nail causes it to separate from the nailbed (nail dystrophy).

Approximately 15% to 20% of people with psoriasis develop arthritic symptoms referred to as psoriatic arthritis (PsA) (see Chapter 23). PsA usually affects one or more joints of the fingers or toes, or sometimes the sacroiliac joints,

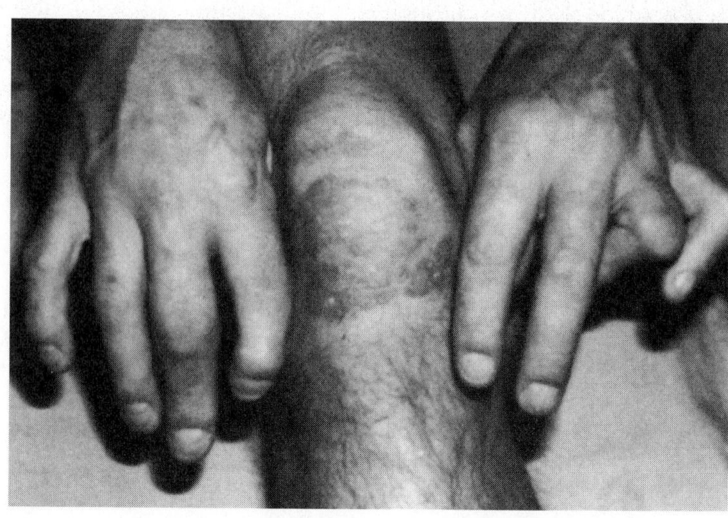

Figure 8–14. Deforming asymmetrical oligoarticular (affecting only a few areas) arthritis of the hands in a person with plaque psoriasis of the knee. (*From Callen JP, Jorizzo J (eds): Dermatological Signs of Internal Disease, ed 2. Philadelphia, WB Saunders, 1995, p 44.*)

and may progress to spondylitis. These clients report morning stiffness that lasts more than 30 minutes. Joint symptoms show no consistent linkage to the course of the cutaneous manifestations of psoriasis but rather demonstrate remissions and exacerbations similar to those of rheumatoid arthritis. No other systemic effects of psoriasis have been reported (Norris et al., 1995).

Medical Management

Diagnosis. Diagnosis depends on the previous history, clinical presentation, and, if needed, skin biopsy. Typically, the serum uric acid level is elevated due to accelerated nucleic acid degradation, but without the corresponding gout usually associated with increased uric acid levels. Psoriasis must be distinguished from eczema, seborrheic dermatitis, and lichen-like papules.

Treatment *(Beck and Morison, 1994).* There is no cure for psoriasis but treatment options exist that adequately suppress the disease process and sometimes provide a short period of remission. Various forms of local or systemic treatment routinely offered fall into five general categories: (1) topical preparations, (2) phototherapy, (3) vitamin A analogues, (4) antimetabolites, and (5) 5-lipoxygenase inhibitors. Topical therapeutic agents include corticosteroids; occlusive ointments (e.g., petroleum jelly, salicylic acid preparations, urea-containing topical ointments); oatmeal baths, emollients, and open wet dressings to relieve pruritus; and tar preparations.

Corticosteroids are the most commonly prescribed therapy for psoriasis but it should be noted that the incidence of side effects has increased with the use of the superpotent fluorinated preparations. Only weak preparations, such as 0.5% or 1.0% hydrocortisone should be used on the face, perineum, or other sensitive areas (e.g., the flexor surfaces of the arms, abdomen).[8] Crude *coal tar*, one of the oldest remedies for psoriasis, is assumed to work by an antimitotic effect (helps retard rapid cell production). This treatment consists of the daily application of 2% to 5% crude coal tar combined with a tar bath and UV light.[9] Exposure to UV light (*phototherapy*), such as UVB or natural sunlight, also helps retard rapid cell production. Widespread involvement may improve with whole-body irradiation with UV light. PUVA refers to the combination of an orally administered photosensitizing drug (Psoralen) plus exposure to 1 to 1½ hours of UVA radiation. It is more effective for thick plaque-type psoriasis, pustular psoriasis, and generalized erythroderma.[10]

Other treatment regimens include the retinoid etretinate (Tegison), methotrexate, a folic acid antagonist used in severe cases to inhibit DNA synthesis, and other antimitotic medications such as hydroxyurea and azathioprine; sulfasalazine (Azulfidine), a 5-lipoxygenase inhibitor; aspirin and local heat to alleviate the pain of PsA; physical and occupational therapy geared toward functional outcome; and nonsteroidal anti-inflammatory drugs (NSAIDs) for severe cases.

Prognosis. Psoriasis usually recurs at intervals and lasts for increasingly longer periods. Spontaneous cure is uncommon and the risk of infection is high owing to the greater than normal amounts of staphylococci present on psoriatic plaques. People with psoriasis who are human immunodeficiency virus (HIV)–positive are at high risk of infection from self-inoculation. As many as 20% of clients who develop PsA may sustain early and severe joint damage with accompanying deformity and disability (Gladman et al., 1987).

Special Implications for the Therapist **8–10**

PSORIASIS

Steroid cream application must be in a thin film, rubbed gently into the skin until all the cream disappears. All topical medications, especially those containing anthralin and tar, should be applied with a downward motion to avoid rubbing them into the hair follicles causing inflammation (folliculitis). Apply medication only to the affected lesions, avoiding contact with normal surrounding skin.

Gloves must be worn when applying the cream since anthralin stains and injures the skin. After application, the client must dust himself or herself with powder to prevent anthralin from rubbing off on the clothes. Mineral oil followed by soap and water can be used to remove the anthralin; the skin should never be rubbed vigorously, but a soft brush can be used to remove the scales.

Any side effects, especially allergic reactions to anthralin, atrophy and acne from steroids, and burning, itching, and nausea, must be reported to the physician immediately. Squamous cell epitheliomas may develop from PUVA. Cytotoxins from methotrexate therapy may cause hepatic or bone marrow toxicity.

Psoriatic Arthritis

Clinically, PsA differs from rheumatoid arthritis in the more frequent involvement of the distal interphalangeal joints, asymmetrical distribution of affected joints, presence of spondyloarthropathy (including the presence of both sacroiliitis and spondylitis), and characteristic extra-articular features (e.g., psoriatic skin lesions, iritis, mouth ulcers, urethritis, colitis, aortic valve disease). Joints are less tender in PsA, which may lead to underestimation of the degree of inflammation (Buskila et al., 1992). Pain and stiffness of inflamed joints is usually increased by prolonged immobility and alleviated by physical activity. Evidence of inflammation is pain on stressing the joint, tenderness at the joint line, and the presence of effusions (Mader and Gladman, 1993; Gladman et al., 1990; see also Rheumatic Disorders, Chapter 23).

Psychological Considerations

Psoriasis can result in psychological problems because the skin lesions may cause the person to feel contagious and "untouchable." Additionally, the smell of some topical preparations and the stain may add to the psychological reaction. Assure the client that psoriasis is not contagious. Flare-ups can be controlled with

[8] The major concerns with all corticosteroid preparations are dermal atrophy, skin fragility, fast relapse times, and in rare cases, adrenal suppression resulting from systemic absorption (Beck and Morison, 1994). See also Corticosteroids, Chapter 4.

[9] The disadvantages of this treatment are the extended time commitments required by the client and the associated mess. More recently, the use of liquor carbonis detergens (LCD) has replaced the use of crude coal tar (Beck and Morison, 1994).

[10] PUVA also has its disadvantages as a treatment option, including premature skin aging, nonmelanoma skin and other cancers, and premature cataract formation. This type of therapy is contraindicated in pregnancy (Beck and Morison, 1994).

treatment and stress control can help prevent recurrences.

Lupus Erythematosus

Definition. Lupus erythematosus is a chronic inflammatory disorder of the connective tissues. It appears in several forms, including discoid lupus erythematosus (DLE), which affects only the skin, and systemic lupus erythematosus (SLE), which affects multiple organ systems including the skin and can be fatal (see Chapter 5). *Lupus* is the Latin word for wolf, referring to the belief in the 1800s that the skin erosion of this disease was caused by a wolf bite. The characteristic rash of lupus is red, hence erythematosus (Matassarin-Jacobs, 1993).

Discoid Lupus Erythematosus

Definition. DLE is marked by chronic skin eruptions that if left untreated can lead to scarring and permanent disfigurement.

Incidence and Etiology. It is estimated that approximately 60% of persons with DLE are women in their late 20s or older. Approximately 1 in 20 persons with DLE later develop SLE. The disease is rare in children. The exact cause of DLE is unknown, but evidence suggests an autoimmune defect. There appears to be interrelated immunologic, environmental, hormonal, and genetic factors involved.

Risk Factors and Pathogenesis. Clients with DLE should avoid prolonged exposure to the sun, fluorescent lighting, or reflected sunlight. They are encouraged to wear protective clothing, use sunscreening agents, and avoid engaging in outdoor activities during periods of intense sunlight. Just how the sun causes skin rash flare-ups remains unknown. One theory is that the DNA of people with lupus, when exposed to sunlight, becomes more antigenic (able to induce a specific immune response). This antigenicity causes accelerated antigen-antibody reactions and thus more deposition of immune complexes in the skin at the dermal-epidermal junction. The photosensitivity is most commonly associated with lupus erythematosus and not other rheumatologic diseases.

Clinical Manifestations. DLE lesions are raised, red, scaling plaques with follicular plugging and central atrophy. The raised edges and sunken centers give them a coinlike appearance (Fig. 8–15). Although these lesions can appear anywhere on the body, they usually erupt on the face, scalp, ears, neck, and arms or any part of the body that is exposed to the sunlight. Hair tends to become brittle or may fall out in patches. Facial plaques sometimes assume the classic butterfly pattern with lesions appearing on the cheeks and the bridge of the nose. The rash may vary in severity from a sunburned appearance to discoid (plaquelike) lesions (Arnold et al., 1990; Norris et al., 1995).

Medical Management

Diagnosis, Treatment, and Prognosis. The client history and appearance of the rash itself are diagnostic. Skin biopsy of the lesions may be performed. Skin rashes occur in 74% of cases of SLE (Lahita, 1992). The client must report any changes in the lesions to the attending physician. Drug treatment consists of topical, intralesional, or systemic medication, as in SLE. The lesions can resolve completely or may cause hypo- or hyperpigmentation, atrophy, and scarring.

Systemic Lupus Erythematosus

Systemic lupus erythematosus is a chronic, systemic, inflammatory disorder of the connective tissues which affects multiple organs, including the skin, joints, kidneys, heart, blood-forming organs, nervous system, and serous membranes (membranes lining the walls of the body cavities and enclosing contained organs).

Symptoms commonly include malaise, overwhelming fatigue, arthralgia, fever, arthritis, skin rashes, photosensitivity, anemia, hair loss, Raynaud's phenomenon (fingers turning white or blue in response to temperature changes), and urologic symptoms associated with kidney involvement.

The most recognized skin manifestation of SLE is the

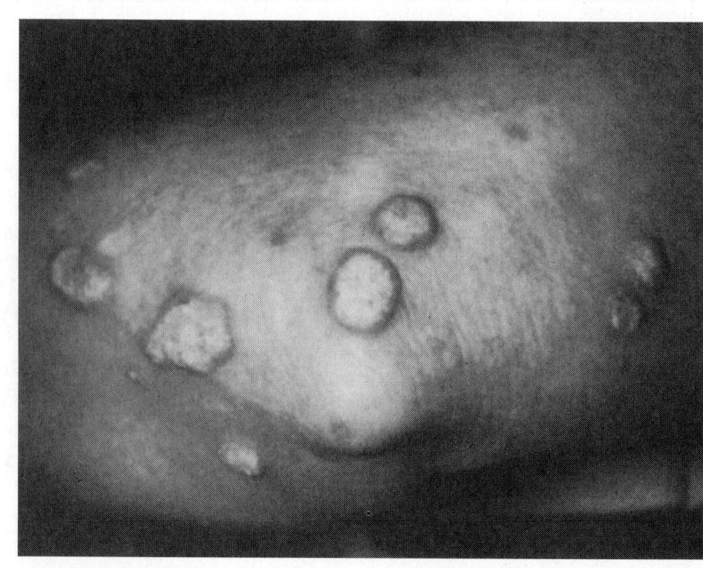

Figure **8–15.** Wartlike lesions referred to as hypertrophic lupus erythematosus present in a person with typical discoid lupus erythematosus (DLE). They simulate warts, keratoacanthoma (benign, crater-like papular lesion), or squamous cell carcinoma. (*From Callen JP, Jorizzo J (eds): Dermatological Signs of Internal Disease, ed 2. Philadelphia, WB Saunders, 1995, p 5.*)

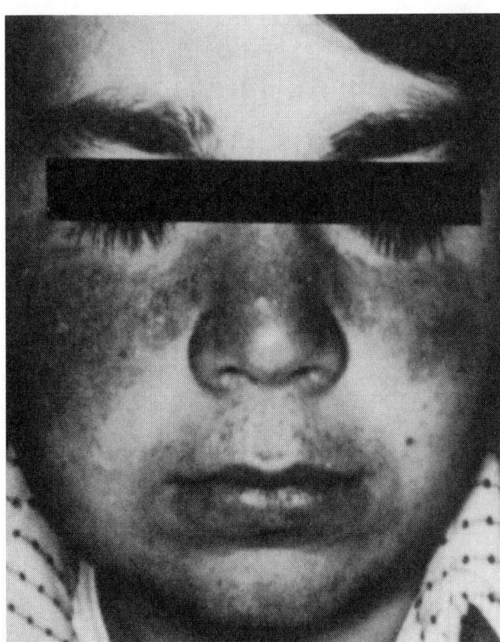

Figure **8–16.** Butterfly rash of systemic lupus erythematosus across the bridge of the nose and the cheeks. (*From Callen JP, Jorizzo J (eds): Dermatological Signs of Internal Disease, ed 2. Philadelphia, WB Saunders, 1995, p 9.*)

classic butterfly rash over the nose and cheeks (Fig. 8–16) commonly precipitated by exposure to sunlight (UV rays). This classic rash over the nose and cheeks occurs in up to 81% of affected people (Gladman and Urowitz, 1993). Other skin manifestations may point to the presence of vasculitis (inflammation of cutaneous blood vessels) leading to infarctive lesions in the digits (see Fig. 4–1), necrotic leg ulcers, or digital gangrene (Arnold et al., 1990).

The medical management of SLE is discussed in Chapter 5. Skin lesions require topical treatment, maintaining an optimal wound environment (moist enough to allow tissue healing, but not swamplike) while preventing further deterioration or infection. Most often, topical corticosteroid creams are used. The disease process can cause loss of skin integrity and subsequent loss of function. The survival rate has improved dramatically in recent years although death can occur from renal failure when there is kidney involvement causing progressive changes in the glomeruli, cardiac involvement with deposition of immune complexes in the coronary vessels, myocardium, and pericardium, or cerebral infarct.

Special Implications for the Therapist **8–11**

LUPUS ERYTHEMATOSUS

Clients with DLE or SLE with skin involvement require careful assessment, supportive measures, and emotional support. Skin lesions should be checked thoroughly at each visit. The client should be urged to get plenty of rest, follow energy conservation guidelines, and practice good nutrition. The therapist can be instrumental in teaching and assisting with skin care and prevention of skin breakdown, range-of-motion (ROM) exercises, prevention of orthopedic deformities, ergonomic and postural training, and relief of joint pain. Persons with lupus erythematosus exposed to the long-term effects of corticosteroids should be followed carefully. See specific side effects and Special Implications for the Therapist: Corticosteroids, Chapter 4.

Systemic Sclerosis

Definition and Overview. Systemic sclerosis (SSc, progressive systemic sclerosis, PSS, scleroderma[11]) is a diffuse connective tissue disease that causes fibrosis of the skin, joints, blood vessels, and internal organs. SSc is a chronic disease, lasting for months, years, or a lifetime, and is classified according to the degree and extent of skin thickening (Table 8–7).

SSc presents in two basic forms: systemic scleroderma and localized scleroderma. *Systemic scleroderma* can take one of three forms: diffuse (dSSc) (15% to 20% of cases), limited (lSSc) (75% to 80%), and an overlap form with either diffuse or limited skin thickening (see Table 8–7). Although the diffuse form is less common than the limited form, it is by far the more debilitating because of the more frequent renal and pulmonary involvement. Some measurable degree of heart, lung, or kidney involvement, or any combination of these, can be found in the majority of people with SSc (Medsger, 1993). Diffuse scleroderma is characterized by involvement of all body parts, including the skin. In most people, this involvement tends to progress slowly, if at all (Greenwald et al., 1987), but if involvement is to become severe, it tends to do so early, within the first 5 years (Steen and Medsger, 1990). The severity of the disease depends on the number of organs affected and the extent of the effect.

Limited systemic scleroderma is also called the CREST syndrome from its manifestations (calcinosis, Raynaud's phenomenon, esophageal dysmotility, sclerodactyly, and telangiectasia; see Fig. 8–2). Persons with this form of SSc have a much lower incidence of serious internal organ involvement, although pulmonary hypertension and esophageal disease are not uncommon. Skin tightness is limited to the hands and face (excluding the trunk).

Localized scleroderma affects primarily the skin in one or many different areas without visceral organ involvement and is therefore a benign form of this disease. Localized scleroderma should not be confused with limited cutaneous scleroderma. The latter is a form of systemic rather than localized disease. There is further differentiation of localized scleroderma into *morphea* characterized by hard oval-shaped patches on the skin, generally on the trunk. These patches are usually white with a purple ring around them. *Linear* refers to the bandlike lesions that occur in the areas of the arms, legs, and forehead. The bones and muscles beneath these areas may also be affected. Ultimately, ROM and a child's growth are greatly affected. Linear scleroderma often occurs in childhood (Arnold et al., 1990).

Other forms include *chemically induced localized scleroderma*, *eosinophilic myalgia syndrome* (previously associated with inges-

[11] The presence of a distinctive, widespread vascular lesion characterized by endothelial abnormalities as well as by proliferative reaction of the vascular intima was a significant factor in changing terminology from scleroderma to systemic sclerosis or SSc (LeRoy and Silver, 1993; Goetz, 1945).

TABLE 8-7 CLASSIFICATION OF SCLERODERMA AND SCLERODERMA-LIKE SYNDROMES

I. Systemic sclerosis
  A. With diffuse skin thickening—symmetrical, widespread thickening of skin affecting the distal and proximal extremities, face, and trunk; rapid progression of skin changes; early appearance of visceral involvement (GI tract, lungs, heart, kidneys)
  B. With limited skin thickening—symmetrical skin involvement restricted to the distal extremities and face; slow progression of skin changes; late appearance of visceral involvement, including distinctive types such as pulmonary arterial hypertension and biliary cirrhosis; prominence of cutaneous telangiectasias and subcutaneous calcinosis (CREST syndrome)
  C. Overlap—either diffuse or limited skin thickening in association with features of one or more other connective tissue diseases (e.g., systemic lupus erythematosus, polymyositis, dermatomyositis)
II. Chemically induced systemic sclerosis–like conditions
III. Localized forms of scleroderma
  A. Morphea
  B. Linear scleroderma
  C. Eosinophilic fasciitis
IV. Chemically induced localized forms of scleroderma
  A. Toxic oil syndrome
  B. Eosinophilia-myalgia syndrome
  C. Epoxy resin–induced fibrosis
  D. Scleroderma following autologous bone marrow transplantation (graft-vs.-host disease)
V. Diseases with skin changes resembling scleroderma (pseudoscleroderma)
  A. May be associated with diabetes mellitus
  B. Acromegaly
  C. Amyloidosis (primary and myeloma-associated)
  D. Phenylketonuria
  E. Carcinoid syndrome
  F. Infiltrating carcinomas

GI, gastrointestinal; CREST, calcinosis, Raynaud's phenomenon, esophageal dysmotility, sclerodactyly, telangiectasia.
Adapted from Medsger TA, Steen V: Systemic sclerosis and related syndromes: Clinical features and treatment. *In* Schumacher HR, Klippel JH, Koopman WJ (eds): Primer on the Rheumatic Diseases, ed 10. Atlanta, Arthritis Foundation, 1993, p 121.

tion of L-tryptophan), *toxic oil syndrome* (associated with ingestion of contaminated rapeseed oil), and *graft-vs.-host disease*.

Incidence. The annual incidence of SSc based on epidemiologic studies of hospital records and death certificates is 20 cases per million. Until recently, SSc was considered a rare disease but more recent studies report a prevalence as much as five times greater than the highest prevalence rate previously reported (Maricq et al., 1989). This condition affects women two to three times more often than men, the female-to-male ratio peaking at 15:1 during the childbearing years. The disease itself usually manifests itself between ages 30 to 50 and rarely occurs during childhood.

Etiology and Risk Factors. The cause of scleroderma is unknown. It has been suggested that an autoimmune mechanism is the underlying cause because specific autoantibodies occur in the sera of these clients. Certain host factors such as age and immunogenetic background may play a role in determining susceptibility to or expression of this illness (LeRoy and Silver, 1993). Vascular changes, vasospasm, sclerosis, or toxic damage may be involved in conjunction with the autoimmune dysfunction.

The occasional onset after trauma suggests the possibility of trophoneurosis (a trophic disorder consequent to disease or injury to nerves). Chemicals, especially from occupational exposure to silica, vinyl chloride, or various organic solvents, may also induce scleroderma-like changes (Owens and Medsger, 1988). The onset of scleroderma immediately following a severe emotional shock is in some cases a manifestation and result of a psychosomatic disturbance that causes vascular spasm (Arnold et al., 1990).

Pathogenesis. The relentless deposition of extracellular matrix in the intima of blood vessels, the pericapillary space, and the interstitium of the skin is distinctive for SSc and distinguishes it from other autoimmune disorders (LeRoy and Silver, 1993). There are three stages in the clinical development of scleroderma: the *edematous stage*, the *sclerotic stage*, and the *atrophic stage*. In the edematous stage, bilateral nonpitting edema is present in the fingers and hands, and rarely, in the feet. The edema can progress to the forearms, arms, upper chest, abdomen, back, and face. After a few weeks to several months, edema is replaced by thick, hard skin.

The replacement of edema takes place in the sclerotic stage, when the skin becomes tight, smooth, and waxy and seems bound down to underlying structures. Accompanying changes include a loss of normal skin folds and skin hyperpigmentation and hypopigmentation.

The skin changes may stabilize for periods (years) and may then either progress to the third stage or soften and return to normal. Actual atrophy of skin may occur, particularly over joints at sites of flexion contractures, such as the proximal interphalangeal joints and the elbows. Such thinning of the skin contributes to the development of ulcerations at these sites. Softening and return to normal of the skin may occur to some extent. Improvement typically begins centrally, so

TABLE 8-8 CHARACTERISTICS LIKELY TO BE SEEN IN CLIENTS WITH SYSTEMIC SCLEROSIS EARLY AND LATE IN THE DISEASE COURSE

	LIMITED DISEASE	DIFFUSE DISEASE

Early (≤5 yr)	Rapidly progressive
	  Renal crisis (5%)
	  Interstitial lung disease (severe in 10%–15%)
	Slowly progressive
	  Raynaud's phenomenon
	  Cutaneous ulceration
	  Esophageal dysmotility
		Rapidly progressive
		  Skin thickening
		  Heart involvement (severe in 10%–15%)
		  Interstitial lung disease (severe in 15%)
		Renal crisis (15%–20%)
		  Contractures, joint pain
		  Cutaneous ulcerations
		  Esophageal dysmotility
		  Gastrointestinal complications

Late (>5 yr)	Slowly progressive
	  Raynaud's phenomenon
	  Cutaneous ulcerations
	  Esophageal dysmotility
	  Gastrointestinal complication
	Very late
	  Pulmonary artery hypertension
	  Biliary cirrhosis
		Improvement
		  Skin thickening
		  Musculoskeletal pain
		Slowly progressive
		  Heart, lung, kidney involvement
		  Raynaud's phenomenon
		  Cutaneous ulceration
		  Esophageal dysmotility
		  Gastrointestinal complications

Modified from Clements PJ: Systemic sclerosis: Natural history and management strategies. J Musculoskel Med 11(11):43–50, 1994.

that the last areas to become classically involved are the first to show regression (Medsger and Steen, 1993).

Not all people pass through all the stages. Subcutaneous calcification (calcinosis) is a late-developing complication that is considerably more frequent in lSSc. Sites of trauma are often affected, such as the fingers, forearms, elbows, and knees. These calcifications vary in size from tiny deposits to large masses ulcerating the overlying skin (Fye and Sack, 1994; Medsger and Steen, 1993).

Clinical Manifestations

Raynaud's Phenomenon. Scleroderma affects everyone in a different fashion. Each previously mentioned form affects the body in different ways (Table 8–8). SSc typically begins with Raynaud's phenomenon (blanching, cyanosis, and erythema of the fingers and toes in response to stress or exposure to cold). Raynaud's phenomenon may precede SSc by months or years; it appears almost universally in lSSc and in approximately 75% of cases of dSSc. Progressive phalangeal resorption may shorten the fingers. Compromised circulation, which results from abnormal thickening of the arterial intima, may cause slowly healing ulcerations on the tips of the fingers or toes that may lead to gangrene.

Skin. Other symptoms include pain, stiffness, and swelling of the fingers and joints. Skin thickening produces taut, shiny skin over the entire hand and forearm. As tightening progresses, contractures may develop. Flexion contractures are especially severe in people with dSSc (Fig. 8–17). Facial skin may also become tight and inelastic and the face takes on a stretched and masklike appearance, with thin lips and a pinched nose.

Joints and Tendons. Polyarthralgias affect both small and large joints and are especially frequent early in dSSc; polyarthritis is unusual. Tenosynovial involvement is characterized by the presence of carpal tunnel syndrome and by coarse, leathery friction rubs palpated during motion over the extensor and flexor tendons of the fingers, distal forearms, knees, ankles, and other sites (Schumacher, 1973). These rubs are found almost exclusively in persons with dSSc and their presence points to the subsequent development of widespread scleroderma long before it occurs.

Skeletal Muscle. Most persons with dSSc have disuse atrophy of muscle due to limited joint motion secondary to skin, joint, or tendon involvement. A small percentage of people may have overlap syndromes and demonstrate marked weakness and inflammatory myopathy indistinguishable from polymyositis or dermatomyositis.

Viscera. Gastrointestinal (GI) dysfunction causes frequent reflux, heartburn, dysphagia, and bloating after meals. Other effects include abdominal distention, diarrhea, constipation, and malodorous floating stools. In advanced disease, cardiac and pulmonary fibrosis produces dysrhythmias and dyspnea. Renal involvement is usually accompanied by malignant arterial hypertension, the main cause of death in dSSc.

Medical Management

Diagnosis. A thorough physical examination and history are the first steps to a definitive diagnosis. Laboratory tests (skin biopsy, urinalysis, and blood studies including erythrocyte sedimentation rate, presence of rheumatoid factor, and presence of antinuclear antibodies[12]) are used to determine the extent of involvement and rule out other disease processes. Other tests may include chest films and pulmonary

[12] Distinctive serum autoantibodies are found in over 90% of cases (Medsger, 1994).

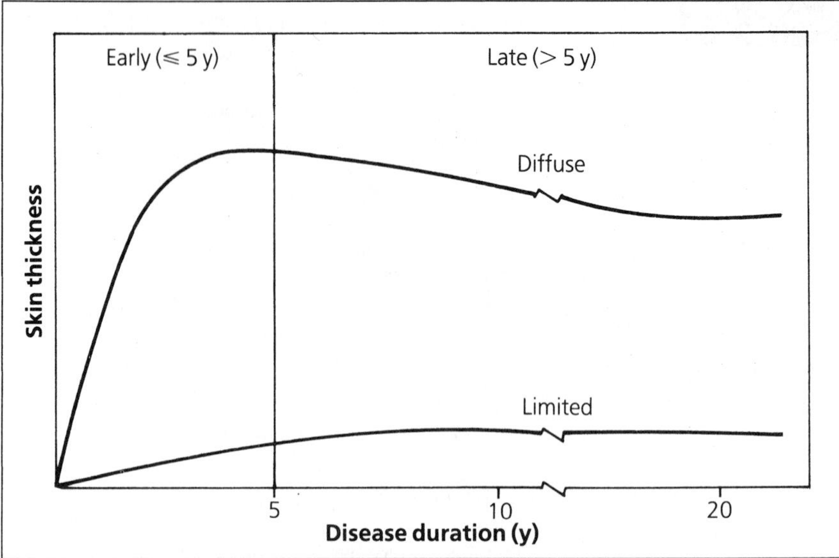

Figure 8-17. The progression of skin thickening in systemic sclerosis is greatest in the early period (first 5 years), especially in those with diffuse disease. (*From Clements PJ: Systemic sclerosis: Natural history and management strategies. J Musculoskel Med 11(11):43–50, 1994.*)

function studies, GI series, and electroencephalogram (ECG). Unfortunately, no one test will prove the presence of scleroderma.

Treatment. Presently there is no cure for SSc. Each treatment program is individualized to manage the specific disease process. Treatment ranges from merely symptomatic for a person with only limited skin involvement after 5 years to aggressive treatment for a person with early, diffuse skin involvement. When organ involvement occurs, it most often develops early in the disease course, and in the acute phase requires aggressive management. The program may include medications (e.g., immunosuppressants, penicillamine,[13] anti-inflammatory drugs), exercises, joint protection techniques, skin protection techniques, and stress management (Clements, 1994). See also Raynaud's Phenomenon, Chapter 10. Home blood pressure monitoring can screen for acute hypertension signalling a renal crisis; treatment with angiotensin converting enzyme (ACE) inhibitors (see Chapter 10) may be lifesaving.

Prognosis. The prognosis in SSc is principally dependent on the intensity and rapidity of involvement of the lungs, heart, gut, and kidneys. Spontaneous recovery is common in children, but approximately 30% of clients with SSc die within 5 years of onset. Persons with dSSc who have lived beyond the 5-year mark with no significant visceral involvement are unlikely to experience such organ involvement. Those in whom significant visceral disease developed early can expect a slowing in its progression or at least a stabilization of its course. This 5-year mark is also a time when skin softening begins and musculoskeletal aches and pains begin to ease (Medsger, 1993). Treatment with ACE inhibitors, started early, now prevents previously fatal complications (acute hypertension and renal failure). Localized scleroderma may reach an endpoint beyond which the disease does not progress.

[13] Penicillamine, a disease-modifying drug, is a penicillin-derivative immunomodulating agent that has been shown to improve the skin by interfering with cross-linking of collagen and prolonging survival in people with early, rapidly progressive SSc (Gimenez and Siegal, 1991).

Special Implications for the Therapist **8-12**

SYSTEMIC SCLEROSIS

Skin Ulcers

Local management of digital tip ulcers may include an occlusive dressing to promote wound healing and protect against trauma and infection. Commercial occlusive dressings are particularly helpful with larger noninfected ulcers. Infected ulcers are treated with a trial of oral antistaphylococcal antibiotics and may require surgical debridement of necrotic tissue. Local skin care requires avoidance of excessive bathing or using moisturizing creams containing glycerin. (See also Special Implications for the Therapist: Peripheral Vascular Disease; and Raynaud's Phenomenon, Chapter 10).

Muscle

Myositis (muscle inflammation) is treated with corticosteroids and sometimes requires the addition of immunosuppressive drugs, whereas fibrotic myopathy (fibrotic tissue laid down within the muscle) is best managed with strengthening and ROM exercises. The efficacy of using soft tissue mobilization or similar techniques has not been investigated. Caution must be used when attempting such treatment because the skin of these people is usually very sclerosed and sensitive to pressure. Aquatic therapy is an excellent choice for clients with this condition.

Joint and Tendons

Joint and tendon sheath involvement is common and may be treated successfully with NSAIDs. In early dSSc, tenosynovitis can be very painful, limiting joint movement. In addition to NSAIDs, early aggressive therapy is important in preventing or minimizing contractures. Active and passive stretching exercises are necessary but difficult in the presence of extreme pain. Analgesia is required to optimize participation in an exercise program. Dynamic splinting has not been found effective in preventing flexion contractures. Carpal tunnel syndrome, which often occurs prior to the diagnosis of scleroderma, usually responds well to conservative therapy without requiring surgery.

Exercise

For clients with scleroderma, regular exercise will assist with keeping the skin and joints flexible, maintaining better blood flow, and preventing contractures. Protecting swollen and painful joints from stresses and strains is also an important factor. This may require teaching activities of daily living (ADL) without causing strain on the joint(s). There may be a necessity for lightweight splints to provide joint protection.

Psychological Considerations

Persons with early dSSc with or without organ involvement are often anxious because their bodies are changing rapidly and in unexpected ways. They may or may not understand the grave nature of the disease. Since persons with dSSc are at greatest risk for early visceral disease and early mortality, education about the disease is important as is identifying where they are in the natural history of SSc. They should be encouraged to take their blood pressure at home at least three times a week, since this is the best method of screening for acute hypertension. The therapist may screen blood pressure as well.

For a detailed discussion, see Medsger and Steen, 1993.

Polymyositis and Dermatomyositis

Definition and Overview. Polymyositis (PM) and dermatomyositis (DM) are diffuse, inflammatory myopathies that produce symmetrical weakness of striated muscle, primarily the proximal muscles of the shoulder and pelvic girdles, neck, and pharynx (Norris et al., 1995; Plotz et al., 1993). These related illnesses belong to the family of rheumatic diseases. Seven types of inflammatory muscle disease have been distinguished (Table 8–9) (Oddis and Medsger, 1991). These diseases often progress slowly, with frequent exacerbations and remissions.

Incidence. These diseases are not very common in the United States, affecting approximately 5 to 10 persons per million; the incidence appears to be increasing (Oddis et al., 1990). Myositis can affect people of any age, but mostly adults between 45 and 65 years and children between 5 and 15 years are affected. Twice as many women as men are affected with the exception of DM associated with malignancy, which is most common in men over age 40.

Etiology. The cause of these conditions remains unknown, although there appears to be some autoimmune mechanism whereby the T cells inappropriately recognize muscle fiber antigens as foreign and attack muscle tissue. Autoantibodies are present in most cases (Love et al., 1991). PM and DM may be drug-induced; possibly triggered by a virus; or associated with other disorders as listed in Table 8–9.

TABLE 8-9 Classification of Inflammatory Myopathies

Type I	Primary idiopathic polymyositis
Type II	Primary idiopathic dermatomyositis
Type III	Dermatomyositis or polymyositis associated with malignancy (lung, breast, and others)
Type IV	Childhood polymyositis or dermatomyositis
Type V	Polymyositis associated with other connective tissue diseases Sjögren's syndrome Mixed connective tissue disease Rheumatoid arthritis Systemic lupus erythematosus Scleroderma
Type VI	Inclusion body myositis
Type VII	Miscellaneous (eosinophilic myositis, localized nodular myositis)

From Plotz PH, Leff RL, Miller FW: Inflammatory and metabolic myopathies. *In* Schumacher HR, Klippel JH, Koopman WJ (eds): Primer on the Rheumatic Diseases, ed 10. Atlanta, Arthritis Foundation, 1993, p 127.

Pathogenesis. If these conditions are caused by an autoimmune reaction, diffuse or focal muscle fiber degeneration is followed by regeneration of new muscle cells, producing remission. Muscle biopsy reveals focal or diffuse inflammatory infiltrates consisting primarily of lymphocytes and macrophages surrounding muscle fibers and small blood vessels. Muscle cells show evidence of degeneration and regeneration and fiber atrophy is often most severe at the periphery of the muscle bundle. Extensive interstitial fibrosis and fatty replacement are common in longstanding cases.

Clinical Manifestations. Symmetrical proximal muscle weakness is the dominant feature of these diseases, although it is variable in its onset, progression, and severity. In some people, symptoms appear suddenly, progress rapidly, and quickly result in a bedridden state, sometimes requiring ventilatory assistance and tube feeding. More typically, weakness, malaise, and weight loss develop insidiously over months or even years, with some people either unable to identify the onset of the disease or unaware of the gradual disability developing.

Cardiac involvement is not uncommon and contributes significantly to mortality. Nearly half of all people with PM or DM have dysrhythmias, congestive heart failure, conduction defects, ventricular hypertrophy, or pericarditis. Pulmonary disease can result from weakness of the respiratory muscles, intrinsic lung pathology, or aspiration. Swallowing difficulties, nasal regurgitation, and esophageal dysphagia and reflux are common, especially in severe cases.

Polymyositis. Polymyositis begins acutely or insidiously with muscle weakness, tenderness, and discomfort. The proximal muscles of the shoulder and pelvic girdles are affected more often than the distal muscles, usually in a symmetrical pattern, but asymmetry is common. The legs are affected more often than the arms, and the anterior thigh is more frequently involved than the posterior thigh. Initially, the muscles may be slightly swollen, but as the disease progresses muscular atrophy and induration become more noticeable, reflecting the deposition of fibrous tissue. Some persons have a mild peripheral neuropathy with loss of deep tendon reflexes.

Early signs of muscle weakness may include impaired functional status such as difficulty climbing stairs, getting up from a chair, reaching into an overhead cupboard, combing the hair, lifting the head from a pillow, difficulty with balance, or a tendency to fall, often resulting in a fracture. Other muscular effects may include decreased deep tendon reflexes, contractures, arthralgias, arthritis, an inability to move against resistance (e.g., pushing open a heavy door, opening a car door), proximal dysphagia (difficulty swallowing), and dysphonia (difficulty speaking).

Dermatomyositis. When a rash is associated with polymyositis, it is referred to as dermatomyositis. A characteristic purplish rash appears on the eyelids, accompanied by periorbital edema (puffy eyelids). The rash may progress to the anterior neck, upper chest and back, shoulders, arms, and may appear around the nail beds. Gottron's papules (red or violet, smooth or scaly patches) may appear on the dorsal surface of the interphalangeal or metacarpal joints, elbows, knees, or medial malleoli. Although the disease usually begins with erythema and swelling of the face and eyelids, cutaneous manifestations can develop concomitantly with muscle involvement or even afterward. In some persons, muscle involvement is minimal, whereas in others it may progress to wasting and contractures associated with extreme disability (Wooldridge, 1995).

Medical Management

Diagnosis. The diagnosis of myositis is often difficult because it resembles closely several other diseases and the pathology can be localized, sometimes resulting in nondiagnostic biopsies. Laboratory studies to evaluate muscle enzymes, biopsy to assess muscle fibers, and electromyography (EMG) to measure the electrical activity of the muscles are all necessary to properly diagnose myositis. Magnetic resonance imaging (MRI) can reveal muscle inflammation and may help to select the site to biopsy in difficult cases (Fraser et al., 1991).

Treatment. The treatment must be individualized; the components include medication, exercise, and rest. High-dose daily oral systemic corticosteroid therapy is the usual initial pharmacologic treatment for PM or DM. Steroids reduce the inflammation, shorten the time to normalization of muscle enzymes, and reduce morbidity. Persons who do not respond well to steroids or who are unable to tolerate the high dosages required may be treated with immunosuppressive drugs.

Prognosis. The adult prognosis varies depending on age and progression of the disease process. Generally, the prognosis worsens with age. The 7-year survival rate for adults is approximately 60%, with death often occurring from associated malignancy, respiratory disease, heart failure, or side effects of therapy (corticosteroids and immunosuppressants). The prognosis for children is guarded if left untreated; it progresses rapidly to disabling contractures and muscular atrophy.

Special Implications for the Therapist **8-13**

POLYMYOSITIS AND DERMATOMYOSITIS

The therapist plays a pivotal role in the management of myositis. Manual muscle testing and tests of functional abilities are useful tools in following disease progression and therapeutic response over a long period. The individualized exercise program can help improve muscle strength.

It is suggested that the medication regimen be well established prior to beginning exercise. In the early stages of treating myositis, the muscle fibers are fragile and could be damaged further, causing rhabdomyolysis (disintegration of muscle fibers) from exercises and other forms of therapy. The therapist treating a client with myositis should keep in close contact with the physician who will be using physical examination and laboratory tests to determine the most opportune time for initiating a graded exercise program. Often heat, whirlpools, and massages are very effective adjunctive treatments. Pool therapy may be initiated sooner than other forms of exercise.

If the person is confined to bed, protection from footdrop and contractures and prevention of pressure ulcers are essential. If the client has a skin rash, the therapist should caution about the possibility of infection from scratching. If antipruritic medications do not relieve severe itching, tepid sponges or compresses can be applied. If the client is receiving corticosteroids, observe for side effects (weight gain, acne, edema, hypertension, purplish stretch marks [striae], or easy bruising). Long-term use of steroids lowers resistance to infection, may induce diabetes, and is associated with loss of potassium in the urine and gastric irritation (see Table 4–7 and Corticosteroids, Chapter 4). If side effects are marked, advise against abruptly discontinuing corticosteroids until the client consults with the physician first. A low sodium diet will help prevent fluid retention.

THERMAL INJURIES

Cold Injuries *(Norris et al., 1995)*

Cold injuries result from overexposure to cold air or water and occur in two major forms: localized injuries (such as frostbite) and systemic injuries (such as hypothermia). Untreated or improperly treated frostbite can lead to gangrene and may necessitate amputation requiring therapy and rehabilitation. Hypothermia is a medical emergency and is not discussed further here.

Etiology and Risk Factors. Frostbite results from prolonged exposure to dry temperatures far below freezing. The risk of serious cold injuries is increased by lack of insulating body fat, wet or inadequate clothing, old age, homelessness, drug abuse, cardiac disease, and smoking.

Pathogenesis and Clinical Manifestations. Localized cold injuries occur when ice crystals form in the tissues and expand extracellular spaces. With compression of cells, cell membranes rupture, interrupting enzymatic and metabolic activities. Increased capillary permeability accompanies the release of histamine, resulting in aggregation of red blood cells and microvascular occlusion.

Frostbite may be deep or superficial. Superficial frostbite affects the skin and subcutaneous tissue, especially of the face, ears, extremities, and other exposed body areas. Although it may go unnoticed at first, upon returning to a warm place, frostbite produces burning, tingling, numbness, swelling, and a mottled, blue-gray skin color. When the affected area begins to rewarm, the person will feel pain. Deep frostbite extends beyond subcutaneous tissue and usually affects the hands or feet. The skin becomes white until it has thawed and then turns purplish blue. Deep frostbite produces pain, blisters, tissue necrosis, and gangrene (Fig. 8–18).

Medical Management

Diagnosis. Diagnosis is usually made based on the history and presenting symptoms. Additional studies may include arteriography or scintiscanning to determine the extent of injury or to open vasoconstricted vessels.

Treatment. In a localized cold injury, treatment consists of warming the injured part without rubbing or massaging the area to avoid further tissue damage, and supportive measures (e.g., analgesics for pain, proper positioning to avoid weight bearing with gauze between the toes to prevent maceration). Debridement of blisters is controversial. Bulky dressings may be applied to permit drainage and provide protection. A bed cradle may be needed to keep the weight of bedcovers off the affected part(s). Other treatment measures may include vasodilators or nerve block.

In the case of a developing compartment syndrome a fasciotomy may be performed to increase circulation by lowering edematous tissue pressure. If gangrene occurs, amputation may be necessary. Smoking causes vasoconstriction and slows healing; the client should be advised to quit smoking, at least during the recovery period.

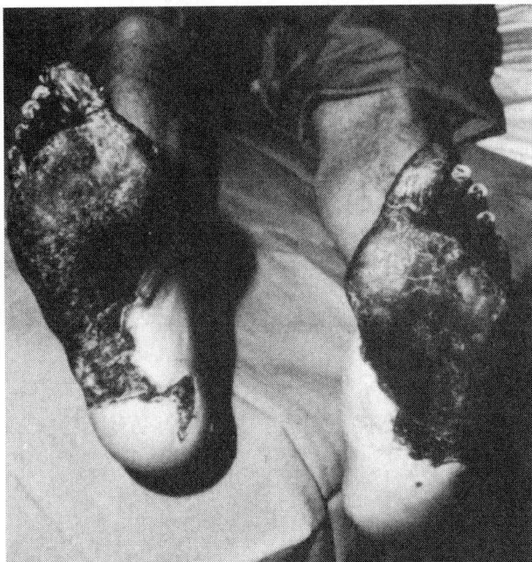

Figure **8–18.** Frostbite of the feet. Blackened areas in the photo show tissue necrosis and gangrene, the result of deep frostbite that extends beyond the subcutaneous tissue. (*From Norris J, McMahon E, Fandek N, et al (eds): Professional Guide To Diseases, ed 5. Springhouse, Pa, Springhouse, 1995, p 298.*)

Prognosis. The prognosis depends on the extent of localized cold injury and development of any complications such as compartment syndrome, necrosis, or gangrene. Long-term effects may include increased sensitivity to cold, burning and tingling upon reexposure to cold, and increased sweating of the affected area.

Future cold injuries may be prevented through the use of windproof, water-resistant, many-layered clothing, moisture-wicking socks, a head covering, mittens instead of gloves, and heat-generating devices in pockets or battery-operated socks.

Special Implications for the Therapist **8–14**

COLD INJURIES

Local cold injury subsequent to prolonged exposure may not be seen in a therapy practice until complications such as necrosis and gangrene result in amputation. Whirlpool with gentle agitation directed away from the affected area may be prescribed as part of the rewarming procedure. Water temperature is based on tissue temperature and should be determined in conjunction with the medical staff.

Use of cryotherapy as a modality among the general population can result in localized tissue damage requiring documentation (such as filing an accident report) and possible medical evaluation and treatment. Massage may cause further tissue damage and should not be carried out until local tissue has healed.

Burns *(Carrougher, 1993)*

Definition and Overview. Injuries that result from direct contact or exposure to any thermal, chemical, electrical, or radiation source are termed *burns*. Burn injuries occur when energy from a heat source is transferred to the tissues of the body. The depth of injury is a function of temperature or source of energy (e.g., radiation) and duration of exposure.

The severity of burn injury is assessed with respect to the risk of mortality and the risk of cosmetic or functional disability (American Burn Association, 1984). Factors that influence injury severity include burn depth, burn size (percentage of total body surface area [TBSA]), burn location, age, general health, and mechanism of injury. Burn depth can be divided into categories based on the elements of the skin that are damaged (Fig. 8–19). Most burn wounds that require medical intervention are a combination of partial- and full-thickness burns.

Burn size is determined by one of two techniques: the "rule of nines" (Fig. 8–20) and the Lund and Browder method (Fig. 8–21). The rule of nines is based on the division of the body into anatomic sections, each of which represents 9% or a multiple of 9% of the TBSA. This is an easy method to quickly assess the percentage of TBSA injured and is most commonly used in emergency departments where the initial evaluation takes place. The Lund and Browder method modifies the percentages for body segments and provides a more accurate estimate of burn size according to age. For the most accurate estimate of burn size, the burn diagram should be confirmed following the initial wound debridement (Lund and Browder, 1994).

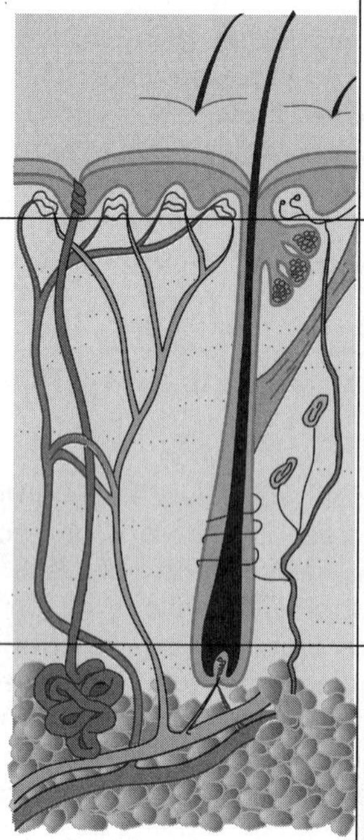

Layer	Burn depth	APPEARANCE	SENSATION	COURSE
EPIDERMIS	SUPERFICIAL BURN	Mild to severe erythema; skin blanches with pressure	Painful Hyperesthetic Tingling Pain eased by cooling	Discomfort lasts about 48 hours Desquamation in 3–7 days
DERMIS	PARTIAL-THICKNESS BURN	Large thick-walled blisters covering extensive area (vesiculation) Edema; mottled red base; broken epidermis; wet, shiny, weeping surface	Painful Sensitive to cold air	Superficial partial-thickness burn heals in 14–21 days Deep partial-thickness burn requires 21–28 days for healing Healing rate varies with burn depth and presence or absence of infection
SUBCUTANEOUS TISSUE	FULL-THICKNESS BURN	Variable, e.g., deep red, black, white, brown Dry surface Edema Fat exposed Tissue disrupted	Little pain Insensate	Full-thickness dead skin suppurates and liquefies after 2–3 weeks Spontaneous healing may be impossible but small areas may be left alone to form scarring without grafting (called secondary intent) Requires removal of eschar and subsequent split- or full-thickness skin grafting Hypertrophic scarring and wound contractures likely to develop without preventive measures

Figure 8–19. Burn injury classification according to depth of injury.

Incidence. In the United States, 2 million people seek medical attention every year for injuries caused by burns; of these, 70,000 are hospitalized with severe injuries and 6000 are fatalities. Burn injuries are the third leading cause of accidental death in all age groups. Males tend to be injured more frequently than females, except for the elderly (older than 70 years) (Feller, 1982).

Etiology. Burn injuries are categorized according to their mechanism of injury: thermal, chemical, electrical, or radiation. *Thermal* burns are caused by exposure to or contact with sources such as flames, hot liquids, steam, semisolids (tar), or hot objects. *Chemical* burns are caused by tissue contact, ingestion, inhalation, or injection with strong acids, alkalis, or organic compounds. Chemical burns can result from contact with certain household cleaning agents and various chemicals used in industry, agriculture, and the military. *Electrical* burns are caused by heat that is generated by the electrical energy as it passes through the body. Electrical burns can result from contact with exposed or faulty electrical wiring, high-voltage power lines, or lightning. *Radiation* burns are the least common burn injury and are caused by exposure to a radioactive source. These types of injuries have been associated with the use of ionizing radiation in industry or from therapeutic radiation sources in medicine. A sunburn from prolonged exposure to UV rays is also considered a type of radiation burn.

Risk Factors. Data collected from the National Burn Information Exchange indicates that 75% of all burn injuries result from the actions of the injured person, occurring most often in the home. The population over 70 years is at the highest risk for burn injury.

Pathogenesis

Cutaneous Burn. The pathophysiologic changes that occur immediately following a cutaneous burn injury depend on the extent or size of the burn. For smaller burns, the body's response to injury is localized to the injured area. With more extensive burns (25% or more of the TBSA), the response is systemic, potentially affecting all major systems of the body. The systems more obviously affected include the cardiovascular, renal, gastrointestinal, immune, and respiratory systems.

Cardiovascular changes occur immediately following a burn injury as vasoactive substances (catecholamines, histamine, serotonin, leukotrienes, prostaglandins) are released from the injured tissue causing an increase in capillary permeability. Extensive burns result in generalized body edema in both burned and nonburned tissues and a decrease in circulating intravascular blood volume. Heart rate increases in response

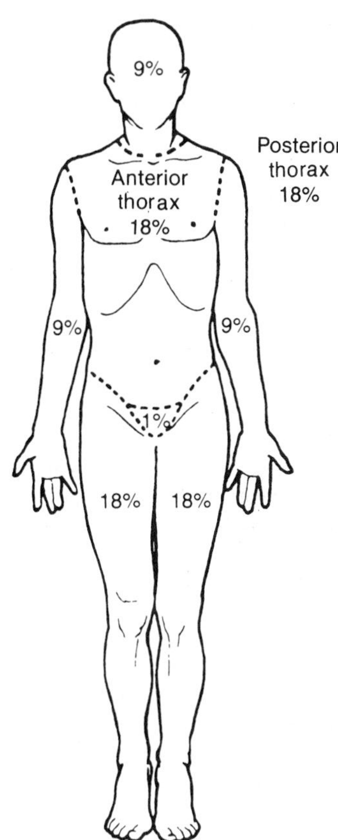

Figure **8–20.** The "rule of nines" provides a quick method for estimating the extent of a burn injury.

to catecholamine release and to the hypovolemia, but overall cardiac output falls. If the intravascular space is not replenished with IV fluids, hypovolemic (burn) shock and death may result. Within 18 to 36 hours postburn, capillary permeability decreases and continues to return to normal for several weeks following the injury. Cardiac output returns to normal and then increases approximately 24 hours after the injury to meet the hypermetabolic needs of the body. The body begins to reabsorb the edema fluid and excretes the excess fluid over the ensuing days and weeks. See also Common Causes of Fluid and Electrolyte Imbalances, Chapter 4.

The *renal* and *gastrointestinal systems* are affected as the body responds initially by shunting blood from the kidneys and intestines leading to oliguria (decreased urine output) and intestinal dysfunction, respectively, in clients with burns greater than 25% of TBSA. *Immune system function* is depressed increasing the risk of infection and life-threatening sepsis. The *respiratory system* may respond with pulmonary artery hypertension and decreased lung compliance, even when there has been no inhalation injury.

Smoke Inhalation. Smoke inhalation may result in injury secondary to inhalation of carbon monoxide, smoke poisoning from the inhalation of byproducts of combustion, or direct thermal burns to the pulmonary airways. See Noxious Gases, Fumes, and Smoke Inhalation, Chapter 12.

Electrical and Chemical Burns. In electrical burns, heat is generated as the electricity travels through the body, resulting in internal tissue damage. However, entrance and exit wounds may be significant, distracting medical personnel from internal injury. Cutaneous burn injuries associated with electrical burns may be negligible, but soft tissue and muscle damage may be extensive, particularly in high-voltage electrical injuries. However, it is possible for electrical burns to ignite the person's clothes causing thermal burns as well. The voltage, type of current (direct or alternating), contact site, and duration of contact are important factors in the amount and type of damage sustained. Alternating current is more dangerous than direct and is often associated with cardiopulmonary arrest, ventricular fibrillation, and tetanic muscle contractions. Other significant injuries such as long-bone or vertebral compression fractures, spinal cord injury, or traumatic brain injury can occur if the victim falls upon electrical contact (Pruit and Goodwin, 1990). Chemical burns are associated with systemic toxicity from cutaneous absorption. See also, Chapter 3.

Clinical Manifestations. Appearance, sensation, and course of injury of superficial, partial-thickness, and full-thickness burns are outlined in Figure 8–19. Burn location influences injury severity in that burns of certain areas of the body are commonly associated with specific complications. For example, burns of the head, neck, and chest frequently have associated pulmonary complications. Burns involving the face may have associated corneal abrasions. Burns of the hands and joints can result in permanent physical and vocational disability requiring extensive therapy and rehabilitation. Circumferential burns of extremities may produce a tourniquet-like effect and lead to total occlusion of circulation.

Theoretically, with a full-thickness burn the nerve endings have been destroyed and no pain should be associated with this type of injury. However, most full-thickness burns occur with superficial and partial-thickness burns in which nerve endings are intact and exposed. Excised eschar (dead tissue produced by a burn) and donor sites expose nerve fibers as well. As peripheral nerves regenerate, painful sensation returns. Consequently, people with burn injuries often experience severe pain that is related to the size and depth of the burn (Atchison, 1991).

The clinical course of the (major) burn client can be divided into three phases: the emergent and resuscitation phase, the acute phase, and the rehabilitation phase (Burgess, 1991). The *emergent phase* begins at the time of injury and concludes with the restoration of capillary permeability, usually 48 to 72 hours following injury. The *resuscitation period* begins with initiation of fluid resuscitation measures and ends when capillary integrity returns to near-normal levels and the large fluid shifts have decreased. The *acute phase* of recovery begins when the person is hemodynamically stable, capillary permeability is restored, and diuresis has begun, usually 48 to 72 hours after the initial injury occurred. The acute phase continues until wound closure is achieved. The *rehabilitation phase* represents the final phase of burn care, often overlaps the acute care phase, and lasts well beyond the period of hospitalization. This phase focuses on gaining independence through achievement of maximal functional recovery.

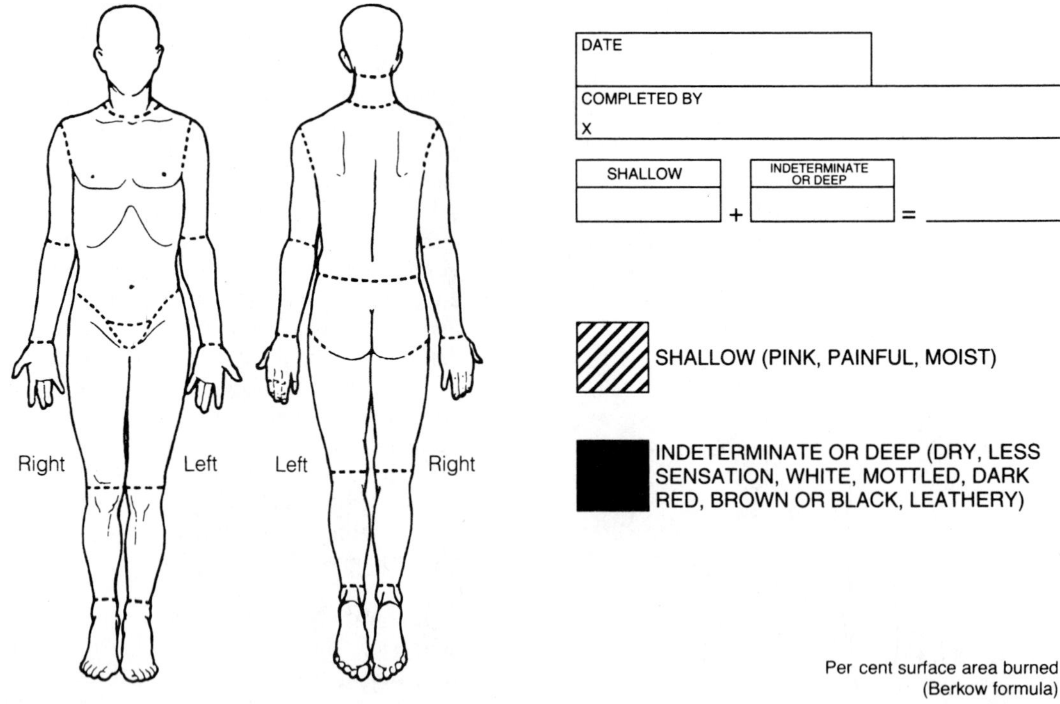

AREA	1 YEAR	1 to 4 YEARS	5 to 9 YEARS	10 to 14 YEARS	Y 15 YEARS	ADULT	SHALLOW	INDETER-MINATE OR DEEP
Head	19	17	13	11	9	7		
Neck	2	2	2	2	2	2		
Ant. Trunk	13	13	13	13	13	13		
Post.Trunk	13	13	13	13	13	13		
R. Buttock	2½	2½	2½	2½	2½	2½		
L. Buttock	2½	2½	2½	2½	2½	2½		
Genitalia	1	1	1	1	1	1		
R. U. Arm	4	4	4	4	4	4		
L. U. Arm	4	4	4	4	4	4		
R. L. Arm	3	3	3	3	3	3		
L. L. Arm	3	3	3	3	3	3		
R. Hand	2½	2½	2½	2½	2½	2½		
L. Hand	2½	2½	2½	2½	2½	2½		
R. Thigh	5½	6½	8	8½	9	9½		
L. Thigh	5½	6½	8	8½	9	9½		
R. Leg	5	5	5½	6	6½	7		
L. Leg	5	5	5½	6	6½	7		
R. Foot	3½	3½	3½	3½	3½	3½		
L. Foot	3½	3½	3½	3½	3½	3½		
TOTAL								

Figure **8–21.** A sample chart for recording the extent and depth of a burn injury using the Lund and Browder formula.

The multiple organ system response that occurs following a burn injury may result in the multiple organ dysfunction syndrome and death. See discussion in Chapter 4.

Medical Management

Treatment. The emergency department therapist may be involved in wound care for minor burns consisting of cleansing; removal of any damaging agents (chemicals, tar, etc.); debridement of loose, nonviable tissue, being careful not to break any blisters; and application of topical antimicrobial creams or ointment and a sterile dressing. Instructions for home care include observation for clinical manifestations of infection and active ROM exercises to maintain normal joint function, decrease edema formation, and decrease possible scar formation.

Treatment of major burns includes lifesaving measures (ABCs: *a*irway, *b*reathing, *c*irculation) immediately after the injury followed by restorative care (e.g., infection control, wound care, skin grafts, pain management) during the acute phase until wound closure is achieved. Therapists are closely involved early in the acute phase of recovery to maximize functional recovery and cosmetic outcome. Therapeutic interventions include wound care, positioning and immobilization following skin grafting to prevent unwanted movement and shearing of grafts, scar and contracture prevention, exercise, ambulation, and ADL. Elasticized garments help reduce scar hypertrophy and may be worn for months to 2 years after hospitalization.

Skin grafts may be used as a temporary measure to minimize fluid and protein loss from the burn surface, prevent infection, and reduce pain. Types of temporary grafts include *allografts* (homografts), which are usually cadaver skin; *xenografts* (heterografts), which are typically pigskin; and *biosynthetic grafts*, which are a combination of collagen and synthetics. To treat a full-thickness burn, an *autograft* (the person's own skin) may be required. The transplanted skin graft will be used intact over areas where appearance or joint movement is important but the graft may be meshed (fenestrated) to cover up to three times its original size. A new method called *test-tube skin graft* has been developed for burns that cover the entire body surface. Small full-thickness biopsy provides epidermal cells that are cultured into smooth sheets of skin and then grafted onto burns (Norris et al., 1995).

Prognosis. Burn care has improved in recent decades, resulting in a lower mortality rate for victims of burn injuries (Feller, 1980). The client's age affects the severity and outcome of the burn. Mortality rates are higher for children less than 4 years of age and for clients over 65 (Linn, 1980). Factors such as obesity, alcoholism, and cardiac disorders affecting general health, especially disorders that impair peripheral circulation such as peripheral vascular disease, have been observed to increase the complication and mortality rates for clients with burns (Heimbach, 1983; Jones, 1989).

Special Implications for the Therapist **8-15**

BURNS

In light of statistics showing that the population over 70 years old is at highest risk of burn injury, prevention of burn accidents, especially in this population, is an important part of client education. Reviewing simple cooking precautions may be helpful, for example, do not leave burners in use unattended, do not use high heat, do not wear clothing with loose sleeves or belts (especially bathrobes), use front burners whenever possible, and avoid leaning over front burners when using back burners.

Unless employed in an emergency department, most therapists do not begin to treat the burn client until the acute phase (as soon as the person is physiologically stable), continuing treatment through much of the rehabilitation phase. The therapist will direct treatment to encourage deep breathing and facilitate lung expansion; promote wound healing; reduce dependent edema formation and promote venous return; prevent or minimize deformities and hypertrophic scarring; increase ROM, strength, and function; increase independence in daily activities and self-care; and encourage emotional and psychological well-being. Specific debridement and wound care procedures are beyond the scope of this book.

Throughout the acute and rehabilitation phases of burn care, the therapist must remain alert to the development of medical complications such as ileus, gastric ulcers, respiratory distress, infection, and impaired circulation. Notify the nursing staff of any new or unusual findings observed during assessment and treatment (Table 8–10).

The amount of body surface area exposed during wound care must be minimized to prevent hypothermia as heat is lost in open wounds and after hydrotherapy by evaporation. Hydrotherapy treatment must be limited to 30 minutes or less with water temperature in the 98° to 102° F range. External heat shields or radiant heat lamps can provide a source of external heat. Clients excluded from hydrotherapy are generally those who are hemodynamically unstable and those with new grafts (Carrougher and Marvin, 1989).

People with burns are at high risk of infection because of the significant loss of skin barrier and impaired immune response. Infection control techniques must be practiced carefully at all times (see Appendix A: Summary of Universal Precautions). Skin donor sites require the same care and precautions as other partial-thickness wounds in order to promote healing and prevent infection.

Arrange any therapy likely to elicit a painful response to coincide with medications (allow 45 minutes for oral, 30 minutes for intramuscular (IM), 5 to 10 minutes for IV administration). Combining relaxation techniques, music therapy, distraction, and other techniques with wound care may be helpful. Burned areas must be maintained in positions of physiologic function within the limits imposed by associated injuries, grafting, and other therapeutic devices (see Table 8–11 for positioning recommendations). Burned areas are prone to develop contractures requiring close

TABLE 8-10 ASSESSING MEDICAL COMPLICATIONS IN THE BURN-INJURED ADULT

Urinary	Visible red or dark-brown urine (catheter)
Respiratory	Signs of respiratory distress Restlessness Confusion Labored breathing Tachypnea (>24 respirations/min) Dyspnea $PaO_2 < 90$ mm Hg; $O_2 < 95\%$
Peripheral vascular	Pulses absent on palpation Capillary refill (unburned area) > 2 sec Numbness or tingling Increased pain with active range-of-motion exercises Increased edema, changes in skin color
Infection	Discoloration of wounds or drainage, odor, delayed healing Headache, chills, anorexia, nausea Change in vital signs Paralytic ileus, confusion, restlessness, hallucinations
Gastrointestinal	Paralytic ileus (painful, distended abdomen) Stress-induced gastric ulcer (epigastric pain, abdominal distention, loss of appetite, nausea)

TABLE 8-11 Therapeutic Positioning for the Burn-Injured Client

Burned Area	Therapeutic Position	Positioning Techniques
Neck		
Anterior	Extension	No pillow; small towel roll beneath cervical spine to promote neck extension
Circumferential	Neutral toward extension	No pillow
Posterior or asymmetrical	Neutral	No pillow
Shoulder, axilla	Arm abduction to 90–110 degrees	Splinting; arms positioned away from body and supported on arm troughs; elbow splint
Elbow	Arm extension	Elbow splint; elbow(s) positioned in extension with slight bend at elbow (≤10 degrees of elbow flexion) Arms supported on arm troughs with the forearm in slight pronation
Hand		
Wrist	Wrist extension	Hand splint
Metacarpophalangeal (MCP) joints	MCP flexion at 90 degrees	Hand splint
Proximal or distal interphalangeal (PIP/DIP) joints	PIP/DIP extension	Hand splint
Thumb	Thumb abduction	Hand splint with thumb abduction
Web spaces	Finger abduction	Web spacers of gauze, foam, or thermoplastics to decrease webbing formation
Hip	Hip extension	Supine with the head of bed flat and legs extended Trochanter roll to maintain neutral rotation (toes pointing toward ceiling)
Knee	Knee extension	Supine with knees extended and toes pointing toward ceiling Prone with feet extended over end of mattress Sitting with legs extended and elevated Knee splint
Ankle	Neutral	Padded footboard Ankle positioning devices (avoid position of ankle inversion or eversion)

Modified from Carrougher GJ: Nursing care of clients with burn injury. *In* Black JM, Matassarin-Jacobs E (eds): Luckmann and Sorensen's Medical-Surgical Nursing, ed 4. Philadelphia, WB Saunders, 1993, p 2008.

assessment of ROM and muscle strength. Encourage active ROM exercises at least every 2 hours while the person is awake unless this is contraindicated by a recent grafting procedure. Provide honest, positive reinforcement throughout treatment, being aware that each individual will progress through stages of denial, grief, and acceptance of injury and recovery. During the rehabilitation phase, chronic pain protocols may be helpful (see Box 2–12).

MISCELLANEOUS SKIN DISORDERS

Pressure Ulcers

Definition. A pressure ulcer (bed sore, decubitus ulcer) is a lesion caused by unrelieved pressure resulting in damage to underlying tissue. Pressure ulcers usually occur over bony prominences such as the sacrum, heels, ischial tuberosities, and greater trochanters and are graded or staged to classify the degree of tissue damage observed (Table 8–12). It should be noted that this staging classification is only for pressure ulcers. Other types of ulcers, such as arterial, venous, or diabetic ulcers (see Table 10–20), are staged using partial- and full-thickness classifications (technically defined by stages II, III, or IV of the Agency for Health Care Policy and Research pressure ulcer guidelines, but still referred to as partial- or full-thickness ulcers).

Etiology and Risk Factors. The primary risk factors for the development of pressure ulcers are (1) interface pressure (externally); (2) friction (rubbing of the skin against another surface); (3) shearing forces (two layers sliding against each other in opposite directions causing damage to the underlying tissues); and (4) maceration (softening caused by excessive moisture).

Bed- and chairbound clients and those with impaired ability to reposition themselves should be assessed for additional factors that increase the risk of developing pressure ulcers. These factors include decreased mobility or immobility; con-

TABLE 8–12 Stages of Pressure Ulcers

Stage I
Nonblanchable erythema of intact skin; the heralding lesion of skin ulceration.
Note: Reactive hyperemia can normally be expected to be present for one-half to three-fourths as long as the pressure occluded blood flow to the area; it should not be confused with a stage I pressure ulcer.

Stage II
Partial-thickness skin loss involving epidermis or dermis, or both. The ulcer is superficial and presents clinically as an abrasion, blister, or shallow crater.

Stage III
Full-thickness skin loss involving damage or necrosis of subcutaneous tissue that may extend down to, but not through, underlying fascia. The ulcer presents clinically as a deep crater with or without undermining of adjacent tissue.

Stage IV
Full-thickness skin loss with extensive destruction, tissue necrosis, or damage to muscle, bone, or supporting structures (e.g., tendon or joint capsule).
Note: Undermining and sinus tracts may also be associated with stage IV pressure ulcers.

Modified from Pressure ulcers in adults: Prediction and prevention. Clinical practice guideline, No. 3. Rockville, Md, US Department of Health and Human Services, AHCPR Publication No. 92-0047, 1992.

tractures; increased muscle tone; loss of sensation; incontinence; obesity; nutritional factors;[14] chronic disease accompanied by anemia, edema, renal failure, or sepsis; and altered level of consciousness.

Pressure contributes to other types of ulcers (e.g., arterial, venous, diabetic) and likewise, the underlying cause of the other types of ulcers can contribute to the development of pressure ulcers (see Table 10–20). However, pressure ulcers are a separate entity from these other types of ulcers. A systemic risk assessment evaluating both sensation and physiologic risk of pressure ulcers can be made using a validated risk assessment tool such as the Braden Scale (Table 8–13).

Pathogenesis. Pressure is the external factor causing ischemia and tissue necrosis. Continuous pressure on soft tissues between bony prominences and hard or unyielding surfaces compresses capillaries and occludes blood flow. Normal capillary blood pressure at the arterial end of the vascular bed averages 32 mm Hg. When tissues are externally compressed, that pressure may be exceeded, reducing blood supply to, and lymphatic drainage of, the affected area (HHS, 1992, 1995).

If the pressure is relieved, a brief period of rebound capillary dilation (called reactive hyperemia) occurs and no tissue damage develops. If the pressure is not relieved, the endothelial cells lining the capillaries become disrupted by platelet aggregation, forming microthrombi that occlude blood flow and cause anoxic necrosis of surrounding tissues. Necrotic tissue predisposes to bacterial invasion and subsequent infection preventing healthy granulation of scar tissue (Hockenberger and Black, 1993).

Clinical Manifestations. Pressure ulcers usually occur over bony prominences as opposed to lower extremity ulcers from chronic venous insufficiency, for example. Superficial sores are more common on the sacrum as a result of shearing or friction forces (parallel to the skin). Deep sores develop closer to the bone as a result of tissue distortion and vascular occlusion from pressure that is perpendicular to the tissue (over heels, trochanters, and ischia). Deep lesions often go undetected until they penetrate the skin, but by then significant subcutaneous damage has occurred.

The wounds are generally red, brown black, or yellow (Fig. 8–22) and the infection is usually localized and self-limiting. Proteolytic enzymes from bacteria and macrophages dissolve necrotic tissues and cause a foul-smelling discharge that appears like, but is not, pus (Huether and Kravitz, 1994).

Pressure ulcers are often painful in individuals who do not have loss of sensation from spinal cord trauma or neuropathy. The presence of necrotic tissue produces an inflammatory response with hyperemia, fever, and increased white blood cell count. If the ulceration is large, toxicity and pain lead to loss of appetite, debilitation, and renal insufficiency. Individuals who are immunosuppressed or who have diabetes mellitus may develop infection and inflammation of adjacent tissues (cellulitis) or septicemia (Huether and Kravitz, 1994).

Medical Management

Diagnosis. Prevention is the key to this condition starting with assessment of people at high risk for the development of pressure ulcers. In fact, risk prediction should be an ongoing assessment carried out by all health care professionals. In addition to the Braden Scale (see Table 8–13), laboratory data on hemoglobin, hematocrit, albumin, total protein, and lymphocytes should be assessed by the physician. The diagnosis is reached by determining the cause of loss of skin integrity. The pressure ulcer is then staged (see Table 8–12). Wound culture and sensitivity testing of the exudate in the ulcer identify infecting organisms and help determine the oral antibiotics that may be needed. Topical antibiotics are not effective.

Treatment. The pressure ulcer is cleaned thoroughly; spontaneous healing will occur more quickly when the ulcer is kept moist with an occlusive dressing (Monk et al., 1988).[15] The use of antiseptics such as hydrogen peroxide or iodine is controversial at this time as these can be damaging to marginal granulation tissue. Successful healing requires continued adequate relief of pressure and absence of infection. The presence of necrotic tissue in a wound may provide an optimal environment for bacteria to grow, hence the importance of removing necrotic material from a wound as rapidly as possible. Therapeutic intervention may include hydrotherapy, electrical stimulation, ultrasound, or any combination

[14] Nutritional factors may include malnutrition or inadequate nutrition leading to weight loss and subsequent reduction of subcutaneous tissue and muscle bulk.

[15] Many plastic surgeons continue to advocate the initial use of wet-to-dry dressing (application of open wet dressing, allowing it to dry on the ulcer, and mechanically debriding exudate by removal of the dressing) for debridement. As there is a risk of removing viable tissue, as well as bleeding, with this procedure, this procedure no longer has universal approval.

TABLE 8-13 Braden Scale: Risk Predictors for Skin Breakdown

SENSORY PERCEPTION (ability to respond to discomfort)	1. Completely limited: Unresponsive to painful stimuli, either because of state of unconsciousness or severe sensory impairment, which limits ability to feel pain over most of body surface.	2. Very limited: Responds only to painful stimuli (but not verbal commands) by opening eyes or flexing extremities. Cannot communicate discomfort verbally, OR has a sensory impairment which limits the ability to feel pain or discomfort over ½ body surface.	3. Slightly limited: Responds to verbal commands by opening eyes and obeying some commands, but cannot always communicate discomfort or needs, OR has some sensory impairment which limits ability to feel pain or discomfort in one or two extremities.	4. No impairment: Responds to verbal commands by obeying. Can communicate needs accurately. Has no sensory deficit which would limit ability to feel pain or discomfort.
MOISTURE (degree to which skin is exposed to moisture)	1. Very moist: Skin is kept moist almost constantly by perspiration and urine. Dampness is detected every time patient is moved or turned. Linen must be changed more than one time each shift.	2. Occasionally moist: Skin is frequently, but not always, kept moist; linen must be changed 2–3 times every 24 hr.	3. Rarely moist: Skin is rarely moist more than 3–4 times a week, but linen does require changing at that time.	4. Never moist: Perspiration and incontinence is never a problem; linen changed at routine intervals only.
ACTIVITY (degree of physical activity)	1. Bedfast: Confined to bed.	2. Chairfast: Ability to walk severely impaired or nonexistent and must be assisted into chair or wheelchair. Is confined to chair or wheelchair when not in bed.	3. Walks occasionally: Walks occasionally during day, but for very short distances, with or without assistance. Spends majority of each shift in bed or chair.	4. Walks frequently: Walks a moderate distance at least once every 1–2 hr during waking hours.
MOBILITY (ability to change and control body position)	1. Completely immobile: Unable to make even slight changes in position without assistance.	2. Very limited: Makes occasional slight changes in position without help but unable to make frequent or significant changes in position independently.	3. Slightly limited: Makes frequent though slight changes in position without assistance but unable to make or maintain major changes in position independently.	4. No limitations: Makes major and frequent changes in position without assistance.
NUTRITION (usual food intake pattern)	1. Very poor: Never eats a complete meal. Rarely eats more than ⅓ of any food offered. Intake of protein is negligible. Takes even fluids poorly. Does not take a liquid dietary supplement, OR is NPO or maintained on clear liquids or IV feeding for more than 5 days.	2. Probably inadequate: Rarely eats a complete meal and generally eats only about ½ of any food offered. Protein intake is poor. Occasionally will take a liquid dietary supplement, OR receiving less than optimum amount of liquid diet or tube feeding.	3. Adequate: Eats over ½ of most meals. Eats moderate amount of protein source 1–2 times daily. Occasionally will refuse a meal. Will usually take a dietary supplement if offered, OR is on tube feeding or TPN, which probably meets most nutritional needs.	4. Excellent: Eats most of every meal. Never refuses a meal. Frequently eats between meals. Does not require a dietary supplement.
FRICTION AND SHEAR	1. Problem: Requires moderate to maximum assistance in moving. Complete lifting without sliding against sheets is impossible. Frequently slides down in bed or chair, requiring frequent repositioning with maximum assistance. Either spasticity, contractures, or agitation leads to almost constant friction.	2. Potential problem: Moves feebly independently or requires minimum assistance. Skin probably slides against bedsheets or chair to some extent when movement occurs. Maintains relatively good position in chair or bed most of the time but occasionally slides down.	3. No apparent problem: Moves in bed and in chair independently and has sufficient muscle strength to lift up completely during move. Maintains good position in bed or chair at all times.	

Source: Black JM, and Matassarin-Jacobs E (eds): Luckmann and Sorensen's Medical-Surgical Nursing, ed 4. Philadelphia, WB Saunders, 1993, p 393.
Key: A score of 15 to 16 (15 to 18 if > 75 yr) indicates minimum risk; 13 to 14, moderate risk; ≤ 12, high risk.
Used with permission of Barbara Braden, Ph.D., R.N., F.A.A.N., Professor and Dean, Graduate School, Creighton University, Omaha, 1996.

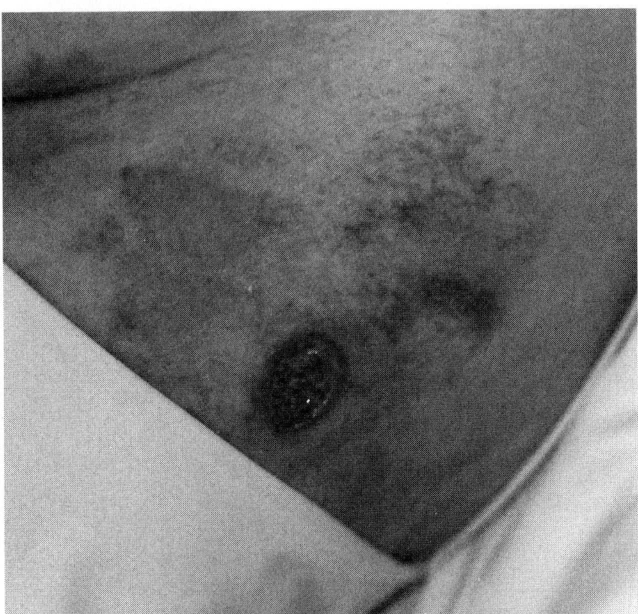

Figure **8–22.** Pressure ulcer. (*Courtesy of Pam Unger, P.T., Community General Hospital, Center for Wound Management, Reading, Pa, 1995.*)

of these. An appropriate wound covering is then applied to provide an optimal wound environment.

Large deep pressure ulcers may require chemical debridement using proteolytic enzyme agents or surgical debridement of necrotic tissue and opening of deep pockets for drainage. A variety of skin grafting techniques may be used if the wound is closed. In stage III ulcers, undamaged tissue near the wound is rotated to cover the ulcer. In stage IV ulcers, musculoskeletal flaps (a single unit of skin with its underlying muscle and vasculature), as well as a variety of other skin grafting techniques, may be used effectively to close the wound (Hockenberger and Black, 1993).

Prognosis. Most clients have multiple complicating medical factors which contribute to the poor healing. Each client responds differently to a course of therapy. Provided there is no infection, good blood supply, the pressure has been eliminated, and the client has no medical complications, the wound should heal successfully. The presence of any of these factors alters the prognosis negatively.

Special Implications for the Therapist **8–16**

PRESSURE ULCERS

The therapist plays a pivotal role in the prevention and management of pressure ulcers. Not only is the therapist an expert in the delivery of therapeutic modalities but appropriate positioning, management of tissue load (mechanical factors acting on the tissues), and good mobility are essential to the success of the intervention.

High-risk clients should be identified, possibly using the Braden Scale (see Table 8–13), but all people in the acute care, home health, or long-term health care setting should be evaluated for risk levels and reassessed every 3 months for changes in status. The high-risk client will need frequent position changes (at least every 2 hours). A trapeze bar, turning sheet, or transfer board can be used to prevent shearing injury to the skin. Frequent shifting of body weight prevents ischemia by redistributing the weight and allowing blood to recirculate. Static or dynamic pressure reducing devices using air, gel or water, foam, or other substances are commercially available. Reducing pressure on the skin must be accompanied by adequate fluid and nutrition intake (see also Table 8–14).

The person who is incontinent presents an additional challenge to keeping the skin clean and dry. Stool or urine becomes an irritant and places the person at additional risk for skin breakdown. Contamination of an already existing wound by wound drainage, perspiration, urine, or feces is also a concern for the incontinent and immobile population. Cleaning should be carried out using a mild agent that minimizes irritation and dryness of the skin. Avoid harsh alkali soaps, alcohol-based products that can cause vasoconstriction, tincture of benzoin (may cause painful erosions), hexachlorophene (may irritate the CNS), and petrolatum gauze. During cleaning or wound care, the force and friction applied to the skin should be minimized.

Pigmentary Disorders *(Goldstein and Odom, 1995)*

Definition and Overview. Skin color or pigmentation is determined by the deposition of melanin, a dark polymer found in the skin, as well as in the hair, ciliary body, choroid of the eye, pigment layer of the retina, and certain nerve cells. Melanin is formed in the melanocytes in the basal layer of the epidermis and is regulated (dispersion and aggregation) through the release of melatonin, a pineal hormone. *Hyperpigmentation* is the abnormally increased pigmentation resulting from increased melanin production. *Hypopigmentation* is the abnormally decreased pigmentation resulting from decreased melanin production.

Pigmentary disorders (either hyperpigmentation or hypopigmentation) may be primary or secondary. Secondary pigmentary changes occur as a result of damage to the skin such as irritation, allergy, infection, excoriation, burns, or dermatologic therapy such as curettage, dermabrasion, chemical peels, or freezing with liquid nitrogen.

Etiology and Risk Factors. The formation and deposition of melanin can be affected by external influences such as exposure to heat, trauma, solar or ionizing radiation, heavy metals, and changes in oxygen potential. These influences can result in hyperpigmentation, hypopigmentation, or both. Local trauma may destroy melanocytes temporarily or permanently, causing hypopigmentation, sometimes with hyperpigmentation in surrounding skin.

Other pigmentary disorders may occur from exposure to exogenous pigments such as carotene, certain metals, and tattooing inks. Carotenemia occurs as a result of excessive carotene in the blood, usually from ingesting certain foods (e.g., carrots, yellow fruit, egg yolk). It may also occur in diabetes mellitus and in hypothyroidism. Exposure to metals such as silver can cause argyria, a poisoning marked by a

TABLE 8–14 Guidelines for Prevention of Pressure Ulcers in Adults

- All clients at risk should have a systematic skin inspection at least once a day, paying particular attention to the bony prominences. Results of skin inspection should be documented.
- Skin should be cleaned at the time of soiling and at routine intervals. The frequency of skin cleaning should be individualized according to need and client preference. Avoid hot water, and use a mild cleaning agent that minimizes irritation and dryness of the skin. During the cleaning or wound care process, minimize the force and friction applied to the skin.
- Minimize environmental factors leading to skin drying such as low humidity (<40%) and exposure to cold. Dry skin should be treated with moisturizers.
- Massage should NOT be carried out over bony prominences in the population at risk (Olson, 1989). Indirect soft tissue mobilization techniques or massaging the tissue around and toward the area must be performed with caution.
- Skin injury caused by friction and shear forces should be minimized through proper positioning, transferring, and turning techniques. Friction injuries may be reduced by the use of lubricants such as cornstarch and creams, protective films such as transparent film dressings and skin sealants, protective dressings such as hydrocolloids, and protective padding.
- Maintain current activity level, mobility, and range of motion. Evaluate the potential for improving the person's mobility and activity status and institute rehabilitation efforts.
- Interventions and outcomes should be monitored and documented.
- Any person in bed who is assessed to be at risk of developing pressure ulcers should be repositioned at least every 2 hr if consistent with overall treatment goals.
- For persons in bed, positioning devices such as pillows or foam wedges should be used to keep bony prominences (e.g., knees and ankles) from direct contact with one another.
- Persons in bed who are completely immobile should be provided with devices that completely relieve pressure on the heels. Do not use doughnut-type devices.
- When side-lying position is used in bed, avoid positioning directly on the greater trochanter.
- Maintain the head of the bed at the lowest degree of elevation consistent with medical conditions and other restrictions. Limit the amount of time the head of the bed is elevated.
- Use lifting devices such as a trapeze, hydraulic lift, slide board, or linen to move (rather than drag) persons in bed who cannot assist during transfers and position changes.
- Any person assessed to be at risk of developing pressure ulcers should be placed, when lying in bed, on a pressure-reducing surface, such as foam, static air, alternating air, gel, or water mattresses.
- Any person at risk of developing a pressure ulcer should avoid uninterrupted sitting in any chair or wheelchair. He or she should be repositioned, shifting the points under pressure at least every hour, or be put back to bed if consistent with overall management goals. Persons who are able should be taught to shift weight every 15 min.
- For chairbound persons, the use of a pressure-reducing device is indicated. Do not use doughnut-type devices.

Modified from Panel of the Prediction and Prevention of Pressure Ulcers in Adults: Pressure ulcers in adults: Prediction and prevention: Clinical practice guidelines. CPR Publication No. 92-0050. Rockville, Md, Agency for Health Care Policy and Research, Public Health Service, US Department of Health and Human Services, 1992.

permanent ashen-gray discoloration of the skin, conjunctivae, and internal organs. Gold, when given chronically for rheumatoid arthritis, can also cause pigmentary changes.

Clinical Manifestations

Hyperpigmentation. Primary disorders in this category include pigmented nevi, mongolian spots, juvenile freckles (ephelides), lentigines (also called liver spots) from sun exposure, café au lait spots associated with neurofibromatosis, and hypermelanosis caused by increased melanocyte-stimulating hormone (e.g., Addison's disease).

Secondary hyperpigmentation most commonly occurs after another dermatologic condition, such as acne (e.g., postinflammatory hyperpigmentation seen in dark-skinned people). *Melasma*, a patterned hyperpigmentation of the face, can occur as a result of steroid hormones, estrogens, and progesterones, as occurs during pregnancy and in 30% to 50% of women taking oral contraceptives. Secondary hyperpigmentation may also develop as a phototoxic reaction to medications, oils in perfumes, and chemicals in the rinds of limes, citrus fruits, and celery.

Hypopigmentation and Depigmentation. The disorder most commonly seen by a therapist in this category is vitiligo. In *vitiligo*, pigment cells (melanocytes) are destroyed resulting in small or large circumscribed areas of depigmentation often having hyperpigmented borders, and enlarging slowly (Fig. 8–23). This condition may be associated with hyperthyroidism, hypothyroidism, pernicious anemia, diabetes mellitus, Addison's disease, and carcinoma of the stomach.

Hypopigmentation can also occur on black skin from the use of liquid nitrogen. Intra-articular injections of high concentrations of corticosteroids may also cause localized temporary hypopigmentation.

Blistering Diseases

Definition, Incidence, and Etiology. On occasion, blistering diseases may be seen in a therapy practice when severe

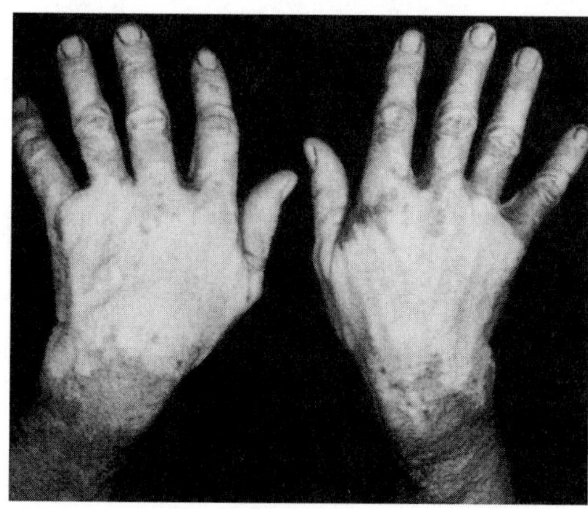

Figure **8–23.** Vitiligo. (*From Callen JP, Jorizzo J (eds): Dermatological Signs of Internal Disease, ed 2. Philadelphia, WB Saunders, 1995, p 191.*)

enough to warrant localized treatment (usually similar to wound care, ulcer care, or burn care). Blisters occur on skin and mucous membranes in a condition called *pemphigus*, which is an uncommon intraepidermal blistering disease in which the epidermal cells separate from one another. This disease occurs almost exclusively in middle-aged or older adults of all races and ethnic groups.

The exact cause is unknown but one type of pemphigus is especially likely to be associated with other autoimmune diseases, and drug-induced pemphigus from penicillamine and captopril has been reported. Paraneoplastic pemphigus (arising from the metabolic effects of cancer on tissues remote from the tumor) is a recently described syndrome that has a distinct clinical and histologic presentation. This form of pemphigus has a poor prognosis because of the underlying malignancy.

Clinical Manifestations. Blistering diseases are characterized by the formation of bullae, or blisters. These bullae appear spontaneously, often on the oral mucous membranes or scalp, and are relatively asymptomatic. Erosions and crusts may develop over the blisters causing toxemia and a "mousy" odor. The lesions become extensive and the complications of the disease, especially infection, can lead to great toxicity and debility. Disturbances of electrolyte balance are also common due to fluid losses through the involved skin in severe cases. See Fluid and Electrolyte Balance, Chapter 4.

Medical Management. Medical management may include hospitalization (bedrest, IV antibiotics and feedings) when the disease is severe. For others, treatment may be with corticosteroids (e.g., prednisone), and local measures. The course of this disorder tends to be chronic in most people and high-dose corticosteroids can mask the signs and symptoms of infection. If untreated, this condition is usually fatal within 2 months to 5 years as a result of infection.

Sarcoidosis

Sarcoidosis is a multisystemic disorder characterized by the formation of granulomas, inflammatory lesions containing mononuclear phagocytes usually surrounded by a rim of lymphocytes. These granulomas may develop in the lungs, liver, bones, or eyes (see Table 12–15) and may be accompanied by skin lesions (see Fig. 12–13). In the United States, sarcoidosis occurs predominantly among blacks, affecting twice as many women as men. Acute sarcoidosis usually resolves within 2 years. Chronic, progressive sarcoidosis, which is uncommon, is associated with pulmonary fibrosis and progressive pulmonary disability (Norris et al., 1995). See Chapter 12 for a complete discussion of this condition.

References

Abrams WB, Beers MH, Berkow R (eds): The Merck Manual of Geriatrics, ed 2. Rahway, NJ, Merck, 1995.

ACS (American Cancer Society): Cancer Statistics 1995. Atlanta, Author, 1997.

American Burn Association: Guidelines for service standards and severity classification in the treatment of burn injury. Bull Am Coll Surg 69(10):24–28, 1984.

Amonette RA, Leffell DJ, Robins P: Actinic Keratosis: What You Should Know About This Common Precancer. New York, Skin Cancer Foundation, 1993.

Ananthaswamy HN, Pierceall WE: Molecular alterations in human skin tumors. Prog Clin Biol Res 376:61–84, 1992.

Arnold HL, Odom RB, James WD (eds): Andrews' Diseases of the Skin: Clinical Dermatology, ed 8. Philadelphia, WB Saunders, 1990.

Atchison NE: Pain during burn dressing change in children: Relationship to burn area, depth, and analgesic regimens. Pain 47:41–45, 1991.

Balch CM, Milton CW, Milton GW, et al (eds): Cutaneous Melanoma, ed 2. Philadelphia, JB Lippincott, 1992.

Barth A, Morton DL: The role of adjuvant therapy in melanoma management. Cancer 75 (suppl 2):726–734, 1995.

Beck LA, Morison WL: Psoriasis. *In* Stein JH (ed): Internal Medicine, ed 4. St Louis, Mosby–Year Book, 1994, pp 2532–2535.

Bellet RE, Mastrangelo DB, Maguire HC: Primary cutaneous melanoma. *In* Kahn BS, Love RR, Sherman R, et al (eds): Concepts in Cancer Medicine. New York, Grune & Stratton, 1983.

Berd D, Maguire HC Jr, Mastrangelo MJ: Treatment of human melanoma with a hapten-modified autologous vaccine. Ann N Y Acad Sci 690:147–152, 1993.

Black, HS, Thomby JI, Wolf JE, et al: Evidence that a low-fat diet reduces the occurrence of non-melanoma skin cancer. Int J Cancer 62:165–169, 1995.

Bouffard D, Wong T-Y, Hernandez M, Mihm MO: Suspicion of early desmoplastic melanoma. Melanoma Lett 11(3):1, 1993.

Burgess M. Initial management of a patient with extensive burn injury. Crit Care Nurs Clin North Am, 3:165–179, 1991.

Burstein JM, Sober AJ: Melanoma in dark-skinned people. Melanoma Lett, 11(2):3–4, 1993.

Buskila D, Langevitz P, Gladman DD, et al: Patients with rheumatoid arthritis are more tender than those with psoriatic arthritis. J Rhematol 19:1115–1119, 1992.

Callaghan S: Skin considerations with silicone-type interfaces. Adv Phys Ther 7:22–23, 1996.

Carrougher GJ: Nursing care of clients with burn injury. *In* Black JM, Matassarin-Jacobs E (eds): Luckmann and Sorensen's Medical-Surgical Nursing, ed 4. Philadelphia, WB Saunders, 1993, pp 1985–2012.

Carrougher GJ, Marvin J: Mechanical debridement: Views from University of Washington Burn Center at Harborview. Seattle, Washington (editorial). J Burn Care Rehabil 10:271–272, 1989.

Cesarman E, Chang Y, Moore PS, et al: Kaposi's sarcoma–associated herpesvirus-like DNA sequences in AIDS-related body cavity–based lymphomas. N Engl J Med 332:1186–1191, 1995.

Clark RE: Alternatives to surgery for nonmelanomas. Skin Cancer Found J 12:17, 82–83, 1994.

Clements PJ: Systemic sclerosis: Natural history and management strategies. J Musculoskel Med 11(11):43–50, 1994.

Dinehart SM: Skin cancer and the sexes. Sun Skin News 10(2):1–3, 1993.

Farrington E: Varicella zoster vaccine (Varivax). Pediatr Nurs 21:358–361, 1995.

Feller I: Burn epidemiology: Focus on youngsters and the aged. J Burn Care Rehabil 3:285–288, 1982.

Feller I: Improvements in burn care, 1965–1979. JAMA 244:2074–2078, 1980.
Fraser DD, Frank JA, Dalakas, M, et al: Magnetic resonance imaging in the idiopathic inflammatory myopathies. J Rheumatol 18:1693–1700, 1991.
Friedman RJ, Rigel DS, Silverman MK, et al: Malignant melanoma in the 1990s: The continued importance of early detection and the role of the physician examination and self-examination. Cancer 41:201–226, 1991.
Fye KH, Sack KE: Rheumatic disease. *In* Stites DP, Terr AI, Parslow TG (eds): Basic and Clinical Immunology, ed 8. Norwalk, Conn, Appleton & Lange, 1994, pp 387–411.
Geller A, Koh HK, Miller D, et al: Death rates of malignant melanoma among white men—United States. MMWR 41:20–21,27, 1992.
Gilchrest BA: How suntans lead to skin cancer. Sun Skin News 12(1):1–2, 1995.
Gilchrest BA, Zhal S, Eller MS, et al: Treatment of human melanocytes and S91 melanoma cells with the DNA repair enzyme T4 endonuclease V enhances melanogenesis after ultraviolet irradiation. J Invest Dermatol 101:666–672, 1993.
Gill, EP, Shandera WX: Infectious diseases: Viral and rickettsial. *In* Tierney LM, McPhee SJ, Papadakis MA (eds): Current Medical Diagnosis and Treatment, ed 34. Norwalk, Conn, Appleton & Lange, 1995, pp 1128–1161.
Gimenez SA, Siegal SH: A 15-year prospective study of treatment of rapidly progressive systemic sclerosis with D-penicillamine. J Rheumatol 18:1496, 1991.
Gladman DD, Farewell V, Buskila D, et al: Reliability of measurements of active and damaged joints in psoriatic arthritis. J Rheumatol 17:62–64, 1990.
Gladman DD, Shuckett R, Russell, ML, et al: Psoriatic arthritis (PsA): An analysis of 220 patients. Q J Med 62:127–141, 1987.
Gladman DD, Urowitz P: Systemic lupus erythematosus. *In* Schumacher HR, Klippel JH, Koopman WJ (eds): Primer on the Rheumatic Diseases, ed 10. Atlanta, Arthritis Foundation, 1993, p 23.
Goetz RH: The pathology of progressive systemic sclerosis (generalized scleroderma) with special reference to changes in the viscera. Clin Proc 4:337, 1945.
Goldstein SM, Odom RB: Skin and Appendages. *In* Tierney LM, McPhee SJ, Papadakis MA (eds): Current Medical Diagnosis and Treatment, ed. 34. Norwalk, Conn, Appleton & Lange, 1995, pp 80–143.
Greenwald GI, Tashkin DP, Gong H, et al: Longitudinal changes in lung function and respiratory symptoms in progressive systemic sclerosis. Prospective study. Am J Med 83:83–92, 1987.
Halpern A: P.T.s can help patients by recognizing signs of skin disorders. Presented at the Hospital of the University of Pennsylvania (HUP), 1993.
Heimbach DM: Smoke inhalation: Current concepts. *In* Wachtel TL (ed): Current Topics in Burn Care. Rockville, Md, Aspen, 1983.
HHS (US Department of Health and Human Services): Pressure ulcers in adults: Predilection and prevention. AHCPR Publication No. 92-0047. Rockville, Md, USDHHS, 1992.
HHS (US Department of Health and Human Services): Pressure ulcer treatment. AHCPR Publication No. 95-0652. Rockville, Md, USDHHS 1995.
Ho RC: Medical management of stage IV malignant melanoma. Cancer 75 (suppl 2):735–741, 1995.
Hockenberger S, Black JM: Wound healing. *In* Black JM, Matassarin-Jacobs E (eds): Luckmann and Sorensen's Medical-Surgical Nursing, ed 4. Philadelphia, WB Saunders, 1993, pp 373–398.
Huether SE, Kravitz M: Structure, function, and disorders of the integument. *In* McCance KL, Huether SE (eds): Pathophysiology: The Biologic Basis for Disease in Adults and Children, ed 2. St. Louis, Mosby–Year Book, 1994, pp 1512–1560.
HWHW (Harvard Women's Health Watch): Melanoma. 2(2):2, 1994.
Jones JD: Alcohol use and burn injury. J Burn Care Rehabil 12:148–152, 1989.
Jones JS, Hoerie D, Rieske R: Stethoscopes: A potential vector of infection? Ann Emerg Med 26:296–299, 1995.
Kolibasova K, Tothova I, Baumgartner J: Eradication of *Helicobacter pylori* as the only successful treatment in rosacea. Arch Dermatol 132:1393, 1996.
Kruger S, Garbe C, Buttner P, et al: Epidemiologic evidence for the role of melanocytic nevi as risk markers and direct precursors of cutaneous malignant melanoma. J Am Acad Dermatol 26:920–926, 1992.
Kurban RS, Kurban AK: Common skin disorders of aging. Geriatrics 48:30–42, 1993.
Lahita RG: What is Lupus? New York, Lupus Foundation of America, 1992.
LeRoy EC, Silver RM: Systemic sclerosis and related syndromes: Epidemiology, pathology, and pathogenesis. *In* Schumacher HR, Klippel JH, Koopman WJ (eds): Primer on the Rheumatic Diseases, ed 10. Atlanta, Arthritis Foundation, 1993, pp 118–120.
Linn BS: Age differences in the severity and outcome of burns. J Am Geriatr Soc 28:118–123, 1980.
Love LA, Leff RL, Fraser DD, et al: A new approach to the classification of idiopathic inflammatory myopathy: Myositis-specific autoantibodies define useful homogeneous patient groups. Medicine (Baltimore) 70:360–374, 1991.
Lund CC, Browder NC: The estimation of areas of burn. Surg Gynecol Obstet 79:352–358, 1994.
Mader R, Gladman DD: Psoriatic arthritis: Making the diagnosis and treating early. J Musculoskel Med 10(5):18–28, 1993.
Marghoob AA, Koff AW, Rigel DS, et al: Risk of cutaneous malignant melanoma in patients with "classic" atypical-mole syndrome. A case-control study. Arch Dermatol 130:993–998, 1994.
Maricq HR, Weinrich MC, Keil JE, et al: Prevalence of scleroderma spectrum disorders in the general population of South Carolina. Arthritis Rheum 32:998–1006, 1989.
Matassarin-Jacobs E: Nursing care of clients with connective tissue disorders. *In* Black JM, Matassarin-Jacobs E (eds): Luckmann and Sorensen's Medical-Surgical Nursing, ed 4. Philadelphia, WB Saunders, 1993, pp 593–614.
Medsger TA: Systemic sclerosis (scleroderma). *In* Stein JH (ed): Internal Medicine, ed 4. St. Louis, Mosby–Year Book, 1994, pp 2443–2449.
Medsger TA: Systemic sclerosis (scleroderma), localized forms of scleroderma, and calcinosis. *In* McCarty DJ, Koopman WJ (eds): Arthritis and Allied Conditions, ed 12. Philadelphia, Lea & Febiger, 1993, pp 1253–1292.
Medsger TA, Steen V: Systemic sclerosis and related syndromes: Clinical features and treatment. *In* Schumacher HR, Klippel JH, Koopman WJ (eds): Primer on the Rheumatic Diseases, ed 10. Atlanta, Arthritis Foundation, 1993, pp 120–126.
Miller DL, Weinstock MA: Nonmelanoma skin cancer in the United States: Incidence. J Am Acad Dermatol 30(5 pt 1):774–778, 1994.
Monk BE, Graham-Brown RAC, Sarkany I: Skin Disorders in the Elderly. Oxford, Blackwell, 1988.
Moore PS, Chang Y: Detection of herpesvirus-like DNA sequences in Kaposi's sarcoma in patients with and without HIV infection. N Engl J Med 332:1181–1185, 1995.
Nicol NH: Nursing care of clients with integumentary disorders. *In* Black JM, Matassarin-Jacobs E (eds): Luckmann and Sorensen's Medical-Surgical Nursing, ed 4. Philadelphia, WB Saunders, 1993, pp 1955–1984.
Norris J, McMahon E, Fandek N, et al (eds): Professional Guide to Diseases, ed 5. Springhouse, Pa, Springhouse, 1995.
Oddis CV, Conte CG, Steen VD, et al: Incidence of polymyositis-dermatomyositis: A 20 year study of hospital diagnosed cases in Allegheny County, PA 1963–1982. J Rheumatol 17:1329–1334, 1990.
Oddis CV, Medsger TA: Chronic inflammatory myopathies: Polymyositis and dermatomyositis. J Musculoskel Med 8(3):26–37, 1991.
Olson, B: Effects of massage for prevention of pressure ulcers. Decubitus 2:32–37, 1989.
O'Toole M (ed): Miller-Keane Encyclopedia and Dictionary of Medicine, Nursing, and Allied Health, ed 5. Philadelphia, WB Saunders, 1992.
Owens GR, Medsger TA Jr: Systemic sclerosis secondary to occupational exposure. Am J Med 85:114–116, 1988.
Pion IA, Rigel DS, Garfinkel L, et al: Occupation and the risk of malignant melanoma. Cancer 75(suppl 2):637–644, 1995.
Plotz PH, Leff RL, Miller FW: Inflammatory and metabolic myopathies. *In* Schumacher HR, Klippel JH, Koopman WJ (eds): Primer on the Rheumatic Diseases, ed 10. Atlanta, Arthritis Foundation, 1993, pp 127–131.
Pruit BA Jr, Goodwin CW Jr: Burn injury. *In* Moore EE (ed): Early Care of the Injured Patient. Philadelphia, Decker, 1990, pp 286–306.
Rigel DS: The gender-related issues in malignant melanoma. Hawaii Med J 52:124, 146, 1993.

Roizman B: New viral footprints in Kaposi's sarcoma. N Engl J Med 332:1227–1228, 1995.
Safai B: Pathophysiology and epidemiology of epidemic Kaposi's sarcoma. Semin Oncol 14(suppl 3):7, 1987.
Salopek TG, Marghoob AA, Slade JM: An estimate of the incidence of malignant melanoma in the United States. Based on a survey of members of the American Academy of Dermatology. Dermatol Surg 21:301–305, 1995.
Sato T, Maguire HC Jr, Mastrangelo MJ, Berd D: Human immune response to DNP-modified autologous cells after treatment with a DNP-conjugated melanoma vaccine. Clin Immunol Immunopathol 74:35–43, 1995.
Schneider JS, Moore DH, Sagebiel RW: Risk factors for melanoma incidence in prospective follow-up: The importance of atypical dysplastic nevi. Arch Dermatol 130:1002–1007, 1994.
Schumacher HR: Joint involvement in progressive systemic sclerosis (scleroderma). Am J Clin Pathol 60:593–600, 1973.
Shadomy H, Utz J: Infections due to gram-positive bacteria. *In* Fitzpatrick T (ed): Dermatology in General Medicine, ed 4. New York, McGraw-Hill, 1993.
Simoes EAF: Immunization. *In* Hathaway WE, Hay WW, Groothuis JR, Paisley JW (eds): Current Pediatric Diagnosis and Treatment, ed 12. Norwalk, Conn, Appleton & Lange, 1995, pp 229–256.
Steen VD, Medsger TA Jr: Epidemiology and natural history of systemic sclerosis. Rheum Dis Clin North Am 16:1–10, 1990.
Truhan AP: Sun protection in childhood. Clin Pediatr (Phila) 30(12):676–681, 1991.
Vossaert KA, Silverman MK, Kopf AW, et al: Influence of gender on survival in patients with stage I malignant melanoma. J Am Acad Dermatol 26(3 pt 2):429–440, 1992.
Waldow SM, Lobraico RV, Kohler IK, et al: Photodynamic therapy for treatment of malignant cutaneous lesions. Laser Surg Med 7:451–456, 1987.
Washington CV: Skin Cancer. *In* Isselbacher KJ, Braunwald E, Wilson JD, et al (eds): Harrison's Principles of Internal Medicine, ed 13. New York, McGraw-Hill, 1994, pp 1866–1867.
Wooldridge WE: A rash followed by muscle weakness. Case study. J Musculoskel Med 12(1):71–72, 1995.
Wong DL (ed): Whaley and Wong's Essentials of Pediatric Nursing, ed 4. St. Louis, Mosby–Year Book, 1993.

SECTION 2

chapter 9

The Endocrine and Metabolic Systems

Catherine C. Goodman

ENDOCRINE SYSTEM

The endocrine system is composed of various glands located throughout the body (Fig. 9–1). These glands are capable of synthesizing and releasing special chemical messengers called *hormones*, which are transported by the bloodstream to the cells and organs on which they have a specific regulatory effect (Table 9–1). The endocrine system in conjunction with the nervous system controls and integrates body function to maintain homeostasis. Whereas the nervous system sends its messages along nerve fibers, eliciting swift and selective neural responses, the endocrine system sends its messages in the form of hormones via the bloodstream. Hormonal effects have a slower onset than neural effects, but they maintain a longer duration of action. The actions of the endocrine system may be localized to one area or generalized to all the cells of the body (Butts-Krakoff, 1993).

The endocrine system has five general functions: (1) differentiation of the reproductive and central nervous system of the developing fetus; (2) stimulation of sequential growth and development during childhood and adolescence; (3) coordination of the male and female reproductive systems; (4) maintenance of optimal internal environment throughout the lifespan; and (5) initiation of corrective and adaptive responses when emergency demands occur (Huether, 1994).

The endocrine system meets the nervous system at the hypothalamic-pituitary interface. The hypothalamus, the main integrative center for the endocrine and autonomic nervous systems, controls the function of endocrine organs by neural and hormonal pathways. Although the communicative and integrative roles of the endocrine and nervous systems are similar, the precise ways in which each system functions differ.

Hypothalamic Control *(Norris, 1995)*

Neural pathways connect the hypothalamus to the posterior pituitary (or neurohypophysis), providing the hypothalamus direct control over both the anterior and posterior portions of the pituitary gland (Fig. 9–2). Disorders of the hypothalamic-pituitary axis are usually clinically manifested either by syndromes of hormone excess or deficiency or by visual impairment from optic nerve compression because of the location of the hypothalamus and pituitary (Benson and Rosenthal, 1993).

Neural stimulation to the posterior pituitary provokes the secretion of two effector hormones: antidiuretic hormone (ADH) and oxytocin. The hypothalamus also exerts hormonal control at the anterior pituitary through releasing and inhibiting factors. Hypothalamic hormones stimulate the pituitary to release tropic (stimulating) hormones, such as adrenocorticotropic hormone (ACTH), thyroid-stimulating hormone (TSH), luteinizing hormone (LH), and follicle-stimulating hormone (FSH) (see Fig. 9–2). At the same time, effector hormones such as growth hormone and prolactin are released or inhibited, affecting the adrenal cortex, thyroid, and gonads. Endocrine pathology develops as a result of dysfunction of releasing, tropic, or effector hormones or when defects occur in the target tissue.

In addition to hormonal and neural controls, a negative feedback system regulates the endocrine system. The mechanism may be simple or complex. Simple feedback occurs when the level of one substance regulates the secretion of a hormone. For example, low serum calcium levels stimulate parathyroid hormone (PTH) secretion; high serum calcium levels inhibit it. Complex feedback occurs through the hypothalamic-pituitary–target organ axis. For example, following an injury or major stress, secretion of the hypothalamic corticotropin-releasing hormone (CRH) releases pituitary ACTH, which in turn stimulates adrenal cortisol secretion. Subsequently, a rise in serum cortisol inhibits ACTH by decreasing CRH secretion (see Fig. 9–2). Steroid therapy disrupts the hypothalamic-pituitary-adrenal (HPA) axis by suppressing hypothalamic-pituitary secretion. Abrupt withdrawal of exogenous steroid can induce life-threatening adrenal crisis when the HPA axis does not have enough time to recover enough to stimulate cortisol secretion.

Hormonal Effects *(Norris, 1995)*

In response to the hypothalamus, the *posterior pituitary* secretes oxytocin and ADH. Oxytocin stimulates contraction of the uterus and is responsible for the milk let-down reflex in lactating women. ADH controls the concentration of body fluids by altering the permeability of the kidney's distal convoluted tubules and collecting ducts to conserve water. The secretion of ADH depends on plasma volume and osmolality as monitored by hypothalamic neurons. Circulatory shock and severe hemorrhage are the most powerful stimulators of ADH; other stimulators include pain, emotional stress, trauma, morphine, tranquilizers, certain anesthetics, and positive-pressure breathing.

The *anterior pituitary* secretes prolactin, which stimulates milk production, and human growth hormone (HGH), which affects most body tissues. HGH stimulates growth by increasing protein synthesis and fat mobilization and by decreasing carbohydrate utilization. Hyposecretion of HGH results in dwarfism; hypersecretion causes gigantism in children and acromegaly in adults.

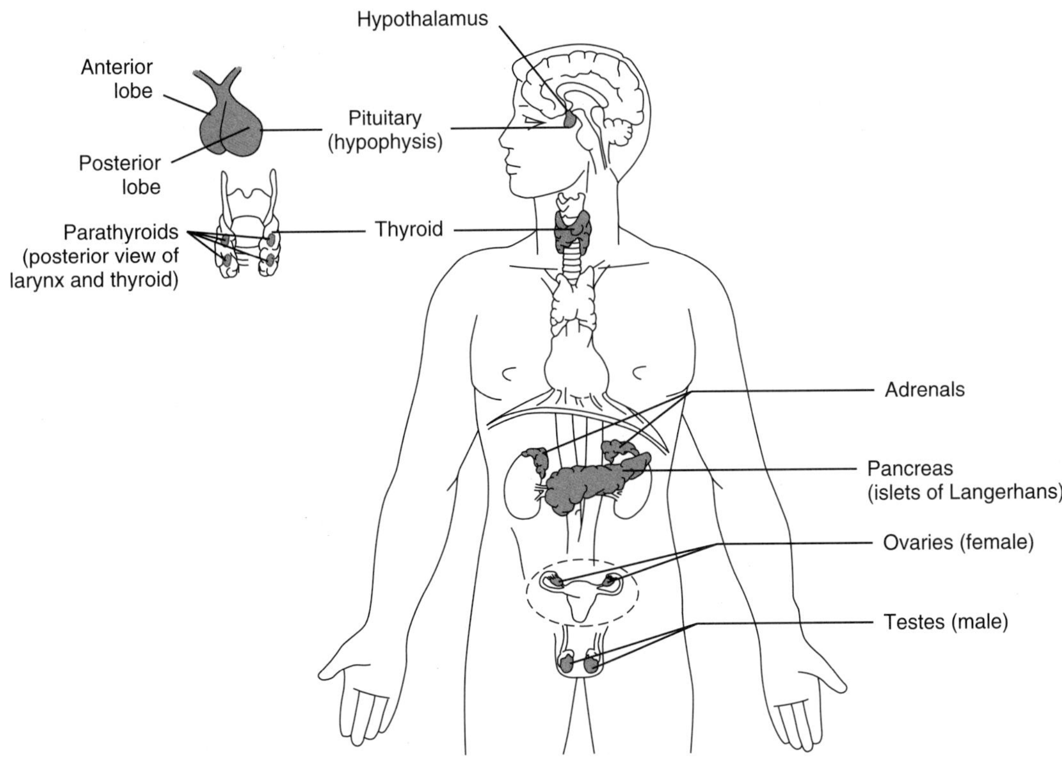

Figure 9–1. Endocrine glands.

The *thyroid gland* secretes the iodinated thyroid hormones thyroxine (T_4) and triiodothyronine (T_3).[1] Thyroid hormones, necessary for normal growth and development, act on many tissues to regulate our basal metabolism (i.e., the rate at which we convert food and oxygen into energy) and to increase metabolic activity and protein synthesis. Deficiency of thyroid hormone causes varying degrees of hypothyroidism, from a mild, clinically insignificant form to the life-threatening extreme, myxedema coma. Congenital hypothyroidism causes a condition in children referred to as *cretinism* (now considered an undesirable term). Hypersecretion of thyroid hormone causes hyperthyroidism and, in extreme cases, thyrotoxic crisis. Excessive secretion of TSH causes thyroid gland hyperplasia, resulting in goiter. Other causes of goiter are also discussed later in this chapter (see Thyroid Gland).

The *parathyroid glands* secrete PTH, which regulates calcium and phosphate metabolism. PTH elevates serum calcium levels by stimulating resorption of calcium and phosphate from bone, reabsorption of calcium and excretion of phosphate by the kidneys, and, by combined action with vitamin D, absorption of calcium and phosphate from the gastrointestinal (GI) tract. Hyperparathyroidism results in hypercalcemia; hypoparathyroidism causes hypocalcemia. Altered calcium levels may also result from nonendocrine causes, such as metastatic bone disease. Pathologic changes in calcium affecting bone bring these conditions to the therapist's attention.

[1] For reference values of thyroid hormone levels mentioned throughout this chapter, see Table 36–16.

The *endocrine pancreas* produces glucagon from the α-cells and insulin from the β-cells. Glucagon, the hormone of the fasting state, releases stored glucose to raise the blood glucose level. Insulin, the hormone of the nourished state, facilitates glucose transport, promotes glucose storage, stimulates protein synthesis, and enhances free fatty acid uptake and storage. Insulin deficiency causes diabetes mellitus; insulin excess can be exogenous (i.e., a person with diabetes may receive more insulin than is required) or insulin excess may result from a tumor of the β-cells called insulinoma. Whatever the cause of excess insulin, hypoglycemia (abnormally low level of glucose in the blood) is the result.

The *adrenal cortex* secretes mineralocorticoids, glucocorticoids, and sex steroids. Aldosterone, a mineralocorticoid, regulates the reabsorption of sodium and the excretion of potassium by the kidneys and is intimately involved in the regulation of blood pressure. An excess of aldosterone (aldosteronism) can result primarily from hyperplasia or from adrenal adenoma or secondarily from many conditions, such as congestive heart failure or cirrhosis. The *adrenal medulla* is an aggregate of nervous tissue that produces the catecholamines epinephrine and norepinephrine, which are involved in the fight-or-flight response. (See Neuroendocrine Response to Stress.)

The *testes* and *ovaries* are also endocrine glands responsible for synthesizing and secreting hormones (see discussion in Chapters 16 and 17).

Endocrine Pathology

Dysfunctions of the endocrine system are classified as hypofunction and hyperfunction. The source of hypofunction and hyperfunction may be inflammation or tumor originating in

TABLE 9-1 Endocrine Glands: Secretion, Target, and Actions

When reading a client's chart, it is important to know basic hormone functions or effects that may have an impact on therapy treatment. At least 30 different hormones have been identified, but only those most common to therapy clients are included here.

Gland	Hormone	Target	Basic Action
Pituitary Gland			
Anterior lobe	Somatotropin (growth hormone [GH])	Bones, muscles, organs	Retention of nitrogen to promote protein anabolism
	Thyroid stimulating hormone (TSH)	Thyroid	Promotes secretory activity
	Follicle stimulating hormone (FSH)	Ovaries, seminiferous tubules	Promotes development of ovarian follicle, secretion of estrogen, and maturation of sperm
	Luteinizing hormone	Follicle, interstitial cell	Promotes ovulation and formation of corpus luteum, secretion of progesterone, and secretion of testosterone
	Prolactin (luteotropic hormone)	Corpus luteum, breast	Maintains corpus luteum and progesterone secretion; stimulates milk secretion
	Adrenocorticotropic hormone (ACTH)	Adrenal cortex	Stimulates secretory activity
Posterior lobe	Antidiuretic hormone (ADH)	Distal tubules of kidney	Reabsorption of water
	Oxytocin	Uterus	Stimulates contraction
Thyroid	Thyroxine (T_4) and triiodothyronine (T_3)	Widespread	Regulate oxidation rate of body cells and growth and metabolism; influence gluconeogenesis, mobilization of fats, and exchange of water, electrolytes, and protein
	Calcitonin	Skeleton	Calcium and phosphorus metabolism
Parathyroids	Parathyroid hormone (PTH)	Bone, kidney, intestinal tract	Essential for calcium and phosphorus metabolism and calcification of bone
Adrenal Gland			
Cortex	Mineralocorticoid (aldosterone)	Widespread, primarily kidney	Maintains fluid/electrolyte balance; reabsorbs sodium chloride; excretes potassium
	Glucocorticoids (cortisol)	Widespread	Concerned with food metabolism and body response to stress; preserves carbohydrates and mobilizes amino acids; promotes gluconeogenesis; suppresses inflammation
	Sex hormones (testosterone, estrogen, progesterone)	Gonads	Ability to influence secondary sex characteristics
Medulla	Epinephrine	Widespread	Vasoconstriction with increased blood pressure; increased blood glucose via glycolysis; stimulates ACTH production
	Norepinephrine	Widespread	Vasoconstriction
Pancreas	Insulin	Widespread	Increased utilization of carbohydrate, decreased lipolysis, and protein catabolism; decreased blood glucose
	Glucagon	Widespread	Hyperglycemic factor; increases blood glucose via glycogenolysis
Gonads			
Ovaries	Estrogen	Widespread	Secondary sex characteristics; maturation and sexual function
	Progesterone	Uterus, breast	Preparation for and maintenance of pregnancy; development of mammary gland secretory tissue
Testes	Testosterone	Widespread	Secondary sex characteristics; maturation and normal sex function

From Goodman CC, Snyder TE: Differential Diagnosis in Physical Therapy, ed 2. Philadelphia, WB Saunders, 1995, pp 327–328.

the hypothalamus or in the pituitary gland. Inflammation may be acute or subacute but is usually chronic, resulting in glandular hypofunction. Chronic endocrine abnormalities (e.g., deficiencies of cortisol, thyroid hormone, or insulin) are common health problems requiring life-long hormone replacement for survival. Endocrine gland tumors (e.g., thyroid carcinoma) result in ectopic hormone production and affect the musculoskeletal system. (See Chapter 7 for a discussion of paraneoplastic syndromes associated with this phenomenon.)

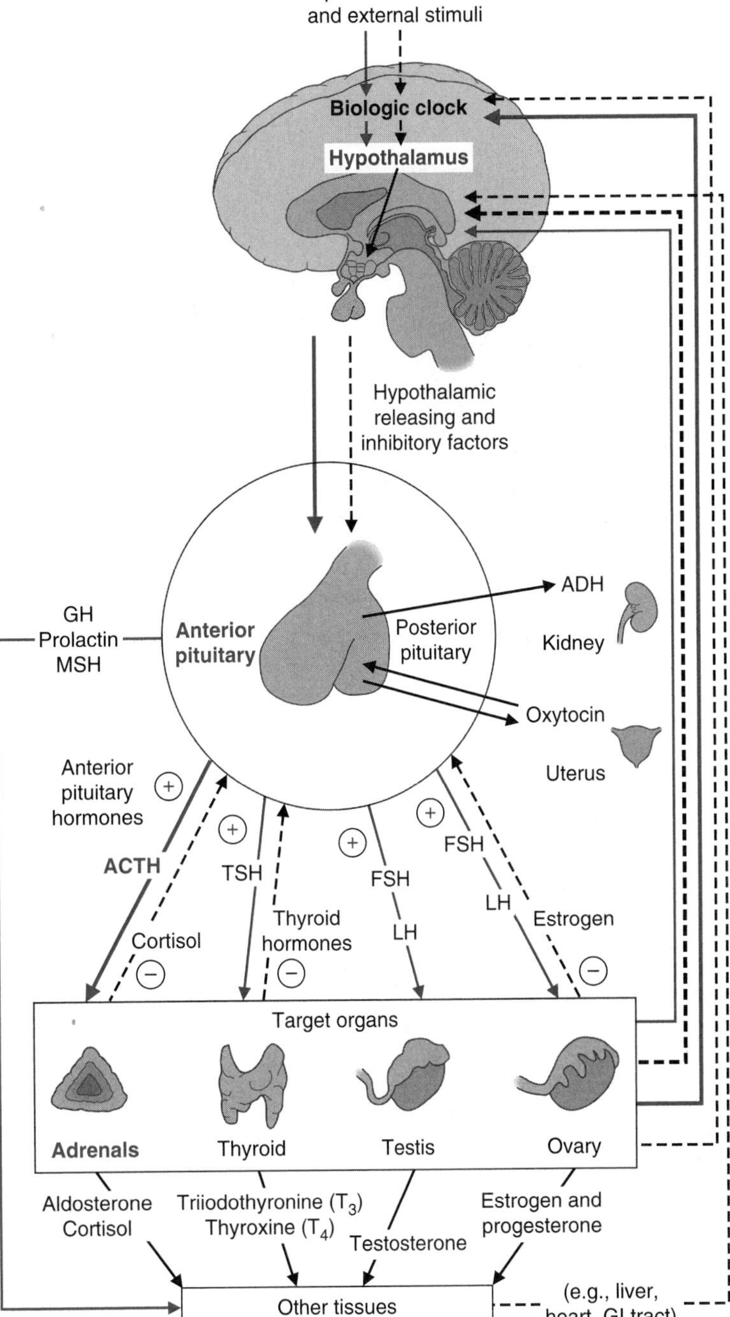

Figure **9–2.** Control of the endocrine system by the nervous system. One example of the complex feedback loops described in the text is highlighted here. The hypothalamus controls the pituitary gland through releasing and inhibiting factors. The anterior lobe of the pituitary gland then releases tropic (stimulating) hormones that act on target glands (thyroid, adrenals, gonads). Endocrine pathology occurs when dysfunction occurs in releasing, tropic, or effector hormones, or when defects occur in the target tissue.

Neuroendocrine Response to Stress[2]

(McCance and Shelby, 1994)

The concept that stress of any kind (emotional, physical, psychological, spiritual) may influence immunity and resistance to disease has been the subject of investigation for many years. The endocrine system, together with the immune system and the nervous system, mounts an integrated response to respond to stressors. Recent evidence to support a psychoneuroimmunologic basis for disease is discussed elsewhere in this text (see Chapters 2 and 5).

Hormones of the neuroendocrine system affect components of the immune system, and mediators produced by immune components regulate the neuroendocrine response. The sympathetic nervous system is aroused during the stress

[2] Only a brief review of the neuroendocrine response to stress contributing to disease is presented in this section. The reader is referred to a more specific text for detailed description of the endocrine system.

TABLE 9–2 Physiologic Effects of Cortisol

Functions Affected	Physiologic Effects
Protein metabolism	Increases protein synthesis in the liver and depresses protein synthesis in muscle, lymphoid tissue, adipose tissue, skin, and bone; increases plasma level of amino acids
Carbohydrate and lipid metabolism	Diminishes peripheral uptake and utilization of glucose; increases output of glucose from the liver; enhances the elevation of blood glucose promoted by other hormones
Lipid metabolism	Breakdown of fat in the extremities (lipolysis) and production of fat in the face and trunk (lipogenesis)
Inflammatory effects	Decreases circulating eosinophils, lymphocytes, and monocytes; increases release of polymorphonuclear leukocytes from the bone marrow; decreases accumulation of leukocytes at the site of inflammation; delays healing; essential for vasoconstrictive action of norepinephrine
Digestive function	Promotes gastric secretion
Urinary function	Enhances urinary excretion
Connective tissue function	Decreases proliferation of fibroblasts in connective tissue (and thus delays healing)
Muscle function	Maintains normal contractility and maximal work output for skeletal and cardiac muscle
Bone function	Decreases bone formation
Vascular system and myocardial function	Maintains normal blood pressure; permits increased responsiveness of arterioles to the constrictive action of adrenergic stimulation; optimizes myocardial performance
Central nervous system function	Modulates perceptual and emotional functioning (mechanism unknown); essential for normal arousal and initiation of activity

Adapted from McCance KL, Huether SE (eds): Pathophysiology: The Biologic Basis for Disease in Adults and Children, ed 2. St Louis, Mosby–Year Book, 1994, p 307.

response and causes the medulla of the adrenal gland to release catecholamines, such as epinephrine, norepinephrine, and dopamine, into the bloodstream. Simultaneously, the pituitary gland releases a variety of hormones, including antidiuretic hormone (from the posterior pituitary gland), prolactin, growth hormone, and adrenocorticotropic hormone (ACTH) from the anterior pituitary gland.

Catecholamines

Catecholamines are organic compounds that play an important role in the body's physiologic response to stress. Their release at sympathetic nerve endings increases the rate and force of muscular contraction of the heart, thereby increasing cardiac output; constricts peripheral blood vessels, resulting in elevated blood pressure; elevates blood glucose levels by hepatic and skeletal glycogenolysis;[3] and promotes an increase in blood lipids by increasing the catabolism (breakdown) of fats. These well-known metabolic effects of adrenal catecholamines prepare the body to take physical action in the "fight-or-flight" phenomenon. Stressors commonly associated with catecholamine release include exercise, thermal changes, and acute emotional states.

Cortisol

Cortisol is the principal glucocorticoid hormone released from the adrenal cortex, also known as *hydrocortisone* when synthesized pharmaceutically. Cortisol has multiple functions (Table 9–2), but it primarily regulates the metabolism of proteins, carbohydrates, and lipids to cause an elevation in blood glucose level. These effects on glucose level and fat metabolism result in increased blood glucose and plasma lipids levels and promotes the formation of ketone bodies when insulin secretion is insufficient. For this reason, glucocorticoids (including cortisol) are referred to as anti-insulin diabetogenic hormones (O'Toole, 1992; McCance and Shelby, 1994).

Cortisol is essential to norepinephrine-induced vasoconstriction and other physiologic phenomena necessary for survival under stress. The production of glucose promoted by cortisol provides a source of energy for body tissues (nerve cells in particular), and the pooling of amino acids from catabolized proteins may ensure amino acid availability for protein synthesis at sites where replacement is critical, such as muscle or cells of damaged tissue.

Another effect of cortisol is that of dampening the body's inflammatory response to invasion by foreign agents. This anti-inflammatory protective mechanism of cortisol help preserve the integrity of body cells at the site of the inflammatory response and provides the basis for the major therapeutic use of this steroid. Cortisol also inhibits fibroblast proliferation and function at the site of an inflammatory response and accounts for the poor wound healing, increased susceptibility to infection, and decreased inflammatory response that are often seen in individuals with chronic glucocorticoid excess. Whether cortisol-induced effects are adaptive or destructive depends on the intensity, type, and duration of the stressor and the subsequent concentration and length of cortisol exposure.

Other Hormones

Other hormones such as endorphins, growth hormone, prolactin, and testosterone may be released as part of the response to stressful stimuli. *Endorphins*, a term derived from *endogenous* and *morphine*, are a group of opiate-like peptides produced naturally by the body at neural synapses in the central nervous system. These hormones serve to modulate the transmission of pain perceptions by raising the pain threshold and producing sedation and euphoria (O'Toole, 1992).

[3] Glycogenolysis is the splitting up of glycogen, a starch stored primarily in the liver but also in the muscles, yielding glucose.

As its name implies, *growth hormone* stimulates and controls the rate of skeletal and visceral growth by directly influencing protein, carbohydrate, and lipid metabolism. GH levels increase in the blood after a variety of physically or psychologically stressful stimuli, such as surgery, fever, physical exercise or the anticipation of exhausting exercise, cardiac catheterization, electroshock therapy, or gastroscopy (Berne and Levy, 1990).

Prolactin stimulates the growth of breast tissue and sustains milk production in postpartum mammals. Prolactin levels in plasma increase with a variety of stressful stimuli, including such procedures as gastroscopy, proctoscopy, pelvic examination, and surgery, but they show little change after exercise. *Testosterone*, a hormone that regulates male secondary sex characteristics and sex drive (libido), decreases after stressful stimuli such as anesthesia, surgery, marathon running, and acute illness (e.g., respiratory failure, burns, congestive heart failure). Decreased testosterone during these circumstances restrains growth and reproduction to preserve energy for protective responses (Chrousos and Gold, 1992).

Aging and the Endocrine System *(Gambert, 1995)*

The exact effects of aging on the endocrine system are not clear and in particular, the question of whether changes in endocrine function are a cause of aging or a natural consequence of aging remains unresolved. The endocrine system has never been implicated as the direct cause of aging. Coexisting age-related variables such as acute and chronic nonendocrine disease, use of medications, alterations in diet, changes in body composition and weight, and changes in sleep-wake cycle affecting the endocrine system confuse the picture.

It is certain that aging is associated with a higher incidence of disorders or diseases of the endocrine system, including diabetes mellitus, hypothyroidism, and an increased incidence of atypical endocrine diseases during later life. Cellular damage associated with aging, genetically programmed cell change, and chronic wear and tear may contribute to endocrine gland dysfunction or alterations in responsiveness of target organs (as a result of changes with aging and disease, the target organs may lose their ability to respond to hormones). Loss of self-regulation leading to autoimmune or immunodeficiency disorders may occur.

Other endocrine changes that may be associated with aging comprise the *neuroendocrine theory of aging* and include altered biologic activity of hormones, altered circulating levels of hormones, altered secretory responses of endocrine glands, altered metabolism of hormones, and loss of circadian control of hormone release. These changes are postulated to occur as a result of a genetic program that is encoded in the brain and then controlled and relayed to peripheral tissues through hormonal and neural agents (Huether, 1994). This theory suggests that cells are programmed to function only for a given time. Menopause as a result of programmed changes in the reproductive system is an example of this theory.

The relationship between aging and the structure and function of the endocrine system cannot be separated from the changes in the central nervous system. The neurons involved in the cascade of hormonal secretion are influenced by a complex network of neurons from the brainstem, limbic system, diencephalon, and neocortex. As the nervous system ages, a progressive reduction takes place in the body's capacity to maintain homeostasis in the face of environmental stress. The overall effect of the changes in aging in the neuroendocrine system is a progressive resistance to the inhibitory feedback of the end-organ hormonal secretion (see Fig. 9–2). Thus, although the initial response to a stressful stimulus may be appropriate, as the body ages, there is an increased likelihood that the response may be persistent and ultimately inappropriate or even harmful (Carnevali and Patrick, 1993).

Anatomic Changes with Aging

The *pituitary gland* undergoes both anatomic and histologic changes associated with aging. By age 80 years, the weight of the anterior pituitary lobe (adenohypophysis) is reduced approximately 75% from its peak during young adulthood. The blood supply is reduced, and a higher incidence of adenomas and cysts is described during later life.

The *thyroid gland* becomes relatively smaller and fibrotic, and its position becomes lower-lying and retrosternal with age. As with the pituitary gland, blood supply to the thyroid gland is decreased. Secretion of thyroid hormones may diminish with age. The *parathyroid gland* demonstrates tissue changes with advancing age, but there appears to be no major change in parathyroid hormone (PTH) levels. Hyperparathyroidism occurs primarily in persons older than 50 years and may result from hyperplasia of all four parathyroid glands or a tumor (usually an adenoma).

The *adrenal glands* have more fibrous tissue with aging, but because of compensatory feedback mechanisms, there appears to be no relative alteration in functional cortisol levels. The most common cause of hypercortisolism occurs in conjunction with the use of corticosteroids for medical conditions. As previously mentioned, since steroid use can suppress the pituitary-adrenal axis, adrenal insufficiency can occur following discontinuation of steroid therapy.

Changes in the *reproductive glands* have clearly been shown to have physiologic effects, most notably on the cardiovascular system and the skeleton (ovary) and muscle mass and libido (testis). These effects are discussed elsewhere (see Chapters 16, 17, and 20).

Hormonal Changes with Aging

Much of the available data regarding changes in hormonal levels and function are contradictory. It is well known that the female reproductive system undergoes changes as part of the normal aging process. Menopause not only leads to changes in the genitourinary tract but also accelerates the loss of minerals from bone and leads to an alteration in the lipid composition in the mature woman. Male hormones have been linked to preservation of muscle mass as well as to an increased tendency toward developing certain diseases (e.g., benign prostatic hypertrophy, liver disease) during later life.

Loss of body hair, changes in the skin's collagen content and thickness, an increase in the percentage of body fat, a decrease in lean body mass, a decrease in bone mass, and a decrease in protein synthesis are signs of endocrinopathy that may be associated with decreased growth hormone levels (Corpas et al., 1993). With the decline of growth hormone secretion, sleep cycles are disrupted (Carnevali and Patrick, 1993), and the potential for sequelae associated with sleep deprivation (e.g., depression, fibromyalgia) is well known.

Interactions between the endocrine and immune systems also influence the aging process. Declining hormonal levels are accompanied by increased activity of tumor-suppressor genes in the aging population unless these genes have been mutated so that suppressor function is lost. In fact, the most common somatic mutation of human cancers is the loss of a tumor-suppressor gene as a result of exposures to a lifetime of mutagens. In the presence of decreased hormonal levels, loss of the tumor-suppressor gene accounts for the increased probability of tumors with advancing age, again demonstrating the link between the endocrine and immune systems (Weinberg, 1991).

Signs and Symptoms of Endocrine Disease

Signs and symptoms of endocrine pathology vary depending on the gland affected and whether the pathology is as a result of an excess (hyperfunction) or insufficiency (hypofunction) of hormonal secretions (Goodman and Snyder, 1995). In a therapy setting, the most common signs and symptoms associated with endocrine pathology are observed in the musculoskeletal system.

Growth and development of connective tissue structures are strongly influenced, and sometimes controlled, by various hormones and metabolic processes. When these processes are altered, structural and functional changes can occur in various connective tissues, producing musculoskeletal signs and symptoms as well as other systemic signs and symptoms of endocrine dysfunction (Table 9–3).

Musculoskeletal System

Rheumatoid arthritis is often the primary indicator of an underlying endocrine disease. For example, about 25% of clients with hyperparathyroidism present with "rheumatism." Diabetes mellitus is associated with a variety of rheumatic syndromes, such as the stiff-hand syndrome and limited joint motion syndrome. Although rheumatic symptoms can appear suddenly in people with an endocrine disorder, an insidious onset is much more common (Bland, 1994).

Muscle weakness, atrophy, myalgia, and *fatigue* that persist despite rest may be early manifestations of thyroid or parathyroid disease, acromegaly, diabetes, Cushing's syndrome, or osteomalacia. In endocrine disease, most proximal muscle weakness is usually painless and unrelated to either the severity or the duration of the underlying disease. Any compromise of muscle energy metabolism aggravates and perpetuates trigger points such as are associated with myofascial pain syndrome (see Chapter 23) or tender points in muscle associated with fibromyalgia syndrome (see Chapter 5).

Carpal tunnel syndrome (CTS)[4] (see discussion, Chapter 34) resulting from median nerve compression at the wrist is a common finding in people with certain endocrine and metabolic disorders (Stevens, 1992) (see Table 34–5). Any increase in the volume of contents of the carpal tunnel impinges on the median nerve (e.g., neoplasm, calcium, gouty tophi deposits, edema, tenosynovitis). Tenosynovitis (inflammation of the tendon sheaths) occurs with some infectious processes (see Table 34–5) as well as with many musculoskeletal conditions. Fluid infiltrating the tunnel may soften the transverse carpal ligament, which can make the bony arch flatten and compress the nerve (Gleeson and Pauls, 1993). Thickening of the transverse carpal ligament may also occur with systemic disorders such as acromegaly or myxedema.

Rheumatoid arthritis (RA) has been shown to occur significantly more often in people with CTS than would be expected in the general population of the same age and sex (Linos et al., 1980). In large studies, RA is usually listed as one of the three most common causes of CTS (Hybbinette and Mannerfelt, 1975; Yamaguchi et al., 1965). Amyloidosis (sometimes associated with RA or accompanying multiple myeloma) may affect nerves, muscles, tendons, and ligaments, especially the carpal tunnel area of the wrist. These deposits of insoluble fragments of monoclonal protein, which resemble starch, cause tissues to become waxy and immobile, resulting in poor tendon and nerve gliding and median nerve pressure (see Amyloidosis, Chapter 23).

Carpal tunnel syndrome in diabetic persons represents one form of diabetic neuropathy caused by ischemia-related microvascular damage of the median nerve. This ischemia then causes increased sensitivity to even minor pressure exerted in the carpal tunnel area (Louthrenoo and Schumacher, 1990). Vitamin B_6 deficiency may also be a factor in the development of CTS for the person with diabetes (Ellis et al., 1991).

CTS occurring during pregnancy may be caused by extra fluid and/or fat (Wand, 1990), diabetes (gestational or previously diagnosed), vitamin deficiencies, or other causes unrelated to the pregnancy itself (e.g., rheumatoid arthritis, job-related biomechanical stress). The fact that many women develop CTS at or near menopause may suggest that the soft tissues about the wrist may be affected in some way by hormones (Grossman et al., 1961; Phalen, 1966).

Periarthritis (inflammation of periarticular structures including the tendons, ligaments, and joint capsule) and *calcific*

TABLE 9–3 Signs and Symptoms of Endocrine Dysfunction

Neuromusculoskeletal	Systemic
Signs and symptoms associated with rheumatoid arthritis	Excessive or delayed growth
Muscle weakness	Polydipsia
Muscle atrophy	Polyuria
Myalgia	Mental changes (nervousness, confusion, depression)
Fatigue	Changes in hair (quality and distribution)
Carpal tunnel syndrome	Changes in skin pigmentation
Synovial fluid changes	Changes in distribution of body fat
Periarthritis	Changes in vital signs (elevated body temperature, pulse rate, increased blood pressure)
Chondrocalcinosis	Heart palpitations
Spondyloarthropathy	Increased perspiration
Osteoarthritis	Kussmaul's respirations (deep, rapid breathing)
Hand stiffness	Dehydration or excessive retention of body water
Arthralgia	

[4] In endocrine disorders, CTS is frequently bilateral, which is one characteristic that distinguishes it from overuse syndromes and other causes of CTS.

tendinitis occur most often in the shoulders of people who have endocrine disease. *Chondrocalcinosis* is the deposition of calcium salts in the joint cartilage; when accompanied by attacks of goutlike symptoms, it is called pseudogout. In 5% to 10% of people with chondrocalcinosis, there is an associated underlying endocrine or metabolic disease, such as hypothyroidism, hyperparathyroidism, or acromegaly (Louthrenoo and Schumacher, 1990). People diagnosed with fibromyalgia may also have altered thyroid function (see Fibromyalgia, Chapter 5) and present with shoulder impingement secondary to chondrocalcinosis.

Spondoarthropathy (disease of joints of the spine) and *osteoarthritis* occur in individuals with various endocrine or metabolic diseases, including hemochromatosis (disorder of iron metabolism with excess deposition in the tissues; also known as bronze diabetes and iron storage disease), ochronosis (metabolic disorder caused by alkali deposits, resulting in discoloration of body tissues), acromegaly, and diabetes mellitus.

Hand stiffness and hand pain, as well as arthralgias of the small joints of the hand, can occur with endocrine and metabolic diseases. In persons with hypothyroidism, flexor tenosynovitis with stiffness is a common finding. This condition often accompanies CTS (Louthrenoo and Schumacher, 1990).

Special Implications for the Therapist **9–1**

OVERVIEW OF ENDOCRINE AND METABOLIC DISEASE

Disorders of the endocrine and metabolic systems may present with recognizable clinical signs and symptoms (see Table 9–3). Clients with a variety of endocrine and metabolic disorders report symptoms of fatigue, muscle weakness, and, occasionally, muscle or bone pain (Louthenroo and Schumacher, 1990). Painless muscle weakness associated with endocrine and metabolic disorders usually involves proximal muscle groups, and these as well as other symptoms such as periarthritis and calcific tendinitis respond to treatment of the underlying endocrine pathology.

In most cases, the person who has received a diagnosis of an endocrine or metabolic disorder has undergone a combination of clinical and laboratory tests. This person may be in the care of a therapist for some other unrelated musculoskeletal problem that can be affected by symptoms associated with hormone imbalances.

Other clinical presentations of musculoskeletal symptoms, such as CTS, rheumatoid arthritis, or adhesive capsulitis, may be referred to the therapist without accurate diagnosis of the underlying endocrine pathology. The therapist must always remain alert to the client's report of systemic signs and symptoms (usually a constellation of symptoms, rather than an isolated few) preceding, accompanying, or developing with the current musculoskeletal problems.

Additionally, the lack of progress in therapy should signal to the therapist the possibility of a systemic origin of musculoskeletal symptoms. Failure to recognize a metabolic cause of symptoms may result in prolonged, ineffective therapy, visits to a variety of therapists, and, occasionally, one or more unsuccessful surgical procedures (Sonkin, 1994).

Any client who is taking diuretics must be monitored for signs or symptoms of potassium depletion or fluid dehydration (see Chapter 4) before initiating exercise and then throughout the duration of exercise. Cortisol suppresses the body's inflammatory response, masking early signs of infection. Any unexplained fever without other symptoms in the immunocompromised client must be reported to the physician.

SPECIFIC ENDOCRINE DISORDERS

Pituitary Gland

The pituitary gland, or hypophysis, is a small (1 cm in diameter) oval gland located at the base of the skull in an indentation of the sphenoid bone (see Figs. 9–1 and 9–2). It is often referred to as the "master gland" because of its role in regulating other endocrine glands. It is joined to the hypothalamus by the pituitary stalk (neurohypophyseal tract) and is influenced by the hypothalamus through releasing and inhibiting factors. The pituitary consists of two parts: the anterior pituitary (adenohypophysis) and the posterior pituitary (neurohypophysis) lobes. The anterior pituitary secretes six different hormones (ACTH, TSH, LH, FSH, human growth hormone, and prolactin) (see Fig. 9–2).

The posterior pituitary is a downward offshoot of the hypothalamus and contains many nerve fibers; it produces no hormones of its own. The hormones ADH (also called vasopressin) and oxytocin are produced in the hypothalamus and then stored and released by the posterior pituitary. These hormones pass down nerve fibers from the hypothalamus through the pituitary stalk to nerve endings in the posterior pituitary; they accumulate in the posterior pituitary during less active periods of the body. Transmitter substances, such as acetylcholine and norepinephrine, are thought to activate release of these substances by the posterior pituitary gland when they are stimulated by nerve impulses from the hypothalamus (Schteingart, 1992).

Anterior Lobe Disorders

Disorders of the pituitary gland occur most frequently in the anterior lobe, most often caused by tumors, pituitary infarction, genetic disorders, and trauma. The three principal pathologic consequences of pituitary disorders are hyperpituitarism, hypopituitarism, and local compression of brain tissue by expanding tumor masses (Loriaux, 1993) (see also Chapter 26).

Hyperpituitarism

Overview. Hyperpituitarism is an oversecretion of one or more of the hormones secreted by the pituitary gland, especially growth hormone, resulting in acromegaly or gigantism. It is primarily caused by a hormone-secreting pituitary tumor, typically a benign adenoma. Other syndromes associated with hyperpituitarism include Cushing's disease,[5] amenorrhea, and hyperthyroidism.

[5] Cushing's disease is one form of Cushing's syndrome and results from oversecretion of ACTH by a pituitary tumor, which, in turn, results in oversecretion of adrenocortical hormones (see further discussion: Cushing's Syndrome, this chapter).

Pituitary tumors produce both systemic effects and local manifestations. Systemic effects include (1) excessive or abnormal growth patterns due to overproduction of growth hormone; (2) abnormal milk secretion, called *galactorrhea* (i.e., persistent, spontaneous milk flow without nursing); and (3) overstimulation of one or more of the target glands, resulting in the release of excessive adrenocortical, thyroid, or sex hormones. Local pituitary tumors produce symptoms as the growing mass expands within the bony cranium. Local manifestations may include visual field abnormalities (pressure on the optic chiasma where the optic nerve crosses over), headaches, and somnolence (sleepiness).

Gigantism and Acromegaly. Gigantism, an overgrowth of the long bones, and acromegaly, increased bone thickness and hypertrophy of the soft tissues, result from growth hormone–secreting adenomas of the anterior pituitary gland. Although growth hormone–producing tumors that cause these conditions are rare, they are the second most common type of hyperpituitarism. Gigantism develops in children before the age when the epiphyses of the bones close; people who develop gigantism may grow to a height of 9 feet. Acromegaly is a disease of adults and develops after closure of the epiphyses of the long bones, so the bones most affected are those of the face, jaw, hands, and feet. In adults, acromegaly occurs equally among men and women and usually between ages 30 and 50 years (Loriaux, 1993).

Gigantism develops abruptly, whereas acromegaly develops slowly. Both conditions are characterized by the same skeletal abnormalities because hypersecretion of growth hormone produces cartilaginous and connective tissue overgrowth, resulting in coarsened facial features; protrusion of the jaw (prognathism); thickened ears, nose, and tongue; and broad hands, with spadelike fingers (Fig. 9–3). In gigantism, as the tumor enlarges and invades normal tissue, target organ functions are impaired by the loss of other tropic (stimulating) hormones, such as TSH, LH, FSH, and ACTH. Clients with acromegaly may experience local manifestations such as headache, diplopia, blindness, and lethargy as the tumor compresses brain tissue.

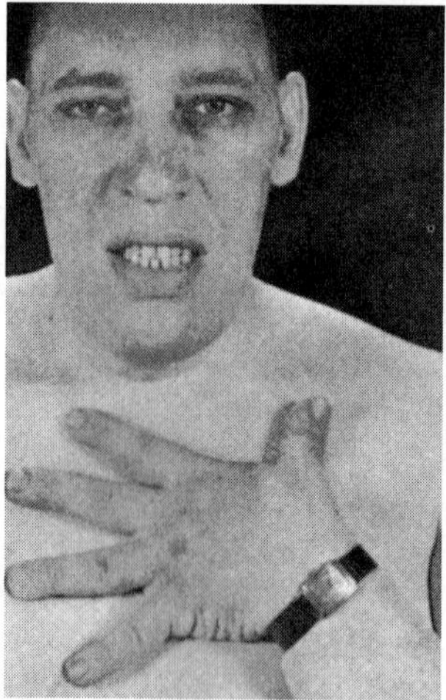

Figure **9–3.** Acromegaly (hyperpituitarism) occurs as a result of excessive secretion of growth hormone after normal completion of body growth. The resulting overgrowth of bone in the face, head, and hands are pictured here. (*From Jarvis C: Physical Examination and Health Assessment. Philadelphia, WB Saunders, 1992, p 219.*)

Medical Management. Pituitary tumors may be treated through implant irradiation of the pituitary gland to destroy the tumor, through surgical hypophysectomy (removal of the tumor and removal of part or all of the pituitary gland), or through the use of drugs that can reduce the levels of growth hormone and decrease tumor size. This type of pharmacologic management may be used if the levels of growth hormone remain high after surgery or until the radiation therapy takes effect. Following surgery, lifetime thyroid, cortisone, and/or gonadal hormone replacement may be necessary.

Special Implications for the Therapist **9–2**

HYPERPITUITARISM

Postoperative Care

Ambulation and exercise are encouraged within the first 24 hours after surgery. Coughing, sneezing, and blowing the nose are contraindicated after surgery, but deep breathing exercises are encouraged. Postoperatively, vital signs and neurologic status must be closely monitored. Any alteration in level of consciousness or visual acuity, falling pulse rate, or rising blood pressure may signal an increase in intracranial pressure due to intracranial bleeding or cerebral edema and must be reported immediately. Observe for signs of meningitis (e.g., severe headache, irritability, nuchal [back of the neck] rigidity), a potential complication of surgery.

The nursing staff will be monitoring blood glucose levels often, as growth hormone levels fall rapidly after surgery, removing an insulin-antagonist effect in many people and possibly precipitating hypoglycemia (low blood glucose level). The therapist is advised to consult with nursing staff to determine the possible need for blood glucose monitoring during or after exercise. The therapist should be familiar with signs and symptoms and special implications of hypoglycemia (see Hypoglycemia, later in the chapter).

Tumors causing visual changes may require the therapist to consciously remain within the client's visual field. Unexpected mood changes can occur, requiring patience and understanding on the part of health-care workers. Although surgical removal of the tumor and/or pituitary gland prevents permanent soft-tissue deformities, bone changes that are already present will not change.

Orthopedic Considerations

Skeletal manifestations, such as arthritis of the hands and osteoarthritis of the spine, may develop with these conditions. Osteophyte formation and widening of the joint space owing to increased cartilage thickening may be seen on x-rays. In late-stage disease, joint spaces become narrowed, and chondrocalcinosis may occasionally be present (Louthrenoo and Schumacher, 1990). CTS is seen in up to 50% of people with acromegaly (Bluestone et al., 1971). The CTS that occurs with this growth disorder is thought to be caused by compression of the median nerve at the wrist from soft tissue hypertrophy or bony overgrowth or by hypertrophy of the median nerve itself.

About half of individuals with acromegaly have thoracic and/or lumbar back pain (Bluestone et al., 1971; Layton et al., 1988). X-ray studies demonstrate increased intervertebral disk spaces and large osteophytes along the anterior longitudinal ligament (ALL).

The therapist may be called on to provide a program that promotes maximum joint mobility, muscle strength, and functional skills. Assistance with activities of daily living (ADL) may be an important aspect of treatment. Home health staff should assess the home to remove any obstacles and recommend necessary adaptive equipment or assistive devices.

Hypopituitarism (Loriaux, 1993)

Hypopituitarism (also panhypopituitarism and dwarfism) results from decreased or absent hormonal secretion by the anterior pituitary gland. Panhypopituitarism refers to a generalized condition caused by partial or total failure of all six of the pituitary's vital hormones (ACTH, TSH, LH, FSH, human growth hormone, and prolactin).

Hypopituitarism and panhypopituitarism are rare disorders that occur as a result of (1) hypophysectomy (removal or destruction of the pituitary by surgery, irradiation, or chemical agents); (2) nonsecreting pituitary tumors; (3) growth hormone deficiency; (4) postpartum hemorrhage (the fall in blood pressure and subsequent hypoxia following delivery causes necrosis of the gland); and (5) functional disorders (in which the pituitary gland does not receive adequate nourishment and dies) such as starvation, anorexia nervosa, severe anemia, and GI tract disorders.

Clinical manifestations are dependent on the age at onset as well as the hormones affected. More than 75% of the pituitary must be obliterated by tumors or thromboses before symptoms develop. Specific disorders resulting from pituitary hyposecretion include *growth hormone deficiency*, with subsequent short stature, delayed growth, and delayed puberty; *secondary adrenocortical insufficiency* from diminished synthesis of ACTH by the pituitary gland, which in turn causes diminished secretion of adrenocortical hormones by the adrenal cortex; *hypothyroidism* (thyroid hormone is dependent on TSH secreted by the pituitary); and *sexual and reproductive disorders* from deficiencies of the gonadotropins (LH and FSH) (Table 9–4).

Treatment for hypopituitarism involves removal (if possible) of the causative factor, such as tumors, and lifetime replacement of the missing hormones.

TABLE 9–4 Clinical Manifestations of Hypopituitarism

Growth hormone deficiency
Short stature
Delayed growth
Delayed puberty
Adrenocortical insufficiency
Hypoglycemia
Anorexia
Nausea
Abdominal pain
Orthostatic hypotension
Hypothyroidism (see also Table 9–7)
Tiredness
Lethargy
Sensitivity to cold
Menstrual disturbances
Gonadal failure
Secondary amenorrhea
Impotence
Infertility
Decreased libido
Absent secondary sex characteristics (children)
Neurologic signs (produced by tumors)
Headache
Bilateral temporal hemianopia
Loss of visual acuity
Blindness

Special Implications for the Therapist **9–3**

HYPOPITUITARISM

Although rarely encountered in a therapy setting, the client with hypopituitarism may report symptoms associated with hormonal deficiencies until hormone replacement therapy is complete. The therapist may observe weakness, fatigue, lethargy, apathy, and orthostatic hypotension (see Special Implications for the Therapist: Orthostatic Hypotension, Chapter 10). Nailbeds and skin may demonstrate pallor associated with anemia (see Special Implications for the Therapist: Anemia, Chapter 11).

Infection prevention requires meticulous skin care following the guidelines outlined in Table 10–22. Impaired peripheral vision associated with bilateral hemianopia (blindness in half of the visual field) requires special consideration. The therapist must be certain to stand where the affected individual can see others and to move slowly in and out of the client's visual field.

Posterior Lobe Disorders

Diabetes Insipidus

Diabetes insipidus, a rare disorder, involves a physiologic imbalance of water secondary to ADH deficiency. Injury or loss of function of the hypothalamus, the neurohypophyseal tract, or the posterior pituitary gland can result in diabetes insipidus (Box 9–1).

Since the major functions of ADH are to promote water resorption by the kidney and to control the osmotic pressure of the extracellular fluid, when ADH production decreases, the kidney tubules fail to resorb water. The end result is excretion of large amounts of dilute urine. Unlike urine in diabetes mellitus, which contains large amounts of glucose, urine in diabetes insipidus is highly dilute and contains no glucose. Other clinical manifestations include polydipsia (ex-

BOX **9–1**
Causes of Diabetes Insipidus

Intracranial or pituitary neoplasm
Metastatic lesions (e.g., breast or lung cancer)
Surgical hypophysectomy or other neurosurgery
Skull fracture or head trauma (damages the neurohypophyseal structures)
Infection (e.g., meningitis, encephalitis)
Granulomatous disease
Vascular lesions (e.g., aneurysm)
Idiopathic
Alcohol
Medications (e.g., phenytoin)
Nephrogenic diabetes insipidus (congenital)

cessive thirst), nocturia (excessive urination at night), and dehydration (e.g., poor tissue turgor, dry mucous membranes, constipation, muscle weakness, dizziness, and hypotension) (see also Box 4–7). Fatigue and irritability may develop secondary to sleep disruption and in association with nocturia.

If a person is conscious and is able to respond appropriately to the thirst mechanism, hydration can be maintained. However, if a person is unconscious or confused and unable to take in necessary fluids to compensate for fluid loss, rapid dehydration, shock, and death can occur. Treatment is usually exogenous replacement of ADH with vasopressin or a synthetic derivative, such as Pitressin, along with administration of diuretics. When this condition is caused by tumor, resection of the tumor can effect a cure.

Special Implications for the Therapist **9–4**

DIABETES INSIPIDUS

The therapist must be alert for possible serious side effects of any type of ADH administration. ADH stimulates smooth muscle contraction of the vascular system (causing increased blood pressure), the GI tract (causing diarrhea), and the coronary arteries (causing angina or myocardial infarction) (Degland and Vallerand, 1993). Increases in blood pressure can cause additional serious problems in some people, particularly those with hypertension or coronary artery disease (CAD) and cerebrovascular disease (CVD). Additionally, after receiving vasopressin, clients need to be assessed for signs and symptoms of water intoxication, which can lead to fluid overload, cerebral edema, and seizures. See also Special Implications for the Therapist: Fluid and Electrolyte Imbalances, Chapter 4.

Syndrome of Inappropriate Antidiuretic Hormone Secretion (SIADH)

SIADH is a disorder associated with excessive release of ADH, which disturbs fluid and electrolyte balance, resulting in a water imbalance. SIADH has a wide variety of causes, including pituitary damage due to infection, trauma, or neoplasm; the stress of surgery or many systemic disorders; and response to certain medications (Box 9–2).

BOX **9–2**
Causes of Syndrome of Inappropriate Antidiuretic Hormone Secretion (SIADH)*

Oat cell carcinoma (accounts for 80% of cases)
Pulmonary disorders
 Pneumonia
 Tuberculosis
 Lung abscess
 Mechanical ventilation (e.g., positive pressure)
Central nervous system disorders
 Brain tumor or abscess
 Cerebrovascular accident
 Head injury
 Guillain-Barré syndrome
 Systemic lupus erythematosus
Other neoplasms (e.g., pancreatic or prostatic cancer, Hodgkin's disease, thymoma)
Infection
Stress (e.g., surgery) or trauma
Medications (e.g., oral hypoglycemic agents, antineoplastic drugs, morphine)
Myxedema
Psychosis

* Listed in descending order.

SIADH is the opposite of diabetes insipidus, so treatment of diabetes insipidus with vasopressin can lead to SIADH if excessive amounts are administered. In SIADH, instead of large fluid losses, water intoxication occurs as a result of fluid retention. Under normal circumstances, ADH regulates serum osmolality.[6] When serum osmolality falls, a feedback mechanism causes inhibition of ADH. This, in turn, promotes increased water excretion by the kidneys to raise serum osmolality to normal. When this feedback mechanism fails and ADH levels are sustained, fluid retention results. Ultimately, serum sodium levels fall, resulting in hyponatremia (sodium depletion) and water intoxication (Loriaux, 1993).

Though fluid retention is the primary symptom, edema is rare unless water overload exceeds 4 L; much of the free water excess is within cellular boundaries. Neurologic and neuromuscular signs and symptoms predominate and are directly related to the swelling of brain tissue and to sodium changes within neuromuscular tissues. Central nervous system dysfunction, characterized by alterations in level of consciousness, seizures, and coma, can occur when serum sodium falls to 120 mEq/L or less. Hyponatremia can result in diminished GI function; this problem is further complicated by the need for fluid restriction.

Correction of life-threatening sodium imbalance is the

[6] Serum osmolality is a measure of the number of dissolved particles per unit of water in serum. In a solution, the fewer the particles of solute in proportion to the number of units of water (solvent), the less concentrated the solution. A low serum osmolality would indicate a higher than usual amount of water in relation to the amount of particles dissolved in it. In other words, serum osmolality provides a measure of hydration of cells. For example, a low serum osmolality accompanies overhydration (i.e., edema); an increased serum osmolality is present in a state of fluid volume deficit. Osmolality is proportional with dilutional or depletional states (true for water and sodium). The normal value for serum osmolality is 270 to 300 mOsm/kg of water (O'Toole, 1992).

first aim of treatment followed by correction of the underlying cause. If SIADH is caused by malignancy, success in alleviating water retention may be obtained by surgical resection, irradiation, or chemotherapy. Otherwise, treatment for SIADH is symptomatic and includes restriction of water intake, careful replacement of sodium chloride, and administration of diuretics. Other pharmaceuticals (e.g., demeclocycline and tetracycline or lithium) may also be used to block the renal response to ADH.

Special Implications for the Therapist **9-5**

SYNDROME OF INAPPROPRIATE ANTIDIURETIC HORMONE SECRETION (SIADH)

Anyone at risk for SIADH (see conditions listed in Box 9–2) should be monitored for sudden weight gain or fluid retention and changes in urination and fluid intake. Observe for headache, lethargy, muscle cramps, restlessness, irritability, convulsions, or weight gain without visible edema (2 lb or more a day). Throughout therapy, the client's cardiovascular status should be assessed regularly so that any unusual alterations can be noted immediately. (See also Special Implications for the Therapist: Fluid Imbalances, Chapter 4.)

Continued need for sodium and fluid restrictions may be necessary for the person discharged to home or who is in a facility other than the acute care setting (hospital). People with unresolved SIADH should avoid the use of aspirin or nonsteroidal anti-inflammatory agents without a physician's approval, because these drugs can increase the hyponatremia.

Thyroid Glands *(Birch, 1993)*

The thyroid gland is located in the anterior portion of the lower neck, below the larynx, on both sides of and anterior to the trachea (see Fig. 9–1). The primary hormones produced by the thyroid are thyroxine (T_4), triiodothyronine (T_3), and calcitonin. Both T_3 and T_4 regulate the metabolic rate of the body and increase protein synthesis. Calcitonin has a weak physiologic effect on calcium and phosphorus balance in the body. Thyroid function is regulated by the hypothalamus and pituitary feedback controls as well as by an intrinsic regulator mechanism within the gland itself (Guyton, 1992).

Disorders of the thyroid gland may be functional abnormalities leading to hyperfunction or hypofunction of the gland or anatomic abnormalities such as thyroiditis, goiter, and tumor. Enlargement of the thyroid gland or neoplasm may or may not be associated with abnormalities of hormone secretion.

Susceptibility to thyroid disease is largely determined by the interaction of genetic makeup, age, and sex. Women, particularly those with a family history of thyroid disease, are much more likely to have thyroid pathology than are men. Although most thyroid conditions cannot be prevented, they respond well to treatment.

Thyroid hormone acts on nearly all body tissues, so excessive or deficient secretion affects various body systems. Alterations in thyroid function produce changes in nails, hair, skin, eyes, GI tract, respiratory tract, heart and blood vessels, nervous tissue, bone, and muscle (Guyton, 1992). Both hyperthyroidism and hypothyroidism can adversely affect cardiac function. Sustained tachycardia in hyperthyroidism and sustained bradycardia with cardiac enlargement in hypothyroidism can result in cardiac failure. Both conditions affect the general rate of metabolism, the muscular system, the nervous system, the gastrointestinal system, and, as mentioned, the cardiovascular system.

Hyperthyroidism

Definition and Overview. Hyperthyroidism is an excessive secretion of thyroid hormone, sometimes referred to as *thyrotoxicosis*, a term used to describe the clinical manifestations that occur when the body tissues are stimulated by increased thyroid hormone. Excessive thyroid hormone creates a generalized elevation of body metabolism, the effects of which are manifested in almost every system.

The most common form of hyperthyroidism is Graves' disease, which increases T_4 production and accounts for 85% of cases of hyperthyroidism. Like most thyroid conditions, hyperthyroidism affects women more than men (4:1), especially women between ages 20 and 40 years.

Rarely, a person with inadequately treated hyperthyroidism may experience what is called a *thyroid storm*. This potentially fatal condition is an acute episode of thyroid overactivity characterized by high fever, severe tachycardia, delirium, dehydration, and extreme irritability or agitation. Stress occurring in the presence of undiagnosed or untreated hyperthyroidism may precipitate such an event. Stressors may include surgery, infection, toxemia of pregnancy, labor and delivery, diabetic ketoacidosis, myocardial infarction, pulmonary embolus, and medication overdose.

Etiology and Risk Factors. Hyperthyroidism may result from both immunologic and genetic factors. It is probably autoimmune in nature, and although it is more common in women with family histories of thyroid abnormalities, major risk factors have not been identified. Hyperthyroidism may also be due to the overfunctioning of the entire gland, or, less commonly, to single or multiple functioning adenomas of thyroid cancer. Rarely, overtreatment of myxedema associated with hypothyroidism (see next section) may result in hyperthyroidism.

Pathogenesis *(Birch, 1993)*. About 60% to 80% of people with Graves' disease have circulating autoantibodies called thyroid-stimulating immunoglobulins (TSI) that react against thyroglobulin (precursor for thyroid hormones). These autoantibodies may be due to a defect in suppressor T-lymphocyte function that allows formation of TSIs. Evidently, TSIs present in the serum of 95% of hyperthyroid clients are autoantibodies that react against a component of the thyroid cell membranes, stimulating enlargement of the thyroid gland and secretion of excess thyroid hormone.

Because the action of thyroid hormone on the body is stimulatory, hypermetabolism results with increased sympathetic nervous system activity. The excessive amounts of thyroid hormone stimulate the cardiac system and increase the number of β-adrenergic receptors. This leads to tachycardia and increased cardiac output, increased stroke volume, and increased peripheral blood flow. The increased metabolism also leads to a negative nitrogen balance, lipid depletion, and a resultant state of nutritional deficiency.

Clinical Manifestations. Because hyperthyroidism is caused by an excess secretion of thyroid hormone, the clinical picture of Graves' disease is in many ways the opposite of that of hypothyroidism with myxedema. The classic symptoms of Graves' disease are mild symmetrical enlargement of the thyroid (goiter), nervousness, heat intolerance, weight loss despite increased appetite, sweating, diarrhea, tremor, and palpitations.

Exophthalmos (abnormal protrusion of the eyes) (Fig. 9–4) is considered most characteristic but is absent in many people with hyperthyroidism. Many other symptoms are commonly present, as this condition affects many body systems (Table 9–5). Complications such as thyroid storm and heart disease can occur (see previous discussion, this section).

Emotions are adversely affected by the increased metabolic activity within the body. Moods may be cyclic, ranging from mild euphoria to extreme hyperactivity or delirium. The excessive hyperactivity leads to extreme fatigue and depression, again followed by episodes of overactivity, in a repetitive cycle.

Hyperthyroidism in the elderly is notorious for presenting with atypical or minimal symptoms. Signs and symptoms are not the usual ones and may be attributed to aging. Many older people actually appear apathetic instead of hyperactive. Cardiovascular abnormalities, such as congestive heart failure, atrial arrhythmias, and varying degrees of heart block, are much more common in the elderly.

Neuromuscular Manifestations. Chronic periarthritis is also associated with hyperthyroidism. Inflammation that involves the periarticular structures, including the tendons, ligaments, and joint capsule, is termed periarthritis. This syndrome is characterized by pain and reduced range of motion. Calcification, whether periarticular or tendinous, may be seen on x-ray studies. Both periarthritis and calcific tendinitis occur most often in the shoulder, and both are common findings in clients who have endocrine disease (Louthrenoo and Schumacher, 1990).

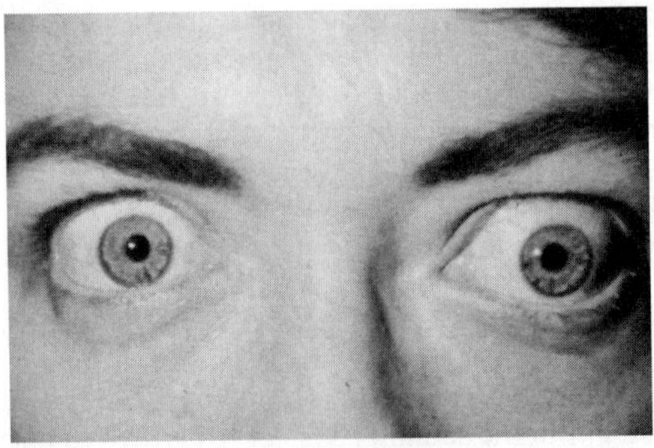

Figure **9–4.** Exophthalmos, or protruding eyes, is a forward displacement of the eyeballs associated with thyroid disease. Because the eyes are surrounded by unyielding bone, fluid accumulation in the fat pads and muscles behind the eyeballs causes protruding eyes and a fixed stare. Without treatment of the underlying cause, the client with severe exophthalmos may be unable to close the eyelids and may develop corneal ulceration or infection, eventually resulting in loss of vision. Note the "lid lag"; the upper eyelid rests well above the limbus (edge of the cornea where it joins the sclera), and white sclera is visible. This is evident when the person moves the eyes from up to down. (*From Jarvis C: Physical Examination and Health Assessment. Philadelphia, WB Saunders, 1992, p 350.*)

Painful restriction of shoulder motion associated with periarthritis has been widely described among clients with hyperthyroidism (Wohlgethan, 1987). The involvement can be unilateral or bilateral and can worsen progressively to become adhesive capsulitis, or frozen shoulder. Acute calcific tendinitis of the wrist also has been described in such clients. Although anti-inflammatory agents may be needed for acute symptoms, chronic periarthritis usually responds to treatment of the underlying hyperthyroidism.[7]

Proximal muscle weakness (most marked in the pelvic girdle and thigh muscles) accompanied by muscle atrophy, known as myopathy, has been described in up to 70% of people with hyperthyroidism (Ramsey, 1965; 1966; 1974). The therapist may first notice problems with coordination or balance or notice weakness of the legs, causing a client difficulty in ambulating, rising from a chair, or climbing stairs. Respiratory muscle weakness can present as dyspnea. The pathogenesis of the weakness is still a subject of controversy; muscle strength seems to return to normal in 6 to 8 weeks after medical treatment, with a slower resolution of muscle wasting. In severe cases, normal strength may not be restored for months.

The incidence of myasthenia gravis is increased in clients with hyperthyroidism, which in turn can aggravate muscle weakness. If the hyperthyroidism is corrected, improvement of the myasthenia gravis follows in about two thirds of affected people (Louthrenoo and Schumacher, 1990).

Medical Management

Diagnosis and Treatment. Diagnosis is based on clinical history, physical presentation, examination findings, and laboratory test results. Treatment is geared toward reducing the excessive secretion of thyroid hormone and preventing and treating complications.

Three major forms of therapy are antithyroid medication, radioiodine, and surgery. Antithyroid medication is recommended for anyone younger than 18 years, for pregnant women, and for anyone who refuses or cannot undergo surgery. Radioiodine therapy (contraindicated in children and pregnant women) with ^{131}I is principally prescribed for middle-aged and elderly clients and is administered orally, dissolved in water. Local irradiation destroys the cells that make T_4, decreasing thyroid hormone secretion and altering symptoms within 6 to 8 weeks. Hypothyroidism with myxedema may occur as a complication of radiotherapy because radioiodine destroys thyroid cells.

Partial or subtotal thyroidectomy (surgical removal of the thyroid) is performed to remove thyroid cancer and to correct extreme cases of hyperthyroidism. The ideal surgical treatment leaves a small portion of the functioning thyroid in order to avoid permanent hormone replacement. Surgical treatment is effective in most people with Graves' disease, although surgical complications, such as vocal cord paralysis or hypoparathyroidism, may develop as a result of nerve damage or inadvertent removal of parathyroid gland tissue, respectively (Birch, 1993).

[7] Physical therapy is not recommended in these cases until after the endocrine problem is resolved. Then therapeutic intervention with ultrasound, joint mobilization, stretching, and strengthening may be indicated to treat any residual dysfunction.

TABLE 9–5 Systemic Manifestations of Hyperthyroidism

CNS Effects	Cardiovascular and Pulmonary Effects	Musculoskeletal Effects	Integumentary Effects	Ocular Effects	Gastrointestinal Effects	Genitourinary Effects
Tremors	Increased pulse rate/ tachycardia/ palpitations	Muscle weakness and fatigue	Capillary dilation (warm, flushed, moist skin)	Exophthalmos	Hypermetabolism (increased appetite with weight loss)	Polyuria (frequent urination)
Hyperkinesis (abnormally increased motor function or activity)	Increased cardiac output	Muscle atrophy	Heat intolerance	Weakness of the extraocular muscles (poor convergence, poor upward gaze)	Diarrhea, nausea, and vomiting	Amenorrhea (absence of menses)
Nervousness	Increased blood volume	Chronic periarthritis	Onycholysis (separation of the fingernail from the nail bed)	Sensitivity to light	Dysphagia	Female infertility
Emotional lability	Dysrhythmias (palpitations)	Myasthenia gravis	Easily broken hair and increased hair loss	Visual loss		Increased risk of spontaneous miscarriage
Weakness and muscle atrophy	Weakness of respiratory muscles (breathlessness, hypoventilation)		Hard, purple area over the anterior surface of the tibia with itching, erythema, and, occasionally, pain	Spasm and retraction of the upper eyelids, lid tremor		Gynecomastia (males)
Increased deep tendon reflexes	Increased respiratory rate					

Adapted from Goodman CC, Snyder TE: Differential Diagnosis in Physical Therapy, ed 2. Philadelphia, WB Saunders, 1995, p 342.

Prognosis. Antithyroid drugs may be tapered and discontinued if there is a possibility of remission. Remission rates are higher in people with mild degrees of hyperthyroidism, small goiters, and for those who are diagnosed early. Even with remission, life-long follow-up is recommended because many remissions are not permanent. Relapses are most likely to occur in the postpartum period (Wilson and Foster, 1992).

After radioiodine treatment, regular life-long medical supervision is required. Frequently, hypothyroidism develops even as long as 1 to 3 years after treatment. Exophthalmos may not be reversed by intervention. In severe cases, the person may be unable to close the eyelids and must have the lids taped shut to protect the eyes. Without intervention, severe exophthalmos can progress to corneal ulceration or infection and loss of vision.

Special Implications for the Therapist **9-6**

HYPERTHYROIDISM

Any time a therapist examines a client's neck and finds unusual swelling, enlargement, or redness, with or without symptoms of pain, tenderness, hoarseness, or dysphagia (difficulty swallowing), a medical referral is required. For the client requiring life-long thyroid hormone replacement therapy, nervousness and palpitations may develop with overdosage (Norris, 1995). A small number of people experience fever, rash, and arthralgias as side effects of antithyroid drugs. The physician should be notified of these or any other unusual symptoms, as it may be possible to use an alternative drug.

Monitoring Vital Signs

Monitoring vital signs is important to assess cardiac function if the involved person is elderly, has coronary artery disease, or presents with symptoms of dyspnea, fatigue, tachycardia, and/or arrhythmia (Small et al., 1992). If the heart rate is more than 100 beats/minute, check the blood pressure and pulse rate and rhythm frequently. The person with dyspnea will be most comfortable sitting upright or in a high Fowler's position (head of the bed raised 18 to 20 in. above a level position with the knees elevated).

Because clients with Graves' disease suffer from heat intolerance (hyperthermia secondary to accelerated metabolic rate), aquatic or pool therapy is potentially contraindicated. Heat intolerance contributes to exercise intolerance and the client may exhibit signs and symptoms of heat stroke even when exercising in a climate-controlled facility. The physician must be made aware of these symptoms (heat intolerance, tachycardia, arrhythmia); strenuous exercise or a conditioning program should be delayed until these symptoms are under control.

Postoperative Care

Postoperatively, the therapist must be careful to avoid palpation or manipulation of the soft tissue surrounding the thyroid to avoid precipitating a thyroid storm. Watch for signs of thyroid storm such as tachycardia, hyperkinesis, fever, and hypertension. Observe for signs of hypoparathyroidism (muscular twitching, tetany, numbness and tingling around the mouth, fingertips, or toes), a complication that results from the accidental removal during surgery of the parathyroid glands. Symptoms can develop 1 to 7 days after surgery.

Any health-care worker in contact with clients who have undergone radioiodine therapy must follow necessary precautions (see Chapter 4). Saliva is radioactive for 24 hours following ^{131}I therapy; health-care professionals in contact with the client while he or she is coughing or expectorating must take precautions.

Side Effects of Radioiodine Therapy

Radioiodine therapy has few immediate side effects. Rarely, anterior neck tenderness may develop 7 to 10 days after therapy, consistent with radiation-induced thyroiditis (Farrar and Toft, 1991). There is a potential for worsening hyperthyroidism soon after radioiodine therapy, secondary to inflammation and release of stored thyroid in the bloodstream. Elderly people and anyone with cardiac disease is usually pretreated with antithyroid agents before receiving radioiodine to prevent this occurrence (McCredie, 1994).

The major adverse reaction from radioiodine is iatrogenic hypothyroidism. This development is so characteristic that it is considered an inevitable consequence of therapy rather than a side effect. Hypothyroidism develops in at least 50% of all cases treated with radioiodine therapy within the first year after therapy, with a gradual increased incidence thereafter. This complication necessitates life-long follow-up with close monitoring of thyroid function.

For further discussion of radiation side effects and precautions for health-care workers coming in contact with a person who has been irradiated, see Chapter 4.

Hyperthyroidism and Exercise

Hyperthyroidism is associated with exercise intolerance, but the exact relationship is unknown. Previous research has shown that cardiac output is either normal or enhanced (e.g., increased heart rate) during exercise in the hyperthyroid state and blood flow to muscles is augmented during submaximal exercise. Thus, cardiovascular and muscular factors do not appear to be responsible for this exercise intolerance (Martin, 1993; McAllister et al., 1995). Fatigue due to the hypermetabolic state and rapid depletion of nutrients may affect exercise capacity (Martin, 1991). Using perceived exertion or exercise tolerance as a guide, exercise parameters (frequency, intensity, duration) remain the same for the person treated for hyperthyroidism as for anyone who does not have this condition.

Hypothyroidism

Definition and Etiology. Hypothyroidism (hypofunction) refers to a deficiency of thyroid hormone in the adult that results in a generalized slowed body metabolism; it is the most common disorder of thyroid function in the United States and Canada. More than 50% of cases occur in families in which thyroid disease is present.

The condition may be classified as either primary or secondary. *Primary hypothyroidism* results from reduced functional thyroid tissue mass or impaired hormonal synthesis or release. *Secondary hypothyroidism* accounts for a small percentage of all cases of hypothyroidism and occurs as a result of inadequate stimulation of the gland because of pituitary or hypothalamic disease (failure to produce TSH and TRH, respectively) (Table 9–6). (Also see discussion of Hashimoto's thyroiditis later in the chapter.)

In the United States and Canada, this disease is commonly due to congenital autoimmune thyroiditis, thyroid ablation via surgery or radioactive iodine therapy, or medication with thiouracil or lithium; rarely it is a result of subacute thyroiditis, iodine deficiency, dietary factors, congenital abnormalities in iodination, or pituitary failure (Sonkin, 1994).

Incidence. Hypothyroidism affects women more than men, in a 4 : 1 ratio. Although hypothyroidism may be congenital and therefore present at birth, the highest incidence is between ages 30 and 60 years. More than 95% of all people with hypothyroidism have the primary form of the disease (Birch, 1993).

Pathogenesis. In primary hypothyroidism, the loss of thyroid tissue leads to a decreased production of thyroid hormone. The thyroid responds by enlarging in an attempt to compensate for hormonal deficiency. Goiter occurs then, as an adaptation to a deficiency of thyroid hormone. Secondary hypothyroidism is most commonly the result of failure of the pituitary to synthesize adequate amounts of TSH.

Decreased levels of thyroid hormone lead to an overall slowing of the basal metabolic rate. This slowing of all body processes leads to achlorhydria (absence of hydrochloric acid from gastric juice), decreased GI tract motility, bradycardia, slowed neurologic functioning, and a decrease in heat production. Lipid metabolism is also altered by hypothyroidism with a resultant increase in serum cholesterol and triglyceride levels and a concomitant increase in arteriosclerosis and coronary heart disease. Thyroid hormones also play a role in the production of red blood cells with the potential for the development of anemia.

Clinical Manifestations. As with all disorders affecting the thyroid and parathyroid glands, clinical signs and symptoms associated with hypothyroidism affect many systems of the body (Table 9–7). Typically, the early clinical features of hypothyroidism are vague and so ordinary as to escape detection (e.g., fatigue, mild sensitivity to cold, mild weight gain [10 to 15 lb], forgetfulness, depression, and dry skin or hair).

As the disorder progresses, myxedema and its associated signs and symptoms appear. Myxedema is a result of an alteration in the composition of the dermis and other tissues, causing connective tissues to be separated by increased amounts of mucopolysaccharides and proteins. This mucopolysaccharide-protein complex binds with water, causing a nonpitting, boggy edema, especially around the eyes, hands, feet, pretibial area, and in the supraclavicular fossae.

Other clinical manifestations associated with myxedema may include decreasing mental stability; dry, flaky, inelastic skin; dry, sparse hair; hoarseness; upper eyelid droop; and thick, brittle nails. Cardiovascular involvement leads to decreased cardiac output, slow pulse rate, and signs of poor peripheral circulation. Anorexia, abdominal distention, menorrhagia, decreased libido, infertility, ataxia, intention tremor, and nystagmus are possible effects of myxedema as well.

Neuromuscular symptoms are among the most frequent manifestations of hypothyroidism. Flexor tenosynovitis with stiffness often accompanies CTS in persons with hypothyroidism (Louthrenoo and Schumacher, 1990). CTS arising from myxedematous tissue in the carpal tunnel area can develop before other signs of hypothyroidism become evident. Most people with CTS associated with hypothyroidism do not require surgical treatment because symptoms of median nerve compression respond to thyroid replacement.

Proximal muscle weakness is common in persons with hypothyroidism, and it is sometimes accompanied by pain. Trigger points are frequently detected on examination, and diffuse muscle tenderness may be the major finding (Sonkin, 1994). Muscle weakness is not always related to either the severity or the duration of hypothyroidism; it can be present several months before a medical diagnosis of hypothyroidism is made. Deep tendon reflexes show delayed relaxation time (i.e., prolonged reflexes), especially in the Achilles tendon.

TABLE 9–6 CAUSES OF HYPOTHYROIDISM

PRIMARY	SECONDARY
Congenital defects	Pituitary tumor
Loss of thyroid tissue	Pituitary insufficiency
Radioiodine treatment (for Hodgkin's disease, throat cancer)	Postpartum necrosis of the pituitary (Sheehan's syndrome)
Surgical removal	
Defective hormone synthesis	
Chronic autoimmune thyroiditis (Hashimoto's disease)	
Iodine deficiency	
Antithyroid drugs	

Medical Management

Diagnosis. A substantial delay in diagnosis due to the vague onset of symptoms is not uncommon. Specific testing, such as radioimmunoassay, confirms hypothyroidism with low T_3 and T_4 levels supported by laboratory findings (e.g., elevated TSH, serum cholesterol, alkaline phosphatase, and triglycerides levels and anemia).

Treatment. The goals of treatment for hypothyroidism are to correct thyroid hormone deficiency, reverse symptoms, and prevent further cardiac and arterial damage. If treatment with (life-long) administration of synthetic thyroid hormone preparations is begun soon after symptoms appear, recovery may be complete. Surgery to remove the thyroid may be a treatment option if the person does not respond to treatment or if a goiter is very large and puts pressure on other structures in the neck.

Prognosis. Severely hypothyroid conditions accompanied by pronounced atherosclerosis (resulting from abnormal lipid metabolism) may cause angina and other symptoms of coronary artery disease. Treatment of hypothyroidism-induced

TABLE 9-7 Systemic Manifestations of Hypothyroidism

CNS Effects	Musculoskeletal Effects	Cardiovascular Effects	Hematologic Effects	Respiratory Effects	Integumentary Effects	Gastrointestinal Effects
Slowed speech and hoarseness	Proximal muscle weakness	Bradycardia	Anemia	Dyspnea	Myxedema (periorbital and peripheral)	Anorexia
Slow mental function (loss of interest in daily activities, poor short-term memory)	Myalgias	Congestive heart failure	Easy bruising	Respiratory muscle weakness	Thickened, cool, and dry skin	Constipation
Fatigue and increased sleep	Trigger points	Poor peripheral circulation (pallor, cold skin, intolerance to cold, hypertension)			Scaly skin (especially elbows and knees)	Weight gain disproportionate to caloric intake
Headache	Stiffness	Severe atherosclerosis			Carotenosis (yellowing of the skin)	Decreased absorption of nutrients
Cerebellar ataxia	Carpal tunnel syndrome	Angina			Coarse, thinning hair	Decreased protein metabolism (retarded skeletal and soft-tissue growth)
Depression	Prolonged deep tendon reflexes (especially Achilles)				Intolerance to cold	Delayed glucose uptake
	Subjective report of paresthesias without supportive objective findings				Nonpitting edema of hands and feet	Decreased glucose absorption
	Muscular and joint edema				Poor wound healing	
	Back pain				Thin, brittle nails	
	Increased bone density					
	Decreased bone formation and resorption					

Adapted from Goodman CC, Snyder TE: Differential Diagnosis in Physical Therapy, ed 2. Philadelphia, WB Saunders, 1995, p 343.

angina can be difficult because thyroid hormone replacement increases the heart's need for oxygen by increasing body metabolism. This increase in metabolism then precipitates angina and aggravates the anginal condition.

Rarely, severe or prolonged hypothyroidism may progress to myxedema coma when aggravated by stress such as surgery, infection, or noncompliance with thyroid treatment. Myxedema coma can be fatal because of the extreme decrease in the metabolic rate, hypoventilation leading to respiratory acidosis, hypothermia, and hypotension.

Special Implications for the Therapist **9-7**

HYPOTHYROIDISM

In the case of myxedematous hypothyroidism, distinctive changes in the synovium can occur, resulting in a viscous noninflammatory joint effusion. Often the fluid contains calcium pyrophosphate dihydrate (CPPD) crystal deposits that may be associated with chondrocalcinosis (i.e., calcium salts in the synovium). When these hypothyroid clients have been treated with thyroid replacement, some have experienced attacks of acute pseudogout caused by the crystals in the periarticular joint structures (found in both the hyaline cartilage and fibrocartilage). Without medical treatment, this condition can lead to permanent joint damage.

CPPD disease (pseudogout) usually affects larger joints, but symptomatic involvement of the spine with deposition of crystals in the ligamentum flavum and atlanto-occipital ligament can result in spinal stenosis and subsequent neurologic syndromes (Ryan, 1993; Delamarter et al., 1993; Salcman et al., 1994). Effective treatment of pseudogout may include joint aspiration to relieve fluid pressure, steroid injection, and nonsteroidal anti-inflammatories (Norris, 1995).* The role of the therapist is much the same as in the treatment of rheumatoid arthritis (see Chapter 23).

Muscular complaints (aches, pain, and stiffness) associated with hypothyroidism are likely to develop into persistent myofascial trigger points. Clinically, any compromise of the energy metabolism of muscle aggravates and perpetuates trigger points. These do not resolve just with specific treatment by a therapist (e.g.,trigger point therapy, myofascial release); they require thyroid replacement as well (Travell and Simons, 1983).

Hypothyroidism and Fibromyalgia

The correlation between hypothyroidism and fibromyalgia syndrome (FMS) is now being investigated (Elsinger et al., 1994; Keenan et al., 1993).† Persons with FMS may have a blunted response to a hypothalamic-releasing hormone (thyrotropin) that stimulates the anterior pituitary to secrete TSH (Ferraccioli, 1990). Reduced high-energy phosphate in muscle, related to impairment of carbohydrate metabolism (glycolysis abnormalities), may explain the chronic fatigue that can approach lethargy; it is noticeable on arising in the morning and is usually worse during midafternoon. These clients are particularly "weather conscious" and have muscular pain that increases with the onset of cold, rainy weather (Layzer, 1985; Travell and Simons, 1983).

Acute Care Setting

Dry, edematous tissues associated with hypothyroidism are more prone to skin breakdown. Prevention of pressure ulcers requires careful monitoring of the usual pressure points (e.g., sacrum, coccyx, scapulae, elbows, greater trochanter, heels, malleoli).

Hypothyroidism and Medication

Clients with cardiac complications are started on small doses of thyroid hormone, as large doses can precipitate heart failure or myocardial infarction by increasing body metabolism, myocardial oxygen requirements, and, consequently, the workload of the heart. Carefully observe for any signs of aggravated cardiovascular disease, such as chest pain and tachycardia. Report any signs of hypertension or congestive heart failure in the elderly person.

After thyroid replacement therapy begins, watch for symptoms of hyperthyroidism (e.g., restlessness, tremor, sweating, dyspnea, excessive weight gain; see also Table 9–5).

Hypothyroidism and Exercise

Activity intolerance, weakness, and apathy secondary to decreased metabolic rate may require developing increased tolerance to activity and exercise once thyroid replacement has been initiated. Increased activity and exercise are especially helpful for the client who is constipated secondary to slowed metabolic rate and decreased peristalsis. Exercise-induced myalgia leading to rhabdomyolysis (disintegration of striated or skeletal muscle fibers with excretion of myoglobin in the urine) has been reported in hypothyroidism. Rhabdomyolysis in this case may occur possibly as a result of poor drug compliance in combination with other aggravating factors, such as exercise (Sekine et al., 1993; Lochmuller et al., 1993). Although they occur infrequently, the therapist should remain alert to any signs or symptoms of rhabdomyolysis (e.g., unexplained muscle pain and weakness) in exercising clients with hypothyroidism. Rhabdomyolysis can progress to renal failure.

Reduction in stroke volume and heart rate associated with hypothyroidism causes lowered cardiac output, increased peripheral vascular resistance to maintain systolic blood pressure, and a variety of ECG changes (e.g., sinus bradycardia, prolonged PR interval, depressed P waves). In animal models, exercise can affect skeletal and cardiac muscle systems independent of thyroid hormone replacement, which supports the role of exercise in improving muscle and cardiovascular function for the person with hypothyroidism (Katzeff et al., 1994; Delp et al., 1995).

What is most important, because changes in lipid and lipoprotein levels occur with exercise, an exercise program can improve the lipid profile. This is especially important for the person with altered lipid metabolism and associated cardiovascular complications (see preceding discussion on clinical manifestations).

---

* Although the synovium contains noninflammatory joint effusion, crystals may loosen, resulting in crystal "shedding" into the joint fluid, thereby causing an inflammatory response.

† Despite the correlation between hypothyroidism and FMS, thyroid dysfunction is seen at least three times more often in women with rheumatoid arthritis (RA) than in women with similar demographic features with noninflammatory rheumatic diseases, such as osteoarthritis and fibromyalgia (Shiroky et al., 1993).

Goiter

Goiter, an enlargement of the thyroid gland, may be a result of lack of iodine, inflammation, or tumors (benign or malignant). Enlargement may also appear in hyperthyroidism, especially Graves' disease. Goiter occurs most often in areas of the world in which iodine, which is necessary for the production of thyroid hormone, is deficient in the diet. Factors that inhibit normal thyroid hormone production result in a negative feedback loop, with hypersecretion of thyroid-stimulating hormone (TSH). The TSH increase results in an increase in thyroid mass (Blevins and Cassmeyer, 1995).

With the use of iodized salt, this problem has almost been eliminated in the United States and Canada. Although the younger population in the United States may be goiter-free, elderly people may have developed goiter during their childhood or adolescent years and may still have clinical manifestations of this disorder. Increased neck size may be observed, and when the thyroid increases to a certain point, pressure on the trachea and esophagus may cause difficulty breathing, dysphagia (difficulty swallowing), and hoarseness.

Thyroiditis

Thyroiditis, inflammation of the thyroid, may be classified as *acute suppurative* (pus-forming), *subacute granulomatous* and *lymphocytic*, or *chronic* (Hashimoto's disease). Acute and subacute thyroiditis are uncommon conditions caused by bacterial (*Streptococcus pyogenes*, *Staphylococcus aureus*, and *Pneumococcus pneumoniae*) and viral agents, respectively. Only the most common form, Hashimoto's thyroiditis, is discussed further.

Hashimoto's (chronic) thyroiditis affects women more frequently than it does men (10:1 ratio) and is most often seen in the 30- to 50-year age group. The disorder has an autoimmune basis, and genetic predisposition appears to play a role in the etiology. It is associated with HLA-DR3, which is also present in other autoimmune conditions (e.g., Graves' disease, systemic lupus erythematosus, rheumatoid arthritis).

Hashimoto's thyroiditis causes destruction of the thyroid gland because of the infiltration of the gland by lymphocytes and antithyroid antibodies. This infiltration results in decreased serum levels of T_3 and T_4, thus stimulating the pituitary gland to increase the production of TSH. The increased TSH causes hyperfunction of the tissue and goiter formation (enlargement of the gland) results. At first, this increase in function helps maintain a normal hormonal level, but eventually, when enough of the gland is destroyed, hypothyroidism develops. Hashimoto's thyroiditis is one of the most common causes of hypothyroidism in women older than 50 years.

Symptoms of chronic thyroiditis include painless (usually) symmetrical enlargement of the gland, which in turn causes pressure on the surrounding structures, subsequently causing dysphagia and respiratory distress. Most clients are euthyroid (have a normally functioning thyroid), about 20% are hypothyroid, and fewer than 5% are hyperthyroid (Birch, 1993). The course of Hashimoto's thyroiditis varies; some persons experience spontaneous remission and others remain stable for years with treatment. Treatment is directed toward correcting any thyroid function abnormalities and reducing the size of the gland. Tablets containing thyroxine (T_4) can help regulate and maintain adequate levels of circulating hormones.

Special Implications for the Therapist **9-8**

THYROIDITIS

Because the symptoms of thyroiditis are related to glandular function, and because the condition may be associated with hypothyroidism or hyperthyroidism, the therapist is referred to the sections relevant to client presentation (see Special Implications for the Therapist: Hypothyroidism or Hyperthyroidism).

Thyroid Cancer

Malignant tumors of the thyroid are rare; they affect women more than men (2 : 1 ratio), mainly between the ages of 40 and 60 years. A past medical history of radiation to the head, neck, or chest (e.g., for an enlarged thymus or tonsils, acne, or Hodgkin's disease) is the most obvious risk factor.

The major manifestation of thyroid cancer is the appearance of a hard, painless nodule in an enlarged thyroid gland. Benign adenomas are usually well encapsulated and are rarely large enough to cause any respiratory symptoms by pressing against the trachea. Malignant transformation of a benign nodule can occur. Thyroid cancers seldom metastasize beyond regional lymph nodes of the neck, resulting in a good prognosis for most people with this condition.

Because more women have thyroid disease, including thyroid cancer, a man with a nodule is regarded with greater suspicion for cancer. Thyroid cancer is diagnosed by fine-needle aspiration and biopsy or open biopsy, laboratory analysis, and radiographic evidence of calcification. Treatment usually involves removal of all or part of the thyroid. Neck resection may be done for metastases to the neck. Chemotherapy and external radiation may be used for metastasis. Major postoperative complications may involve respiratory complications, recurrent laryngeal damage, hemorrhage, and hypoparathyroidism (Birch, 1993). Most thyroid cancers are not highly malignant and with treatment, the person experiences normal life expectancy.

Special Implications for the Therapist **9-9**

THYROID CANCER

A thyroid neoplasm can be the incidental finding in persons being treated for a musculoskeletal condition involving the head and neck. Most thyroid nodules are benign, but as mentioned previously, any time a therapist examines a client's neck and finds an asymptomatic nodule or unusual swelling, enlargement, or redness, with or without symptoms of pain, hoarseness, dyspnea, or dysphagia (difficulty swallowing), a medical referral is required.

Parathyroid Glands

Two parathyroid glands are located on the posterior surface of each lobe of the thyroid gland. These glands secrete parathyroid hormone (PTH), which regulates calcium and phosphorus metabolism. PTH exerts its effect by (1) increasing the release of calcium and phosphate from the bone (bone demineralization); (2) increasing the absorption of calcium and excretion of phosphate by the kidneys; and (3) promoting calcium absorption in the GI tract (Wong, 1993).

Disorders of the parathyroid glands may come to the therapist's attention because these conditions can cause periarthritis and tendinitis. Both types of inflammation may be crystal-induced, with formation of periarticular or tendinous calcification (Moskowitz, 1969). Ruptured tendons due to bone resorption at the insertions have been reported in cases of primary hyperparathyroidism (Preston, 1972).

Hyperparathyroidism (Birch, 1993)

Definition and Incidence. Hyperparathyroidism is a disorder caused by overactivity of one or more of the four parathyroid glands that disrupts calcium, phosphate, and bone metabolism. Women are affected more than men (2 : 1), usually after age 60 years.

Hyperparathyroidism is frequently overlooked in the over-60 population. Symptoms in the early stages for this group are subtle and easily attributed to the aging process, depression, or anxiety. Eventually the symptoms intensify as the level of serum calcium rises, but this situation is accompanied by increased bone damage and other complications.

Etiology and Risk Factors. Hyperparathyroidism is classified as primary, secondary, or tertiary. *Primary hyperparathyroidism* develops when the normal regulatory relationship between serum calcium levels and PTH secretion is interrupted. This occurs when one or more of the parathyroid glands enlarges, increasing PTH secretion and elevating serum calcium levels. The most common cause is an adenoma or hyperplasia of the gland without an identifying injury (e.g., congenital or genetic disorder, multiple endocrine neoplasia).

Secondary hyperparathyroidism occurs when the glands are hyperplastic from malfunction of another organ system. A hypocalcemia-producing abnormality outside the parathyroid gland results in a compensatory response of the parathyroid glands to chronic hypocalcemia. This is usually the result of renal failure (decreased renal activation of vitamin D), but it may also occur with osteogenesis imperfecta, Paget's disease, multiple myeloma, carcinoma with bone metastasis, laxative abuse, and vitamin D deficiency. *Tertiary hyperparathyroidism* occurs when PTH production is overactive in people with normal or low serum calcium levels.

Pathogenesis and Clinical Manifestations. The primary function of parathyroid hormone (PTH) is to maintain a proper balance of calcium and phosphorus ions within the blood. PTH is not regulated by the pituitary or the hypothalamus and maintains normal blood calcium levels by increasing bone resorption and GI absorption of calcium. It also maintains an inverse relationship between serum calcium and phosphate levels by inhibiting phosphate reabsorption in the renal tubules (Norris, 1995). Abnormal PTH production disrupts this balance; symptoms of parathyroidism are related to this release of bone calcium into the bloodstream. Excessive circulating PTH leads to bone damage, hypercalcemia, and kidney damage (Table 9–8).

Bone Damage. Oversecretion of PTH causes excessive osteoclast growth and activity within the bones. Osteoclasts are active in promoting resorption of bone, which then releases calcium into the blood, causing hypercalcemia. This calcium loss leads to bone demineralization, and in time, the bones may become so fragile that pathologic fractures, deformity (e.g., kyphosis of the thoracic spine), and compression fractures of the vertebral bodies occur. If uncontrolled, osteoclast proliferation may cause lytic bone lesions (bone disintegrates, leaving holes) eventually producing a severe bone disease called *osteitis fibrosa cystica* (von Recklinghausen's disease). If hyperparathyroidism is surgically treated early in its course, bone pain may disappear within 48 to 72 hours, and bone lesions may heal completely.

TABLE 9–8 SYSTEMIC MANIFESTATIONS OF HYPERPARATHYROIDISM

EARLY CNS SYMPTOMS	MUSCULOSKELETAL EFFECTS	GASTROINTESTINAL EFFECTS	GENITOURINARY EFFECTS
Lethargy, drowsiness, paresthesias	Mild-to-severe proximal muscle weakness of the extremities	Peptic ulcers	Renal colic associated with kidney stones
Slow mentation, poor memory	Muscle atrophy	Pancreatitis	Hypercalcemia (polyuria, polydipsia, constipation)
Easily fatigued	Bone decalcification (bone pain, especially spine; pathologic fractures; bone cysts)	Nausea, vomiting, anorexia	Kidney infections
Hyperactive deep tendon reflexes	Gout and pseudogout	Constipation	Renal hypertension
Occasionally glove-and-stocking distribution sensory loss	Arthralgias involving the hands	Abdominal pain	
	Myalgia and sensation of heaviness in the lower extremities		
	Joint hypermobility		

Adapted from Goodman CC, Snyder TE: Differential Diagnosis in Physical Therapy, ed 2. Philadelphia, WB Saunders, 1995, p 346.

Hypercalcemia. As excessive parathyroid hormone secretion results in bone resorption and hypercalcemia as just described, hypercalciuria (excessive calcium in the urine) eventually develops. High serum calcium levels also stimulate hypergastrinemia (excess gastrin, a hormone that stimulates secretion of gastric acid and pepsin in the blood), abdominal pain, peptic ulcer disease, and pancreatitis.

Kidney Damage. As serum calcium levels rise in response to excessive PTH levels, large amounts of phosphorus and calcium are excreted and lost from the body. Excretion of these compounds occurs through the renal system, leaving deposits of calcium phosphate within the renal tubules. This produces a kidney condition called *nephrocalcinosis*. Because calcium salts are insoluble in urine, kidney stones composed of calcium phosphate develop. Serious renal damage may not be reversible with parathyroidectomy.

Some people with hyperparathyroidism may be completely asymptomatic, but even asymptomatic clients with elevated serum and PTH levels have been found to have paresthesias, muscle cramps, and loss of pain and vibratory sensation in a stocking-glove distribution (Dorwart, 1993). Others suffer from a wide range of symptoms as a result of skeletal disease, renal involvement, GI tract disorders, and neurologic abnormalities.

Medical Management

Diagnosis. Diagnosis of hyperparathyroidism depends on laboratory and x-ray findings. Serum calcium level is elevated, serum phosphate level is depressed, and urine calcium and phosphorus levels are both high. Skeletal damage can be seen on x-ray as diffuse demineralization of bones, bone cysts, subperiosteal bone resorption, and loss of the laminae durae surrounding the teeth.

Treatment and Prognosis. Treatment for primary hyperparathyroidism is surgical removal (parathyroidectomy). The prognosis is good if the condition is identified and treated early. Medical management may also include lowering severely elevated calcium levels, increasing urinary calcium excretion with diuretics, and long-term management of hypercalcemia with drugs to increase bone resorption of calcium. If present, kidney pathologic lesions or conditions are irreversible and tend to progress even with treatment for excess PTH.

Special Implications for the Therapist **9-10**

HYPERPARATHYROIDISM

The therapist is likely to see skeletal, articular, and neuromuscular manifestations associated with hyperparathyroidism. Chronic low back pain and easy fracturing due to bone demineralization may be compounded by marked muscle weakness and atrophy, especially in the legs (Norris, 1995).

Inflammatory erosive polyarthritis may be associated with chondrocalcinosis and calcium pyrophosphate dihydrate (CPPD) crystal deposits in the synovial fluid in up to 35% of cases of hyperparathyroidism. This erosion, described as *osteogenic synovitis,* occurs as part of the bone destruction that can occur with hyperparathyroidism. When this complication develops, the Achilles, triceps, and obturator tendons are most commonly affected; other affected areas may include hands and wrists (CTS), shoulders, knees, clavicle, and axial skeleton (Terkeltaub, 1994). Concurrent illness and surgery (e.g., parathyroidectomy) are recognized inducers of acute arthritic episodes (Louthrenoo and Schumacher, 1990).

The therapist may be involved in treating the arthritis associated with this (or any other endocrine) condition, but unless the underlying cause is treated first, treatment for the arthritis will be frustrating and poorly effective. Following medical treatment, the therapist's treatment of the residual arthritis is the same as for arthritis, regardless of the cause.

Acute Care

In the acute care setting, auscultate for lung sounds and listen for signs of pulmonary edema in the person receiving large amounts of saline solution IV, especially in the presence of pulmonary or cardiac disease. Monitor the person on digitalis carefully for any toxic effects produced by elevated calcium levels, as clients with hypercalcemia are hypersensitive to digitalis and may quickly develop toxic symptoms (e.g., arrhythmias, nausea, fatigue, visual changes) (see Table 10–9).

These clients are all predisposed to pathologic fractures and must be treated with caution to minimize the risk of injury. Take every safety precaution, assisting carefully with walking, keeping the bed at its lowest position, raising the side rails, and lifting the immobilized person carefully to minimize bone stress. Schedule care to allow the person with muscle weakness recovery time and rest between all activities.

Postoperative Care

Postoperatively, the person should use a semi-Fowler's position with support for the head and neck to decrease edema, which can cause pressure on the trachea. Observe for any signs of mild tetany, such as reports of tingling in the hands and around the mouth. These symptoms should subside quickly but may be prodromal signs of tetany. Watch for increased neuromuscular irritability and other signs of severe tetany and report them immediately. Acute postoperative arthritis may occur secondary to gout or pseudogout.

Early ambulation (although uncomfortable) is essential, because weight-bearing and pressure on bones speed up recalcification. The use of light ankle weights or a light weight-resistive elastic for the lower extremities provides tension at the musculotendinous/bone interface, accomplishing the same response. The same type of exercise program for the upper extremities must be approved by the physician first, as care must be taken not to disturb the surgical site.

Home Health Care

For the person at home, fluids are important, and the use of cranberry or prune juice to increase urine acidity and help prevent stone formation may be recommended. Evaluate the living environment for any potential safety hazards that may predispose the client to injury, such as throw rugs, tub or shower stall without a rubber mat

TABLE 9–9 CHARACTERISTICS OF HYPERPARATHYROIDISM AND HYPOPARATHYROIDISM

HYPERPARATHYROIDISM	HYPOPARATHYROIDISM
Increased bone resorption	Decreased bone resorption
Elevated serum calcium levels	Depressed serum calcium levels
Depressed serum phosphate levels	Elevated serum phosphate levels
Hypercalciuria and hyperphosphaturia	Hypocalciuria and hypophosphaturia
Decreased neuromuscular irritability	Increased neuromuscular activity, which may progress to tetany

From Black JM, Matassarin-Jacobs E (eds): Luckmann and Sorensen's Medical-Surgical Nursing, ed 4. Philadelphia, WB Saunders, 1993, p 1828.

or decals to prevent slipping, missing hand and guard rails wherever necessary, improper lighting (encourage the use of a night-light in dark areas at all times).

Hypoparathyroidism

Definition. Hyposecretion, hypofunction, or insufficient secretion of parathyroid hormone (PTH) are all ways to describe hypoparathyroidism (Birch, 1993). Because the parathyroid glands primarily regulate calcium balance, hypoparathyroidism causes hypocalcemia and produces a syndrome opposite that of hyperparathyroidism with abnormally low serum calcium levels, high serum phosphate levels, and possible neuromuscular irritability (tetany) (Table 9–9).

Etiology and Incidence. Hypoparathyroidism is either iatrogenic, which is most common, or idiopathic. *Iatrogenic* (acquired) causes include accidental removal of the parathyroid glands during thyroidectomy or anterior neck surgery,[8] infarction of the parathyroid glands resulting from an inadequate blood supply to the glands during surgery, strangulation of one or more of the glands by postoperative scar tissue, and, rarely, massive thyroid irradiation. Other secondary causes of hypoparathyroidism may include hemochromatosis, sarcoidosis, amyloidosis, tuberculosis, neoplasms, or trauma.

Idiopathic causes affect children nine times as often as adults and affect twice as many women as men. Like Graves' disease and Hashimoto's thyroiditis, idiopathic hypoparathyroidism may be an autoimmune disorder with a genetic basis.

Pathogenesis. See discussion of pathogenesis of hyperparathyroidism for a description of the regulation of calcium and phosphate by PTH and the parathyroid glands. PTH normally functions to increase bone resorption to maintain a proper balance between serum calcium and phosphate. When parathyroid secretion of PTH is reduced, bone resorption slows, serum calcium levels fall, and severe neuromuscular irritability develops. Calcifications may form in various organs, such as the eyes and basal ganglia. Serum phosphate levels rise without sufficient PTH, as fewer phosphorus ions are secreted by the distal tubules of the kidneys with decreased renal excretion of phosphorus.

Clinical Manifestations. Mild hypoparathyroidism may be asymptomatic, but it usually produces hypocalcemia and high serum phosphate levels that affect the CNS as well as other body systems (Table 9–10). The most significant clinical consequence of hypocalcemia associated with hypoparathyroidism is neuromuscular irritability. In people with chronic hypoparathyroidism, this neuromuscular irritability may result in tetany. Hypocalcemia resistant to PTH, called *pseudohypoparathyroidism*, is associated with shortened metacarpals and metatarsals (Dorwart, 1993).

Acute (overt) tetany begins with a tingling in the fingertips, around the mouth, and, occasionally, the feet. This tingling spreads and becomes more severe, producing painful muscle tension, spasms, grimacing, laryngospasm, and arrhythmias. Trousseau's sign (carpal spasm) and Chvostek's sign (hyperirritability of the facial nerve, producing a characteristic spasm when tapped) are apparent on examination (see Figs. 4–4 and 4–5). In severe cases, a tracheostomy may be required to correct acute respiratory obstruction secondary to laryngospasm.

Medical Management

Diagnosis. Diagnosis of this condition is based on history, clinical presentation, examination, and laboratory values (low serum calcium, high serum phosphate, low or absent urinary calcium). Radioimmunoassay for parathyroid hormone will demonstrate decreased PTH concentration.

Treatment. Acute hypoparathyroidism, with its major manifestation of acute tetany, is a life-threatening disorder. Treatment is directed toward elevation of serum calcium levels as rapidly as possible, prevention or treatment of convulsions, and control of laryngeal spasm and subsequent respiratory obstruction. Treatment of chronic hypoparathyroidism with pharmacologic management is accomplished more gradually than treatment for an acute situation. Surgical intervention is not a treatment choice for hypoparathyroidism and, in fact, is often the cause of this condition (see Etiology, this section).

Prognosis. Full recovery from the effects of hypoparathyroidism is possible when the condition is diagnosed early, before the development of serious complications. Unfortunately, once formed, cataracts and brain (basal ganglion) calcifications are irreversible. Death can occur from respiratory obstruction secondary to tetany and laryngospasms if treatment is not initiated early in acute hypoparathyroidism.

Special Implications for the Therapist **9–11**

HYPOPARATHYROIDISM

Anyone experiencing acute tetany will be receiving acute medical care and will not be a likely candidate for therapy until the condition has resolved with treatment.

[8] Variations in location and color as well as the minute size of parathyroid glands make identification very difficult and may result in glandular damage or accidental removal during thyroid removal or anterior neck surgery.

TABLE 9–10 Systemic Manifestations of Hypoparathyroidism

CNS Effects	Musculoskeletal Effects*	Cardiovascular Effects*	Integumentary Effects	Gastrointestinal Effects
Personality changes (irritability, agitation, anxiety, depression) Convulsions	Hypocalcemia (neuromuscular excitability and muscular tetany, especially involving flexion of the upper extremity) Spasm of intercostal muscles and diaphragm compromising breathing Positive Chvostek's sign	Cardiac arrhythmias Eventual heart failure	Dry, scaly, coarse, pigmented skin Tendency to have skin infections Thinning of hair, including eyebrows and eyelashes Fingernails and toenails become brittle and form ridges	Nausea and vomiting Constipation or diarrhea Neuromuscular stimulation of the intestine (abdominal pain)

* Musculoskeletal and cardiovascular effects are the most common and important for the therapist to be aware of.
Adapted from Goodman CC, Snyder TE: Differential Diagnosis in Physical Therapy, ed 2. Philadelphia, WB Saunders, 1995, p 348.

Chronic Hypoparathyroidism

For the person with chronic hypoparathyroidism, observe carefully for any minor muscle twitching or signs of laryngospasm, as these may signal the onset of acute tetany. Chronic tetany is less severe, usually affects one side only, and may cause difficulty with gait and balance. Gait training and prevention of falls are key components of a therapy program. Hyperventilation may worsen tetany; focus on breathing during exercise is important.

Chronic hypoparathyroidism can lead to cardiac complications (e.g., arrhythmia, heart block, decreasing cardiac output) which necessitates careful monitoring. Calcium prescribed for this condition potentiates* the effect of digitalis, requiring close monitoring of the person receiving both digitalis and calcium for any signs of digitalis toxicity (see Table 10–9).

Home Health Care

Life-long medication, dietary modifications, and medical care are required for the person with chronic hypoparathyroidism. Serum calcium levels must be checked by a physician at least three times a year to maintain normal serum calcium levels. Cheese and milk should be omitted from the diet because they have a high phosphorus content. Other foods high in calcium but low in phosphorus are encouraged.

* When one agent potentiates the effects of another agent, the enhancement is such that the combined effect is greater than the sum of the effects of the individual agents.

Adrenal Glands

The adrenals are two small glands located on the upper part of each kidney (see Fig. 9–1). Each adrenal gland consists of two relatively discrete parts: an outer cortex and an inner medulla. The outer cortex is responsible for the secretion of mineralocorticoids (steroid hormones that regulate fluid and mineral balance), glucocorticoids (steroid hormones responsible for controlling the metabolism of glucose), and androgens (sex hormones).

The centrally located adrenal medulla is derived from neural tissue and secretes epinephrine and norepinephrine, which exert widespread effects on vascular tone, the heart, and the nervous system, as well as affecting glucose metabolism. Together, the adrenal cortex and medulla are major factors in the body's response to stress.

Glandular hypofunction and hyperfunction characterize the major disorders of the adrenal cortex. Underactivity of the adrenal cortex results in a deficiency of glucocorticoids, mineralocorticoids, and adrenal androgens. Overactivity results in excessive production of these same hormones.

Adrenal Insufficiency

Hypofunction of the adrenal cortex can originate from a disorder within the adrenal gland itself (primary adrenal insufficiency) or it may be due to hypofunction of the pituitary-hypothalamic unit (secondary adrenal insufficiency) (Loriaux, 1993). Adrenocortical insufficiency, whether primary or secondary, can be either acute or chronic.

Primary Adrenal Insufficiency (Addison's Disease)

Definition and Overview. Addison's disease is a condition that occurs as a result of a disorder within the adrenal gland itself, named for the physician who first studied and described the associated symptoms. Adrenal insufficiency affects both sexes equally across the lifespan. Primary forms of adrenal insufficiency are uncommon; the therapist is most likely to see secondary adrenal insufficiency as a result of suppression of ACTH by steroid therapy.

Etiology. At one time, most causes of Addison's disease occurred as a complication of tuberculosis, but now most cases are considered idiopathic. Because more than half of all people with idiopathic Addison's disease have circulating autoantibodies that react specifically against adrenal tissue, this condition is considered to have an autoimmune basis. Less frequent causes of primary insufficiency include bilateral adrenalectomy, adrenal hemorrhage or infarction, radiation to the adrenal glands, malignant adrenal neoplasm, infections (e.g., histoplasmosis, cytomegalovirus), and destruction of the adrenal glands by chemical agents (Alspach, 1991).

Risk Factors. Surgery (including dental procedures); pregnancy (especially with postpartum hemorrhage); accident, injury, or trauma; infection; salt loss due to profuse diaphoresis (hot weather or with strenuous physical exertion); or failure to take steroid therapy in persons who have chronic adrenal insufficiency can cause acute adrenal insufficiency, known as an *addisonian crisis*.

Pathogenesis and Clinical Manifestations. This adrenal gland disorder results in decreased production of cortisol (a glucocorticoid) and aldosterone (a mineralocorticoid), two of the primary adrenocortical hormones. Glucocorticoid deficiency causes widespread metabolic disturbances. Glucocorticoids promote gluconeogenesis[9] and have an "anti-insulin" effect. Consequently, when glucocorticoids become deficient, gluconeogenesis decreases, with resultant hypoglycemia and liver glycogen deficiency. The person grows weak, exhausted, hypotensive, and suffers from anorexia, weight loss, nausea, and vomiting. Emotional disturbances can develop, ranging from mild neurotic symptoms to severe depression. Glucocorticoid deficiency also diminishes resistance to stress.

Cortisol deficiency results in a failure to inhibit anterior pituitary secretion of adrenocorticotropic hormone (ACTH). The result is a simultaneous increase in ACTH secretion and melanocyte-stimulating hormone (MSH) (see Fig. 9–2); excessive MSH increases skin and mucous membrane pigmentation. Persons with Addison's disease may have a bronzed or tanned appearance, which is the most striking physical finding with primary adrenal insufficiency (not present in all people with this disorder).

This change in pigmentation may vary in the white population from a slight tan or a few black freckles to an intense generalized pigmentation. The change in pigmentation is most commonly observed over extensor surfaces, such as the backs of the hands (metacarpophalangeal joints), elbows, knees, creases of the hands, lips, and mouth. Increased pigmentation of scars formed after the onset of the disease is common. Members of darker-skinned races may develop a slate-gray color that is obvious only to family members.

Aldosterone deficiency causes numerous fluid and electrolyte imbalances. Aldosterone normally promotes conservation of sodium and therefore conserves water and excretion of potassium. A deficiency of aldosterone causes increased sodium excretion, dehydration (see symptoms listed in Box 4–9), hypotension (low blood pressure causing orthostatic symptoms, see Chapter 10), and decreased cardiac output affecting heart size (decrease in size). Eventually, hypotension becomes severe and cardiovascular activity weakens, leading to circulatory collapse, shock, and death. Excess potassium retention (>7 mEq/L) can result in arrhythmias and possible cardiac arrest.

Other clinical effects include decreased tolerance for even minor stress, poor coordination, fasting hypoglycemia (due to decreased gluconeogenesis), and a craving for salty food. Addison's disease may also retard axillary and pubic hair growth in females, decrease the libido (from decreased androgen production), and, in severe cases, cause amenorrhea (absence of menstruation) (Norris, 1995).

Medical Management

Diagnosis, Treatment, and Prognosis. Diagnosis of Addison's disease depends primarily on blood and urine hormonal assays. Medical management is primarily pharmacologic, consisting of life-long administration of synthetically manufactured corticosteroids. If untreated, Addison's disease is ultimately fatal. Adrenal crisis requires immediate hospitalization and treatment.

[9] *Gluconeogenesis* (formerly called *glyconeogenesis*) is the synthesis of glucose from noncarbohydrate sources, such as amino acids; it occurs primarily in the liver and kidneys whenever the supply of carbohydrates is insufficient to meet the body's energy needs.

Special Implications for the Therapist **9-12**

PRIMARY ADRENAL INSUFFICIENCY (ADDISON'S DISEASE)

With pharmacologic therapy, listlessness and exhaustion should gradually lessen and disappear, making exercise possible. Stress should be minimized and infectious illnesses monitored by a physician. Any signs of infection, such as sore throat or burning on urination (see Table 6–1), should be reported to the physician. The client may be directed by the physician to increase medication dosage during times of stress and self-limiting illnesses (e.g., colds and flu). The therapist may need to advise the person to check with the physician if illness or any of the listed risk factors develop at home or during outpatient care.

Clients with Addison's disease should be carefully assessed for signs or hypercortisolism, which can result from excessive long-term cortisol therapy (see Tables 4–7 and 4–8). Assess for signs of sodium and potassium imbalance as well. If steroid replacement therapy is inadequate or too high, changes in amounts of sodium and water are observed (see Table 4–14). Persons receiving glucocorticoid alone may need mineralocorticoid therapy if signs of orthostatic hypotension or electrolyte abnormalities develop.

Elderly persons with Addison's disease often experience more pronounced symptoms if their adrenal function has decreased with aging. These people may be more sensitive to the side effects of steroid therapy, such as osteoporosis, hypertension, and diabetes, when these conditions already exist. The therapist must not overlook the presence of these other conditions when providing treatment.

Anyone with identified Addison's disease should wear an identification bracelet and carry an emergency kit containing hydrocortisone. Steroids administered in the late afternoon or evening may cause stimulation of the CNS and insomnia in some people. Anyone reporting sleep disturbances should be encouraged to discuss this with the physician.

Secondary Adrenal Insufficiency

Secondary adrenal insufficiency is caused by other conditions outside the adrenals, such as hypothalamic or pituitary tumors, removal of the pituitary, or other causes of hypopituitarism, or rapid withdrawal of corticosteroid drugs. Long-term exogenous corticosteroid stimulation suppresses pituitary ACTH secretion and results in adrenal gland atrophy.

Clinical manifestations of secondary disease are somewhat different from symptoms of primary adrenal insufficiency. Whereas most symptoms of primary adrenal insufficiency arise from cortisol and aldosterone deficiency, symptoms of secondary disease are related to cortisol deficiency only. Because the gland is still intact, aldosterone is secreted normally, but the lack of stimulation from ACTH results in deficient cortisol secretion. Arthralgias, myalgias, and tendon calcification can occur, which resolve with treatment of the underlying condition.

Hyperpigmentation is not part of the clinical presentation, as ACTH and MSH levels are low. Additionally, because aldosterone secretion may continue at fairly normal levels in secondary adrenal hypofunction, this condition does not necessarily cause accompanying hypotension and electrolyte abnormalities (Norris, 1995).

As with primary adrenal insufficiency, treatment involves replacement of ACTH and monitoring for fluid and electrolyte imbalances. Too much cortisol replacement can result in the development of Cushing's syndrome (see next section).

Adrenocortical Hyperfunction

Hyperfunction of the adrenal cortex can result in excessive production of glucocorticoids, mineralocorticoids, and androgens. The three major conditions of adrenocortical hyperfunction are Cushing's syndrome (glucocorticoid excess), Conn's syndrome or aldosteronism (aldosterone excess), and adrenal hyperplasia (adrenogenital syndrome). This last, a rare congenital condition, is not discussed further in this text.

Cushing's Syndrome

Definition and Overview. *Hypercortisolism* (hyperfunction of the adrenal gland) is a general term for increased secretion of cortisol by the adrenal cortex. When corticosteroids are administered externally, a condition of hypercortisolism called *Cushing's syndrome* occurs, producing a group of associated signs and symptoms. Hypercortisolism caused by excess secretion of ACTH (e.g., from pituitary stimulation) is called *Cushing's disease;* the clinical presentation is the same as for Cushing's syndrome.

Etiology and Incidence. The primary causes of Cushing's syndrome include pituitary hypersecretion and pituitary or adrenocortical tumors, but therapists are more likely to treat people who have developed iatrogenic Cushing's syndrome. This condition occurs after these individuals have received large doses of cortisol (also known as hydrocortisone) or cortisol derivatives. Exogenous steroids are administered for a number of inflammatory and other disorders (see Box 4–5). Cushing's syndrome occurs mainly in women, with an average age at onset of 20 to 40 years, although it can be seen up to age 60 years.

Pathogenesis and Clinical Manifestations. When the normal function of the glucocorticoids becomes exaggerated, multiple physiologic responses occur (Table 9–11; see also Table 4–7). Overproduction of cortisol causes liberation of amino acids from muscle tissue with resultant weakening of protein structures (specifically muscle and elastic tissue). The end result may include a protuberant abdomen (Fig. 9–5) with striae ("stretch marks"), poor wound healing, generalized muscle weakness, and marked osteoporosis that is made worse by an excessive loss of calcium in the urine. In severe cases of prolonged Cushing's syndrome, muscle weakness and demineralization of bone may lead to pathologic fractures and wedging of the vertebrae, kyphosis (Fig. 9–6), osteonecrosis (especially of the femoral head), bone pain, and back pain.

The effect of increased circulating levels of cortisol on the muscles varies from slight to very marked. There may be so much muscle wasting that the condition simulates muscular dystrophy. Marked weakness of the quadriceps muscle often prevents affected people from rising out of a chair unassisted. Cortisone-induced myopathies are discussed in Chapter 4.

Whenever corticosteroids are administered, the increase in serum cortisol levels triggers a negative feedback signal to the anterior pituitary gland to stop its secretion of ACTH. This decrease in ACTH stimulation of the adrenal cortex results in adrenocortical atrophy during the period of exogenous corticosteroid administration. If these medications are stopped suddenly rather than reduced gradually, the atrophied adrenal gland will not be able to provide the cortisol necessary for physiologic needs. A life-threatening situation known as *acute adrenal insufficiency* can develop, requiring emergency cortisol replacement (see addisonian crisis discussion).

TABLE 9-11 PATHOPHYSIOLOGY OF CUSHING'S SYNDROME

PHYSIOLOGIC EFFECT	CLINICAL RESULT
Persistent hyperglycemia	"Steroid diabetes"
Protein tissue wasting	Weakness due to muscle wasting; capillary fragility resulting in ecchymoses; osteoporosis due to bone matrix wasting
Potassium depletion	Hypokalemia (Table 4–14), cardiac arrhythmias, muscle weakness, renal disorders
Sodium and water retention	Edema and hypertension
Hypertension	Predisposes to left ventricular hypertrophy, congestive heart failure, cerebrovascular accidents
Abnormal fat distribution	Moon-shaped face; dorsocervical fat pad; truncal obesity, slender limbs, thinning of the skin with striae on the breasts, axillary areas, abdomen, and legs
Increased susceptibility to infection; lowered resistance to stress	Absence of signs of infection; poor wound healing
Increased production of androgens	Virilism in women (e.g., acne, thinning of scalp hair, hirsutism or abnormal growth and distribution of hair)
Mental changes	Memory loss, poor concentration and thought processes, euphoria, depression ("steroid psychosis," see Chapter 4)

Data from Black JM, Matassarin-Jacobs E (eds): Luckmann and Sorensen's Medical-Surgical Nursing, ed 4. Philadelphia, WB Saunders, 1993, p 1843.

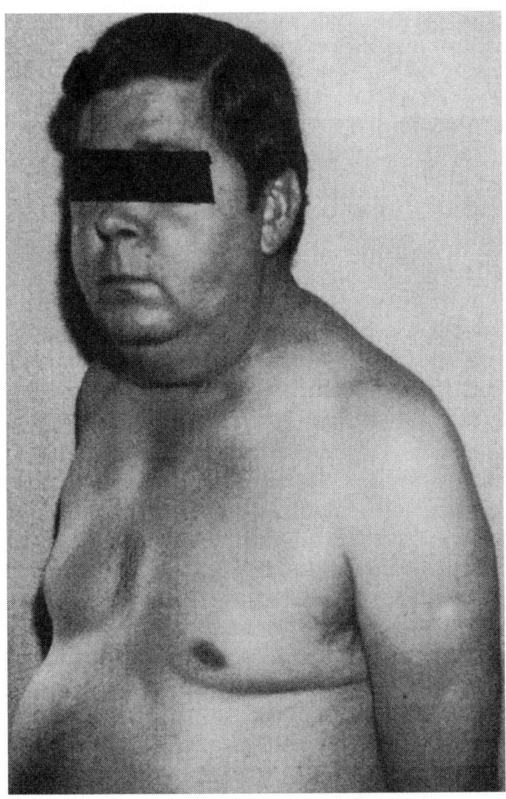

Figure **9–5.** Central obesity of Cushing's syndrome. (*From Callen JP, Jorizzo J (eds): Dermatological Signs of Internal Disease, ed 2. Philadelphia, WB Saunders, 1995, p 204.*)

Medical Management

Diagnosis, Treatment, and Prognosis. Although there is a classic "cushingoid" appearance in persons with hypercortisolism (Fig. 9–7), diagnostic laboratory studies are used to confirm the diagnosis. Treatment to restore hormone balance and reverse Cushing's syndrome may require radiation, drug therapy, or surgery, depending on the underlying cause (e.g., resection of pituitary tumors). Prognosis depends on the underlying cause and the ability to control the cortisol excess.

Special Implications for the Therapist **9–13**

CUSHING'S SYNDROME

See Adverse Effects of Corticosteroids, Chapter 4.

Conn's Syndrome

Definition and Overview. Conn's syndrome, or primary aldosteronism, occurs when an adrenal lesion results in hypersecretion of aldosterone, the most powerful of the mineralocorticoids. Its primary role is to conserve sodium, and it also promotes potassium excretion. The major cause of primary aldosteronism (an uncommon condition present most often in women aged 30 to 50 years) is a benign, aldosterone-secreting tumor called *aldosteronoma*. Rarely, Conn's syndrome develops as a consequence of adrenocortical carcinoma or excessive ingestion of English black licorice or licorice-like substances (Loriaux, 1993).

Secondary hyperaldosteronism can also occur as a consequence of pathologic lesions that stimulate the adrenal gland to increase production of aldosterone. For example, conditions that reduce renal blood flow (e.g., renal artery stenosis), induce renal hypertension (e.g., nephrotic syndrome, ingestion of oral contraceptives), and edematous disorders (e.g., cardiac failure, cirrhosis of the liver with ascites) can cause secondary hyperaldosteronism.

Pathogenesis and Clinical Manifestations. Aldosterone affects the tubular reabsorption of sodium and water and the excretion of potassium and hydrogen ions in the renal tubular epithelial cells; an excess of aldosterone enhances sodium reabsorption by the kidneys. This leads to the development of hypernatremia (excess sodium in blood, indicating water loss exceeding sodium loss), hypervolemia (fluid volume excess, increase in the volume of circulating fluid or plasma in the body), hypokalemia (low blood levels of potassium), and metabolic alkalosis (see discussion of these conditions, Chapter 4). With the hypervolemia and hypernatremia, the blood pressure increases, often to very high levels, and renin produc-

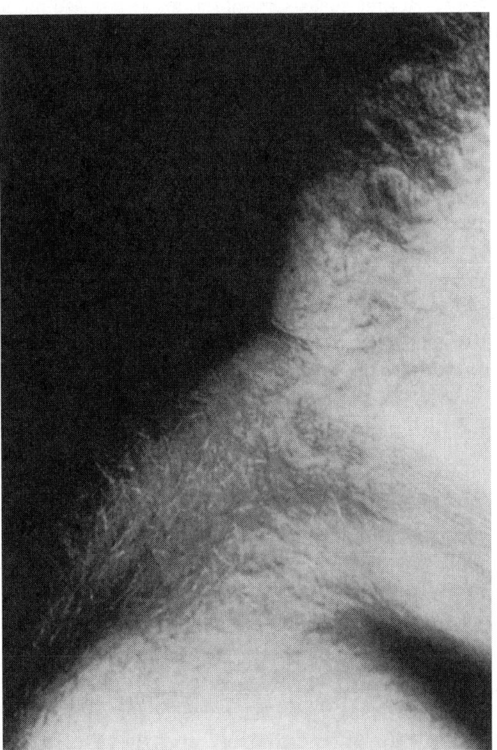

Figure **9–6.** "Buffalo hump" and hypertrichosis (excessive hairiness; hirsutism) in a male with Cushing's syndrome. This hump is a painless accumulation of fat that can also occur idiopathically in (usually) women. There may be a familial pattern (i.e., affected women report a similar anatomic change in their mothers). In the case of steroid-induced changes, this condition resolves when the individual stops taking the medication; in such cases, therapeutic intervention by the therapist has no permanent effect. Idiopathic fat deposits and underlying postural changes can be altered with postural correction and soft tissue and joint mobilization techniques. No studies have substantiated whether these changes are long term. (*From Callen JP, Jorizzo J (eds): Dermatological Signs of Internal Disease, ed 2. Philadelphia, WB Saunders, 1995, p 204.*)

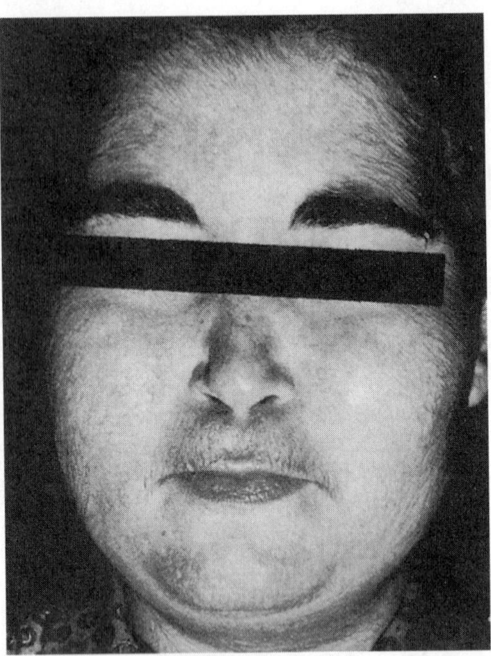

Figure **9–7.** Round facies sometimes referred to as "moon face," telangiectasia, and hirsutism in a woman with Cushing's disease. (*From Callen JP, Jorizzo J (eds): Dermatological Signs of Internal Disease, ed 2. Philadelphia, WB Saunders, 1995, p 204.*)

tion is suppressed. This hypertension can lead to cerebral infarctions and renal damage.

Without intervention, complications of chronic hypertension develop in the presence of hypertension, hypernatremia, and hypokalemia, such as visual disturbances, heart failure, renal damage, and cerebrovascular accident. Hypokalemia results from excessive urinary excretion of potassium causing muscle weakness; intermittent, flaccid paralysis; paresthesias; or cardiac arrhythmias (see Table 4–14).

This excessive urinary excretion of potassium (hypokalemia) leads to polydipsia (excessive thirst). Diabetes mellitus is common because hypokalemia interferes with normal insulin secretion. Finally, hypokalemia leads to metabolic alkalosis, which can cause a decrease in ionized calcium levels, resulting in tetany and respiratory suppression.

Medical Management

Diagnosis, Treatment, and Prognosis. Diagnosis of primary hyperaldosteronism is based on low serum potassium, alkalosis, and elevated urinary or plasma aldosterone levels. Radiographic studies can reveal cardiac hypertrophy resulting from chronic hypertension. Radionuclide scanning techniques using radiolabeled substances allow visualization of any tumors present.

The goals of treatment are to reverse hypertension, correct hypokalemia, and prevent kidney damage. Usually, surgical removal of the aldosterone-secreting tumor (may require adrenalectomy) completely resolves the hypertension within 1 to 3 months. However, without early diagnosis and treatment, renal complications from long-term hypertension may be progressive. Pharmacologic treatment to increase sodium excretion and treat the hypertension and hypokalemia is a nonsurgical alternative.

Special Implications for the Therapist **9–14**

CONN'S SYNDROME

The therapist treating someone with hyperaldosteronism, primary or secondary, may observe signs of tetany (muscle twitching, Chvostek's sign; see Fig. 4–5) and hypokalemia-induced cardiac dysrhythmias, paresthesias, or muscle weakness. If these are encountered in an acute care setting, the medical team is usually well aware of such symptoms and is working to establish a fluid-electrolyte balance. When such signs and symptoms are observed in the outpatient setting, the client must seek medical attention.

Pancreas (Islets of Langerhans)

The pancreas lies behind the stomach, with the head and neck of the pancreas located in the curve of the duodenum and the body extending horizontally across the posterior abdominal wall (see Figs. 9–1 and 13–1). It has two functions, acting as both an endocrine gland (secreting the hormones insulin and glucagon) and an exocrine gland (producing digestive enzymes). The cells of the pancreas that function in the endocrine capacity are the islets of Langerhans.

The islets of Langerhans have three major functioning cells: (1) the α-cells produce glucagon, which increases the blood glucose levels by stimulating the liver and other cells to release stored glucose (glycogenolysis); (2) the β-cells produce insulin, which lowers blood glucose levels by facilitating the entrance of glucose into the cells for metabolism; and (3) the δ (delta)-cells produce somatostatin, which is believed to regulate the release of insulin and glucagon (Wong, 1993) (Table 9–12).

Diabetes Mellitus *(Butts-Krakoff and Black, 1993)*

Definition and Overview. Diabetes mellitus (DM) is a chronic, systemic disorder characterized by hyperglycemia (excess glucose in the blood) and disruption of the metabolism of carbohydrates, fats, and proteins. Insulin, produced in the pancreas, normally maintains a balanced blood glucose level. In DM, either not enough insulin is produced or the insulin that is produced is ineffective, resulting in high blood glucose levels. Over time, DM results in serious small- and large-vessel vascular complications and neuropathies.

There are two types of diabetes: insulin-dependent DM (IDDM), caused by an absolute deficiency of insulin (previously called type I or juvenile-onset diabetes, affecting children and young adults) and non–insulin-dependent DM (NIDDM), caused by resistance to insulin's action in the peripheral tissues (previously called type II or adult-onset diabetes). A comparison of the primary differences between the two types of diabetes is shown in Table 9–13.

Incidence. According to the American Diabetes Association, more than 12 million Americans have been diagnosed with diabetes, and approximately 7 million more people have undiagnosed cases. Diabetes, with its severe complications of heart disease, stroke, kidney disease, blindness, and loss of limbs, is the most common endocrine disorder, ranked as the third cause of death from disease in the United States; it is the leading cause of blindness and renal failure in adults.

TABLE 9-12 Regulation of Glucose Metabolism

Location	Regulating Function
α-Cells (islets of Langerhans)	Secrete glucagon; increase blood glucose level
β-Cells (islets of Langerhans)	Secrete insulin (glucose-regulating hormone); decrease blood glucose level
δ-Cells (islets of Langerhans)	Secrete somatostatin; regulate the release of insulin and glucagon
Adrenal medulla	Responds to stress; secretes epinephrine, which stimulates liver and muscle glycogenolysis to increase the blood glucose level
Adrenocorticotropic hormone (ACTH)	Increases blood glucose levels
Glucocorticoids	Increase blood glucose levels by promoting the flow of amino acids to the liver where they are synthesized into glucose
Human growth hormone (HGH)	Limits storage of fat; favors fat catabolism; inhibits carbohydrate catabolism, raising blood glucose levels
Thyroid-stimulating hormone (TSH)	Mixed effect on carbohydrate metabolism; may raise or lower blood glucose levels

Black, Native American, and Hispanic Americans are three times more likely to develop DM than are white Americans, with increasing incidence being associated with advancing age. Nearly one third of all Americans with DM are older than 60 years; males and females are affected equally. Ninety percent of all cases of DM are NIDDM. IDDM and secondary causes (e.g., medications, genetic disease, hormonal changes) account for the remaining 10%.

Since the mid-1970s, the incidence of diabetes has steadily increased as a result of prolonged life expectancy; increased incidence of obesity; and reduced mortality resulting in increased live births to people with IDDM, whose children are predisposed to future development of IDDM.

Insulin-Dependent Diabetes Mellitus

Etiology and Risk Factors. Both genetic and environmental factors seem to precipitate IDDM. Current research investigation is exploring the causes of IDDM. Environmental factors are suspected in that the highest incidence of new cases of IDDM occurs during the winter months, possibly related to certain viruses. Infection with polio-related viruses and coxsackievirus B may be the most likely trigger of the autoimmune response. How these viruses initiate and accelerate this process remains unclear (Hyoty et al., 1995; Helfand et al., 1995).

After infection with the virus, the β-cells in the pancreas, where insulin is secreted, inappropriately express an antigen. The antigens on these β-cells are recognized as foreign or nonself and are destroyed by circulating T cells. T cells may even attract the superantigen proteins derived from viruses and activate a wide variety of T cells that attack the surface of the pancreas cells. The discovery of pancreas cells with high levels of the protein that is found only in a retrovirus may make it possible to develop a vaccine that could make the immune system eliminate T cells that would otherwise attack the insulin cells (Conrad et al., 1994).

Hereditary factors are suspected, because siblings of affected persons have 10 times the risk of developing diabetes over the general population. Certain HLA antigens (HLA-DR3 and HLA-DR4; see Chapter 5) on specific chromosomes appear to predispose persons to the development of IDDM. A possible autoimmune basis may be present, as some trigger causes the body to develop islet cell antibodies and anti-insulin antibodies. These antibodies attack the β-cells of the

TABLE 9-13 Differences Between IDDM and NIDDM

Features	IDDM (Type I) (Ketosis-Prone)	NIDDM (Type II) (Ketosis-Resistant)
Age at onset	Usually <20 yr	Usually >40 yr
Proportion of all cases	<10%	>90%
Type of onset	Abrupt (acute or subacute)	Gradual
Etiology	Possible viral/autoimmune, resulting in destruction of islet cells	Obesity-associated insulin receptor resistance
HLA association	Yes	No
Insulin antibodies	Yes	No
Seasonal trend	Fall and winter	None
Body weight at onset	Normal or thin, obesity uncommon	Majority are obese (80%)
Endogenous insulin production	Decreased (little or none)	Variable (above or below normal)
Ketoacidosis	May occur	Rare
Treatment	Diet and insulin	Diet, oral hypoglycemic agents or insulin, exercise

Adapted from Goodman CC, Snyder TE: Differential Diagnosis in Physical Therapy, ed 2. Philadelphia, WB Saunders, 1995, p 350.

pancreas, where insulin is produced, and attack the insulin molecules as well.

Non–Insulin-Dependent Diabetes Mellitus

Etiology and Risk Factors. Heredity, obesity, and increasing age appear to play a major role in the development of NIDDM. Viruses and HLA antigens do not seem to be a part of the source of NIDDM. Eighty percent or more of all persons with NIDDM are obese and the remaining 20% are considered to be above their ideal weight. Although the exact link between obesity and diabetes remains undetermined, it is known that overweight people require more insulin for metabolizing the food they eat. Hyperglycemia (excess blood glucose) develops when the pancreas cannot secrete enough insulin to match the body's needs or when the number of insulin receptor sites is decreased or altered, as often occurs with obesity. Increasing age may be a risk because the pancreas becomes more sluggish with age in people who are already predisposed to diabetes.

Risk factors (Box 9–3) may include prolonged physiologic or emotional stress, pregnancy, medications, chronic or recurrent pancreatitis, other endocrine disease (e.g., Cushing's syndrome, hyperaldosteronism, acromegaly), and genetic disorders (e.g., myotonic dystrophy and other muscle disorders, cystic fibrosis) (Betts et al., 1995).

Prolonged stress causes prolonged elevation of stress hormone levels (cortisol, epinephrine, glucagon, and growth hormone), which raises blood glucose levels, which in turn places increased demands on the pancreas. Pancreatic disease interfering with pancreatic function can alter the ability of the β-cells to secrete insulin. Pregnancy causes weight gain and increases levels of estrogen and placental hormones, which antagonize insulin. Medications such as thiazide diuretics, adrenal corticosteroids, and oral contraceptives are known to antagonize the effects of insulin (Norris, 1995). Any condition that interferes with muscle function interferes with the uptake and disposal of glucose in skeletal muscle, thereby influencing whole-body glucose homeostasis.

Pathogenesis. Insulin is a hormone secreted by the β-cells of the pancreas that functions to transport glucose into the cell for use as energy and storage as glycogen, i.e., it turns food into energy. It also stimulates protein synthesis and free fatty acid storage in the fat deposits. In DM, insulin is either insufficient in amount or ineffective in action. Insulin deficiency compromises the body tissues' access to essential nutrients for fuel and storage (Norris, 1995). When glucose levels are elevated normally (e.g., after eating a meal), β-cells increase secretion of insulin to transport and dispose of the glucose into peripheral tissues, thereby lowering blood glucose levels and reestablishing blood glucose homeostasis. Defects in the pancreas, liver, or skeletal muscle, singularly or collectively, can contribute to abnormal glucose homeostasis (DeFronzo, 1988).

Without insulin, three major metabolic problems occur: (1) decreased utilization of glucose, (2) increased fat mobilization, and (3) impaired protein utilization. *Decreased utilization of glucose* occurs because insulin is unavailable to transport glucose. Normally, after a meal, the blood glucose level rises. A large amount of this glucose is taken up by the liver for storage or for use by other tissues, such as skeletal muscle and fat. When insulin function is impaired, the glucose in the general circulation is not taken up or removed by these tissues; thus, it continues to accumulate in the blood. Because new glucose has not been "deposited" in the liver, the liver synthesizes more glucose and releases it into the general circulation, which increases the already elevated blood glucose level (Eaks and Cassmeyer, 1995).

Cells that require insulin as a carrier for glucose, such as skeletal and cardiac muscle, and adipose tissue are affected most, whereas nerve tissue, erythrocytes, and the cells of the intestines, liver, and kidney tubules, which do not require insulin for glucose transport, are affected the least. In an attempt to restore balance and normal levels of glucose, the kidney excretes the excess glucose resulting in glucosuria (sugar in the urine). Glucose excreted in the urine acts as an osmotic diuretic and causes excretion of increased amounts of water. This process results in fluid volume deficit (FVD) (see Chapter 4). The conscious person becomes extremely thirsty and drinks large amounts of water (polydipsia).

Increased fat mobilization occurs because the body can rely on fat stores for energy when glucose is not available. The process of fat metabolism leads to the formation of breakdown products called ketones, which accumulate in the blood and are excreted through the kidneys and lungs. Ketones can be measured in the blood and the urine to indicate the presence of diabetes. Ketones interfere with acid-base balance by producing hydrogen ions. The pH can fall, and the affected person can develop metabolic acidosis (see Chapter 4). When ketones are excreted, osmotic pressure is increased with an increase in fluid loss. Sodium is also eliminated, which results in sodium depletion and further acidosis. When the renal threshold for ketones is exceeded, the ketones appear in the urine as acetone (ketonuria). When fats are used for a primary source of energy, the body lipid level can rise to five times the normal amount. This elevated level can lead to atherosclerosis and its subsequent cardiovascular complications (see Chapter 10).

Impaired protein utilization occurs because the transport of amino acids (the chief constituent of proteins) into cells requires insulin. Normally, proteins are constantly being broken down and rebuilt. Without insulin to transport amino

BOX **9–3**
Risk Factors for Diabetes Mellitus

Ethnic or racial origins: black, Native American, Hispanic
Positive family history (sibling or parent)
Obesity
Increasing age (>40 yr)
Physical inactivity
Pregnancy
Previous history of gestational diabetes
Delivery of a baby weighing >9 lb at birth
Medications
- Steroid therapy
- Oral contraceptives
- Antihypertensive diuretics (e.g., furosemide, thiazides, ethacrynic acid)

Prolonged physiologic or emotional stress
Chronic or recurring pancreatitis
Other diseases or disorders (see text)

acids, thereby contributing to protein synthesis, the balance is altered and there is increased protein catabolism. Catabolism of body proteins and resultant protein loss hamper the inflammatory process and diminish the tissue's ability to repair itself.

Clinical Manifestations

Cardinal Signs and Symptoms. The excretion of glucose and ketones leads to increased urine output and thirst. Extra food is eaten but cannot be metabolized, which leads to hunger and weight loss. These processes result in four cardinal signs of diabetes (Table 9–14). The person with IDDM usually presents with these cardinal signs and symptoms, sometimes with complications such as ketoacidosis (see next section).

People with NIDDM may also develop these cardinal signs and symptoms, but the aging population may not recognize the abnormal thirst or frequent urination as abnormal for their age. More commonly, they may experience visual blurring, neuropathic complications (e.g., foot pain), or infections. NIDDM is commonly diagnosed while the client is hospitalized or receiving medical care for another problem. Frequently the person presents with one of the long-term side effects of DM, such as neuropathy, retinopathy, or nephropathy.

Long-term effects of diabetes may include microvascular problems resulting in retinopathy (retinal disease), nephropathy (kidney disease), and peripheral (motor and sensory) and autonomic neuropathy. Neuropathy in diabetes is thought to be related to the accumulation in the nerve cells of sorbitol, a byproduct of improper glucose metabolism. This accumulation then results in abnormal fluid and electrolyte shifts and nerve-cell dysfunction (Strowig and Raskin, 1992). The combination of this metabolic derangement and the diminished vascular perfusion to nerve tissues contributes to the severe problem of diabetic neuropathy (Leon, 1993). (See detailed discussion of diabetic neuropathy, Chapter 34.)

TABLE 9–14 CARDINAL SIGNS OF DIABETES

CLINICAL MANIFESTATIONS	PATHOPHYSIOLOGIC BASES
Polyuria (excessive urination)	Water not reabsorbed from renal tubules because of osmotic activity of glucose in the tubules
Polydipsia (excessive thirst)	Polyuria causes severe dehydration, which causes thirst
Polyphagia (excessive hunger)	Tissue breakdown and wasting cause a state of starvation that compels the person to eat excessive amounts of food
Weight loss (IDDM)	Glucose is not available to the cells; body breaks down fat and protein stores for energy
Fatigue	Energy deficiency and protein catabolism

Adapted from Black JM, Matassarin-Jacobs E (eds): Luckmann and Sorensen's Medical-Surgical Nursing, ed 4. Philadelphia, WB Saunders, 1993, p 1778.

Atherosclerosis. It is well known that because of the increased fat metabolism associated with IDDM, atherosclerosis begins earlier and is more extensive among people with diabetes than in the general population. Atherosclerosis and the accompanying large-vessel changes result in skin and nail changes, poor tissue perfusion, decreased or absent pedal pulses, and impaired wound healing. Atherosclerosis combined with peripheral neuropathy and the subsequent foot deformities increases the risk for ulceration of skin and underlying tissues (Woolridge, 1996).

Infection. Because hyperglycemia impairs resistance to infection, diabetes may result in skin and urinary tract infections and vaginitis. Glucose content of the epidermis and urine encourages bacterial growth (Norris, 1995).[10]

Neuromusculoskeletal Problems. Neuromusculoskeletal complications are common, often involving the hands, shoulders, spine, and feet. Sensory, motor, and autonomic neuropathy is a common phenomenon. The loss of sensation in diabetic neuropathy predisposes joints to repeated trauma and progressive joint destruction. This progression results in the development of neuropathic joints and forefoot osteolysis (Kaye, 1994).

Sensory, Motor, and Autonomic Neuropathy. Neuropathy may affect the central nervous system, peripheral nervous system, or autonomic nervous system (see also Chapter 34). The most common form of diabetic neuropathy is a *sensory polyneuropathy*, usually affecting the hands and feet and causing symptoms that range from mild tingling, burning, or numbness to a complete loss of sensation (usually feet).

Chronic progressive degeneration of the stress-bearing portion of a joint associated with loss of proprioceptive sensation in the joint produces a condition called Charcot's disease, Charcot's arthropathy, or neuropathic arthropathy. Diabetes is the most common cause of neuropathic joints (Bland, 1994). The tarsal and tarsometatarsal joints are most commonly involved, but neuropathy of ankles or knees can also occur. In the nondiabetic population, the arm and knee are most often affected. A neuropathic joint is swollen, warm, and edematous, but pain is minimal because of the underlying altered sensation.

Motor neuropathy produces weakness (bilateral but asymmetrical proximal muscle weakness, called diabetic amyotrophy) and deformity (e.g., claw toes, severe flatfoot with valgus of the midfoot, collapse of the longitudinal arch) that contribute to biomechanical changes in foot function resulting in abnormal patterns of loading (Brodsky and Negrine, 1995). Pain and erythema of the forefoot may constitute forefoot osteolysis, sometimes considered another form of neuroarthropathy distinguished from cellulitis or osteomyelitis by laboratory values (leukocyte count) and roentgenographic appearance.

Autonomic neuropathy may manifest itself in several ways, including loss of normal regulation of sweating (skin becomes

[10] It is important that the health-care team assess the presence of macrovascular or peripheral vascular disease (which can be present in diabetes) and diabetic foot disease, which is caused by neuropathy, a microvascular problem. Improving circulation may be a goal with macrovascular or peripheral vascular disease (see Chapter 10), whereas foot care and orthoses are more appropriate treatments for microvascular-caused neuropathy (see Chapter 34).

dry and cracked with a buildup of callus), temperature control, and blood flow in the limbs. Skin changes such as these can create more openings for bacteria to enter. The combination of all three types of neuropathy can ultimately lead to gangrene and possible amputation, largely preventable with proper care (see Special Implications for the Therapist: Diabetes and Foot Care, this section).

Upper Extremity. In the hand, the *syndrome of limited joint mobility* (SLJM or LJM) and the stiff hand syndrome are unique to diabetes. SLJM is characterized by painless stiffness and limitation of the finger joints (Fig. 9–8). Flexion contractures typically progress to result in loss of dexterity and grip strength. The SLJM is an underdiagnosed complication of diabetes, largely because this type of loss of hand range of motion is considered a common normal sign of aging (Swedler et al., 1995). The severity of this syndrome in diabetes is correlated with the duration of disease, duration and quantity of insulin therapy, and smoking. Joint contractures may also develop in larger joints, such as the elbows, shoulders, knees, and spine (Schulte et al., 1993).

The *stiff hand syndrome* is often confused with or included in SLJM, but it has a distinct pathogenesis and clinical presentation. The stiff hand syndrome occurs uniquely with diabetes and is seen more frequently with IDDM (type I) disease and poor blood glucose control. Paresthesias, which eventually become painful, are accompanied by subcutaneous tissue changes such as stiffness and hardness. Vascular insufficiency may be the underlying cause or may be secondary to neuropathy, nodular tenosynovitis, and osteoarthritis.

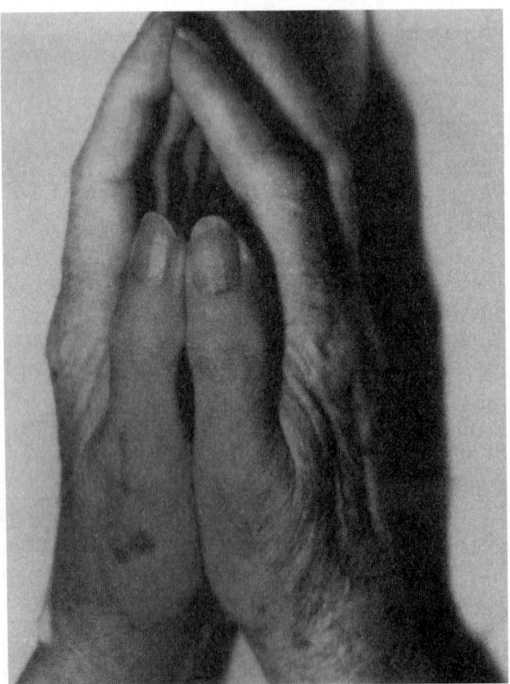

Figure 9–8. The prayer sign. The individual is unable to press the palms flat against each other, a diagnostic sign for the syndrome of limited joint mobility in diabetic persons. Other conditions can also result in loss of extension with a positive prayer sign. (*From Kaye T: Watching for and managing musculoskeletal problems in diabetes. J Musculoskel Med 11:25–37, 1994.*)

Dupuytren's contracture is characterized by the formation of a flexion contracture and thickening band of palmar fascia (Fig. 9–9) usually involving the third and fourth digits in the diabetic population (rather than the fourth and fifth digits in the nondiabetic population) (Holt, 1981). Pain and decreased range of motion are the primary presentation. Painless nodules develop in the distal palmar crease, often in line with the ring finger, that slowly mature into a longitudinal cord that is readily distinguishable from a tendon. The skin overlying the nodules is usually puckered.

Flexor tenosynovitis (also called chronic stenosing tenosynovitis) is another rheumatologic condition seen more commonly in diabetic persons. Tenosynovitis is caused by accumulation of fibrous tissue in the tendon sheath and can cause aching, nodularity along the flexor tendons, and contracture. Locking of the digit, called trigger finger, can occur in flexion or extension and may be associated with crepitus or pain. In the diabetic population, tenosynovitis is found predominantly in women and affects the thumb, middle, and ring fingers most often.

Diabetes is the systemic disease most often seen in connection with *peripheral neuropathy of the hand,* including CTS. The clinical presentation of CTS is the same for the person with diabetes as for the person without diabetes, although in diabetes CTS is more likely to be a neuropathic process than an entrapment problem. Both neuropathy and compression within the carpal tunnel may exist together.

Adhesive capsulitis (also known as periarthritis or frozen shoulder) is characterized by diffuse shoulder pain and loss of motion in all directions, often with a positive painful arc test and limited joint accessory motions. The pattern is slightly different from that of typical adhesive capsulitis, in which regional tightness in the anteroinferior joint capsule primarily compromises external rotation, followed by loss of abduction and, less often, internal rotation and flexion. The pattern in diabetes is one of significant global tightness with external and internal rotation equally limited in the dominant shoulder, followed by limitations in abduction and hyperextension. External rotation and hyperextension are most limited in the nondominant shoulder, followed by internal rotation and abduction (Schulte et al., 1993). The pathogenesis of the capsular thickening and adherence to the humeral head remains unknown. The long head of the biceps tendon may become "glued down" in its tendon sheath on the anterior humeral head (Swedler et al., 1995).

Adhesive capsulitis may be accompanied by vasomotor instability of the hand known as *reflex sympathetic dystrophy* (RSD; formerly called shoulder-hand syndrome). This condition is characterized by severe pain, swelling, and trophic skin changes of the hand[11] (e.g., thinning and shininess of the skin with loss of wrinkling, sometimes with increased hair growth). Skin and subcutaneous tissue atrophy and tendon flexion contractures develop. The natural history of this condition ranges from spontaneous remission to permanent loss of function. (See further discussion: Reflex Sympathetic Dystrophy, Chapter 34.)

[11] Skin changes in diabetic hand arthropathy, as well as skin changes because of RSD, may occur in association with adhesive capsulitis. Other skin changes associated with diabetes include *scleroderma diabeticorum*, an asymptomatic thickening of the skin that may lead to a peau d'orange appearance, usually involving the posterior neck, upper back, and shoulders (Swedler et al., 1995).

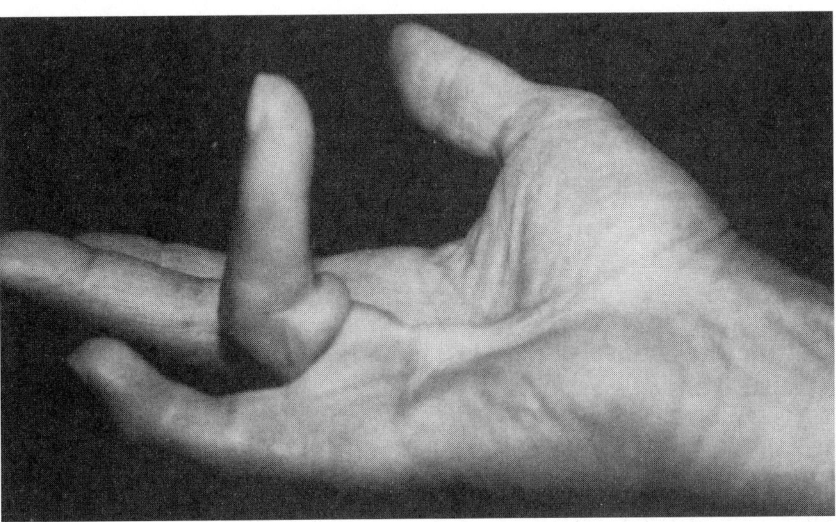

Figure **9–9.** Dupuytren's contracture. Painless nodules develop in the distal palmar crease, often in line with the ring finger, that slowly mature into a longitudinal cord that is readily distinguishable from a tendon. The skin overlying the nodules is usually puckered. The contracture may be symptomatic (painful), but with or without pain it results in impaired hand function. (*From Kaye T: Watching for and managing musculoskeletal problems in diabetes. J Musculoskel Med 11:25–37, 1994.*)

Spine. Diffuse idiopathic skeletal hyperostosis (DISH; also known as ankylosing hyperostosis) is a condition of the spine seen most often in people with NIDDM (type II) diabetes, although it can occur in a person who does not have diabetes. In DISH, osteophytes develop into bony spurs, typically right-sided syndesmophytes, that may join to form bridges (Fig. 9–10). The thoracic spine is most commonly involved. In contrast to ankylosing spondylitis, the sacroiliac joints are spared, and vertebral body osteoporosis is absent. Calcaneal and olecranon spurs may develop, and new bone may form around hips, knees, and wrists.

People with DISH may be asymptomatic or they may experience back pain and stiffness without limitations in range of motion. Dysphagia may develop if there is extensive cervical spine involvement. The pathogenesis of DISH is unknown and there does not appear to be any correlation between the degree of diabetic control and the extent of hyperostosis.

Osteoporosis. Generalized osteoporosis usually develops within the first 5 years after the onset of diabetes mellitus and is more severe in persons with IDDM. It is hypothesized that bone matrix formation may be inadequate in the absence of normal circulating insulin levels. Results of bone density studies in persons with NIDDM are conflicting, with some studies demonstrating decreased bone density and others indicating increased bone density. This may be understood from the point of view that people with NIDDM have decreased circulating insulin levels because of β-cell exhaustion, and others are hyperinsulinemic because of insulin resistance (Kaye, 1994).

As in any case of osteoporosis, regardless of the underlying cause, this condition places the person at greater risk for fractures. With the additional loss of sensation associated with diabetes, minor trauma easily produces injury. Microfractures can occur in already weakened bone and cartilage and may remain unrecognized because of the lack of pain appreciation. A vicious circle is started, leading to further damage.

Joints with less movement transmit abnormal forces through the foot to injure already damaged joints. This is especially true during gait, when large forces are placed on the midtarsal and tarsometatarsal joints. Obesity further increases

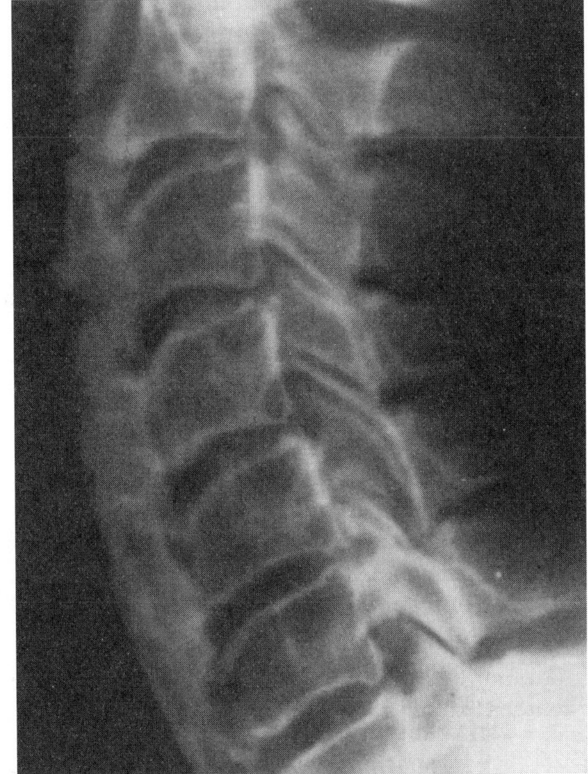

Figure **9–10.** DISH (diffuse idiopathic skeletal hyperostosis; ankylosing hyperostosis) associated with NIDDM. This condition can occur with other conditions such as ankylosing spondylitis. Although the dense anterior bony bridging of the cervical vertebrae is pictured on this lateral roentgenogram, the thoracic spine is most commonly involved in diabetes. This type of DISH can be distinguished from ankylosing spondylitis by the preservation of sacroiliac joints, a site of typical involvement in ankylosing spondylitis. (*From Kaye T: Watching for and managing musculoskeletal problems in diabetes. J Musculoskel Med 11:25–37, 1994.*)

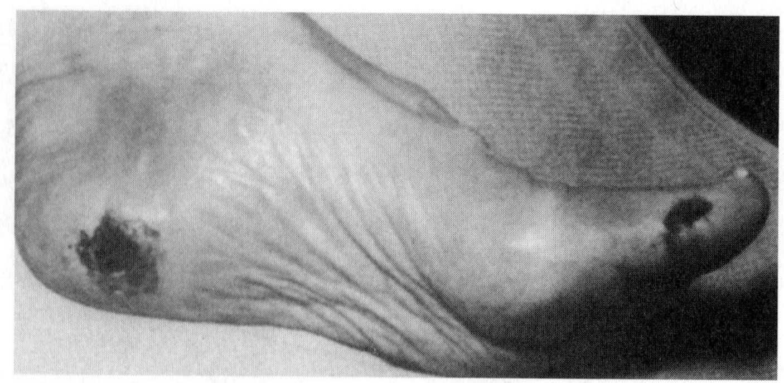

Figure **9–11.** Neurotrophic ulcers associated with diabetic neuropathy. (*From Callen JP, Jorizzo JL (eds): Dermatological Signs of Internal Disease. Philadelphia, WB Saunders, 1995, p 187.*)

these forces and in the presence of any preexisting gait abnormalities or deformities, and both create additional stress that compounds the condition. For example, if the foot is excessively pronated, increased shearing force is placed on the medial forefoot; excessive supination gives rise to intensified lateral pressures; and equinus is characterized by increased forefoot loading and in-toeing (Sammarco, 1994).

Ulceration. Neuropathy occurring as a result of improper glucose metabolism and diminished vascular perfusion to nerve tissues places the diabetic person at risk for the development of ulcers. Diabetic foot ulcers are primarily caused by repetitive stress on the insensitive skin with increased pressure. Changes in pressure and gait, fat atrophy, and muscle weakness are all mechanical factors that, along with sensory neuropathy, influence the development of plantar skin abnormalities, especially ulceration (Sammarco, 1994).

Body weight and activity level increase the force that the foot must transmit, and this may also increase pressure, especially in the presence of an underlying bony prominence or foot imbalance. As a result, shear forces increase and become a factor in skin breakdown. In addition, previously healed ulcers leave scars that transmit force to underlying tissues in a more concentrated manner and hold the fat pad locally so that it cannot function physiologically. As a result, it cannot transmit shear forces, and it becomes damaged easily.

The normal response to damaged areas is to spare them from pressure because they are painful. However, in the insensitive diabetic foot, this normal alteration of weight-bearing surface, pressure, and duration does not take place, resulting in subcutaneous and cutaneous necrosis and skin breakdown.

The skin itself is likely to contribute to ulceration because the collagen and keratin[12] may be glycosylated (saturated with glucose) with increased cross-linking, which makes the skin stiff. Keratin builds up in response to the increased pressure, covering the openings of unhealed ulcers, and cannot be removed as readily as normal keratin. The areas most commonly affected by foot ulcers are the plantar areas of the metatarsal heads, the toes, and the plantar area of the hallux (Fig. 9–11). In the Charcot foot, the incidence of ulceration beneath the talus and navicular bones becomes more common because of the rigid rocker-bottom deformity.

Medical Management

Diagnosis. Diagnostic assessment may include a variety of testing procedures such as blood glucose, blood glucose finger-stick, fasting blood sugar, glucose tolerance test, glycosylated hemoglobin, and urine ketone levels, to name just a few (see Table 35–10). Frequent self-monitoring by performing a direct blood sampling (finger-stick technique) is an important management tool in the long-term treatment of this disease.

Treatment. At the present time, there is no known cure for diabetes. The goal of overall care for persons with diabetes is control or regulation of blood glucose. Researchers in two separate locations[13] are currently investigating a drug that would prevent the formation of fat cells, thereby reducing the problem of obesity before diabetes can develop (P.T. Bulletin, 1996).

In other recent developments, a new orally active hypoglycemic agent (troglitazone) has been shown to be effective in both IDDM and NIDDM subsets. Although the exact mechanism of action of this drug remains unknown, it appears to improve the effectiveness of insulin in various types of cells, thereby lowering blood glucose levels (Khoursheed et al., 1995; Reusch, 1995). Other future potential research results may identify the major genes that allow the development of diabetes, which could then be biologically manipulated so that a person will not become fat even in the presence of overeating.

IDDM requires exogenous insulin administration and dietary management to achieve blood glucose control. Although exercise has not been proven to provide increased glycemic control for the person with IDDM, it should be taken into account as part of the total picture. The insulin dosage schedule varies depending on the individual's age, level of compliance, and severity of diabetes (sometimes referred to as how "brittle" the diabetes is) (Tables 9–15 and 9–16). Poorly controlled diabetes is ideally treated with more frequent administration of insulin (e.g., four times per day) whereas other individuals may receive insulin once or twice daily, sometimes mixing different types of insulin (e.g., short-acting [regular] with intermediate-acting [NPH] insulin). From a therapist's point of view, the client receiving more frequent dosages is less likely to develop hypoglycemia, especially when beginning an exercise program.

[12] A protein that is the principal constituent of epidermis, hair, and nails.

[13] Salk Institute for Biological Studies, La Jolla, Calif; Glaxo, Inc., Triangle Park, NC.

TABLE 9-15 INSULIN DOSAGE SCHEDULE

INSULIN TYPE	INSULIN PREPARATION	ONSET	PEAK (HR)	DURATION (HR)
Short-acting	Insulin injection (regular)	30–60 min	2–4	4–12
	Prompt insulin zinc suspension (semilente)	1–3 hr	2–8	12–16
Intermediate-acting	Isophane insulin suspension and regular insulin	30 min	4–12	24
	NPH, isophane insulin suspension	3–4 hr	6–12	24–48
	Insulin zinc suspension (lente)	1–3 hr	8–12	24–48
Long-acting	Extended insulin zinc suspension (ultralente)	4–6 hr	18–24	36

Courtesy of Michael B. Koopmeiners, M.D., Associate Professor, Institute of Physical Therapy, St. Augustine, Fla, 1996.

An insulin pump is now available to deliver fixed amounts of regular insulin continuously, thereby more closely imitating the release of the hormone by the islet cells. This lightweight device is conveniently worn on a belt or a shoulder holster; a waterproof design makes swimming (especially competitive swimming) possible. Although this type of insulin administration provides better control, it has some disadvantages. It cannot be removed for more than 1 hour, reactions to the needle are common, and like any other mechanical device, it is subject to malfunction (Wong, 1993).

NIDDM is most often treated with diet and exercise, sometimes in conjunction with oral hypoglycemic drugs (OHDs); insulin is occasionally required. Several types of OHDs are available, including those used to stimulate islet cells to increase endogenous insulin secretion and enhance insulin receptor binding (sulfonylureas), those that act by slowing the digestion of sugars in the intestine (acarbose), those referred to as insulin-resistance reducers (troglitazone [Rezulin]), and those[14] used to improve hepatic and peripheral tissue sensitivity to insulin (metformin [Glucophage]), thereby increasing the effectiveness of insulin found in the body (Dunn and Peters, 1995; Epstein, 1995).

Medical treatment of long-term diabetic complications may include dialysis or kidney transplantation for renal failure and vascular surgery for large-vessel disease. The therapist is often involved in prevention and wound care for diabetic ulcers, which sometimes necessitate amputation. Topical application of growth factors on wounds without infection and with at least a minimal level of vascularization has been introduced (Gillam and Da Camara, 1993; Ganio et al., 1993). This idea is based on the normal healing process of a wound that includes certain growth factors, derived from platelets in the blood. Because diabetic persons have poor circulation, growth factor does not reach the wound; this procedure provides exogenous growth factor.

Some people with IDDM are now receiving pancreas transplants, but life-long immunosuppression and its complications make this treatment option less than ideal. Research is being conducted on the use of transplanted pancreatic islet cells rather than the entire pancreas (Ricordi, 1995; Carroll et al., 1994).

TABLE 9-16 THERAPEUTIC REGIMENS FOR INSULIN

INSULIN SCHEDULE	INDICATIONS
Single daily injections	Primarily for elderly clients Long-term complications less likely Usually use intermediate- or long-acting insulin May be combined with short-acting insulin to maximize control
Twice-daily injections	Used in people with reasonably stable activity and diet Combined short- and intermediate-acting insulin
Multiple injections	Used in younger people (more flexible to fit their lifestyle) Frequently use one-time long-acting dose to establish baseline effect
Infusion pump	Used after diabetic crisis, after surgery, during labor Short-acting insulin
Intraperitoneal	Used in people with peritoneal dialysis for renal failure Insulin added to dialysis fluid

Courtesy of Michael B. Koopmeiners, M.D., Associate Professor, Institute of Physical Therapy, St. Augustine, Fla, 1996.

Prognosis. Diabetes control depends on the proper interaction between three factors—(1) food, (2) insulin or oral medication to lower blood glucose, and (3) activity (e.g., sedentary or exertional) or exercise. When diabetes is successfully regulated, complications of hyperglycemia and hypoglycemia can be avoided with minimal disruption to a normal lifestyle. However, diabetes can be fatal even with medical treatment, or it can cause major permanent disabilities and seriously impair functional abilities. In fact, about 50% of myocardial infarctions and 75% of strokes are attributable to diabetes, and it is the leading cause of new blindness as well as a contributory cause to renal failure and peripheral vascular disease.

[14] The advantage of this OHD is that it does not stimulate activity with concomitant weight gain. However, diarrhea develops for 2 to 3 weeks in approximately one third of people using this drug. One potentially serious side effect (rare) is lactic acidosis, a life-threatening buildup of lactic acid in the blood. This condition can be fatal in people with kidney or liver disease or alcoholism. The main clinical feature of lactic acidosis is hyperventilation.

Special Implications for the Therapist **9-15**

DIABETES MELLITUS

Client education is the key to therapeutic, nonsurgical treatment of the neuromusculoskeletal complications associated with diabetes. Extensive self-management is the focus of the educational program.* Exercise is a key component of the overall treatment plan. The client must be taught the importance of assessing glucose levels before and after exercise and to judge what carbohydrate and insulin requirements are suitable for the activity or workout (see Diabetes and Exercise, this section).

People with diabetes and peripheral neuropathy have a high incidence of injuries (e.g., falls, fractures, sprains, cuts, bruises) during walking or standing and a low level of perceived safety (Cavanagh et al., 1992; Mueller et al., 1989). Suggested strategies for appropriate clinical treatment to reduce these complications are available (Mueller et al., 1994).

Complications of Insulin Therapy

Hypoglycemia. Insulin therapy can result in hypoglycemia (low blood glucose, also called an insulin reaction); tissue hypertrophy, atrophy, or both, at the site of injection; insulin allergy; erratic insulin action; and insulin resistance. Symptoms of hypoglycemia are related to two body responses; increased sympathetic activity and deprivation of CNS glucose supply (Table 9–17). The clinical picture may be varied from a report of headache and weakness to irritability and lack of muscular coordination (much like drunkenness) to apprehension, inability to respond to verbal commands, and psychosis.

Symptoms can occur when the blood glucose level drops to 70 mg/dL or less. In diabetes, an overdose of insulin, late or skipped meals, or overexertion in exercise may cause hypoglycemic reactions. Immediately provide carbohydrates in some form (e.g., fruit juice, honey, hard candy, commercially available glucose tablets or gel); a blood glucose test should be performed as soon as the symptoms are recognized. The unconscious person needs immediate medical attention; to prevent aspiration, fluids should not be forced.

It is important to note that clients can exhibit signs and symptoms of hypoglycemia when their elevated blood glucose level drops rapidly to a level that is still elevated (e.g., 400 to 200 mg/dL). The rapidity of the drop is the stimulus for sympathetic activity–based symptoms; even though a blood glucose level appears elevated, affected individuals may still have hypoglycemia (Eaks and Cassmeyer, 1995).

When a person with diabetes mentions the presence of nightmares, unexplained sweating, and/or headache causing sleep disturbances, this may be an indication of hypoglycemia during nighttime sleep (most often related to the use of intermediate and long-acting insulins given more than once a day). These symptoms should be reported to the physician.

Erratic insulin action (i.e., low blood glucose followed by high blood glucose) can occur as a result of a variety of factors such as overeating, irregular meals, irregular exercise, irregular rest periods, chronic overdosage of insulin (Somogyi effect),† emotional or psychological stress, failure to administer insulin, or intermittent use of hyperglycemic or hypoglycemic drugs (e.g., aspirin, phenylbutazone, steroids, birth control pills, alcohol). The therapist may be a helpful source of education to help clients remember the many factors affecting their condition.

Lipogenic Effect of Insulin. Frequent injections of insulin at the same site can cause thickening of the subcutaneous tissues (hypertrophy or lipohypertrophy) and a loss of subcutaneous fat (atrophy or lipoatrophy) resulting in a dimpling of the skin that is lumpy and hard or spongy and soft. These abnormal tissue changes may cause decreased absorption of the injected insulin and poor glucose control.

The client is usually instructed to choose an injection site that is easily accessible (e.g., thighs, upper arms, abdomen, lower back) and relatively insensitive to pain (away from the midline of the body). Sites of injection should be rotated, and rotation within each area is recommended. An individual can rotate within an area using 1 in. of the surrounding tissue at a time. The client who is going to exercise should avoid injecting sites or muscles that will be exercised heavily that day, because exercise increases the rate of absorption. Following a definite injection plan can help avoid tissue damage.

Diabetic Ketoacidosis. The therapist must always be alert for signs of ketoacidosis (e.g., acetone breath, dehydration, weak and rapid pulse, Kussmaul's respirations) progressing to hyperosmolar coma (polyuria, thirst, neurologic abnormalities, stupor). Immediate medical care is essential. If it is not clear whether the symptoms are the result of hypoglycemia or hyperglycemia (Table 9–18), the health-care worker is advised to administer fruit juice or honey. This procedure will not harm the hyperglycemic person but could potentially save the hypoglycemic person. (See discussion in next section.)

Diabetes and Exercise

An overwhelming body of evidence now exists that acute muscle contractile activity and chronic exercise

TABLE 9-17 Clinical Signs and Symptoms of Hypoglycemia

Sympathetic Activity	CNS Activity
Pallor	Headache
Perspiration*	Blurred vision
Piloerection (erection of the hair)	Slurred speech
Increased heart rate (tachycardia)	Numbness of the lips and tongue
Heart palpitation	Confusion
Nervousness* and irritability	Euphoria
Weakness*	Convulsion*
Shakiness/trembling	Coma
Hunger	

* Signs most often reported by clients.

From Phipps W, Cassmeyer VL, Sands JK, et al (eds): Medical-Surgical Nursing: Concepts and Clinical Practice, ed 5. St Louis, Mosby–Year Book, 1995, p 1330.

TABLE 9-18 COMPARISON OF MANIFESTATIONS OF HYPOGLYCEMIA AND HYPERGLYCEMIA

VARIABLE	HYPOGLYCEMIA	HYPERGLYCEMIA
Onset	Rapid (minutes)	Gradual (days)
Mood	Labile, irritable, nervous, weepy	Lethargic
Mental status	Difficulty concentrating, speaking, focusing, coordinating	Dulled sensorium, confused
Inward feeling	Shaky, hungry, headache, dizziness	Thirst, weakness, nausea/vomiting, abdominal pain
Skin	Pallor, sweating	Flushed, signs of dehydration (see Box 4–9)
Mucous membranes	Normal	Dry, crusty
Respirations	Shallow	Deep, rapid (Kussmaul's respirations)
Pulse	Tachycardia	Less rapid, weak
Breath odor	Normal	Fruity, acetone
Neurologic	Tremors; late: dilated pupils, convulsion	Diminished reflexes, paresthesias
Blood values		
Glucose	Low: <60 mg/dL	High: ≥250 mg/dL
Ketones	Negative	High/large
pH	Normal	Low: ≤7.25
Hematocrit	Normal	High
Urine values		
Output	Normal	Polyuria (early) to oliguria (late)
Glucose	Negative	High
Ketones	Negative/trace	High

From Wong DL: Whaley and Wong's Essentials of Pediatric Nursing, ed 4. St Louis, Mosby–Year Book, 1993, p 1004.

improve skeletal muscle glucose transport and whole-body glucose homeostasis in the person with NIDDM (Table 9–19). Therapists must recognize, understand, and utilize the role of skeletal muscle in glucose homeostasis because of the high prevalence of people with underlying skeletal muscle insulin resistance or impaired skeletal muscle glucose disposal such as occurs with inactivity, bedrest, limb immobilization, or denervation (Sinacore and Gulve, 1993[‡]).

A program of planned exercise including all the elements of fitness (flexibility, muscle strength, cardiovascular endurance) can greatly benefit persons with diabetes, especially those with NIDDM. Exercise increases carbohydrate metabolism (which lowers the blood glucose level); aids in maintaining optimal body weight; increases high-density lipoproteins (HDLs); and decreases triglycerides, blood pressure, and stress and tension (Table 9–20).

Many people with diabetes may not be able to exercise intensely to a calculated heart rate because of preexisting heart conditions, deconditioning, age, neuropathies, arthritis, or other joint problems. Some people with autonomic neuropathy may have "silent myocardial infarctions" without angina. The first symptom may be shortness of breath due to congestive heart failure. Decrease in nerve innervation to the heart associated with this type of neuropathy may prevent a normal increase in heart rate with stress or exercise, requiring careful observation and monitoring of vital signs during exercise.

Exercise in IDDM (Type I). The person with IDDM tends to be thin, may be poorly nourished, and, because of the islet cell deficiency, always needs exogenous insulin for adequate control of blood glucose. Exercise can increase strength and facilitate maintenance of weight as well as provide other important benefits (see Table 9–20), but, unfortunately, exercise has not been proven to provide increased glycemic control for the person with IDDM. Hyperglycemia after exertion can be profound and prolonged for days owing to insulin deficiency. Further exercise can lead to impaired glucose uptake, and without exogenous insulin, diabetic ketoacidosis can occur. For the person with IDDM, exercise is viewed as adjunctive therapy and is secondary in importance to proper insulin management and consistency in dietary regulation (Hough, 1994).

The person with well-controlled IDDM may commonly work out for approximately 30 to 45 minutes of sustained intense aerobic exercise without problems. Lack of adequate glycogen stores (i.e., decreased glycogen stores in the liver and, to a lesser extent, in skeletal muscle) leads to impaired aerobic exercise endurance when compared with the nondiabetic person.

Hypoglycemia is a common occurrence in persons with IDDM who are exercising. In those who do not have diabetes, plasma insulin levels decrease during exercise and insulin counterregulatory hormones (glucagon and epinephrine) promote increased hepatic glucose production, which matches the amount of glucose used during exercise. For the person with IDDM, plasma insulin concentrations may not fall during exercise and may even increase if exercise occurs within 1 hour of insulin injection. These sustained insulin levels during exercise enhance peripheral glucose uptake and stimulate glucose oxidation by exercising muscle. For this reason, insulin should not be injected into muscles or at sites close to areas involved in exercise within 1 hour of exercise.

Moderate periods of exercise provide beneficial

TABLE 9-19 Diabetes Mellitus: Key Points to Remember

General Guidelines

Although "safe" blood glucose levels are between 100 and 250 mg/dL (i.e., the person is not likely to experience diabetic ketoacidosis), the goal of therapy may be toward tighter control (e.g., in a young person with IDDM, 80 to 120 mg/dL) or moderate control (e.g., in an adult with NIDDM, up to 150 mg/dL). A measurement over 120 mg/dL should still be monitored closely in any age group

If the blood glucose level is ≤70 mg/dL, a carbohydrate snack should be given and the glucose retested in 15 minutes to ensure an appropriate level. Food eaten in response to blood glucose levels between 70 and 100 mg/dL is symptom-dependent (i.e., if a person's blood glucose is 80 mg/dL but there are no signs or symptoms of hypoglycemia, no snack is necessary)

Observe carefully for signs or symptoms of diabetic ketoacidosis: acetone breath, dehydration, weak and rapid pulse, Kussmaul's respirations

Administer fruit juice or honey to anyone with diabetes who is in a hypoglycemic state. If uncertain whether the person is hypoglycemic or hyperglycemic, provide juice or honey anyway

Exercise must be carefully planned in conjunction with food intake and administration of insulin or oral hyperglycemic agents

Do *not* exercise during peak insulin times. The peak activity of insulin occurs at different times depending on the type, dose, and time of the insulin injection (see explanation in text)

When under stress, the person with diabetes will have increased insulin requirements and may become symptomatic even though the disease is usually well-controlled in normal circumstances

Avoid exercising late at night if this has not been gradually and consistently incorporated into the overall lifestyle. Delayed hypoglycemic reactions can occur during sleep hours following heavy, unaccustomed exercise late in the evening

Before Exercise

Glucose levels must be monitored immediately before exercise

Do *not* exercise when blood glucose levels are at or near 250 mg/dL (equivalent to 250 mg/100mL)

Do *not* exercise without eating at least 2 hr before exercise (exercise about 1 hr *after* a meal is best, but individual variations must be determined)

Do *not* inject short-acting insulin in muscles or sites close to areas involved in exercise within 1 hr of exercise because insulin is absorbed much more quickly in an active extremity

Clients with IDDM may have to reduce the insulin dose or increase food intake when initiating an exercise program

Ketosis can be checked by means of a urine test before exercise (e.g., if the blood glucose is close to 250 mg/dL). If the test is positive (i.e., showing large numbers of ketones in the urine), exercise should be delayed until the urine test shows negative or low numbers of ketones. The person should administer added insulin. Delay exercise until glucose and ketones are under control

Do not use drugs that may contribute to exercise-induced hypoglycemia (e.g., β-blockers, alcoholic beverages, diuretics, estrogens, phenytoin)

Menstruating women need to increase their insulin during menses, especially those who are inactive or who do not exercise on a regular basis

During Exercise

It is best to exercise regularly (5 times/wk or at least every other day) and consistently at the same time each day

Duration of exercise is optimal at 40 to 60 min, although as little as 20 to 30 min of continuous aerobic exercise is beneficial in improving glucose homeostasis (Bogardus et al., 1984)

During prolonged activities, a readily absorbable carbohydrate snack (e.g., fruit) is recommended for each 30 minutes of activity

Following exercise, a more slowly absorbed carbohydrate snack (e.g., bread, pasta, crackers) helps prevent delayed-onset hypoglycemia

Activities should be stopped with the development of any symptoms of hypoglycemia, and blood glucose tested

Replace fluid losses adequately

Monitor blood glucose every 30 min during prolonged exercise

Anyone with diabetes should not exercise alone. Health-care workers, partners, teammates, and coaches must understand the possibility of hypoglycemia and how to manage it

After Exercise

Glucose levels must be monitored 15 min after exercise, especially if exercise is not consistent

Increase caloric intake for 12 to 24 hr after activity, according to intensity and duration of exercise

Reduce insulin, which peaks in the evening or night, according to intensity and duration of exercise

---

effects, but longer periods may result in hypoglycemia. The greatest risk of severe hypoglycemia occurs 6 to 14 hours after strenuous exercise. Muscle and hepatic glycogen must be restored during periods of rest. Insulin and caloric intake must be adjusted after strenuous exercise to avoid severe nocturnal hypoglycemia.

Exercise in NIDDM (Type II). In contrast, people with NIDDM are often obese and exercise is a major contributor in controlling hyperglycemia. Exercise can improve short-term insulin sensitivity and reduce insulin resistance, making it possible to prevent NIDDM in those persons at risk and to improve glycemic control in

TABLE 9-20 BENEFITS AND POTENTIAL RISKS OF EXERCISE IN DIABETES MELLITUS

BENEFITS	POTENTIAL RISKS*
Improves cardiovascular function Improves maximum oxygen uptake Improves insulin binding and sensitivity Lowers insulin requirements (NIDDM) Improves sense of well-being and quality of life Promotes other healthy lifestyle activities Increases carbohydrate metabolism Improves blood glucose control† Reduces hypertension May help with weight reduction Improves lipid profile Reduces stress	Hypoglycemia in people taking oral hypoglycemics or insulin Worsening of hyperglycemia Cardiovascular disease, such as myocardial infarction, arrhythmias, excessive increases in blood pressure during exercise, postexercise orthostatic hypotension, or sudden death Microvascular disease, such as retinal hemorrhage or increased proteinuria Degenerative joint disease Orthopedic injury related to neuropathy

* These are potential risks over the long term. In general, the benefits of regular exercise outweigh the risks (Hough, 1994).
† Not confirmed for insulin-dependent diabetes mellitus (IDDM).
Data from Christakos CN, Fields KB: Exercise in diabetes: Minimize the risks and gain the benefits. J Musculoskel Med 12:16–25, 1995 [benefits]; and Hough DO: Diabetes mellitus in sports. Sports Med 78:423–431, 1994 [risks].

those with diabetes. These effects disappear a few days after exercise is discontinued (Hough, 1994).

Hypoglycemia is not a common problem for the person with NIDDM because endogenous insulin levels can usually be maintained. Control of blood glucose levels by lowering the medication dose or increasing carbohydrate intake (or both) before exercise can prevent hypoglycemia.

General Exercise Considerations. For anyone with diabetes, IDDM or NIDDM, the exercise prescription must take into account any of the complications present, especially cardiovascular changes, autonomic and sensory neuropathy, and retinopathy. Generally, individuals with autonomic neuropathy have a poor ability to perform aerobic exercise owing to decreased maximal heart rate and increased resting heart rate. Persons with a generalized form of autonomic neuropathy may have hypotensive episodes after exercising, especially those who are deconditioned. They also demonstrate a predisposition toward dehydration in the heat and poor exercise tolerance in cold environments. Silent myocardial infarction during exercise and postexercise hypotension are likely problems. Exercise is contraindicated in anyone with a severe form of autonomic neuropathy unless it is specifically approved by a physician (Box 9–4). This includes anyone with vasomotor instability, angina, and a history of myocardial infarction (Hough, 1994).

Muscle damage, with accompanying insulin resistance and impaired glucose uptake and disposal, can occur when untrained individuals begin to exercise (Sinacore and Gulve, 1993). For this reason, clients with diabetes must start any new activity at a well-tolerated intensity level and duration, gradually increasing over a period of weeks or even months. Unplanned exercise can be dangerous for people taking insulin or oral hypoglycemic agents. During periods of exercise, muscles are stimulated to take up glucose to supply the fuel to the working muscles, causing blood glucose levels to fall abruptly. However, anyone with blood glucose levels at or near 300 mg/dL should *NOT* exercise, because vigorous activity can also raise the blood glucose level by releasing stored glycogen. Exercise or therapy sessions should be scheduled so as to avoid peak insulin times (see Table 9–15) and to avoid periods of fasting (e.g., missed meal, just before the next meal).

Exercise in the morning is recommended to avoid hypoglycemia due to fluctuations in insulin sensitivity caused by factors such as diurnal variations in growth hormone. Growth hormone levels remain low in the afternoon, and less gluconeogenesis occurs. Too-vigorous exercise late in the day or evening could lead to delayed hypoglycemia during sleep, which is a dangerous time for this (Christakos and Fields, 1995; Vitug et al., 1988).

Some thought should be given to the specific type of exercise selected. For the able-bodied and/or the

BOX **9–4**
Contraindications to Exercise in Diabetes Mellitus

Poor control of blood glucose levels
Unevaluated or poorly controlled associated conditions:
- Retinopathy
- Hypertension
- Neuropathy (autonomic or peripheral)
- Nephropathy

Recent photocoagulation or surgery for retinopathy
Dehydration
Extreme environmental temperatures (hot or cold)

Adapted from Campaigne BN: Exercise in the management of diabetes mellitus. *In* Goldberg L, Elliot DL: Exercise for Prevention and Treatment of Illness. Philadelphia, FA Davis, 1994, p 181.

person with good control and without significant diabetic complications, more choices may be possible. Even for the person with IDDM in good control, sports in which hypoglycemia may be life-threatening (e.g., scuba diving, rock climbing, parachuting) should be discouraged.

Walking should be accomplished with care toward proper footwear for the person who does not already have evidence of peripheral neuropathy. Swimming may be a good choice, once again taking care to provide meticulous foot care (see also Diabetes and Physical Agents, this section). Wearing boat shoes (specially designed shoes for water wear available in many local stores) can help prevent scraping the feet along the sides or bottom of the pool. Care must be taken to gently dry the feet, especially between the toes, after swimming; to prevent infection, anyone with abrasions or open sores should not enter a swimming pool environment.

Intermittent, high-intensity activities (e.g., racquetball, baseball)§ or contact sports (e.g., basketball or soccer) should be avoided to prevent trauma (especially to the feet or eyes). Strength training programs should be encouraged unless retinopathy is present (weightlifting is contraindicated in anyone with retinopathy; see Box 9–4). Outdoor activities must be evaluated carefully, taking into consideration the weather extremes (hot or cold) and the person's ability to maintain distal circulation. Stationary indoor equipment (many types are now available) may be the best overall choice.

Balancing Insulin, Food, and Exercise. As mentioned, insulin should be injected in sites away from the part of the body involved in exercising. Because glucose can enter the cells without insulin during exercise, food should be eaten if the person is exercising more than usual. Conversely, when exercising less often, a lighter diet or more insulin is required.

Glucose levels should be monitored before and after exercise (or therapy activities), remembering that the effect of exercise can be felt up to 12 to 24 hours later. After exercise, available glucose is important for the replenishment of muscle glycogen stores. Bouts of hypoglycemia can be delayed until hours after completion of exercise (Wallberg-Hendriksson, 1992). The insulin-dependent person must regulate activity so that the rate of energy expenditure balances the amount and type of insulin and food intake (Table 9–21). Women who are menstruating will need to increase their insulin during menses.

Glucose monitoring is not as crucial for a person who has an established pattern of activities and/or exercise. When a new activity is introduced, such as occurs in an exercise or rehabilitation program, monitoring blood glucose levels is recommended until the individual's response to the change is known and predictable in maintaining stable blood glucose levels.

Diabetes and Musculoskeletal Complications

The treatment of musculoskeletal problems outlined in Clinical Manifestations (previous discussion, this section) does not differ from treatment for these same conditions in the nondiabetic population. Hand function can be maintained and disease progression delayed with hand therapy, especially for the stiff hand syndrome. SLJM does not always benefit from therapy, but treatment should be tried (Kaye, 1994).

Treatment for CTS must take into account the neuropathic as well as the entrapment components in the person with diabetes; surgical decompression may not be beneficial because of the neuropathic component. Nonsurgical efforts should be the focus of treatment. In conditions such as adhesive capsulitis and RSD, a successful outcome is more likely with early medical and therapeutic intervention.

Early aggressive therapy for the adhesive capsulitis usually results in restoration of functional motion, even though full range of motion may not be achieved. For either of these conditions, the client must understand the importance of a self-directed exercise program established by the therapist to prevent recurrence of symptoms and to maintain functional outcomes.

Diabetes and Foot Care *(Brodsky and Negrine, 1995)*

Disorders of the feet constitute a source of increasing morbidity in diabetics. Foot problems are a leading cause of hospital admission in people with diabetes, and diabetes is the most common reason for lower limb amputation. Half of those cases are preventable with proper foot care (Betts, 1993). Treatment of the underlying diabetes has little effect on any joint disease already present. The most beneficial treatment includes stabilizing the joint, minimizing trauma, maintaining muscular strength, and daily foot care (Kaye, 1994).

Assess for signs of diabetic neuropathy (e.g., numbness or pain in hands or feet, footdrop¶) and teach each person with diabetes proper foot and skin care (see Table 10–22). Note the location of any foot ulcerations for possible causes that can be corrected. For example, ulcers on the medial or lateral borders of the feet may be caused by ill-fitting shoes, whereas ulcers on top of the foot may be caused by deformities such as hammer (claw) toes. Ulcers appearing on the bottom of the foot may be caused by the pressure exerted during standing and other weight-bearing activities. The presence of corns or calluses is an indication that footwear fits poorly and should be carefully evaluated by the therapist. Additionally, cartilage requires insulin for glucose uptake, metabolism of carbon dioxide, and collagen synthesis. Lacking an adequate supply, the articular cartilage in the person with diabetes does not tolerate repetitive trauma, compression, and motion, making proper footwear all the more important (Sammarco, 1994).

Although the management of the diabetic foot (Charcot joint) sometimes requires surgery, most people can be treated nonsurgically with appropriate cast, shoe, and orthotic techniques. When a neuropathic joint is detected early, complete avoidance of weight-bearing for 8 weeks may prevent progression of disease (Kaye, 1994). Because wound healing (surgical and nonsurgical) is impaired in the diabetic foot, surgery can be accompanied by increased risks of poor healing and infection. Sympathectomy, arthrodesis, and joint immobilization have not been proved helpful (Kroop

TABLE 9-21 Making Food Adjustments for Exercise: General Guidelines

Type of Exercise and Examples	If Blood Glucose Is:*	Increase Food Intake by:	Suggestions of Food to Use
Exercise of short duration and low to moderate intensity (walking a half mile or leisurely bicycling for <30 min)	<100 mg/dL	10–15 g of carbohydrate per hour of exercise	1 fruit or 1 starch/bread exchange
	≥100 mg/dL	Not necessary to increase food	
Exercise of moderate intensity (1 hr of tennis, swimming, jogging, leisurely bicycling, golfing)	<100 mg/dL	25–50 g of carbohydrate before exercise, then 10–15 g per hour of exercise	½ meat sandwich with a milk or fruit exchange
	100–180 mg/dL	10–15 g of carbohydrate	1 fruit or 1 starch/bread exchange
	180–300 mg/dL	Not necessary to increase food	
	≥300 mg/dL	Do not begin exercise until blood glucose is under better control	
Strenuous activity or exercise (about 1 to 2 hr of football, hockey, racquetball, or basketball games; strenuous bicycling or swimming; shoveling heavy snow)	<100 mg/dL	50 g carbohydrate; monitor blood glucose carefully	1 meat sandwich (2 slices of bread) with a milk and fruit exchange
	100–180 mg/dL	25–50 g carbohydrate, depending on intensity and duration	½ meat sandwich with a milk or fruit exchange
	180–300 mg/dL	10–15 g carbohydrate	1 fruit or starch/bread exchange
	≥300 mg/dL	Do not begin exercise until blood glucose is under better control	

* 100 mg/dL = 100 mg/100 mL. The 100 mg/dL is a general guideline. There are wide individual variations in this area. The timing of food intake may be symptom-dependent. Some individuals may experience symptoms of hypoglycemia when the blood glucose is 150 mg/dL, others not until the level is below 80 mg/dL, and so on.

From Franz MJ, Norstrom J: Diabetes Actively Staying Healthy (DASH): Your Game Plan for Diabetes and Exercise. Minneapolis, International Diabetes Center, 1990.

and Simon, 1994). This underscores the importance of therapists' providing nonsurgical alternatives such as appropriate shoes, insoles, and orthoses for these problems.** The presence of a previous history of plantar ulceration may alert the therapist to the need to teach the client how to control activity levels to lessen shear forces on scars from previous ulcers.

The detrimental effects of cigarette smoking on wound healing and peripheral circulation are well documented (see discussion of substance abuse in Chapter 2). Substance abuse of any kind can impair or slow the rehabilitation process, especially delaying wound healing. Client education in this area is an important aspect of treatment.

Diabetes and Physical Agents *(Betts et al., 1995)*

The application of heat causes local vasodilation and hyperemia (excess blood to an area) necessitating burn precautions in this population. In a therapy practice, heat application may take the form of hot packs, paraffin, hydrotherapy, fluidotherapy, infrared radiation, ultrasound, or aquatic (pool) therapy. Heat from the use of hot baths, whirlpools, saunas, or sun beds have been shown to accelerate the absorption of subcutaneous injections of insulin, presumably by increasing skin blood flow (Cuppers, 1980; Koivisto, 1980; Husband and Gill, 1984). To reduce the risk of hypoglycemia, local application of heat to the site of a recent insulin injection should be avoided.

The use of cryotherapy (cold) with its effects of vasoconstriction and decreased skin blood flow would logically be expected to slow or delay insulin absorption from the injection site. Studies to confirm this conclusion are not currently available. Information about the effect of massage on tissue absorption of insulin is limited (Linde, 1986) and inconclusive at this time.

Diabetes and Aquatic Therapy†† *(Charness, 1996)*

A rise in ambient (surrounding) temperature such as a client might experience in an indoor, warm, and humid pool setting, also causes an increase in insulin absorption from subcutaneous injection sites. The insulin disappearance rate may be as much as 50% to 60% greater with an increase of 15 degrees in ambient temperature (Koivisto et al., 1981).

Additionally, the ease of movement in the water allows increased activity without the same perceived intensity of exertion for the same amount of work performed outside the water. The combination of increased temperatures and increased activity can result in hypoglycemia. The therapist and client must work closely together to maintain a balance of activity, food intake, and insulin dosage.

Prior to pool therapy, the client must not miss any meals or snacks and must measure blood glucose levels. A snack or beverage such as orange juice should be readily available throughout the therapy session for anyone developing symptoms of hypoglycemia. Glucose testing should be performed following completion of the pool program. Exercise can have a positive effect in reducing blood glucose levels in persons with NIDDM, but sudden drops in blood glucose levels following exercise should be avoided.

With careful management, the individual should be able to adjust food intake and exercise tolerance to avoid having to increase insulin dosage. Throughout the pool program, the therapist must closely monitor each individual with diabetes for any signs of hypoglycemia. The affected individuals must be cautioned to carry out self-monitoring as well, and to respond to the earliest perceived symptoms.

---

* *Diabetes Self-Management* magazine is an invaluable asset for anyone with diabetes: available by title at P.O. Box 51125, Boulder, CO 80321–1125.

† The Somogyi effect occurs when the blood glucose level decreases to the point at which stress hormones (epinephrine, growth hormone, and corticosteroids) are released, causing a rebound hyperglycemia. Treatment consists of increasing the amount of food eaten and/or decreasing the insulin (Wong, 1993).

‡ See Sinacore and Gulve (1993) for an excellent, detailed review of the pathways for glucose transport into skeletal muscle and the pathophysiology of insulin action in skeletal muscle as it contributes to disturbances of whole-body glucose metabolism.

§ More specific recommendations for the long-distance runner and other athletes are available (see Hough, 1994; Landry, 1994; Robbins, 1989).

¶ For a description of an easy and reliable method to test for protective sensation using the Semmes-Weinstein monofilaments, see Mueller (1996). This test is an easily used clinical indicator for identifying people who are at risk for developing foot ulcers and requiring subsequent amputations. The results of this test provide a definitive idea of who can benefit most from preventive care, education, and prescription of appropriate therapeutic footwear (Mueller, 1996).

** For an excellent discussion of how to provide a good fit in shoes, including proper shoe lacing patterns to match foot type, as well as a review of the "Diabetic Shoe Bill," see Bottomley JM: 'Diabetic Shoe Bill' provides assistance in Medicare part B. The ADVANCE Magazine for Physical Therapists, Dec 12, 1994, pp. 20, 23. For more specific information on this Medicare provision, contact a durable medical equipment (DME) dealer or the DME Regional Center, Nashville, Tenn (615) 251–8182.

†† The Aquatics Section of the American Physical Therapy Association (APTA) has a 20-page bound, annotated bibliography with relevant articles related to pool therapy including the use of aquatics with medical conditions such as diabetes mellitus. This document is available through the management company for the section: PRADCOM (334) 990–8612. The cost is $5.00 for APTA Aquatic Section members; $10.00 for APTA nonsection members; and $20.00 for non-APTA members.

Insulin Resistance Syndrome

A syndrome of insulin resistance has been proposed to explain the frequent association of hypertension, carbohydrate intolerance, abdominal obesity, dyslipidemia, and accelerated atherosclerosis associated with NIDDM. Although a primary insufficiency of insulin secretion is the pathology in the development of NIDDM, obesity is a major risk factor for the development of this type of DM, owing in part to the associated insulin resistance. In offspring of people with NIDDM, insulin resistance appears inherited and may be the best predictor of future diabetic state (Garber, 1994). *Syndrome X* is sometimes referred to as the *insulin resistance syndrome;* but these are two separate entities (see further discussion of syndrome X in Chapter 10).

Hyperglycemia

Two primary life-threatening metabolic conditions can develop if uncontrolled or untreated DM progresses to a state of severe hyperglycemia (400 mg/dL). These are diabetic ketoacidosis (DKA) and hyperglycemic, hyperosmolar, nonketotic coma (HHNK). Between diabetic ketoacidosis and hyperosmolar nonketotic coma is a continuum of metabolic abnormalities. Emphasis of treatment differs in the two disorders. HHNK primarily requires hydration and potassium replacement; administration of insulin is more important in DKA (Fish, 1994).

Diabetic Ketoacidosis

Definition and Overview. A common condition, DKA can occur when complications develop from severe insulin deficiency. Most episodes of DKA occur in persons with previously diagnosed IDDM. However, the condition may occur in new cases of IDDM and in persons with NIDDM (under stressful conditions in the latter, such as during a myocardial infarction). It is characterized by the triad of hyperglycemia, acidosis, and ketosis (Lipsky, 1994).

Etiology. Causes of DKA commonly include taking too little insulin; omitting doses of insulin; failing to meet an increased need for insulin due to surgery, trauma, pregnancy, stress, puberty, or infection; and development of insulin resistance caused by insulin antibodies. Other precipitating causes are listed in Box 9–5.

The most common precipitating factor is infection, which occurs in up to half of all cases and may seem like a trivial condition, such as mild cellulitis or upper respiratory tract infection. Omission of insulin, either because of noncompliance or because people mistakenly believe that insulin is not required on "sick days" when they are not eating well, is another important and preventable cause of DKA. In approximately 15% to 30% of cases, no identifiable cause can be determined (Sanson and Levine, 1989).

Pathogenesis. The initiating metabolic defect in diabetic ketoacidosis is an insufficient or absent level of circulating insulin. Insulin may be present, but not in a sufficient amount for the increase in glucose due to the stressor (see Box 9–5).

BOX 9–5
Precipitating Causes of Diabetic Ketoacidosis*

- Inadequate insulin under stressful conditions
- Infection
- Missed insulin doses
- Trauma
- Medications
  - β-Blockers
  - Calcium channel blockers
  - Pentamidine (NebuPent, Pentam)
  - Steroids
  - Thiazides (diuretics)
- Alcohol abuse (inability to manage insulin due to mentation change; alcoholic ketoacidosis)
- Hypokalemia
- Myocardial ischemia
- Surgery
- Pregnancy
- Renal failure
- Stroke

* Listed in descending order.

From Lipsky MS: Management of diabetic ketoacidosis. Am Fam Physician 49:1608, 1994.

Inadequate insulin creates a biologic "alarm state," which triggers the excess secretion of counterregulatory hormones, particularly glucagon. The abnormal insulin-to-glucagon ratio, along with excess circulating catecholamine, cortisol, and growth hormone levels, initiates a host of complex metabolic reactions, leading to hyperglycemia, acidosis, and ketosis.

When the body lacks insulin and cannot use carbohydrates for energy, it resorts to fats and proteins. The process of catabolizing fats for fuel gives rise to incomplete lipid metabolism, dehydration, metabolic acidosis, and electrolyte and acid-base imbalances. (See more complete discussion in previous section on pathogenesis of diabetes mellitus.)

Clinical Manifestations. The signs and symptoms of DKA vary, ranging from mild nausea to frank coma (Table 9–22). Common symptoms are thirst, polyuria, nausea, and weakness that have progressed over several days. This condition can also develop quickly, with symptoms progressing to coma over the course of only a few hours.

Other symptoms may include dry mouth; hot, dry skin; fruity (acetone) odor to the breath, indicating the presence of ketones; overall weakness, possible paralysis; confusion, lethargy, or coma; and deep, rapid respirations (Kussmaul's respirations). Fever is seldom present even though infection is common. Severe abdominal pain, possibly accompanied by nausea and vomiting, easily mimics an acute abdominal disorder.

Medical Management

Diagnosis, Treatment, and Prognosis. Prevention of DKA through client education is the key to avoiding this serious condition. Once DKA is suspected, the diagnosis must be established quickly, with immediate treatment following diagnostic confirmation (blood glucose level >250 mg/dL, pH <7.3, bicarbonate level <15 mEq/L, serum ketones).

Treatment includes fluid administration, insulin therapy, and correction of metabolic abnormalities, as well as correction of any underlying illnesses (e.g., infection). Prior to the discovery of insulin in the 1920s, DKA was almost universally fatal. This complication is still potentially lethal with an average mortality rate between 5% and 10% (Lipsky, 1994).

Special Implications for the Therapist 9–16

DIABETIC KETOACIDOSIS (DKA)

The therapist will be an active member of the health-care team, emphasizing to anyone with IDDM the need for regular, daily self-monitoring of blood glucose, adherence to the diabetes management program, and early recognition of and intervention for mild ketosis. The therapist must also be able to recognize early signs and symptoms of DKA as well as signs of infection, a major cause of DKA (see Table 6–1). The first sign of an infection in a foot or leg or an upper respiratory, urinary tract, or vaginal infection should be reported immediately to the physician.

DKA can cause major potassium deficits accompanied by muscular weakness that can progress to flaccid quadriparesis. The weakness is initially most prominent in the legs, especially the quadriceps, and then extends to the arms with involvement of the respiratory muscles. (See Chapter 4 for further discussion of hypokalemia as well as a discussion of the other conditions associated

TABLE 9–22 Clinical Symptoms of Life-Threatening Glycemic States

Hyperglycemia		Hypoglycemia
Diabetic Ketoacidosis (DKA)	Hyperglycemic, Hyperosmolar, Nonketotic Coma (HHNK)	Insulin Shock
Gradual Onset*	**Gradual Onset**	**Sudden Onset**
Headache	Thirst	Pallor
Thirst	Polyuria leading quickly to decreased urine output	Perspiration
Hyperventilation	Volume loss from polyuria leading quickly to renal insufficiency	Piloerection
Fruity odor to breath	Severe dehydration	Increased heart rate
Lethargy/confusion/coma	Lethargy/confusion	Palpitations
Abdominal pain and distention	Seizures	Irritability/nervousness
Dehydration	Coma	Weakness
Polyuria	Abdominal pain and distention	Hunger
Flushed face	Blood glucose level >300 mg/dL	Shakiness
Elevated temperature		Headache
Blood glucose level >300 mg/dL		Double/blurred vision
Serum pH <7.30		Slurred speech
		Fatigue
		Numbness of lips/tongue
		Confusion
		Convulsion/coma
		Blood glucose level <70 mg/dL

* Less gradual than HHNK.

From Goodman CC, Snyder TE: Differential Diagnosis in Physical Therapy, ed 2. Philadelphia, WB Saunders, 1995, p 356.

with DKA, such as dehydration, metabolic acidosis, and electrolyte and acid-base imbalances.)

Hyperglycemic, Hyperosmolar, Nonketotic Coma

Overview. Hyperglycemic, hyperosmolar, nonketotic coma (HHNK) is another acute complication of diabetes, a variation of diabetic ketoacidosis. HHNK is characterized by extreme hyperglycemia (800 to 2000 mg/dL), mild or undetectable ketonuria, and the absence of acidosis. It is most commonly seen in older persons with NIDDM (Butts-Krakoff, 1993).

The precipitating factors of HHNK may be much the same as those for DKA, such as infections, medications (see Box 9–5), or stress. HHNK may be the first indication of undiagnosed diabetes and it may occur in the case of someone who is receiving total parenteral nutrition (hyperalimentation) or who is on renal dialysis and is receiving solutions containing large amounts of glucose.

The major difference between HHNK and DKA is the lack of ketonuria with HHNK. Because there is some residual ability to secrete insulin in NIDDM, the mobilization of fats for energy is avoided. When adequate insulin is lacking, blood becomes concentrated with glucose. Because glucose molecules are too large to pass into cells, osmosis of water occurs from the interstitial spaces and cells to dilute the glucose in the blood. Osmotic diuresis occurs, and eventually the cells become dehydrated.

Clinical manifestations of HHNK are polyphagia, polydipsia, polyuria, glucosuria, dehydration, abdominal discomfort, hyperventilation, changes in sensorium, coma, hypotension, and shock (see Table 9–22). Lactic acidosis can also develop. Treatment is with careful fluid replacement so as to avoid congestive heart failure and intercerebral swelling in the elderly, who often have other cardiovascular or renal disorders.

Special Implications for the Therapist **9–17**

HYPERGLYCEMIC, HYPEROSMOLAR, NONKETOTIC COMA

The therapist should be alert to any signs of HHNK in the aging adult who may have a previous diagnosis of NIDDM. Early recognition and treatment to restore fluid and electrolyte balance are important for a good prognosis in this condition. (See also Special Implications for the Therapist: Diabetes Mellitus, 9–15.)

METABOLIC SYSTEM

As noted earlier, the endocrine system works with the nervous system to regulate and integrate the body's metabolic activities. Metabolism is the physical and chemical (physiologic) processes that allow cells to utilize food to continually rebuild body cells and transform food into energy. Metabolism is broken down into two phases: the anabolic (tissue-building) and catabolic (energy-producing) phases. The *anabolic phase* converts simple compounds derived from nutrients into substances the body cells can use, whereas the *catabolic phase* is a destructive phase when these organized substances are reconverted into simple compounds with the release of energy necessary for the proper functioning of body cells (Guyton, 1992).

The body gets most of its energy by metabolizing carbohydrates, especially glucose. A complex interplay of hormonal and neural controls regulates the homeostasis of glucose metabolism. Hormone secretions of five endocrine glands dominate this regulatory function (see Table 9–12). The rate of metabolism can be increased by exercise, elevated body temperature (e.g., high fever, prolonged exertional exercise), hormonal activity (e.g., thyroxine, insulin, epinephrine), and increased digestive action following the ingestion of food.

Fluid and Electrolyte Balance

Fluid and electrolyte balance is a key component of cellular metabolism. Homeostasis, maintaining the body's chemical and physical balance, involves the proper functioning of body fluids to preserve osmotic pressure, acid-base balance, and anion-cation balance. The goal of metabolism and homeostasis is to maintain the complex environment of body fluid that nourishes and supports every cell (Norris, 1995).

Body fluids, classified as intracellular and extracellular, contain two kinds of dissolved substances: those that dissociate (separate) in solution (electrolytes) and those that do not. For example, when dissolved in water, glucose does not break down into smaller particles, but sodium chloride dissociates into sodium cations (positively charged) and chloride anions (negatively charged). The composition of these electrolytes in body fluids is electrically balanced so the positively charged cations (sodium, potassium, calcium, and magnesium) equal the negatively charged anions (chloride, bicarbonate, sulfate, phosphate, carbonic acid). Although these particles are present in relatively low concentrations, any deviation from their normal levels can have profound physiologic effects.

Because many situations in the body cause both normal and abnormal fluid shifts, it is important to have a clear understanding of fluid compartments. The recognition of pathologic conditions such as edema, dehydration, ketoacidosis, and various types of shock can depend on the understanding of these concepts. In the healthy body, fluids and electrolytes are constantly lost or exchanged between compartments. This balance must be maintained for the body to function properly. The amount used in these functions depends on such factors as humidity; body and environmental temperature; physical activity; metabolic rate; and fluid loss from the GI tract, skin, respiratory tract, and renal system. Normal balance is achieved through fluid intake and dietary consumption. Alterations in fluid and electrolyte balance are discussed more completely in Chapter 4.

Acid-Base Balance

The proper balance of acids and bases in the body is essential to life. The body maintains the pH of extracellular fluid (fluid found outside cells) between 7.35 and 7.45 through a complex chemical regulation of carbonic acid by the lungs and base bicarbonate by the kidneys. The pH is essentially a measure of hydrogen ion concentration in body fluid. Nutritional deficiency or excess, disease, injury, or metabolic disturbance can interfere with normal homeostatic mechanisms and cause a lowering of pH called *acidosis* or a rise in pH called *alkalosis*.

Various bodily functions operate to keep the pH at a relatively constant level. Acid-base regulatory mechanisms include chemical buffer systems, the respiratory system, and the renal system. These systems interact very closely to maintain a normal acid-base ratio of 20 : 1 bicarbonate to carbonic acid. The consequences of an acid-base metabolism disorder can result in many signs and symptoms encountered by the therapist. These conditions are discussed more completely in Chapter 4.

Aging and the Metabolic System

Aging as measured by loss of physiologic function has not yet been defined precisely so that the distinction between "usual," "normal," and "ideal" metabolic changes remains as yet undetermined. Cross-sectional studies[15] of the aging population have shown that several physiologic parameters such as body weight, basal metabolism, renal clearance, and cardiovascular function decline with age (Shock, 1962; Shock et al., 1984). Protein-calorie nutritional status has pervasive effects on metabolic regulatory systems; nutritional status often declines with age, which contributes to metabolic dysfunction (Abrams et al., 1995).

Because the respiratory and renal systems are largely responsible for maintaining acid-base balance, changes in these systems associated with aging also have an impact on metabolic function. A common measure for metabolic loss in tissues is the decline in VO_2max, the maximum oxygen extraction capacity of the lungs (Hagberg, 1987; Abrams et al., 1995) (see also Chapters 12, Aging and the Pulmonary System, and 15, Aging and the Renal System).

Mitochondria, the principal site of adenosine triphosphate (ATP) synthesis (also containing DNA and RNA) is the cellular site of energy production from oxygen. As a result of normal metabolic activity, reactive free radical derivatives of oxygen are generated[16] (see Chapter 3, Physical Agents), producing destructive oxidation of membranes, proteins, and DNA. The major defenses against such destruction are the protective enzymes, which remove the reactive free radicals and remove, repair, and replace cell constituents. Impairment of cellular function and metabolism occurs as proteins and DNA (which turn over slowly or not at all) are damaged over time (Brink and Reichel, 1995).

Signs and Symptoms of Metabolic Disease

Clinical manifestations of metabolic disorders vary depending on the specific pathology present. Fluid and electrolyte disorders, disorders of acid-base metabolism leading to metabolic (nonrespiratory) alkalosis or acidosis, and their associated signs and symptoms are discussed in Chapter 4.

SPECIFIC METABOLIC DISORDERS

Hereditary metabolic disorders such as the amyloid diseases are discussed in Chapter 23, *metabolic bone disease* is discussed in Chapter 20, and *disorders of purine and pyrimidine metabolism* resulting in gout and pseudogout are discussed in Chapter 23.

Metabolic Bone Disease

Metabolic disorders involving the connective tissue may result in pathologic loss of bone mineral density such as occurs in osteomalacia or osteoporosis or acceleration of both deposition and resorption of bone as seen in Paget's disease. These disorders differ in pathogenesis and treatment and are discussed in Chapter 20.

Metabolic Neuronal Diseases

Metabolic neuronal diseases are rare and are not likely seen in a therapy practice. Phenylketonuria (PKU) and Wilson's disease are the two most often encountered and are only briefly discussed in this section.

Phenylketonuria

PKU is a congenital disease due to a defect in the metabolism of the amino acid phenylalanine. This condition is hereditary and is transmitted recessively through apparently healthy parents, who only show signs of the disease on testing. The lack of an enzyme (phenylalanine hydroxylase) necessary for the conversion of the amino acid phenylalanine into tyrosine results in an accumulation of phenylalanine in the blood with excretion of phenylpyruvic acid in the urine. If untreated, the condition results in mental retardation and other manifestations such as tremors, poor muscular coordination, excessive perspiration, mousy odor (due to skin and urinary excretion of phenylpyruvic acid), and seizures.

Although PKU cannot be cured, a simple screening test for PKU can be administered to newborns and is required by law in most states in the United States and in all provinces in Canada. Currently, between 160 and 400 of the 4 million babies born in the United States each year are affected. The recent practice of discharging newborns in 24 hours is resulting in an increase in the number of babies at risk of PKU.

Testing within the first 24 hours of life has a high false-negative rate. The American Academy of Pediatrics has recommended that babies receiving PKU tests within the first 24 hours be retested by 2 weeks of age to decrease the possibility of missing this disorder. Only 13 states within the United States require retesting within the first month of life (Sinai et al., 1995). Restriction of the infant's diet to control the effects of PKU is prescribed on an individual basis with the additional administration of a dietary protein substitute (Lofenalac).

Wilson's Disease

Wilson's disease, also known as *hepatolenticular degeneration*, is a progressive disease inherited as an autosomal recessive trait (both parents must carry the abnormal gene). This condition produces a defect in the metabolism of copper, with accumulation of copper in the liver, brain, kidney, cornea, and other tissues. Although the pathogenesis of Wilson's disease is still uncertain, it seems likely that defective biliary excretion of copper is involved.

[15] The Baltimore Longitudinal Study of Aging is an ongoing multidisciplinary study of biomedical and psychological aging. Over 1000 men and women are currently active, returning to the Gerontology Research Center (National Institute on Aging, NIH) every 2 years (Costa and McCrae, 1993).

[16] These processes produce ions and free radicals (unstable oxygen molecules robbed of electrons). Free radicals attempt to replace their missing electrons by scavenging the body and taking electrons from healthy cells, causing a chain reaction called *oxidation*. The balance of radical and non-radical reactive oxygen can be upset by many exogenous (outside) factors such as cigarette smoke, air pollution, anticancer drugs, ultraviolet lights, pesticides and other chemicals, uncontrolled diabetes, radiation, and emotional stress (Cooper, 1994).

The disease is characterized by the presence of Kayser-Fleischer rings around the iris of the eye (from copper deposits), cirrhosis of the liver (see Chapter 14), and degenerative changes in the brain, particularly the basal ganglia. Liver disease is the most likely manifestation in the pediatric population and neurologic disease is most common in young adults. Cerebellar intoxication from deposition of copper in the brain results in athetoid movements and an unsteady gait. Other CNS symptoms may include pill-rolling tremors in the hands, facial and muscular rigidity, dysarthria, and emotional and behavioral changes. Musculoskeletal effects occur in severe disease and may include muscle atrophy and wasting, contractures, deformities, osteomalacia, and pathologic fractures (Norris, 1995).

Treatment is pharmacologic (e.g., lifetime administration of vitamin B_6 and D-penicillamine) and is aimed at reducing the amount of copper in the tissues by promoting its urinary excretion. Managing hepatic disease is also important; if left untreated, Wilson's disease progresses to fatal hepatic failure.

Special Implications for the Therapist **9-18**

WILSON'S DISEASE *(Norris, 1995)*

For the person with Wilson's disease, physical or vocational rehabilitation may be required. In the advanced stage of this disease, self-care is promoted to prevent further mental and physical deterioration. An exercise schedule is essential to encourage consistent focus on rehabilitation. Sensory deprivation or overload should be avoided and prevention of injuries that could occur as a result of neurologic deficits is important (see Table 10-22).

References

Abrams WB, Beers MH, Berkow R: The Merck Manual of Geriatrics, ed 2. Rahway, NJ, Merck & Co., 1995.

Alspach J: Core Curriculum for Critical Care Nursing. Philadelphia, WB Saunders, 1991.

Benson EA, Rosenthal NR: Endocrinologic and related metabolic disorders. *In* Ramsey PG, Larson EG (eds): Medical Therapeutics, ed 2. Philadelphia, WB Saunders, 1993, pp 428–463.

Berne RM, Levy MN: Principles of Physiology. St Louis, Mosby–Year Book, 1990.

Betts EF, Betts JJ, Betts CJ: Pharmacologic management of hyperglycemia in diabetes mellitus: Implications for physical therapy. Physical Therapy 75:415–425, 1995.

Betts JJ: Diabetes and Exercise: Putting Theory into Practice. APTA combined sections meeting. Cincinnati, 1993.

Birch C: Nursing care of clients with thyroid and parathyroid disorders. *In* Black JM, Matassarin-Jacobs E (eds): Luckmann and Sorensen's Medical-Surgical Nursing, ed 4. Philadelphia, WB Saunders, 1993, pp 1809–1836.

Bland JH: 'Arthritis' symptoms: Is it endocrine disease? J Musculoskel Med 11:34–46, 1994.

Blevins DR, Cassmeyer VL: Management of persons with problems of the pituitary, thyroid, parathyroid and adrenal glands. *In* Phipps W, Cassmeyer VL, Sands JK, Lehman MK (eds): Medical-Surgical Nursing: Concepts and Clinical Practice, ed 5. St Louis, Mosby–Year Book, 1995, pp 1200–1280.

Bluestone R, Bywaters EGL, Hartog M, et al: Acromegalic arthropathy. Ann Rheum Dis 30:243–258, 1971.

Brink JJ, Reichel W: Cell biology and physiology of aging. *In* Reichel W: Care of the Elderly: Clinical Aspects of Aging, ed 4. Baltimore, Williams & Wilkins, 1995, pp 472–475.

Brodsky JW, Negrine JP: Orthotic solutions for recalcitrant Charcot deformity. Biomechanics 11:65–68, 1995.

Butts-Krakoff D: Structure and function: Assessment of clients with metabolic disorders. *In* Black JM, Matassarin-Jacobs E (eds): Luckmann and Sorensen's Medical-Surgical Nursing, ed 4. Philadelphia, WB Saunders, 1993, pp 1757–1774.

Butts-Krakoff D, Black JM: Nursing care of clients with endocrine disorders of the pancreas. *In* Black JM, Matassarin-Jacobs E (eds): Luckmann and Sorensen's Medical-Surgical Nursing, ed. 4. Philadelphia, WB Saunders, 1993, pp 1775–1808.

Carnevali DL, Patrick M (eds): Aging changes in structure and function. *In* Nursing Management for the Elderly, ed. 3. Philadelphia, JB Lippincott, 1993, pp 113–140.

Carroll PB, Fontes P, Rao AS, et al: Simultaneous solid organ, bone marrow, and islet allotransplantation in type 1 diabetic patients. Transplant Proc 26:3523–3524, 1994.

Cavanagh PR, Derr JA, Ulbrecht JS, et al: Problems with gait and posture in neuropathic patients with insulin-dependent diabetes mellitus. Diabet Med 9:469–474, 1992.

Charness A: Personal communication (President, Aquatics Section, American Physical Therapy Association; faculty, Medical College of Pennsylvania, Philadelphia), 1996.

Christakos CN, Fields KB: Exercise in diabetes: Minimize the risks and gain the benefits. J Musculoskel Med 12:16–25, 1995.

Chrousos GP, Gold PW: The concepts of stress and stress system disorders: Overview of physical and behavioral homeostasis. JAMA 267:1244–1252, 1992.

Conrad B, Weidmann E, Trucco G, et al: Evidence for superantigen involvement in insulin-dependent diabetes mellitus aetiology. Nature 371:351–355, 1994.

Cooper KH: Antioxidant Revolution. Nashville, Thomas Nelson Publishers, 1994.

Corpas E, Harman SM, Blackman MR: Human growth hormone and aging. Endocrinol Rev 14:20–39, 1993.

Costa PT Jr, McCrae RR: Psychological research in the Baltimore Longitudinal Study of Aging. J Gerontol 26:138–141, 1993.

Cuppers HJ: Sauna-induced acceleration in insulin absorption? Br Med J 281:621–622, 1980.

DeFronzo RA: The triumvirate: Beta-cell, muscle, liver-A collusion responsible for NIDDM. Diabetes 37:667–687, 1988.

Degland J, Vallerand A: Davis Drug Guide for Nurses. Philadelphia, FA Davis, 1993.

Delamarter RB, Sherman JE, Carr J: Lumbar spinal stenosis secondary to calcium pyrophosphate crystal deposition (pseudogout). Clin Orthop 289:127–130, 1993.

Delp MD, McAllister RM, Laughlin MH: Exercise training alters aortic vascular reactivity in hypothyroid rats. Am J Physiol 268(4 pt 2): H1428–1435, 1995.

Dorwart BB: Arthropathies associated with endocrine diseases. *In* Schumacher HR (ed): Primer on the Rheumatic Diseases, ed 10. Atlanta, Arthritis Foundation, 1993, pp 242–243.

Drugs for obesity, diabetes forseen. PT Bull 11:18, 1996.

Dunn CJ, Peters DH: Metformin: A review of its pharmacological properties and therapeutic use in non-insulin dependent diabetes mellitus. Drugs 49:721–749, 1995.

Eaks GA, Cassmeyer V: Management of persons with diabetes mellitus and hypoglycemia. *In* Phipps W, Cassmeyer VL, Sands JK, Lehman MK (eds): Medical-Surgical Nursing: Concepts and Clinical Practice, ed 5. St Louis, Mosby–Year Book, 1995, pp 1281–1354.

Ellis JM, Folkers K, Minadea M, et al: A deficiency of vitamin B_6 is a plausible molecular basis of the retinopathy of patients with diabetes mellitus. Biochem Biophys Res Commun 179:615–619, 1991.

Elsinger J, Plantamura A, Ayavou T: Glycolysis abnormalities in fibromyalgia. J Am Coll Nutr 13:144–148, 1994.

Epstein S: Role of metformin in type II diabetes. Cleve Clin J Med 62:278–279, 1995.

Farrar JJ, Toft AD: Iodine-131 treatment of hyperthyroidism: Current issues. Clin Endocrinol 35:207–212, 1991.

Ferraccioli G: Neuroendocrinologic findings in fibromyalgia syndrome. J Rheumatol 17:869–873, 1990.

Fish LH: Diabetic ketoacidosis: Treatment strategies to avoid complications. Postgrad Med 96:75–96, 1994.

Gambert SR: Endocrinology and aging. *In* Reichel W (ed): Care of the Elderly: Clinical Aspects of Aging, ed 4. Baltimore, Williams & Wilkins, 1995, pp 365–372.

Ganio C, Tenewitz FE, Wilson RC, et al: The treatment of chronic nonhealing wounds using autologous platelet-derived growth factors. J Foot Ankle Surg 32:263–268, 1993.

Garber AJ: Diabetes mellitus. *In* Stein JH (ed): Internal Medicine, ed 4. St Louis, Mosby–Year Book, 1994, pp 1391–1424.

Gillam AJ, Da Camara CC: Treatment of wounds with procuren. Ann Pharmacother 27:1201–1203, 1993.

Gleeson PB, Pauls J: Carpal tunnel syndrome during pregnancy and lactation. PT Magazine 9:52–54, 1993.

Goodman CC, Snyder TE: Differential Diagnosis in Physical Therapy, ed 2. Philadelphia, WB Saunders, 1995.

Gotlin RW, Chase HP, Klingensmith GJ: Endocrine disorders. *In* Hathaway WE, Hay WW, Groothuis JR, et al: Current Pediatric Diagnosis and Treatment, ed 11. Norwalk, Conn, Appleton & Lange, 1993, pp 841–884.

Grossman LA, Kaplan HJ, Ownby FD, et al: Carpal tunnel syndrome—initial manifestations of systemic disease. JAMA 176:259–261, 1961.

Guyton A: Human Physiology and Mechanisms of Disease, ed 5. Philadelphia, WB Saunders, 1992.

Hagberg JM: Effect of training on the decline of VO_2max with aging. Fed Proc 46:1830–1833, 1987.

Helfand RF, Gary HE Jr, Freeman CY, et al: Serologic evidence of an association between enteroviruses and the onset of type 1 diabetes mellitus. J Infect Dis 172:1206–1211, 1995.

Holt PJL: Rheumatologic manifestations of diabetes mellitus. Clin Rheum Dis 7:723–746, 1981.

Hough DO: Diabetes mellitus in sports. Sports Med 78:423–437, 1994.

Huether SE: Mechanisms of hormonal regulation. *In* McCance KL, Huether SE: Pathophysiology: The Biologic Basis for Disease in Adults and Children. St Louis, Mosby–Year Book, 1994, pp 626–655.

Husband DJ, Gill GV: "Sunbed seizures": A hypoglycemic hazard for insulin-dependent diabetics. Lancet 22:1477, 1984.

Hybbinette CH, Mannerfelt L: The carpal tunnel syndrome: A retrospective study of 400 operated patients. Acta Orthop Scand 46:610–620, 1975.

Hyoty H, Hiltunen M, Knip M, et al: A prospective study of the role of coxsackie B and other enterovirus infections in the pathogenesis of IDDM. Diabetes 44:652–657, 1995.

Katzeff HL, Ojamaa KM, Klein I: Effects of exercise on protein synthesis and myosin heavy chain gene expression in hypothyroid rats. Am J Physiol 267:E63–67, 1994.

Kaye T: Watching for and managing musculoskeletal problems in diabetes. J Musculoskel Med 11:25–37, 1994.

Keenan GF, Ostrov BE, Goldsmith DP, et al: Rheumatic symptoms associated with hypothyroidism in children. J Pediatr 123:586–588, 1993.

Khoursheed M, Miles PD, Gao KM, et al: Metabolic effects of troglitazone on fat-induced insulin resistance in the rat. Metabolism 44:1489–1494, 1995.

Koivisto VA: Sauna-induced acceleration in insulin absorption from subcutaneous injection site. Br Med J 280:1411–1413, 1980.

Koivisto VA, Fortney S, Hendler R, et al: A rise in ambient temperature augments insulin absorption in diabetic patients. Metabolism 30:402–404, 1981.

Kroop SF, Simon LS: Joint and bone manifestations of diabetes mellitus. *In* Kahn CR, Weir GC (eds): Joslin's Diabetes Mellitus. Philadelphia, Lea & Febiger, 1994, pp 912–920.

Landry GL, Allen DB: Diabetes mellitus and exercise. Clin Sports Med 11:403–418, 1992.

Layton MW, Fudman EJ, Barkan A, et al: Acromegalic arthropathy: Characteristics and response to therapy. Arthritis Rheum 31:1022–1027, 1988.

Layzer RB: CNS (Contemporary Neurology Series): Neuromuscular Manifestations of Systemic Disease. Philadelphia, FA Davis, 1985.

Leon A: Diabetes, *In* Skinner J (ed): Exercise Testing and Exercise Prescription for Special Cases: Theoretical Basis and Clinical Application, ed 2. Philadelphia, Lea & Febiger, 1993, pp 153–183.

Linde B: Dissociation of insulin absorption and blood flow during massage of a subcutaneous injection site. Diabetes Care 9:57–574, 1986.

Linos A, Worthington JW, O'Fallon WM, et al: The epidemiology of rheumatoid arthritis in Rochester, Minnesota: A study of incidence, prevalence, and mortality. Am J Epidemiol 111:87–98, 1980.

Lipsky MS: Management of diabetic ketoacidosis. Am Fam Physician 49:1607–1612, 1994.

Lochmuller H, Reimers CD, Fischer P, et al: Exercise-induced myalgia in hypothyroidism. Clin Invest 71:999–1001, 1993.

Loriaux TC: Nursing care of clients with adrenal, pituitary, and gonadal disorders. *In* Black JM, Matassarin-Jacobs E (eds): Luckmann and Sorensen's Medical-Surgical Nursing, ed 4. Philadelphia, WB Saunders, 1993, pp 1837–1862.

Louthrenoo W, Schumacher HR: Musculoskeletal clues to endocrine or metabolic disease. J Musculoskel Med 7:33–56, 1990.

Ludwig-Beymer P, Huether SE: Alterations of hormonal regulation. *In* McCance KL, Huether SE: Pathophysiology: The Biologic Basis for Disease in Adults and Children, ed 2. St Louis, Mosby–Year Book, 1994, pp 656–710.

Martin WH: Mechanisms of impaired exercise capacity in short duration experimental hyperthyroidism. J Clin Invest 88:2047–2053, 1991.

Martin WH: Triiodothyronine, beta-adrenergic receptors, agonist responses, and exercise capacity. Ann Thorac Surg 56(suppl 1):S24–34, 1993.

McAllister RM, Sansone JC Jr, Laughlin MH: Effects of hyperthyroidism on muscle blood flow during exercise in rats. Am J Physiol 268 (1 pt 2):H330–335, 1995.

McCance KL, Shelby J: Stress and disease, *In* McCance KL, Huether SE (eds): Pathophysiology: The Biologic Basis for Disease in Adults and Children, ed 2. St Louis, Mosby–Year Book, 1994, pp 299–320.

McCredie C: Hyperthyroidism and its implications for the physical therapist (unpublished paper). Indianapolis, Krannert Graduate School of Physical Therapy, University of Indiana, 1994.

Moskowitz RW: Crystal-induced inflammation associated with chronic renal failure treated with periodic hemodialysis. Am J Med 47:450–460, 1969.

Mueller MJ: Identifying patients with diabetes mellitus who are at risk for lower-extremity complications: Use of Semmes-Weinstein monofilaments. Phy Ther 76:68–71, 1996.

Mueller MJ, Diamond JE, Delitto A, et al: Insensitivity, limited joint mobility, and plantar ulcers in patients with diabetes mellitus. Phys Ther 69:453–462, 1989.

Mueller MJ, Minor SD, Sahrmann SA, et al: Differences in the gait characteristics of patients with diabetes and peripheral neuropathy compared with age-matched controls. Phys Ther 74:299–312, 1994.

Norris J (ed): Professional Guide to Diseases, ed 5. Springhouse, Pa, Springhouse Corporation, 1995.

O'Toole M (ed): Miller-Keane Encyclopedia and Dictionary of Medicine, Nursing, and Allied Health, ed 5. Philadelphia, WB Saunders, 1992.

Phalen GS: The carpal tunnel syndrome: Seventeen years' experience in diagnosis and treatment of six hundred and fifty-four hands. J Bone Joint Surg Am 48:211–228, 1966.

Preston ET: Avulsion of both quadriceps tendons in hyperparathyroidism. JAMA 221:406–407, 1972.

Ramsey ID: Muscle dysfunction in hyperthyroidism. Lancet 2:931, 1966.

Ramsey ID: Thyrotoxic myopathy—electromyography. Q J Med 34:255, 1965.

Ramsey ID: Thyroid Disease and Muscle Dysfunction. Chicago, Year Book Medical Publishers, 1974.

Reusch, JE: New directions in treating insulin resistance. Hosp Prac 30:9–10, 1995.

Ricordi C: The structure of scientific revolutions: A cell transplant perspective. Cell Transplant 4:357–360, 1995.

Robbins C: Managing the diabetic athlete. Phys Sports Med 17:45–54, 1989.

Ryan LM: Calcium pyrophosphate dihydrate crystal deposition and other crystal deposition diseases. Curr Opin Rheumatol 5:517–521, 1993.

Salcman M, Khan A, Symonds DA: Calcium pyrophosphate arthropathy of the spine: Case report and review of the literature. Neurosurgery 34:915–918, 1994.

Sammarco GJ: The biomechanics of the diabetic foot. Biomechanics 1:47–51, 1994.

Sanson TH, Levine SN: Management of diabetic ketoacidosis. Drugs 38:289–300, 1989.

Schteingart D: Principles of endocrine and metabolic function, *In* Price S, Wilson L (eds): Pathophysiology: Clinical Concepts of Disease Processes. St Louis, Mosby–Year Book, 1992, pp 831–839.

Schulte L, Roberts MS, Zimmerman C, et al: A quantitative assessment of limited joint mobility in patients with diabetes. Arthritis Rheum 36:1429–1443, 1993.

Sekine N, Yamamoto M, Michikawa M, et al: Rhabdomyolysis and acute

renal failure in a patient with hypothyroidism. Intern Med 32:269–271, 1993.
Shiroky JB, Cohen M, Ballachey ML: Thyroid dysfunction in rheumatoid arthritis: A controlled prospective survey. Ann Rheum Dis 52:454–456, 1993.
Shock NW: The science of gerontology, *In* Jeffers EC: Council on Gerontology: Proceedings of Seminars, 1959–1961. Durham, NC, Duke University Press, 1962, pp 123–140.
Shock NW, Greulich RC, Andres R, et al: Normal human aging: The Baltimore longitudinal study of aging. Washington DC, US Government Printing Office, 1984, pp 174–179.
Sinacore DR, Gulve EA: The role of skeletal muscle in glucose transport, glucose homeostasis, and insulin resistance: Implications for physical therapy. Phys Ther 73:878–891, 1993.
Sinai LN, Kim SC, Casey R, et al: Phenylketonuria screening: Effect of early newborn discharge. Pediatrics 96(4 pt 1):605–608, 1995.
Small D, Gibbons W, Levy RD, et al: Exertional dyspnea and ventilation in hyperthyroidism. Chest 101:1268–1273, 1992.
Sonkin LS: Myofascial pain due to metabolic disorders: Diagnosis and treatment, *In* Rachlin ES (ed): Myofascial Pain and Fibromyalgia: Trigger Point Management. St Louis, Mosby–Year Book, 1994, pp 45–59.
Stevens JC: Conditions associated with carpal tunnel syndrome. Mayo Clinic Proc 67:541–548, 1992.
Strowig S, Raskin P: Glycemic control and diabetic complications. Diabetes Care 15:1126–1138, 1992.
Swedler WI, Baak S, Lazarevic MB, et al: Rheumatic changes in diabetes: Shoulder, arm, and hand. J Musculoskel Med 12:45–52, 1995.
Terkeltaub RA: Identifying and managing calcium pyrophosphate deposition disease. J Musculoskel Med 11:29–37, 1994.
Travell JG, Simons DG: Myofascial Pain and Dysfunction: The Trigger Point Manual, vol I. Baltimore, Williams & Wilkins, 1983.
Vitug A, Schneider SH, Ruderman NB: Exercise and type I diabetes mellitus. Exerc Sport Sci Rev 16:285–304, 1988.
Wallberg-Hendriksson H: Exercise and diabetes mellitus. Exerc Sport Sci Rev 20:339–368, 1992.
Wand JS: Carpal tunnel syndrome in pregnancy and lactation. J Hand Surg Am 15:93–95, 1990.
Weinberg RA: Tumor suppressor genes. Science 254:1138–1146, 1991.
Wilson JD, Foster DW: Williams Textbook of Endocrinology, ed 8. Philadelphia, WB Saunders, 1992.
Wohlgethan JR: Frozen shoulder in hyperthyroidism. Arthritis Rheum 30:936–939, 1987.
Wong DL: Whaley and Wong's Essentials of Pediatric Nursing, ed 4. St Louis, Mosby–Year Book, 1993.
Woolridge WE: An ulcer that would not heal (case study): J Musculoskel Med 13:59–60, 1996.
Yamaguchi DM, Lipscomb PR, Soule EH: Carpal tunnel syndrome. Minn Med 48:22–33, 1965.

SECTION 2

chapter 10

The Cardiovascular System

Catherine C. Goodman

The cardiovascular system functions in coordination with the pulmonary system to circulate oxygenated blood through the arterial system to all cells. This system then collects deoxygenated blood from the venous system and delivers it to the lungs for reoxygenation (Fig. 10–1).

Pathologic conditions of the cardiovascular system are varied, multiple, and complex. In this chapter, cardiovascular structure and function are presented according to how diseases affect each individual part, including diseases of the heart muscle, cardiac nervous system, heart valves, pericardium, and blood and lymphatic vessels. Other factors such as surgery, pregnancy, and complications from other pathologic conditions (e.g., collagen vascular diseases,[1] acquired immunodeficiency syndrome [AIDS], cancer treatment, metabolic diseases) can also adversely affect the normal function of the cardiovascular system. Discussion of these additional factors is limited in this chapter (see specific chapters for each subject).

SIGNS AND SYMPTOMS OF CARDIOVASCULAR DISEASE

Cardinal symptoms of cardiac disease (Box 10–1) usually include chest, neck and/or arm pain or discomfort, palpitations, dyspnea, syncope (fainting), fatigue, cough, and cyanosis. Edema and leg pain (claudication) are the most common symptoms of the vascular component of cardiovascular pathology. Symptoms of cardiovascular involvement should be reviewed by system as well (Table 10–1).

Chest pain or discomfort is a common presenting symptom of cardiovascular disease and must be evaluated carefully. Chest pain may be cardiac or noncardiac in origin and may radiate to the neck, jaw, upper trapezius, upper back, shoulder, or arms (most commonly the left arm). Radiating pain down the arm is in the pattern of ulnar nerve distribution. Noncardiac chest pain can be caused by an extensive list of disorders and is not covered in this text. Cardiac-related chest pain may arise secondary to angina, myocardial infarction (MI), pericarditis, endocarditis, mitral valve prolapse, or dissecting aortic aneurysm. Location and description (frequency, intensity, and duration) vary according to the underlying pathology (see each individual condition).

Chest pain is often accompanied by associated signs and symptoms such as nausea, vomiting, diaphoresis, dyspnea, fatigue, pallor, or syncope. Cardiac chest pain or discomfort can also occur when coronary circulation is normal, as in the case of anemia causing lack of oxygenation of the myocardium (heart muscle) during physical exertion.

Palpitations, the presence of an irregular heartbeat, may also be referred to as arrhythmia or dysrhythmia, which may be caused by a relatively benign condition (e.g., mitral valve prolapse, "athlete's heart," caffeine, anxiety, exercise) or a severe condition (e.g., coronary artery disease [CAD], cardiomyopathy, complete heart block, ventricular aneurysm, atrioventricular valve disease, mitral or aortic stenosis). Palpitations have been described as a bump, pound, jump, flop, flutter, or racing sensation of the heart. Associated symptoms may include lightheadedness or syncope. Palpated pulse may feel rapid or irregular, as if the heart has "skipped" a beat.

Dyspnea, also referred to as breathlessness or shortness of breath, can be cardiovascular in origin, but it may also occur secondary to pulmonary pathology (see also Chapter 12), fever, certain medications, or obesity. Early onset of dyspnea may be described as a sensation of having to breathe too much or as an uncomfortable feeling during breathing after exercise or exertion. Shortness of breath with mild exertion (dyspnea on exertion [DOE]), when caused by an impaired left ventricle that is unable to contract completely, results in the lung's inability to empty itself of blood. Pulmonary congestion and shortness of breath then ensue. With severe compromise of the cardiovascular or pulmonary systems, dyspnea may occur at rest.

The severity of dyspnea is determined by the extent of disease; the more severe the heart disease, the more readily episodes of dyspnea occur. More extreme dyspnea includes paroxysmal nocturnal dyspnea (PND) and orthopnea. PND, which is sudden, unexplained episodes of shortness of breath, awakens a person sleeping in a supine position, because the amount of blood returning to the heart and lungs from the lower extremities increases in this position. This type of dyspnea frequently accompanies congestive heart failure (CHF). During the day, the effects of gravity in the upright position and the shunting of excessive fluid to the lower extremities permits more effective ventilation and perfusion of the lungs, keeping the lungs relatively fluid-free, depending on the degree of CHF. Orthopnea is the term used to describe breathlessness that is relieved by sitting upright, using pillows to prop the head and trunk. Orthopnea can occur anytime during the day or night.

Cardiac syncope (fainting or in a milder form, lightheadedness) can be caused by reduced oxygen to the brain. Cardiac conditions resulting in syncope include arrhythmias, orthostatic hypotension, poor ventricular function, CAD, and vertebral artery insufficiency. Lightheadedness as a result of orthostatic hypotension (sudden drop in blood pressure) may occur with any quick change in a prolonged position (e.g.,

[1] Collagen vascular disorders are now more commonly referred to as *diffuse connective tissue diseases*. See Box 10–13 for a specific listing of these diseases.

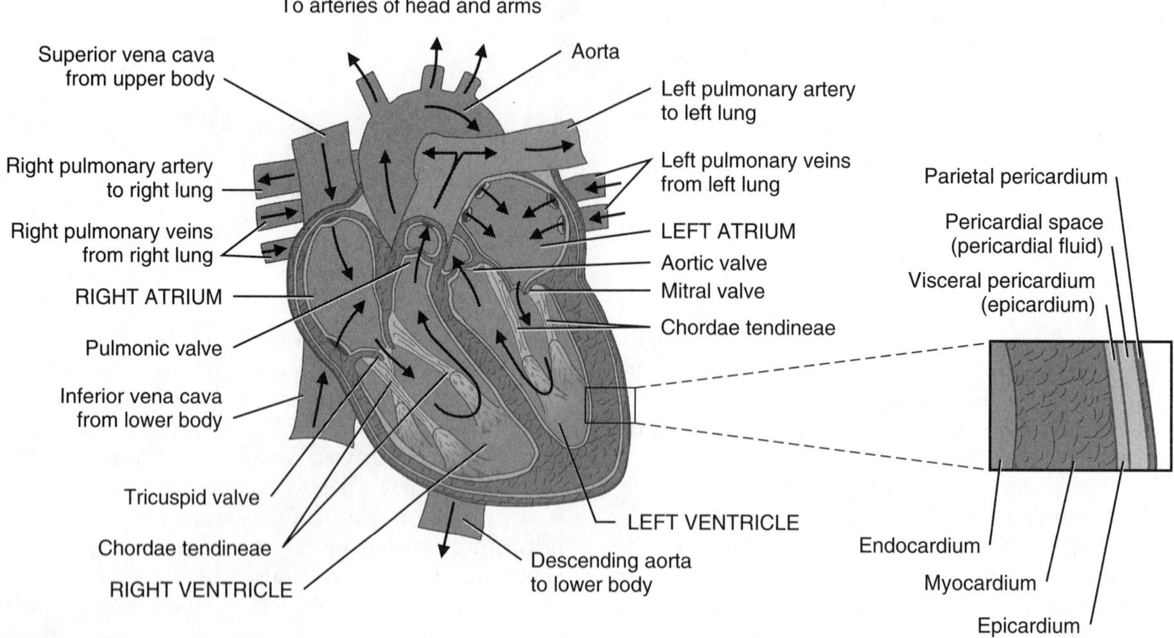

Figure **10-1.** *A*, Structure and circulation of the heart. Blood entering the left atrium from the right and left pulmonary veins flows into the left ventricle. The left ventricle pumps blood into the systemic circulation through the aorta. From the systemic circulation, blood returns to the heart through the superior and inferior venae cavae. From there, the right ventricle pumps blood into the lungs through the right and left pulmonary arteries. *B*, Sagittal view of the layers of heart.

going from a supine position to an upright posture or standing up from a sitting position) or with physical exertion involving increased abdominal pressure (e.g., straining with a bowel movement, lifting). Any client with aortic stenosis is more likely to experience lightheadedness as a result of these activities. Noncardiac conditions such as anxiety and emotional stress can cause hyperventilation and subsequent lightheadedness (vasovagal syncope). During the period of initiation and regulation of cardiac medications (e.g., vasodilators), side effects such as orthostatic hypotension may occur.

Fatigue provoked by minimal exertion indicates a lack of energy that may be cardiac in origin (e.g., CAD, aortic valve dysfunction, cardiomyopathy, or myocarditis), or it may occur secondary to neurologic, muscular, metabolic, or pulmonary pathology. Often fatigue of cardiac nature is accompanied by associated symptoms such as dyspnea, chest pain, palpitations, or headache.

Cough (see also Chapter 12) is usually associated with

BOX 10-1
Most Common Signs and Symptoms of Cardiovascular Disease

- Chest pain or discomfort
- Neck and/or arm pain or discomfort
- Palpitation
- Dyspnea
- Syncope
- Fatigue
- Cough
- Cyanosis
- Edema
- Claudication

TABLE 10-1 Cardiovascular Signs and Symptoms by System

System	Symptom
General	Weakness Fatigue Weight change Poor exercise tolerance
Integumentary	Pressure ulcers Loss of body hair
Central nervous system	Headaches Impaired vision Dizziness or syncope
Respiratory	Labored breathing Productive cough
Cardiovascular	Chest pain Palpitations Edema Claudication
Genitourinary	Urinary frequency Nocturia Concentrated urine Decreased urinary output
Musculoskeletal	Myalgias Muscular fatigue Edema
Gastrointestinal	Nausea and vomiting

pulmonary conditions but may occur as a pulmonary complication of cardiovascular pathology. Left ventricular dysfunction, including mitral valve dysfunction as a result of pulmonary edema or left ventricular CHF, may result in a cough when aggravated by exercise, metabolic stress, supine position, or PND. The cough is often hacking and may be productive of large amounts of frothy, blood-tinged sputum. In the case of CHF, cough develops because a large amount of fluid is trapped in the pulmonary tree, irritating the lung mucosa.

Cyanosis is a bluish discoloration of the lips and nailbeds of the fingers and toes that accompanies inadequate blood oxygen levels (reduced amounts of hemoglobin). Although cyanosis can accompany cardiac, pulmonary, hematologic, or central nervous system (CNS) disorders, visible cyanosis most often accompanies cardiac and pulmonary problems.

Edema is the hallmark of right ventricular failure; it is usually bilateral and dependent and is accompanied by jugular venous distention (JVD), cyanosis (lips and appendages), and abdominal distention from ascites (see Fig. 14–7). Right upper quadrant pain, described as constant, aching, or sharp, may occur secondary to an enlarged liver with this condition. Right heart failure and subsequent edema can also occur as a result of cardiac surgery, venous valve incompetence or obstruction, cardiac valve stenosis, CAD, or mitral valve dysfunction. Noncardiac causes of edema may include pulmonary hypertension, kidney dysfunction, cirrhosis, burns, infection, lymphatic obstruction, or allergic reaction.

Claudication or leg pain occurs with peripheral vascular disease (PVD) (arterial or venous), often occurring simultaneously with CAD. Claudication can be more functionally debilitating than other associated symptoms, such as angina or dyspnea, and may occur in addition to these other symptoms. The presence of pitting edema along with leg pain is usually associated with vascular disease. Other noncardiac causes of leg pain (e.g., sciatica, pseudoclaudication,[2] anterior compartment syndrome, gout, peripheral neuropathy) must be differentiated from pain associated with PVD.

Special Implications for the Therapist **10–1**

SIGNS AND SYMPTOMS OF CARDIOVASCULAR DISEASE

(Cohen and Michel, 1988)

The evaluation and treatment of clients with cardiac symptoms described goes beyond the scope of this text, and the clinician is referred to any of the specific cardiopulmonary texts available. *Special implications* included in this chapter should be supplemented by other such materials. As a general guideline, the therapist monitors the unstable cardiac client (whether or not an initial ECG readout is available) during initial exercise to keep intensity lower than the threshold at which cardiac symptoms appear.

Cervical disk disease and arthritic changes can mimic atypical *chest pain* requiring screening for medical disease. However, pain of cardiac origin can be experienced in the shoulder because the heart (and diaphragm) are supplied by the C5–6 spinal segment, which refers visceral pain to the corresponding somatic area. Chest pain attributed to trigger points and other noncardiac causes are discussed in detail elsewhere (Goodman and Snyder, 1995).

Palpitations lasting for hours or occurring in association with pain, shortness of breath, fainting, or severe lightheadedness require medical evaluation. Palpitations in any person with a history of unexplained sudden death in the family require medical referral. Clients describing "palpitations" or similar phenomena may not be experiencing symptoms of heart disease. Palpitations can be considered physiologic (i.e., when fewer than 6 occur per minute, this may be considered within the normal function of the heart) or they may occur as a result of an overactive thyroid, secondary to caffeine sensitivity, as a side effect of some medications, and through the use of drugs such as cocaine. Encourage the client to report any such symptoms to the physician if this has not already been brought to the physician's attention.

Dyspnea may be a sign of poor physical conditioning, obesity, and asthma or allergies. Anyone who cannot climb a single flight of stairs without feeling moderately to severely winded or who awakens at night or experiences shortness of breath when lying down should be evaluated by a physician. Anyone with known cardiac involvement in whom progressively worse dyspnea develops must also notify the physician of these findings.

Dyspnea relieved by specific breathing patterns (e.g., pursed-lip breathing) or by specific body positions (e.g., leaning forward on arms to lock the shoulder girdle) is more likely to be pulmonary than cardiac in origin. Because breathlessness can be a terrifying experience, any activity that provokes the sensation is avoided, which quickly reduces functional activities. Pulmonary rehabilitation can favorably influence both exertional and clinically assessed dyspnea. The therapist is key in preventing this vicious circle and in delaying decline of function in the cardiopulmonary population (Reardon et al., 1994) (see Chapter 12).

Syncope without any warning period of lightheadedness, dizziness, or nausea may be a sign of heart valve or arrhythmia problems. Sudden death can occur; therefore, medical referral is recommended for any unexplained syncope, especially in the presence of heart or circulatory problems or if the client has any risk factors for heart attack or stroke. Examination of the cervical spine may include vertebral artery tests for compression of the vertebral arteries (see Aspinall, 1989; Magee, 1997; and Rivett, 1995, for specific test procedures).* If signs of eye nystagmus, changes in pupil size, or report of visual disturbances and symptoms of dizziness or lightheadedness occur, care must be taken with any subsequent treatment.

Fatigue beyond expectations during or after exercise, especially in a client with a known cardiac condition, must be closely monitored. It should be remembered

[2] Low back pain associated with *pseudoclaudication* often indicates spinal stenosis. The typical person affected is approximately 60 years old and bothered less by back pain than by a discomfort occurring in the buttock, thigh, or leg that (like true claudication) is brought on by walking but (unlike claudication) can also be elicited by prolonged standing. The discomfort associated with pseudoclaudication is frequently bilateral and improves with rest or with flexion of the lumbar spine (Hellman, 1994).

that β-blockers prescribed for cardiac problems can also cause unusual fatigue symptoms. For the client experiencing fatigue without a prior diagnosis of heart disease, monitoring vital signs may indicate a failure of the blood pressure to rise with increasing workloads. Such a situation may indicate inadequate cardiac output† to meet the demands of exercise. However, poor exercise tolerance is often the result of deconditioning, especially in the elderly population. Further testing (e.g., exercise treadmill test) may be helpful in determining whether fatigue is related to cardiac problems.

Edema in the form of a 3-lb or greater weight gain or gradual, continuous gain over several days with swelling of the ankles, abdomen, and hands, and shortness of breath, fatigue, and dizziness may be red flag symptoms of CHF. When such symptoms persist despite rest, medical referral is required. Edema of a cardiac origin may require ECG monitoring during exercise or activity (the physician may not want the client stressed when extensive ECG changes are present), whereas edema of peripheral origin requires treatment of the underlying cause.

Claudication may occur in the absence of physical findings, but it is usually accompanied by skin discoloration and trophic changes (e.g., thin, dry, hairless skin) in the presence of vascular disease. Core temperature, peripheral pulses, and skin temperature should be assessed. Cool skin is more indicative of vascular obstruction; warm to hot skin may indicate inflammation or infection. Abrupt onset of ischemic rest pain or sudden worsening of intermittent claudication may be due to thromboembolism and must be reported to the physician immediately.

If persons with intermittent claudication have normal-appearing skin at rest, exercising the extremity to the point of claudication usually produces marked pallor of the skin over the distal third of the extremity. This postexercise cutaneous ischemia occurs in both upper and lower extremities and is due to selective shunting of the available blood to the exercised muscle and away from the more distal parts of the extremity (Garrison, 1975).

* The effect of these tests, known as the *vertebral basal artery test, vertebral artery compression test, Wallenberg test,* or the *de Kleyn hanging head test,* on blood flow velocity was recently reviewed. It was suggested that other factors such as individual sensitivity to extreme head positions, age, and vestibular responsiveness could affect the results of this test for vertebral artery compression (Thiel et al., 1994).

† Cardiac output is the amount of blood that the heart is able to pump per minute and is directly affected by stroke volume (the amount the ventricle pumps out with each heartbeat) and the heart rate (the number of heartbeats per minute) (Grimes and Cohen, 1994).

AGING AND THE CARDIOVASCULAR SYSTEM

Cardiovascular disease, especially coronary atherosclerosis, is the most common cause of hospitalization and death in the elderly population in the United States. With the aging of America, by the year 2030, nearly 50% of all Americans will be 45 years old or older. By that time the number of people 65 years and older will more than double and the 85 years and older population is expected to triple (USDHHS, 1991). With this increase in a population of older persons, cardiovascular disease is likely to be even more of a major health problem in the future (Eaker et al., 1993).

Although the specific organ changes associated with aging are discussed here, disease and lifestyle may have a greater impact on cardiovascular function than aging. The heart itself undergoes some changes associated with advancing age, such as moderate thickening of the left ventricular wall (exaggerated in hypertensive clients) and increased left atrial size. Thickening of the cardiac tissue occurs as a result of myocyte enlargement or replacement by fibrous tissue but overall enlarging or atrophy of the aging heart is not representative of normative aging. Decreased ventricular filling compensated by increased systolic blood pressure occur as a result of the changes in the ventricular wall. Left ventricular functioning is compromised in the presence of stress such as vigorous exercise or disease. Arrhythmia or hypertension may occur as a result.

The vasculature changes with aging as the arterial walls stiffen with age and the aorta becomes dilated and elongated. Much controversy exists regarding the effects of normal aging on the cardiovascular system because of the presence of atherosclerosis in the majority of the elderly population. The incidence and severity of atherosclerosis does increase with aging, and this contributes to changes in vasculature function. Calcium deposition and changes in the amount and loss of elasticity in elastin and collagen most often affect the larger and medium-sized vessels (Lakatta, 1990; McCance and Richardson, 1994).

Resting cardiac function (e.g., cardiac output, heart rate) shows minimal age-related changes; a small increase in stroke volume may occur (Rodeheffer et al., 1984). Changes in functional capacity are more apparent during exercise than at rest. The maximum heart rate or the highest heart rate during exercise does decline with age, possibly because of a decreased cardiovascular response to catecholamines (see p. 342). The effect of the Frank-Starling mechanism[3] is unaltered with age and is used effectively during exercise to maintain cardiac output through a higher stroke volume (Weisfeldt et al., 1992).

Most researchers have reported a decline in maximum oxygen uptake, heart rate, and reduced maximal cardiac output with aging during exercise, even in athletes (Stratton et al., 1994; Weisfeldt et al., 1992). These cardiovascular alterations parallel changes that occur with deconditioning or disuse, including the decrease in maximal oxygen intake and maximal cardiac output. It has been hypothesized that these functions would normalize with increased activity (Bortz, 1982).

Significant cardiovascular improvements induced by training occur in both the young and the old supporting the hypothesis that age-related cardiovascular changes are simply the result of inactivity (Stratton et al., 1994). In older people,

[3] The Frank-Starling law states that the greater the myocardial fiber length (or stretch), the greater will be its force of contraction. The more the left ventricle fills with blood, the greater will be the quantity of blood ejected into the aorta. This is like a rubber band: the more it is stretched, the stronger it recoils or snaps back. Thus, a direct relationship exists between the volume of blood in the heart at the end of diastole (the length of the muscle fibers) and the force of contraction during the next systole.

aerobic exercise training lowers heart rate at rest, reduces levels of heart rate and plasma catecholamine levels at the same absolute submaximal workload, and, at least in men, improves left ventricular performance during peak exercise (Seals et al., 1994). It may be that the effect of training is relatively greater in older subjects.

DISEASES AFFECTING THE HEART MUSCLE

Ischemic Heart Disease

Coronary arteries carry oxygen to the myocardium. When these arteries become narrowed or blocked, the areas of the heart muscle supplied by that artery become ischemic and injured, and infarction may result. Major disorders of the myocardium owing to insufficient blood supply are collectively known as ischemic heart disease or CHD, also CAD.

Cardiovascular diseases continue to be the number one cause of death in the United States (see Table 2–1) accounting for 42% of the more than 2.2 million deaths in adults each year. Eleven million Americans who are alive today have a history of angina pectoris, myocardial infarction, or both. As many as 1.5 million Americans will have a myocardial infarction each year; a third of them will die (AHA, 1992). More than 750,000 persons annually experience significant cardiac symptoms as a result of CAD requiring surgical intervention for heart disease. Approximately 400,000 bypass procedures, 300,000 angioplasty operations, 58,000 repairs to damaged heart valves, and 2,000 heart transplants took place in 1991 (National Hospital Discharge Survey, 1991).

Non-atherosclerotic causes of coronary artery obstruction and subsequent ischemic heart disease (Box 10–2) are uncommon; each of these conditions is discussed more completely elsewhere in this chapter. Connective tissue disorders are associated with dissection of the coronary arteries (Andreoli et al., 1993). Radiotherapy for left-sided breast cancer may present as an independent risk factor in the long-term development (15 to 20 years after radiotherapy) of ischemic heart disease. There is a need to optimize adjuvant radiotherapy for early breast cancer by considering the dose both to the cancer as well as to the heart (Gyenes et al., 1994).

BOX 10–2
Nonatherosclerotic Causes of Coronary Artery Obstruction

- Kawasaki's disease
- Coronary embolism
  - Infective endocarditis
  - Prosthetic valves
  - Cardiac myxomas
  - Cardiopulmonary bypass
  - Coronary arteriography
- Syndrome X
- Insulin resistance syndrome (hyperinsulinemia)
- Trauma to coronary arteries
  - Penetrating
  - Nonpenetrating
- Arteritis
  - Syphilis
  - Polyarteritis nodosa
  - Lupus erythematosus
  - Rheumatoid arthritis
- Connective tissue diseases
- Radiotherapy

TABLE 10–2 Risk Factors and Coronary Artery Disease

Modifiable Risk Factors	Nonmodifiable Risk Factors	Contributing Factors
Physical inactivity	Age	Obesity
Cigarette smoking	Male sex	Discriminatory medicine
Elevated serum cholesterol	Family history	Response to stress
High blood pressure	Race	Personality
		Diabetes
		Hormonal status
		Alcohol consumption

Adapted from Reigle J, Ringel KA: Nursing care of clients with disorders of cardiac function. *In* Black JM, Matassarin-Jacobs E (eds): Luckmann and Sorensen's Medical-Surgical Nursing, ed 4. Philadelphia, WB Saunders, 1993, p 1140.

Arteriosclerosis

Arteriosclerosis represents a group of diseases characterized by thickening and loss of elasticity of the arterial walls, often referred to as "hardening of the arteries." Arteriosclerosis can be divided into three types: (1) *atherosclerosis*, in which plaques of fatty deposits form in the inner layer or intima of the arteries; (2) *Mönckeberg's arteriosclerosis*, involving the middle layer of the arteries with destruction of muscle and elastic fibers and formation of calcium deposits; and (3) *arteriolosclerosis* or *arteriolar sclerosis*, characterized by thickening of the walls of small arteries (arterioles) (O'Toole, 1992).

All three forms of arteriosclerosis may be present in the same person, but in different blood vessels. Frequently the terms arteriosclerosis and atherosclerosis are used interchangeably, although technically atherosclerosis is the most common form of arteriosclerosis.

Atherosclerosis *(O'Toole, 1992)*

Etiology and Risk Factors. In 1948, the US government decided to investigate the etiology, incidence, and pathology of CAD by studying residents of a typical small town in the United States, Framingham, Mass (O'Toole, 1992). Results from this ongoing research have identified important modifiable and nonmodifiable risk factors associated with death caused by coronary heart disease. Since that time, an additional category, *contributing factors*, has been added (Table 10–2). Three modifiable risk factors (cigarette smoking, high blood cholesterol levels, and high blood pressure) can be controlled, and many other risk factors can be managed (e.g., obesity, lack of exercise, diabetes, stress, and response to stress[4]). Some risk factors cannot be altered, such as age, sex, race, and family history of heart disease.

[4] One study has been published showing no correlation between heart disease and job stress, dispelling the presumption that the development of heart disease is related to job stress (Hlatky et al., 1995). Stress as a manageable risk factor may be further evaluated in future studies.

Modifiable Risk Factors. *Cigarette smoking* increases heart rate and blood pressure; decreases the oxygen-carrying capacity of blood; increases poisonous gases and elements of the blood such as carbon monoxide, cyanide, formaldehyde, and carbon dioxide; causes narrowing of blood vessels; and increases the work of the heart. Smoking enhances the process of atherosclerosis by a direct effect on the blood vessel wall, increasing the tendency for blood clot formation. People who quit smoking will lose their increased risk of heart attack (more than double that of a nonsmoker) in 24 months (Waller, 1989).

Elevated serum cholesterol levels (between 200 and 240 mg/dL) places a person at greater risk for heart disease; this risk doubles when cholesterol levels exceed 240 mg/dL and the ratio of total cholesterol to high-density lipoprotein (HDL) cholesterol is more than 4.0. Cholesterol levels are influenced by heredity, diet, exercise, heavy alcohol consumption, obesity, medications, menopausal status (Posner et al., 1993), and smoking.

High levels of triglycerides and low levels of HDL[5] produce twice as many cases of CAD as any other lipid abnormality. This trait is associated with increased insulin resistance (see syndrome X, later in this chapter), higher blood glucose levels, higher uric acid levels, hypertension, and obesity (Castelli, 1992). Clinical trials have demonstrated that therapy to lower low-density lipoprotein levels can delay progression of coronary stenosis and reduce recurrent cardiac episodes (Rosenson et al., 1994).

Hypertension, or high blood pressure, causes the heart to work harder and may injure the arterial walls, making them prone to atherosclerosis. Hypertension is aggravated by obesity and is associated with diabetes and regular alcohol use. It can be initiated or aggravated by the use of oral contraceptives, especially in women who smoke. Women who have undetected or uncontrolled hypertension are five times more likely to experience angina, heart attack, or sudden death than women with normal blood pressure (Kannel et al., 1993).

Physical inactivity or a sedentary lifestyle has not been established as a direct cause of CAD, but it has been observed that people who seldom exercise do not recover from heart attacks as quickly or as easily as do physically active people. The Centers for Disease Control and Prevention have proclaimed that inactivity is a major risk factor equal to cholesterol, cigarette smoking, and high blood pressure (CDC, 1987). Because a higher proportion of US adults lead a sedentary lifestyle (60%) than suffer from hypertension (10%), hypercholesterolemia (excessive cholesterol in the blood) (10%), or smoke a pack or more of cigarettes a day (18%), increasing the general population's physical activity level may have a greater effect on reducing the incidence of ischemic heart disease than the modification of the other three risk factors.

Regular aerobic exercise lowers resting pulse rate and blood pressure, improves the ratio of "good" to "bad" cholesterol, and helps prevent and control diabetes and osteoporosis (Diethrich and Cohen, 1992a). Possible mechanisms by which physical training can exert a favorable influence on the atherosclerotic or thrombotic processes are reviewed and are available for the interested reader (see Goldberg and Elliot, 1994a; Kavanagh, 1994).

Nonmodifiable Risk Factors. The risk of CAD increases with increasing age, and the person older than 40 years is more likely to become symptomatic. Sex as a nonmodifiable risk factor is reflected in the fact that heart disease is more prevalent among men; women generally develop CAD 10 years later than men and heart attacks another 10 years later, because of the "biologic protection factor" provided premenopausally by estrogen (Barrett-Conner and Bush, 1991; Colditz et al., 1987; Lobo, 1990). By age 45 years, heart disease affects 1 woman in 9. By age 65 years, this ratio becomes 1 in 3, more closely approximating rates among men (Lerner and Kannel, 1986; AHA, 1992). These statistics represent the outcome when no hormone replacement is initiated. (See also hormonal status in following text.)

A *family history* (i.e., one or more members of the immediate family) of cardiovascular disease is associated with increased incidence of heart disease. For selected individuals, genetic predisposition, especially abnormalities in lipoprotein metabolism, can play a very important role in their risk of development of atherosclerosis (Haskell and Durstine, 1993).

Certain *races* have a higher rate of heart disease. The risk of heart disease is higher among blacks, who are three times more likely to have extremely high blood pressure, a major risk factor for CAD. Native Americans have an unusually high rate of diabetes and obesity, although lower total and LDL cholesterol levels appear to offset the difference.

Contributing Factors. *Obesity* (see Chapter 2) alone can lead to CAD, as the excess weight makes the heart work harder to pump blood throughout the body. Obesity is commonly associated with diabetes mellitus, high blood pressure, and high fat (triglycerides and cholesterol) levels.

Emotional stress raises the heart rate and blood pressure, which takes some time to return to normal after the stress reaction subsides. The personality trait most likely to affect the heart is hostility associated with anger. The long-held belief that anger can be an immediate trigger of heart attacks has been verified in one study (Mittleman et al., 1994).[6] In addition to activating the "fight-or-flight" response of the sympathetic nervous system to perceived adversity, the calming response of the parasympathetic nervous system is weak in persons who are hostile. In these individuals, the parasympathetic counterbalance does not stop the effects of adrenaline on the heart. These emotions trigger the stress response, increasing blood pressure and heart rate and altering platelet function. Increasing evidence suggests that behavioral therapy may benefit cardiac clients by improving medical outcome (Ketterer, 1993; Ketterer et al., 1993; Williams and Williams, 1994). (See also Special Implications for the Therapist: Stress, Chapter 2.)

Discriminatory medicine is the idea that women are treated less aggressively than men for heart problems; this concept has been strongly debated. On the one hand, it has been

[5] Total cholesterol is broken into HDL, or "good" cholesterol, which carries cholesterol away from the cells, and low-density lipoprotein (LDL), or "bad" cholesterol, which carries cholesterol to the cells. Lipoproteins are complexes that help dissolve, transport, and utilize the cholesterol molecule. For reference values see Table 35–12.

[6] Although some studies have indicated that anger rather than competitiveness or time urgency is the "toxic" component of the so-called type A behavior that increases men's risk for heart attack, there is no evidence at this time that either anger or anxiety raises women's risk of CHD (Harvard Women's Health Letter, 1994).

suggested that a woman's symptoms are more likely to be misinterpreted, overlooked, or dismissed as psychosomatic, and that women are less likely to receive high-tech tests, such as angiograms (Diethrich and Cohen, 1992). On the other hand, lower rates of cardiac catheterization among women may be related to women's lower rate of positive exercise test results (Mark et al., 1994; 1991) and older age at time of symptomatic presentation rather than bias based on sex.

Diabetes (see also Chapter 9), when uncontrolled, creates excess blood glucose that can be transformed into triglycerides, which, along with cholesterol, promote the development of atherosclerosis. Kidney disease accompanied by hypertension is a serious complication affecting the cardiovascular system among people with diabetes. The incidence of cardiovascular disease among diabetic men is about twice that of nondiabetic men and about three times higher among diabetic women than nondiabetic women (Kannel and McGee, 1979). More than 80% of persons who have diabetes die of some form of cardiovascular disease.

Hormonal status in the menopausal or postmenopausal woman is now known to be a likely contributing risk factor in the development of CAD. The mechanism through which a protective effect is mediated by estrogen has not been explained completely. It is possible that estrogen exerts a beneficial effect on risk by lowering thrombotic tendency. Most recently, researchers have located estrogen receptors, molecules that attract and bind to that hormone, in the cells of the smooth muscle layer of blood vessels (Karas et al., 1994; Losordo et al., 1994). Atherosclerosis may develop because blood vessel cells cannot extract needed estrogen from the blood without the necessary receptors.

Exogenous (externally administered) estrogen has been reported to improve plasma lipid profiles (Vaziri et al., 1993; Walsh et al., 1991), carbohydrate metabolism (Barrett-Connor and Laakso, 1990; Busby et al., 1992), and vascular reactivity (Clarkson et al., 1993; Collins et al., 1993), but the benefits expected from these changes do not fully account for the marked decrease in cardiovascular disease that has been observed. Understanding the effects of estrogen in the development of cardiovascular disease in postmenopausal women may change this risk factor through the use of hormone replacement therapy (Nabulsi et al., 1993). The use of estrogen for postmenopausal replacement therapy almost never raises the blood pressure, so the concerns about hypertension associated with hormone replacement should not interfere with the use of this therapy (Kaplan, 1995).

There has been some indication that moderate *alcohol consumption* decreases the risk of heart disease because of an associated elevated level of an enzyme called tissue-type plasminogen activator, or t-PA, which helps to keep blood flowing smoothly by dissolving clots (Beilin et al., 1996; Seigneur, 1990). The highest levels of endogenous t-PA antigen have been found among daily consumers of alcohol, and the lowest levels were found among subjects who never (or rarely) consumed alcohol (Ridker et al., 1994).[7]

However, in concentrations equal to 2 to 4 glasses of beer, alcohol causes direct coronary artery constriction (Morley and Bove, 1990). This vasoconstriction may explain the relationship between ethanol and sudden coronary ischemia that is seen clinically. Additionally, the depressive effect of excessive alcohol on the function of myocardial cells decreases myocardial contractility and can be very disabling. Chronic abuse of alcohol is also related to a higher incidence of hypertension, which places greater stress on a heart already compromised by CAD (Miller and Morley, 1993). Chemical dependency is also associated with increased stress on the diseased heart.

Pathogenesis. In the normal artery, the endothelial lining is tightly packed with cells that allow for the smooth passage of blood and act as a protective covering against harmful substances circulating in the bloodstream. In the earliest stage of atherosclerosis, fatty streaks form along the intima; these are widely scattered at first, but as the disease progresses they become more numerous and can eventually cover the entire intimal surface of an artery (Fig. 10–2).

The exact mechanism by which the development of CAD can be explained has yet to be determined. In general, most of the current theories include the following major events in the development of an atherosclerotic plaque (Haskell and Durstine, 1993; Weschler, 1991): *Arterial wall damage* occurs either from injury caused by harmful substances in the blood or by physical wear and tear as a result of high blood pressure. This injury to the blood vessel wall permits the *infiltration* of macromolecules (especially cholesterol) from blood through the damaged endothelium to the underlying smooth muscle cells. Naked collagen acts like fly-paper for platelets, causing them to aggregate at the site of injury and plug up the wound. Although platelet activation is a normal response to injury, in atherosclerosis, once they adhere, platelets also release chemicals that alter the structure of the blood vessel wall, so that what starts out as a small erosion in the wall can end up a swollen mound of platelets, muscle cells, and fibrous clots (coronary thrombosis), called *proliferation*, which obstructs the flow of blood through the vessel. This cycle of injury, platelet activation, and lipid deposition can lead to complete blockage of a vessel and result in *ischemia* and *necrosis* of tissue supplied by the obstructed blood vessel.

Clinical Manifestations. Atherosclerosis by itself does not necessarily produce symptoms. For manifestations to develop, there must be a critical deficit in blood supply to the heart. Often symptoms of CAD do not appear until the lumen of the coronary artery narrows by 75% (Reigle and Ringel, 1993). Pain and dysfunction referable to the region supplied by an occluded artery may occur. When atherosclerosis develops slowly, collateral circulation develops to meet the heart's needs.

Complications from CAD occur because it is a progressive disorder, which results in more severe cardiac disease if it is not prevented or untreated. Common sequelae of CAD include peripheral vascular disease, angina pectoris, MI or heart attack, or sudden death. Additionally, heart failure, conduction disturbances, chronic arrhythmias, aneurysm, and intestinal infarction may occur.

Medical Management

Diagnosis. Studies to determine the site and extent of necrosis associated with CAD include laboratory analysis to

[7] Although a small amount of daily alcohol taken with meals may elevate levels of HDL cholesterol, most researchers oppose recommending drinking as a public health measure to fight heart disease, and stress that no one, particularly people with a personal or family history of alcohol abuse, should drink alcohol to improve cholesterol. It should always be remembered that heavy alcohol consumption and binge drinking increase risk of blood clot formation, cardiac arrhythmia, elevated blood pressure, and cardiovascular disease.

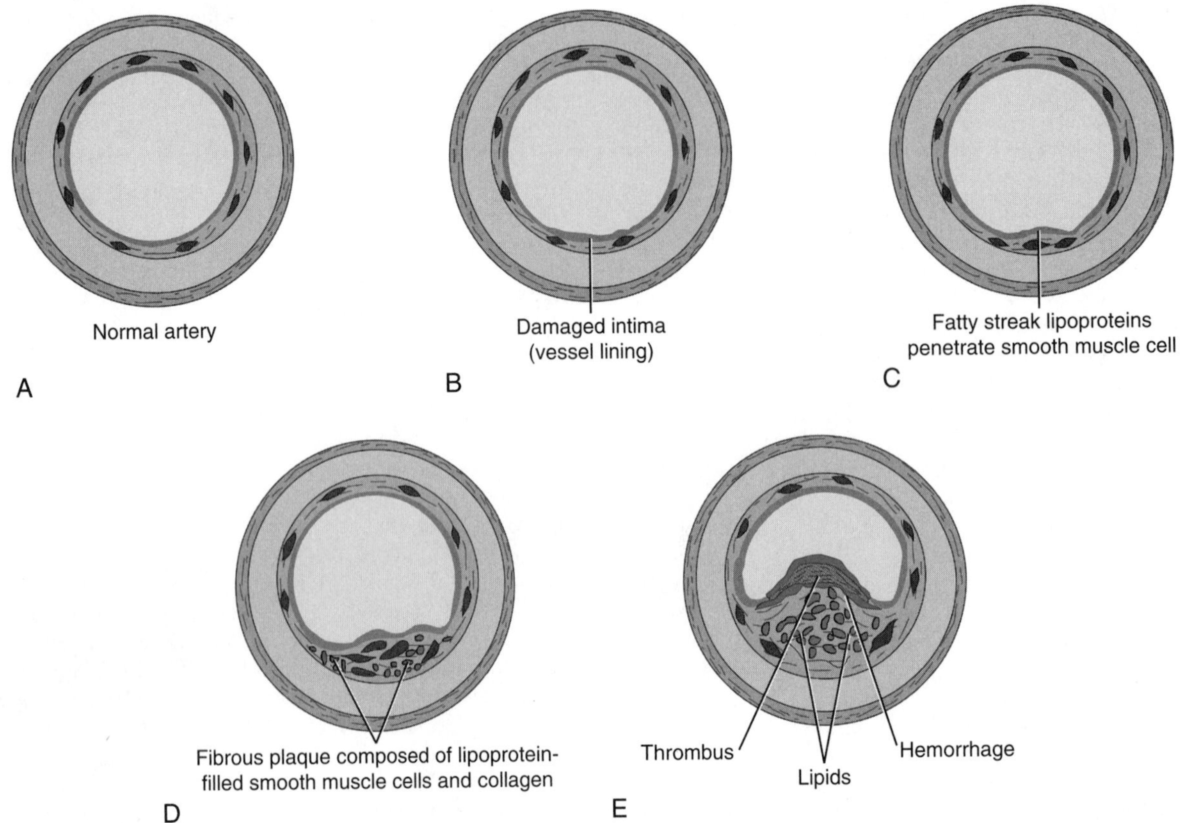

Figure **10–2.** A, Cross section of a normal artery. *B*, Atherosclerosis begins with an injury to the endothelial lining of the artery (intimal layer) that makes the vessel permeable to circulating lipoproteins. C, Penetration of lipoproteins into the smooth muscle cells of the intima produces "fatty streaks." *D*, A fibrous plaque large enough to decrease blood flow through the artery develops. *E*, Calcification with rupture or hemorrhage of the fibrous plaque is the final advanced stage. Thrombosis may occur, further occluding the lumen of the blood vessel.

evaluate elevation of certain enzyme levels (creatine kinase [CK], aspartate aminotransferase [AST], alanine aminotransferase [ALT], lactic dehydrogenase [LDH]) ECG, nuclear scanning, and angiography (see Chapter 35, Tables 35–13 to 35–15). Serum cholesterol must be determined because of its importance as a modifiable risk factor.

Coronary arteriography is the most reliable anatomic test to assess the degree of obstructive coronary disease and left ventricular contractility. Advances are being made in nonangiographic means of demonstrating coronary artery morphology, such as magnetic resonance angiography (Reagan et al., 1994).

The standard exercise stress test has now been compared with variance cardiography, a new, higher-resolution ECG that is a noninvasive, stress-free (administered at rest) method of identifying CAD with equally accurate results in men and women (Nowak et al., 1993; Sylven et al., 1994). Another procedure, exercise echocardiography, has been reported to be more accurate in detecting heart disease in women than in men and as compared with angiography, thallium exercise testing, and exercise ECG (Anderson et al., 1995).

Treatment. Whenever possible, prevention of CAD is the goal for persons with a high risk profile. Fatty streaks consisting of lipid-laden macrophages, T lymphocytes, and smooth-muscle cells are capable of regressing and disappearing entirely before progressing to form a fibrous plaque if cholesterol and fat intake are reduced (Ross, 1994; Wissler and Vesselinovitch, 1976). Modifying risk factors whenever possible can also decrease the risk of CAD, especially cessation of cigarette smoking, controlling diet, and managing diabetes and hypertension. Pharmacologic management is used to reduce the risk of clotting, to treat hypertension, and to decrease serum cholesterol level when it exceeds 200 mg/dL.

Treatment is directed toward the specific blood vessel occlusion and is dependent on complications, for example, occlusive disease of the peripheral vasculature, arterial disease in diabetic clients, occlusive cerebrovascular disease, or visceral artery insufficiency (intestinal ischemia) (see discussion of each individual complication).

Surgical management of atherosclerosis of the coronary arteries may include percutaneous transluminal coronary angioplasty (PTCA) (Fig. 10–3), coronary artery bypass graft (CABG, pronounced *cabbage*) (Fig. 10–4), and most recently, coronary stents (Figs. 10–5 and 10–6). Approximately 30% of persons undergoing angioplasty or bypass surgery require repeated procedures within 3 years for restenosis; stents have reduced the need for repeat surgery (Fischman et al., 1994; Goldberg, 1994).

Other newer surgical techniques such as arthrectomy (similar to angioplasty, but plaque is removed instead of compressed) and the use of laser-assisted balloon angioplasty

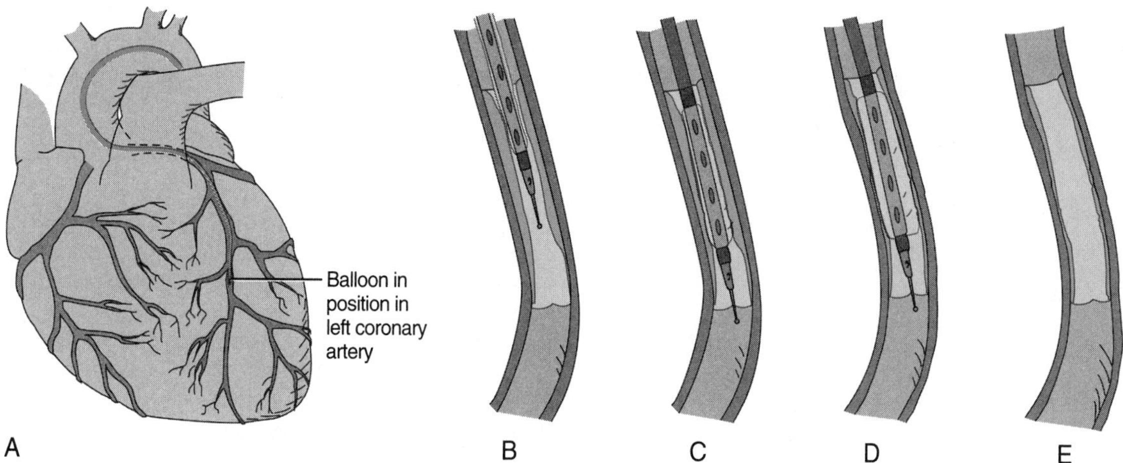

Figure **10–3.** Percutaneous transluminal coronary angioplasty (PTCA) can open an occluded coronary artery without opening the chest, an important advantage over bypass surgery. *A*, Once coronary angiography has been performed to determine the presence and location of an arterial occlusion, a guide catheter is threaded through the femoral artery into the left coronary artery. *B*, When the angiography shows the guide catheter positioned at the site of occlusion, the uninflated balloon is centered in the obstruction. *C*, A smaller double-lumen balloon catheter is inserted through the guide catheter. *D*, The balloon is inflated and deflated until the angiogram confirms arterial dilation with a reduced pressure gradient in the vessel. *E*, The balloon is removed and the artery is left unoccluded.

(LABA, a laser beam at the tip of a catheter), show promise for the future but carry higher rates of major complications, especially for women (Casale, 1993; Elliott et al., 1995). Intravascular ultrasound, a technology that combines echo with catheterization, may eventually allow diagnosis and therapy to be combined as the cardiologist uses a camera on the tip of a catheter to precisely target atherosclerotic blockage.

Although surgical intervention has been a mainstay for the treatment of CAD (see statistics in incidence earlier in this section), researchers are questioning the necessity of heart surgery and studying the benefits of pharmacologic treatment combined with exercise and lifestyle changes. Results from the Stanford Coronary Risk Intervention Project (SCRIP) conducted over 4 years have demonstrated that

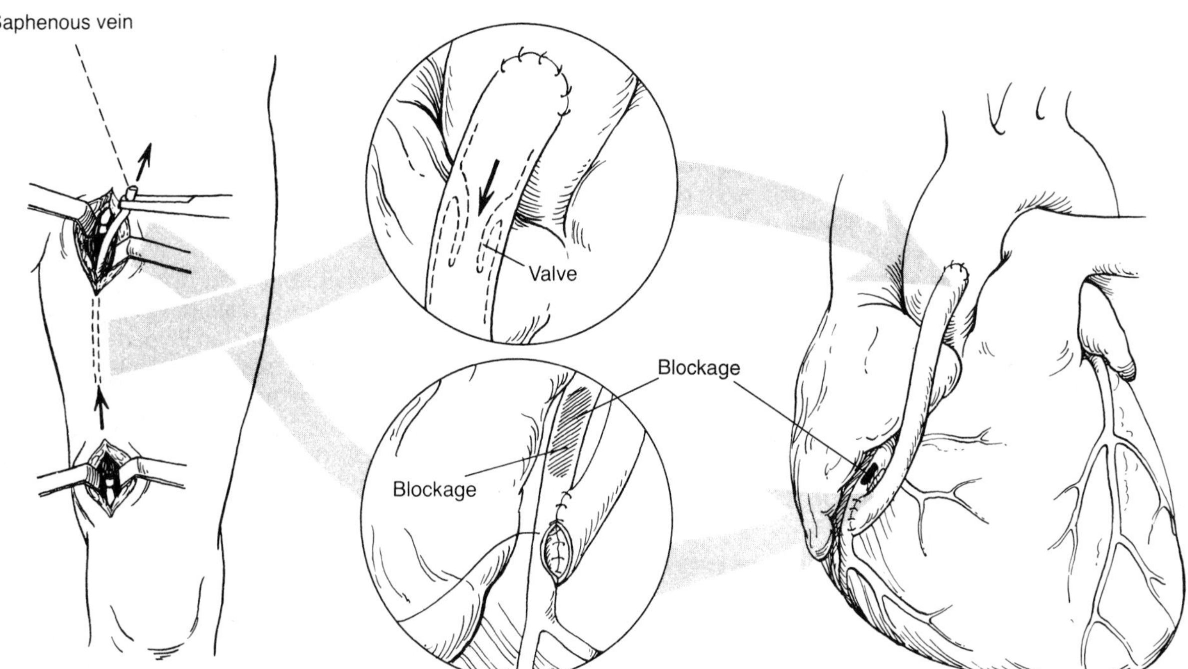

Figure **10–4.** Coronary bypass surgery. This procedure uses a section of the saphenous vein as a graft to route blood around areas of blockage. Bypassing the clogged vessel provides an alternative route for blood to reach the heart muscle. The internal mammary artery can be used as an alternate vein site for grafting. (*From Black JM, Matassarin-Jacobs E (eds): Luckmann and Sorensen's Medical-Surgical Nursing, ed 4. Philadelphia, WB Saunders, 1993, p 1145.*)

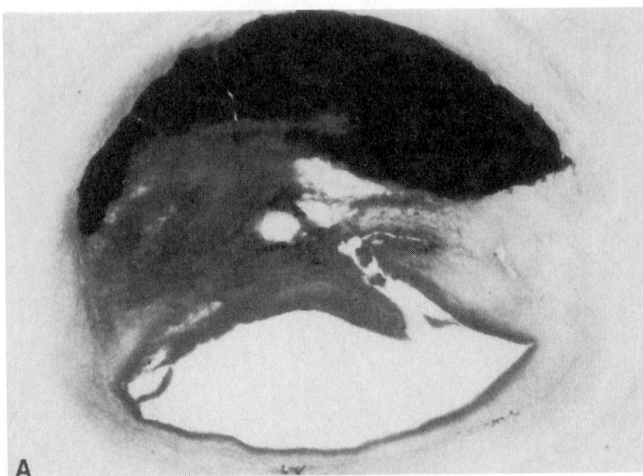

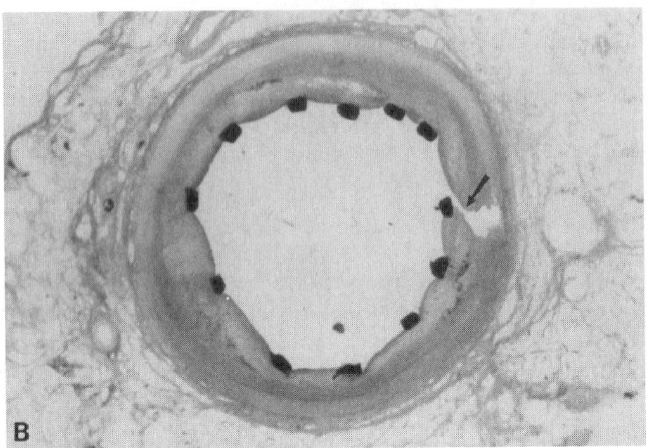

Figure **10–5.** A, Cross section of a severely occluded coronary artery. B, Stent in place to maintain opened vessel allowing blood to pass through freely. (*Courtesy of Thomas Jefferson University, Philadelphia.*)

intensive multifactor risk reduction favorably alters the rate of luminal narrowing in coronary arteries of men and women with coronary artery disease and decreases hospitalizations for clinical cardiac events (Haskell et al., 1994). Other ongoing investigations of postinfarction survival include the International Study of Infarct Survival (ISIS) and Thrombolysis in Myocardial Infarction (TIMI).

Numerous other trials (e.g., Leiden Intervention Trial, Heidelberg Diet and Exercise Study, St. Thomas' Atherosclerosis Regression Study, Cholesterol Lowering Atherosclerosis Study [CLAS]) have focused on the effect of diet-induced reductions in LDL cholesterol and the resultant changes in CAD. Restricting the intake of saturated fat and cholesterol has a favorable result in changing the course of coronary atherosclerosis. In addition, dietary and lifestyle interventions slowed CAD progression, decreased the incidence and severity of angina, and reduced the number of cardiac events. The effect of exercise alone without dietary changes was not evaluated (Rosenson, 1994).

Prognosis. Fatality rates for CHD remain low before age 35 years, but these figures increase exponentially until age 75 years, with men generally experiencing mortality at approximately twice the rate of women *until* age 65 years. Total CHD mortality in women *after* age 65 years now exceeds that of men (CDC, 1989).

Prognosis depends on the site and extent of necrosis, but nearly 500,000 deaths each year in the United States are attributable to CAD. Of the nearly 20,000 persons eligible for heart transplants, only 2,000 a year receive a new heart. Advanced atherosclerosis is usually fatal if vessels to the brain or heart are affected. Use of the balloon-expandable stent is associated with a low restenosis rate and a favorable clinical outcome with event-free survival rate at 1 year. The need for repeat revascularization is also significantly reduced (Fenton et al., 1994; Savage et al., 1994).

Although surgical procedures are considered safe, complications can occur, and women are at greater risk for complica-

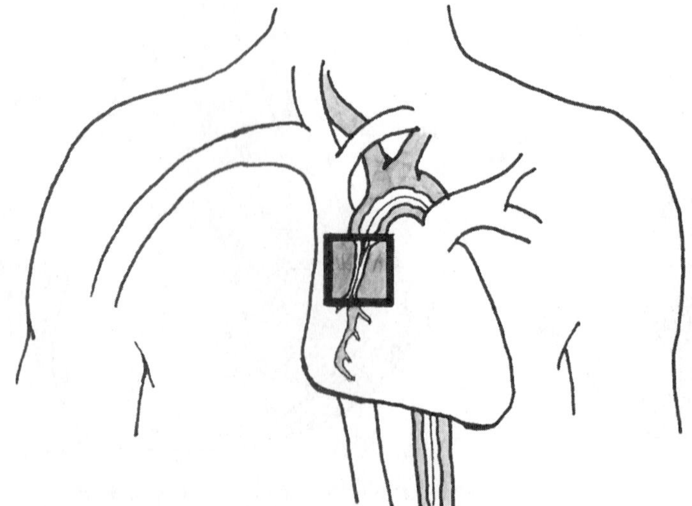

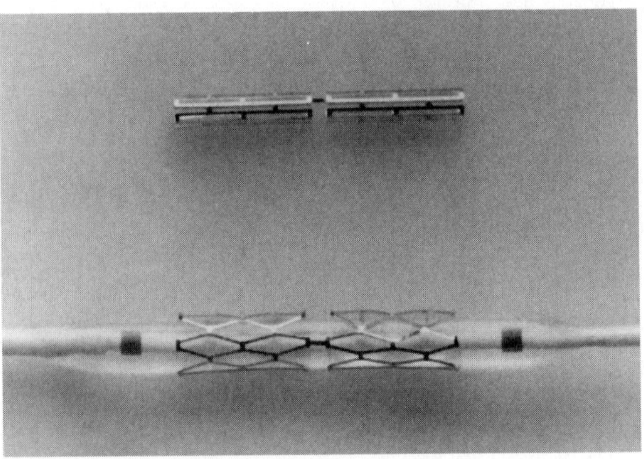

Figure **10–6.** Blocked coronary artery can be held open using a balloon-expandable device called a coronary stent. (*Courtesy of Thomas Jefferson University, Philadelphia.*)

tions and have a higher mortality rate. Most studies attribute the higher mortality rate to the fact that they more often undergo the surgery during an emergency, they are usually older at the time of diagnosis than men, they are more likely to have other complicating conditions (e.g., hypertension or diabetes), and they may have smaller, more delicate coronary arteries, making surgery more difficult (Elefteriades, 1993).

Special Implications for the Therapist **10-2**

CORONARY ARTERY DISEASE (ATHEROSCLEROSIS)

Postoperative Considerations

Chest physical therapy is recommended routinely for persons who have had abdominal or cardiothoracic surgery, but the efficacy of chest physical therapy for reducing complications after coronary artery surgery has been repeatedly studied and has not been proved. It has been suggested that postoperative chest physical therapy should be limited to clients with postsurgical complications. The necessity for prophylactic chest physical therapy after routine coronary artery surgery should be reviewed further (Stiller et al., 1994).

Home monitoring of symptoms for the first 5 to 6 weeks after surgery is essential (Box 10–3). Discharge instructions for the cardiovascular surgical population may vary according to physician and institution, but some general guidelines apply (Box 10–4).

Exercise

People recovering from cardiac surgery, despite an excellent hemodynamic result, may be disabled by persistent left ventricular hypertrophy and years of presurgical restricted activity and deconditioning. Exercise rehabilitation is an important part of the recovery process (Carstens et al., 1983; Newell, 1980). Easy fatigability related to muscular weakness lessens with increased physical activity. Exercise-induced symptoms of angina and light-headedness or syncope disappear immediately after surgery with a successful result.

The exercise capacity of clients soon after MI and bypass surgery is determined by the same parameters as in healthy individuals or for other cardiac problems, including time since MI, age, physical training status, and amount of myocardial dysfunction that occurs with exercise. CNS dysfunction (e.g., impaired cognition) is a common consequence of otherwise uncomplicated surgery that may affect exercise capacity. As yet, the cause of this neurologic phenomenon has not been

BOX **10-3**

Home Monitoring After Cardiovascular Surgery

The physician should be contacted if the client experiences one or more of these symptoms:

- Sudden shortness of breath
- Palpitations (>6/min)
- Increased swelling of the feet and ankles
- Chest pain unrelated to the chest incision
- Fever ≥100°F
- Persistent drainage or change in drainage from any incision
- Increased swelling, tenderness, and redness around any of the incision areas
- Dizziness
- Change in pulse of >20 beats/min (unrelated to exercise)
- Extreme tiredness or weakness
- Weight gain of 3 lb/day for 2–3 days
- No improvement in client condition

Adapted from Lawrence KE, Eutsey DE: Cardiovascular Patient Education Resource Manual: Exercise and Physical Fitness. 4:15. Gaithersburg, Md, Aspen, 1994.

BOX **10-4**

Discharge Instructions after Cardiovascular Surgery

Showers: Permitted 10 days after surgery. Avoid tub baths or soaking in water until incisions are healed; avoid extremely hot water

Incisions: The incision should be kept dry but can be gently washed with mild soap and warm water (directly over the tapes); lotions, creams, oils, or powders are not permitted until the wound is completely healed unless prescribed by the physician

Care of surgical leg (for bypass graft involving the leg): Avoid crossing the legs, which impairs circulation; avoid sitting in one position or standing for prolonged periods. Elevate the involved leg when sitting or lying down. Swelling should decrease after leg elevation but may recur when standing. Progressive edema must be reported to the physician

Elastic stockings: Worn for at least 2 wk after discharge during the daytime and removed at bedtime

Rest: A balance of rest and exercise is an essential part of the recovery process. Resting between activities and short naps are encouraged. Resting may include sitting quietly or reading for 20 to 30 min

Walking: Walking increases circulation throughout the body and to the heart muscle and is encouraged. Activity must be increased gradually. Pacing of activities throughout the day, combined with energy conservation, is important

Stairs: Climbing stairs is permitted unless the physician indicates otherwise

Sexual relations: Sexual relations can be resumed when the client feels physically comfortable (usually 2 to 4 wk after discharge; see also text discussion)

Driving: Driving, outdoor bicycling, or motorcycle riding is not permitted for 6 wk after surgery to protect the sternum and to allow time for the bone to heal. Riding as a passenger in an automobile is permitted

Lifting: Pressure or strain on the sternum must be avoided. Preventing separation of the sternum may require handheld assistance in place of assistive devices (e.g., walker, quad cane) during early postoperative recovery. Lifting, pushing, or pulling is restricted to anything under 10 lb for 6 wk after surgery. For example, this includes avoiding lifting or carrying children, groceries, suitcases; mowing the grass; vacuuming; and moving furniture

Stop any activity immediately if dyspnea, palpitations, chest pain or discomfort, or dizziness or fainting develop. Notify the physician if symptoms do not subside with rest in 20 min.

Adapted from Lawrence KE, Eutsey DE: Cardiovascular Patient Education Resource Manual: Postsurgical Concerns. 3:52–53. Gaithersburg, Md, Aspen Publications, 1994.

determined. It is known that increased age is a predisposing factor in the decline in cognitive function, but impaired cognition following surgery is not associated with age-related changes in cerebral blood flow autoregulation or the effects of mean arterial pressure during the procedure. Hypotension and rapid rewarming after cardiac surgery in the elderly may be key components (Newman et al., 1994; 1995a).

Specific exercise considerations following CABG surgery are available (see Haskell and Durstine, 1993). A program to increase the strength and flexibility of the pectoral and leg muscles should be performed. Special exercises to improve chest wall function include deep breathing, shoulder shrugs and adduction, arm circles and lifts, trunk motion, and wall pushups. During this time, elastic stockings are usually worn to prevent fluid accumulation at the site of the leg incisions (Haskell and Durstine, 1993).

Regular dynamic exercise is considered adjunctive therapy for lipid management along with dietary management and reduction of excess weight. The benefits of participation in a program of endurance-type training for persons with CAD is well known. Both short- and long-term endurance exercise can contribute to an improvement in blood lipid abnormalities (Leon, 1993; Leighton, 1997). Resistive exercise training has been reported to raise HDL cholesterol levels in some, but not all, studies (Goldberg, 1989; Wood et al., 1988).

The increased risk that exercise may precipitate cardiovascular complications and silent symptoms of ischemia, arrhythmias, abnormal blood pressure, and heart responses to exercise and fatigue necessitate special considerations for the formulation and execution of physical conditioning programs. Specific exercise and training guidelines are available (Goldberg and Elliot, 1994b; Haskell and Durstine, 1993; Hillegass and Sadowsky, 1994). Indications for stopping an exercise test can be used as precautions during therapy or exercise (Table 10–3; see also Box 10–7). Therapists in all settings are encouraged to read the complete American Heart Association *Exercise Standards* (Fletcher et al., 1990).

TABLE 10-3 Indications for Discontinuing or Modifying Exercise

Symptoms
New-onset anginal chest pain
Easily provoked angina
Increasing episodes, intensity, or duration of angina (unstable angina)
Discomfort in the upper body, including chest, arm, neck, or jaw
Fainting or lightheadedness
Severe dyspnea
Severe fatigue or muscle pain
Nausea or vomiting
Back pain during exercise
Bone or joint pain or discomfort during or after exercise
Severe leg claudication
Clinical Signs
Pallor; peripheral cyanosis; cold, moist skin
Staggering gait, ataxia
Confusion or blank stare in response to inquiries
Resting heart rate >130 beats/min, <40 beats/min
More than 6 arrhythmias (irregular heart beats) per hour
Uncontrolled diabetes mellitus (blood glucose >250 mg/dL)
Oxygen saturation <85% (98% is normal)
Acute infection or fever >100° F
Inability to converse during activity
Blood pressure (BP) abnormalities
Fall in systolic BP with increase in workload; specifically, a decrease of 10 mm Hg or more below any previously recorded BP accompanied by other signs or symptoms
Rise in systolic blood pressure above 250 mm Hg or diastolic pressure above 120 mm Hg
Other
Person indicates need or desire to stop

From Fletcher GF, Froelicher VG, Hartley H et al: AHA Medical/Scientific Statement. Exercise standards: A statement for health professionals from the American Heart Association. Circulation 82:2286, 1990.

Monitoring During Exercise

More than half of all ischemic episodes are not accompanied by angina. Ask any client with CAD or CAD risk factors to report all unusual sensations, not just episodes of chest pain or discomfort. Exercise testing should be performed before beginning an exercise program, but if this has not been accomplished and baseline measurements are unavailable for use in planning exercise, monitor the heart rate and blood pressure and note any accompanying symptoms during exercise (see Appendix B).

Almost all antihypertensive agents, including diuretics that may have a dual action of peripheral dilatation and volume depletion, can have a profound effect on postexercise blood pressure (Miller and Morley, 1993). In some healthy people, when exercise is terminated abruptly, precipitous drops in systolic blood pressure can occur owing to venous pooling. Some people with CAD have higher levels of systolic blood pressure that exceed peak exercise values; a proper cooldown after vigorous exercise is important to prevent such an occurrence (Fletcher et al., 1990).

Several drugs used in the treatment of CAD are known to alter the heart rate. For example β-adrenergic blocking agents used in the treatment of angina and hypertension cause a reduction in resting and exercise heart rate. Anyone taking these medications may not be able to achieve a target heart rate above 90 beats/min. A safe rate of exercise will allow the heart rate to return to the resting level 2 minutes after stopping exercise. Avoid increases of more than 20 beats/min over the resting rate.

More detailed information on the effects of various drugs on the exercise response during training in clients with CAD can be found in *Exercise Guidelines for Exercise Testing and Prescription* by the American College of Sports Medicine (ACSM, 1995).

Angina Pectoris

Definition and Incidence. As blood vessels become obstructed by the formation of atherosclerotic plaque, the blood supply to tissues supplied by these vessels becomes restricted. When the cardiac workload exceeds the oxygen supply to myocardial tissue, ischemia occurs, causing temporary chest pain or discomfort, called *angina pectoris*. The exact incidence of angina is unknown, though it is considered common, especially in people aged 65 years and older, and occurs more often in men.

Overview. There are several types of anginal pain (Box 10–5). *Chronic stable angina*, classified as classic, exertional angina, occurs at predictable levels of physical or emotional stress and responds promptly to rest or to nitroglycerin. No pain occurs at rest and the location, duration, intensity, and frequency of chest pain are consistent over time (60 days). *New onset* describes angina that has developed for the first time within the last 60 days. *Nocturnal angina* may awaken a person from sleep with the same sensation experienced during exertion. During sleep, this type of angina is associated with exertion, usually caused by increased heart rate associated with dreams or in response to underlying CHF.

Postinfarction angina occurs after MI when residual ischemia triggers an episode of angina. *Preinfarction angina* or *unstable angina*, also known as *progressive angina* or *crescendo angina*, is unpredictable and is characterized by an abrupt change (increase) in the intensity and frequency of symptoms or decreased threshold of stimulus. This angina lasts longer than 15 minutes and is a symptom of worsening cardiac ischemia.

Prinzmetal's, *vasospastic*, or *variant angina* produces symptoms similar to those of typical angina, but it is caused by coronary artery spasm. These spasms periodically squeeze arteries shut and keep the blood from reaching the heart. In this type of angina, coronary arteries are usually clear of plaque or free of physiologic changes that cause obstruction of the vessels. The pattern of Prinzmetal's angina is characterized by early morning occurrence, frequently at the same time each day, and it occurs at rest (i.e., it is unrelated to exertion). Prinzmetal's angina is more common in women younger than 50 years; it is often associated with various types of arrhythmias or conduction effects (Sokolow et al., 1990).

Decubitus or *resting angina* is considered atypical; it occurs most often among the elderly when at rest and frequently occurs at the same time every day. This type of anginal chest pain is atypical in that it is paroxysmal in nature, not brought on by exercise, and not relieved by rest, but it is reduced when the person sits or stands up.

Syndrome X is an unusual form of ischemic heart disease used to describe *microvascular angina* or angina without obvious coronary atherosclerosis (Drexler and Schroeder, 1994). It is more prevalent among women, particularly those who have undergone hysterectomy.[8] Microvascular angina associated with syndrome X affects the microcirculatory system, a network of tiny blood vessels that branch from the large coronary vessels and that provide oxygen to each of the millions of myocardial cells. Why these vessels spasm and cause decreased blood flow remains undetermined; the cause may be a decrease in estrogen during menopause or a specific trigger from within the heart.

Syndrome X is sometimes referred to as the insulin resistance syndrome, characterized by a constellation of interrelated CHD risk factors, including dyslipidemia (improper lipids[9]), obesity, elevated systolic blood pressure, and hyperinsulinemia (excess insulin in the blood) (Edwards et al., 1994; Reaven, 1994; Wajchenberg et al., 1994; Williams, 1994). There may be some overlap between syndrome X (microvascular angina) and insulin resistance syndrome (also called hyperinsulinemia syndrome), but they are two separate entities.

BOX 10–5
Types of Angina Pectoris

- Chronic (stable) angina
- New-onset angina
- Nocturnal angina
- Postinfarction angina
- Preinfarction angina (unstable)
- Prinzmetal's (variant) angina
- Resting angina (decubitus)

TABLE 10–4 Causes of Myocardial Ischemia

Decreased Oxygen Supply	Increased Oxygen Demand
Vessels	
Atherosclerotic narrowing	Hyperthyroidism
Inadequate collateral circulation	Arteriovenous fistula
Spasm due to smoking, emotion, or cold	Thyrotoxicosis
Coronary arteritis	Exercise/exertion
Hypertension	Emotion/excitement
Hypertrophic cardiomyopathy	Digestion of large meal
Circulatory Factors	
Arrhythmias (↓ blood pressure)	
Aortic stenosis	
Hypotension	
Bleeding	
Blood Factors	
Anemia	
Hypoxemia	
Polycythemia (↑ viscosity)	

From Goodman CC, Snyder TE: Differential Diagnosis in Physical Therapy, ed 2. Philadelphia, WB Saunders, 1995, p 88.

Etiology and Risk Factors. Any condition that alters the blood (oxygen) supply or demand of the myocardium can cause ischemia (Table 10–4). Increased oxygen needs of the heart, increased cardiac output, or reduced blood flow to the heart can cause angina. CAD accounts for 90% of all cases

[8] This includes a total abdominal hysterectomy (TAH) or TAH with bilateral salpingo-oophorectomy (BSO).

[9] Dyslipidemias constitute elevations of LDL cholesterol (hypercholesterolemia) as well as abnormalities in the metabolism of triglyceride-rich lipoproteins (hypertriglyceridemia) and lipoprotein (hypoalphalipoproteinemia) (Rosenson et al., 1994).

of angina, although other conditions affecting normal vessels can also cause angina. Disorders of circulation, such as relative hypotension secondary to spinal anesthesia, antihypertensive drugs, or blood loss, can also result in decreased blood return to the heart and subsequent ischemic pain.

Four known triggers are associated with the onset of angina: (1) vigorous exercise or exertion, especially involving thoracic or upper extremity muscles or walking rapidly uphill (Mittleman et al., 1993); (2) exposure to cold or wind; (3) psychological or emotional stress; or (4) a large meal (or any of these in combination). The threshold for angina is often lower in the morning or after strong emotion; the latter can provoke attacks in the absence of exertion. Angina may also occur less commonly during sexual activity, at rest, or at night during sleep (Massie, 1994).

Pathogenesis. Angina is a symptom of ischemia usually brought on by an imbalance between cardiac workload and oxygen supply to myocardial tissue usually secondary to coronary artery disease (see previous discussion on pathogenesis of atherosclerosis). Platelet aggregations associated with atherosclerosis release prostaglandin, which is capable of causing vessel spasm and can create a repeated cycle of spasm and pain.

Myocardial pain occurs as a result of metabolites within the ischemic segment of the myocardium. Buildup of lactic acid or abnormal stretching of the myocardium irritates myocardial fibers. These afferent sympathetic fibers enter the spinal cord from levels C3 to T4 (Fig. 10–7), accounting for the variety and locations and radiation pattern of anginal pain (Haak et al., 1994). The effects of temporary ischemia are reversible; if blood flow is restored, no permanent damage or necrosis of the heart muscle occurs.

Clinical Manifestations. Angina is characterized by temporary pain or, more often, discomfort that starts suddenly in the chest (substernal or retrosternal) and sometimes radiates to other parts of the body, most commonly to the left shoulder and down the ulnar border of the arm to the fingers. Pain or discomfort may also be referred to any dermatome from C3 to T4, presenting at the back of the neck, lower jaw, teeth, left upper back, interscapular area, the abdomen, occasionally, and possibly down the right arm (Fig. 10–8).

The sensation described is often referred to as "squeezing," "burning," "pressing," "heartburn," "indigestion," or "choking." It is usually mild to moderate (rarely reported as severe); it usually lasts 1 to 3 minutes, sometimes 3 to 5 minutes, but can persist up to 15 to 20 minutes following a heavy meal, extreme anger, or in association with unstable angina. Symptoms are usually relieved by rest or nitroglycerin.

Recognizing symptoms of myocardial ischemia in women is more difficult, as the symptoms are less reliable and do not follow the classic pattern described. Many women describe the pain in ways consistent with unstable angina, suggesting that they first become aware of their chest discomfort or have it diagnosed only after it reaches more advanced stages. Some experience a sensation similar to that of inhaling cold air, rather than the more typical shortness of breath. Other women notice only weakness and lethargy, and some have observed isolated pain in the midthoracic spine or throbbing and aching in the right biceps muscle (Diethrich and Cohen, 1992).

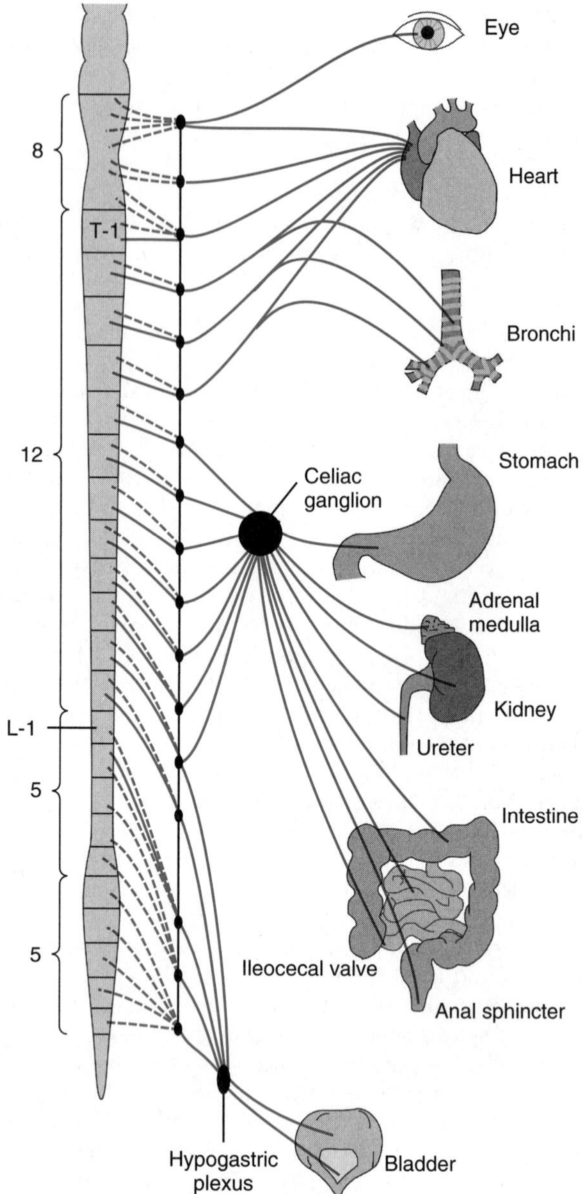

Figure **10–7.** Diagram of the autonomic nervous system. The visceral afferent fibers mediating cardiac pain travel with the sympathetic nerves (represented by solid lines) and enter the spinal cord from multiple levels (C3 to T4). Parasympathetic nervous system is represented by *dashed lines*. This multisegmental innervation results in a variety of pain patterns associated with myocardial ischemia and infarction.

Medical Management

Diagnosis. The diagnosis of angina pectoris is strongly suspected by history and is supported if sublingual nitroglycerin shortens an attack and if prophylactic nitrates permit greater exertion or prevent angina entirely (Massie, 1994). Medical evaluation includes examination for signs of diseases that may produce angina or contribute to or accompany atherosclerotic disease (see previous discussion on clinical manifestations).

ECG is normal in about 25% to 30% of people with angina, so the *exercise tolerance test* (ETT) is a more useful noninvasive

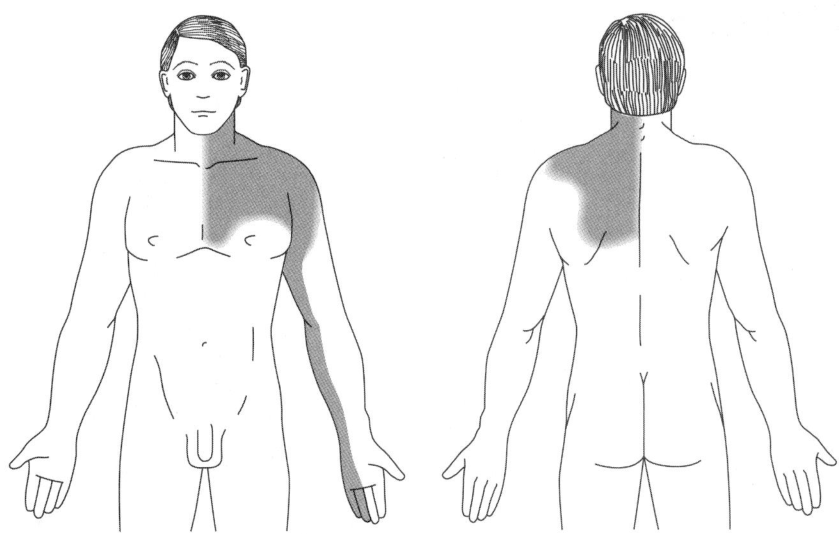

Figure **10–8.** Pain patterns associated with angina. *Left,* Area of substernal discomfort projected to the left shoulder and arm over the distribution of the ulnar nerve. Referred pain may be present only in the left shoulder or in the shoulder and along the arm only to the elbow. *Right,* Occasionally, anginal pain may be referred to the back in the area of the left scapula or the interscapular region. Isolated midthoracic spine or biceps muscle pain experienced by some women is not shown (see text for complete description).

procedure for evaluating the ischemic response to exercise in the client with angina. (See also discussion of Atherosclerosis Diagnosis: Variance Cardiography.) *Coronary angiography* may be used to determine the anatomic location and extent of CAD, but it is a more expensive diagnostic tool and carries increased associated risk. The results of this test aid in determining whether the obstructions can be corrected surgically.

Radioisotope imaging with thallium 201 is another technique used to diagnose CAD. This isotope enters myocardial cells and is taken up by tissue adequately perfused by blood supply. Areas of infarction appear as regions of diminished isotope activity or no activity (a "cold spot"). In coronary disease, resting abnormalities usually represent infarction, and those that occur with exercise usually indicate stress-induced ischemia (Haak et al., 1994; Massie, 1994).

Echocardiography to image the left ventricle and assess ventricular function may indicate ischemia or prior infarction. This test may be done during supine exercise or immediately following upright exercise.

Treatment. Short-acting sublingual nitroglycerin is the drug of choice for the acute attack, usually relieving symptoms within 1 to 2 minutes. Nitroglycerin oral spray is also available in a metered delivery system, which is especially useful for anyone having difficulty handling or swallowing pills. The spray is also easy to use in the dark and is more rapid-acting.

Prevention of attacks is the first step after the acute attack subsides. Treatment of underlying disorders such as hypertension is essential. The client is also encouraged to avoid situations and stressors that precipitate angina. This usually requires modifying all possible risk factors through changes in lifestyle and modifications of life-long habits.

Pharmacologic treatment may include other vasodilators such as long-acting nitrates (e.g., oral sustained-release nitroglycerin, transdermal nitroglycerin patches, nitroglycerin ointment), β-blockers (i.e., β-adrenergic receptor blockers), and calcium-channel blockers (Table 10–5; see also Table 10–12). Intravascular thrombosis is a key element in the pathophysiology of unstable angina and its progression to MI. Thrombolytic therapy using aspirin and/or heparin is an important part of treatment for unstable angina.

Revascularization procedures are recommended for persons who do not become ischemia-free on medical therapy, especially the client with progressive unstable angina. Surgical treatment such as PTCA has been shown to relieve angina, but it does not halt the progress of atherosclerosis or prolong life. CABG can diminish the probability of ischemia leading to necrosis and lethal infarction.

Prognosis. Myocardial ischemia leaves the heart vulnerable to arrhythmias and MI, which can be fatal. About a third of all people who experience angina pectoris die suddenly from MI or arrhythmias (O'Toole, 1992). Prognosis is dependent on type of angina, ability to prevent angina, and severity of underlying disease, such as hypertension or atherosclerosis.

Special Implications for the Therapist **10–3**

ANGINA PECTORIS

See also Special Implications for the Therapist: CAD.

Identifying Angina

Referred pain from the external oblique abdominal muscle and the pectoral major muscle can cause the sensation referred to as "heartburn" in the anterior chest wall, which mimics angina. When active trigger points are present in the left pectoralis major muscle, the referred pain is easily confused with that from coronary insufficiency (Travell and Simons, 1983). Physical therapy to eliminate the trigger points can aid in the diagnostic process.

Anterior chest wall syndrome with localized tenderness of intercostal muscles, Tietze's syndrome with inflammation of the chondrocostal junctions, intercostal neuritis, and cervical or thoracic spine disease involving the dorsal nerve roots can all produce chest pain that mimics angina. Evaluation of range of motion, palpation of soft tissue structures, and analysis of relieving or aggravating factors usually differentiates these conditions from true angina (Goodman and Snyder, 1995). Likewise, heartburn from indigestion, hiatal hernia, peptic ulcer, esophageal spasm, and gallbladder disease can also cause angina-like

TABLE 10-5 Medications Commonly Used for Angina Pectoris*

Vasodilators (Nitrates)	β-Blockers	Calcium Channel Blockers
Nitroglycerin	Acebutolol (Sectral)	Amlodipine (Norvasc)
Isosorbide dinitrate (Isordil, Iso-Bid)	Atenolol (Tenormin)	Diltiazem (Cardizem)
	Betaxolol (Kerlone)	Felodipine (Plendil)
	Carteolol (Cartol)	Nicardipine (Cardene)
	Esmolol (Brevibloc)	Nifedipine (Procardia)
	Labetalol (Normodyne, Trandate)	Verapamil (Calan, Isoptin)
	Metoprolol (Lopressor)	
	Nadolol (Corgard)	
	Penbutolol (Levatol)	
	Pindolol (Visken)	
	Propranolol (Betachron, Inderal)	
	Timolol (Blocadren)	

* Only the most commonly used medications are listed here. The reader is encouraged to use appropriate drug references to become familiar with actions and side effects of these (and other) medications.

symptoms that require a medical evaluation for an accurate diagnosis.

The development of unstable angina also requires immediate medical referral and may be reported as the onset of angina at rest, occurrence of typical angina at a significantly lower level of activity than usual, changes in the typical anginal pattern (e.g., symptoms occurring more frequently), or changes in blood pressure (decrease) or heart rate (increase) with levels of activity previously well tolerated (Hillegass and Sadowsky, 1994).

Nitroglycerin

Nitroglycerin may be used prophylactically 5 minutes before activities likely to precipitate angina. This is especially true in the treatment or exercise setting of the person with chronic, stable, exertional angina. This procedure must be performed by physician order and cannot be decided solely by the therapist and client. Clients must be reminded that they are not to alter their prescribed drug schedule without consulting their health care provider and that nitrates should be taken as prescribed. For example, taking sublingual nitroglycerin orally markedly decreases its effectiveness (Grimes and Cohen, 1994).

Nitroglycerin tablets are inactivated by light, heat, air, and moisture, and they should be stored in the refrigerator in a tight-fitting amber container. Nitroglycerin has a short shelf life and needs to be replaced about every 3 months. A potent nitroglycerin tablet should produce a burning sensation under the tongue when taken sublingually (if it does not, check the expiration date).

A person experiencing angina should reduce the pace or, if necessary, stop all activity and sit down for a few minutes until the symptoms disappear. Exercise can be reinitiated at a reduced intensity, and interval-type training may be required (i.e., slow activity alternating with activity requiring more effort).

Clients should be seated when taking nitroglycerin to avoid syncope and falls. For anginal pain or discomfort that is not relieved by rest or relieved by up to three nitroglycerin doses in 10 to 15 minutes (i.e., the initial dose followed by a second dose 5 minutes later and a third dose 5 minutes after the second dose), the physician should be contacted. Until the angina is controlled and coronary blood flow re-established, the client is at risk of myocardial damage from myocardial ischemia.

Orthostatic Hypotension

Orthostatic hypotension (see discussion later in this chapter) is one of the most common side effects of prophylactic medications for angina. Caution on the part of the therapist is required when exercising or ambulating clients who receive these medications. If the person becomes hypotensive, have him or her assume a supine position with legs elevated to increase venous return and to ensure cerebral blood flow. Support hose may be recommended, and the person should be reminded to change positions slowly to minimize the effects of orthostatic hypotension. Headache, weakness, increasing pulse, or other unusual signs or symptoms should be reported to the physician. In a home health setting, the home should be evaluated for potentially hazardous conditions. All clients should be encouraged to avoid hazardous activities until their condition is stabilized by medication, especially in the presence of dizziness.

Monitoring Vital Signs

Exercise testing should be performed before a client begins an exercise program, but if this has not been accomplished and baseline measurements are unavailable for use in planning exercise, monitor the heart rate and blood pressure and note any accompanying symptoms during exercise (see Appendix B). Exercise and activity should be performed below the anginal threshold. The therapist must document heart rate and blood pressure when the ischemia began (as evidenced by symptoms of angina) to establish these parameters. Angina occurring after a myocardial infarction is not considered "normal" and should be reported to the physician. Exercise testing is

BOX **10–6**
Causes of Myocardial Infarction

Coronary thrombus (blood clot)
- Atherosclerosis
- Rheumatic heart disease
- Endocarditis
- Aortic stenosis
- Prosthetic mitral or aortic valve

Prolonged vasospasm
Hypotension (inadequate myocardial blood flow)
Dislodged calcium plaque from calcified aortic or mitral valve
Excessive metabolic demand
Vasculitis
Aortic root or coronary artery dissection
Aortitis
Cocaine use

recommended before a client resumes an exercise program (Hillegass, 1995).

Myocardial Infarction

Definition and Incidence. MI, also known as a heart attack or coronary, is the development of ischemia with resultant necrosis of myocardial tissue. Any prolonged obstruction depriving the heart muscle of oxygen can cause an MI.

Myocardial infarction occurs in 1,500,000 persons each year and represents the leading cause of death (500,000 deaths annually) in the adult American population. On the basis of data from the Framingham Study, approximately 45% of all heart attack clients are younger than 65 years, and 5% younger than 40 years. This condition is very common in males and postmenopausal females (Haak et al., 1994; Reigle and Ringel, 1993).

Etiology and Risk Factors. Etiology and risk factors are the same as for all forms of CAD, especially angina pectoris (see previous discussion on angina pectoris). Eighty percent to 90% of MIs result from coronary thrombus at the site of a preexisting atherosclerotic stenosis. Other causes are listed in Box 10–6.

Silent ischemia is highly prevalent among people with diabetes; plasminogen activator inhibitor (PAI-1)[10] has been identified as a risk factor for MI in diabetics as well as for postmenopausal women not receiving hormone replacement therapy. Research now shows that diabetic clients have higher PAI activity than nondiabetic clients, both at hospital admission for acute MI and at follow up 1 year later. Raised PAI activity may predispose diabetic clients to MI and may also impair pharmacologic and spontaneous reperfusion after acute MI, contributing to the poor outcome in this population (Gray et al., 1993a; 1993b).

Smokers have more than twice as many heart attacks as nonsmokers, and sudden cardiac death occurs 2 to 4 times more frequently in smokers. After an infarction, smokers have a poorer chance of recovery than nonsmokers (Lawrence and Eutsey, 1994).

Pathogenesis. The myocardium receives its blood supply from the two large coronary arteries and their branches (Fig. 10–9). One or more of these blood vessels may become occluded by a clot that forms suddenly when an atheromatous plaque ruptures through the sublayers of a blood vessel, or when the narrow, roughened inner lining of a sclerosed artery becomes completely filled with thrombus (clot) (O'Toole, 1992).

The most common site involved is the left ventricle, the chamber of the heart with the greatest workload. Thrombosis of the descending branch of the *left coronary artery* is the most common location of infarction and affects the anterior left ventricle (Fig. 10–10). Occlusion of the *left circumflex artery* produces anterolateral or posterolateral infarction. *Right coronary artery* thrombosis leads to infarction of the posteroinferior portion of the left ventricle and may involve the right ventricular myocardium and interventricular septum. The arteries supplying the atrioventricular node and the sinus node more commonly arise from the right coronary artery; thus, atrioventricular block at the nodal level and sinus node dysfunction occur more frequently during inferior infarctions. However, because there are great individual variations in coronary anatomy and because associated lesions and collateral vessels may confuse the picture, prediction of coronary anatomy from the infarct location may be inaccurate (Massie, 1994).

When the myocardium has been completely deprived of oxygen, cells die and the tissue becomes necrotic in an area called the *zone of infarction* (Fig. 10–11). In response to this necrosis, leukocytes aid in removing the dead cells, and fibroblasts form a connective tissue scar within the area of infarction. Usually the formation of fibrous scar tissue is complete within 6 to 8 weeks (Table 10–6). Immediately surrounding the area of infarction is a less seriously damaged area of injury called the *zone of hypoxic injury*. This zone is able to return to normal, but it may also become necrotic if blood flow is not restored. With adequate collateral circulation, this area may regain its function within 2 to 3 weeks. Adjacent to the zone of hypoxic injury is another reversible zone called the *zone of ischemia*. Ischemic and injured myocardial tissue cause characteristic ECG changes; as the myocardium heals, the ST segment and T waves gradually return to normal, but abnormal Q waves may persist (Haak et al., 1994).

Oxygen deprivation is accompanied by electrolyte disturbances, particularly loss of potassium, calcium, and magnesium from cells. Myocardial cells deprived of necessary oxygen and nutrients lose contractility, thereby diminishing the pumping ability of the heart. Normally the myocardium takes up varying quantities of catecholamines (epinephrine and norepinephrine), which are released when significant arterial occlusion occurs. Released catecholamines predispose the individual to serious imbalances of sympathetic and parasympathetic function, irregular heartbeats (arrhythmia), and heart failure.

Clinical Manifestations. The most notable symptom of MI is a sudden sensation of pressure, often described as prolonged "crushing chest pain," occasionally radiating to the arms, throat, neck (as high as the occipital area), and back (Fig.

[10] PAI is a naturally occurring substance that inhibits another natural substance, t-PA. t-PA is an enzyme released endogenously as part of the body's defense against thrombosis; it lyses fibrin and dissolves forming blood clots. The effect of PAI on t-PA is to *prevent* clot destruction in the bloodstream (Gebara et al., 1995).

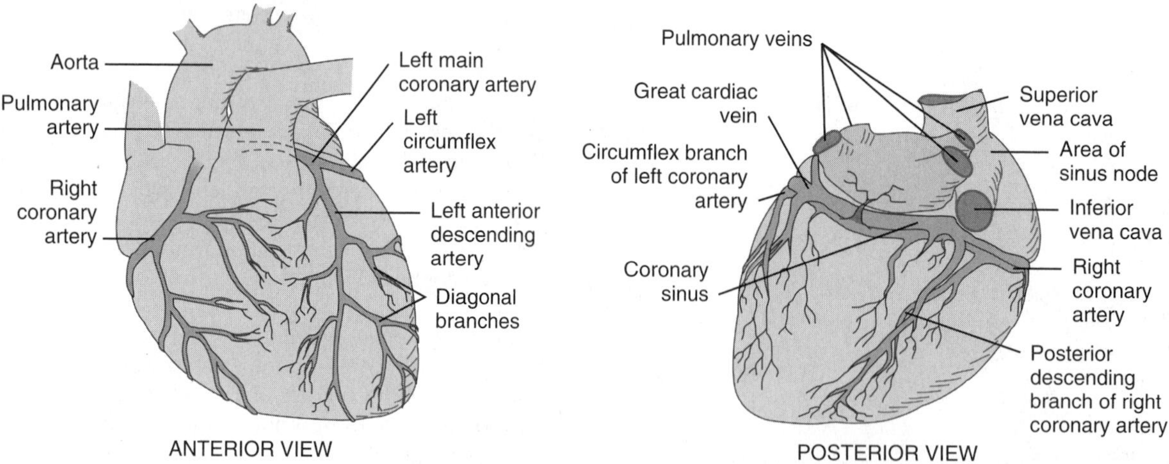

Figure **10–9.** Areas of myocardium affected by arterial insufficiency of specific coronary arteries. The right and left coronary arteries branch off the aorta just above the aortic valve and normally supply the myocardium with oxygenated blood. The most commonly affected arteries and the area of myocardium supplied are listed in order of decreasing occurrence.

Coronary Artery Supply	Area of Myocardium Involved
Left coronary artery (LCA), left anterior descending (LAD) branch	Anterior
Right coronary artery (RCA)	Posterior
RCA	Inferior
LCA, LAD branch	Anteroseptal
Circumflex artery, marginal branch, or LCA, diagonal branch	High lateral
Usually LCA, left anterior branch, may be RCA, posterior descending branch	Apical

10–12). The pain is constant, lasting 30 minutes up to hours and may be accompanied by pallor, shortness of breath (SOB), and profuse perspiration. Catecholamine release resulting in sympathetic stimulation may produce diaphoresis and peripheral vasoconstriction that cause the skin to become cool and clammy. Nausea and vomiting may occur because of reflex stimulation of vomiting centers by pain fibers. Fever may develop in the first 24 hours and persist for a week because of inflammatory activity within the myocardium.

Angina pectoris pain can be similar, but it is less severe, does not last for hours, and is relieved by cessation of activity, rest, or nitrates. It is possible to have a painless infarction without acute symptoms, especially among the elderly and in diabetic persons. As many as 25% of infarctions are detected on routine ECG without the person's recalling any acute episode.

Postinfarction complications include arrhythmias, congestive heart failure, cardiogenic shock, pericarditis, rupture of the heart, thromboembolism, recurrent infarction, and sudden death. Arrhythmias caused by ischemia, hypoxia, autonomic nervous system imbalances, lactic acidosis, electrolyte imbalances, drug toxicity, or alterations of impulse conduction pathways or conduction defects are the most common complication of acute MI, affecting more than 90% of individuals.

Medical Management

Diagnosis. Diagnosis of MI is based on the presenting symptoms and evidence of impaired heart function found by physical examination, ECG, and laboratory results. Serum measurements of cardiac enzymes are specific for infarction and serum lactic acid dehydrogenase is specific for myocardial damage. Serial enzyme levels are assessed for several days, as elevation of certain enzymes will be noted at characteristic times; 24 to 48 hours of negative enzyme elevations rule out MI (see Tables 35–13 and 35–14) (Massie, 1994).

A new blood test to confirm heart attack in clients within 2 hours may replace unnecessary diagnostic expenditures described. The new test uses a rapid assay of the subforms of creatine kinase MB (CK-MB), one of the cardiac enzymes specific for MI. Fewer than 30% of persons admitted to coronary care units (CCUs) have had an MI; this test may dramatically reduce the cost of treating heart attacks by allowing physicians to quickly discharge people with noncardiac chest pain (Puleo et al., 1994).

Infarcted tissue is electrically silent and does not contribute to the ECG. Most clients with acute infarction have ECG changes, although this test provides only a crude estimate of the magnitude of infarction. When diagnosis by ECG and enzymes is not possible (e.g., when people seek medical attention post-MI), scintigraphic studies (radionuclide imaging) can show areas of necrotic myocardium and diminished perfusion. These tests, which use radiotracers, do not distinguish old damage from recent infarction, and false-positive results can occur.

Other test procedures may include echocardiography, which is useful in assessing the ability of the heart walls to contract and relax, and transesophageal echocardiography (TEE), a technique that provides a clearer image of the heart, including the posterior wall, valvular anatomy, and thoracic aortic structure and pathology (Blanchard et al., 1994; DeMaria et al., 1994; Wolfe, 1989). Magnetic resonance imaging (MRI) to evaluate structural defects of the heart and positron emission tomography (PET) to evaluate cardiac me-

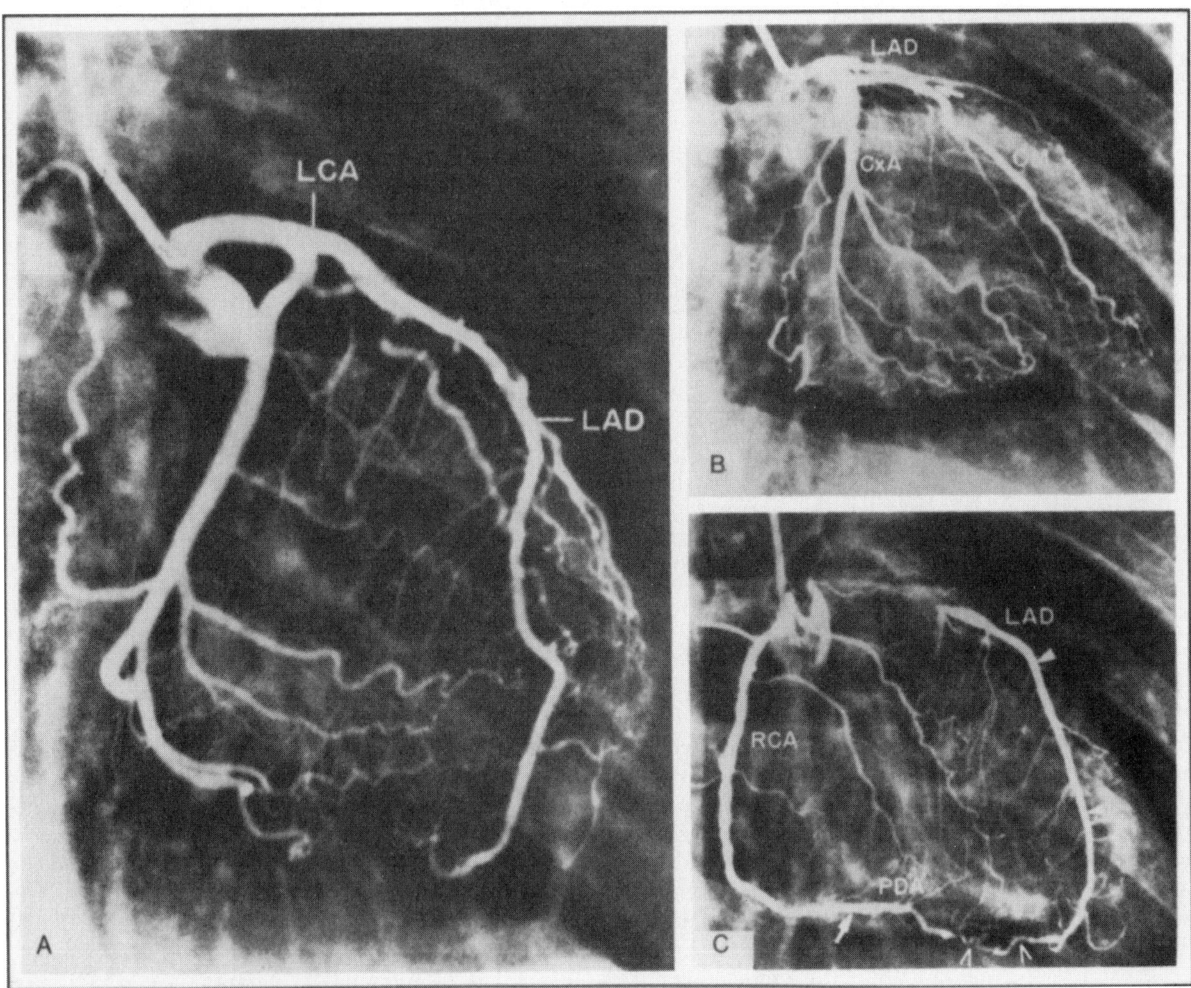

Figure 10–10. A, Angiogram of a normal left coronary artery (LCA). B, Angiogram of a totally obstructed left anterior descending (LAD) coronary artery. C, Angiogram of the right coronary artery (RCA) and its major branch, the posterior descending artery (PDA) (same heart as in B). The LAD is seen because of collateral vessels connecting the LAD and the RCA system. (*From Boucek R, Morales A, Romanelli R, et al: Coronary Artery Disease: Pathologic and Clinical Assessment. Baltimore, Williams & Wilkins, 1984, pp 4, 9.*)

tabolism and assess tissue perfusion may be used, but these tests have very limited usefulness at the present time.

Another new technique being investigated is the use of a contrast agent called EchoGen, used in conjunction with an ultrasound procedure. This agent infiltrates healthy heart muscle, but not muscle that has been deprived of blood or oxygen. Existing contrast agents only image the heart chambers, which provides information about the flow of blood through the chamber but not about the structure of the heart muscle itself (Pugh et al., 1996).

Treatment. CCU monitoring accompanied by bed rest, followed by gradual return to activities, is the mainstay of initial treatment. The first 6 hours after the onset of pain is the crucial period for salvage of the myocardium. Coronary arteriography and PTCA may be performed in persons who present within 3 hours after infarction, although the results of this approach have not been entirely successful (Grines, 1993; Woo, 1992).

Pain relief is essential, usually accomplished by pharmacologic means. Pharmacologic intervention is also used to limit infarction size, reduce vasoconstriction, prevent thrombus formation, and augment repair. MI caused by intracoronary thrombi can be relieved by infusion of thrombolytic agents (e.g., streptokinase, urokinase, t-PA[11]) that dissolve clots, promote vasodilation, and reduce infarct size (Granger, 1992; Tiefenbrunn, 1992). This treatment must be performed within 3 to 6 hours after the onset of infarction and can reestablish blood flow in approximately 3 minutes.

After a thrombolytic agent is administered, intravenous (IV) heparin therapy is usually continued for 5 to 7 days. Adjunctive aspirin administration causes a significant further reduction in mortality rate when administered during the acute phase (Popma and Topol, 1991; Yusuf, 1990). Recently, safe upper dosage limits for heparin were established; exceeding these limits almost doubles a person's risk of severe stroke (Topol et al., 1994). A new class of anti-thrombotic agents

[11] Tissue plasminogen activator (t-PA), a naturally occurring enzyme that acts directly on blood clots to dissolve them, is now a genetically engineered drug used in thrombolytic therapy. However, a single dose of recombinant t-PA (rt-PA) costs about $2000, whereas other drugs are much cheaper (e.g., streptokinase costs about $300).

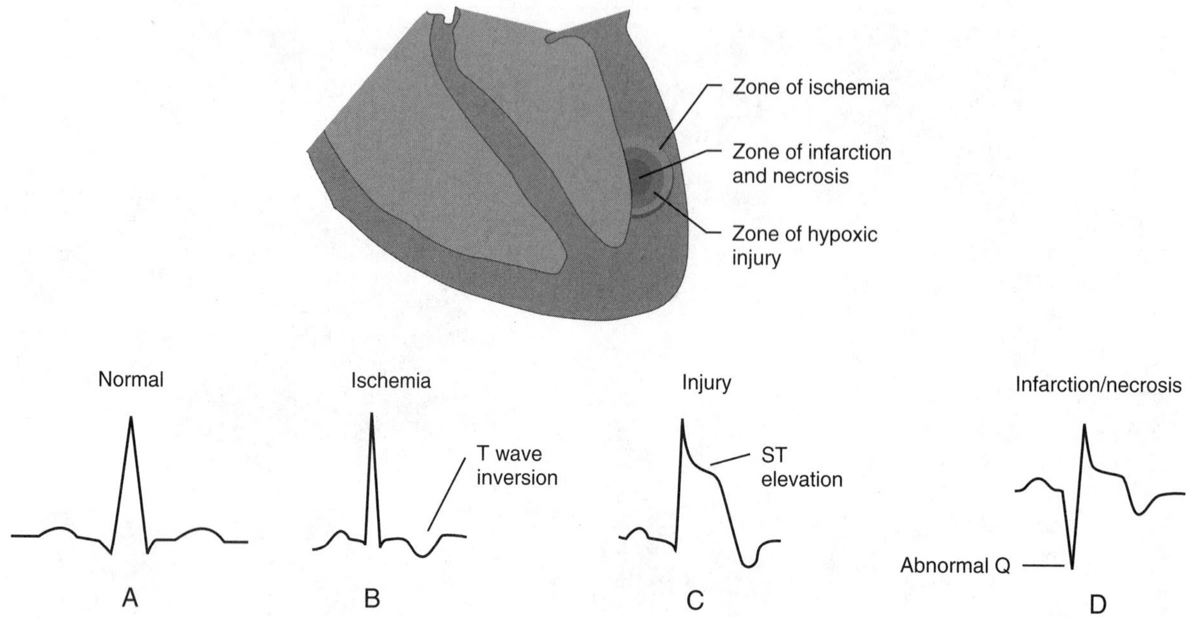

Figure **10–11.** ECG alterations associated with the three zones of MI.

that directly inactivate clot-bound thrombin may replace heparin. These newer antithrombotics that inhibit thrombin generation and thrombin activity at various strategic points within the coagulation cascade are in the early stages of development (Ward et al., 1997; Muller et al., 1996).

Postinfarction management includes identification and modification of risk factors (Fig. 10–13), treatment of underlying pathology, continued use of prophylactic pharmacologic agents, and cardiac rehabilitation utilizing exercise programs. Exercise has been recommended as a means of increasing pain tolerance, increasing the stimulus required to induce angina, alleviating depression, reducing anxiety, and possibly inducing collateral circulation (Todd, 1991). Increasing evidence suggests that combining a low-fat diet and intensive exercise training can improve myocardial perfusion by regression of coronary atherosclerosis (Ornish, 1990; Schuler, 1992).

Exercise training may be contraindicated for some people

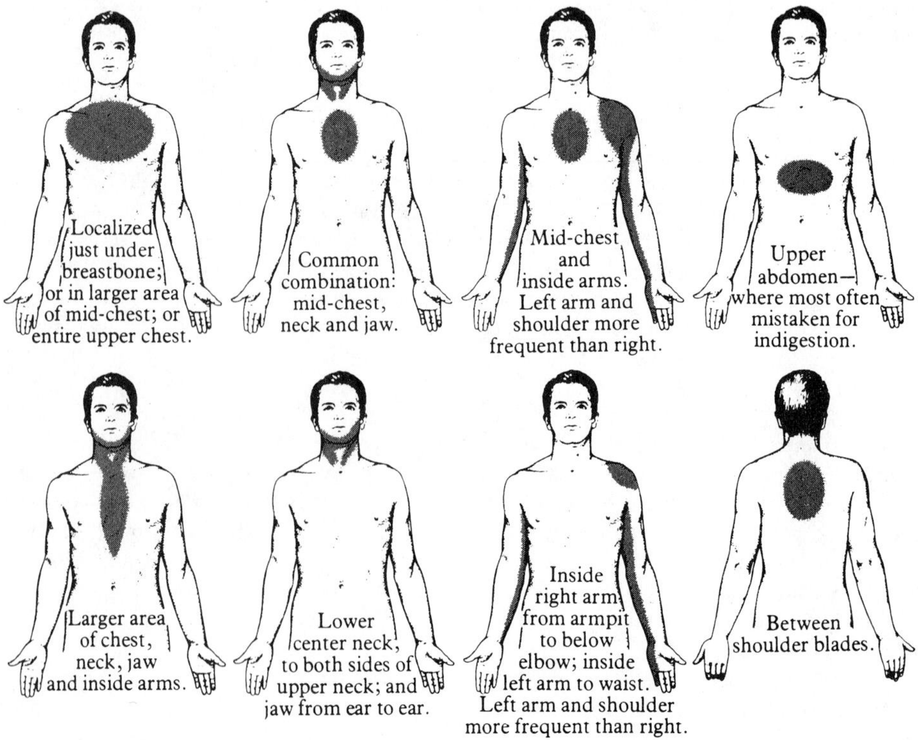

Figure **10–12.** Early warning signs of a heart attack. Multiple segmental nerve innervation shown in Figure 10–7 accounts for the varied pain patterns possible. (*From Goodman CC, Snyder TE: Differential Diagnosis in Physical Therapy; ed 2. Philadelphia, WB Saunders, 1995, p 125.*)

TABLE 10-6 Tissue Changes After Myocardial Infarction

Time After MI	Tissue Changes
6–12 hr	No gross changes; healing process has not begun
18–24 hr	Inflammatory response; intercellular enzyme release
2–4 days	Visible necrosis; proteolytic enzymes remove debris; catecholamines, lipolysis and glycogenolysis elevate plasma glucose and increase free fatty acids to assist depleted myocardium recovery from anaerobic state
4–10 days	Debris cleared; collagen matrix laid down
10–14 days	Weak, fibrotic scar tissue with beginning revascularization; area vulnerable to stress
6 wk	Scarring usually complete; tough, inelastic scar replaces necrotic myocardium; unable to contract and relax like healthy myocardial tissue

Adapted from McCance KL, Huether SE: Pathophysiology: The Biologic Basis for Disease in Adults and Children, ed 2. St Louis, Mosby–Year Book, 1994, p 1028.

(Box 10–7; see also Table 10–3). Medical clearance must be obtained for entry into an exercise training program. Exercise testing is the most useful tool to establish guidelines for exercise training in apparently healthy adults and is mandatory for people with known or suspected cardiovascular disease.

It is still unclear whether exercise training improves prognosis, and the efficacy of supervised training after MI is still questioned as well. Only marginal physical performance improvements and no long-term psychological benefits 6 months after a twice weekly supervised training program have been reported (Holmbäck et al., 1994). Previous results from the Toronto Program report that more is gained from weekly attendance at a formal class for 18 months than from attending three times weekly for 6 months (Kavanagh, 1982).

Prognosis. The size and anatomic location of the infarction, together with the amount of damage from previous infarctions, determines the acute clinical picture, the early complications, and the long-term prognosis. The first 24 hours after onset of symptoms is the time of highest risk for sudden death. The sooner someone reaches the hospital, the better the prognosis. Eighty percent of those suffering from an acute MI survive the initial attack when transported to a CCU.

Factors negatively affecting prognosis include age (clients older than 80 years have a 60% mortality); evidence of other cardiovascular diseases, respiratory diseases, or uncontrolled diabetes mellitus; anterior location of MI (30% mortality rate); and hypotension (clients whose systolic blood pressure is less than 55 mm Hg have a 60% mortality rate).

Sex differences on the outcome of coronary angioplasty have been investigated. Compared with men, women have similar procedural success rates, need for coronary artery bypass surgery, and mortality rates at coronary angioplasty. During the follow-up period, there are no significant differences in the requirement for coronary bypass surgery, repeat angioplasty, reinfarction, or death between the sexes. Women do have significantly more recurrent angina following bypass surgery and coronary angioplasty (Welty et al., 1994).

Fifty percent of persons who completely recover from their first coronary will die within 5 years, and 75% will die within 10 years from massive infarctions (Stewart, 1992). Most deaths occur outside the hospital owing to complications (see Clinical Manifestations). Forty percent to 50% of deaths occur because of arrhythmias, 30% of deaths occur as a result of CHF at the time of the infarction or up to weeks later, and 10% of deaths are attributed to cardiogenic shock.

Special Implications for the Therapist **10-4**

MYOCARDIAL INFARCTION

Early Post-MI Considerations

Although the myocardium must rest, bed rest puts the client at risk for development of hypovolemia, hypoxemia, muscle atrophy, and pulmonary embolus. Developing a program of progressive physical activity with adequate pacing and rest periods begins within 24 hours for the acute care client in uncomplicated cases. Gentle movement exercises, deep breathing, and coughing are usually begun immediately as a prophylactic measure.

Early therapeutic exercise helps prevent cardiopulmonary complications, venous stasis, joint stiffness, and muscle weakness. Relaxation is often promoted with low-intensity activity. Activities that increase intrathoracic or intra-abdominal pressure, such as breath-holding and Valsalva maneuvers (see Box 13–1), can precipitate bradycardia followed by increased venous return to the heart, causing possible cardiac overload. For this reason, these actions are contraindicated during all activities with CAD, and should not be performed in any stage of their rehabilitation program (Dean, 1996).

The therapist must continually monitor for signs of impending infarction, including generalized or localized pain anywhere over the thorax, upper limbs, and neck; palpitations; dyspnea; lightheadedness; syncope; sensation of indigestion; hiccups; and nausea (see Clinical Manifestations, this section). Specific aspects of cardiac rehabilitation and postoperative care are beyond the scope of this text. Other more specific texts are available to guide the therapist in this area (Frownfelter and Dean, 1996; Hillegass and Sadowsky, 1994; Irwin and Tecklin, 1995; Karavangh, 1994). See also the Agency for Health Care Policy and Research Clinical Guidelines for Cardiac Rehabilitation (1995).

Incisional pain or discomfort from cardiac surgery may cause a person to exhibit rapid, shallow respirations in an attempt to ease the discomfort. If analgesics are prescribed to prevent severe discomfort, the drug can be administered before therapy to better enable the person to do deep breathing exercises. This problem is of limited duration and usually resolves when the incision heals. The therapist must beware that analgesics also mask pain response, making it possible for the client to overexert himself or herself.

During the first 6 weeks post-MI, the client is cautioned to avoid saunas, hot tubs, whirlpools, and

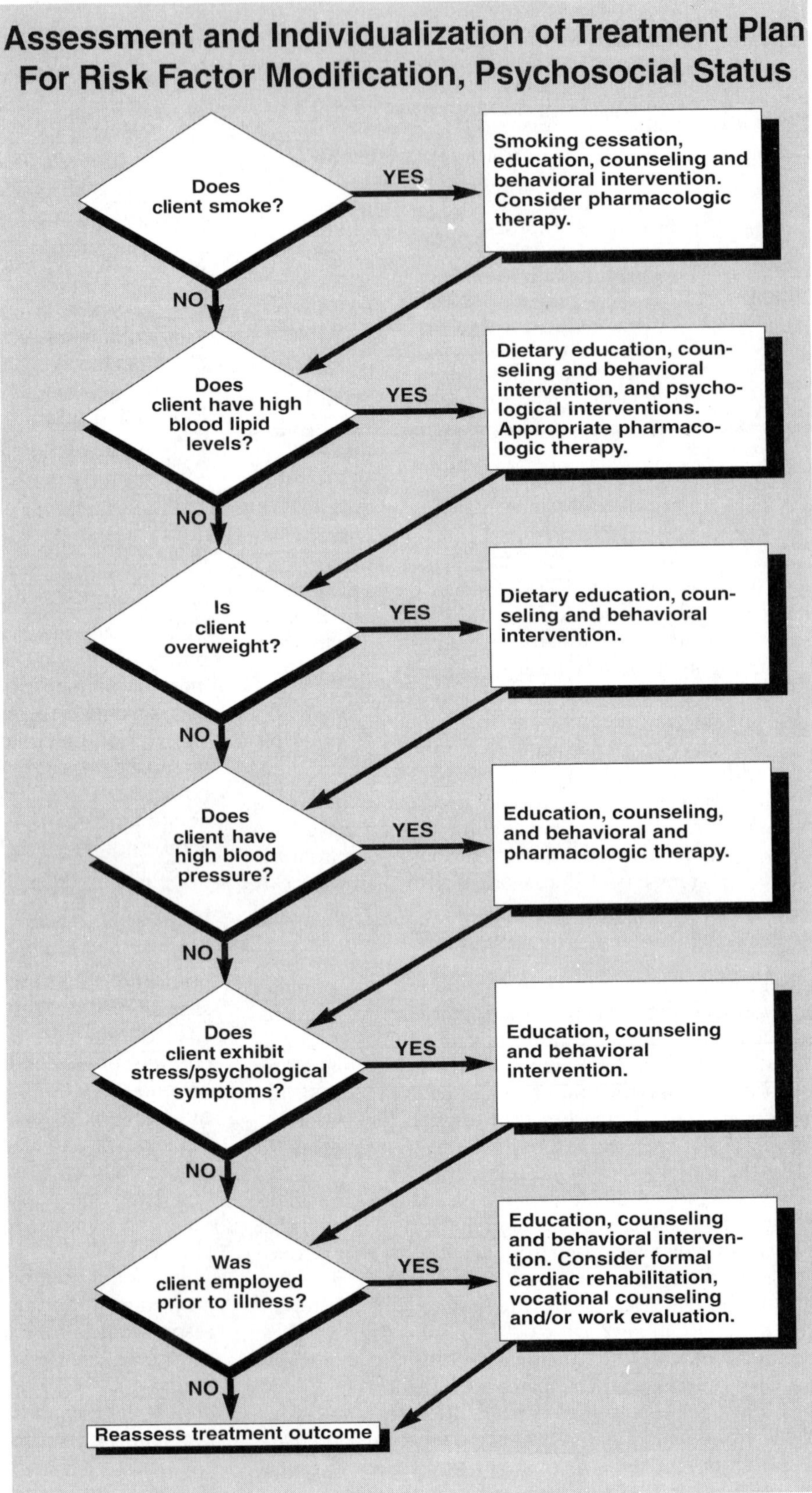

Figure **10–13.** Assessing and modifying risk factors is an important part of the prevention and treatment plan for heart disease. The new Agency for Health Care Policy and Research clinical guidelines formulated for cardiac rehabilitation services covers all of the essential elements of cardiac rehabilitation and is available for $8.00 by calling the Government Printing Office (stock No. 01702600154–9); telephone: (202) 512–1800. (*From the Agency for Health Care Policy and Research: Clinical Guideline No. 17, Cardiac Rehabilitation.* Columbia, Md, 1995.)

BOX 10-7
Contraindications to Exercise Post-Myocardial Infarction

Acute MI (<1–2 days after an MI without physician approval)
Unstable angina; easily provoked angina
New ECG signs and symptoms of MI
Any symptom of MI (e.g., nausea, dyspnea, lightheadedness, chest pain)
PaO_2 <60
O_2 saturation <86%
Hemoglobin <8 g/dL; hematocrit <26%
Severe aortic outflow obstruction
Suspected or known dissecting aneurysm
Acute myocarditis or pericarditis
Uncontrolled complex arrhythmias
Active severe CHF; resting respiratory rate >45 breaths/min
Recent pulmonary embolism or thrombophlebitis
Untreated 3rd-degree heart block
Severe systemic hypertension unresponsive to medication
Uncontrolled diabetes
Acute infections
Digoxin toxicity

Adapted from Kavanaugh T: Cardiac Rehabilitation. *In* Goldberg L, Elliot DL: Exercise for Prevention and Treatment of Illness. Philadelphia, FA Davis, 1994, p 55.

excessively warm swimming pools. Early rehabilitation lasting 2 to 3 weeks is often followed by exercise testing, at which time water therapy may be permissible per physician approval (see Guidelines for Aquatic Therapy, Appendix B).

Monitoring Vital Signs

When used to minimize discomfort initially, pain medications such as morphine may also depress the respiratory drive. The CCU therapist must monitor corresponding vital signs. The home health therapist must monitor pulse and blood pressure measurements for hypotension because of the side effects precipitated by antihypertensive medications, vasodilators, and other antianginal agents. (See also Special Implications for the Therapist: Angina Pectoris.) Initial ambulation and activities at home should be roughly equivalent to levels achieved at the hospital at the time of discharge, depending on the client's physiologic response to the transition from hospital to home.

The client must increase activities gradually to avoid overtaxing the heart as it pumps oxygenated blood to the muscles. The metabolic equivalent system provides one way of measuring the amount of oxygen needed to perform an activity: 1 metabolic equivalent of the task (MET) equals 3.5 mL of oxygen per kilogram of body weight per minute; 1 MET is approximately equivalent to the oxygen uptake a person requires when resting. Early mobilization activities after acute MI should not exceed 1 to 2 MET (e.g., brushing teeth, eating). By comparison, people who can exercise to 8 or more MET (oxygen uptake of 28 mL/kg/min or more) can perform most daily physical activities.

As activity level increases, the therapist must monitor heart rate, blood pressure, and fatigue, adjusting activity level accordingly. During phase I (acute hospital) care, the heart rate should not rise more than 25% above resting level, and blood pressure must not rise more than 25 mm Hg above resting level. The normal increase in systolic blood pressure is 7.5 mm Hg/MET (Naughton and Haider, 1973). When systolic blood pressure falls or fails to increase as the intensity of exercise increases, exercise intensity should be immediately reduced. A drop in systolic blood pressure during exercise below standing rest value is associated with increased risk of lethal arrhythmia in clients with a prior MI or myocardial ischemia (Fletcher et al., 1990).

Oxygen may be used to help reduce myocardial work and eliminate dyspnea. Blood gas analysis is usually performed within an hour of initiating oxygen therapy to establish a baseline of arterial saturation. By monitoring blood gases, oxygen dose can be altered to regulate blood gases and acid base balance. Oxygen saturations levels must be monitored by the therapist during exercise or treatment because these activities may increase myocardial oxygen demand (Dean, 1996) (see Table 35–21).

The client with chronic obstructive pulmonary disease (COPD) who receives oxygen therapy must be monitored very closely for symptoms of decreased ventilation such as headache, giddiness, tinnitus (ringing in the ears), nausea, weakness, and vomiting. Frequently persons with COPD retain carbon dioxide (CO_2) making the use of oxygen a deadly drug. CO_2 levels are elevated in the COPD client, eliminating the drive to breathe normally that is initiated by rising levels of CO_2. The only drive to breathe in the COPD client is hypoxia (reduced oxygen levels). The administration of oxygen in a person with CO_2 retention can further depress the respiratory drive, resulting in death.

Exercise

Traditionally, isometric exercises have been contraindicated, and resistance training or weightlifting has been excluded from the cardiac client's program. (See Special Implications for the Therapist: Cardiac Transplantation). Although weight training is not an isometric (static) exercise, it is similar during maximal lifts.* However, cardiac clients have undertaken supervised and prescribed weight-training programs without ill effects, especially if regimens incorporate moderate levels of resistance and high numbers of repetitions (Butler et al., 1987; Keleman, 1986; Salvidar, 1983; Vander, 1986). Thrombolytic agents reduce the client's blood-clotting ability, necessitating special care to avoid tissue trauma during therapy (e.g., resistive exercises, soft tissue or scar mobilization).

Exercise may induce cardiac arrhythmias under several conditions, including diuretic and digitalis therapy; recent ingestion of caffeine may exacerbate arrhythmias. Exercise-induced arrhythmias are generated by enhanced sympathetic tone, increased myocardial oxygen demand, or both.

The immediate postexercise period is particularly dangerous because of high catecholamine levels associated with a generalized vasodilation. Sudden termination of muscular activity is accompanied by diminished venous return and may lead to a reduction in coronary perfusion while heart rate is elevated (Fletcher et al., 1990). A careful cooldown period is required with continued monitoring of vital signs postexercise.

Sexual Activity

People with cardiac disease, both men and women, are prone to sexual dysfunction. Often their concerns are voiced to the therapist. Problems may be caused by medications, anxiety, depression, or limited physical capacity. The most common drugs to cause loss of sexual desire or ability to reach orgasm are the antihypertensives. Fear of death during sexual intercourse, fear of another infarction caused by sexual activity, and diminished sexual ability caused by illness and aging may occur. The sexual partner may have many similar fears and may want to be included in any information provided about return to sexual function.

Sexual intercourse is physiologically equivalent to such activities as a brisk walk or climbing a flight of stairs. It has been equated to 5 MET of work on an exercise stress test. Advice to clients should be based on consultation with the physician. Some general guidelines include the following: (1) when the client can sustain a heart rate of 110 to 120 beats/min with no shortness of breath or anginal pain, he or she can resume sexual activity; (2) sexual activity should be resumed gradually, and only after activities such as walking moderate distances or climbing stairs comfortably have been accomplished; (3) sexual activity causes the least amount of stress when it occurs in familiar surroundings with the usual partner; (4) gradual foreplay helps the heart prepare for coitus; (5) positions requiring isometric contractions should be avoided; (6) eating a large meal or drinking alcohol before sexual activity should be avoided (Kinney and Packa, 1995).

*A static muscle contraction that involves 70% or more of maximum effort results in a disproportionate increase in heart rate and blood pressure for the absolute level of oxygen uptake, which is potentially harmful for the ischemic heart (Kavanaugh, 1994). For some people, use of a cane or walker is an isometric use of muscles that can increase heart rate, and careful monitoring of vital signs and indications of perceived exertion are required.

Congestive Heart Failure

Definition and Overview. CHF is a condition in which the heart is unable to pump sufficient blood to supply the body's needs (see also Chapter 12). Heart failure is not a disease but rather represents a group of clinical manifestations caused by inadequate pump performance from either the cardiac valves or the myocardium. It may be chronic over many years, requiring management by oral medications, or it may be acute and life-threatening, requiring more dramatic medical management to maintain an adequate cardiac output.

Failure may occur on both sides of the heart or may predominantly affect the right or left side. Strictly classified, left ventricular failure is referred to as *congestive heart failure;* acute right ventricular failure, seen almost exclusively in association with massive pulmonary embolism, is labeled *cor pulmonale.*

Cor pulmonale is heart disease, but it arises from an underlying pulmonary pathology; therefore, it is discussed in Chapter 12. Right-sided heart dysfunction secondary to either left-sided heart failure, vascular dysfunction, or congenital heart disease is excluded in the definition of cor pulmonale.

Incidence. CHF is a common complication of ischemic and hypertensive heart disease, occurring most often in the elderly. In the United States, heart failure develops in an estimated 400,000 individuals annually: it is the most common inpatient diagnosis in persons older than 65 years (Francis, 1990). This condition is on the increase as the population ages and more people survive heart attacks.

Etiology and Risk Factors. People with preexisting heart disease are at greatest risk for the development of CHF. Many cardiac conditions predispose individuals to CHF (Table 10–7), because when the heart is stressed, compensatory mechanisms may be inadequate. For example, a faster redistribution of blood volume and increased demand for oxygen by the myocardium occurs with increased activity, such as exercise, resulting in heart failure.

Risk factors for CHF include any condition that precipitates or exacerbates stress on the already diseased heart. Pregnancy is a risk factor for any woman with rheumatic valvular disease. In some cases, Paget's disease (see Chapter 20) increases myocardial workload. This disease causes vascular proliferation in the bones. When the disease involves over one third of the skeleton, a high cardiac output state exists and may tax the compromised heart (Reigle and Ringel, 1993). Medications such as steroids or nonsteroidal anti-inflammatory drugs (NSAIDs) (Van den Ouweland et al., 1988; Yost and Morgan, 1994) and drug toxicity are also risk factors.

For the person with chronic, stable heart failure, acute exacerbations may occur caused by alterations in therapy, client noncompliance with therapy, excessive salt and fluid intake, arrhythmias, excessive activity, pulmonary emboli, infection, or progression of the underlying disease (Massie, 1994).

Pathogenesis and Clinical Manifestations. Over the last decade, major advances have occurred in our understanding of heart failure, involving the complex interactions that take

TABLE 10-7 Etiology and Risk Factors Associated with Congestive Heart Failure

Etiology	Risk Factors*
Myocardial infarction	Emotional stress
Hypertension	Fever
Valvular heart disease	Infection
Congenital heart disease	Anemia
Pericarditis	Thyroid disorders
Myocarditis	Pregnancy
Cardiomyopathy	Paget's disease
Chronic alcoholism	Pulmonary disease
Atrioventricular malformation	Medications (e.g., steroids, NSAIDs)
Thyrotoxicosis (arrhythmia)	Drug toxicity
	Renal disease

* Risk factors for new onset or exacerbation of previous CHF.

place between the adrenergic nervous system, the renin-angiotensin axis, the peripheral circulation, and other vasoactive substances in response to impaired cardiac function (O'Toole, 1992). Even so, knowledge of this complex and increasingly prevalent clinical syndrome remains far from complete.

When the heart fails to propel blood forward normally, the body utilizes three compensatory mechanisms; these are effective for a short time but eventually become insufficient to met the oxygen needs of the body. First, the failing heart attempts to maintain a normal output of blood by enlarging its pumping chambers so that they can hold a greater volume of blood. This lengthening of the muscle fibers, called *ventricular dilation*, increases the amount of blood ejected from the heart. This compensatory mechanism has limits, because contractility of ventricular muscle fibers ceases to increase when they are stretched beyond a certain point.

During this first compensatory phase, the right ventricle, which is not yet affected by CHF, continues to pump more blood into the lungs. Congestion occurs in the pulmonary circulation with accumulation of blood in the lungs. The immediate result is shortness of breath (most common symptom), and if the process continues, actual flooding of the air spaces of the lungs occurs, with fluid seeping from the distended blood vessels; this is called *pulmonary congestion* or *pulmonary edema* (Urden et al., 1992). Congestion in the vascular system interferes with the movement of body fluids in and out of the various fluid compartments resulting in fluid accumulation in the tissue spaces and progressive edema.

Second, the heart begins to increase its muscle mass to strengthen the force of its contractions. This results in *ventricular hypertrophy* and a need for more oxygen. Eventually, the coronary arteries cannot meet the oxygen demands of the enlarged myocardium, and the person may experience angina pectoris owing to ischemia.

Third, a *sympathetic nervous system response* occurs to increase the stimulation of the heart muscle, causing it to pump more often. As a muscle, the heart is regulated by autonomic (involuntary) innervation. In response to failing contractility of the myocardial cells, the sympathetic nervous system activates adaptive processes that increase the heart rate, increase peripheral vascular resistance via venous and arteriolar constriction (to maintain vital organ perfusion), and retain urine.

Sympathetic stimulation also reduces renal blood flow, and the kidneys respond by retaining water and sodium, which further exacerbates tissue edema. The expanded blood volume increases the load on an already compromised heart. These mechanisms are responsible for the symptoms of diaphoresis, cool skin, tachycardia, cardiac arrhythmias, and oliguria (reduced urine excretion).

When the combined efforts of these three compensatory mechanisms achieve a normal level of cardiac output, the client is said to have *compensated* CHF. When these mechanisms are no longer effective and the disease progresses to the final stage of impaired heart function, the client has *decompensated* CHF.

This condition ranges from mild congestion with few symptoms to life-threatening fluid overload and total heart failure (Table 10–8). Symptoms usually develop very gradually so that many people do not recognize or report signals of serious disease. The elderly in particular may wrongly associate early symptoms with a lack of fitness or as a sign of aging (Alliance for Aging Research, 1993). Confusion and impaired thinking can characterize heart failure in elderly people.

TABLE 10-8 CLINICAL MANIFESTATIONS OF HEART FAILURE

LEFT VENTRICULAR FAILURE	RIGHT VENTRICULAR FAILURE
Progressive dyspnea (exertional first)	Progressive failure
Paroxysmal nocturnal dyspnea	Dependent edema (ankle or pretibial first)
Orthopnea	Jugular vein distention
Productive spasmodic cough	Abdominal pain and distention
Pulmonary edema	Weight gain
Extreme breathlessness	Right upper quadrant pain (liver congestion)
Anxiety	Cardiac cirrhosis
Frothy pink sputum	Ascites
Nasal flaring	Jaundice
Accessory muscle use	Anorexia, nausea
Rales	Cyanosis (nail beds)
Tachypnea	Psychological disturbances
Diaphoresis	
Cerebral hypoxia	
Irritability	
Restlessness	
Confusion	
Impaired memory	
Sleep disturbances	
Fatigue, exercise intolerance	
Muscular weakness	
Renal changes	

Left Heart Failure

Failure of the left ventricle causes either pulmonary edema or a disturbance in the respiratory control mechanisms. The degree of respiratory distress varies with the client's position, activity, and level of emotional or physical stress, but any of the symptoms listed under pulmonary edema may occur.

Dyspnea is subjective and does not always correlate with the extent of heart failure, but exertional dyspnea occurs in all clients to some degree. Time for dyspnea to subside is an indication of progress or deterioration in a client's status, and it can be measured for documentation. Paroxysmal nocturnal dyspnea resembles the frightening sensation of awakening with suffocation. Once the client is in the upright position, relief from the attack may not occur for 30 minutes or longer. *Orthopnea* is a more advanced stage of dyspnea. The client often assumes a "three-point position," sitting up with both hands on the knees and leaning forward. In severe heart failure, the client may resort to sleeping upright in a chair or recliner.

Fatigue and muscular weakness are often associated with left ventricular failure, as dyspnea develops along with weight gain and a faster resting heart rate, which decrease the person's ability to exercise. Inadequate cardiac output leads to decreased peripheral blood flow and blood flow to skeletal muscle. The resultant tissue hypoxia and slowed removal of metabolic wastes cause the person to tire easily (Minotti et al., 1991). Disturbances in sleep and rest patterns may aggravate fatigue; muscle atrophy is common in advanced CHF (Lipkin et al., 1988).

Renal changes can occur in both right- and left-sided heart failure, but they are more evident with left-sided failure. During the day, the client is upright, decreased cardiac output reduces blood flow to the kidneys, and the formation of urine is reduced (oliguria). Sodium and water not excreted in the urine are retained in the vascular system, adding to the blood volume.

Diminished blood supply to the renal system causes the kidney to secrete renin, which indirectly stimulates the secretion of aldosterone from the adrenal gland. Aldosterone acts on the renal tubules, causing them to increase reabsorption of sodium and water, further increasing fluid volume. At night, urine formation increases with the recumbent position as blood flow to the kidney improves. *Nocturia* may interfere with effective sleep patterns, which contributes to fatigue as mentioned.

Right Ventricular Failure

Failure of the right ventricle results in peripheral edema and venous congestion of the organs (see Table 10–8) (see also Chapter 12, Cor Pulmonale). *Dependent edema* is one of the early signs of right ventricular failure, although significant CHF can be present in the absence of peripheral edema. In CHF, fluid is retained because the pressoreceptors of the body sense a decreased volume of blood as a result of the heart's inability to pump an adequate amount of blood. The pressoreceptors subsequently relay a message to the kidneys to retain fluid so that a greater volume of blood can be ejected from the heart to the peripheral tissues (Pastan and Braunwald, 1992). Unfortunately this compounds the problem and makes the heart work even harder, which further decreases its pumping ability. The retained fluid commonly accumulates in the extracellular spaces of the periphery (Braunwald, 1992).

Edema is usually symmetrical and occurs in the dependent parts of the body, where venous pressure is the highest. In ambulatory persons, edema begins in the feet and ankles and ascends up the lower legs (pretibial areas). It is most noticeable at the end of a day and often decreases after a night's rest. In the recumbent person, pitting edema may develop in the presacral area and, as it worsens, progress to the medial thighs and genital area.

Jugular venous distention also results from fluid overload. As fluid is retained and the heart's ability to pump is further compromised, the retained fluid "backs up" into both the lungs and the venous system, of which the jugular veins are the simplest to identify and evaluate. This distention may be observed in all positions[12] in individuals with marked CHF (Cahalin, 1994).

As the liver becomes congested with venous blood it becomes enlarged, and *abdominal pain* occurs. If this occurs rapidly, stretching of the capsule surrounding the liver causes severe discomfort, and the person may notice either a constant aching or a sharp *right upper quadrant pain*. In chronic CHF, long-standing congestion of the liver with venous blood and anoxia can lead to ascites (see Fig. 14–7) and jaundice, which are symptoms of liver damage. *Anorexia, nausea,* and *bloating* develop secondary to venous congestion of the gastrointestinal tract. Anorexia and nausea may also result from digitalis toxicity, which is a common problem as digitalis is usually prescribed for CHF.

Cyanosis of the nail beds appears as venous congestion reduces peripheral blood flow. Clients with CHF often feel anxious, frightened, and depressed. Fears may be expressed as frightening nightmares, insomnia, acute anxiety states, depression, or withdrawal from reality.

Medical Management

Diagnosis. Diagnosis is based on the clinical picture and depends on where symptoms are on the continuum of mild to severe. Echocardiogram is the main diagnostic tool; noninvasive cardiac testing such as ECG, chest radiography, and echocardiography (Aronow, 1994) are secondary tools that can determine left ventricular size and function well enough to confirm the diagnosis. Cardiac catheterization is not routinely performed, but it may be useful in certain cases (e.g., atherosclerotic heart disease, which is potentially correctable). For people with severe pulmonary disease, radionuclide angiography may be used to measure left ventricular ejection fraction and permits analysis of regional wall motion.

Arterial blood gases are drawn to measure oxygen saturation. Liver enzymes (e.g., AST, alkaline phosphatase) are often elevated (see Tables 35–15 and 35–21); liver involvement with hyperbilirubinemia commonly occurs, resulting in jaundice.

Treatment. In the past, heart failure progressed despite therapy, and life expectancy was significantly shortened. Nonpharmacologic interventions such as diet, medications, and exercise that alter interactions between the heart and the periphery are now accepted therapeutic approaches. Alterations in lifestyle reduce symptoms and the need for additional medication (Rich, 1993).

Traditionally, the diagnosis of CHF was a contraindication for participation in exercise training. In fact, it is clear that activity restriction should be avoided (Minotti and Massie, 1992), as exercise programs have proved to quantitatively achieve similar results to those attained with most effective drug treatments (Kostis et al., 1994; Leier, 1993). These findings have shifted attention away from treating the heart toward exercising the muscles. Whenever possible, physical activity and exercise is prescribed per client tolerance (Coats et al., 1990; 1992; Koch, et al., 1992; Sullivan et al., 1989).

Physical training for clients with CHF results in an increase in muscular strength and better adaptation to effort owing to the effect of training on peripheral muscles (e.g., decreased vascular resistance in the muscles, delay in the onset of anaerobic metabolism). Improvements in peak oxygen consumption are probably related to increased oxygen uptake in the exercising muscles, because the function of the left ventricle is not improved (Coats et al., 1990; Sullivan et al., 1988). Studies are under way to determine the specific benefit of aerobic exercise for persons with CHF (Kitzman, 1995).

At the present time, acute CHF is usually treated in a hospital setting, where major reversible causes of CHF are treated first. Treatment focus is toward initial stabilization with diuretics to assist in the elimination of water and sodium in the urine (Cohn, 1994a), parenteral vasodilators to reduce resistance to the flow of blood being pumped from the heart

[12] Distention of the neck veins that are normally empty when the head is elevated to a 45-degree angle.

(Cohn, 1994b), and inotropic agents (e.g., digoxin, digitoxin) to strengthen the force of myocardial contractions. Persons with CHF are placed on a sodium-restricted diet, sometimes with limited fluid intake. Emotional and physical rest during the initial phases of treatment as an intervention are also important in diminishing the workload of the heart.

Angiotensin-converting enzyme (ACE) inhibitors have become standard therapy for heart failure in their ability to block the renin-angiotensin-aldosterone system, increasing renal blood flow and decreasing renal vascular resistance, thereby enhancing diuresis. ACE inhibitors reduce left ventricular filling pressure and moderately increase cardiac output. Vasodilator therapy in combination with ACE inhibitors prolongs life in persons with moderate to severe heart failure (Cohn, 1994c; Mujais, 1992; Om and Hess, 1993).

Surgical treatment may include CABG for underlying myocardial ischemia and infarction (see Fig. 10–4); reconstruction of incompetent heart valves; venoarterial bypass, which assists the heart by diverting blood to a pump that returns it to the arterial tree; counterpulsation, which uses an external pump or balloon to adjust the aortic blood pressure; and use of an artificial heart or cardiac transplantation.

Cardiac transplantation is now more common for treatment of heart failure. Transplantation is successful for selected individuals, usually those who are treated early in the course of heart failure, before advanced symptoms develop. Reform of the selection process is recommended to identify people who, though not critically ill, will not survive without early transplantation (O'Connell, 1992; Stevenson, 1993).

Other newer specialized treatment may include dialysis and ultrafiltration (mechanical removal of fluid) for persons unresponsive to diuretic therapy because of severe CHF or insensitivity to diuretics. Mechanical removal of fluid may be associated with the risk of complications (e.g., pneumothorax, infection, peritonitis, cardiac arrhythmias). Cardiovascular collapse may occur if too much fluid is removed or if removal takes place too rapidly (Cahalin, 1994). In the future, emphasis on the management of heart failure will continue to shift from attempts to alter hemodynamics and symptoms to attempts to interfere with the natural history of the disease (Cohn, 1994d; Kubo and Cohn, 1994).

Prognosis. Treatment of CHF remains difficult, and the prognosis is poor, even with recent advances in pharmacologic treatment. To achieve the maximum benefit from drug therapy, symptoms must be recognized as early as possible and treatment initiated. Because this condition often develops gradually, treatment is delayed, full resolution is not usually possible, and CHF becomes a chronic disorder (Rector and Cohn, 1994).

Annual mortality rates range from 10% in stable clients with mild symptoms to over 50% in people with advanced, progressive symptoms. About 40% to 50% of clients with heart failure die suddenly, probably owing to ventricular arrhythmias.

Exercise capacity may be the most powerful predictor of survival in the CHF client (Szlachcic et al., 1985). Poor prognostic signs include severe left ventricular dysfunction, severe symptoms and limitation of exercise capacity, secondary renal insufficiency, and elevated plasma catecholamine levels. Survival rates for cardiac transplantation in persons with CHF are greater than 85% at 1 year.

Special Implications for the Therapist **10–5**

CONGESTIVE HEART FAILURE

Early Considerations

Clients hospitalized with severe CHF require a therapy program to maintain pulmonary function and prevent complications of bed rest (e.g., skin breakdown, venous stasis, venous thrombus, pulmonary emboli). An important aspect of treatment includes functional assessment (Box 10–8) and physical exercise within the limitations set by the physician. See also established guidelines for exercise training in CHF (Cahalin, 1994). Physical therapy assessment of cardiopulmonary status is beyond the scope of this text. The clinician is referred to any of the specific examination and assessment texts available (Frownfelter and Dean, 1996; Hillegass and Sadowsky, 1994; Jarvis, 1992; Swartz, 1994).

Monitoring Vital Signs

Progressing activities from bed rest to transfers or ambulation requires vital sign assessment immediately after the major activity and 3 minutes later to assess for return to baseline. Oxygen may be administered by mask or cannula; team members must consult with respiratory therapy staff to determine appropriate oxygen levels during exercise.

Monitor the client for signs of increasing peripheral edema by assessing jugular neck vein distention, peripheral edema in the legs or sacrum, and any report of right upper quadrant pain. In the outpatient or home health setting, the client is advised to call the nurse or physician if shoes, belt, or pants become too tight to fasten, usual activities of daily living or tasks become difficult, extra sleep is needed, or urination at night becomes more frequent. Monitoring blood pressure is essential to detect heart failure; observe for decreasing

BOX **10–8**

Functional and Therapeutic Classification of Heart Disease

Class I: Cardiac disease present but no limitation on physical activity. Ordinary physical activity does not cause undue fatigue, palpitation, dyspnea, or anginal pain

Class II: Slight limitation on physical activity. Comfortable at rest, but ordinary physical activity results in fatigue, palpitation, dyspnea, or anginal pain

Class III: Marked limitation of physical activity. Comfortable at rest, but less than ordinary physical activity causes fatigue, palpitation, dyspnea, or anginal pain

Class IV: Unable to carry on any physical activity without discomfort. Symptoms of cardiac insufficiency or of the anginal syndrome may be present even at rest. If any physical activity is undertaken, discomfort is increased

From Criteria Committee of the New York Heart Association: Nomenclature and Criteria for Diagnosis of Diseases of the Heart and Great Vessels, ed 9. Boston, Little, Brown, 1994, pp 253–256.

blood pressure and report any change in status to the nurse or physician immediately.

Positioning

Positioning is important and the client is taught to use a high Fowler's position (head of the bed elevated at least 20 in. above the level) or chair to reduce pulmonary congestion, facilitate diaphragmatic expansion and ventilation, and ease dyspnea. The legs are maintained in a dependent position as much as possible to decrease venous return. Range of motion to decrease venous pooling and monitoring for the development of thrombophlebitis (e.g., unilateral swelling, calf pain, pallor) are required.

Exercise

The American College of Sports Medicine guidelines (1991) suggest that CHF clients entering an exercise program should start with moderate intensity exercise (40% to 60% Vo_2max [see explanation of Vo_2max, Chapter 12]) for a duration of 2 to 6 minutes, followed by 2 minutes of rest. Blood pressure and heart rhythm should be routinely monitored at rest, during peak exercise, and after cooldown. The goal is to gradually increase the intensity and duration of exercise. Others (Cortes and Goetz, 1994) advocate starting CHF clients at a low to moderate exercise intensity (<40% Vo_2max) with a shorter duration of exercise initially and a shorter rest period (<2 minutes). Refer to Hanson, 1994, for further information on exercise testing and training in persons with CHF.

The therapist should keep in mind that some older CHF clients are unable to increase their exercise intensity or duration despite starting very slowly. These people do not achieve the goal of increased endurance and often leave the program owing to increased symptoms and exercise intolerance. Maintaining or even improving functional activities and independence at home may be a more appropriate goal for this group.

Medications

Diuretics can produce mild to severe electrolyte imbalance requiring special consideration (see Chapter 4). Digitalis toxicity is a life-threatening condition that occurs in one of every five clients and may present with systemic or cardiac manifestations. Any sign or symptom of digitalis toxicity should be reported to the physician (Table 10–9). Digitalis toxicity can cause a dip in the ST segment on ECG; whenever possible, the ECG should be monitored during exercise. Activity should not increase the magnitude of the altered ST segment. In addition, NSAIDs, including over-the-counter drugs such as ibuprofen, increase fluid retention independently and significantly blunt the action of diuretics and other cardiovascular drugs (especially ACE inhibitors), exacerbating preexisting CHF and causing isolated lower extremity edema (Rich, 1993; Yost and Morgan, 1994).

The major consideration for exercise in clients taking ACE inhibitors is the possibility of hypotension and accompanying arrhythmias. These problems should be reported to the physician and can be addressed by maintaining proper hydration and by altering dosages and the simultaneous use of other medications (Miller and Morley, 1993).

TABLE 10–9 SIGNS AND SYMPTOMS OF DIGITALIS TOXICITY

Gastrointestinal tract	Anorexia, nausea, vomiting, diarrhea, abdominal cramps
Central nervous system	Headache, fatigue, lethargy, depression, restlessness, irritability, drowsiness
Cardiovascular system	Bradycardia, ventricular tachycardia
Eyes	Flickering flashes of light; "colored vision" usually yellow or blue, halo vision, photophobia, blurring, diplopia, scotomata (blind spots in visual field)

From Reigle J, Ringel KA: Nursing care of clients with disorder of cardiac function. *In* Black JM, Matassarin-Jacobs E (eds): Luckmann and Sorensen's Medical-Surgical Nursing, ed 4. Philadelphia, WB Saunders, 1993, p 1172.

Hypertensive Cardiovascular Disease

Hypertensive cardiovascular disease includes hypertensive vascular disease, hypertensive heart disease, pulmonary hypertension, and pulmonary heart disease. The latter two conditions affecting the heart are caused by an underlying pulmonary pathology and are discussed in Chapter 12.

Hypertension (Hypertensive Vascular Disease)

Definition. Hypertension, or high blood pressure, is defined by the World Health Organization (WHO) as a persistent elevation of systolic blood pressure above 140 mm Hg and of diastolic pressure above 90 mm Hg measured on at least two separate occasions at least 2 weeks apart (i.e., sustained elevation of blood pressure above a predetermined level).

Overview. Hypertension can be classified according to type (systolic or diastolic), cause, and degree of severity (Table 10–10). *Primary* (or essential) hypertension is also known as

TABLE 10–10 BLOOD PRESSURE LEVELS FOR ADULTS*

CATEGORY	SYSTOLIC (mm Hg)	DIASTOLIC (mm Hg)
Normal	<130	<85
High normal	130–139	85–89
Hypertension		
Stage 1 (mild)	140–159	90–99
Stage 2 (moderate)	160–179	100–109
Stage 3 (severe)	180–209	110–119
Stage 4 (very severe)	≥210	≥120

* For adults aged 18 years and older not taking antihypertensive drugs and not acutely ill.

From the Fifth Report of the Joint National Committee on Detection, Evaluation, and Treatment of High Blood Pressure (JNCW). Arch Intern Med 153:154–183, 1993.

BOX **10–9**
Risk Factors of Primary (Essential) Hypertension

Modifiable
- High sodium intake (causes water retention, increasing blood volume)
- Obesity (associated with increased intravascular volume)
- Hypercholesterolemia and increased serum triglycerides levels
- Smoking (nicotine restricts blood vessels)
- Chronic abuse of alcohol (increases plasma catecholamines)
- Continuous emotional stress (stimulates sympathetic nervous system)
- Sedentary lifestyle

Nonmodifiable
- Positive family history
- Age (advanced)
- Sex (male)
- Race (black)

Adapted from Walsh E: Management of persons with vascular problems. *In* Phipps W, Cassmeyer VL, Sands JK, et al (eds): Medical-Surgical Nursing: Concepts and Clinical Practice, ed 5. St Louis, Mosby–Year Book, 1995, p 920.

idiopathic hypertension and accounts for 90% to 95% of all cases of hypertension. *Secondary* hypertension accounts for only 5% to 10% of cases and results from an identifiable cause (see Etiology). Intermittent elevation of blood pressure interspersed with normal readings is called *labile* hypertension or *borderline* hypertension. Malignant hypertension is a syndrome of markedly elevated blood pressure (diastolic blood pressure above 125 mm Hg) with target organ damage (e.g., retinal hemorrhages, papilledema, heart failure, encephalopathy, renal insufficiency).

Incidence and Risk Factors. The incidence of hypertension varies considerably among different groups in the American population, but it is estimated that 20% to 35% of the population is affected. This means that 1 in 3, or an estimated 60 million, Americans have high blood pressure. Risk factors for hypertension may be modifiable or nonmodifiable (Box 10–9). Hypertension occurs slightly more often in men than in women and at an earlier age. After age 50 years, hypertension begins to develop in more women than men.

Hypertension is twice as prevalent and more severe among blacks as whites. This phenomenon has been attributed to heredity, reduced access to health care, greater environmental stress, and greater salt intake, although the actual cause is not clear (Andreoli, 1993).[13] In all groups the incidence of hypertension increases with age, with a poorer prognosis for people whose hypertension begins at a young age.

Hypertension itself represents a significant risk factor for the development of coronary heart disease, stroke, and CHF.

Etiology. Primary or essential hypertension has no established etiology. Although a familial association with hypertension has been documented, no specific genetic defect has been shown to be causal in animal or human studies. Small arteries branching from the aorta, called arterioles, regulate blood pressure. Any condition that can narrow the opening of these arterioles can increase the blood pressure in the arteries. A variety of specific diseases or problems, such as chronic renal failure, renal artery stenosis, or endocrine disease, can cause secondary hypertension (Table 10–11).

The influence of NSAIDs on blood pressure in normotensive and hypertensive persons remains in question. At the very least it has been determined that there is always the potential for NSAIDs to interact with antihypertensive agents, most notably diuretics, β-receptor antagonists, and ACE inhibitors (Yost and Morgan, 1994). Given the high prevalence of NSAID use by elderly persons, especially for conditions like arthritis, gout, and other similar problems, the association between this drug use and blood pressure must be observed carefully (Gurwitz et al., 1994).

Pathogenesis *(Walsh, 1995).* Blood pressure is regulated by two factors: blood flow and peripheral vascular resistance. Blood flow is determined by cardiac output (strength, rate, rhythm of heartbeat, and blood volume). The resistance to flow is primarily determined by the diameter of blood vessels and, to a lesser degree, by the viscosity of blood.

Increased peripheral resistance as a result of the narrowing of the arterioles is the single most common characteristic of hypertension. Constriction of the peripheral arterioles may be controlled by two mechanisms, each with several components: (1) sympathetic nervous system activity and (2) activation of the renin-angiotensin system. In the case of the sympathetic nervous system, norepinephrine is released in response to psychogenic stress or baroreceptor activity. The blood vessels constrict, which increases peripheral resistance. At the same time, epinephrine is secreted by the adrenal medulla,

TABLE **10–11** CAUSES OF SECONDARY HYPERTENSION

Coarctation of the aorta	Acute stress
Pheochromocytoma (a rare, catecholamine-secreting tumor)	Surgery
Alcohol abuse	Psychogenic hyperventilation
Pregnancy induced	Alcohol withdrawal
Thyrotoxicosis	Burns
Increased intracranial pressure from tumors or trauma	Pancreatitis
Collagen disease	Sickle cell crisis
Endocrine disease	Neurologic disorders
Acromegaly	Brain tumor
Cushing's disease	Respiratory acidosis
Diabetes	Encephalitis
Hypothyroidism	Sleep apnea
Hyperthyroidism	Guillain-Barré syndrome
Renal disease (e.g. connective tissue diseases, diabetic nephropathy)	Quadriplegia
Effects of drugs (e.g. oral contraceptives, cyclosporine, cocaine)	Lead poisoning

Adapted from Kaplan NM: Systemic hypertension: mechanisms and diagnosis. *In* Braunwald E: Heart Disease: A Textbook of Cardiovascular Medicine, ed 4. Philadelphia, WB Saunders, 1992, p 820.

[13] From a pathogenetic point of view, recent research findings have suggested that β-adrenergic receptor downregulation is characteristic of hypertension in whites, whereas heightened vascular α-receptor sensitivity or early vascular hypertrophy may be a feature of hypertension in blacks (Sherwood et al., 1995).

resulting in increased force of cardiac contraction, increased cardiac output, and vasoconstriction.

Within the renin-angiotensin system, vasoconstriction results in decreased blood flow to the kidney. Whenever blood flow to the kidney diminishes, renin is secreted and angiotensin is formed, causing vasoconstriction within the renal system and increased total peripheral resistance. Angiotensin also stimulates the secretion of aldosterone, which promotes sodium and water retention by the kidney tubules, causing an increase in intravascular volume. All of these factors increase blood pressure.

With prolonged hypertension, the elastic tissue in the arterioles is replaced by fibrinous collagen tissue. The thickened arteriole wall becomes less distensible, offering even greater resistance to the flow of blood. This process leads to decreased tissue perfusion, especially in the target organs of high blood pressure (i.e., heart, kidneys, brain). Atherosclerosis is also accelerated in persons with high blood pressure.

Clinical Manifestations. Hypertension is frequently asymptomatic (except for elevated blood pressure when measured) especially in the early stages; this creates a significant health care risk for affected people. When symptoms do occur, they may include headache (usually occipital and present in the morning, worse on waking and slowly improving with activity), vertigo and flushed face, spontaneous epistaxis, blurred vision, and nocturnal frequency.

Progressive hypertension may be characterized by cardiovascular or cerebral symptoms such as dyspnea, orthopnea, chest pain, and leg edema (cardiovascular) or nausea, vomiting, drowsiness, confusion, and fleeting numbness or tingling in the limbs (cerebral).

Medical Management

Diagnosis. Blood pressure varies over the course of any single day depending on exertion, emotional state, ingestion of food, medications, and the presence of risk factors described previously. Thus, it is important that blood pressure be measured at several different times and under consistent circumstances before a diagnosis of hypertension is made.

No tests are specific for essential hypertension. Studies used in the routine evaluation of hypertension may include a complete blood count (CBC); urinalysis; serum potassium, cholesterol, and creatinine assays; fasting blood glucose level; ECG; and chest radiography. Other more specific tests may be needed for secondary hypertension.

Treatment. Once diagnosed, hypertension requires ongoing management, despite the absence of symptoms. The goal is to achieve and maintain arterial blood pressure (without side effects) below 140/90 mm Hg. Treatment of the underlying disorder is necessary with secondary hypertension. Nonpharmacologic intervention through lifestyle modification is widely advocated as initial therapy for primary hypertension.

This program may include sodium restriction, weight reduction, smoking cessation, a regular program of aerobic exercise,[14] restriction of alcohol and caffeine, modification of dietary fat, and administration of nutritional supplements (e.g., potassium, calcium, magnesium). Dietary potassium deficiency may have a role in increasing blood pressure; individuals may also become hypokalemic from increased urinary magnesium excretion during diuretic therapy and require additional potassium (Linas, 1991).

Magnesium and calcium influence vascular tone as magnesium acts to relax blood vessels and calcium assists in blood vessel contraction. A proper balance of these two substances is essential, as they compete for entry into the cell. When magnesium is low, an abnormally large amount of calcium enters the cells so that blood vessels begin to lose their ability to relax. Progressive vasoconstriction and subsequent spasms result in elevated blood pressure and eventual ischemia. Muscle weakness with depressed tendon reflexes may accompany this condition. A fall in serum potassium level also enhances the effects of digitalis, increasing the risk of digoxin toxicity.

Elderly individuals, blacks, and hypertensive individuals are more sensitive to change in dietary sodium chloride than are other individuals. A reduction of sodium intake alone may be enough to control blood pressure in persons with mild hypertension and may reduce the medication requirements in those who require drug therapy. It is also recommended that individuals with high blood pressure limit their intake of alcohol to 1 oz/day (1 oz of 100-proof whiskey, 4 oz of red wine, or 8 oz of beer)(JNVC, 1993).

Obesity has long been associated with hypertension and is an independent risk factor for CAD as well (Taylor, 1987). Regular exercise enhances weight loss and reduces blood pressure independent of weight loss. (For further discussion see Special Implications: Exercise, in this section.)

When to initiate the use of antihypertensive medications remains controversial, particularly in cases of mild hypertension. Presence of other cardiovascular risk factors, presence of target organ damage, and length of time that elevated blood pressure has been present are evaluated in making this treatment decision. Other factors must be taken into consideration in the use of antihypertensive medications. The presence of other disease processes that may be affected adversely by specific antihypertensives, prohibitive cost to the individual, altered quality of life by adverse side effects, and drug interaction with other prescribed medications are a few of these important considerations. Compliance with the treatment program is the most important factor in treating hypertension.

Antihypertensive medications can be classified by mode of action as diuretics, adrenergic inhibitors, vasodilators, ACE inhibitors, and calcium antagonists (Table 10–12). More than 50% of cases of mild hypertension can be controlled with one drug; a combination of medications may be required for others.

Diuretics are often the first step in the pharmacologic treatment of hypertension. Although these drugs decrease plasma volume, potassium depletion and renal complications may require the use of β-blockers, calcium channel blockers, or ACE inhibitors. Black people are generally more responsive to calcium antagonists and diuretics than to β-blockers or ACE inhibitors. Elderly persons with hypertension are generally equally responsive to all classes of antihypertensive medications, but they have an increased likelihood of side effects.

Prognosis. Hypertension is a major risk factor for atherosclerosis (see Atherosclerosis), implicating hypertension as a

[14] Moderate aerobic exercise alone should not be considered a replacement for pharmacologic therapy in nonobese people with mild hypertension (Blumenthal et al., 1991).

TABLE 10-12 Common Cardiovascular Medications

Medications (Trade/Generic Names)	Indications and Side Effects
Angiotensin-Converting Enzyme Inhibitors Capoten/captopril Lotensin/benazepril Vasotec/enalapril maleate	**Indication:** To treat high blood pressure and heart failure; prevent constriction of blood vessels and retention of sodium and fluid **Side Effects:** Cough, rash, loss of taste, weakness, headaches, palpitations,* swelling of feet or abdomen,* dizziness,† fainting†
α-Blockers Hytrin/terazosin HCl Minipress/prazosin HCl	**Indication:** To lower blood pressure by dilating blood vessels **Side Effects:** Headache, palpitations, fatigue, nausea, weakness, drowsiness, palpitations,* dizziness,† fainting†
Antiarrhythmics Cardioquin/quinidine Procan/procainamide HCl Rythmol/propafenone HCl	**Indication:** To alter conduction patterns in the heart **Side Effects:** Nausea, palpitations, vomiting, rash,* insomnia,* dizziness,† symptoms of CHF (shortness of breath, swollen ankles, coughing up blood)†
Anticoagulants Coumadin/warfarin sodium Platelet inhibitors Aspirin Persantine/dipyridamole	**Indication:** To prevent blood clot formation **Side Effects:** Easy bruising, stomach irritation (aspirin and persantine),* joint or abdominal pain,† difficulty in breathing or swallowing,† paralysis,† unexplained swelling, unusual or uncontrolled bleeding†
Central α-Agonists Aldomet/methyldopa Catapres/clonidine Wytensin/guanabenz acetate	**Indication:** To lower high blood pressure by dilating the blood vessels **Side Effects:** Drowsiness, depression, sexual dysfunction, fatigue, dry mouth, stuffy nose, fever, upset stomach, change in bowel habits, weight gain, fluid retention, dizziness†
β-Blockers Inderal/propranolol HCl Lopressor/metoprolol tartrate Tenormin/atenolol	**Indications:** To block sympathetic conduction at β-receptors and decrease blood pressure, dysrhythmias, and angina **Side Effects:** Insomnia, nausea, fatigue, slow pulse, weakness, increased cholesterol and blood glucose levels, nightmares,* sexual dysfunction,* asthmatic attacks,† dizziness†
Calcium Channel Blockers Procardia/nifedipine Cardizem/diltiazem HCl	**Indications:** To dilate coronary arteries to lower blood pressure and suppress some dysrhythmias **Side Effects:** Fluid retention, palpitations, headache, flushes, rash,* dizziness†
Digitalis Compounds Lanoxin/digoxin Crystodigin/digitoxin	**Indications:** To strengthen the heart's pumping force and decrease electrical conduction **Side Effects:** Fatigue, weakness, headache, irregular heart rhythms, nausea, vomiting, bradycardia†
Diuretics Thiazide diuretics (e.g., Diuril/chlorothiazide) Potassium-sparing diuretics (e.g., Aldactone/spironolactone) Loop diuretics (e.g., Lasix/furosemide)	**Indications:** To increase the excretion of sodium and water and control high blood pressure and fluid retention **Side Effects:** Drowsiness, dehydration, electrolyte imbalances, gout, nausea, pain, hearing loss, blood glucose abnormalities, elevated cholesterol and lipoprotein levels, muscle cramps,* dizziness,† light-headedness†
Lipid-Lowering Drugs Lopid/gemfibrozil Mevacor/lovastatin Questran/cholestyramine Zocor/simvastatin Nia-Bid, Niacor, Nicobid/niacin	**Indication:** To interfere with the metabolism of blood fats in various ways by lowering cholesterol, low-density lipoproteins, and/or triglyceride levels in the blood **Side Effects:** Nausea, vomiting, diarrhea, constipation, flatulence, and abdominal discomfort
Nitrates Nitrostat, Nitro-Bid/nitroglycerin Iso-Bid, Isodril/isosorbide dinitrate	**Indication:** For dilation of coronary arteries **Side Effects:** Headache, dizziness, orthostatic hypotension,* tachycardia*
Vasodilators Nitroglycerin Isosorbide dinitrate	**Indication:** To dilate the peripheral blood vessels (used in combination with diuretics) **Side Effects:** Headache, drowsiness, nausea, vomiting, diarrhea, hair growth (minoxidil only), increased heart rate,* swollen ankles,* dizziness,† difficulty in breathing†

* Call doctor when possible.
† Call doctor immediately.
Adapted from Goodman CC, Snyder TE: Differential Diagnosis in Physical Therapy, ed 2. Philadelphia: WB Saunders, 1995, pp 145–146.

common cause of death in the United States. Among black Americans, hypertension is also the most common fatal familial disease. Most of the mortality and morbidity associated with hypertension is attributed to an increased risk for a variety of cardiovascular disorders (Benditt and Schwartz, 1994).

More than half of persons with angina pectoris, sudden death, stroke, and thrombotic occlusion of the abdominal aorta or its branches have hypertension. Three fourths of people with dissecting aortic aneurysm, intracerebral hemorrhage, or rupture of the myocardial wall also have elevated blood pressure. If it is untreated, nearly half of people with hypertension die of heart disease, a third die of stroke, and 10% to 15% die of renal failure.

When a person with hypertension achieves the target blood pressure, it must be emphasized that blood pressure control does not equal cure. Adherence to treatment and follow-up monitoring must be continued on an ongoing basis (JNCV, 1993). Treatment prolongs life and antihypertensive medications have dramatically reduced the mortality rate associated with hypertension. Unfortunately, the cost of antihypertensives, side effects, and lack of symptoms sometimes lead to poor compliance with treatment.

Special Implications for the Therapist **10-6**

HYPERTENSION (HYPERTENSIVE VASCULAR DISEASE)

See also Special Implications for the Therapist: Coronary Artery Disease, earlier in this chapter.

It is estimated that hypertension remains undiagnosed in nearly half of the 60 million Americans who have it. It is possible that many people referred to therapy will be hypertensive without knowing it. Cardiac pathology may be unknown, requiring the therapist to remain alert for risk factors that require medical screening. A baseline blood pressure measurement should be taken on two or three separate occasions, and any unusual findings should be reported to the physician.

A sudden increase in blood pressure such as occurs with any increase in intra-abdominal pressure (e.g., Valsalva maneuver; see also Box 13–1) during exercise or stabilization exercises can be dangerous for already hypertensive persons. The therapist must alert individuals with hypertension to this effect and teach proper breathing techniques during all activities.

Medications

Whenever a health care provider knows that a client has been prescribed antihypertensive medications, appropriate follow-up questions as to whether the client is taking the medication and taking it as prescribed must be addressed. Many people take the medication only when symptoms are perceived and are at risk for the complications described previously (especially during an exercise program, when oxygen demands of the myocardium increase).

People with coronary artery disease taking NSAIDs may also be at slight risk for a myocardial event during times of increased myocardial oxygen demand (e.g., exercise or fever) (Yost and Morgan, 1994). Additionally, elderly people taking NSAIDs and antihypertensive agents must be monitored carefully. Regardless of the NSAID chosen, it is important to check blood pressure within the first few weeks in which therapy or exercise is initiated, and periodically thereafter (Radack and Deck, 1987).

Exercise

The mechanisms by which exercise lowers blood pressure are still unknown (Blumenthal et al., 1995). A regular program of aerobic exercise, introduced gradually, facilitates cardiovascular conditioning, may assist in weight reduction, and may provide some benefit in reducing blood pressure. Exercising using primarily the lower extremities (e.g., cycling, walking) can also reduce blood pressure (Kelly et al., 1994). The amount of time required to lower resting blood pressure by physical activity has not been established. Diastolic blood pressure reduction seems to be related to the duration of the exercise program (i.e., the longer the program, the more likely the hypotensive effect). Blood pressure reduction has occurred after just several weeks to 6 months of regular training (Harris and Holly, 1987). On the other hand, blood pressure will return to its previous elevated level if training is discontinued (Bjorntorp, 1982).

Most individuals with mild to moderate hypertension have blood pressure elevations during exercise similar to those of normotensive individuals. Higher ending levels merely reflect elevated resting systolic pressures. In hypertensive individuals, both systolic and diastolic pressures are reduced below resting values immediately following dynamic exercise. Systolic blood pressure can be lowered for 60 to 90 minutes; diastolic blood pressure often returns to preexercise levels within 1 hour (Goldberg and Elliot, 1994c).

Heavy isometric exercises and heavy weightlifting may be harmful, as the blood pressure often rises because of vasovagal reflexes that occur. Generally, antihypertensive drugs have not been found to affect the blood pressure response to isometric exertion (Williams, 1988). However, the use of isometric exercise to lower blood pressure has not been studied in hypertensive individuals; a fall in resting blood pressure has been observed in normotensive individuals after repetitive isometric contractions equal to 30% of maximal capacity (Wiley et al., 1992).

Insulin levels can be modified by exercise. Hypertensive persons, even with average body weight and normal glucose tolerance, can be relatively insulin resistant (Ferrannini, 1987). (See also Chapter 9, Special Implications for the Therapist: 9–15).

Exercise Training Guidelines

The intensity of exercise required to produce health benefits and decrease blood pressure has been confused with the level of exercise necessary to improve physical fitness. Health benefits can be achieved without large gains in fitness. Encouraging people to increase their level of total energy expenditure is the key to increasing activity levels, rather than emphasizing physical fitness.

The type, intensity, duration, and frequency of training, as well as progression, should be assessed regularly. A pre-exercise evaluation and exercise testing may be prescribed by the physician. This information is helpful in establishing submaximal and maximal blood pressure responses. Monitoring vital signs before, during, and after exercise or activity is essential. Any person with an exaggerated systolic blood pressure response (over 250 mm Hg) or failure to reduce diastolic pressure (below 90 mm Hg) should be referred to the physician for reevaluation.

Training intensity does not need to be high, and it appears that low-intensity activity (65% to 70% of maximum heart rate) three times per week is as effective as high intensity activity in blood pressure reduction. Training intensity should be based on maximum heart rate using the calculated formulas (see Appendix B), or measured during a maximal exercise test. After 12 to 16 weeks, if the blood pressure is adequately controlled, the physician may reduce the antihypertensive medication slowly to determine the long-term effect of training on blood pressure.

Several resources are available for determining the appropriate exercise program for the hypertensive client whether symptomatic or asymptomatic (American College of Sports Medicine, 1991; Goldberg and Elliot, 1994b).

Exercise and Antihypertensive Drugs

Antihypertensive medications reduce resting blood pressure levels and may influence blood pressure changes during submaximal and maximal exertion, which affects exercise capacity. Vasodilators selectively inhibit an increase in heart rate. Clinically, this means that when the person increases his or her activity or exercise level, the normal physiologic response of increased heart rate is blunted. Sudden changes in position (e.g., supine to standing) should be avoided, as this may result in orthostatic hypotension (see Special Implications for the Therapist: 10–8 [Orthostatic Hypotension], this chapter).

The following brief description of the impact of various drug classes (all vasodilators) on exercise may assist the therapist in prescribing activities for those who require pharmacologic agents and provide insight into therapeutic decisions for active hypertensive individuals. Any side effects noted may indicate that a medication adjustment is needed and should be brought to the physician's attention (see Table 10–12).

Vasodilators such as *nitroglycerin* and other *nitrates* act as a prophylactic for angina by dilating the coronary arteries and improving collateral cardiac circulation, increasing oxygen to the heart muscle, and decreasing the blood pressure, thereby decreasing symptoms of angina. *β-Adrenoreceptor antagonists* (β-blockers) diminish catecholamine-induced elevations of heart rate, myocardial contractility, and blood pressure. These effects reduce myocardial oxygen requirements during exertion and stress, thereby preventing angina and allowing the person to exercise for longer periods before the onset of angina. The intended action of β-blockers may prevent normal blood pressure and heart rate responses to exercise; therefore, using heart rate as an index for monitoring response to exercise is not recommended. Although β-blockers are effective antihypertensives, most of them adversely alter aerobic capacity so that exercise capacity is reduced (Ades, 1988; Tesch, 1985). An exercise prescription should be based on exercise stress test results using recommended guidelines (see American College of Sports Medicine, 1991; Peel and Mossberg, 1995). Side effects of β-blockers include bronchospasm, which causes difficulty breathing, or chest tightness, which mimics angina; orthostatic hypotension; syncope; headache; or fatigue and weakness.

Diuretics have been first-line antihypertensive agents for many years, but few studies have observed the effect of diuretic therapy on exercise performance. Existing evidence reveals that peak blood pressures induced by physical activity may not always be controlled with diuretics (Lee et al., 1979; Rosendorff et al., 1984). Diuretic therapy can result in hypokalemia accompanied by muscular cramps and skeletal muscle fatigue. (See also Chapter 4.) Potassium-sparing diuretics may cause hyperkalemia, which can in turn cause arrhythmias. Exercise tolerance may be reduced with arrhythmias because of a decrease in left ventricular filling time. Prolonged exercise in the heat is not recommended for people taking diuretics because of the cumulative effects of heat, exercise, and diuretics on blood volume and electrolytes. The length of time an individual who is taking a diuretic can safely exercise in the heat varies with the heat index and the physical condition of the person (Peel and Mossberg, 1995).

Calcium plays a role in the electrical excitation of cardiac cells and in the mechanical contraction of the myocardial and vascular smooth muscle cells (Haak et al., 1994). *Calcium channel antagonists* inhibit calcium ion influx across the cell membrane during cardiac depolarization, relax coronary vascular smooth muscle, dilate coronary and peripheral arteries, and increase myocardial oxygen delivery in people with vasospastic angina.* This class of vasodilators decreases peripheral vascular resistance at rest and during physical activity, thereby altering exercise tolerance by affecting heart rate and blood pressure during exercise. During exercise, calcium channel antagonists have been observed to reduce systolic and diastolic pressure at submaximal loads (Szlachcic, 1987), but higher systolic blood pressures measured during maximal exercise were not lowered (Goldberg and Elliot, 1989). Side effects of calcium antagonists (e.g., drowsiness, dizziness, headache, peripheral edema, tachycardia, or bradycardia) may interfere with a client's ability to participate in an exercise program.

ACE inhibitors reduce blood pressure by lowering peripheral vascular resistance. The effects of ACE inhibition during physical activity have not been well studied. During isometric exercise, blood pressure and heart rate do not appear to be affected (Williams, 1988). ACE inhibitors do not alter $\dot{V}O_2max$ (Leon, 1986).

Use of calcium antagonists and ACE inhibitors in hypertension has increased dramatically in the past 10 years, whereas the use of less expensive agents, such as diuretics and β-blockers, has declined. The authors of one study (Manolio et al., 1995) suggest that in the absence of convincing evidence that the more expensive medications reduce stroke and coronary disease and prevent heart disease in the hypertensive population, physicians should return to the use of less expensive but just as effective diuretics and β-blockers.

Monitoring During Exercise

Therapists often treat people who are diagnosed with conditions that are highly correlated with hypertension, such as stroke, obesity, diabetes mellitus, alcoholism, coronary artery disease, pregnancy, and others (see Table 10–11). Monitoring tolerance to exercise by observing for unusual symptoms and measuring blood pressure before, during, and after therapy are important steps in identifying a potential cardiovascular event (Hillegass, 1994a). Many factors can cause an increase in blood pressure (see Appendix B).

* The use of calcium channel blockers for angina and hypertension is increasing and may ultimately equal that of the β-blockers.

Hypertensive Heart Disease

Definition and Overview. The term *hypertensive heart disease* is used when the heart is enlarged as a result of persistently elevated blood pressure (hypertension) (see previous discussion). Left ventricular hypertrophy (LVH) and diastolic dysfunction are found in 10% to 30% of the adult population with chronic hypertension, and it may present with many of the signs and symptoms of CHF. Both the prevalence and the severity of the disease are greater in blacks than in whites. In all adults, it increases progressively with age.

Medical Management

Diagnosis, Treatment, and Prognosis. Cardiac enlargement viewed on x-ray and ECG changes of LVH are diagnostic of hypertensive heart disease. Treatment is as for hypertension unless heart failure develops, in which case treatment is as for heart failure (see each section for more discussion). The most common cause of death in hypertensive heart disease is CHF, accounting for 40% of all deaths from hypertension (Jennings et al., 1994).

Special Implications for the Therapist **10-7**

HYPERTENSIVE HEART DISEASE

See Special Implications for the Therapist: Coronary Artery Disease, Congestive Heart Failure, and Hypertensive Vascular Disease (all in this chapter).

Orthostatic (Postural) Hypotension

Definition and Etiology. The term *orthostatic (postural) hypotension* signifies a decrease of 20 mm Hg or greater in systolic blood pressure or a drop of 10 mm Hg or more of both systolic and diastolic arterial blood pressure with a concomitant pulse increase of 15 beats/min or more on standing from a supine or sitting position. When a normal individual stands up, the gravitational changes on the circulation are compensated for by several mechanisms, including the circulatory and autonomic nervous systems. Postural reflexes are slowed as part of the aging process for some, but not all, persons.

BOX **10-10**

Causes of Orthostatic Hypotension

- Volume depletion (e.g., diabetes mellitus, sodium or potassium depletion)
- Venous pooling (e.g., pregnancy, varicosities of the legs)
- Side effects of medication (e.g., antihypertensives) (see Table 10–12)
- Prolonged immobility
- Starvation
- Performing the Valsalva maneuver
- Sluggish normal regulatory mechanisms (e.g., anatomic variation, altered body chemistry)
- Secondary to other conditions (e.g., endocrine or metabolic disorders, diseases of the central or peripheral nervous system)

Orthostatic hypotension may be acute and temporary or chronic. The *acute* or temporary type is caused by sluggish normal regulatory mechanisms as a result of conditions listed in Box 10–10. A general result of treatment for hypertension may be hypotension. Additionally, many elderly people with systolic hypertension have postural hypotension that may require management before the hypertension is addressed (Kaplan, 1994). *Chronic* orthostatic hypotension may occur secondary to a specific disease, such as endocrine disorders, metabolic disorders, or diseases of the central or peripheral nervous system.

Pathogenesis. Normal aging is associated with various changes that may lead to postural hypotension. Cardiac output falls with age; in the elderly with hypertension, it is even lower. When elderly subjects are put under passive postural stress (60-degree upright tilt), their stroke volume falls even further. These "normal" changes obviously predispose the elderly to postural hypotension from any process that further reduces fluid volume or vascular integrity. For example, pooling of blood after eating may lead to profound hypotension, called *postprandial hypotension*. Additionally, as systolic pressure rises from atherosclerosis, baroreceptor sensitivity and vascular compliance are reduced further, increasing the likelihood of postural hypotension (Kaplan, 1994).

Clinical Manifestations and Medical Management. Orthostatic hypotension is often accompanied by dizziness, blurring or loss of vision, and syncope or fainting. Tilt study or tilt-table test may be used to assess hypotension by monitoring blood pressure and pulse while tilting a person from horizontal supine to 60 degrees upright. This test has proved very valuable in determining the cause of dizziness or syncope and can reveal irregularities in the vascular regulating system. There is no curative treatment for orthostatic hypotension of unknown cause; whenever the underlying disorder causing hypotension is corrected, symptoms cease.

Special Implications for the Therapist **10-8**

ORTHOSTATIC HYPOTENSION

Many of the medications used to treat hypertension can result in hypotension, especially when combined with therapy treatments or exercise that result in vasodilation. Of particular concern are heat treatments, such as the whirlpool or Hubbard tank. In addition, moderate to vigorous exercise of large muscle groups can produce significant vasodilation and can result in hypotension. This is particularly true following exercise, when venous return diminishes as exercise abruptly ceases. A cooldown period is essential, and safety measures must be employed (Watchie, 1994).

Stationary standing, as is performed in many activities of daily living, can produce hypotension. Some elderly individuals may experience unexpected and unexplained falls associated with orthostatic hypotension. The cause of such falls may be circulatory impairment that causes a drop in blood pressure on standing upright quickly, an early sign of some other illness, or effects of medication.

Anyone who is considered borderline hypotensive when tested in the supine position should have blood pressures measured and pulses counted in a sitting position with the legs dangling. If no change occurs when this is done, repeat the measurements with the person standing, if possible. A drop in systolic pressure of 10 to 20 mm Hg or more associated with an increase in pulse rate of more than 15 beats/min suggests depleted intravascular volume (Fig. 10–14). Some normovolemic persons with peripheral neuropathies or those taking antihypertensive medications may demonstrate an orthostatic fall in blood pressure, but without associated increase in pulse rate (Tierney, 1994).

Anyone with orthostatic hypotension, especially persons taking antihypertensive agents, should be instructed to rise slowly from the bed or chair after a long period of recumbency or sitting to avoid loss of balance and prevent falls. Dorsiflexing the feet before standing often promotes venous return to the heart, accelerates the pulse, and increases blood pressure. If the person becomes hypotensive, he or she should assume a supine position with legs elevated to increase venous return and to ensure cerebral blood flow. The use of elastic stockings may also help with venous return. Elevating the head of the bed 5 to 20 degrees prevents the nocturnal diuresis and supine hypertension caused by nocturnal shifts of interstitial fluid from the legs to the rest of the circulation. Eating small meals may help to avoid postprandial (after eating) hypotension. The physician should be notified if the person remains symptomatic after these measures have been taken (Lipsitz, 1990).

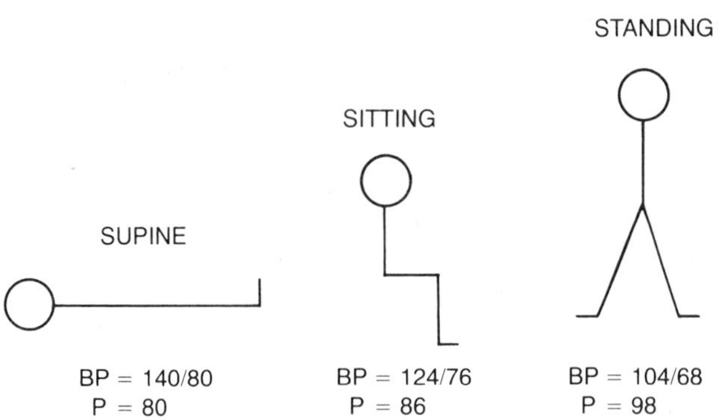

Figure 10–14. Assessing postural hypotension. After measuring the blood pressure (BP) and pulse in the supine position, leave the BP cuff in place and assist the person to sit. Remeasure the BP within 15 to 30 seconds. Assist the person to stand, and measure again. A BP drop of more than 20 mm Hg systolic and more than 10 mm diastolic accompanied by a 10% to 20% increase in heart rate (pulse) indicates postural hypotension. Sample measurements are given. (*From Black JM, Matassarin-Jacobs E (eds): Luckmann and Sorensen's Medical-Surgical Nursing, ed. 4. Philadelphia, WB Saunders, 1993, p 1111.*)

Myocardial Disease

Myocarditis

Myocarditis is a relatively uncommon inflammatory condition of the muscular walls of the heart (myocardium); it is most often a result of bacterial or viral infection, but it also includes those inflammatory processes related to infectious and noninfectious causes of ischemic heart disease. Other possible causes of myocarditis include chest radiation for treatment of malignancy, sarcoidosis, and drugs, such as lithium and cocaine.

The therapist is most likely to treat the person with systemic lupus erythematosus (SLE) (see Chapter 5), who may have a type of myocarditis called *lupus carditis* (see also Collagen Vascular Diseases: Lupus Carditis, this chapter). SLE is a multisystem autoimmune disease characterized by a release of autoantibodies into the circulation, with a subsequent inflammatory process that can target the heart and vasculature.

Clinical evidence of cardiac involvement among people with SLE has been reported in from 18% to 56% of cases (Chang, 1982). Clinical manifestations may include mild continuous chest pain or soreness in the epigastric region or under the sternum, palpitations, fatigue, and dyspnea, and onset may follow a viral upper respiratory illness in the population at large as well as in persons with SLE. Complications include heart failure, arrhythmias, dilated (congestive) cardiomyopathy (see next section), and sudden death.

Myocarditis usually resolves with treatment of the underlying condition or cause; specific antimicrobial therapy is prescribed if an infectious agent can be identified. Management of myocarditis in SLE is usually with NSAIDs, but corticosteroids and immunosuppressive agents may be required (Spiera and Rothschild, 1995). Myocarditis that progresses to dilated cardiomyopathy with heart failure is frequently fatal without heart transplantation.

Special Implications for the Therapist **10-9**

MYOCARDITIS

Active myocarditis is considered a contraindication for therapy, because this condition can progress very quickly and stress must be avoided; each case is evaluated by the physician. If an impairment of myocardial contractility is present, diastolic blood pressure may be elevated to maintain stroke volume. Disruptions leading to lethal cardiac arrhythmias cannot

TABLE 10–13 COMPARISON OF CARDIOMYOPATHIES

	Type of Cardiomyopathy		
	Dilated	Hypertrophic	Restrictive
Etiology/risk factors	Alcoholism, pregnancy, infection, toxins, nutritional deficiency, hypertension Idiopathic	Inherited defect of muscle growth and development	Infiltrative disease Amyloidosis Sarcoidosis Hemochromatosis
Pathology	Cardiac enlargement; myocardial fiber degeneration	Left ventricular hypertrophy; rigid walls	Endocardial scarring of the ventricles; rigid walls
Chamber size	Increased	Normal or decreased	Decreased or normal
Myocardial mass	Increased	Increased	Normal or increased
Endocardial thickness	Normal or increased	Increased	Increased
Contractility	Decreased	Increased or decreased	Normal or decreased
Clinical manifestations	Fatigue, weakness, chest pain, palpitations	Dyspnea, angina pectoris, fatigue, dizziness, palpitations; exercise intolerance	Exercise intolerance; dyspnea, fatigue; neck vein distention, peripheral edema, ascites
Cardiovascular complication	Left ventricular failure	Left ventricular failure	Right ventricular failure

Adapted from Haak SW, Richardson SJ, Davey SS: Alterations of cardiovascular function. *In* McCance KL, Huether SE (eds): Pathophysiology: The Biologic Basis for Disease in Adults and Children, ed 2. St Louis, Mosby–Year Book, 1994, pp 1035 and 1037.

be predicted. See also Special Implications for the Therapist: Rheumatic Fever and Endocarditis.

Cardiomyopathy

Definition and Overview. Cardiomyopathy is actually part of a group of conditions affecting the heart muscle itself, so that contraction and relaxation of myocardial muscle fibers is impaired. Cardiomyopathies are not caused by other heart or systemic disease, so by definition, cardiomyopathy excludes structural and functional abnormalities due to valvular disorders, CAD, hypertension, congenital defects, and pulmonary vascular disorders.

Cardiomyopathies are classified as *dilated, hypertrophic,* or *restrictive* on the basis of general features of presentation and pathophysiology (Table 10–13). Considerable overlap can occur between these three classifications within the same person (see Pathogenesis).

Incidence and Risk Factors. The cause of most cardiomyopathies is unknown; cardiomyopathy can affect persons of any age and is often seen in young adults in the second and third decades. The actual incidence is also unknown, but the disease may be more common than was previously realized. Delayed-onset cardiotoxic effects of chemotherapeutic agents may appear as chronic cardiomyopathy. Risk factors for the development of this type of cardiomyopathy include increasing doses of chemotherapeutic agents and previous mediastinal radiation (Watchie, 1992).

Dilated cardiomyopathy occurs most often in black men between ages 40 and 60 years. About half of the cases of dilated cardiomyopathy are idiopathic, and the remainder result from some known disease process (e.g., rheumatic fever, myasthenia gravis, progressive muscular dystrophy, hemochromatosis, amyloidosis, sarcoidosis). Risk factors for dilated cardiomyopathy may include long-term alcohol abuse, systemic hypertension, cigarette smoking, infections, and pregnancy.[15]

Hypertrophic cardiomyopathy appears to be genetically transmitted as an autosomal dominant trait on chromosome 14 (DeSanctis, 1990) and *restrictive cardiomyopathy* occurs as a result of myocardial fibrosis (e.g., amyloidosis, sarcoidosis, hemochromatosis), hypertrophy, infiltration or defect in myocardial relaxation (Wynne and Braunwald, 1992).

Pathogenesis. The exact pathogenesis of cardiomyopathy is unknown; the risk factors mentioned previously seem to lower the threshold for the development of cardiomyopathy. For example, heavy consumption of alcohol is thought to cause dilated cardiomyopathy through three mechanisms: direct toxic effect of alcohol or of its metabolites; effects of nutritional deficiencies, especially thiamine deficiency; and toxic effects of beverage additives, such as cobalt (Haak et al., 1993).

Dilated cardiomyopathy results from extensively damaged myocardial muscle fibers and is characterized by cardiac enlargement. The heart ejects blood less efficiently than normal, so that a large volume of blood remains in the left ventricle after systole, which results in ventricular dilation with enlargement and dilation of all four chambers and eventually leads to CHF (Fig. 10–15).

Hypertrophic cardiomyopathy is distinguished by inappropriate and excessive left ventricular hypertrophy (thickening of the interventricular septum) and normal or even enhanced

[15] Peripartum cardiomyopathy is a rare but very serious disease that results in heart failure. It may appear for no apparent reason during the last month of pregnancy or shortly after delivery; incidence is higher among multiparous women older than 30 years, particularly those with malnutrition or pre-eclampsia. Estimates vary, but the occurrence may be one in every 1300 to 4000 deliveries. Maternal death from CHF, blood clots, and infection and stillbirth can occur. Symptoms of orthopnea, cough, palpitations, and high blood pressure may not occur until several weeks after delivery (Pashkow and Libov, 1993).

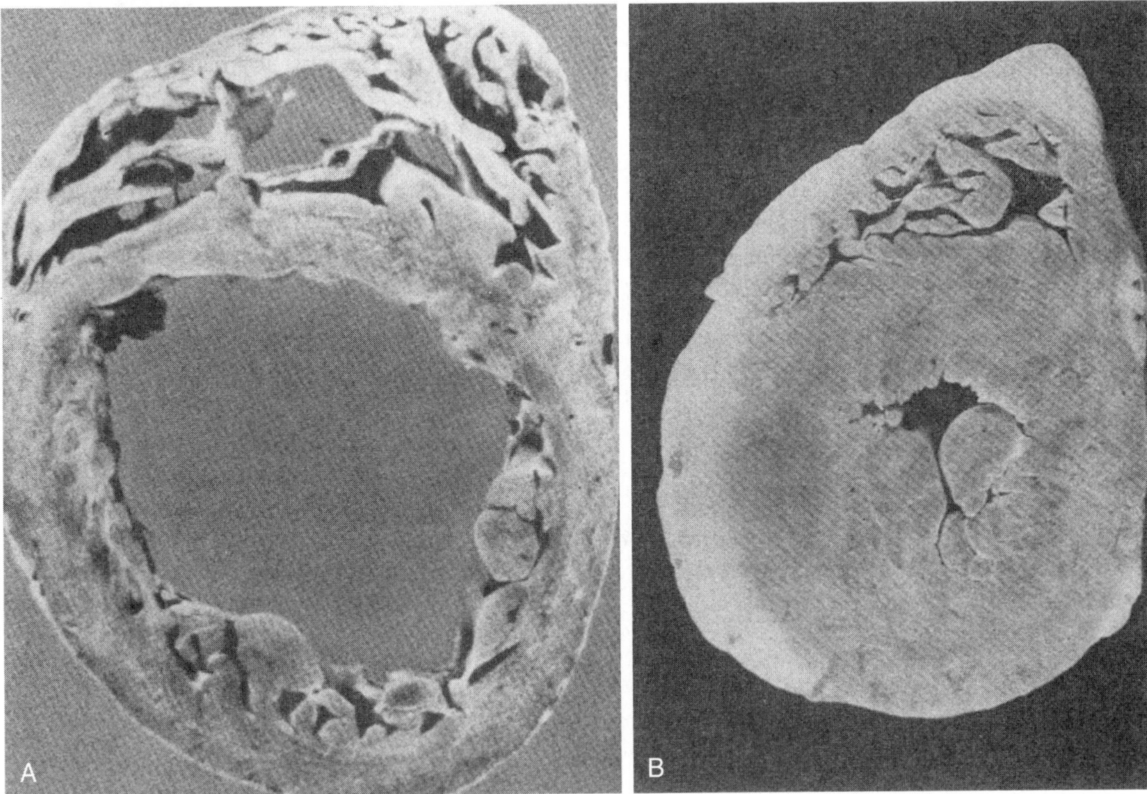

Figure 10–15. A, Cross-sectional view of dilated cardiomyopathy. B, Hypertrophied heart. (*From Kinney M: Comprehensive Cardiac Care, ed 7. St Louis, Mosby–Year Book, 1991, pp 346, 349.*)

cardiac muscle contractile function. Over time, the overgrowth of the wall leads to rigidity in the wall, increasing resistance to blood flow from the left atrium. *Restrictive cardiomyopathy* is the least common form; it is identified by marked endocardial scarring (fibrosis) of the ventricles, and the resulting rigidity impairs diastolic filling (Wynne and Braunwald, 1992).

Clinical Manifestations. Generally, the symptoms of cardiomyopathy are the same as for heart failure (e.g., dyspnea, orthopnea, tachycardia, palpitations, peripheral edema, distended jugular vein) (see Table 10–13). *Dilated cardiomyopathy* is characterized by fatigue and weakness; chest pain (unlike angina) may occur. Blood pressure is usually normal or low. *Hypertrophic cardiomyopathy* is frequently asymptomatic, sudden death being the presenting sign. The most common symptom is dyspnea due to high pulmonary pressures produced by the elevated left ventricular diastolic pressure; symptoms are often exacerbated during strenuous exercise. *Restrictive cardiomyopathy* causes clinical manifestations related to decreasing cardiac output. As cardiac output falls and intraventricular pressures rise, signs of CHF appear. The earliest manifestations may include exercise intolerance, fatigue, and shortness of breath followed by other symptoms listed in Table 10–13 (Ott, 1993).

Medical Management

Diagnosis and Treatment. Diagnosis requires exclusion of other causes of cardiac dysfunction, especially causes of CHF and arrhythmias. Catheterization to assess arteries and valves, echocardiography, chest radiography, blood chemistries, and ECG are specific tests performed.

The specific treatment of cardiomyopathy is determined by the underlying cause and may include physical, dietary, pharmacologic, mechanical, and surgical intervention. In the case of *dilated* cardiomyopathy, only transplantation and specific vasodilator therapy (hydralazine plus nitrates) have prolonged life (Wenger, 1990). Idiopathic dilated cardiomyopathy has no known cause; therefore, there is no specific therapy. In contrast to the other forms of cardiomyopathy, the progression of myocardial dysfunction of dilated cardiomyopathy may be stopped or reversed if alcohol consumption is reduced or stopped early in the course of the disease (Wynne and Braunwald, 1992). Currently, controlled clinical studies (i.e., not yet approved by the FDA for general use) are investigating the efficacy of long-term β-blocker therapy for cardiomyopathy.

Hypertrophic cardiomyopathy is treated with β-adrenergic blockers (e.g., propranolol) to reduce myocardial contractility and workload. Calcium channel blocking agents (e.g., verapamil) may be used to relieve symptoms and improve exercise intolerance. *Restrictive cardiomyopathy* has no specific treatment interventions. The goal is to control CHF through the use of diuretics, vasodilators, and salt restriction.

Prognosis. Seventy-five percent of persons diagnosed with *idiopathic dilated cardiomyopathy* die within 5 years after the onset of symptoms because diagnosis does not usually occur until advanced stages (Wynne and Braunwald, 1992). Persons with *hypertrophic cardiomyopathy* can lead long, relatively asymptomatic lives; some people have a history of gradually progressive symptoms, but others experience sudden death, especially during exercise, as the initial diagnostic event. *Restrictive cardiomyopathy* may cause sudden death due to arrhythmia or a more progressive course may occur, with eventual heart failure. Treatment rarely results in long-term improvement.

Many persons with various types of cardiomyopathy experience a stabilization or even an improvement in symptoms, but the end result of cardiomyopathy is sudden death or a fatal progression toward heart failure. No cure exists, outside of cardiac transplantation. Heart transplantation shows a 1-year survival rate of over 80% and a 3-year survival of 70% for *dilated cardiomyopathy*. The 1-year survival rate without transplant is 5%.

Special Implications for the Therapist **10-10**

CARDIOMYOPATHY

Cardiomyopathy associated with cardiotoxicity following chemotherapy is often clinically silent because of the clients' low levels of physical activity. An evaluation to screen for potential cardiopulmonary dysfunction is essential with these clients. The evaluation should include an assessment of current physical activity levels, exercise tolerance, and monitoring of heart rate and rhythm, blood pressure, respiratory responses, and any other signs and symptoms of exercise intolerance (e.g., dyspnea, fatigue, lightheadedness or dizziness, pallor, palpitations, and chest discomfort) (Watchie, 1992). Using a rating of perceived exertion scale (Table 10–14) is often useful during the evaluation and for establishing initial exercise guidelines toward improving endurance.

Sudden death occurs more often in younger people who have cardiomyopathy, and it may be avoided by eliminating strenuous exercise (e.g., running, competitive sports) when a diagnosis has been established. Rest improves cardiac function and reduces heart size. The therapist can provide valuable information regarding energy conservation techniques (see Box 7–1) to assist persons with continued independence in activities of daily living and possibly even to improve activity tolerance. This is especially true for the person awaiting a cardiac transplant.

For the person who has been hospitalized and has not ambulated yet, the therapist will need to assess tolerance to activities in bed before ambulating. During activities, monitor pulse, respirations, blood pressure, and color. The heart rate, systolic blood pressure, and respiratory rate normally increase in proportion to the exercise (movement) intensity whereas the diastolic blood pressure changes minimally (±10 mm Hg).

Abnormal responses include either blunted or excessive rises in heart rate or systolic blood pressure, excessive increases in diastolic blood pressure or respiratory rate, a fall in systolic blood pressure with increasing activity, or increasing irregularity of the pulse (Åstrand and Rodahl, 1977). These signs may be the result of cardiopulmonary toxicity or simply the result of deconditioning. Increasing irregularity in the pulse with pairs or runs of faster beats or more than six isolated irregular beats per minute must be reported to the physician (Watchie, 1992). If the person is receiving diuretics, monitor for signs of too-vigorous diuresis (e.g., muscle cramps, orthostatic hypotension). If the person becomes hypotensive, use a supine position with legs elevated to increase venous return and to ensure cerebral blood flow.

Improved activity tolerance may be demonstrated by minimal change in pulse or blood pressure during activities with minimal fatigue after the activity. Pulse, respirations, and blood pressure should return to a normal range within 3 minutes of the end of the activity. Discontinue any activity that results in chest pain, severe dyspnea, cyanosis, dizziness, hypotension, or sustained tachycardia.

During the early stages of the disease, many people find it difficult to accept activity restrictions and need encouragement to follow guidelines for activity restriction. Clients should avoid poorly tolerated activities; combine rest with activity; understand that physical and emotional stress exacerbate the disease; learn correct breathing techniques, as Valsalva maneuvers decrease the inflow of venous blood and impair outflow and should be avoided; understand that alcohol depresses myocardial contractility and should be eliminated.

TABLE 10-14 BORG SCALE OF PERCEIVED EXERTION*

NUMERICAL RATING	VERBAL RATING
0	Nothing at all
0.5	Very, very weak
1	Very weak
2	Weak
3	Moderate
4	Somewhat strong
5	Strong
6	
7	Very strong
8	
9	
10	Very, very strong
•	Maximal

* Using a perceived exertion scale is a useful approach to activity prescription. The individual is asked to identify a desirable rating of perceived exertion and uses that level of intensity as a daily guideline for activity. A suggested rating of perceived exertion for most healthy individuals is 3 to 5 (moderate to heavy); for the compromised person, a more moderate level of perceived exertion may be recommended by the physician.

Adapted from Borg GA: Psychosocial bases of perceived exertion. Med Sci Sports Exerc 472:194–381, 1982.

Trauma *(Andreoli et al., 1993)*

Nonpenetrating

Any blunt chest trauma, which is especially common in steering wheel impact from an automobile accident, may produce myocardial contusion, resulting in myocardial hemorrhage with little if any myocardial scar once healing is complete.

Large contusions may lead to myocardial scars, cardiac rupture, CHF, or formation of aneurysms.

The chest pain of myocardial contusion is similar to that of MI and is often confused with musculoskeletal pain from soft tissue consequences of chest trauma. Myocardial contusion is usually treated similarly to MI, with initial monitoring and subsequent progressive ambulation and cardiac rehabilitation. (See Special Implications for the Therapist: Myocardial Infarction.)

Penetrating

Penetrating cardiac injuries are most often due to external objects, such as bullets or knives, and sometimes from bony fragments secondary to chest injury. Iatrogenic causes of cardiac penetrating injury include perforation of the heart during catheterization and cardiac trauma from cardiopulmonary resuscitation.

Complications include arrhythmias, aneurysm formation, death from infection (e.g., bacterial endocarditis or infection from a retained foreign body), a form of pericarditis associated with this type of injury, ventricular septal defects, and foreign body embolus. Specific information related to wound ballistics is available (see Bergren, 1993; DiMaio, 1985; Ordog, 1988; Swan, 1989).

Myocardial Neoplasms

Tumors involving the heart are rare, but they may be primary or metastatic and benign or malignant. The most common primary tumor (usually benign) is a *myxoma,* arising most often from the endothelial surface of the left atrium; tumors located in other cardiac chambers account for 10% of myxomas. Other benign cardiac tumors (also rare) include lipoma, papilloma, fibroelastoma, rhabdomyoma, and fibroma. Malignant cardiac neoplasms may include angiosarcoma, rhabdomyosarcoma, mesothelioma, fibrosarcoma, and malignant lymphoma.

Cardiac neoplasms come to the attention of a therapist when (1) progressive interference with mitral valve function results in exercise intolerance or exertional dyspnea; (2) embolus causes a stroke; or (3) systemic manifestations occur, including muscle atrophy, arthralgias, malaise, or Raynaud's phenomenon.

Treatment is surgical excision with subsequent cardiac rehabilitation as required by the postoperative cardiovascular condition. Secondary tumors that have metastasized to the heart from elsewhere are not usually considered curable and are treated with radiation and chemotherapy.

Congenital Heart Disease

Overview and Incidence. Congenital heart disease is an anatomic defect in the heart that develops in utero during the first trimester and is present at birth. Congenital heart disease affects about 8 of every 1000 babies born in the United States, making this the most common category of congenital structural malformation. Other than prematurity, it is the major cause of death in the first year of life. Children with congenital heart disease are also more likely to have extracardiac defects, such as tracheoesophageal fistula, diaphragmatic hernias, and renal abnormalities.

There are two categories of congenital heart disease: *cyanotic* and *acyanotic* (Table 10–15). In clinical practice this system of classification is problematic, because children with acyanotic defects may develop cyanosis and those with cyanotic defects may be pink and have more clinical signs of CHF (Wong, 1993).

Cyanotic defects result from obstruction of blood flow to the lungs or mixing of desaturated blue venous blood with fully saturated red arterial blood within the chambers of the heart. Most acyanotic defects involve primarily left-to-right shunting through an abnormal opening.

Etiology. Only 8% of all congenital heart defects are known to be associated with a single mutant gene or chromosomal abnormalities; the remaining causes are either unknown or are attributable to multiple factors, such as diabetes, alcohol consumption, viruses, maternal rubella infection during the first trimester, and drugs, such as thalidomide (Wolfe and Wiggins, 1993).

Pathogenesis. The heart begins to form from a tubelike structure during the fourth week after conception. As development progresses, the tube lengthens and forms chambers, septa, and valves. Anything that interferes with this developmental process during the first 8 to 10 weeks of pregnancy can result in a congenital defect (Fig. 10–16).

Cyanotic

In *transposition of the great vessels* (TGV), no communication exists between systemic and pulmonary circulations so that the pulmonary artery leaves the left ventricle and the aorta exits from the right ventricle. *Tetralogy of Fallot* (TOF) consists of four classic defects: (1) pulmonary stenosis, (2) ventricular septal defect (VSD), (3) aortic communication with both ventricles, and (4) right ventricular hypertrophy. *Tricuspid atresia* is a failure of the tricuspid valve to develop, with a lack of communication from the right atrium to the right ventricle. Blood flows through an atrial septal defect or a patent ductus ovale to the left side of the heart and through a ventricular septal defect to the right ventricle and out to the lungs. There is complete mixing of unoxygenated and oxygenated blood in the left side of the heart, resulting in systemic desaturation and varying amounts of pulmonary obstruction.

Acyanotic

VSD is an abnormal opening between the right and left ventricles that may vary in size from a small pinhole to complete absence of the septum, resulting in a common ventricle. *Atrial septal defect* is an abnormal opening between the atria, allowing blood from the high-pressure left atrium to flow into the lower-pressure right atrium. *Coarctation of the aorta* is a localized narrowing near the insertion of the ductus arteriosus, resulting in increased pressure proximal to the defect (head and upper extremities) and decreased pressure distal to the obstruction (body and lower extremities). *Patent ductus arteriosus* is a failure of the fetal ductus arteriosus (artery connecting the aorta and pulmonary artery) to close within the first weeks of life. The continued function of this vessel allows blood to flow from the high-pressure aorta to the low-pressure pulmonary artery, causing a left-to-right shunt.

TABLE 10–15 CONGENITAL HEART DISEASE

DEFECT	INCIDENCE	CLINICAL MANIFESTATIONS	PROGNOSIS
Cyanotic			
Transposition of the great vessels	16%; 3:1 male-to-female ratio	Depends on size and type of defects; cyanosis; CHF	Undetermined as yet with new surgical treatment
Tetralogy of Fallot	10%–15%*	*Infants:* Acutely cyanotic at birth or progressive cyanosis first year *Children:* Increasing cyanosis, digital clubbing; poor growth and development	At risk for sudden lethal arrhythmias; mild obstruction progresses with age; reduced life expectancy
Tricuspid atresia	<1%; relatively rare	Newborn cyanosis; tachycardia; dyspnea; digital clubbing (older child)	Unreported; depends on success of treatment
Acyanotic			
Ventricular septal defect	25%; single most common CHD	Asymptomatic with small defect; CHF (age 1–6 mo); history of frequent respiratory infections; poor growth and development; dyspnea, fatigue, and exercise intolerance (older child)	No physical restrictions
Atrial septal defect	10%; 2:1 female-to-male ratio	Asyptomatic; growth failure; CHF (older child)	No physical restrictions if corrected; frequent complications in adults
Coarctation of the aorta	6%; 3:1 male-to-female ratio	High blood pressure (BP) and bounding pulses in arms; weak or absent femoral pulses; cool lower extremities with lower BP *Infants:* CHF *Children:* Headaches, fainting, epistaxis (hypertension); exercise intolerance, easy fatigability	Good if survive to childhood; exercise testing recommended prior to participation in athletics; reduced life expectancy
Patent ductus arteriosus	12%; spontaneous closure in normal term infants by day 4; common in children born to mothers affected by rubella during first trimester; increased incidence in infants born at high altitudes (over 10,000 ft); present in 20%–60% of premature infants weighing <1500 g	Asymptomatic; CHF	Closure may occur up to age 2 yr; poor prognosis for large defect without transplantation
Aortic stenosis	5% of all CHD	Asymptomatic; exercise intolerance, dizziness, and chest pain with prolonged standing	Good with early detection and surgical treatment; exercise testing recommended prior to participation in athletics

* Figures account for percentage of all CHD

Clinical Manifestations. The most common signs and symptoms include cyanosis and signs of CHF (e.g., dyspnea, pulmonary edema, and fatigue). See Table 10–15 for clinical manifestations of each particular defect. Complications may include heart failure, pulmonary edema, pneumonia, hypoxia, and sudden death. There is often a risk of bacterial endocarditis and pulmonary vascular obstructive disease later in life.

Medical Management

Diagnosis, Treatment, and Prognosis. Clinical diagnosis relies on detection of signs and symptoms, auscultation and detection of heart murmur, ECG, echocardiography, and cardiac catheterization. Prenatal screening for maternal rubella antibodies provides important information for further diagnostic testing.

Curative or palliative (provides relief of symptoms) surgi-

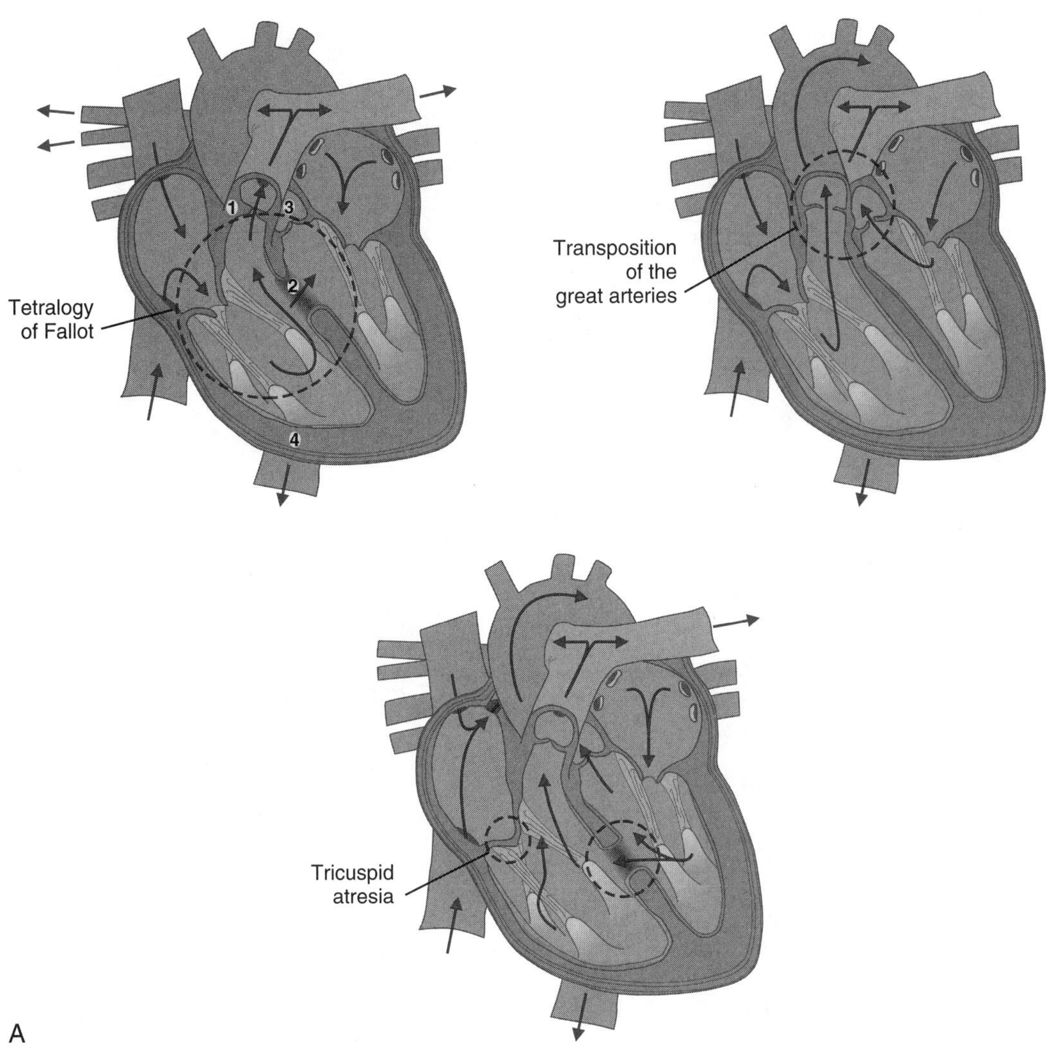

Figure 10–16. A, Major cyanotic defects: tetralogy of Fallot, transposition of the great arteries, tricuspid atresia.
Illustration continued on following page

cal correction is now available for more than 90% of persons with congenital heart disease. The risk for most surgical procedures is low (between 1% and 5%).

Special Implications for the Therapist **10–11**

CONGENITAL HEART DISEASE

Therapists need to be alert to signs of CHF in children with congenital heart disease and in infants with suspected congenital heart disease. Signs of CHF indicate a worsening clinical condition; the earlier these are detected, the sooner treatment can be initiated. (See also Special Implications for the Therapist: Congestive Heart Failure.)

Young children with tetralogy of Fallot instinctively learn to squat, getting into the flat-footed baseball catcher's stance when they are fatigued. This posture increases the tension in the leg muscles, reduces blood flow to the leg muscles, and raises peripheral resistance and blood pressure (Cumming, 1993a).

Most children with significant heart defects will have had heart surgery before they start school. In general, anyone who has had successful surgery is allowed unrestricted sports activity. The therapist should evaluate for soft tissue restriction at the site of the healed scar (either sternal or thoracic) which may affect breathing capacity. Data on exercise capacity after specific types of surgical procedures are available (Cumming, 1993a).

Twenty or 30 years ago, diagnosis of congenital defects was much more difficult, and many anomalies went undetected. Adults with undiagnosed congenital defects may develop exercise intolerance, shortness of breath, palpitations, blood pressure irregularities, or

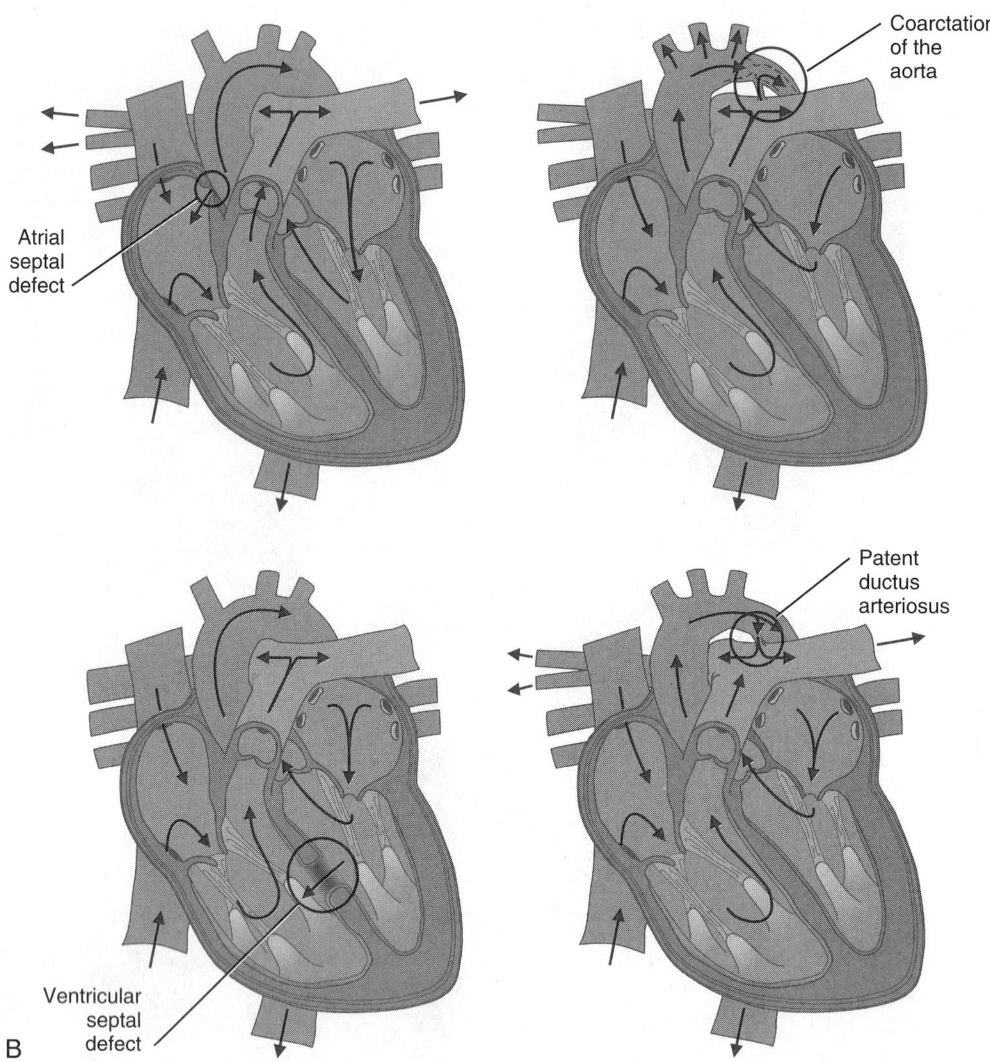

Figure **10–16.** *Continued.* B, Major acyanotic defects: atrial septal defect, coarctation of the aorta, ventricular septal defect, patent ductus arteriosus.

symptoms of CHF, which should alert the therapist of the need for medical referral.

DISEASES AFFECTING THE CARDIAC NERVOUS SYSTEM

Arrhythmias: Disturbances of Rate or Rhythm

Definition and Overview. Normally the heart rhythm is generated by the sinoatrial (SA) node, the internal pacemaker located in the upper right portion of the heart. The signal from the SA node travels through the cardiac conduction system, causing the atrial (supraventricular) and ventricular chambers of the heart to contract and relax at regular rates that are necessary to maintain circulation at different levels of activity. An arrhythmia (dysrhythmia) is a disturbance of heart rate or rhythm caused by an abnormal rate of electrical impulse generation by the SA node or the abnormal conduction of impulses.

Arrhythmias are usually classified according to their origin as ventricular or supraventricular (atrial), according to the pattern (fibrillation or flutter), or according to the speed or rate at which they occur (tachycardia or bradycardia). Arrhythmias vary in severity from mild, asymptomatic disturbances that require no treatment (e.g., sinus arrhythmia, in which the heart rate increases and decreases with respiration) to catastrophic ventricular fibrillation, which requires immediate resuscitation. The clinical significance depends on the effect on cardiac output and blood pressure, which is partially influenced by the site of origin.

Etiology and Incidence. Arrhythmias may be congenital or may result from one of several factors, including hypertrophy of heart muscle fiber secondary to hypertension or valvular heart disease or degeneration of conductive tissue that is necessary to maintain normal heart rhythm (called *sick sinus syndrome*). Arrhythmias can occur when a portion of the heart is temporarily deprived of oxygen, disturbing the normal pathway of the heartbeat. Toxic doses of cardioactive drugs, such as digoxin and other cardiac glycosides, may also lead to arrhythmias.

The number of rate or rhythm disturbances appears to be increasing, particularly arrhythmias after heart attacks. Improved cardiac care has increased the number of survivors of cardiac incidents who may suffer subsequent complications, such as arrhythmias.

Pathogenesis and Clinical Manifestations.

Rate. The heart beats an average of 60 to 100 beats/min; an arrhythmia is considered any significant deviation from the normal range. Whether change in heart rate (number of contractions of the cardiac ventricles per period of time) produces symptoms at rest or on exertion depends on the underlying state of the cardiac muscle and its ability to alter its stroke output to compensate.

Rate arrhythmias are of two basic types: tachycardia and bradycardia. *Tachycardia* occurs when the heart beats too fast (more than 100 beats/min). Tachycardia develops in the presence of increased sympathetic stimulation, such as occurs with fear, pain, emotion, exertion, or exercise, or with ingestion of artificial stimulants, such as caffeine, nicotine, and amphetamines. Tachycardia is also found in situations in which the demands for oxygen are increased, such as fever, CHF, infection, anemia, hemorrhage, myocardial injury, and hyperthyroidism (Hillegass, 1994b). Usually no symptoms are perceived by the individual with tachycardia, and medical treatment is directed toward the underlying cause.

Bradycardia (less than 60 beats/min) is normal in well-trained athletes, but it is also common in individuals taking β-blockers, those who have had traumatic brain injuries or brain tumors, and those experiencing increased vagal stimulation (e.g., from suctioning or vomiting) to the physiologic pacemaker. Organic disease of the sinus node, especially in elderly persons and persons with heart disease, can also cause sinus bradycardia. Bradycardia is usually asymptomatic, but when it is caused by a pathologic condition, the person may experience fatigue, dyspnea, syncope, dizziness, angina, or diaphoresis. Medical treatment is not usually required unless symptoms interfere with function or are drug- or angina-induced; atropine or a mechanical pacemaker can be used to re-establish a more normal heart rate.

Rhythm. Arrhythmias as variations from the normal rhythm or movement of the heart (especially the heartbeat) are detected when they become symptomatic or during monitoring for another cardiac condition. Abnormalities of cardiac rhythm and electrical conduction can be lethal (sudden cardiac death), symptomatic (syncope, near syncope, dizziness, chest pain, dyspnea, or palpitations), or asymptomatic. They are dangerous because they reduce cardiac output so that perfusion of the brain or myocardium is impaired, or they tend to deteriorate into more serious arrhythmias with the same consequences.

The many different types of abnormal cardiac rhythms are usually classified according to their origin (atrial or ventricular), but only the most common ones are included here. Complete discussion of all other cardiac arrhythmias is available (see Hillegass, 1994b).

Sinus arrhythmia is an irregularity in rhythm that may be a normal variation in athletes, children, and elderly people or may be caused by an alteration in vagal stimulation. Sinus arrhythmia may be respiratory (increases and decreases with respiration) or nonrespiratory, associated with infection, drug toxicity (e.g., digoxin, morphine), and fever. Treatment for the respiratory type of sinus arrhythmia is not necessary; all other sinus arrhythmias are treated by providing treatment for the underlying cause.

Atrial fibrillation, involuntary, irregular muscular contractions of the atrial myocardium, is the most common chronic arrhythmia; it occurs most often in rheumatic heart disease, dilated cardiomyopathy, atrial septal defect, hypertension, mitral valve prolapse, and hypertrophic cardiomyopathy. Atrial fibrillation can also occur in people without cardiac disease (e.g., thyrotoxicosis, medications, or alcohol intoxication or withdrawal). Atrial fibrillation can result in cardiac failure, cardiac ischemia, and arterial emboli, the latter from the poorly contracting left atrium.

Ventricular fibrillation, involuntary incoordinated muscular contractions of the ventricular muscle, is a frequent cause of cardiac arrest. Treatment with an electrical device called a defibrillator is used to depolarize the muscle, thus ending the irregular contractions and allowing the heart to resume normal regular contractions.

Heart block is a disorder of the heartbeat caused by an interruption in the passages of impulses through the heart's electrical system. Causes include CAD, hypertension, myocarditis, overdose of cardiac medications (such as digitalis), and aging. Depending on the degree of the heart block, it can cause dizziness, fainting, or possibly stroke. Heart block can affect people at any age, but this condition primarily affects the elderly. Mild cases do not require treatment; medication and pacemakers are the two primary forms of treatment for symptomatic cases.

Medical Management

Diagnosis. ECG is the most common test procedure to document arrhythmias, but if the person is not experiencing symptoms, the heartbeat may look normal. Tape-recorded ambulatory ECG, called *Holter monitoring* (Fig 10–17), permits monitoring of all cardiac cycles over a prescribed period of time (usually 24 hours) and may be used to document arrhythmias. It is especially helpful in recording sporadic arrhythmias that an office or stress-test ECG might miss. Holter monitoring may also be used by persons recovering from MIs, receiving antiarrhythmic medications, or using pacemakers.

If a serious arrhythmia is suspected, an electrophysiologic study (EPS) can be performed. This test is an invasive study, similar to cardiac catheterization, that uses wires to electronically stimulate the heart in an attempt to reproduce the arrhythmia.

Treatment and Prognosis. In the past, antiarrhythmic drugs have been credited with significantly reducing mortality by reducing the irritability of the heart cells responsible for rhythm disturbances. For example, treatment of atrial fibrillation with digoxin to control the heart rate has been used to reduce risk of stroke and other embolic complications. When conversion to normal sinus rhythm is not possible, anticoagulation treatment may be initiated to reduce thromboembolic complications. New data have more clearly shown the risks of antiarrhythmic drug therapy while indicating that the benefit previously ascribed to these drugs may not exist (Echt et al., 1991; Roden, 1994).

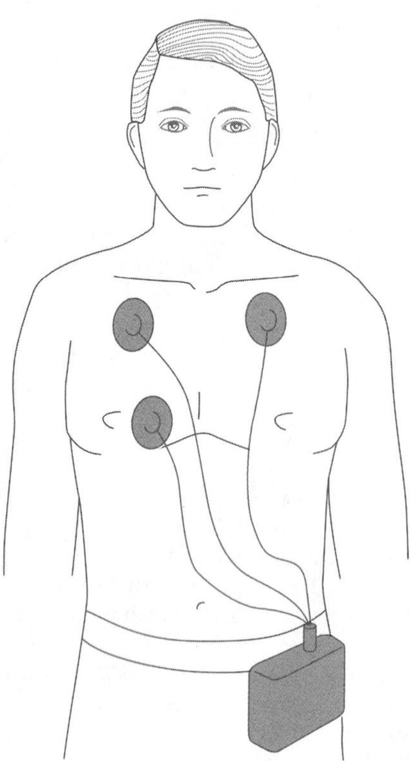

Figure 10–17. Cardiac monitoring may be used to evaluate effects of medical treatment and allows continuous observation of the heart's electrical activity in people with symptomatic arrhythmia or any cardiac abnormality that might lead to life-threatening arrhythmias. The Holter monitor is usually strapped around the person's waist, securely but comfortably. If the belt is not snug enough, the weight of the monitor pulls on the electrodes. A three-electrode system consists of a positive electrode, negative electrode, and ground electrode.

Some tachycardias can be treated with radio-wave ablation, a nonsurgical but invasive technique that uses catheterization to thread wires into the heart through which radio waves can be aimed at the heart tissue where the arrhythmia originates. One complication of this technique is the potential destruction of the sinoatrial node (the heart's own internal pacemaker), which necessitates surgical implantation of an artificial pacemaker for some people.

Pacemakers, implants designed to replace the heartbeat by delivering a battery-supplied electrical stimulus through leads attached to electrodes in contact with the heart, may be used in cases of bradycardia, heart block, or refractory tachycardia.[16] Pacemakers initiate the heartbeat when the heart's intrinsic conduction system fails or is unreliable. In the case of life-threatening arrhythmias that do not respond to other types of treatment, a device called an *implantable cardioverter defibrillator* (ICD) may be implanted. The ICD uses an electric shock to restart the heart rhythm.

[16] This refers to a condition in which the heart is beating very quickly, but only a portion of those beats are functional; many more beats just "echo," or make a beat but without contractile force behind the blood flow. Functionally, the heartbeat is actually very slow.

Conduction Disturbance

Sick Sinus Syndrome

Sick sinus syndrome, or "brady tachy syndrome," is a complex cardiac arrhythmia associated with CAD or drug therapy (e.g., digitalis, calcium channel blockers, β-blockers, antiarrhythmics). Sick sinus syndrome as a result of degeneration of conductive tissue necessary to maintain normal heart rhythm occurs most often among the elderly. A variety of other heart diseases and other conditions (e.g., cardiomyopathy, sarcoidosis, amyloidosis) also may result in sinus node dysfunction. Sick sinus syndrome is characterized by bradycardia alone, bradycardia alternating with tachycardia, or bradycardia with atrioventricular block resulting in cerebral manifestations of lightheadedness, dizziness, and near or true syncope.

Sinus node dysfunction is suspected in elderly persons experiencing episodes of syncope or near syncope, especially in the presence of heart palpitations. An accurate diagnosis is made with ECG, often requiring a 24-hour Holter monitoring to document the arrhythmias described. Treatment for the symptomatic person varies according to the specific arrhythmia manifestations and may include antiarrhythmic agents alone or combined with a permanent-demand pacemaker or withdrawal of agents that may be responsible.

Special Implications for the Therapist **10–12**

ARRHYTHMIAS

Anytime a person's pulse is abnormally slow, rapid, or irregular, especially in the presence of known cardiac involvement, documentation and notification of the physician is necessary. Predisposing factors for arrhythmias include fluid and electrolyte imbalance (see Chapter 4) and drug toxicity (see Table 10–9 and Special Implications for the Therapist: Cardiomyopathy). To prevent postoperative cardiac arrhythmias, consult carefully with respiratory therapy to provide adequate oxygen during activities that increase the heart's workload.

Clients describing "palpitations" or similar phenomena may not be experiencing symptoms of arrhythmic heart disease. Palpitations can occur as a result of an overactive thyroid, secondary to caffeine sensitivity, as a side effect of some medications, from decreased estrogen levels, and through the use of drugs such as cocaine. Encourage the client to report any such symptoms to the physician if this has not already been brought to the physician's attention.

Exercise and Arrhythmias *(Peel and Mossberg, 1995)*

Exercise often increases arrhythmias because of the increase in activity of the sympathetic nervous system and the increase in circulating catecholamines (Podrid et al., 1992). Exercise may induce cardiac arrhythmias under several conditions, including diuretic and digitalis therapy, or recent ingestion of caffeine may exacerbate arrhythmias. Exercise-induced arrhythmias are generated by enhanced sympathetic tone, increased myocardial oxygen demand, or both. Most people with chronic obstructive pulmonary disease (COPD) who have mild arrhythmias at rest do not tend to have increased arrhythmias during exercise. At times, the arrhythmias may disappear with exercise and increased perfusion (Frownfelter, 1987).

Medications that are effective in controlling arrhythmias at rest may not be effective during exertion or stress. In addition, side effects of antiarrhythmic agents may be more apparent during exercise. For example, decreases in either exercise performance or blood pressure during exercise may occur. Because of their effects on the electrophysiologic characteristics of cardiac cells, these medications have the potential to cause abnormal rhythms. The effect of slowing the impulse through the myocardium may manifest itself during exercise as a partial or complete heart block.

Individuals with known arrhythmias and clients who are taking antiarrhythmic medications may need to be evaluated under conditions of graded exercise to ensure that the arrhythmia remains under control during activity. Monitoring heart rate and blood pressure during activity and palpation of peripheral pulses is essential in the absence of ECG. Continued monitoring and observation during the recovery period is also important because arrhythmias often occur during recovery rather than during peak exercise (Jelinek and Lown, 1974). If the exercise is stopped abruptly and the individual remains upright, pooling of blood in the lower body occurs. The decreased venous return and subsequent decreased blood flow to the heart may facilitate an irregular rhythm. By continuing to exercise at a low intensity during recovery, a sudden decrease in venous return is avoided.

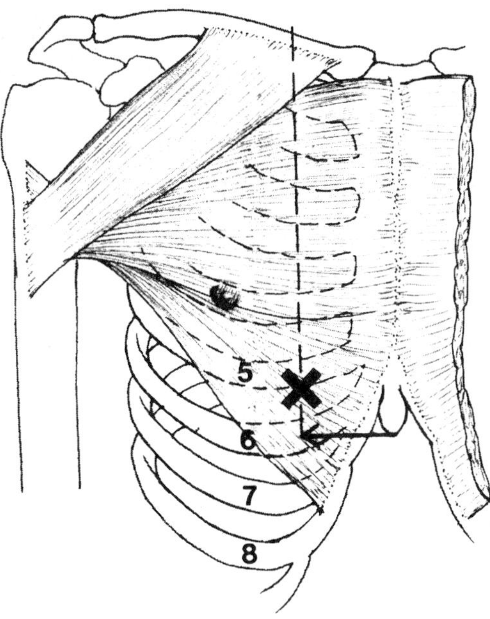

Figure 10–18. Location of the "cardiac arrhythmia" trigger point (X) below the lower border of the fifth rib in the vertical line that lies midway between the sternal margin and the nipple line. On this line, the sixth rib is found at the level of the tip of the xiphoid process (*arrow*). (*From Travell JG, Simons DG: Myofascial Pain and Dysfunction: The Trigger Point Manual, I. Baltimore, Williams & Wilkins, 1983, p 579.*)

Trigger Points

People who experience episodes of supraventricular tachycardia, supraventricular premature contractions, or ventricular premature contractions without evidence of heart disease should be checked for an active trigger point in the right pectoralis major muscle between the fifth and sixth ribs (Fig. 10–18).* Inactivation of the trigger point promptly restores normal sinus rhythm when an ectopic (i.e., produced in a tissue where it is not normally found) supraventricular rhythm is present, and often eliminates recurrences of paroxysmal arrhythmia of frequent premature contractions for a long period (Travell and Simons, 1983).

Pacemaker

For the client wearing a pacemaker, the first 6 weeks after surgery may be characterized by fatigue, during which time activity restrictions apply. Most people can drive, but strenuous activities using the arms (e.g., housework, golf, tennis, lifting more than 10 lb) are contraindicated. Once the incision is fully healed and the pacemaker is stable, scar mobilization is permissible. The usual precautions for scar mobilization apply, including mobilizing the tissue in the direction of the scar before using any cross transverse techniques, and mobilizing toward the scar rather than away from the scar to avoid overstretching the healing tissue.

Problems with pacemakers are uncommon, but any unusual deviation from the set heartbeat expected or the development of unusual symptoms such as dyspnea, dizziness or lightheadedness, and syncope or near syncope must be reported immediately to the physician. It is important that the therapist understand the underlying problem as well as the type of pacemaker the client is using before monitoring the client's response to an exercise program. More detailed information regarding types of pacemakers and pacemaker implantation is available (see Sadowsky, 1994; Reigle and Ringel, 1993; see also information from pacemaker manufacturer).

Heart rate is limited to the programmed level, and individuals with fixed-rate ventricular synchronous devices require monitoring by blood pressure and perceived exertion scales, with close attention to symptoms of cerebral ischemia. Newer, improved pacemakers produce the cardiac output needed for exercise, making it possible for individuals with pacemakers to be physically active at work and during recreation. Exercise may be limited only by the underlying heart disease and left ventricular function. If the pacemaker recipient has undergone exercise testing safely, aerobic conditioning and endurance training can be initiated, although precaution is still advised regarding vigorous upper-body activities (Kavanagh, 1994).

* Edeiken and Wolferth (1936) identified this "trigger zone" as a hypersensitive spot in the skeletal musculature of the chest responsible for referred chest pain that persisted following an acute myocardial infarction (Kennard and Haugen, 1995). Subsequent authors noted that tender spots in the left pectoralis major muscle ("pectoral myalgia") referred pain to the chest in a manner that confusingly simulated the pain of coronary insufficiency in people

with no history or evidence of cardiac disease (Good, 1950; Gutstein, 1938; Kelly, 1944; Rinzler and Travell, 1948). Travell and Simons (1983) suggest that other authors recognized the non-cardiac nature of this pain, but were unaware of its trigger point (TP) origin (DeMaria et al., 1980; Epstein et al., 1979; Pasternak et al., 1980).

DISEASES AFFECTING THE HEART VALVES

Heart problems that occur secondary to impairment of valves may be caused by infection such as endocarditis, congenital deformity, or disease (e.g., rheumatic fever or coronary thrombosis). Three types of valve deformities may affect aortic, mitral, tricuspid, or pulmonic valves (Fig. 10–19): *stenosis*, *insufficiency*, or *prolapse* (see also Congenital Heart Disease).

Stenosis is a narrowing or constriction that prevents the valve from opening fully and may be caused by scars or abnormal deposits on the leaflets. Valvular stenosis causes obstruction to blood flow and the chamber behind the narrow valve must produce extra work to sustain cardiac output.

Insufficiency (also referred to as regurgitation) occurs when the valve does not close properly and causes blood to flow back into the heart chamber. The heart gradually dilates in response to the increased volume of work; severe degrees of incompetence are possible in the absence of symptoms. *Prolapse* affects only the mitral valve and occurs when enlarged leaflets bulge backward into the left atrium.

Valve conditions increase the workload of the heart and require the heart to pump harder to force blood through a stenosed valve or to maintain adequate flow if blood is seeping back. These conditions may be asymptomatic or may cause easy fatigue. As stenosis or insufficiency progress, symptoms of heart failure (breathlessness or dyspnea) develop (Urden et al., 1992). The person with valvular disease from any cause is predisposed to infective endocarditis.

Mitral Stenosis *(Massie, 1994)*

Etiology and Pathogenesis. Nearly all people with mitral stenosis have underlying rheumatic heart disease even though a history of rheumatic fever is often absent. Because the mitral valve is thickened, it opens in early diastole with a "snap" that is audible on auscultation, then closes slowly with a resultant murmur. The anterior and posterior leaflets are fixed like a funnel with an opening in the center, and they move together, rather than in opposite directions. When the valve has narrowed sufficiently, left atrial pressure rises to maintain

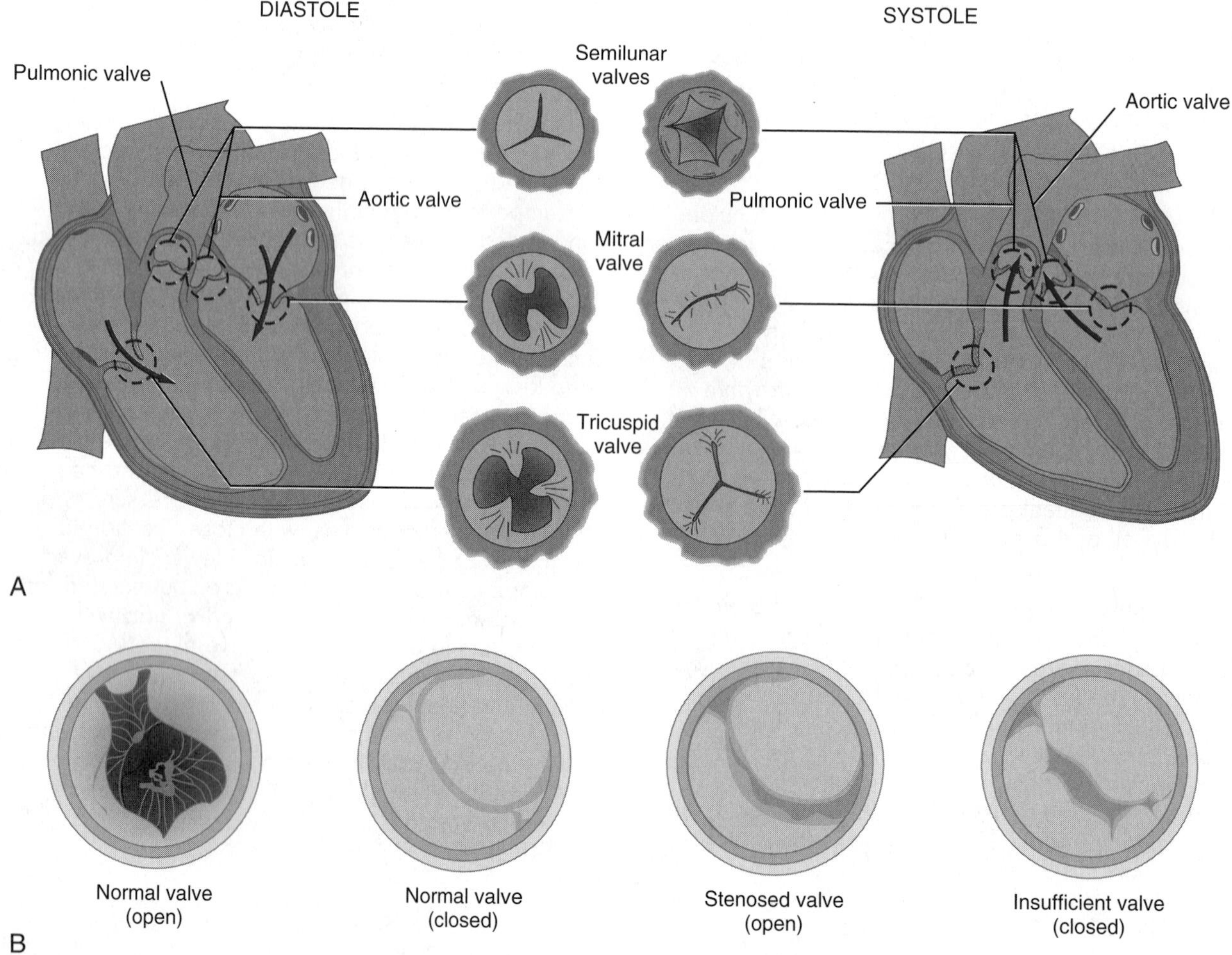

Figure 10–19. Valves of the heart. *A*, The pulmonic, aortic, mitral, and tricuspid valves are shown here as they appear during diastole (ventricular filling) and systole (ventricular contraction). *B*, Normal position of the valve leaflets, or cusps, when the valve is open and closed; fully open position of a stenosed valve; closed regurgitant valve showing abnormal opening for blood to flow back into.

normal flow across the valve and to maintain a normal cardiac output. This results in a pressure difference between the left atrium and the left ventricle during diastole.

Clinical Manifestations. In mild cases, left atrial pressure and cardiac output remain normal, and the person is asymptomatic. In moderate stenosis, dyspnea and fatigue appear as the left atrial pressure rises. With severe stenosis, left atrial pressure is high enough to produce pulmonary venous congestion at rest and reduce cardiac output with resulting dyspnea, fatigue, and right ventricular failure. Lying down at night further increases the pulmonary blood volume, causing orthopnea and PND.

Medical Management

Diagnosis, Treatment, and Prognosis. Echocardiography is the most valuable technique for assessing mitral valve stenosis and providing information about the condition of the valve and left atrial size. Doppler techniques (measuring blood flow using ultrasound) can be used to determine the severity of the problem.

Because mitral stenosis may be asymptomatic, treatment is delayed until symptoms develop. The onset of atrial fibrillation accompanied by more severe symptoms may be treated pharmacologically (digoxin, antiarrhythmic agents, anticoagulants). Surgery may be indicated in the presence of uncontrollable pulmonary edema, severe dyspnea limiting function, pulmonary hypertension, arrhythmia, or systemic emboli uncontrolled by anticoagulation treatment. Surgical procedures include valve repair (commissurotomy to break apart the adherent leaves) or replacement with an artificial valve.[17]

Mitral stenosis may be present for a lifetime, with few or no symptoms, or it may become severe in a few years. Operative mortality rates are low; problems associated with prosthetic valves may occur because of thrombosis, leaking, endocarditis, or degenerative changes in tissue valves.

Mitral Regurgitation *(Massie, 1994)*

Etiology and Pathogenesis. There are many possible causes of mitral regurgitation, but mitral valve prolapse accounts for approximately half of all cases. Other secondary causes include infective endocarditis (valve perforation), dilated cardiomyopathy, rheumatic disease, rupture of the chordae tendineae, and, rarely, cardiac tumors.

During left ventricular systole, the mitral leaflets do not close normally, and blood is ejected into the left atrium as well as through the aortic valve. In acute regurgitation, left atrial pressure rises abruptly, possibly leading to pulmonary edema. When regurgitation is a chronic condition, the left atrium enlarges progressively; the degree of enlargement usually reflects the severity of regurgitation.

Clinical Manifestations. For many years the left ventricular end-diastolic pressure and the cardiac output may be normal at rest, even with considerable increase in left ventricular volume. Eventually, left ventricular overload may lead to left ventricular failure. People with mitral regurgitation experience exertional dyspnea, because of increased left atrial pressure, and exercise-induced fatigue, because of reduced cardiac output. Atrial fibrillation may also develop.

Medical Management

Diagnosis, Treatment, and Prognosis. The diagnosis is primarily clinical (auscultation), but it can be confirmed and quantified by echocardiography. Other testing procedures may include cardiac catheterization to assess the regurgitation, left ventricular function, and pulmonary artery pressure; coronary arteriography to determine the cause of the lesion and for preoperative evaluation; and nuclear medicine techniques to measure left ventricular function and estimate the severity of regurgitation.

Persons with chronic lesions who are asymptomatic may not receive treatment for many years. In fact, life expectancy may be unaffected. Surgical intervention may be recommended when activity becomes severely limited or if left ventricular function is measured by less than 40% ejection fraction (for explanation of ejection fraction see footnote 26). Acute mitral regurgitation often requires emergency surgery, but the surgical risk is high and the outcome poor.

Mitral Valve Prolapse

Incidence and Etiology. In a little more than 10% of the American population, a slight variation in the shape or structure of the mitral valve occurs that could cause prolapse. This structural variation has many other names, including floppy valve syndrome, Barlow's syndrome, and click-murmur syndrome. Incidence appears to be increasing, possibly attributable to nutritional changes and ever-increasing stress levels in our society, or possibly a result of better diagnostic testing and more accurate documentation (Frederickson, 1992).

The cause remains unknown, although there may be a genetic component; abnormalities in connective tissue protein have been identified at the gene level, but the exact genetic defect remains undetermined (Lavie and Savage, 1987; Andersen and Devereux, 1994). Results of family studies of people with mitral valve prolapse favor an autosomal dominant pattern of transmission for primary mitral valve prolapse with nearly 100% gene expression by females (Devereux et al., 1982). This condition usually occurs in isolation; however, it can be associated with a number of other conditions, such as rheumatic fever, endocarditis, myocarditis, atherosclerosis, SLE, muscular dystrophy, acromegaly, adult polycystic kidney disease, and cardiac sarcoidosis.

Pathologic evidence of thrombotic lesions on segments of endothelium at the junction between the mitral leaflets and the left atrial wall have been found in people with mitral valve prolapse who have had a stroke. Unfortunately, no clinical clues have been found to help identify people at increased risk for future stroke (Andersen and Devereux, 1994).

Pathogenesis. Mitral valve prolapse appears to be the result of connective tissue abnormalities in the valve leaflets. Normally, when the lower part of the heart contracts, the mitral valve remains firm and prevents blood from leaking back into the upper chambers. In mitral valve prolapse, the slight variation in shape of the mitral valve allows one part

[17] About 60,000 heart valve replacement operations are performed in the United States annually. Most replacements are either mechanical valves or pig valves treated to prevent rejection. As "nonliving" structures, these replacement valves cannot utilize the body's own mechanisms for growth and repair, which limits their durability and longevity. Research to grow replacement heart valves from a person's own cells is being investigated (Breuer, 1995).

of the valve, the leaflet, to billow back into the left atrium during contraction of the ventricle. One or both of the valve leaflets may bulge into the left atrium during ventricular systole. Usually the amount of blood that leaks back into the left atrium is not significant, but in a small number of people, it develops into mitral regurgitation.

Clinical Manifestations. More than half of all people with mitral valve prolapse are asymptomatic, another 40% experience occasional symptoms that are mildly to moderately uncomfortable, and only 1% suffer severe symptoms and lifestyle restrictions. Although the malformation occurs during gestation, it usually remains unnoticed until young adulthood. The person usually becomes aware of symptoms suddenly and there does not appear to be any correlation between the severity of symptoms and the severity of the prolapse.

Symptoms include profound fatigue that cannot be correlated with exercise or stress, cold hands and feet, shortness of breath, chest pain, and heart palpitations. The most common triad of symptoms associated with mitral valve prolapse is profound fatigue, palpitations, and dyspnea. Fatigue may not be related to exertion, but deconditioning from prolonged inactivity may develop, further complicating the picture.

Chest pain associated with mitral valve prolapse may be a direct result of an imbalance in the autonomic nervous system called *dysautonomia*. As the autonomic nervous system is being formed in utero, the mitral valve is also being formed. If there is a slight variation in the structure of the heart valve, there is also a slight variation in the function or balance of the autonomic nervous system. This imbalance results in inadequate relaxation between respirations and eventually causes the chest wall muscles to go into spasm. The chest pain is sharp, lasts several seconds, and is usually felt to the left of the sternum. It is intermittent pain, which may occur frequently for a few weeks and then disappear completely, only to return again some weeks later.

Frequently occurring musculoskeletal findings in clients with mitral valve prolapse include joint hypermobility, temporomandibular joint (TMJ) syndrome, pectus excavatum, mild scoliosis, straight thoracic spine, and myalgias. The increased joint mobility that has been identified in a small proportion of persons with mitral valve prolapse does not appear to lead to either severe arthritis or to frequent joint dislocations (Devereux et al., 1986).

Migraine headaches, orthostatic hypotension, anxiety, depression, and panic attacks may also occur. Minor symptoms associated with mitral valve prolapse may include tremors, swelling of the extremities, sleep disturbances, low back pain, irritable bowel syndrome, excessive perspiration or inability to perspire, rashes, muscular fasciculations, visual changes or disturbances, difficulty in concentrating, memory lapses, and dizziness.

Medical Management

Diagnosis, Treatment, and Prognosis. Mitral valve prolapse is characterized by a symptomatic clinical presentation and clicking noise on auscultation in late systole, with or without sounds of valvular leak (murmur). Echocardiography may be used to confirm the diagnosis, and ECG and/or Holter monitoring (see Fig. 10–17) to show arrhythmias may be used.

Treatment includes reassurance, β-blockers to control arrhythmias, exercise program to improve overall cardiovascular function, counseling to eliminate caffeine, alcohol, and cigarette use, and administration of prophylactic antibiotics before any invasive procedure (including dental work) to prevent infective endocarditis. Rarely, surgical replacement of the valve may be recommended when severe structural problems are present that contribute to reduced activity or deterioration of left ventricular function.

Mitral valve prolapse is not life threatening, and only rarely does it significantly alter a person's lifestyle. Serious complications, such as severe mitral regurgitation, infectious endocarditis, stroke, and sudden death, do occur in a minority of cases (Devereux et al., 1989).

Aortic Stenosis *(Massie, 1994)*

Etiology and Pathogenesis. Aortic valvular stenosis is more commonly caused by progressive valvular calcification either superimposed on a congenitally bicuspid valve or, in the elderly, involving a previously normal valve following rheumatic fever. Over 80% of affected persons are men. Preschool and school-aged children are more likely to have a bicuspid valve; teenagers and young adults present with three leaves, but these are partially fused.

The orifice of the aortic semilunar valve narrows, causing diminished blood flow from the left ventricle into the aorta. Outflow obstruction increases pressure within the left ventricle as it tries to eject blood through the narrow opening, causing decreased cardiac output, left ventricular hypertrophy, and pulmonary vascular congestion (Haak et al., 1994).

Clinical Manifestations. In adults, aortic stenosis is usually asymptomatic until middle or old age. Characteristic sounds on auscultation may be heard, but cardiac output is maintained until the stenosis is severe and left ventricular failure, angina pectoris, or exertional syncope develops. Sudden death may occur, even in previously asymptomatic individuals.

Medical Management

Diagnosis, Treatment, and Prognosis. The clinical assessment of aortic stenosis can be difficult, especially in the older person. Echo-Doppler, also called Doppler ultrasonography, is diagnostic in most cases. ECG may show left ventricular hypertrophy, and x-ray or fluoroscopy may show a calcified aortic valve.

Surgical treatment is usually required for the symptomatic person and should be strongly considered for the asymptomatic person because of the risk of sudden death. Surgical procedures may include valve replacement with a mechanical prosthesis or bioprosthesis (made with biological material); recently, balloon valvuloplasty (splitting the stenotic valve with a balloon-tipped catheter that is introduced into the valve and inflated) has been used in treatment for aortic stenosis, delaying indefinitely the need for further surgical intervention.

The prognosis for aortic stenosis is poor without surgery. The onset of angina, exercise-induced syncope, or cardiac failure represents a poor prognostic outcome resulting in death. Surgical mortality is low for valve replacement for people younger than 70 years. Mortality rises to 10% after age 70 years. Bioprostheses may develop degenerative changes, requiring replacement in 7 to 10 years.

Aortic Regurgitation (Insufficiency)

Etiology and Pathogenesis. In the past, aortic regurgitation occurred secondary to rheumatic fever, but antibiotics have reduced the number of rheumatic-related cases. Nonrheumatic causes account for most cases today, including congenitally bicuspid valves, infective endocarditis (valve destruction by bacteria), and hypertension. Aortic regurgitation may also occur secondary to aortic dissection (see Fig. 10–26), ankylosing spondylitis, Reiter's syndrome, and Marfan's syndrome.

When cardiac systole ends, the aortic valve should completely prevent the flow of aortic blood back into the left ventricle. A leakage during diastole is referred to as *aortic regurgitation* or *aortic insufficiency*. When aortic regurgitation develops gradually, the left ventricle compensates by both dilation and enough hypertrophy to maintain a normal wall thickness-to-cavity ratio, thereby preventing development of symptoms. Eventually the left ventricle fails to stand up under the chronic overload, and symptoms develop (Cumming, 1993b).

Clinical Manifestations. Long-standing aortic regurgitation may remain asymptomatic even as the deformity increases, causing a decrease in diastolic blood pressure and enlargement of the left ventricle. Exertional dyspnea, fatigue, and excessive perspiration with exercise are the most frequent symptoms, but paroxysmal nocturnal dyspnea and pulmonary edema may also occur. Angina pectoris or atypical chest pain may be present.

Medical Management

Diagnosis, Treatment, and Prognosis. ECG, chest x-ray, echocardiography, Doppler and scintigraphic studies (use of internally administered radioactive imaging agent to visualize the area), and cardiac catheterization may be part of the diagnostic procedures. Scintigraphic studies can quantify left ventricular function and functional reserve during exercise and provides a useful predictor of prognosis.

Acute aortic regurgitation may lead to left ventricular failure, and surgical replacement of the valve is required. Chronic regurgitation carries a poor prognosis without surgery when significant symptoms develop. Medical therapy may include vasodilators to reduce the severity of regurgitation and diuretics and digoxin to stabilize or improve symptoms.

Tricuspid Stenosis and Regurgitation

Tricuspid stenosis occurs in people with severe mitral valve disease (usually rheumatic in origin) and is uncommon. Exercise testing and rehabilitation does not occur until after valve surgery. Tricuspid regurgitation may occur secondary to carcinoid syndrome, SLE, infective endocarditis among injection drug users, and in the presence of mitral valve disease. Surgical repair is more common than valvular replacement for tricuspid valve disease.

Special Implications for the Therapist **10–13**

VALVULAR HEART DISEASE *(Cumming, 1993b)*

People with mild valvular malfunction have no symptoms and can usually exercise vigorously and take part in intense sports activities without adverse effects. Although exercise will not improve the mechanical function of a valve, improvement in submaximal cardiac capacity can occur. Exercise is usually stopped for the same reason as it is in healthy adults (i.e., when respiratory distress is obvious or when the person expresses a desire to stop).

Pulmonary edema can be produced by exercising beyond a certain point in people with valvular disease, especially those with mitral stenosis. Pulmonary congestion induced by exercise may cause coughing rather than dyspnea, and exercise should be stopped if coughing becomes significant. Heart failure may occur secondary to chronic, progressive valvular disease. Slight puffiness of the ankles at the end of the day, nocturia, mild nocturnal dyspnea, unexpected weight gain, or more than the usual amount of fatigue can be minor symptoms that are passed over unless specifically sought. Such symptoms must be reported to the physician. (See also Special Implications for the Therapist: Congestive Heart Failure.)

Fatigue, weakness, and pallor are signs of an inadequate cardiac output for the demands of the exercise. These signs and symptoms are partly subjective and it is a clinical decision as to how far to allow these people to continue in exercising. Chest pain may indicate myocardial ischemia or pulmonary hypertension, or it may be a noncardiac symptom arising from the chest wall. Follow precautions for angina pectoris. Discontinue exercise when any signs of reduced cerebral blood flow develop, such as severe facial pallor, confusion, dizziness, and unsteady gait. (See also Table 10–3.)

Tolerance to symptoms and current exercise habits are important determinants in progressing an exercise program. Some people with valvular disease avoid physical activity as much as possible and never exercise to the point of developing any symptoms of dyspnea, fatigue, or muscular discomfort. These symptoms develop at light loads in people unaccustomed to any physical activity, regardless of the severity of the valvular disease. Other people force themselves to ignore mild (or even moderate to severe) symptoms to stay on the job or finish a task started.

The status of the myocardium is another important variable in exercise impairment relative to valvular heart disease. Severe aortic regurgitation is well tolerated for many years until myocardial weakness occurs. In all forms of heart disease, the healthy myocardium can compensate and maintain the systemic blood flow at or near normal levels. For the client with valvular disease and myocardial disease or associated CAD, this compensation is not possible, and a lower exercise capacity results.

Stenosis

Valvular stenosis develops or progresses gradually, and because the normal valve orifice is larger than is necessary, stenosis is usually severe before exercise symptoms occur (Cumming, 1993b). In other words, a normal valve is larger than is needed for normal functioning and therefore has excess "capacity." Stenosis only becomes symptomatic when the condition encroaches on critical cross-sectional diameter of the opening. Stress testing may be performed prior to initiation of an exercise program; with or without those test results, clients should be monitored closely, possibly using the perceived exertion or dyspnea scales mentioned earlier in this chapter. The client may not complain of dyspnea from lung congestion, only muscular fatigue on exertion due to a low cardiac output.

Because of reduced cardiac output, muscle perfusion is reduced and lactate is produced at low workloads. Maximal heart rate may be reduced when dyspnea is the cause of premature termination of exercise. Exercise systolic blood pressure (SBP) may reach only 130 mm Hg because of low output. Exercise capacity in clients with mitral stenosis can be improved by slowing heart rate and prolonging diastolic filling period with the use of β-blocking agents.

In the case of symptomatic aortic stenosis, clients are not candidates for exercise programs because of the danger of sudden death. Persons who are asymptomatic must be carefully screened before increasing their physical activity, and for most, exercise intensity should be mild. In people with impaired left ventricular function, cardiac output fails to increase normally with exercise, causing fatigue. Angina with exercise is a common symptom when the aortic stenosis is severe.

Regurgitation

Exercise capacity may be unaffected in cases of mild regurgitation. Mitral regurgitation increases when aortic blood pressure is increased, as occurs during isometric contractions. Light to moderate rhythmic and repetitive exercise is recommended because of a reduction in peripheral resistance in place of isotonic exercise, which increases the heart rate.

Persons with aortic regurgitation caused by weakening of the aortic wall (Marfan's or Ehlers-Danlos syndromes) must avoid all strenuous exercise.

Prolapse

Most people with mitral valve prolapse can participate in all sports activities, including intense competitive sport. Exercise is a key component in the treatment of mitral valve prolapse (not to alter function of the prolapsed valve, but to improve overall cardiovascular function) and although many clients are referred to an exercise physiologist, the physical therapist may also encounter requests for conditioning and exercise programs. Many times, symptoms of fatigue and dyspnea cause a person to limit physical activity, leading to deconditioning and contributing to a cycle of even more fatigue and shortness of breath.

Caution is advised in the use of weight training for the client with mitral valve prolapse; gradual buildup using light weights and increased repetitions is recommended. Some people with mitral valve prolapse syndrome are prone to exercise-induced arrhythmias, which can (rarely) result in sudden death. Any time tachycardia develops in someone with known mitral valve prolapse, immediate medical referral is necessary.

Postoperative Considerations

Postoperative considerations are the same as for people who have had abdominal or cardiothoracic surgery (see Boxes 10–3 and 10–4). After uncomplicated valve ballooning, a return to normal activities is possible within 5 to 7 days. Gradual walking programs can be initiated at home 10 to 30 days after surgery, or the client may enroll in a structured cardiac rehabilitation program.

The degree of improvement in exercise capacity depends on the degree of residual dysfunction, presence or absence of arrhythmia, age of the subject, and the effort made to improve exercise capacity. People with mechanical prosthetic valves receive lifelong anticoagulant therapy (not required for bioprostheses) and may not tolerate vigorous, weight-bearing activities. Mechanical prostheses have fixed openings that place some limitation, at least theoretically, on cardiac performance during maximal effort (Kavanagh, 1994). Because stress testing can be normal, exercise Doppler echocardiography has been used to help prescribe physical activity in clients with prosthetic valves (Alonzo et al., 1993).

Infective Endocarditis

Infective, or bacterial, endocarditis is an infection of the endocardium, the lining inside of the heart, including the heart valves. It is categorized as either acute or subacute, depending on the clinical course, organisms, and condition of the valves. Endocarditis can occur at any age but rarely occurs in children; half of all clients diagnosed are older than 50 years. Endocarditis is more prevalent among men than women (Hunder, 1992).

Etiology and Risk Factors. Endocarditis is frequently caused by bacteria (particularly streptococci or staphylococci) normally present in the mouth, respiratory system, or gastrointestinal tract, or as a result of abnormal growths on the closure lines of previously damaged valves (e.g., rheumatic disease).

In addition to previous valvular damage, persons with prosthetic heart valves, injection drug users, immunocompromised clients, women who have had a suction abortion or pelvic infection related to intrauterine contraceptive devices, and postcardiac surgical clients are at high risk for developing endocarditis. Congenital heart disease and degenerative heart disease, such as calcific aortic stenosis, may also cause endocarditis.

Hospital-acquired infective endocarditis has become more common as a result of iatrogenic endocardial damage produced by surgery, intracardiac pressure-monitoring catheters, ventriculoatrial shunts, and hyperalimentation lines that reach the right atrium. Portals of entry for microorganisms are also provided by wounds, biopsy sites, pacemakers, intravenous and arterial catheters, indwelling urinary catheters, and intratracheal airways (Durack, 1994).

Pathogenesis. As an infection, endocarditis causes inflammation of the cardiac endothelium and most commonly damages the mitral valve, followed by the aortic and tricuspid valves. Bloodborne microorganisms adhere to the damaged endocardial surface, reproduce, and multiply, forming growths called *vegetations*. These vegetations, consisting of fibrin and platelets, may separate from the valve, embolize, and cause septic infarction in the myocardium, kidney, brain, spleen, abdomen, or extremities.

Clinical Manifestations. Endocarditis can develop insidiously, with symptoms remaining undetected for months, or it can cause symptoms immediately, as in the case of acute bacterial endocarditis. Clinical manifestations can be divided into three groups (Table 10–16) (Durack, 1994). It causes varying degrees of valvular dysfunction and may be associated with manifestations involving any number of organ systems including lungs, eyes, kidneys, bones, joints, and central nervous system. The "classic" findings of fever, cardiac murmur, and petechial lesions of the skin, conjunctiva, and oral mucosa are not always present (Haak et al., 1994).

Up to 45% of people with infective endocarditis initially have musculoskeletal symptoms including arthralgia (most common), arthritis, low back pain, and myalgias. Half of these people will have only musculoskeletal symptoms without other manifestations of endocarditis. The early onset of joint pain and myalgia is more likely if the person is older and has had a previously diagnosed heart murmur.

Proximal joints are most often affected, especially the shoulder, followed by knee, hip, wrist, ankle, metatarsophalangeal and metacarpophalangeal joints, and acromioclavicular joints (order of declining incidence). Most often one or two joints are painful, and symptoms begin suddenly accompanied by warmth, tenderness, and redness. Symmetrical arthralgia in the knees or ankles may lead to a diagnosis of rheumatoid arthritis (RA) but as a rule, morning stiffness is not as prevalent in clients with endocarditis as in those with RA or polymyalgia rheumatica.

Almost one third of clients with endocarditis have low back pain, which may be the primary symptom reported. Back pain is accompanied by decreased range of motion and spinal tenderness. Pain may affect only one side, and it may be limited to the paraspinal muscles. Endocarditis-induced back pain may be very similar to that associated with a herniated lumbar disk, as it radiates to the leg and may be accentuated by raising the leg or by sneezing, coughing, or laughing; however, neurologic deficits are usually absent in persons with endocarditis.

Endocarditis may produce destructive changes in the sacroiliac joint characterized by pain localized over the sacroiliac, probably as a result of seeding of the joint by septic emboli. Widespread diffuse myalgia may occur during periods of fever, but these are not appreciably different from the general myalgia seen in clients with other febrile illnesses. More commonly, myalgia is restricted to the calf or thigh. Bilateral or unilateral leg myalgias occur in approximately 10% to 15% of all persons with endocarditis.

The cause of back pain and leg myalgia associated with endocarditis has not been determined. Concurrent aseptic meningitis is a possible hypothesis; emboli that break off from the infected cardiac valves is supported by biopsy evidence of muscle necrosis or vasculitis in clients with endocarditis. Rarely, other musculoskeletal symptoms, such as osteomyelitis, nail clubbing, tendinitis, hypertrophic osteoarthropathy, bone infarcts, and ischemic bone necrosis, may occur.

TABLE 10–16 Clinical Manifestations of Infective Endocarditis

Systemic Infection	Intravascular Involvement	Immunologic Reaction
Fever	Dyspnea	Arthralgia
Chills	Chest pain	Proteinuria
Sweats	Cold and painful extremities	Hematuria
Malaise	Petechiae	Acidosis
Weakness	Splinter hemorrhages	Arthritis
Anorexia		
Weight loss		
Myalgia		

Medical Management

Diagnosis, Treatment, and Prognosis. Blood cultures to identify specific pathogens in the presence of septicemia are required to determine appropriate antibiotic treatment, which is the primary medical treatment. Echocardiography may be used to confirm the diagnosis and is useful in showing underlying valvular lesions and quantifying their severity.

Although it is easily prevented (for the at-risk person) by taking antibiotics before and after procedures such as dental cleaning, genitourinary instrumentation, and open cardiovascular surgery, endocarditis is difficult to treat and can result in serious heart damage or death. Potential complications are many, including CHF and arterial, systemic, or pulmonary emboli. Relapse can occur up to 2 or more weeks after treatment. Surgical valve replacement may be necessary, depending on the response to treatment, sites of infection, recurrent infection, or infection of a prosthetic valve.

Special Implications for the Therapist **10–14**

INFECTIVE ENDOCARDITIS

Physical exertion beyond normal activities of daily living are usually limited for the person receiving antibiotic therapy for endocarditis and during the following weeks of recovery. The therapist is not likely to treat a person diagnosed during this acute phase of endocarditis. However, because early symptoms of endocarditis may be primarily musculoskeletal in nature, the person may come to a therapist, so screening for this disease is important. For any client with known risk factors or a recent history of endocarditis, the therapist must be alert for signs of endocarditis, indications of complications (easy fatigue associated with heart failure or peripheral emboli), lack of response to therapy treatment, or signs indicating relapse. Often, the client thinks the symptoms are recurrent bouts of the flu.

Rheumatic Fever and Heart Disease

(Williams, 1991)

Overview, Incidence, and Etiology. Rheumatic fever is one form of endocarditis (infection), caused by streptococcal group A bacteria, that can be fatal or may lead to rheumatic heart disease (10% of cases), a chronic condition caused by scarring and deformity of the heart valves (Fig. 10–20). It is called rheumatic fever because two of the most common symptoms are fever and joint pain (O'Toole, 1992).

The infection generally starts with "strep throat" in chil-

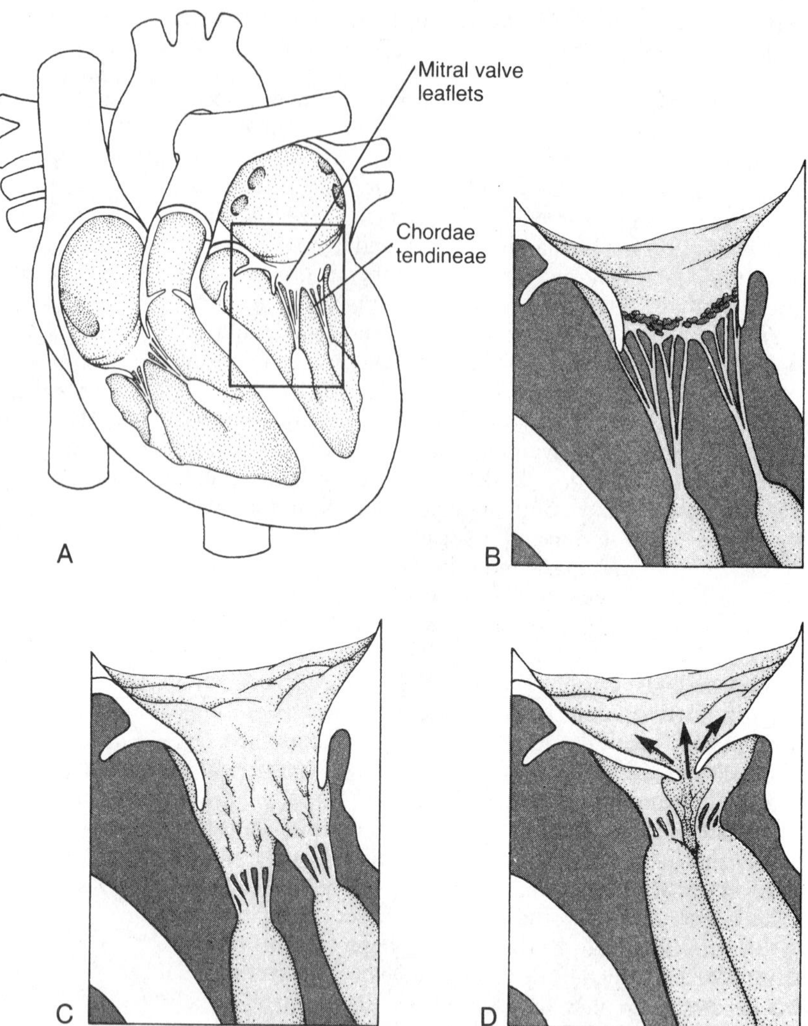

Figure 10–20. Cardiac valvular disease caused by rheumatic fever. A, Inflammation of the membrane over the mitral (and aortic) valves may cause edema and accumulation of fibrin and platelets on the chordae tendineae. B, This accumulation of inflammatory materials produces rheumatic vegetations that affect the support provided by the chordae tendineae to the atrioventricular valves. C, In this view, the mitral valve leaflets have become thickened with scar tissue and calcified. The chordae tendineae often fuse. D, As a result, the scarred valve fails to close tightly (mitral stenosis) and regurgitation or backflow of blood into the atrium develops. Prolonged, severe stenosis with mitral regurgitation leads to symptoms of CHF. (*Adapted from Goodman CC, Snyder TE: Differential Diagnosis in Physical Therapy, ed 2. Philadelphia, WB Saunders, 1995, p 100.*)

dren between ages 5 and 15 years and damages the heart in approximately 50% of cases. The aggressive use of specific antibiotics in the United States had effectively reduced the incidence of rheumatic fever and removed it as the primary cause of valvular damage. However, in 1985, a series of epidemics of rheumatic fever were reported in several widely diverse geographic regions of the continental United States, affecting children, young adults aged 18 to 30 years, and, occasionally, middle-aged persons (Odio, 1986; Veasy et al., 1987; Wald et al., 1987).

Currently, the prevalence and incidence of cases have not approximated the 1985 record, but they have remained above previous levels. The cause for the resurgence of rheumatic fever is unknown, but some theories are that a new, more virulent strain of the bacteria has become resistant to antibiotics, or that perhaps streptococcal bacteria strains follow periodic cycles that are seen in other diseases, such as measles (Williams, 1991). Additionally, a noted number of increasing cases has been attributed to the increased number of new immigrants to the United States.

Pathogenesis. The exact pathogenesis is unclear, but rheumatic fever produces a diffuse, proliferative, and exudative inflammatory process in the connective tissue of certain structures. In the case of the heart valves, this inflammatory process occurs through an autoimmune reaction involving antibodies that cross-react with cardiac proteins. Antigens to streptococcal cells bind to receptors on the heart, brain cells, muscles, and joints, which begins the autoimmune response; thus, rheumatic fever is classified as an autoimmune disease.

All layers of the heart (epicardium, endocardium, myocardium, and pericardium) (see Fig. 10–1) may be involved, including the valves. Endocardial inflammation causes swelling of the valve leaflets, with secondary erosion along the lines of leaflet contact. Small, beadlike clumps of vegetation containing platelets and fibrin are deposited on eroded valvular tissue and on the chordae tendineae;[18] the mitral and aortic valves are most commonly affected. Over time, scarring and shortening of the involved structures occurs, and the leaflets adhere to each other as the valves lose their elasticity. As many as 25% of clients will have mitral valvular disease

[18] *Chordae* refers to the tendinous cords connecting the two atrioventricular (AV) valves (tricuspid valve between the right atrium and right ventricle and the mitral valve between the left atrium and left ventricle) to the appropriate papillary muscles in the heart ventricles; the chordae tendineae in effect "anchor" the valve leaflets. This support to the AV valves during ventricular systole helps prevent prolapse of the valve into the atrium.

25 to 30 years later, with fibrosis and calcification of valves, fusion of commissures (union or junction between adjacent cusps of the heart valves) and chordae tendineae, and mitral stenosis with "fish-mouth" deformity (Fig. 10–21).

Clinical Manifestations *(Haak et al., 1994)*. Although "strep throat" is the most common manifestation of the streptococcal virus, streptococcal infections can also affect the skin and, less commonly, the lungs. In some cases of strep throat the initial triggering sore throat or pharyngitis does not cause extreme illness, if any discomfort at all. However, the major manifestations of acute rheumatic fever are usually carditis, acute migratory polyarthritis, and chorea, which may occur singly or in combination. In the acute, full-blown sequelae, shortness of breath and increasing nocturnal cough also occur. A ring or crescent-shaped rash with clear centers on the skin of the limbs or trunk (erythema marginatum) is present in fewer than 2% of persons with an acute episode. Subcutaneous nodules may occur over bony prominences and along the extensor surfaces of the arms, heels, knees, or back of the head, but these do not interfere with joint function.

Carditis. Carditis is most likely to occur in children and adolescents. Mitral or aortic semilunar valve dysfunction (see Pathogenesis) may result in a previously undetected murmur. Chest pain caused by pericardial inflammation and characteristic heart sounds may occur.

Polyarthritis. The most typical clinical profile of a child or young adult with acute rheumatic fever is an initial cold or sore throat followed 2 or 3 weeks later by sudden or gradual onset of painful migratory joint symptoms in knees, shoulders, feet, ankles, elbows, fingers, or neck. Fever (99° to 103° F) and palpitations and fatigue are also present. Malaise, weakness, weight loss, and anorexia may accompany the fever.

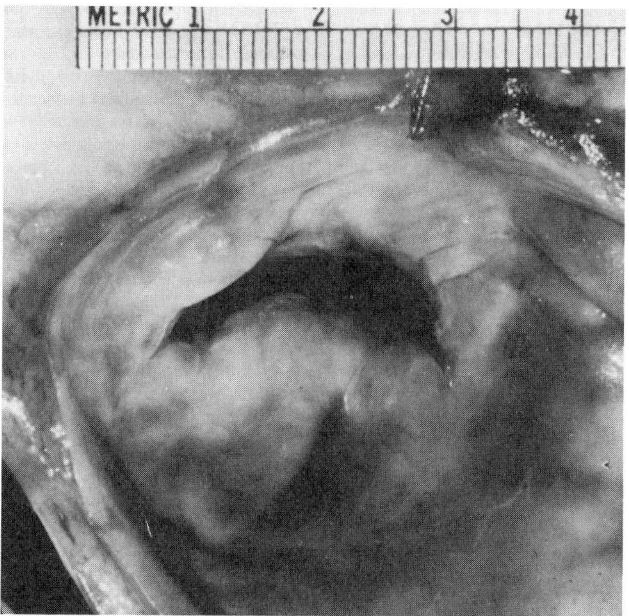

Figure 10–21. When viewed from the atrial aspect, a severely stenotic mitral valve has a narrowed orifice that has the appearance of a classic "fishmouth" deformity. (*From Kissane JM (ed): Anderson's Pathology. St Louis, Mosby–Year Book, 1990.*)

The migratory arthralgias usually involve two or more joints simultaneously or in succession and may last only 24 hours, or they may persist for several weeks. In adults, only a single joint may be affected. Joints that are sore and hot and contain fluid completely resolve, followed by acute synovitis, heat, synovial space tenderness, swelling, and effusion present in a different area the next day. The persistence of swelling, heat, and synovitis in a single joint or joints for more than 2 to 3 weeks is extremely unusual in acute rheumatic fever.

Chorea. Rheumatic chorea (also called Sydenham's chorea or St. Vitus' dance) occurs in 3% of cases 1 to 3 months after the streptococcal infection and is always preceded by polyarthritis. Chorea in a child, teenager, or young adult is almost always a manifestation of acute rheumatic fever.[19] The chorea develops as rapid, purposeless, nonrepetitive movements that may involve all muscles except the eyes. This pattern of movement may last for 1 week, several months, or even several years without permanent impairment of the central nervous system (Berkow and Fletcher, 1992; Williams, 1991).

Medical Management

Diagnosis and Treatment. In acute rheumatic fever, Jones criteria may be used for diagnosis (Table 10–17) and throat culture for group A streptococci is usually positive; chronic valvular disease is assessed by auscultation, echocardiography, and cardiac catheterization.

Penicillin is administered therapeutically and prophylactically and can prevent the development of rheumatic fever if administered within the first 9 days of infection (Harris, 1991). Aspirin may be used to treat the joint manifestations and as a general antiinflammatory agent. Corticosteroids are used when there is clear evidence of rheumatic carditis. Children with acute chorea are generally treated with some form of CNS depressant, such as phenobarbital. Commissurotomy and prosthetic valve replacement may be necessary for valvular dysfunction associated with chronic rheumatic disease.

Prognosis. Initial episodes of rheumatic fever last weeks to months, but 20% of children affected have recurrences within 5 years; relapses increase the risk of heart damage that leads to rheumatic heart disease, with mitral or aortic stenosis or insufficiency due to progressive valve scarring. Mortality rate for acute rheumatic fever is low (1% to 2%) but persistent rheumatic activity with complications (enlarged heart, atrial fibrillation, arterial embolism, heart failure, pericarditis) are associated with a long-term morbidity and mortality.

Special Implications for the Therapist **10–15**

RHEUMATIC FEVER

The increased incidence of streptococcal group A bacteria in the adult population may result in cases of sudden or gradual onset of painful migratory joint symptoms affecting the knees, shoulders, feet, ankles, elbows, fingers, or neck. Anytime an adult presents with

[19] Other causes of chorea are SLE, thyrotoxicosis, and cerebrovascular accident, but these are uncommon and unlikely in a child.

TABLE 10-17 JONES CRITERIA FOR DIAGNOSIS OF RHEUMATIC FEVER (1992 UPDATE)

MAJOR MANIFESTATIONS	MINOR MANIFESTATIONS	SUPPORTING EVIDENCE OF STREPTOCOCCAL INFECTION
Carditis	Previous rheumatic fever or rheumatic heart disease	Recent scarlet fever
Polyarthritis	Arthralgia	Positive throat culture for group A *Streptococcus*
Chorea	Fever	Other positive laboratory tests
Erythema marginatum	Elevated appearance of C-reactive protein	
Subcutaneous nodules	Leukocytosis	
	ECG changes	

Dajani AS, Ayoub A, Burman FZ, et al: American Heart Association Medical/Scientific Statement: Guidelines for the diagnosis of rheumatic fever: Jones Criteria, 1992 update. Circulation 87:302–307, 1993.

intermittent or migratory joint symptoms, the client's temperature must be taken. The therapist should ask about the recent history or presence of rash anywhere on the body, sore throat, or cold. The sore throat or cold symptoms may be mild enough that the person does not seek medical care of any kind. The presence of fever accompanied by a clinical presentation of migratory arthralgias or a positive history of recent illness described requires medical evaluation.

As many as 25% of people affected by rheumatic fever develop mitral valve dysfunction 25 to 30 years later. Adults who experience exercise intolerance or exertional dyspnea of unknown cause and who have a previous history of childhood rheumatic fever may be experiencing the effects of mitral valve prolapse. Dyspnea associated with mitral valve prolapse is most commonly accompanied by fatigue and palpitations. This history in combination with this triad of symptoms requires evaluation by a physician.

In the case of a confirmed diagnosis of rheumatic fever–related mitral valve involvement, exercise will not improve the mechanical function of the valve, but improvement in cardiovascular function can occur. (See previous discussion on Valvular Heart Disease: Special Implications for the Therapist: 10–13.)

DISEASES AFFECTING THE PERICARDIUM

The pericardium consists of two layers: the inner visceral layer, which is attached to the epicardium; and an outer parietal layer (see Fig. 10–1). The pericardium stabilizes the heart in its anatomic position despite changes in body position and reduces excess friction between the heart and surrounding structures. It is composed of fibrous tissue that is loose enough to permit moderate changes in cardiac size, but that cannot stretch fast enough to accommodate rapid dilation or accumulation of fluid without increasing intracardiac pressure.

The pericardium may be a primary site of disease and is often involved by processes that affect the heart; it may also be affected by diseases of the adjacent tissues (Massie, 1994). Three conditions primarily affect the pericardium: acute pericarditis, constrictive pericarditis, and pericardial effusion. These three diseases are grouped together for ease of understanding in the following section.

Pericarditis

Definition and Overview. Pericarditis or inflammation of the pericardium may be a primary condition or may be secondary to a number of diseases and circumstances (Box 10–11). It may occur as a singular acute event or it may recur and become a chronic condition called *constrictive pericarditis*.

Incidence and Etiology. The most common types of pericarditis encountered by the therapist will be those present in association with connective tissue diseases (e.g., SLE, rheumatoid arthritis), postmyocardial infarction, renal failure,

BOX 10–11
Causes of Pericarditis

- Infections
  - Viral
  - Bacterial: tuberculosis, *Staphylococcus*, *Streptococcus*, *Meningococcus*, pneumonia
  - Parasitic
  - Fungal
- Myocardial injury
  - MI
  - Cardiac trauma: blunt or penetrating pericardium; rib fracture
  - Post cardiac surgery
- Hypersensitivity
  - Collagen diseases: rheumatic fever, scleroderma, SLE, rheumatoid arthritis
  - Drug reaction
  - Radiation/cobalt therapy
- Metabolic disorders
  - Uremia
  - Myxedema
  - Chronic anemia
- Neoplasm
  - Lymphoma, lung or breast cancer
- Aortic dissection

Adapted from Ott B: Nursing care of clients with cardiac structure disorders. *In* Black JM, Matassarin-Jacobs E (eds): Luckmann and Sorensen's Medical-Surgical Nursing, ed 4. Philadelphia, WB Saunders, 1993, p 1221.

after open heart surgery, and after radiation therapy. Other types encountered less often include viral pericarditis (e.g., Epstein-Barr, hepatitis, and HIV) and neoplastic pericarditis (from spread to the pericardium of adjacent lung cancer or invasion by breast cancer, Hodgkin's disease, or lymphoma).

Pathogenesis. Many causes of pericarditis affect both the pericardium and the myocardium (myopericarditis) with varying degrees of cardiac dysfunction. Constrictive pericarditis is characterized by a fibrotic, thickened, and adherent pericardium that is compressing the heart. The heart becomes restricted in movement and function (cardiac tamponade). Diastolic filling of the heart is reduced, venous pressures are elevated, cardiac output is decreased, and eventual cardiac failure may result.

When fluid accumulates within the pericardial sac it is referred to as *pericardial effusion*. Blunt chest trauma or any cause of acute pericarditis can lead to pericardial effusion. Rapid distention or excessive fluid accumulation from this condition can also compress the heart and reduce ventricular filling and cardiac output.

Clinical Manifestations. The presentation and course of pericarditis is determined by the underlying etiology. For example, pericarditis may occur 2 to 5 days after infarction due to an inflammatory reaction to myocardial necrosis, or it may occur within the first year after radiation initiates a fibrinous and fibrotic process in the pericardium. Often there is pleuritic chest pain that is made worse by lying down and by respiratory movements and is relieved by sitting upright or leaning forward. The pain is substernal and may radiate to the neck, shoulders, upper back, upper trapezius, left supraclavicular area, epigastrium, or down the left arm. Other symptoms may include fever, joint pain, dyspnea, or difficulty swallowing.

Pericardial effusion may be characterized by the symptoms described above when associated with an acute inflammatory process or it may be asymptomatic and painless (e.g., uremic or neoplastic effusion). Symptoms of constrictive pericarditis develop slowly and usually include progressive dyspnea, fatigue, weakness, edema, and ascites.

Medical Management

Diagnosis. Clinical examination, including clinical presentation, auscultation, and client history, may be diagnostic. A classic sign of pericarditis is the pericardial friction rub heard on auscultation. This sound is produced by inflamed, roughened layers of the pericardium that create friction as their surfaces rub together during heart movement. Other diagnostic tools include chest x-ray (showing enlarged cardiac shadow), characteristic ECG changes (showing evidence of an underlying inflammatory process), and laboratory studies (e.g., elevated sedimentation rate or elevated white blood count [nonspecific indicators of inflammation] and elevated cardiac enzymes [post-MI]). Echocardiography is the most accurate technique for diagnosing pericardial effusion.

Treatment. Treatment is two-fold, directed toward (1) prevention of long-term complications and (2) the underlying cause. For example, while treating the underlying infection, symptomatic treatment is provided for idiopathic, viral, or radiation pericarditis; anti-inflammatory drugs are given for pericarditis associated with connective tissue disorders; chemotherapy is given for neoplastic pericarditis; or dialysis is performed for uremic pericarditis. Analgesics may be prescribed for the pain and fever. Pericardiocentesis (surgical drainage with a needle catheter through a small subxiphoid incision) may be performed if cardiac compression from pericardial effusion does not resolve.

Treatment for constrictive pericarditis is both medical and surgical, including digitalis preparations, diuretics, sodium restriction, and pericardiectomy (surgical excision of the damaged pericardium).

Prognosis. The prognosis in most cases of acute viral pericarditis is excellent when there is no (or only minimal) myocardial involvement, as this is frequently a self-limited disease. Without treatment, shock and death can occur from decreased cardiac output with cardiac involvement.

Constrictive pericarditis is a progressive disease without spontaneous reversal of symptoms. Most people become progressively disabled over time. Surgical removal of the pericardium is associated with a high mortality rate when progressive calcification and fibrosis are present (Brockington, 1990).

Special Implications for the Therapist: **10-16**

PERICARDITIS

Pericardial pain can masquerade as a musculoskeletal problem, presenting as just upper back, neck, or upper trapezius pain. In such cases, the pain may be diminished by holding the breath or aggravated by swallowing or neck or trunk movements, especially side bending or rotation (Schlant and Alexander, 1994). Pain is also aggravated by respiratory movements, such as deep breathing, coughing, and laughing. The therapist must screen for medical disease by assessing aggravating and relieving factors and by asking the client about a history of fever, chills, upper respiratory tract infection (recent cold or "flu"), weakness, heart disease, or recent MI (heart attack).

Special precautions depend on the underlying cause of the pericarditis. Mild cases require treatment per client tolerance, and the therapist observes for any symptoms of CHF. A mild pericarditis can quickly progress to a severe condition that requires medical evaluation. The clinician is referred to each individual section in this text representing the etiology of pericarditis for treatment precautions.

DISEASES AFFECTING THE BLOOD VESSELS AND THE LYMPHATIC VESSELS

The Blood Vessels

Diseases affecting the blood vessels usually result in some form of peripheral vascular disease (PVD) (Table 10–18). PVD can affect the arterial, venous, or lymphatic circulatory systems (see The Lymphatic Vessels). Arterial and venous disorders are presented here based on the underlying pathology (i.e., whether the condition is caused by occlusion, inflammation, vasomotor disturbances, or neoplastic diseases).

TABLE 10–18 PERIPHERAL VASCULAR DISEASES

INFLAMMATORY DISORDERS	OCCLUSIVE DISORDERS	VENOUS DISORDERS	VASOMOTOR
Polyarteritis nodosa Arteritis Allergic or hypersensitivity angiitis Kawasaki's disease Thromboangiitis obliterans (Buerger's disease)	Arteriosclerosis obliterans Thromboangiitis obliterans Arterial thrombosis Arterial embolism	Thrombophlebitis Varicose veins Chronic venous insufficiency	Raynaud's disease Reflex sympathetic dystrophy (RSD)

Special implications related to arterial and venous disorders, whether of an inflammatory or occlusive (including thrombotic) nature, are compiled rather than listed at the end of each individual section (see Special Implications for the Therapist: 10–18).

Occlusive Diseases

Occlusive diseases of the blood vessels are a common cause of disability and usually occur as a result of atherosclerosis. Other causes of arterial occlusion may include trauma, thrombus or embolism, vasculitis, vasomotor disorders such as Raynaud's and reflex sympathetic dystrophy, arterial punctures, polycythemia, and chronic mechanical irritation of the subclavian artery being compressed by a cervical rib. For each individual case, see the discussion of the underlying cause of the occlusion to understand etiology, risk factors, and pathogenesis.

Atherosclerotic occlusive disease can also affect other vessels throughout the body other than the cardiac blood vessels. For example, occlusive disease affecting the intestines results in acute intestinal ischemia or *ischemic colitis* (see Chapter 13), depending on the location of the occlusion. *Occlusive cerebrovascular disease* (see Chapter 28) as a result of atherosclerosis accounts for many episodes of weakness, dizziness, blurred vision, or sudden cerebrovascular accident (CVA) or stroke. Extracranial arterial ischemia (e.g., common carotid bifurcation, vertebral artery) accounts for over half of these types of strokes.

Arterial Thrombosis and Embolism

Occlusive diseases may be complicated by arterial thrombosis and embolism (Fig. 10–22). Chronic, incomplete arterial obstruction usually results in the development of collateral vessels before complete occlusion threatens circulation to the extremity. Arterial embolism is generally a complication of ischemic or rheumatic heart disease, with or without MI. Signs and symptoms of pain, numbness, coldness, tingling or changes in sensation, skin changes (pallor or mottling), weakness, and muscle spasm occur in the extremity distal to the block (Fig. 10–23). Treatment may include immediate or delayed embolectomy, anticoagulation therapy (e.g., heparin), and protection of the limb.

Thromboangiitis Obliterans (Buerger's Disease)

This condition is discussed as a vasculitis in a subsequent section (see Inflammatory Diseases) but is mentioned here as an occlusive disorder because the inflammatory lesions of the peripheral blood vessels are accompanied by thrombus formation and vasospasm occluding blood vessels.

Arteriosclerosis Obliterans

Definition and Overview. Arteriosclerosis obliterans, defined as arteriosclerosis in which proliferation of the intima has caused complete obliteration of the lumen of the artery, is also known as *atherosclerotic occlusive disease*, *chronic occlusive arterial disease*, *obliterative arteriosclerosis*, and *peripheral arterial disease*. It is the most common occlusive disease and accounts for about 95% of cases. This disease is most often seen in elderly clients and is commonly associated with diabetes mellitus (Kisner and Colby, 1996) (see Chapter 9).

Etiology and Risk Factors. Atherosclerosis as the underlying cause of occlusive disease, with its known etiology and associated risk factors, is discussed earlier in the chapter. The most common risk factors in arteriosclerosis obliterans are smoking, hypertension, hyperlipidemia (increased lipids), obesity, and diabetes. Atherosclerosis leading to arteriosclerosis obliterans develops more often and earlier in people with diabetes mellitus, especially if the person smokes.

Pathogenesis. See also Pathogenesis: Atherosclerosis.

Clinical Manifestations. Occlusive disease of the *aorta* and *iliac arteries* usually begins just proximal to the bifurcation of the common iliac arteries, causing changes in both lower extremities (Fig. 10–24; Table 10–19). Bilateral, progressive, intermittent claudication (pain, ache, or cramp in the muscles causing limping) is almost always present in the calf muscles and is usually present in the gluteal and quadriceps muscles. The distance a person can walk before the onset of pain is indicative of the degree of circulatory inadequacy (e.g., 2 blocks or more is mild; 1 block is moderate; ½ block or less is severe). The primary symptom may only be a sense of weakness or "tiredness" in these same areas; both the pain and weakness or fatigue are relieved by rest.

Occlusive disease of the *femoral* and *popliteal arteries* usually occurs at the point at which the superficial femoral artery passes through the adductor magnus tendon into the popliteal space. Occlusion of these regions is also marked by intermittent claudication of the calf and foot that may radiate to the ipsilateral[20] popliteal region and lower thigh. There are definite changes of the affected lower leg and foot as listed in Table 10–19.

Occlusive disease of the *tibial* and *common peroneal arteries*, as well as the pedal vessels and small digital vessels, occurs slowly and progressively over months or years. The eventual

[20] Although symptoms occur ipsilateral to the occlusion anywhere distal to the bifurcation of the aorta, most people have bilateral disease and, therefore, bilateral symptoms.

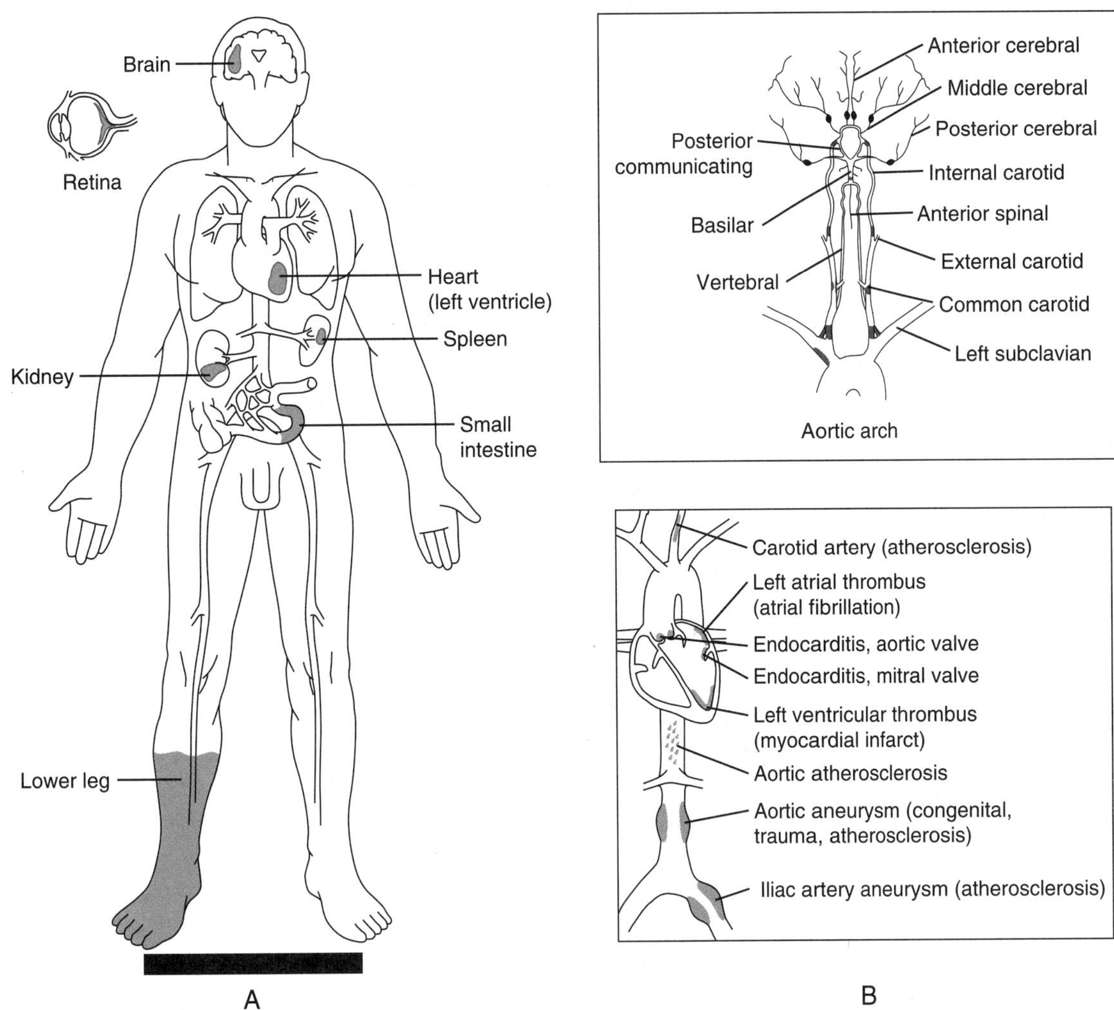

Figure **10–22.** A, Common sites of infarction from arterial emboli. B, Sources of arterial emboli.

outcome depends on the vessels that are occluded and the condition of the proximal and collateral vessels. Pain at rest is indicative of more severe involvement, which may mimic deep venous thrombosis (DVT), but relief from the occlusive disease can sometimes be obtained by dangling the uncovered leg over the edge of the bed. This dependent position would increase symptoms of DVT, which is usually treated by leg elevation. Exercise may cause pedal pulses to disappear in some people.

Medical Management

Diagnosis. Diagnosis is based on client history and clinical examination. Diagnostic tools may include Doppler ultrasonography to accurately determine arterial blood pressure, transcutaneous oximetry to evaluate pressure and oxygenation, and radiographic films of the lower leg and foot to show calcification of the vessels. Aortography may be used to view the level and extent of the occlusion and to determine the condition of the vessels distal to the block (including the thigh and leg arteries); magnetic resonance angiography is used to show the same information, but without using a contrast medium.

Treatment. A conservative approach to care includes a program of dietary management to decrease cholesterol and fat, pain control, and daily walking to improve collateralization and function. Careful attention must be given to preventive skin care (see Table 10–22) to avoid even minor injuries, infections, or ulcerations. Low-dose aspirin may be administered as an antiplatelet agent.

Cessation of smoking is essential and may be required by the physician before surgery is considered. Surgical treatment (bypass graft) or angioplastic treatment is indicated if claudication interferes with essential activities or work. Persons with localized occlusions of the aorta and iliac arteries less than 10 cm in length, with relatively normal vessels proximally and distally, are good candidates for angioplasty or stenting (see Figs. 10–3, 10–5, and 10–6). Conversely, people with multisegmented arterial disease with more involved symptoms are likely to require surgical treatment and are at greater risk of amputation. Endovascular intervention includes a variety of catheter-based surgical techniques that are being improved by laser techniques.

Prognosis. Occlusive diseases are not life threatening un- less a thrombus breaks off from the blood vessel wall ar ried to the heart, brain, or lungs as an embolism more slowly through the veins than through

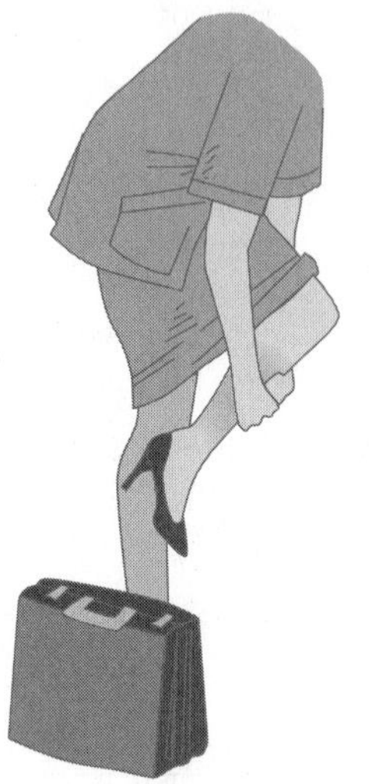

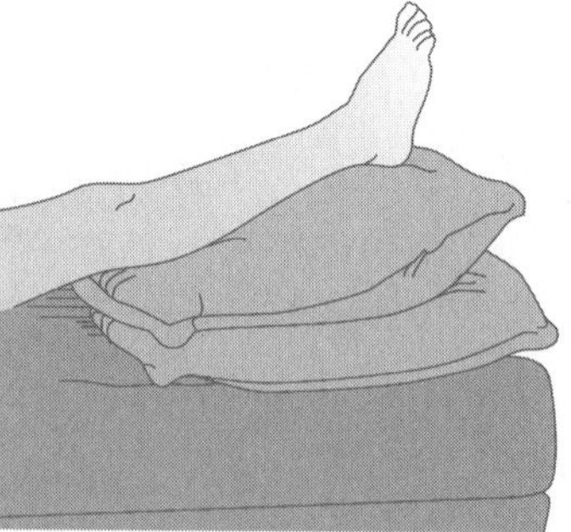

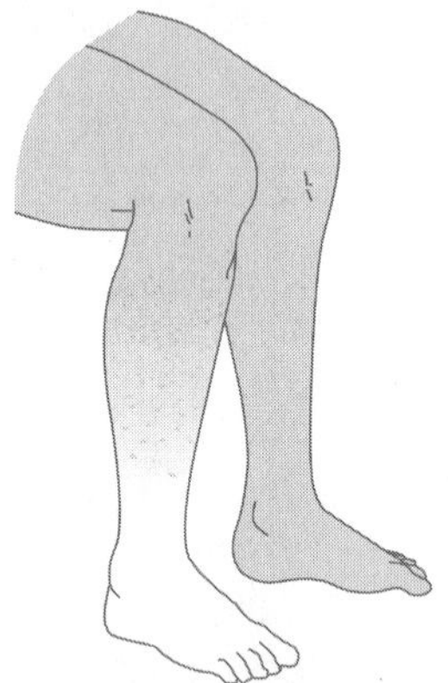

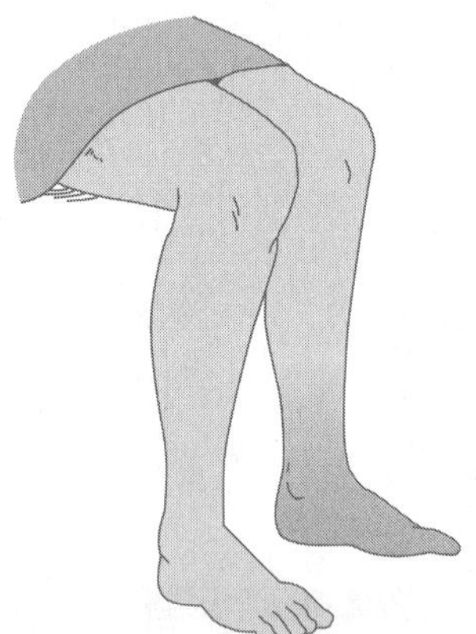

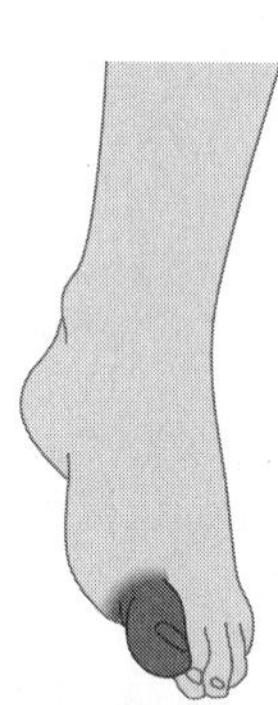

Figure 10–23. Signs and symptoms of arterial insufficiency.

thrombosis is more common in the veins as a result of coagulation promoted by stasis. Progressive disability from pain, ulceration, gangrene, and loss of function or limbs are more likely to occur than death as a result of peripheral occlusive diseases. Frequently, persons with peripheral vascular disease also have coronary artery disease and may die from MI.

Occlusive arterial disease for the person with diabetes is further complicated by very slow healing, and healed areas may break down easily. Diabetic neuropathy with diminished or absent sensation of the toes or feet often occurs, predisposing the person to injury or pressure ulcers that may progress because of poor blood flow and subsequent loss of sensation (Table 10–20) (Tierney, 1994) (see Chapter 9).

Aneurysm

Overview and Incidence. An aneurysm is an abnormal stretching (dilation) in the wall of an artery, a vein, or the heart. When the vessel wall becomes weakened from trauma, congenital vascular disease, infection, or atherosclerosis, a saclike formation develops. A *false aneurysm* can occur when the wall of the blood vessel is ruptured and blood escapes into surrounding tissues, forming a clot (Fig. 10–25; see also Fig. 10–26).

Aneurysms are of various types (either arterial or venous) and are named according to the specific site of formation. The most common site for an arterial aneurysm is the aorta, forming a *thoracic aneurysm* (which involves the ascending, transverse, or first part of the descending portion of the aorta) or an *abdominal aneurysm* (which generally involves the aorta between the renal arteries and iliac branches). *Peripheral arterial aneurysms* affect the femoral and popliteal arteries.

Incidence increases with increasing age, usually beginning after age 50 years. Aneurysms occur much more often in men than in women, and half of affected persons are hypertensive.

Etiology and Pathogenesis. Although atherosclerosis is responsible for most arterial aneurysms (plaque formation erodes the vessel wall), any injury to the middle or muscular layer of the arterial wall (tunica media) can predispose the vessel to stretching of the inner and outer layers of the artery and formation of a sac.

This stretching produces infarct expansion, a weak and thin layer of necrotic muscle, and fibrous tissue that bulges with each systole. With time, the aneurysm becomes more fibrotic, but it continues to bulge with each systole, thus acting as a reservoir for some of the stroke volume (Haak et al., 1994).

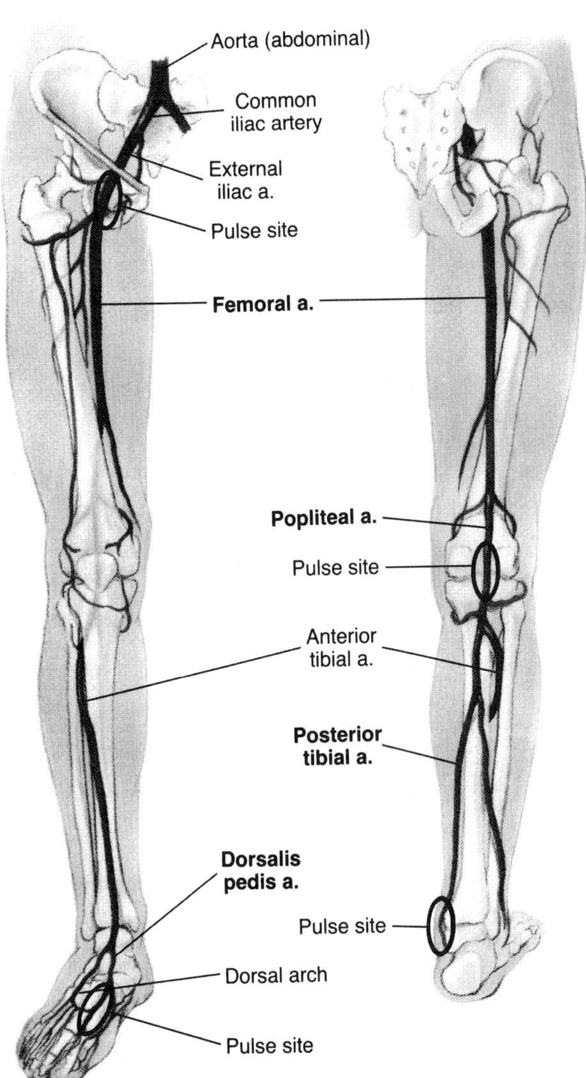

Figure 10–24. Arteries in the leg. The abdominal aorta branches (aortic bifurcation) into the right and left *common iliac artery*. This artery passes through the pelvic cavity and under the inguinal ligament to become the major artery supplying the leg, called the *femoral artery*. The femoral artery travels down the thigh until, at the lower thigh, it courses posteriorly, where it becomes the *popliteal artery*. Below the knee, the popliteal artery divides into the anterior tibial artery and posterior tibial artery. The *anterior tibial artery* travels down the front of the leg onto the dorsum of the foot, where it becomes the *dorsalis pedis*. In the back of the leg, the *posterior tibial artery* travels down behind the malleolus and forms the *plantar arteries* in the foot. (*From Jarvis C: Physical Examination and Health Assessment. Philadelphia, WB Saunders, 1992, p 635.*)

TABLE 10–19 ARTERIAL OCCLUSIVE DISEASE

SITE OF OCCLUSION	SIGNS AND SYMPTOMS
Aortic bifurcation	Sensory and motor deficits Muscle weakness Numbness (loss of sensation) Paresthesias (burning, pricking) Paralysis Intermittent claudication (lower back, gluteal muscles, quadriceps, calves; relieved by rest) Cold, pale legs with decreased or absent peripheral pulses
Iliac artery	Intermittent claudication (buttock, hip, thigh; relieved by rest) Diminished or absent femoral or distal pulses Impotence in males
Femoral and popliteal artery	Intermittent claudication (calf and foot; may radiate) Leg pallor and coolness Dependent rubor Blanching of feet on elevation No palpable pulses in ankles and feet Gangrene
Tibial and common peroneal artery	Intermittent claudication (calf; feet occasionally) Pain at rest (severe disease); possibly relieved by dangling affected leg Same skin and temperature changes in lower leg and foot as described above Pedal pulses absent; popliteal pulses may be present

Other less common causes of aneurysm include Marfan's disease (congenital defects of the arterial wall), infection (bacterial infection, syphilis, polyarteritis), and hereditary abnormalities of connective tissue. Hypertension seems to enhance aneurysm formation.

Thoracic Aortic Aneurysm

Thoracic aortic aneurysms account for approximately 10% of all aortic aneurysms and occur most frequently in hypertensive men between the ages of 40 and 70 years. Marked elevation of blood pressure may facilitate rapid disruption and rupture of the aortic wall when a small tear in the intima occurs (Bauwens and Paine, 1983). A dissecting aneurysm (actually a hematoma) usually affects the thoracic aorta as a result of hemorrhage that causes a lengthwise splitting of the arterial wall, creating a false vessel (Fig. 10–26).

Clinical Manifestations. Aneurysms may be asymptomatic; when they do occur, manifestations depend largely on the size and position of the aneurysm and its rate of growth. Substernal, back, or neck pain may occur. Dissection over the aortic arch and into the descending aorta may be experienced as extreme pain felt at the base of the neck and/or along the back into the interscapular areas. When pressure from a large volume of blood is placed on the trachea, esophagus, laryngeal nerve, or superior vena cava, symptoms of dyspnea, cough, dysphagia, hoarseness, or edema of the neck, arms, and distended neck veins may occur, respectively.

Abdominal Aortic Aneurysm

Abdominal aortic aneurysms occur about four times more often than thoracic aneurysms, and the incidence is increas-

TABLE 10–20 COMPARISON OF ARTERIAL, VENOUS, AND DIABETIC ULCERS

	ARTERIAL ULCER	VENOUS ULCER	DIABETIC ULCER
Etiology	Arteriosclerosis obliterans Atheroembolism	Valvular incompetence History of DVT Venous hypertension	Combination of arterial disease and peripheral neuropathy Repetitive unrecognized trauma
Location	Distal appendages (toes) Bone prominences (anterior tibial) Lateral malleolus	Medial aspect of distal third of lower extremity Behind medial malleolus	Same areas in which arterial ulcers appear Areas where peripheral neuropathy occurs (pressure points on plantar aspect of foot, toes, heels)
Clinical manifestations	Painful, especially with legs elevated Pulses poor quality or absent Claudication, rest pain Atrophic changes History of minor nonhealing trauma	Not often painful; comfortable with legs elevated Normal arterial pulses Eczema or stasis dermatitis Edema Dark pigmentation	Not painful; loss of sensation Sepsis common Pulses may be present or diminished (arteries become calcified)

Adapted from Dennison PD, Black JM: Nursing care of clients with peripheral vascular disorders. *In* Black JM, Matassarin-Jacobs E: Luckmann and Sorensen's Medical Surgical Nursing, ed 4. Philadelphia, WB Saunders, 1993, p 1264.

ing, probably because of the increasing number of elderly persons (Grand Rounds, 1993). The natural course of an untreated abdominal aortic aneurysm is expansion and rupture in one of several places, including the peritoneal cavity, the mesentery, retroperitoneum, into the inferior vena cava, or into the duodenum or rectum. The most common site for an abdominal aortic aneurysm is just below the renal arteries, and it may involve the bifurcation of the aorta (Fig. 10–27).

Clinical Manifestations. Most abdominal aortic aneurysms are asymptomatic, but intermittent or constant pain in the form of mild to severe midabdominal or lower back discomfort is present in some form in 25% to 30% of cases. Groin or flank pain may be experienced because of increasing pressure on other structures.

Rupture is most likely to occur in aneurysms that are 5 cm or larger, causing intense flank pain with referred pain to the back at the level of the rupture. Pain may radiate to the lower abdomen, groin, or genitalia. Back pain may be the only presenting symptom before rupture occurs.

Peripheral Aneurysm

The most common site for peripheral arterial aneurysm is the popliteal space in the lower extremities. Most are caused by atherosclerosis and occur bilaterally in men. *Popliteal aneurysm* presents as a pulsating mass, 2 cm or more in diameter, and causes ischemic symptoms in the lower limbs (e.g., intermittent claudication, rest pain, thrombosis and embolization resulting in gangrene). *Femoral aneurysm* presents as a pulsating mass in the femoral area on one or both sides.

Medical Management

Diagnosis, Treatment, and Prognosis. Clinical diagnosis of abdominal and peripheral aneurysms includes palpation of a pulsating mass. Radiography, ultrasonography, computed tomography (CT) and magnetic resonance imaging (MRI), arteriography, and aortography may be used for investigation. Surgical treatment before rupture provides a good diagnosis; frequently, aneurysms are discovered only at autopsy. Aneurysm rupture is associated with a high mortality.

Special Implications for the Therapist **10–17**

ANEURYSM

For the person who has had a surgically repaired aneurysm, activities are restricted and are only gradually reintroduced. The therapist may be involved in bedside exercises and early mobility, which are especially important to prevent thromboembolism as a result of venous stasis during prolonged bed rest and immobility.

Activities that require pushing, pulling, straining, or lifting more than 10 lb are restricted for 6 to 10 weeks postoperatively. The acute care therapist should review proper lifting techniques prior to discharge, even though the client will not be able to provide a return demonstration.

Anterior or abdominal soft tissue mobilization for persons with back pain who have postoperative abdominal scars may require indirect techniques. This precaution is especially true for the person with a previous abdominal aneurysm, the person with a known nonoperative aneurysm (less than 5 cm), or the person with an undiagnosed aneurysm.

The therapist must always palpate the abdomen for a pulsating mass prior to performing anterior or abdominal therapy. It is possible to palpate the width of the pulse beginning at the abdominal midline and progressing laterally. The pulse should be characterized by a uniform width on either side of the abdominal midline until the umbilicus is reached, at which point the aortic bifurcation results in expansion of the pulse width. Throbbing pain that increases with exertion should alert the therapist to the need to monitor vital signs and palpate pulses.

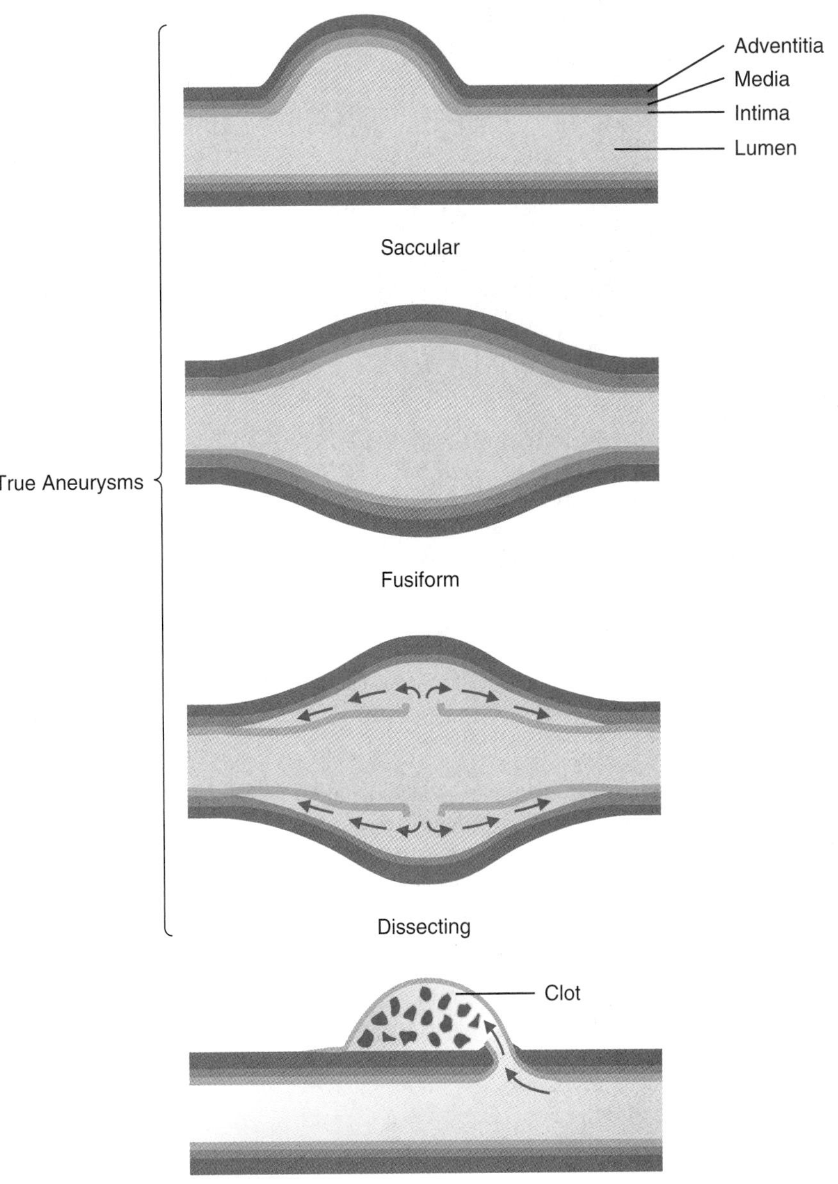

Figure **10–25.** Longitudinal sections showing types of aneurysms. In a true aneurysm, layers of the vessel wall dilate in one of the following ways: *saccular*, a unilateral outpouching; *fusiform*, a bilateral outpouching; or *dissecting*, a bilateral outpouching in which layers of the vessel wall separate, with creation of a cavity. In a false aneurysm, the wall ruptures, and a blood clot is retained in an outpouching of tissue.

Inflammatory Diseases

Inflammatory conditions of the blood vessels are often discussed as immunologic conditions because inflammation and damage to large and small vessels results in end-stage organ damage. Vasculitis (e.g., arteritis, such as polyarteritis nodosa and giant cell arteritis, Kawasaki's disease, and thromboangiitis obliterans) is the most commonly encountered inflammatory blood vessel disease in a therapy practice. Vascular inflammation is a central feature of many rheumatic diseases, especially rheumatoid arthritis and scleroderma. (See also Rheumatoid Vasculitis, Chapter 4.)

Vasculitis is actually a group of disorders that share in a common pathologic result of necrotizing inflammation of the blood vessels involving arteries (arteritis), veins (venulitis), or a combination of both (Table 10–21). Immune complexes to each disorder are deposited in the blood vessels resulting in varying symptoms, depending on the organs affected.

Polyarteritis Nodosa

Overview and Etiology. Polyarteritis nodosa refers to a condition consisting of multiple sites of inflammatory and destructive lesions in the arterial system; the lesions are small masses of tissue in the form of nodes or projections (nodosum). The cause of polyarteritis nodosa is unknown, although hepatitis B is present in 50% of cases, and polyarteritis occurs more commonly among intravenous drug abusers and other groups who have a high prevalence of hepatitis B (see Hepatitis B, Chapter 14). Any age can be affected but it is more common among young men.

Clinical Manifestations. Polyarteritis nodosa affects small and medium-sized blood vessels, resulting in a variety of clinical presentations, depending on the specific site of the blood vessel involved. Some of the more likely symptoms include abrupt onset of fever, chills, tachycardia, arthralgia, and myositis with muscle tenderness.

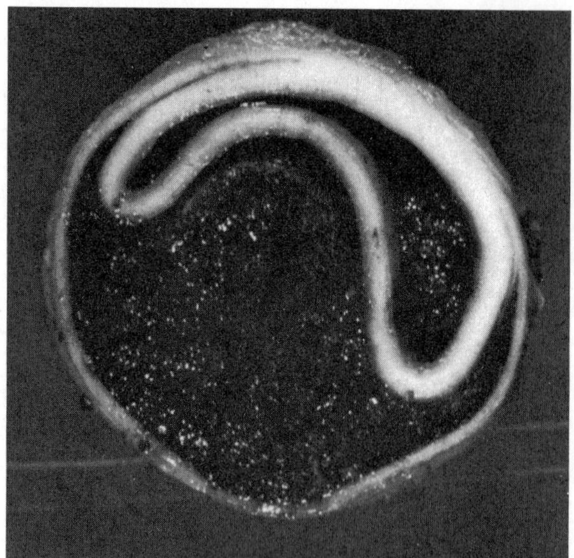

Figure 10–26. Dissecting aneurysm. Cross section of the aorta with dissecting aneurysm showing true aortic lumen (above and right) compressed by dissecting column of blood that separates the media and creates a false lumen. (*From Kissane JM (ed): Anderson's Pathology. St Louis, Mosby–Year Book, 1990.*)

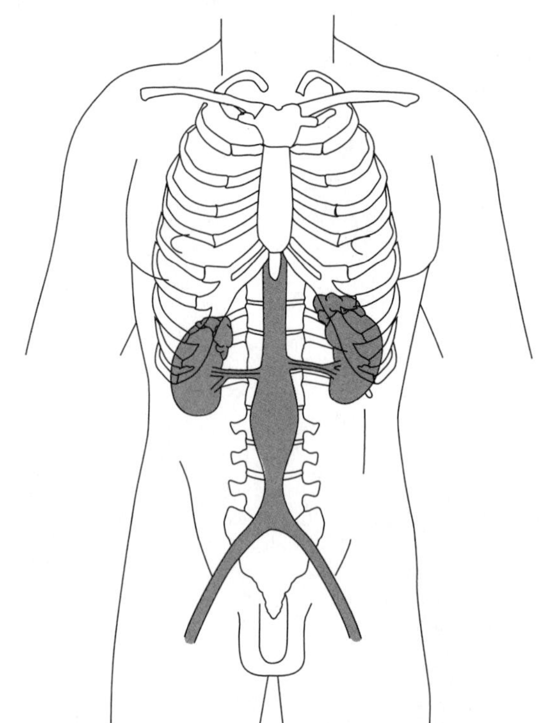

Figure 10–27. Aortic aneurysm. More than 95% of aortic aneurysms are located below the renal arteries and extend to the umbilicus, causing low back pain. Early warning signs of an impending rupture may include an abdominal heartbeat when lying down or a dull ache (intermittent or constant) in the midabdominal left flank or lower back.

Any organ of the body may be affected, but most often involved are the kidneys, heart, liver, GI tract, muscles, and testes. Abdominal pain, nausea, and vomiting are common with GI tract involvement. Pericarditis, myocarditis, arrhythmias, and myocardial infarction reflect cardiac involvement. Complications may include aneurysm, hemorrhage, thrombosis, and fibrosis leading to occlusion of the lumen. Multiple asymmetrical neuropathies (motor and sensory distribution) can occur when vasculitis affects the arteries of the peripheral nerves (vasa nervorum). Paresthesias, pain, weakness, and sensory loss occur, involving several or many peripheral nerves simultaneously.

Medical Management

Diagnosis, Treatment, and Prognosis. Diagnosis is made by characteristic laboratory findings, biopsy of symptomatic sites (especially muscle or nerve), and, possibly, visceral angiography. When CNS vasculitis is suspected, angiography is necessary because MRI and CT do not provide sufficient evidence to confirm the diagnosis.

Prolonged use of corticosteroids is necessary to control fever and constitutional symptoms while vascular lesions are healing. Immunosuppressants may be used in conjunction with steroids to improve survival; withdrawal from drugs is often followed by relapse. Treatment of polyarteritis nodosa associated with hepatitis B is more complicated because cytotoxic drugs can exacerbate the hepatic disease (Perazella, 1995). Prognosis is poor without treatment with a 5-year survival rate of only 20%. Treatment with corticosteroids increases survival to 50% and steroids combined with immunosuppressive drugs has improved 5-year survival to 90% (Hellman, 1994).

Arteritis

Overview and Incidence. Arteritis, sometimes called *giant cell arteritis* or *cranial* or *temporal arteritis*, is a vasculitis primarily involving multiple sites of temporal and cranial arteries. It is the most common vasculitis in the United States affecting older people; women are affected twice as often as men. The average age at onset is 70 years, and incidence increases with age.

Etiology and Pathology. The etiology and pathology are unknown, possibly related to cell-mediated autoimmunity directed against arterial antigens. The middle layer of the blood vessel (tunica media) is inflamed, with giant cells distributed along the internal elastica; secondary thrombosis may occur. Healing produces fibrosis of the arterial wall and the affected blood vessel becomes cord-like, thickened, and nodular, which can be observed externally when the temporal artery is involved.

Clinical Manifestations. The onset of arteritis is usually sudden, with severe, continuous, unilateral, throbbing headache and temporal pain as the first symptoms. The pain may radiate to the occipital area, face, or side of the neck. Other symptoms may include enlarged, tender temporal artery; scalp sensitivity; and visual symptoms. Visual disturbances range from blurring to diplopia to visual loss. Irreversible blindness may occur anywhere in the course of the disease from involvement of the ophthalmic artery (Eagle and DeSanctis, 1992). Jaw claudication (i.e., pain in response to chewing, talking, or swallowing) may occur when involvement of the external carotid artery causes ischemia of the masseter muscles; the pain is relieved by rest. Approximately 40% of cases present

TABLE 10-21 VASCULITIS

VASCULITIDES	VESSELS INVOLVED	ORGAN SYSTEMS INVOLVED
Polyarteritis nodosa	Small and medium-sized muscular arteries	Viscera, muscle, testes, nerves, renal
Giant cell arteritis	Large and medium muscular arteries; aorta less common	Extracranial arteries of head and neck; any other artery less common
Hypersensitivity vasculitis	Small vessels (arterioles, capillaries, venules)	Skin, viscera, heart, synovium, GI tract
Kawasaki's disease	Medium muscular arteries; rarely veins	Cardiac; also iliac, renal, internal mamillary
Thromboangiitis obliterans	Intermediate and small arteries and veins	Extremities; distal affected more often than proximal; head, cardiac, viscera involvement very rare

Adapted from Schumacher HR: Primer on Rheumatic Diseases, ed 10. Atlanta, Arthritis Foundation, 1993, p 138.

with nonclassic symptoms of respiratory tract problems (most often dry cough), fever of unknown origin, or painful paralysis of a shoulder (mononeuritis multiplex).

Medical Management

Diagnosis, Treatment, and Prognosis. Diagnosis is made by recognition of the presenting symptoms, and in some cases, arteritis follows polymyalgia rheumatica,[21] a similar condition (see Chapter 23). Biopsy of the temporal artery is often negative given the focal (segmental) nature of the disease. Laboratory findings include elevated erythrocyte sedimentation rate (ESR), reflective of the underlying inflammatory process. Early diagnosis is important to prevent blindness due to obstruction of the ophthalmic arteries. Treatment with corticosteroids is usually very effective, providing symptomatic relief in 3 to 5 days. Arteritis is a self-limiting disease, usually resolving within 6 to 12 months.

Hypersensitivity Angiitis

This form of vasculitis can occur at any age, but it most commonly affects children and young adults. The etiology is unknown, but the disease often follows an upper respiratory tract infection, and allergy or drug sensitivity play a role in some cases. It is usually localized to the small vessels of the skin first appearing on the lower extremities in a variety of possible lesions. A classic triad of symptoms occurs in 80% of cases that includes purpura (bruising and petechiae or round purplish red spots under the skin), arthritis, and abdominal pain. Inflammation and hemorrhage may occur in the synovium and CNS.

Medical management (diagnosis, treatment, and prognosis) are the same as for the other forms of vasculitis already discussed.

Kawasaki Disease

Overview and Etiology. Kawasaki disease, also known as *mucocutaneous lymph node syndrome,* is an acute systemic vasculitis that can occur in any ethnic group but seems most prevalent in Asian populations. Children under the age of 5 years comprise 80% of all cases, and 20% develop cardiac complications. The etiology is unknown, but because seasonal and geographic outbreaks appear to occur, an infectious cause is suspected. Current etiologic theories center on an immunologic response to an infectious, toxic, or antigenic substance (Moller and Neal, 1990).

Pathogenesis. The principal area of pathology is the cardiovascular system. Kawasaki disease progresses pathologically and clinically in stages. During the initial stage of the illness (first 2 weeks) extensive inflammation of the arterioles, venules, and capillaries occurs, which later progresses (stage 2, weeks 2 to 4) to include the main coronary arteries, the heart, and the larger veins. In the final stage the vessels develop scarring, intimal thickening, calcification, and formation of thrombi. If death occurs as a result of this disease (rare) it is usually the result of aneurysm, coronary thrombosis, or severe scar formation and stenosis of the main coronary artery.

Clinical Manifestations. Clinical manifestations present in three phases: acute phase, subacute phase, and convalescent phase. In the *acute phase,* a sudden high fever (lasting over 5 days) that is unresponsive to antibiotics and antipyretics is followed by extreme irritability. During the *subacute phase,* the fever resolves, but the irritability persists along with other symptoms, such as rash (exanthema) of the trunk and extremities with reddened palms and soles of the hands and feet and subsequent desquamation (skin scales off) of the tips of the toes and fingers, peripheral edema, cervical lymphadenopathy ($\geq$1.5 cm, usually unilateral), bilateral conjunctival infection without exudate, and changes in the oral mucous membranes (e.g., erythema, dryness and cracks or fissures of the lips, reddening or "strawberry" tongue). Some children develop large joint arthralgias and GI tract symptoms. During this subacute phase, the person is at risk for cardiac involvement, especially the development of myocarditis, pericarditis, and arteritis that predisposes to the formation of coronary artery aneurysm.

The *convalescent phase* occurs 6 to 8 weeks after onset of Kawasaki disease and is characterized by a resolution of all clinical signs and symptoms. However, during this phase the blood values have not returned to normal. At the end of the convalescent phase, all values return to normal and the child has usually regained his or her usual temperament, energy, and appetite (Wong, 1993).

[21] Although giant cell arteritis and polymyalgia rheumatica may occur as separate entities, there is considerable overlap of clinical and pathologic features so that most epidemiologic surveys group these two conditions together as one disorder. In polymyalgia rheumatica, the most common symptoms are bilateral pain and stiffness of the shoulder and pelvic girdles, especially in the morning, lasting more than 1 hour (MacLennan, 1990).

Medical Management

Diagnosis, Treatment, and Prognosis. Diagnosis is made on the basis of clinical manifestations and associated laboratory tests (there are no specific laboratory tests for Kawasaki disease). Echocardiograms are useful in providing a baseline and for monitoring myocardial and coronary artery status. Treatment includes high-dose intravenous γ-globulin and salicylate therapy to reduce fever and control inflammation and aneurysm formation (Newburger, 1991). Prognosis is good for recovery with treatment, although serious cardiovascular problems (e.g., coronary thrombosis) may occur later in persons with cardiac sequelae.

Thromboangiitis Obliterans (Buerger's Disease)

Overview and Pathogenesis. Thromboangiitis obliterans, also referred to as *Buerger's disease,* is a vasculitis (inflammatory *and* thrombotic process) affecting the peripheral blood vessels (both arteries and veins), primarily in the extremities. The cause is not known but it is most often found in men younger than 40 years who smoke heavily, although the incidence in women is increasing.

The pathogenesis of thromboangiitis obliterans is unknown; general inflammatory concepts apply. The inflammatory lesions of the peripheral blood vessels are accompanied by thrombus formation and vasospasm occluding and eventually obliterating (destroying) small and medium-sized vessels of the feet and hands.

Clinical Manifestations. Clinical manifestations of pain and tenderness of the affected part are caused by occlusion of the arteries, reduced blood flow, and subsequent reduced oxygenation. The symptoms are episodic and segmental, meaning that the symptoms come and go intermittently over time and appear in different asymmetrical anatomic locations. The plantar, tibial, and digital vessels are most commonly affected in the lower leg and foot. Intermittent claudication centered in the arch of the foot or the palm of the hand is often the first symptom.

When the hands are affected, the digital, palmar, and ulnar arteries are most commonly involved. Pain at rest occurs with persistent ischemia of one or more digits. Other symptoms include edema, cold sensitivity, rubor (redness of the skin from dilated capillaries under the skin), cyanosis, and thin, shiny, hairless skin (trophic changes) from chronic ischemia. Paresthesias, diminished or absent posterior tibial and dorsalis pedis pulses, ulceration (see Table 10–19), and eventual gangrene may develop (see Fig. 10–23).

Medical Management

Diagnosis, Treatment, and Prognosis. Arteriography may be used in the diagnosis, but definitive diagnosis of thromboangiitis obliterans is determined by histologic examination of the blood vessels (microabscesses in the vessel wall) in a leg amputated for gangrene.

Treatment should begin with cessation of smoking. All other treatment techniques are aimed at improving circulation to the foot or hand, including pharmacologic intervention (e.g., vasodilators, pain relief) and physical or occupational therapy treatment (see also Medical Management: Atherosclerotic Occlusive Disease). Regional sympathetic ganglionectomy may produce vasodilation, ulcerations require wound care, and amputation may be required when conservative care fails.

Thromboangiitis is not life threatening, but it can result in progressive disability from pain and loss of function secondary to amputation. Cessation of smoking is the key determinant in prognosis.

Venous Diseases

Venous diseases can be acute or chronic; *acute* venous disease includes thrombophlebitis and *chronic* venous disease includes varicose vein formation and chronic venous insufficiency.

Thrombophlebitis

Definition and Overview. Thrombophlebitis is a partial or complete occlusion of a vein by a thrombus (clot) with secondary inflammatory reaction in the wall of the vein. Thrombophlebitis may affect the deep veins (usually of the pelvis and lower extremities) or the superficial veins most commonly affecting the saphenous vein (Fig. 10–28).

Incidence, Etiology, and Risk Factors. Approximately 30% of all people (women more than men) undergoing major general surgical procedures[22] develop clinical manifestations of deep vein thrombophlebitis (DVT) up to 2 weeks postoperatively (Fig. 10–29).

Thrombus formation is usually attributed to venous stasis, hypercoagulability, and/or injury to the venous wall. It is commonly held that at least two of these three conditions must be present for thrombi to form. *Venous stasis* is caused by prolonged immobility (e.g., spinal cord injury, cardiac failure, stroke, fracture) or absence of the calf muscle pump, surgery, obesity, pregnancy, and CHF.

Hypercoagulability often accompanies malignant neoplasms, especially visceral and ovarian tumors. Women older than 30 years who use oral contraceptives and who smoke experience an appreciably higher incidence of thromboembolic complications (Tierney, 1994). *Vein wall trauma* may occur as a result of a direct blow to the leg, intravenous injections, varicose veins, thromboangiitis obliterans (Buerger's disease), fractures and dislocations, certain antibiotics (e.g., chlortetracycline), sclerosing agents, and opaque media-tor radiography.

Pathogenesis. Any trauma to the endothelium of the vein wall exposes subendothelial tissues to platelets in the venous blood, initiating thrombosis. Platelets on the vein wall attract the deposition of fibrin, leukocytes, and erythrocytes, forming a thrombus that may remain attached to the vessel wall or break off and become free-floating as an embolism.

When the thrombus adheres to the vein wall, secondary inflammatory changes develop and the thrombus is eventually invaded by fibroblasts, resulting in scarring of the vein wall and destruction of the valves. Restoration of the central venous canal (recanalization) may occur as a result of the healing process. Although blood flow is restored through the vein, the valves do not recover function, resulting in backflow of

[22] High-risk surgical candidates have a history of recent venous thromboembolism or have undergone extensive pelvic or abdominal surgery for advanced malignancy, CABG, renal transplantation, splenectomy, or major orthopedic surgery to the lower limbs (e.g., hip or knee arthroplasty, surgery for fractured hip, tibial osteotomy) (Denison and Black, 1993; Hull et al., 1992).

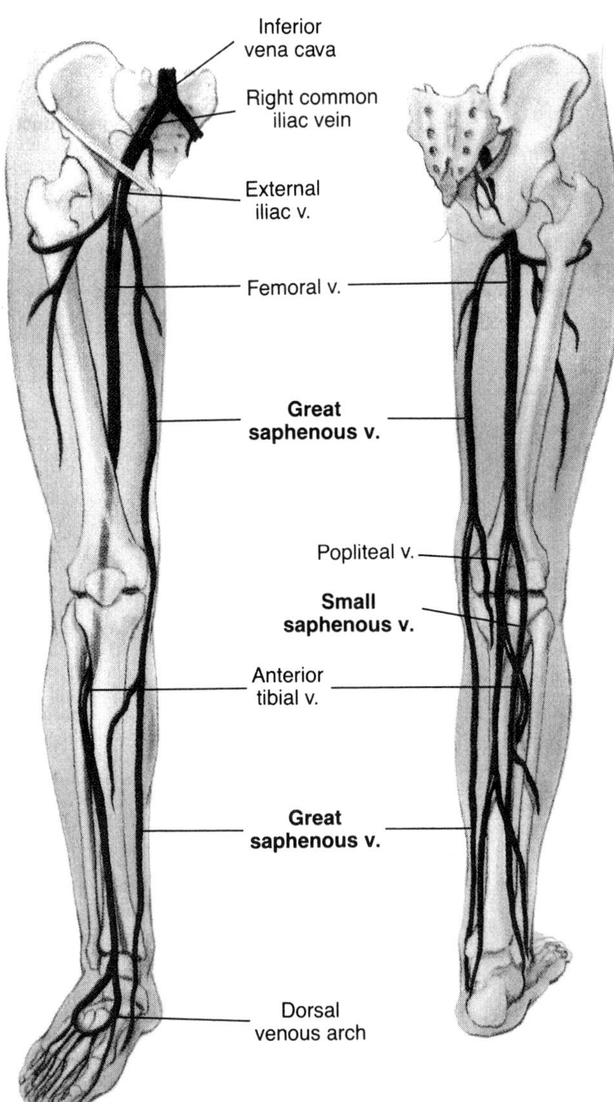

Figure **10–28.** Veins in the leg. The legs have three types of veins: deep veins (*femoral* and *popliteal*) coursing alongside the deep arteries to conduct most of the venous return from the legs; superficial veins, the *great* and *small saphenous veins*, and perforators (not pictured), the connecting veins that join the two sets and route blood from the superficial into the deep veins. The great saphenous vein starts at the medial side of the dorsum of the foot and ascends in front of the medial malleolus, crossing the tibia obliquely and ascending along the medial side of the thigh. The small saphenous vein starts on the lateral side of the dorsum of the foot, ascends behind the lateral malleolus and up the back of the leg, where it joins the popliteal vein. (*From Jarvis C: Physical Examination and Health Assessment. Philadelphia, WB Saunders, 1992, p 637.*)

blood and other secondary functional and anatomic problems (e.g., stasis, venous stasis ulcers, risk of another DVT, or pulmonary embolism from recurrent DVT).

If a thrombus occludes a major vein (e.g., femoral vein, vena cava, axillary vein), the venous pressure and volume rise distally. However, if a thrombus occludes a deep small vein (e.g., tibial, popliteal), collateral vessels develop and relieve the increased venous pressure and volume (Dennison and Black, 1993).

Clinical Manifestation. In the early stages, approximately half of the people with *deep vein thrombosis (DVT)* are asymptomatic for any signs or symptoms in the affected extremity. When symptoms occur, the client may report a dull ache, a tight feeling, or pain in the calf. When symptoms are reported in the entire extremity, the condition is more extensive. Thrombi may be present in both extremities, even though symptoms are unilateral.

Signs are often absent; when present, they may be variable and unreliable, consisting of slight swelling in the involved calf or ankle, slight fever, and, possibly, tachycardia. Any of these symptoms can occur without DVT. An asymmetrical prominence of the subcutaneous vein pattern may be present, such as across the inguinal ligament, indicating an iliofemoral occlusion, or across the front of the shin, indicating a popliteal thrombosis. The skin of the leg and ankle on the affected side may be relatively warmer than on the unaffected side (check for temperature changes with the backs of the fingers). If venous obstruction is severe, the skin may be cyanotic. Pulmonary emboli (see Chapter 12), most often from the large, deep veins of the pelvis and legs, is the most devastating complication of DVT and can occur without apparent warning.

In the case of *superficial thrombophlebitis*, dull pain and local tenderness in the region of the involved vein may be accompanied by signs of superficial induration (firm or hard cord) and redness. Swelling and deep calf tenderness are only present when DVT has developed. Chills and high fever accompany iatrogenic phlebitis secondary to IV catheter insertion; tenderness (not redness) is an early sign of peripheral IV site phlebitis.

Medical Management

Diagnosis. Homans' sign (Fig. 10–30) is commonly assessed during physical examination. Unfortunately, this test is insensitive, nonspecific, and present in fewer than 30% of documented cases of DVT. Additionally, more than half of all people with a positive Homans' sign do not have evidence of venous thrombosis (Dennison and Black, 1993). A positive Homans' sign can also occur with superficial phlebitis, Achilles tendinitis, and gastrocnemius and plantar muscle injury.

Calf muscle strain or contusion may be difficult to differentiate from thrombophlebitis; further diagnostic testing may be required to determine the correct diagnosis. Occasionally, a ruptured Baker cyst may produce unilateral pain and swelling in the calf. A history of arthritis in the knee of the same leg and the disappearance of the popliteal cyst at the time symptoms develop are clues the physician can use to make the differentiation (Tierney, 1994).

History and clinical examination are followed by Doppler ultrasonography as a rapid screening procedure to detect thrombosis; small thrombi in calf veins are easily missed when collateral circulation exists. Venous duplex scanning has replaced contrast venography as the primary diagnostic test of DVT because it allows noninvasive visualization of the vein.

Treatment. Treatment of acute thrombophlebitis is a simultaneous combination of pharmacology (anticoagulants or "blood thinners," such as heparin and warfarin) and symptomatic treatment. Symptomatic treatment includes bed rest for 1nb3 to 5 days to prevent emboli and pressure fluctuations in the venous system that occur with walking; elevation of the

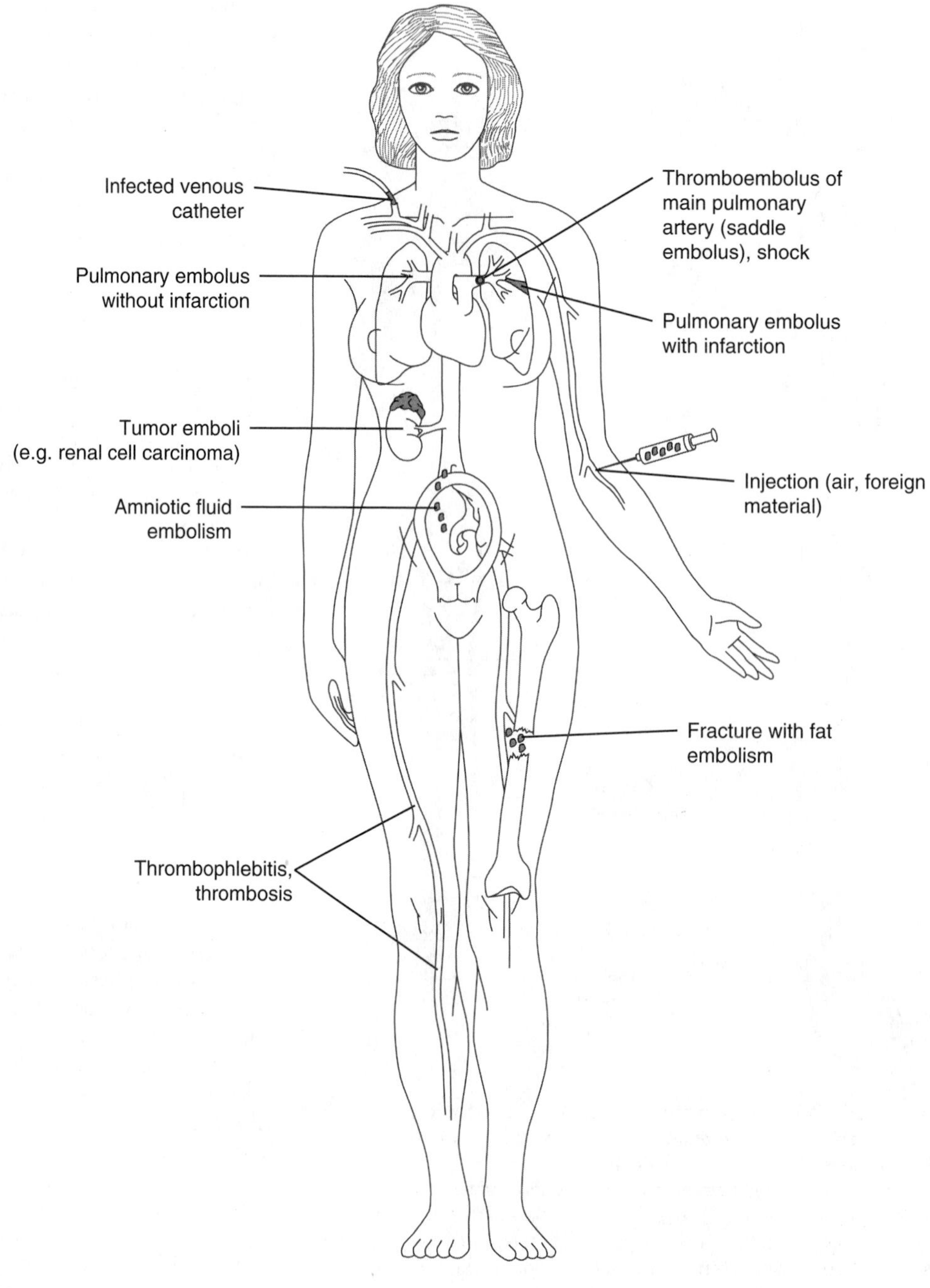

Infected venous catheter

Pulmonary embolus without infarction

Tumor emboli (e.g. renal cell carcinoma)

Amniotic fluid embolism

Thromboembolus of main pulmonary artery (saddle embolus), shock

Pulmonary embolus with infarction

Injection (air, foreign material)

Fracture with fat embolism

Thrombophlebitis, thrombosis

Figure 10–29. Sources and effects of venous emboli.

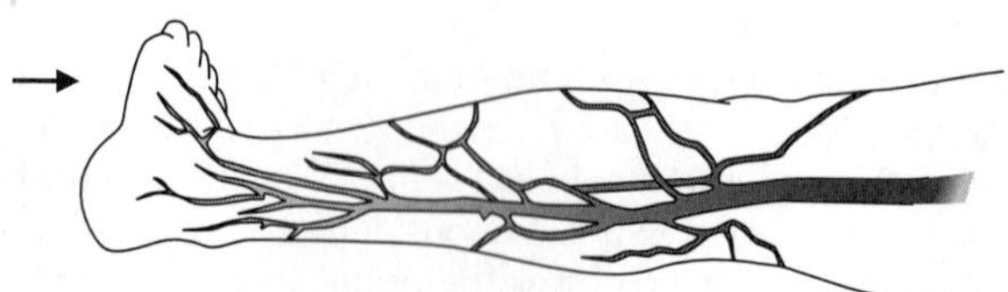

Figure 10–30. Homans' sign. Discomfort in the upper calf during gentle, forced dorsiflexion of the foot with the knee extended is called *Homans' sign*. This response may occur in the presence of thrombophlebitis as a result of the stretch imposed on the affected vessels. Homans' sign is not a specific finding in phlebitis because dorsiflexion may be painfully restricted with a variety of musculoskeletal conditions. However, it is a useful diagnostic clue in the presence of other clinical findings.

leg with the knee flexed until the edema and tenderness subside; and continuous local application of heat to relieve venospasm, produce analgesia, and promote resolution of inflammation. Ambulation (wearing elastic stockings) is permitted if local tenderness and swelling have resolved (usually after 1 week for calf thrombosis and 10 to 14 days for thigh or pelvic thrombosis). Prolonged standing or sitting are still avoided for another 5 to 7 days.

Primary prevention of DVT is important through the prophylactic use of anticoagulants (e.g., low-dose heparin, warfarin, Lovenox [enoxaparin], or aspirin) in people considered at high risk for venous thrombosis. The highest incidence of DVT occurs with abdominal, pelvic, hip, or knee surgery and open prostate procedures.

Prognosis. With treatment and in the absence of complications, a return to normal health and activity can be expected within 1 to 3 weeks for the person with a calf DVT and within 6 weeks for the person with thigh or pelvic DVT. Prognosis depends on the size of the vessel involved, the presence of collateral circulation, and the underlying cause of the thrombosis (e.g., spinal cord injury, stroke, or neoplasm may prevent return to former health).

Varicose Veins

Definition and Incidence. Varicose veins are abnormal dilation of veins, usually the saphenous veins of the lower extremities, leading to tortuosity (twisting and turning) of the vessel, incompetence of the valves (Fig. 10–31), and a propensity to thrombosis. Fifteen percent of adults develop varicosities, with the incidence increasing with age. Women are affected more often than men (secondary to pregnancy) with leg varicosities until age 70 years, when the gender ratio disappears; the condition most often develops between the ages of 30 and 50 years for all persons.

Etiology and Risk Factors. Varicose veins may be an inherited trait but it is unclear whether the valvular incompetence is secondary to defective valves in the saphenous veins or to a fundamental weakness of the walls of the vein leading to dilation of the vessel. Periods of high venous pressure associated with heavy lifting or prolonged sitting or standing are risk factors. Pregnancy often contributes to the development of this condition. Other risk factors include obesity, heart failure, hemorrhoids, constipation, esophageal varices, and hepatic cirrhosis.

Pathogenesis *(O'Toole, 1992).* Blood returning to the heart from the legs must flow upward through the veins, against the pull of gravity. This blood is "milked" upward, principally by the massaging action of the muscles against the veins. To prevent the blood from flowing backward, the veins contain flaplike valves located at frequent intervals, which operate in pairs by closing to stop the reverse movement of the blood.

The vessels most commonly affected by varicosities are located just beneath the skin superficial to the deep fascia and function without the kind of support deep veins of the legs receive from surrounding muscles. Any condition accompanied by pressure changes places a strain on these veins, and the lack of pumping action of the lower leg muscles causes blood to pool. Other sites involved include the hemorrhoidal plexus of the rectum and anal canal (either inside or outside the anal sphincter), submucosal veins of the distal esophagus, and the scrotum (varicocele).

The weight of the blood continually pressing downward against the closed venous valves causes the veins to distend and eventually lose their elasticity. When several valves lose their ability to function properly, the blood collects in the veins, causing the veins to become swollen and distended.

During pregnancy, the uterus may press against the veins coming from the lower extremities and prevent the free flow of returning blood. More force is required to push the blood through the veins, and the increased back-pressure can result in varicose veins.

Clinical Manifestations. The clinical picture is not directly correlated with the severity of the varicosities; extensive varicose veins may be asymptomatic, but minimal varicosities may result in multiple symptoms. The development of varicose veins is usually gradual; the most common symptom reported is a dull, aching heaviness or feeling of fatigue brought on by periods of standing. Cramps of the lower legs may occur, especially at night, and elevation of the legs often provides relief. Itching from an associated dermatitis may also occur above the ankle.

The most visible sign of varicosities is the dilated, tortuous,

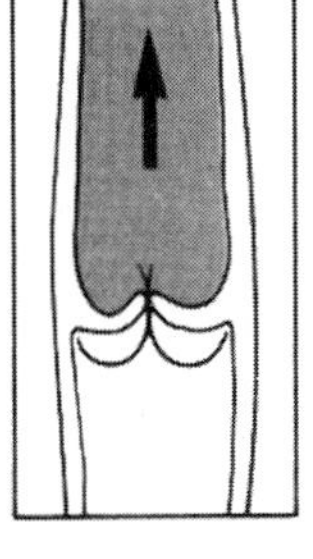

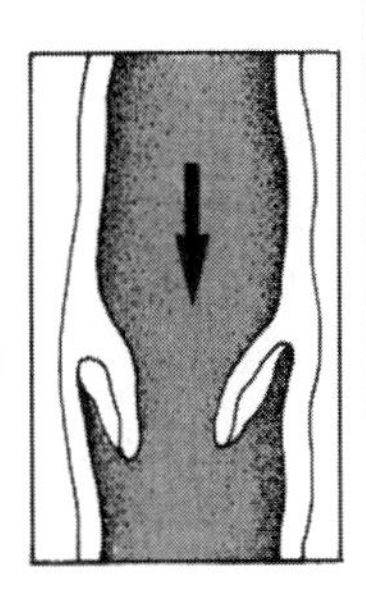

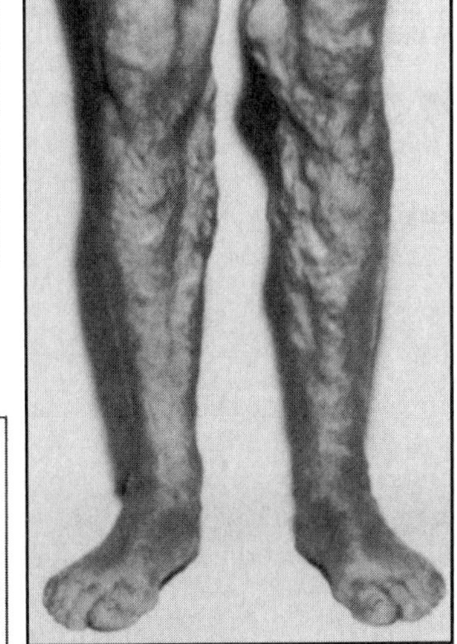

Figure **10–31.** A, Diagrams of normal (*top*) and varicose (*bottom*) veins. B, Person with varicose veins. (A *from O'Toole M (ed): Miller-Keane Encyclopedia and Dictionary of Medicine, Nursing, and Allied Health, ed 5. Philadelphia, WB Saunders, 1992, p 1575.* B *from Jarvis C: Physical Examination and Health Assessment. Philadelphia, WB Saunders, 1992, p 660.*)

elongated veins beneath the skin, which are usually readily visible when the person is standing. Varicosities of long duration may be accompanied by secondary tissue changes, such as a brownish pigmentation of the skin and a thinning of the skin above the ankle. Swelling may also occur around the ankles. Untreated, the veins become thick and hard to the touch; impaired circulation and skin changes may lead to ulcers of the lower legs, especially around the ankles (see Table 10–20). (See also Esophageal Varices, Chapter 13.)

Medical Management

Diagnosis. The physician must distinguish between the symptoms of arteriosclerotic peripheral vascular disease, such as intermittent claudication and coldness of the feet, and symptoms of venous disease, because occlusive arterial disease usually contraindicates the operative treatment of varicosities below the knee. When the two conditions co-exist, the reduced blood flow due to the atherosclerosis may even improve the varicosities by reducing blood flow through the veins.

Visual inspection and palpation identify varicose veins of the legs, and Doppler ultrasonography or the duplex scanner are useful in detecting the location of incompetent valves. Endoscopy or radiographic diagnosis identifies esophageal varices, rectal examination or proctoscopy are used to diagnose hemorrhoids, and palpation identifies varicocele (scrotal swelling).

Treatment. Treatment of mild varicose veins is conservative, consisting of periodic daily rest periods with feet elevated slightly above the heart. Client education as to the importance of promoting circulation is stressed, including instructions to make frequent changes in posture, performance of simple exercises, daily exercise program, and the appropriate use of properly fitting elastic stockings.

When varicosities have progressed past the stage at which conservative care is helpful, surgical intervention and compression sclerotherapy may be considered. The surgical treatment of varicose veins consists of removal of the varicosities and the incompetent perforating veins; this procedure is sometimes referred to as *stripping* the veins. A new procedure for varicose veins, called *ambulatory phlebectomy*, which uses a tumescent technique of local anesthesia in an office setting, is currently being developed. This method eliminates the need for multiple injections along the length of the vein, thereby reducing the pain from local anesthetic infiltration (Cohn et al., 1995).

Sclerotherapy to obliterate and produce permanent fibrosis of the involved veins may be carried out as the primary therapy or after varicose vein surgery for the treatment of residual small varicosities that remain. In this procedure, injections of a hardening, or sclerosing, solution are introduced into the affected veins. Over several months' time, the injected veins atrophy and blood is channeled into other veins. This procedure is not recommended for advanced cases because of the likelihood of recurrence.

Prognosis. Good results with relief of symptoms is usually possible in the majority of cases. Early conservative care for varicose veins during initial stages may help prevent the condition from worsening, but advanced disease may not be prevented from recurring even with surgical treatment or sclerotherapy. A high mortality is associated with ruptured, bleeding esophageal varices (see Chapter 13).

Chronic Venous Insufficiency

Definition and Etiology. Chronic venous insufficiency (CVI), also known as *postphlebitic syndrome*, is defined as inadequate venous return over a long period of time. This condition follows most severe cases of DVT although it is possible to develop chronic venous insufficiency without prior episodes of DVT. CVI may also occur as a result of leg trauma, varicose veins, and neoplastic obstruction of the pelvic veins.

Pathogenesis. Chronic venous insufficiency occurs when damaged or destroyed valves in the veins prevent venous return, thereby increasing venous pressure and producing venous stasis. Without adequate valve function and in the absence of the calf muscle pump, blood flows in the veins bidirectionally, causing high ambulatory venous pressures in the calf veins.

Poor circulation caused by chronic pooling of blood in the veins of the lower extremities prevents adequate cellular oxygenation and removal of waste products. Any trauma, especially pressure, further lowers the oxygen supply by reducing blood flow into the area. Cell death occurs, and necrotic tissue develops into venous stasis ulcers. The cycle of reduced oxygenation, necrosis, and ulceration prevents damaged tissue from obtaining necessary nutrients, causing delayed healing and persistent ulceration. Poor circulation impairs immune and inflammatory responses, leaving venous stasis ulcers susceptible to infection.

Clinical Manifestations. CVI is characterized by progressive edema of the leg; thickening, coarsening, and brownish pigmentation of skin around the ankles; and venous stasis ulceration (see Table 10–20). Venous insufficiency ulcers constitute approximately 80% of all lower extremity ulcers. These ulcers characteristically are shallow wounds with a white creamy to fibrous slough over a base of good granulation tissue. They generally produce little pain and a moderate to large amount of drainage. The wounds typically have irregular borders, often with signs of reepithelialization. Frequently, moderate to severe edema is present in the limb; in long-standing cases, this edema becomes hardened to a dense, woody texture (Burks, 1995). The skin of the involved extremity is usually thin, shiny, and cyanotic. Dermatitis and cellulitis may develop later in this condition.

Medical Management. The physician will differentiate between CVI and other causes of edema and ulceration of the lower extremities using client history and clinical examination and diagnostic tests to rule out or confirm superimposed acute phlebitis. Arterial and venous insufficiency may coexist in the same person.

Treatment goals and techniques are as for varicose veins (increase in venous return and reduction of edema); venous valvular reconstructive surgery is now available for those clients who meet stringent diagnostic requirements (Kistner et al., 1995). More frequent periods of leg elevation above the level of the heart are encouraged throughout the day with the foot of the bed elevated 6 in. at night. Venous stasis ulcers require ongoing treatment, usually involving the therapist (e.g., primary intervention for edema reduction and topical ulcer and wound care) (for more detailed information see Davis et al., 1992; McCulloch, 1995; McCulloch et al., 1994).

The prognosis is poor for resolution of CVI, with chronic venous stasis ulcers causing loss of function and progressive disability. Recurrent episodes of acute thrombophlebitis may occur, and noncompliance with the treatment program is common.

Vasomotor Disorders

Vasomotor disorders of the blood vessels causing headaches and reflex sympathetic dystrophy (RSD) are discussed in section IV: Pathology of the Neurologic System (Chapters 24 through 34).

Raynaud's Disease and Raynaud's Phenomenon

Definition and Overview. Intermittent episodes of small artery or arteriole constriction of the extremities causing temporary pallor and cyanosis of the digits (fingers more often than toes) and changes in skin temperature is called *Raynaud's phenomenon*. These episodes occur in response to cold temperature or strong emotion such as anxiety or excitement. When this condition is a primary vasospastic disorder it is called (idiopathic) *Raynaud's disease*. If the disorder is secondary to another disease or underlying cause, the term *Raynaud's phenomenon* is used.

Incidence and Etiology

Raynaud's Disease. Eighty percent of persons with Raynaud's disease are women between the ages of 20 and 49 years. The exact etiology of Raynaud's disease remains unknown, but it appears to be caused by hypersensitivity of digital arteries to cold, release of serotonin, and congenital predisposition to vasospasm. Raynaud's disease accounts for 65% of all people affected by this condition. Raynaud's disease is usually experienced as more annoying than medically serious.

Raynaud's Phenomenon. Epidemiologists estimate that this condition is a problem for 10% to 20% of the general population; it affects women 20 times more frequently than men, usually between the ages of 15 and 40 years. Raynaud's phenomenon as a condition secondary to another disease (called *secondary Raynaud's*) is often associated with Buerger's disease or connective tissue disorders (collagen vascular diseases), such as Sjögren's syndrome, scleroderma, polymyositis and dermatomyositis, mixed connective tissue disease, SLE, and rheumatoid arthritis (see Box 10–13). Raynaud's phenomenon can be a sign of occult (hidden) neoplasm, especially suspected when it presents unilaterally.

Raynaud's phenomenon may also occur with change in temperature such as occurs when going from a warm outside environment to an air-conditioned room. Raynaud's phenomenon may also be associated with occlusive arterial diseases and neurogenic lesions, such as thoracic outlet syndrome, or with the effects of long-term exposure to cold (occupational or frostbite), trauma, or use of vibrating equipment such as jackhammers. Injuries to the small vessels of the hands may produce Raynaud's phenomenon. The trauma can be a result of repetitive stress that comes from using crutches for extended periods, typing on a computer keyboard, or even playing the piano.

Several medications (e.g., β-blockers, ergot alkaloids prescribed for migraine headaches, antineoplastics used in chemotherapy) have also been implicated. Because nicotine causes small blood vessels to constrict, smoking can trigger attacks in persons who are predisposed to this phenomenon.

Pathogenesis and Clinical Manifestations. Scientists theorize that Raynaud's phenomenon is associated with a disturbance in the control of vascular reflexes. Although the causes differ for Raynaud's disease and Raynaud's phenomenon, the clinical manifestations are the same, based on a pathogenesis of arterial vasospasm in the skin. It begins with the release of chemical messengers, which cause blood vessels to constrict and remain constricted. The flow of oxygenated blood to these areas is reduced, and the skin becomes pale and cold. The blood in the constricted vessels, which has released its oxygen to the tissues surrounding the vessels, pools in the tissues, producing a bluish or purplish color.

The skin color progresses from blue to white to red. First, ischemia from vasospastic attacks causes cyanosis, numbness, and the sensation of cold in the digits (thumbs usually remain unaffected). The affected tissues become numb or painful. For unknown reasons, the flow of chemical that triggered the process eventually stops. The vessels relax, and blood flow is restored. The skin becomes white (characterized by *pallor*) and then red (characterized by *rubor*) as the vasospasm subsides and the capillaries become engorged with oxygenated blood. Oxygen-rich blood returns to the area, and as it does so, the skin becomes warm and flushed. The person may experience throbbing, paresthesia, and slight swelling as this occurs.

Sensory changes such as numbness, stiffness, diminished sensation, and aching pain often accompany vasomotor manifestations. Initially, no abnormal findings are present between attacks, but over time, frequent, prolonged episodes of vasospasm causing ischemia interfere with cellular metabolism, causing the skin of the fingertips to thicken and the fingernails to become brittle. In severe, chronic Raynaud's phenomenon, the underlying condition may have produced scars in the vessels, reducing the vessel diameter and, therefore, blood flow. When attacks occur, they are often more severe, resulting in prolonged loss of blood to fingers and toes, which can produce painful skin ulcers; rarely, gangrene may develop. Episodes of Raynaud's disease are often bilateral, progressing distally to proximally along the digits. Raynaud's phenomenon may be unilateral, involving only 1 or 2 fingers, but this clinical presentation warrants physician differential diagnosis, as it can be associated with cancer (Fig. 10–32).

Medical Management

Diagnosis and Prognosis. Diagnosis is usually made by clinical presentation and past medical history. Raynaud's disease is diagnosed by a history of symptoms for at least 2 years with no progression and no evidence of underlying cause (Berkow and Fletcher, 1992). Raynaud's disease must be differentiated from the numerous possible disorders associated with Raynaud's phenomenon.

Untreated and uncontrolled Raynaud's may damage or destroy the affected digits. Rarely, necrosis, ulceration, and gangrene result. Even with treatment, the person with Raynaud's disease or phenomenon may experience disability and loss of function.

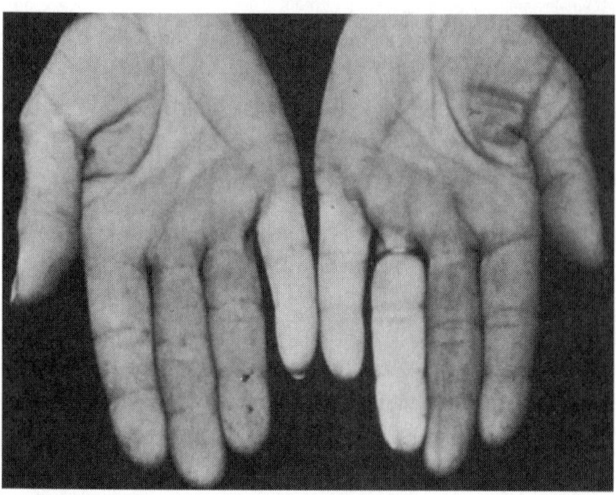

Figure **10-32.** Raynaud's disease or phenomenon. White (pallor) from arteriospasm and resulting deficit in blood supply may initially involve only 1 or 2 fingers, as shown here. Cold and numbness or pain may accompany the pallor or cyanosis stage. Subsequent episodes may involve the entire finger and may include all the fingers. Toes are affected in 40% of cases. (*From Jarvis C: Physical Examination and Health Assessment. Philadelphia, WB Saunders, 1992, p 658.*)

Treatment

Raynaud's Disease. Treatment for this disease is limited to prevention or alleviation of the vasospasm because no underlying cause or condition has been discovered. Clients are encouraged to avoid stimuli that trigger attacks, such as cool or cold temperatures, changes in temperature, and emotional stress, and to eliminate use of nicotine, which has a constricting effect on blood vessels.

Physical or occupational therapy is often prescribed and should include client education about managing symptoms through protective skin care and cold protection (Table 10–22), biofeedback, stress management and relaxation techniques, whirlpool or other gentle heat modalities, and exercise. Pharmacologic management may include vasodilators and nonaddicting analgesics for pain.

When conservative care fails to provide relief from symptoms and the condition progresses clinically, sympathetic blocks followed by intensive therapy may be helpful. Sympathectomy may be necessary for persons who are only temporarily benefited by the sympathetic blocks.

Raynaud's Phenomenon. Treatment for Raynaud's phenomenon consists of appropriate treatment for the underlying condition or removing the stimulus causing vasospasm. The clinical care described for Raynaud's disease may also be of benefit.

Special Implications for the Therapist **10-18**

PERIPHERAL VASCULAR DISEASE

Prevention of complications is an important aspect of therapy for the client with peripheral vascular disease (PVD). Preventing edema, providing proper skin care, and avoiding constrictive clothing and trauma are important. In addition to the skin changes caused by edema that lead to ulceration, edema may also cause soft tissues to compress local nerves, resulting in neuralgia. Properly fitted anti-embolic hose, Jobst stockings, or other commercially available compressive garments can reduce edema and assist venous return.

PVD can be confusing, with the wide range of diseases affecting veins and/or arteries, the etiology of which is sometimes occlusive, sometimes inflammatory, and, occasionally, as in the case of Buerger's disease, both occlusive and inflammatory. The basic point to keep in mind is how arterial disease differs (significantly) from venous disease in clinical presentation, pathogenesis, and treatment.

In *venous disorders,* the tissues are oxygenated but the blood is not moving, and stasis occurs. With venous occlusion, the skin is discolored rather than pale (ranging from angry red to deep blue-purple), edema is prominent, and pain is most marked at the site of occlusion, although extreme edema can render all the skin of the limb quite tender (Haak et al., 1994). The goal of therapy is to create compressive pumping forces to move fluid volume and reduce edema. For this reason, heat or cold, compressive stockings, massage and activity (e.g., ankle pumps, heel slides, quad sets, ambulation) are part of the treatment protocol.

In the case of *acute arterial disease,* the tissues are not oxygenated and ischemia can result in local trauma or burns; gangrene can develop quickly. The goal is to increase oxygen without increasing demand or need for oxygen. Claudication occurs when the activity causes increased oxygen demand in an already compromised area. Treatment and movement are minimized; heat and massage are contraindicated,* and the person is instructed in the use of positions that will increase blood flow to the tissues involved (e.g., head elevated with legs slightly lower than supine horizontal).

Chronic arterial disease can be treated in therapy concentrating on improving collateral circulation and increasing vasodilation. Specific protocols for daily graded ambulation, Buerger-Allen exercises, and vasodilation by iontophoresis and reflex heating are outlined elsewhere (Kisner and Colby, 1996). (See also Arteriosclerotic Obliterans, below.) Improving exercise duration and decreasing claudication, preventing joint contractures and muscle atrophy, preventing skin ulcerations, and promoting healing of any pressure ulcers are also part of the therapy plan of care. See Table 10–23 for a comparison of acute and chronic arterial disease.

Inflammatory Disorders

Vasculitis (Inflammatory Disease of Arteries and Veins). The therapist's role in treatment of vasculitis may be primarily for relief of painful muscular and joint symptoms when present and in the prevention of functional loss in the case of neuropathies.

For the client with thromboangiitis obliterans (Buerger's disease), exercise must be graded to avoid claudication and the client must be instructed in a home program for preventive skin care (see Table 10–22). Gangrene can occur as a result of prolonged ischemia from vessel obliteration; clients are typically treated for

TABLE 10-22 Guidelines for Skin Care and Protection

Temperature Protection

- Wear layers of clothing made of natural fibers, such as cotton, to draw moisture away from the skin; in cold weather, wear a hat and scarf because heat is lost through the scalp
- Wear thick mittens, which are warmer than gloves, and socks purchased from an outdoor clothing or ski shop designed to wick moisture away while retaining body heat
- Avoid air-conditioning; wear warmer clothes, layer light clothing, or wear a sweater or jacket in air-conditioning; be careful when going into an air-conditioned environment after being out in the heat, or vice versa
- Test water temperature before bathing or showering or have a member of the family test first; use other portion of the body to test if insensitivity exists in hand or foot
- Use a heating pad, hot water bottle, or an electric blanket to warm the sheets of your bed before getting into bed, but *DO NOT* apply these directly to the skin and do not sleep with any electric device left on; if necessary wear light socks and mittens or gloves to bed
- Keep household temperatures at a constant, even, and comfortable temperature
- Keep protective covering available at all times, even in the summer
- Avoid contact with extremes of temperature such as oven, dishwasher (hot dishes), refrigerator, or freezer; wear thick oven mitts whenever reaching into the oven, refrigerator, or freezer
- Wear rubber gloves whenever cleaning, washing dishes, or rinsing and/or peeling vegetables under water
- Avoid holding ice, ice-cold fruit, hot or cold drinks, or frozen foods; wear protective gloves whenever making contact with any of these items

Skin Care

- Take care of your skin and give your hands and feet extra care and protection; examine hands and feet daily; at the first sign of bruising, skin changes (e.g., cracking, calluses, blisters, redness), swelling, infection, or ulcer, immediately contact a member of your health care team (e.g., nurse, physical therapist, physician)
- Circulation problems tend to create dry skin and delay healing; keep your skin clean and well moisturized; wash with a mild, creamy, or moisturizing liquid soap or gel; clean carefully between fingers and toes; *DO NOT* soak them
- Avoid perfumed lotions and do not put lotion on sores or between toes
- Observe carefully for *any* activities that might put pressure on your fingertips, such as using a manual typewriter, playing a musical instrument (e.g., guitar, piano), and doing crafts or needlework
- Do not go barefoot indoors or outdoors; this includes getting up at night; avoid wearing open-toed shoes, pointy-toed shoes, high heels, or sandals; always wear absorbent socks or socks that wick perspiration away from skin; avoid nylon material (including pantyhose material); avoid stockings with seams or with mends; change socks or stockings daily
- Make sure shoes provide good support without being too tight, avoid shoes that cause excessive foot perspiration, and alternate shoes throughout the week (i.e., do not wear the same shoes every day)
- Avoid hot tubs and prolonged baths; dry carefully between toes; water temperature should be between 90° and 95° F
- Use heel protectors, sheepskin, and other protective devices whenever recommended

Other Tips

- (For Raynaud's disease or phenomenon) Avoid situations that precipitate excitement, anxiety, or feelings of fear; teach yourself how to recognize early signs of these emotions and use relaxation techniques to reduce stress
- (For Raynaud's disease or phenomenon) When you have an attack, gently rewarm fingers or toes as soon as possible; place your hands under your armpits, wiggle fingers or toes, move or walk around to improve circulation; if possible, run warm (*NOT* hot) water over the affected body part until normal color returns
- Do not use razor blades; use electric razors
- Avoid medications and substances (e.g., nicotine, caffeine in chocolate, tea, coffee, and soft drinks) that can cause blood vessels to narrow; discuss all medications with your physician
- Maintain good circulation; do not stay in one position for more than 30 min; use breathing and stretching exercises whenever confined to a desk, chair, car, or bed for more than 30 min
- Do not wear constricting or tight clothing, especially tight socks; avoid elastic around wrist or ankles
- Do not wear jewelry such as watches or bracelets to bed at night
- Leave a night light on in dark areas; turn on lights in dark areas and hallways
- Do not sit with legs crossed

Table continued on following page

TABLE 10-22 GUIDELINES FOR SKIN CARE AND PROTECTION (*Continued*)

- Avoid sunburn
- Do not scratch insect bites; do not scratch areas of itchy skin
- Do not do "bathroom surgery" on corns or calluses; do not use chemical agents for the removal of corns or calluses; see your doctor

CARE OF NAILS

- Use clippers, not scissors; *DO NOT* use razor blades; cut toenails straight across but file fingernails in a rounded fashion to the tips of your fingers
- Take care of your nails; use cuticle softener or moisturizing cream or lotion around cuticles; push the cuticles back very gently with a cotton swab soaked in cuticle remover; *DO NOT* push cuticles back with a sharp object and *DO NOT* cut the cuticles with scissors or nail clippers
- Use lamb's wool between overlapping toes

wound care and postoperatively after amputation. (See Arteriosclerosis Obliterans, below.)

It is often the case that a client with some other primary orthopedic or neurologic diagnosis has also been medically diagnosed with vasculitis. (See Rheumatoid Vasculitis, Chapter 4, and Special Implications features for clients with associated cardiovascular involvement, such as atherosclerosis, myocarditis, pericarditis, or aneurysm.)

Arterial Disease

Arteriosclerotic Obliterans (Arterial Occlusive Disease). In prescribing an exercise program for someone with claudication secondary to occlusive disease, exercise tolerance must be determined. A training heart rate should be based on the exercise tolerance test (ETT) because persons with PVD frequently have CAD as well. Frequently, symptoms of claudication occur before a training heart rate is reached, but the heart rate should be monitored and should not exceed the training heart rate, even in the absence of symptoms. Anginal chest pain is a red flag to decrease intensity (Ward et al., 1992).

A progressive conditioning program, including walking for fixed periods, is essential, even if the initial length of walking time is only 1 minute. Walking is the optimal exercise for people with PVD because walking can improve functional capacity. The relative ischemia that occurs in the calf muscles during walking may aid in the development of collateral vessels. The person should walk to the point of claudication and then rest until the pain subsides. This sequence should be repeated until the person has completed 20 to 30 minutes of exercise (Ward et al., 1992). A walking program to near maximal pain of at least 6 months should be part of the standard medical care for people with intermittent claudication (Gardner and Poehlman, 1995).

The client is encouraged to gradually build up tolerance and is precautioned to rest for any episodes of claudication. Claudication is influenced by the speed, incline, and surface of the walk and should be modified

TABLE 10-23 COMPARISON OF ACUTE AND CHRONIC ARTERIAL SYMPTOMS

SYMPTOM ANALYSIS	ACUTE ARTERIAL SYMPTOMS	CHRONIC ARTERIAL SYMPTOMS
Location	Varies; distal to occlusion; may involve entire leg	Deep muscle pain, usually in calf, may be lower leg or dorsum of foot
Character	Throbbing	Intermittent claudication, feels like cramp, numbness and tingling, feeling of cold
Onset and duration	Sudden onset (within 1 hr)	Chronic pain, onset gradual following exertion
Aggravating factors		Activity such as walking or stairs; elevation
Relieving factors		Rest (usually within 2 min); dangling (severe involvement)
Associated symptoms	6 Ps: pain, pallor, pulselessness, paresthesia, poikilothermia (coldness), paralysis (severe)	Cool pale skin
At risk	History of vascular surgery, arterial invasive procedure, abdominal aneurysm, trauma including injured arteries, chronic atrial fibrillation	Older adults, more males than females, inherited predisposition, history of hypertension, smoking, diabetes, hypercholesterolemia, obesity, vascular disease

Adapted from Jarvis C: Physical Examination and Health Assessment. Philadelphia, WB Saunders, 1992, p 658.

whenever possible to improve exercise tolerance. After exercise, numbness in the foot as well as pain in the calf may occur. The foot may be cold and pale, which is an indication that the circulation has been diverted to the arteriolar bed of the leg muscles (Layzer, 1985). Many people with claudication are already receiving β-blockers for angina or hypertension (see also Special Implications for the Therapist: Angina and Hypertension.)

When arterial thrombosis and/or embolism are suspected, the affected limb must be protected by proper positioning below the horizontal plane and protective skin care provided. Heat or cold application and massage are contraindicated, and family members must also be notified of these restrictions.

Venous Disorders

Thrombophlebitis. Prevention is the key to treatment of thrombophlebitis, both prevention of thrombus formation and to prevent thrombi from becoming emboli. Populations at risk, especially postoperative, postpartum, and immobilized clients, should be identified by the medical staff and observed carefully.

Preventive therapy includes active and passive range of motion exercise, early ambulation for brief but regular periods whenever possible, coughing and deep-breathing exercises, and proper positioning. The person at risk must be taught the importance of avoiding one position for prolonged periods and to avoid pillows under the legs postoperatively to facilitate venous return. At the same time, elevation of the legs just above the level of the heart aids blood flow by gravitational force and prevents venous stasis as a contributing factor to the formation of new thrombi. Placing the foot of the bed in a Trendelenburg position (6 in. elevation with slight knee bend to prevent popliteal pressure) decreases venous pressure and helps relieve pain and edema. Sitting in a chair in the early postoperative period should be avoided. Therapy staff may assist the nursing staff in applying and monitoring (rewrap every 4 to 8 hours) elastic wraps from toe to groin. After thrombosis of a deep calf vein, elastic support hose should be worn for at least 6 to 8 weeks, and ideally for life.

The person at risk for DVT secondary to fracture and subsequent immobility involving a lower extremity cast should be carefully evaluated when the cast is removed. Normally, calf muscle atrophy is easily observed when the cast is removed. Normal calf size (less than 1 cm difference between left and right) without atrophy on cast removal may signal swelling associated with DVT.

For the client with diagnosed thrombophlebitis, the therapist should monitor and report any signs of pulmonary embolism, such as chest pain, hemoptysis, cough, diaphoresis, dyspnea, and apprehension. Clients with a history of DVT may develop chronic venous insufficiency even years later and therefore must be monitored periodically for life.

Anyone receiving anticoagulant therapy (e.g., Coumadin [warfarin]) must be monitored for manifestations of bleeding as evidenced by blood in the urine, stool, or along the gums or teeth; subcutaneous bruising; or flank pain. Bleeding under the skin and easy bruising in response to the slightest trauma can occur when platelet production is altered. This condition necessitates extreme care in the therapy setting, especially any treatment requiring soft tissue mobilization, manual therapy, or the use of any equipment, including modalities and weight-training devices. (See discussion Platelets, Chapter 35; see also Table 35–7.)

Chronic Venous Insufficiency. An assessment of the legs should be performed frequently to observe for stasis ulcers, skin changes (e.g., color, texture, temperature), impaired growth of nails, and discrepancy in size of extremities, including observations and measurements for edema. In the home health setting, the client should be instructed to contact a member of the medical team if any edema or change in the condition of the extremity occurs. When a stasis ulcer of any size is detected, treatment is initiated.

The client should be advised to avoid prolonged standing and sitting; crossing the legs; sitting too high for feet to touch the floor or too deep, causing pressure against the popliteal space; and wearing tight clothing (including girdles and elastic waistbands) or support hose or stockings that extend above the knee, which act as a tourniquet at the popliteal fossa. Thigh-high elastic stockings are recommended, but they must be worn properly to avoid bunching behind the knee.

Physical therapy is most often requested for clients with chronic venous insufficiency who have venous insufficiency ulcers with infection. Whirlpool beyond an initial 1 to 2 treatments is contraindicated, as the increased blood volume and dependent position (underlying causes of wound) can make the edema worse. Limited hydrotherapy (maximum temperature 80° F.) may be indicated to remove loose debris and toxic antiseptics, to moisten dried exudate, or to facilitate debridement when pulsatile debridement devices are unavailable (Burks, 1995; Haynes et al., 1994; LaRaus, 1995). (For specific wound care management see Gogia, 1995; Krasner, 1990; and McCulloch et al., 1995.)

Arterial obstruction in the presence of venous insufficiency may not be readily recognized. Wounds associated with chronic venous insufficiency that do not demonstrate healing within 2 weeks of beginning wound care may undergo a noninvasive arterial Doppler study (*ankle-brachial index*) to determine the level of circulation. This index is the result of a vascular diagnostic test comparing the systolic blood pressure between the ankle and brachial pulses. An index result of 1.0 indicates an adequate arterial blood supply; an index less than 1.0 indicates insufficient blood flow to the distal regions for healing to occur. An index less than 0.8 is used to determine the need for surgical intervention.

Raynaud's Disease and Phenomenon. Prevention of episodes of Raynaud's is important. The affected individual must be encouraged to keep warm, avoid air-conditioning, and dress warmly in the winter (e.g., protect the extremities as well as the head, chest, and back to maintain overall body temperature). Aquatic therapy is often helpful in diminishing symptoms, but again, the individual must be careful when moving from place to place with extreme temperature changes (e.g., from outside winter temperatures into a warm pool area and back outside). The use of antihypertensives for Raynaud's can result in postural hypotension; the physician should be notified of these findings to alter the dosage.

* The home health therapist must be alert to the possibility of hot water bottles, heating pads, electric blankets, and hot foot soaks being used by the client without physician approval. This precaution is especially true for people with diabetic-associated peripheral neuropathies and for paraplegics. Encourage the person with vascular disease to prevent becoming chilled by keeping the thermostat at home set at 70° to 72°F and to avoid prolonged exposure to cold outdoors (e.g., prewarming the car, dressing properly in layers, especially protecting hands and feet).

Vascular Neoplasms *(Benditt and Schwartz, 1994)*

Malignant vascular (i.e., involving the blood vessels) neoplasms are rare and may include angiosarcoma, hemangiopericytoma, and Kaposi's sarcoma. (See also Myocardial Neoplasm, this chapter.) *Angiosarcomas* (hemangiosarcomas) can occur in either sex and at any age, most commonly appearing as small, painless, red nodules on the skin, soft tissue, breast, bone, liver, and spleen. Almost half of all people with angiosarcoma die of the disease

Hemangiopericytoma arises from the smooth muscle cells that are external to the walls of capillaries and arterioles. Most commonly located on the lower extremities and retroperitoneum (space between the peritoneum lining of the walls of the abdominal and pelvic cavities and the posterior abdominal wall) these tumors are composed of spindle cells with a rich vascular network. Metastasis to the lungs, bone, liver, and lymph nodes occurs in 10% to 50% of cases, but the majority of hemangiopericytomas are removed surgically without having invaded or metastasized.

Kaposi's sarcoma in association with AIDS most likely occurs as a result of loss of immunity. One form of the tumor resembles a simple hemangioma with tightly packed clusters of capillaries, most often visible on the skin. Although Kaposi's sarcoma is malignant and may be widely spread in the body, it is not usually a cause of death.

Arteriovenous Malformations

Arteriovenous (AV) malformations are congenital vascular malformations that result from a localized maldevelopment of part of the primitive vascular plexus and consist of abnormal arteriovenous communications without intervening capillaries. AV malformations vary in size, ranging from massive lesions that are fed by multiple vessels to lesions too small to identify. AV malformations may occur in any blood vessel, but the most common sites include the brain, GI tract, and skin. Approximately 10% of cases present with aneurysms. Small AV malformations are more likely to bleed than large ones, and once bleeding occurs, repeated episodes are likely. Clinical presentation depends on the location of the malformation and may relate to hemorrhage from the malformation or an associated aneurysm or to cerebral ischemia due to diversion or stasis of blood (Aminoff, 1994).

The Lymphatic Vessels

The lymphatic system is part of the circulatory system that collects excess tissue fluid and plasma that has leaked out of capillaries into the interstitial space and returns it to the bloodstream. The lymphatic system consists of lymphatic vessels and lymph nodes and functions to remove impurities from the circulatory system and to produce cells of the immune system (lymphocytes) that are vital in fighting bacteria and viruses. The lymph nodes are also part of the lymphoid system, the organs and tissues of the immune system. These lymphoid organs are primary (thymus and bone marrow) and secondary (spleen, lymph nodes, tonsils, and Peyer's patches of the small intestine) (see Fig. 11–1).

All of the lymphoid organs link the hematologic and immune systems in that they are sites of residence, proliferation, differentiation, or function of lymphocytes and mononuclear phagocytes (mononuclear phagocyte system)(McCance and Cipriano, 1994).

Three forms of lymph vascular insufficiency may occur. The first, *dynamic insufficiency*, occurs when the lymphatic load exceeds the lymphatic transport capacity. In this situation, the anatomy of the lymphatic system and its function are normal but are overwhelmed. A second form of insufficiency of the lymph vascular system is caused by a reduction of the lymphatic transport capacity below the level of a normal lymphatic protein load. This reduction results in low lymph flow failure called *mechanical insufficiency*. A third form of lymph vascular insufficiency occurs when the lymphatic system has a reduced transport capacity, leading to an overflowing of lymph. This form is called *safety valve insufficiency* (Foldi et al., 1989; Granda, 1994).

Diseases of the Lymphatic Channels

Disorders of the lymphatic system may result from inflammation of a lymphatic vessel (*lymphangitis*), inflammation of one or more lymph nodes (*lymphadenitis*), an increased amount of lymph (*lymphedema*) or enlargement of the lymph nodes (*lymphadenopathy*). Lymph nodes act as defense barriers and are secondarily involved in virtually all systemic infections and in many neoplastic disorders arising elsewhere in the body.

The specific node or nodes affected in an infectious disease depend on the location of the infection, the nature of the invading organism, and the severity of the disease. For example, infections involving the pharynx, salivary glands, and scalp often cause tender enlargement of the neck nodes, referred to as *reactive cervical lymphadenopathy*. *Generalized lymphadenopathy* (enlargement of two or three regionally separated lymph node groups) is usually due to inflammation, neoplasm, or immunologic reactions (Dennison and Black, 1993).

These two types of lymphadenopathy are normal reactions to infection that result in large and tender lymph nodes, but the node is not necessarily infected (warm or reddened as with lymphadenitis; see next section). The presence of lymphadenopathy is usually more significant in persons older than 50 years. Lymphadenopathy in people under 30 years is due to benign causes in approximately 80% of cases, whereas in people over 50 years, lymphadenopathy is due to benign causes in only 40% of cases (Haynes, 1994).

Lymphadenitis

Infections elsewhere in the body can lead to lymphadenopathy as described previously. When the lymph node becomes overwhelmed by the infection, the lymph node itself can become infected, which is called *lymphadenitis*. Lymphadenitis can be classified as acute or chronic; acutely inflamed lymph nodes are most common locally in the cervical region in association with infections of the teeth or tonsils or in the axillary or inguinal regions secondary to infections of the extremities. In acute lymphadenitis, the lymph nodes are enlarged, tender, warm, and reddened. In the case of chronic lymphadenitis, long-standing infection from a variety of sources results in scarred lymph nodes with fibrous connective tissue replacement. The nodes are enlarged and firm to palpation but not warm or tender. The management of lymphadenitis is treatment of the underlying disorder (Dennison and Black, 1993).

Lymphangitis

Lymphangitis, an acute inflammation of the subcutaneous lymphatic channels, usually occurs as a result of hemolytic streptococci or staphylococci (or both) entering the lymphatic channels from an abrasion or local trauma, wound, or infection (usually cellulitis). The involvement of the lymphatics is often first observed by a red streak under the skin (referred to in lay terms as *blood poisoning*), which radiates from the infection site in the direction of the regional lymph nodes. The red streak may be very obvious or it may be very faint and easily overlooked, especially in dark-skinned people. The nodes most frequently affected are submandibular, cervical, inguinal, and axillary, in that order. Involved nodes are usually tender and enlarged (>3 cm).

Systemic manifestations may include fever, chills, malaise, and anorexia. Other symptoms may present in association with the underlying infection located elsewhere in the body. Streptococcal bacteremia from any cause can result in suppurative arthritis (inflammatory with pus formation), osteomyelitis, peritonitis, meningitis, or visceral abscesses. When cellulitis results in lymphangitis, throbbing pain occurs at the site of bacterial invasion.

Medical Management

Diagnosis. Lymphangitis may be confused with superficial thrombophlebitis, but the erythema associated with lymphangitis is first seen as a red streak under the skin radiating toward the regional lymph nodes, whereas the erythema associated with thrombosis is usually over the thrombosed vein with local induration and inflammation. However, suppurative thrombophlebitis may develop if bacteria are introduced during IV therapy, especially when the needle or catheter is left in place for more than 48 hours. The physician will also differentiate cellulitis from soft tissue infections (e.g., gangrene, necrotizing fasciitis) that require early and aggressive incision and resection of necrotic infected tissue.

Laboratory tests are often not required but may include blood culture, often positive for staphylococcal or streptococcal species, and culture and sensitivity studies on the wound exudate or pus.

Treatment and Prognosis. Antibiotic therapy may be accompanied by general measures such as heat, elevation, immobilization of the infected area, and analgesics for pain. Appropriate wound care may include drainage of the pus from an infected wound when it is clear that an abscess is associated with the site of initial infection. An area of cellulitis should not be excised, because the infection may be spread by attempted drainage when pus is not present (Tierney, 1994).

Treatment as described should be effective against the invading bacteria within a few days. Delayed or inadequate therapy can lead to massive infection with septicemia and its subsequent sequelae.

Special Implications for the Therapist **10-19**

LYMPH NODES

Palpable lymph nodes do not always indicate serious or ongoing disease. Some degree of inguinal lymphadenopathy is relatively common, reflecting prior episodes of infection in the lower extremities. Similarly, minor enlargement of cervical nodes may be residual from previous pharyngeal or dental infections. Lymphadenopathy in certain anatomic areas such as preauricular or postauricular (in front of or behind the ear), supraclavicular, deltopectoral, and pectoral regions should be viewed with greater suspicion because these areas are not usually enlarged as a result of local subclinical infections or trauma (Swartz, 1995).

Intraoral infection may cause an inflamed cervical node, leading to spasm of the sternocleidomastoid muscle and causing neck pain. Palpation may appear to aggravate a primary spasm, as if the spasm were originating in the muscle, when in fact a lymph node under the muscle is the source of symptoms. In such cases, past history is an important part of the client's evaluation process to identify the need for medical referral or follow-up.

Supraclavicular and inguinal nodes are common metastatic sites for cancer. Nodes involved with metastatic cancer are usually hard and fixed to the underlying tissue. In acute infections, nodes are tender asymmetrically, enlarged, and matted together, and the overlying skin may be red and warm (erythematous). Changes in size (>1 cm), shape (matted together), and consistency (rubbery or firm) of lymph nodes in more than one area that persist for more than 4 weeks or the presence of *painless* enlarged lymph nodes should be reported to the physician.

Lymphedema

Definition and Overview. Lymphedema is not a disease of the lymphatic channels but is rather a symptom of lymphatic transport malfunction that results in an accumulation of lymphatic and edema fluid. Lymphedema as a symptom is briefly discussed earlier in the chapter but owing to the prevalence of this condition in the physical or occupational therapy practice, greater detail is provided here.

Lymphedema is categorized as primary or secondary. *Primary lymphedema* is defined as impaired lymphatic flow owing to congenital malformation of the lymphatic vessels (lymph vessel aplasia, hypoplasia, or hyperplasia) and accounts for approximately 10% of all lymphedema. *Secondary lymphedema* is acquired and represents the most common type of lym-

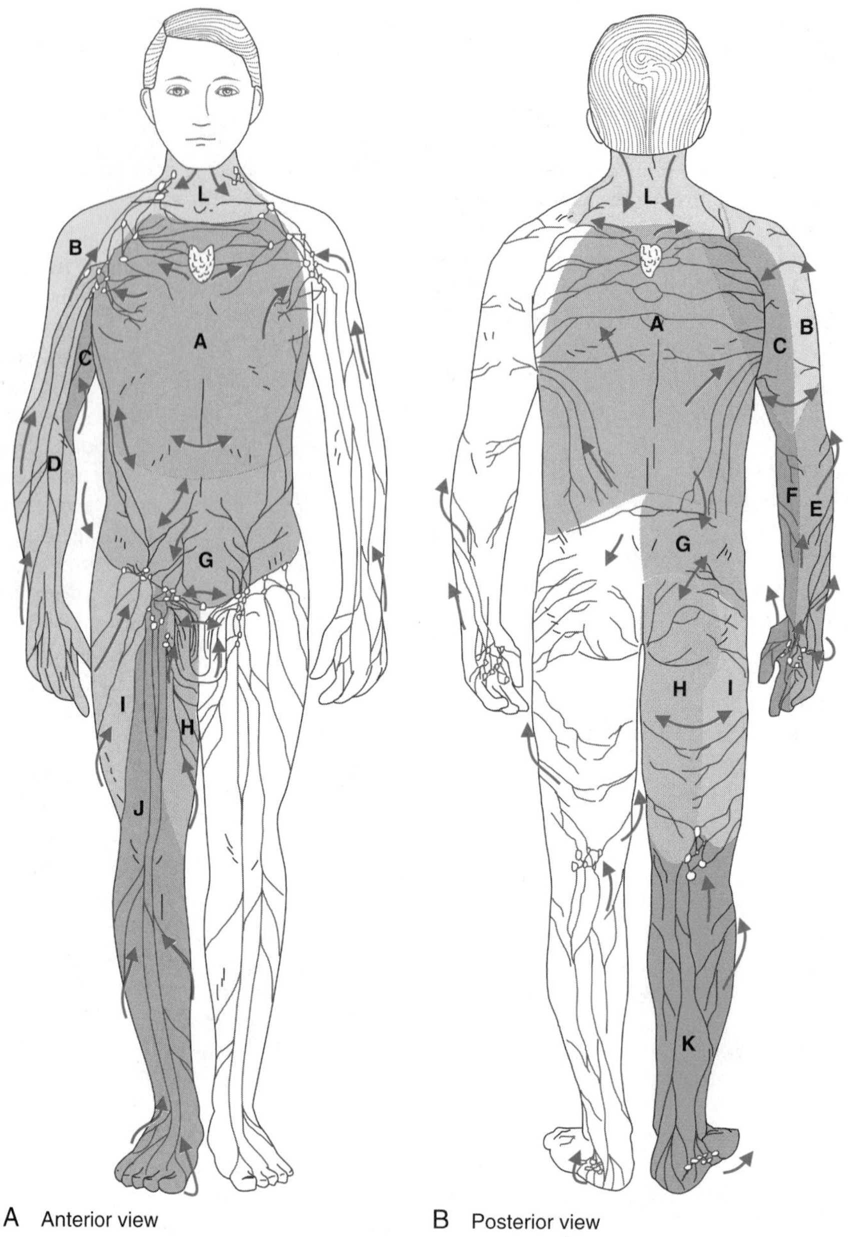

Figure **10–33.** Lymphotomes of the lymphatic system. *Arrows* indicate the direction of flow. Letters designate various lymphotomes. A, Anterior view. B, posterior view. (*From Foldi M, Kubik S: Lehrbuch der Lymphologie für Mediziner und Physiotherapeuter mit Anhang, Praktische Linweise fur die Physiotherape. Stuttgart, Gustav Fischer Verlag, 1989.*)

phedema; it is caused by known precipitating factors (Boris et al., 1994).

Etiology and Incidence. The most common causes of secondary lymphedema in the United States are surgical removal of the lymph nodes, fibrosis secondary to radiation, and traumatic injury to the lymphatic system. The incidence of lymphedema varies greatly in different geographic areas, and overall statistics are unavailable at this time. Over a decade ago, the World Health Organization (WHO) reported 140 million cases throughout the world (WHO, 1984).

The incidence of postmastectomy lymphedema alone has been estimated as approximately 3,300,000; this figure is extrapolated from previous statistics that 1 in 9 women[23] will develop breast cancer over a lifetime (based on life expectancy of 80 years) and that 32% of these women will develop lymphedema (Casley-Smith and Casley-Smith, 1991; Lerner and Requena, 1986).

Pathogenesis. Under normal conditions, the lymphatic circulation starts with the collection of interstitial fluid by the initial lymphatic vessels. These drain into progressively larger vessels within a distinct anatomic region called the *lymphotome* (Fig. 10–33).

Lymphedema fluid contains high concentrations of protein, water, and macrophages. The primary mechanisms causing lymphedema are interference with lymphatic drainage, protein filtration impairment, and defects in proteolysis and/or macrophage activity. When venous or lymphatic vessels or both are impaired, the lymph fluid may exceed the lymphatic transport capacity. As a result, an abnormal amount of protein

[23] This statistic is now 1 in 8 women over a lifetime, which would increase the overall incidence of postmastectomy lymphedema.

fluid collects in the tissues of the extremity. If untreated, this stagnant, protein-rich fluid not only causes tissue channels to increase in size and number, but also reduces oxygen through the transport system, interferes with wound healing, and provides a culture medium for bacteria that can result in various infections. A chronic inflammatory condition stemming from this accumulation of fluid eventually results in fibrosis of tissues, which increases vulnerability to injury (Thiadens, 1995).

Detailed explanation of the anatomic, pathologic, microscopic, and physiologic mechanisms of lymphedema are available (see Casley-Smith et al., 1985; Foldi and Casley-Smith, 1983; Kubik, 1985).

Clinical Manifestations. Swelling, pain, decreased range of motion and coordination, paresthesia, and loss of functional mobility are the typical manifestations of lymphedema and can be quite severe (Fig. 10–34). Lymphedema also affects psychological well-being; many persons with lymphedema consider themselves unsightly and withdraw from society. Medical complications of lymphedema include lymphangitis, cellulitis, ulceration, thrombosis, and, rarely, lymphangiosarcoma.

Medical Management

Diagnosis. Lymphedema is easily observed on examination, but lymphoscintigraphy using radioactive agents can provide a two-dimensional image of the distribution of lymph flow, including speed of lymph flow, lymph node uptake, and presence of backflow.

Treatment. Treatment includes physical and/or occupational therapy, surgical intervention, and pharmacologic management. Diuretics continue to be recommended by some practitioners, but these should be used cautiously as they may have little effect on reducing lymphedema, and long-term use can cause harmful side effects. Antibiotics are widely used to treat local infections or to prevent recurrent chronic infections (Thiadens, 1995).

Experimental medications such as benzo-α-pyrones (benzopyrones) can reduce the volume of high-protein edema by stimulating proteolysis by macrophages. Once excess protein is eliminated, the fluid that edema causes is no longer retained. 5,6-benzo-α-pyrone has been tested effective (especially when combined with physical therapy but is not available yet in the United States[24] (Smith et al., 1993). Although benzopyrones rapidly reduce acute edema secondary to accidental or surgical trauma, they do not rapidly reduce chronic forms of lymphedema (Piller et al., 1988).

Physical therapy may include techniques such as elevation, manual lymphatic drainage,[25] compressive garments, pneumatic compressive machines, heat application, range of motion exercises, and mobilization of the nervous system (Butler, 1991). Pneumatic compression does influence the reabsorption of fluids but it does not influence the reabsorption of proteins. Residual proteins cause recurrence of the edema and acceleration of fibrosclerotic hardening of the tissues. Although rare, there have been documented cases of infection and necrosis requiring amputation secondary to compressive treatment (Bastien et al., 1989; Callam et al., 1988). The application of heat has been reported to reduce lymphedema (Chang et al., 1989; Liu and Olszewski, 1993), although this approach remains controversial.

The goal of noninvasive treatment is to increase lymphatic drainage from obstructed areas into normal lymphotomes by (theoretically) opening collateral vessels. Although it removes lymph from the tissues, it also reportedly dilates the lymph vessels, increases their contractility, and breaks up tissue fibrosis. Treatment for lymphedema involves a combination of techniques including attention to skin hygiene, manual lymph drainage, specific compressive bandaging, custom compression garments individually prescribed after limb stabilization, and individual-specific exercises utilizing lymphotome anatomy to open collateral pathways, prevent infection, and improve function.

Prognosis. Untreated lymphedema becomes irreversible and progressive; the earlier treatment is initiated, the more beneficial it is likely to be in the long run. With a home program of maintenance therapy, more than half the persons treated can maintain the reduction initially obtained with noninvasive treatment (Foldi, 1994; Boris et al., 1994). Radiation may impair the availability of collateral pathways and impair the success of treatment. Further investigation is warranted.

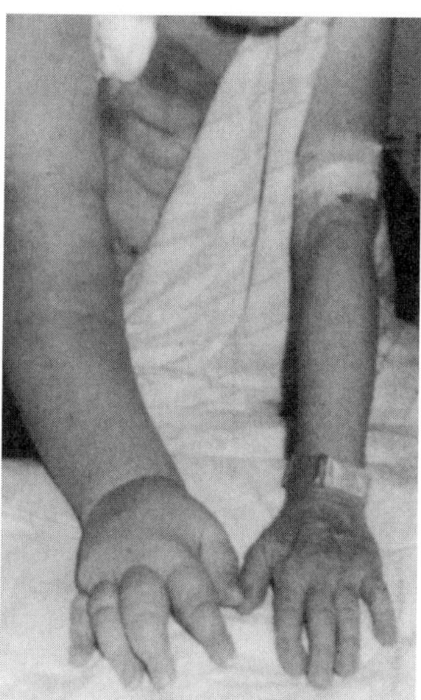

Figure **10–34.** Lymphedema. Unilateral arm swelling from obstructed lymph channels secondary to removal of axillary nodes with radical mastectomy. Overlying skin is indurated (hard) and lymphedema is nonpitting. (*From Jarvis C: Physical Examination and Health Assessment. Philadelphia, WB Saunders, 1992, p 658.*)

[24] Benzopyrones in the powder or cream form can be purchased in Germany or Australia, but deaths have been reported in association with their use. The use of bioflavinoids is considered an acceptable alternative in the US and Canada.

[25] Manual lymphatic drainage (MLD) is a form of gentle connective tissue massage that stimulates the weakened lymphatic system by pushing the stagnant fluid through the vessels. This action allows the venous system to resorb the fluid and helps develop collateral channels through which the lymph can begin to flow (Thiadens, 1995).

Special Implications for the Therapist **10-20**

LYMPHEDEMA

Persons with lymphedema must be monitored closely. For the client with lymphedema associated with infection, once antibiotics have been administered and the infection has been controlled, compression techniques including compression garments, gradient pumps, and manual lymph drainage can be applied to reduce swelling (Specific precautions for lymphedema are listed in Box 10–12.)

Some clinicians discourage the use of pumps because the high pressures involved cause edematous fluid to be pushed distally to the foot or hand or genitalia, where the lymphatics are not functioning properly. Others argue that the use of a programmable pump provides customized pressures and gradients for each clinical situation. When compression is used, the pressure applied with a compression device must not exceed 40 mm Hg, in accordance with the physiologic tolerance of the lymphatic system. High-intensity pneumatic compression is only used under exceptional circumstances, such as when the lymphatic system is so altered that there is no possibility of physiologic function (Vaillant-Newman, 1995).

Jewelry, constrictive clothing, heavy lifting, and the use of pumps that apply the same amount of pressure over the arm should be avoided. The latter precaution is made because evenly distributed pressure in an extremity, distal to proximal, can overpressurize the lymphatic system and cause increased swelling from the collapse of lymph vessels.

A lymph vessel from the breast may pierce the pectoralis major muscle, terminating in the subclavicular lymph nodes. Entrapment of this lymph duct by passage between tense fibers of an involved pectoralis major muscle may cause edema of the breast. These signs of entrapped lymphatic drainage and breast tenderness are relieved by extinction of the related pectoralis major muscle trigger points or muscle tension (Travell and Simons, 1983). Assessment of trigger points is an important part of any client evaluation when presenting symptoms include lymphedema.

BOX **10-12**

Life-long Precautions for Clients with Lymphedema

- No blood pressure measurements taken on involved extremity
- No needle sticks or blood drawing on the involved extremity
- Immediate treatment for all wounds no matter how minor (insect bites, paper cuts, hangnail, blister, burn), e.g., cleansing, antibiotic ointment, and bandaging
- Protect hands and feet at all times (e.g., socks and supportive shoewear, rubber gloves for cleaning, long oven mitts, garden gloves for any outdoor work)
- Use extreme caution when cutting fingernails or cuticles; creams are best for removing cuticles
- Keep the skin supple by applying oil or bland cream; perfumed lotions and creams can be irritating
- Use electric razors to remove unwanted hair; never use a razor blade
- Avoid constricting jewelry; clothing, especially tight underwear, socks or stockings; and elastic around wrists and ankles
- Avoid lifting heavy weights or carrying heavy objects; no heavy handbags with over-the-shoulder straps
- Proper nutrition with low-salt, low-caffeine diet; avoid smoking and drinking alcoholic beverages
- Changes in pressure gradient during air travel require use of compression garments and salt-free diet
- Avoid overheating local body parts or rise in core body temperature: use pyrogenic medications, even with low-grade fever; avoid saunas, hot tubs, hot pads, hot packs; close monitoring is required during intensive exercise or marathon running
- Do not use sun-tanning salons; keep the limb protected from the sun and avoid sunburn
- Beware that chemicals such as those used in the application of artificial fingernails may cause an edematous response in some people

Other resources for information about lymphedema include the National Lymphedema Network (1-800-514-3259) and a helpful publication that is available from the Indiana Chapter of the American Cancer Society (ACS), *Reach to Recovery: What You Should Know About Lymphedema Risks After Breast Cancer.*

OTHER CARDIAC CONSIDERATIONS

Cardiac Transplantation

Although cardiac transplantation is a treatment for cardiac disease, it is included because it applies to multiple cardiac conditions discussed throughout this chapter.

Overview and Incidence. In 1960, Lower and Shumway developed the technique for heart transplantation that remains the basis of standard clinical surgical transplant technique worldwide. The first human heart procedure was performed in South Africa by Christiaan Barnard (1967), followed shortly by the first United States transplant by Norman Shumway at Stanford in 1968 (Hunt et al., 1994). Since that time, more than 20,000 heart transplantations have been performed. The advent of endomyocardial biopsy technique to allow for early rejection detection and FDA approval of cyclosporine (1983) has made treatment even more successful. In the United States, approximately 2,000 heart transplants are performed each year.

Heart transplantation has been *heterologous* (or xenograft) (i.e., from a nonhuman primate, extremely rare now) or, more commonly, *homologous* (or allograft) (i.e., from another human). *Orthotopic* homologous cardiac transplantation refers to the surgical placement (grafting) of the donor heart into the normal anatomic site. In the *heterotopic* homologous cardiac transplantation, the recipient's diseased heart is left intact and the donor heart is placed in parallel with anastomoses between the two right atria, pulmonary arteries, left atria, and aorta.

Transplant Candidates *(Tanio and Eisen, 1993).* People accepted as candidates for heart transplantation are expected to have a limited survival if they do not have surgery. Potential recipients of cardiac transplants must have end-stage heart disease with severe heart failure to be considered for a donor heart. Anyone with an ejection fraction[26] of less than 20% is also considered a potential candidate for transplantation. Other selection criteria are being debated such as the issue of transplantation in people with diabetes. Currently, most centers accept candidates with well-controlled diabetes who have no microvascular disease. Age cutoff is also controversial. Although the upper age limit for transplant recipients has been 55 to 65 years, some centers are now willing to transplant hearts into older people who are healthy in all other respects.

Absolute contraindications for transplantation include any presurgical evidence of uncontrolled malignancy or infection. Relative contraindications vary from one center to another, but in general they include irreversible moderate to severe hepatic or renal dysfunction; pulmonary vascular resistance irreversible by intensive vasodilator therapy; moderate to severe chronic lung disease; peripheral or cerebrovascular disease; active peptic ulcer disease; high likelihood of noncompliance with postoperative medical therapy; psychiatric instability; and a history of active substance abuse. Combined heart/lung transplantation may be considered in candidates with severe irreversible pulmonary hypertension.

Left Ventricular Assistive Device. Despite the success of new immunosuppressive regimens, few people who are dying of heart failure will actually have the opportunity to receive a heart transplant.Researchers are actively pursuing engineering a mechanical device called a *left ventricular assist device* (LVAD) to help keep people alive while they await heart transplant. The left ventricular assist system is a pneumatic device that consists of an implanted blood pump connected by a cable to an external computerized console (Fig. 10–35) (Frazier, 1993; Frazier et al., 1994).

The LVAD provides circulatory support by pumping blood through the body until a donor is available, improving rehabilitation and quality of life (McCarthy et al., 1994a). Studies to determine the capabilities of the LVAD at rest and during exercise are under way (Branch et al., 1994).

Based on the success of the pneumatically powered LVAD, researchers at the Texas Heart Institute have begun conducting clinical studies of a vented electric (VE), referred to as a second-generation, device. Like the pneumatic device, the VE device is implanted intraperitoneally (i.e., placed in the left upper quadrant, sutured to the anterior abdominal wall[27]), but the electric pump is powered through a percutaneous lead that is connected to two rechargeable batteries worn in a shoulder holster, so that the client is not tethered to a control console and remains fully mobile (Fig. 10–36).

This technology may eventually allow selected persons to receive long-term (permanent) support as a substitute for cardiac transplantation. The recipient is often home in 6 weeks with follow-up home health care. Device-related complications have been minimal, with a lower rate of infectious complications in the first 6 months after transplantation in those persons who have undergone bridge to transplantation (Birovljev et al., 1992). In the future, studies may be done to determine the efficacy of removing the cardiac assistive device after prolonged heart rest provides cardiac recovery. Survival with the natural recovered heart may be possible in some people.

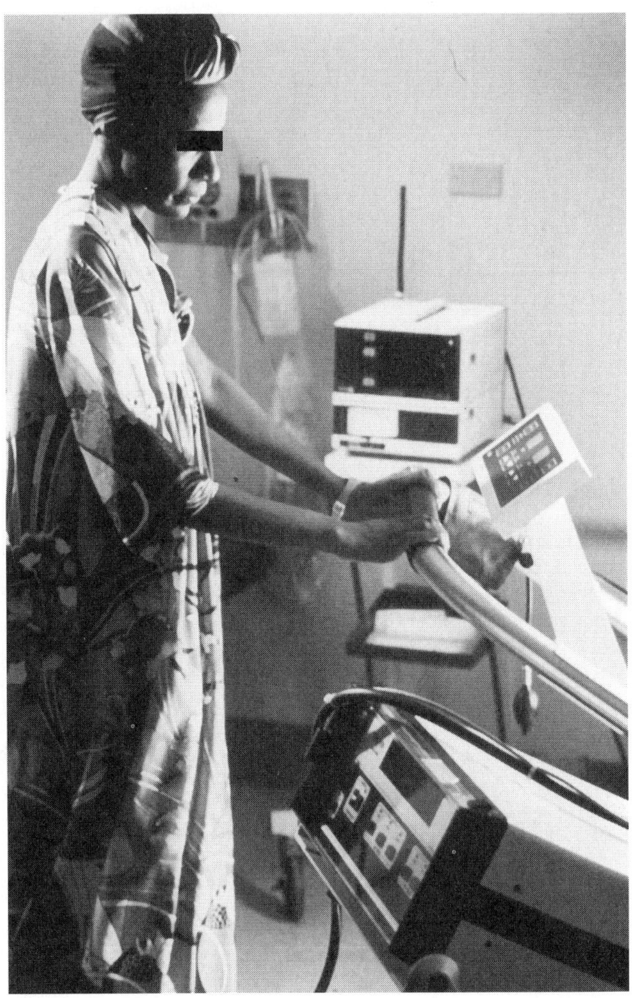

Figure 10–35. The left ventricular assist system, a pneumatic blood-pumping device connected by a cable to an external computerized console, implanted for 344 days in this 42-year-old woman. (*Courtesy of Thermo Cardiosystems, Inc. (TCI), Woburn, Mass.*)

Pathogenesis. To perform a transplant, the heart is denervated and lacks autonomic neural control but has normal contractility (systolic function) and normal to high-normal contractile reserve, possibly because of undetected episodes of allograft rejection or coronary artery disease (Hartmann, 1993). After surgical transplantation, an external pacemaker is used to generate a heart rate of 120 beats/min. This is gradually decreased over the first 7 days until the subcutaneous pacemaker wires are pulled out gently.

The transplanted heart usually begins functioning at 60 to 70 beats/min; later resting heart rate is in the 90 to 95 beats/min range because parasympathetic tone is not functioning to moderate the heart rate. Heart rate peaks a minute after activity or exercise is stopped and may take an hour after exercise to return to resting levels. During rest, heart rate and

[26] The amount of blood the ventricle ejects is called the *ejection fraction;* the normal ejection fraction is about 60% to 75%. A decreased ejection fraction is a hallmark finding of ventricular failure.

[27] Preperitoneal insertion has been evaluated by placing the implant in a pocket formed below the rectus abdominis and internal oblique muscles and above the posterior rectus sheath separating the device from the abdomen, thus avoiding problems posed by intra-abdominal LVAD insertion (McCarthy et al., 1994b).

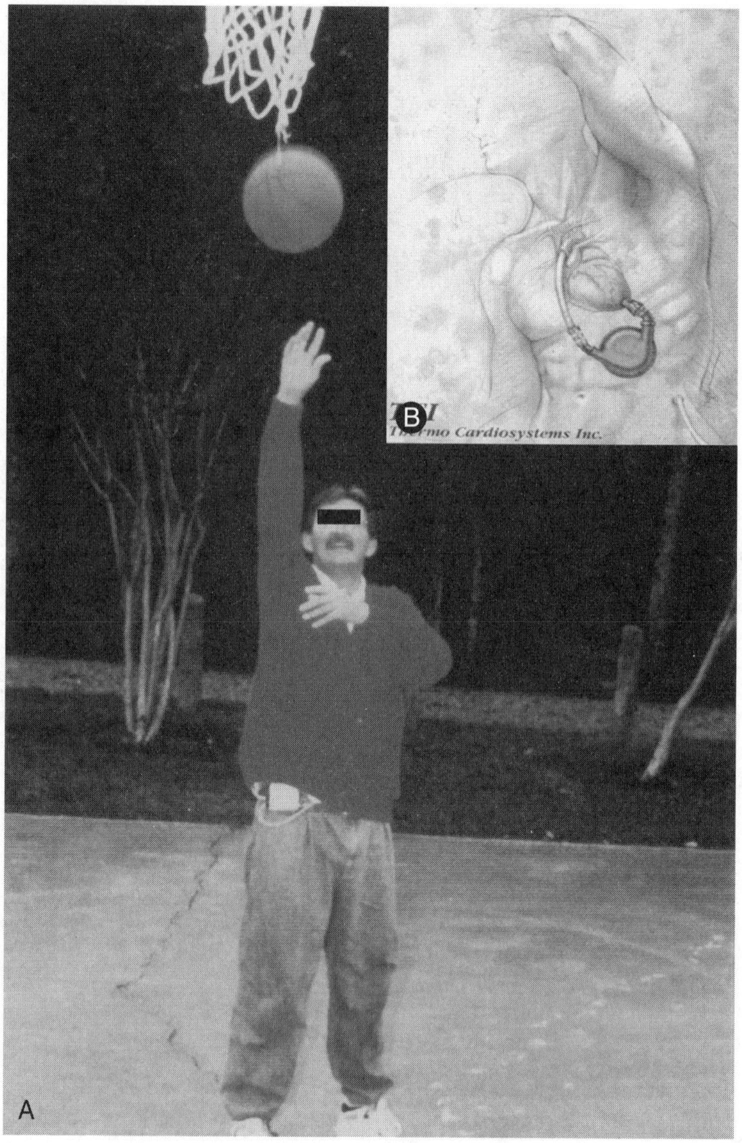

Figure **10–36.** A, Electric devices, called *vented electric* (VE) *devices*, are now available. This second-generation device is powered by rechargeable batteries worn in a shoulder holster or belt-bag around the waist, allowing complete freedom of movement as the person is not tethered to a control console.
B, Diagram of placement of device. (*Courtesy of Thermo Cardiosystems, Inc. (TCI), Woburn, Mass.*)

blood pressure increase (as compared to the nontransplanted heart) and cardiac output drops to the low end of the normal range.

Although the denervation eliminates the sympathetic and parasympathetic nervous system input to the heart, the Bainbridge reflex,[28] catecholamine response[29] and Starling's law (see Aging and the Cardiovascular System early in this chapter) allow for increased stroke volume. In other words, a strong initial increase in venous return associated with increased activity is responsible for early increases in heart rate; within 5 to 6 minutes after warmup, catecholamines are activated and heart rate continues to increase. During exercise, the transplanted heart continues to depend on large muscle contraction to facilitate venous return and maintain cardiac output. Increases in cardiac output are lower and increases in the heart rate are slower than normal for the transplanted heart.

[28] The Bainbridge reflex causes heart rate to increase as venous return to the heart stimulates volume receptors in the atria to trigger an increased heart rate.

[29] Catecholamines such as epinephrine and norepinephrine result in sympathetic stimulation to increase rate and force of muscular contraction of the heart, thereby increasing cardiac output and to constrict peripheral blood vessels, resulting in elevated blood pressure. Five to six minutes after warmup the effect of the catecholamines causes an increase in heart rate.

Complications. Complications may occur during the waiting period before the cardiac transplantation takes place. The supply of donor hearts is limited so that more than half of persons waiting die before an available heart can be transplanted; women die more often than men, possibly because of delayed diagnosis and more advanced heart disease at the time of diagnosis (Sineath, 1995).

During surgery, centrifugal heart-lung bypass machines have malfunctioned in an undetermined number of cases (Kolff, 1990). This is an intraoperative complication that can occur in any open heart surgery and is not specific to transplantation. Complications may occur if the donor heart has been preserved on ice in an ischemic state for more than 6 hours; it must be warmed up slowly and without air bubbles that may form in the cardiac blood vessels during the time the bypass machine is being removed.

The most common post-transplant complications are acute or chronic organ rejection (see Graft-vs-Host Disease, Chapter 5) and infections, especially pulmonary infections (Rose et al., 1992). Rapidly progressive transplant CAD may occur and affect distal, small subendocardial arteries in an extensive, diffuse, obliterative process (Young, 1992); reports have also been made of generalized polyneuropathy accompanying solid organ rejection of the heart and kidneys. The neuropathy affects proximal and distal muscles and demonstrates hyporeflexia or areflexia (Amato et al., 1993).

Other complications occur as a result of long-term use of cyclosporine to prevent organ rejection (see Isoimmune Disease, Chapter 5). For example, a unique form of osteoporosis characterized by the most severe vertebral osteopenia occurs in younger persons who have their transplanted hearts longer. Significant osteopenia may already be present before cardiac transplantation in the presence of risk factors such as physical inactivity and dietary calcium deficiency (Shane et al., 1993).

Medical Management *(Tanio and Eisen, 1993)*

Diagnosis of Rejection. Diagnosis of postoperative organ rejection is made by endomyocardial biopsy. This is an invasive procedure with complications of its own, so efforts are being made to develop a superior, noninvasive approach based on echocardiography, radionuclide scanning, magnetic resonance spectroscopy, or peripheral blood studies. At present, none of these modalities is sensitive and specific enough to permit widespread clinical use for the detection of rejection.

Because the heart has been denervated as a result of the surgical procedure, clients lack a consistent or predictable "anginal" warning system for myocardial ischemia. Some clients experience angina inconsistently and without clear explanation or predictability. Only transplanted hearts in situ less than 3 to 4 months should be considered completely denervated. Periodic exercise testing and/or coronary angiography are used to assess the development and progression of CAD in the transplanted heart.

Treatment of Rejection. While waiting for a heart transplantation, transplant candidates are treated with drugs or intraaortic balloon pumps, but these treatments only provide temporary help to sustain life until a donor heart is available. Early postoperative management care is centered on prevention and treatment of acute rejection of the donor heart, primarily through the use of immunosuppressive drugs. Most centers advocate the routine use of daily "triple therapy," consisting of prednisone, azathioprine, and cyclosporine. Treatment has its own complications, ranging from infection to malignancy.

As management improves in these respects and people live longer, the accelerated form of atherosclerosis (transplant CAD) peculiar to grafted arteries is increasingly prevalent. Recent research advocates the use of calcium channel blockers as antiatherosclerotic therapy based on their ability to retard the development of atherosclerosis (Drexler and Schroeder, 1994; Waters and Lesperance, 1994).

Prognosis. In general, people tolerate the transplant procedure well, and the graft resumes normal function promptly. Recipients are often extubated and out of bed into a chair 2 to 3 days after surgery. Worldwide results of cardiac transplantation are excellent with 1-year and 5-year survival rates of 80% to 90%, owing to improved immunosuppression and more careful screening of donor hearts; the 10-year overall survival rate is approximately 73%. Most posttransplant recipients rate their quality of life as good to excellent.

Early cardiac graft failure (morbidity) has been reported to occur in 4% to 25% of persons undergoing orthotopic heart transplantation (Hauptman et al., 1994). Infection and acute and/or chronic rejection are still the major causes of death in heart transplant recipients. Accelerated atherosclerosis develops rapidly postoperatively and contributes to complications causing death.

Special Implications for the Therapist (Butler, 1992; Butler, 1995a) **10-21**

CARDIAC TRANSPLANTATION

Early Posttransplant Considerations

Because most cardiac transplant recipients have experienced months of restricted activity prior to surgery, pulmonary hygiene and general strengthening are important aspects of early treatment. Preoperative gradual physical deconditioning responds well to a preoperative and postoperative endurance exercise program. Specific guidelines for exercise prescription are available (Butler, 1995b).

Postoperative reports of chest pain may be due to the sternal incision and musculoskeletal manipulation during surgery. Chest pain secondary to myocardial ischemia or coronary insufficiency is not as likely in the early postoperative months because the heart has been denervated. Any other symptoms of ischemia, such as dyspnea, lightheadedness, faintness, or increase in perceived exertion, should be attended to and reported.

Physical therapy initiated in the coronary care unit (CCU) focuses on restoring mobility, increasing strength, and improving balance and reflexes; heel slides, ankle pumps, and bedside standing are included in the early postoperative protocol. Pulmonary hygiene and breathing exercises are essential to prevent atelectasis (particularly left lower lobe atelectasis) especially in the case of implantation of an artificial heart, because of the location of the device. Frequent, slow, rhythmic reaching, turning, bending, and stretching of the trunk and all extremities many times throughout the day helps alleviate the surgical pain-tension cycle and facilitates pulmonary function.

Progressive ambulation can be initiated as soon as the client can transfer. Sternal precautions are standard postoperative orders; preventing separation of the sternum may require handheld assistance in place of assistive devices (e.g., walker, quad cane) initially. When the client can ambulate 1000 feet, the treadmill (1 mile/hour) or exercise cycle (0.5 RPEs [rating of perceived exertion]) can be used (see Table 10–14), usually around the fourth postoperative day, if there are no complications (Kavanagh, 1994).

Whether to use the treadmill or bicycle is usually an individual decision made by the client based on personal preference; presence of orthopedic problems must be taken into consideration. Resistive elastic or small weights and aerobic training are introduced between 4 and 6 weeks postoperatively. Pushing or pulling activities and lifting more than 10 lb are contraindicated in the first 4 to 6 weeks.

Effects of Immunosuppressants

Prolonged use of immunosuppressives such as prednisone may result in decreased bone density; joint deterioration in a small number of people and other complications may also occur (Howe and Edwards, 1995) (see Chapter 4). Specific to cardiac transplantation, cyclosporine-induced hyperuricemia may occur 3 to 4 years after initiation of cyclosporine, especially in people with a history of gout before transplantation. It is characterized by early symptoms of gout, including arthralgias and monoarthritis affecting the first metatarsophalangeal joint, knees, ankles, heels, and insteps. Over time, upper extremity joints become involved, progressing to polyarticular chronic arthritis. There is a greater occurrence of early involvement of atypical joints (other than knees and feet) in people taking cyclosporine with the development of tophi around the time of initial symptoms (Fig. 10–37). Treatment is as for primary gout (see Chapter 23).

Exercise

The use of lower extremity–derived aerobic exercise to improve hemodynamics, normalize heart rate, improve oxygen uptake and delivery, and decrease diastolic blood pressure has been documented (Kavanagh, 1991; Shephard, 1991). Because of the physiologic changes unique to heart transplant clients, a thorough warmup prior to exercise is required to stimulate catecholamine release and give the heart necessary time to prepare for peak activity. Factors such as lower increases in peak heart rate, systolic blood pressure, stroke volume, and cardiac output produce a lower maximum exercise tolerance when compared with that of someone of the same age who has not had a heart transplant.

Likewise, a cooldown period is essential; resting heart rate should be around 100 beats/min before leaving the clinic. Cyclosporine raises the resting heart rate, but dosages are eventually decreased. Everyone reacts differently, even to the same amounts of this medication; watch for a decreased resting heart rate as the dosage is decreased, keeping in mind that the normal resting heart rate of a transplanted heart remains in the range of 90 to 99 beats/min.

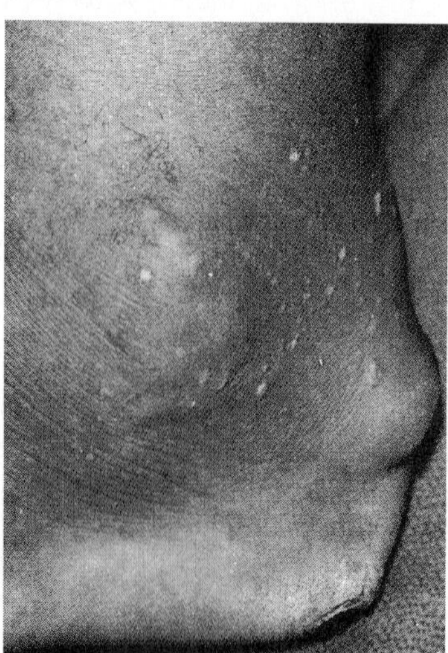

Figure **10–37.** Tophus, a chalky deposit of sodium urate present in the Achilles tendon and foot in a cardiac transplant recipient. These tophi form most often around the joints in cartilage, bone, bursae, and subcutaneous tissue, producing a chronic foreign body inflammatory response. (*From Howe S, Edwards NL: Controlling hyperuricemia and gout in cardiac transplant recipients. Musculoskel Med 12:15–24, 1995.*)

Monitoring During Exercise

Exercise tolerance must be monitored closely during the early weeks after surgery. Ischemic damage during transport of the donor heart or subclinical damage associated with early rejection in combination with the denervated status of the heart may only become apparent during exercise. The therapist is encouraged to use perceived exertion scales such as the dyspnea index (Temes, 1994) or Borg scale (Barr, 1994; Borg, 1982; Pollock and Wilmore, 1990) (see Table 10–14), monitor changes in diastolic pressure (see below), and rely on measurements of oxygen uptake to set exercise limits.

As the transplanted heart is less compliant, exercise in an upright position is preferred to increase venous return, improve heart compliance, increase heart rate, and improve cardiac performance (Bonzheim et al., 1992; Mettauer, 1991; Rudas, 1990). This reduced compliance or "stiffness" of the heart requires increased blood pressure to fill the ventricles. Consequently, the transplanted heart has a reduced cardiac output and therefore a reduced reserve. This reduced reserve will be most evident during exercise, requiring close monitoring for increased diastolic blood pressure (±10 to 15 mm Hg*). Most recipients receiving cyclosporine are more hypertensive, whereas individuals taking calcium channel blockers may experience decreased blood pressure. Any diastolic measurement consistently over 90 mm Hg should be reported to the physician, keeping in mind that kidney function and medications affect this measurement.

Isometric exercise puts a volume stress rather than a pressure stress on the heart and cannot be graduated. For this reason, isometric exercise *may* be considered to be contraindicated†; it should be initiated only with the physician's approval and performed with extreme caution only after considerable dynamic warmup to raise the heart rate (Fletcher et al., 1990). Exercise should be stopped or decreased in intensity if the diastolic pressure exceeds 120 mm Hg (Amundsen, 1979).

* Other sources indicate an increase/decrease greater than 20 mm Hg or a diastolic blood pressure greater than 120 mm Hg at rest (Butler, 1995b). Each physician/center will have known protocols for these guidelines available through the nursing staff.

† This contraindication is under consideration at this time; research for the transplanted population likely will be reported in the near future.

Cardiogenic Shock

Shock is acute, severe circulatory failure associated with a variety of precipitating conditions. Regardless of the cause, shock is associated with marked reduction of blood flow to vital organs, eventually leading to cellular damage and death. See Table 11-1 for categories and causes of shock.

The therapist may see a client in one of three stages of shock. The first stage, *compensated hypotension*, is characterized by reduced cardiac output that stimulates compensatory mechanisms that alter myocardial function and peripheral resistance. During this stage, the body tries to maintain circulation to vital organs such as the brain and the heart and clinical symptoms are minimal. Blood pressure may remain normotensive.

In stage 2, compensatory mechanisms for dealing with the low delivery of nutrients to the body are overwhelmed, and tissue perfusion is decreased. Early signs of cerebral, renal, and myocardial insufficiency are present. *Cardiogenic shock* (inadequate cardiac function) may result from disorders of the heart muscle, valves, or the electrical pacing system. Shock associated with MI or other serious cardiac disease carries a high mortality rate. The therapist is only likely to see this type of client in a CCU setting.

Stage 3 is characterized by severe ischemia with damage to tissues by toxins and antigen-antibody reactions. The kidneys, liver, and lungs are especially susceptible; ischemia of the GI tract allows invasion by bacteria with subsequent infection.

Clinical manifestations of shock may include (early stages): tachycardia; increased respiratory rate; and distended neck veins. In early septic shock (vascular shock caused by infection), there is hyperdynamic change with increased circulation so that the skin is warm and flushed and the pulse is bounding rather than weak.

In the second phase of shock (late septic shock) hypofusion (reduced blood flow) occurs with cold skin and weak pulses; hypotension (systolic blood pressure of 90 mm Hg or less[30]); mottled extremities with weak or absent peripheral pulses; and collapsed neck veins. This phase is usually irreversible; the client is unresponsive, and cardiovascular collapse eventually occurs.

Treatment is directed toward both the manifestations of shock and its cause.

Special Implications for the Therapist **10-22**

CARDIOGENIC SHOCK

The therapist in an acute care or home health setting may be working with a client who is demonstrating signs and symptoms of impending shock. Careful monitoring of vital signs and clinical observations will alert the therapist to the need for medical intervention (see early signs of shock listed in previous section). The client in question may demonstrate normal mental status or may become restless, agitated, and confused.

For the acute care therapist, people hospitalized with shock are critically ill and are usually unresponsive. Cardiopulmonary and musculoskeletal function as well as prevention of further complications will be the focus of physical therapy care. Treatment for the immobile person in shock, which is directed toward positioning, skin care, and pulmonary function, must be short but in duration effective, to avoid fatiguing the person.

[30] Some healthy adults may have blood pressure levels this low without ill effects or with only minor symptoms of orthostatic hypotension when changing positions quickly.

The Cardiac Client and Surgery

Persons with previously diagnosed cardiac disease undergoing general or orthopedic surgery are at risk for additional postoperative complications. Anesthesia and surgery are often associated with marked fluctuations of heart rate and blood pressure, changes in intravascular volume, myocardial ischemia or depression, arrhythmias, decreased oxygenation, and increased sympathetic nervous system activity (Massie, 1994). Additionally, changes in medications, surgical trauma, wound healing, infection, hemorrhage, and pulmonary insufficiency may overwhelm the diseased heart. All of these factors place an additional stress on the cardiac client during the perioperative period.

Special Implications for the Therapist **10-23**

CARDIAC CLIENT AND SURGERY

Therapy for these clients is only altered by the need for more deliberate and careful monitoring of the person's response to activity and exercise. Postoperative rehabilitation may take longer because of the underlying cardiac condition and any complications that may arise as a result of cardiovascular compromise. Careful observation for DVT must be ongoing during the first 1 to 3 weeks postoperatively. Anyone with polycythemia or thrombocytopenia is at increased risk for hemorrhage, necessitating additional special precautions (see Chapter 11).

The Cardiac Client and Pregnancy

Normal physiologic changes during pregnancy can exacerbate symptoms of underlying cardiac disease, even in previously asymptomatic individuals. The most common cardiovascular complications of pregnancy are peripartum cardiomyopathy, aortic dissection, and pregnancy-related hypertension. Peripartum cardiomyopathy or cardiomyopathy of pregnancy is discussed briefly earlier in the text (see Cardiomyopathy). Pregnancy predisposes to aortic dissection, possibly because of the accompanying connective tissue changes. Dissection usually occurs near term or shortly postpartum in the arteries (including coronary arteries) or the aorta (Massie, 1994). Treatment and special implications are the same as for aneurysm. Pregnancy-related hypertension is discussed in Chapter 17.

The Heart in Collagen Vascular Diseases

Collagen vascular diseases (now more commonly referred to as *diffuse connective tissue disease*) (Box 10–13) often involve the heart, although cardiac symptoms are usually less prominent than other manifestations of the disease (Jennings et al., 1994).

BOX 10-13
Collagen Vascular Diseases

Ankylosing spondylitis
Dermatomyositis
Localized (cutaneous) scleroderma
Mixed connective tissue disease
Polyarteritis nodosa
Polymyalgia rheumatica
Polymyositis
Rheumatoid arthritis (RA)
Sjögren's syndrome
Systemic lupus erythematosus (SLE)
Systemic sclerosis (scleroderma)
Temporal arteritis

Lupus Carditis

SLE is a multisystem clinical illness (see Chapter 5) characterized by an inflammatory process that can target all parts of the heart, including the coronary arteries, pericardium, myocardium, endocardium, conducting system, and valves (Spiera and Rothschild, 1995; Stevens and Ziminski, 1992). Lupus cardiac involvement may include pericarditis, myocarditis, endocarditis, or a combination of the three.

Pericarditis is the most frequent cardiac lesion associated with SLE, presenting with the characteristic substernal chest pain that varies with posture, becoming worse in recumbency and improving with sitting or bending forward. In some people, pericarditis may be the first manifestation of SLE.

Myocarditis (see also Myocardial Disease) is a serious complication reported to occur in less than 10% of people with SLE. The simultaneous involvement of cardiac and skeletal muscle may occur more commonly than previously suspected. More sensitive diagnostic techniques now make early detection of occult myocarditis possible. Myocarditis in association with SLE occurs most often as left ventricular dysfunction and conduction abnormalities with varying degrees of heart block (Borenstein et al., 1978).

Lupus endocarditis occurs in up to 30% of persons affected by SLE. Major lesions associated with lupus endocarditis include the formation of multiple noninfectious wartlike elevations (verrucae) around or on the surface of the cardiac valves, most commonly the mitral and tricuspid valves. Other types of valvular disease associated with SLE include mitral and aortic regurgitation or stenosis.

Cardiac disease can occur as a direct result of the autoimmune process responsible for SLE or secondary to hypertension, renal failure, hypercholesterolemia (excess serum cholesterol), drug therapy for SLE, and, more rarely, infection (infective carditis).

Rheumatoid Arthritis

On rare occasions, the heart is involved as a part of rheumatoid arthritis (RA), a chronic, systemic, inflammatory disorder that can affect various organs but predominantly involves synovial tissues of joints (see Chapter 23). When the heart is affected, rheumatoid granulomatous inflammation with fibrinoid necrosis may occur in the pericardium, myocardium, or valves. Involvement of the heart in RA does not compromise cardiac function.

Ankylosing Spondylitis

Ankylosing spondylitis is a chronic, progressive inflammatory disorder affecting fibrous tissue primarily in the sacroiliac joints, spine, and large peripheral joints (see Chapter 23). A characteristic aortic valve lesion develops in as many as 10% of persons with long-standing ankylosing spondylitis. The aortic valve ring is dilated, and the valve cusps are scarred and shortened. The functional consequence is aortic regurgitation (see Aortic Regurgitation).

Scleroderma

Scleroderma or systemic sclerosis is a rheumatic disease of the connective tissue characterized by hardening of the connective tissue (see Chapter 8). Involvement of the heart in persons with scleroderma is second only to renal disease as a cause of death in scleroderma. The myocardium exhibits intimal sclerosis (hardening) of small arteries, which leads to small infarctions and patchy fibrosis. As a result, CHF and arrhythmia are common. Cor pulmonale may occur secondary to interstitial fibrosis of the lungs, and hypertensive heart disease may occur as a result of renal involvement.

Polyarteritis Nodosa

Polyarteritis refers to a condition of multiple sites of inflammatory and destructive lesions in the arterial system; the lesions consist of small masses of tissue in the form of nodes or projections (nodosum) (see previous discussion in this chapter). The heart is involved in up to 75% of cases of polyarteritis nodosa. The necrotizing lesions of branches of the coronary arteries result in MI, arrhythmias, or heart block. Cardiac hypertrophy and failure secondary to renal vascular hypertension occurs.

Special Implications for the Therapist **10-24**

COLLAGEN VASCULAR DISEASES

Treatment of the collagen vascular diseases described must take into consideration the possibility of cardiac involvement. The physician has usually diagnosed concomitant cardiac disease, but complete health care records are not available to the therapist. If the therapist identifies signs or symptoms of cardiac origin, the client may be able to confirm previous diagnosis of the condition. In such cases, careful monitoring may be all that is required. However, the alert therapist may be the first health care provider to identify signs or symptoms of underlying dysfunction during onset, necessitating medical referral. (See each collagen vascular disease for discussion of individual implications.)

Cardiac Complications of Cancer Treatment

(Watchie, 1992)

Chest radiation for any type of cancer (e.g., Hodgkin's disease, non-Hodgkin's lymphoma, lung cancer, breast cancer) exposes the heart (and lungs) to varying degrees and doses of radiation. Cardiac toxicity may occur following chest irradiation and the administration of many chemotherapeutic agents. Previous mediastinal radiation and increasing cumulative doses of chemotherapy or irradiation are known risk factors for the development of cardiotoxicity.

The most common manifestations of cardiotoxicity are cardiac arrhythmias or acute or chronic pericarditis. Other cardiac problems that may develop include myocardial fibrosis with a resultant restrictive cardiomyopathy, conduction disturbances, accelerated and radiation-induced CAD, and valvular dysfunction.

Although only a small percentage of persons develop serious problems or obvious symptoms of cardiotoxicity, many people have functional limitations that are not clinically apparent because they are physically inactive.

Special Implications for the Therapist **10–25**

CARDIAC COMPLICATIONS OF CANCER TREATMENT

Any client referred to therapy who has completed oncologic treatment should be assessed for potential cardiac (and pulmonary) dysfunction, including questions about previous and current activity levels, evaluation of exercise tolerance or endurance, monitoring of heart rate and rhythm, blood pressure, and respiratory responses. Any symptoms of exercise intolerance (shortness of breath, lightheadedness or dizziness, fatigue, pallor, palpitations, and chest pain or discomfort) must be noted. (See also Special Implications for the Therapist: Pericarditis and Cardiomyopathy.) Specific exercise guidelines have also been outlined for the inclusion of gradual endurance training as a part of the treatment plan for anyone with cardiotoxicity secondary to oncologic treatment (Watchie, 1992). (See also Radiation Injuries, Chapter 4.)

References

Ades PA: Hypertension, exercise, and beta-adrenergic blockade. Ann Intern Med 109:629–634, 1988.

Agency for Health Care Policy and Research: Clinical Guideline No. 17, Cardiac Rehabilitation. Columbia, Md, 1995. (Copies are available for $8.00 from the Government Printing Office (202) 512–1800. Order: stock No. 01702600154–9.

Alliance for Aging Research: Awareness and Knowledge of Congestive Heart Failure among Adults Age 50 and Over. New York, The Gallup Organization, Nov 1993.

Alonzo G, Aros F, Bello MC, et al: The prescription of physical exercise in the individual with aortic prostheses: The role of Doppler exercise study. Rev Esp Cardiol 46:727–734, 1993.

Amato AA, Barohn RJ, Sahenk Z, et al: Polyneuropathy complicating bone marrow and solid organ transplantation. Neurology 43:1513–1518, 1993.

American College of Sports Medicine: Guidelines for Exercise Testing and Prescription, ed 5. Baltimore, Williams & Wilkins, 1995.

American Heart Association: 1993 Heart and Stroke Facts Statistics. Dallas, American Heart Association, 1992.

Aminoff MJ: Nervous system. *In* Tierney LM, McPhee SJ, Papadakis MA (eds): Current Medical Diagnosis and Treatment. Norwalk, Conn, Appleton & Lange, 1994, pp 798–854.

Amundsen LR: Assessing exercise tolerance: A review. Phys Ther 59:534–537, 1979.

Andersen HS, Devereux RB: Mitral valve prolapse: Guidelines for diagnosis and management. J Musculoskel Med 11:38–50, 1994.

Anderson TJ, Marwick T, Williams J, et al: Tests for Detecting Heart Disease in Women. Presented at the American College of Cardiology Annual Meeting, New Orleans, 1995.

Andreoli TE, Bennett JC, Carpenter CCJ, et al: Cecil Essentials of Medicine, ed 3. Philadelphia, WB Saunders, 1993.

Aronow WS: Echocardiography should be performed in all elderly patients with congestive heart failure. J Am Geriatr Soc 42:1300–1302, 1994.

Aspinall W: Clinical testing for the craniovertebral hypermobility syndrome. J Orthop Sports Phys Ther 12:180–181, 1989.

Åstrand P-O, Rodahl K: Textbook of Work Physiology: Physiological Basis of Exercise, ed 2. New York, McGraw-Hill, 1977.

Barr RN: Pulmonary rehabilitation. *In* Hillegass E, Sadowsky S: Essentials of Cardiopulmonary Physical Therapy. Philadelphia, WB Saunders, 1994, p 685.

Barrett-Connor E, Bush TL: Estrogen and coronary heart disease in women. JAMA 265:1861–1867, 1991.

Barrett-Connor E, Laakso M: Ischemic heart disease risk in postmenopausal women: Effects of estrogen use on glucose and insulin levels. Arteriosclerosis 10:531–534, 1990.

Bastien MR, Goldstein BG, Lesher JL, et al: Treatment of lymphedema with a multicompartmental pneumatic compression device. J Am Acad Dermatol 20:853–854, 1989.

Bauwens DB, Paine R: Thoracic pain. *In* Blacklow RS (ed.): MacBryde's Signs and Symptoms, ed 6. Philadelphia, JB Lippincott, 1983, pp 139–164.

Beilin LJ, Puddey IB, Burke V: Alcohol and hypertension: Kill or cure? J Hum Hypertens 10(suppl 2):S1–5, 1996.

Benditt EP, Schwartz SM: Blood vessels. *In* Rubin E, Farber JL (eds): Pathology, ed 2. Philadelphia, JB Lippincott, 1994, pp 454–501.

Bergren CT: Wound Ballistics and Medical Consequences: A Health Care Providers Handbook. US Air Force Publication, San Antonio, 1993.

Berkow R, Fletcher AJ (eds): The Merck Manual of Diagnosis and Therapy, ed 16. Rahway, NJ, Merck Sharp & Dohme, 1992.

Birovljev S, Radovancevic B, Burnett SM, et al: Heart transplantation after mechanical circulatory support: Four years' experience. J Heart Lung Transplant 11:240–245, 1992.

Bjorntorp P: Hypertension and exercise. Hypertension 4(suppl 3):56–59, 1982.

Blanchard DG, Kimura BJ, Dittrich HC, et al: Transesophageal echocardiography of the aorta. JAMA 272:546–551, 1994.

Blumenthal JA, Siegel WC, Appelbaum M: Failure of exercise to reduce blood pressure in patients with mild hypertension. JAMA 266:2098–2104, 1991.

Blumenthal JA, Thyrum ET, Gullette ED, et al: Do exercise and weight loss reduce blood pressure in patients with mild hypertension? NC Med J 56:92–95, 1995.

Bonzheim SC, Franklin BA, DeWitt C, et al: Physiologic responses to recumbent versus upright cycle ergometry, and implications for exercise prescription in patients with coronary artery disease. Am J Cardiol 69:40–44, 1992.

Borenstein DG, Fye B, Arnett FC, et al: The myocarditis of systemic lupus erythematosus: Association with myositis. Ann Intern Med 89:619–625, 1978.

Borg GAV: Psychophysical bases of perceived exertion. Med Sci Sports Exerc 14:377–387, 1982.

Boris M, Weindorf S, Lasinski B: Lymphedema reduction by noninvasive complex lymphedema therapy. Oncology 8:95–110, 1994.

Bortz WM: Disuse and aging. JAMA 248:1203–1208, 1982.

Branch KR, Dembitsky WP, Peterson KL, et al: Physiology of the native heart and Thermo Cardiosystems left ventricular assist device complex at rest and during exercise: Implications for chronic support. J Heart Lung Transplant 13:641–650, 1994.

Braunwald E: Clinical aspects of heart failure. *In* Braunwald E, Grossman W (eds): Heart Disease: A Textbook of Cardiovascular Medicine, ed 4. Philadelphia, WB Saunders, 1992, pp 444–463.

Breuer C: Treatment for Heart Valve Disease. Presented at the American Chemical Society, Anaheim, Calif, 1995.

Brockington GM: Constrictive pericarditis. Cardiol Clin 8:645, 1990.

Burks R: Effective treatment of venous insufficiency ulcers. Acute Care Perspectives Summer 1995, pp 1–4.

Busby MJ, Bellantoni MF, Tobin JD, et al: Glucose tolerance in women: The effects of age, body composition, and sex hormones. J Am Geriatr Soc 40:497–502, 1992.

Butler BB: Personal communication. May 1995a.

Butler BB: Physical therapy in heart and lung transplantation. *In* Irwin S,

Tecklin J (eds): Cardiopulmonary Physical Therapy, ed 3. St Louis, Mosby–Year Book, 1995b, pp 404–422.

Butler BB: Physiologic Changes Unique to Heart Transplant Patients: Treatment Precautions. American Physical Therapy Association, Combined Sections Meeting, San Francisco, 1992.

Butler D: Mobilization of the Nervous System. New York, Churchill Livingstone, 1991.

Butler RM, Beierwaltes WH, Rogers FJ: The cardiovascular response to circuit weight training in patients with cardiac disease. J Cardpulm Rehabil 7:402–409, 1987.

Cahalin LP: Cardiac muscle dysfunction. *In* Hillegass E, Sadowsky S (ed): Essentials of Cardiopulmonary Physical Therapy. Philadelphia, WB Saunders, 1994, pp 123–188.

Callam MJ, Ruckley CV, Dale JJ, et al: Hazards of compression treatments of the leg. Br Med J 295:1382, 1988.

Canobbio MM: Cardiovascular Disorders. St Louis, Mosby–Year Book, 1990.

Carstens V, Behrenbeck DW, Hilger HH: Exercise capacity before and after cardiac valve surgery. Cardiology 70:41–49, 1983.

Casale P: The pros and cons of atherectomy. *In* Pashkow FJ, Libov C: The Woman's Heart Book. New York, Penguin Books, 1993, pp 209–211.

Casley-Smith JR, Casley-Smith JR: The frequency of lymphedema. *In* Casley-Smith JR, Casley-Smith JR (eds): Lymphedema. Adelaide, Australia, The Lymphedema Association of Australia, 1991, pp 74–77.

Casley-Smith JR, Foldi M, Ryan TJ, et al: Summary of the 10th International Congress of Lymphology, working group discussions and recommendations. Lymphology 18:175–180, 1985.

Casley-Smith JR, Morgan RG, Piller NB: Treatment of lymphedema of the arms and legs with 5, 6 benzo-alpha-pyrone. N Engl J Med 329:1158–1163, 1993.

Castelli WP: Epidemiology of triglycerides: A view from Framingham. Am J Cardiol 70:3H–9H, 1992.

Centers for Disease Control and Prevention: Protective effect of physical activity on coronary heart disease. MMWR 36:426–430, 1987.

Centers for Disease Control and Prevention: Chronic disease reports: Deaths from coronary heart disease—United States, 1986. MMWR, 38:285, 1989.

Chang RW: Cardiac manifestations of SLE. Clin Rheum Dis 8:197–206, 1982.

Chang TS, Han LY, Gan JL, et al: Microwave: An alternative to electric heating in the treatment of peripheral lymphedema. Lymphology 22:20–24, 1989.

Clarkson TB, Williams JK, Adams MR: Experimental effects of estrogens and progestins on the coronary artery wall. *In* Wenger NK, Speroff L, Packard B (eds): Proceedings of an NHLBI Conference: Cardiovascular Health and Disease in Women. Greenwich, Conn, Le Jacq Communications, 1993, pp 169–174.

Coats AJS, Adamopoulos S, Meyer TE, et al: Effects of physical training in chronic heart failure. Lancet 335:63, 1990.

Coats AJS, Adamopoulos S, Radaelli A, et al: Controlled trial of physical training in chronic heart failure: Exercise, performance, hemodynamics, ventilation, and autonomic function. Circulation 85:2119–2131, 1992.

Cohen M, Michel TH: Cardiopulmonary Symptoms in Physical Therapy Practice. New York, Churchill Livingstone, 1988.

Cohn JN: Physiological rationale for co-treatment with diuretics in heart failure. Br Heart J 72(2 suppl):S63–67, 1994a.

Cohn JN: Vasodilators in heart failure. Drugs 47(suppl 4):47–58, 1994b.

Cohn JN: Treatment of infarct related heart failure: Vasodilators other than ACE inhibitors. Cardiovasc Drugs 8:119–122, 1994c.

Cohn JN: Has the problem of heart failure been solved? Am J Cardiol 73:40C–43C, 1994d.

Cohn MS, Seiger E, Goldman S: Ambulatory phlebectomy using the tumescent technique for local anesthesia. Dermatol Surg 21:315–318, 1995.

Colditz G, Walter B, Willetts W, et al: Menopause and the risk of coronary heart disease in women. N Engl J Med 316:1105–1110, 1987.

Collins P, Rosano GMC, Jiang C, et al: Cardiovascular protection by estrogen: A calcium antagonist effect? Lancet 341:1264–1265, 1993.

Cortes CW, Goetz JM: Guidelines for exercise training in the older cardiac patient. Cardiovasc Rev Rep 15:52–58, 1994.

Cumming GR: Children with heart disease. *In* Skinner JS: Exercise Testing and Exercise Prescription for Special Cases, ed 2. Philadelphia, Lea & Febiger, 1993a, pp 291–315.

Cumming GR: Valvular and congenital heart disease in adults. *In* Skinner JS: Exercise Testing and Exercise Prescription for Special Cases, ed 2. Philadelphia, Lea & Febiger, 1993b, pp 317–338.

Dahlman T, Lindvall N, Hellgren M: Osteopenia in pregnancy during long-term heparin treatment: A radiologic survey post partum. Br J Obstet Gynecol 97:221–228, 1990.

Davis LB, McCulloch JM, Neal MB: The effectiveness of Unna boot and semipermeable film vs. Unna boot alone in the healing of venous ulcers. Ostomy Wound Manage 38:19–21, 1992.

Dean E: Guidelines for the delivery of cardiopulmonary physical therapy: Intensive care. *In* Frownfelter D, Dean E, (eds): Principles and Practices of Cardiopulmonary Physical Therapy, ed 3. St Louis, Mosby–Year Book, 1996, pp 565–616.

DeMaria A, Klein A, Belli G, et al: Transesophageal echocardiography: Why and when to use it. Cleve Clin J Med 61:211–218, 1994.

DeMaria AN, Lee G, Amsterdam EA, et al: The anginal syndrome with normal coronary arteries. JAMA 244:826–828, 1980.

Dennison PD, Black JM: Nursing care of clients with peripheral vascular disorders. *In* Black JM, Matassarin-Jacobs E (eds): Luckmann and Sorensen's Medical-Surgical Nursing, ed 4. Philadelphia, WB Saunders, 1993, pp 1253–1314.

DeSanctis RW: Cardiomyopathies. Sci Am Med 1(I–XIV):1–23, 1990.

Devereux RB, Brown WT, Kramer-Fox R, et al: Inheritance of mitral valve prolapse: Effect of age and sex on gene expression. Ann Intern Med 97:826–832, 1982.

Devereux RB, Kramer-Fox R, Brown WT, et al: Relation between clinical features of mitral valve prolapse syndrome and echocardiographically documented mitral valve prolapse. J Am Coll Cardiol 8:763–772, 1986.

Devereux RB, Kramer-Fox R, Kligfield P: Mitral valve prolapse: Etiology, clinical manifestations, and management. Ann Intern Med 111:305–317, 1989.

Diethrich EB, Cohen C: Women and Heart Disease. New York, Random House, 1992.

DiMaio VJM: Gunshot Wounds: Practical Aspects of Firearms, Ballistics, and Forensic Techniques. New York, Elsevier, 1985.

Drexler H, Schroeder JS: Unusual forms of ischemic heart disease. Curr Opin Cardiol 9:457–464, 1994.

Durack DT: Infective and noninfective endocarditis. *In* Schlant RC, Alexander RW (eds): Hurst's The Heart, ed 8. New York, McGraw-Hill, 1994, pp 1681–1709.

Eagle KA, DeSanctis RW: Diseases of the aorta. *In* Braunwald E (ed): Heart Disease: A Textbook of Cardiovascular Medicine, ed 4. Philadelphia, WB Saunders, 1992, pp 1528–1557.

Eaker E, Chesebro JH, Sacks FM, et al: Cardiovascular Disease in Women: AHA Medical Scientific Statement: Special Report. Dallas, American Heart Association, 1993.

Echt DS, Liebson PR, Mitchell LB, et al: Mortality and morbidity in patients receiving encainide, flecainide, or placebo: The Cardiac Arrhythmia Suppression Trial (CAST): Mortality in the entire population enrolled. N Engl J Med 324:781–788, 1991.

Edeiken J, Wolferth CC: Persistent pain in the shoulder region following myocardial infarction. Am J Med Sci 191:201–210, 1936.

Edwards KL, Austin MA, Newman B, et al: Multivariate analysis of the insulin resistance syndrome in women. Arterioscler Thromb Vasc Biol 14:1940–1945, 1994.

Elefteriades JA: Bypass risks for women. *In* Pashkow FJ, Libov C: The Woman's Heart Book. New York, Penguin Books, 1993, pp 214–215.

Elliott JM, Berdan LG, Holmes DR, et al: One-year follow-up in the coronary angioplasty versus excisional atherectomy trial (CAVEAT I). Circulation 91:2158–2166, 1995.

Epstein SE, Gerber LH, Borer JS: Chest wall syndrome: A common cause of unexplained cardiac pain. JAMA 241:2793–2797, 1979.

Fenton SH, Fischman DL, Savage MP, et al: Long-term angiographic and clinical outcome after implantation of balloon-expandable stents in aortocoronary saphenous vein grafts. Am J Cardiol 74:1187–1191, 1994.

Ferrannini E: Insulin resistance in essential hypertension. N Engl J Med 317:350–357, 1987.

Fischman DL, Savage MP, Goldberg S: Coronary stent placement in patients with de-novo and restenotic native coronary artery lesions. Coron Artery Dis 5:571–574, 1994.

Fletcher GF, Froelicher VF, Hartley H, et al: Exercise standards: A statement for health professionals from the American Heart Association. Circulation 82:2286–2322, 1990.

Foldi M, Casley-Smith JR (eds): Lymphangiology. Stuttgart, Schattauer, 1983, pp 195–210.

Foldi M: Treatment of lymphedema. Lymphology 27:1–5, 1994.

Francis GS: Congestive heart failure. *In* Rakel R (ed): Conn's Current Therapy 1990. Philadelphia, WB Saunders, 1990, p 242.

Frazier OH: Chronic left ventricular support with a vented electric assist device. Ann Thorac Surg 55:273–275, 1993.

Frazier OH: First use of an untethered, vented electric left ventricular assist device for long-term support. Circulation 89:2908–2914, 1994.

Frazier OH, Macris MP, Myers TJ, et al: Improved survival after extended bridge to cardiac transplantation. Ann Thorac Surg 57:1416–1422, 1994.

Frederickson L: Confronting Mitral Valve Prolapse Syndrome. New York, Warner Books, 1992.

Frownfelter D, Dean E (eds): Principles and Practices of Cardiopulmonary Physical Therapy, ed 3. St Louis, Mosby–Year Book, 1996.

Gardner AW, Poehlman ET: Exercise rehabilitation for the treatment of claudication pain. A meta-analysis. JAMA 274:975–980, 1995.

Garrison GE: Peripheral arterial insufficiency. Hosp Med 11:64–79, 1975.

Gebara OCE, Mittleman MA, Sutherland P, et al: Association between increased estrogen status and increased fibrinolytic potential in the Framingham Offspring Study. Circulation 91:1952–1958, 1995.

Gogia PP (ed): Clinical Wound Management. Thoroughfare, NJ, Slack, 1995.

Goldberg JA: Aerobic and resistive exercise modify risk factors for coronary heart disease. Med Sci Sports Exerc 21:669–674, 1989.

Goldberg JA, Elliot DL: Comparison of labetalol and verapamil at rest and during maximal exercise among hypertensives. Med Sci Sports Exerc 21:S87, 1989.

Goldberg L, Elliot DL: The use of exercise to improve lipid and lipoprotein levels. *In* Goldberg L, Elliot DL (eds): Exercise for Prevention and Treatment of Illness. Philadelphia, FA Davis, 1994a, pp 189–210.

Goldberg L, Elliot DL: Exercise for Prevention and Treatment of Illness. Philadelphia, FA Davis, 1994b.

Goldberg L, Elliott DL: Exercise as treatment for essential hypertension. *In* Goldberg L, Elliott DL (eds.) Exercise for Prevention and Treatment of Illness. Philadelphia, FA Davis, 1994c, pp 27–47.

Goldberg S: A randomized comparison of coronary-stent placement and balloon angioplasty in the treatment of coronary artery disease. N Engl J Med 331:496–501, 1994.

Good MG: The role of skeletal muscles in the pathogenesis of diseases. Acta Med Scand 138:285–292, 1950.

Goodman CC, Snyder TE: Differential Diagnosis in Physical Therapy, ed 2. Philadelphia, WB Saunders, 1995.

Grand Rounds: Abdominal aortic aneurysm. Lancet 341:215–220, 1993.

Granda C: Nursing management of patients with lymphedema associated with breast cancer therapy. Cancer Nursing 17:229–235, 1994.

Granger CB: Thrombolytic therapy for acute myocardial infarction: A review. Drugs 44:293, 1992.

Gray RP, Yudkin JS, Patterson DL: Plasminogen activator inhibitor: A risk factor for myocardial infarction in diabetic patients. Br Heart J 69:228–232, 1993a.

Gray RP, Yudkin JS, Patterson DL: Enzymatic evidence of impaired reperfusion in diabetic patients after thrombolytic therapy for acute myocardial infarction: A role for plasminogen activator inhibitor? Br Heart J 70:530–536, 1993b.

Grimes K, Cohen M: Cardiac medications. *In* Hillegass E, Sadowsky S: Essentials of Cardiopulmonary Physical Therapy. Philadelphia, WB Saunders, 1994, pp 481–529.

Grines CL: A comparison of immediate angioplasty with thrombolytic therapy for acute myocardial infarction. N Engl J Med 328:673, 1993.

Gurwitz JH, Avorn J, Bohn RL, et al: Initiation of antihypertensive treatment during nonsteroidal anti-inflammatory drug therapy. JAMA 272:781–786, 1994.

Gutstein M: Diagnosis and treatment of muscular rheumatism (cases IX and 52). Br J Phys Med 1:302–321, 1938.

Gyenes G, Gornander T, Carlens P, et al: Morbidity of ischemic heart disease in early breast cancer 15–20 years after adjuvant radiotherapy. Int J Radiat Oncol Biol Phys 28:1235–1241, 1994.

Haak SW, Richardson SJ, Davey SS: Alterations of cardiovascular function. *In* McCance KL, Huether SE (eds): Pathophysiology: The Biologic Basis for Disease in Adults and Children, ed 2. St Louis, Mosby–Year Book, 1994, pp 1000–1084.

Hanson P: Exercise testing and training in patients with chronic heart failure. Med Sci Sports Exerc 26:527–537, 1994.

Harris ED: Acute rheumatic fever. Sci Am Med 3(15–VII):1–4, 1991.

Harris KA, Holly RG: Physiological response to circuit weight training in borderline hypertensive subjects. Med Sci Sports Exerc 19:246–252, 1987.

Hartmann A: Serial evaluation of left ventricular function by radionuclide ventriculography at rest and during exercise after orthotopic heart transplantation. Eur J Nucl Med 20:146, 1993.

Haskell WL, Alderman EL, Fair JM, et al: Effects of intensive multiple risk factor reduction on coronary atherosclerosis and clinical cardiac events in men and women with coronary artery disease: The Stanford Coronary Risk Intervention Project (SCRIP). Circulation 89:975–990, 1994.

Haskell WL, Durstine JL: Coronary heart disease. *In* Skinner JS (ed): Exercise Testing and Exercise Prescription for Special Cases, ed 2. Philadelphia, Lea & Febiger, 1993, pp 251–273.

Hauptman PJ, Aranki S, Mudge GH, et al: Early cardiac allograft failure after orthotopic heart transplantation. Am Heart J 127:179–186, 1994.

Haynes BF: Enlargement of lymph nodes and spleen. *In* Isselbacher KJ, Braunwald E, Wilson JD, et al (eds): Harrison's Principles of Internal Medicine, ed 13. New York, McGraw-Hill, 1994, pp 323–329.

Haynes LH, Brown MH, Handley BC, et al: Comparison of Pulsevac and sterile whirlpool regarding the promotion of tissue granulation (abstract). Phys Ther 74 (suppl 5):S4, 1994.

Hellman DB: Arthritis and musculoskeletal disorders. *In* Tierney LM, McPhee SJ, Papadakis MA (eds): Current Medical Diagnosis and Treatment. Norwalk, Conn, Appleton & Lange, 1994, pp 664–710.

Hillegass E: Are You Prescribing Exercise Safely? Activity and Exercise for Patients with Medical Diagnoses. Billings, Montana Physical Therapy Association Spring Meeting, May 19–20, 1995.

Hillegass E, Sadowsky S: Essentials of Cardiopulmonary Physical Therapy. Philadelphia, WB Saunders, 1994.

Hillegass E: Cardiopulmonary assessment. *In* Hillegass E, Sadowsky S: Essentials of Cardiopulmonary Physical Therapy. Philadelphia, WB Saunders, 1994a, pp 553–595.

Hillegass E: Electrocardiography. *In* Hillegass E, Sadowsky S: Essentials of Cardiopulmonary Physical Therapy. Philadelphia, WB Saunders, 1994b, pp 355–401.

Hlatky MA, Lam LC, Lee KL, et al: Job strain and the prevalence and outcome of coronary artery disease. Circulation 92:327–333, 1995.

Holmbäck AM, Säwe U, Fagher B: Training after myocardial infarction: Lack of long-term effects on physical capacity and psychological variables. Arch Phys Med Rehabil 75:551–554, 1994.

Howe S, Edwards NL: Controlling hyperuricemia and gout in cardiac transplant recipients. J Musculoskel Med 12:15–24, 1995.

Hull RD, Kakkar VV, Raskob GE: Prevention of venous thrombosis and pulmonary embolism. *In* Fuster V, Verstraete M (ed): Thrombosis in Cardiovascular Disorders. Philadelphia, WB Saunders, 1992, pp 451–464.

Hunder GG: When musculoskeletal symptoms point to endocarditis. J Musculoskel Med 9:33–40, 1992.

Hunt SA, Schroeder JS, Billingham ME: Cardiac transplantation. *In* Schlant RC, Alexander RW (eds): Hurst's the Heart, 8th ed. New York, McGraw-Hill, Inc., 1994, pp 629–636.

Irwin S, Tecklin JS: Cardiopulmonary Physical Therapy, ed 3. St Louis Mosby–Year Book, 1995.

Jarvis C: Physical Examination and Health Assessment. Philadelphia, WB Saunders, 1992.

Jelinek MV, Lown B: Exercise stress testing for exposure of cardiac arrhythmia. Prog Cardiovasc Dis 16:497–522, 1974.

Jennings RB, Steenbergen C, and Hackel DB: The heart. *In* Rubin E, Farber JL (eds): Pathology, ed 2. Philadelphia, JB Lippincott, 1994, pp 502–555.

Joint National Committee on Detection, Evaluation, and Treatment of High Blood Pressure: The Fifth Annual Report. Arch Intern Med 153:154–183, 1993.

Kannel WB, Garrison RJ, Dannenberg AL: Secular blood pressure trends in normotensive persons: The Framingham Study. Am Heart J 125:1154–1158, 1993.

Kannel WB, McGee DL: Diabetes and cardiovascular disease: The Framingham Study. JAMA 241:2035–2038, 1979.

Kaplan NM: Clinical Hypertension, ed 6. Baltimore, Williams & Wilkins, 1994.

Kaplan NM: The treatment of hypertension in women. Arch Intern Med 155:563–567, 1995.
Karas RH, Patterson BL, Mendelsohn ME: Human vascular smooth muscle cells contain functional estrogen receptor. Circulation 89:1943–1949, 1994.
Kavanagh T: Cardiac rehabilitation. *In* Goldberg L, Elliot DL: Exercise for Prevention and Treatment of Illness. Philadelphia, FA Davis, 1994, pp 48–82.
Kavanagh T: Exercise training in patients after heart transplantation. Herz 16:243–250, 1991.
Kavanagh T: The Toronto Rehabilitation Centre's Cardiac Exercise Program. J Cardiac Rehabil 2:496–502, 1982.
Keene A: Physical examination. *In* Black JM, Matassarin-Jacobs E (eds): Luckmann and Sorensen's Medical-Surgical Nursing, ed 4. Philadelphia, WB Saunders, 1993, pp 215–246.
Kelemen MH: Circuit weight training in cardiac patients. J Am Coll Cardiol 7:38–42, 1986.
Kelly G, McClellan P, Johnson C: Antihypertensive effects of aerobic exercise. Am J Hypertens 7:115–119, 1994.
Kelly M: Pain in the chest: Observations on the use of local anaesthesia in its investigation and treatment. (cases V, VII, and IX) Med J Aust 1:4–7, 1944.
Kennard MA, Haugen FP: The relation of subcutaneous focal sensitivity to referred pain of cardiac origin. J Am Soc Anesthesiol 16:297–311, 1955.
Ketterer MW, Lovallo WR, Lumley MA: Quantifying the density of Friedman's pathogenic emotions (AIAI). Int J Psychosom 40:22–28, 1993.
Ketterer MW: Secondary prevention of ischemic heart disease: The case for aggressive behavioral monitoring and intervention. Psychosomatics 34:478–484, 1993.
Kinney MR, Packa DR: Andreoli's Comprehensive Cardiac Care, ed 8. St Louis, Mosby–Year Book, 1995.
Kisner C, Colby LA: Therapeutic Exercise: Foundations and Techniques, ed 3. Philadelphia, FA Davis, 1996.
Kistner RL, Eklof B, Masuda EM: Deep venous valve reconstruction. Cardiovasc Surg 3:129–140, 1995.
Kitzman DW: Prospective Aerobic Reconditioning Intervention Study (P.A.R.I.S.). Personal communication, February 1995.
Koch M, Douard H, Broustet J-P: The benefit of graded physical exercise in chronic heart failure. Chest 101:231S–235S, 1992.
Kolff J: Beware centrifugal pumps: Not a one-way street, but a potentially dangerous "siphon." Ann Thorac Surg 50:512, 1990.
Kostis JB, Rosen RC, Cosgrove NM, et al: Nonpharmacologic therapy improves functional and emotional status in congestive heart failure. Chest 106:996–1001, 1994.
Krasner D (ed): Chronic Wound Care. King of Prussia, Pa, Health Management Publications, 1990.
Kubik S: The Lymphatic System. New York, Springer, 1985.
Kubo SH, Cohn JN: Approach to treatment of the patient with heart failure in 1994. Adv Intern Med 39:485–515, 1994.
Lakatta EG: Normal changes of aging. *In* Abrams WB, Berkow R (eds): The Merck Manual of Geriatrics: Rahway, NJ, Merck & Co., 1990, pp 310–325.
LaRaus SN: Whirlpool: An overused treatment. Acute Care Perspect Summer 1995, pp 15–17.
Lavie D, Savage D: Prevalence and clinical features of mitral valve prolapse. Am Heart J 113:1281, 1987.
Lawrence KE, Eutsey DE: Cardiovascular Patient Education Resource Manual. Aspen Publishers. Gaithersburg, Md, 1994.
Layzer RB: Neuromuscular Manifestations of Systemic Disease. Philadelphia, FA Davis, 1985.
Lee WR, Fox LM, Slotkoff LM: Effects of antihypertensive therapy on cardiovascular response to exercise. Am J Cardiol 44:325–328, 1979.
Leier CV: Nonpharmacologic considerations in the management of patients with CHF: Activity and exercise. CHF Index Rev 5:1–15, 1993.
Leighton RF: Aerobic exercise: How does it affect serum lipids? J Musculoskel Med 14(2):50–61, 1997.
Leon AS: Diabetes. *In* Skinner JS (ed): Exercise Testing and Exercise Prescription for Special Cases, ed 2. Philadelphia, Lea & Febiger, 1993, pp 153–183.
Leon AS: Enalapril alone and in combination with hydrochlorothiazide in the treatment of hypertension: Effect on treadmill exercise performance. J Cardipulm Rehabil 6:251–256, 1986.
Lerner D, Kannel W: Patterns of coronary heart disease morbidity and mortality in the sexes: A 26-year follow up on the Framingham population. Am Heart J 111:383–390, 1986.
Lerner R, Requena R: Upper extremity lymphedema secondary to mammary cancer treatment. Am J Clin Oncol 9:481–487, 1986.
Linas SL: The role of potassium in the pathogenesis and treatment of hypertension. Kidney Int 39:771–786, 1991.
Lipkin DP, Jones DA, Round JM, et al: Abnormalities of skeletal muscle in patients with chronic heart failure. Int J Cardiol 18:187–195, 1988.
Lipsitz LA: Hypotension. *In* Abrams WB, Berkow R (eds): The Merck Manual of Geriatrics. Rahway, NJ, Merck & Co, 1990, pp 348–352.
Liu NF, Olszewski W: The influence of local hyperthermia on lymphedema and lymphedematous skin of the human leg. Lymphology 26:28–37, 1993.
Lobo R: Estrogen and cardiovascular disease. Ann NY Acad Sci 592:286–294, 1990.
Losordo DW, Kearney BA, Kim EA, et al: Variable expression of the estrogen receptor in normal and atherosclerotic coronary arteries of premenopausal women. Circulation 89:1501–1510, 1994.
MacLennan WJ: Giant cell (temporal) arteritis and polymyalgia rheumatica (PMR). *In* Abrams WB, Berkow R (eds): The Merck Manual of Geriatrics, Rahway, NJ, Merck & Co, 1990, pp 703–710.
Magee DJ: Orthopedic Physical Assessment, ed 3. Philadelphia, WB Saunders, 1997.
Manolio TA, Cutler JA, Furberg CD, et al: Trends in pharmacologic management of hypertension in the United States. Arch Intern Med 155:829–837, 1995.
Mark DB, Shaw LK, DeLong ER, et al: Absence of sex bias in the referral of patients for cardiac catheterization. N Engl J Med 330:1101–1116, 1994.
Mark DB, Shaw LK, Harrell FE, et al: Prognostic value of a treadmill exercise score in outpatients with suspected coronary artery disease. N Engl J Med 325:849–853, 1991.
Massie BM: Cardiovascular disease. *In* Tierney LM, McPhee SJ, Papadakis MA (eds): Current Medical Diagnosis and Treatment. Norwalk, Conn, Appleton & Lange, 1994, pp 280–366.
McCance KL, Cipriano PF: Structure and function of the hematologic system. *In* McCance KL, Huether S: Pathophysiology: The Biologic Basis for Disease in Adults and Children, ed 2. St Louis, Mosby–Year Book, 1994, pp 830–859.
McCance KL, Richardson SJ: Structure and function of the cardiovascular and lymphatic systems. *In* McCance KL, Huether SE (eds): Pathophysiology: The Biologic Basis for Disease in Adults and Children, ed 2. St Louis Mosby–Year Book, 1994, pp 943–999.
McCarthy PM, James KB, Savage RM, et al: Implantable left ventricular assist device: Approaching an alternative for end-stage heart failure: Implantable LVAD Study. Circulation 90:1183–1186, 1994a.
McCarthy PM, Wang N, Vargo R: Preperitoneal insertion of the HeartMate 1000 IP implantable left ventricular assist device. Ann Thorac Surg 57:634–638, 1994b.
McCulloch JM: Intermittent pneumatic compression improves venous ulcer healing: A randomized study. Adv Wound Care 7:22–26, 1994.
McCulloch JM, Kloth LC, Feedar JA: Wound Healing: Alternatives in Management, ed 2. Philadelphia, FA Davis, 1995.
Mettauer B: Cardiorespiratory and neurohormonal response to incremental maximal exercise in patients with denervated transplanted hearts. Transplant Proc 23:1178–1181, 1991.
Miller HS, Morley DL: Low functional capacity. *In* Skinner JS (ed): Exercise Testing and Exercise Prescription for Special Cases, ed 2. Philadelphia, Lea & Febiger, 1993, pp 339–349.
Minotti JR, Massie BM: Exercise training in heart failure patients: Does reversing the peripheral abnormalities protect the heart? Circulation 85:2323, 1992.
Minotti JR, Christoph I, Oka R, et al: Impaired skeletal muscle function in patients with congestive heart failure: Relationship to systemic exercise performance. J Clin Invest 88:2077–2082, 1991.
Mittleman MA, Maclure M, Sherwood JB, et al: Triggering of myocardial infarction onset by episodes of anger (abstract). Circulation 89:936, 1994.
Mittleman MA, Maclure M, Tofler GH, et al: Triggering of acute myocardial infarction by heavy physical exertion: Protection against triggering by regular exertion. N Engl J Med 329:1677–1683, 1993.

Moller JH, Neal WA: Fetal, Neonatal, and Infant Cardiac Disease. Norwalk, Conn, Appleton & Lange, 1990.

Morley D, Bove AA: Moderate concentrations of ethanol constrict human coronary arteries. Clin Res 88:431A, 1990.

Mujais SK: Principles and clinical uses of diuretic therapy. Prog Cardiovasc Dis 35:221, 1992.

Muller DW, Gordon D, Topol EJ, et al: Sustained-release local hirulog therapy decreases early thrombosis but not neointimal thickening after arterial stenting. Am Heart J 131(2):211–218, 1996.

Nabulsi AA, Folsom AR, White A, et al: Association of hormone-replacement therapy with various cardiovascular risk factors in postmenopausal women. N Engl J Med 328:1069–1075, 1993.

National Hospital Discharge Survey: Annual Summary. Atlanta, Centers for Disease Control and Prevention, 1991.

Naughton J, Haider R: Methods of exercise testing. *In* Naughton J, Hellerstein HK (eds): Exercise Testing and Exercise Training in Coronary Heart Disease. New York, Academic Press, 1973.

Newburger J: A single intravenous infusion of gammaglobulin as compared with four infusions in the treatment of acute Kawasaki syndrome. N Engl J Med 324:1623–1639, 1991.

Newell J: Physical training after heart valve replacement. Br Heart J 44:638–649, 1980.

Newman MF, Croughwell ND, Blumenthal JA, et al: Effect of aging on cerebral autoregulation during cardiopulmonary bypass: Association with postoperative cognitive dysfunction. Circulation 90:243–249, 1994.

Newman MF, Kramer D, Croughwell ND, et al: Differential age effects of mean arterial pressure and rewarming on cognitive dysfunction after cardiac surgery. Anesth Analg 81:236–242, 1995a.

Nowak J, Hagerman I, Glen M, et al: Electrocardiogram signal variance analysis in the diagnosis of coronary artery disease—a comparison with exercise stress test in an angiographically documented high prevalence population. Clin Cardiol 16:671–682, 1993.

O'Connell JB: Cardiac transplantation: Recipient selection, donor procurement, and medical follow-up. Circulation 86:1061, 1992.

Odio A: The incidence of acute rheumatic fever in a suburban area of Los Angeles: A ten-year study. West J Med 144:179–184, 1986.

Om A, Hess MC: Inotropic therapy of the failing myocardium. Clin Cardiol 16:5, 1993.

Ordog GJ: Management of Gunshot Wounds. New York, Elsevier, 1988.

Ornish D: Can lifestyle changes reverse coronary heart disease? The Lifestyle Heart Trial. Lancet 336:129–133, 1990.

O'Toole M (ed): Miller-Keane Encyclopedia and Dictionary of Medicine, Nursing, and Allied Health, ed 5. Philadelphia, WB Saunders, 1992.

Ott B: Nursing care of clients with disorders of cardiac function. *In* Black JM, Matassarin-Jacobs E (eds): Luckmann and Sorensen's Medical-Surgical Nursing, ed 4. Philadelphia, WB Saunders, 1993, pp 1211–1252.

Pashkow FJ, Libov C: The Woman's Heart Book. New York, Penguin Books, 1993.

Pastan SO, Braunwald E: Renal disorders and heart disease. *In* Braunwald E (ed): Heart Disease: A Textbook of Cardiovascular Medicine, ed 4. Philadelphia, WB Saunders, 1992, pp 1856–1874.

Pasternak RC, Thibault GE, Savoia M, et al: Chest pain with angiographically insignificant coronary arterial obstruction. Am J Med 68:813–817, 1980.

Peel C, Mossberg KA: Effects of cardiovascular medications on exercise response. Physical Therapy 75:387–396, 1995.

Perazella MA: Abdominal pain, hypertension, and renal failure (case study). J Musculoskel Med 12:69–70, 1995.

Piller NB, Morgan RG, Casley-Smith JR: A double-blind cross-over trial of o-(beta hydroxyethyl)-rutosides (benzo-pyrones) in the treatment of lymphedema of the arms and legs. Br J Plast Surg 41:20–27, 1988.

Podrid PJ, Bumio F, Fogel RI: Evaluating patients with ventricular arrhythmias: Role of the signal-averaged electrocardiogram, exercise test, ambulatory electrocardiogram, and electrophysiologic studies. Cardiol Clin 10:371–395, 1992.

Pollock ML, Wilmore JH: Exercise in Health and Disease: Evaluation and Prescription for Prevention and Rehabilitation, ed 2. Philadelphia, WB Saunders, 1990.

Posner BM, Cupples LA, Miller DR, et al: Diet, menopause, and serum cholesterol levels in women: The Framingham Study. Am Heart J 125:483–489, 1993.

Popma JJ, Topol EJ: Adjuncts to thrombolysis for myocardial reperfusion. Ann Intern Med 115:34, 1991.

Puelo PR, Meyer D, Wathen C, et al: Use of rapid assay of subforms of creatine kinase-MB to diagnose or rule out myocardial infarction. N Engl J Med 331:561–566, 1994.

Pugh CR, Arger PH, Sehgal CM: Power, spectral, and color flow Doppler enhancement by a new ultrasonographic contrast agent. J Ultrasound Med 15(12):843–852, 1996.

Radack K, Deck C: Do nonsteroidal antiinflammatory drugs interfere with blood pressure control in hypertensive patients? Gen Intern Med 2:108–112, 1987.

Reagan K, Boxt LM, Katz J: Introduction to coronary arteriography. Radiol Clin North Am 32:419–433, 1994.

Reardon J, Awad E, Normandin E, et al: The effect of comprehensive outpatient pulmonary rehabilitation on dyspnea. Chest 105:1046–1052, 1994.

Reaven GM: Syndrome X: Six years later. J Intern Med 736(suppl): 13–22, 1994.

Rector TS, Cohn JN: Prognosis in congestive heart failure. Annu Rev Med 45:341–350, 1994.

Reigle J, Ringel KA: Nursing care of clients with disorders of cardiac function. *In* Black JM, Matassarin-Jacobs E (eds): Luckmann and Sorensen's Medical-Surgical Nursing, ed 4. Philadelphia, WB Saunders, 1993, pp 1139–1210.

Rich MW: Congestive heart failure in the elderly: Nonpharmacologic aspects of management. Cardiovasc Rev Rep 14:32–37, 1993.

Ridker PM, Vaughan DE, Stampfer MJ, et al: Association of moderate alcohol consumption and plasma concentration of endogenous tissue-type plasminogen activator. JAMA 272:929–933, 1994.

Rinzler SH, Travell J: Therapy directed at the somatic component of cardiac pain (cases 1 and 3). Am Heart J 35:248–268, 1948.

Rivett DA: The premanipulative vertebral artery testing protocol: A brief review. Physiother 23:9–12, 1995.

Rodeheffer RJ, Gerstenblith G, Becker LC, et al: With exercise cardiac output is maintained with advancing age in healthy subjects: Cardiac dilatation and increased stroke volume compensate for a diminished heart rate. Circulation 69:203–213, 1984.

Roden DM: Risks and benefits of antiarrhythmic therapy. N Engl J Med 331:785–791, 1994.

Rose AG, Viviers L, Odell JA: Autopsy-determined causes of death following cardiac transplantation: A study of 81 patients and literature review. Arch Pathol Lab Med 116:1137–1141, 1992.

Rosendorff C, Goodman C, Coull A: Effect of antihypertensive therapy on left ventricular function and myocardial perfusion at rest and during exercise. J Hypertens 2(suppl 2):63–68, 1984.

Rosenson RS, Frauenheim WA, Tangney CC: Dyslipidemias and the secondary prevention of coronary heart disease. Dis Mon 40:369–464, 1994.

Rosenson RS: Reversing coronary artery disease: Diet-based strategies. Physician Sports Med 22:59–64, 1994.

Ross R: Factors affecting atherogenesis. *In* Schlant RC, Alexander RW (eds): Hurst's the Heart, ed 8. New York, McGraw-Hill, 1994, pp 989–1008.

Rudas L: Comparison of hemodynamic responses during dynamic exercise in the upright and supine postures after orthotopic cardiac transplantation. J Am Coll Cardiol 16:1367–1373, 1990.

Sadowsky HS: Thoracic surgical procedures, monitoring, and support equipment. *In* Hillegass E, Sadowsky S: Essentials of Cardiopulmonary Physical Therapy. Philadelphia, WB Saunders, 1994, pp 437–477.

Salvidar M: Safety of a low-weight, low-repetition strength training program in patients with heart disease. Med Sci Sports Exerc 15:119, 1983.

Savage MP, Fischman DL, Schatz RA, et al: Long-term angiographic and clinical outcome after implantation of a balloon-expandable stent in the native coronary circulation. J Am Coll Cardiol 24:1207–1212, 1994.

Schlant RC, Alexander RW (eds): Hurst's the Heart, ed 8. New York, McGraw-Hill, 1994, pp 208, 463.

Schuler G: Myocardial perfusion and regression of coronary heart disease in patients on a regimen of intensive physical exercise and low fat diet. J Am Coll Cardiol 19:34–42, 1992.

Seals DR, Taylor JA, Ng AV, et al: Exercise and aging: Autonomic control of the circulation. Med Sci Sports Exerc 26(5):568–576, May 1994.

Seigneur M: Effect of the consumption of alcohol, white wine, and red wine on platelet function and serum lipids. J Appl Cardiol 5:215–222, 1990.

Shabetai R: Beneficial effects of exercise training in compensated heart failure. Circulation 78:774–775, 1988.
Shane E, Rivas MDC, Silverberg S, et al: Osteoporosis after cardiac transplantation. Am J Med 94:257–264, 1993.
Shepard RJ: Responses to acute exercise and training after cardiac transplantation: A review. Can J Sports Sci 16:9–22, 1991.
Sherwood A, May CW, Siegel WC, et al: Ethnic differences in hemodynamic responses to stress in hypertensive men and women. Am J Hypertens 8:552–557, 1995.
Sineath L: Unpublished data. 1995.
Sokolow M, McIlroy MB, Cheitlin MD: Clinical Cardiology, ed 5. Norwalk, Conn, Appleton & Lange, 1990.
Spiera H, Rothschild J: When systemic lupus erythematosus involves the heart. J Musculoskel Med 12:54–69, 1995.
Stevens MB, Ziminski CM: Heart disease in systemic lupus erythematosus. J Musculoskel Med 9:41–46, 1992.
Stevenson LW: Advanced congestive heart failure: Inpatient treatment and selection for cardiac transplantation. Postgrad Med 94:97–112, 1993.
Stewart SL: Acute MI: A review of pathophysiology, treatment, and complications. J Cardiovasc Nurs 6:1–25, 1992.
Stiller K, Montarello J, Wallace M: Efficacy of breathing and coughing exercises in the prevention of pulmonary complications after coronary artery surgery. Chest 105:741–747, 1994.
Stratton JR, Levy WC, Cerqueira MD, et al: Cardiovascular responses to exercise: Effects of aging and exercise training in healthy men. Circulation 89:1648–1655, 1994.
Sullivan MJ, Higginbotham MB, Cobb FR: Exercise training in patients with chronic heart failure delays ventilatory anaerobic threshold and improves submaximal exercise performance. Circulation 79:324–329, 1989.
Sullivan MJ, Higginbotham MB, Cobb FR: Exercise training in patients with severe left ventricular dysfunction: Hemodynamic and metabolic effects. Circulation 78:506–551, 1988.
Swan KG: Gunshot Wounds: Pathophysiology and Management. St Louis, Mosby–Year Book, 1989.
Swartz M: Textbook of Physical Diagnosis: History and Examination, ed 2. Philadelphia, WB Saunders, 1994.
Swartz MN: Lymphadenitis and lymphangitis. *In* Mandell GL, Bennett JE, Dolin R (ed): Principles and Practices of Infectious Diseases, ed 4. 1995, pp 936–944.
Sylven C, Hagerman I, Ylen M, et al: Variance ECG detection of coronary artery disease—a comparison with exercise stress test and myocardial scintigraphy. Clin Cardiol 17:132–140, 1994.
Szlachcic J: Diltiazem versus propranolol in essential hypertension: Responses of rest and exercise blood pressure and effects on exercise capacity. Am J Cardiol 59:393–399, 1987.
Szlachcic J, Massie BM, Kramer BL, et al: Correlates and prognostic implication of exercise capacity in chronic congestive heart failure. Am J Cardiol 55:1037–1042, 1985.
Tanio JW, Eisen HJ: Medical aspects of cardiac transplantation: Management update. Hosp Pract 28:61–74, 1993.
Taylor S: Coronary artery disease risk factor management in the hypertensive patient. Am J Cardiol 59:2G–8G, 1987.
Temes WC: Cardiac rehabilitation. *In* Hillegass E, Sadowsky S: Essentials of Cardiopulmonary Physical Therapy. Philadelphia, WB Saunders, 1994, pp 633–675.
Tesch PA: Exercise performance and beta-blockade. Sports Med 2:389–412, 1985.
Thiadens SRJ: Lymphedema: An Information Booklet, ed 4. San Francisco, National Lymphedema Network, 1995.
Thiel H, Wallace K, Donut J, et al: Effect of various head and neck positions on vertebral artery blood flow. Clin Biomechanics 9:105–110, 1994.
Tiefenbrunn AJ: Clinical benefits of thrombolytic therapy in acute myocardial infarction. Am J Cardiol 69:3A–11A, 1992.
Tierney LM: Blood vessels and lymphatics. *In* Tierney LM, McPhee SJ, Papadakis MA (eds): Current Medical Diagnosis and Treatment. Norwalk, Conn, Appleton & Lange, 1994, pp 385–414.
Todd IC: Effects of daily high-intensity exercise on myocardial perfusion in angina pectoris. Am J Cardiol 68:1593–1599, 1991.
Topol EJ, Fuster V, Harrington RA, et al: Recombinant hirudin for unstable angina pectoris. Circulation 89:1557–1566, 1994.
Travell JG, Simons DG: Myofascial Pain and Dysfunction: The Trigger Point Manual, vol. 1. Baltimore, Williams & Wilkins, 1983.
Urden L, Davie J, Thelan L: Essentials of Critical Care Nursing. St Louis, Mosby–Year Book, 1992.
US Senate Special Committee on Aging: Aging America: Trends and Projections. Washington, DC, United States Department of Health and Human Services, 1991.
Vaillant-Newman A: Definitions to Know with Lymphedema. Princeton, NJ, American Society for the Advancement of Lymphedema Management, 1995.
Van den Ouweland FA, Gribrau FW, Meyboon RH: Congestive heart failure due to nonsteroidal anti-inflammatory drugs in the elderly. Age Aging 17:8–16, 1988.
Vander LB: Acute cardiovascular responses to Nautilus exercise in cardiac patients: Implications for exercise training. Ann Sports Med 2:165–169, 1986.
Vaziri SM, Evans JC, Larson MG, et al: The impact of female hormone usage on the lipid profile: The Framingham Offspring Study. Arch Intern Med 153:2200–2206, 1993.
Veasy LG, Wiedmeier SE, Orsmond GS, et al: Resurgence of acute rheumatic fever in the intermountain area of the United States. N Engl J Med 316:421–427, 1987.
Wajchenberg BL, Malerbi DA, Rocha MS, et al: Syndrome X: A syndrome of insulin resistance: Epidemiological and clinical evidence. Diabetes Metab Rev 10:19–29, 1994.
Wald ER, Dashefsky B, Feidt C, et al: Acute rheumatic fever in Western Pennsylvania and the Tristate area. Pediatrics 80:371–374, 1987.
Waller BF: Atherosclerotic and nonatherosclerotic coronary artery factors in acute myocardial infarction. Cardiovasc Clin 20:29–104, 1989.
Walsh BW, Schiff I, Rosner B, et al: Effects of postmenopausal estrogen replacement on the concentrations and metabolism of plasma lipoproteins. N Engl J Med 325:1196–1204, 1991.
Walsh E: Management of persons with vascular problems. *In* Phipps W, Cassmeyer VL, Sands JK, et al (eds): Medical-Surgical Nursing: Concepts and Clinical Practice, ed 5. St Louis, Mosby–Year Book, 1995, pp 885–928.
Ward A, Taylor PA, Ahlquist L, et al: Exercise and exercise intervention. *In* Ockene RS, Ockene JD: Prevention of Coronary Heart Disease. Boston, Little, Brown, 1992, pp 267–298.
Ward SR, Sutton JM, Pieper KS, et al: Effects of thrombolytic regimen, early catheterization, and predischarge angiographic variables on six-week ventricular function. The TAMI Investigators. Thrombolysis and Angioplasty in Acute Myocardial Infarction. Am J Cardiol 79(5):539–544, 1997.
Watchie J: Cardiopulmonary complications of cancer treatment. Clin Manage 12:92–95, July/August 1992.
Watchie J: Cardiopulmonary implications of specific diseases. *In* Hillegass E, Sadowsky, S: Essentials of Cardiopulmonary Physical Therapy. Philadelphia, WB Saunders, 1994, pp 285–323.
Waters D, Lesperance J: Calcium channel blockers and coronary atherosclerosis: From the rabbit to the real world. Am Heart J 128:1309–1316, 1994.
Weisfeldt ML, LaKatta EG, Gerstenblith G: Aging and the heart. *In* Braunwald E (ed): Heart Disease: A Textbook of Cardiovascular Medicine, ed 4. Philadelphia, WB Saunders, 1992, pp 1656–1669.
Welty FK, Mittleman MA, Healy RW, et al: Similar results of percutaneous transluminal coronary angioplasty for women and men with postmyocardial infarction ischemia. J Am Coll Cardiol 23:35–39, 1994.
Wenger NK: Cardiomyopathy and specific heart muscle disease. *In* Hurst JW, Schlant RC (eds): The Heart, ed 7. New York, McGraw-Hill, 1990, pp 1278–1347.
We're not like men. Harvard Women's Health Watch 2:6, October 1994.
Weschler R: Diabetes and heart disease: Researchers define the connection. Countdown: Juvenile Diabetes Foundation International, Winter 1991, pp 14–22.
World Health Organization: Lymphatic filariasis: Report of a WHO expert committee. WHO Tech Rep Ser 702:1–112, 1984.
Wiley RL, Dunn CL, Cox RH, et al: Isometric exercise training lowers resting blood pressure. Med Sci Sports Exerc 24:749–754, 1992.
Williams B: Insulin resistance: The shape of things to come. Lancet 344:521–524, 1994.
Williams GH: Converting-enzyme inhibitors in the treatment of hypertension. N Engl J Med 319:1517–1525, 1988.
Williams RC: Recognizing and managing rheumatic fever in the 90s. J Musculoskel Med 8:18–27, 1991.
Williams V, Williams R: Anger Kills: Seventeen Strategies for

Controlling the Hostility that can Harm your Health. New York, Harper-Perennial, 1994.
Wissler RW, Vesselinovitch D: Studies of regression of advanced atherosclerosis in experimental animals and man. Ann NY Acad Sci 275:363–378, 1976.
Wolfe CL (ed): Cardiac imaging: Diagnosis and assessment of cardiac disorders. Cardiol Clin 7:483–737, 1989.
Wong D: Whaley & Wong's Essentials of Pediatric Nursing, ed 4. St Louis, Mosby–Year Book, 1993.
Woo MA: Clinical management of the patient with acute myocardial infarction. Nurs Clin North Am 27:189–203, 1992.
Wood PD, Stefanick ML, Dreone DM, et al: Changes in plasma lipids and lipoproteins in overweight men during weight loss through dieting compared with exercise. N Engl J Med 319:1173–1179, 1988.
Wynne J, Braunwald E: The cardiomyopathies and myocarditides. *In* Braunwald E (ed): Heart Disease: A Textbook of Cardiovascular Medicine, ed 4. Philadelphia, WB Saunders, 1992, pp 1394–1450.
Yost JH, Morgan GJ: Cardiovascular effects of NSAIDs. J Musculoskel Med 11:22–34, 1994.
Young JB: Cardiac allograft arteriopathy: An ischemic burden of a different sort. Am J Cardiol 70:9F–13F, 1992.
Yusuf S: Routine medical management of acute myocardial infarction: Lessons from overview of recent randomized controlled trials. Circulation 82(2 suppl):11–117, 1990.

SECTION 2

chapter 11

The Hematologic System

Catherine C. Goodman

Hematology is the branch of science that studies the form and structure of blood and blood-forming tissues. Two major components of blood are examined: plasma and formed elements (erythrocytes or red blood cells [RBCs], leukocytes or white blood cells [WBCs], and platelets or thrombocytes). Delivery of these formed elements throughout the body tissues is necessary for cellular metabolism, defense against injury and invading microorganisms, and acid-base balance. The formation and development of blood cells, which usually takes place in the red bone marrow, is controlled by hormones and feedback mechanisms that maintain an ideal number of cells.

The lymphatic system comprises lymphatic vessels and the lymph nodes. Lymphatic vessels are discussed as part of the cardiovascular system (see Chapter 10), but the lymph nodes are included in this chapter as part of the hematopoietic (blood-forming) system.

The lymph nodes are also part of the lymphoid system, which consists of organs and tissues of the immune system. Lymph fluid passes through these nodes, or valves, which are located in the lymph channels at 1- to 2-cm intervals. As the fluid passes through the nodes, it is purified of harmful bacteria and viruses. Networks of the lymphatic system are situated in several areas of the body and may be considered primary (thymus and bone marrow) or secondary (spleen, lymph nodes, tonsils, and Peyer's patches of the small intestine) (Fig. 11–1). All of the lymphoid organs link the hematologic and immune systems in that they are sites of residence, proliferation, differentiation, or function of lymphocytes[1] and mononuclear phagocytes (mononuclear phagocyte system)[2] (McCance and Cipriano, 1994).

SIGNS AND SYMPTOMS OF HEMODYNAMIC DISORDERS

Hemodynamic disorders are characterized by edema and congestion, infarction, thrombosis and embolism, lymphedema, and hypotension and shock (Box 11–1). *Edema* is the accumulation of excessive fluid within the interstitial tissues or within body cavities. *Congestion* is the accumulation of excessive blood within the blood vessels of an organ or tissue (Harruff, 1994). The forms of lymphedema include cerebral edema, inflammatory edema, peripheral dependent edema, or pulmonary edema. Congestion may be localized, as with a venous thrombosis, or generalized, as with heart failure (i.e., congestive heart failure [CHF]), which results in congestion in the lungs, lower extremities, and abdominal viscera.

Infarction is a localized region of necrosis caused by reduction of arterial perfusion below a level required for cell viability. Such a situation occurs as a result of arterial obstruction due to atherosclerosis, arterial thrombosis, or embolism, when oxygen supply fails to meet the oxygen requirements of organs with end-arteries such as the gastrointestinal (GI) tract and heart and, less often, the kidneys and spleen. Cerebral cortical neurons (cerebral infarction) and myocardial cells (myocardial infarction) are most vulnerable to ischemia, although protective collateral blood flow develops in the heart through anastomoses. A common cause of infarction of the lower extremity is diabetes, often causing gangrene and necessitating amputation.

A *thrombus* is a solid mass of clotted blood within an intact blood vessel or chamber of the heart. An *embolus* is a mass of solid, liquid, or gas that moves within a blood vessel to lodge at a site distant from its place of origin (see Fig. 10–22). Most emboli are thromboemboli. Thrombosis (development of a thrombus or clot) results from pathologic activation of the hemostatic mechanisms involving platelets, coagulation factors, and blood vessel walls. Endothelial injury, alteration in blood flow (stasis and turbulence), and hypercoagulability of the blood promote thrombosis and thromboembolism (Harruff, 1994).

Lymphedema, or chronic swelling of an area owing to accumulation of interstitial fluid (edema), occurs in hematolymphatic disorders secondary to obstruction of lymphatic vessels or lymph nodes. Obstruction may be of an inflammatory or mechanical nature from trauma, regional lymph node resection or irradiation, or extensive involvement of regional nodes by malignant disease. Women who have been treated surgically for breast cancer with lymph node dissection, mastectomy, and/or radiation therapy are at double the risk of developing lymphedema.

When the obstruction that slows the lymph fluid exceeds the pumping capacity of the system, the fluid accumulates in the tissues in the extremity, causing edema in one or more limbs. This accumulation of fluid may become a source for bacterial growth, leading to infection, fibrosis, and possible loss of functional limb use (see also Lymphedema, Chapter 10).

Shock occurs when the hemodynamic changes diminish arterial blood circulation and the organs and tissues do not receive adequate oxygen to meet their metabolic needs. Shock may be classified by cause as hypovolemic, cardio-

[1] Lymphocytes are any of the nonphagocytic leukocytes (WBCs) found in the blood, lymph, and lymphoid tissues that make up the body's immunologically competent cells. They are divided into two classes: B and T lymphocytes (see section on leukocytosis in this chapter; see also Chapter 5 for further discussion).

[2] Macrophage and monocyte cells capable of ingesting microorganisms and other antigens.

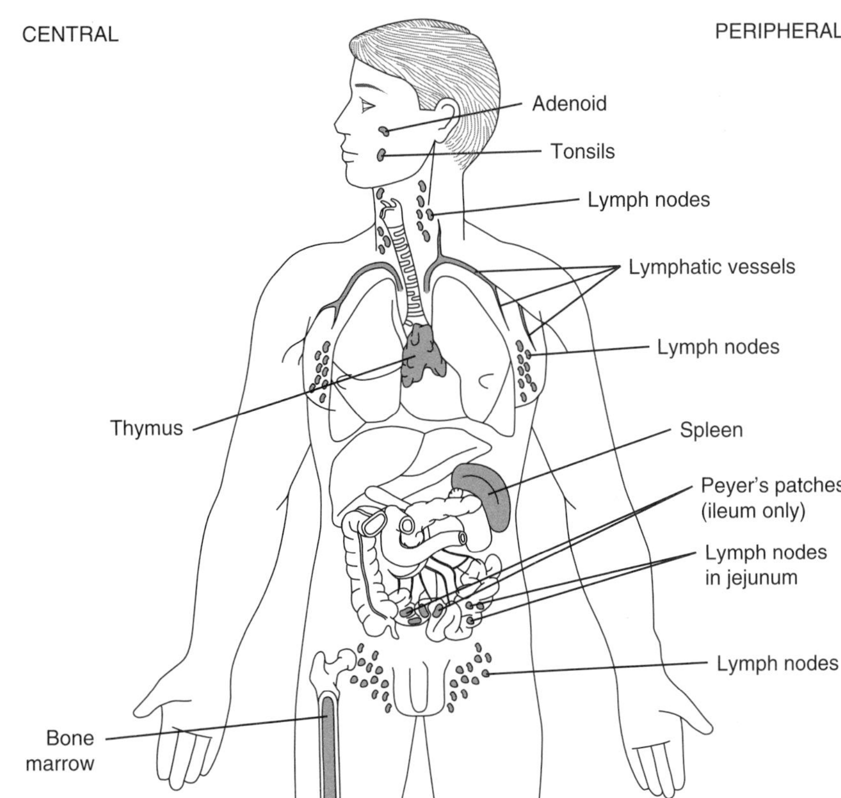

Figure **11–1.** Organs of the immune system referred to as *lymphoid tissues*. Central lymphoid tissues (bone marrow and thymus) are the central sites of B- and T-cell differentiation, respectively. Immature lymphocytes migrate through the central lymphoid tissues and later reside as mature lymphocytes in the peripheral lymphoid tissues.

genic, obstructive, septic (also called endotoxin shock, urosepsis, and gram-negative sepsis), or neurogenic (Table 11–1). Signs of shock include rapid, weak pulse; hypotension (systolic blood pressure of 90 mm Hg or less); cool, pale, moist skin and mottled extremities with weak or absent peripheral pulses.

In early septic shock, hyperdynamic change accompanies increased circulation so that the skin is warm and flushed and the pulse is bounding rather than weak. In the second phase of shock (late septic shock), hypoperfusion (reduced blood flow) occurs, characterized by cold skin and weak pulses; this phase is usually irreversible and the client is unresponsive. Eventually, cardiovascular collapse occurs.

BOX **11–1**

Most Common Signs and Symptoms of Hemodynamic Disorders

- Edema
  - Lymphedema
  - Cerebral edema
  - Inflammatory edema
  - Peripheral dependent edema
  - Pulmonary edema
- Congestion
- Infarction (brain, heart, GI tract, kidney, spleen)
- Thrombosis
- Embolism
- Shock

Special Implications for the Therapist **11–1**

HEMODYNAMIC DISORDERS

Precautions and treatment protocols for the client with lymphedema are discussed in Chapter 10 (see Box 10–12).

Clients in whom *shock* develops may exhibit orthostatic changes in vital signs. A drop in systolic blood pressure of 10 to 20 mm Hg or more associated with an increase in pulse rate of more than 15 beats/min may indicate a depleted intravascular volume. The therapist is unlikely to see a client with acute hypovolemia; he or she is likely to encounter hypovolemia as a result of dehydration as in the case of the long-distance runner or the client with severe diarrhea or slow GI tract bleeding. The elderly population is especially vulnerable to development of unknown slow intestinal bleeding, especially with the use of aspirin or nonsteroidal anti-inflammatory drugs (NSAIDs).

Clients with peripheral neuropathies or clients taking medications such as certain antihypertensive drugs may be normovolemic and experience an orthostatic fall in blood pressure, but without associated increase in pulse rate. The elderly client is likely to experience orthostatic changes as a natural consequence of aging. If any doubt exists, the client should be placed in the supine position with legs elevated to maximize cerebral blood flow (Tierney, 1994). The Trendelenburg position, in which the head is lower than the rest of the body, is no

TABLE 11-1 ETIOLOGIES OF SHOCK

CATEGORY OF SHOCK	CAUSES
Hypovolemic	Hemorrhage (loss of blood, shock) Vomiting Diarrhea Dehydration secondary to: Decreased fluid intake Diabetes mellitus (diuresis during diabetic ketoacidosis or severe hyperglycemia) Diabetes insipidus Inadequate rehydration of long-distance runner Addison's disease Burns Pancreatitis, peritonitis, bowel obstruction
Cardiogenic	Arrhythmias Acute valvular dysfunction Acute myocardial infarction Severe congestive heart failure Cardiomyopathy
Obstructive	Massive pulmonary embolism Pulmonary hypertension Tension pneumothorax Obstructive valvular disease (aortic or mitral stenosis) Cardiac tumor (atrial myxoma)
Septic	Gram-negative or other overwhelming infections
Neurogenic	Spinal cord injury Pain Trauma Fright Vasodilator drugs

Adapted from Andreoli TE, Bennett JC, Carpenter CC, et al.: Cecil Essentials of Medicine, ed 3. Philadelphia, WB Saunders, 1993, p 43.

longer used because of the client's increased difficulty breathing in this position.

AGING AND THE HEMATOPOIETIC SYSTEM

Although blood composition changes little with age, the percentage of the marrow space occupied by hematopoietic (blood-forming) tissue declines progressively from birth until age 30 years. Between ages 30 and 70 years, the amount of hematopoietic bone marrow tissue reaches a plateau with levels declining again after age 70 years. The second decline may be relative to an increase in bone marrow fat or owing to an actual decrease in the blood-forming elements; the exact cause is as yet unknown.

Other changes include decreased total serum iron, total iron-binding capacity, and intestinal iron absorption; increased fragility of plasma membranes; increased platelet adhesiveness[3]; and increased total body and bone marrow iron. Age-related changes in the peripheral blood include slightly decreased hemoglobin and hematocrit, although levels remain within the normal adult range.

Low hemoglobin levels noted in elderly people are often caused by iron deficiency as a result of impaired incorporation of iron into RBCs. This depletion of iron stores and subsequent anemia is usually secondary, a result of other conditions such as chronic GI blood loss, anemia of chronic disease (diabetes mellitus, rheumatoid arthritis, kidney failure, CHF), or decreased iron intake.

Aging is also associated with a decreased number of lymph nodes and diminished size of remaining nodes, decreased function of lymphocytes, and decline in cellular immunity owing to altered T-cell function (see Effects of Aging on the Immune System in Chapter 5). The effect of aging on quantity, form, and structure of lymphocytes is not well documented.

BOX 11-2
Signs and Symptoms of Blood Transfusion Reaction

Local burning sensation at site of transfusion
Facial flushing
Chills and fever
Headache
Low back pain
Rash
Red urine
Allergic reaction: hives, wheezing, anaphylaxis

BLOOD TRANSFUSIONS *(Andreoli et al., 1993)*

In the last decade, advances in treating hematologic/immunologic disorders through blood transfusions and bone marrow transplantation have provided new success in long-term treatment and a cure for some previously fatal disorders.

Modern blood banking and transfusion medicine have developed techniques to administer only the blood component needed by the client, such as packed RBCs for anemia or platelets for bleeding disorders. Clients in a therapy setting who have undergone numerous surgical procedures (e.g., traumatic injuries) or elective orthopedic or cardiac procedures may also receive autologous blood transfusions (re-infusion of a person's own blood) when significant blood loss or hemorrhage occurs.

When autologous transfusion is unavailable or inappropriate, the therapist must be alert for any signs of adverse reaction. Among the most common transfusion reactions are antigen-antibody reactions resulting from blood type incompatibility with clumping of cells, hemolysis, and release of cellular elements into the serum. Signs and symptoms indicating such a reaction are listed in Box 11–2 (O'Toole, 1992).

Other complications may include transmission of disease, iron overload, air embolism, circulatory overload when blood is administered rapidly in large amounts, and hyperkalemia

[3] Platelet morphology (form and structure) does not appear to change with age, but platelet count and platelet function have been found to vary from normal to increased or decreased.

(from an excess of potassium in donor blood that is several days old). These complications are rare, but they occur most often in clients with either cardiac or renal disease, in whom they may cause flaccid paralysis, which affects the muscles of respiration and eventually the heart, which can lead to cardiac arrest.

Hepatitis remains a serious hazard of blood transfusion, despite the reduction in transmission of hepatitis B. Up to 4% of persons who receive blood products develop hepatitis. People with hemophilia who received coagulation factor concentrates prior to 1984 have been at highest risk among transfusion recipients because of exposures to pooled blood products prepared from thousands of donors. The availability of nonhuman plasma factors has virtually eliminated the transmission of viruses among hemophiliacs.

Acquired immunodeficiency syndrome (AIDS) has developed in a small percentage of people receiving transfusion of RBCs, platelets, or commercial coagulation factor concentrates. By the end of 1991, about 4000 persons in the United States with no risk factors other than transfusion had developed AIDS out of 180,000 total reported cases of AIDS.

The risk of human immunodeficiency virus (HIV) infection by transfusion is low overall, calculated at 1 in 10^6 transfusions. The risk of HIV transmission by blood transfusion has been continually reduced through the elimination of high-risk individuals from blood donor pools, use of more sensitive screening for anti-HTLV-III (human T-cell lymphotropic virus III) antibodies, and screening for HTLV-I, a retrovirus that causes adult T cell leukemia/lymphoma, and for HIV-2, which causes AIDS. AIDS has also been reported in infants following neonatal exchange, but the majority of pediatric cases (3000 by the end of 1990) were associated with maternal transmission from HIV-positive mothers.

Special Implications for the Therapist **11-2**

BLOOD TRANSFUSIONS

Most blood transfusion reactions occur during the actual transfusion and are not of consequence to the therapist. Occasionally, a client may develop a delayed allergic reaction observed as hives, which may be brought to the therapist's attention following local modality treatment. The therapist may also be the first to recognize early signs of hepatitis (jaundice), especially changes in sclerae or skin color or reported changes in urine (dark or tea-colored) and stools (light-colored or white).

DISORDERS OF ERYTHROCYTES

The Anemias

Definition. Anemia is a reduction in the oxygen-carrying capacity of the blood owing to an abnormality in the quantity or quality of erythrocytes (RBC). The World Health Organization (WHO) has defined anemia in terms of the level of hemoglobin: less than 14 g/dL for men and less than 12 g/dL for women. Different ranges exist for men and women, for infants and growing children, and for different metabolic and physiologic states.[4] Anemia is present if the hematocrit is less than 41% in adult males or 37% in adult females.

Overview. Anemia is not a disease but is rather a symptom of many other disorders, such as dietary deficiency (nutritional anemia), acute or chronic blood loss (iron deficiency), congenital defects of hemoglobin (sickle cell diseases), exposure to industrial poisons, diseases of the bone marrow, chronic inflammatory, infectious, or neoplastic disease, or any other disorder that upsets the balance between blood loss through bleeding or destruction of blood cells and production of blood cells (O'Toole, 1992).

There are many types of anemia; not all are discussed in this text. The most common anemias observed in a therapy setting fall into four broad disease-related categories: (1) iron deficiency associated with chronic GI blood loss secondary to NSAID use; (2) chronic diseases or inflammatory diseases, such as rheumatoid arthritis or systemic lupus erythematosus; (3) neurologic conditions (pernicious anemia); and (4) infectious diseases, such as tuberculosis or AIDS, and neoplastic disease or cancer (bone marrow failure). Anemia with neoplasia may be a common complication of chemotherapy or as a consequence of bone marrow metastasis.

Anemias are classified according to etiology (Table 11–2) or morphology (form/structure) (Box 11–3). Descriptions of anemias based on erythrocyte morphology refer to the size and hemoglobin content of the RBC. In some anemias, variations occur in size (e.g., anisocytosis) or shape (e.g., poikilocytosis) of erythrocytes (Mansen et al., 1994).

Etiology and Incidence. Anemia results from (1) excessive blood loss, (2) increased destruction of erythrocytes, or (3) decreased production of erythrocytes. It is the most common hematologic abnormality, with iron-deficiency anemia from dietary lack or from GI or genitourinary tract blood loss being the most common type of anemia. *Excessive blood loss* from the GI tract may be associated with peptic ulcers, hiatal hernia, gastritis, gastric carcinoma, hemorrhoids, diverticula, ulcerative colitis, or salicylate use, which account for many causes of hemorrhagic anemia.

Conditions associated with *destruction of erythrocytes* occur as a result of a variety of underlying factors (e.g., secondary to hemoglobinopathy, hereditary conditions, enzyme deficiencies, parasites). Chronic diseases such as rheumatoid arthritis, tuberculosis, or cancer may cause destruction of erythrocytes or may interfere with the production of erythrocytes.

Although anemia can occur at any age, there is an increased risk of *decreased production of erythrocytes* associated with iron deficiency anemia. Iron, protein, vitamin B_{12}, and other vitamins and minerals are needed for the production of hemoglobin and the formation of erythrocytes. Growing children, lower socioeconomic groups, the elderly (as a result of economic constraints, lack of interest in food preparation, and poor dentition), menstruating women, and pregnant

[4] These "normal" values must be evaluated on an individual basis; "normal" levels may be inadequate if tissue oxygen delivery is impaired by pulmonary insufficiency, cardiac disorders, or an increase in hemoglobin oxygen affinity, whereas "low" levels may be appropriate if tissue oxygen requirements are decreased, as in the case of hypothyroidism (Price and Solomon, 1993).

TABLE 11–2 CAUSES OF ANEMIA

EXCESSIVE BLOOD LOSS (HEMORRHAGE)
Trauma, wound
Gastrointestinal cancer
Bleeding peptic ulcer
Excessive menstruation
Bleeding hemorrhoids
DESTRUCTION OF ERYTHROCYTES
Mechanical or autoimmune hemolysis
Hemoglobinopathies (e.g., sickle cell diseases)
Enzyme defects (e.g., glucose-6-phosphate dehydrogenase deficiency)
Parasites (e.g., malaria)
Hypersplenism
Hereditary spherocytosis
Chronic diseases (e.g., rheumatoid arthritis, tuberculosis, cancer)
DECREASED PRODUCTION OF ERYTHROCYTES
Nutritional deficiency (e.g., iron, vitamin B_{12}, folic acid deficiency)
Cellular maturational defects (e.g., thalassemias, cytotoxic or antineoplastic drugs)
↓ Bone marrow stimulation (e.g., hypothyroidism, ↓ erythropoietin production)
Bone marrow failure (e.g., leukemia, aplasia)
Bone marrow replacement (myelophthisis; usually replacement by neoplasm)
Inborn or acquired metabolic defect; myelodysplastic syndrome (sideroblastic anemia)

Adapted from Goodman CC, Snyder TE: Differential Diagnosis in Physical Therapy, ed 2. Philadelphia, WB Saunders, 1995, p 196.

women are the most common groups to develop iron deficiency anemia.

The most common cause of vitamin B_{12} deficiency is pernicious anemia. Loss of intrinsic factor may contribute to a vitamin B_{12} deficiency. Intrinsic factor, a protein secreted by gastric parietal cells, normally binds with vitamin B_{12} for transport. Destruction of intrinsic factor production sites may occur with gastrectomy (see Aging and the Gastrointestinal System, Chapter 13).

Other causes of vitamin B_{12} deficiency include bacterial overgrowth in the lumen of the intestine (competes for vitamin B_{12}), surgical resection of the ileum (eliminates the site of vitamin B_{12} absorption), and, more rarely, dietary deficiency (e.g., strict vegetarian diet), tapeworm infection, and severe Crohn's disease. The latter condition can cause sufficient destruction of the ileum to retard vitamin B_{12} absorption (Linker, 1994).

Folic acid deficiency is a very common cause of decreased production of erythrocytes. Folic acid deficiency has many causes, but it usually results from inadequate dietary intake, chronic alcoholism, malabsorption syndromes, anorexia, and consumption of overcooked food. Long-term use of anticonvulsants (e.g., primidone, diphenylhydantoin, phenobarbital), antimetabolites administered for cancer and leukemia, and certain oral contraceptives may interfere with folate absorption (Pavel et al., 1993).

Bone marrow disorders constitute the most likely source of anemia caused by decreased production of erythrocytes in a therapy practice. Aplastic anemia, marrow replacement with fibrotic tissue or tumor (myelophthisis and myelodysplastic syndromes), acute leukemia, or infiltrative disease (e.g., lymphoma, myeloma, carcinoma) fall into this etiologic category.

BOX 11–3
Anemia Classified by Morphology

Normocytic (normal size)
Macrocytic (abnormally large)
Microcytic (abnormally small)
Normochromic (normal amounts of hemoglobin)
Hyperchromic (high concentration of hemoglobin)
Hypochromic (low concentration of hemoglobin)
Anisocytosis (various sizes)
Poikilocytosis (various shapes)

Pathogenesis. The underlying pathogenesis is multifactorial and depends on the condition causing the anemia. Only the anemias most commonly encountered by the therapist are discussed here, using the three etiologic categories from Table 11–2 as a guideline. Oxygen is transported throughout the body by the RBCs, which contain hemoglobin. Hemoglobin consists of two parts: heme (iron) and globin (a protein). Anemia may occur when levels of hemoglobin are reduced, either from a lack of heme or a lack of iron. Conditions such as folic acid deficiency, a lack of vitamin B_{12}, or a malabsorption disorder can also result in anemia despite normal amounts of iron.

Excessive blood loss, as occurs with GI bleeding in the client with a history of long-term use of aspirin or NSAIDs, is the most commonly encountered cause of anemia seen in a therapy practice. Slow, chronic GI blood loss from medication or any GI disorder can result in iron-deficiency anemia (see also Chapter 13).

Anemia associated with *destruction of erythrocytes* most often includes autoimmune disorders, such as systemic lupus erythematosus, and the lymphoproliferative diseases, such as leukemia and lymphoma. These anemias are called *autoimmune hemolytic anemia.* The immune system produces antibodies that clump (agglutinate) a person's own RBCs together. These are then recognized by the immune system as non-self or foreign bodies and are phagocytized in the spleen, thereby reducing the available RBCs (and available hemoglobin). Medications such as penicillin, quinidine, quinine, and methyldopa can also cause autoimmune hemolytic anemia.

Hemoglobinopathy-related anemias (e.g., sickle cell anemia, thalassemias) develop as a result of destroyed erythrocytes, but these diseases are discussed elsewhere in this chapter.

Anemia of chronic disease is characterized by modestly reduced RBC survival; the bone marrow fails to compensate for the slightly decreased RBC life span. Normally, iron is released from disintegrating RBCs and recirculates within the bloodstream. In the chronic inflammatory process, inflammatory cytokines cause an increase of ferritin (an iron storage complex formed in the intestinal mucosa) in macrophages, thereby hindering release of iron. Failure to increase RBC production is largely caused by this trapping of iron within the reticuloendothelial system,[5] preventing its transfer to the bone marrow for use (Linker, 1994).

The pathogenesis of the most commonly encountered anemias associated with *decreased production of erythrocytes* is as follows: In the case of pernicious anemia caused by a deficiency of vitamin B_{12}, poor diet rarely causes the vitamin deficiency; rather it is a result of defective intestinal absorption. After being ingested, vitamin B_{12} becomes bound to intrinsic factor, a protein secreted by gastric parietal cells. Any condition that destroys gastric parietal cells also results in decreased intrinsic factor, which is required for absorption of vitamin B_{12}.

In anemia due to folic acid deficiency associated with alcoholism, high levels of alcohol in the blood partially block the response of the bone marrow to folic acid, which thereby interferes with erythropoiesis. The common occurrence of folic acid deficiency during the growth spurts of childhood and adolescence and during the third trimester of pregnancy is explained by the increased demands for folate required for DNA synthesis in these circumstances. Pregnant women need six times the normal amount of folic acid to meet the needs of the developing fetus.

Anemias of bone marrow failure are not completely understood. It is known that in the case of neoplasm, when radiation therapy is used, mitosis (cell division) is inhibited, which affects synthesis of RBCs. Antimetabolites used in cancer therapy also cause bone marrow failure by blocking the synthesis of purines or nucleic acids required for synthesis of protein within the cell.

Because bone marrow transplantation may be curative for aplastic anemia, it is hypothesized that the defect associated with that type of anemia must be intrinsic to the hematopoietic cells, perhaps consisting of damage to the stem cells with a resultant inability to regenerate and repopulate the bone marrow.

Clinical Manifestations. Mild anemia often causes only minimal and usually vague symptoms such as fatigue until hemoglobin concentration and hematocrit fall below half of normal. As the anemia progresses, general signs and symptoms caused by the inability of anemic blood to supply the body tissues with enough oxygen may include weakness; dyspnea on exertion; easy fatigue; pallor or yellowness of skin, especially the palms of the hands, fingernails,[6] mucosa, and conjunctiva; tachycardia; increased angina in pre-existing coronary artery disease (CAD); leg ulcers (sickle cell); and, occasionally, koilonychia (Fig. 11–2).

Central nervous system (CNS) symptoms develop in 75% of clients with pernicious anemia. Subacute degeneration of the spinal cord caused by vitamin B_{12} deficiency can occur in pernicious anemia, characterized by pyramidal and posterior column deficits. CNS manifestations may include headache, drowsiness, dizziness, fainting, slow thought processes, decreased attention span, apathy, depression, and irritability. Polyneuropathy, mental changes, or optic neuropathy may occur.

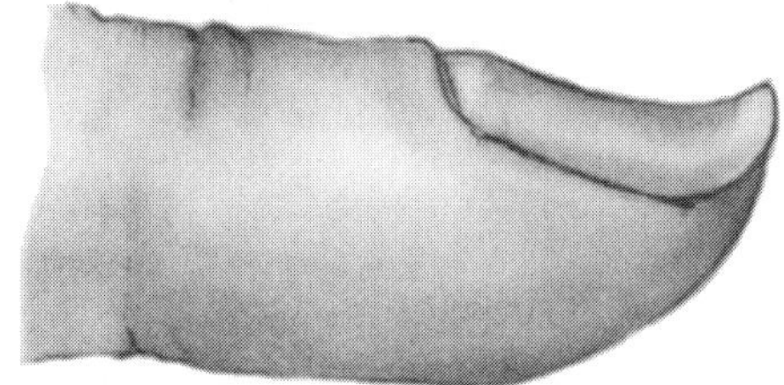

Figure **11–2.** Koilonychia, sometimes called spoon-shaped nails or spoon nails. They are thin, depressed nails with lateral edges turned up, concave from side to side. They may be idiopathic, congenital, or a hereditary trait, and are occasionally due to iron deficiency anemia. (*From Jarvis C: Physical Examination and Health Assessment. Philadelphia, WB Saunders, 1992, p 271.*)

Complications depend on the specific type of anemia; severe anemia can cause heart failure and hypoxic damage to the liver and kidney, with all the signs and symptoms associated with either of those conditions. Anemia in the presence of any coronary obstruction results in low blood oxygen levels. The decreased oxygen perfusion of the heart precipitates angina more quickly and more often.

Medical Management

Diagnosis. The clinical picture cannot be depended on for confirmation of the suspected diagnosis because symptoms may not be recognized until hemoglobin concentration is reduced to half of normal. Personal and family history may point to congenital anemia, and a physical examination may elicit signs of primary hematologic diseases, such as lymphadenopathy, hepatosplenomegaly, skin and mucosal changes, or bone tenderness (Pavel et al., 1993).

To determine the specific type of anemia present, the hematologist examines a bone marrow specimen and a peripheral blood smear and calculates red cell indices (and, in some cases, the rate of RBC destruction). Laboratory diagnosis may include a complete blood cell count (CBC), determination of serum iron, serum ferritin, reticulocyte count, sickle cell screen, hemoglobin electrophoresis, Coombs' test, glucose-6-phosphate dehydrogenase (G6PD) (an enzyme) assay, and osmotic fragility (for further explanation of laboratory tests, see Chapter 35).

Treatment and Prognosis. Treatment of anemia is directed toward alleviating or controlling the causes, relieving the symptoms, and preventing complications. It is critical that the underlying cause of anemia be determined. For example, endoscopy to identify the source of GI blood loss for a client with a long-term history of NSAID use would indicate the need to stop taking the medication.

Treating the underlying cause can include bone marrow transplantation to replace damaged marrow; vitamin B_{12}, folic acid, or iron supplemental therapy for nutritional deficits; oxygen therapy to prevent hypoxia; corticosteroids and androgens to stimulate marrow to produce RBCs; splenectomy to decrease the destruction of RBCs; anti-T lymphocyte antibodies and other immunosuppressive agents for the treatment of aplastic anemia; and erythropoietin replacement.

[5] The reticuloendothelial system is a network of cells and tissues found throughout the body, especially in the blood, general connective tissue, spleen, liver, lungs, bone marrow, and lymph nodes. Some of the reticuloendothelial cells found in the blood are concerned with blood cell formation and destruction and the metabolism of iron and pigment. These cells have a significant role in inflammation and immunity.

[6] Pallor in dark-skinned people may be observed by the absence of the underlying red tones that normally give brown or black skin its luster. The brown-skinned individual demonstrates pallor with a more yellowish-brown color, and the black-skinned person will appear ashen or gray (Jarvis, 1992).

Occasionally, treatment can include RBC transfusion to replace acute or chronic blood loss, especially chronic blood loss with cardiac complications in the presence of angina. Blood transfusion does not change the underlying cellular pathology, so this treatment has no long-term curative benefit.

The recent development of recombinant human erythropoietin (epoietin alfa or Epogen) has been introduced in the treatment of anemia associated with chronic renal failure and anemia secondary to zidovudine (AZT) therapy in HIV-infected persons. Human erythropoietin stimulates erythropoiesis and may elevate RBC counts enough to decrease the need for blood transfusions in these two groups (Deglin and Vallerand, 1993).

The prognosis for anemia depends on the etiology and potential treatment for the underlying cause. For example, the prognosis is good for anemia related to nutritional deficiency, but poor for hemolytic anemia. Likewise, treatment is aimed at correcting the underlying pathogenesis.

Special Implications for the Therapist **11-3**

THE ANEMIAS

Exercise and Anemia

Exercise for any anemic person should be first approved by the physician. Diminished exercise tolerance may be expected in anyone with anemia, depending on the cause of the anemia. Increased physical activity increases the demand for oxygen, which may not be adequately available in the circulating blood. For the sedentary elderly person, decreased activity can mask exercise intolerance; observe carefully for any changes in mental status.

Research has shown that people with chronic renal failure who have severe anemia are able to exercise but must do so at a lower intensity than that of the normal population. The maximum oxygen consumption (VO_{2max}) for the anemic client is at least 20% less than that for the normal population. Exercise testing and prescribed exercise(s) in anemic clients must be initiated with extreme caution and should proceed very gradually to tolerance and/or perceived exertion levels (Painter, 1993).

Precautions

Knowing the underlying cause of the anemia may be very helpful in identifying red flag symptoms indicating need for alteration of the program or medical referral. For example, GI blood loss associated with NSAID use may worsen suddenly, precipitating a crisis in a therapy setting. It is not uncommon for clients to present with both anemia and cardiovascular disease, precipitating angina (see also Special Implications for the Therapist: Angina). Splenomegaly associated with some types of anemia requires precautions in performing soft tissue techniques in the left upper quadrant (especially up and under the rib cage); indirect techniques away from the spleen are indicated.

Bleeding under the skin and easy bruising in response to the slightest trauma often occur when platelet production is altered (thrombocytopenia) secondary to hypoplastic or aplastic anemia. This condition necessitates extreme care in the therapy setting, especially any treatment requiring manual therapy or the use of any equipment, including modalities and weight-training devices.

Decreased oxygen delivery to the skin results in impaired healing and loss of elasticity, delaying wound healing and healing of other musculoskeletal injuries. If the anemia is caused by vitamin B_{12} deficiency (e.g., pernicious anemia, pregnancy, hyperthyroidism), the nervous system is affected. Alteration of the structure and function of the peripheral nerves, spinal cord (myelin degeneration), and brain may occur. Paresthesias (especially numbness mimicking carpal tunnel syndrome), gait disturbances, extreme weakness, spasticity, and abnormal reflexes can result. Permanent neurologic damage unresponsive to vitamin B_{12} therapy can occur in extreme cases when intervention has been delayed.

Monitoring Vital Signs

Systolic blood pressure may not be affected, but diastolic pressure may be lower than normal, with an associated increase in the resting pulse rate. Resting cardiac output is usually normal in people with anemia, but cardiac output increases with exercise more than in nonanemic persons. As the anemia becomes more severe, resting cardiac output increases and exercise tolerance progressively decreases until dyspnea, tachycardia, and palpitations occur at rest (Goodman and Snyder, 1995).

DISORDERS OF LEUKOCYTES

Alterations in the blood leukocyte (WBC) concentration and in the relative proportions of the several leukocyte types are recognized as measures of the reaction of the body to disease processes and noxious agents. In many instances, these alterations give useful indications of the nature of the pathologic process, and may be seen in association not only with acute infections, but also with many chronic ailments treated by the therapist (Athens, 1993).

Leukocytes may be classified in two main groups: granular (basophils, eosinophils, neutrophils) and nongranular (lymphocytes, monocytes). Granulocytes (granular leukocytes) contain lysing agents within their granules that are capable of digesting various foreign materials. Lymphocytes produce antibodies and react with antigens, thus initiating the immune response to fight infection. Monocytes are the largest circulating blood cells and represent an immature cell until they leave the blood and travel to the tissues. Once migrated, monocytes form macrophages when activated by foreign substances, such as bacteria (Mansen et al., 1994).

Leukocytosis *(Athens, 1993)*

Leukocytosis may occur as a result of a variety of causes (Box 11–4) and may also occur as a normal protective response to physiologic stressors, such as strenuous exercise, emotional changes, temperature changes, anesthesia, surgery, pregnancy, and some drugs, toxins, and hormones.

Leukocytosis develops within 1 or 2 hours after the onset

BOX 11–4
Causes of Leukocytosis

Bacterial infections
Inflammation or tissue necrosis (e.g., infarction, myositis, vasculitis)
Metabolic intoxications (e.g., uremia, eclampsia, acidosis, gout)
Neoplasms (e.g., bronchogenic carcinoma, lymphoma, melanoma)
Acute hemorrhage
Splenectomy
Acute appendicitis
Pneumonia
Intoxication by chemicals
Acute rheumatic fever

From Griffin JP: Hematology and Immunology. Norwalk, Conn, Appleton-Century-Crofts, 1986, p 151.

of acute hemorrhage and is greater when the bleeding occurs internally (i.e., into the peritoneal cavity, pleural space, or joint cavity or as a result of a skull fracture with associated intracranial bleed or subarachnoid hemorrhage) than when the bleeding is external.

Leukocytosis is a common finding in and characterizes many infectious diseases recognized by a count of more than 10,000 WBCs/mm^3 (see Table 35–9). Leukocytosis can be associated with an increase in circulating neutrophils (neutrophilia), which are recruited in large numbers early in the course of most bacterial infections. Most commonly, leukocytosis results from an increase in the number of neutrophils; thus the term is often, but incorrectly, considered to be synonymous to neutrophilia. Leukocytosis owing to eosinophilia, monocytosis, or basophilia is relatively rare.

Rapidly growing neoplasms may cause neutrophilia, presumably as a result of necrosis within areas that have outgrown their blood supply. When the liver, GI tract, or bone marrow is involved, the counts may be especially high. Some tumors can also release hormone-like substances that cause leukocytosis.

Clinical Manifestations. Clinical signs and symptoms of leukocytosis are usually associated with symptoms of the conditions listed in Box 11–4 and may include fever, symptoms of localized or systemic infection, and symptoms of inflammation or trauma to tissue.

Medical Management

Diagnosis, Treatment, and Prognosis. Major leukocyte functions are accomplished in the tissues so that the leukocytes in the blood are in transit from the site of production or storage to the tissues, even in normal persons. Variations in the blood concentrations of each leukocyte type may be of brief duration and easily missed or may persist for days or weeks (Athens, 1993). Laboratory tests for detecting leukocyte abnormalities include total leukocyte count, leukocyte differential cell count (see Chapter 35), peripheral blood morphology, and bone marrow morphology.

Treatment is directed toward the underlying cause of the change in leukocytes and control of any infections. Prognosis is dependent on the etiology of the leukocytosis.

Leukopenia

Leukopenia, or reduction of the number of leukocytes in the blood below 5000/μL (see Chapter 35), can be caused by a variety of factors such as anaphylactic shock and systemic lupus erythematosus. It can occur in many forms of bone marrow failure, such as that following antineoplastic chemotherapy or radiation therapy, in overwhelming infections, in dietary deficiencies, and in autoimmune diseases (Pagana and Pagana, 1992). Unlike leukocytosis, leukopenia is never beneficial. As the leukocyte count decreases, the risk for infection increases.

Mild reduction in the WBC count can be caused by viral infections. Leukopenia from bone marrow radiation dramatically increases the risk of infection. The nadir, or the lowest point that the WBC reaches, usually occurs 7 to 14 days after chemotherapy or radiation therapy.

Clinical Manifestations. Clinical signs and symptoms of leukopenia may include sore throat, cough, high fever, chills, sweating, ulcerations of mucous membranes (e.g., mouth, rectum, vagina), frequent or painful urination, and persistent infections.

Medical Management

Diagnosis and Treatment. As with leukocytosis, diagnosis is by laboratory testing for leukocyte abnormalities. Treatment is directed toward elimination of the cause of the reduced leukocytes and control of any infections. Pharmacologic therapy includes the use of antibiotics, antifungal agents, and colony-stimulating drugs such as filgrastim (Neupogen). This drug is a glycoprotein that binds to and stimulates immature neutrophils to divide and differentiate and also activates mature neutrophils. This drug markedly assists in decreasing the incidence of infection in people who have received bone marrow-depressing antineoplastic agents (Deglin and Vallerand, 1993).

Basophilia[7]

Basophils have a high content of heparin (anticoagulant) and histamine and have an important role in acute systemic allergic reactions. In the presence of bacteria or other infectious agents, the basophils erupt and distribute chemicals that trigger inflammation. At this point, neutrophils, eosinophils, or monocytes arrive to engulf or phagocytose the alien particle. Little else is known about the function of basophil cells.

Basophilia is quite rare; it is seen as a response to inflammation and hypersensitivity reactions of the immediate type. Other conditions associated with basophilia include infection (e.g., measles, chicken pox), myeloproliferative disorders (e.g., polycythemia vera, Hodgkin's disease, hemolytic anemia), and endocrine disorders (e.g., myxedema, antithyroid therapy).

Basopenia

Basopenia, a decrease in circulating basophils, can occur in hyperthyroidism, in acute infections, and in long-term ther-

[7] The remaining categories (e.g., basophilia/basopenia, eosinophilia/eosinopenia, neutrophilia/neutropenia, and so on) are all types of leukocytosis or leukopenia. The specific type is determined when the leukocyte differential (WBC count) determines the percentage of each type of granular and nongranular leukocyte.

apy with steroids. Other physiologic conditions associated with basopenia include pregnancy, ovulation, and stress.

Eosinophilia/Eosinopenia

Eosinophils, usually active in the later stages of inflammation, have some phagocytic properties, but they are generally weaker than neutrophils. One of the primary functions of eosinophils is to surround and engulf antigen-antibody complexes formed during an allergic response. They are also able to defend against parasitic infections (Jennings, 1992).

Eosinophilia (abnormally large number of eosinophils in the blood) can occur as a result of allergic reactions such as asthma or hay fever, pernicious anemia, drug reactions, and neoplastic conditions, such as leukemia. Increased levels of eosinophils have been identified with *eosinophilia-myalgia syndrome*, which is associated with ingestion of tryptophan taken for insomnia and back pain (Ashinsky, 1990; Silver, 1994).

Eosinopenia, a decrease in circulating eosinophils, occurs when eosinophils migrate into inflammatory sites; it may also be seen in Cushing syndrome or as a result of stress caused by surgery, shock, trauma, burns, or mental distress.

Neutrophilia

Granulocytes assist in initiating the inflammatory response and they defend the body against infectious agents by phagocytosing bacteria and other infectious substances. Generally, the neutrophils (the most plentiful of the granulocytes) are the first phagocytic cells to reach an infected area, followed by monocytes; neutrophils and monocytes work together to phagocytose all foreign material present.

Granulocytosis (an excess of granulocytes in the blood) or *neutrophilia* (increased number of neutrophils in the blood) are terms used to describe the early stages of infection or inflammation. The capacity of corticosteroids or alcohol to diminish the accumulation of neutrophils in inflamed areas may be due to their ability to reduce cell adherence.

The many potential causes of neutrophilia include inflammation or tissue necrosis (e.g., after surgery from tissue damage, severe burns, myocardial infarction, pneumonitis, rheumatic fever, rheumatoid arthritis), acute infection (e.g., *Staphylococcus*, *Streptococcus*, *Pneumococcus*), drug- or chemical-induced (e.g., epinephrine, steroids, heparin, histamine), metabolic (e.g., acidosis associated with diabetes, gout, thyroid storm, eclampsia), and neoplasms of the liver, GI tract, or bone marrow. Physiologic neutrophilia may also occur as a result of exercise, extreme heat/cold, third-trimester pregnancy, and emotional distress.

Neutropenia

Neutropenia is the condition associated with a reduction in circulating neutrophils (less than 2000/mL). This may occur in severe, prolonged infections (e.g., influenza, hepatitis B, malaria, measles, mumps, rubella) when production of granulocytes cannot keep up with demand. Neutropenia may also occur in the presence of decreased bone marrow production, such as happens with radiation, chemotherapy, leukemia, and aplastic anemia. Increased destruction of neutrophils may also result in neutropenia (e.g., splenomegaly, hemodialysis).

Lymphocytosis/Lymphocytopenia

Lymphocytosis is rare in acute bacterial infections and occurs most commonly in acute viral infections, especially those caused by the Epstein-Barr virus (EBV). Other causes include endocrine disorders (e.g., thyrotoxicosis, adrenal insufficiency) and malignancies (e.g., acute and chronic lymphocytic leukemia).

Lymphocytopenia may be attributed to abnormalities of lymphocyte production associated with neoplasms and immune deficiencies and destruction of lymphocytes by drugs, viruses, or radiation. In some individuals, there is no known cause. Lymphocytopenia associated with heart failure and other acute illnesses may be caused by elevated levels of cortisol, but this is not yet well understood (Athens, 1993). Most recently, lymphocytopenia associated with AIDS has become a major problem (see Acquired Immunodeficiency Syndrome, Chapter 5).

Monocytosis/Monocytopenia

Monocytosis, an increase in monocytes, is most often seen in chronic infections such as tuberculosis, subacute endocarditis, myeloproliferative disorders, Hodgkin's disease, and as a normal physiologic response in newborns. In malignant neoplasms, such as carcinoma of the ovary, stomach, or breast, monocytosis is a frequent finding. Monocytosis is present in more than 50% of people with collagen vascular disease (see Box 10–13). Monocytosis is usually seen in the late stages of recovery from bacterial infections, when monocytes are needed to phagocytose surviving microorganisms and debris.

Monocytopenia, a decrease in monocytes, is rare, and not much is known about the condition because of the small numbers of monocytes generally present in the blood. Monocytopenia has been identified with hairy cell leukemia and prednisone therapy.

Special Implications for the Therapist **11-4**

LEUKOCYTES (WBCs)

It is important for the therapist to be aware of the client's most recent WBC count prior to and during the course of treatment if that person is immunosuppressed. At that time, the client is extremely susceptible to opportunistic infections and severe complications. The importance of good handwashing and hygiene practices cannot be overemphasized when treating immunocompromised clients. Some centers recommend that persons with a WBC count of less than 1000/mm^3 or a neutrophil count of less than 500/mm^3 should wear a protective mask. Therapists should ensure that these persons are provided with equipment that has been disinfected according to universal precautions (Grant, 1994). (See also Appendix A and Winningham Contraindications for Aerobic Exercise in Chemotherapy Clients, Table 7–3.)

NEOPLASTIC DISEASES OF THE BLOOD AND LYMPH SYSTEMS

Hematologic malignancies include diseases in any hematologic tissue (e.g., bone marrow, spleen, thymus) that arise from changes in stem cells as well as metastases to the bone marrow. The primary hematologic disorders are the immuno-

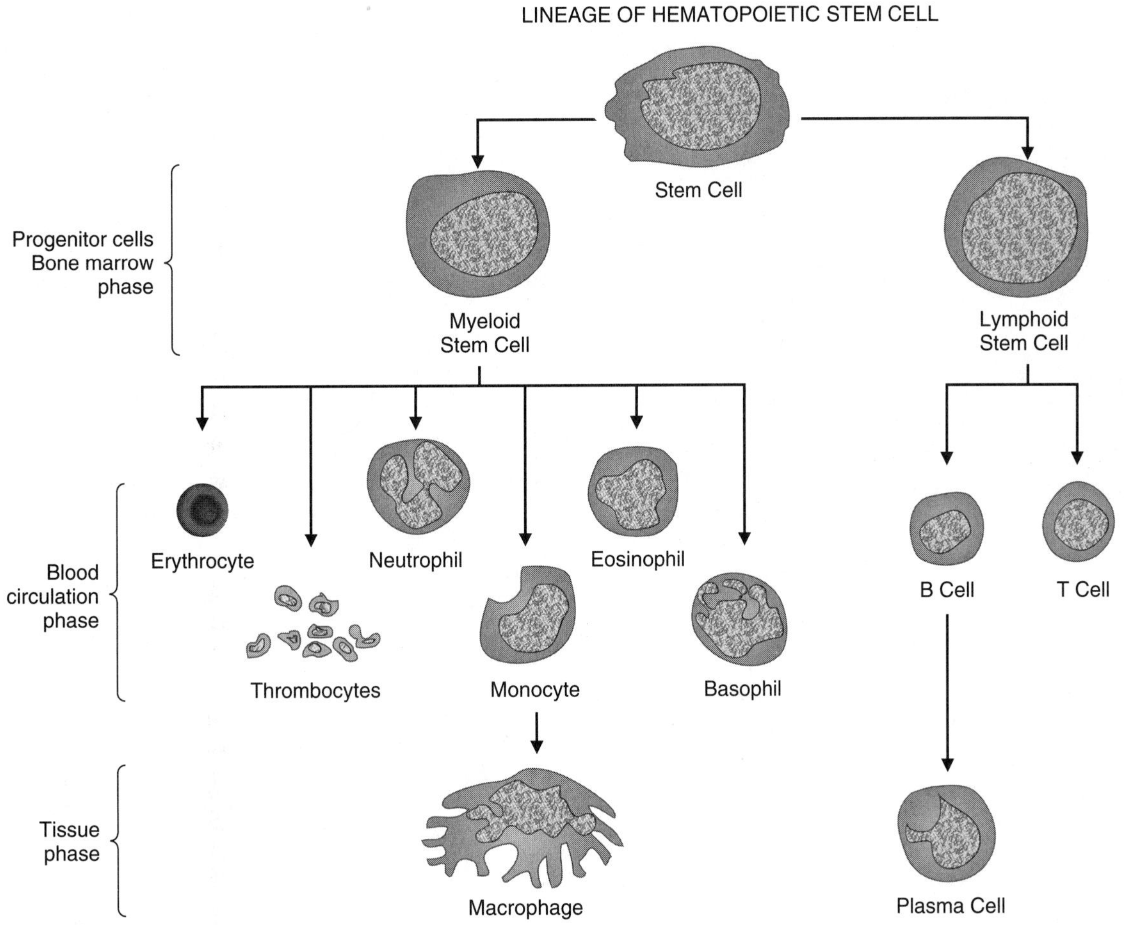

Figure **11–3.** A stem cell is any precursor cell or "mother" cell that has the capacity for both replication and differentiation, giving rise to different blood cell lines. This figure shows the origin, development, and structure of thrombocytes, leukocytes, and erythrocytes from pluripotent (able to develop into different cells) stem cells. The process of hematopoiesis (formation and development of blood cells) usually takes place in the bone marrow.

proliferative diseases, such as multiple myeloma, and the myeloproliferative disorders, such as polycythemia vera, thrombocytopenia, the leukemias, and myelofibrosis with myeloid metaplasia (MMM). Evidence suggests that all of these diseases arise from single cell mutations specific to that disease. These cellular mutations produce malignant clones (genetically identical cells) that have a growth advantage over normal cells in the marrow (Andreoli et al., 1993).

Cancers arising from the major lymphoid cells of the body (lymph nodes and the spleen) are called *malignant lymphomas*. Origin of malignancy in this case is not the source of differentiation (i.e., lymphoma gets its name from the cells affected rather than from the origin of disease, and is categorized as either Hodgkin's disease or non-Hodgkin's lymphoma).

Bone Marrow and Stem Cell Transplantation

Bone marrow transplantation (BMT) is included in this section because it is often a treatment choice for many of the neoplastic diseases of the blood and lymph systems. Both BMT and the more recent technique of stem cell transplantation are discussed.

Bone Marrow Transplantation

Definition and Overview. BMT is the intravenous infusion of hematopoietic progenitor cells (Fig. 11–3) to reestablish marrow function in a person with damaged or defective bone marrow. Acute and chronic leukemias, aplastic anemia, and congenital immunologic defects are the primary indications for the use of bone marrow transplantation. Other uses are listed in Box 11–5. BMT may be the actual treatment for the disorder or, when used in the presence of malignancy, BMT allows higher doses of chemotherapy to be used for more effective tumor elimination. The bone marrow transplantation is then used to offset the lethal effects of the chemotherapy on the bone marrow.

Approximately 8 people per million receive one of three types of BMT in the United States each year. These three types of transplants are determined by the source of donated bone marrow. *Allogeneic* transplantation is one in which the bone marrow comes from an HLA-matched[8] donor (usually a sibling); *syngeneic* transplant is from an identical twin; and an *autologous* BMT comes from the recipient, from whom it

[8] The genes for the human leukocyte antigen (HLA), the human major histocompatibility complex, are located on the short arm of chromosome 6; siblings have a 25% chance of being a match. Nonrelated clients have less than a 1 in 5000 chance of having identical HLA types. Graft rejection and graft-vs-host disease rates are inversely related to the degree of HLA compatibility. The National Bone Marrow Donor Registry has now typed 100,000 persons as potential donors for unrelated people who require transplant (McCullough et al., 1989).

BOX 11-5
Indications for Autologous Bone Marrow Transplantation

Hematologic malignancies
- Acute leukemia
- Lymphoma
- Hodgkin's disease
- Multiple myeloma

Solid tumors*
- Testicular cancer
- Small cell lung cancer
- Ewing sarcoma
- Neuroblastoma

* Scientific evidence as to the use of autologous bone marrow transplant in breast and ovarian cancer is controversial. Current research results are not yet conclusive; investigation is ongoing.
From Jagannath S, Barlogie B, Tricot G: Hematopoietic stem cell transplantation. Hosp Pract 28:79–86, 1993.

has been harvested during remission or after cancer cells have been killed. Autologous BMTs are the most common type of transplant performed, and are often referred to as a "rescue."

Unlike allogeneic transplantation, autologous bone marrow transplantation (ABMT) can be performed in older persons with relative safety owing to the freedom from graft-vs-host disease as a complication (see Complications, following). A primary concern with ABMT is the possible presence of viable tumor cells in the graft. Numerous methods have been developed to remove contaminating tumor cells from the graft in a process referred to as *purging* (Gribben et al., 1991).

The transplant process consists of several phases: conditioning, harvest, marrow infusion, pre-engraftment, and engraftment. Conditioning refers to the immunosuppression treatment regimen of chemotherapy, radiation therapy (RT), or both, used to eradicate all malignant cells, provide a state of immunosuppression, and create space in the bone marrow for the engraftment of the new marrow. Marrow is usually infused 48 to 72 hours after the last dose of chemotherapy or RT (Jassak et al., 1993).

Stem Cell Transplantation

It is impossible to discuss BMT without introducing the recently developed concept of hematopoietic stem cell transplantation, now widely used in place of autologous marrow transplantation and even of allogeneic bone marrow transplantation (Henon, 1993).

Peripheral blood stem cell transplantation (PBSCT) is the process of removing circulating stem cells (see Fig. 11–3) from the peripheral blood through apheresis (blood is withdrawn from the donor, a portion is separated and retained, and the remainder is retransfused into the donor) and returning these cells to the person after dose-intensive chemotherapy. Peripheral blood stem cells can then reconstitute bone marrow function after high-dose chemotherapy and/or radiotherapy even more rapidly than bone marrow stem cells.

Injury to hematopoietic stem cells from cytotoxic chemotherapy, radiation, or disease disables immune and blood cell production and can lead to death from bleeding or infection. However, only a few hematopoietic stem cells are required for repopulation of bone marrow (Jagannath et al., 1993).

Hematopoietic growth factors, called *colony-stimulating factors* (CSF), are naturally occurring glycoproteins used to help collect blood stem cells (Appelbaum, 1993). Growth factors move the stem cells from the bone marrow into the peripheral blood and can result in a temporary 10- to 100-fold increase in the numbers of circulating stem cells at the time of bone marrow recovery (Jagannath et al., 1993). The redistribution of stem cells has permitted successful harvests requiring only a few leukapheresis procedures (selective removal of leukocytes from withdrawn blood, which is then retransfused into the donor).

Clinical indications for blood stem cell transplant as the preferred option over an ABMT are still being evaluated and determined (Korbling et al., 1994). Which technique becomes the treatment of choice depends on the disease and the point in the blood-forming process (hematopoiesis) at which cells can be harvested for a successful outcome. Taking cells from the bone marrow goes all the way to the beginning of the blood-formation process, whereas cells taken from the blood come from the last step of the hematopoietic process.

The most striking advantage of blood stem cell transplants over ABMTs is the shortened period of total aplasia of bone marrow after chemotherapy. This reduction in the period of aplasia may allow repeated myeloablative treatment cycles in solid tumors, thereby reducing mortality (Korbling et al., 1994). Additionally, blood-derived grafts may contain fewer malignant cells than do the bone marrow cells. The preliminary results have been so encouraging that PBSCT has quickly replaced ABMT in myeloma, Hodgkin's disease, and non-Hodgkin's lymphoma (Mijovic et al., 1994).

Complications of Bone Marrow and Stem Cell Transplantation. The complications of PBSCT are essentially the same as those of BMT, but hematologic recovery after PBSCT is much more rapid (10 to 12 days, and as early as 7 days), thereby significantly shortening the period of postchemotherapy neutropenia (decreased neutrophils, a type of granular leukocyte used to fight infection) and thrombocytopenia (decreased platelets in peripheral blood). This in turn reduces platelet and RBC transfusion and facilitates earlier discharge from the hospital (Richel et al., 1993). In most cases, PBSCT can be performed on an outpatient basis.

Cardiac or pulmonary toxicity may occur as a result of the irradiation and immunosuppressive drugs used to prepare recipients for the transplantation. Interstitial pneumonitis, an inflammation of the lungs, is a common complication, especially among allogeneic transplantations, which leaves the client susceptible to obstructive small airways disease. Arrhythmias may be the first sign that a chemotherapeutic agent is becoming cardiotoxic.

Infections and hemorrhagic complications during the period of bone marrow anaplasia and emerging immune competence and graft-vs-host disease (see Immunologic System, Chapter 5) are the most life-threatening complications of transplantation, and they may be fatal. Infections include early bacterial infections or later opportunistic infections, especially cytomegalovirus (CMV) interstitial lung disease. Recurrence of malignancy is always a possibility. Other complications of transplantation include sterility, cystitis, cataract formation, cardiomyopathy, and veno-occlusive liver disease. Neuromuscular changes, such as peripheral neuropathies, muscle cramping, and steroid myopathies, may also develop.

Prognosis. Enormous progress has been made in understanding the biology, therapy, and prophylaxis strategies of transplantation and in extending the range of potential marrow donors to include unrelated persons. Dramatic advances have occurred in the prevention of serious infection, including CMV infection, formerly a cause of a high rate of mortality.

Recent advances in use of recombinant hematopoietic growth factors and autologous peripheral stem cells are currently reducing morbidity and mortality and significantly shortening the length of hospitalization and the cost of transplantation (Rowe et al., 1994). As it becomes increasingly possible to remove hematopoietic stem cells from a person, replace a defective gene or add a missing one, and then transplant the altered cells, ABMT may become a common treatment for genetic disorders as well (Armitage, 1994).

Although the success rates of transplantation have been improving over time, the prognosis still depends on the underlying disease, associated risk of relapse (e.g., leukemia), the development of graft-vs-host disease based on the level of match between donor and recipient, and the age of the recipient. The success of allogeneic marrow grafting is inversely proportional to the age of the recipient. Most marrow transplant centers do not perform transplants in persons older than 50 years, but some groups do make treatment decisions on the basis of a person's estimated physiologic age rather than chronologic age. These age restrictions do not apply to syngeneic or autologous transplants, because these persons will not develop graft-vs-host disease. However, persons older than 50 years do not tolerate intensive treatment as well as do younger persons (Thomas, 1994). There is no effective therapy for severe graft-vs-host disease, and persons stricken with it rarely recover.

Graft rejection is evident if the bone marrow fails to produce peripheral blood cells after several weeks. Late recurrence of leukemia is still a major concern and represents inadequate eradication of the leukemic clone by the initial cytotoxic treatment (Andreoli et al., 1993).

Overall, the success rates for transplantation are about 60% to 70% in aplastic anemia, with 40% to 75% survival at 1 year in various forms of leukemia and even more variable rates in immune deficiency diseases (Adelman and Terr, 1994). Children treated early with BMT from an HLA-identical sibling are now reported to have a survival rate of greater than 80% (Casper, 1990).

Special Implications for the Therapist **11-5**

BONE MARROW AND STEM CELL TRANSPLANTATION

Infection

Myelosuppression as a result of specific chemotherapeutic agents or drug combinations is the number one factor that predisposes the client to infection. Until bone marrow function returns, the BMT or PBSCT client is extremely susceptible to life-threatening infection, which requires all staff to practice interventions to minimize or prevent infection, such as good handwashing technique (Wujcik, 1993a).

Therapists and nursing staff must work closely together to prevent infection, recognize early signs of infection or rejection, and reinforce the educational program (which is complex and is often taught in a short time under less-than-ideal conditions) (Bova and Matassarin-Jacobs, 1993). Expanding the lungs regularly during common movements, such as getting out of bed or turning, while coughing, and during exercise, is an important part of minimizing infections.

Monitoring Vital Signs

Vital signs must be monitored before, during, and after exercise to assess each BMT or PBSCT client for an abnormal response. At this time, no data show the effects of drug interventions or the physiologic responses to transplant procedures in recovery or over the long term. Monitoring responses over time during the recovery process can alert the therapist to any developing cardiopulmonary compromise.

The concept of routine monitoring applies to clients who are seemingly healthy post-transplant and may provide helpful information about when to advance an exercise program. Knowledge of past medical history and/or preexisting conditions that could affect physical conditioning is essential. Preexisting conditions in the presence of extended periods of inactivity can contribute to further physical deconditioning.

Normal changes in vital signs include an increased heart rate and increased systolic blood pressure proportional to the workload, with minimal change in diastolic blood pressure (no more than ±10 mm Hg). Hypertension or the use of antihypertensive medications (or other medications) can alter the normal response of blood pressure to exercise. Clients may be deconditioned with a less-than-normal ("sluggish") blood pressure response. (See Appendix B.)

Graft-vs-Host Disease

Early symptoms of graft-vs-host reaction (see discussion, Chapter 5) usually appear within 10 to 30 days post-transplant and may include rash, hepatomegaly, and diarrhea. Although some cardiopulmonary abnormalities can only be detected by echocardiography, early warning symptoms of cardiopulmonary complications, such as progressive dyspnea, sensation of heart palpitations, irregular heartbeats, chest pain or discomfort, or increasing fatigue, may be reported by the client or observed by the therapist. The physician must be notified of such changes and modifications made to the exercise program for mildly to moderately abnormal responses.

Post-transplantation Exercise

Extremely abnormal responses may require consultation with the physician before therapy is initiated or continued. These clients may need continuous monitoring over many therapy sessions rather than just using symptoms as a guide to exercise tolerance once a baseline is established. Exercise may begin approximately 1 month post-PBSCT, depending on the medical and physical condition both prior to the transplant and after transplant and chemotherapy. Exercise following BMT may be delayed as much as 3 or 4 months owing to the intensity of the course of treatment required.

Interval activity training (see Appendix B) combined with energy-conservation techniques (see Box 7–1) is an important component of therapy as the client's blood counts drop (including hemoglobin count, resulting in anemia), thereby reducing the body's capacity for exertion or aerobic activity. For all transplant clients, the duration of beginning exercise should be until fatigue begins; then add 1 to 2 minutes per day. Until the duration is at least 20 minutes of continuous exercise, the person is best advised to exercise to the point of initial fatigue twice a day. The goal is to perform at least 30 minutes of non-stop activity daily before reducing exercise frequency to 3 to 5 times weekly. Clients trying to control blood pressure or lose weight should work for a longer duration, 30 to 45 minutes, at a lower intensity (e.g., 50% to 65% of predicted maximum heart rate) (Watchie, 1994).

Decreased platelet counts increase the client's susceptibility to bleeding from minor injuries. Safety education is important, and assistive devices may be needed. (See also Special Implications for the Therapist; Thrombocytopenia, this chapter.)

The Leukemias

Overview. Leukemia is a malignant neoplasm of the blood-forming cells, specifically replacement of the bone marrow by a malignant clone (genetically identical cell) of lymphocytic or granulocytic cells. The disease may be acute or chronic, based on its natural course; acute leukemias have a rapid clinical course, resulting in death in a few months without treatment, whereas chronic leukemias have a more prolonged course.

Acute leukemia is an accumulation of neoplastic, immature lymphoid or myeloid cells in the bone marrow and peripheral blood, tissue invasion by these cells, and associated bone marrow failure. *Chronic leukemia* is a neoplastic accumulation of mature lymphoid or myeloid elements of the blood that usually progresses more slowly than an acute leukemic process (Abrams et al., 1995).

Leukemia occurs with varying frequencies at different ages. In general, it occurs more often in adults—about 29,300 cases/year in adults compared to 2500 cases/year in children (American Cancer Society, 1993).

Pathogenesis. Leukemia develops in the bone marrow and is characterized by abnormal multiplication and release of WBC precursors. Causal risk factors in combination with a genetic predisposition can alter nuclear DNA. The leukemic cell is then unable to mature and respond to normal regulatory mechanisms. With rapid proliferation of leukemic cells, the bone marrow becomes overcrowded with WBCs, which then spill over into the peripheral circulation. Crowding of the bone marrow by leukemic cells inhibits normal blood cell production.

Clinical Manifestations. Leukemia is not limited to the bone marrow and peripheral blood. Abnormalities in one or more organ systems can result from the infiltration and replacement of any tissue of the body with nonfunctional leukemic cells or metabolic complications related to leukemia (Devine and Larson, 1994; Schiffer, 1993).

The three main symptoms that occur as a consequence of this infiltration and replacement process are (1) *anemia* and reduced tissue oxygenation from decreased erythrocytes, (2) *infection* from neutropenia as leukemic cells are functionally unable to defend the body against pathogens, and (3) *bleeding tendencies* from decreased platelet production (thrombocytopenia) (Fig. 11–4) (Wong, 1993).

Medical Management

Diagnosis. Leukemia is a complex disease that requires careful identification of the subtype for appropriate treatment. Molecular probes can be used to establish a morphologic diagnosis of acute or chronic leukemia and to predict a person's response to therapy (Cline, 1994). These analyses are sufficiently sensitive to detect one leukemic cell among 100,000 or even in 1 million normal cells. Because of this extreme sensitivity, molecular markers have generally been used to determine the presence or absence of a few leukemic cells remaining after intensive therapy, so-called *residual disease* (Lo Coco et al., 1992).

Treatment. Future clinical and laboratory investigation will likely lead to the development of new, even more effective treatments specifically for different subsets of leukemia. The development of new chemotherapeutic and biologic agents combined with refined dose and schedule has already contributed to the clinical success of treatment. Intensive consolidation of chemotherapy without maintenance therapy (e.g., repeated intensive chemotherapy, high-dose chemoradiotherapy with allogeneic bone marrow transplantation, or high-dose chemotherapy with autologous bone marrow transplantation) is a common treatment strategy in the United States to combat the substantial numbers of leukemic cells that remain after induction chemotherapy has been used.

Knowledge of the molecular mechanisms of leukemia has important implications for treatment. A more complete understanding of the pathogenetic mechanisms in leukemia will lead to new strategies for circumventing the molecular lesions. One approach is to use gene therapy to nullify the effects of an abnormal oncogene or to replace a tumor-suppressor gene missing in leukemic cells (Szczylik et al., 1991).

Other treatment techniques under investigation include insertion of the multiple-drug–resistance gene into normal marrow cells to invest them with enhanced resistance to cytotoxic drugs used in the treatment of leukemia. Attempts to induce leukemic cells to relinquish their malignant phenotype and enter a program of normal cellular differentiation and death have also been made (Sorrentino et al., 1992).

Acute Leukemia

Overview. Acute leukemias are categorized according to the cellular morphology, histochemical staining, and immunologic markers (Table 11–3). When leukemia is classified according to its morphology (i.e., the predominant cell type and level of maturity), the following descriptors are used: *lympho-* for leukemias involving the lymphoid or lymphatic system, *myelo-* for leukemias of myeloid or bone marrow ori-

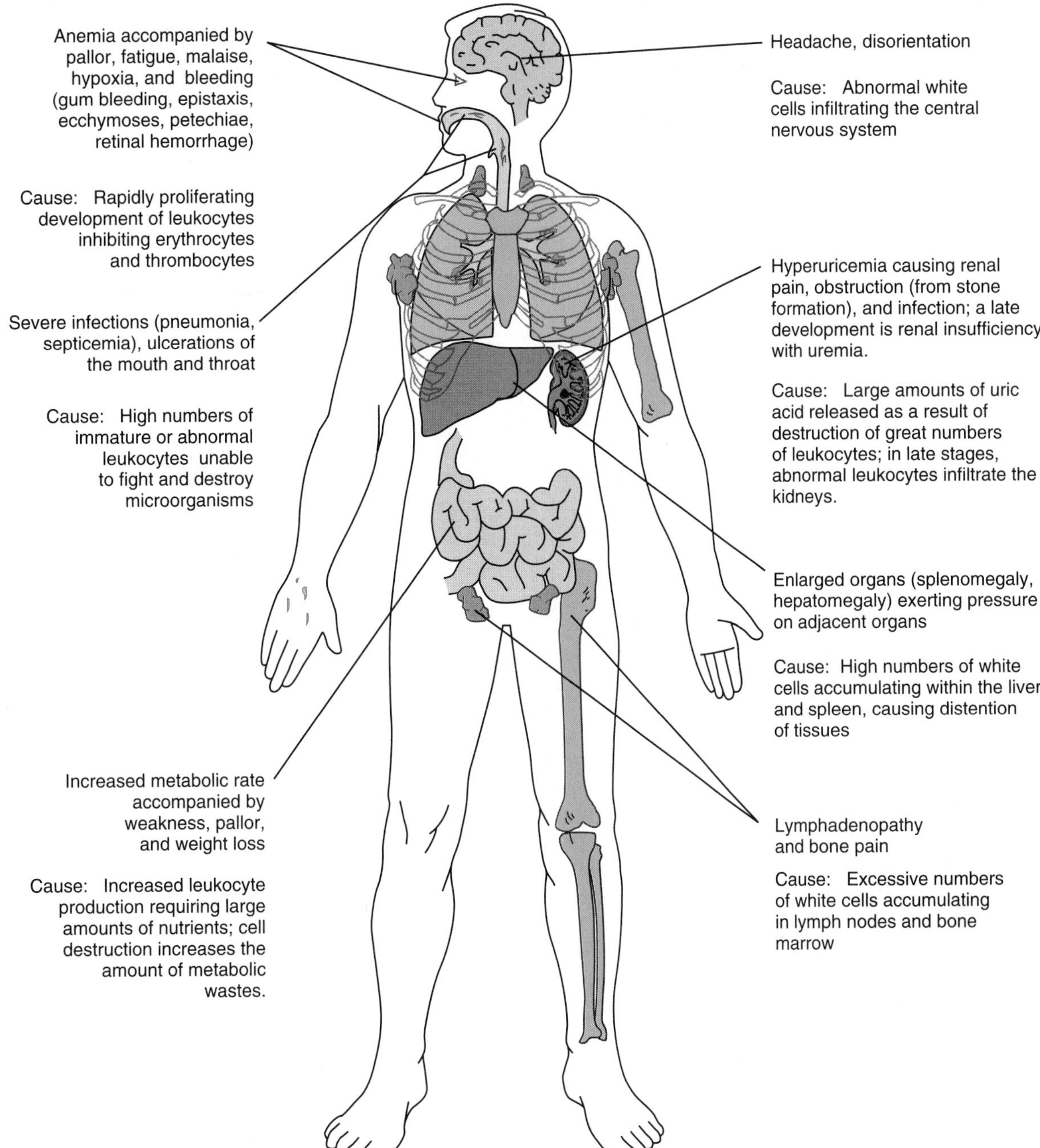

Figure **11–4.** Pathologic basis for the clinical manifestations of leukemia. (*Redrawn with permission from Black JM, Matassarin-Jacobs E (eds): Luckmann and Sorensen's Medical-Surgical Nursing, ed 4. Philadelphia, WB Saunders, 1993, p 1358.*)

gin,[9] *-blastic* and *acute* for leukemia involving immature cells, and *-cytic* and *chronic* for leukemia involving mature cells. If classified immunologically, T-cell, B-cell, or null-cell leukemias are described.

The two major forms of acute leukemia are *acute lymphocytic leukemia* (ALL) and *acute nonlymphocytic leukemia* (ANLL).[10] Lymphocytic leukemia involves the lymphocytes and lymphoid organs and nonlymphocytic leukemia involves hematopoietic stem cells that differentiate into myeloid cells (monocytes, granulocytes, erythrocytes, and platelets) (see Fig. 11–3).

Incidence. Acute leukemia is primarily a disease of the

[9] Clear distinctions between acute myeloid and lymphoid leukemia may not be as important as was once thought; the disordered differentiation inherent in these diseases frequently leads to co-expression of myeloid and lymphoid characteristics on the same cell (Borson and Loeb, 1994).

[10] Acute nonlymphocytic leukemia (ANLL) was formerly known as acute myelogenous leukemia or AML. Other synonyms for ANLL include granulocytic, myelocytic, monocytic, myelogenous, monoblastic, and monomyeloblastic.

TABLE 11-3 OVERVIEW OF LEUKEMIA

	ALL	ANLL (AML)	CLL	CML
Incidence (% of all leukemias)	20	20	25–40	15–20
Adults	20	85	100	95–100
Children	80–85	10–20	—	3
Age (yr)	Peak: 3–7 65+ (older adults)	15–40; incidence increases with age from 40–80+	50+	25–60
Etiology	? Unknown; chromosomal abnormality; environmental factors; Down syndrome (high incidence)	Benzene; alkylating agents; radiation; myeloproliferative disorders; aplastic anemia	Chromosomal abnormalities; slow accumulation of CLL lymphocytes	Philadelphia chromosome; radiation exposure
Prognosis	Adults: poor Children: 60% with aggressive treatment	Poor even with treatment 10%–15% survival	2–10 yr survival Median survival: 6 yr	Poor; 2–8 yr Median survival: 3–4 yr

ALL, acute lymphocytic leukemia; ANLL, acute nonlymphocytic leukemia; CLL, chronic lymphocytic leukemia; CML, chronic myelocytic leukemia.

elderly, present equally between the sexes. The incidence across all age groups is 15 per 100,000 persons, but this begins to rise at age 40 years and by age 80 years, incidence is approximately 160 per 100,000. ANLL constitutes 20% of all leukemias: 85% of adult acute leukemias and 20% of childhood leukemias. Eighty percent of children with acute leukemia have the lymphocytic type (ALL). Even so, the incidence of acute lymphocytic leukemia is still four times higher in the elderly than in children (Abrams et al., 1995).

Etiology and Risk Factors. The etiology of acute leukemia is unknown in most cases. Most of the genetic defects that increase the likelihood of leukemia are acquired rather than inherited, but little is known about the environmental factors that induce these defects. The occurrence of certain leukemias early in childhood has led to the suggestion that there may be changes in genes that are inherited or acquired in utero, but such changes have yet to be fully identified (Cline, 1994).

Predisposing environmental factors may include exposure to ionizing radiation (e.g., atomic bomb survivors, diagnostic radiologists, or people with thymus enlargement, ankylosing spondylitis, or acne who received RT early in this century); occupational exposure to the chemical benzene; long-term, low-dose exposure to drugs, such as alkylating agents and nitrosourea used in chemotherapy; presence of primary immune disorders; and infection with the human leukocyte virus (HTLV-1) (Linker, 1994).

Chronic bone marrow disorders, such as the myelodysplastic syndromes, polycythemia vera, and aplastic anemia, are sometimes followed by a rapidly progressive leukemic phase. Other acquired disorders that progress to acute leukemia include chronic myelocytic leukemia (CML), Hodgkin's disease, multiple myeloma, ovarian cancer, and chronic lymphocytic leukemia (CLL). In fact, therapy-related ANLL (t-ANLL)[11] is the most frequently reported secondary cancer as a result of high doses of chemotherapy for Hodgkin's disease, multiple myeloma, ovarian cancer, non-Hodgkin's lymphoma, and breast cancer (Fraser and Tucker, 1988).

[11] The reader may still see this reported in the literature as t-AML.

Pathogenesis. The molecular analysis of ALL has produced new insights into the pathogenesis of this disease. This disease is heterogenous (i.e., can be produced by genes at more than one location) (Levitt and Lin, 1996). ALL, which accounts for 80% of all childhood leukemias, is caused by the malignant proliferation of precursor lymphocytes, called *lymphoblasts* (Wujcik, 1993b). ANLL involves neoplastic proliferation of multipotent or committed hematopoietic precursor cells. In the case of therapy-related ANLL, alkylating agents (cytotoxic drugs and radiation) react directly with DNA and induce ANLL, primarily through partial chromosomal deletions or loss of whole chromosomes. The chromosome changes provide the altered cells with a proliferative advantage compared with normal cells (Pedersen-Bjergaard and Rowley, 1994).

Clinical Manifestations. Acute leukemia frequently presents as an apparent infection with an acute onset and high fever (see Fig. 11–4). Bleeding due to thrombocytopenia usually occurs in the skin and mucosal surfaces, manifested as gingival bleeding, epistaxis, mid-cycle menstrual bleeding, or heavy bleeding associated with menstruation.

Bone pain, especially of the sternum, ribs, and tibia, caused by expanded leukemic marrow and joint pain from leukemic infiltration or hemorrhage into a joint, may be initial symptoms (more common finding in children than adults). Involvement of the synovium may lead to symptoms suggestive of a rheumatic disease, especially in children with ALL. Leukemic infiltration, hemorrhage into a joint, synovial reaction to an adjacent tumor mass, or crystal-induced synovitis may result in arthritis symptoms as well. In the elderly, the disease can present insidiously with progressive weakness, pallor, a change in sense of well-being, and delirium.

Neurologic manifestations are unusual at initial diagnosis of ANLL, but they occur with increasing frequency over time and may be due to either leukemic infiltration or cerebral bleeding. Cranial nerve palsies most often involve the sixth and seventh cranial nerves. Headache, vomiting, papilledema, facial palsy, blurred vision, auditory disturbances, and meningeal irritation can occur if leukemic cells infiltrate the cerebral or spinal meninges. Because chemotherapeutic agents do not pass the blood-brain barrier, leukemia cells can grow easily in the brain (Mansen et al., 1994).

Medical Management

Diagnosis. Leukemic cells react differently when exposed to various chemicals leading toward a histochemical diagnosis (e.g., chemical markers in the cells are used to differentiate between ALL and ANLL). Chromosomal studies are becoming an important tool in the differential diagnosis of ALL, and cell-surface antigens have made it possible to further differentiate ALL into immunologic classes.

In the acutely ill client who presents with symptoms that indicate abnormal bone marrow function (infection, thrombocytopenia, anemia, bone pain), diagnosis is quickly confirmed by bone marrow aspiration and biopsy. Blood smear, hemoglobin, platelet counts, and blood uric acid assays are usually all abnormal. Lumbar puncture may be performed to investigate any CNS involvement.

Treatment. The diagnosis of acute leukemia is a medical emergency, especially if the WBC count is high (greater than 100,000/μL), placing the person at risk for cerebral hemorrhage caused by leukostasis (obstruction of and damage to blood vessels plugged with rigid blasts). Treatment decisions are based on ALL subtypes. For example, persons with T-cell ALL can be cured with chemotherapy alone, whereas in the case of B-cell ALL with certain chromosomal abnormalities bone marrow transplantation is recommended if an HLA-match is unavailable (Levitt and Lin, 1996).

ANLL has been treated initially for 4 to 6 weeks with intensive combination chemotherapy, called *remission induction therapy*, to eradicate the neoplastic cells and restore normal hematopoiesis. Supportive care, including transfusion and antibiotics, may be required during the recovery period (Burnett and Eden, 1997). Relatively few studies have been conducted to determine the optimum treatment strategy for the older person with ANLL. At the present time, intensive chemotherapy is considered if the older person's overall status and desires are consistent with this approach (Auerbach, 1994).

Prognosis. If left untreated, all leukemias are fatal. Over the last 30 years, a dramatic improvement has been seen in survival of individuals with ALL, owing to the effectiveness of improved treatment. Survival rate has improved from a 4-year survival rate of 4% in the 1960s to a 75% 5-year survival rate in the 1990s (American Cancer Society, 1992; Borson and Loeb, 1994). Only 25% achieve long-term disease-free survival, and the prognosis for clients with ALL is less favorable if any of the following factors exist: (1) presentation in younger or older age groups, (2) male sex, (3) high leukocyte count (over 100,000) at the time of diagnosis, (4) CNS involvement, and (5) chromosomal abnormalities (Pavel et al., 1993).

New probes for specific chromosomal DNA and sensitive techniques for the detection of immunoglobulin and T-cell receptor gene rearrangements may allow detection and quantification of minimal residual disease after treatment or early detection of remission (Arenson, 1993).

Chronic Leukemia

Overview. Chronic leukemia has two major groups: chronic myelocytic leukemia (CML) and chronic lymphocytic leukemia (CLL). Other less common forms include prolymphocytic leukemia (terminal transformation of CLL), large lymphocytic leukemia, and hairy cell leukemia (also called *leukemic reticuloendotheliosis*, accounting for only 1% to 2% of adult leukemias).

Incidence, Etiology, and Risk Factors. CML accounts for 15% of all leukemias. CLL is the most common type in Western society, accounting for 25% to 40% of all leukemias and increasing with advancing age. Ninety percent of all affected persons are older than 50 years, and men are affected twice as often as women.

Although its etiology is unknown, the incidence of CML is increased in people with radiation exposure. It is the only form of leukemia with a known genetic predisposition (Philadelphia chromosome; Ph). The specific genetic anomaly is a translocation that fuses the long arm of chromosome 22 to chromosome 9 in all three hematopoietic cell lines; this form of leukemia is more common in families, and especially those with immunologic abnormalities.

The cause of CLL is also unknown. Unlike other hematologic malignancies, there is no increased incidence following radiation exposure, nor is there a known retroviral association (Morrison, 1994) but investigation continues as to a possible viral cause. Chronic viral infections such as Epstein-Barr virus are considered possible causes of chronic leukemia.

Pathogenesis. CML originates in the pluripotent hematopoietic stem cell[12] and involves overproduction of myeloid (bone marrow) cells. The Ph chromosome was the first consistent chromosomal anomaly identified in a cancer, and is now detected in all cases of chronic myelocytic leukemia. The molecular defect in CLL is unknown. In general, it is characterized by the proliferation of early B lymphocytes.

In the case of the Ph chromosome associated with CML, the accidental fusion disrupts the normal pathway and results in a dysregulated proliferation signal (Cline, 1994). The Ph chromosome is present in more than 95% of CML cases as well as in 25% of cases of adult ALL, 10% of cases of childhood leukemia, and 5% of cases of ANLL (Morrison, 1994).

Clinical Manifestations. Chronic leukemia may be asymptomatic or it may present with fatigue or lymphadenopathy found in the cervical, axillary, and supraclavicular areas. Other less common sites of involvement include the gut mucosa, lungs, skin, and bone. The most common initial symptoms are splenomegaly, extreme fatigue, malaise, weight loss, low-grade fever, night sweats, easy bruisability, bone pain, and decreased exercise tolerance.

The duration of the chronic phase is about 3 years. In most persons a gradual transition occurs called the *accelerated phase* from the chronic to the acute phase over a median

---

[12] Remember that this cell has the ability to develop into any one of several blood cells (see Fig. 11–3).

time of 4 years (Kantarjian et al., 1987; Cannellos, 1990). Infections complicate the disease course of more than 75% of clients.

Medical Management

Diagnosis. Presenting signs and symptoms are often quite nonspecific. Abnormal bleeding and symptomatic splenomegaly are clinical signs pointing to CML, but CML must be differentiated from other myeloproliferative disease. As with other leukemias, laboratory findings, including blood and bone marrow testing, will assist in establishing the diagnosis. The Ph chromosome is almost invariably present and may be detected in either the peripheral blood or the bone marrow (Linker, 1994).

Treatment. Recombinant human α-interferon in the chronic phase of CML may induce hematologic remission, and suppress the Ph chromosome. At present, allogeneic bone marrow transplantation in highly selected clients with CML (those younger than 40 years who have a suitable matched donor) offers the only chance of producing long-term disease-free survival and possible cure (Andreoli et al., 1993; Clift et al., 1993).

There is no known cure for CLL, and treatment is usually based on clinical staging. Initial stages of chronic leukemia do not require treatment, because the complications of chemotherapy may be more harmful than the leukemia. Treatment is palliative during the symptomatic stage. A new class of drugs (purine analogues) has had a major impact on both response rates and remissions in CLL (Borson and Loeb, 1994).

Prognosis. The chronic forms of leukemia usually remain stable for years and then transform to a more overtly malignant disease. Once the disease has progressed to the accelerated or blast phase, survival is measured in months. Approximately 60% of young adults who have successful allogeneic bone marrow transplantation appear to be cured (McGlave, 1990).

Despite treatment advances, the median survival of CLL clients remains 4 to 6 years. Death is usually due to disease progression with infectious or hemorrhagic complications (Morrison, 1994).

Special Implications for the Therapist **11-6**

LEUKEMIA

Precautions

The period following chemically induced remission is critical for each client who is now highly susceptible to spontaneous hemorrhage and defenseless against invading organisms. The usual precautions for thrombocytopenia and infection control must be adhered to strictly. The importance of strict handwashing technique with an antiseptic solution cannot be overemphasized. The therapist should be alert to any sign of infection and report any potential site of infection, such as mucosal ulceration, skin abrasion, or a tear (even a hangnail). Precautions are as for anemia, outlined earlier in this chapter.

Neuropathy can occur as a result of the neurotoxic effects of chemotherapy. For the client on bed rest, prevention of pressure ulcers through client and family education and positioning with appropriate protection (e.g., footboard to prevent footdrop, protective coverings such as sheepskin and eggshell foam) are important. For the mobile client, safety standards must be followed during ambulation because of weakness and numbness of the extremities that may occur after treatment. Drug-induced mood changes, ranging from feelings of well-being and euphoria to depression and irritability, may occur; depression and irritability may also be associated with the cancer. Anticipating these and other potential side effects of medications used in the treatment of leukemia can help the therapist better understand client reactions during therapy.

Joint Involvement

Arthralgias or arthritis occur in approximately 12% of adults with chronic leukemia, 13% of adults with acute leukemia, and up to 60% of children with acute lymphoblastic leukemia. Articular symptoms are the result of leukemic infiltrates of the synovium, periosteum, or periarticular bone, or of secondary gout or hemarthrosis (Andreoli et al., 1993). Asymmetrical involvement of the large joints is most commonly observed. Pain that is disproportionate to the physical findings may occur, and joint symptoms are often transient (Gilkeson and Caldwell, 1990).

Hodgkin's Disease

Definition and Overview. Hodgkin's disease is a neoplastic disease of lymphoid tissue with the primary histologic finding of giant Reed-Sternberg cells in the lymph nodes. These cells are part of the tissue macrophage system and have twin nuclei and nucleoli that give it the appearance of "owl eyes." The Reed-Sternberg cell is probably the malignant cell, with the surrounding cells representing tissue reaction. Although this malignancy originates in the lymphoid system and primarily involves the lymph nodes, it can metastasize to any tissue and often metastasizes to non-nodal or extralymphatic sites, such as the spleen, liver, bone marrow, and lungs.

Hodgkin's disease is staged (determination of anatomic extent) according to the microscopic appearance of the involved lymph nodes, the extent and severity of the disorder, and the prognosis. The classic TNM (for *tumor*, *node*, *metastasis*) system of staging is being replaced by the Ann Arbor staging classification (Table 11–4) because it is not always possible to determine the primary tumor site (Beahrs et al., 1992). The stages are subdivided by the absence (A) or presence (B) of fever (more than 38°C, or 102°F), night sweats, or weight loss (more than 10% of body weight in the last 6 months) (Press et al., 1993).

At diagnosis, about 10% to 15% of clients will have disease limited to a single lymph node region (stage I), and another 10% to 15% of clients will have bone marrow or extensive extranodal disease (stage IV). The majority of people diagnosed with Hodgkin's disease will have stage II or III disease at presentation (70% to 80%) (Weinshel and Peterson, 1993).

Incidence. Hodgkin's disease is primarily a disease of young adults but children and the elderly can be affected. Incidence

TABLE 11-4 MODIFIED ANN ARBOR STAGING CLASSIFICATION FOR HODGKIN'S DISEASE*

Stage I:	Involvement of a single lymph node region or a single lymphoid structure referred to as an extralymphatic site I_E (e.g., spleen, thymus, Waldeyer's ring)
Stage II:	Involvement of 2 or more lymph node regions on the same side of the diaphragm
Stage III:	Involvement of lymph node regions or structures on both sides of the diaphragm
Stage IV:	Diffuse involvement of extralymphatic sites, with or without lymph node enlargement

* For all stages: A = asymptomatic; B = constitutional symptoms.
From Weinshel EL, Peterson BA: Hodgkin's disease. CA Cancer J Clin 43:333, 1993.

rates differ according to age with an overall incidence of approximately 2.6 per 100,000 (slightly lower for women). In the United States, about 7900 cases of Hodgkin's disease were diagnosed in 1994 compared with 43,000 cases of non-Hodgkin's disease. The overall incidence of Hodgkin's disease has remained stable for many years.

Hodgkin's disease peaks at two different ages: during the second to third decades and during the sixth to seventh decades; overall a progressive increase in incidence occurs with advancing age. By age 80 years, the incidence is approximately 40/100,000. A greater incidence is seen in geographic bands, including the United States, the Netherlands, and Denmark.

Etiology. The cause of Hodgkin's disease is unknown, although persons with long-term autoimmune disease or immunosuppression secondary to illness, cytotoxic drugs, or drug abuse have an increased incidence. Other risk factors may include a history of viral infection (mononucleosis or Epstein-Barr virus), environmental exposures, and/or genetically determined factors (Kennedy, 1993).

Most recently, evidence to support a familial link has been reported (Mack et al., 1995). Data from this study indicated that genetic susceptibility, rather than environmental factors, is responsible for the familial clustering of Hodgkin's disease. However, an environmental factor such as a virus could still play a role by triggering the disease in persons who are genetically susceptible.

Pathogenesis. Hodgkin's disease is considered a clonal disorder because abnormal chromosomes are present in multiple cells from the lymph nodes. The origin of these abnormal cells (Reed-Sternberg cells) and the kinds of molecular events that result in malignant transformation remain unknown. The identity of the normal counterpart of the Reed-Sternberg cell may be an activated lymphoid cell with features of lymphocytes and reticulum cells. It is possible that the cell of origin (T cell, B cell, or monocytic) varies depending on the specific case studied and that multiple pathologic processes may lead to the development of Hodgkin's disease (Weinshel and Peterson, 1993).

Normal lymphoid tissue is replaced by the malignant lymphoma, resulting in immunodeficiency and infections. Without treatment, the entire node is replaced by malignant tissue with subsequent necrosis. The bone marrow may be replaced, resulting in pancytopenia (depression of all the cellular blood elements) and subsequent bleeding and infection. Tumor bulk may obstruct or invade vital organs, ultimately causing death (Abrams et al., 1995).

Clinical Manifestations *(Fig. 11–5)*. Asymptomatic lymphadenopathy (enlarged, firm, nontender, movable nodes) of the cervical (Fig. 11–6), axillary, inguinal, and retroperitoneal areas may be discovered on routine examination; but constitutional symptoms of fever, night sweats, pruritus, anorexia, or weight loss may be present in about 40% of the population with lymphoma. Some clients report that lymph node tenderness increases with ingestion of alcohol.

Hodgkin's disease follows an anatomic distribution of nodal involvement, referred to as the *contiguous spread model*, so that a client with cervical adenopathy may also have supraclavicular or mediastinal adenopathy. Pelvic adenopathy or liver involvement is unlikely in the case of isolated cervical adenopathy. All symptoms occur with greater frequency in older clients and in people with a poor prognosis based on histologic findings (Weinshel and Peterson, 1993).

When enlarged lymph nodes obstruct or compress adjacent structures, local symptoms may occur, such as edema of the face, neck, or right arm secondary to superior vena cava compression or renal failure secondary to urethral obstruction. When enlarged lymph nodes obstruct the inferior vena cava, significant dependent edema of the lower extremities may occur.

Pulmonary symptoms of nonproductive cough, dyspnea, chest pain, and cyanosis may occur secondary to mediastinal lymph node enlargement extending to the lung parenchyma with invasion of the pleura. Obstruction of the bile ducts as a result of liver damage causes bilirubin to accumulate in the blood and discolor the skin.

Dissemination of disease from lymph nodes to bone may cause compression of the spinal cord, leading to paraplegia. Spinal cord involvement is more common in the dorsal and lumbar regions than in the cervical area. Compression of nerve roots of the brachial, lumbar, or sacral plexus can cause nerve root pain. Epidural involvement causes back and neck pain with hyperreflexia. Retroperitoneal nodes can involve vertebral bodies and nerves. Extremity involvement is characterized by pain, nerve irritation, and obliteration of the pulse.

Special Problems

Pregnancy and Hodgkin's Disease. Since the mean age at diagnosis of Hodgkin's disease is 32 years, it is not uncommon for women to develop Hodgkin's disease while pregnant. Pregnancy has no adverse impact on the natural course of Hodgkin's disease, and Hodgkin's disease has no effect on the course of gestation, delivery, or the incidence of prematurity or spontaneous abortions. The risk of metastatic involvement of the fetus by Hodgkin's disease is negligible (Ward and Weiss, 1989).

The management of Hodgkin's disease during pregnancy must be individualized. Many women have been successfully treated while pregnant without adverse effects on the fetus. In cases of disease onset early in pregnancy, the recommendation may be made to consider a therapeutic abortion. Women presenting in later pregnancy are often able to have therapy delayed until after delivery (Weinshel and Peterson, 1993).

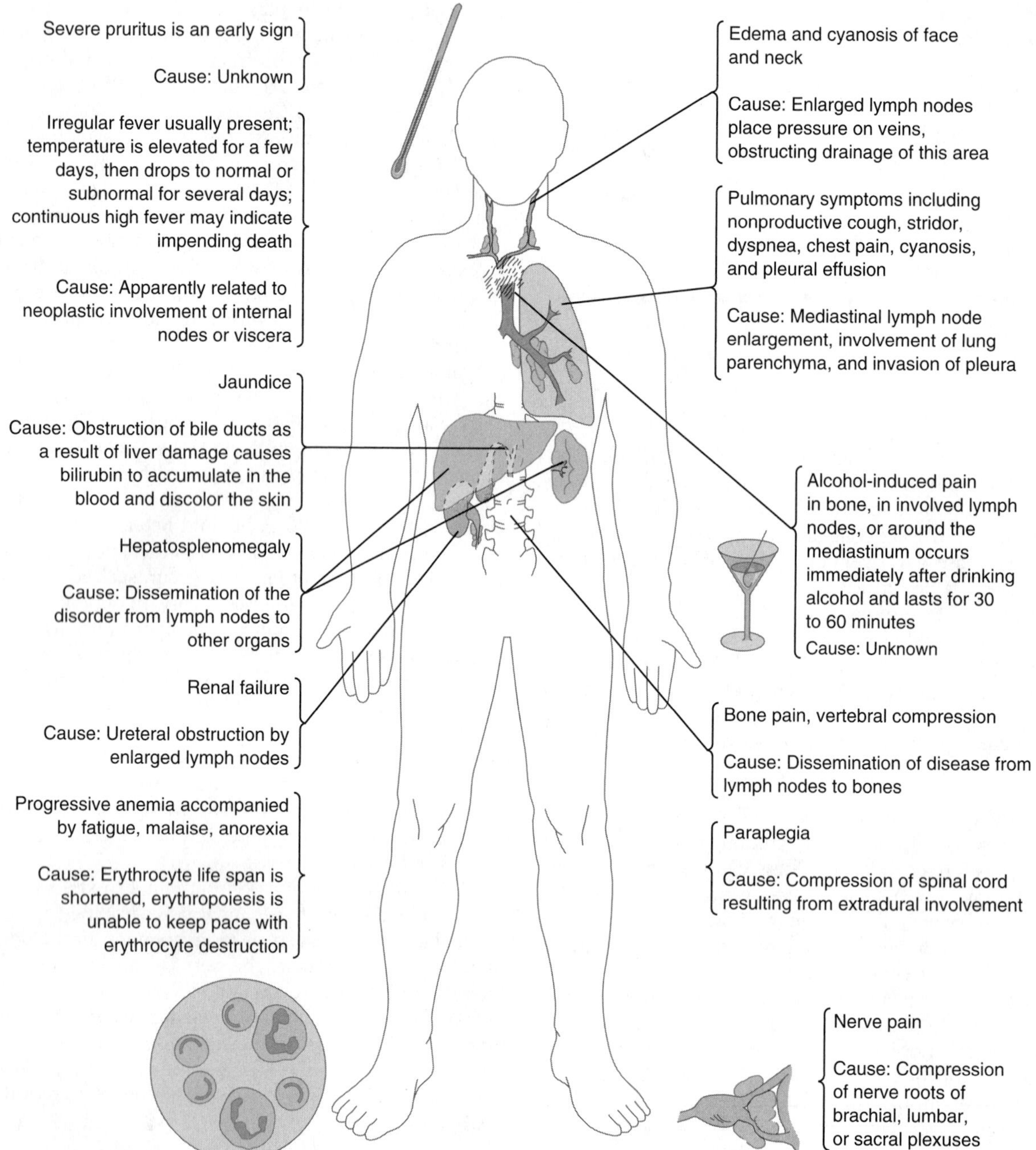

Figure **11–5.** Pathologic basis for the clinical manifestations of Hodgkin's disease. (*Redrawn with permission from Black JM, Matassarin-Jacobs E (eds): Luckmann and Sorensen's Medical-Surgical Nursing, ed 4. Philadelphia, WB Saunders, 1993, p 1370.*)

Hodgkin's Disease in the Elderly. This disease in the elderly person appears to have a different course when compared with that in younger clients. Older people tend to present with more advanced stages and a worse prognosis. Their health is often complicated by other medical problems, causing difficulty in tolerating aggressive chemotherapy. The prognosis for the older person with Hodgkin's disease is worse, and treatment is more problematic (Kennedy et al., 1992).

Hodgkin's Disease in AIDS. The incidence of Hodgkin's disease in young men is relatively high, irrespective of the AIDS epidemic, but HIV-positive clients are at increased risk, and those who develop Hodgkin's disease usually present with aggressive, advanced-stage disease and systemic symptoms. Treatment with standard chemotherapy can produce long-term remissions, but the chemotherapy is poorly tolerated and the incidence of opportunistic infections is increased. Overall survival is shortened by AIDS-related complications and refractory disease (Prior et al., 1986).

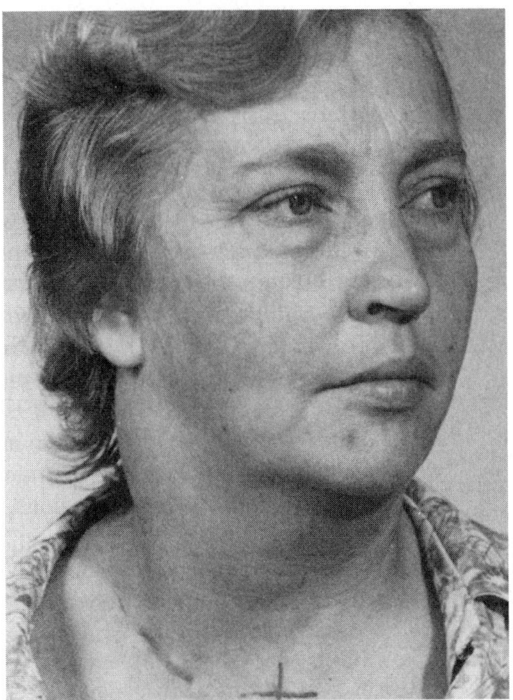

Figure **11-6.** Enlarged cervical lymph node associated with Hodgkin's disease. (*From del Regato J, Spjut HJ, Cox JD: Cancer: Diagnosis, Treatment, and Prognosis, ed 6. St Louis, Mosby-Year Book, 1985.*)

Medical Management

Diagnosis. Diagnosis depends on identification of Reed-Sternberg cells in lymph node tissue or at other sites. Diagnosis may be delayed by several years owing to the insidious nature of lymphadenopathy. Because of the multiple organs that can be involved, diagnosis requires a complete physical examination in addition to routine blood chemistry profile and tests to determine the extent or the stage of the disease.

Accurate staging is essential for planning the treatment protocol and is accomplished with computed tomographic (CT) scan, possible exploratory laparotomy with splenectomy, liver biopsy (if the findings will significantly alter stage and therapy), multiple node biopsies, and, possibly, a lymphogram. Needle biopsy is not adequate for diagnosis, as it does not yield sufficient tissue to exclude other diseases and to subclassify the disease; the excisional lymph node biopsy is required.

Treatment. Cure of Hodgkin's disease is the primary treatment goal through the use of radiation therapy, chemotherapy, and, in some cases, both. The specific treatment is guided by the stage of the disease at diagnosis. External-beam radiation therapy is used with stages I and II unless chemotherapy is required to shrink the bulk of disease before curative radiation therapy. Radiation therapy alone for stages I to III provides a 10-year freedom-from-relapse rate of 80% and a 10-year survival rate of 90% (Hoppe, 1990; Lee et al., 1990). For persons who have relapse after radiation therapy, standard combination chemotherapy is the usual second-line treatment of choice.

Clinical stage III or IV is too widespread for successful radiation treatment only and requires treatment with chemotherapy. Combination chemotherapy, called MOPP (for nitrogen mustard [*m*echlorethamine], vincristine [*O*ncovin], *p*rocarbazine, and *p*rednisone), is one of the best treatment programs for stage III or IV Hodgkin's disease. Therapy consists of at least six 14-day cycles with 14-days' rest between cycles. The duration of chemotherapy is 6 to 12 months or at least 2 months following complete remission. A 94% 10-year survival rate for persons with stage III disease is recorded with this treatment (Longo et al., 1986). Stage IV disease treatment with MOPP has shown a long-term disease-free survival rate of 50% (Wiernik, 1988).

The introduction of bone marrow transplantation offers further potential for cure with complete remission rates of 40% to 70% with a 5-year relapse-free survival rate of 20% to 40% (Vose et al., 1990; Reece et al., 1991). Newer studies have used peripheral blood stem cells with or without colony stimulating factor (Korbling et al., 1990).

Side effects of radiation treatment may include sore throat, dysphagia, nausea, and diarrhea. Delayed effects may also occur, including pneumonitis, suppressed ovarian function (if the ovaries are not moved out of the radiation field prior to treatment), and hypothyroidism (if the thyroid is present in the radiation field). Graves' disease and thyroid cancer can occur. The risk of late complications with irradiation may persist for more than 25 years after the treatment (Hancock et al., 1991) (see Adverse Drug Reactions, Chapter 4).

Side effects of the MOPP program include nausea, vomiting, and bone marrow suppression. Long-term effects may include sterility, leukemia (usually within 2 to 10 years), or secondary neoplasm directly related to radiation exposure (primarily lung cancer, but also sarcoma, melanoma, and stomach and breast tumors).

Prognosis. The long-term prognosis for clients with Hodgkin's disease depends on several factors including age at diagnosis, disease stage at diagnosis, suitability of treatment administered (Mausch et al., 1990), and rapidity of response to chemotherapy; B symptoms (see Table 11-4) decrease the survival figures at each stage. With successful treatment (primary radiation therapy and salvage combination chemotherapy for relapse after radiation therapy) almost 70% of clients are long-term survivors.

Despite significant advances in radiation techniques and combination chemotherapy, 20% to 50% of clients will be resistant to therapy or relapse after primary therapy. Persons who suffer relapse from primary radiation therapy (stage I to II) have a similar or even better prognosis than those with advanced stage (stage III to IV) disease treated with chemotherapy. The most important prognostic factors following relapse are the extent of disease at the time of relapse and age greater than 50 years (Weinshel and Peterson, 1993).

Most relapses occur within the first 3 years after completion of therapy. Early relapse of less than 1 year from a complete remission after first-line MOPP therapy carries a complete remission rate of about 20% to 40% with alternative chemotherapy. In such cases, a failure-free survival rate of about 10% to 25% is seen at 3 to 5 years (Buzaid et al., 1987; Canellos, 1991).

Late first-time relapses can occur in up to 10% of clients

at risk more than 3 years after the first remission was induced by irradiation (Herman et al., 1985). In late relapses from a complete remission that lasted at least 12 months, a high response rate is still seen (50% to 90% complete remission) with further chemotherapy. In this group, the 5-year failure-free survival rate is 10% to 50% (Buzaid et al., 1987). Very late relapses are uncommon.

Elderly persons in advanced stages of disease are unable to tolerate maximal radiation and chemotherapy doses, which decreases their chances for survival. Treatment of older persons may also be less effective owing to a biologic difference in Hodgkin's disease in older persons (Kennedy, et al., 1992). Untreated, clients with Hodgkin's disease have a life expectancy of 5 years (Weinshel and Peterson, 1993).

Special Implications for the Therapist **11-7**

HODGKIN'S DISEASE

The therapist may palpate enlarged painless lymph nodes during a cervical, spine, shoulder, or hip examination. Lymph nodes are evaluated on the basis of size, consistency, mobility, and tenderness. Lymph nodes up to 1 cm in diameter of soft to firm consistency that move freely and easily without tenderness are considered within normal limits. Lymph nodes greater than 1 cm in diameter that are firm and rubbery in consistency or tender are considered suspicious. Enlarged lymph nodes associated with infection are more likely to be tender than slow-growing nodes associated with cancer.

Because lymph nodes enlarge in response to infections throughout the body, referral to a physician is not necessary on finding enlarged lymph nodes unless the nodes persist for more than 4 weeks or involve more than one area. However, the physician should be notified of these findings and the client advised to have the lymph nodes checked at the next follow-up visit with the physician. As always, *changes* in size, shape, tenderness, and consistency should raise a red flag. Supraclavicular nodes are common metastatic sites for occult lung, breast, and testicular cancers, whereas inguinal nodes implicate tumors arising in the legs, perineum, prostate, or gonads (Press et al., 1993).

Requirements for infection control and treatment subsequent to the cytotoxic effects on the CNS are outlined previously in the section The Leukemias.

Malignant Lymphomas

Overview. Lymphomas, or non-Hodgkin's lymphoma (NHL), are solid tumors arising from cells of the lymphatic system (lymphoid cells). Malignant transformation can occur at any stage of B or T lymphocyte differentiation. The lymph nodes are usually involved first and any extranodal lymphoid tissue, particularly the spleen and thymus, and GI tract may also be involved. The bone marrow is commonly involved by lymphoma cells, but this is rarely the primary site of a lymphoma.

Lymphomas are classified according to cell size, growth pattern, T- and B-cell markers, and clinical grade. Low-grade lymphomas are clinically indolent (slow-growing and painless) and include small cell lymphocytic and most follicular lymphomas; intermediate lymphomas include diffuse and most large cell lymphomas; and high-grade lymphomas are clinically aggressive and include large cell immunoblastic, lymphoblastic, and Burkitt's lymphomas.

Clinical staging of NHL is done according to the same criteria for Hodgkin's disease with two exceptions: NHLs are more likely to present in an extranodal site and the progression of the NHL does not follow the orderly anatomic progression typical of Hodgkin's disease. Stage I and II NHLs are rare, because the disease is much more likely to be disseminated at the time of diagnosis.

Incidence. In the past, NHL constituted only 3% of all malignancies in the United States and was uncommon except in groups with a predisposition. Recent recognition by epidemiologists and clinicians that the incidence of NHL has been undergoing a universal increase without identifiable cause has been reported. This increase has occurred since the early 1970s among all age groups (except the very young), whites and blacks, both United States and international populations, and both sexes (Devesa and Fears, 1990). Three factors that may contribute to the rise of NHL have been suggested: the increased incidence of HIV, effects of immunosuppressant drugs taken by increasing numbers of people receiving organ transplants, and improved diagnostic techniques.

Malignant lymphomas are the most common neoplasm of adults between the ages of 20 and 40 years. The reported epidemic preceded that of HIV infection, but with the increasing incidence of AIDS, the number of cases of NHL has also sharply increased. Certain kinds of malignant lymphomas (lymphoblastic and Burkitt's) occur in children.

Etiology and Risk Factors. Predisposing factors for lymphoma include infection and immunologic defects resulting from illness or from medical treatment, such as kidney or cardiac transplants. A wide variety of primary and secondary immunodeficiencies, including collagen vascular diseases and AIDS, have been associated with an increased incidence of lymphomas. This phenomenon may reflect a decrease in the host's surveillance mechanism against transformed cells or from prolonged exposure to oncogenic agents, such as Epstein-Barr virus, as a consequence of failure to mount an adequate immune response (Arenson, 1993). The recently reported increased incidence occurring before the HIV phenomenon remains unaccounted for (Mueller, 1994).

Although the occurrence of lymphoma may be associated with autoimmune diseases, low-dose methotrexate therapy used for classic and juvenile rheumatoid arthritis carries an increased risk of lymphoproliferative disease (Zimmer-Galler and Lie, 1994). Other risk factors include viruses, cancer treatment with alkylating agents, and occupational exposure to chemicals such as herbicides and benzene.

Pathogenesis. Although the exact cause of NHL is unknown, studies using techniques of molecular biology have provided some clues to the pathogenesis of NHL. The malignant lymphomas develop from the malignant transformation of a single lymphocyte that is arrested at a specific stage of B or T lymphoid cell differentiation (Shipp, 1994; Terhune and Cooper, 1993). Because immunosuppressed persons have a greater incidence of the disease, an immune mechanism is suspected. Unlike in Hodgkin's disease, T cell function is minimally affected (30%), but B cell abnormalities are more common in NHL (70%). In children, virtually all malignant lymphomas are high-grade, aggressive neoplasms (Rubin and Farber, 1994).

Clinical Manifestations. The NHLs are variable in clinical presentation and course, varying from indolent disease to rapidly progressive disease. Lymphadenopathy is the first symptom of NHL with painless enlargement of isolated or generalized lymph nodes of the cervical, axillary, inguinal, and femoral (pelvic) chains. This development occurs slowly and progressively over an extended period (months to years).

Extranodal sites of involvement may include the nasopharynx, GI tract, bone, thyroid, testes, and soft tissue. Abdominal lymphoma may cause abdominal fullness, GI obstruction or bleeding, ascites, back pain, and leg swelling. NHL presenting as polyarthritis has been reported (McDonagh et al., 1994). Constitutional symptoms, which may include fever, night sweats, pallor, fatigue, and weight loss, are present with high-grade lymphomas.

Lymphomas are frequently associated with lesions of the CNS and may be AIDS-associated primary CNS lymphoma or non-AIDS associated CNS lymphoma. Clients with NHL associated with AIDS may have symptoms isolated to the CNS but the clinical and radiographic presentation, clinical characteristics, and prognosis differ substantially between AIDS-associated CNS lymphoma and non–AIDS-associated CNS lymphoma. Recent advances in the treatment of lymphoma in clients without AIDS have not largely affected lymphoma clients with AIDS (Fine and Mayer, 1993).

Medical Management

Diagnosis and Treatment. Accurate diagnosis is important because of the other clinical conditions that can mimic malignant lymphomas (e.g. tuberculosis, systemic lupus erythematosus, lung and bone cancer). Molecular genetic techniques that take advantage of the clonal nature of this malignancy are now being applied to better characterize and diagnose the lymphomas (Terhune and Cooper, 1993).

However, at the present time, a biopsy is still required to confirm the underlying cause of persistent enlargement of lymph nodes present on clinical examination. Fine-needle aspiration is starting to be used in place of biopsy, but fine-needle aspiration has not replaced biopsy as the primary diagnostic procedure. Chest x-ray and CT scan of the abdomen and pelvis may be helpful in staging. Spleen and bone marrow may be examined for staging and peripheral blood may be tested, but blood abnormalities are not present until the disease is in an advanced stage.

Aggressive chemotherapy is administered for high-grade lymphomas and conservative therapy is used for low-grade lymphomas; localized disease may be treated with irradiation. The low-grade lymphomas are indolent and unaffected by therapy; treatment is palliative until the disease progresses, necessitating treatment (usually 1 to 3 years). Disseminated large-cell (intermediate grade) lymphomas are curable in 50% of cases using combination chemotherapy. Autologous BMT may be used for clients with high-risk aggressive lymphomas; combined with aggressive chemotherapy, BMT (or PBSCT) can be curative even in older clients with NHL.

Advances in irradiation of the CNS supplemented with corticosteroids and intrathecally and intravenously administered chemotherapeutic agents have resulted in improvement in the poor prognosis for persons with large-cell lymphoma (Buettner and Bolling, 1993).

Prognosis. Individuals with NHL survive for long periods when involvement is only regional. The presence of diffuse disease reduces survival time. The low-grade lymphomas are usually systemic and widespread, and cure cannot be achieved, whereas intermediate- and high-grade lymphomas are more likely to present as treatable and even curable localized disorders. The prognosis for persons with high-grade lymphomas depends on their response to chemotherapy, except high-grade NHL associated with AIDS, which has an extremely poor prognosis.

Multiple Myeloma

Definition and Overview. Multiple myeloma (MM), also called *plasma cell myeloma,* is a primary malignant neoplasm of plasma cells arising most often in bone marrow. This bone tumor initially affects the bone marrow of the vertebrae, ribs, skull, pelvis, and femur. Later, organs such as the spleen, liver, and kidney are damaged. The extent, clinical course, complications, and sensitivity to treatment vary widely among affected persons.

Incidence and Etiology. The incidence of multiple myeloma has doubled in the past two decades with an annual incidence of approximately 12,500 cases in the United States (Wingo et al., 1995). Myeloma occurs less frequently than the most common cancers (e.g., breast, lung, or colon); its incidence is similar to that of Hodgkin's disease (Anderson, 1994).

This disease can develop at any age, but it peaks among persons between 50 and 70 years; black men are affected twice as frequently as white men. The incidence of multiple myeloma in blacks is almost twice that in whites. It is slightly more common in men than in women. Risk factors and the cause of multiple myeloma are unknown, but in the last decade, plasma cell malignancy has become another AIDS-associated neoplasm (Kumar et al., 1994).

Pathogenesis. Malignant plasma cells arise from B cells that produce abnormally large amounts of one class of immunoglobulin (usually IgG, occasionally IgA, and rarely any others). The abnormal immunoglobulin produced by the malignant transformed plasma cell is called the *M-protein.*

The M-protein is responsible for many of the clinical manifestations of the disease. Infiltration and destruction of organs, especially bone, by the neoplastic plasma cells results in pain. In addition to bone destruction, multiple myeloma is characterized by disruption of RBC, leukocyte, and platelet production, which results from plasma cells crowding the bone marrow. Impaired production of these cell forms causes anemia, increased vulnerability to infection, and bleeding tendencies.

Clinical Manifestations. The onset of multiple myeloma is usually gradual and insidious. Many people pass through a long presymptomatic period that lasts from 5 to 20 years. Most often, the initial symptom is bone pain, particularly in the pelvis, spine, and ribs.

Bone pain occurs when plasma cells infiltrate the bone

marrow with subsequent destruction of bone. Initially, the bone pain may be mild and intermittent or it may develop suddenly as a severe pain in the back, rib, leg, or arm, often the result of an abrupt movement or effort that has caused a spontaneous (pathologic) bone fracture (Linker, 1994). The pain is often radicular and sharp to one or both sides and is aggravated by movement (Salmon and Cassady, 1993).

Symptoms associated with bone pain usually subside within days to weeks after initiation of systemic chemotherapy, but if the disease progresses, more and more areas of bone destruction develop. Drainage of calcium and phosphorus from damaged bones eventually leads to the development of renal stones, particularly in immobilized clients; renal failure may occur (Pavel et al., 1993). To rid the body of the excess calcium (hypercalcemia), the kidneys increase the output of urine, which can lead to serious dehydration if intake of fluids is inadequate. Symptoms of hypercalcemia may include confusion, increased urination, loss of appetite, abdominal pain, constipation, and vomiting (see further discussion of Hypercalcemia, Chapter 4).

Amyloidosis (deposits of insoluble fragments of a protein resembling starch) develops in approximately 10% of people with multiple myeloma. These deposits cause tissues to become waxy and immobile and may affect nerves, muscles, and ligaments, especially the carpal tunnel area of the wrist. Carpal tunnel syndrome with pain, numbness, or tingling of the hands and fingers may develop.

More serious neurologic complications may develop in 10% to 15% of clients with multiple myeloma when vertebral body collapse or extradural extension of the tumor occurs. Spinal cord compression is usually observed early or in the late relapse phase of the disease. Back pain associated with spinal cord compression is usually present as the initial symptom, with radicular pain that is aggravated by coughing or sneezing. Motor or sensory loss and bowel/bladder dysfunction are signs of more extensive compression. Paraplegia is a late, irreversible event (Salmon and Cassady, 1993).

Medical Management

Diagnosis. In approximately 20% of people diagnosed with multiple myeloma, screening laboratory studies may reveal an increased serum protein concentration indicating multiple myeloma (Alexanian et al., 1988). Plasma cells circulating in the peripheral blood can be detected by use of sensitive immunofluorescence, flow cytometric studies, or molecular genetic techniques. The detection of these cells is clinically important because they correlate with disease activity. As multiple myeloma progresses, the plasma cells appear in greater numbers in the peripheral blood (Witzig, 1994). The presence of abnormal immunoglobulin in the urine (Bence Jones protein) is also diagnostic of multiple myeloma.

Treatment. All clients with multiple myeloma should be monitored, but not all require treatment. Symptoms, physical findings, and laboratory data are taken into consideration (Press et al., 1993). For many years, standard treatment for multiple myeloma has been intermittent cycles of melphalan plus prednisone (MP) or a combination of alkylating agents. Clinical results were good with temporary disease control in 50% of cases but relapse occurred in less than 2 years with low survival rate (Oken, 1994).

Multiple myeloma continues to be one of the most difficult cancers to treat effectively. No available treatment is curative, but now about two-thirds of symptomatic people treated initially with low-dose combination chemotherapy achieve a stable response. These responses are associated with elimination of bone pain and symptom-free status for months without further treatment (MacLennan et al., 1994). Treatment of complications, such as fractures, anemia, hypercalcemia, renal failure, and recurrent bacterial infections, is also part of the picture.

In persons who have a response to chemotherapy, the primary goal is to prolong the duration of remission with the fewest side effects. Interferon inhibits the growth of plasma cells in vitro and has been used to prolong remission. Long-term interferon therapy is costly and has side effects, such as fatigue, mental depression, and anorexia, to which older people are more susceptible.

Allogeneic (matched donor) bone marrow transplantation is possible for only 5% to 10% of people with multiple myeloma who are younger than 50 years (median age, 65 to 70 years) and have an HLA-compatible sibling. The advantage of this type of BMT is that the graft contains no tumor cells that can provoke a relapse. However, there is a significant early and high rate of mortality (40%), and risk of graft-vs-host disease and relapse is common (Kyle, 1993; Gahrton et al., 1991). This treatment is reserved for persons with a poor prognosis after standard therapy.

Autologous (harvested from recipient) bone marrow transplantation (ABMT) has broader applicability because the age limit is higher and a matched donor is unnecessary. It is not suitable for persons older than 70 years or who have major medical problems or relapsing disease. Eradication of multiple myeloma may not occur, even with large doses of chemotherapy and irradiation, when infused ABMT or peripheral blood stem cells (PBSCT) have been contaminated by myeloma cells or by their precursors, which will cause relapse (Tricot et al., 1996).

Complications associated with standard treatment (prolonged alkylating agent therapy prior to transplantation) include myelodysplastic syndromes and acute myeloid leukemia. Stem cell–damaging treatment should be avoided so as not to compromise the peripheral bone stem cells and to reduce the risk of these complications (Govindarajan et al., 1996). Future treatment under investigation includes peripheral stem cell grafting, posttransplant immunotherapy, gene therapy, new drugs, new ways of delivering radiotherapy to specific sites, and radiopharmaceuticals that concentrate at involved marrow sites.

Prognosis. If untreated, unstable multiple myeloma can result in skeletal deformities, particularly of the ribs, sternum, and spine. Diffuse osteoporosis develops, accompanied by a negative calcium balance. Prognosis is affected by the presence of renal failure, hypercalcemia, or extensive bony disease; infection and renal failure are the most common causes of death (Fang, 1993).

Despite 30 years of clinical trial research conducted by three major cooperative groups under the auspices of the National Cancer Institute, the prognosis for multiple myeloma has not improved probably due to marked resistance of tumor cells, even at diagnosis, to commonly employed cytotoxic drugs (Alexanian et al., 1994; Barlogie et al., 1997). For those persons with multiple myeloma who receive radiation or chemotherapy treatment, the median duration of remission is approximately 2 years and the median survival is approximately 3 years. Fewer than 10% live longer than 10 years; relapse occurs on average in a little under 2 years, and despite response to second-line chemotherapy, the disease often recurs (Alexanian and Dimopoulos, 1994).

Early data from studies of autologous transplantation indicate that overall survival of newly diagnosed and refractory multiple myeloma treated with transplantation appears superior to that of treatment with conventional chemotherapy. Such therapy can be administered safely in people up to 70 years old (Barlogie et al., 1997; Jagannath et al., 1994).

Most clients with myeloma ultimately suffer relapse. Autotransplantation as currently performed is not curative in a substantial proportion of people treated. Future improvements with transplantation may be achieved by providing tumor-free grafts and posttransplant treatment aimed at eradicating minimal residual disease (Tricot et al., 1996).

Special Implications for the Therapist **11-8**

MULTIPLE MYELOMA

Adequate hydration and mobility help minimize the development of hypercalcemia. Any symptoms of hypercalcemia (see Clinical Manifestations) must be reported to the physician; the client should seek immediate medical care as this condition can be life-threatening. (For the client with amyloidosis, anemia, or renal failure, see Special Implications for the Therapist for each of these conditions.)

A laminectomy may be required when spinal cord compression occurs. The client with multiple myeloma who develops signs of cord compression must be referred to the physician. Emergency magnetic resonance imaging (MRI) is required to locate the area of cord compression. Immediate radiation and high-dose glucocorticoid therapy usually relieve the compression, avoiding the need for a laminectomy (Alexanian and Dimopoulos, 1994). Orthopedic back braces are generally poorly tolerated; however, newer lightweight supports with Velcro fasteners may be more useful (Salmon and Cassady, 1993).

(For clients receiving BMT or PBSCT treatment, see Bone Transplantation, this chapter.)

Myeloproliferative Disorders

Uncontrolled expansion of all bone marrow elements results in a group of clinical conditions known as *myeloproliferative disorders*, which can be characterized as a malignant disease because increased production of bone marrow elements, such as erythroid, myeloid, and platelet lines, results from a neoplastic transformation of a hematopoietic stem cell or precursor cell that develops into a specific bone marrow cell.

The four diseases commonly grouped together as the myeloproliferative disorders are polycythemia vera, myelofibrosis with myeloid metaplasia, essential thrombocytopenia, and chronic myelogenous leukemia (CML). These disorders are grouped together because the disease may evolve from one form into another; all of the myeloproliferative disorders may progress to acute myelogenous leukemia. Polycythemia vera, thrombocytopenia, and CML are included in this text (polycythemia because of the thrombosis or stroke associated as a complication, thrombocytopenia because of the risks during exercise, and CML because it is the most common myeloproliferative disorder) (discussed previously).

TABLE 11-5 LABORATORY VALUES ASSOCIATED WITH POLYCYTHEMIA

	MEN	WOMEN
Hemoglobin (g/dL)	>17.5	>15.5
Erythrocytes ($\times 10^{12}$/L)	>6.0	>5.5
Hematocrit (%)	42–52	37–47

From Goodman CC, Snyder TE: Differential Diagnosis in Physical Therapy, ed 2. Philadelphia, WB Saunders, 1995, p 199.

Polycythemia Vera

Definition and Overview. Polycythemia vera, also known as erythrocytosis, is a neoplastic disease of the bone marrow stem cell primarily affecting the erythroid cells, which produce erythrocytes, but causing overproduction of all three hematopoietic cell lines. Polycythemia vera may be primary or secondary (see Etiology for differentiation); it is characterized by an excessive number of erythrocytes leading to an increased concentration of hemoglobin, increased hematocrit (measure of the volume of packed RBCs), and an increased hemoglobin level (Table 11–5).

Etiology and Pathogenesis. Polycythemia is considered *primary* when caused by a precursor cell abnormality. *Secondary* polycythemia is a physiologic condition resulting from a decreased oxygen supply to the tissues associated with high altitudes, heavy tobacco smoking, and chronic heart and lung disorders. In secondary polycythemia, the body attempts to compensate for the reduced oxygen by producing more hemoglobin and more erythrocytes.

The etiology of primary polycythemia vera is unknown, but it occurs in older persons between 50 and 60 years, equally distributed between the sexes. Primary (absolute) polycythemia (increased red cell mass) is relatively uncommon, whereas secondary (relative) polycythemia (normal red cell mass but decreased plasma volume) is more likely encountered. The increased concentration of erythrocytes causes increased blood viscosity with potential decreased cerebral blood flow, decreased cardiac output, and a tendency toward clotting (thrombosis) when the hematocrit level exceeds 60%.

Clinical Manifestations. Clinically, symptoms are related to expanded blood volume, increased blood viscosity, and clogging of microcirculatory blood vessels. The client may demonstrate increased skin coloration (ruddy complexion of face, hands, feet, ears, and mucous membranes) and elevated blood pressure. Gout is sometimes a complication of secondary polycythemia, and a typical attack of acute gout may be the first symptom.[13]

[13] The metabolic consequences of increased cell turnover associated with this condition result in increased waste products, including increased uric acid, which may lead to gout.

The symptoms of both primary and secondary polycythemia are much the same; they are often insidious in onset and characterized by vague complaints, and diagnosis may not be made until a secondary complication, such as stroke or thrombosis, occurs. Other symptoms may include headache, dizziness, epistaxis, irritability, blurred vision, fainting, feeling of fullness in the head, disturbances of sensation in the hands and feet,[14] splenomegaly, general malaise and fatigue, backache, weight loss, easy bruising, and intolerable pruritus (itching), especially after bathing with warm water.

Medical Management

Diagnosis. Diagnosis is made by history, examination, and laboratory analysis. WBC and platelet count are elevated in most persons with polycythemia vera and are normal in most persons with secondary polycythemia. A specific test (chromium-labeled red cell mass) is used to distinguish between absolute polycythemia (increased red cell mass) and relative polycythemia (normal red cell mass but decreased plasma volume).

Treatment. Treatment goals are to reduce erythrocytosis and blood volume, control symptoms, and prevent thrombosis. The primary treatment for polycythemia vera is phlebotomy to remove excess blood, but this does not stop the rapid regeneration of erythrocytes and may cause iron deficiency, necessitating supplemental iron administration. More serious cases may be treated with myelosuppression; the current choice of chemotherapy in polycythemia vera is the antimetabolite hydroxyurea, which does not appear to be associated with an increased incidence of acute leukemia. Treatment for secondary polycythemia is directed toward the underlying condition as well as toward treatment of symptoms, such as controlling the uric acid levels that produce gout.

Prognosis. The prognosis for polycythemia vera is good, and median survival is 10 years with appropriate treatment. Without proper treatment, the mortality rate (18 months from the time of symptomatic onset) is 50%. The risk for stroke, myocardial infarction, and thromboembolism is high for persons with this condition; thrombosis or hemorrhage is the major cause of death. Late in the course of this disease, bone marrow may be replaced with fibrous tissue (myelofibrosis), red cell production may decrease, and anemia and marked splenomegaly may develop.

Special Implications for the Therapist **11-9**

POLYCYTHEMIA VERA

Although polycythemia vera is associated with high altitudes, heavy smoking, and chronic heart conditions, clients with COPD have the highest potential risk for secondary polycythemia. Clients with chronic pulmonary conditions do not ventilate adequately, and the body attempts to compensate for the reduced oxygen by producing more RBCs.

Thrombosis occurs more often in clients with polycythemia, which requires the therapist to be alert to any possible signs of deep vein thrombosis (DVT) (see discussion of thrombophlebitis, Chapter 10). Watch for complications such as hypervolemia, thrombocytosis, and signs of impending cerebrovascular accident (e.g., decreased sensation, numbness, transitory paralysis, fleeting blindness, headache, and epistaxis).

If the person has symptomatic splenomegaly, follow precautions for soft tissue techniques required in the left upper quadrant (especially up and under the rib cage). These procedures must be secondary or indirect techniques away from the spleen.

DISORDERS OF HEMOSTASIS

Hemostasis is the arrest of bleeding after blood vessel injury and involves the interaction between the blood vessel wall, the platelets, and the plasma coagulation proteins. Disorders of hemostasis are caused by defects in platelet number or function or to problems in the formation of a blood clot (coagulation). Simply stated, any interruption of the coagulation cascade (Fig. 11–7) results in a bleeding or a clotting disorder.

Normal platelet function and a platelet count greater than 100,000/μL in the peripheral blood are needed for normal hemostasis. Alterations of platelets and coagulation affect hemostasis, either by preventing hemostasis or by causing hemostasis to occur when it is not needed. When this process is pathologically exaggerated, thrombosis occurs.

Platelets (thrombocytes) are not cells; they are granular, disk-shaped, nonnucleated cell fragments. Approximately two thirds of all platelets are contained in the circulatory system, and the remainder are present in the spleen as a reserve pool. Platelet life span is approximately 6 to 10 days. Platelets also derive from the stem cells and are essential to hemostasis and coagulation.

Hemostasis results from the adhesion and aggregation capabilities of platelets to plug small breaks in blood vessels. Most physiologic and pathologic coagulation is initiated by the exposure of blood to tissue factor (previously called *thromboplastin* or *coagulation factor III*). Platelets release tissue factor (thromboplastin),[15] which converts prothrombin into thrombin in the first step of the coagulation mechanism. In the second step of the coagulation process, thrombin promotes the conversion of fibrinogen into fibrin (Lottman and Thompson, 1995).

Bleeding caused by platelet disorders is characterized by mucosal and skin bleeding (petechiae), purpura,[16] and pro-

---

[14] Blockage of the capillaries supplying the digits of either the hands or the feet may cause a peripheral vascular neuropathy with decreased sensation, burning, numbness, or tingling. This same small blood vessel occlusion can also contribute to the development of cyanosis and clubbing of the digits. If untreated, the worst case scenario may include gangrene requiring amputation.

[15] Tissue factor is found in places not normally exposed to blood flow, where the presence of blood is pathologic. It is present in significant amounts in the brain, subendothelium, smooth muscle, uterus, and epithelium. Tissue factor is not found in skeletal muscle or synovium, the usual locations for spontaneous bleeding in people with hemophilia (Wheeler and Rubenstein, 1994).

[16] Purpura is a hemorrhagic condition that occurs when there are not enough normal platelets to plug damaged vessels or prevent leakage from even minor injury to normal capillaries. Purpura is characterized by movement of blood into the surrounding tissue (extravasation), under the skin and through the mucous membranes, producing spontaneous ecchymoses (bruises) and petechiae (small red patches) on the skin. When accompanied by a decrease in the circulating platelets, it is called *thrombocytopenic purpura*. In the acute form, there may be bleeding from any of the body orifices, such as hematuria, nosebleed, vaginal bleeding, and bleeding gums (O'Toole, 1992).

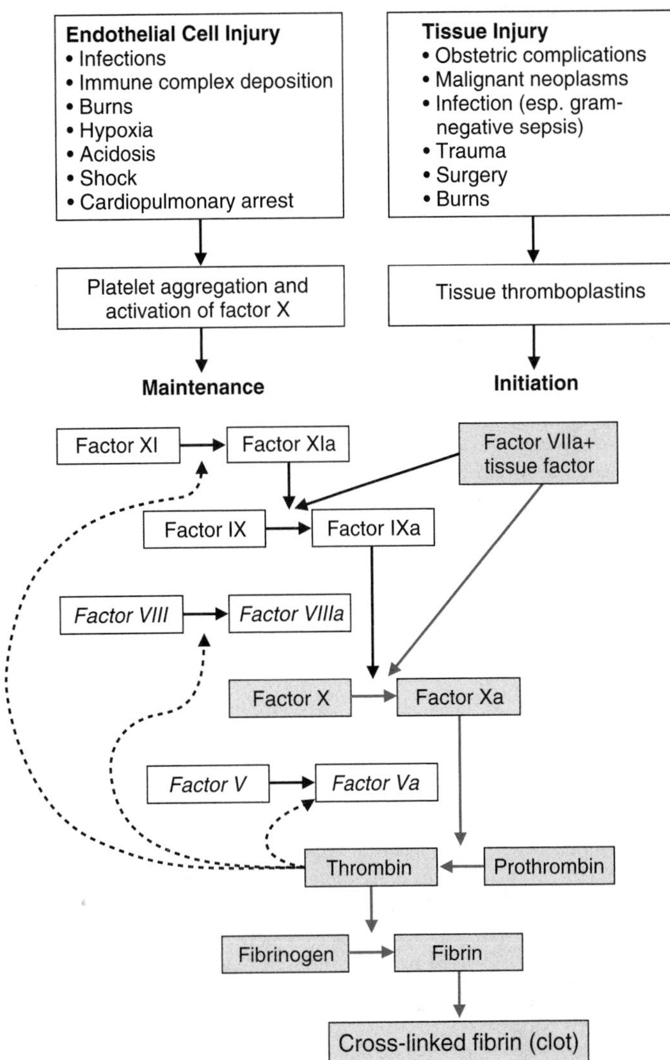

Figure **11-7.** Formation of a blood clot. This schematic diagram of the coagulation cascade reflects recent changes in the understanding of coagulation. Most coagulation is initiated by the combination of factor VIIa and tissue factor, now called the *initiation* (or tissue factor) *pathway* (formerly called the *extrinsic pathway*). The response is amplified and maintained by a positive feedback loop of thrombin-activating enzymes (*dotted arrows*) called the *maintenance pathway* (formerly the *intrinsic pathway*). Factors Va and VIIIa are co-factors, not enzymes, and are shown in italics. (*Adapted from Wheeler A, Rubenstein EB: Current management of disseminated intravascular coagulation.* Oncology 8:74, 1994.)

longed oozing of blood after trauma or surgery (Andreoli et al., 1993). Other common problems include epistaxis, gum bleeding, menorrhagia (excessive menstruation), and GI bleeding.

Coagulation disorders caused by a deficiency of one or more clotting factors result in more serious bleeding, such as deep muscle hematoma and spontaneous hemarthrosis. Conversely, vascular abnormalities that stimulate clotting produce disorders called *thromboembolic disease*, in which coagulation occurs unnecessarily.

Abnormalities in the number of circulating platelets, either an increase in the number of platelets, called *thrombocytosis*, or a decrease in the number of platelets, called *thrombocytopenia*, can interrupt normal blood coagulation and prevent hemostasis.

Thrombocytosis

Thrombocytosis, an increase in the number of circulating platelets (>400,000/mm^3) may be primary or secondary; it usually remains asymptomatic until the platelet count exceeds 1 million/mm^3. Thrombocytosis may occur as a normal physiologic response (mobilization of platelets from the spleen or lung under the influence of epinephrine) to stress, infection, trauma, surgery, splenectomy, exercise, and ovulation. Abnormal thrombocytosis is caused by accelerated platelet production in the bone marrow.

Primary thrombocytosis (hemorrhagic thrombocythemia) is a myeloproliferative disorder in which megakaryocytes (giant cell of the bone marrow) overproliferate in association with other conditions such as chronic nonlymphoblastic leukemia, polycythemia vera, and myelofibrosis (replacement of hematopoietic bone marrow with fibrous tissue).

Secondary thrombocytosis occurs after splenectomy because platelets that normally would be stored in the spleen remain in the circulating blood. The increase in platelets may be gradual, so that thrombocytosis does not occur for up to 3 weeks after splenectomy (Mansen et al., 1994). Other forms of secondary (reactive) thrombocytosis occur as a result of conditions such as infection (e.g., tuberculosis), inflammatory disease (e.g., rheumatoid arthritis), and malignancy, and resolve with treatment of the underlying pathology.

Blood viscosity is increased by the high platelet count, which causes intravascular clumping or thrombosis, particularly of peripheral blood vessels and especially in the fingers or toes. In severe episodes, thrombosis of hepatic, mesenteric, or pulmonary vessels may occur. Other symptoms may include

TABLE 11-6 CAUSES OF THROMBOCYTOPENIA

ADULT	CHILD
Bone marrow failure or infiltration	Phototherapy
Radiation	Congenital or hereditary disorders
Aplastic anemia	Trisomy 13 or 18
Leukemia	Metabolic disorders
Metastatic cancer	Perinatal aspiration syndromes
Cytotoxic agents (chemotherapy)	Immunologic
Drug hypersensitivities (e.g., gold, sulfonamides, ethanol/alcohol, aspirin, quinidine, quinine, antibiotics [penicillins and cephalosporins])	Idiopathic thrombocytopenic purpura
Blood transfusions	Drug-induced
Nutritional deficiency	Infection-induced
Prosthetic heart valves	Post-transfusion
Hypersplenism	Autoimmune or lymphoproliferative disorders
Viral and bacterial infections	Neonatal immune thrombocytopenia
Complication of heparin therapy	Post-transplant
Autoantibody-mediated platelet injury (called idiopathic thrombocytopenic purpura)	Allergy and anaphylaxis
	Nonimmunologic
	Hemolytic anemia
	Thrombotic thrombocytopenic purpura
	Catheters, prostheses, cardiopulmonary bypass
	Congenital or acquired heart disease
	Persistent pulmonary hypertension
	Sequestration
	Hypersplenism
	Hypothermia

splenomegaly and easy bruising. Treatment may not be necessary or the condition may resolve with treatment of the underlying condition, as with secondary thrombocytosis. When thrombosis and hemorrhage occur, treatment with phlebotomy or chemotherapy agents is used to lower the platelet count.

Special Implications for the Therapist **11-10**

THROMBOCYTOSIS

The same precautions and screening for symptomatology apply for thrombocytosis as for deep vein thrombosis. Anyone who has had a splenectomy has increased susceptibility to infection. Observe carefully for any signs of infection (see Table 6–1).

Thrombocytopenia

Thrombocytopenia, a decrease in the platelet count below 150,000/mm^3 of blood, is caused by inadequate platelet production from the bone marrow, increased platelet destruction outside the bone marrow, or splenic sequestration. Thrombocytopenia is a common complication of leukemia or metastatic cancer (bone marrow infiltration) and aggressive cancer chemotherapy (cytotoxic agents). Thrombocytopenia may also be a presenting symptom of aplastic anemia (bone marrow failure); other causes are listed in Table 11–6.

Primary bleeding sites include bone marrow or spleen; secondary bleeding occurs from small blood vessels in the skin, mucosa (e.g., nose, uterus, GI tract, urinary tract, and respiratory tract), and brain (intracranial hemorrhage). Symptoms include petechiae and/or purpura in the skin and mucosa, easy bruising, epistaxis, melena, hematuria, excessive menstrual bleeding, and gingival bleeding.

Diagnosis requires the recognition of a bleeding disorder with laboratory examination of blood and bone marrow to confirm the suspected diagnosis. Treatment depends on the precipitating cause (e.g., splenectomy for splenic sequestration, treatment of underlying leukemia, or cessation of cytotoxic drugs until platelet count elevates). Other treatment methods for immune-related thrombocytopenia (e.g., idiopathic thrombocytopenic purpura, or ITP) may include use of cortocosteroids (e.g., prednisone),[17] attenuated androgens (danazol), and plasmapheresis, a procedure that removes blood from the body, separates the portion containing the antiplatelet antibodies, then returns the "cleansed" blood to the body (Jennings, 1992).

The prognosis is variable depending on the underlying cause; it is poor when associated with leukemia or aplastic anemia but good with conditions amenable to treatment.

Special Implications for the Therapist **11-11**

THROMBOCYTOPENIA

Thrombocytopenia can cause bleeding into the muscles or joints, and the severe consequences of this condition may be encountered by the therapist. The therapist must be alert for obvious skin or mucous membrane symptoms of thrombocytopenia, such as severe bruising,

[17] Prednisone therapy decreases the affinity of splenic macrophages for antibody-coated platelets. High-dose prednisone therapy also reduces the binding of antibody to the platelet surface, and long-term therapy may decrease antibody production (Linker, 1994).

external hematomas, and the presence of petechiae. Such symptoms usually indicate a platelet level below 100,000/mm³. Instruct the client to watch for signs of thrombocytopenia, to immediately apply ice and pressure to any external bleeding site, and to avoid aspirin and aspirin-containing compounds without a physician's approval because of the risk of increased bleeding.

Strenuous exercise or any exercise that involves straining or bearing down could precipitate a hemorrhage, particularly of the eyes or brain. See Table 11–7 for specific exercise guidelines for thrombocytopenia. Exercise prescription is highly individualized and should take into account intensity, duration, and frequency that is appropriate for the individual's condition, age, and previous activity level.

Blood pressure cuffs and similar devices must be used with caution. When used, elastic support stockings must be thigh-high, never knee-high. Mechanical compression with a pneumatic pump and soft tissue mobilization are contraindicated unless approved by the physician.

Anyone who has had a splenectomy has increased susceptibility to infection. Practice good handwashing and observe carefully for any signs of infection (see Table 6–1). (See also Special Implications for the Therapist: Anemia: 11–3.)

Effects of Aspirin and Other NSAIDs on Platelet Function

Acquired disorders of platelet function can occur through the use of aspirin and other NSAIDs that inactivate platelet cyclooxygenase. This key enzyme is required for the production of thromboxane A_2, a potent inducer of platelet aggregation and constrictor of arterial smooth muscle.

A single dose of aspirin can suppress normal platelet aggregation for 48 hours or longer (up to a week) until newly formed platelets have been released. Platelets are anucleate and cannot synthesize new enzyme; once inactivated by aspirin or other NSAIDs, platelets remain inactive for the rest of their lifespan. Other NSAIDs have antiplatelet effects lasting less than 24 hours. The use of aspirin or an aspirin-containing compound is usually contraindicated prior to any surgical procedure.

Symptoms from this phenomenon are mild and may consist of easy bruising and bleeding confined to the skin. Prolonged oozing after surgery involving dental or reconstructive plastic surgery may occur.

TABLE 11-7 EXERCISE GUIDELINES FOR THROMBOCYTOPENIA

PLATELET COUNTS (Cells/mm³)	EXERCISE
150,000–450,000 (normal range)	Normal activity (unrestricted)
50,000–150,000	Progressive resistive exercise (see below) Swimming Low bench stepping Bicycling (no grade; flat only)
30,000–50,000	Active range-of-motion (ROM) exercise Moderate exercise: Stationary bicycling Walking as tolerated Aquatic (pool) therapy
20,000–30,000	Light exercise: Active ROM exercise only Walking as tolerated Aquatic (pool) therapy with physician approval
<20,000	Active ROM Activity restricted to activities of daily living; walking with physician approval

Disseminated Intravascular Coagulation

Definition and Overview. Disseminated intravascular coagulation (DIC), sometimes referred to as *consumption coagulopathy*, is a thrombotic disease caused by overactivation of the coagulation cascade (i.e., normal coagulation gone awry). It is an acquired disorder of platelet function, with diffuse or widespread coagulation occurring within arterioles and capillaries all over the body.

DIC is actually a paradoxical condition in which clotting and hemorrhage occur simultaneously within the vascular system. Uncontrolled activation occurs of both the coagulation sequence, causing widespread formation of thromboses (clots) in the microcirculation, and the fibrinolytic system, leading to consumption of platelets, fibrin (protein essential to clotting), and coagulation factors (element essential to normal blood clotting). Hemorrhage may occur from the kidneys, brain, adrenals, heart, and other organs.

Incidence and Etiology. DIC is common, particularly after shock, sepsis, obstetric complications, leukemia and other neoplasms, and massive trauma. The incidence is estimated at 1 in every 900 to 2400 adult admissions in large urban hospitals (Bell, 1992). The oncology client may develop this syndrome as a result of either the neoplasm itself or of the treatment for the neoplasm. DIC may occur as a result of a variety of predisposing conditions that activate the clotting mechanisms (Table 11–8).

Pathogenesis. The development of DIC is generally associated with three complex pathologic processes (see Fig. 11–7): (1) endothelial damage; (2) release of tissue thromboplastin (TTP); and (3) direct activation of factor X (Mansen et al., 1994). *Damage to the endothelium* (e.g., from sepsis, hypoxia, cardiopulmonary arrest) can precipitate DIC by activating the maintenance (intrinsic clotting) pathway. *Excessive amounts of TTP* in the circulation activate the initiation (extrinsic clotting) pathway by stimulating the release of factor VIIa and tissue factor. Release of TTP is associated with numerous conditions, particularly with various types of trauma such as burns, head injury, myocardial infarction, surgery, obstetric accidents, and malignancies. *Activation of factor X* (proteolytic effect) is stimulated by substances released into the bloodstream from pancreatic and hepatic enzymes and from snake venom.

Once either the maintenance (intrinsic) or initiation (extrinsic) clotting cascade is stimulated, widespread coagulation

TABLE 11-8 Conditions that May Precipitate Disseminated Intravascular Coagulation

Shock

Cirrhosis

Necrotizing enterocolitis

Purpura fulminans

Glomerulonephritis

Acute fulminant hepatitis

Acute bacterial and viral infections, fungal

Release of tissue factor (see Fig. 11–7)
- Fat emboli (fracture)
- Snake bites
- Hemolytic processes (e.g., infection, transfusion reaction, immunologic disorders)
- Liver disease
- Acute pancreatitis
- Neoplasm
  - Acute leukemias
  - Prostatic cancer
  - Pancreatic cancer
  - Stomach cancer
  - Bronchogenic cancer
  - Giant cavernous hemangioma
- Tissue damage
  - Trauma (especially head injury)
  - Pulmonary embolism
  - Myocardial infarction
  - Aspirin poisoning
  - Heat stroke
  - Extensive burns
  - Transplant rejection
  - Surgery (extensive procedures; malignant hyperthermia)
  - Fresh water near-drowning

Obstetric conditions
- Abruptio placentae
- Eclampsia
- Retained placenta
- Retained dead fetus
- Septic abortion
- Amniotic fluid embolism

Adapted from Pavel J, Plunkett A, Sink B: Nursing care of clients with hematologic disorders. *In* Black JM, Matassarin-Jacobs E (eds): Luckmann and Sorensen's Medical-Surgical Nursing, ed 4. Philadelphia, WB Saunders, 1993, p 1378.

occurs throughout the body, leading to thrombotic events within the vasculature. The normal inhibitory mechanisms become overwhelmed so that clotting can occur unrestricted. As a result of the widespread clotting that occurs, the clotting factors become used up and hemorrhage occurs. This leads to the two primary pathophysiologic alterations of DIC: thrombosis in the presence of hemorrhage.

Clinical Manifestations. The tendency toward excessive bleeding can appear suddenly, with little warning, and can rapidly progress to severe or even fatal hemorrhage. Thrombosis may occur in various sites distant to the tumor or its metastases.

Signs of DIC include continued bleeding from a venipuncture site, occult and internal bleeding, and, in some cases, profuse bleeding from all orifices. Other less obvious and more easily missed signs are generalized sweating, cold and mottled fingers and toes (due to capillary thrombi and hypoxia), and petechiae (O'Toole, 1992).

Medical Management

Diagnosis, Treatment, and Prognosis. Diagnosis is made based on clinical presentation in combination with client history, especially the presence of any of the conditions listed in Table 11–8. The diagnosis is confirmed by laboratory blood tests.

Treatment is always directed toward the underlying cause. The hemorrhagic or thrombotic symptoms may be alleviated by blood products or anticoagulants, but the coagulopathy will continue until the causative process is reversed (Phillips, 1994).

In certain conditions (e.g., retained dead fetus), or when the primary disease cannot be treated, intravenous injections of heparin may be used to inhibit the clotting process by blocking thrombin activity and raising the level of the depleted clotting factors. There is some controversy in the use of heparin as it can be a cause of bleeding itself, especially in the presence of peptic ulcer, postoperative bleeding, or central nervous system bleeding.

The mortality rate for DIC is 50% to 80% and can reach 90% if shock or infection is the precipitating event. Survival depends largely on control of the primary underlying condition. Many clinicians view treatment of DIC as futile, and the terminal outcome as unavoidable (Wheeler and Rubenstein, 1994). However, with aggressive individualized treatment, survival rates as high as 76% have been reported in cases of fulminant DIC (Bick and Kunkel, 1992).

Special Implications for the Therapist **11-12**

DISSEMINATED INTRAVASCULAR COAGULATION

Clients with DIC are treated by the therapist in oncology or intensive care units. DIC is either the consequence of malignancy or the end result of multisystem organ failure after trauma affecting multiple systems (e.g., severe trauma or burns). Clients are in critical condition and require bedside care.

Care must be taken to avoid dislodging clots and causing fresh bleeding (see Special Implications for the Therapist: Peripheral Vascular Disease (Thromboembolism): 11–18. Monitor the results of serial blood studies, particularly hematocrit, hemoglobin, and coagulation times. To prevent injury, bed rest during bleeding episodes is required.

Sickle Cell Disease

Sickle cell disease (SCD) is a generic term for a group of inherited, autosomal recessive disorders characterized by the presence of an abnormal form of hemoglobin (hemoglobin S, or Hb S) within the erythrocytes. The presence of Hb S can cause RBCs to change from their usual biconcave disk shape to a crescent or sickle shape during deoxygenation. Hb S is formed by a single genetic mutation; sickle cell disease occurs when an individual inherits the mutant gene from each parent, so that almost all of the hemoglobin consists of Hb S.

Sickle cell diseases include sickle cell anemia, sickle β-thalassemia syndromes (Hb S β'-thalassemia), and hemoglobinopathies such as Hb SC disease, Hb SD disease, and Hb S O_{Arab}. Approximately 50,000 individuals have sickle cell disease in the United States; the number in Africa is correspondingly higher.

The two primary pathophysiologic features of sickle cell disorders are chronic hemolytic anemia and vasoocclusion resulting in ischemic injury. When a sickled cell reoxygenates, the cell resumes a normal shape, but after repeated cycles of "sickling and unsickling," the erythrocyte is permanently damaged and hemolyzes. This hemolysis is responsible for the anemia that is a hallmark of sickle cell disease (Agency for Health Care Policy and Research, 1993). A brief discussion of thalassemias is presented, but only the most severe disorder, sickle cell anemia, is fully discussed in this text.

Sickle Cell Anemia

The anemia associated with sickle cell disease is merely a result (symptom) of the disease and is not the disease itself. Consistent with this idea, the term *sickle cell disease* is used throughout the discussion of sickle cell anemia.

Definition and Incidence. Sickle cell anemia is a hereditary, chronic form of hemolytic anemia in which the rupture of erythrocytes (forming sickle cells) releases hemoglobin prematurely into the plasma, thereby reducing the delivery of oxygen to the tissues. It is a worldwide health problem, affecting many races, countries, and ethnic groups, and is the most common inherited hematologic disorder.

The World Health Organization estimates that each year more than 250,000 babies are born worldwide with this inherited blood disorder. About one in 400 black newborns in the United States has sickle cell anemia, and 1 in 12 black Americans carries the sickle cell trait. The disease is also prevalent in many Spanish-speaking regions of the world, such as South America, Cuba, and Central America, and among the Hispanic community in the United States. There are reported incidences of sickle cell disease in Mediterranean countries such as Turkey, Greece, and Italy (Gaston, 1990).

Etiology. The cause of sickle cell disease and its worldwide incidence is the result of several factors. The sickle cell trait may have developed as a single genetic mutation that provided a selective advantage against severe forms of falciparum malaria. Anyone who carries the inherited trait for sickle cell disease but does not have the actual illness is protected against this form of malaria. In countries with malaria, children born with sickle cell trait survived and then passed the gene for sickle cell disease to their offspring. As populations migrated, the sickle cell trait and sickle cell anemia moved throughout the world.

Several theories purport to explain the origination of sickle cell disease but its actual origin is unknown. It is known that there are four separate types of genetic mutations; each is related to the severity of illness and each is associated with a different geographic location, including different locations in Africa, in Eastern Saudi Arabia, and in India (Powars and Hiti, 1993).

Risk Factors. Because sickle cell disease is inherited as an autosomal recessive trait, both parents of an offspring must have the sickle hemoglobin gene. When both parents have sickle cell trait, they have a 25% chance with each pregnancy of having a child with sickle cell anemia. If one parent has sickle cell trait and the other has a β-thalassemic disorder, they are at the same risk for having a child with a sickle β-thalassemia syndrome. In couples in which one individual has sickle cell trait and one has hemoglobin C trait, the chance of having a child with Hb SC disease is also 25% with each pregnancy. If one parent has sickle cell anemia and the other has the sickle cell trait, the risk of having a child with sickle cell anemia is 50% (Fig. 11–8). Individuals with sickle cell trait should receive nondirective genetic counseling (i.e., counselees are given objective information without personal bias and without provision of specific recommendations) after hemoglobin electrophoresis and other measurements have been performed on each prospective parent (Charache et al., 1991).

Sickle cell disease is characterized by a series of "crises" that result from early destruction of the abnormal cells and obstruction of blood flow to the tissues. Stress from viral or bacterial infection, hypoxia, dehydration, emotional disturbance, extreme temperatures (hot or cold), or fatigue may precipitate a crisis. Additionally, a crisis may be precipitated by the presence of acidosis; exposure to low oxygen tensions as a result of strenuous physical exertion, climbing to high altitudes, flying in nonpressurized planes, or undergoing anesthesia without receiving adequate oxygenation; pregnancy; trauma; and increased body temperature (fever). Any of these factors may shorten release time of oxygen, thereby precipitating a crisis (Adams and Zanderer, 1993).

Pathogenesis. The sickle cell defect occurs in hemoglobin, the oxygen-carrying constituent of erythrocytes. Hemoglobin contains four chains of amino acids, the compounds that make up proteins. Two of the amino acid chains are known

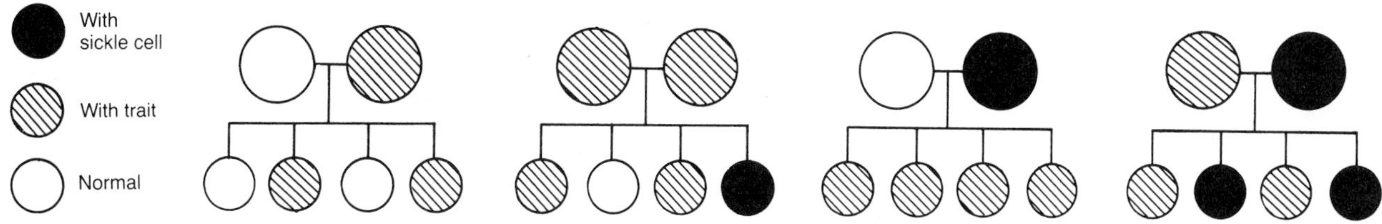

Figure **11–8.** Statistical probabilities of inheriting sickle cell anemia. (*From Page J: Blood: The River of Life. Washington, DC, Torstar Books, 1981.*)

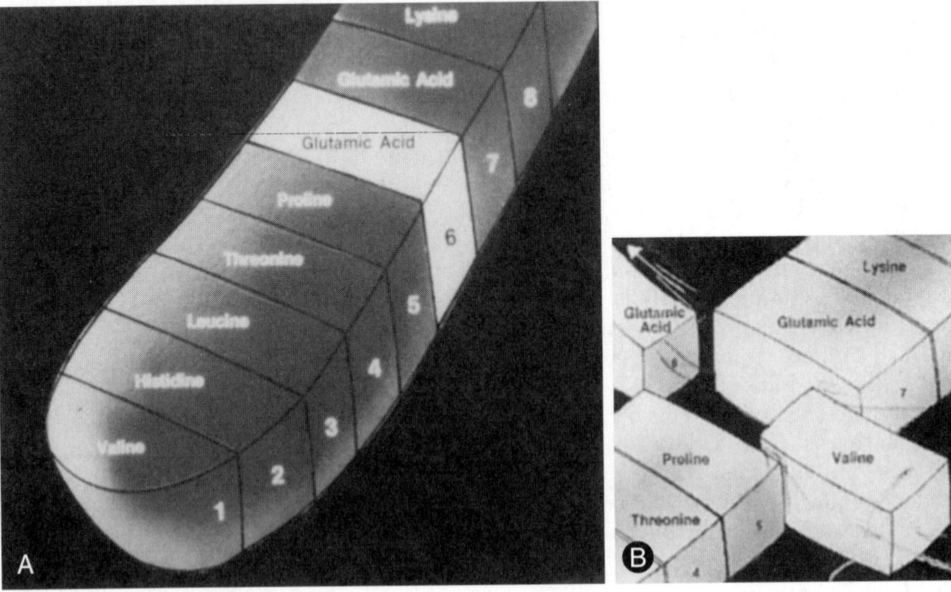

Figure **11–9.** A structural defect in the hemoglobin molecule (A). This single amino acid substitution from glutamic acid to valine at the sixth position in the β chain of hemoglobin (B) has some devastating consequences. (*From Gaston, M: Sickle Cell Anemia, NIH publication No. 90–3058. Bethesda, Md, National Institutes of Health, June 1990, p 4.*)

as α chains, and two are called β chains. In normal hemoglobin, the amino acid in the sixth position on the β chains is glutamic acid. In persons with sickle cell disease, the sixth position is occupied by another amino acid, valine (Fig. 11–9). Using DNA recombinant technology, the genetic locus for the β globin has now been identified on chromosome 11.

This single point mutation of valine for glutamic acid results in a loss of two negative charges that causes surface abnormalities. The sickle hemoglobin transports oxygen normally, but after releasing oxygen, hemoglobin molecules that contain the β chain defect stick to one another instead of remaining separate, and form long, rigid rods or tubules inside RBCs. The rods cause the normally smooth, doughnut-shaped RBCs to take on a sickle or curved shape and to lose their vital ability to deform and squeeze through tiny blood vessels (Fig. 11–10).

The two cardinal pathophysiologic features of sickle cell disorders are chronic hemolytic anemia and vasoocclusion resulting in ischemic tissue injury. Hemolytic anemia is caused by abnormal properties of Hb S and/or by repeated cycles of sickling and unsickling, which interact to produce irreversible red cell membrane changes and erythrocyte destruction.

The sickled cells, which become stiff and sticky, clog small blood vessels, depriving tissue from receiving an adequate blood supply. Occlusion of the microcirculation increases hypoxia, which causes more erythrocytes to sickle; thus is a vicious circle precipitated, which is compounded if dehydration is present. This accumulation of sickled erythrocytes obstructing blood vessels produces tissue injury. The organs at greatest risk are those with venous sinuses, in which blood flow is slow and oxygen tension and pH are low (spleen,

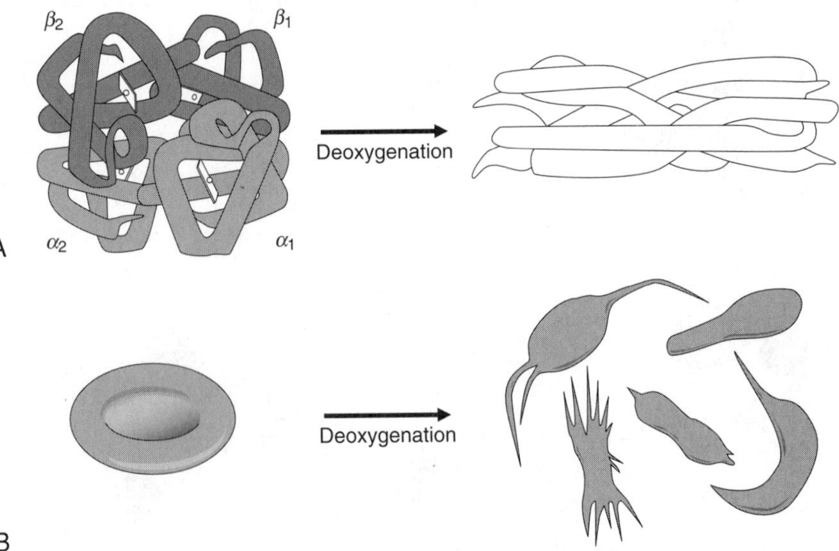

Figure **11–10.** A, The molecular structure of hemoglobin (Hb) contains a pair of α polypeptide chains and a pair of β chains, each wrapped around a heme group (an iron atom in a porphyrin ring). The quaternary structure of the hemoglobin molecule enables it to carry up to four molecules of oxygen. A, In the folded β chain molecule, the sixth position contacts the α chain. The amino acid substitution at the sixth position of the β chain occurring in sickle cell anemia causes the hemoglobins to aggregate into long chains, altering the shape of the cell (Hb S). B, The change of the RBC from a biconcave disk to an elongated or crescent (sickle) shape occurs with deoxygenation.

kidney, bone marrow), or those with a limited terminal arterial supply (eye, head of the femur). No tissue or organ is spared from this injury (Charache et al., 1991).

The earlier the oxygen is released, the more severe (clinically) is the sickle cell disease. The release time can be shortened even more by the risk factors mentioned. Occlusion of small blood vessels throughout the body causes infarcts, such as in the spleen, bone, kidney, and lung; bone marrow expands to compensate for increased red cell hemolysis, leading to osteoporosis and eventually osteosclerosis (Harruff, 1994).

Clinical Manifestations. Intravascular sickling and hemolysis can begin by 6 to 8 weeks of age, but clinical manifestations do not usually appear until the infant is at least 6 months old, at which time the postnatal decrease in Hb F (normal fetal hemoglobin, which inhibits sickling) and increased production of Hb S leads to the increased concentration of Hb S (Andrews and Mooney, 1994).

Acute manifestations of symptoms, called *crises*, usually fall into one of four categories: vasoocclusive or thrombotic, aplastic, sequestration, or, rarely, hyperhemolytic (marked increase in red cell hemolysis associated with drugs or infections) (Fig. 11–11). Pain caused by the blockage of sickled RBCs forming sickle cell clots is the most common symptom of sickle cell disease, occurring unpredictably in any organ, bone, or joint of the body, wherever and whenever a blood

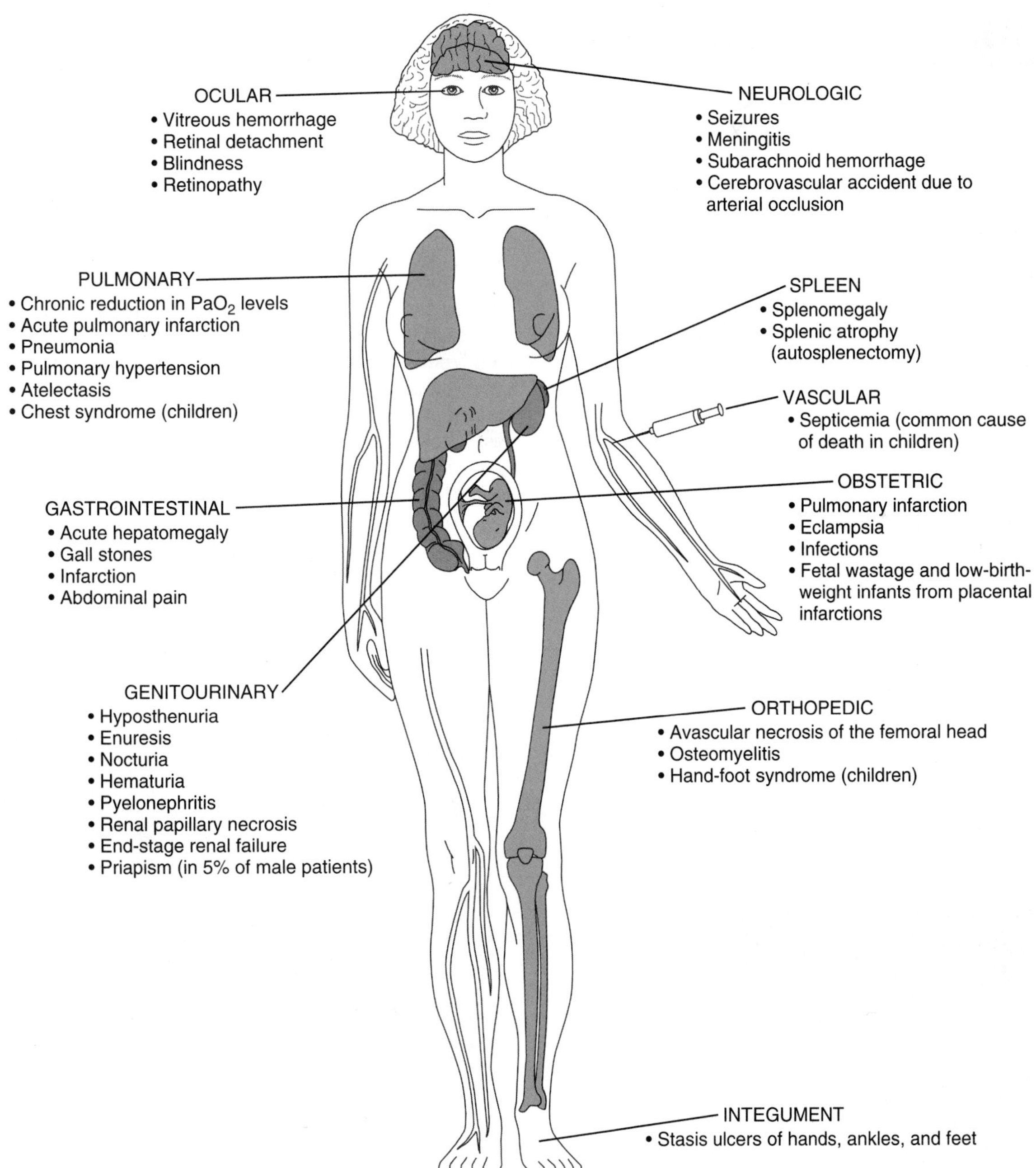

Figure **11–11.** Clinical manifestations and possible complications associated with sickle cell disease.

clot develops. The frequency, duration, and intensity of the painful episodes varies widely (Table 11–9). Some persons experience painful episodes only once a year; others may have as many as 15 to 20 episodes annually. The vasoocclusive crises causing ischemic tissue damage may last 5 or 6 days, requiring hospitalization and subsiding gradually. Older clients more often report extremity and back pain during vascular crises.

Aplastic crisis caused by diminished RBCs results in profound anemia characterized by pallor, fatigue, jaundice, and irritability. This anemia occurs because sickled RBCs last only 10 to 20 days in the bloodstream, rather than the normal 120-day lifespan. The sickled RBCs are removed faster from the circulation than the bone marrow can produce them.

In a sequestration crisis, sickled cells undergoing hemolysis in the spleen get trapped, causing blood pooling, infarction of splenic vessels, and splenomegaly. The spleen may become completely fibrotic, called *autosplenectomy*, owing to repeated blood vessel obstruction. Overwhelming infection may occur due to functional asplenia (i.e., the spleen is physically present but not functioning).

TABLE 11–9 Clinical Manifestations of Sickle Cell Anemia

Pain
- Abdominal
- Chest
- Headaches

Bone and joint crises
- Low-grade fever
- Extremity pain
- Back pain
- Periosteal pain
- Joint pain, especially shoulder and hip

Vascular complications
- Cerebrovascular accidents
- Chronic leg ulcers
- Avascular necrosis of the femoral head
- Bone infarcts

Pulmonary crises
- Bacterial pneumonia
- Pulmonary infarction

Neurologic manifestations
- Convulsions
- Drowsiness
- Coma
- Stiff neck
- Paresthesias
- Cranial nerve palsies
- Blindness
- Nystagmus

Hand-foot syndrome
- Fever
- Pain
- Dactylitis

Splenic sequestration crisis
- Liver and spleen enlargement
- Spleen atrophy

Renal complications
- Enuresis
- Nocturia
- Hematuria
- Pyelonephritis
- Renal papillary necrosis
- End-stage renal failure (elderly population)

Adapted from Goodman CC, Snyder TE: Differential Diagnosis in Physical Therapy, ed 2. Philadelphia, WB Saunders, 1995, p 202.

Complications. Other complications include neurologic manifestations, hand-foot syndrome, renal involvement, bacterial infections (e.g., pneumococcal pneumonia, *Salmonella* osteomyelitis), iron overload, cholelithiasis, chronic leg ulcers (present in about 75% of older children or adults), retinopathy, and priapism (persistent penile erection).

Hand-and-foot syndrome (dactylitis) occurs when a microinfarction (clot) occludes the blood vessels that supply the metacarpal and metatarsal bones, causing ischemia; it may be the infant's first problem caused by sickle cell disease. It presents with low-grade fever and symmetric, painful, diffuse, nonpitting edema in the hands and feet, extending to the fingers and toes (Fig. 11–12). This is a fairly common phenomenon seen almost exclusively in the young infant and child. Despite radiographic changes and swelling, the syndrome is almost always self-limiting, and bones usually heal without permanent deformity (Charache et al., 1991).

In the CNS, unlike other areas of the body, there is a tendency for sickle cell crisis to involve large vessels. Cerebrovascular accidents (CVAs) are a frequent and severe manifestation of sickle cell disease, affecting 6% to 12% of all people with sickle cell disease, and most commonly occurring in the pediatric population. Careful neurologic examination frequently reveals hemiplegia or other mild neurologic deficits. Angiography or EEG may show more extensive changes than are seen clinically, suggesting that "silent" strokes are not uncommon.

It is important for the therapist to recognize signs of com-

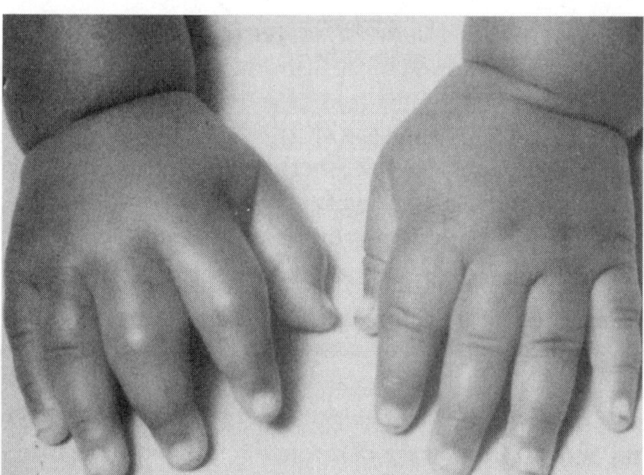

Figure **11–12.** Dactylitis. Painful swelling of the hands or feet can occur when a clot forms in the hands or feet. This problem, known as *hand-and-foot syndrome*, occurs most often in children affected by sickle cell disease. (*From Gaston M: Sickle Cell Anemia, NIH publication No. 90–3058. Bethesda, Md, National Institutes of Health, June 1990, p 8.*)

plications, especially signs of chest syndrome and stroke. Stroke is a relatively infrequent complication in the young infant; the median age for occurrence of stroke in children is 7 years. Infection or trapped red blood cells in the lung can cause acute chest syndrome. Report signs of chest syndrome or stroke immediately (Table 11–10).

Medical Management

Diagnosis. It is recommended that all infants should be screened for sickle cell disease regardless of race or ethnic background (universal screening) (Agency for Health Care Policy and Research, 1993). This recommendation is based on several factors. First, twice-daily oral prophylactic penicillin reduces both morbidity and mortality from pneumococcal infections in infants with sickle cell anemia and sickle β'-thalassemia. Second, although sickle cell disease is more prevalent in certain racial and ethnic groups, it is not possible to define accurately an individual's heritage by physical appearance or surname. Screening targeted to specific racial and ethnic groups, therefore, will miss some affected infants, subjecting them to an increased risk of early mortality. Universal screening is the best, most reliable, and most cost-effective screening method to identify affected infants (Sickle Cell Disease Guideline Panel, 1993).

The diagnosis of sickle cell trait or any of the other sickle syndromes depends on the demonstration of sickling under reduced oxygen tension. A sickle turbidity test (Sickledex) can confirm the presence of Hb S in peripheral blood, and hemoglobin electrophoresis (separation and identification of hemoglobin under the influence of an applied electric field) is used to determine the amount of Hb S in erythrocytes. Electrophoresis is used to screen blood for sickle cell trait and will also detect sickle cell disease and heterozygosity (carrier state) for other hemoglobin disorders, such as Hb C (Charache et al., 1991).

Safe and accurate methods for performing prenatal diagnosis for sickle cell disease are possible as early as the 10th gestational week. Analyses of DNA from fetal cells obtained by amniocentesis or chorionic villus sampling can be performed at the 16th gestational week. The sickle and Hb C genes can be detected directly in fetal DNA samples, as can most Hb S β-thalassemia genes.

TABLE 11-10 COMPLICATIONS ASSOCIATED WITH PEDIATRIC SICKLE CELL ANEMIA

CHEST SYNDROME	STROKE
Severe chest pain	Jerking or twitching of the face, legs, or arms
Fever of ≥38.8°C (≥102°F)	Convulsions or seizures
Very congested	Unusual or strange behavior
Cough	Inability to move an arm and/or a leg
Dyspnea	Ataxia or unsteady gait (do not assume these are guarding responses to pain)
Tachypnea	Stutter or slurred speech
Sternal or costal retractions	Distal muscular weakness in the hands, feet, or legs
	Changes in vision
	Severe, unrelieved headaches
	Severe vomiting

Treatment. A large number of anti-sickling regimens are being investigated; although some have been shown to be effective in vitro, unacceptable toxicity prevents their use in humans at this time. There is no treatment to cure sickle cell diseases beyond supportive care (e.g., rest, oxygen, administration of intravenous fluids and electrolytes, physical and occupational therapy for joint and bone involvement). Splenic or hepatic sequestration requires aggressive rehydration and transfusion.

Prenatal and neonatal screening can identify this disorder and significantly reduce morbidity and mortality through the use of prophylactic antibiotics. Infants with documented sickle cell disease (sickle cell anemia or Hb S β'-thalassemia) should be started on twice daily oral prophylactic penicillin as soon as possible, but not later than at 2 months of age (Agency for Health Care Policy and Research, 1993). Preventive measures (see Risk Factors) are used to reduce the incidence of crises. Medications, such as analgesics or corticosteroids, are sometimes administered to relieve musculoskeletal pain.

Exchange transfusions to reduce Hb S levels below 40% may be used therapeutically for neurologic, cardiac, or retinal symptoms; hypoxemia; severe prolonged or infarctive crises; acute splenic sequestration (in infants); and chronic leg ulcers. These transfusions also can be used prophylactically during pregnancy or before general anesthesia, but they carry the risk of hepatitis, red cell sensitization, hemosiderosis (increased iron storage), and transfusion reactions.

Bone marrow transplantation cures sickle cell disease, but the risks associated with the procedure prevent its widespread use. In severe cases, bone marrow transplantation may be considered.

Investigators at the National Institutes of Health, Bethesda, Md, and Johns Hopkins University School of Medicine, Baltimore, are investigating the use of fetal hemoglobin as a treatment possibility. Fetal hemoglobin is produced during fetal development and for the first 6 months after birth. Hb F has some ability to prevent sickling and reduce hemolysis; some adults with sickle cell disease who naturally make substantial amounts of Hb F have less pain and better spleen function than others with sickle cell disease who do not have elevated levels of Hb F.

Drugs such as hydroxyurea, which stimulate Hb F production, are now being tested as a possible treatment for sickle cell anemia. The drug has some serious side effects, and researchers are looking for safer drugs (Charache et al., 1996; Charache et al., 1995; Steinberg et al., 1997).[18] Progress in understanding globin gene regulation is now being combined with advances in retrovirus-mediated gene transfer toward the goal of providing gene therapy for hemoglobinopathies (Stamatoyannopoulos, 1992).

Prognosis. Historically, sickle cell disease has been associ-

[18] At the time of this writing, drug trials were ended early and physicians were notified by the National Institutes of Health of test results. Dramatic reduction of painful episodes, fewer hospitalizations, decreased need for transfusions, and fewer cases of acute chest syndrome occurred with the use of hydroxyurea. Hydroxyurea is only recommended for adults with acute sickle cell anemia because this potent drug may pose a risk of leukemia, and the long-term effects remain unknown.

ated with high mortality in early childhood due to overwhelming bacterial infections, splenic sequestration crises, and the acute chest syndrome. Since the mid-1970s, comprehensive medical care has reduced morbidity and mortality in children with sickle cell disease.

There is no cure for sickle cell disease; it is a devastating condition with recurrent crises leading to death at ages as young as 30 years. However, many persons with sickle cell disease have lived into their 40s, 50s, and 60s. The sickle cell clots can be life-threatening, depending on their location. For example, a blood clot in the brain can cause a stroke. Recovery may be complete in some cases, but serious neurologic damage is more likely to occur, and repeated CVAs may lead to increased neurologic involvement, permanent paralysis, or death. Permanent damage from blood clots to the heart, kidney, lungs, liver, or eyes (blindness), can occur. Clients who survive until 50 years or older usually develop progressive renal damage with fatal uremia.

Special Implications for the Therapist **11-13**

SICKLE CELL DISEASE

During a sickle cell crisis, the therapist may be involved in pain control or management. Precautions include avoiding stressors that can precipitate a crisis, such as overexertion, dehydration, and the use of cryotherapy for painful, swollen joints. (See also Special Implications for the Therapist: Splenomegaly: 11–15.)

Should a person with sickle cell disease experience an isolated musculoskeletal injury (e.g., sprained ankle) in the absence of any sickle cell crisis, careful application of ice can be undertaken. The sickle cell pain crises can be successfully managed using whirlpool at a slightly warmer temperature (102 to 104°F), facilitating muscle relaxation through active movement in the water. Combined used of medications, psychological support, relaxation techniques, biofeedback, and imagery is a useful treatment protocol to lessen the effects of painful crises (Hockey, 1994).

Joint effusions in sickle cell disease can occur secondary to long bone infarctions with extension of swelling, and septic arthritis. Clients with sickle cell disease may also have coexistent rheumatic or collagen vascular disease or osteoarthritis, necessitating careful evaluation to determine the presence of marked inflammation or fever before initiating treatment procedures.

Persistent thigh, buttock, or groin pain in an adult with known sickle cell disease may be an indication of aseptic necrosis of the femoral head. Blood supply to the hip is just adequate, even in healthy persons, so the associated microvascular obstruction can leave the hip especially vulnerable to ischemia and necrosis. Total hip replacement may be indicated in cases in which severe structural damage occurs.

Sickle Cell Trait

Sickle cell trait is not a disease, but is rather a heterozygous condition in which the individual has the mutant gene from only one parent (β^s gene), and the normal gene (β^A globin gene), resulting in the production of both Hb S and Hb A with a predominance of Hb A (60%) over Hb S (40%). One in 12 black Americans (8%) has the sickle cell trait, and many other races and nationalities also carry the genetic defect. The gene has persisted because heterozygotes gain slight protection against falciparum malaria.

Under normal circumstances, sickle cell trait is rarely symptomatic; symptoms may occur with conditions associated with marked hypoxia and at high altitudes. There appears to be no increased risk for individuals with sickle cell trait who undergo general anesthesia and no increased risk of sudden death for those who participate in athletics, and a normal life expectancy is predicted.

The Thalassemias

Definition. The thalassemias are a group of inherited, chronic hemolytic anemias predominantly affecting people of Mediterranean or southern Chinese ancestry (*thalassa* means "sea," referring to early cases of sickle cell disease reported around the Mediterranean). American blacks and people from central Africa and southern Asia can also be affected by thalassemia (Pavel et al., 1993).

Overview and Pathogenesis. The thalassemias are characterized by production of extremely thin, fragile erythrocytes, called *target cells*. Normal postnatal hemoglobin is composed of two α and two β polypeptide chains (see Fig. 11–10). Unlike the α and β polypeptide chains in sickle cell anemia, the polypeptide chains in the thalassemias are completely normal in structure, but they are insufficient in number because of a genetic alteration (e.g., deletion, nonsense mutation) that affects globin synthesis. The defective polypeptide unit is unbalanced and unstable and disintegrates, damaging RBCs and resulting in anemia.

Thalassemia is classified as α-thalassemia or β-thalassemia because either α or β chains can be affected by diminished synthesis. β-Thalassemia is more common and is the center of discussion in this section. It is called *classic thalassemia* or simply thalassemia. Some β-thalassemia genes produce no β globin chains and are termed β'-thalassemia. Other β globin genes produce some β, but in diminished quantities, and are termed β^+-thalassemia.

The severity of thalassemia depends on whether the afflicted client is homozygous or heterozygous for the thalassemia trait; homozygotes may develop *thalassemia major* (Cooley's anemia) or *thalassemia intermedia*, both characterized by profound anemia. Heterozygotes may develop *thalassemia minor* or *thalassemia trait*, characterized by mild anemia.

Clinical Manifestations. The onset of thalassemia major is usually insidious and is not recognized until the latter half of infancy. The clinical manifestations of thalassemia are primarily attributable to (1) defective synthesis of hemoglobin, (2) structurally impaired RBCs, and (3) shortened life span of erythrocytes (Wong, 1993).

The symptoms of thalassemia major resemble those of other hemolytic anemias (e.g., jaundice, cholelithiasis, leg ulcers, and enlarged spleen). Bony changes can occur in older children if untreated. Ineffective erythropoiesis causes extreme expansion of marrow space into long bones, skull, and facial bones, causing a thickening of the cranium and a mongoloid appearance or facies. Extramedullary hematopoiesis in the liver, spleen, and around the spinal vertebrae, may also develop. Growth abnormalities and cortical bone fragility result, with an increased rate of fractures. Thalassemia minor is usually asymptomatic, except for a mild anemia.

Medical Management

Diagnosis. Diagnosis is by laboratory testing, and results may include target cells (abnormally thin, fragile cells) and other bizarrely shaped RBCs in the circulation and elevated serum bilirubin and fecal and urinary urobilinogen levels (from the severe hemolysis of abnormal cells). Electrophoresis is usually diagnostic when Hb F or Hb A is elevated.

Treatment. Thalassemia minor is usually so mild that treatment is not required. Treatment for thalassemia major is by transfusion therapy; packed RBCs may be given on a regular transfusion schedule monthly or bimonthly, when the hemoglobin falls below 3 to 4 g/dL, or every 15 days to maintain the hemoglobin at 12 to 15 g/dL. When transfused cells are being rapidly destroyed by the spleen, splenectomy may be necessary. A major postsplenectomy complication may be severe and overwhelming infection requiring prophylactic antibiotics. Experimental approaches to therapy now include BMT (Lucarelli, 1990) and agents that increase Hb F production, such as 5-azacytidine and hydroxyurea (see Sickle Cell Anemia: Treatment) (Andreoli et al., 1993).

Repeated transfusions may result in iron overload, which may cause diabetes mellitus, hypofunction of the thyroid, parathyroid, and adrenal glands, and, eventually, myocardial hemosiderosis (accumulation of iron in the myocardium) and cardiac arrhythmias. Excessive iron can be somewhat removed from the blood by chelating agents, such as deferoxamine (Desferal), which binds iron ions to form water-soluble complexes that are removed by the kidneys.

Prognosis. Thalassemia minor does not affect life expectancy, but clients who carry the thalassemia trait need genetic counseling. Until recently, the outlook for clients with thalassemia major has been poor, with lethal, severe hemolytic anemia and subsequent iron overload and dysfunction of almost all organ systems. Children are significantly delayed in growth and development; delay of puberty is universal, and many die before puberty.

Treatment with blood transfusion and early chelation therapy has improved life expectancy from early puberty to early adulthood. In a large study from Italy, the probability of a 3-year event-free survival was 94% when BMT was performed prior to the development of hepatomegaly or portal fibrosis (Lucarelli, 1990).

Death from *hydrops fetalis* (the absence of all α globin production with progressive hemolysis causing fetal hypoxia, cardiac failure, generalized edema) can occur in homozygous α-thalassemia; it consistently results in stillbirth or death in utero.

Hemophilia

Overview. Hemophilia is a bleeding disorder inherited as a sex-linked autosomal recessive trait (males are affected and females are the carriers) in two-thirds of all cases. It is the most common inherited coagulation (blood-clotting) disorder and is caused by an abnormality of plasma-clotting proteins necessary for blood coagulation. There are two primary types of hemophilia: *hemophilia* A, or classic hemophilia (which constitutes 80% of all cases of hemophilia), and *hemophilia* B, or Christmas disease (which affects about 15% of all people with hemophilia). Other less common deficiencies (hemophilia C, a factor XI deficiency) and deficiencies of other clotting factors (I, II, V, VII, X, or XIII) are transmitted autosomally; they therefore affect males and females equally. These are not fully discussed in this text.

The level of severity is classified according to the percentage of clotting factor, which is determined through blood tests:[19] mild (5% to 50%), moderate (1% to 5%), and severe (<1%) (Table 11–11). For persons with *mild* hemophilia, spontaneous hemorrhages are rare, and joint and deep muscle bleeding are uncommon. Surgical, dental, or other injury or trauma precipitates symptoms that must be treated the same as for severe hemophilia. For those people with *moderate* hemophilia, spontaneous hemorrhage is not usually a problem, but major bleeding episodes can occur after minor trauma. People with *severe* hemophilia may bleed spontaneously or with only slight trauma.

Bleeding is prolonged in hemophilia, but the blood flow is not any faster than would occur in a normal person with the same injury. Generally, severity of bleeding among people with inherited bleeding disorders depends on the type of disorder, degree of factor deficiency, and other less identifiable factors. Individually, the level of severity remains constant throughout a person's life. The level of clotting factor is always the same among affected family members, and clinical symptoms are usually similar (though bleeding patterns may be slightly different) among family members.

Individuals, primarily those with severe hemophilia, who were treated before current purification techniques for factor concentrates (prior to 1985) may have been exposed to the human immunodeficiency virus (HIV). In 1991, approximately 70% of persons with hemophilia had seroconverted to HIV positive; by the end of 1993, seroprevalence was estimated at 42%, with some of the decrease being accounted

TABLE 11-11 HEMOPHILIA STATISTICS SHEET

ESTIMATED % OF HEMOPHILIA BY SEVERITY

	No. of Bleeds/yr	Factor VIII	Factor IX
Mild	0–1	15%	20%
Moderate	12	15%	30%
Severe	52	70%	50%

PERCENTAGE OF PERSONS WITH HEMOPHILIA WHO ARE HIV POSITIVE*

	Factor VIII	Factor IX
Mild	20.3%	6.7%
Moderate	47.8%	24.6%
Severe	69.6%	48.6%

* Figures are based on 1991 census; 1993 data reports that 49% of active clients are known to have received potentially contaminated products; 42% of those clients are HIV positive.

From HANDI Publication. New York, National Hemophilia Foundation, 1994.

[19] Normal concentrations of coagulation factors are between 50% and 150%.

for by deaths, test refusal, and unknown test status (CDC, 1993).

Transmission of hepatitis is equally serious, and about 90% of persons with hemophilia who received clotting factor before the mid-1980s test positive for hepatitis C, the world's leading cause of transfusion-associated viral disease (Ewenstein, 1994). Data suggest that current improved methods of viral inactivation through pasteurization and solvent-treatment, as well as monoclonal and recombinant technology, have resulted in a reduced risk of hepatitis transmission (NHF, 1993). Younger clients with hemophilia have received the hepatitis B vaccination, but older clients usually have hepatitis B, with its long-term sequelae.

Incidence. Hemophilia affects approximately 1 in 10,000 males from all races and socioeconomic groups, including the Amish, Pacific Islanders, Chinese, Japanese, Vietnamese, Native Americans, Latinos, black Americans, and others (Odubiyi, 1994). Approximately 20,000 people in the United States have been diagnosed with hemophilia: approximately 10,000 with hemophilia A, 3000 with hemophilia B, and 6600 with von Willebrand disease and other bleeding disorders. Thirty-five percent of the known cases of hemophilia are in children younger than 13 years, approximately 15% are in persons between 13 and 19 years, and approximately 50% are in persons 20 years and older (CDC, 1993).

Etiology. In this sex-linked (X chromosome) recessive disorder, the female carries the defective gene and the male presents with the disease (Fig. 11–13). Female hemophilia carriers have a 50% chance of transmitting the gene to their daughters and a 50% chance of transmitting the disease to their sons. Males with hemophilia transmit the gene to all of their daughters (obligate carrier) but to none of their sons (Pavel et al., 1993). Although in two thirds of the cases of hemophilia there is a known family history, this disorder can occur in families (approximately one third) without a previous history of blood-clotting disorders because of spontaneous genetic mutation (Miller, 1992).

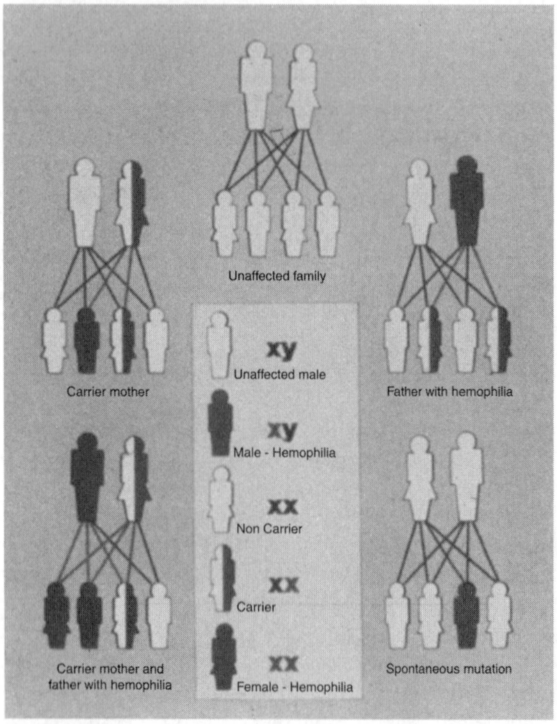

Figure **11–13.** Inheritance patterns in hemophilia. (*From The School Program Presentation Guide. New York, National Hemophilia Foundation, 1990.*)

Women and Bleeding Disorders. The hemophilia community is just beginning to recognize the needs of females affected by inherited bleeding disorders. Approximately 3000 women in the United States have an active bleeding disorder. Most women with a bleeding disorder fall into one of three groups: (1) asymptomatic carriers, (2) those with von Willebrand disease,[20] and (3) those with a factor deficiency that is not a sex-linked defect. Women with bleeding disorders experience excessive uterine bleeding during their menstrual cycle with possible oozing from the ovary after ovulation mid-cycle. Heavy menstrual flow is frequently the symptom that initiates a coagulation evaluation.

There are cases in which a female carrier of the hemophilia gene has abnormal bleeding when the level of clotting factor is low enough to cause significant problems with coagulation, especially following trauma or surgery. Most women who have a bleeding disorder have von Willebrand disease, but isolated cases of mild bleeding problems in carrier women may be caused by extreme expression of the affected gene. Abnormal bleeding from bruising, dental extractions, miscarriage, prolonged postpartum hemorrhage, nosebleeds, and minor trauma (such as cuts with prolonged oozing) may be overlooked because of the misconception that bleeding disorders do not occur in women (Paper, 1993).

Pathogenesis. Hemophilia A, the most common of the congenital coagulation disorders, is due to a deficiency of the procoagulant protein factor VIII (antihemophilic factor, or AHF). AHF is produced by the liver and is necessary for the formation of thromboplastin in phase I of blood coagulation (see Fig 11–7). The genetic pattern of hemophilia is very different from that of disorders such as sickle cell disease, in which every affected individual has the identical genetic defect. The presence of such variable defects in the same gene probably accounts for the differences in severity of hemophilia between families. Many different genetic lesions cause factor VIII deficiency, such as gene deletions, with all or part of the gene missing, or missense and nonsense mutations, which cause the clotting factor to be made incorrectly or not at all; 25% to 30% of cases are due to new mutations (Miller, 1992).

New, sensitive methodologies have provided researchers information that the rate at which factor VIII gene mutations are occurring is rapidly increasing. Gene deletions and point mutations (a single base in the DNA is mutated to another base) are the two most common types of defects. Approximately 50 deletion mutations in the gene for factor VIII have been identified at the molecular level, and about 34

[20] von Willebrand disease occurs equally in males and females, with bleeding primarily from mucous membranes; joint bleeding is rare but can occur in severe cases. Individuals with von Willebrand disease have a 50% chance of having children with the same disorder. The child will have one chromosome with the normal clotting gene and one with the von Willebrand disease gene. Those who do not get the von Willebrand disease gene from their parents will be unaffected, as will their children. (Moyer and Weinblatt, 1994).

independent deletion mutations in the factor IX gene have been found to be the cause of hemophilia B (Furie and Furie, 1992). Future studies should lead to the discovery of a wide range of defects as well as to potential new mutations. Advances in understanding of the protein will also provide new insights into the effects of particular mutations (Gitschier, 1991).

Clinical Manifestations. Clinically, hemophilia A can only be distinguished from hemophilia B by specific factor assays. Spontaneous bleeding as a result of hemophilia is uncommon the first year of life, but hematoma formation may result from injections or after firm holding, such as occurs when a child is held under the arms or by the elbow and lifted. Easy bruising, bleeding from the mouth or tongue, hematomas of the head, and hemarthrosis (bleeding into the joints), frequently occur during early ambulation. By age 3 to 4 years, 90% of children with severe hemophilia have had an episode of persistent bleeding (Andrews and Mooney, 1994).

Early signs and symptoms of a bleeding disorder include slow, persistent bleeding from circumcision, immunizations, and other minor trauma (e.g., cuts, scratches); excessive bruising from minor trauma; delayed hemorrhage (hours to days after injury) following a minor injury; severe hemorrhaging from the gums after dental extraction; bleeding after brushing teeth; severe nosebleeds; gastric hemorrhage; and recurrent bleeding into subcutaneous tissue and muscles and around peripheral nerves and joints.

Bleeding into the joint spaces (hemarthrosis) is one of the most common clinical manifestations of hemophilia, most often affecting the synovial joints: knee, ankle, elbow, hip, shoulder, and wrist (in order of most common occurrence). Bleeding in the synovial joints of the feet, hands, temporomandibular joint, and spine is less common. Muscle hemorrhages can be more insidious and massive than joint bleeding and can occur anywhere, most commonly in the flexor muscle groups (e.g., iliopsoas, gastrocnemius, forearm flexors).

Recurrent hemarthrosis results in chronic synovitis, hemophiliac arthropathy with flexion contractures and joint fixation from the muscle bleeds, and incompletely absorbed blood in the joints. When blood is introduced into the joint, the synovial membrane responds by producing an increased number of synovial villi and vascular hyperplasia in an attempt to resorb the blood. The synovium becomes hypertrophied with formation of fingerlike projections of tissue extending onto the articular surface. The mechanical trauma of normal weight-bearing motion may then impinge and further injure the pathologic synovium. A vicious circle is established as the synovium attempts to cleanse the joint of blood and debris, becoming more hypertrophic and susceptible to still further bleeding (Holdredge and Cotta, 1989).

Erosive damage of the cartilage follows these changes in the synovium with narrowing of the joint space (Fig. 11–14), erosions at the joint margins, and subchondral cyst formation. Collapse of the joint, joint sclerosis, and eventual spontaneous ankylosis may occur. In later stages of joint degeneration, chronic pain, severe loss of motion, muscle atrophy, crepitus, and joint deformities occur (Gill et al., 1989) (Tables 11–12 and 11–13).

Intramuscular hemorrhage that is visible in superficial areas such as the calf or forearm will also result in pain and limitation of motion of the affected part. Less obvious intramuscular hemorrhage, such as occurs in the iliopsoas, may result in groin pain, pain on extension of the hip, and reflexive flexion of the hip and thigh (see Figs. 13–10 and 13–11). A large iliopsoas hemorrhage can cause displacement of the kidney and ureter and can compress the femoral nerve.

In general, compression of peripheral nerves and blood vessels by hematoma may result in severe pain, anesthesia of the innervated part, loss of perfusion, permanent nerve damage, and even paralysis. The femoral, ulnar, and median nerves are most commonly affected. CNS hemorrhage may include intracranial hemorrhage and, rarely, intraspinal hemorrhage.

Complications occur in 20% to 33% of persons with moderately severe or severe factor VIII deficiency who develop "inhibitors," antibodies that destroy the infused factor. Inhibitors are much less frequent among persons with hemophilia B or factor IX deficiency, affecting only 1% to 4% (DiMichele, 1995).

The risk of developing an inhibitor does not remain the same during the lifetime of a person with hemophilia. Young children with severe hemophilia A are at the highest risk of inhibitor development after relatively few exposure days

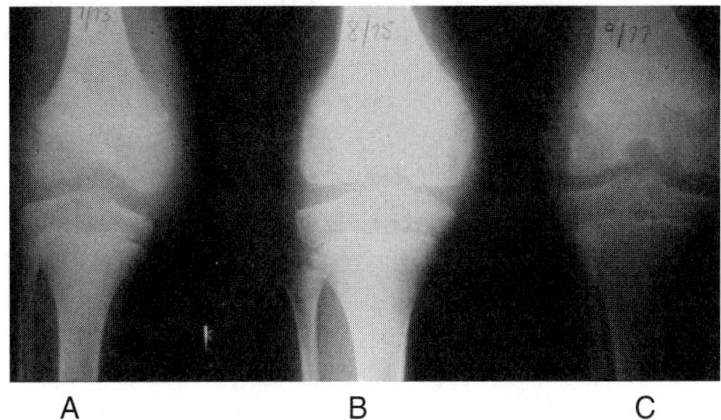

Figure **11–14.** Stages of hemophilic arthropathy according to the Arnold-Hilgartner scale. A, Stage I (1973). *B*, Stage III (1975). C, Stage IV (1977). (*Courtesy of Mountain States Regional Hemophilia Center, Colorado State Treatment Program, Denver, 1995.*)

TABLE 11–12 ARNOLD-HILGARTNER HEMOPHILIC ARTHROPATHY STAGES

I. No skeletal abnormalities; soft tissue swelling
II. Osteoporosis and overgrowth of epiphysis; no erosions; no narrowing of cartilage space
III. Early subchondral bone cysts, squaring of the patella; intercondylar notch of distal femur and humerus widened; cartilage space remains preserved
IV. Finding of stage III more advanced; cartilage space narrowed significantly
V. End stage; fibrous joint contracture, loss of joint cartilage space, marked enlargement of the epiphyses and substantial disorganization of the joints

From Arnold WD, Hilgartner MW: Hemophilic arthropathy. J Bone Joint Surg Am 59:287–305, 1977.

TABLE 11-13 Petterson Radiologic Classification of Hemophilic Arthropathy

Type of Change	Finding	Score*
Osteoporosis	Absent	0
	Present	1
Enlarged epiphysis	Absent	0
	Present	1
Irregular subchondral surface	Absent	0
	Surface partially involved	1
	Surface totally involved	2
Narrowing of joint space	Absent	0
	Present; joint space >1 mm	1
	Present; joint space <1 mm	2
Subchondral cyst formation	Absent	0
	1 Cyst	1
	>1 Cyst	2
Erosions at joint margins	Absent	0
	Present	1
Gross incongruence of articulating bone ends	Absent	0
	Slight	1
	Pronounced	2
Joint deformity (angulation and/or displacement between articulating bones)	Absent	0
	Slight	1
	Pronounced	2

* Note: Possible joint score is 0–13 points.
From Petterson H, Ahlberg A, Nilsson IM: A radiologic classification of hemophilic arthropathy. Clin Orthop 149:152–159, 1980.

(Scharrer and Neutzling, 1993). The newer purification procedures provide factor concentrates that are safe in terms of inhibitor production and do not elicit higher rates of inhibitor production to either factor VIII or factor IX (Mariani et al., 1994).

Medical Management

Diagnosis. Effective treatment is based on an accurate diagnosis of the deficient clotting factor and its level in the blood. This requires a battery of common blood tests for bleeding time, PTT, and tests to monitor the liver, kidney, immune function, and hepatitis status. It is also important for women in families of members with hemophilia to identify their carrier status through factor level analysis and gene testing (Moyer and Weinblatt, 1994).

If possible, genetic studies to determine carrier status should be completed before pregnancy. However, prenatal diagnosis of hemophilia A and B is possible if a specific mutation has been found or if linkage studies have provided enough information about carrier status in the family. If one of these two criteria have been met, prenatal diagnosis can be performed through either chorionic villus sampling (CVS) at 10 to 12 weeks' pregnancy or amniocentesis at approximately 16 weeks' gestation. Both tests have associated risks and benefits (Moyer and Weinblatt, 1994).

Treatment. Currently, there is no known cure or prenatal treatment for hemophilia. Primary treatment goals for the hemophiliac client during bleeding episodes are to stop any bleeding that is occurring as quickly as possible and to infuse the missing factors until the bleeding stops. Treatment with infusion of the missing factor at a 40% to 50% level is recommended prior to minor surgery and dental extractions or in case of minor injury (Pavel et al., 1993), and it may be recommended prior to physical or occupational therapy treatment. Infusion at 80% to 100% may be recommended prior to major surgery or in the case of head or abdominal trauma.

Permanent prophylaxis of recombinant factors for severe hemophilia (i.e., factor infusion given on a regularly scheduled basis to maintain a blood factor level every other day of the person's life) is a recommended approach to treatment that is now accepted in European countries but is limited in the United States by the cost of such products.

Standard treatment based on infusion of heat-treated factor VIII concentrates (human plasma-derived clotting factor) has now been replaced by administration of purified recombinant factor VIII products (KoGENate and Recombinate) (Linker, 1994; Soutar, 1994). Unlike human plasma-derived factors made from plasma pooled from thousands of donors, recombinant factor VIII is now derived from a nonhuman source. With recombinant factor, human viruses will not be easily transmitted through factor use, and the chance of any other contaminants being transmitted appears unlikely (National Hemophilia Foundation, 1993).

Comprehensive medical management of hemophilia may involve the use of drugs to control pain in acute bleeding and chronic arthropathies. The common pain reliever aspirin and any of its derivatives cannot be used by persons with hemophilia because these agents inhibit platelet function.[21] Some anti-inflammatory nonsteroidal drugs contain derivatives of aspirin and must be used cautiously. Corticosteroids are used occasionally for the treatment of chronic synovitis. Acetaminophen (Tylenol) is a suitable aspirin substitute for pain control, especially in children.

Adults with severe hemophilia who have debilitating joint arthropathy may have received methadone in the past for chronic pain management. This treatment is accompanied by the medical and psychological complications of a habit-forming drug. Today, aggressive infusion treatment and/or prophylactic infusion have eliminated the need for this pharmacologic approach.

Chronic hepatitis (for those who received clotting factor before the mid-1980s) treated with recombinant interferon alfa given subcutaneously may result in normalized liver function in 50% of clients, but 50% of responders relapse on stopping treatment. Liver transplantation is successful in people who have hemophilia with advanced liver disease (Makris and Preston, 1993). Younger children are now vaccinated against hepatitis A and B.

Physical therapy treatment (see Special Implications for the Therapist: 11–14) has been effective in reducing the number of bleeding episodes through protective strengthening of the musculature surrounding affected joints, muscle reeducation, and gait training, and through client education.

[21] More precisely, platelets do form an initial clot, but no factor VIII or IX is available to stabilize the clot.

Physical therapy is used during episodes of acute hemorrhage to control pain and additional bleeding and to maintain positioning and prevent further deformity (Cotta et al., 1986).

Prognosis. Tremendous improvement has been made in carrier detection and prenatal diagnosis to provide early treatment and prevent complications. Medical treatment prolongs life and improves quality of life associated with improved joint function, but longevity and quality of life can be significantly reduced by HIV and hepatitis. Mortality among people with hemophilia A has tripled since 1979 owing to the transmission of HIV through plasma infusion. Since the AIDS virus was not isolated until 1984, approximately 9000 people with hemophilia (50% of all persons with hemophilia) have become HIV-infected in the United States and another 2000 people who had hemophilia have already died of AIDS. Other virally transmitted diseases affecting people infused prior to 1984 include hepatitis B and C, cytomegalovirus (CMV), and Epstein-Barr virus (EBV).

Fortunately, improvements in blood screening tests, more stringent donor exclusion criteria, improved viral inactivation methods, and the introduction of recombinant hemophilia therapies have combined to dramatically reduce the rate of new bloodborne viral infections among people with hemophilia, especially those children born in the last decade (Ewenstein, 1994). Additionally, home infusion therapy provides immediate treatment with clotting factor for joint and muscle bleeds recognized early. Early treatment has significantly reduced the morbidity formerly associated with hemophilia (Wong, 1993).

Gene therapy for hemophilia A and B, now in the developmental stage, holds promise of a cure. The genes for factors VIII and IX have been cloned and transfer techniques of their cDNA into cells have been developed. Thus far, successful in vivo therapy has been demonstrated in a hemophiliac animal model, with conversion to a less severe hemophiliac state (Lozier and Brinkhous, 1994).

Special Implications for the Therapist **11-14**

HEMOPHILIA

Only a brief discussion of treatment for the adult or child with hemophilia can be included in this text. For a more detailed treatment protocol, the reader is referred to other more specific references (Boone, 1990; Gill et al., 1989; Holdredge, 1990; Holdredge and Cotta, 1989; Riske, 1995).

Hemophilia and Exercise

A regular exercise program, including appropriate sports activities and therapeutic strengthening and stretching exercises for affected extremities, is an important part of the comprehensive care of the individual with hemophilia (Harris, 1996). Exercise not only promotes physical wellness in the form of improved work capacity and enhanced joint function, it may also be beneficial for decreasing the frequency of bleeds (Nelson, 1994).

The therapist must be alert to recognize any signs of early bleeding episodes (Table 11–14). Factor replacement self-infusion should be instituted whenever possible by the client along with supportive measures by the therapist following the RICE principle (*r*est, *i*ce, *c*ompression [applying pressure to the area for at least 10 to 15 minutes] and *e*levation [immobilizing and elevating the body part above the heart level while applying the ice]).

Initiation of exercise after a bleed must be delayed and rehabilitation progress is typically slower for individuals with factor VIII and factor IX deficiency who develop factor inhibitors. Prognosis for full return of function is diminished in such cases. Clients may die of bleeding because they cannot be adequately supported with factor replacement. A review of research related to exercise and hemophilia is available (Nelson, 1994).

An overall therapy program includes family and client education early on for prevention, conditioning, wellness, and use of developmentally appropriate toys and activities. Specific guidelines are available (Harris, 1996; Holdredge and Cotta, 1989). As orthopedic problems occur, a problem-oriented program is developed specific to the pathology. Generally, a therapy program includes exercises to strengthen muscles and improve coordination; methods to prevent and reduce deformity; methods to influence abnormal muscle tone and pathologic patterns of movement; techniques to decrease pain; functional training related to everyday activities; special techniques such as manual traction and mobilization; massage; and physiotechnical modalities such as cold, heat (including ultrasound), and electric modalities (Heijnen and Timmermans, 1990).

Specific Exercise Guidelines

When active bleeding stops, isometric muscle exercise should be initiated to prevent atrophy of articular musculature. This exercise is especially critical with recurrent knee hemarthroses to prevent the visible atrophy of the quadriceps femoris muscle. As pain and edema diminish, the client should begin gentle active range-of-motion exercises followed by slowly progressing strengthening exercises. As a prophylactic measure, clients with severe hemophilia generally need to self-infuse with clotting factor when participating in a strengthening program. Unfortunately, this self-infusion may be limited because of reduction in reimbursement for the very expensive clotting factor (Nelson, 1994).

In some individuals, increased stress levels result in increased frequency of spontaneous bleeding. Biofeedback may be considered especially helpful for these clients who experience spontaneous bleeding during emotional upsets and periods of depression.

Orthopedic/Surgical Interventions

At times, even with optimal infusion therapy and aggressive hemophilia care, a joint becomes a chronic problem (Funk, 1995). In such cases, orthopedic or surgical intervention may be indicated to alleviate pain and deformity and to restore the joint to a more functional state. This may include prescription for an orthosis or a knee or ankle splint or serial casting to increase range of motion. Joint aspiration may be

TABLE 11-14 Clinical Signs and Symptoms of Hemophilia Bleeding Episodes

Acute Hemarthrosis	Muscle Hemorrhage	GI Involvement	CNS Involvement
Aura, tingling, or prickling sensation Stiffening into the position of comfort Decreased range of motion Pain Swelling Tenderness Heat	Gradually intensifying pain Protective spasm of muscle Limitation of movement at the surrounding joints Muscle assumes a position of comfort (usually shortened) Loss of sensation	Abdominal pain and distention Melena (blood in stool) Hematemesis (vomiting blood) Fever Low abdominal/groin pain due to bleeding into wall of large intestine or iliopsoas muscle Hip flexion contracture due to spasm of the iliopsoas muscle secondary to retroperitoneal hemorrhage	Impaired judgment Decreased visual and spatial awareness Short-term memory deficits Inappropriate behavior Motor deficits: spasticity, ataxia, abnormal gait, apraxia, decreased balance, loss of coordination

Adapted from Goodman CC, Snyder TE: Differential Diagnosis in Physical Therapy, ed 2. Philadelphia, WB Saunders, 1995, p 208.

recommended to relieve a tense, severe hemarthrosis, although opinion differs as to whether removal of blood from the joint decreases the risk of increased joint damage.

Synovectomy (removal of the joint synovium) is recommended to stop a target joint from its cycle of bleeding. This procedure is not usually done to improve range of motion or to decrease pain, but rather to prevent further damage to the joint caused by bleeding. Synovectomy is best performed before joint degeneration has progressed beyond a stage II on the Arnold-Hilgartner scale (see Table 11–12). Several surgical techniques are available for this procedure, including an open synovectomy through an incision in the joint capsule and an arthroscopic synovectomy, which is less invasive to the joint capsule and quadriceps mechanism and requires less rehabilitation. Another option for treatment includes injection of a radioactive isotope (usually ^{32}P in the United States), which causes scarring to the synovium to arrest bleeding. Each of these procedures has unique advantages and disadvantages and may be more appropriate for one type of client than another.

Arthroplasty (joint replacement) is indicated when a joint shows end-stage damage and has become extremely painful. Client age, range of motion, and level of pain and function are determinants as to the timing of this procedure. Knees, hips, and shoulders are most commonly aided through arthroplasty with restoration of pain-free joint movement. *Arthrodesis* (joint fusion) may be performed in a joint with advanced, painful arthropathy untreatable by arthroplasty. Joint fusion can relieve or eliminate pain to provide improved quality of life, but it also causes permanent loss of joint motion. Arthrodesis can be a very effective way to provide the individual with a more stable base for weight-bearing activities.

Osteotomy (removal of a section of bone) may be done to correct angular deformities in a joint and may be considered prior to arthroplasty to reduce the stresses placed on a joint caused by poor alignment. Other less common interventions may include excision of a hemophilia pseudotumor or removal of cysts or exostoses.

ALTERATIONS IN SPLENIC FUNCTION

Most pathology of the spleen occurs as a result of disorders elsewhere in the body. When primary anatomic alterations cause splenomegaly (splenic enlargement), the underlying dysfunction may include splenic rupture (trauma), tumors, cysts, and vascular anomalies such as infarction (blockage) or aneurysm (dilation of blood vessel wall forming a sac) (Mansen et al., 1994).

Hypersplenism, hyperactivity of the spleen, is the most common primary physiologic alteration. Hyposplenism, decreased function, may occur secondary to disease or removal of the spleen (splenectomy); congenital absence (asplenia) is rare.

Splenomegaly

Incidence and Etiology. The spleen's involvement in the lymphopoietic and mononuclear phagocyte systems predisposes it to multiple conditions causing splenomegaly (Table 11–15). Persons of any age can be affected, but adults have a greater likelihood of developing any of the conditions listed.

Pathogenesis. The spleen may become enlarged by an increase in the number of cellular elements, by the deposition of extracellular material (as occurs in amyloidosis), or in the presence of extracellular hemopoiesis that accompanies reactive bone marrow disorders and neoplasm.

Splenic macrophages accumulate in chronic infections, hemolytic anemias, and storage diseases with a corresponding increase in the size of the spleen. Thickening of the arteries and central arterioles of the white pulp of the spleen occurs in systemic lupus erythematosus, and chronic passive congestion of the red pulp is common in people with portal hypertension due to cirrhosis, thrombosis of the portal or splenic veins, or right-sided heart failure. Congestive splenomegaly is characterized by slow passage of blood from the spleen and with more turbulence than when it enters.

TABLE 11-15 CAUSES OF SPLENOMEGALY

Infections
  Acute
  Subacute
  Chronic

Immunologic-inflammatory disorders
  Rheumatoid arthritis
  Felty syndrome
  Immune thrombocytopenia
  Lupus erythematosus
  Sarcoidosis

Hemolytic anemias

Splenic vein hypertension
  Cirrhosis
  Splenic or portal vein thrombosis or stenosis
  Right-sided cardiac failure

Primary or metastatic neoplasm
  Leukemia
  Lymphoma
  Hodgkin's disease
  Myeloproliferative syndromes
  Sarcoma
  Carcinoma

Storage diseases
  Gaucher disease
  Niemann-Pick disease
  Mucopolysaccharidoses

Miscellaneous
  Amyloidosis
  Thyrotoxicosis

From Rubin E, Farber JL: Pathology, ed 2. Philadelphia, JB Lippincott, 1994, p 1043.

Clinical Manifestations. A large palpable splenic mass in the left upper quadrant under the costal margin may be accompanied by pain during the acute phase of splenomegaly. Other signs depend on the etiology (e.g., ascites associated with cirrhosis, pallor with anemia, fever with infection). Lymphadenopathy (disease of the lymph nodes) often occurs with splenomegaly in association with any inflammatory or infectious condition.

Medical Management

Diagnosis, Treatment, and Prognosis. Clinical diagnosis is based on history and physical examination; x-rays, ultrasound, CT, or MRI may be used to determine if the enlargement is diffuse or localized, solid or cystic. Underlying hematologic disorder or infection may be confirmed with laboratory studies. Medical treatment depends on the underlying condition; a splenectomy may reverse anemia or other cytopenias (deficiency of any blood elements).

Special Implications for the Therapist **11-15**

SPLENOMEGALY

Because splenomegaly is often associated with conditions characterized by rapid destruction of blood cells, it is important to follow the usual precautions for anyone with poor clotting abilities (e.g., see Thrombocytopenia, Anemia: 11-3). The client must be taught proper breathing techniques in conjunction with ways to avoid activities or positions that could traumatize the abdominal region or increase intracranial, intrathoracic, or intra-abdominal pressure.

The person with a small or absent spleen is more susceptible to streptococcal infection, which calls for prevention techniques such as good handwashing (see Appendix A). For the client with an enlarged spleen, any soft tissue techniques required in the left upper quadrant (especially up and under the rib cage) must be secondary or indirect techniques away from the spleen.

References

Abrams WB, Beers MH, Berkow R: The Merck Manual of Geriatrics, ed 2. Rahway, NJ, Merck & Co., 1995.

Adams P, Zanderer B: Sickle cell anemia. Med Surg Nurs Q 1:1–21, 1993.

Adelman DC, Terr A: Allergic and immunologic disorders. *In* Tierney LM, McPhee SJ, Papadakis MA (eds): Current Medical Diagnosis and Treatment, ed 33. Norwalk, Conn, Appleton & Lange, 1994, pp 640–663.

Agency for Health Care Policy and Research: Sickle Cell Disease: Comprehensive Screening and Management in Newborns and Infants, publication no. 93–0563. Rockville, Md, Department of Health and Human Services, 1993.

Alexanian R, Barlogie B, Dixon D: Prognosis of asymptomatic multiple myeloma. Arch Intern Med 148:1963–1965, 1988.

Alexanian R, Dimopoulos M: The treatment of multiple myeloma. N Engl J Med 330:484–489, 1994.

Alexanian R, Dimopoulos M, Smith T, et al: Limited value of myeloblative therapy for late multiple myeloma. Blood 83:512–516, 1994.

American Cancer Society: Cancer Facts and Figures, 1992. New York, ACS, 1992.

Anderson KC: The Jagannath et al. article reviewed. Oncology 8:104–106, 1994.

Andreoli TE, Bennett JC, Carpenter CC, et al: Cecil Essentials of Medicine, ed 3. Philadelphia, WB Saunders, 1993.

Andrews MM, Mooney KH: Alterations in hemolytic function in children. *In* McCance KL, Huether S (eds): Pathophysiology: The Biologic Basis for Disease in Adults and Children, ed 2. St Louis, Mosby–Year Book, 1994, pp 908–942.

Appelbaum FR: The use of colony stimulating factors in marrow transplantation. Cancer 72(suppl):3387–3392, 1993.

Arenson EB: Neoplastic diseases. *In* Hathaway WE, Hay WW, Groothuis JR, et al (eds): Current Pediatric Diagnosis and Treatment, ed 11. Norwalk, Conn, Appleton & Lange, 1993, pp 1094–1113.

Armitage JO: Bone marrow transplantation. N Engl J Med 330:827–838, 1994.

Ashinsky D: Eosinophilia-myalgia syndrome linked to tryptophan. Postgrad Med 88:193–195, 1990.

Athens JW: Variations of leukocytes in disease. *In* Lee GR, Bithell TC, Foerster J, et al (eds): Wintrobe's Clinical Hematology, ed 9. Philadelphia, Lea & Febiger, 1993, pp 1564–1588.

Auerbach M: Acute myeloid leukemia in patients more than 50 years of age: Special considerations in diagnosis, treatment, and prognosis. Am J Med 96:180–185, 1994.

Barlogie B, Jagannath S, Epstein J, et al: Biology and therapy of multiple myeloma in 1996. Semin Hematol 34(1 suppl):67–72, 1997.

Beahrs OH, Henson DE, Hutter RVP, et al. (eds): American Joint Committee on Cancer (AJCC) Manual: Staging of Cancer, ed 4. Philadelphia, JB Lippincott, 1992.

Bell TN: Coagulation and disseminated intravascular coagulation. *In* Huddleston VB (ed): Multisystem Organ Failure: Pathophysiology and Clinical Implications. St Louis, Mosby–Year Book, 1992, pp 57–81.

Bick RL, Kunkel LA: Disseminated intravascular coagulation syndromes. Int J Hematol 55:1–26, 1992.

Boone DC: A perspective on conservative management of musculoskeletal problems: Is it time for the next crusade? Hemophilia World 6:1, 1990.

Borson R, Loeb V: Acute and chronic leukemias in adults. CA Cancer J Clin 44:323–325, 1994.

Bova C, Matassarin-Jacobs E: Nursing care of clients with altered immune systems. *In* Black JM, Matassarin-Jacobs E: Luckmann and Sorensen's Medical-Surgical Nursing, ed 4. Philadelphia, WB Saunders, 1993, pp 549–578.

Buettner H, Bolling JP: Intravitreal large-cell lymphoma. Mayo Clin Proc 68:1011–1015, 1993.

Burnett AK, Eden OB: The treatment of acute leukemia. Lancet 349:270–275, 1997.

Buzaid AC, Lippman SM, Miller TP: Salvage therapy of advanced Hodgkin's disease: Critical appraisal of curative potential. Am J Med 83:523–532, 1987.

Canellos GP: Clinical characteristics of the blast phase of chronic granulocytic leukemia. Hematol Oncol Clin North Am 4:359–367, 1990.

Canellos GP: Is there an effective salvage therapy for advanced Hodgkin's disease? Ann Oncol 2(suppl 1):1–7, 1991.

Casper JT: Bone marrow transplantation for severe aplastic anemia in children. Am J Pediatr Hematol Oncol 12:434, 1990.

Centers for Disease Control and Prevention: Minimal Data Set (MDS) for Risk Reduction. Atlanta, CDC, 1993.

Charache S: Experimental therapy of sickle cell disease: Use of hydroxyurea. Am J Pediatr Hematol Oncol 16:62–66, 1994.

Charache S, Barton FB, Moore RD: Hydroxyurea and sickle cell anemia. Clinical utility of a myelosuppressive "switching" agent. Medicine (Baltimore) 75(6):300–326, 1996.

Charache S, Lubin B, Reid CD (eds): Management and Therapy of Sickle Cell Disease, NIH publication No. 91–2117. Rockville, Md, US Department of Health and Human Services, 1991.

Charache S, Terrin ML, Moore RD, et al: Effect of hydroxyurea on the frequency of painful crises in sickle cell anemia. N Engl J Med 332:1317–1322, 1995.

Clift RA, Appelbaum FR, Thomas ED: Treatment of chronic myeloid leukemia by marrow transplantation. Blood 82:1954–1956, 1993.

Cline MJ: The molecular basis of leukemia. N Engl J Med 330:328–336, 1994.

Cotta S, Jutra M, McQuarrie A: Physical Therapy in Hemophilia. New York, The National Hemophilia Foundation, 1986.

Deglin J, Vallerand A: Davis's Drug Guide for Nurses, ed 3. Philadelphia, FA Davis, 1993.

Devesa SS, Fears T: Non-Hodgkin's lymphoma time trends: United States and international data. Cancer Res 52(suppl):5432s–5440s, 1990.

Devine SM, Larson RA: Acute leukemia in adults: Recent developments in diagnosis and treatment. CA Cancer J Clin 44:326–352, 1994.

DiMichele DM: Inhibitors in hemophilia: A primer. NHF Community Alert 2:1–6, 1995.

Ewenstein B: Hepatitis C: New understanding about an old viral enemy. The Community Alert 1:1, 1994.

Fang LS: Renal diseases. *In* Ramsey PG, Larson EB (eds): Medical Therapeutics, ed 2. Philadelphia, WB Saunders, 1993, pp 192–237.

Fine HA, Mayer RJ: Primary central nervous system lymphoma. Ann Intern Med 119:1093–1104, 1993.

Fraser MC, Tucker MA: Late effects of cancer therapy: Chemotherapy related malignancy. Oncol Forum 15:67–77, 1988.

Funk SM: Unpublished paper. Denver, Mountain States Regional Hemophilia Center, 1995.

Furie B, Furie BC: Molecular and cellular biology of blood coagulation. N Engl J Med 326:800–806, 1992.

Gahrton G, Tura S, Ljungman P, et al: Allogeneic bone marrow transplantation in multiple myeloma. N Engl J Med 325:1267–1273, 1991.

Gaston M: Sickle Cell Anemia, publication No. 90–3058. Washington, DC, National Institutes of Health 1990.

Gilkeson GS, Caldwell DS: Rheumatic associations with malignancy. J Musculoskel Med 7:64–79, 1990.

Gill JC, Thometz J, Scott JP, et al: Musculoskeletal problems in hemophilia. *In* Hilgartner M, Pochedly C (eds): Hemophilia in the Child and Adult. New York, Raven Press, 1989, pp 27–41.

Gitschier J: The molecular basis of hemophilia A. Ann NY Acad Sci 614:89–96, 1991.

Goodman CC, Snyder TE: Differential Diagnosis in Physical Therapy, ed 2. Philadelphia, WB Saunders, 1995.

Grant J: Corticosteroid side effects: Implications for PT. PT Magazine 2:56–60, 1994.

Gribben JG, Freedman AA, Neuberg D, et al: Immunologic purging of marrow assessed by PCR before autologous bone marrow transplantation for B-cell lymphoma. N Engl J Med 325:1525–1533, 1991.

Hancock SL, Cox RS, McDougall IR: Thyroid diseases after treatment of Hodgkin's disease. N Engl J Med 325:599–605, 1991.

Harris N (ed): Hemophilia and Sports. New York, The National Hemophilia Foundation, 1996.

Harruff RC: Pathology Facts. Philadelphia, JB Lippincott, 1994.

Heijnen L, Timmermans H: When should you call the physical therapist? Hemophilia World 6:3, 1990.

Henon PR: Peripheral blood stem cell transplantation: Critical review. Int J Artif Organs 16(suppl 5):64–70, 1993.

Herman TS, Hoppe RT, Donaldson SS, et al: Late relapse among patients treated for Hodgkin's disease. Ann Intern Med 102:292–297, 1985.

Hockey EG: Personal communication. 1994.

Holdredge SA: Physical therapy management. Hemophilia World 6:4–7, 1990.

Holdredge SA, Cotta S: Physical therapy and rehabilitation in the care of the adult and child with hemophilia. *In* Hilgartner M, Pochedly C (eds): Hemophilia in the Child and Adult. New York, Raven Press, 1989, pp 235–262.

Hoppe RT: Radiation therapy in the management of Hodgkin's disease. Semin Oncol 17:704–715, 1990.

Jagannath S, Barlogie B, Tricot G: Hematopoietic stem cell transplantation. Hosp Pract 28:79–86, 1993.

Jagannath S, Vesole DH, Tricot G, et al: Hemopoietic stem cell transplants for multiple myeloma. Oncology 8:89–106, 1994.

Jarvis C: Physical Examination and Health Assessment. Philadelphia, WB Saunders, 1992.

Jassak PF, Petty J, Krol MA: Treatment modalities for neoplastic disorders. *In* Black JM, Matassarin-Jacobs E (eds): Luckmann and Sorensen's Medical-Surgical Nursing, ed 4. Philadelphia, WB Saunders, 1993, pp 501–526.

Jennings B: Nursing role in management: Hematological problems. *In* Lewis S, Collier I (eds): Medical-Surgical Nursing: Assessment and Management of Clinical Problems. St Louis, Mosby–Year Book, 1992, pp 664–714.

Kantarjian HM, Keating MJ, Talpaz M, et al: Chronic myelogenous leukemia in blast crisis. Am J Med 83:445–454, 1987.

Kennedy BJ: Hodgkin's disease. CA Cancer J Clin 43:325–326, 1993.

Kennedy BJ, Loeb V Jr, Peterson V, et al: Survival in Hodgkin's disease by stage and age. Med Pediatr Oncol 20:100–104, 1992.

Korbling M, Holle R, Haas R, et al: Autologous blood stem-cell transplantation in patients with advanced Hodgkin's disease and prior radiation to the pelvic site. J Clin Oncol 8:978–985, 1990.

Korbling M, Juttner C, Henon P, et al: Blood versus bone marrow transplants. *In* Gale RP, Juttner CA, Henon P (eds): Blood Stem Cell Transplants. New York, Cambridge University Press, 1994.

Kumar S, Kumar D, Schnadig VJ, et al: Plasma cell myeloma in patients who are HIV-positive. Am J Clin Pathol 102:633–639, 1994.

Kyle RA: Newer approaches to the management of multiple myeloma. Cancer 72(suppl 11):3489–3494, 1993.

Lee CK, Aeppli DM, Bloomfield CD, Levitt SH: Curative radiotherapy for laparotomy-staged IA, IIA, IIIA, Hodgkin's disease: An evaluation of the gains achieved with radical radiotherapy. Int J Radiat Oncol Biol Phys 19:547–549, 1990.

Levitt L, Lin R: Biology and treatment of adult acute lymphoblastic leukemia. West J Med 164(2):143–155, 1996.

Linker CA: Blood. *In* Tierney LM, McPhee SJ, Papadakis MA (eds): Current Medical Diagnosis and Treatment, ed 33. Norwalk, Conn, Appleton & Lange, 1994, pp 415–466.

Lo Coco F, Diverior D, Pandolfi PP, et al: Molecular evaluation of residual disease as a predictor of relapse in acute promyelocytic leukemia. Lancet 340:1437–1438, 1992.

Longo DL, Young RC, Wesley M, et al: Twenty years of MOPP therapy for Hodgkin's disease. J Clin Oncol 4:1295–1306, 1986.

Lottman MS, Thompson KS: Assessment of the hematologic system. *In* Phipps WJ, Cassmeyer VL, Sands JK, et al (eds): Medical-Surgical Nursing, ed 5. St Louis, Mosby–Year Book, 1995, pp 931–940.

Lozier JN, Brinkhous KM: Gene therapy and the hemophilias. JAMA 271:47–51, 1994.

Lucarelli G: Bone marrow transplantation in patients with thalassemia. N Engl J Med 322:417–421, 1990.

Mack TM, Cozen W, Shibata DK, et al: Concordance for Hodgkin's disease in identical twins suggesting genetic susceptibility to the young-adult form of the disease. N Engl J Med 332:413–418, 1995.

MacLennan IC, Drayson M, Dunn J: Multiple myeloma. Br J Med 308:1033–1036, 1994.

Makris M, Preston FE: Chronic hepatitis in hemophilia. Blood Rev 7:243–250, 1993.

Mansen TJ, McCance KL, Field R: Alterations of leukocyte, lymphoid, and hemostatic function. *In* McCance KL, Huether S (eds): Pathophysiology: The Biologic Basis for Disease in Adults and Children, ed 2. St Louis, Mosby–Year Book, 1994, pp 878–907.

Mariani G, Di Nucci GD, Arcieri P: Immunopurified clotting factor concentrates. Nouv Rev Fr Hematol 36(suppl 1):S61–65, 1994.

Mausch P, Larson D, Osteen R, et al: Prognostic factors for positive surgical staging in patients with Hodgkin's disease. J Clin Oncol 8:257–265, 1990.

McCance KL, Cipriano PG: Structure and function of the hematologic system. *In* McCance KL, Huether S (eds): Pathophysiology: The Biologic Basis for Disease in Adults and Children, ed 2. St Louis, Mosby–Year Book, 1994, pp 830–860.

McCullough J, Hansen J, Perkins H, et al: The National Marrow Donor Program: How it works, accomplishments to date. Oncology 3:63–68, 1989.

McDonagh JE, Clarke F, Smith SR, et al: Non-Hodgkin's lymphoma presenting as polyarthritis. Br J Rheumatol 33:79–84, 1994.

McGlave P: Bone marrow transplants in chronic myelogenous leukemia: An overview of determinants of survival. Semin Hematol 27:23, 1990.

McIntosh S, Rooks Y, Ritchey AK, et al: Fever in young children with sickle cell disease. J Pediatr 96:199–204, 1980.

Mijovic A, Pagliuca A, Mufti GJ: Autologous blood stem transplantation in hematological malignancies. Leuk Lymphoma 13:33–40, 1994.

Miller C: Inheritance of Hemophilia. New York, National Hemophilia Foundation, 1992.

Morrison VA: Chronic leukemias. CA Cancer J Clin 44:353–377, 1994.

Moyer S, Weinblatt VJ: The science of being a carrier. HANDI Q 5:6–7, 1994.

Mueller N: Another view of the epidemiology of non-Hodgkin's lymphoma. Oncology 8:83, 1994.

National Hemophilia Foundation: AIDS Update. Revised Recommendations by Medical and Scientific Advisory Council Concerning HIV Infection, AIDS and Hepatitis in the Treatment of Hemophilia Following the FDA Approval of Recombinant Factor VIII, Medical bulletin No. 176. New York, June 7, 1993.

Nelson J: Hemophilia and exercise. PT Magazine 2:60–66, 1994.

Odubiyi M: Cultural awareness in the world of hemophilia. HANDI Q, 5:1–7, 1994.

Oken MM: Standard treatment of multiple myeloma. Mayo Clin Proc 69:781–786, 1994.

O'Toole M (ed): Miller-Keane Encyclopedia and Dictionary of Medicine, Nursing, and Allied Health, ed 5. Philadelphia, WB Saunders, 1992.

Pagana K, Pagana T: Mosby's Diagnostic and Laboratory Test Reference. St Louis, Mosby–Year Book, 1992.

Painter P: End stage renal disease. *In* Skinner J (ed): Exercise Testing and Exercise Prescription for Special Cases: Theoretical Basis and Clinical Application, ed 2. Philadelphia, Lea & Febiger, 1993, pp 351–362.

Paper R: Females bleed too! HANDI Q 4:1–3, 1993.

Pavel J, Plunkett A, Sink B: Nursing care of clients with hematologic disorders. *In* Black JM, Matassarin-Jacobs E (eds): Luckmann and Sorensen's Medical-Surgical Nursing, ed 4. Philadelphia, WB Saunders, 1993, pp 1335–1402.

Pedersen-Bjergaard J, Rowley JD: The balanced and the unbalanced chromosome aberrations of acute myeloid leukemia may develop in different ways and may contribute differently to malignant transformation. Blood 83:2780–2786, 1994.

Phillips MD: The Wheeler and Rubenstein article reviewed. Oncology 8:73–75, 1994.

Powars D, Hiti A: Sickle cell anemia: Beta S gene cluster haplotypes as genetic markers for severe disease expression. AJDC 147:1197–1202, 1993.

Press OW, Collins C, Mortimer J, et al: Oncologic therapeutics. *In* Ramsey PG, Larson EB (eds): Medical Therapeutics, ed 2. Philadelphia, WB Saunders, 1993, pp 374–427.

Price RH, Solomon LR: Hematology and transfusion medicine. *In* Ramsey PG, Larson EB (eds): Medical Therapeutics, ed 2. Philadelphia, WB Saunders, 1993, pp 346–373.

Prior E, Goldberg AF, Conjalka MS, et al: Hodgkin's disease in homosexual men: An AIDS-related phenomenon? Am J Med 81:1085–1088, 1986.

Reece DE, Barnett MJ, Connors JM, et al: Intensive chemotherapy with cyclophosphamide, carmustine, and etoposide followed by autologous bone marrow transplantation for relapsed Hodgkin's disease. J Clin Oncol 9:1871–1879, 1991.

Richel DJ, Van der Wall E, Slaper J, et al: Peripheral blood stem cell (PBSC) mobilization and transplantation (PSCT) in patients with malignant lymphomas and solid tumors. Int J Artif Organs 16(suppl 5):71–75, 1993.

Riske B: The Hemophilia Nursing Handbook. New York, National Hemophilia Foundation, 1995.

Rowe JM, Ciobanu N, Ascensao J, et al: Recommended guidelines for the management of autologous and allogeneic bone marrow transplantation. Ann Intern Med 120:143–158, 1994.

Rubin E, Farber JL: Pathology, ed 2. Philadelphia, JB Lippincott, 1994.

Salmon SE, Cassady JR: Plasma cell neoplasms. *In* DeVita VT, Hellman S, Rosenberg SA (eds): Cancer: Principles and Practice of Oncology, ed 4. Philadelphia, JB Lippincott, 1993, pp 1984–2025.

Samuels-Reid JH: Common problems in sickle cell disease. Am Fam Physician 49:1477–1480, 1994.

Scharrer I, Neutzling O: Incidence of inhibitors in haemophiliacs: A review of the literature. Blood Coagul Fibrinolysis 4:753–758, 1993.

Schiffer CA: Acute myeloid leukemia in adults. *In* Holland JF, Frei E, Bast RC, (eds): Cancer Medicine, ed 3. Philadelphia, Lea & Febiger, 1993, pp 1907–1933.

Shipp MA: Prognostic factors in aggressive non-Hodgkin's lymphoma: Who has high-risk disease? Blood 83:1165–1173, 1994.

Sickle Cell Disease Guideline Panel: Sickle Cell Disease: Screening, Diagnosis, Management, and Counseling in Newborns and Infants. Clinical Practice Guideline No. 6, AHCPR publication No. 93-0562. Rockville, Md, Agency for Health Care Policy and Research, 1993.

Silver RM: The eosinophilia-myalgia syndrome. Clin Dermatol 12:457–465, 1994.

Sorrentino BP, Brandt SJ, Bodine D, et al: Selection of drug-resistant bone marrow cells in vivo after retroviral transfer of human MDR1. Science 257:99–103, 1992.

Soutar RL: Recent advances in the development and use of plasma concentrates. Br J Hosp Med 51:119–122, 1994.

Stamatoyannopoulos JA: Future prospects for treatment of hemoglobinopathies. West J Med 157:631–636, 1992.

Steinberg MH, Lu ZH, Barton FB: Fetal hemoglobin in sickle cell anemia: Determinants of response to hydroxyurea. Blood 89:1078–1088, 1997.

Szczylik C, Skorksi T, Nicolaides NC, et al: Selective inhibition of leukemia cell proliferation by BCR-ABL antisense oligodeoxynucleotides. Science 253:562–565, 1991.

Terhune MH, Cooper KD: Gene rearrangements and T-cell lymphomas. Arch Dermatol 129:1484–1490, 1993.

Thomas ED: Bone marrow transplantation. *In* Isselbacher KJ, Braunwald E, Wilson JD, et al (eds): Harrison's Principles of Internal Medicine, ed 13. New York, McGraw-Hill, 1994, pp 1793–1798.

Tierney LM: Blood vessels and lymphatics. *In* Tierney LM, McPhee SJ, Papadakis MA (eds): Current Medical Diagnosis and Treatment, ed 33. Norwalk, Conn, Appleton & Lange, 1994, pp 385–414.

Tricot G, Jagannath S, Vesole D, et al: Hematopoietic stem cell transplants for multiple myeloma. Leuk Lymphoma 22(1-2):25–36, 1996.

Vose JM, Bierman PJ, Armitage JO: Hodgkin's disease: The role of bone marrow transplantation. Semin Oncol 17:749–757, 1990.

Ward FT, Weiss RB: Lymphoma and pregnancy. Semin Oncol 16:397–409, 1989.

Watchie J: Cardiopulmonary Issues in Bone Marrow Transplantation. American Physical Therapy Association, Combined Sections Meeting, New Orleans, Feb 3, 1994.

Weinshel EL, Peterson BA: Hodgkin's disease. CA Cancer J Clin 43:327–346, 1993.

Wheeler A, Rubenstein EB: Current management of disseminated intravascular coagulation. Oncology 8:69–79, 1994.

Wiernik PH: Chemotherapy of Hodgkin's disease. Principles Pract Oncol 2:1–12, 1988.

Wingo PA, Tong T, Bolden S: Cancer statistics, 1995. CA Cancer J Clin 45:8–30, 1995.

Witzig TE: Detection of malignant cells in the peripheral blood of patients with multiple myeloma: Clinical implications and research applications. Mayo Clin Proc 69:903–907, 1994.

Wong D: Whaley and Wong's Essentials of Pediatric Nursing, ed 4. St Louis, Mosby–Year Book, 1993.

Wujcik D: Infection control in oncology patients. Nurs Clin North Am 28:639–650, 1993a.

Wujcik D: Leukemia. *In* Groenwald S, Frogge M, Goodman B, et al (eds): Cancer Nursing: Principles and Practice, ed 3. Boston, Jones & Bartlett, 1993b, pp 1149–1173.

Zimmer-Galler I, Lie JT: Choroidal infiltrates as the initial manifestation of lymphoma in rheumatoid arthritis after treatment with low-dose methotrexate. Mayo Clin Proc 69:258–261, 1994.

SECTION 2

chapter 12

The Respiratory System

Catherine C. Goodman

The primary function of the respiratory system is to provide oxygen to, and remove carbon dioxide from, the bloodstream. The respiratory system can be divided into three main portions: the upper airway, the lower airway, and the terminal alveoli (Fig. 12–1). The upper airway consists of the nasal cavities, sinuses, pharynx, tonsils, and larynx. The lower airway consists of the conducting airways, including the trachea, bronchi, bronchioles, and alveoli (Fig. 12–2). The alveoli or air sacs at the end of the conducting airways in the lower respiratory tract are the primary lobules, sometimes called the acini, of the lung. The lungs are the major organs of respiration, providing gas exchange and thereby supplying the blood and body tissues with oxygen and disposing of waste carbon dioxide.

SIGNS AND SYMPTOMS OF PULMONARY DISEASE *(Davey and McCance, 1994)*

Pulmonary disease is often classified as acute or chronic, obstructive or restrictive, infectious or noninfectious, and is associated with many common signs and symptoms. The most common of these are cough and dyspnea. Other manifestations include chest pain, abnormal sputum, hemoptysis, cyanosis, digital clubbing, and altered breathing patterns (Box 12–1, Table 12–1).

Cough as a physiologic response occurs frequently in healthy people, but a persistent dry cough is commonly caused by a tumor, congestion, or hypersensitive airways (allergies). A productive cough with purulent *sputum* may indicate infection, whereas a productive cough with nonpurulent sputum is nonspecific and just indicates irritation. *Hemoptysis* (coughing and spitting blood) indicates pathology—infection, inflammation, abscess, tumor, or infarction.

Dyspnea, or shortness of breath (SOB), usually indicates inadequate ventilation (i.e., hyperventilation with anxiety) or insufficient amounts of oxygen in the circulating blood. Dyspnea is usually caused by diffuse and extensive rather than focal pulmonary disease, pulmonary embolism being the exception. Factors contributing to the sensation of dyspnea include increased work of breathing, respiratory muscle fatigue, decreased breathing reserve, and strong emotions, particularly anxiety and anger. Dyspnea when the person is lying down is called *orthopnea* and is caused by redistribution of body water. Fluid shift leads to increased fluid in the lung, which leads to orthopnea. The abdominal contents also exert pressure on the diaphragm, decreasing the efficiency of the respiratory muscles.

Chest pain originates in the pleurae, airways, or the chest wall and is caused by pulmonary disorders, including pleurisy, pneumonia, pulmonary infarct, tumor, and spontaneous pneumothorax. Pulmonary pain patterns are usually localized in the substernal or chest region over involved lung fields which may include the anterior chest, side, or back. However, pulmonary pain can radiate to the neck, upper trapezius, costal margins, thoracic back, scapulae, or shoulder. Shoulder pain caused by pulmonary involvement may radiate along the medial aspect of the arm mimicking other neuromuscular causes of neck or shoulder pain. Musculoskeletal causes of chest (wall) pain must be differentiated from pain of cardiac, pulmonary, epigastric, and breast origins before therapy begins.

Extensive disease may occur in the periphery of the lung without occurrence of pain until the process extends to the parietal pleura (Fig. 12–3). Pleural irritation then results in sharp, localized pain that is aggravated by any respiratory movement. Clients usually note that the pain is alleviated by autosplinting, that is, lying on the affected side, which diminishes the movement of that side of the chest (Scharf, 1989; Snider, 1994).

Cyanosis, a bluish discoloration of the skin and mucous membranes, may be central, that is, caused by decreased oxygen saturation of hemoglobin in arterial blood, or peripheral, with slow blood circulation in fingers and toes. Central cyanosis is best observed in buccal (cheek) mucous membranes and lips. Peripheral cyanosis is observed in nail beds. Cyanosis can be caused by decreased arterial oxygenation, pulmonary or cardiac right-to-left shunts, decreased cardiac output, cold external temperature, or anxiety.

Decreased oxygenation does not always cause cyanosis. For example, severe anemia and carbon monoxide poisoning can cause inadequate oxygenation of tissues without causing cyanosis. Persons with polycythemia (increase in red blood cells) may have cyanosis when oxygenation is adequate because polycythemia causes hemoglobin concentrations to be higher than normal.

Clubbing, thickening and widening of the terminal phalanges of the fingers and toes, results in a painless clublike appearance recognized by the loss of the angle between the nail and the nail bed (Fig. 12–4). Any condition that interferes with oxygenation may cause clubbing, including cystic fibrosis, lung cancer, bronchiectasis, pulmonary fibrosis, congenital heart disease, and lung abscess. Although 75% to 85% of clubbing is due to pulmonary disease and resultant hypoxia (diminished availability of blood to the body tissues), clubbing does not always indicate lung disease. It is sometimes present

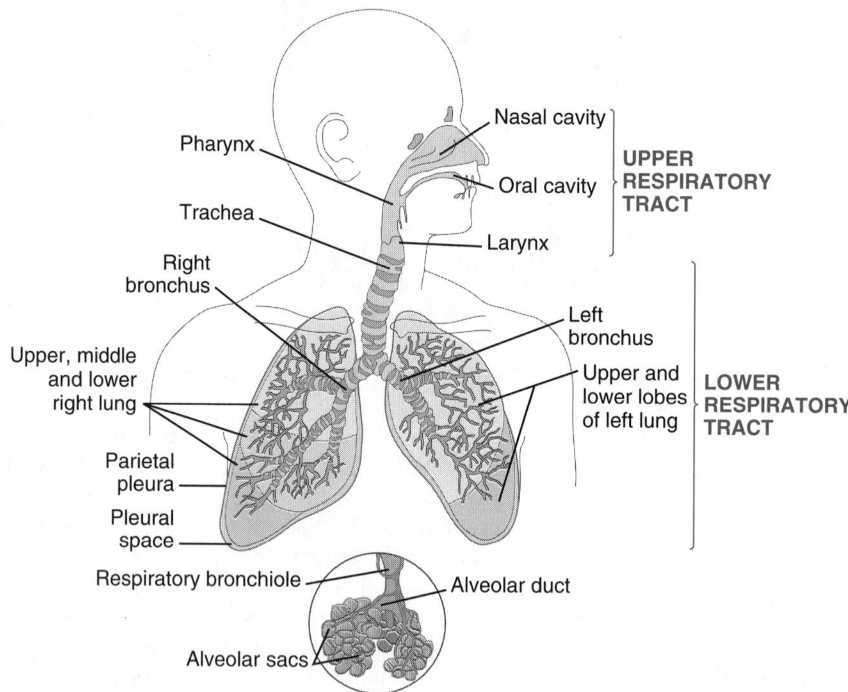

Figure **12–1.** Structures of the upper and lower respiratory tracts. The upper respiratory tract consists of the nasal cavity, pharynx, and larynx; the lower respiratory tract includes the trachea, bronchi, and lungs. The *circle* shows the acinus, the terminal respiratory unit, which consists of the respiratory bronchioles, alveolar ducts, and alveolar sacs. This is the portion of the lungs where oxygen and carbon dioxide are exchanged.

in heart disease and disorders of the liver and gastrointestinal tract (O'Toole, 1992).

Altered breathing patterns, including changes in the rate, depth, regularity, and effort of breathing, occur in response to any condition affecting the pulmonary system (see Table 12–1). Breathing patterns can vary depending on the neuromuscular or neurologic disease or trauma, or disease present (Table 12–2).

Neuromuscular. Some of the neuromuscular diseases with respiratory compromise include inflammatory polyneuropathy, Guillain-Barré syndrome, amyotrophic lateral sclerosis (ALS), myasthenia gravis, poliomyelitis, and severe kyphoscoliosis, whatever the cause (e.g., idiopathic ankylosing spondylitis, Marfan syndrome, poliomyelitis, cerebral palsy).

Disruption of the neuromuscular chain of command, malnutrition, metabolic disturbance, fever, or decreased blood or oxygen supply cause hypoxemia (deficient oxygenation of the blood), acidosis,[1] or low cardiac output, which in turn reduces energy supplies and results in respiratory muscle dysfunction and hypoventilation.

Nocturnal respiratory abnormalities such as hypoventilation may further jeopardize the ventilatory pump when combined with skeletal muscle atonia associated with any neuromuscular cause. Sleep disturbances associated with fibromyalgia syndrome or chronic fatigue syndrome, or sleep apnea of any origin may result in hypoventilation. Typical clinical findings include paradoxical motion (reverse breathing) of the rib cage and abdomen, increased respiratory rate, and inability to take deep breaths.

Neurologic Disease or Trauma. Breathing pattern abnormalities seen with head trauma, brain abscess, diaphragmatic paralysis of chest wall muscles and thorax (e.g., generalized myopathy or neuropathy), heat stroke, spinal meningitis, and encephalitis can include *apneustic breathing, ataxic breathing,* or *Cheyne-Stokes respiration* (CSR). Apneustic breathing localizes damage to the midpons and is most commonly due to a basilar artery infarct. Ataxic, or Biot's, breathing is caused by disruption of the respiratory rhythm generator in the medulla.

Spinal cord injuries above C3 result in loss of phrenic nerve innervation, necessitating a tracheostomy and mechanical ventilation. Clients with generalized weakness, as in the Guillain-Barré syndrome, some myopathies or neuropathies, or incomplete spinal cord injuries, may show a tendency toward a specific breathing pattern called "lateral breathing.[2]"

Systemic Disease. CSR may be evident in the well elderly as well as in compromised clients. The most common cause of CSR is severe congestive heart failure (see Chapter 10), but it can also occur with renal failure, meningitis, drug overdose, and increased intracranial pressure. It may be a normal breathing pattern in infants and aging persons during sleep (Jarvis, 1992).

[1] For a discussion of respiratory acidosis, see Chapter 4; see also Tables 4–17 and 35–9.

[2] In the supine position, the chest becomes flattened anteriorly with excessive flaring of the lower ribs. The person breathes into the lateral plane of respiration because the weakened diaphragm and intercostal muscles cannot effectively oppose the force of gravity in the anterior plane. The chest expands primarily in the lateral plane, where gravity is eliminated (Massery, 1996).

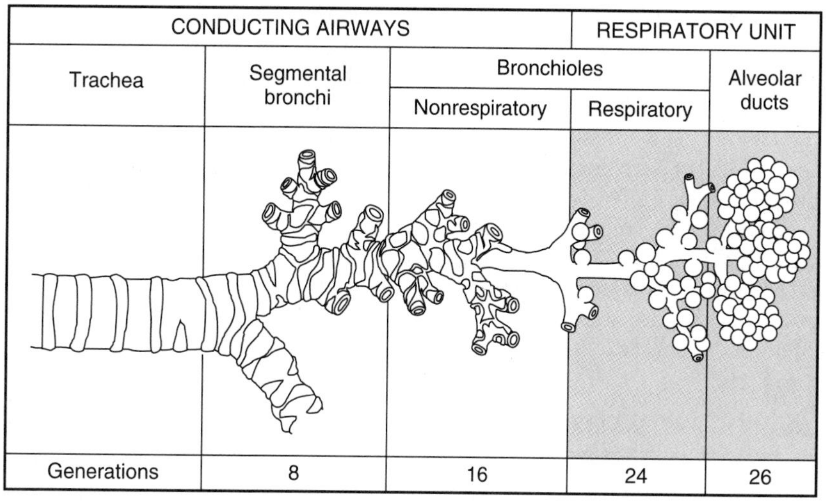

CONDUCTING AIRWAYS				RESPIRATORY UNIT
Trachea	Segmental bronchi	Bronchioles		Alveolar ducts
		Nonrespiratory	Respiratory	
Generations	8	16	24	26

Figure **12–2.** Structures of the lower airway. The first 16 generations of the airways branching in human lungs are purely conducting; transitional airways lead into the final respiratory zone consisting of alveoli where gas exchange takes place.

Special Implications for the Therapist **12–1**

SIGNS AND SYMPTOMS OF PULMONARY DISEASE

Many people with neuromusculoskeletal conditions have potential for impaired ventilation and altered breathing patterns. Clinical observation of the client as he or she breathes is important (Table 12–3) and can alert the therapist to respiratory pathology. Assessment of the three muscle groups (abdominal and intercostal muscles and the diaphragm) involved in normal ventilatory function may be required. Enhancing motor performance and improving a client's functional level involves improving pulmonary potential. This can be accomplished using techniques to improve ventilation during therapy. The reader is referred to more specific texts for treatment techniques (Massery, 1994; Frownfelter and Dean, 1996).

High blood pressure in the pulmonary circulation (pulmonary hypertension) can cause pain during exercise that is often mistaken for cardiac pain (angina pectoris). For the therapist, musculoskeletal causes of chest pain must be differentiated from pain of cardiac, pulmonary, epigastric, and breast origins before treatment begins (Goodman and Snyder, 1995). The therapist involved in chest therapy and pulmonary rehabilitation must recognize precautions for and contraindications to treatment in the medical client (Table 12–4).

BOX **12–1**

Most Common Signs and Symptoms of Pulmonary Disease

- Cough
- Dyspnea
- Abnormal sputum
- Chest pain
- Hemoptysis
- Cyanosis
- Digital clubbing
- Altered breathing patterns

CONDITIONS CAUSED BY PULMONARY DISEASE OR INJURY

Hypoxemia and pulmonary edema are two of the most common conditions caused by pulmonary disease or injury. *Hypoxemia,* deficient oxygenation of arterial blood, may lead to *hypoxia,* a broad term meaning diminished availability of

TABLE **12–1** DESCRIPTIONS OF ALTERED BREATHING PATTERNS

Hyperventilation	Abnormally prolonged and deep breathing
Kussmaul's respiration	A distressing dyspnea characterized by increased respiratory rate (>20/min), increased depth of respiration, panting, and labored respiration typical of air hunger
Cheyne-Stokes respiration	Repeated cycle of deep breathing followed by shallow breaths or cessation of breathing
Hypoventilation	Reduction in the amount of air entering the pulmonary alveoli, which causes an increase in the arterial CO_2 level
Apneustic	Gasping inspiration followed by short expiration
Biot's respiration (ataxia)	A haphazard random distribution of deep and shallow breaths
Wheezing	Breathing with a rasp or whistling sound resulting from constriction or obstruction of the throat, pharynx, trachea, or bronchi

Modified from O'Toole M (ed): Miller-Keane Encyclopedia and Dictionary of Medicine, Nursing, and Allied Health, ed 5. Philadelphia, WB Saunders, 1992.

oxygen to the body tissues (O'Toole, 1992). Hypoxemia is caused by respiratory alterations (Table 12–5), whereas hypoxia may occur anywhere in the body caused by alterations of other systems that have no relation to changes in the pulmonary system. Signs and symptoms of hypoxemia vary depending on the level of oxygenation in the blood (Table 12–6) (Davey and McCance, 1994).

Pulmonary edema, accumulation of fluid in the tissues and air spaces of the lung, is most commonly caused by heart disease, especially left ventricular failure, but it is also a complication of pulmonary disease and other systemic conditions. Pulmonary edema is discussed in detail later under Parenchymal Disorders.

AGING AND THE PULMONARY SYSTEM

Aging affects not only the physiologic functions of the lungs (ventilation and gas exchange) but also the ability of the respiratory system to defend itself. More than any other organ, the lung is susceptible to infectious processes and environmental and occupational pollutants (see Environmental and Occupational Diseases, this chapter). These factors, combined with the normal aging process, contribute to the decline of lung function. Most of the changes that occur with aging affect the lower airway, but in the upper airway the movement of the cilia slows and becomes less effective in sweeping away mucus and debris. This reduced ciliary action predisposes the aging client to increased respiratory infections.

Loss of an effective cough reflex contributes to an increased susceptibility to pneumonia and postoperative atelectasis in the elderly. Contributing factors which result in the loss of an effective cough reflex include conditions more common in older age such as reduced consciousness, use of sedatives, impaired esophageal motility, dysphagia, and neurologic diseases.

With increasing age, especially after age 55 years, there is an overall decrease in the functional ability of the lungs to move air in and out. In the lower airways, symptomatic airways obstruction (AO) occurs. It is unclear whether the increasing rate of ventilatory functional decline with age results from a progressive, lifelong process or occurs abruptly in brief steps leading to AO. Airway obstruction increases the risk of death from chronic obstructive pulmonary disease (COPD), heart disease, and lung cancer (Abrams et al., 1995).

The lung tissue (parenchyma) changes in size and shape, becoming rounder with a loss of alveolar wall tissue and elastic tissue fibers in the alveolar walls. The reduced alveolar surface area and airways available for gas diffusion account for reduced lung function. The lung bases become less ventilated due to closing off of a number of airways. This increases the person's risk of dyspnea with exertion beyond the usual workload (Jarvis, 1992).

Respiratory muscle strength weakens in all people after age 40 and there is increased stiffness of the chest wall as the rib articulations and cartilage ossify and become less flexible. Other changes include the loss of elastic recoil of the lungs from a reduction of elastic fibers in the lung tissue, and alterations in gas exchange. All of these changes contribute to the increased work of breathing, meaning that the elderly person must have more ventilation for the same oxygenation than the younger person (Protas, 1993). These changes are influenced by environmental factors, respiratory disease, body size, and race (Crapo, 1993).

Special Implications for the Therapist **12-2**

AGING AND THE PULMONARY SYSTEM

It does not appear that healthy older people are limited in exercise capacity by pulmonary function, that is, lung

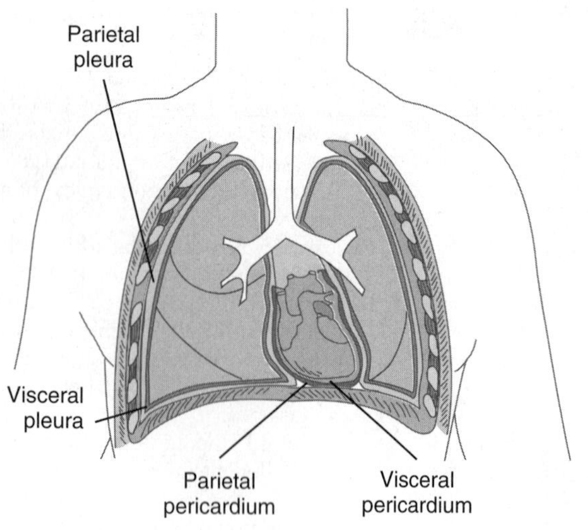

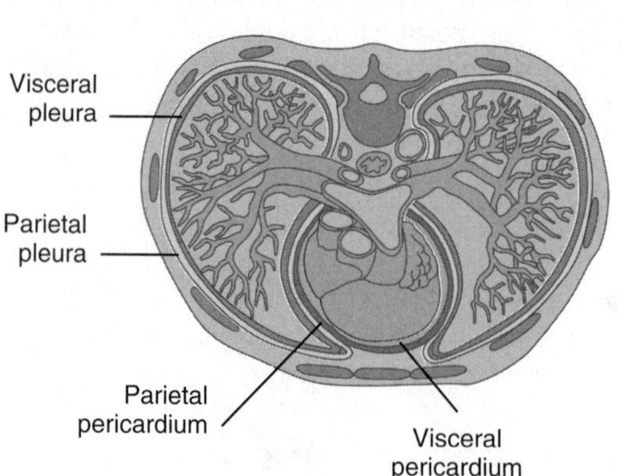

Figure **12-3.** Chest cavity and associated structural linings shown in anterior (*A*) and cross-sectional (*B*) views. For instructional purposes the layers are depicted larger than actually found in the human body.

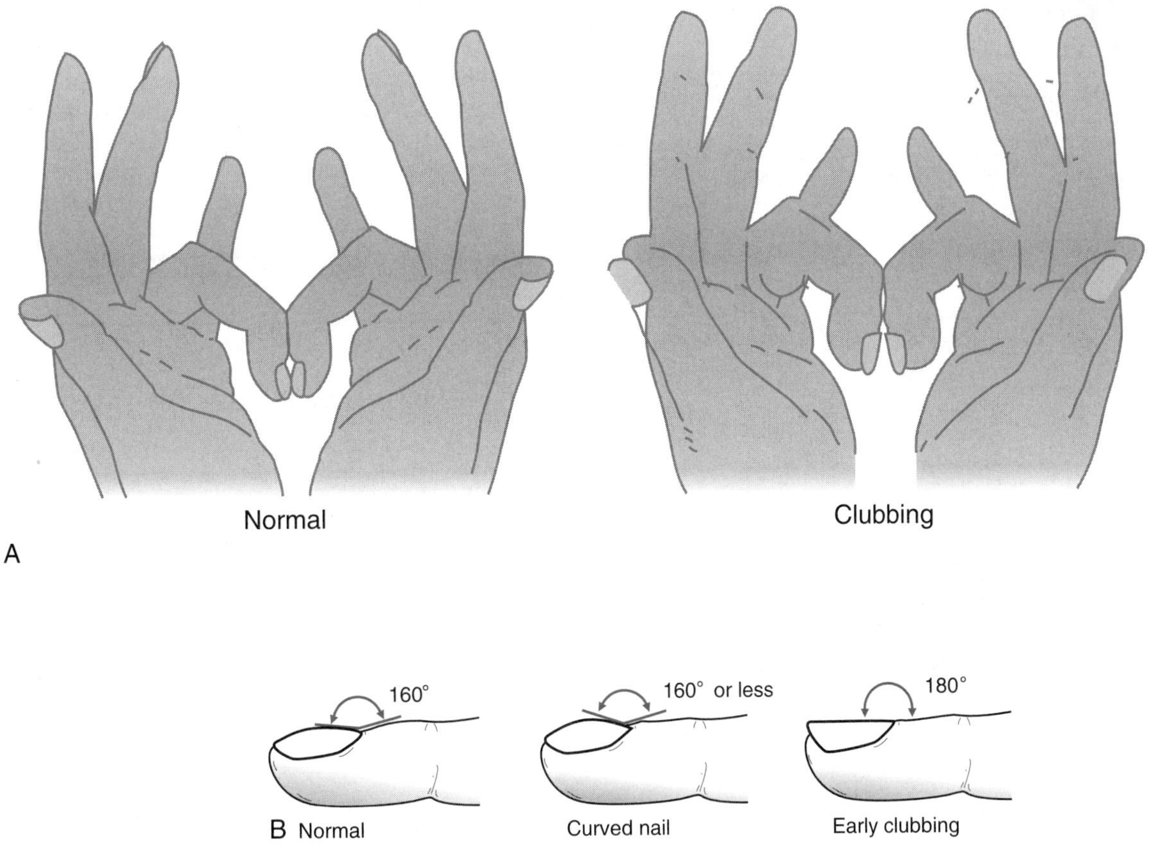

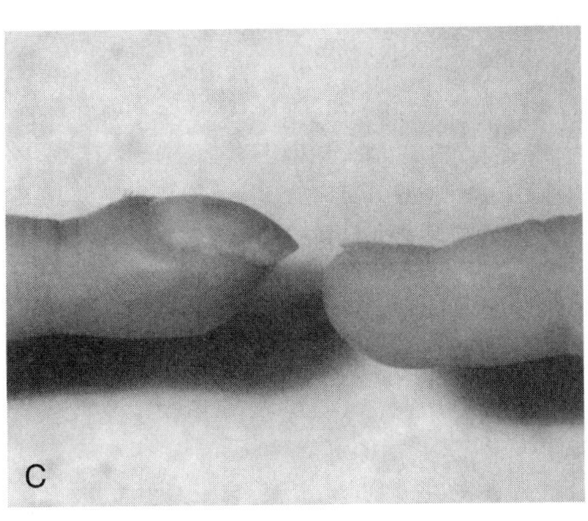

Figure **12-4.** A, Assessment of clubbing by the Schamrath method. The client places the fingernails of opposite fingers together and holds them up to a light. If a diamond shape can be seen between the nails, there is no clubbing. B, The profile of the index finger is examined and the angle of the nail base is noted; it should be about 160 degrees. The nail base is firm to palpation. Curved nails are a variation of normal with a convex profile and may look like clubbed nails, but the angle between the nail base and the nail is 160 degrees or less. In early clubbing, the angle straightens out to 180 degrees and the nail base feels spongy to palpation. C, Photograph of advanced clubbing of the finger (*left*) compared with normal finger (*right*). (*From Swartz MH: Textbook of Physical Diagnosis: History and Examination. Philadelphia, WB Saunders, 1989, plate IX [A].*)

function or ventilation does not limit exercise performance (Brown and Kohrt, 1993; Hagberg et al., 1988; Kohrt et al., 1991; Makrides et al., 1990; Yerg et al., 1985). However, clients with obstructive lung disease have a significant loss of vital capacity before functional loss is evident and may experience shortness of breath at relatively low exercise intensities. In fact, the older person with obstructive lung disease may be limited in exercise by shortness of breath rather than by reduced cardiovascular capacity (Protas, 1993).

Exercise capacity or exercise tolerance does decrease in the elderly as the $Pa{O_2}$ (measure of oxygen in arterial blood) decreases. The level of habitual physical activity* is one factor favorably influencing O_2 delivery. The ability to deliver O_2 to the tissues is called maximal O_2 consumption, or $V{O_2}max$. This measurement reflects the integration of three components of the delivery system that transports O_2 from the outside air to the working muscles: pulmonary ventilation, blood circulation, and muscle tissue. When the ventilation/perfusion imbalance is further compromised by age-associated reductions in cardiac output, the $Pa{O_2}$ (and thus O_2 delivery) may be reduced even more.

Regular exercise can substantially slow the decline in maximal O_2 delivery caused by cardiovascular deconditioning related to age or lowered levels of

TABLE 12-2 Breathing Patterns and Associated Conditions

Hyperventilation	Kussmaul's	Cheyne-Stokes
Anxiety	Strenuous exercise	Congestive heart failure
Acute head injury	Metabolic acidosis	Renal failure
Blood oxygenation		Meningitis
Fever		Drug overdose
		Increased intracranial pressure
		Infants (normal)
		Elderly during sleep (normal)
Hypoventilation	**Apneustic**	**Biot's (Ataxia)**
Fibromyalgia syndrome	Midpons lesion	Exercise
Chronic fatigue syndrome	Basilar artery infarct	Shock
Sleep apnea		Cerebral hypoxia
Muscle fatigue		Heat stroke
Muscle weakness		Spinal meningitis
Malnutrition		Head injury
Fever		Brain abscess
		Encephalitis

TABLE 12-3 Clinical Inspection of the Respiratory System

Respiratory rate, depth, and effort of breathing
- Tachypnea
- Dyspnea
- Gasping respirations

Breathing pattern
- Paradoxical breathing
- Kussmaul's respiration
- Cheyne-Stokes respiration
- Hypoventilation
- Hyperventilation
- Wheezing
- Pursed-lip breathing
- Prolonged expiration

Cyanosis
Pallor or redness of skin during activity
Clubbing (toes, fingers)
Nicotine stains on fingers and hands
Retraction of intercostal, supraclavicular, or suprasternal spaces
Use of accessory muscles
Nasal flaring
Tracheal tug
Chest wall shape and deformity
- Barrel chest
- Pectus excavatum
- Pectus carinatum
- Kyphosis
- Scoliosis

Cough
Sputum: frothy, red-tinged, green, or yellow

habitual physical activity. Decreases in respiratory muscle strength and endurance occurring with age can be enhanced with exercise (Chen and Kuo, 1989; Yerg et al., 1985). The total muscle mass decline with increasing age accounts for the age-related decrease in aerobic exercise capacity. This decrease in exercise capacity can also be slowed by exercise training.

* Daily physical activity can be assessed using the following categories: sedentary; sedentary with some daily activity; active through occupation or recreational activity; and trained athlete.

INFECTIOUS AND INFLAMMATORY DISEASES

Pneumonia

Overview and Etiology. Pneumonia is an inflammation affecting the parenchyma of the lungs and can be caused by (1) a bacterial, viral, or mycoplasmal infection; (2) inhalation of toxic or caustic chemicals, smoke, dusts, or gases; or (3) aspiration of food, fluids, or vomitus. It may be primary or secondary; it often follows influenza.

The common feature of all types of pneumonia is an inflammatory pulmonary response to the offending organism or agent. This response may involve one or both lungs at the level of the lobe (lobar pneumonia) or more distally at the bronchioles and alveoli (bronchopneumonia). Bronchopneumonia denotes patchy and diffuse areas of involvement, is a less severe form, is seen more frequently than lobar pneumonia, and is common in clients postoperatively and in clients with chronic bronchitis, particularly when these two situations coexist (Cronin, 1993).

Incidence. Pneumonia is a commonly encountered disease with more than 1 million cases diagnosed each year accounting for about 10% of admissions to adult medical services. In one form or another, pneumonia continues to be a leading cause of death in the United States during people's productive years. Bacterial pneumonia is especially prevalent in the elderly and occurs during epidemics of viral respiratory infections. Viral pneumonia, though common, is not usually life-threatening except in the immunocompromised client.

Risk Factors. Infectious agents responsible for pneumonia are typically present in the upper respiratory tract and cause no harm unless resistance is lowered by some other factor. There are many host conditions that promote the growth of pathogenic organisms, including cigarette smoking and chronic bronchitis, poorly controlled diabetes mellitus, uremia, dehydration, poor nutrition or malnutrition, and prior existing critical illnesses such as chronic renal failure, chronic lung disease, or acquired immunodeficiency syndrome (AIDS). Additionally, the stress of hospitalization, confinement to a nursing facility or intensive care unit, surgery, tracheal intubation, and treatment with antineoplastic chemotherapy or immunosuppressive drugs promotes rapid colonization with pathogenic organisms (Reynolds, 1994).

Infants, the elderly, and persons with altered consciousness (e.g., caused by alcoholic stupor, head injury, seizure disorder,

TABLE 12-4 PRECAUTIONS FOR AND CONTRAINDICATIONS TO CHEST THERAPY* IN THE MEDICAL CLIENT

PRECAUTIONS	CONTRAINDICATIONS
Fragile ribs (e.g., metastatic bone cancer, osteoporosis, flail chest, rib fractures, osteomyelitis of the ribs)	Untreated tension pneumothorax; treat when chest tube has been inserted and client is stable
Burns, open wounds, skin infections in thoracic area	Hemoptysis
Pulmonary edema, congestive heart failure	Unstable cardiovascular system
Large pleural effusion	Hypotension
Pulmonary embolism (controversial)†	Uncontrolled hypertension
Symptomatic aneurysm or decrease in circulation of the main blood vessels	Acute myocardial infarction
Platelet count between 20,000 and 50,000/mm³	Arrhythmias
Postoperatively	Conditions prone to hemorrhage (platelet count <20,000/mm³ must have physician's approval)
Neurosurgery (positioning may cause increased intracranial pressure; can begin gentle breathing exercises)	Unstabilized head and neck injury
Esophageal anastomosis (gastric juices may affect suture line)	Intracranial pressure >20 mm Hg
Orthopedic clients who are limited in positioning	
Recent spinal fusion	
Surgical complications (e.g., pericardial sac tear)	
Recent skin grafts or flaps	
Resected tumors (avoid tumor area)	
Recently placed pacemaker	
Aged or nervous clients who become agitated or upset with therapy	
Acute spinal injury or recent spinal surgery such as laminectomy (precaution: logroll and position with care to maintain vertebral alignment)	

* Chest therapy refers to postural drainage including percussion and vibration.
† A question remains whether there may be a recurrence (repeat emboli in the medically unstable client, that is, one whose blood level of anticoagulants is not yet adequate to prevent a possible second embolus from dislodging) with movement in positioning the client for postural drainage. However, allowing the client to lie still can contribute to the development of further venous stasis.
Adapted from AARC Clinical Practice Guideline. Postural drainage therapy. Respir Care 36:1418–1426, 1991.

TABLE 12-5 CAUSES OF HYPOXEMIA

MECHANISM	COMMON CLINICAL CAUSE
Ventilation/perfusion mismatch	Asthma Chronic bronchitis Pneumonia
Decreased oxygen content	High altitude Low oxygen content Enclosed breathing space (suffocation)
Hypoventilation	Lack of neurologic stimulation of the respiratory center Oversedation Drug overdose Neurologic damage Chronic obstructive pulmonary disease
Alveolocapillary diffusion abnormality	Emphysema Fibrosis Edema
Shunting	Adult respiratory distress syndrome (ARDS) Hyaline membrane disease (ARDS in newborn) Atelectasis

Adapted from Davey SS, McCance KL: Alterations of pulmonary function. *In* McCance KL, Huether SE (eds): Pathophysiology: The Biologic Basis for Disease in Adults and Children, ed 2. St Louis, Mosby–Year Book, 1994, p 1152.

drug overdose, general anesthesia) are most vulnerable owing to inactivity and immobility causing pooling of normal secretions in the airways, thereby facilitating bacterial growth (O'Toole, 1992). People with severe periodontal disease, structural disease of the oropharynx, or with cough reflexes impaired by drugs, alcohol, or neuromuscular disease are at increased risk for the development of pneumonia due to aspiration.

Pathogenesis. Although a common disease, pneumonia is relatively rare in healthy people because of the effectiveness of the respiratory host defense system and the fact that healthy lungs are generally kept sterile below the first major bronchial divisions (Reynolds, 1994). In the compromised person, the normal release of biochemical mediators by alveolar mast cells as part of the inflammatory response does not eliminate invading pathogens. The multiplying microorganisms release damaging toxins stimulating full-scale inflammatory and immune responses with damaging side effects (Davey and McCance, 1994).

Endotoxins released by some microorganisms damage bronchial mucous and alveolocapillary membranes. Inflammation and edema cause the acini and terminal bronchioles to fill with infectious debris and exudate so that air cannot enter the alveoli, leading to ventilation/perfusion abnormalities. With the appearance of an inflammatory response, clinical illness usually occurs. Production of interleukin-1 (IL-1) and tumor necrosis factor by alveolar macrophages can contribute to many of the systemic effects of pneumonia such as fever, chills, malaise, and myalgias (Reynolds, 1994).

TABLE 12-6 SIGNS AND SYMPTOMS OF HYPOXEMIA

Pa_{O_2} (mm Hg)	SIGNS AND SYMPTOMS
80–100	Normal
60–80	Moderate tachycardia, possible onset of respiratory distress
50–60	Malaise Lightheadedness Nausea Vertigo Impaired judgment Incoordination Restlessness
35–50	Marked confusion Cardiac dysrhythmias Labored respiration
25–35	Cardiac arrest Decreased renal blood flow Decreased urine output Lactic acidosis Poor oxygenation Lethargy Loss of consciousness
<25	Decreased minute ventilation* secondary to depression of the respiratory center

Pa_{O_2}, partial pressure of arterial oxygen.
* The total expired volume of air per minute.
Adapted from Frownfelter DL, Dean E: Principles and Practice of Cardiopulmonary Physical Therapy, ed 3. St Louis, Mosby–Year Book, 1996, p 237.

Resolution of the infection with eventual healing occurs with successful containment of the pathogenic microorganisms. However, little is known about the actual processes that halt the acute inflammatory reaction in pneumonia and initiate recovery.

Aspiration Pneumonia. The risk of aspiration pneumonia occurs when anatomic defense mechanisms are impaired, as occurs with seizures; depressed central nervous system (CNS); recurrent gastroesophageal reflux; neuromuscular disorders, especially with suck-swallow dysfunction; anatomic abnormalities (laryngeal cleft, tracheoesophageal fistula); and debilitating illnesses. Chronic aspiration often causes recurrent bouts of acute febrile pneumonia. Although any region may be affected, the right side, especially the right upper lobe in the supine person, is commonly affected (Larsen et al., 1993).

Viral Pneumonia. Viral pneumonia is usually mild and self-limiting, often bilateral and panlobular, but confined to the septa rather than the intra-alveolar spaces as is more likely with bacterial pneumonia. Viral pneumonia can be a primary infection creating an ideal environment for a secondary bacterial infection or it can be a complication of another viral illness such as measles or chickenpox. The virus destroys ciliated epithelial cells and invades goblet cells and bronchial mucous glands. Bronchial walls become edematous and infiltrated with leukocytes. The destroyed bronchial epithelium sloughs throughout the respiratory tract, preventing mucociliary clearance.

Bacterial Pneumonia. Destruction of the respiratory epithelium by infection with the influenza virus may be one mechanism whereby influenza predisposes people to bacterial pneumonia. The lung parenchyma, especially the alveoli in the lower lobes, is the most common site of bacterial pneumonia. When bacteria reach the alveolar surfaces, most are rapidly ingested by phagocytes. Once phagocytosis has occurred, intracellular killing proceeds, but at a slower rate for bacteria than for other particles.

In pneumonia caused by staphylococci, gram-negative bacteria, or pneumococcal pneumonia (*Streptococcus pneumoniae*), alveolar edema creates a medium for multiplication of bacteria and aids in spreading infection into adjacent portions of the lung. The involved lobe fills with exudate causing solidification of the tissue, called consolidation (see Fig. 12–12). The next stage is called *red hepatization* in which alveoli fill with blood cells, fibrin, edematous fluid, and pneumococci, giving lung tissue a red color. This passes into the *gray hepatization* stage in which affected tissues turn gray because of fibrin deposition over the pleural surfaces and fibrin and leukocytes (neutrophils) in the consolidated alveoli.

As the condition resolves, neutrophils degenerate and macrophages appear in the alveolar spaces, which ingest the fibrin threads, and the remaining bacteria in the respiratory bronchioles are then transported by lung lymphatics to regional lymph nodes. The infection is usually limited to one or two lobes.

Clinical Manifestations. Most cases of pneumonia are preceded by an upper respiratory infection, frequently viral. Signs and symptoms of pneumonia include sudden and sharp pleuritic chest pain aggravated by chest movement and accompanied by a hacking, productive cough with rust-colored or green, purulent sputum. Other symptoms include dyspnea, tachypnea accompanied by decreased chest excursion on the affected side, cyanosis, headache, fatigue, fever and chills, and generalized aches and myalgias that may extend to the thighs and calves. Elderly people with bronchopneumonia may remain afebrile because of the changes in temperature regulation as part of the normal aging process and may present with altered mental status because of changes in oxygenation.

Medical Management

Diagnosis. The clinical presentation of pneumonias caused by different pathogenic microorganisms overlap considerably, requiring microscopic examination of respiratory secretions in making a differential diagnosis. Gram stain, color, odor, and cultures are part of the sputum analysis. A blood culture may help identify the bacteria and if positive identification of the bacteria cannot be obtained, it is assumed to be viral. Chest films show infiltrates that may involve a single lobe (lobar pneumonia from staphylococci) or may be more diffuse as in the case of bronchopneumonia (usually streptococci). Physical examination, including percussion and auscultation of the chest, may reveal signs of lung consolidation such as dullness, inspiratory crackles, or bronchial breath sounds.

Treatment. The primary treatment for many forms of pneumonia is antibiotic therapy. Treatment with specific antibiotics is based on the history and whether the pneumonia was community-acquired, hospital-acquired, or nursing home–acquired and on the medical status and overall condition of the client (e.g., otherwise healthy or debilitated). Viral pneumonia is treated symptomatically unless secondary bacterial pneumonia develops. Hospitalization may be required for the immunocompromised client.

The Centers for Disease Control and Prevention (CDC) recommend adherence to universal precautions for clients with pneumonia. At the very least, careful handwashing by all personnel involved is essential for reducing the transmission of infectious agents. Adequate hydration, and pulmonary hygiene, including deep breathing, coughing, and chest therapy, should be instituted in all clients hospitalized with pneumonia. Mechanical ventilation and supplemental oxygen may be needed to maintain adequate gas exchange in severely compromised clients. If severe pneumonia progresses to adult respiratory distress syndrome (ARDS), positive end-expiratory pressure (PEEP) is added to ventilatory support measures.

Preventive measures are important and include early ambulation in postoperative clients and postpartal women unless contraindicated. Proper positioning to prevent aspiration during the postoperative period and for all people who are immobilized or who have a poor gag reflex is important. A vaccine is recommended for the elderly; for people with chronic disorders of the lungs, heart, liver, or kidneys; for individuals with poorly controlled diabetes mellitus; and for those with a compromised immune system. Immunization can provide protection from pneumococcal disease for a period of 3 to 5 years in 80% of vaccinated persons (O'Toole, 1992).

Prognosis. Pneumonia ranks sixth among the causes of death in the United States and currently accounts for almost 40% of hospital deaths. It is a potentially lethal illness that is readily reversible with early diagnosis and treatment.

Special Implications for the Therapist **12-3**

PNEUMONIA

Occasionally, a lower lobe infection can irritate the diaphragmatic surface so that pain referred to the shoulder is the presenting symptom. For the client with a known diagnosis of pneumonia, the breathing pattern and the position assumed in bed can indicate the client's discomfort, reveal tachypnea, and demonstrate splinting of the chest to minimize pleuritic pain (i.e., lying on the affected side reduces the pleural rubbing that often causes discomfort) (Reynolds, 1994).

Lobes affected by pneumonia will remain vulnerable to further infection for some time, especially in the bedridden, debilitated, or neuromuscularly compromised population. Chest physical therapy is not usually helpful in adults with uncomplicated pneumonias. However, the client, family, or caretakers should be instructed in breathing exercises and a positional rotation program with frequent positional changes to prevent secretions from accumulating in dependent positions.

Pneumocystis carinii Pneumonia

Definition and Incidence. *Pneumocystis carinii* pneumonia (PCP) is a progressive, often fatal pneumonia and represents the most frequently occurring opportunistic infection in persons with AIDS. Eighty percent of people with AIDS develop PCP during the course of their illness. PCP has been shown to be the first indicator of conversion from human immunodeficiency virus (HIV) infection to the designation of AIDS in 60% of cases (Flaskerud and Ungvarski, 1992).

Etiology and Risk Factors. The origin of the organism is unknown. It is possibly acquired from the environment, infected humans, or animals or fungi or protozoa (Rubin and Farber, 1994). Other people at risk for the development of PCP include anyone who is immunosuppressed for renal transplantation, by chemotherapy for lymphoma or leukemia, by steroid therapy, or by malnutrition (Harruff, 1994).

Pathogenesis and Clinical Manifestations. Infection begins with the attachment of the *Pneumocystis* trophozoite (the feeding stage of a sporozoan parasite) to the alveolar lining cell. The trophozoite feeds on the host cell, enlarges, and transforms into the cyst form which ruptures to release new trophozoites, repeating the cycle. If the process is uninterrupted by the immune system or antibiotic therapy, the affected alveoli progressively fill with organisms and proteinaceous fluid until consolidation disrupts gas exchange, slowly suffocating the person.

The physiologic response to PCP includes hyperthermia, impaired gas exchange, altered respiratory function, and altered nutrition. Symptoms of PCP develop slowly and present as fever and progressive dyspnea, accompanied by a nonproductive cough. Fatigue, tachypnea, weight loss, and other manifestations of underlying immunosuppressive disease may be present (Henry and Holzemer, 1992).

Medical Management

Diagnosis, Treatment, and Prognosis. Diagnosis is important because effective pharmacologic treatment is available. In most cases, diagnosis is made by radiograph and bronchoscopy or sputum induction for analysis of alveolar material.

The increasing seroprevalence of HIV among women of reproductive age, the risks of vertical transmission of HIV, and the fact that PCP is the most common infection seen in people progressing to AIDS have led to recommendations for routine prenatal HIV infection counseling and testing. Treatments considered during pregnancy include the antiretroviral agent zidovudine and prophylactic agents to prevent PCP (Sperling and Stratton, 1992).

Mortality from the first episode of PCP averages 20%. All people who recover from PCP are at risk for recurrent episodes of the disease as long as the underlying immunosuppressive condition persists. Persons with AIDS have the highest recurrence rate (50% at 1 year) (Walzer, 1991). Prophylaxis effectively prevents and reduces the incidence of future episodes (Zackrison and Tsou, 1991).

Special Implications for the Therapist **12–4**

***Pneumocystis carinii* PNEUMONIA**

Implement universal precautions to prevent contagion. Teach the client energy conservation techniques (see Box 7–1) as well as deep-breathing exercises.

Pulmonary Tuberculosis

Definition. Tuberculosis (TB, formerly known as "consumption") is an infectious, inflammatory systemic disease that affects the lungs and may disseminate to involve lymph nodes and other organs. It is caused by infection with *Mycobacterium tuberculosis* and is characterized by granulomas, caseous (resembling cheese) necrosis, and subsequent cavity formation.

Overview. TB may be primary or secondary. The first or primary infection with the tubercle bacillus is usually asymptomatic and almost always (99%) remains quiet after the development of a hypersensitivity to the microorganism. The primary infection usually involves the middle or lower lung area with lesions consisting of exudation in the lung parenchyma. These lesions quickly become caseous and spread to the bronchopulmonary lymph nodes, where they gain access to the bloodstream and predispose the person to the subsequent development of chronic pulmonary and extrapulmonary TB at a later time.

Secondary TB develops as a result of either endogenous or exogenous reinfection by the tubercle bacillus. This is the most common form of clinical TB. In the United States, development of secondary TB is almost always the result of endogenous reinfection which occurs when the primary lesion becomes active as a result of debilitation or lowered resistance.

Incidence. Despite improved methods of detection and treatment, TB remains a global health problem with an estimated 10 million Americans infected, 10 million new cases diagnosed each year worldwide, and 3 million deaths attributable to tuberculosis annually (Perez-Stable and Hopewell, 1989; Daniel, 1994).

Before the development of anti-TB drugs in the late 1940s, TB was the leading cause of death in the United States. Drug therapy, along with improvements in public health and general living standards, resulted in a marked decline in incidence. However, recent influxes of immigrants from developing Third World nations, rising homeless populations, prolonged life span, and the emergence of HIV led to an increase in reported cases in the mid-1980s, reversing a 40-year period of decline (Cronin, 1993). Overall, between 1985 and 1992 there was a 20% increase in new TB cases in the United States.

Increases in TB cases in many areas are related to the high risk of TB among persons infected with HIV. According to the American Lung Association, at least 100,000 people in the United States are infected with both HIV and TB (American Lung Association, 1993). The risk of progression to active disease is markedly increased for persons with HIV infection (Selwyn et al., 1989; Huebner et al., 1992).

Additionally, multidrug-resistant TB (MDRTB) is an iatrogenic disease now emerging as a major infectious disease problem throughout the world. The AIDS pandemic, the increased incidence of TB in populations without easy access to anti-TB medications (e.g., the homeless, the economically disadvantaged), the deterioration of the public health infrastructure, and inadequate training of health-care providers in the epidemiology of TB are some of the factors contributing to the increased incidence of MDRTB (Riley, 1993).

Previously, only about 10% of new TB cases were believed to be caused by recent bacteria transmission with the rest resulting from reactivation of latent infections. New techniques to track the spread of specific strains of TB bacteria have revealed that 30% to 40% of new TB cases result from recent transmission of TB bacteria from a person with active infection (Alland et al., 1994).

Etiology. The causative agent is the tubercle bacillus, commonly transmitted in the United States by inhalation of infected airborne particles, known as droplet nuclei, which are produced when the infected persons sneeze, laugh, speak, sing, or cough. Casual contact or brief exposure to a few bacilli will not result in transmission of sufficient bacilli to infect a person. Rather, household contact of many months is required for transmission. In some other parts of the world, bovine TB carried by unpasteurized milk and other dairy products from tuberculous cattle is more prevalent.

The tubercle bacillus is capable of surviving for months in sputum that is not exposed to sunlight. Within the body it can lie dormant for decades and then become reactivated years after an initial infection. This secondary TB infection (endogenous reinfection) can occur at any time the person's resistance is lowered (e.g., alcoholism, immunosuppression, silicosis, advancing age, cancer) (O'Toole, 1992).

The elderly people of today were children when transmission of tubercle bacilli occurred more often. Now reactivation of the disease is developing in their later years with an increasing portion of elderly persons who have never been infected acquiring new infections in nursing homes (Daniel, 1994).

Risk Factors. Although TB can affect anyone, certain segments of the population have an increased risk of contracting the disease, including (1) elderly people, who constitute nearly half of the newly diagnosed cases of TB in the United States; (2) racial and ethnic groups, such as Native Americans, and blacks, especially the economically disadvantaged or homeless; (3) immigrants from Southeast Asia, Ethiopia, Mexico, and Latin America, (4) clients dependent on alcohol, or on other drugs because of malnutrition, debilitation, and poor health; (5) infants and children under the age of 5 years; (6) current or past prison inmates; (7) diabetes mellitus; (8) endstage renal disease; and (9) people with reduced immunity (e.g., those with HIV infection, with malnutrition, or on cancer chemotherapy or prolonged corticosteroid therapy) (Dooley et al., 1990).

Environmental factors that enhance transmission include contact between susceptible persons and an infectious person in relatively small, enclosed spaces (e.g., recent concern has been expressed about airline travel); inadequate ventilation that results in insufficient dilution or removal of infectious droplet nuclei (e.g., older buildings such as hospitals, prisons, government buildings, universities); and recirculation of air containing infectious droplet nuclei. Adequate ventilation is the most important measure to reduce the infectiousness of the environment. Mycobacteria are susceptible to ultraviolet irradiation (i.e., sunshine), so outdoor transmission of infection rarely occurs.

Pathogenesis. Infection occurs when a susceptible person inhales droplet nuclei containing M. *tuberculosis*, and bacilli become established in the alveoli of the lungs and spread throughout the body. In the lungs, a proliferation of epithelial cells surround and encapsulate the multiplying bacilli in an attempt to wall off the invading organisms, thus forming a typical tubercle. Two to 10 weeks after initial human infection with the bacilli, acquired cell-mediated immunity usually limits further multiplication and spread of the TB bacilli.

Researchers have recently identified a segment of DNA that allows the TB organism to invade macrophages where they lie dormant for years before leaving the macrophage cells to invade the lungs or other parts of the body. Finding this genetic fragment may provide information needed to block the microorganisms from entering human cells. The DNA segment identified probably represents only one of several mechanisms that permit the TB invasion (Arruda et al., 1993).

The presence of antigen concentrations at the initial site of infection brings about necrosis and eventually fibrosis and calcification of the tissues, which arrests the infection and renders the disease inactive, or *latent*. Residual lesions are often visible on chest radiograph and sites remain potential lesions for reactivation years later. If the infection is not controlled, the person develops symptoms of progressive primary TB (CDC, 1990; O'Toole, 1992).

Tubercle bacilli can spread to other parts of the body by way of the blood, producing a condition called *miliary tuberculosis*, most common in people 50 years or older and in very young children with unstable or underdeveloped immune systems. Erosion of blood vessels by the primary lesion can cause a large number of bacilli to enter the circulatory system where they are carried to all areas of the body and may lodge in any organ, especially the kidneys, bone growth plates, lymph nodes, and meninges. Untreated, these tiny lesions spread and produce large areas of infection (e.g., TB pneumonia, tubercular meningitis).

Clinical Manifestations. Most symptoms associated with TB do not appear in the early, most curable stage of the disease. Often symptoms are delayed until a year or more after initial exposure to the bacilli. Long before the symptoms appear, TB may be detected by a simple skin test. Symptoms suggestive of tuberculosis include productive cough of more than 3 weeks' duration, especially when accompanied by other symptoms such as weight loss, fever, night sweats, fatigue, malaise, and anorexia.

Complications associated with TB include pleurisy with effusion, intestinal infections, tuberculous pneumonia or laryngitis, and sudden lung atelectasis indicating that a deep tuberculous cavity in the lung has perforated or created an opening into the pleural cavity allowing air and infected material to flow to it. Tuberculous spondylitis (Pott's disease), a rare complication of extrapulmonary TB, is discussed in Chapter 21.

Medical Management

Diagnosis. Diagnostic measures for identifying tuberculosis include history, physical examination, tuberculin skin test, chest radiograph, and microscopic examination and culture of sputum. The tuberculin skin test determines whether the body's immune response has been activated by the presence of the bacillus. The skin and other tissue become sensitized to the protein part of the tubercle bacilli. A positive reaction causes a swelling or hardness at the site of infection and develops 3 to 10 weeks after the initial infection. A positive skin test reaction indicates the presence of a TB infection but does not show whether the infection is dormant or is causing a clinical illness (Cronin, 1993). Other diagnostic methods, such as bronchoscopy or biopsy, may be indicated in some cases.

Because of the dormant properties of the tubercle bacillus, anyone infected with TB should have periodic TB testing performed. In the case of someone with known TB, the skin test will always test positive, requiring periodic screening[3] with chest x-ray studies. The tuberculin skin test is the only method currently available that demonstrates infection with M. *tuberculosis* in the absence of active TB (CDC, 1990).

Tuberculosis may be more difficult to diagnose in persons with HIV infection; the diagnosis may be overlooked because of an atypical clinical or radiographic presentation or the simultaneous occurrence of other pulmonary infections (e.g., PCP). Additionally, the diagnosis may be further compounded by impaired responses to tuberculin skin tests (Dooley et al., 1990) and lack of methods for rapid detection of resistant strains of M. *tuberculosis* (Riley, 1993).

Treatment. All cases of active disease are treated, and certain cases of inactive disease are treated prophylactically. Treatment may be initiated with only a positive skin test even if a chest film and sputum analysis show no evidence of the disease. In this way, the disease is less likely to reactivate later in life when the immune system is more likely to be compromised.

Pharmacologic treatment through medication is the primary treatment of choice and renders the infection noncontagious and nonsymptomatic. Treatment is problematic with homeless people and people who abuse alcohol and use injection drugs because this population is often noncompliant with the recommended 6- to 9-month treatment regimen. Treatment has been further complicated by multidrug-resistant TB present in at least 13 states (Snider and Roper, 1992; Edlin et al., 1992).

Chemotherapy using a variety of chemical agents may be used and often two or more drugs are used simultaneously to prevent the emergence of drug-resistant mutants. New drug treatments now include combinations of all primary anti-TB medications (e.g., rifampin; isoniazid; pyrazinamide [Rifater]) taken in one dose to replace the traditional treatment requir-

[3] Previously, an annual examination was recommended, but currently screening is based on symptomatic presentation (if asymptomatic, testing is not required) and job exposure (i.e., those health-care workers treating persons with active TB or AIDS or HIV infection are at increased risk of exposure).

ing multiple drugs daily. Treatment regimens do not differ for pulmonary and extrapulmonary tuberculosis.

Preventing the transmission of tuberculosis by using such simple measures as covering the mouth and nose with a tissue when coughing and sneezing reduces the number of organisms excreted into the air. Adequate room ventilation and preventing overcrowding such as in homeless shelters and prisons are well-known preventive measures. Preventive drug therapy is under investigation (Claremont et al., 1991; CDC, 1989).

Vaccination with BCG (bacille Calmette-Guérin), a freeze-dried preparation of a live, attenuated strain of *Mycobacterium bovis*, is used for children. It is at least 60% effective in preventing dissemination of tuberculosis in children if they become infected with TB. There is no evidence at present regarding the efficacy of vaccination in HIV-infected children, and the World Health Organization does not recommend its unlimited use. It is recommended for any tuberculin-negative infant living in a household in which repeated exposure to untreated or ineffectively treated TB cases occurs (Mann et al., 1992).

Prognosis. Untreated, tuberculosis is 50% to 80% fatal, and the median time period to death is 2½ years. Noncompletion of treatment among inner city residents and the homeless presents an additional factor in the prognosis and subsequent failure to eradicate TB (Brudney and Dobkin, 1991; Daniel, 1994). Mortality from multidrug-resistant TB exceeds 80% in persons infected with HIV but is also high in persons free of HIV (Riley, 1993).

Special Implications for the Therapist 12-5

PULMONARY TUBERCULOSIS

Health-care workers should be particularly alert to the need for preventing tuberculosis transmission in settings in which persons with HIV infection receive care, especially settings in which cough-inducing procedures are being performed. Precautions must be followed by all health-care personnel having contact with clients diagnosed with TB (Table 12–7; see also Appendix A: Summary of Universal Precautions).

For the therapist evaluating a client with pulmonary TB, a thorough chest assessment and musculoskeletal evaluation should be performed (Gallantino and Bishop, 1994). Chest expansion may be decreased because of diffuse fibrotic changes in progressive disease. Tracheal deviation may be present if there is a significant loss of volume in the upper lobes. Postural adaptations may have developed in late stages of the disease because of poor breathing patterns (Gallantino and Bishop, 1994). Other areas of assessment should include overall posture, gait, muscle strength, balance, and functional mobility.

People with TB typically have a poor nutritional status and a progressive weight loss that may have secondary effects on the musculoskeletal system, such as postural defects and trigger point irritability. The effects of isolation result in disuse atrophy, and cardiopulmonary and physical deconditioning, including progressive dyspnea. Finding the balance between exercise and clinical limitations is always a challenge for the therapist

TABLE 12-7 GUIDELINES FOR THERAPISTS FOR PREVENTING TRANSMISSION OF TUBERCULOSIS (TB)

All new employees (and student therapists) should be screened with the tuberculin skin test.
Doors to isolation rooms must be kept closed.
Clients infected with TB must cover mouth and nose with tissues when coughing, sneezing, or laughing.
Cough-inducing procedures should not be performed on TB clients unless absolutely necessary; such procedures should be performed using local exhaust, in a high-efficiency particulate air (HEPA)–filtered booth or individual TB isolation room. After completion of treatment, such persons should remain in the booth or enclosure until the cough subsides.
Clients must wear a mask when leaving the room.
Anyone entering the room must wear a protective mask, called a high-efficiency particulate (HEPA) respirator, properly.
Therapists must be adequately trained in the use and disposal of masks and should use a particulate respirator (PR, a special mask)* whenever the client is undergoing cough-inducement or aerosol-generating procedures.
The therapist must check the condition of both the facepiece and face seal each time the PR is worn.
Gloves are worn when touching infective material.
Disinfect the stethoscope between treatment sessions.
Staff and employees attending clients in all settings must be tested for TB: every 6 months for high-risk therapists; other personnel annually.
Handwashing is required before and after contact with the client.
Isolation precautions must be continued until a clinical and bacteriologic response to medical treatment has been demonstrated.
Environmental surfaces (e.g., walls, crutches, bedrails, walkers, etc.) are not associated with transmission of infections; only routine cleaning of such items is required.
Therapists with current pulmonary or laryngeal tuberculosis should be excluded from work until adequate treatment is instituted, cough is resolved, and sputum is free of bacilli on 3 consecutive smears.
All tuberculosis control recommendations for inpatient facilities apply to hospices and home health services.
Home health personnel can reinforce client education about the importance of taking medications as prescribed unless adverse effects are observed.

* There are several types of face masks designated as "particulate respirators;" all National Institute for Occupational Safety and Health (NIOSH)–certified respirators are acceptable protection for health-care workers against *Mycobacterium tuberculosis*. The respiratory protection standard set by the Occupational Safety and Health Administration (OSHA) requires a NIOSH-certified respirator; when such a respirator is used, the law requires that a training and fit-test program be present. For an in-depth discussion of respirator recommendations, see Jarvis et al., 1995.

Guidelines for preventing the transmission of *M. tuberculosis* in health-care facilities, 1994. MMWR 43(RR-13):1–132, 1994.

and specific research related to exercise and the client with TB is only in the preliminary stages (Sandoval et al., 1991; Gallantino and Bishop, 1994). Specific guidelines for evaluation of medical status during exercise are offered by Gallantino and Bishop (1994).

Side effects of the medication can lead to peripheral neuritis which may be brought to the attention of the therapist. This and any other complication such as hepatitis, hemoptysis, optic neuritis, or purpura should be reported to the physician.

Extrapulmonary TB is much less common than pulmonary TB. Treatment of Pott's disease follows the same chemotherapy regimen, with prompt response. Immobilization and avoidance of weight bearing may be required to relieve pain, with attention to maintaining strength and range of motion (see further discussion in Chapter 21).

Lung Abscess

Definition. Described as a localized accumulation of purulent exudate within the lung, an abscess usually develops as a complication of pneumonia, especially aspiration and staphylococcal pneumonia, from aspiration of bacteria from the oropharynx along with foreign material or vomitus, or from septic embolus from lung or heart valve. Septic pulmonary emboli from staphylococcal endocarditis of the tricuspid or pulmonary valves is most often a complication of the use of illicit injection drugs. An abscess may also form when a neoplasm becomes necrotic and contains purulent material that does not drain from the area because of partial or complete obstruction.

Risk Factors. Alcoholism is the single most common condition predisposing to lung abscess. Other predisposed persons include those with altered levels of consciousness due to drug use or alcohol use as mentioned, seizures, general anesthesia, or CNS disease; impaired gag reflex due to esophageal disease or neurologic disorders; poor dentition and periodontal care; and those with tracheal or nasogastric tubes, which disrupt the mechanical defenses of the airways (Stauffer, 1994).

Pathogenesis. As with all abscesses, a lung abscess is a natural defense mechanism in which the body attempts to localize an infection and wall off the microorganisms so these cannot spread throughout the body. As the microorganisms destroy the local parenchymal tissue (including alveoli, airways, and blood vessels), an inflammatory process causes alveoli to fill with fluid, pus, and microorganisms (*consolidation*). Death and decay of consolidated tissue may progress proximally until the abscess drains into the bronchus, spreading the infection to other parts of the lung and forming cavities (*cavitation*).

Clinical Manifestations. Clinical signs and symptoms of abscess formation almost always include cough productive of foul-smelling sputum, and persistent fever. Other characteristic features include chills, dyspnea, pleuritic chest pain, cyanosis, and clubbing of fingernails which can develop over a short period of time. Cavitation causes severe cough with copious amounts of purulent sputum and sometimes hemoptysis.

Medical Management

Diagnosis. Radiographic appearance of a thick-walled solitary cavity surrounded by consolidation suggests lung abscess but must be differentiated from TB, mycosis, cancer, infarction, and Wegener's granulomatosis. Cavitary lesions in the apex of the upper lobes are frequently due to TB rather than bacterial abscess. Sputum analysis and culture or material from bronchoscopy may be diagnostic.

Treatment and Prognosis. Treatment includes drainage by percutaneous thoracoscopy, specific antibiotics, and good nutrition. Chest physical therapy may be helpful if the abscess communicates with the main-stem bronchi; percussion helps promote drainage of associated secretions. Other measures are similar to the treatment of pneumonia. Bronchoscopy may be used to drain the abscess. Prognosis is good if the underlying cause can be treated by antibiotics, leaving only a residual lung scar. However, mortality remains in the range of 5% to 10% and is influenced by the severity of the primary disease that initially caused consolidation.

Pneumonitis

Pneumonitis, an inflammation of lung tissue, is covered in this chapter (see Environmental and Occupational Diseases) under its most common presentation as Hypersensitivity Pneumonitis. Other causes of pneumonitis include lupus pneumonitis associated with systemic lupus erythematosus (SLE), aspiration pneumonitis associated with inspiration of acidic gastric fluid, and interstitial pneumonitis associated with AIDS.

Pneumonitis is an acute, localized inflammation of the lung without the toxemia associated with lobar pneumonia. Histologically, pneumonitis or an inflammatory reaction causes alveolitis with accumulation of an exudate and is most often due to infection. With spread to the interstitium around alveoli, consolidation and a degree of impaired gas exchange may occur in the involved lung tissue. With successful inactivation of the infecting agent, resolution occurs with restoration of normal lung structure (Reynolds, 1994).

Acute Bronchitis

Acute bronchitis is an inflammation of the trachea and bronchi (tracheobronchial tree) that is of short duration and self-limiting with few pulmonary signs. It may result from chemical irritation such as smoke, fumes, or gas, or it may occur with viral infections such as influenza, measles, chickenpox, or whooping cough. These predisposing conditions may become apparent during the therapist's interview with the client.

Symptoms of acute bronchitis include the early symptoms of an upper respiratory infection of a common cold, which progress to fever, a dry, irritating cough, sore throat, possible laryngitis, and chest pain from the effort of coughing. Later the cough becomes more productive of purulent sputum, followed by wheezing. There may be constitutional symptoms including moderate fever with accompanying chills, back pain, muscle pain and soreness, and headache (O'Toole, 1992).

Clients with viral bronchitis present with a nonproductive cough that frequently occurs in paroxysms and is aggravated by cold, dry, or dusty air. Bacterial bronchitis (common in clients with chronic obstructive pulmonary disease, or COPD) causes restrosternal (behind the sternum) pain that is aggravated by coughing.

Treatment is conservative and symptomatic with cough suppressants, rest, humidity, and nutrition and hydration. Prognosis is usually good with treatment and although acute bronchitis is usually mild, it can become complicated in people with chronic lung or heart disease and in elderly clients because they are more susceptible to secondary infections.

Pneumonia is a critical complication (Liles and Ramsey, 1993).

OBSTRUCTIVE DISEASES

Chronic Obstructive Pulmonary Disease

Definition. Chronic obstructive pulmonary disease, also called chronic obstructive lung disease, refers to a number of disorders that affect movement of air in and out of the lungs, particularly within the small airways. The most important of these disorders are obstructive bronchitis, emphysema, and asthma. Although these three diseases may occur independently, they most commonly coexist. Although the term *COPD* is most often used, specialists in pulmonary medicine use the term *chronic air flow limitation* (CAL) as a more accurate description of the disease process (Cronin, 1993). In this chapter, the terms COPD and CAL are used interchangeably.

Incidence and Risk Factors. COPD/CAL is second only to heart disease as a cause of disability in adults under 65 years of age. Smoking is the most common cause of COPD/CAL; this condition rarely occurs in nonsmokers. This disorder usually presents at age 55 to 60 years and 1 in 14 people over the age of 45 years is affected (Johnson, 1988). More men are affected than women, but the incidence in women is increasing with the concomitant increase in smoking by women.

Morbidity and mortality rates for COPD/CAL increase with the effects of exposure to irritating gases, dusts, or allergens; chronic irritation; and pollution in urban environments. Other contributing factors include chronic respiratory infections (e.g., sinusitis), the aging process, heredity, and genetic predisposition.

Pathogenesis. The pathogenesis of each component of COPD/CAL (i.e., chronic obstructive bronchitis, emphysema, and asthma) is discussed separately in their respective sections. A broad overview of COPD/CAL is shown in Figure 12–5.

Medical Management

Diagnosis. Physical examination and air flow limitation on pulmonary function testing (see Table 35–19) are assessment tools in determining the presence and extent of COPD/CAL. Clinical examination, x-ray studies, and laboratory findings usually enable the physician to distinguish COPD/CAL from other obstructive pulmonary disorders such as bronchiectasis, cystic fibrosis (CF), and central airway obstruction. Laboratory analysis may include blood gas measurements to indicate the level of functional impairment or the presence of hypoxia or hypercapnia (excess carbon dioxide in blood), sputum culture, or presence of IgE antibodies against specific allergens. Skin testing for allergens that trigger attacks is most useful in young clients with extrinsic asthma.

Thoracic computed tomography (CT) scanning may detect emphysema not apparent on the chest film, but it is very costly and rarely indicated for this purpose. Most cases of emphysema involve a history of cigarette smoking, chronic cough and sputum production, and dyspnea.

Treatment. The main goals for the client with COPD/CAL are to improve oxygenation and decrease carbon dioxide retention. These are accomplished by (1) reducing airway edema secondary to inflammation (asthma), (2) facilitating the elimination of bronchial secretions, (3) preventing and treating respiratory infection, (4) increasing exercise tolerance, (5) controlling complications, (6) avoiding airway irritants and allergens, and (7) relieving anxiety and treating depression, which often accompany COPD/CAL (Cronin, 1993).

Specific treatment approaches include smoking cessation, pharmacologic management, pulmonary hygiene, exercise, control of complications, avoiding irritants, psychological support, and dietary management. Surgical treatment for COPD/CAL is uncommon, but bullectomy (removal of large bullae that compress the lung and add to dead space) may benefit clients who have repeated spontaneous pneumothorax. Lung transplantation has been successful for up to at least 3 to 4 years in people with COPD/CAL (Mal et al., 1989), although long-term follow-up has been limited. Single-lung transplantation is currently recommended in most cases; after this procedure, exercise tolerance is only slightly less than after double-lung transplantation (Ferguson and Cherniack, 1994).

Common classifications of medications used in the treatment of COPD/CAL include bronchodilators, steroids, antibiotics, expectorants, mast cell membrane stabilizers, and antihistamines. Although the benefits of pneumococcal vaccine are debated, vaccination is recommended for all people with COPD/CAL (Spika et al., 1990). Annual prophylactic vaccination against influenza is also recommended (Ferguson and Cherniack, 1994). Narcotics, tranquilizers, and sedatives are used with caution because these depress the respiratory center. Oxygen is used when the client has severe hypoxemia, exertional or at rest (Pa_{O_2} below 40 mm Hg) (Cronin, 1993).

Chest physical therapy remains a standard adjunct to treatment of COPD/CAL, including breathing exercises, postural drainage, physical training, a program to improve posture, and strengthening of respiratory musculature. For the motivated child with asthma, breathing exercises and controlled breathing are of value in preventing overinflation and improving the strength of respiratory muscles and the efficiency of the cough (Wong, 1993).

Prognosis. The prognosis for chronic bronchitis and emphysema is poor as these are chronic, progressive, and debilitating diseases. The death rate from COPD/CAL has increased 22% in the last decade, especially among elderly men. COPD/CAL is the fifth leading cause of death in the United States and the mortality rate 10 years after diagnosis is greater than 50%.

COPD/CAL is largely preventable and many believe that early recognition of small airways obstruction with appropriate treatment and cessation of smoking may prevent relentless progression of this disease. Early treatment of airway infections and vaccination against influenza and pneumococcal disease may provide symptomatic improvement but have no effect on the progression of the disease (Stauffer, 1994).

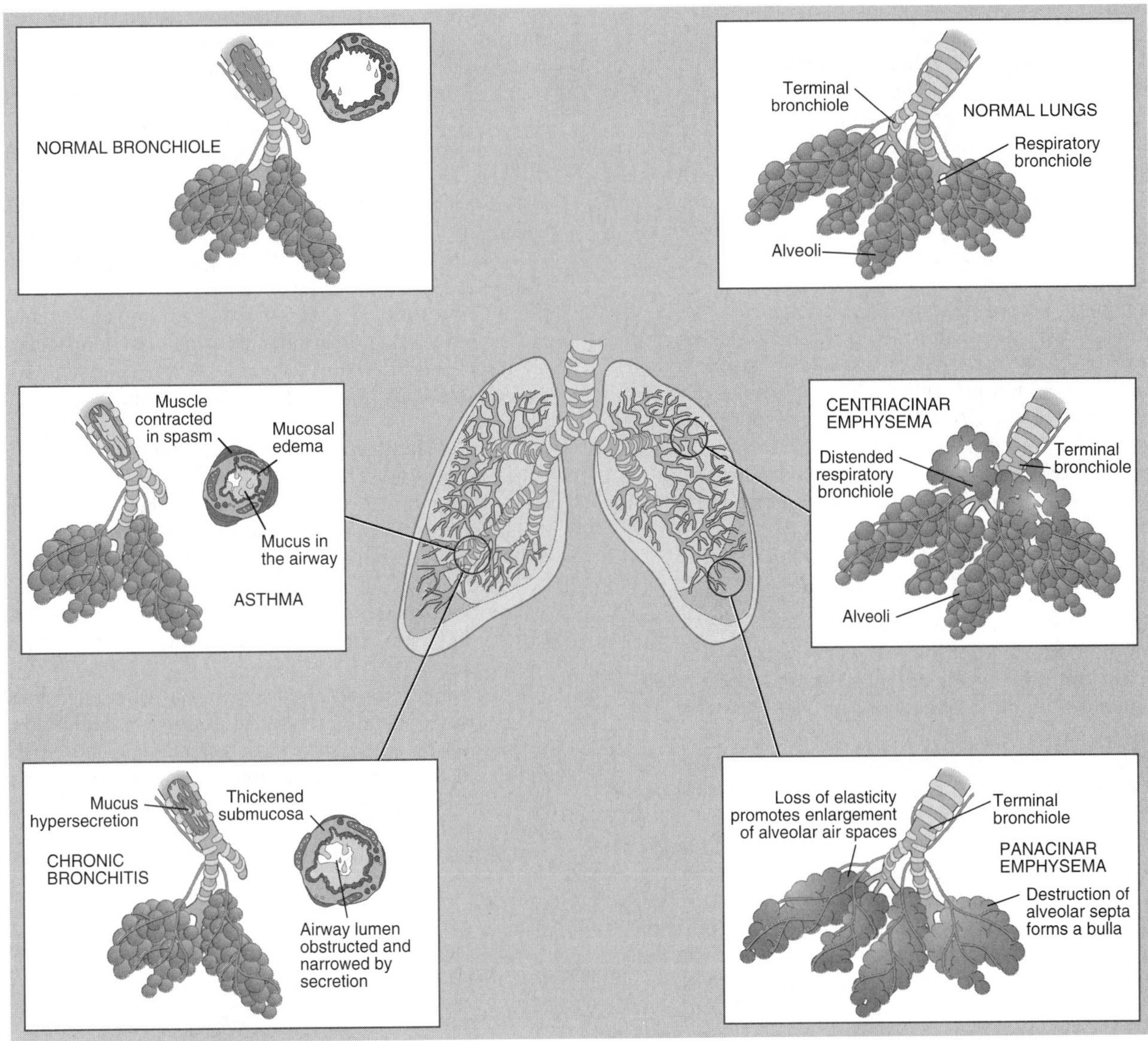

Figure 12–5. What happens in chronic obstructive lung disease/chronic air flow limitation (COPD/CAL).

Special Implications for the Therapist **12–6**

CHRONIC OBSTRUCTIVE PULMONARY DISEASE

Clients with COPD/CAL must be encouraged to remain active, with specific attention directed toward activities they enjoy. Training in pacing and energy conservation (see Box 7–1) allows even those with limited exercise tolerance to increase their daily activities (Ferguson and Cherniack, 1994). To strengthen the muscles of respiration, teach the person with COPD/CAL to take slow, deep breaths and to exhale through pursed lips. To help mobilize secretions, teach effective coughing techniques using diaphragmatic breathing. If secretions are thick, urge the client to drink fluids throughout the day.

People with chronic airflow obstruction report disabling dyspnea when performing seemingly trivial tasks with unsupported arms. Some of the muscles of the upper torso and shoulder girdle share both a respiratory and a positional function for the arms, resulting in functional limitations in many clients with lung disease during unsupported upper extremity activities. Simple arm elevation results in significant increases in metabolic and ventilatory requirements in clients with chronic air flow limitations. Pulmonary rehabilitation that includes upper extremity training (progressive resistance exercises, PREs) reduces metabolic and ventilatory requirements for arm elevation (Martinez et al., 1993). This type of program may allow clients with COPD/CAL to perform sustained upper extremity activities with less dyspnea (Couser et al., 1993; Couser et al., 1992).

Exercise

Exercise does not improve lung function but is used to enhance cardiovascular fitness and train skeletal muscles to function more effectively. Exercise training increases the maximal oxygen consumption and the workload achieved, reduces the ventilation and heart rate for a given workload consistent with cardiopulmonary conditioning (Casaburi et al., 1991), and fosters a sense of well-being. Progressively increased walking is the most common form of exercise for COPD/CAL. Swimming is a preferred exercise option for clients with bronchial asthma (see following discussion). Therapists working with these clients should encourage them to maintain hydration by drinking fluids to prevent mucous plugs from hardening and to take prescribed medications.

Any person with COPD/CAL with cardiac arrhythmias before exercise should be carefully monitored with exercise training. Blood pressure and pulse should be observed at rest and in response to exercise. Most people with COPD who have mild arrhythmias at rest do not tend to have increased arrhythmias during exercise. Arrhythmias may disappear with exercise and increased perfusion (Frownfelter, 1987). See also Exercise and Arrhythmias, Chapter 10.

Exercise and Medications

The majority of pulmonary medications are used to promote bronchodilation and improve alveolar ventilation and oxygenation.These effects should improve an individual's ability to exercise and more effectively obtain the effects of training. However, the many side effects of pulmonary medications may interfere with normal adaptations to habitual exercise so that exercise tolerance and conditioning may not occur (Cahalin and Sadowsky, 1995). For example, corticosteroids mask or impede the beneficial effects of exercise. Anyone with pulmonary disease taking prolonged corticosteroids may develop steroid myopathy (see Chapter 4) and muscular atrophy not only in the peripheral skeletal muscles but also in the muscle fibers of the diaphragm (Dekhuijzen et al., 1993; Janssens and Decramer, 1989).

Chronic Obstructive Bronchitis

Definition and Overview. *Chronic bronchitis* is clinically defined as a condition of productive cough lasting for at least 3 months (usually the winter months) per year for 2 consecutive years. If obstructive lung disease characterized by a decreased FEV_1/FVC ratio[4] less than 75% is combined with chronic cough, chronic obstructive bronchitis is diagnosed. Initially, only the larger bronchi are involved, but eventually all airways become obstructed, especially during expiration.

Pathogenesis. Irritants such as cigarette smoke, long-term dust inhalation, or air pollution cause mucous hypersecretion and hypertrophy (increased number and size) of mucus-producing cells in the large bronchi. The swollen mucous membrane and thick sputum obstruct the airways, causing wheezing and a subsequent cough as the person tries to clear the airways. Additionally, impaired ciliary function reduces mucous clearance and increases client susceptibility to infection. Infection results in even more mucus production with bronchial wall inflammation and thickening.

As airways collapse, air is trapped in the distal portion of the lung causing reduced alveolar ventilation, hypoxia, and acidosis. This downward spiral continues as the client now has poor tissue oxygenation (hypoxemia and resultant decreased PaO_2) and an abnormal ventilation/perfusion (V/Q) ratio. As compensation for the hypoxemia, polycythemia (overproduction of erythrocytes) occurs. Cyanosis from insufficient arterial oxygenation and peripheral edema from ventricular failure result (Fig. 12–6). If left untreated, hypoxemia will lead to cor pulmonale and congestive heart failure.

Clinical Manifestations. The symptoms of chronic bronchitis are persistent cough and sputum production (worse in the morning and evening than at midday). The increased secretion from the bronchial mucosa and obstruction of the respiratory passages interferes with the flow of air to and from the lungs. The result is shortness of breath, prolonged expiration, persistent coughing with expectoration, and recurrent infection. Infection may be accompanied by fever and malaise.

Over time, reduced chest expansion, wheezing, cyanosis, and decreased exercise tolerance develop. Additionally, the obstruction present results in decreased alveolar ventilation and increased partial pressure of arterial carbon dioxide ($PACO_2$). Hypoxemia (deficient oxygenation of the blood) leads to polycythemia (overproduction of erythrocytes) and cyanosis. If not reversed, hypoxemia leads to pulmonary hy-

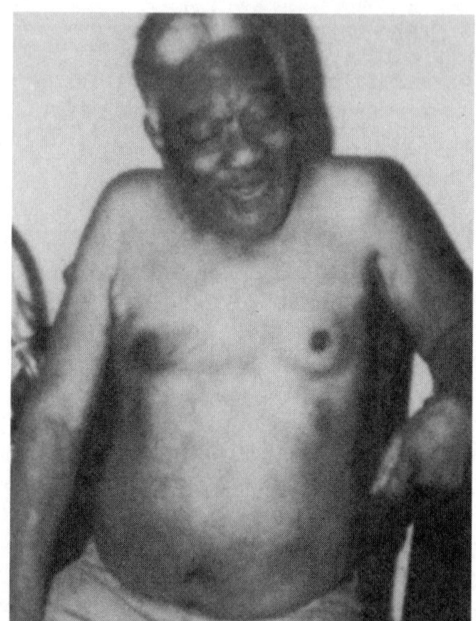

Figure **12–6.** The person with chronic bronchitis may develop cyanosis and pulmonary edema causing a characteristic look. The person's shoulders are raised and muscles are tensed from shortness of breath and the increased work of breathing. In addition, slight gynecomastia (breast development) and petechiae present in the midsternal area are both side effects of large-dose oral corticosteroid therapy. (*From Kersten LD: Comprehensive Respiratory Nursing. Philadelphia, WB Saunders, 1989.*)

[4] FEV_1 is the forced expiratory volume, a measure of the greatest volume of air a person can exhale during forced expiration; the subscript is added to indicate the percentage of the vital capacity that can be expired in 1 second. FVC is forced vital capacity, a measure of the greatest volume of air that can be expelled when a person performs a rapid, forced expiratory maneuver. This usually takes about 5 seconds (O'Toole, 1992).

pertension and eventually cor pulmonale and congestive heart failure. Severe disability or death is the final clinical picture.

Medical Management

See Medical Management and Special Implications for the Therapist in previous section, Chronic Obstructive Pulmonary Disease.

Emphysema

Definition and Overview. *Emphysema* is defined as a pathologic accumulation of air in tissues, particularly in the lungs. There are three types of emphysema (see Fig. 12–5). *Centrilobular* emphysema, the most common type, produces destruction in the bronchioles, usually in the upper lung regions. Inflammation develops in the bronchioles, but usually the alveolar sac (distal to respiratory bronchioles) remains intact. *Panlobular* emphysema destroys the air spaces of the entire acinus and most commonly involves the lower lung. These forms of emphysema, collectively called *centriacinar* emphysema, occur most often in smokers. *Paraseptal* (or panacinar) emphysema destroys the alveoli in the lower lobes of the lungs resulting in isolated blebs along the lung periphery. Paraseptal emphysema is believed to be the likely cause of spontaneous pneumothorax (Cronin, 1993).

Etiology. Cigarette smoking is the major etiologic factor in the development of emphysema and has been shown to increase the numbers of alveolar macrophages and neutrophils in the lung,[5] enhance protease[6] release, and impair the activity of antiproteases. However, other factors must determine susceptibility to emphysema, because less than 10% to 15% of smokers develop clinical evidence of airways obstruction (Andreoli et al., 1993).

In many cases, emphysema occurs as a result of prolonged respiratory difficulties, such as chronic bronchitis that has caused partial obstruction of the smaller divisions of the bronchi. Emphysema can also occur without serious preceding respiratory problems as in the case of a defect in the elastic tissue of the lungs or in aged persons whose lungs have lost their natural elasticity (O'Toole, 1992).

A small number of clients with COPD/CAL have an inherited deficiency of alpha$_1$-antitrypsin (AAT), a nonspecific proteolytic enzyme inhibitor. AAT deficiency is suspected in persons who develop emphysema before age 40 and in nonsmokers who develop the disease. Panacinar emphysema occurs in the elderly and in clients with AAT deficiency.

Pathogenesis. Emphysema is a disorder in which destruction of alveolar walls leads to permanent enlargement of the acini. Eventually there is a loss of elasticity in the lung tissue so that inspired air becomes trapped in the lungs, making breathing difficult, especially during the expiratory phase. Obstruction results from changes in lung tissues, rather than from mucus production as in chronic bronchitis (which is why steroids are usually not helpful in this condition).

The permanent overdistention of the air spaces with destruction of the walls (septa) between the alveoli is accompanied by partial airway collapse and loss of elastic recoil. Pockets of air form between the alveolar spaces (blebs) and within the lung parenchyma (bullae). This process leads to increased ventilatory dead space, or areas that do not participate in gas or blood exchange. The work of breathing is increased because there is less functional lung tissue for exchange of oxygen and carbon dioxide. As the disease progresses, there is increasing dyspnea and pulmonary infection. Eventually, cor pulmonale (right-sided congestive heart failure) develops (Cronin, 1993).

Clinical Manifestations. Marked exertional dyspnea that progresses to dyspnea at rest is characteristic of emphysema owing to the irreversible destruction reducing elasticity of the lungs and increasing the effort to exhale trapped air. Cough is uncommon, with little sputum production. The client is often thin, has tachypnea with prolonged expiration, and must use accessory muscles for ventilation. To increase lung capacity, the client often leans forward with arms braced on the knees supporting the shoulders and chest. The combined effects of trapped air and alveolar distention change the size and shape of the client's chest, causing a barrel chest, and increased expiratory effort. The normal arterial oxygen levels and dyspnea give clients a classic appearance (Fig. 12–7).

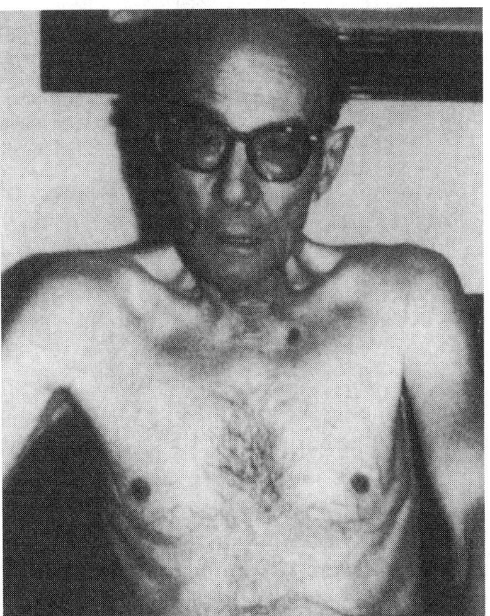

Figure **12–7.** The person with emphysema presents with classic findings. Use of respiratory accessory (intercostal, neck, shoulder) muscles and cachectic appearance (wasting due to ill health) reflect two factors: (1) shortness of breath, the most disturbing symptom, and (2) the tremendous increased work of breathing necessary to increase ventilation and maintain normal arterial blood gases. (*From Kersten LD: Comprehensive Respiratory Nursing. Philadelphia, WB Saunders, 1989.*)

[5] Neutrophils, the most numerous type of leukocytes (white blood cells), increase dramatically in number in response to infection and inflammation. However, neutrophils not only kill invading organisms but may also damage host tissues when there are too many.

[6] Proteases, or proteolytic enzymes, are enzymes that destroy cells (proteins). The airway goblet cells and serous cells of bronchial glands normally secrete a protein called secretory leukoprotease inhibitor, which is capable of inhibiting neutrophils. The cellular interactions associated with smoking result in inactivation of protease inhibitors. This results in an imbalance between proteases and antiproteases (in favor of proteases), allowing even more cellular destruction than warranted by the inflammatory process already present.

As emphysema progresses, there is a loss of surface area available for gas exchange. In the final stages, cardiac complications, especially enlargement and dilation of the right ventricle, may develop (O'Toole, 1992). The overloaded heart reaches its limit of muscular compensation and begins to fail (cor pulmonale).

Medical Management

Diagnosis and Treatment. Diagnosis is made on the basis of history (usually cigarette smoking), physical examination, chest film, and pulmonary function tests. The most important factor in the treatment of emphysema is cessation of smoking. Human lungs benefit no matter when someone quits smoking; quitting smoking is the most effective way of preventing lung function decline due to emphysema (and chronic bronchitis). Pursed-lip breathing causes resistance to outflow at the lips, which in turn maintains intrabronchial pressure and improves the mixture of gases in the lungs (Anthonisen et al., 1994). This type of breathing should be encouraged to help the client get rid of the stale air trapped in the lungs. See also Chronic Obstructive Pulmonary Disease; Medical Management; and Special Implications for the Therapist 12–6.

Asthma

Definition and Overview. *Asthma* is defined as an inflammatory condition with secondary bronchospasm marked by recurrent attacks of dyspnea, with wheezing due to the spasmodic constriction of the bronchi (Jacobs, 1994). Asthma is a complex disorder involving biochemical, autonomic, immunologic, infectious, endocrine, and psychological factors in varying degrees in different individuals. This condition can be divided into two main types according to causative factors: extrinsic (allergic) and intrinsic (nonallergic), but other recognized categories include adult-onset, exercise-induced, aspirin-sensitive, *Aspergillus* hypersensitivity, and occupational (Table 12–8).

TABLE 12-8 Types of Asthma

Classification	Initiating Factors
Extrinsic	IgE-mediated external allergens Foods Pollen, dust, molds, smoke, exhaust Animal dander
Intrinsic	Unknown; secondary to respiratory infections
Adult-onset	Unknown
Exercise-induced	Alteration in airway temperature and humidity; mediator release
Aspirin-sensitive (associated with nasal polyps)	Aspirin and other nonsteroidal anti-inflammatory drugs
Allergic bronchopulmonary aspergillosis	Hypersensitivity to *Aspergillus* species (not infection)
Occupational	Metal salts (platinum, chrome, nickel) Antibiotic powder (penicillin, sulfathiazole, tetracycline) Toluene diisocyanate (TDI) Flour Wood dusts Cotton dust (byssinosis) Animal proteins Smoke inhalation (firefighters)

Adapted form Andreoli TE, Bennett JC, Carpenter CC, et al: Cecil Essentials of Medicine, ed 3. Philadelphia, WB Saunders, 1993, p 144.

Incidence and Risk Factors Asthma as one component of COPD/CAL is the most common chronic disease in adults (10% incidence) and children (5% incidence) and the prevalence, morbidity, and mortality of asthma are increasing in the United States. According to a recent study released by the CDC (CDC, 1995), the incidence of asthma cases and asthma deaths increased at least 40% between 1982 and 1992.

The reason for the increase nationwide is unknown, but one explanation may be that the accuracy of the diagnosis of asthma is changing with increasing chart documentation among physicians (Osborne et al., 1992; Vollmer et al., 1993). Researchers at the CDC postulate that air pollution, airtight homes, and windowless offices may also be risk factors contributing to the significant rise in incidence (CDC, 1995).

Asthma is found most often in urban, industrialized settings; in colder climates; and among the urban disadvantaged (areas of poverty). Overcrowded living conditions with repeated exposure to cigarette smoke, dust, cockroaches, and mold may be contributing factors. It is estimated that asthma goes unrecognized as an adverse factor affecting performance in 1 in 10 athletes.

Asthma can occur at any age, although it is more likely to occur for the first time before the age of 5 years. In childhood, it is three times more common and more severe in boys; however, after puberty, the incidence in the sexes is equal (Skobeloff et al., 1992).

Etiology Asthma occurs in families, which indicates that it is an inherited disorder. Recent findings suggest a possible link between asthma and the interleukin-4 (IL-4) gene which regulates the production of immunoglobulin E (IgE).[7] Asthma is influenced by two genetic tendencies: one associated with the capacity to develop allergies (atopy) and the other with the tendency to develop hyperresponsiveness of the airways independent of atopy. Apparently, environmental factors interact with inherited factors to cause attacks of bronchospasm. Asthma can develop when predisposed persons are infected by viruses or exposed to allergens or pollutants (Davey and McCance, 1994).

Extrinsic asthma, also known as atopic or allergic asthma, is due to an allergy to specific triggers; usually the offending allergens are foods or environmental antigens suspended in the air in the form of pollen, dust, molds, smoke, automobile exhaust, and animal dander. In this type of asthma, mast cells, sensitized by IgE antibodies, degranulate and release bronchoactive mediators following exposure to a specific anti-

[7] The higher the level of IgE in the blood, the greater the likelihood of asthma. Variations in the amount of IgE people produce are closely linked to the gene for IL-4, a molecule that causes immune cells to switch on production of IgE (Marsh et al., 1995).

gen. More than half of the cases of asthma in children and young adults are of this type.

Intrinsic asthma, or nonallergic asthma, has no known allergic cause or trigger, has an adult onset (usually over 40 years of age), and is most often secondary to chronic or recurrent infections of the bronchi, sinuses, or tonsils and adenoids. This type of asthma may develop from a hypersensitivity to the bacteria, or more commonly, viruses causing the infection. Other factors precipitating intrinsic asthma include drugs (aspirin, β-adrenergic antagonists), environmental irritants (occupational chemicals, air pollution), cold dry air, exercise, and emotional stress.

Occupational asthma is defined as variable airways narrowing, causally related to exposure in the working environment to specific airborne dusts, gases, acids, molds, dyes, vapors, or fumes (Cartier, 1994). Occupational asthma has received considerable attention recently as the most frequent occupational lung disease worldwide (Cullinan et al., 1993; Kimura and Takahashi, 1994; Beckett, 1994; Meredith, 1993; Chan-Yeung, 1994; Gottlieb et al., 1993; Quirce, et al., 1994).

Pathogenesis. The airways are the site of an inflammatory response consisting of cellular infiltration, epithelial disruption, mucosal edema, and mucous plugging. The release of inflammatory mediators produces bronchial smooth muscle spasm, vascular congestion, increased vascular permeability, edema formation, production of thick, tenacious mucus, and impaired mucociliary function. Several mediators also cause thickening of airway walls and increased contractile response of bronchial smooth muscles. These changes in the bronchial musculature, combined with the epithelial cell damage caused by eosinophil infiltration, result in the airway hyperresponsiveness characteristic of asthma (McFadden and Gilbert, 1992).

Once the airway is in spasm, mucus plugs the airway, trapping distal air. Ventilation/perfusion mismatch, hypoxemia, and increased workload of breathing follow. Most attacks of asthmatic bronchospasm are short-lived, with freedom from symptoms between episodes, although airway inflammation is present, even in asymptomatic persons (Davey and McCance, 1994).

Clinical Manifestations. Clinical signs and symptoms of asthma differ in presentation (Table 12–9), degree (Table 12–10), and frequency among clients, but typically an attack of asthma is characterized by dyspnea and a wheezing type of respiration. The person usually assumes a classic sitting position, leaning forward so as to use all the accessory muscles of respiration. The skin is usually pale and moist with perspiration, but in a severe attack there may be cyanosis of the lips and nail beds. In the early stages of the attack coughing may be dry, but as the attack progresses, the cough becomes more productive of a thick, tenacious, mucoid sputum (O'Toole, 1992).

During full remission, clients are asymptomatic and pulmonary function tests are normal. At the beginning of an attack, there is a sensation of chest constriction, inspiratory and expiratory wheezing, nonproductive coughing, prolonged expiration, tachycardia, and tachypnea. Other symptoms may include fatigue, a tickle in the back of the throat accompanied

TABLE 12–9 Clinical Manifestations of Bronchial Asthma

Cough
Hacking, paroxysmal, exhausting, irritative, involuntary, nonproductive
Becomes rattling and productive of frothy, clear, gelatinous sputum
Main or only symptom
Tickle in the back of the throat accompanied by a cough

Respiratory-Related Signs
Shortness of breath; may occur at rest
Prolonged expiratory phase
Audible wheeze on inspiration and expiration or on expiration only; never on inspiration only
Often appears pale
May have a malar flush and red ears
Lips deep dark-red color
May progress to cyanosis of nail beds, around mouth and lips
Restlessness
Apprehension
Anxious facial expression
Itching around nose, eyes, throat, chin, scalp
Sweating may be prominent as attack progresses
May sit upright with shoulders in a hunched-over position, hands on the bed or chair, and arms braced (older children)
Speaks with short, panting broken phrases

Chest
Coarse, loud breath sounds
Prolonged expiration
Generalized inspiratory and expiratory wheezing; increasingly high-pitched

With Repeated Episodes
Barrel chest
Elevated shoulders
Use of accessory muscles of respiration
Skin retraction (clavicles, ribs, sternum)
Facial appearance: flattened malar bones, circles beneath the eyes, narrow nose, prominent upper teeth, nostrils flaring

Adapted from Wong DL: Whaley and Wong's Essentials of Pediatric Nursing, ed 4. St Louis, Mosby–Year Book, 1993, p 736.

TABLE 12–10 Stages of Asthma

Stage	Symptoms
Mild	Symptoms reverse with cessation of activity
Moderate	Audible wheezing Use of accessory muscles of respiration Leaning forward to catch breath
Severe	Blue lips and fingernails Tachypnea (30–40 breaths/min) despite cessation of activity Cyanosis-induced seizures Skin and rib retraction

Adapted from Goodman CC, Snyder TE: Differential Diagnosis in Physical Therapy, ed 2. Philadelphia, WB Saunders, 1995, p 160.

by a cough in an attempt to clear the airways, and nostril flaring (advanced). The severity of asthma may be classified as mild, moderate, or severe, depending on the symptoms.

An acute attack that cannot be altered with routine care is called *status asthmaticus*. This is a medical emergency requiring more vigorous measures and despite treatment can be fatal. With severe bronchospasm, the workload of breathing increases 5 to 10 times, which can lead to acute cor pulmonale. When air is trapped, a severe paradoxical pulse develops as venous return is obstructed; blood pressure drops over 10 mm Hg during inspiration.

Pneumothorax commonly develops. If status asthmaticus continues, hypoxemia worsens and acidosis begins. If the condition is untreated or not reversed, respiratory or cardiac arrest will occur. An acute asthma episode may constitute a medical emergency requiring emergency management with β-adrenergic drugs and intravenous theophylline and corticosteroids.

Medical Management

Diagnosis. Pulse oximetry, pulmonary function studies, arterial blood gas (ABG) analysis, complete blood count with differential, and chest films may be used in assessing for both the presence and the severity of asthma (see Chapter 35 for a description of and reference values for these tests).

Treatment. Most people require bronchodilator therapy to control symptoms; those with mild symptoms may use metered dose inhaler (MDI) devices to administer sympathomimetic bronchodilators on an "as needed" basis. These type of inhalers activate β-agonist receptors on smooth muscle cells in the respiratory tract, the end result being relaxation of bronchial smooth muscle (bronchodilation).

Those people who experience moderate to severe asthma may require daily administration of anti-inflammatory agents such as corticosteroids to prevent asthma attacks. It is important that people with asthma know the difference between medications that must be taken daily to prevent asthma symptoms, and medications that relieve symptoms once they begin.

Prognosis. The outlook for clients with *bronchial asthma* is excellent despite the recent increase in the death rate. Childhood asthma may disappear; in fact, approximately half of all children with asthma "outgrow" the disease by their middle teens; adult asthma may progress to COPD. Attention to general health measures and use of pharmacologic agents permit control of symptoms in nearly all cases. *Status asthmaticus* can result in respiratory or cardiac arrest and possible death (see previous discussion). If ventilation becomes necessary, prognosis for recovery is poorer.

Special Implications for the Therapist **12-7**

ASTHMA

Many people with asthma do not even know they have the disease. Some think they simply have chronic bronchitis, colds, or allergies. Anyone who reports coughing or feeling of tightness in the chest when others smoke near them and especially anyone who gasps for breath after exercise should be referred to a physician for evaluation of these symptoms.

Exercise and Medication

Bronchospasm can occur during exercise (especially in exercise-induced asthma) if the person with asthma has a low oxygen blood level prior to exercise. For this reason, it is helpful to take bronchodilators by MDI 20 to 30 minutes before exercise, performing mild stretching and warmup exercises during that time period to avoid bronchospasm with higher workload exercise. Increased exercise should be accompanied by good bronchodilator coverage to promote bronchodilation and improve alveolar ventilation and oxygenation. Exercise guidelines for adults with asthma can be modified from recommendations for children with asthma (Table 12–11).

Many clients have found that using their inhalers in this way before exercise permits them to exercise without onset of symptoms. Proper administration of an MDI is essential and the therapist should observe the client self-administer the medication at least one time. The person should empty the lungs of air, place the metered device 3 to 5 in. away from the mouth, and discharge the canister into the mouth while inhaling slowly and deeply. The client holds the breath for 5 to 10 seconds, exhales waits 5 to 10 minutes, and administers a second metered dose using the same technique. A 4- to 6-in. spacer that fits over the end of the inhaler and is then placed into the mouth may be used to maintain the correct distance away while both administering the dose deeper into the lungs and avoiding spraying the eyes.

The first dose induces dilation of the bronchial tubes, relaxing smooth muscles in the airways; the second dose dilates the bronchioles (smaller airways). Metabolism of certain drugs administered can be altered by exercise, tobacco, marijuana, or phenobarbital, (all of which increase drug metabolism. Cimetidine (Tagamet) erythromycin, troleandomycin, or the presence of a viral infection may decrease drug metabolism. If a client develops signs of asthma or any bronchial activity during the exercise, the physician must be informed. Medication dosage can then be altered to maintain optimal physical performance. Excessive use of inhaled β-adrenergic agents (using three or more full canisters monthly) requires physician referral for further evaluation (Stauffer, 1994).

Exercise-Induced Asthma

Exercise-induced bronchospasm (EIB), or exercise-induced asthma (EIA) does not represent a unique syndrome but rather an example of the airway hyperactivity common to all persons with asthma. EIA is an acute, reversible, usually self-terminating airway obstruction that develops 5 to 15 minutes after strenuous exercise when the person no longer breathes through the nose, warming and humidifying the air, but opens the mouth. Breathing cold, dry air through the mouth degranulates mast cells that release bronchoconstrictive mediators inducing EIB. EIB/EIA lasts 15 to 60 minutes after the onset.

If an asthma attack should occur during therapy, first

TABLE 12-11 EXERCISE GUIDELINES FOR CHILDREN WITH ASTHMA

RECOMMENDATION	BENEFIT
General exercise, school-based physical education	Maintains motor function, strength, stamina, and coordination; prevents or reverses side effects of medication (e.g., corticosteroids) Raises threshold for strenuous exercise before mouth breathing and EIB occur
Low-impact exercise (aerobics, weight training, stationary bike)	Permits exercise without increased bronchospasm
Warmup before aerobic activity	Helps control airway reactivity; gradually desensitizes mast cells reducing release of bronchoconstrictive mediators
Exercise in a trigger-free environment (i.e., avoid cold, pollution or increased pollen outdoors; exercise indoors; avoid tobacco smoke; swimming program is ideal)	Prevents bronchospasm; controls symptoms
Take prescribed medication properly before exercise or activity producing bronchospasm	Prevents bronchospasm
Monitor FEV_1/FVC ratio before, during, and after physical activity* Decrease of 10% requires slowing activity Drop of 15%–20% from initial measurement requires cessation of exercise	Determines whether shortness of breath is due to exercise or if air flow is decreasing due to bronchospasm

EIB, exercise-induced bronchospasm; FEV_1/FVC, ratio of forced expiratory volume in 1 second to forced vital capacity.
* Peak flowmeters can be used to obtain this information. Determine the child's normal range of lung function by having the child blow in the meter in the morning and evening for 1 week. The average level measured varies from person to person and is influenced by sex and height. The physician should establish a peak flow protocol against which lung function can be compared to determine if deterioration has occurred.

assess the severity of the attack. Place the person in the high Fowler's position and encourage diaphragmatic and pursed-lip breathing. If the client has a bronchodilator available, provide whatever assistance is necessary for that person to self-administer this medication. Help the person to relax while assessing the person's response to the medication.

Usually the episode subsides spontaneously in 30 minutes to 1 hour. The severity of an attack increases as the exercise becomes increasingly strenuous. The problem is rare in activities that require only short bursts of energy (such as baseball, sprints, gymnastics, skiing) rather than those that involve endurance exercise (e.g., soccer, basketball, distance running). Swimming, even long-distance swimming, is well tolerated by people with EIA, partly because they are breathing air fully saturated with moisture, but the type of breathing required may also play a role. Exhaling under water, which is essentially pursed-lip breathing, is of benefit because it prolongs each expiration and increases the end-expiratory pressure within the respiratory tree (Wong, 1993).

Monitoring Vital Signs

Monitoring vital signs can alert the therapist to important changes in bronchopulmonary function. Developing or increasing tachypnea may indicate worsening asthma; tachycardia may indicate worsening asthma or drug toxicity. Other signs of toxicity, such as diarrhea, headache, and vomiting, may be misinterpreted as influenza. Hypertensive blood pressure readings may indicate asthma-related hypoxemia.

Auscultate the lungs frequently, noting the degree of wheezing and the quality of air movement. In this way, any change in respiratory status will be more readily perceived. If the client does not have a productive cough in the presence of rhonchi (dry rattling in the bronchial tube), teach effective coughing techniques.

Status Asthmaticus

Therapy can augment the medical management of the client with status asthmaticus. In coordination with the individual's medications, the therapist helps to remove secretions; promotes relaxed, more efficient breathing; enhances ventilation/perfusion matching; reduces hypoxemia; and teaches the client to coordinate relaxed breathing with general body movement. Caution needs to be observed to avoid stimuli that bring on bronchospasm and deterioration (e.g., aggressive percussion, forced expiration maneuvers, aggressive "bagging"). Certain body positions may have to be avoided because of client intolerance or exacerbation of symptoms in those positions (Dean et al., 1996).

Bronchiectasis

Definition. This form of obstructive lung disease is actually an extreme form of bronchitis. There is chronic dilation of the bronchi and bronchioles that develops when the supporting structures (bronchial walls) are weakened by chronic inflammatory changes associated with secondary infection.

Incidence and Etiology. The incidence of bronchiectasis is low in the United States because of improved control of bronchopulmonary infections. However, any condition producing a narrowing of the lumen of the bronchioles may create bronchiectasis, including TB, adenoviral infections, and pneumonia. Bronchiectasis also develops in people with immunodeficiencies involving humoral immunity, recurrent aspiration, and abnormal mucociliary clearance (immotile cilia syndromes). Cystic fibrosis causes about half of all cases of bronchiectasis. Sinusitis, dextrocardia (heart located on right side of chest), Kartagener's syndrome (alterations in ciliary activity), defective development of bronchial cartilage (Williams-Campbell syndrome), and endobronchial tumor predispose a person to bronchiectasis.

Pathogenesis. Abnormal bronchial dilation characteristic of bronchiectasis is accompanied by accumulation of "wet" secretions which plug the airway and cause bronchospasm, producing even more purulent mucus. Destruction or fragmentation of the bronchial wall with resultant fibrosis may further obstruct and obliterate the bronchial lumen (Fig. 12–8). In response to these changes, large anastomoses develop between the bronchial and pulmonary blood vessels to increase the blood flow through the bronchial circulation. These anastomoses are responsible for the hemoptysis present in persons with bronchiectasis. Complications such as an abnormality in ventilation/perfusion and resultant hypoxemia may occur.

Clinical Manifestations. The most immediate symptom of bronchiectasis is persistent coughing, with large amounts of purulent sputum production (worse in the morning). Weight loss, anemia and other systemic manifestations such as low-grade fever, hemoptysis, fatigue, weakness, nasal congestion, and drainage from sinusitis are also common. Clubbing may occur and the breath and sputum may become foul-smelling with advanced disease.

Medical Management

Diagnosis. Diagnosis is made using x-ray studies, laboratory tests including sweat chloride test for CF, electron microscopy of bronchial biopsy for immotile cilia, and sputum culture analyses (Harruff, 1994). Bronchograms (chest films with contrast media) are less commonly used; CT scanning may detect moderate to severe cases (Stauffer, 1994).

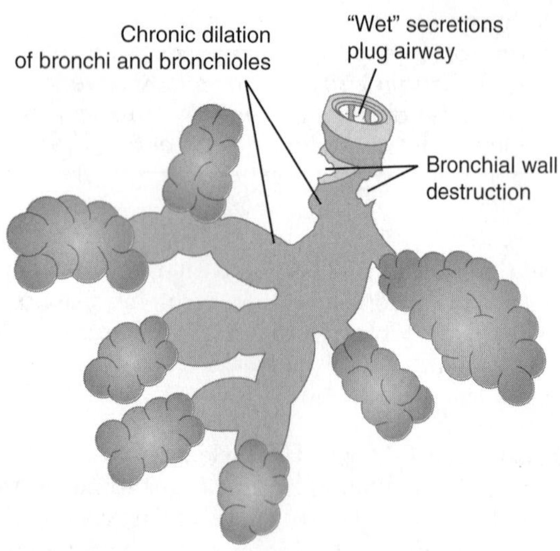

Figure **12–8.** Airway pathology in bronchiectasis.

Treatment. The goals of treatment are removal of secretions and prevention of infection. The principal treatment is pulmonary physical therapy, bronchodilators, and antibiotics selected on the basis of sputum smears and cultures. Hydration is important and oxygen may be administered. Surgical resection is reserved for the few clients with localized bronchiectasis and adequate pulmonary function who fail to respond to conservative management or for the person with massive hemoptysis. Long-term care is the same as for any person with COPD/CAL.

Prognosis. The overall prognosis is often poor and although bronchiectasis is usually localized to a lung lobe or segment, persistent, nonresolving infection may cause the disorder to spread to other parts of the same lung. Complications of bronchiectasis include recurrent pneumonia, lung abscesses, metastatic infections in other organs (e.g., brain abscess), and respiratory failure (Harruff, 1994). Good pulmonary hygiene and avoidance of infectious complications in the involved areas may reverse some cases of bronchiectasis.

Special Implications for the Therapist **12-8**

BRONCHIECTASIS

Chest physical therapy for the person with bronchiectasis may include postural drainage and chest percussion of involved lobes performed several times a day. The best times to do this are early morning and just before bedtime. Family members can be instructed in how to provide this care at home. Coughing and deep-breathing exercises to promote good ventilation and removal of secretions should follow positional or percussive therapy.

Bronchiolitis

Definition and Overview. Bronchiolitis is a commonly occurring acute, diffuse, and often severe inflammation of the lower airways (bronchioles) caused by a viral infection. Once classified as a type of chronic interstitial pneumonia, *bronchiolitis obliterans* in the adult has been reclassified as five clinical types (Epler et al, 1985): (1) toxic fume bronchiolitis obliterans, (2) postinfectious bronchiolitis obliterans, (3) bronchiolitis obliterans associated with connective tissue disease and organ transplantation, (4) bronchiolitis obliterans associated with localized lung lesions, and (5) idiopathic bronchiolitis obliterans with organizing pneumonia (BOOP).

Toxic fume bronchiolitis obliterans follows 1 to 3 weeks after fume inhalation or exposure to noxious gases such as oxides of nitrogen and phosgene. Bronchiolitis obliterans is the most important clinical complication in heart-lung transplant recipients and may represent a form of allograft rejection (Epler, 1988). It is a rare complication of allogeneic (human-to-human) bone marrow transplantation. Bronchiolitis obliterans may occur in association with rheumatoid arthritis, polymyositis, and dermatomyositis. Penicillamine therapy has been implicated as a possible cause of bronchiolitis obliterans in clients with rheumatoid arthritis (Stauffer, 1994).

Incidence and Etiology. In adults, bronchiolitis usually occurs with chronic bronchitis; children under 2 years of age are most commonly affected with a peak incidence at approximately 6 months. Most cases in children are associated with pulmonary infections such as respiratory syncytial virus (RSV), parainfluenza viruses, adenoviruses, pertussis (whooping cough), or associated with measles. Primarily present in winter and spring, it is easily spread by hand-to-nose or nose-to-eye transmission. *Exudative bronchiolitis*, inflammation of the bronchioles with exudation of gray tenacious sputum, is often associated with asthma.

Pathogenesis. Variable degrees of obstruction occur in response to infection as the bronchiolar mucosa swells and the lumina fill with mucus and exudate. These changes occur as the walls of the bronchi and bronchioles are infiltrated with inflammatory cells. Hyperinflation, obstructive emphysema from partial obstruction, and patchy areas of atelectasis may occur distal to the inflammatory lesion as the disease progresses.

Clinical Manifestations. Bronchiolitis begins as a simple upper respiratory infection (URI) with serous nasal discharge and mild fever. Cough, respiratory distress, and cyanosis occur initially, followed by a brief period of improvement. Dyspnea, paroxysmal cough, sputum production, and wheezing with marked use of accessory muscles follow as the disease progresses. Apnea may be the first indicator of RSV infection in very young infants. Severe disease may be followed by a rise in arterial carbon dioxide tension ($Pa{CO_2}$) (hypercapnia), leading to respiratory acidosis and hypoxemia (Wong, 1993).

Bronchiolitis obliterans associated with organ transplantation is not preceded by typical features of chronic graft-vs.-host disease (see Chapter 5), but has the same clinical course of dyspnea, air flow obstruction, and poor response to medical treatment (Epler, 1988).

Medical Management

Diagnosis and Treatment. Diagnosis of bronchiolitis is made on the basis of clinical findings, the child's age, the season, and the epidemiology of the community. On chest radiographs bronchiolitis is difficult to differentiate from bacterial pneumonia. RSV can be positively identified using an enzyme-linked immunosorbent assay (ELISA) from direct aspiration of nasal secretions.

There is no specific treatment for bronchiolitis and medical therapy is controversial. Treatment modalities may include steroids, humidified air, hydration, and physical therapy for postural drainage, coughing, and deep-breathing exercises. Antibiotics may be used initially when bacterial cause of illness has not been ruled out or for secondary infections. Mist therapy combined with oxygen by hood or tent to alleviate dyspnea and hypoxia may be used with children.

Prognosis. The disease lasts about 3 to 10 days in children and the majority of children with bronchiolitis can be managed at home with a good prognosis. Hospitalization is usually recommended for children with complicating conditions such as underlying lung or heart disease, associated debilitated states, poor hydration, or questionable care at home. Some children deteriorate rapidly and die within weeks; others may follow a more chronic course.

In the adult, acute bronchiolitis usually has a good prognosis. The prognosis for chronic bronchiolitis is poor, as in COPD/CAL (Harruff, 1994).

Special Implications for the Therapist **12-9**

BRONCHIOLITIS

RSV is the most common cause of pediatric acute bronchiolitis and pneumonia. For this reason, any staff member with evidence of URI serves as a potential reservoir of RSV and should be excluded from direct contact with high-risk infants. All persons who come within 3 feet of an RSV client must wear a gown and mask with an eye shield and keep hands away from the face, especially the eyes, nose, and mouth. Hands must be washed before and after caring for any client and after handling potentially contaminated client care equipment. Universal precautions (see Appendix A) must be strictly carried out (Filippell and Rearick, 1993).

Because RSV is readily transmitted by close contact with personnel, families, and other children by both direct contact (especially lifting or holding) and through contact with objects handled by the child, precautions against cross-infection are important. The primary routes of inoculation for the organisms are large-droplet inhalation through the nose and eyes. When contact is made with mucous discharge or drainage from the eye, nose, or mouth, the therapist is reminded to wear an exterior hospital gown and to discard the gown (or change clothing) when leaving. Pregnant female personnel or visitors should be advised of the risk of potential physical defects in the developing embryo from contact with RSV (CDC, 1988).

Sleep Apnea

Definition. *Sleep apnea syndrome* is defined as episodes of cessation of breathing occurring at the transition from NREM (non–rapid eye movement) to REM (rapid eye movement) sleep, with repeated wakening and excessive daytime sleepiness. *Adult sleep apnea* is arbitrarily defined as more than five cessations of air flow for at least 10 seconds each per hour of sleep (O'Toole, 1992).

There are three types of apnea: central, obstructive, and mixed. *Central apnea* is caused by altered chemosensitivity and cerebral respiratory control. In this type of apnea, there is no central drive to respiration, no diaphragmatic movement, and no air flow. This is seen in infants under 40 weeks' conceptual age. In *obstructive apnea* there is respiratory effort but no air flow because of upper airway obstruction. *Mixed apnea* is a central apnea that is immediately followed by an obstructive event (O'Toole, 1992).

Incidence. Sleep apnea syndrome occurs most often in middle-aged, obese males. More than 1% of the general population is affected, with a dramatic increase in the elderly (Andreoli et al., 1993). The incidence of obstructive sleep apnea may be much higher because the signs and symptoms of chronic sleep disruption are often overlooked in spite of their debilitating consequences (Wiegand and Zwillich, 1994). The female hormone progesterone, a respiratory stimulant, may protect premenopausal women from sleep-disordered breathing (Block, 1980).

Etiology and Risk Factors. The cause of sleep apnea syndrome is unclear in many clients. Snoring, a prerequisite for this syndrome, runs in families, suggesting a possible inherited link (Douglas et al., 1993). People with anatomically narrowed upper airways such as occurs in micrognathia, macroglossia (large tongue), obesity, and adenoid, uvula, soft palate, or tonsillar hypertrophy are predisposed to the development of obstructive sleep apnea. Alcohol or sedatives before sleeping may precipitate or worsen the condition.

Pathogenesis. There are several hypotheses as to the pathogenesis of sleep apnea syndrome. Collapse or obstruction of the airway may occur with the inhibition of muscle tone that characterizes REM sleep. When loss of normal pharyngeal muscle tone allows the larynx to collapse passively during inspiration, upper airway obstruction occurs.

Apneas may occur hundreds of times each night and are usually due to upper airway obstruction with continued respiratory efforts that result in paradoxical motion of the rib cage and abdomen. This causes progressive asphyxia, which increasingly stimulates breathing efforts against the collapsed airway until the person is awakened.

Clinical Manifestations. Daytime symptoms may include morning sluggishness and headaches, daytime fatigue, daytime somnolence, cognitive impairment, recent weight gain, and impotence. Bed partners usually report loud cyclical snoring, breath cessation, restlessness, and often thrashing movements of the extremities during sleep. Personality changes, irritability, depression, judgment impairment, work-related problems, memory loss, and difficulty concentrating may be observed.

Medical Management

Diagnosis. Diagnosis is confirmed by monitoring (polysomnography) the subject during sleep for periods of apnea and lowered blood oxygen levels. The physician must differentiate sleep apnea syndrome from seizure disorder, narcolepsy, or psychiatric depression. A hemoglobin level is obtained and thyroid function tests are performed.

Treatment. Obstructive and mixed types of sleep apnea syndrome can be treated. Since many clients with sleep apnea are overweight, weight loss is recommended. The most common treatment for obstructive sleep apnea is nasal continuous positive airway pressure (CPAP), used during sleep. The positive pressure from the CPAP prevents the airway from obstructing but this treatment technique may not be tolerated by 25% of clients (Eveloff et al., 1994). Only about 75% of clients using CPAP continue its use after 1 year. Weight loss may be curative, but only a small percentage of people maintain their weight loss and symptoms return with weight gain (Andreoli et al., 1993).

Surgery is recommended if an airway obstruction can be determined as the cause of the sleep apnea. Neurogenic causes of sleep apnea are more difficult to control. Medications to stimulate breathing have not been beneficial and alcohol and hypnotic medications should be avoided. In a limited number of cases, administration of oxygen during the night is helpful, but polysomnography must be used to assess the effects of oxygen therapy.

Other treatment ideas include surgical procedures to correct anatomic deformity or tracheostomy with insertion of a special tube that can be plugged during the day for normal use of the airway and opened at night to bypass upper airway obstruction. Mechanical devices inserted into the mouth at bedtime to hold the jaw forward and prevent pharyngeal occlusion appear promising in preliminary studies (Stauffer, 1994; Della Bella, 1993; Eveloff et al., 1994).

Prognosis. Evidence indicates that chronic, heavy snoring may be associated with increased long-term cardiovascular and neurophysiologic morbidity. Cardiac and vascular morbidity may include systemic hypertension, cardiac arrhythmias, pulmonary hypertension, cor pulmonale, left ventricular dysfunction, stroke, and sudden death. Recognition and appropriate treatment of obstructive sleep apnea and related disorders will often significantly enhance the client's quality of life, overall health, productivity, and safety on the highway (Wiegand and Zwillich, 1994).

Special Implications for the Therapist **12-10**

SLEEP APNEA

Because of the possible cardiovascular complications associated with clients who have obstructive sleep apnea, vital signs should be monitored before, during, and after submaximal or maximal exercise. The client should not be left in the supine position for prolonged periods of time, even while awake.

There has been one case report of dysphagia and sleep apnea associated with cervical osteophytes due to diffuse idiopathic skeletal hyperostosis (DISH) (Hughes et al., 1994). As this syndrome is studied more closely, a definitive correlation between cervical lesions and sleep disturbances may be documented. Physical therapy may be explored in developing treatment protocols when the musculoskeletal structures of the mandible contribute to the problem.

RESTRICTIVE LUNG DISEASE

Overview. Restrictive lung disorders are a major category of pulmonary problems including any condition that limits lung expansion. Pulmonary function tests are characterized by a decrease in lung volume or total lung capacity (TLC).

There are many causes of restrictive lung diseases that are covered in other sections of this chapter or book. Over 100 identified interstitial lung diseases can cause restrictive lung disease. Extrapulmonary causes may include neurologic (e.g., head or spinal cord injury, amyotrophic lateral sclerosis, myasthenia gravis, Guillain-Barré syndrome, muscular dystrophy, poliomyelitis) and neuromuscular disorders (e.g., ankylosing spondylitis, kyphosis or scoliosis, chest wall injury or deformity), obesity, or obstructive sleep disorders.

Clinical Manifestations. Clinical presentation varies according to the cause of the restrictive disorder. Generally, clients with restrictive lung disease exhibit a rapid, shallow respiratory pattern. Chronic hyperventilation occurs in an effort to overcome the effects of reduced lung volume and compliance. Exertional dyspnea progresses to dyspnea at rest. As the disease progresses, respiratory muscle fatigue may occur, leading to inadequate alveolar ventilation and carbon dioxide retention. Hypoxemia is a common finding, especially in the later stages of restrictive disease (Cronin, 1993).

Medical Management

Treatment and Prognosis. The management of restrictive lung disease is based in part on the underlying cause. Treatment goals are toward adequate oxygenation, maintaining an airway, and obtaining maximal function. For example, persons with spinal deformities may be helped with corrective surgery and obese persons may experience improved breathing after weight loss. Corticosteroids may help control inflammation and reduce further impairment, but previously damaged alveolocapillary units cannot be regenerated or replaced. Some clients with endstage disease may be candidates for single-lung transplantation. Most restrictive lung diseases are not reversible and the disease progresses to include pulmonary hypertension, cor pulmonale, severe decreased oxygenation, and eventual ventilatory failure.

Special Implications for the Therapist **12-11**

RESTRICTIVE LUNG DISEASE

A primary problem for clients with restrictive lung disease secondary to generalized weakness and neuromuscular disease is ineffective cough. Pulmonary physical therapy to facilitate cough and effective dislodging of secretions to the central airways may be exhausting for the client. Rest periods must be incorporated in the treatment.

A person with restrictive lung disease will be more adversely affected by the restriction on lung function in the recumbent position, emphasizing the importance of routine positioning for immobile clients and active or active-assisted movements whenever possible.

Pulmonary Fibrosis

Definition and Overview. Pulmonary fibrosis is an excessive amount of fibrous or connective tissue in the lung, predominantly fibroblasts and small blood vessels that progressively remove and replace normal tissue. It may be *idiopathic pulmonary fibrosis* (cause unknown) or fibrosis in the lung can be caused by healing scar tissue after active disease such as TB, systemic sclerosis, ARDS, or following inhalation of toxic substances such as coal dust or asbestos. There has been some question as to whether low-dose methotrexate (MTX) treatment for rheumatoid arthritis can cause chronic, progressive interstitial pulmonary fibrosis (Phillips et al., 1987; Kaplan and Waite, 1978). The most recent information available suggests that acute lung injury is more likely than pulmonary fibrosis in people receiving MTX therapy (Cash, 1994).

Fibrosis causes a marked loss of lung compliance. Gradually, increasing alveolar fibrosis leads to a shrunken and firm lobe and the lung becomes stiff and difficult to ventilate. The diffusing capacity of the alveolocapillary membrane decreases due to thickening, causing hypoxemia. Diffuse pulmonary fibrosis has a very poor prognosis (Davey and McCance, 1994).

Radiation Lung Disease

See Radiation Injuries, Chapter 4.

Systemic Sclerosis Lung Disease

Definition. Systemic sclerosis (SS), or scleroderma, is an autoimmune disease of connective tissue characterized by excessive collagen deposition in the skin and internal organs (Silver, 1990). This condition is discussed in detail in Chapter 8.

Incidence. Clinically, more than half of all people with SS develop interstitial lung disease, although autopsy results suggest a prevalence of 75%. The lungs, owing to a rich vascular supply and abundant connective tissue, are a frequent target organ, second to the esophagus in visceral involvement. Skin changes generally precede visceral alterations and lung involvement rarely presents symptoms first, but eventually pulmonary symptoms develop.

Pathogenesis and Clinical Manifestations. On open lung biopsy, early lesions show capillary congestion, hypercellularity of alveolar walls, increased fibrous tissue in the alveolar septa, and interstitial edema with fibrosis. As a result, initial symptoms of dyspnea on exertion and nonproductive cough develop. As fibroblast proliferation and collagen deposition progress, fibrosis of the alveolar wall occurs and the capillaries are obliterated. Clinically, the client demonstrates more severe dyspnea and has a greater risk of deterioration in pulmonary function.

Medical Management

Diagnosis. Traditional tests such as pulmonary function tests and chest radiographs are insensitive and not predictive of outcome. Thin-section CT is very sensitive for early diagnosis of SS lung involvement and some investigators use bronchoalveolar lavage (BAL) to identify alveolitis in clients with SS (Silver et al., 1984).

Treatment. Successful treatment of SS pulmonary disease remains an area for further development. Pharmacologic treatment using low-dose prednisone (as opposed to high-dose corticosteroids used with idiopathic pulmonary fibrosis) is recommended because of the possible association of high-dose corticosteroids with renal failure in clients with SS. Organ transplantation is not feasible in client with endstage lung disease secondary to SS.

Prognosis. SS lung disease is unpredictable and may be a mild, prolonged course or it may progress rapidly to respiratory failure and death. Lung disease is becoming the most frequent cause of death from SS. With the advent of angiotensin converting enzyme inhibitors, renovascular hypertension can usually be treated successfully and its complications avoided. Thus, more clients are at risk for lung disease and its complications. As the pulmonary fibrosis advances, cor pulmonale characterized by peripheral edema may develop.

Chest Wall Disease or Injury

Flail chest occurs as a result of sternum or multiple rib fracture. By definition, a flail chest consists of fractures of two or more adjacent ribs on the same side, and possibly the sternum, with each bone fractured into two or more segments (O'Toole, 1992). The fractured rib segments are detached (free-floating) from the rest of the chest wall.

Clinical Manifestations. It is common for a fractured rib end to tear the pleura and lung surface, thereby producing hemopneumothorax. Fractures of this type result in instability of a portion of the chest wall, causing paradoxical movement of the chest with breathing. During inspiration, the unstable portion of the chest wall moves inward, and during expiration the chest wall moves outward with unequal chest expansion impairing movement of gas in and out of the lungs (Fig. 12–9). Other clinical manifestations of flail chest include excruciating pain, severe dyspnea, hypoventilation, cyanosis, and hypoxemia, which leads to respiratory failure without intervention.

Medical Management. Initial treatment follows the ABCs of emergency treatment (*a*irway, *b*reathing, *c*irculation) to treat the pneumothorax, thereby enabling the person to breathe deeply and to effectively clear secretions. Treatment for any cardiovascular collapse is then followed by pain control. Intermittent positive-pressure breathing may be used to enhance lung expansion. Treatment may require internal fixation by controlled mechanical ventilation until the chest wall has stabilized, which may take 14 to 21 days or more (Davey and McCance, 1994). Whenever pulmonary function is adequate, intubation is avoided to help reduce infection, the most common complication associated with morbidity and mortality in clients with flail chest (LoCicero and Mattox, 1989). Pharmacologic treatment may include muscle relaxants or musculoskeletal paralyzing agents (e.g., pancuronium bromide) to reduce the risk of separation of the healing costochondral junctions.

Hemothorax, blood in the pleural cavity following chest trauma, must be removed through a chest tube. The tube is usually positioned in the sixth intercostal space in the posterior axillary line.

Special Implications for the Therapist **12-12**

CHEST WALL DISEASE OR INJURY

The emergency room therapist is the most likely therapist to evaluate and treat someone with a flail chest. Once the person has been stabilized and moved to the acute care setting, therapists may come into contact with this person during the recovery period. Chest physical therapy has a significant role in facilitating chest tube drainage but must be used carefully in the presence of any rib fractures. Percussion and vibration techniques are contraindicated directly over fractures but can be used over other lung segments. Rib or chest taping and ultrasound over the site of the fracture should not be used. Once the fractures have healed, rib mobilization and soft tissue mobilization for the intercostals may be necessary to restore normal respiratory movements.

Frequent turning and position changes, as well as deep-breathing and coughing exercises, are important. A semi-Fowler's position may help with lung reexpansion necessary to prevent atelectasis. In the case of flail chest from injury, simultaneous cardiac damage may have occurred necessitating the same care as for a person who has suffered a myocardial infarction (see Special Implications for the Therapist: Myocardial Infarction, 10–4).

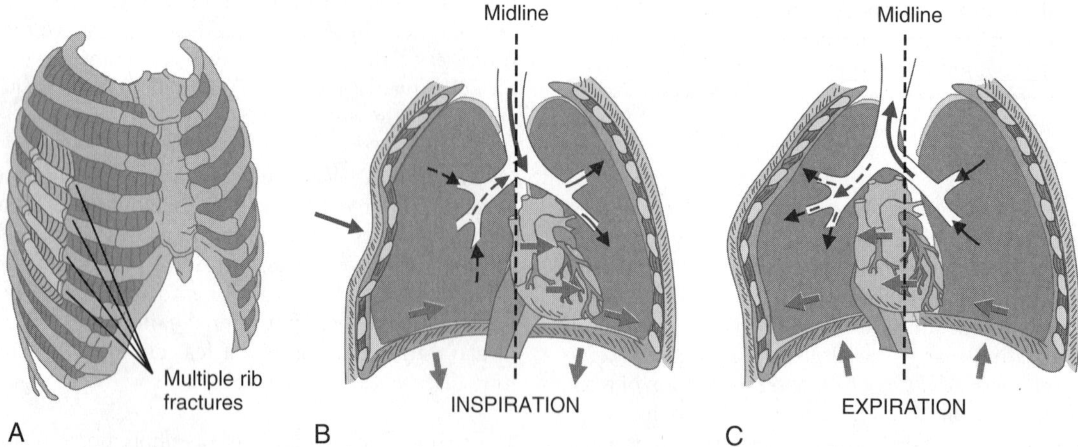

Figure **12-9.** Flail chest. *Solid arrows* indicate air movement; *open arrows*, structural movement. *A*, A flail chest consists of fractured rib segments that are detached (free-floating) from the rest of the chest wall. *B*, On inspiration, the flail segment of ribs is "sucked" inward. The affected lung and mediastinal structures shift to the unaffected side. This compromises the amount of inspired air in the unaffected lung. *C*, On expiration, the flail segment of ribs "bellow" outward. The affected lung and mediastinal structures shift to the affected side. Some air within the lungs is shunted back and forth between the lungs instead of passing through the upper airway.

ENVIRONMENTAL AND OCCUPATIONAL DISEASES

The relationship between occupations and disease has been observed, studied, and documented for many years. An in-depth discussion of this broad topic is included in section 1 (see Chapter 2). In this chapter, only environmental and occupational diseases related to the lung are discussed.

Occupational diseases can be divided into three major categories: (1) inorganic dusts (pneumoconioses), (2) organic dusts (hypersensitivity pneumonitis), and (3) fumes, gases, and smoke inhalation. These three categories have pathologic characteristics in common, including involvement of the pulmonary parenchyma with a fibrotic response.

Pneumoconioses

Definition. Any group of lung diseases resulting from inhalation of particles of industrial substances, particularly inorganic dusts such as that from iron ore or coal with permanent deposition of substantial amounts of such particles in the lung, are included in the generic term of *pneumoconiosis* ("dusty lungs"). Clinically common pneumoconioses include coal worker's pneumoconiosis, silicosis, and asbestosis. Other types of pneumoconiosis include talc, beryllium lung disease (berylliosis), aluminum pneumoconiosis, cadmium worker's disease, and siderosis (inhalation of iron or other metallic particles).

Incidence. Obviously occurring in occupational groups, pneumoconiosis is most common among miners, sandblasters, stonecutters, asbestos workers, and insulators. There is an increasing incidence with age due to cumulative effects of exposure. Exposure while washing clothes soiled with these toxic substances has caused mesothelioma (malignancy associated with asbestos exposure) and berylliosis (beryllium lung disease associated with exposure to beryllium used in the manufacture of fluorescent lamps before 1950) (Harruff, 1994). Beryllium is used today as a metal in structural materials employed in aerospace industries, in the manufacture of industrial ceramics, and in atomic reactors, so exposure is still possible.

Silicosis, formerly called potter's asthma, stonecutter's cough, miner's mold, and grinder's rot, is most likely to be contracted in today's industrial jobs involving sandblasting in tunnels, hard-rock mining (extraction and processing of ores), and preparation and use of sand. It can occur in anyone habitually exposed (usually over a period of 10 years) to the dust contained in silica and any miner is subject to it. Usually, silicosis is associated with extensive or prolonged inhalation of free silica (silicon dioxide) particles in the crystalline form of quartz.

Risk Factors. Not all clients exposed to occupational inhalants will develop lung disease. Harmful effects depend on the (1) type of exposure; (2) duration and intensity of exposure; (3) presence of underlying pulmonary disease; (4) smoking history; and (5) particle size and water solubility of the inhalant. The larger the particle, the lower the probability of its reaching the lower respiratory tract; highly water-soluble inhalants tend to dissolve and react in the upper respiratory tract, whereas poorly soluble substances may travel as far as the alveoli (Cronin, 1993).

Pathogenesis. Dust particles that are not filtered out by the nasociliary mechanism or mucociliary escalator (MCE) may be deposited anywhere in the respiratory tract and lungs, especially the small airways and alveoli. Each disease has its own pathogenesis, but in general the most dangerous dust particles measure 2 μm or less and are deposited in the smallest bronchioles and the acini (see Fig. 12–2). The particles are ingested by alveolar macrophages and most of the phagocytosed particles ascend to the mucociliary lining and are expectorated or swallowed. Some migrate into the interstitium of the lung and then into the lymphatics. Fibroblast stimulating factor secreted by activated macrophages mediates excessive fibrosis. In *coal worker's pneumoconiosis*, ingestion of inhaled coal dust[8] by alveolar macrophages leads to the formation of coal macules, which appear on the radiograph as diffuse small opacities (or white areas) in the upper lung.

In the pathogenesis of *silicosis*, groups of silicon hydroxide on the surface of the particles form hydrogen bonds with phospholipids and proteins, an interaction that is presumed to damage cellular membranes and thereby kill the macrophage. The dead macrophages release free silica particles and fibrogenic factors. The released silica is then reingested by macrophages and the process is amplified (Rubin and Farber, 1994). Anywhere from 10 to 40 years after initial exposure to silica, small rounded opacities called silicotic nodules form throughout the lung. These fibrotic nodules scar the lungs and make them receptive to further complications (e.g., TB, bronchitis, and emphysema).

Asbestosis is characterized by inhalation of asbestos fibers, a fibrous magnesium and calcium silicate nonburning compound used in roofing materials, insulation for electric circuits, brake linings, and many other products that must be fire-resistant. As with the other pneumoconioses, asbestos particles are engulfed by macrophages. Once activated, macrophages then release inflammatory mediators resulting in nodular interstitial fibrosis that can be seen on radiographs along with thickened pleura. After an interval of 10 to 20 years between exposure and further complications, calcified pleural plaques on the dome of the diaphragm or lateral chest wall develop. The lower lungs are more often involved than the upper lungs in asbestosis (Rom et al., 1991).

Clinical Manifestations. Symptoms of pneumoconioses include progressive dyspnea, chronic cough, and expectoration of mucus containing the offending particles. In rare cases, rheumatoid arthritis coexisting primarily with coal worker's pneumoconiosis, but also silicosis and asbestosis, causes *Caplan's syndrome*, a condition characterized by the presence of rheumatoid nodules in the periphery of the lung.

Simple silicosis is usually asymptomatic and has no effect on routine pulmonary function tests. As the disease progresses, mucus tinged with blood, loss of appetite, chest pain, and general weakness may occur. In complicated silicosis, dyspnea, and obstructive and restrictive lung dysfunction occur. Asbestosis is characterized by dyspnea, inspiratory crack-

[8] Anthracite or hard coal is associated with a higher incidence of black lung than is bituminous or soft coal.

les (on auscultation), and sometimes clubbing and cyanosis (Stauffer, 1994). As in the case of the other pneumoconioses, the simple or uncomplicated form of coal worker's pneumoconiosis is uncommon, but the chronic form is often associated with chronic bronchitis and infections.

Medical Management

Diagnosis. Diagnosis is by history of exposure (which may be minimal with asbestosis and far removed in time from the onset of disease; the person may even be unaware of the exposure), sputum cytology, lung biopsy, chest film showing nodular or interstitial fibrosis, and pulmonary function studies. Other pulmonary imaging techniques used in conjunction with the initial chest radiograph include conventional CT, high-resolution CT, and gallium scintigraphy (Leonard and Templeton, 1992). High-resolution CT scanning is the best imaging method in asbestosis because of its ability to detect parenchymal fibrosis and define the presence of coexisting pleural plaques.

Treatment. Prevention is the first line of defense against occupational diseases. Workplace-based education, preemployment screening, yearly physical examinations, surveillance and exposure reduction, and elimination are essential components of a strategy to prevent occupational lung disorders (Markowitz, 1992; Saric, 1992). Precautions such as the use of face masks, protective clothing, and proper ventilation are essential. Regular chest films are recommended for all workers exposed to silica as a means of early detection. In 1971, asbestos became the first material to be regulated by the Occupational Safety and Health Administration (OSHA). The Environmental Protection Agency has proposed a total ban but there remains much controversy over the lack of scientific basis for this policy.

The dust deposits are permanent so treatment is toward relief of symptoms. Corticosteroids may produce some improvement in silicosis. While there is no cure for any of the pneumoconioses, the complications of chronic bronchitis and cor pulmonale must be treated.

Prognosis. The devastating feature of pneumoconioses is that there may be no obvious symptoms until the disease is in an advanced state. Once fully developed, prognosis is poor for most occupational lung diseases, with progressive and disabling results. Simple silicosis is not ordinarily associated with significant respiratory dysfunction unless complicated by emphysema and chronic bronchitis due to cigarette smoking. Although now uncommon, acute silicosis, resulting from heavy exposure to silica, rarely responds to treatment, and progresses rapidly over a few years when it occurs. The increased incidence of TB among people with silicosis presents an additional negative factor to the prognosis.

Exposure to asbestos may result in neoplasm. Both bronchogenic carcinoma and mesotheliomas of the pleura and peritoneum have been linked to asbestos. The exposure typically occurs 20 years before the development of bronchogenic carcinoma and approximately 30 to 40 years before the appearance of mesothelioma. Mesothelioma is terminal with no effective treatment.

Coal worker's pneumoconiosis was once thought to cause severe disability, but it is now clear that black lung causes minor impairment of pulmonary function at its worst. When coal miners have severe air flow obstruction, it is usually due to smoking (Rubin and Farber, 1994).

Special Implications for the Therapist **12-13**

PNEUMOCONIOSES

Steam inhalation and chest physical therapy techniques, such as controlled coughing and segmental bronchial drainage with chest percussion and vibration, help clear secretions. Exercise tolerance must be increased slowly over a long period of time beginning with increasing regular activities of daily living. Daily activities should be planned carefully to conserve energy (see Box 7–1), to decrease the work of breathing, and to afford frequent rest periods. Progression from increasing tolerance for daily activities to a conditioning program may precede an actual exercise program. In severe cases, oxygen may be necessary for any increase in activity level or exercise and the person may not progress beyond self-care skills.

Hypersensitivity Pneumonitis

Exposure to organic dusts may result in hypersensitivity pneumonitis, also called extrinsic allergic alveolitis. The alveoli and distal airways are most often involved as a result of exposure to more than 30 known environmental antigens. Most of the diseases are named according to the specific antigen or occupation and involve organic materials such as molds (e.g., mushroom compost, moldy hay, sugar cane, or logs left unprotected from moisture), fungal spores (e.g., stagnant water in air conditioners and central heating units), plant fibers or wood dust (particularly redwood and maple), cork dust, coffee beans, bird feathers, and serum.

Regardless of the specific antigen involved in the pathogenesis of hypersensitivity pneumonitis, the pathologic alterations in the lung are similar. A combination of immune complex–mediated and cell-mediated hypersensitivity reactions occurs, although the exact mechanism of these processes is still unknown. Most characteristic is the presence of scattered, poorly formed granulomas that contain foreign body giant cells. Mild fibrosis may occur, usually in the alveolar walls (Rubin and Farber, 1994).

The diagnosis of hypersensitivity pneumonitis of an organic origin is made by history of exposure, pulmonary function studies, and clinical manifestations, which commonly include abrupt onset of dyspnea, fever, chills, and a nonproductive cough. The symptoms typically remit within 24 to 48 hours but return on reexposure, and with time may become chronic. Initially, symptoms can be reversed by removing the worker from the exposure (the only adequate treatment), by modifying the materials handling process, or by using protective clothing and masks.

Hypersensitivity pneumonitis may present as acute, subacute, or chronic pulmonary disease depending on the frequency and intensity of exposure to the antigen. The prognosis is poor with repeated exposure to these organic dusts, resulting in nonreversible interstitial fibrosis (Pearlstein, 1987).

Noxious Gases, Fumes, and Smoke Inhalation

Exposure to toxic gases and fumes is an increasing problem in modern industrial society. Any time oxygen in the air is replaced by another toxic or nontoxic agent, asphyxia (deficient blood oxygen; increased carbon dioxide in blood and tissues) occurs. Such is the case when products manufactured from manmade compounds are heated at high temperatures releasing fumes. For example, workers who use heating elements to seal meat in plastic wrappers and workers involved in the manufacture of plastics and packaging materials made of polyvinyl chlorides, are exposed to these fumes.

The most common mechanism of injury is local irritation, the specific type and extent depending on the type and concentration of gas, and the duration of exposure. For example, highly soluble gases such as ammonia rapidly injure the mucous membranes of the eye and upper airway, causing an intense burning pain in the eyes, nose, and throat. Insoluble gases, such as nitrogen dioxide, encountered by farmers, cause diffuse lung injury (Andreoli et al., 1993).

Metal fume fever is a systemic response to inhalation of certain metal oxides, such as zinc oxide used in brass founding and chrome and copper plating. Symptoms include fever, myalgias, and malaise. *Polymer fume fever,* associated with heating of polymers, may cause high fever, chills, malaise, dry cough, and headache. With brief exposures, the symptoms associated with these two syndromes are self-limiting, but prolonged exposure results in chronic cough, hemoptysis, and impairment of pulmonary function.

Chemical pneumonitis can result from exposure to toxic fumes. The acute reaction may produce diffuse lung injury characterized by air space disease typical of pulmonary edema. In its chronic form, bronchiolitis obliterans develops (McLoud, 1991).

Smoke inhalation injury produces direct mucosal injury secondary to hot gases, tissue anoxia due to combustion products, and asphyxia as oxygen is consumed by fire. Thermal injury seen in the upper airway is characterized by edema and obstruction. Incomplete combustion of industrial compounds produces ammonia, acrolein, sulfur dioxide, and other substances in today's fires.

Environmental tobacco smoke (ETS) exposure is associated with rhinitis symptoms of runny nose and nasal congestion in some people. Other symptoms following exposure to sidestream tobacco smoke may include headache, chest discomfort or tightness, and cough (Willes et al., 1992; Bascom et al., 1991).

Near Drowning *(Wallace, 1994)*

Definition. *Near drowning* refers to surviving (24 hours or longer) the physiologic effects of hypoxemia and acidosis that result from submersion in fluid. Near drowning occurs in three forms: (1) "dry drowning," inhalation of little or no fluid with minimal lung injury because of laryngeal spasm (10% to 15% of cases); (2) "wet drowning," aspiration of fluid with asphyxia or secondary changes due to aspiration (85%); and (3) recurrence of respiratory distress secondary to aspiration pneumonia or pulmonary edema within 1 to 2 days after a near-drowning incident (Norris, 1995). Recovery is rapid if respiration and circulation are restored before permanent neurologic damage occurs. Death may occur from asphyxia secondary to reflex laryngospasm and glottic closure.

Incidence and Risk Factors. Drowning is the most common cause of death in those under 25 years old and the third leading cause of accidental death among all age groups. Nearly 80% of drowning victims are males; other risk factors include epilepsy, mental retardation, heart attack, alcohol consumption while swimming or boating, head or spinal cord injury at the time of the accident, failure to use personal flotation devices, increased use of hot tubs and spas, and lack of proper swimming training or overestimation of endurance by those who can swim.

Pathogenesis. The complications of near drowning fall into two categories: the effects of prolonged *anoxia* on the brain and kidney which as end organs may experience complications that are irreversible (determining the final prognosis), and acute lung injury from *aspiration* of fluids. When aspiration accompanies drowning, severe pulmonary injury often occurs, resulting in persistent arterial hypoxia and metabolic acidosis even after ventilation has been restored.

In the past, a distinction was made between the effects of saltwater and freshwater drowning (e.g., cardiovascular function, changes in blood volume, and serum electrolyte concentrations), but it is now known that hypoxia is the most important determinant of survival in human near drowning regardless of the type of water involved. Regardless of the amount of water aspirated, the duration of submersion and the water temperature determine the pathologic events.

Hypoxia results in global cell damage; different cells tolerate variable lengths of anoxia. Neurons, especially cerebral cells, sustain irreversible damage after 4 to 6 minutes of submersion. The heart and lungs can survive up to 30 minutes. The extent of CNS injury tends to correlate with the duration of hypoxia, but hypothermia accompanying the incident may reduce the cerebral oxygen requirements and help reduce CNS injury.

Clinical Manifestations. The clinical features in near drowning are variable and the person may be unconscious, semiconscious, or awake but apprehensive. Pulmonary and neurologic symptoms predominate with cough, tachypnea, and possible development of ARDS (see earlier discussion in this chapter) with progressive respiratory failure. Other pulmonary complications include pulmonary edema, bacterial pneumonia, pneumothorax, or pneumomediastinum secondary to resuscitation efforts. Fever occurs in the presence of aspiration during the first 24 hours but can occur later in the presence of infection.

Early neurologic manifestations include seizures, especially during resuscitative measures, and altered mental status, including agitation, combativeness, or coma. Speech, motor, or visual abnormalities may occur and may improve gradually and resolve over several months.

Medical Management

Treatment. Nearly 90% of near-drowning victims who live long enough to receive hospital care will survive, indicating the need for extensive resuscitative efforts. Restoration of ventilation and circulation by means of resuscitation at the scene of the accident is the primary goal of treatment to restore oxygen delivery and prevent further hypoxic damage. Other treatment is largely supportive, with antibiotics for pulmonary infection, maintenance of fluid and electrolyte balance, possible transfusion for significant anemia, and management of acute renal failure.

Comatose near-drowning victims frequently have elevated intracranial pressure caused by cerebral edema and loss of cerebrovascular autoregulation. Reduction of cerebral blood flow adds ischemic injury to already damaged brain tissue. In order to reserve cerebral function in such cases, cerebral resuscitation (controlled hyperventilation, deliberate hypothermia, use of barbiturates, glucocorticoids, and diuretics) may be performed.

Prognosis. The prognosis depends in large part upon the extent and duration of the hypoxic episode. People have survived as long as 70 minutes of immersion with complete recovery, but up to 20% of all near-drowning victims will have permanent sequelae, many of which are ultimately fatal. If laryngospasm is finally overcome and the person aspirates water or if aspiration of vomitus occurs during resuscitative measures, prognosis is worse than without these complications.

Coincident head trauma or subdural hematoma presents additional prognostic complications. Neurologic injury is the most serious and least reversible complication in those successfully resuscitated. Little, if anything, has been shown to help, and it carries a grave prognosis (Andreoli et al., 1993).

Special Implications for the Therapist **12–14**

NEAR DROWNING

All near-drowning victims should be admitted to a hospital inpatient setting for observation over 24 to 48 hours because of the possibility of delayed drowning syndrome with confusion, substernal pain, and adventitious breath sounds (rales or rhonchi). The therapist is often involved early on in the case management, providing bedside care much the same as for a person with traumatic brain injury (TBI) or spinal cord injury (SCI). It is not uncommon for a near-drowning accident to be associated with either TBI or SCI.

Evaluate cardiopulmonary status, monitor vital signs and observe respirations. To facilitate breathing, elevate the head of the bed slightly if possible; observe for signs of infection (see Table 6–1); and check for any areas of skin pressure or factors precipitating pressure ulcers. Provide passive or active-assistive exercise according to the person's functional abilities and progress as quickly as possible given the medical status.

In the rehabilitation setting, large doses of steroids are administered early in the treatment of TBI and SCI clients to control cerebral or spinal cord edema. Suppression of the inflammatory reaction in persons receiving large doses of steroids may be so complete as to mask the clinical signs and symptoms of major diseases, perforation of a peptic ulcer, or spread of infection. See also Corticosteroids, Chapter 4.

CONGENITAL DISORDERS

Cystic Fibrosis

Definition and Overview. Cystic fibrosis is an inherited disease of the exocrine glands affecting the hepatic, digestive, male reproductive (the vas deferens is functionally disrupted in nearly all cases), and respiratory systems (Fig. 12–10). The majority of morbidity and mortality is caused by lung disease and almost all persons develop obstructive lung disease associated with chronic infection that leads to progressive loss of pulmonary function (Larsen et al., 1993).

Incidence. CF is the most common inherited genetic disease in the white population, affecting approximately 30,000 children and young adults (equal sex distribution) in the United States. More than 1000 new cases are diagnosed each year. The disease is inherited as an autosomal recessive trait meaning that both parents must be carriers so that the child inherits a defective gene from each one. In the United States, 5% of the population, or 12 million people, carry a single copy of the CF gene. The family with a child who has CF has a 25% chance (1:4) for another child with CF and a 50% (1:2) chance that a child will be a carrier. The chance that a healthy sibling will be a carrier is 66% (2:3).

Etiology. In recent years there have been major advances in understanding the genetics and pathophysiology of the disease. In 1985, the CF gene was located on the long arm of chromosome 7. In 1989, the gene for CF was cloned[9] and abnormalities in the CF transmembrane conductance regulator (CFTR) protein were attributed to CF. In healthy people, this CFTR protein provides a channel by which chloride (a component of salt) can pass in and out of cells. Clients with CF have a defective copy of the gene that normally enables cells to construct that channel. As a result, salt accumulates in the cells lining the lungs and digestive tissues, making the surrounding mucus abnormally thick and sticky. A mutation, a deletion of phenylalanine (a specific amino acid of the CF gene), is present in the majority of CF cases, making the apical membrane of CF airway epithelia impermeable to chloride (Welsh et al., 1993; Drumm and Collins, 1993).

Today, affected children are studied using polymerase chain reaction (PCR) techniques to search for identifiable mutations. Over 400 mutations in the CFTR gene have been described in cases of CF, but not all of the mutations have been identified, so mass screening cannot yet identify individuals carrying the gene for CF who would otherwise test "negative" (Sujansky et al., 1993; Dean and Santis, 1993).

Pathogenesis. The basic biochemical defect in CF is still unknown but it does appear that impermeability of epithelial cells to chloride is the primary problem resulting in (1) dehydrated and increased viscosity of mucous gland secretions, primarily in the lungs, pancreas, intestine, and sweat glands; (2) elevation of sweat electrolytes (sodium chloride); and (3) pancreatic enzyme deficiency. The dehydration resulting in

[9] Clones are identical copies of genes used to study the DNA sequence which allows scientists to determine the nature and function of the protein encoded by the gene. Cloning opens up the possibility of gene therapy for a disorder.

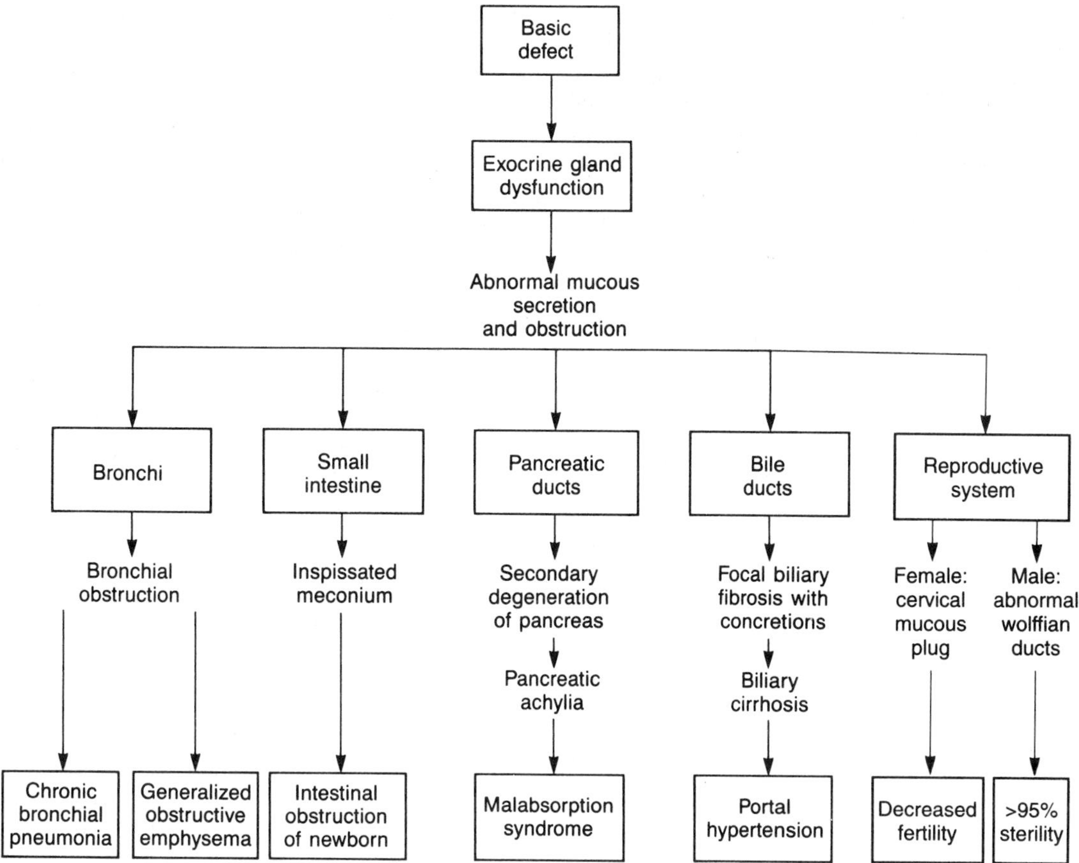

Figure 12–10. Various effects of exocrine gland dysfunction in cystic fibrosis. (*From Wong, DL: Whaley and Wong's Essentials of Pediatric Nursing, ed 4. St Louis, Mosby–Year Book, 1993, p 743.*)

TABLE 12–12 RESPIRATORY DISEASES: SUMMARY OF DIFFERENCES

DISEASE	PRIMARY AREA AFFECTED	RESULT
Acute bronchitis	Membrane lining bronchial tubes	Inflammation of lining
Bronchiectasis	Bronchial tubes (bronchi or air passages)	Bronchial dilation with inflammation
Pneumonia	Alveoli (air sacs)	Causative agent invades alveoli with resultant outpouring from lung capillaries into air spaces and continued healing process
Chronic bronchitis	Larger bronchi initially; all airways eventually	Increased mucus production (number and size) causing airway obstruction
Emphysema	Air spaces beyond terminal bronchioles (alveoli)	Breakdown of alveolar walls; air spaces enlarged
Asthma	Bronchioles (small airways)	Bronchioles obstructed by muscle spasm, swelling of mucosa, thick secretions
Cystic fibrosis	Bronchioles	Bronchioles become obstructed and obliterated; later, larger airways become involved Mucous plugs cling to airway walls, leading to bronchitis, bronchiectasis, atelectasis, pneumonia, or pulmonary abscess

From Goodman CC, Snyder TE: Differential Diagnosis in Physical Therapy, ed 2. Philadelphia, WB Saunders, 1995.

thick, viscous mucous gland secretions causes the mechanical obstruction responsible for the multiple clinical manifestations of CF.

Bronchial and bronchiolar obstruction by the abnormal mucus predisposes the lung to infection and causes patchy atelectasis with hyperinflation. The disease progresses from mucous plugging and inflammation of small airways (bronchiolitis) to bronchitis, followed by bronchiectasis, pneumonia, fibrosis, and the formation of large cystic dilations that involve all bronchi. A summary of differences among these various respiratory diseases is provided (Table 12–12). Recurrent pneumothorax, hemoptysis, pulmonary hypertension, and cor pulmonale are serious and life-threatening complications of severe and diffuse CF pulmonary disease (Huether, 1994).

Clinical Manifestations. Almost all clinical manifestations of CF are a result of overproduction of extremely viscous mucus and pancreatic enzyme deficiency. A complete list of clinical manifestations by organ and in order of progression is given in Table 12–13. The consistent finding of abnormally high sodium and chloride concentrations in the sweat is a unique characteristic of CF. Parents frequently observe that their infants taste "salty" when they kiss them (Wong, 1993).

TABLE 12–13 CLINICAL MANIFESTATIONS OF CYSTIC FIBROSIS

Early Stages	**Meconium Ileus**
Persistent coughing	Abdominal distention
Persistent wheezing	Vomiting
Recurrent pneumonia	Failure to pass stools
Excessive appetite, poor weight gain	Rapid development of dehydration
Salty skin and sweat	**Gastrointestinal Manifestations**
Bulky foul-smelling stools	Large, bulky, loose, frothy, foul-smelling stools
Pulmonary Manifestations	Voracious appetite (early)
Initial	Anorexia (late)
Wheezy respirations	Weight loss
Dry, nonproductive cough	Marked tissue wasting, muscle atrophy
Progressive involvement	Failure to thrive or grow
Increased dyspnea	Distended abdomen
Decreased exercise tolerance	Thin extremities
Paroxysmal cough	Sallow (yellowish) skin
Tachypnea	Anemia
Obstructive emphysema	**Pancreatic Manifestations**
Patchy areas of atelectasis	Vitamin deficiency (vitamins A, D, E, K)
Advanced stage	Iron deficiency anemia
Barrel chest	Malnutrition
Kyphosis	Diabetes mellitus
Pectus carinatum	
Cyanosis	
Clubbing (fingers and toes)	
Recurrent bronchitis	
Recurrent bronchopneumonia	
Pneumothorax	
Hemoptysis	
Right-sided heart failure secondary to pulmonary hypertension	

Adapted from Wong DL: Whaley and Wong's Essentials of Pediatric Nursing, ed 4. St Louis, Mosby–Year Book, 1993, p 743.

Pancreas. Approximately 85% of clients have pancreatic insufficiency with thick secretions blocking the pancreatic ducts causing dilation of the small lobes of the pancreas, degeneration, and eventual progressive fibrosis throughout. The blockage also prevents essential pancreatic enzymes from reaching the duodenum, thus impairing digestion and absorption of nutrients. Clinically, this process results in bulky, frothy (undigested fats due to a lack of amylase and tryptase enzymes), foul-smelling stools (decomposition of proteins producing compounds such as hydrogen sulfide and ammonia).

As the life expectancy for people with CF has improved, the incidence of diabetes has increased because pancreatic damage can eventually affect the beta cells. Hyperglycemia may adversely influence weight, pulmonary function, and development of microvascular complications (Hayes et al., 1994).

Gastrointestinal. The earliest manifestation of CF, *meconium ileus* is present in approximately 10% to 15% of newborns; the small intestine is blocked with thick, putty-like, tenacious meconium. Prolapse of the rectum is the most common gastrointestinal complication associated with CF, occurring most often in infancy and childhood. Children of all ages are susceptible to intestinal obstruction from thickened, dried, or impacted stools (inspissated meconium). Advances in investigative techniques have led to increasing reports of Crohn's disease in persons with CF (Lloyd-Still, 1994).

Pulmonary. Chronic cough and purulent sputum production are symptomatic of lung involvement. The child is unable to expectorate the mucus because of its increased viscosity. This retained mucus provides an excellent medium for bacterial growth, placing the individual at increased risk of infection. Reduced oxygen–carbon dioxide exchange causes variable degrees of hypoxia, clubbing (see Fig. 12–4), cyanosis, hypercapnia, and resultant acidosis. Chronic pulmonary infection and malabsorption lead to secondary manifestations of barrel chest, pectus carinatum, and kyphosis (Huether, 1994).

Medical Management

Diagnosis. Now that the gene responsible for CF has been identified, prenatal diagnosis and screening of carriers is possible as part of genetic counseling. The tests only detect mutations already observed, accounting for 70% of all CF carriers. Routine screening procedures are not employed at this time and testing is reserved for families in which there is a member affected with CF (Tizzano and Buchwald, 1992). A new genetic test (prenatal CF carrier screening) has been available for several years but has not been widely used because of its cost ($100 to $200) (Lieu et al., 1994).

About half of all children with CF present in infancy with failure to thrive, respiratory compromise, or both. The age at presentation can vary and some people are not diagnosed until adulthood. CF is traditionally diagnosed using the sweat test; a positive test occurs when the sodium chloride concentration is greater than 60 mEq/L (reference value: 40 mEq/L). Although elevated sweat electrolytes are associated with other conditions, a positive sweat test coupled with the clinical picture usually confirms the diagnosis (Larsen et al., 1993). Seventy-two-hour stool fat measurements are used to determine the extent of pancreatic function. Stools may also be examined for absence of pancreatic enzymes, particularly trypsin and chymotrypsin.

Treatment. A multidisciplinary approach must be taken in treating CF toward the goal of promoting a normal life for the individual. Medical management is toward alleviating symptoms and includes the use of antibiotics, aggressive pulmonary therapy with drugs to thin mucous secretions, chest physical therapy, humidified air, supplemental oxygen, and adequate hydration and nutrition with pancreatic enzymes administered before or with meals.

Drug therapy for CF has been primarily directed at treating infections with antibiotics and supplementing digestive enzymes and vitamins. Pharmacotherapy to date has included broad-spectrum antimicrobials to protect the respiratory epithelium from damage and aggressive nutritional management with microencapsulated pancreatic enzymes. A recent report has shown that ibuprofen (the generic name for the drug found in Advil, Motrin, and Nuprin) slows the deterioration of the lungs by reducing inflammation and breaking the cycle of mucous buildup, infection, and inflammatory destruction (Konstan et al., 1995).

The identification of the mutated CF gene has been followed by the first phase of somatic gene therapy in 1993 and new pharmacologic approaches are being explored to improve treatment. Finding a way to deliver the normal copy of the gene into the lung or intrahepatic biliary epithelial (IBE) cells remains a challenge (Grubman et al., 1995). It is possible that delivery through an aerosolized technique will incorporate sufficient quantities of the CFTR gene into the cells to offset the presence of the abnormal protein. The expectation is that the normal CFTR will reverse the physiologic defect in CF cells.

In the future, current therapeutic measures, such as intravenous antimicrobial treatment, will be improved by the additional delivery of new drugs to the bronchial tree by aerosol. Antibiotics, as well as protease inhibitors delivered by aerosol, should help to prevent damage by infection and inflammation and increase the probability of successful somatic gene therapy in this disease (Suter, 1994).

Amiloride and recombinant human DNAase administered by aerosol have the potential to improve mucociliary clearance; aerosolized amiloride is being tested to modify the basic defect in the chloride ion channel. Dornase alfa, a new mucolytic, is used to reduce sputum viscosity and increase mucociliary clearance. Leukoprotease inhibitors are currently being evaluated for reducing the acute inflammatory reaction in the lung (Wallace et al., 1993).

Double-lung or heart-lung transplants have been attempted on children with CF with advanced pulmonary vascular disease and who are severely disabled by dyspnea and hypoxia. Long-term survival has yet to be determined, but improved quality of life has been achieved.

Prognosis. The prognosis has steadily improved over the past 20 years, so that the median survival is now 28 years; more than 50% of children with CF live into adulthood. Children whose presenting symptoms were gastrointestinal at diagnosis have a good clinical course; those whose initial symptoms at diagnosis were pulmonary frequently demonstrate subsequent clinical deterioration. Pulmonary failure is still the most common cause of death. Males have a more favorable prognosis than females (Wong, 1993). New agents and gene therapy may substantially change the morbidity and mortality of this disease.

Special Implications for the Therapist **12-15**

CYSTIC FIBROSIS

Malnutrition and deterioration of lung function are closely interrelated and interdependent in the child with CF. Each affects the other, leading to a spiral decline in both. The occurrence of malnutrition during childhood seems to be associated with impaired growth and repair of the airway walls. In children, when growth in body length occurs, prevention of malnutrition is associated with better lung function. When adequate nutrition is combined with physical training, improved body weight, respiratory muscle function, lung function, and exercise tolerance occurs with increase in both respiratory and other muscle mass (Heijerman, 1993).

An exercise program not only improves the ability to clear accumulated lung secretions but increasing exercise tolerance delays the onset of dyspnea and increases feelings of well-being, thereby potentially improving self-image, self-confidence, and quality of life for the person with CF.

The therapist will also be involved with postural drainage and chest physical therapy carried out several times a day or as often as the child is able to tolerate it without undue fatigue. Chest therapy should not be performed before or immediately after meals, so treatment must be scheduled to avoid mealtimes. Aerosol therapy to deliver medication to the lower respiratory tract should be administered just before chest therapy to maximize the effectiveness of both treatments. Breathing exercises, improving posture, mobilizing the thorax through active exercise, and manual therapy are part of promoting good breathing patterns.

PARENCHYMAL DISORDERS

Atelectasis

Definition. Atelectasis is the collapse of normally expanded and aerated lung tissue at any structural level (e.g., lung parenchyma, alveoli, pleura, chest wall, bronchi) involving all or part of the lung. Most cases are categorized as either obstructive-absorptive or compressive. Atelectasis is a sign of disease since it is always secondary to another lesion such as obstruction of a bronchus, decreased motion secondary to paralysis or pleural disease, or loss of ability for pulmonary expansion due to pleural disease, diaphragmatic disease, and masses in the thorax.

Etiology and Pathogenesis. The primary cause of atelectasis is obstruction of the bronchus serving the affected area. It develops when there is interference with the natural forces that promote lung expansion. Absorption atelectasis is collapse resulting from removal of air from obstructed or hypoventilated alveoli. If a bronchus is obstructed, atelectasis occurs as air in the alveoli is slowly absorbed into the bloodstream.

The obstructive-absorptive type is caused by tumors, mucus, or foreign material obstructing bronchi. Failure to breathe deeply postoperatively (i.e., because of muscular guarding and splinting from pain or discomfort with an upper abdominal incision), oversedation, immobility, coma, or neuromuscular disease interferes with the natural forces that promote lung expansion, leading to obstructive atelectasis.

Insufficient pulmonary surfactant, as occurs in respiratory distress syndrome, inhalation of anesthesia, high concentrations of oxygen, lung contusion, aspiration of gastric contents or smoke inhalation, or increased elastic recoil as a result of interstitial fibrosis (e.g., silicosis, radiation pneumonitis) can also interfere with lung distention. When atelectasis is caused by inhalation of concentrated oxygen or anesthetic agents, quick absorption of these gases into the bloodstream can lead to collapse of alveoli in dependent portions of the lung (Huether, 1994).

Although atelectasis is usually caused by bronchial obstruction, direct compression can also cause atelectasis. The compressive type is due to air (pneumothorax), blood (hemothorax), or fluid (hydrothorax) filling the pleural space. Abdominal distention that presses on a portion of the lung can also collapse alveoli causing atelectasis. *Right middle lobe syndrome* refers to atelectasis secondary to compression of the bronchus to the right middle lobe by lymph nodes containing metastatic cancer (Rubin and Farber, 1994)

Clinical Manifestations. When sudden obstruction of the bronchus occurs, there may be dyspnea, tachypnea, cyanosis, elevation of temperature, drop in blood pressure, substernal retractions, or shock. In the chronic form of atelectasis, the client may be asymptomatic with gradual onset of dyspnea and weakness.

Medical Management

Diagnosis. Atelectasis is suspected in penetrating or other chest injuries. X-ray examination may show a shadow in the area of collapse. If an entire lobe is collapsed, the radiograph will show the trachea, heart, and mediastinum deviated toward the collapsed area, with the diaphragm elevated on that side (O'Toole, 1992). Chest auscultation and physical assessment add to the clinical diagnostic picture. Blood gas measurements may show decreased oxygen saturation.

Treatment and Prognosis. Once atelectasis occurs, treatment is directed toward removing the cause whenever possible. Suctioning or bronchoscopy may be employed to remove airway obstruction. Chronic atelectasis may require surgical removal of the affected segment or lobe of lung. Antibiotics are used to combat infection accompanying secondary atelectasis. Reexpansion of the lung is often possible, but the final prognosis depends on the underlying disease.

Special Implications for the Therapist **12-16**

ATELECTASIS

Atelectasis is a common postoperative complication of thoracic or high abdominal surgery. Left lower lobe atelectasis is common following cardiac surgery. Within a few hours postsurgery, atelectasis becomes increasingly resistant to reinflation. This complication is exacerbated in people receiving narcotics. One of the underlying goals of acute care therapy is to prevent atelectasis in the high-risk client. Diminished respiratory movement as a result of postoperative pain is often addressed by the therapist (Thomas and McIntosh, 1994). Frequent, gentle position changes, deep breathing, coughing, and early ambulation help promote drainage of all lung segments.

Deep breathing and effective coughing enhance lung expansion and prevent airway obstruction. Deep breathing is beneficial because it promotes the ciliary clearance of secretions, stabilizes the alveoli by redistributing surfactant, and permits collateral ventilation of the alveoli, through Kohn's pores in the alveolar septa. Kohn's pores, which open only during deep breathing, allow air to pass from well-ventilated alveoli to obstructed alveoli, minimizing their tendency to collapse and facilitating removal of the obstruction (Huether, 1994). To minimize postoperative pain during deep-breathing and coughing exercises, teach the client to hold a pillow tightly over the incision.

Pulmonary Edema

Definition and Incidence. Pulmonary edema or pulmonary congestion is an excessive fluid in the lungs which may accumulate in the interstitial tissue, in the air spaces (alveoli), or in both. Pulmonary edema is a common complication of many disease processes. It occurs at any age but with increasing incidence in aged people with heart failure.

Etiology and Risk Factors. Most cases of pulmonary edema are due to left ventricular failure, acute hypertension, or mitral valve disease, but noncardiac conditions, especially kidney or liver disorders prone to the development of sodium and water retention, can also produce pulmonary edema. Noncardiac causes of pulmonary edema include intravenous narcotics, increased intracerebral pressure, high altitude, sepsis, medications, inhalation of smoke or toxins (e.g., ammonia), transfusion reactions, shock, and disseminated intravascular coagulation.

Other risk factors include hyperaldosteronism, Cushing's syndrome, use of glucocorticoids, use of hypotonic fluids to irrigate nasogastric tubes, and transurethral resection of the prostate with sodium-free irrigation during and after surgery. Pulmonary edema itself is a major predisposing factor in the development of pneumonia that complicates heart failure and ARDS.

Pathogenesis. Pulmonary edema occurs as a result of (1) fluid overload, (2) disruption of capillary permeability, (3) decreased serum and albumin, and (4) lymphatic obstruction (Fig. 12–11). In any condition creating a fluid volume excess (fluid overload), the fluid pressure is even greater than usual at the arterial end of the capillary. Fluid is pushed into the tissue spaces with greater force because venous pressure

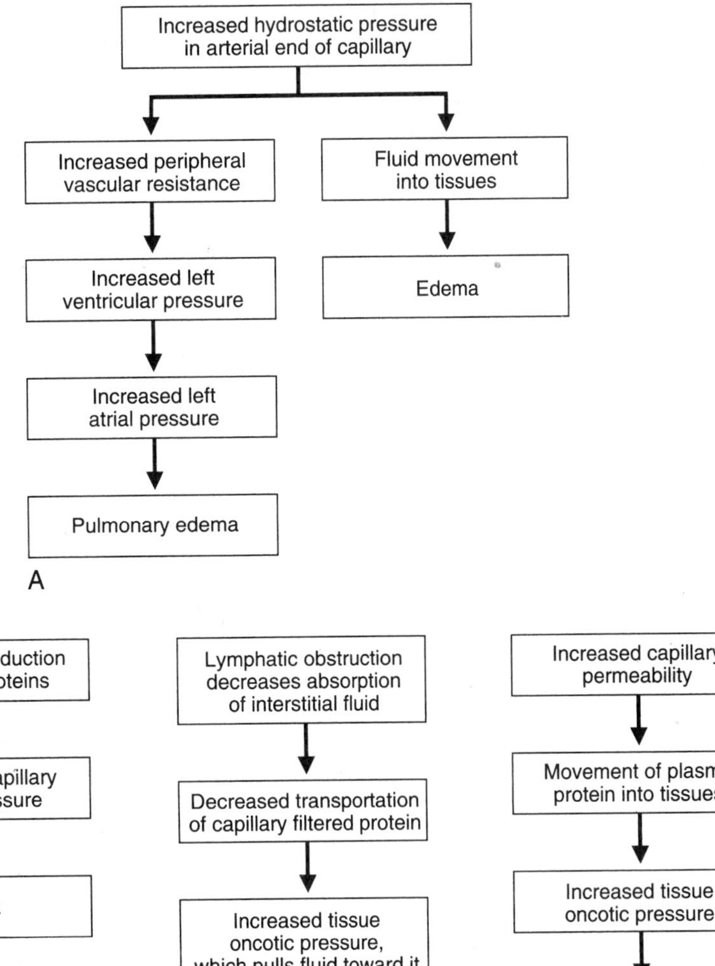

Figure 12-11. Mechanisms of pulmonary edema formation: A, Fluid overload. B, Decreased serum and albumin. C, Lymphatic obstruction. D, Tissue injury. (*From Black JM, Matassarin-Jacobs E (eds): Luckmann and Sorensen's Medical-Surgical Nursing, ed 4. Philadelphia, WB Saunders, 1993, p 266.*)

also exceeds oncotic pressure.[10] When osmotic pressure in the venous end of the capillary exceeds interstitial pressure, fluid cannot return to the bloodstream and peripheral and pulmonary edema may result. Fluid overload may also occur from decrease in sodium and water excretion associated with renal disorders (Kee, 1993).

[10] A brief review of this concept may be necessary for an understanding of many pulmonary conditions. The reader is referred to a physiology text (Guyton AC: Human Physiology and Mechanisms of Disease, ed 5. Philadelphia, WB Saunders 1992.) for an in-depth discussion. Fluid movement in the lung (as in all vessels) is governed by vascular permeability and the balance of the hydrostatic and oncotic pressures across the capillary endothelium as described by the Starling equation. Hydrostatic forces favor fluid filtration, whereas oncotic pressure promotes reabsorption. Normally, filtration forces dominate and fluid continuously moves from the vascular space into the interstitium. Extravascular water does not accumulate because the lung lymphatics effectively remove the filtered fluid and return it to the circulation. When the capacity of the lymphatic system is exceeded, if the rate of fluid filtration exceeds its functional capabilities, water accumulates in the loose interstitial tissues around the airways, pulmonary arteries, and, eventually, the alveolar walls (alveolar edema) (Andreoli et al., 1993).

As the fluid pressure increases in the tissues, it also increases in the left ventricle, which increases pressure in the left atrium. From the atrium, fluid will be forced backward across the alveolocapillary membrane of the lungs, resulting in pulmonary edema. Pulmonary edema is commonly seen when the left side of the heart is distended and fails to pump adequately. If the right side of the heart fails, peripheral edema occurs through the same process. Left-sided heart failure leads to right-sided failure (and vice versa), so both pulmonary and peripheral edema may exist simultaneously.

Disruption of capillary permeability is the cause of pulmonary edema in acute lung injury associated with ARDS, inhalation of toxic gases, aspiration of gastric contents, viral infections, and uremia. In these conditions, destruction of endothelial cells or disruption of the tight junctions between them alter capillary permeability.

In clients with cirrhosis of the liver, the serum protein and albumin levels are reduced in the vascular fluids. This results in less fluid reabsorption from the tissue spaces and peripheral edema and ascites occur.

Finally, when lymphatic channels are obstructed, tissue oncotic pressure rises and results in edema. This obstruction can occur as a result of tumor infiltration, but most often occurs in association with cardiogenic causes of pulmonary edema. When hemodynamic alterations (changes in the movement of blood and the forces involved) in the heart increase the perfusion pressure in the pulmonary capillaries, effective lymphatic drainage is blocked.

Clinical Manifestations. Clinical manifestations of pulmonary edema occur in stages. During the initial stage, clients may be asymptomatic or they may complain of restlessness and anxiety and the feeling that they are developing a common cold. Other signs include a persistent cough, slight dyspnea, diaphoresis, and intolerance to exercise.

As fluid continues to fill the pulmonary interstitial spaces, the dyspnea becomes more acute, respirations increase in rate, and there is audible wheezing. If the edema is severe, the cough becomes productive of frothy sputum tinged with blood, giving it a pinkish hue. If the condition persists, the person becomes less responsive and consciousness decreases (O'Toole, 1992).

Medical Management

Diagnosis. Pulmonary edema is usually recognized by its characteristic clinical presentation. Cardiogenic pulmonary edema is differentiated from noncardiac causes by the history and physical examination; an underlying cardiac abnormality can usually be detected clinically or by the electrocardiogram (ECG), chest film, or echocardiogram.

A chest film may show increased vascular pattern, and increased opacity of the lung, especially at the bases, and pleural effusion. There are no specific laboratory tests diagnostic of pulmonary edema; when the condition progresses enough to cause liver involvement the physician may observe the hepatojugular reflex (positional or palpatory pressure on the liver results in distention of the jugular vein). Blood gas measurements indicate the degree of functional impairment, and sputum cultures may indicate accompanying infection.

Treatment. Prevention is a key component with persons at increased risk for the development of pulmonary edema. Preventive measures may be as simple as lowering salt intake or pharmacologic treatment such as the use of digoxin and diuretics.

Once pulmonary edema has been diagnosed, treatment is aimed at enhancing gas exchange, reducing fluid overload, and strengthening and slowing the heartbeat. Oxygen by mask or through mechanical ventilation is used along with diuretics, diet, and fluid restriction to remove excess alveolar fluid. Morphine to relieve anxiety and reduce the effort of breathing may be used for people who do not have narcotic-induced pulmonary edema. Other pharmacologic-based treatment may include aminophylline to help dilate the bronchi and increase cardiac output, and a preparation of digitalis to strengthen contractions of the heart and increase cardiac output.

Prognosis. The prognosis depends on the underlying condition. The presence of pulmonary edema is a medical emergency requiring immediate interventions to prevent further respiratory distress. It is often reversible with clinical management.

Special Implications for the Therapist **12-17**

PULMONARY EDEMA

Symptoms of pulmonary edema that may come to the therapist's attention include engorged neck and hand veins (due to peripheral vascular fluid overload), pitting edema of the extremities, and, of course, the paroxysmal nocturnal dyspnea so common with this condition. One of the first signs of dyspnea may be an increased difficulty breathing when lying down, relieved by sitting up (orthopnea).

With liver involvement, positional or palpatory pressure on the liver may result in right upper quadrant or right shoulder pain as well as jugular vein distention (JVD). The JVD may be best observed with the person positioned sitting 30 to 45 degrees up from a fully supine position. Any liver involvement requires precautions when performing any soft tissue mobilization techniques to the anterior abdomen, including the diaphragm. Indirect techniques or mobilization away from the liver is recommended.

Gradual exercise intolerance usually occurs as the dyspnea progresses. The client may comment about weight gain or difficulty fastening clothes. Check for peripheral edema in the immobile or bedridden client. In this group of people, edema can occur in the sacral hollow rather than in the feet and legs, because the sacrum is the lowest place on the trunk. Care must be taken to prevent pressure ulcers in this area.

When working with a client already diagnosed with pulmonary edema, the sitting position is preferred with legs dangling over the side of the bed or plinth. This facilitates respiration and reduces venous return. If oxygen is being administered, check with the nursing staff or respiratory therapy for oxygen settings. It may be necessary to increase oxygen levels prior to exercise.

Adult Respiratory Distress Syndrome

Definition. ARDS is a group of symptoms which accompany acute respiratory failure following a systemic or pulmonary insult. It is also called shock lung, wet lung, stiff lung, adult hyaline membrane disease, posttraumatic lung, or diffuse alveolar damage (DAD).

Incidence. ARDS has only been identified within the last 25 years, affecting a reported 150,000 people per year in the United States. This figure has been challenged and part of the reason for the uncertainty of numbers is the lack of uniform definitions for ARDS and the heterogeneity of diseases underlying ARDS (Bernard et al., 1994). The incidence has increased as improvements in intensive care have allowed more people to survive the catastrophic illnesses that precede ARDS. Any age can be affected, but often young adults with traumatic injuries develop ARDS.

Etiology and Risk Factors. ARDS occurs as a result of injury to the lung by a variety of unrelated causes; the most common are listed in Table 12–14.

Pathogenesis. Alveolocapillary units, alveolar spaces, alveolar walls, and lungs are the site of initial damage (thus the name "diffuse alveolar damage"). Although the mechanism of lung injury varies with the cause, damage to capillary endothelial cells and alveolar epithelial cells is common in ARDS regardless of cause. Damage to these cells inactivates surfactant and allows fluids, proteins, and blood cells to leak from the capillary bed into the pulmonary interstitium and alveoli. The increased vascular permeability and inactivation of surfactant lead to interstitial and alveolar pulmonary edema and alveolar collapse (Stauffer, 1994).

Pulmonary edema decreases lung compliance and impairs oxygen transport. The loss of surfactant leads to atelectasis and further impairment in lung compliance and oxygen transport (gas exchange). These are only the pulmonary manifestations of what is now recognized as a more systemic process called multiple organ dysfunction syndrome (MODS), formerly called multiple organ failure (MOF). See Chapter 4 for discussion of MODS.

Clinical Manifestations. The clinical presentation is relatively uniform regardless of cause and occurs within 12 to 48 hours of the initiating event. The earliest sign of ARDS is usually an increased respiratory rate characterized by shallow, rapid breathing. Pulmonary edema caused by alveolar filling with exudate causes solidification of the tissue (consolidation). The subsequent alveolar collapse decreases lung compliance, causing dyspnea, hyperventilation and the changes observed on chest radiographs (Fig. 12–12).

As breathing becomes increasingly difficult, the individual may gasp for air, exhibit skin retractions, and cyanosis. Unless the underlying disease is reversed rapidly, especially in thepresence of sepsis (toxins in the blood), the condition quickly progresses to full-blown MODS involving kidneys, liver, gut, CNS, and the cardiovascular system.

TABLE 12-14 CAUSES OF ADULT RESPIRATORY DISTRESS SYNDROME (ARDS)*

Severe trauma (e.g., multiple bone fractures)
Septic shock
Pancreatitis
Cardiopulmonary bypass surgery
Diffuse pulmonary infection
Burns
High concentrations of supplemental oxygen
Aspiration of gastric contents
Massive blood transfusions
Embolism: fat, thrombus, amniotic fluid, venous air
Near drowning
Radiation therapy
Inhalation of smoke or toxic fumes
Indirect: chemical mediators released in response to systemic disorders (e.g., viral infections, pneumonia)
Drugs (e.g., aspirin, narcotics, lidocaine, phenylbutazone, hydrochlorothiazide, most chemotherapeutic and cytotoxic agents)

* Listed in order of decreasing frequency.

Medical Management

Diagnosis. Since ARDS is a collection of symptoms rather than a specific disease, differential diagnosis is through a process of diagnostic elimination. Cardiogenic pulmonary edema and bacterial pneumonia must be ruled out because there are specific treatments for those disorders. By definition, respiratory failure in the proper clinical setting (history and physical findings) constitutes ARDS. Physical examination, blood gas analysis to assess the severity of hypoxemia, microbiologic cultures to identify or exclude infection, and radiographs may be part of the diagnostic process.

Treatment. Specific treatment is administered for any underlying conditions (e.g., sepsis, pneumonia). Otherwise, treatment is based on early detection, and treatment goals are supportive and toward prevention of complications. Supportive therapy to maintain adequate blood oxygen levels may include administration of humidified oxygen by a tight-fitting face mask allowing for CPAP. Mechanical ventilation with PEEP may be necessary if hypoxemia does not respond adequately to these measures.

Sedation to reduce anxiety and restlessness during ventilation is required in some cases. If tachypnea, restlessness, or respirations out of phase with the ventilator ("bucking") cannot be managed by sedation, pharmacologic paralysis (e.g., pancuronium bromide, curare) may be induced (Cronin, 1993).

Many studies are underway investigating new methods of prevention or treatment of ARDS. Prophylactic immunotherapy, antibodies against endotoxin, inhalation of nitric oxide, and inhibition of various inflammatory mediators are among the possibilities being tested (Rossaint, et al., 1994; St. John and Dorinsky, 1993).

Prognosis. The final outcome is difficult to predict at the onset of disease, but the mortality rate for ARDS is close to 65% despite therapy (Raffin, 1987; Harruff, 1994). The major cause of death in ARDS is nonpulmonary MODS, often with sepsis. If ARDS is accompanied by sepsis, the mortality rate may reach 90%. Median survival in such cases is 2 weeks (Stauffer, 1994). The mortality rate increases with age and clients older than 60 years of age have a mortality rate as high as 90% (Rubin and Farber, 1994).

Most survivors are asymptomatic within a few months and have almost normal lung function 1 year after the acute illness. Lung fibrosis is the most common post-ARDS complication which may resolve completely, may result in respiratory dysfunction, and in some cases, pulmonary hypertension, or may result in death.

Special Implications for the Therapist **12-18**

ADULT RESPIRATORY DISTRESS SYNDROME

ARDS requires careful monitoring and supportive care. Assess the client's respiratory status frequently and observe for retractions on inspiration, the use of

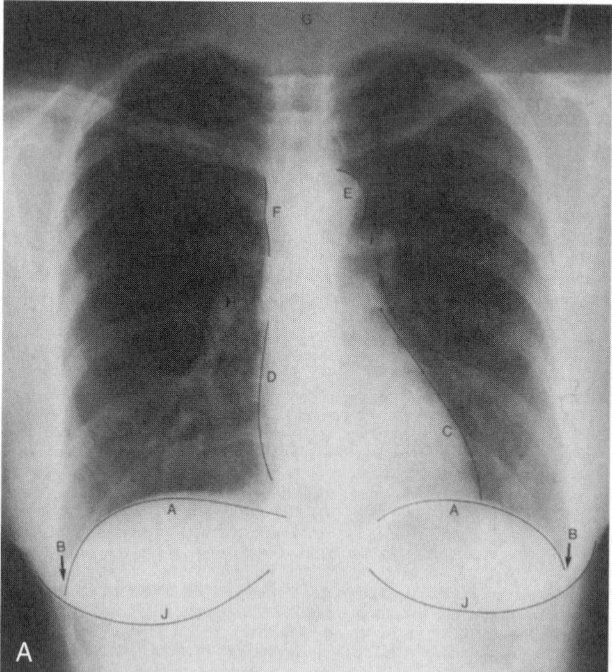

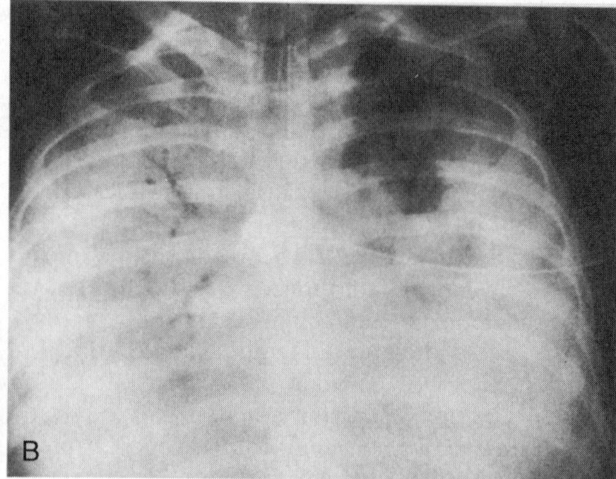

Figure **12–12.** A, Normal chest film taken from a posteroanterior (PA) view. The backward *L* in the upper right corner is placed on the film to indicate the left side of the chest. Some anatomic structures can be seen on the x-ray study and are outlined: *A*, diaphragm; *B*, costophrenic angle; C, left ventricle, *D*, right atrium; *E*, aortic arch; *F*, superior vena cava; G, trachea; *H*, right bronchus; *I*, left bronchus; *J*, breast shadows. (*From Black JM, Matassarin-Jacobs E (eds): Luckmann and Sorensen's Medical-Surgical Nursing, ed 4. Philadelphia, WB Saunders, 1993, p 935.*) B, This chest film shows massive consolidation from pulmonary edema associated with adult respiratory distress syndrome (ARDS) following multisystem trauma. (*From Fraser RG, Paré JA, Paré PD, et al: Diagnosis of Diseases of the Chest, ed 3. Philadelphia, WB Saunders, 1990.*)

accessory muscles of respiration, and developing or worsening dyspnea. On auscultation, listen for adventitious (rales or rhonchi) or diminished breath sounds and report any clear, frothy sputum that may indicate pulmonary edema.

Closely monitor heart rate and blood pressure watching for arrhythmias (see Special Implications for the Therapist: Arrhythmias: 10–12) that may result from hypoxemia, acid-base disturbances, or electrolyte imbalance. With pulmonary artery catheterization, know the desired pulmonary capillary wedge pressure (PCWP)* level and check the readings; report any significant elevations (see Table 35–20) or changes in waveform that indicate the catheter has become wedged. Empty condensation from the tubing of the ventilator to ensure maximum oxygen delivery during therapy.

Oxygenation in clients with ARDS may sometimes be improved by turning them from the supine to the prone position, although mechanical ventilation may prevent the use of this positioning. The sitting position optimizes lung capacity, so the use of a reclining chair at bedside should be considered. Improvement in lung function by means of continuous body positioning called kinetic positioning (KIN) has been reported (Pape et al., 1994). Without this capability, frequent changes in position and passive range-of-motion exercises (or active-assisted if possible) must be carried out by staff and family members.

* Pulmonary artery catheterization measures left ventricular pressure and diastolic pressure. PCWP can indicate left ventricular failure coinciding with the onset of pulmonary congestion and pulmonary edema. PCWP can also register insufficient volume and pressure in the left ventricle indicating hypovolemic shock in other conditions.

Postoperative Respiratory Failure

Postoperative respiratory failure can result in the same pathophysiologic and clinical manifestations as ARDS, but without the severe progression to MODS (see previous discussion of ARDS). Risk factors include surgical procedures of the thorax or abdomen, limited cardiac reserve, chronic renal failure, chronic hepatic disease, infection, period of hypotension during surgery, sepsis, and smoking, especially in the presence of preexisting lung disease. In the pediatric population, a difficult respiratory course may result in necrotizing enterocolitis (NEC), a postoperative gastrointestinal complication related to ischemia of the bowel. This condition occurs when oxygen depletion in the heart or brain causes blood to be shunted away from less vital organs, such as the intestine.

The most common postoperative pulmonary problems include atelectasis, pneumonia, pulmonary edema, and pulmonary emboli. Prevention of any of these problems involves frequent turning, deep breathing, humidified air to loosen secretions, antibiotics for infection as appropriate, supplemental oxygen for hypoxemia, and early ambulation.

If respiratory failure develops, mechanical ventilation may be required and treatment is very similar to that for ARDS.

Lung Transplantation

Overview. The first lung transplant was performed in 1963 on a 58-year-old man with bronchogenic carcinoma; he survived for 18 days. Other lung transplants were attempted without success because of lung rejection, anastomotic complications, or infection in the transplant recipients. In the early 1980s, human heart-lung transplantation was successfully performed for the treatment of pulmonary vascular disease. Lung transplantation involving the replacement of one of the diseased lungs with a lung from a cadaver donor is most often combined with heart transplantation because of the poor results with just lung transplants. After this procedure, single-lung transplantation for the treatment of endstage interstitial lung disease and obstructive lung disease was developed. More recently, the technique of double-lung transplantation has come into existence (Jenkinson and Levine, 1994).

Transplant Candidates. Single-lung transplantation is still relatively uncommon, but the success rate is increasing with advancing surgical techniques and immunosuppressants used as antirejection medications. Single-lung transplantation may be a possible treatment option in selected clients with unresponsive chronic respiratory failure (e.g., emphysema, pulmonary fibrosis, pulmonary hypertension) and in carefully selected individuals with endstage lung involvement related to systemic disease (e.g., sarcoidosis, systemic sclerosis) or chemotherapy-induced fibrosis (Levine et al., 1994). One-year survival for single-lung transplantation is approximately 60%; survival for combined heart-lung transplantation is approximately 65%.

It is difficult to find lungs of appropriate size for double-lung transplantation in teenagers and small adults. Lung transplants in many young people with CF have been successful, but they usually require bilateral transplantation to reduce the risk of infecting a single-lung transplant from the remaining native lung. Many more are waiting for lung transplantation (Bisson et al., 1994).

Postoperative Complications. Postoperative complications of primary lung transplantation include airway disorders (bronchial stricture, stenosis, or anastomoses), infection, and acute or chronic rejection. Ischemia appears to be the most important factor influencing airway healing. Low-pressure bronchial blood flow from the pulmonary artery may be affected by low cardiac output, reperfusion edema, or rejection; mucosal injury may be further increased by prolonged positive-pressure ventilation. With the early use of steroids and continued technical modifications in the surgical procedure, early stenosis and obstructions are increasingly prevented (Griffith et al., 1994; Shennib and Massard, 1994).

Rejection. Transplant failure is primarily due to histoincompatibility and lack of effective immunosuppressive drugs to prevent rejection. Pretransplant serologic testing is employed to avoid transmitting infectious agents (e.g., cytomegalovirus [CMV], hepatitis viruses) from donor to recipient. In order to minimize rejection and improve chances of survival, blood types and tissue types are matched as closely as possible between donor and recipient.

In the case of organs such as the lungs, as well as the kidney, heart, liver, and pancreas, a generous blood supply in the recipient is essential to survival. As blood is drained from the transplanted organ into the host's general circulation, the body recognizes the transplanted tissue cells as foreign invaders (antigens) and immediately sets up an immune response by producing antibodies. These antibodies are capable of inhibiting metabolism of the cells within the transplanted organ and eventually actively cause their destruction (O'Toole, 1992).

Some people in rejection will be asymptomatic, but when present, clinical manifestations of rejection may present as dyspnea, fatigue, fever and chills, prolonged need for ventilatory support, and changes in x-ray findings. Signs and symptoms of infection may also appear as changes in vital signs, local infections at intravenous access sites and incision lines, and changes in respiratory status such as excessive secretions, tachypnea, dyspnea, and fatigue.

Medical Management

Treatment. Control of the immune response in the recipient is attempted by the use of immunosuppressive agents and antimetabolites, which tend to suppress the growth of rapidly dividing cells, and cyclosporin, which inhibits T cell function. Corticosteroids are used for their anti-inflammatory effect and pharmacologic prophylaxis is employed to prevent complications such as PCP. There is a need to balance the use of drugs to avoid rejection while preventing fatal infection. Complications following surgery are treated individually.

Following surgery, the client is observed for excessive bleeding. Pulmonary edema may develop in the denervated transplanted lung so fluids are restricted and the client is placed on continuous mechanical ventilation with PEEP for the first 24 to 48 hours.

Special Implications for the Therapist 12-19

LUNG TRANSPLANTATION

The therapist working with transplantation candidates is usually treating people who may be very close to death. In the preoperative therapy program, functional goals are the primary focus with attention directed toward functional mobility, identifying and maintaining or improving strength or motion deficits, and improving breathing patterns whenever possible.

Following the initial surgery, the client is at high risk of infection and transplant rejection requiring protective isolation (reverse isolation) (see Table 6–4). Early postoperative therapy involves maintaining range of motion, skin care, bed positioning, and progressing functional mobility. Initially, the client is very weak and may have difficulty learning and remembering all the instructions provided during the early posttransplant rehabilitation phase.

The client is usually weaned from a ventilator within 24 hours but some people may remain on a ventilator for up to a month or more. Client education, including pulmonary hygiene and postural drainage, is augmented by breathing, and strengthening exercises. Coughing and deep breathing must be relearned because the lung is denervated; this is especially true in the case of bilateral lung transplantation. Diaphragmatic breathing is encouraged as the client usually has a history of previous respiratory problems and the thoracic cage remains stiff and noncompliant. Flexibility and mobility of the thoracic cage may be improved with thoracic stretching and rib mobilization; scar mobilization may be appropriate to increase tissue mobility. Postoperative trigger points often respond well to ice and appropriate stretching (Travell and Simons, 1983).

During this time, the therapist must be alert and observe carefully for any signs of organ rejection as evidenced by fever, fatigue, exercise intolerance, reduced vital capacity, and decreased oxygen saturation (O_2 saturation should be consistently maintained above 90% and often values of 97% to 100% are recommended). Supplemental oxygen can be used during therapy if resting levels of oxygen saturation are too low. Any signs of rejection should be reported to the physician immediately.

Treatment progresses from bed mobility and sitting tolerance to standing tolerance, transfers, and gait training. General strengthening, including the trunk muscles; conditioning; and endurance remain an integral part of therapy. When the ventilator is removed, therapy continues with aggressive strengthening per physician approval. At this point, the client is often receiving therapy as an outpatient 5 days a week until the greatest risk of infection has passed (1 to 3 months) and may be able to tolerate resistive exercises and modified aerobics, including stair climbing, bench stepping, and Swiss ball techniques. When working with clients who have received a heart-lung transplant, the same rehabilitation protocol is followed with monitoring of both systems.

Client education regarding the importance of consistently following a home program to increase and maintain METs (metabolic equivalents, multiples of resting O_2 consumption) level with exercise is essential. When approved by the physician, a daily walking program can help minimize weight gain, muscle atrophy, osteoporosis, and edema (effect of cyclosporin on kidneys). Physician referral is essential for any reports of pain or increased edema. Risk of rejection, kidney failure, side effects of medication, and infection remain lifelong concerns. A simple cold can progress quickly to life-threatening pneumonia. Transplant recipients remain at risk for stress fractures, especially of the vertebrae, femoral neck, pubic ramus, and tibia associated with prolonged (lifelong) use of prednisone.

Psychosocially, the client may develop alterations in self-concept related to changes in appearance from the side effects of medications such as steroids and immunosuppressants (see Chapter 4), a change in lifestyle, or a change in work ability and performance (Cronin, 1993).

Sarcoidosis

Definition. A systemic disease of unknown cause involving any organ, sarcoidosis is characterized by granulomatous inflammation present diffusely throughout the body. These granulomas consist of a collection of macrophages surrounded by lymphocytes taking a nodular form. The lungs and lymph nodes are most commonly involved. In fact, granulomatous inflammation of the lung is present in 90% of clients with sarcoidosis (Stauffer, 1994). Secondary sites include the skin, eyes, liver, spleen, heart, and small bones in the hands and feet.

Incidence. Sarcoidosis occurs predominantly in the third and fourth decades (between the ages of 20 and 40 years) and has a slightly higher incidence in women than men. It is present worldwide with some interesting differences in prevalence among racial and ethnic groups. It is 14 times more frequent in blacks in the southern United States.

Pathogenesis. The pathogenesis of sarcoidosis is unknown but there appears to be an exaggerated cellular immune response on the part of the helper T lymphocytes to a foreign antigen whose identity remains unclear. Increasing evidence points to a triggering agent that may be genetic, infectious, immunologic, or toxic. Abnormalities of immune function, as well as autoantibody production, including rheumatoid factor and antinuclear antibodies, are seen in sarcoidosis and in connective tissue diseases, suggesting a common immunopathogenetic mechanism (Enzenauer and West, 1992).

A series of interactions between the excessive accumulation of T lymphocytes and monocytes and macrophages leads to the formation of noncaseating (i.e., do not undergo necrotic degeneration) granulomas in the lung and other organs which are characteristic of the disease (Weissler, 1994). Granuloma formation may regress with therapy or as a result of the disease's natural course, but may also progress to fibrosis and restrictive lung disease (Cronin, 1993).

Clinical Manifestations. Signs and symptoms may develop over a period of a few weeks to a few months and include dyspnea, cough, fever, malaise, weight loss, skin lesions (Fig. 12–13), and erythema nodosum (multiple, tender, nonulcerating nodules). It may be entirely asymptomatic presenting with abnormal findings on routine chest radiographs. Sarcoidosis may present with extrapulmonary symptoms referable to bone marrow, skin, eyes, peripheral nerves (neurosarcoidosis), liver, or heart (Table 12–15).

Respiratory symptoms of dry cough and dyspnea without constitutional symptoms[11] occur in over half of all people with sarcoidosis, and up to 15% develop progressive fibrosis (Rubin and Farber, 1994). Chest pain, hemoptysis, or pneumothorax may be present.

Medical Management

Diagnosis. There is no specific test other than history for sarcoidosis so diagnosis is based on clinical examination, radiographic and laboratory test findings, and biopsy of easily accessible granulomas (e.g., skin lesions, salivary gland, or palpable lymph nodes). When lung involvement is suspected, further testing may be required. Other granulomatous diseases (e.g., TB, berylliosis, lymphoma, carcinoma, and fungal disease) must be ruled out.

[11] Symptoms of systemic illness, including fatigue, weakness, malaise, weight loss, sweating, and fever.

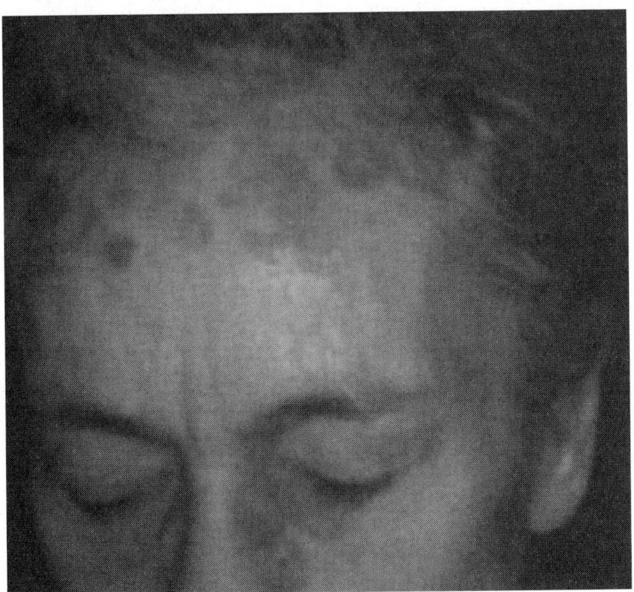

Figure 12–13. Cutaneous sarcoidal granuloma associated with sarcoidosis. This extrapulmonary sign (present in approximately 10% to 35% of documented systemic sarcoidosis cases) results from the presence of the granulomas in the tissues. The most common presentation is papular lesions noted on the head and neck, particularly the periorbital region, although they may appear in other areas of the body (including scars). The papules may be flesh-colored, red, or slightly hyperpigmented as shown here. In blacks, the papules may be hypopigmented. (*From J Musculoskel Med 12:73–74, 1995 [case study].*)

TABLE 12–15 Clinical Manifestations of Sarcoidosis

Pulmonary
Asymptomatic with abnormal chest film
Gradually progressive cough and shortness of breath
Pulmonary fibrosis with pulmonary insufficiency
Laryngeal and endobronchial obstruction
Extrapulmonary
Löfgren's syndrome: fever, arthralgias, bilateral hilar adenopathy, erythema nodosum
Heerfordt's syndrome (uveoparotid fever): fever, swelling of parotid gland and uveal tracts, seventh cranial nerve palsy
Erythema nodosum
Peripheral lymphadenopathy/splenomegaly
Eyes: Excessive tearing, swelling, uveitis, iritis, glaucoma, cataracts
Skin: lupus pernio or skin plaques (see Fig. 12–13)
Central nervous system: cranial nerve palsies, subacute meningitis, diabetes insipidus
Joints: polyarticular and monarticular arthritis
Bones: Punched-out cystic lesions in phalangeal and metacarpal bones
Heart: paroxysmal arrhythmias, conduction disturbances
Kidney: hypercalcemia with nephrocalcinosis or nephrolithiasis
Liver: granulomatous hepatitis

Adapted from Andreoli TE, Bennett JC, Carpenter CC, et al: Cecil Essentials of Medicine, ed 3. Philadelphia, WB Saunders, 1993, p 154.

CNS involvement in sarcoidosis poses a difficult diagnostic problem. Although neurologic involvement may occur long before the onset of symptoms, contrast-enhanced CT does not always reveal parenchymal and meningeal involvement. Recently gadolinium-enhanced magnetic resonance imaging (MRI) has shown increased sensitivity in detecting CNS involvement, but these findings are not specific for sarcoidosis (Kadakia et al., 1993).

Treatment. Treatment may not be required, especially in those clients who are asymptomatic, but the long-term use of corticosteroids is the treatment of choice for those clients who have impaired lung function with pulmonary granulomas. Corticosteroids are quite effective in reducing the acute granulomatous inflammation, but their efficacy in altering the long-term prognosis is unproven. Other agents, such as methotrexate, chloroquine, indomethacin, and azathioprine, are used for symptomatic skin involvement (Andreoli et al., 1993).

People with sarcoidosis who smoke are encouraged to quit because smoking aggravates impaired lung function. Prolonged exposure to direct sunlight should be avoided because vitamin D aids absorption of calcium, which can contribute to elevated serum and urinary calcium levels and the formation of kidney stones.

Prognosis. The prognosis is usually favorable, with complete resolution of symptoms and chest radiographic changes within 1 to 2 years. Most clients do not manifest clinically significant sequelae. However, because it is a multisystem disease that can cause complex problems, it can have a variable prognosis ranging from spontaneous remissions to progressive lung disease with pulmonary fibrosis in active sarcoidosis. In such cases, respiratory insufficiency and cor pulmonale may eventually occur. In 65% to 70% of cases there are no residual manifestations, 20% are left with permanent lung or ocular changes, and 10% of all cases die. Active sarcoidosis responds well to the administration of corticosteroids (Rubin and Farber, 1994).

Special Implications for the Therapist **12–20**

SARCOIDOSIS

There is a distinct arthritic component associated with sarcoidosis which is variously reported in from 10% to 35% of people who develop extrapulmonary involvement. The arthritic symptoms may develop early as the first manifestation of the disease or late in the disease and are usually accompanied by erythema nodosum. When further complicated by bilateral hilar adenopathy (enlargement of hilum or "roots" of the lung where the main bronchi enter the lungs), this triad of symptoms is called *Löfgren's syndrome.* Recurrent Löfgren's syndrome is extremely rare (Johard and Eklund, 1993).

The knees or ankles are the most common sites of acute arthritis. Distribution of joint involvement is usually polyarticular and symmetrical and the arthritis is commonly self-limiting after several weeks or months. Occasionally, the arthritis is recurrent or chronic, but even then, joint destruction and deformity are rare.

Treatment of arthritis in sarcoidosis is usually as for any other form of arthritis (Enzenauer and West, 1992).

Therapists should be alert to any presenting signs or symptoms of increased disease activity associated with sarcoidosis, especially exertional dyspnea which progresses to dyspnea at rest, chest pain, joint swelling, or increased fatigue and malaise reducing the client's functional level or ability to participate in therapy.

Cranial nerve palsies (especially facial palsy), multiple mononeuropathy, and less commonly, symmetrical polyneuropathy may all occur. Symmetrical polyneuropathy can affect either motor or sensory fibers solely or both disproportionately. Improvement may occur with the use of corticosteroids (Aminoff, 1994).

For clients receiving steroid therapy, increased side effects of the medication should be reported to the physician. For example, long-term use of steroids lowers resistance to infection, may induce diabetes, and is associated with weight gain, loss of potassium in the urine, and gastric irritation (see Table 4–7; Chapter 4).

Lung Cancer

Overview. Lung cancer, a malignancy of the epithelium of the respiratory tract, is the most frequent cause of cancer death in the United States. The term *lung cancer,* also known as *bronchogenic carcinoma,* excludes other pulmonary tumors such as sarcomas, lymphomas, blastomas, hematomas, and mesotheliomas.

Types of Lung Cancer. There are at least a dozen different types of tumors included under the broad heading of lung cancer. Clinically, lung cancers are classified as small cell lung cancer (SCLC, 25% of all lung cancers) and non-SCLC (NSCLC, 75% of all lung cancers). Within these two broad categories, there are four major types of primary malignant lung tumors: SCLC includes small cell carcinoma (oat cell carcinoma); NSCLC includes squamous cell carcinoma, adenocarcinoma, and large cell carcinoma. The characteristics of these four lung cancers are summarized in Table 12–16.

Staging. Cancers of the lung are staged at the time of their initial presentation. The American Joint Committee for Cancer's tumor, nodes, metastasis (TNM) staging system is used (see explanation in Chapter 7). Tumors confined to the lung without any metastases, regional or distant, are classified as stage I, and tumors associated with only hilar or peribronchial lymph node involvement (N1) are classified as stage II. Locally advanced tumors with mediastinal or cervical lymph node metastases and those with extension to the chest wall, mediastinum, diaphragm, or carina are classified as stage III tumors. Finally, tumors presenting with distant metastases (M1) are classified as stage IV (Martini, 1993).

SCLC is usually not considered a surgical disease requiring staging but rather is designated as "limited" or "extensive" disease. Limited disease is defined by involvement of one lung, the mediastinum, and either or both ipsilateral and contralateral supraclavicular lymph nodes (i.e., disease that can be encompassed in a single radiation therapy port). Spread beyond the lung, mediastinum, and supraclavicular lymph nodes is considered extensive disease (Hinson and Perry, 1993).

Metastasis. Carcinomas of the lung of all types metastasize most frequently to the regional lymph nodes, particularly the hilar and mediastinal nodes. The most frequent site of extranodal metastases is the adrenal gland. Lung cancer can also metastasize to the brain, bone, and liver before presenting symptomatically. Brain metastases constitute nearly one third of all observed recurrences in people with resected NSCLC of the adenocarcinoma type (Martini, 1993). Metastases to the brain usually result in CNS symptoms of confusion, gait disturbances, headaches, or personality changes.

As a form of secondary malignancy, the lungs are the most frequent site of metastases from other types of cancer. Any tumor cell dislodged from a primary neoplasm can find its way into the circulation or lymphatics, which are filtered by the lungs. Carcinoma of the kidney, breast, pancreas, colon, and uterus are especially likely to metastasize to the lungs (Mitchell, 1992)

Incidence. The lung cancer incidence and mortality rates have risen steadily and from the mid-1950s to the mid-1980s, lung cancer has been the most common cause of death from cancer in men. In 1987, lung cancer overtook breast cancer to become the most common cause of death from cancer among women in the United States. The American Cancer Society projects 177,000 new cases of lung cancer in 1996 (98,900 men, 78,100 women) (Parker et al., 1996).

The encouraging news is that as a result of a decline in smoking by men, the incidence in males has been decreasing since 1985 (Miller et al., 1993). Mortality rates have stabilized since the late 1980s and if present trends continue, there should be a decline in lung cancer mortality in men by the end of this decade. Among women, both incidence and mortality continue to rise although at a slower rate than in the 1970s. Although the percentage of women smokers has declined, it has not decreased as much as in men (Garfinkel, 1994).

Deaths from lung cancer increase at ages 35 to 44 years with a sharp increase between ages 45 and 55. Incidence continues to increase up until age 74, after which the incidence levels off and decreases among the very old.

Risk Factors. Cigarette smoking (more than 20 cigarettes a day) remains the greatest risk factor for lung cancer; 85% to 90% of all lung cancers occur in smokers.[12] The statistics point to the fact that lung cancer is the most preventable of all cancers. The elimination of cigarette smoking would virtually eliminate SCLC (Hinson and Perry, 1993).

There are 43 known carcinogens and promoting substances found in cigarette smoke (Seale and Beaver, 1992). For this reason, the risk of lung cancer is increased in a smoker who is also exposed to other carcinogenic agents such as radioactive isotopes, polycyclic aromatic hydrocarbons and arsenicals, vinyl chloride, metallurgic ores, and mustard gas. Other occupational or environmental risk factors associated with lung cancer include diesel exhaust, benzopyrene and radon particles associated with uranium mining, and ionizing radiation. Exposure to excess levels of radon gas contained in the soil and ground water of residential homes in the United States accounts for 20,000 cases of lung cancer annually.

The rare nonsmoker who develops lung cancer usually

[12] The cancer death rates for pipe and cigar smokers are about equal to those of cigarette smokers for cancer of the larynx, oral cavity, and esophagus.

TABLE 12-16 CHARACTERISTICS OF LUNG CANCER

TUMOR TYPE	INCIDENCE	GROWTH RATE	METASTASIS	TREATMENT
Small Cell Lung Cancer (SCLC)				
Small cell (oat cell)	25%	Very rapid	Very early; to mediastinum or distal lung	Chemotherapy; surgical resectability is poor Radiation therapy successful if tumor limited to lung
Non–Small Cell Lung Cancer (NSCLC)				
Squamous cell (epidermal)	30%	Slow	Localized; metastasis late, usually to hilar lymph nodes	Surgical resectability is good if stage I or II Chemotherapy and radiation therapy for symptomatic relief only
Adenocarcinoma	30%–35%	Slow to moderate	Early; metastasis throughout lung or to other organs	Surgical resectability is good if localized stage I or II Radiation therapy for palliation Moderately good response to chemotherapy
Large cell (anaplastic)	5%–10%	Rapid	Early and widespread metastasis to kidney, liver, adrenals	Surgical resectability is poor if involvement is widespread; better prognosis if stage I or II Chemotherapy of limited use; radiation therapy is palliative

Adapted from Black JM, Matassarin-Jacobs E (eds): Luckmann and Sorensen's Medical-Surgical Nursing, ed 4. Philadelphia, WB Saunders, 1993, p 1062.

has an adenocarcinoma. Studies suggest that passive smoking (i.e., smoke inhaled from the environment surrounding an active smoker) may be responsible for up to 5% of all lung cancers (Lesmes and Donofrio, 1992; White et al., 1991; Davila and Williams, 1993).

Whether occupational factors increase the risk of cancer development in the nonsmoker is still unclear. The inhalation of asbestos fibers is associated with higher cancer risks for both smokers and nonsmokers. The rate of lung cancer in people who live in urban areas is 2.3 times greater than that of those living in rural areas, possibly implicating air pollution as a risk factor in lung cancer. The exact role of air pollution is still unknown (Cronin, 1993).

The presence of other lung diseases such as pulmonary fibrosis, scleroderma, and sarcoidosis may increase the risk of developing lung cancer. COPD or fibrosis of the lungs inhibits the clearance of carcinogens from the lungs, thereby increasing the risk of alteration of DNA with resultant malignant cell growth (Glover and Maskowski, 1994; Davila and Williams, 1993).

Pathogenesis. The pathogenesis of lung cancer is still unknown. Increasing evidence suggests that a predisposition to lung cancer may be inherited. As mentioned, there is a clear etiologic relationship between cigarette smoking and the development of SCLC (Hinson and Perry, 1993). The effects of smoking include structural, functional, malignant, and toxic changes. DNA-mutating agents in cigarettes produce alterations in both oncogenes and tumor-suppressor genes (Carbone, 1992).

All lung cancers are thought to arise from a common bronchial precursor cell, with differentiation then proceeding along various histologic pathways. Perhaps the histologic changes (thickening of bronchial epithelium, mucous gland hypertrophy, and alveolar cell rupture) that occur more frequently in smokers than nonsmokers predispose the lungs to changes leading to metaplasia and, eventually, carcinoma. As the details of the carcinogenic process are unraveled, one goal is to identify intermediate (preneoplastic) markers of exposure and inherent predisposition that will help assess the risk of lung cancer (Davila and Williams, 1993).

When the cells become so dense that there is almost no cytoplasm present and the cells are compressed into an ovoid mass, the tumor is called *small cell carcinoma* or *oat cell carcinoma*. This type of lung cancer is located centrally, most often near the hilum of the lung. *Squamous cell carcinomas* arise in the central portion of the lung near the hilum, projecting into the major or segmental bronchi. These tumors may be difficult to differentiate from TB or an abscess because they often undergo central cavitation (formation of a cavity or hollow space).

Adenocarcinoma tends to arise in the periphery, usually in the upper lobes at different levels of the bronchial tree. An individual tumor may reflect the cell structure of any part of the respiratory mucosa from the large bronchi to the smallest bronchioles. Because of this, adenocarcinoma refers to a heterogeneous group of neoplasms that have in common the formation of glandlike structures (Rubin and Farber, 1994). Adenocarcinoma is further subdivided into four categories: acinar, papillary, bronchioloalveolar, and solid carcinoma.

Large cell carcinomas are so poorly differentiated that they cannot be classified with the other three categories above and require special diagnostic testing procedures to differentiate from other lung pathology.

Clinical Manifestations. Symptoms of early-stage, localized lung cancer do not differ much from pulmonary symptoms associated with smoking, so the person does not seek medical attention. Symptoms may depend on the location within the pulmonary system, whether centrally located, peripheral, or in the apices of the lungs. Systemic symptoms such as anorexia, fatigue, and weight loss are common, especially with advanced disease.

Small cell carcinoma is most often associated with ectopic hormone production, production of hormones by tumors of nonendocrine origin, or production of an inappropriate hormone by an endocrine gland. Neuroendocrine cells containing neurosecretory granules exist throughout the tracheobronchial tree (MacKay et al., 1991). This phenomenon is important because resulting signs and symptoms may be the first manifestation of underlying cancer. For example, adrenocorticotropic hormone (ACTH) secretion leads to Cushing's syndrome in lung cancer clients with signs and symptoms related to this condition.

Centrally located pulmonary tumors usually obstruct air flow, producing symptoms such as coughing, wheezing, stridor, pneumonia, hemoptysis, and dyspnea. As obstruction increases, bronchopulmonary infection (obstructive pneumonitis) often occurs distal to the obstruction. Centrally located tumors cause chest pain with perivascular nerve or peribronchial involvement that can refer pain to the shoulder, scapulae, upper back, or arm.

The less common peripheral pulmonary tumors often do not produce signs or symptoms until disease progression produces localized, sharp, and severe pleural pain increased on inspiration, limiting lung expansion; cough and dyspnea are present. Pleural effusion may develop and limit lung expansion even more.

Tumors in the apex of the lung called *Pancoast's tumors* occur both in squamous cell and adenocarcinomatous cancers. Symptoms do not occur until the tumors invade the brachial plexus (see Special Implications for the Therapist, this section).

Medical Management

Diagnosis. Most early lung cancers are detected on routine chest film in clients presenting for unrelated medical conditions without pulmonary symptoms. CT scans are routinely done to assess for metastasis to the mediastinum, liver, and adrenals. Less than 1% of lung cancers are detected at an occult stage before radiographic abnormalities occur. Diagnosis is usually established on sputum cytology for participants in a lung cancer detection program or on bronchoscopy in persons presenting with hemoptysis and a normal chest film. Localization of occult lung tumors is done by fiberoptic bronchoscopy which allows examination to the sixth or seventh branch of the bronchial tree (Martini, 1993).

Other routine procedures include evaluation of serum chemistries to look for electrolyte abnormalities (see Chapter 4), especially those associated with paraneoplastic syndrome (see Chapter 7), evaluation of renal and hepatic function, hematologic profiles, and ECG analysis.

Treatment. Surgery with lymph node resection when appropriate, radiation therapy, and chemotherapy are all treatment choices. Surgery is the treatment of choice in early-stage NSCLC and may include wedge resection, segmentectomy, or lobe resection for small peripheral tumors. In more centrally located tumors, lobectomy or pneumonectomy is the treatment of choice.

Surgical resection in the treatment of SCLC is not usually considered and seems most effective for clients in the early stages of SCLC, after chemotherapy (Ginsberg, 1989). For clients with more advanced disease, surgery causes unnecessary risk and stress, with no valid benefits (Cronin, 1993). Laser therapy is a surgical treatment used when the tumor mass is causing nonresectable bronchial obstructions and when accessible by bronchoscope.

SCLC is quite sensitive to radiation therapy, which, in conjunction with chemotherapy, is now routinely administered to those with limited disease (Perry et al., 1989; Pignon et al., 1992). Radiation therapy called intraoperative brachytherapy uses radiation implants as a potentially curative treatment in clients with locally advanced disease. Intraoperative brachytherapy by various techniques delivers higher doses of radiation to the tumor without damage to the normal lung (Nori, 1993).

Systemic brachytherapy with radiolabeled antibodies may be a treatment approach in the future. Combined modality therapy will be the most important area of investigation during the next several years (Hilaris, 1994). Currently, radiation therapy may be used in combination with surgery or chemotherapy to improve treatment outcomes.

Chemotherapy is commonly used in clients treated with surgery or radiation who experience recurrent disease or distant metastasis. The decision to use chemotherapy is made on an individual basis, depending on the client's previous history, current condition, and acceptance of the risks and side effects involved.

In the future, tumor growth may be halted by replacement or substitution of mutated tumor suppressor gene functions or biochemical modulation of oncogene products. New forms of immunotherapy may also be targeted specifically toward mutant oncogenes in cancer cells (Carbone, 1992).

Prognosis. The curability of lung cancer remains poor. The prognosis is also influenced by the stage of the disease at presentation and by the treatment that can be given. Curative treatment requires effective control of the primary tumor before metastasis occurs. Radiation therapy when used alone has been unsuccessful in attaining long-term survival. Chemotherapy is usually combined with surgery or irradiation for more advanced tumors. Once metastasis has occurred, surgical therapy is limited and treatment is palliative.

Currently, with treatment, only 10% to 13% of people with lung cancer survive beyond 5 years after diagnosis (Boring et al., 1994). Survival without treatment is rarely possible, and most untreated persons die within 1 year of diagnosis, with a median survival of less than 6 months. The key to increasing the survival rate is early detection, but by the time the tumor is detectable on chest film (1 cm in diameter), invasion and metastasis usually have already occurred.

Other factors thought to confer poor prognosis include male sex, age greater than 70 years, prior chemotherapy, elevated serum lactic dehydrogenase levels, low serum sodium, and elevated alkaline phosphatase levels (see Tables 35–14 and 35–15) (Hansen et al., 1994; Maurer and Pajak, 1987).

Special Implications for the Therapist **12-21**

LUNG CANCER

Metastasis

Metastatic spread of pulmonary tumors to the long bones and to the vertebral column, especially the thoracic vertebrae, is common, occurring in as many as 50% of cases. Local metastases by direct extension may involve the chest wall and may even erode the first and second ribs and associated vertebrae, causing bone pain and paravertebral pain associated with involvement of sympathetic nerve ganglia. Subsequently, chest, shoulder, arm, or back pain can be the presenting symptom, but usually with accompanied pulmonary symptoms. The client may not associate the musculoskeletal symptoms with the pulmonary symptoms, so the therapist must always remember to screen for medical disease.

Apical (Pancoast's) tumors do not usually cause symptoms while confined to the pulmonary parenchyma, but once they extend into the surrounding structures, the brachial plexus (C8–T1) may become involved presenting as a form of thoracic outlet syndrome (TOS). This nerve involvement produces sharp pleuritic pain in the axilla, shoulder (radiating in an ulnar nerve distribution down the arm), and subscapular area of the affected side, with atrophy and weakness of the upper extremity muscles. Therapy for the TOS is an important part of the palliative treatment for this condition (see also Thoracic Outlet Syndrome, Chapter 34).

Trigger points of the serratus anterior muscle also mimic the distribution of pain caused by C8 nerve root compression and must be ruled out by palpation, lack of neurologic deficits, and possible elimination with appropriate trigger point therapy. Pancoast's tumors may also masquerade as subacromial bursitis (Snider, 1994).

Paraneoplastic Syndromes

Paraneoplastic syndromes (remote effects of a malignancy; see discussion in Chapter 7) occur in 10% to 20% of lung cancer clients. These usually result from the secretion of hormones by the tumor acting on target organs producing a variety of symptoms, most commonly digital clubbing, osteoarthropathies, or rheumatologic disorders such as polymyositis, lupus, and dermatomyositis. Occasionally, symptoms of paraneoplastic syndrome occur before detection of the primary lung tumor or as the first sign of recurrence presenting as a neuromusculoskeletal condition (Goodman and Snyder, 1995).

Chemotherapy and Radiation Treatment

Side effects of chemotherapy, including nausea and vomiting, require careful scheduling of therapy to optimize treatment success. In the presence of cancer pain, pain medication should be timed to allow maximum comfort during therapy (e.g., approximately 30 to 60 minutes prior to therapy).

Loss of appetite with accompanying weight loss may result in muscle weakness and decreased physical endurance requiring more frequent rest periods. The therapist may be able to assist the client with reduced functional status exhibiting other symptoms such as dyspnea and fatigue by teaching diaphragmatic breathing techniques, use of relaxation techniques for overused respiratory accessory muscles, and positioning for easing the work of breathing (e.g., sitting upright leaning forward slightly with elbows resting on knees).

Energy conservation (see Box 7–1) should be addressed by teaching the client to schedule strenuous activities at times of day when energy levels are the highest, alternating strenuous tasks with easier ones, utilizing frequent rest breaks, planning activities to minimize the use of stairs or walking long distances, workload reduction (encourage the client to perform elective tasks, especially household chores, less often and in the sitting position whenever possible) (Hamburgh, 1992).

Other concerns addressed by the therapist may include regaining strength and endurance following chemotherapy or radiation therapy, mobility training for those clients with gait and balance disturbances, instruction for sleeping postures and bed mobility for clients with bone pain from metastasis, and in late-stage cancer, prevention or treatment of contractures or skin breakdown.

DISORDERS OF THE PULMONARY VASCULATURE

Pulmonary Embolism and Infarct

Definition and Incidence. Pulmonary embolism (PE) is the lodging of a blood clot in a pulmonary artery with subsequent obstruction of blood supply to the lung parenchyma. Although a blood clot is the most common cause of occlusion, air, fat, bone marrow (e.g., fracture), foreign intravenous material, vegetations on heart valves that develop with endocarditis, amniotic fluid, and tumor cells (tumor emboli) can also embolize and occlude the pulmonary vessels (Michael, 1990).

PE is common and in the United States the incidence is estimated at approximately 650,000 cases annually. It is the most common cause of sudden death in the hospitalized population (Harruff, 1994).

Etiology and Risk Factors. Three major physiologic risk factors linked with PE are (1) *blood stasis* (e.g., immobilization due to prolonged trips; bed rest, such as with burn cases, obstetric and gynecologic clients; fracture care with casting or pinning; and elderly or obese populations); (2) *endothelial injury* secondary to surgical procedures, trauma, or fractures of the legs or pelvis; and (3) *hypercoagulable states* (e.g., oral contraceptive use, cancer, protein C or S deficiency, and antithrombin-III deficiency).

The most common cause of PE is deep venous thrombosis (DVT) originating in the proximal deep venous system of the lower legs.[13] Other clinical risk factors for PE include congestive heart failure, trauma, age over 50 years, previous history of thromboembolism, malignant disease, infection, diabetes mellitus, inactivity or obesity, pregnancy, clotting abnormalities, and fractures of the hip or femur.

[13] Prior to the introduction of routine prophylaxis with heparin or warfarin sodium (Coumadin), the incidence of DVT following hip fracture, total hip replacement, or other surgeries involving the abdomen, pelvis, prostate, hip, or knee was extremely high (30% to 50%) with 20% of all clients having a clot in the iliofemoral vein (Michael, 1990).

Pathogenesis. Any level of the pulmonary artery, from the main trunk to the distal branches, are sites for emboli to lodge. Each embolus is a cylindrical mass of fresh or organizing thrombus comprised of alternating bands of red cells, fibrin strands, and leukocytes with a rim of fibroblasts at the periphery (Harruff, 1994).

The embolism causes an area of blockage, but actual pulmonary infarction is uncommon due to the dual circulation of the lungs. PE leads to ventilation/perfusion mismatch, which leads to hypoxia, but the pulmonary arteries bringing in oxygenated blood will keep the lungs from infarction. The greater risk is that a clot will embolize to the lung from the popliteal or iliofemoral vein (approximately 50%) or from the calf veins (less than 5%) (Michael, 1990).

Discharge of thrombus into the pulmonary artery with mechanical obstruction of the pulmonary vascular bed causes vasoconstriction, increased pulmonary vascular resistance, pulmonary hypertension, and right ventricular failure (in severe cases).

Clinical Manifestations. Clients may be asymptomatic in the presence of small thromboemboli. The clinical findings in acute pulmonary thromboembolism depend on the size of the embolus and the individual's preexisting cardiopulmonary status. PE as a result of DVT can occur without warning. The DVT can become a thromboembolism by becoming dislodged from the venous wall, traveling through the venous return to the lungs, thus becoming a PE.

A *DVT* may present up to 2 weeks postoperatively as tenderness, leg pain, swelling (a difference in leg circumference of 1.4 cm in men and 1.2 cm in women is significant), and warmth. One exception to this presentation is the person who has been immobilized for a prolonged period of time in a cast. Removal of the cast normally presents with a leg that would measure less in circumference (muscle atrophy) than the uninvolved leg. Equal leg circumference should be a clinical red flag for medical evaluation.

DVT from any cause may be accompanied by a positive Homans' sign (deep calf pain on slow dorsiflexion of the foot or gentle squeezing of the affected calf; see Fig. 10–30), but Homans' sign is not specific for this condition because it also occurs with Achilles tendinitis and gastrocnemius and plantar muscle injury (Jarvis, 1992). Only half the people with DVT experience pain with this test in the presence of a thrombus.

Other signs of DVT may include subcutaneous venous distention, discoloration, a palpable cord (superficial thrombus),[14] and pain upon placement of a blood pressure cuff around the calf (considerable pain with the cuff inflated to 160 to 180 mm Hg). At least half the cases of DVT are symptomatic, but in up to 30% of clients with clinical evidence of DVT, no DVT is demonstrable (Mengert and Albert, 1993).

Signs and symptoms of *PE* are nonspecific and vary greatly, depending on the extent to which the lung is involved, the size of the clot, and the general medical condition of the individual. Sudden death may be the presentation but dyspnea, pleuritic chest pain, and persistent cough are the most common symptoms. Inflammatory reaction of the lung parenchyma or ischemia caused by obstruction of small pulmonary arterial branches causes pleuritic chest pain that is sudden in onset and aggravated by breathing. Other symptoms include hemoptysis, apprehension, diaphoresis, tachypnea, and fever. The presence of hemoptysis indicates that alveolar damage has occurred (Cronin, 1993).

[14] The femoral vein, which is part of the larger deep system of veins, may be palpable along the inner aspect of the thigh extending from the knee to the groin. This is distinguishable from a superficial phlebitis which is usually superficial, localized, and limited in length to a small area.

Medical Management

Diagnosis. PE is difficult to diagnose because the signs and symptoms are nonspecific. PE may mimic pneumonia, myocardial infarction, pneumothorax, and even rib fractures. The physician must also differentiate conditions that can mimic thromboembolism to the calf such as cellulitis, muscle strain or rupture, lymphangitis, and rupture of a Baker's cyst (Stauffer, 1994).

Circumstances such as the onset of chest pain or dyspnea in hospitalized, postsurgical, or trauma cases are highly suspicious of PE. A ventilation/perfusion lung scan, pulmonary angiography, and ECG are used to confirm the diagnosis.

Because the history and physical examination are neither sensitive nor specific in detecting thrombi in the deep veins of the lower extremities, duplex ultrasonography has become the mainstay of diagnosis. Other specific tests such as contrast venography or impedance plethysmography (IPG) may be conducted (Stauffer, 1994).

Treatment. Given the mortality of PE and the difficulties involved in its clinical diagnosis, prevention of DVT and PE is crucial. Primary prevention of DVT through the prophylactic use of anticoagulants is important for persons undergoing total hip replacement, major knee surgery, abdominal or pelvic surgery, prostate surgery, and neurosurgery.

Heparin (anticoagulant) is the most common agent for prophylaxis as it prolongs the clotting time and allows the body time to resolve the existing clot, thereby preventing further development of the thrombus; it does not reduce the immediate embolic risk or enhance clot lysis. Warfarin (Coumadin), an oral anticoagulant, is used simultaneously with heparin or during the transition from intravenous to oral anticoagulant. Prophylaxis and treatment are different (see further discussion under thrombophlebitis, Chapter 10).

Thrombolytic therapy (a controversial, expensive treatment used with massive embolism) to lyse pulmonary thromboemboli in situ is accomplished through the use of streptokinase, urokinase, and recombinant tissue plasminogen activator, which enhance fibrinolysis by activating plasminogen, generating plasmin. Plasmin directly lyses thrombi both in the pulmonary artery and in the venous circulation and has a secondary anticoagulant effect (Stauffer, 1994).

Surgical implantation of a Greenfield filter in the vena cava may be used to prevent PE by filtering the blood and preventing clots from moving past the screen. There is an increased risk of dependent edema as a result of obstruction of the filter with this procedure.

Prognosis. PE is the primary cause of death for as many as 100,000 people each year (perhaps double that amount), and a contributory factor in another 100,000 deaths annually. About 10% of victims die within the first hour, but prognosis for survivors (depending on underlying disease and on proper diagnosis and treatment) is generally favorable. Clients with

PE who have cancer, congestive heart failure, or chronic lung disease have a higher risk of dying within 1 year than do clients with isolated PE (Carson et al., 1992).

Small emboli resolve without serious morbidity, but large or multiple emboli (especially in the presence of severe underlying cardiac or pulmonary disease) have a poorer prognosis. PE may recur despite heparin therapy, most commonly in people with massive PE or in whom anticoagulant therapy has been inadequate (Michael, 1990). PE is the leading cause of pregnancy-related mortality in the United States.

Special Implications for the Therapist **12-22**

PULMONARY EMBOLISM AND INFARCTION

A careful review of the client's medical history may alert the therapist to the presence of predisposing factors for the development of a PE. Although frequent changing of position, exercise, and early ambulation are necessary to prevent thrombosis and embolism, sudden and extreme movements should be avoided. Under no circumstances should the legs be massaged to relieve "muscle cramps," especially when the pain is located in the calf and the person has not been up and about (O'Toole, 1992).

Restrictive clothing, crossing the legs, and prolonged sitting or standing should be avoided. Elevating the legs, bending the bed at the knees, or propping pillows under the knees can produce venous stasis and should be done with caution to avoid severe flexion of the hips, which will slow blood flow and increase the risk of new thrombi (Mengert and Albert, 1993).

After a PE, long-term treatment with an oral anticoagulant such as warfarin continues for 4 to 6 months for those at high risk of recurrence. Long-term use requires careful monitoring for signs of bleeding such as bloody stool, blood in urine, or large ecchymoses. If the person mentions any of these symptoms to the therapist, the client should be instructed to contact the physician immediately. Medications should not be changed without the physician's approval; the use of additional medications, especially over-the-counter preparations for colds, headaches, rheumatic pain, and so on, must be approved by the physician. See also Special Implications for the Therapist: Peripheral Vascular Disease, 10-17, in Chapter 10.

Pulmonary Hypertension

Definition and Incidence. Pulmonary hypertension is high blood pressure in the pulmonary arteries defined as a rise in pulmonary artery pressure of 5 to 10 mm Hg above normal (normal is 15 to 18 mm Hg).[15] Pulmonary hypertension may be *primary* or *secondary*; primary includes elevated pulmonary vascular resistance in the absence of other disease of the heart or lungs.

Primary pulmonary hypertension is rare, usually occurring in women between 20 and 40 years of age (pregnant women have the highest mortality). It may have no known cause (idiopathic) and may be hereditary in isolated cases. Secondary hypertension occurs as a complication of another disease, usually a respiratory or cardiovascular disorder (especially left-sided heart failure in the elderly) (Table 12-17).

Pathogenesis. *(Davey and McCance, 1994)* Primary pulmonary hypertension is characterized by diffuse narrowing of the pulmonary arterioles caused by hypertrophy of smooth muscle in the vessel walls and formation of fibrous lesions around the vessels. What causes these changes is unknown.

Secondary pulmonary hypertension is caused by any respiratory or cardiovascular disorder that increases the volume or pressure of blood entering the pulmonary arteries or narrows or obstructs the pulmonary arteries (see Table 12-17). Increased volume or pressure overloads the pulmonary circulation while narrowing or obstruction elevates the blood pressure by increasing resistance to flow within the lungs.

If hypertension persists, hypertrophy occurs in the medial smooth muscle layer of the arterioles. The larger arteries

TABLE 12-17 Causes of Pulmonary Hypertension

Primary or Idiopathic	Secondary
Altered immune mechanisms	Primary cardiac disease
Silent pulmonary emboli	Congenital (patent ductus arteriosus, atrial septal defect, ventricular septal defect, persistent fetal circulation)
Oral contraceptives	Acquired (rheumatic valvular disease, mitral stenosis,* myxoma, left ventricular failure)
Injection drug abuse	Pulmonary vasoconstriction due to hypoxia
Collagen vascular disease (loss of vessels)	Chronic hypoxia (e.g., chronic obstructive lung disease)
Sickle cell disease	Obesity
	Smoke inhalation
	Valvular heart disease
	High altitude (reactive hypertension)
	Neuromuscular disease
	Sleep apnea syndrome
	Chronic liver disease
	Hypoventilation (persistent or intermittent)
	Reduction of pulmonary vascular bed (must impair 50%-75% of vascular bed)
	Pulmonary emboli*
	Vasculitis
	Widespread interstitial lung disease (sarcoidosis, systemic sclerosis)
	Tumor emboli
	Pulmonary artery stenosis
	Pulmonary venous hypertension

* Most common causes.

Adapted from Smeltzer SC, Bare BG: Brunner and Suddarth's Textbook of Medical-Surgical Nursing, ed 7. Philadelphia, JB Lippincott, 1992, p 585.

[15] There is no definitive set of values used to diagnose pulmonary hypertension, but the National Institutes for Health (NIH) requires a resting mean artery pressure of 25 mm Hg or greater.

stiffen, and hypertension progresses until pulmonary artery pressure equals systemic blood pressure. The result is right ventricular hypertrophy and eventual cor pulmonale.

Clinical Manifestations. Signs and symptoms of secondary pulmonary hypertension are difficult to recognize in the early stages when the symptoms of the underlying disease are more prominent. When pulmonary artery pressure is equal to systemic blood pressure, pulmonary hypertension may be detected. The most common symptoms are fatigue, chest discomfort, tachypnea, cyanosis, and progressive dyspnea, beginning with exercise and later occurring with minimal activity or at rest.

Medical Management

Diagnosis. Sometimes the first indication of pulmonary hypertension is seen on a chest radiograph or ECG. The x-ray study may show rib scalloping (erosion of the inferior aspect of the ribs) from dilation of the arteries supplying the ribs. A reading of left ventricular hypertrophy (LVH) on the ECG report is also indicative of pulmonary hypertension.

The physician must differentiate primary pulmonary hypertension from chronic pulmonary heart disease (cor pulmonale), recurrent pulmonary emboli, mitral stenosis, and congenital heart disease. Exclusion of secondary causes is performed by echocardiography and lung scanning and sometimes by pulmonary angiogram. A chest film will show some characteristic changes such as enlarged main pulmonary arteries with reduced peripheral branches, but is not diagnostic alone. Diagnosis of pulmonary hypertension can only be made with right-sided heart catheterization.

Treatment. Usually treatment includes oxygen therapy to decrease hypoxemia and resulting pulmonary vascular resistance. Digitalis (to increase cardiac output) and diuretics (to decrease intravascular volume and extravascular fluid accumulation) are used for right ventricular failure. Secondary pulmonary hypertension is treated by treating the underlying cause.

Heart-lung transplantation is being used more often for primary pulmonary hypertension with improved results because of the availability of cyclosporin to prevent rejection. Candidates for heart-lung transplants are usually in the advanced stages of the disease with predicted survival at less than 1 year. Usually these individuals have failed to respond to vasodilator drugs. To date, recurrence of the disease has not been reported in a transplant recipient (Rich, 1994).

Prognosis. The prognosis in primary pulmonary hypertension is poor. Some individuals may live 5 to 6 years from the time of diagnosis, but most people have a downhill course over a shorter period of time (2 to 3 years) with a fatal outcome (D'Alonzo et al., 1991). The cause of death is usually right ventricular failure or sudden death; sudden death occurs late in the disease process.

Secondary pulmonary hypertension can be reversed if the underlying disorder is successfully treated. If the hypertension has persisted long enough for the medial smooth muscle layer to hypertrophy, secondary pulmonary hypertension is no longer reversible.

Special Implications for the Therapist **12-23**

PULMONARY HYPERTENSION

Because pulmonary vascular resistance increases dramatically with exercise, clients with pulmonary hypertension must be closely monitored when participating in activities or therapy that requires increased physical stress. Monitor PCWP in anyone with a pulmonary artery catheter (see Special Implications for the Therapist: ARDS). Maintenance of adequate systemic blood pressure is essential and the therapist must be familiar with the medications and potential side effects used, especially if blood pressure is altered pharmacologically. See Appendix B, Guidelines for Activity and Exercise.

Secondary pulmonary hypertension may occur in clients with connective tissue diseases such as scleroderma because the disease affects the vasculature of several organs, including the lungs (pulmonary fibrosis) and kidneys. The arterioles usually demonstrate intimal proliferation with progressive luminal occlusion. The development of hypertension often indicates the onset of an accelerated scleroderma renal crisis. Medical treatment is toward control of the blood pressure.

Cor Pulmonale *(Newman and Ross, 1994)*

Definition and Incidence. Cor pulmonale, also called pulmonary heart disease, is the enlargement of the right ventricle secondary to pulmonary hypertension that occurs in diseases of the thorax, lung, and pulmonary circulation. It is a term that describes the pathologic effects of lung dysfunction as it affects the right side of the heart. Right-sided heart dysfunction secondary to either left-sided heart failure, vascular dysfunction, or congenital heart disease is excluded in the definition of cor pulmonale.

Chronic cor pulmonale occurs most frequently in adult male smokers, although the incidence in women is increasing as heavy smoking in females becomes more prevalent. The actual prevalence of cor pulmonale is difficult to determine because cor pulmonale does not occur in all cases of chronic lung disease and because routine physical examination and laboratory tests are relatively insensitive to the presence of pulmonary hypertension. It has been estimated that cor pulmonale accounts for 5% to 10% of organic heart disease.

Etiology and Risk Factors. Pulmonary vascular diseases and respiratory diseases (e.g., emphysema, chronic bronchitis) are the primary causes of cor pulmonale. Emphysema and chronic bronchitis cause over 50% of cases of cor pulmonale in the United States. When a PE has been sufficiently massive to obstruct 60% to 75% of the pulmonary circulation, acute cor pulmonale can occur, but cor pulmonale can also be caused by COPD.

Cor pulmonale can also develop under conditions of sustained elevations in intrathoracic pressure associated with mechanical ventilation (and PEEP). The intrathoracic vessels narrow leading to reduced cardiac output and possible cor pulmonale. Chronic widespread vasculitis, as occurs in association with the collagen-vascular disorders (e.g., rheumatoid arthritis, SLE, dermatomyositis, polymyositis, Sjögren's syndrome, CREST syndrome accompanying scleroderma), can also cause chronic cor pulmonale. Occasionally, widespread radiation pneumonitis can be the underlying cause of cor pulmonale.

Other (uncommon) causes include pneumoconiosis, pulmonary fibrosis, kyphoscoliosis, pickwickian syndrome, lymphangitic infiltration from metastatic carcinoma, and obliterative pulmonary capillary. The feature common to all these conditions which predisposes to cor pulmonale is hypoxia.

Pathogenesis. As pulmonary hypertension creates chronic pressure overload in the right ventricle, cor pulmonale develops. Normally, the ventricle is a thin-walled (heart) muscle able to meet an increase in volume and pressure, but chronic pressure overload from hypertension causes the tissue to hypertrophy. In the case of acute cor pulmonale due to emboli, loosely adherent, soft, thrombus forms undetected in the veins of the legs or pelvis (phlebothrombosis or thrombophlebitis). The thrombus suddenly breaks loose and lodges at or near the bifurcation of the main pulmonary artery. Whether caused by ventricular hypertrophy or embolic obstruction, there is a marked fall in pressure necessary to drive blood through the compromised vascular bed since the right ventricle is compromised.

Clinical Manifestations. Evidence of cor pulmonale may be obscured by primary respiratory disease and appear only during exercise testing. The heart appears normal at rest, but with exercise, cardiac output falls and the ECG shows right ventricular hypertrophy. The predominant symptoms are related to the pulmonary disorder and include chronic productive cough, exertional dyspnea, wheezing respirations, easy fatigability, and weakness.

Sudden severe, central chest pain can occur caused by acute dilation of the root of the pulmonary artery and secondary to right ventricular ischemia. The person may collapse, often with loss of consciousness, and death may occur within minutes if the thrombus is large and does not dislodge. If the thrombus is small or moves more peripherally in response to pounding on the chest or chest compression during resuscitation, acute cor pulmonale develops rather than sudden death (Sokolow et al., 1990).

Low cardiac output causes pallor, sweating, hypotension, anxiety, impaired consciousness, and a rapid pulse of small amplitude. The specific signs associated with cor pulmonale include exercise-induced peripheral cyanosis, clubbing (see Fig. 12–4), distended neck veins, and bilateral dependent edema (Newman and Ross, 1994).

Medical Management

Diagnosis. Diagnosis is made on the basis of physical examination, radiologic studies, and ECG or echocardiogram, sometimes both. Pulmonary function tests usually confirm the underlying lung disease. Laboratory findings may include polycythemia present in cor pulmonale secondary to COPD.

The diagnosis of acute cor pulmonale may be difficult to confirm in light of the emergency procedures required to manage the acute life-threatening situation. Physical examination may not reveal any specific diagnostic signs and the ECG and chest film may not be diagnostic in the early stages of cor pulmonale.

Treatment. The primary goal of medical treatment is to reduce the workload of the right ventricle. This is accomplished by lowering pulmonary artery pressure as in the treatment of pulmonary hypertension. Oxygen administration, salt and fluid restriction, and diuretics are essential along with treatment of the underlying chronic pulmonary disease.

Surgical removal of embolic material is a controversial procedure performed only when a confirmed diagnosis of massive PE with accessible thrombus in the main pulmonary artery or its branches is available. There is no specific surgical treatment available for most causes of chronic cor pulmonale. Heart-lung transplantation for clients with primary pulmonary hypertension is a proven therapy in the early stages of development.

Prognosis. Since cor pulmonale generally occurs late during the course of COPD/CAL and other irreversible disease, the prognosis is poor. Once congestive signs appear, the average life expectancy is 2 to 5 years, but survival is significantly longer when uncomplicated emphysema is the cause (Massie, 1994). Although cor pulmonale can be caused by obstructive and restrictive lung diseases, restrictive lung diseases have a lower life expectancy once they reach the stage of cor pulmonale.

Special Implications for the Therapist **12–24**

COR PULMONALE

Those people who are bedridden must be repositioned frequently to prevent atelectasis. Breathing exercises should be carried out frequently throughout the day. Diaphragmatic and pursed-lip breathing exercises should be reviewed for anyone with COPD. Teach the client (or family member) how to detect edema in the lower extremities, especially the ankles, by pressing the skin over the shins for 1 to 2 seconds looking for a lasting finger impression. Watch for signs of digitalis toxicity (see Table 10–9), such as complaints of anorexia, nausea, vomiting, or yellow halos around visual images.

Since pulmonary infection exacerbates COPD and cor pulmonale, all health-care workers must practice careful handwashing and follow universal precautions. Early signs of infection (e.g., increased sputum production, change in sputum color, chest pain or chest tightness, fever) must be reported to the physician immediately. Watch for signs of respiratory failure such as change in pulse rate; deep, labored respirations; and increased fatigue produced by exertion.

Collagen Vascular Disease

Collagen vascular diseases, now more commonly referred to as diffuse connective tissue diseases (see Box 10–13), are often associated with pulmonary manifestations, including exudative pleural effusion, pulmonary nodules, rheumatoid nodules in association with coal worker's pneumoconiosis (Caplan's syndrome), interstitial fibrosis, and pulmonary vasculitis.

All of these pulmonary conditions have been associated with rheumatoid arthritis, all except the nodules and pleural effusion have been seen with SLE, and pleuritis and pneumonitis have been observed in Sjögren's syndrome, polymyositis, and dermatomyositis. Pulmonary fibrosis or pulmonary hypertension or both, are commonly part of the clinical picture associated with scleroderma. Polymyalgia rheumatica and temporal arteritis may demonstrate granulomatous inflammation of the pulmonary parenchyma.

Approximately half of clients with SLE develop lung disease, primarily pleuritis, pleural effusion, or acute pneumonitis. Pulmonary involvement may not be evident clinically, but pulmonary function tests reveal abnormalities in many persons with SLE. Lupus pneumonitis causes recurrent episodes of fever, dyspnea, and cough. Interstitial pneumonitis leading to fibrosis occurs in a small proportion of people with SLE; the inflammatory phase may respond to treatment, whereas the fibrosis does not. Occasionally, pulmonary hypertension develops. Rarely are ARDS and massive intra-alveolar hemorrhage fatal pulmonary complications (Hahn, 1994; Orens et al., 1994).

Interstitial lung disease (ILD) can develop before joint involvement becomes evident in rheumatoid arthritis, particularly in men. People with rheumatoid arthritis who are receiving treatment with methotrexate or gold may develop ILD that represents a drug hypersensitivity. Penicillamine therapy in clients with rheumatoid arthritis has been implicated in causing bronchiolitis obliterans (Reynolds, 1994).

Bilateral upper lobe fibrosis may develop late in ankylosing spondylitis. Lung involvement varies in systemic sclerosis, but there is radiographic evidence of pulmonary disease in a majority of clients. Cutaneous scleroderma can involve the anterior chest wall and abdomen, causing restrictive lung function. General dryness and lack of airways secretions cause the major problems of hoarseness, cough, and bronchitis in Sjögren's syndrome and interstitial lung disease is possible. Only 5% to 10% of clients with polymyositis and dermatomyositis develop ILD, but weakness of respiratory muscles contributing to aspiration pneumonitis is common.

DISORDERS OF THE PLEURAL SPACE

Pleurisy

Definition and Etiology. Pleurisy (pleuritis) is an inflammation of the pleura caused by infection, injury (e.g., rib fracture), or tumor. It may be a complication of lung disease, particularly of pneumonia, but also TB, lung abscesses, influenza, SLE, rheumatoid arthritis, or pulmonary infarction (O'Toole, 1992).

Clinical Manifestations. The symptoms develop suddenly, usually with a sharp, sticking chest pain that is worse on inspiration, coughing, sneezing, or movement associated with deep inspiration. Other symptoms may include cough, fever, chills, and rapid shallow breathing (tachypnea). The visceral pleura is insensitive; pain results from inflammation of the parietal pleura. Because the latter is innervated by the intercostal nerves, chest pain is usually felt over the site of the pleuritis, but pain may be referred to the lower chest wall, abdomen, neck, upper trapezius muscle, and shoulder (Berkow and Fletcher, 1992). On auscultation, a pleural rub can be heard (sound caused by the rubbing together of the visceral and costal pleurae).

Pathogenesis. There are two types of pleurisy: wet and dry. The membranous pleura that encases each lung is composed of two close-fitting layers; between these layers is a lubricating fluid. If the fluid content remains unchanged by the disease, the pleurisy is said to be dry. If the fluid increases abnormally, it is a wet pleurisy, or pleurisy with effusion (Fig. 12–14). Inflammation of the part of the pleura that covers the diaphragm is called *diaphragmatic pleurisy* and occurs secondary to pneumonia. When the central portion of the diaphragmatic pleura is irritated, sharp pain may be referred to the neck, upper trapezius, or shoulder. Stimulation of the peripheral portions of the diaphragmatic pleura results in sharp pain felt along the costal margins, which can be referred to the lumbar region by the lower thoracic somatic nerves (Fig. 12–15).

Wet pleurisy is less likely to cause pain because there usually is no chafing. The fluid may interfere with breathing by compressing the lung. If the excess fluid of wet pleurisy becomes infected with formation of pus, the condition is known as purulent pleurisy or empyema. Pleurisy causes pleura to become reddened and covered with an exudate of lymph, fibrin, and cellular elements and may lead to pleural effusion.

In *dry pleurisy*, the two layers of membrane may become congested and swollen and rub against each other, which is painful. Although only the outer layer causes pain, (the inner layer has no pain nerves), the pain may be severe enough to require the use of a strong analgesic.

Medical Management. Treatment is usually with aspirin and time, or if severe and unresponsive, nonsteroidal anti-inflammatory drugs (NSAIDs). Antibiotics may be prescribed for a specific infection. Sclerosing therapy for chronic or recurrent pleurisy may be recommended.

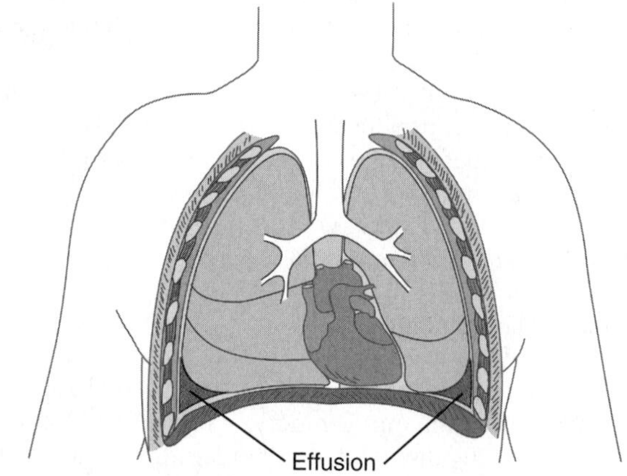

Figure **12–14.** *Pleural effusion*, a collection of fluid in the pleural space between the membrane encasing the lung and the membrane lining the thoracic cavity, as seen on upright x-ray examination. *Pleurisy* (pleuritis) is an inflammation of the visceral and parietal pleurae. When there is an abnormal increase in the lubricating fluid between these two layers, it is called *pleurisy with effusion*.

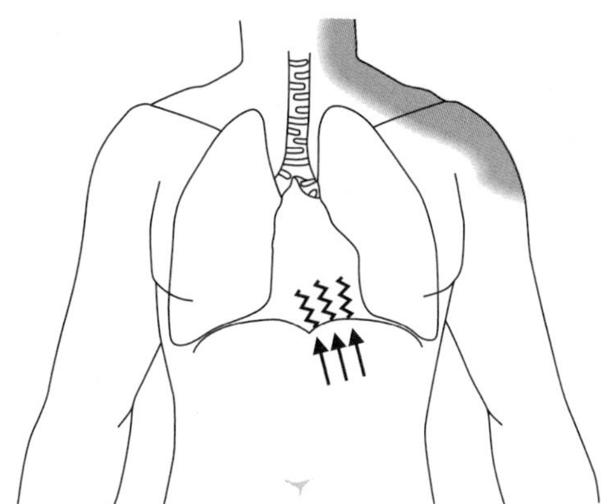

Figure **12–15.** Diaphragmatic pleurisy. Irritation of the peritoneal (outside) or pleural (inside) surface of the central area of the diaphragm refers sharp pain to the neck, supraclavicular fossa, and upper trapezius muscle. The pain pattern is ipsilateral to the area of irritation. Irritation to the peripheral portion of the diaphragm refers sharp pain to the costal margins and lumbar region (not shown).

Special Implications for Therapy **12–25**

PLEURISY

Bed rest is an important part of the care plan for the client with pleurisy. Therapy in the acute care setting should be coordinated to provide as much uninterrupted rest as possible. Breathing and coughing exercises are important but often avoided because of the pain these respiratory movements cause. To minimize discomfort, apply firm pressure with hands or a pillow to the site of the pain during deep breathing and coughing.

Pneumothorax

Definition. Pneumothorax is an accumulation of air or gas in the pleural cavity caused by a defect in the visceral pleura or chest wall. The result is collapse of the lung on the affected side. There are several types of pneumothorax, including spontaneous, tension, open, traumatic, and iatrogenic (Fig. 12–16).

Incidence. Pneumothorax is common, especially with trauma or after medical or surgical procedures that puncture the chest wall. Following chest trauma, both air and blood are likely to escape into the pleural space. This is called hemopneumothorax. Pneumothorax can develop at any age; spontaneous pneumothorax is especially common in healthy adults, usually tall, slender men between the ages of 20 and 40 years.

Pathogenesis. When air enters the pleural cavity the lung collapses and a separation between the visceral and parietal pleurae (see Fig. 12–3) occurs destroying the negative pressure of the pleural space. This disruption in the normal equilibrium between the forces of elastic recoil and the chest wall causes the lung to recoil by collapsing toward the hilum. The result is shortness of breath and mediastinal shift toward the unaffected side compressing the opposite lung. The causative pleural defect may be in the visceral pleura (lung lining) or the parietal pleura (chest wall lining). The pleural space fills with air and the lung becomes atelectatic with collapsed alveolar air spaces.

Spontaneous pneumothorax occurs when there is an opening on the surface of the lung allowing leakage of air from the airways or lung parenchyma into the pleural cavity. Most often this happens when an emphysematous bleb (blister-like formation) or bulla (larger vesicle) or other weakened area on the lung ruptures. The cause of this overdistention and rupture is unknown, and can occur during sleep, at rest, or during exercise. Spontaneous pneumothorax can progress to become a tension pneumothorax.

Tension pneumothorax is a dangerous form of pneumothorax that occurs when air in the pleural space cannot escape through the rupture and cannot regain entry into the bronchus. In tension pneumothorax, the site of pleural rupture acts as a one-way valve, permitting air to enter on inspiration but preventing its escape by closing up during expiration. Under these conditions, continuously increasing air pressure in the pleural cavity may cause progressive collapse of the lung tissue. Air pressure in the pleural space pushes against the already recoiled lung, causing compression atelectasis, and against the mediastinum, compressing and displacing the heart and great vessels. Venous return and cardiac output decrease.

Open pneumothorax occurs when air pressure in the pleural space equals barometric pressure because air that is drawn into the pleural space during inspiration (through the damaged chest wall and parietal pleura or through the parietal pleura and damaged visceral pleura) is forced back out during expiration (Davey and McCance, 1994).

Trauma pneumothorax is a secondary pneumothorax with the entry of air directly through the chest wall or by laceration of the lung caused by penetrating or nonpenetrating chest trauma, such as a rib fracture, stab, or bullet wound that tears the pleura. Bleb or bulla rupture associated with COPD can also introduce air into the pleural space. Other causes of this type of pneumothorax include TB, sarcoidosis, lung abscess, ARDS, and PCP. The pathogenesis is similar to spontaneous pneumothorax.

Iatrogenic pneumothorax develops as a result of direct puncture or laceration of the visceral pleura during attempts at central line placement, percutaneous lung aspiration, thoracentesis, or closed pleural biopsy. Direct alveolar distention can occur with anesthesia, cardiopulmonary resuscitation, or mechanical ventilation with PEEP.

Clinical Manifestations. Dyspnea is the first and primary symptom of pneumothorax, but other symptoms may include a sudden sharp pleural chest pain, fall in blood pressure, weak and rapid pulse, and cessation of normal respiratory movements on the affected side of the chest. If the pneumothorax is large or if there is a tension pneumothorax, it may push the mediastinum toward the unaffected lung, causing the chest to appear asymmetrical. The pain may be referred to the ipsilateral shoulder (corresponding shoulder on the same side as the pneumothorax), across the chest, or over the abdomen.

Clinical manifestations of tension pneumothorax include severe hypoxemia, dyspnea, and hypotension (low blood pressure) in addition to the other signs and symptoms of pneumothorax already mentioned. Increased intrathoracic pressure

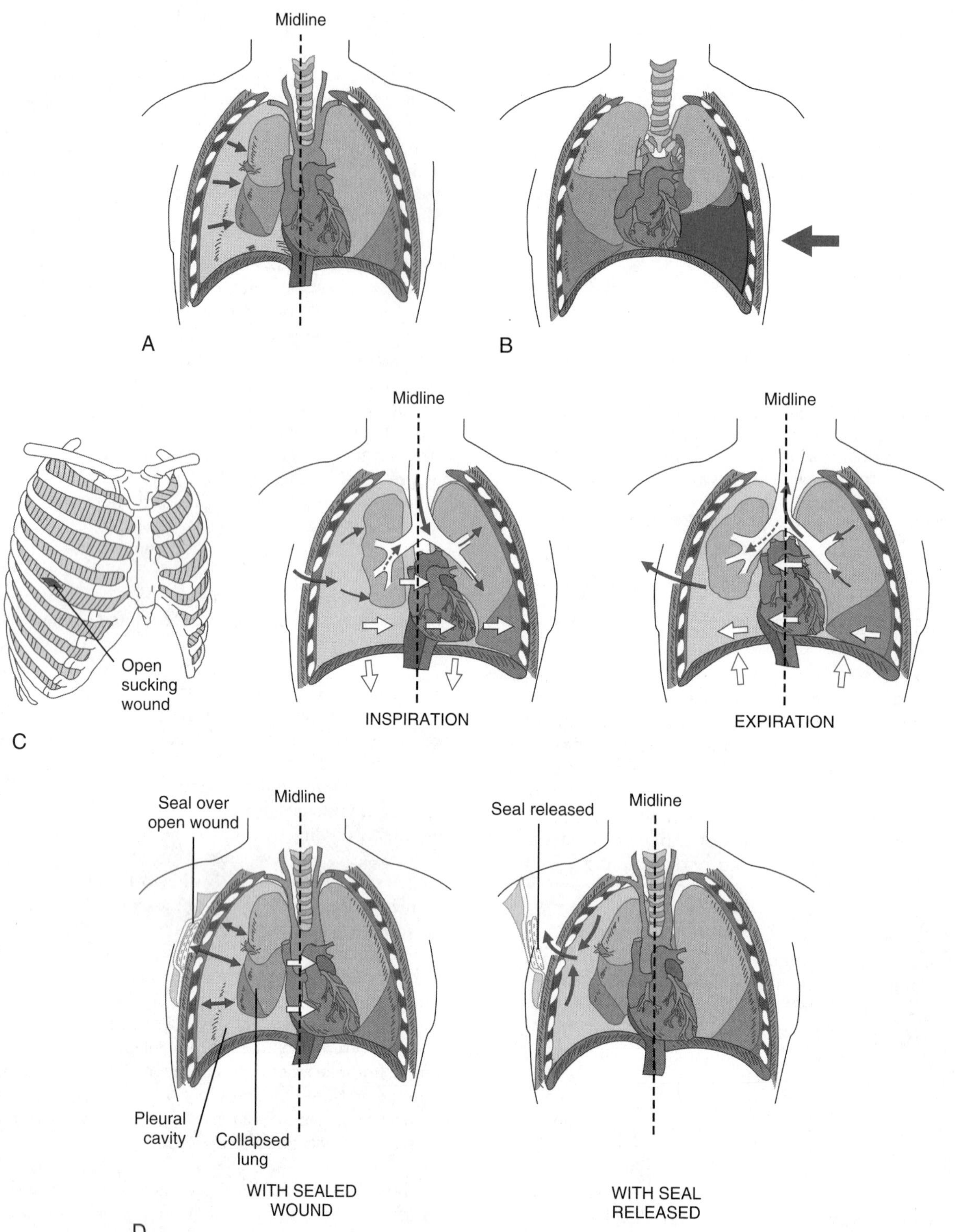

Figure 12–16. *A*, Pneumothorax. Lung collapses as air gathers in the pleural space between the parietal and visceral pleurae. *B*, Massive hemothorax, blood in the pleural space (*arrow*) below the right lung, causing collapse of lung tissue. C, Open pneumothorax (sucking chest wound). *Solid arrows* indicate air movement; *open arrows*, structural movement. A chest wall wound connects the pleural space with atmospheric air. During inspiration, atmospheric air is "sucked" into the pleural space through the chest wall wound. Positive pressure in the pleural space collapses the lung on the affected side and "pushes" the mediastinal contents toward the unaffected side. This reduces the volume of air in the unaffected side considerably. During expiration, air escapes through the chest wall wound, lessening positive pressure in the affected side and allowing the mediastinal contents to "swing" back toward the affected side. Movement of mediastinal structure from side to side is called mediastinal flutter. *D*, Tension pneumothorax. If an open pneumothorax is covered (e.g., with a dressing), it forms a seal, and tension pneumothorax with a mediastinal shift develops. A tear in lung structure continues to allow air into the pleural space. As positive pressure builds in the pleural space, the affected lung collapses, and the mediastinal contents shift to the unaffected side. Tension pneumothorax is corrected by removing the seal (i.e., dressing), allowing air trapped in the pleural space to escape.

from a tension pneumothorax may result in neck vein distention. Untreated tension pneumothorax may quickly produce life-threatening shock and bradycardia.

Medical Management

Diagnosis and Treatment. Diagnosis is made by chest film. There are no specific laboratory tests, but blood gas measurements indicate the degree of respiratory impairment. Depending on the size of the pneumothorax, no specific treatment is required for spontaneous pneumothorax beyond bed rest and the administration of oxygen to relieve dyspnea. Repair or closure of the pleural defect with evacuation of air from the pleural space is rarely necessary, although a chest tube may be inserted.

Emergency aspiration of air (via chest tube) from the pleural cavity is necessary in tension pneumothorax when progressive collapse of the lung tissue occurs. Thoracotomy (incision of the chest wall) is occasionally required to control bleeding, remove large volumes of blood clots, and treat coexisting complications of trauma.

Prognosis. There is a low mortality rate with idiopathic pneumothorax, but a corresponding 15% mortality for pneumothorax associated with underlying lung disease. From 30% to 50% of affected persons experience a recurrence and after one recurrence, subsequent episodes are much more likely (Pierson, 1991). The physiologic events associated with tension pneumothorax are life-threatening, requiring immediate treatment.

Pleural Effusion

Definition. Pleural effusion is the collection of fluid in the pleural space (between the membrane encasing the lung and the membrane lining the thoracic cavity) where there is normally only a small amount of fluid to prevent friction as the lung expands and deflates (see Fig. 12–14). Pleural fluid normally seeps continually into the pleural space from the capillaries lining the parietal pleura and is then reabsorbed by the visceral pleural capillaries and lymphatics.

Incidence and Etiology. The causes of pleural effusions are best considered in terms of the underlying pathophysiology: *transudates* due to abnormalities of hydrostatic or osmotic pressure (e.g., congestive heart failure, cirrhosis with ascites, nephrotic syndrome, peritoneal dialysis) and *exudates*,[16] resulting from increased permeability or trauma (e.g., infection, primary or secondary malignancy, PE, trauma). Any condition that interferes with either the secretion or drainage of this fluid will lead to pleural effusion (Cronin, 1993). Pleural effusion is common with heart failure and lymphatic obstruction due to neoplasm.

Less common causes include drug-induced effusion, pancreatitis, collagen-vascular diseases (SLE and rheumatoid arthritis), intra-abdominal abscess, or esophageal perforation. A person of any age can be affected, but it is more common in the elderly owing to the increased incidence of heart failure and cancer.

Pathogenesis. The most common mechanism of pleural effusion is migration of fluids and other blood components through the walls of intact capillaries bordering the pleura. When stimulated by biochemical mediators of inflammation, junctions in the capillary endothelium separate slightly, enabling leukocytes and plasma proteins to migrate out into affected tissues. Rupture of a blood vessel or leakage of blood from an injured vessel causes a form of pleural effusion called *hemothorax* (see Fig. 12–16) (Davey and McCance, 1994).

Malignancy effusion is usually a local effect of the tumor, such as lymphatic obstruction or bronchial obstruction with pneumonia or atelectasis. Lymphatic blockage from any cause can result in drainage of the contents of lymphatic vessels into the pleural space. It can also be a result of systemic effects of tumor elsewhere, but in either case malignant cells in the pleural effusion of a person with lung cancer indicates an inoperable situation.

Clinical Manifestations. Clinical manifestations of pleural effusion will depend on the amount of fluid present and the degree of lung compression. A small amount of effusion may be discovered only by chest x-ray examination. Large effusions cause clinical manifestations related to their volume and the rate at which they accumulate in the pleural space causing restriction of lung expansion. Clients usually present with dyspnea on exertion which becomes progressive. They may develop nonspecific chest discomfort; sometimes the chest pain is pleuritic, a sharp, stabbing pain exacerbated by coughing or breathing. Other symptoms characteristic of the underlying cause of pleural effusion may be the primary clinical picture (e.g., weight loss and fever with TB or cancer, signs of heart failure).

Medical Management

Diagnosis. Examination of the pleural fluid (diagnostic thoracentesis: surgical puncture and drainage of the thoracic cavity) includes analysis of pH; specific gravity; protein; stains and cultures for bacteria, TB, and fungi; eosinophilia count; and glucose concentration to aid in the differential diagnosis. Chest pain must be differentiated from pain of pericardial or musculoskeletal origin. Chest radiographs and physical examination with possible CT scan are necessary components of the diagnostic process.

Treatment. Treatment may not be required when the individual is asymptomatic, or if only mildly symptomatic, thoracentesis may be all that is necessary. In the case of an underlying disease process (e.g., congestive heart failure or renal pathology associated with transudates), treatment is aimed toward that condition. Drainage of the fluid for exudate-caused effusion provides symptomatic improvement but does not significantly alter lung volumes or gas exchange. Removal of fluid associated with malignancy is considered only if the individual is symptomatic and could benefit from thoracentesis. Repeated thoracentesis is avoided as significant protein loss can occur and the fluid reaccumulates in 1 to 3 days.

Some (exudate) pleural effusions resolve with antibiotic therapy. Recurrent (exudate) pleural effusions may be treated

[16] An *exudate* is a fluid with a high content of protein and cellular debris that has escaped from blood vessels and has been deposited in tissues or on tissue surfaces, usually as a result of inflammation. *Transudate* is a fluid substance that has passed through a membrane or has been forced out from a tissue; in contrast to an exudate, a transudate is characterized by high fluidity and a low content of protein, cells, or solid matter derived from cells.

by pleurectomy (surgically stripping the parietal pleura away from the visceral pleura) and pleurodesis (sclerosing substance introduced into the pleural space to create an inflammatory response that scleroses tissues together). Both of these procedures have negative effects that must be taken into consideration.

Prognosis. Prognosis depends on the underlying disease; in cancer, recurrent pleural effusion may be associated with the terminal stage of disease. Tumor-related effusion generally implies a poor prognosis.

Special Implications for the Therapist **12-26**

PLEURAL EFFUSION

After thoracentesis, encourage deep-breathing exercises to promote lung expansion and watch for respiratory distress or pneumothorax (sudden onset of dyspnea, cyanosis). Prevent chest tube kinking by carefully coiling the tubing on top of the bed and securing it to the bed linen, leaving room for the client to turn. Position changes must be performed carefully to avoid disturbing the surgical site or the chest tube. The therapist may apply firm support with both hands to the surgical site and chest tube area to help lessen muscle pull and pain as the client coughs. If the person has open drainage through a rib resection or intercostal tube, use hand and dressing precautions.

Pleural Empyema

Pleural empyema (infected pleural effusion) is an accumulation of pus that occurs occasionally as a complication of pleurisy or some other respiratory disease, usually pneumonia. It is a normal response to infection but may also occur following external contamination (penetrating trauma, chest tube placement, or other surgical procedure) or esophageal perforation.

Symptoms include dyspnea, coughing, ipsilateral pleural chest pain, malaise, tachycardia, cough, and fever. In addition to chest films, thoracentesis may be done to confirm the diagnosis and determine the specific causative organism. The condition is treated with chest tube drainage, antibiotics, rest, and sedative cough mixtures (O'Toole, 1992). See Special Implications for the Therapist: Pleural Effusion: 12–26.

References

Abrams WB, Beers MH, Berkow R: The Merck Manual of Geriatrics, ed 2. Rahway, NJ, Merck, 1995.

Alland D, Kalkut GE, Moss AR, et al: Transmission of tuberculosis in New York City. An analysis by DNA fingerprinting and conventional epidemiologic methods. N Engl J Med 330:1710–1716, 1994.

American Lung Association: Lung Disease Data 1993. Washington, DC, Author, 1993.

Aminoff MJ: Nervous system. *In* Tierney LM, McPhee SJ, Papadakis MA (eds): Current Medical Diagnosis and Treatment. Norwalk, Conn, Appleton & Lange, 1994, pp 798–854.

Andreoli TE, Bennett JC, Carpenter CC, et al: Cecil Essentials of Medicine, ed 3. Philadelphia, WB Saunders, 1993.

Anthonisen NR, Connett JE, Kiley JP, et al: Effects of smoking intervention and the use of an inhaled anticholinergic bronchodilator on the rate of decline of FEV_1. JAMA 272:1497–1505, 1994.

Arruda S, Bomfim G, Knights R, et al: Cloning of an M. *tuberculosis* DNA fragment associated with entry and survival inside cells. Science 261:1454–1457, 1993.

Bascom R, Kulle T, Kagey-Sobotka A, Proud D: Upper respiratory tract environmental tobacco smoke sensitivity. Am Rev Respir Disease 143:1304–1311, 1991.

Beckett WS: Epidemiology of occupational asthma. Eur Respir J 7:161–164, 1994.

Berkow R, Fletcher AJ (eds): The Merck Manual of Diagnosis and Therapy, ed 16. Rahway, NJ, Merck, 1992.

Bernard GR, Artigas A, Brigham KL, et al: The American-European Consensus Conference on ARDS. Definitions, mechanisms, relevant outcomes, and clinical trial coordination. Am J Respir Crit Care Med 149(3 pt 1):818–824, 1994.

Bisson A, Bonnette P, el Kadi NB, et al. Bilateral pulmonary lobe transplantation. Ann Thora Surg 57:219–221, 1994.

Block AJ: Respiratory disorders during sleep. Part I. Heart Lung 9:1011–1024, 1980.

Boring CC, Squires RS, Tong T, Montgomery S: Cancer statistics, 1994. CA Cancer J Clin 44:7–26, 1994.

Brown M, Kohrt WM: Endurance training of the older adult. *In* Guccione AA (ed): Geriatric Physical Therapy. St Louis, Mosby–Year Book, 1993, pp 201–218.

Brudney K, Dobkin J: Resurgent tuberculosis in New York City: HIV, homeless, and the decline of tuberculosis control programs. Am Rev Respir Dis 144:745–749, 1991.

Cahalin LP, Sadowsky HS: Pulmonary medications. Phys Ther 75:397–414, 1995.

Carbone D: Smoking and cancer. Am J Med 93(suppl 1A):135–175, 1992.

Carson JL, Kelley MA, Duff A, et al: The clinical course of pulmonary embolism. N Engl J Med 326:1240–1245, 1992.

Cartier A: Definition and diagnosis of occupational asthma. Eur Respir J 7:153–160, 1994.

Casaburi R, Patessio A, Loli F, et al: Reductions in exercise lactic acidosis and ventilation as a result of exercise training in patients with obstructive lung disease. Am Rev Respir Dis 143:9–18, 1991.

Cash JM: Does methotrexate cause pulmonary fibrosis? J Musculoskel Med 11:11–12, 1994.

CDC (Centers for Disease Control and Prevention): American Thoracic Society: Diagnostic standards and classification of tuberculosis. Am Rev Respir Dis 142:725–735, 1990.

CDC (Centers for Disease Control and Prevention): Assessing exposures of health care personnel to aerosols of ribavirin—California. MMWR 37:560–563, 1988.

CDC (Centers for Disease Control and Prevention): Asthma—United States, 1982–1992. MMWR 43:952–955, 1995.

CDC (Centers for Disease Control and Prevention): Tuberculosis and human immunodeficiency virus infections: Recommendations of the Advisory Committee for the Elimination of Tuberculosis (ACET). MMWR 38:236–250, 1989.

Chan-Yeung M: Mechanisms of occupational asthma due to western red cedar. Am J Ind Med 25:13–18, 1994.

Chen HI, Kuo CS: Relationship between respiratory muscle function and age, sex, and other factors. J App Physiol 66:943–948, 1989.

Claremont H, Johnson M, Coberly J, et al: Tolerance of short course tuberculosis chemoprophylaxis in HIV-infected individuals. Presented at the Seventh International Conference on AIDS, Florence, Italy, June 1991.

Couser JI Jr, Martinez FJ, Celli BR: Pulmonary rehabilitation that includes arm exercise reduces metabolic and ventilatory requirements for simple arm elevation. Chest 103:37–41, 1993.

Couser JI Jr, Martinez FJ, Celli BR: Respiratory response and ventilatory muscle recruitment during arm elevation in normal subjects. Chest 101:336–340, 1992.

Crapo RO: The aging lung. *In* Mahler DA (ed): Pulmonary Disease in the Elderly Patient. New York, Marcel Dekker, 1993, pp 1–25.

Cronin SN: Nursing care of clients with lower airway disorders. *In* Black JM, Matassarin-Jacobs E (eds): Luckmann and Sorensen's Medical-Surgical Nursing, ed 4. Philadelphia, WB Saunders, 1993, pp 1021–1088.

Cullinan P, Cannon J, Sheril D, et al: Asthma following occupational exposure to *Lycopodium clavatum* in condom manufacturers. Thorax 48:774–775, 1993.

D'Alonzo GE, Barst RJ, Ayres SM, et al: Survival in patients with primary pulmonary hypertension. Ann Intern Med 115:343–349, 1991.

Daniel TM: Tuberculosis. *In* Isselbacher KJ, Braunwald E, Wilson JD, et al (eds): Harrison's Principles of Internal Medicine, ed 13. New York, McGraw-Hill, 1994, pp 710–718.

Davey SS, McCance KL: Alterations of pulmonary function. *In* McCance KL, Huether SE (eds): Pathophysiology: The Biologic Basis for Disease in Adults and Children, ed 2. St Louis, Mosby–Year Book, 1994, pp 1148–1190.

Davila DG, Williams DE: The etiology of lung cancer. Mayo Clinic Proc 68:170–182, 1993.

Dean E: Monitoring systems in the intensive care unit. *In* Frownfelter DL, Dean E (eds): Principles and Practice of Cardiopulmonary Physical Therapy, ed 3. St Louis, Mosby–Year Book, 1996.

Dean E, Hammon WE, Hobson L: Acute medical conditions. *In* Frownfelter DL, Dean E (eds): Principles and Practice of Cardiopulmonary Physical Therapy, ed 3. St Louis, Mosby–Year Book, 1996, pp 469–494.

Dean M, Santis G: Heterogeneity in the severity of cystic fibrosis and the role of CFTR gene mutations. Hum Genet 93:364–368, 1993.

Dekhuijzen PNR, Gayon-Ramirez G, Decramer M: Does corticosteroid treatment affect the respiratory muscles? Eur Respir J 6:465–466, 1993.

Della Bella AM: Snoring eliminated with simple dental appliance. Dental Econ 83:80–81, 1993.

Dooley SW, Castro KG, Hutton MD, et al: Guidelines for preventing the transmission of tuberculosis in health care settings, with special focus on HIV-related issues. MMWR 39:1–29, 1990.

Douglas NJ, Luke M, Mathur R: Is the sleep apnea/hypopnea syndrome inherited? Thorax 48:719–721, 1993.

Drumm ML, Collins FS: Molecular biology of cystic fibrosis. Mol Genet Med 3:33–38, 1993.

Edlin BR, Tokars JI, Grieco MH, et al: An outbreak of multidrug resistant tuberculosis among hospitalized patients with the acquired immune deficiency syndrome. N Engl J Med 326:1514–1521, 1992.

Enzenauer RJ, West SG: Sarcoidosis in autoimmune disease. Semin Arthritis Rheum 22:1, 1992.

Epler GR: Bronchiolitis obliterans and airways obstruction associated with graft-versus-host disease. Clin Chest Med 9:551–556, 1988.

Epler GR, Colby TV, McLoud TC, et al: Bronchiolitis obliterans organizing pneumonia. N Engl J Med 312:152–158, 1985.

Eveloff SE, Rosenberg CL, Carlisle CC, Millman RP: Efficacy of a Herbst mandibular advancement device in obstructive sleep apnea. Am J Respir Crit Care Med 149(4 pt 1):905–909, 1994.

Ferguson GT, Cherniack RM: Management of chronic obstructive pulmonary disease. N Engl J Med 328:1017–1022, 1994.

Filippell MB, Rearick T: Respiratory syncytial virus. Nur Clin North Am 28:651–668, 1993.

Flaskerud J, Ungvarski P: HIV/AIDS, A Guide to Nursing Care, ed 2. Philadelphia, WB Saunders, 1992.

Frownfelter D: Pulmonary rehabilitation. *In* Frownfelter DL: Chest Physical Therapy and Pulmonary Rehabilitation, ed 2. St Louis, Mosby–Year Book, 1987, pp 295–335.

Frownfelter D, Dean E (eds): Principles and Practice of Cardiopulmonary Physical Therapy, ed 3. St Louis, Mosby–Year Book, 1996.

Galantino ML, Bishop KL: The new TB. PT Magazine 2(2):53–60, 1994.

Garfinkel L: Evaluation cancer statistics. CA Cancer J Clin 44:5–6, 1994.

Ginsberg RJ: Surgery and small cell lung cancer: An overview. Lung Cancer 5:232–236, 1989.

Glover J, Maskowski C: Small cell lung cancer: Pathophysiologic mechanisms and nursing implications. Oncol Nurs Forum 21:87–95, 1994.

Goodman CC, Snyder TE: Differential Diagnosis in Physical Therapy, ed 2. Philadelphia, WB Saunders, 1995.

Gottlieb SJ, Garibaldi E, Hutcheson PS, Slavin RG: Occupational asthma to the slime mold *Dictyostelium discoideum*. J Occup Med 35:1231–1235, 1993.

Griffith BP, Magee MJ, Gonzalez IF, et al: Anastomotic pitfalls in lung transplantation. J Thorac Cardiovasc Surg 107:743–753, 1994.

Grubman SA, Fang SL, Mulberg AE, et al: Correction of the cystic fibrosis defect by gene complementation in human intrahepatic biliary epithelial cell lines. Gastroenterology 108:584–592, 1995.

Hagberg JM, Seals DR, Yerg JE, et al: Metabolic responses to exercise in young and older athletes and sedentary men. J App Physiol 65:900–908, 1988.

Hahn BV: Systemic lupus erythematosus. *In* Isselbacher KJ, Braunwald E, Wilson JD, et al (eds): Harrison's Principles of Internal Medicine, ed 13. New York, McGraw-Hill, 1994, pp 1643–1648.

Hamburgh RR: Principles of cancer treatment. Clin Manage 12:37–41, 1992.

Hansen H, Perry MC, Arriagada A, et al: Treatment evaluation: Second IASLC workshop on combined radiotherapy and chemotherapy modalities in lung cancer. Lung Cancer 10(suppl 1):S7–9, 1994.

Harruff RC: Pathology Facts. Philadelphia, JB Lippincott, 1994.

Hayes DR, Sheehan JP, Ulchaker MM, Rebar JM: Management dilemmas in the individual with cystic fibrosis and diabetes. J Am Diet Assoc 94:78–80, 1994.

Heijerman HG: Chronic obstructive lung disease and respiratory muscle function: The role of nutrition and exercise training in cystic fibrosis. Respir Med 87(suppl B):49–51, 1993.

Henry SB, Holzemer WL: Critical care management of the patient with HIV infection who has *Pneumocystis carinii* pneumonia. Heart Lung 21:243–249, 1992.

Hilaris BS: Lung brachytherapy. An overview and current indications. Chest Surg Clin North Am 4:45–53, 1994.

Hinson JA, Perry MC: Small cell lung cancer. CA Cancer J Clin 43:216–225, 1993.

Huebner R, Villarino M, Snider D: Tuberculin skin testing and the HIV epidemic. JAMA 267:409–410, 1992.

Huether SE: Alterations of pulmonary function in children. *In* Huether SE, McCance KL (eds): Pathophysiology: The Biologic Basis for Disease in Adults and Children, ed 2. St Louis, Mosby–Year Book, 1994, pp 1191–1211.

Hughes TA, Wiles CM, Lawrie BW, Smith AP: Case report: Dysphagia and sleep apnoea associated with cervical osteophytes due to diffuse idiopathic skeletal hyperostosis. J Neurol Neurosurg Psychiatry 57:384, 1994.

Jacobs M: Maintenance therapy for obstructive lung disease. How to achieve the best response with the fewest agents. Postgrad Med 95:87–99, 1994.

Janssens S, Decramer S: Corticosteroid-induced myopathy and the respiratory muscles: Report of two cases. Chest 95:1160–1162, 1989.

Jarvis C: Physical Examination and Health Assessment. Philadelphia, WB Saunders, 1992.

Jarvis WR, Bolyard EA, Bozzi CJ, et al: Respirators, recommendations, and regulations: The controversy surrounding protection of health care workers from tuberculosis. Ann Intern Med 122:142–146, 1995.

Jenkinson SG, Levine SM: Lung transplantation. Dis Mon 40:1–38, 1994.

Johard U, Eklund A: Recurrent Löfgren's syndrome in three patients with sarcoidosis. Sarcoidosis 10:125–127, 1993.

Johnson AP: The elderly and COPD. J Gerontol Nurs 14:20, 1988.

Kadakia JK, Collette PM, Sharma OP: Role of magnetic resonance imaging in neurosarcoidosis. Sarcoidosis 10:98–99, 1993.

Kaplan RL, Waite DH: Progressive interstitial lung disease from prolonged methotrexate therapy. Arch Dermatol 114:1800–1802, 1978.

Kee J: Fluid and electrolyte balance. *In* Black JM, Matassarin-Jacobs E (eds): Luckmann and Sorensen's Medical-Surgical Nursing, ed 4. Philadelphia, WB Saunders, 1993.

Kimura I, Takahashi K: Occupational asthma. Nippon Rinsho 3(suppl):398–402, 1994.

Kohrt WM, Malley MT, Coggan AR, et al: Effects of gender, age, and fitness level on response of VO_2max to training in 60- to 71-year olds. J Appl Physiol 71:2004–2011, 1991.

Konstan MW, Byard PJ, Hoppel CL, Davis PB: Effect of high-dose ibuprofen in patients with cystic fibrosis. N Engl J Med 332:848–854, 1995.

Larsen GL, Abman SH, Leland L, et al: Respiratory tract and mediastinum. *In* Hathaway WE, Hay WW, Groothuis JR, Paisley JW (eds): Current Pediatric Diagnosis and Treatment, ed 11. Norwalk, Conn, Appleton & Lange, 1993, pp 466–516.

Leonard JF, Templeton PA: Pulmonary imaging techniques in the diagnosis of occupational interstitial lung disease. Occup Med 7:241–260, 1992.

Lesmes GR, Donofrio KH: Passive smoking: The medical and economic issues. Am J Med 93(1A):38S–42S, 1992.

Levine SM, Anzueto A, Peters J, et al: Single lung transplantation in patients with systemic disease. Chest 105:837–841, 1994.

Lieu TA, Watson SE, Washington AE: The cost-effectiveness of prenatal carrier screening for cystic fibrosis. Obstet Gynecol 84:903–912, 1994.

Liles WC, Ramsey PG: Infectious diseases. *In* Ramsey PG, Larson EB (eds): Medical Therapeutics, ed 2. Philadelphia, WB Saunders, 1993, pp 62–127.

Lloyd-Still JD: Crohn's disease and cystic fibrosis. Dig Dis Sci 39:880–885, 1994.
LoCicero J, Mattox K: Epidemiology of chest trauma. Surg Clin North Am 69:15–19, 1989.
MacKay B, Lukeman JM, Ordonez NG: Tumors of the Lungs. Philadelphia, WB Saunders, 1991.
Makrides L, Heigenhauser GJF, Jones NL: High-intensity endurance training in 20- to 30- and 60- to 70 year old healthy men. J Appl Physiol 69:1792–1798, 1990.
Mal H, Andreassian B, Pamela F, et al: Unilateral lung transplantation in end-stage pulmonary emphysema. Am Rev Respir Dis 140:797–802, 1989.
Mann J, Tarantola DJM, Netter TW (eds): AIDS in the World: A Global Report. Cambridge, Mass, Harvard University Press, 1992, p 162.
Markowitz S: Primary prevention of occupational lung disease: A view from the United States. Isr J Med Sci 28:513–519, 1992.
Marsh DG, Neely JD, Breazeale DR, et al: Genetic basis of IgE responsiveness: Relevance to the atopic diseases. Int Arch Allergy Immunol 107:25–28, 1995.
Martinez FJ, Vogel PD, Dupont DN, et al: Supported arm exercise vs unsupported arm exercise in the rehabilitation of patients with severe chronic airflow obstruction. Chest 103:1397–1402, 1993.
Martini N: Operable lung cancer. CA Cancer J Clin 43:201–213, 1993.
Massery M: Incorporating breathing exercises into physical therapy treatment. Continuing Education Course, 1994. Available from Mary Massery, PT, 3820 Timbers Edge, Glenview Il 60026; (708) 803-0803.
Massery M: The patient with neuromuscular or musculoskeletal dysfunction. *In* Frownfelter DL, Dean E (eds): Principles and Practice of Cardiopulmonary Physical Therapy, ed 3. St Louis, Mosby–Year Book, 1996, pp 679–702.
Massie BM: Cardiovascular disease. *In* Tierney LM, McPhee SJ, Papadakis MA (eds): Current Medical Diagnosis and Treatment, ed 33. Norwalk, Conn, Appleton & Lange, 1994, pp 280–366.
Maurer LH, Pajak TG: Prognostic factors in small cell carcinoma of the lung: A Cancer and Leukemia Group B study. Cancer Treat Rep 71:767–774, 1987.
McLoud TC: Occupational lung disease. Radiol Clin North Am 29:931–941, 1991.
McFadden ER Jr, Gilbert IA: Asthma. N Engl J Med 327:1928–1937, 1992.
Mengert TJ, Albert RK: Pulmonary conditions. *In* Ramsey PG, Larson EB (eds): Medical Therapeutics, ed 2. Philadelphia, WB Saunders, 1993, pp 238–293.
Meredith S: Reported incidence of occupational asthma in the United Kingdom, 1989–90. J Epidemiol Commun Health 47:459–463, 1993.
Michael JR: Pulmonary embolism. *In* Abrams WB, Berkow R (eds): The Merck Manual of Geriatrics. Rahway, NJ, Merck, 1990, pp 451–459.
Miller BA, Ries LAG, Hankey BF, et al: SEER Cancer Statistics Review: 1973–1990. NIH publication no. 93-2789. Bethesda, Md, National Cancer Institute, 1993.
Mitchell J: Nursing in management: Lower respiratory problems. *In* Lewis S, Collier I (eds): Medical-Surgical Nursing, Assessment and Management of Clinical Problems, ed 3. St Louis, Mosby–Year Book, 1992, pp 500–556.
Newman JH, Ross JC: Chronic cor pulmonale. *In* Hurst JW (ed): The Heart, ed 8. New York, McGraw-Hill, 1994, pp 1895–1904.
Nori D: Intraoperative brachytherapy in non-small cell lung cancer. Semin Surg Oncol 9:99–107, 1993.
Norris J (ed): Professional Guide to Diseases, ed 5. Springhouse, Pa, Springhouse, 1995.
Orens JB, Martinez FJ, Lynch JP III: Pleuropulmonary manifestations of systemic lupus erythematosus. Rheum Dis Clin North Am 20:159–193, 1994.
Osborne ML, Vollmer WM, Buist AS: Diagnostic accuracy of asthma within a health maintenance organization. J Clin Epidemiol 45:403–411, 1992.
O'Toole M (ed): Encyclopedia and Dictionary of Medicine, Nursing and Allied Health, ed 5. Philadelphia, WB Saunders, 1992.
Pape HC, Regel G, Borgmann W, et al: The effect of kinetic positioning on lung function and pulmonary haemodynamics in posttraumatic ARDS: A clinical study. Injury 25:51–57, 1994.
Parker SL, Tong T, Bolden S, et al: Cancer statistics, 1996. CA Cancer J Clin 46:5–28, 1996.
Perez-Stable EJ, Hopewell PC: Current tuberculosis treatment regimens: Choosing the right one for your patient. Clin Chest Med 10:323, 1989.
Perry MC, Eaton WL, Propert KJ, et al: Chemotherapy with or without radiation therapy in limited small-cell carcinoma of the lung. N Engl J Med 316:912–918, 1989.
Phillips TJ, Jones DH, Baker H: Pulmonary complications following methotrexate therapy. J Am Acad Dermatol 16:373–375, 1987.
Pierson DJ: Disorders of the pleura, mediastinum, and diaphragm. *In* Wilson JD, Braunwald E, Isselbacher KJ, et al (eds): Harrison's Principles of Internal Medicine, ed 12. New York, McGraw-Hill, 1991, pp 1111–1116.
Pignon J-P, Arriagada R, Ihde DC, et al: A meta-analysis of thoracic radiotherapy for small cell lung cancer. N Engl J Med 327:1618–1624, 1992.
Protas EJ: Physiological change and adaptation to exercise in the older adult. *In* Guccione AA (ed): Geriatric Physical Therapy. St Louis, Mosby–Year Book, 1993, pp 33–46.
Quirce S, Cuevas M, Olaguibel JM, Tabar A: Occupational asthma and immunologic responses induced by inhaled carmine among employees at a factory making natural dyes. J Allergy Clin Immunol 93(1 pt 1):44–52, 1994.
Raffin TA: ARDS: Mechanisms and management. Hosp Pract 22(11):65–80, 1987.
Reynolds HY: Interstitial lung diseases. *In* Isselbacher KJ, Braunwald E, Wilson JD, et al (eds): Harrison's Principles of Internal Medicine, ed 13. New York, McGraw-Hill, 1994, pp 1206–1211.
Rich S: Primary pulmonary hypertension. *In* Isselbacher KJ, Braunwald E, Wilson JD, et al (eds): Harrison's Principles of Internal Medicine, ed 13. New York, McGraw-Hill, 1994, pp 1211–1214.
Riley LW: Drug-resistant tuberculosis. Clin Infect Dis 17(suppl 2): S442–446, 1993.
Rom WN, Travis WD, Brody AR: Cellular and molecular basis of the asbestos-related diseases. Am Rev Respir Dis 143:408, 1991.
Rossaint R, Gerlach H, Falke KJ: Inhalation of nitric oxide—A new approach in severe ARDS. Eur J Anaesthesiol 11:43–51, 1994.
Rubin E, Farber JL: The respiratory system. *In* Rubin E, Farber JL (eds): Pathology, ed 2. Philadelphia, JB Lippincott, 1994, pp 556–617.
Sandoval J, Cicer R, Scoane M, et al: Behavior of the pulmonary circulation at rest and during exercise in miliary tuberculosis. Chest 99:152–254, 1991.
Saric M: Occupational and environmental exposures and nonspecific lung disease—A review of selected studies. Isr J Med Sci 28:509–512, 1992.
Scharf SM: History and physical examination. *In* Baum GL, Wolinsky E (eds): Textbook of Pulmonary Diseases, ed 5. Boston, Little, Brown, 1989, pp 213–226.
Seale DD, Beaver BM: Pathophysiology of lung cancer. Nurs Clin North Am 27:603–613, 1992.
Selwyn PA, Hartel D, Lewis VA, et al.: A prospective study of the risk of tuberculosis among intravenous drug users with human immunodeficiency virus infection. N Engl J Med 320:546–550, 1989.
Shennib H, Massard G: Airway complications in lung transplantation. Ann Thorac Surg 57:506–511, 1994.
Silver RM: Pulmonary manifestations of systemic sclerosis. J Musculoskel Med 7:33–46, 1990.
Silver RM, Metcalf JF, Stanley JH, et al: Interstitial lung disease in scleroderma: Analysis by bronchoalveolar lavage. Arthritis Rheum 27:1254–1262, 1984.
Skobeloff EM, Spivery WH, St Clair SS, Schoffstall JM: The influence of age and sex on asthma admissions. JAMA 268:3437–3440, 1992.
Snider DE, Roper WL: The new tuberculosis. N Engl J Med 332:703–705, 1992.
Snider GL: History and physical examination. *In* Baum GL, Wolinsky E (eds): Textbook of Pulmonary Diseases, ed 5., vol I. Boston, Little, Brown, 1994, pp 243–271.
Sokolow M, McIlroy, MB, Cheitlin MD: Clinical Cardiology, ed 5. Norwalk, Conn, Appleton & Lange, 1990.
Sperling RS, Stratton P: Treatment options for human immunodeficiency virus–infected pregnant women. Obstet Gynecol 79:443–448, 1992.
Spika JS, Fedson DS, Facklam RR: Pneumococcal vaccination: Controversies and opportunities. Infect Dis Clin North Am 4:11–27, 1990.
Stauffer JL: Pulmonary Diseases. *In* Tierney LM, McPhee SJ, Papadakis MA (eds): Current Medical Diagnosis and Treatment, ed 33. Norwalk, Conn, Appleton & Lange, 1994, pp 207–279.

St John RC, Dorinsky PM: Immunologic therapy for ARDS, septic shock, and multiple-organ failure. Chest 103:932–943, 1993.

Sujansky E, Stewart JM, Manchester DK: Genetics and dysmorphology. *In* Hathaway WE, Hay WW, Groothuis JR, Paisley JW (eds): Current Pediatric Diagnosis and Treatment, ed 11. Norwalk, Conn, Appleton & Lange, 1993, pp 906–942.

Suter S: New perspectives in understanding and management of the respiratory disease in cystic fibrosis. Eur J Pediatr 153:144–150, 1994.

Thomas JA, Mcintosh JM: Are incentive spirometry, intermittent positive pressure breathing, and deep breathing exercises effective in the prevention of postoperative pulmonary complications after upper abdominal surgery? A systematic overview and meta-analysis. Phys Ther 74:3–16, 1994.

Tizzano EF, Buchwald M: Cystic fibrosis: Beyond the gene to therapy. J Pediat 120:337–349, 1992.

Travell JG, Simons DG: Myofascial Pain and Dysfunction: The Trigger Point Manual, vol 1. Baltimore, Williams & Wilkins, 1983.

Vollmer WM, Osborne ML, Buist AS: Temporal trends in hospital-based episodes of asthma care in a health maintenance organization. Am Rev Respir Dis 147:347–353, 1993.

Wallace CS, Hall M, Kuhn RJ: Pharmacologic management of cystic fibrosis. Clin Pharmacol Ther 12:657–674, 1993.

Wallace JF: Drowning and near-drowning. *In* Wilson JD, Braunwald E, Isselbacher KJ, et al (eds): Harrison's Principles of Internal Medicine, ed 13. New York, McGraw-Hill, 1994, pp 2479–2480.

Walzer PD: *Pneumocystis carinii* pneumonia. *In* Wilson JD, Braunwald E, Isselbacher KJ, et al (eds): Harrison's Principles of Internal Medicine, ed 12. New York, McGraw-Hill, 1991, pp 799–801.

Weissler JC: Southwestern Internal Medicine Conference: Sarcoidosis: Immunology and clinical management. Am J Med Sci 307:233–245, 1994.

Welsh MJ, Denning GM, Ostedgaard LS, Anderson MP: Dysfunction of CFTR bearing the delta F508 mutation. J Cell Sci Suppl 17:235–239, 1993.

White JR, Froeb HF, Kulik JA: Respiratory illness in nonsmokers chronically exposed to tobacco smoke in the work place. Chest 100:39–43, 1991.

Wiegand L, Zwillich CW: Obstructive sleep apnea. Dis Mon 40:197–252, 1994.

Willes SR, Fitzgerald TK, Bascom R: Nasal inhalation challenge studies with sidestream tobacco smoke. Arch Environ Health 47:223–230, 1992.

Wong DL: Whaley and Wong's Essentials of Pediatric Nursing, ed 4. St Louis, Mosby–Year Book, 1993.

Yerg JE, Seals DR, Hagberg JM, Holloszy JO: Effect of endurance exercise training on ventilatory function in older individuals. J Appl Physiol 58:791–4, 1985.

Zackrison LH, Tsou E: *Pneumocystis carinii:* A deadly opportunist. Am Fam Physician 44:528–541, 1991.

SECTION 2

chapter 13

The Gastrointestinal System

Catherine C. Goodman

The gastrointestinal (GI) tract consists of upper and lower segments with separate functions. The upper GI tract includes the mouth, esophagus, stomach, and duodenum and aids in the ingestion and digestion of food. The lower GI tract includes the small and large intestines (Fig. 13–1). The small intestine accomplishes digestion and absorption of nutrients, whereas the large intestine absorbs water and electrolytes, storing waste products of digestion until elimination.

SIGNS AND SYMPTOMS OF GASTROINTESTINAL DISEASE

Clinical manifestations of GI disease can be caused by a variety of underlying conditions or disorders. The primary condition may be of GI origin, but some GI symptoms are part of a collection of systemic symptoms called *constitutional symptoms* and may be associated with any systemic condition (Table 13–1).

Nausea occurs when nerve endings in the stomach and other parts of the body are irritated and usually precedes vomiting. Intense pain in any part of the body can produce nausea as a result of the nausea-vomiting mechanism of the involuntary autonomic nervous system. Nausea can be caused by strong emotions, but may also accompany psychological disorders, a variety of systemic disorders (e.g., acute myocardial infarction, diabetic acidosis, migraine, hepatobiliary and pancreatic disorders, Ménière's syndrome, and GI disorders), and drugs such as morphine, codeine, excess alcohol, anesthetics, and anticancer drugs.

Vomiting may be caused by anything that precipitates nausea. Complications of vomiting include fluid and electrolyte imbalances, pulmonary aspiration of vomitus, gastroesophageal mucosal tear (Mallory-Weiss Syndrome), malnutrition, and rupture of the esophagus (McQuaid and Knauer, 1994).

Diarrhea (frequent, watery stools) results in poor absorption of water and nutritive elements and electrolytes, fluid volume deficit, and acidosis as a result of potassium depletion (see discussion in Chapter 4). Other systemic effects of prolonged diarrhea are dehydration, electrolyte imbalance, and weight loss. The causes of diarrhea are many and varied (Table 13–2). Drug-induced diarrhea, most commonly associated with antibiotics, may not develop until 6 to 8 weeks after first ingestion of an antibiotic, but if the onset of diarrhea coincides with the use of drugs, it will resolve when the drug is discontinued.

Anorexia, diminished appetite or aversion to food, is a nonspecific symptom that is often associated with nausea, vomiting, and sometimes diarrhea. It may be associated with disorders of other organ systems, including cancer, heart disease, and renal disease (Huether and McCance, 1994). *Anorexia-cachexia*, a systemic response to cancer, occurs as a result of increased metabolic rate caused by the tumor cells and metabolites produced and released by tumor cells into the bloodstream. These effects of tumor cells stimulate the satiety center in the hypothalamus and produce appetite loss, gross alterations of metabolic patterns, and a profound systemic confusion referred to as anorexia-cachexia. A downward spiral of symptoms occurs with appetite loss leading to malnutrition, weight loss, muscular weakness, and a negative nitrogen balance that contributes to the development of cachectic wasting (O'Toole, 1992).

Constipation is a condition in which fecal matter is too hard to pass easily or in which bowel movements are so infrequent that discomfort and other symptoms interfere with daily activities. Constipation may occur as a result of many other factors such as diet, dehydration (including lack of fluid intake), side effects of medication, acute or chronic diseases of the digestive system, inactivity or prolonged bed rest, emotional stress, personality, and lack of exercise (Table 13–3). Although constipation is often described as a condition of old age, it is probably caused by lifestyle factors rather than physiologic decline. Lifelong bowel habits, current diet, lack of fluid intake, and immobility are likely causes of constipation in the elderly (Shamburek and Farrar, 1990).

Dysphagia (difficulty swallowing) may be caused by neurologic conditions, local trauma and muscle damage (including physical assault), or mechanical obstruction. Obstruction may be *intrinsic*, originating in the wall of the esophageal lumen (e.g., tumors, strictures, outpouchings called diverticular herniations), or *extrinsic*, outside the esophageal lumen, such as a tumor or swelling that prevents the passage of food.

Achalasia is a failure to relax the smooth muscle fibers of the GI tract. This especially occurs as a result of failure of the lower esophageal sphincter to relax normally with swallowing. The affected person reports a feeling of fullness in the sternal region and progressive dysphagia. Although the cause of achalasia is not known, the loss or absence of ganglion cells in the myenteric plexus[1] of the esophagus appears to be a part of the cause. Anxiety and emotional tension aggravate the condition and precipitate the attacks. As the condition progresses, there is a dilation of the esophagus above the constriction and loss of peristalsis in the lower two thirds of the esophagus.

Heartburn, dyspepsia, pyrosis, or indigestion, a burning sensation in the esophagus usually felt in the midline below the sternum in the region of the heart, is often a symptom

[1] The myenteric plexus is the nerve plexus lying in the muscular layers of the esophagus, stomach, and intestines.

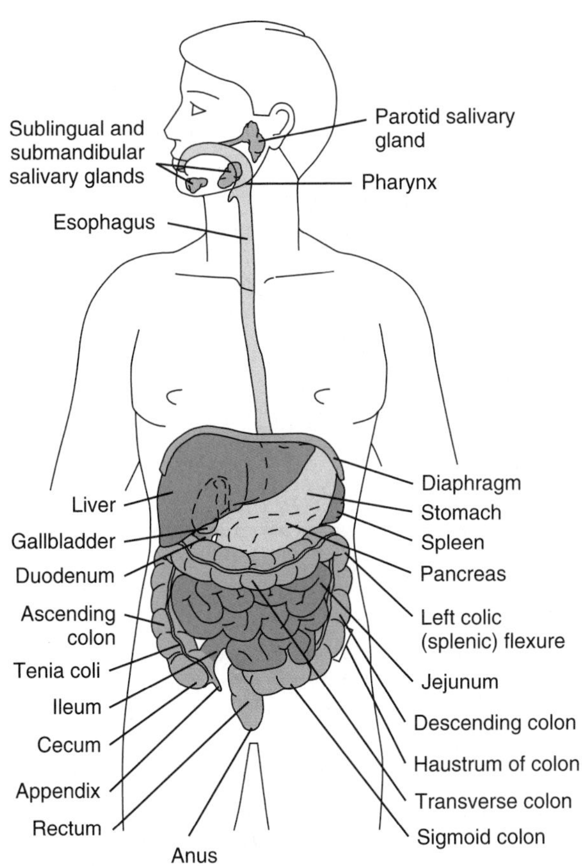

Figure **13-1.** The digestive system.

TABLE 13-1 CLINICAL MANIFESTATIONS OF GASTROINTESTINAL DISEASE

GASTROINTESTINAL SIGNS AND SYMPTOMS	CONSTITUTIONAL SYMPTOMS
Nausea and vomiting	Nausea
Diarrhea	Vomiting
Anorexia	Diarrhea
Constipation	Malaise
Dysphagia	Fatigue
Achalasia	Fever
Heartburn	Night sweats
Abdominal pain	Pallor
Gastrointestinal bleeding	Diaphoresis
Hematemesis	Dizziness
Melena	
Hematochezia	
Fecal incontinence	

of indigestion and occurs when acidic contents of the stomach move backward or regurgitate into the esophagus. The presence of a hiatal hernia, ingestion of certain foods,[2] drugs such as alcohol and aspirin, and movements such as lifting, stooping, or bending over after a large meal may bring on heartburn. Indigestion can also be a potential manifestation of angina associated with coronary artery disease (see Chapter 10).

Emotional stress can stimulate the vagus nerve, which controls the secretory and motility functions of the stomach. Stimulation of this cranial nerve causes the stomach to churn, increases the flow of various gastric juices, and causes contraction and spasm of the pylorus (opening of the stomach into the duodenum). If some of the stomach contents are displaced into the esophagus during this nervous activity, heartburn can occur (O'Toole, 1992).

Abdominal pain accompanies a large number of GI diseases and may be mechanical, inflammatory, ischemic (Table 13–4), or referred. *Mechanical pain* occurs by stretching the wall of a hollow organ or the capsule of a solid organ. *Inflammatory pain* occurs via the release of mediators such as prostaglandins, histamine, and serotonin or bradykinin stimulating sensory nerve endings. *Ischemic pain* occurs as tissue metabolites are released in the area of diminished blood flow (Andreoli et al., 1993). *Referred pain* is usually well localized and may be associated with hyperalgesia and muscle guarding (Auch, 1983; Fields and Martin, 1994). Pain from the spine can also be referred to the abdomen, usually as a result of nerve root irritation or compression. This type of neuromusculoskeletal pain referred to the abdomen is characteristically associated with hyperesthesia over the involved spinal dermatomes and is intensified by motions such as coughing, sneezing, or straining (Silen, 1994).

GI bleeding may be characterized by coffee-ground emesis (blood that has been in contact with hydrochloric acid), hematemesis (vomiting of bright-red blood), melena (black, tarry stools), hematochezia (bleeding from the rectum, or maroon-colored stools), depending on the location of the lesion. Bleeding may not be clinically obvious to the client and may only be diagnosed by a hemoccult test.

The major causes of upper GI bleeding in the therapy population are erosive gastritis common in (1) severely ill people with major trauma or systemic illness, burns, or head injury; (2) peptic ulcers; (3) nonsteroidal anti-inflammatory drugs (NSAIDs) such as aspirin or ibuprofen; and (4) chronic alcohol use. Drugs such as warfarin, heparin, and aspirin used as anticoagulants in the treatment of pulmonary emboli, venous thrombus, or valvular abnormalities do not "cause" gastric erosion and subsequent bleeding but can exacerbate bleeding already present.

Accumulation of blood in the GI tract is irritating and increases peristalsis, causing nausea, vomiting, or diarrhea. The digestion of proteins originating from massive upper GI bleeding is reflected by an increase in blood urea nitrogen (BUN) (see Table 35–11) (Huether and McCance, 1994). Other complications include fatigue, postural hypotension, tachycardia, weakness, or shortness of breath on exertion. Slow, chronic blood loss may result in iron deficiency anemia.

Fecal incontinence (inability to control bowel movements) has both psychological and physiologic contributing factors.

[2] Certain foods act as muscle relaxants. For example, chocolate contains four substances that can relax the lower esophageal sphincter: caffeine, theobromine, theophylline, and fat. Fat-rich foods lower sphincter muscle pressure by release of cholecystokinin from the upper intestinal mucosa. Fat also delays emptying of the stomach, giving more opportunity for this effect to occur. Other implicated foods include spicy and highly seasoned foods, onions, alcohol, peppermint, and spearmint.

TABLE 13-2 CAUSES OF DIARRHEA

MALABSORPTION	NEUROMUSCULAR	MECHANICAL	INFECTIOUS/ INFLAMMATORY	NONSPECIFIC
Pancreatitis	Irritable bowel syndrome	Incomplete obstruction	Viral	Crohn's disease
Pancreatic carcinoma	Diabetic enteropathy	Neoplasm	Bacterial	Ulcerative colitis
Crohn's disease	Hyperthyroidism	Adhesions	Parasitic	Diverticulitis
	Caffeine	Stenosis	Protozoal (*Giardia*)	Diet
		Fecal impaction	Pelvic inflammation	Laxative abuse
		Muscular incompetence		Food allergy
		Postsurgical effect		Antibiotics
		Ileal bypass		Lactose intolerance
		Gastrectomy		Food additives
		Intestinal resection		Food poisoning
		Cholecystectomy		Heavy metal poisoning
		Diverticulitis		Drugs containing magnesium and sorbitol

Adapted from Blacklow RS (ed): MacBryde's Signs and Symptoms, ed 6. Philadelphia: JB Lippincott, 1983, p 381.

Psychological factors include anxiety, confusion, disorientation, and depression. The most commonly observed physiologic causes seen in a therapy practice are neurologic sensory and motor impairment (e.g., stroke and spinal cord injury); anal distortion secondary to traumatic childbirth, sexual assault, hemorrhoids and hemorrhoidal surgery; altered levels of consciousness; and severe diarrhea.

Special Implications for the Therapist **13-1**

SIGNS AND SYMPTOMS OF GASTROINTESTINAL DISEASE

Body fluid loss associated with weight loss, excessive perspiration, or chronic diarrhea and vomiting may cause an imbalance in the body chemistry called an

TABLE 13-3 CAUSES OF CONSTIPATION

NEUROGENIC	MUSCULAR	MECHANICAL	RECTAL LESIONS	DRUGS/DIET
Central nervous system lesions	Amyloidosis	Bowel obstruction	Anal fissure	Analgesics
Cord tumors	Atony	Extra-alimentary tumors	Hemorrhoids	Anesthetic agents
Cortical, voluntary, or involuntary evacuation	Dermatomyositis	Pregnancy	Perirectal abscess	Antacids containing aluminum or calcium
Multiple sclerosis	Duchenne's muscular dystrophy	Colostomy	Rectocele	Anticholinergics
Tabes dorsalis	Hypercalcemia		Stenosis	Anticonvulsants
Traumatic spinal cord lesions	Hyperparathyroidism		Ulcerative proctitis	Antidepressants
	Hypothyroidism			Antihistamines
	Inactivity			Antipsychotics
	Metabolic defects			Barium sulfate
	Potassium depletion			Diuretics
	Severe malnutrition			Hypotensives
	Systemic sclerosis			Iron compounds
				Lack of dietary bulk
				Monoamine oxidase inhibitors
				Myocardial infarction (narcotics for pain control)
				Narcotics
				Opiates
				Parkinson's disease (drugs for)
				Psychotherapeutic drugs
				Renal failure (fluid restriction, phosphate binders)

Adapted from Blacklow RS (ed): MacBryde's Signs and Symptoms, ed 6. Philadelphia, JB Lippincott, 1983, p 378; and Devroede G: Constipation. *In* Sleisenger MH, Fordtran JS (eds): Gastrointestinal Disease, ed 5. Philadelphia, WB Saunders, 1993, pp 837–847.

TABLE 13-4 Causes of Abdominal Pain

Intra-abdominal

Generalized Peritonitis

- Perforated viscus: peptic ulcer
- Primary bacterial peritonitis
  - Pneumococcal
  - Streptococcal
  - Enteric bacillus
  - Tuberculosis
- Nonbacterial peritonitis
  - Ruptured ovarian cyst
  - Ruptured follicle cyst

Localized Peritonitis*

- Appendicitis
- Cholecystitis
- Peptic ulcer
- Regional enteritis (Crohn's disease)
- Colitis: ulcerative, amebic, bacterial
- Abdominal abscess
  - Postoperative
  - Hepatic
  - Pancreatic
  - Splenic
  - Diverticular
  - Tubo-ovarian
- Pancreatitis
- Hepatitis: viral, toxic
- Pelvic inflammatory disease
- Endometriosis
- Lymphadenitis

Pain from Increased Visceral Tension

- Intestinal obstruction
  - Adhesions
  - Hernia
  - Tumor
  - Fecal impaction
- Intestinal hypermotility
  - Irritable colon
  - Gastroenteritis
- Biliary obstruction
  - Gallstone
  - Stricture
  - Tumor
  - Parasites
- Ureteral obstruction: calculi (kidney stones)
- Hepatic capsule distention
  - Acute hepatitis (toxic or viral)
  - Common duct obstruction
  - Budd-Chiari syndrome
- Renal capsule distention
  - Pyelonephritis
  - Ureteral obstruction
- Uterine obstruction
  - Neoplasm
  - Pregnancy/childbirth
- Ruptured ectopic pregnancy
- Rupturing arterial aneurysm
  - Aortic
  - Iliac
  - Visceral

Retroperitoneal Neoplasms

Ischemia

- Intestinal angina or infarction
  - Arterial stenosis
  - Embolism
  - Polyarteritis
- Splenic infarction
- Torsion
  - Gallbladder
  - Spleen
  - Ovarian cyst
  - Testicle
  - Appendix
- Hepatic infarction: toxemia
- Tissue necrosis: uterine fibroid, hepatoma

Extra-abdominal

Thoracic

- Pneumonitis
- Pulmonary embolism
- Pneumothorax
- Empyema
- Myocardial ischemia
- Myocarditis
- Endocarditis
- Esophagitis
- Esophageal spasm
- Esophageal rupture

Neurogenic

- Radiculitis
  - Spinal cord tumors
  - Peripheral nerve tumors
  - Spinal arthritis
  - Herpes zoster
- Tabes dorsalis

Metabolic

- Uremia
- Diabetes mellitus
- Porphyria
- Acute renal insufficiency

Hematologic

- Sickle cell anemia
- Hemolytic anemia

Miscellaneous

- Muscular contusion
- Hematoma
- Tumor
- Toxins
  - Hypersensitivity reactions
  - Insect bites
  - Reptile venoms
  - Drugs
  - Lead poisoning

* Many types of local peritonitis may become generalized by rupture into the free peritoneal cavity.

Modified from Sleisenger MH, Fordtran JS (eds): Gastrointestinal Disease, ed 5. Philadelphia, WB Saunders, 1993, p 155.

electrolyte imbalance and may cause orthostatic changes in blood pressure (i.e., postural drops in blood pressure). Electrolyte changes often include decreased potassium which alters the sodium-potassium pump necessary for normal muscle function (contraction and relaxation). Muscle cramping occurs, which increases a person's risk for musculoskeletal injury during exercise.

The maintenance of arterial pressure during upright posture depends on adequate blood volume, an unimpaired venous return, and an intact sympathetic nervous system. Significant postural hypotension often reflects extracellular fluid volume depletion as occurs with excessive body fluid loss. Monitoring vital signs and observing for accompanying symptoms will promote safe and effective exercise for anyone with the potential for electrolyte imbalance. See discussion in Chapter 4; see also Appendix B: Guidelines for Activity and Exercise.

During an upper quadrant screening, the therapist usually inquires whether the client has difficulty swallowing. Forward head posture or anterior disk protrusion may be a possible cause of difficulty swallowing, but a pathologic condition of the esophagus may be the cause.

GI bleeding can be reduced with regular exercise and people with limited physical activity (e.g., physical disability) are at greater risk for severe GI bleeding (Pahor et al., 1994a and b). An acute ulcer can present as thoracolumbar junction pain. Back pain caused by GI bleeding and perforation associated with an ulcer of long standing may cause painful biomechanical changes in muscular contractions and spinal movement

(Rose and Rothstein, 1982). The clinical presentation may be one with objective musculoskeletal findings to support a diagnosis of back dysfunction when, in fact, the symptoms may be associated with GI bleeding. See also Special Implications for the Therapist: Anemias: 11–3.

People with mechanical low back pain may develop constipation as a result of muscle guarding and splinting that causes reduced bowel motility. Pressure on sacral nerves from stored fecal content may cause an aching discomfort in the sacrum, buttocks, or thighs (Goodman and Snyder, 1995).

Pain in the left shoulder caused by free air or blood in the abdominal cavity is called *Kehr's sign* and may occur with perforation of viscus (e.g., stomach ulcer, diverticular disease), following laparoscopy* (lasting 24 to 48 hours), or rupture of the spleen. Any precipitating trauma or injury, such as a sharp blow during an athletic event, a fall, assault, or automobile accident, may elicit Kehr's sign.

* Laparoscopy, the visual inspection of the peritoneal cavity using an instrument called an endoscope, or other abdominal surgical procedures that introduce air into the abdominal cavity, place pressure on the diaphragm causing shoulder pain (see Fig. 12–15).

AGING AND THE GASTROINTESTINAL SYSTEM

Age-related changes in GI function begin before the age of 50 years. Oral changes may include tooth enamel and dentin wear increasing tooth decay, causing periodontal disease and subsequent tooth loss; and decreased taste buds and diminished sense of smell resulting in altered sense of taste. These oral and sensory changes eventually depress the appetite and make eating less pleasurable. Salivary secretion decreases contribute to dry mouth and when complicated by tooth decay or loss, chewing food and swallowing become more difficult (Abrams et al., 1995; Huether, 1994).

Changes within the alimentary tract include decreases in gastric motility, blood flow, nutrient absorption, and volume and acid content of gastric juice. These changes slow gastric digestion and emptying. Proteins, fats, and minerals, including iron and calcium, and vitamins are absorbed more slowly and in lesser amounts, and carbohydrates are absorbed more slowly.

A decrease in hydrochloric (gastric) acid causes a decrease in the absorption of iron and vitamin B_{12} and leads to an increase in bacteria. Increased bacteria in the gut can lead to diarrhea and infection. Intrinsic factor (IF), a glycoprotein, plays an important role in the absorption of vitamin B_{12}. Decrease in iron and IF deficiency resulting in vitamin B_{12} deficiency may lead to pernicious anemia.

In addition to the effects of aging on the GI system, changes in other organ systems (e.g., endocrine, cardiovascular, and nervous systems) can also affect GI structure and function producing many variations in presentation of illness. Extraintestinal disorders, such as diabetes and the neurologic and vascular changes that occur with age, have a greater effect on the GI tract than the natural process of aging.

Constipation, incontinence, and diverticular disease are the GI problems most commonly seen in elderly people, but each of these disorders has many different underlying causes, and the specific pathogenesis dictates treatment.

THE ESOPHAGUS

Hiatal Hernia

Overview and Definition. A hiatal or diaphragmatic hernia occurs when the cardiac (lower esophageal) sphincter becomes enlarged, allowing the stomach to pass through the diaphragm into the thoracic cavity (Fig. 13–2). Hernias are either *congenital*, resulting from a failure of formation or fusion of the multiple developmental components of the diaphragm,

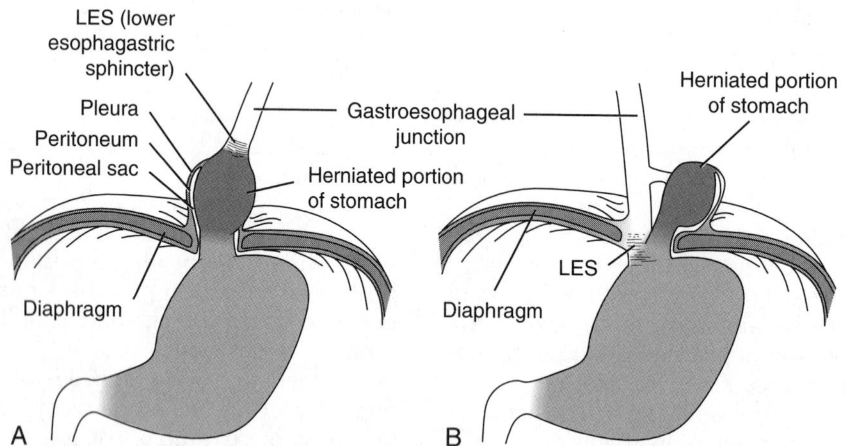

Figure **13–2.** A, Sliding hiatal hernia. Ninety percent of esophageal hiatal hernias are sliding hernias. The stomach and gastroesophageal junction are displaced upward into the thorax (i.e., the stomach and gastroesophageal junction slide up into the thoracic cavity, following the usual path of the esophagus through an enlarged hiatal opening in the diaphragm). *B*, Rolling hiatal hernia. The remaining hiatal hernias are rolling or paraesophageal hernias. The gastroesophageal junction stays below the diaphragm, but all or part of the stomach pushes through into the thorax.

or *acquired,* as a result of penetrating wounds, particularly stab wounds and gunshot wounds; blunt trauma, as occurs in motor vehicle accidents; and less commonly as a result of surgical trauma, empyema, and subphrenic abscess (Harford and McArthur, 1993).

Incidence. Hiatal hernia, be it symptomatic or asymptomatic, is common and the incidence has been estimated as 5 per 1000. The incidence increases with age and may be as high as 60% in people over 60 years of age. Women are affected more often than men and children may have the sliding type, but do not usually exhibit symptoms until they reach middle age (Ruder, 1993b).

Etiology and Risk Factors. As an acquired condition, there are multiple causes and risk factors for the development of hiatal hernia. Anything that weakens the diaphragm muscle or alters the hiatus (the opening in the diaphragm for the passage of the esophagus) and increases intra-abdominal pressure can predispose a person to hiatal hernia. Muscle weakness can be congenital, caused by aging, trauma, surgery, or anything that increases intra-abdominal pressure (Box 13–1).

Pathogenesis and Clinical Manifestations. As part of the stomach herniates through a weakness in the diaphragm, regurgitation and motor impairment result causing the major clinical manifestations associated with this type of hernia. Symptoms vary depending on the type of hernia present and increase in the presence of tight, constrictive clothing or if the person is in a recumbent position.

A sliding hernia may produce heartburn 30 to 60 minutes after a meal, especially if the person is lying down or sleeping in the supine position. Large sliding hernias with reflux may be associated with substernal pain. Rolling hernias are not subject to altered pressure or the resulting reflux, but the person may complain of difficult and painful swallowing.

Medical Management

Diagnosis, Treatment, and Prognosis. Hiatal hernias may be diagnosed by a barium swallow with fluoroscopy, showing the position of the stomach in relation to the diaphragm. This test is not always definitive because the hernia may slide down when the person is placed in the upright position for the radiograph. The primary treatment remains symptomatic control through the use of antacids and elevating the head of the bed. Treatment is essentially the same for gastroesophageal reflux disease (GERD) including histamine H_2-receptor antagonists (see under Gastroesophageal Reflux Disease, this chapter) and the use of sucralfate (Carafate), a GI agent with a coat to protect the stomach. The prognosis is good overall with recurrences expected.

BOX **13–1**
Causes of Increased Intra-abdominal Pressure

- Lifting
- Straining
- Bending over
- Prolonged sitting or standing
- Chronic or forceful cough
- Pregnancy
- Ascites
- Obesity
- Congestive heart failure
- Low fiber diet
- Constipation
- Delayed bowel movement

Special Implications for the Therapist **13–2**

HIATAL HERNIA

For any client with a known hiatal hernia, the flat supine position and any exercises requiring the Valsalva maneuver (which increases intra-abdominal pressure) should be avoided during treatment.

Postoperatively (after surgical repair of the hernia using the thoracic approach), the client may have chest tubes in place requiring careful observation of the tubes during turning and repositioning and chest physical therapy to prevent pulmonary complications.

Prior to discharge, the client must be warned against activities that cause increased intra-abdominal pressure and given safe lifting instructions. A slow return to function over the next 6 to 8 weeks is advised.

Gastroesophageal Reflux Disease

Definition. GERD, or esophagitis, may be defined as an inflammation of the esophagus, which may be the result of reflux (backward flow) of gastric juices, infections, chemical irritants, involvement by systemic diseases, or physical agents such as radiation and nasogastric intubation (Harruff, 1994). Reflux esophagitis is the most common type, with backward or return flow of the stomach and duodenal contents into the esophagus.

Other types of esophagitis, such as infectious esophagitis, may occur with immunosuppression due to viral, bacterial, fungal, or parasitic organisms. Chemical esophagitis is usually a result of accidental poisoning in children or attempted suicide in adults. External irradiation for the treatment of thoracic cancers may include portions of the esophagus and lead to esophagitis and stricture (Rubin and Farber, 1994).

Incidence and Etiology. Although any age can be affected, this condition has an increasing incidence with increasing age. It is estimated that 10% of the population has daily symptoms of GERD and as much as one third of the population has monthly symptoms (Castell, 1986; McQuaid and Knauer, 1994).

A reduction in the pressure of the lower esophageal sphincter (LES), increased gastric pressure, or gastric contents located near the gastroesophageal junction can contribute to the development of esophageal reflux (Table 13–5) (Goyal, 1994). Reflux is often associated with a sliding hiatal hernia, also called a diaphragmatic hernia (see Fig. 13–2). Smooth muscle relaxants used for cardiac conditions, such as β-adrenergics, aminophylline, nitrates, and calcium channel blockers may contribute to incompetence of the LES.

Pathogenesis. Normally, a high-pressure zone exists around the gastroesophageal sphincter which permits the pas-

TABLE 13-5 CAUSES OF GASTROESOPHAGEAL REFLUX DISEASE

DECREASED PRESSURE OF LOWER ESOPHAGEAL SPHINCTER	INCREASED GASTRIC PRESSURE	GASTRIC CONTENTS NEAR JUNCTION
Chocolate	Food (protein)	Recumbency
Peppermint	Pregnancy	Increased intra-abdominal pressure
Caffeine	Obesity	
Fatty foods	Ascites	
Alcohol	Tight clothing	
Nicotine or cigarette smoke	Back supports	
Central nervous system depressants (e.g., morphine, diazepam)	Girdles	
Other medications (e.g., calcium channel blockers, dopamine, theophylline)	Antacids	
Estrogen therapy	Histamines	
Nasogastric intubation		
Scleroderma		
Prolonged vomiting		
Surgical resection (destroys sphincter)		
Position (right or left side-lying; sitting)		

sage of food and liquids but prevents reflux. Any of the predisposing factors listed in Table 13–5 may alter the pressure around the LES, resulting in reflux. Hydrochloric acid or gastric and duodenal contents containing bile acid and pancreatic juice coming in contact with the walls of the esophagus cause inflammation and mucosal ulcerations. Subsequent granulation tissue causes scarring that frequently develops into esophageal strictures.

Clinical Manifestations. Heartburn, reflux, dysphagia, and painful swallowing are the primary symptoms of esophagitis. Pain is usually described as a burning sensation that moves up and down and may radiate to the back, neck, or jaw. Heartburn most often occurs 30 to 60 minutes after a meal and is produced by contact of regurgitated contents with the inflamed esophageal mucosa. Dysphagia is an indication of narrowing of the lumen, usually as a result of edema, spasm, or esophageal strictures. Aggravating factors include recumbency, bending, and meals; relief is obtained with antacids or baking soda, standing and walking, fluids, and avoidance of predisposing factors.

Reflux in the absence of esophagitis may be asymptomatic or accompanied by a sour taste in the mouth; severe reflux may reach the pharynx and mouth and result in laryngitis, morning hoarseness, and pulmonary aspiration. Recurrent pulmonary aspiration can cause aspiration pneumonia, pulmonary fibrosis, or chronic asthma (Goyal, 1994).

Medical Management

Diagnosis and Prognosis. Diagnostic tools include history, barium swallow, esophagoscopy, mucosal biopsy, and evaluation of esophageal motility. A full diagnostic evaluation is not always required when history and current symptoms clearly point to esophagitis; a therapeutic trial of treatment in mild cases may be diagnostic in itself. Response to nitroglycerin may help the physician differentiate between esophagitis and angina pectoris, but the response is not always diagnostic because nitroglycerin can also relieve esophageal spasm.

Prognosis is good for reflux esophagitis with complete symptom resolution, but often variable for the chemical type and poor for infectious esophagitis.

Treatment. The primary treatment is lifestyle modifications such as dietary restrictions; weight loss if obese; avoiding nicotine, alcohol, salicylates, and NSAIDs; remaining upright after meals; and elevation of the head of the bed to reduce nocturnal reflux and enhance esophageal acid clearance. Uncomplicated cases of esophagitis and typical symptoms of heartburn and regurgitation may be treated with antacids (e.g., preparations such as calcium carbonate–magnesium carbonate [Mylanta], or magnesium hydroxide–aluminum hydroxide [Maalox], or H_2-receptor antagonists).[3]

Persistent, unresponsive disease requires endoscopy to document the presence and severity of esophagitis. Surgery is indicated for people who fail or who are noncomplicant with medical therapy and for those people with difficult reflux-induced strictures requiring repeated dilation (McQuaid and Knauer, 1994).

Special Implications for the Therapist **13-3**

GASTROESOPHAGEAL REFLUX DISEASE

Clients with GERD are often treated in therapy for orthopedic and other conditions. Since education and encouragement are essential to the lifestyle modifications necessary to this condition, the knowledgeable therapist can assist the person implement changes related to diet and exercise. Any treatment requiring a supine position should be scheduled before meals and avoided just after eating. Modification of position toward a more upright posture may be required if symptoms persist during therapy.

[3] H_2-receptor antagonists such as cimetidine (Tagamet), ranitidine (Zantac), or famotidine (Pepcid), anticholinergic drugs, and sedatives block the action of H_2-receptors and inhibit histamine-stimulated gastrin release resulting in reduced secretion of gastric acid and pepsin. Less acid contact with the walls of the esophagus reduces inflammation.

See also Special Implications for the Therapist: Hiatal Hernia: Box 13–2. Activities that increase intra-abdominal pressure, such as bending and vigorous exercise; constipation, which often accompanies back pain and other conditions (see Table 13–3); and tight clothing must be avoided.

After surgery using a thoracic approach, chest physical therapy may be indicated. The presence of GERD requires careful positioning to promote drainage of secretions without causing reflux. This is more readily accomplished when the stomach is empty.

Mallory-Weiss Syndrome

Mallory-Weiss syndrome is laceration of the lower end of the esophagus associated with bleeding. The most common cause is severe retching and vomiting as a result of alcohol abuse, eating disorders such as bulimia, or in the case of a viral syndrome. Any event that suddenly raises transabdominal pressure in exercise or lifting can cause such a tear. Diagnosis is made on endoscopy and when treatment is necessary, fluid replacement and blood transfusion, and H_2-receptor antagonists may be administered. Operative intervention may be required if bleeding cannot be brought under control (Kovacs and Jensen, 1991).

Scleroderma Esophagus

Esophageal involvement is common in people with progressive systemic sclerosis caused by the CREST syndrome (*c*alcinosis, *R*aynaud's phenomenon, *e*sophageal motility disorder, *s*clerodactyly, and *t*elangiectasia; see discussion of systemic sclerosis, Chapter 5). The esophageal lesions in systemic sclerosis consist of muscular atrophy of the smooth muscle portion, with weakness of contraction in the lower two thirds of the esophagus and incompetence of the LES. Symptoms include dysphagia to solids and to liquids in the recumbent position. Heartburn and regurgitation occur in the presence of gastroesophageal reflux and esophagitis. Currently, there is no effective treatment for the motor difficulty, but reflux esophagitis and its complications are treated aggressively as described earlier (Goyal, 1994).

Neoplasm

Overview. Esophageal cancer is relatively uncommon and constitutes less than 7% of all GI cancers, usually developing between the ages of 50 and 70 years with a male to female ratio of 3 : 1 (Harruff, 1994; Luk, 1993). Histologically, there are two types of esophageal cancer: squamous cell and adenocarcinoma. In the United States, squamous cell cancer is much more common in blacks than whites. Chronic alcohol and tobacco use are strongly associated with an increased risk of squamous cell carcinoma.

Adenocarcinoma is more common in whites and is increasing dramatically in incidence. Most adenocarcinomas occur in the distal third of the esophagus as a complication of chronic gastroesophageal reflux causing erosion and ulceration eventually leading to metaplasia and neoplastic changes (Luk, 1993).

Etiology and Risk Factors. The direct cause of esophageal cancer is unknown, but geographic differences have led researchers to look for environmental causes. In the Western world, heavy pipe, cigar, and cigarette smoking, and chronic alcohol abuse may be risk factors. The presence of other chronic esophageal disease such as hiatal hernia, reflux, rings, webs, diverticula, stricture from lye ingestion, achalasia, and other head and neck cancers increases the risk of developing esophageal cancer (McQuaid and Knauer, 1994).

Pathogenesis. Chronic inadequate nutrition can impair both the structure and function of the esophagus. Nutritional deprivation, particularly deficiencies of vitamin A and zinc, results in mucosal changes increasing the vulnerability of esophageal mucosa to neoplastic changes. Any change in esophageal function that permits food and drink to remain in the esophagus for prolonged periods of time can result in ulceration and metaplasia. Chronic exposure to irritants such as alcohol and tobacco (inhaled or chewed)[4] can also cause neoplastic transformation (Huether and McCance, 1994). Tumors may be obstructive causing circumferential compression or ulceration with bleeding. Distant metastases may also occur, most commonly involving the liver and lung, but almost any organ can be involved (Rubin and Farber, 1994).

Clinical Manifestations. Dysphagia with or without pain is the predominant symptom of this condition and may not occur until the diameter of the lumen of the esophagus is reduced 30% to 50%. Pain associated with dysphagia is usually described as pressure-like and may radiate posteriorly between the scapulae. Heartburn initiated by eating spicy or highly seasoned foods and by lying down is the most common type of pain. Constant retrosternal chest pain that radiates to the back may occur in the presence of mediastinal extension or spinal nerve compression. Other signs and symptoms include anorexia and weight loss, hoarseness due to laryngeal nerve compression, and tracheoesophageal fistula causing cough and recurrent pneumonia.

Medical Management

Diagnosis. Diagnosis is made by endoscopy with cytology and biopsy. After diagnosis, staging of the disease is performed with chest and abdominal computed tomography (CT) scanning or, if available, endoscopic ultrasonography to determine the most appropriate treatment.

Treatment. Neoplasms are classified as resectable with curative intent, resectable but not curable, and not resectable and not curable. The presence of distant metastases, invasion of the mediastinal muscularis or pleural invasion, or distant lymph node involvement excludes a curative resection. Curative surgery is esophageal reconstruction, which may improve the ability to eat and may prevent local tumor complications (McQuaid and Knauer, 1994). The use of preoperative chemotherapy with radiation is under investigation. Unresectable disease or poor operative candidates may receive radiation therapy, which provides short-term relief of symptoms. Combinations of surgery, radiation therapy, and chemotherapy are under clinical investigation (Herskovic et al., 1992).

---

[4] Nitrosamines are powerful carcinogens believed to be involved as causative agents of cancers of the lung, oral cavity, esophagus, and pancreas associated with the use of tobacco products. Chronic stimulation of nicotinic receptors by nicotine and nitrosamines in smokers is one of the molecular events responsible for stimulation of cell proliferation and ultimately neoplasms.

Prognosis. Prognosis is very poor with median survival of less than 10 months. The first symptoms of esophageal cancer are not usually apparent until the tumor involves the entire esophageal circumference. More important, the tumor by that time has often invaded the deeper layers of the esophagus and adjacent structures and is unresectable. Esophageal cancer metastasizes rapidly and given the continuous nature of lymphatic vessels in the area, removal of lymph nodes with the tumor is impossible, contributing to the poor prognosis.

Special Implications for the Therapist **13-4**

ESOPHAGEAL CANCER

Lymphatic vessels of the esophagus are continuous with mediastinal structures and drain to the lymph nodes from the neck of the celiac axis. Metastasis is via this lymphatic drainage with tumors of the upper esophagus metastasizing to the cervical, internal jugular, and supraclavicular nodes. The therapist may identify changes in lymph nodes, requiring medical referral, during an upper-quarter screening examination.

The usual precautions regarding clients with cancer apply to neoplasms of the GI system. The primary concern is the side effects of chemotherapy-induced bone marrow suppression. An exercise regimen including aerobic exercise at a minimal level enhances the immune system and is incorporated whenever possible. See also Chapter 7.

Esophageal Varices

Esophageal varices are dilated veins in the lower third of the esophagus immediately beneath the mucosa (see Fig. 14–6). Dilation occurs in the presence of portal hypertension, usually secondary to cirrhosis of the liver. All the blood from the intestine drains via the portal vein to the liver before passing into the general circulation. Therefore, any disease of the liver or portal vein which obstructs the flow of blood will cause backpressure resulting in dilated veins. The normal anatomic reaction to this condition is to decompress the portal venous system by opening up bypass veins (anastomoses), most commonly around the lower esophagus and stomach. Unfortunately, rupture and hemorrhage of these dilated veins are common when portal pressure causes the varices to reach a size greater than 5 mm in diameter.

Variceal bleeding usually presents with painless but massive hematemesis with or without melena. Associated signs range from mild postural tachycardia to profound shock, depending on the extent of blood loss and degree of hypovolemia (decreased amount of blood in the body). The clinical picture is frequently consistent with chronic liver disease.

Diagnosis requires differentiation from peptic ulcer, gastritis, and other bleeding sources, often simultaneous conditions in people with cirrhosis secondary to alcoholism (Podolsky and Isselbacher, 1994). Diagnosis is made by fiberoptic endoscopy. Bleeding varices constitutes one of the most common causes of death among people with cirrhosis and other disorders associated with portal hypertension; therefore treatment to replace blood and maintain intravascular volume is essential.

About half of all episodes of variceal hemorrhage cease without intervention, although there is a high risk of rebleeding. Other treatment measures may include vasoconstrictors (vasopressin), endoscopic sclerosing of varices (sclerotherapy, the injection of hardening agents), and balloon tamponade (inflation of an esophageal balloon and compression against the areas of bleeding) (Fig. 13–3).

Special Implications for the Therapist **13-5**

ESOPHAGEAL VARICES

The primary concerns in therapy are to avoid causing rupture of varices and proper handling of clients with known GI bleeding. Carefully instruct the client in proper lifting techniques and avoid any activities that will increase intra-abdominal pressure (see Box 13–1).

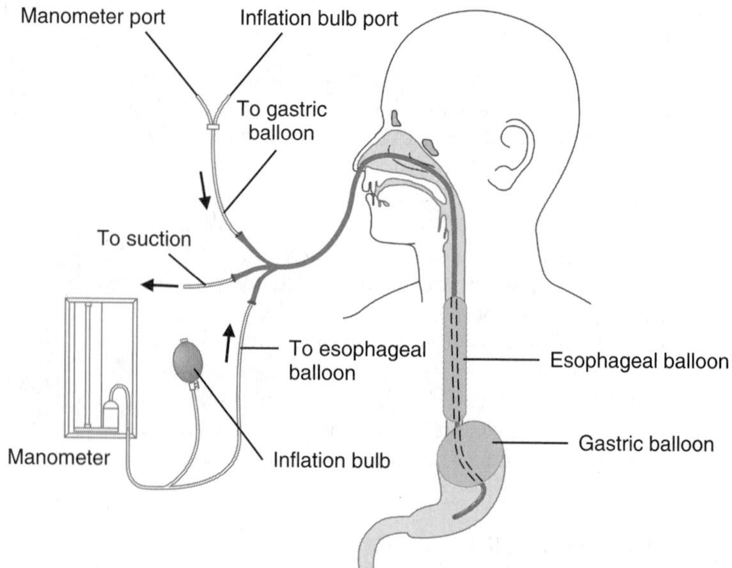

Figure **13-3.** A Sengstaken-Blakemore tube may be used to control ruptured esophageal varices, a potential complication of portal hypertension. This device consists of three tubes: one leading to a balloon that is inflated in the stomach to retain the instrument in place and compress the vessels around the cardia; one leading to a long narrow balloon by which pressure is exerted against the wall of the esophagus; and the third attached to a suction apparatus for aspirating the contents of the stomach. The tubing is removed in 24 hours if the bleeding is controlled.

See also Special Implications for the Therapist: Anemias (11–3) and Portal Hypertension (Chapter 14).

For the client with known esophageal varices, observe closely for signs of behavioral or personality changes. Report increasing stupor, lethargy, hallucinations, or neuromuscular dysfunction. Watch for asterixis (involuntary jerking movements), a sign of developing hepatic encephalopathy (see Fig. 14–1).

To assess fluid retention, inspect the ankles and sacrum for dependent edema. To prevent skin breakdown associated with edema and pruritus, caution the client and family members caring for that person to avoid using soap when bathing and to use moisturizing cleansing agents instead. Precautions must be taken to handle the client gently, turning and repositioning often to keep the skin intact. Rest and good nutrition will conserve energy and decrease metabolic demands on the liver.

Congenital

Tracheoesophageal Fistula

Overview. Tracheoesophageal fistula (TEF) is the most common esophageal anomaly and one of the most common congenital defects, occurring in approximately 1 in 4000 live births with equal sex distribution. In this disorder, the esophagus fails to develop as a continuous passage and abnormal communication between the lower portion of the esophagus and trachea occurs, often combined with some form of esophageal atresia, a condition in which the esophagus ends in a blind pouch (Fig. 13–4). Other associated conditions include congenital heart disease, prematurity, and the VATER complex (*v*ertebral defects, imperforate *a*nus, *t*racheoesophageal fistula, and *r*adial and *r*enal dysplasia).

Etiology and Pathogenesis. As a congenital malformation, the cause is unknown, but abnormalities are postulated to arise from defective differentiation as the trachea separates from the esophagus during the fourth to sixth weeks of embryonic development. Defective growth of endodermal cells leads to atresia (closure or absence of a normal body opening or tubular structure).

In 90% of cases, the esophagus ends in a blind pouch with communication between the distal esophagus and the trachea. Less often, the proximal esophagus communicates with the trachea, or the esophagus is continuous in an H-type fistula.

Clinical Manifestations. The blind end of the proximal esophagus has a capacity of only a few milliliters, so as the infant with esophageal atresia swallows oral secretions, the pouch fills and overflows into the pharynx resulting in excessive drooling and, occasionally, aspiration. If a fistula connects the trachea with the distal esophagus, the abdomen fills with air and becomes distended, which may interfere with breathing. If the fistula connects the proximal esophagus to the trachea, the first feeding after birth will signal a problem. As the infant swallows, the blind end of the esophagus and the mouth fill with fluid which is aspirated into the lungs hen the infant tries to take a breath. This triggers protective cough and choke reflexes with intermittent cyanosis (Danek et al., 1994). Coughing, choking, and cyanosis are called the three Cs of TEF and may occur especially with the H-type fistula, which may not be diagnosed for weeks to months after birth.

Medical Management

Diagnosis and Treatment. Esophageal anomalies are usually diagnosed at birth on the basis of clinical manifestations, but occasionally this condition escapes detection until adulthood when recurrent pulmonary infections call attention to it. Confirmation of the non-H type is made by passing a catheter into the esophagus with radiographs of the chest and abdomen taken with the tube in place to show the level of the blind pouch. Fluoroscopy using radiopaque fluid may also be used to establish the diagnosis.

Surgical treatment to restore esophageal continuity and eliminate the fistula is usually performed shortly after birth. Surgical procedures may be performed in stages for infants who are premature, have multiple anomalies, or who are in poor health. Antibiotics are instituted early owing to the certainty of aspiration pneumonia.

Prognosis. Without early diagnosis and treatment this condition is rapidly fatal. Early detection prevents feedings, which could cause aspiration and its complications. The survival rate is nearly 100% in full-term infants without severe respiratory distress or other anomalies. In premature, low-birth-weight infants with associated anomalies, the incidence of complications is high. The overall mortality is 10% to 15% (Wright, 1991).

THE STOMACH

Gastritis

Definition and Incidence. Gastritis, inflammation of the lining of the stomach (gastric mucosa), is not a single disease but represents a group of the most common stomach disorders. Gastric erosions by definition are limited to the mucosa and do not extend beneath the muscularis mucosae. Based on clinical features, gastritis can be classified as acute or chronic. Other classifications may be made according to clinical, endoscopic, radiographic, or pathologic criteria. *Acute gastritis* may be hemorrhagic or acute-erosive, reflecting the presence of bleeding from the gastric mucosa. Gastric erosions and sites of hemorrhage may be distributed diffusely throughout the gastric mucosa or localized to the body of the stomach (McGuigan, 1994).

Chronic gastritis has two forms classified as types A and B. Type A gastritis is the less common form of chronic gastritis, associated with pernicious anemia and is possibly an autoimmune disorder. The most severe type of chronic gastritis, chronic fundal gastritis, occurs in association with autoimmune diseases such as diabetes, Addison's disease, and thyroid disease, also suggesting an autoimmune mechanism. Type B, the more common form of chronic gastritis, is caused by chronic bacterial infection by *Helicobacter pylori*[5] (Sipponen, 1994).

[5] *Helicobacter pylori* is a gram-negative spiral bacterium that lives in the gastric mucosal layer of humans and induces a chronic inflammatory response that can result in both peptic ulceration and gastric neoplasms (Blaser, 1993).

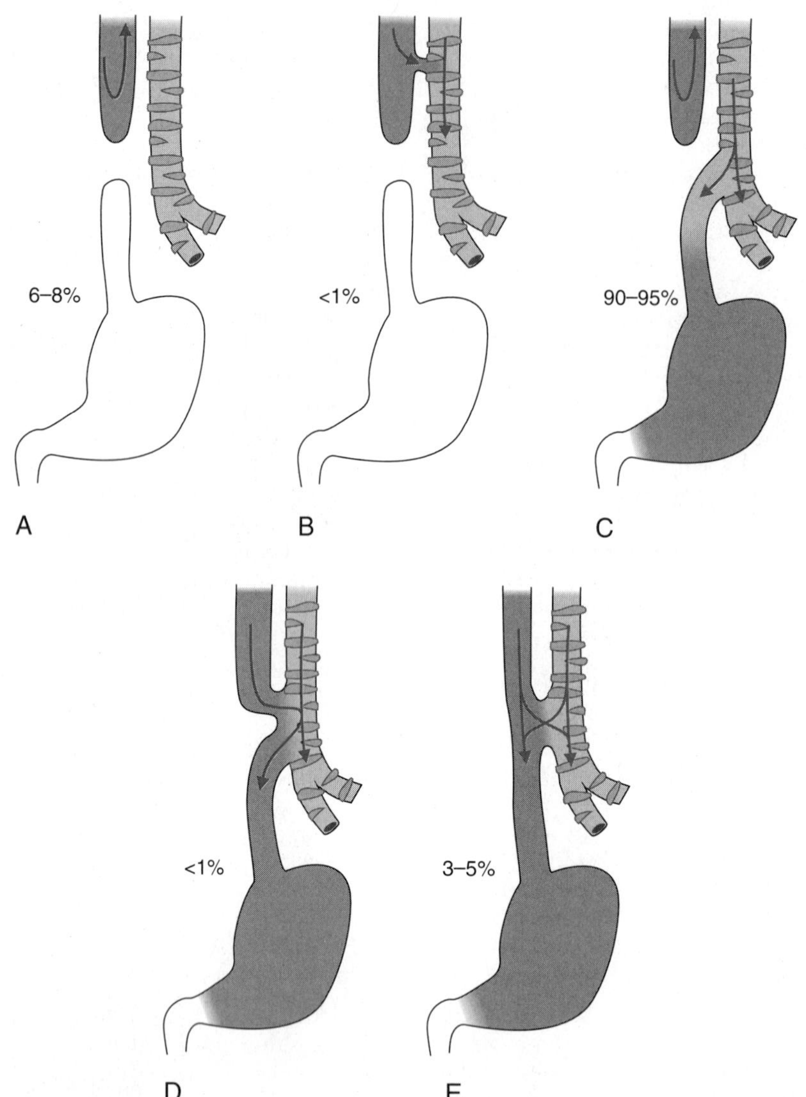

Figure **13–4.** Five types of esophageal atresia and tracheoesophageal fistula. *A*, Simple esophageal atresia. Proximal and distal esophagus end in blind pouches. Nothing enters the stomach; regurgitated food and fluid may enter the lungs. *B*, Proximal and distal esophageal segments end in blind pouches, and a fistula connects the proximal esophagus to the trachea. Nothing enters the stomach; food and fluid enter the lungs. *C*, Proximal esophagus ends in a blind pouch, and a fistula connects the trachea to the distal esophagus. Air enters the stomach; regurgitated gastric secretions enter the lungs through the fistula. *D*, Fistula connects both proximal and distal esophageal segments to the trachea. Air, food, and fluid enter the stomach and lungs. *E*, Simple tracheoesophageal fistula between otherwise normal esophagus and trachea. Air, food, and fluid enter the stomach and lungs. Between 90% and 95% of esophageal anomalies are type C; 6% to 8% are type A; 3% to 5% are type E; and less than 1% are type B or D.

Etiology. Acute erosive gastritis may develop without apparent cause, but is more likely to occur in association with serious illness or with various drugs (Table 13–6). Aspirin or other NSAIDs can produce acute gastric mucosal erosions. GI complications occur only in a small percentage of people taking NSAIDs but the widespread use of these agents results in a substantial number of people affected. Most susceptible persons are those 65 years of age or older, especially those who have a history of ulcer disease. Other risk factors include taking NSAIDs longer than 3 months, taking high-dose or multiple NSAIDs, and concurrent corticosteroid therapy (Lichtenstein et al., 1995). Acute erosive gastritis associated with physiologic stress, often referred to as *stress-induced gastritis*, is associated with hospitalization for severe life-threatening disease, central nervous system (CNS) injury, or trauma (particularly burns but also renal failure, mechanical ventilation, sepsis, and hepatic failure).

There is no persuasive evidence that acute gastric mucosal injury associated with stress, alcohol, aspirin, or other NSAIDs progresses to chronic gastritis. Aging is a primary risk factor in the development of chronic gastritis, but other causes include vitamin deficiencies, abnormalities of the gastric juice, hiatal hernia, alcohol abuse, or a combination of any of these.

Pathogenesis *(Huether and McCance, 1994).* Agents known to injure the gastric mucosa (e.g., aspirin or other NSAIDs, bile acids, pancreatic enzymes, alcohol) alter the mucosal defense

TABLE 13-6 CLASSIFICATION OF GASTRITIS BY ETIOLOGY

Idiopathic
Atrophic gastritis
Chronic erosive gastritis
Chronic nonerosive gastritis
Eosinophilic gastritis
Gastric pseudolymphoma
Hypertrophic hypersecretory gastropathy
Ménétrier's disease (gastric mucosa proliferation)
Medications
Aspirin
Nonsteroidal anti-inflammatory drugs
Corticosteroids
Cytotoxic agents
Chemical Agents
Alcohol
Alkaline reflux
Coffee (with or without caffeine)
Corrosive agents: acids and alkalis
Nicotine, cigarette smoke
Systemic Diseases
Crohn's disease
Sarcoidosis
Physiologic stress
Infectious Agents
Bacteria
Helicobacter pylori
Staphylococcus spp.
Escherichia coli
Salmonella spp.
Syphilis
Tuberculosis
Opportunistic infections

Adapted from Cappell MS: Gastritis: Making the differential diagnosis. Hosp Med 30:45–50, 1994, p 47.

mechanism leading to *acute gastritis*. The mechanism of mucosal injury is unclear and probably multifactorial. The most commonly accepted theory for agent-induced mucosal injury is the suppression of endogenous prostaglandins which normally stimulate the protective secretion of mucus.

There are three phases in the pathogenesis of *chronic gastritis*. Superficial gastritis is the initial stage with inflammation limited to the upper epithelial half of the gastric mucosa. Atrophic gastritis, the second stage, takes place as the inflammatory process extends to the deep portions of the mucosa with progressive distortion and destruction of the gastric glands. Pepsinogen, hydrochloric acid, and intrinsic factor (glycoprotein secreted by the gastric glands) are diminished and the feedback mechanism that normally inhibits gastrin secretions is impaired, causing elevated plasma levels of gastrin.

As mentioned under Aging and the Gastrointestinal System, IF plays an important role in the absorption of vitamin B_{12}. IF deficiency resulting in vitamin B_{12} deficiency may lead to pernicious anemia.

The final stage, gastric atrophy, involves a profound loss of the glandular structures with thinning of the mucosa.

Clinical Manifestations. The most noticeable symptom of acute gastritis is epigastric pain with a feeling of abdominal distention, loss of appetite, and nausea. Pain is much less common with erosive gastritis than with ulcer disease; painless GI hemorrhage is frequently the only clinical manifestation. Additional symptoms may include heartburn, low-grade fever, and vomiting. Occult (no visible evidence) GI bleeding commonly occurs, especially in cases of trauma and in people taking aspirin or other NSAIDs. Chronic gastritis may be asymptomatic or pain may occur after eating accompanied by indigestion.

Medical Management

Diagnosis and Treatment. The diagnosis of gastritis may be made by a careful history, but confirmation is made by upper endoscopic examination, possibly including biopsy because epigastric pain may be due to peptic ulcer, gastroesophageal reflux, gastric cancer, biliary tract disease, food poisoning, and viral gastroenteritis (Cappell, 1994).

Management of this condition requires avoidance of identified irritating substances (e.g., caffeine, nicotine, alcohol) combined with the use of antacids or H_2-blocking agents or both to reduce gastric acid secretion and minimize stomach acidity. Vitamin B_{12} is administered to correct pernicious anemia when it develops secondary to chronic gastritis. Since people taking NSAIDs and those in intensive care units have a high incidence of erosive gastritis, preventive therapy with cimetidine, ranitidine, or misoprostol (Cytotec), a synthetic prostaglandin is used to reduce mucosal injury[6] (Andreoli et al., 1993).

Prognosis. Prognosis is good for both acute and chronic gastritis, especially with removal of the predisposing factor for acute gastritis, and unless gastric-carcinoma develops for chronic gastritis. The risk of gastric cancer is known to be high in people with chronic gastritis and particularly in those with atrophic gastritis (Sipponen, 1994).

Special Implications for the Therapist **13-6**

GASTRITIS

Half of all clients receiving NSAIDs on a chronic basis have acute gastritis (often asymptomatic). The therapist should continue to monitor clients for any symptoms of GI involvement indicating need for medical referral. For the client with known chronic GI bleeding, urge the client to seek immediate attention for recurring symptoms such as hematemesis, nausea, or vomiting.

Urge the client to take prophylactic medications as prescribed by the physician. Steroids should be taken with milk, food, or antacids to reduce gastric irritation; antacids can be taken between meals and at bedtime.

[6] Unfortunately the overuse of these H_2-blocking agents creates an alkaline environment in an immunocompromised person and is the major cause of iatrogenic septic shock. Misoprostol is the only effective agent for preventing NSAID-induced gastroduodenal ulcers. Its effectiveness in reducing complications such as bleeding or perforation during long-term NSAID use is unproven (Lichtenstein et al., 1995).

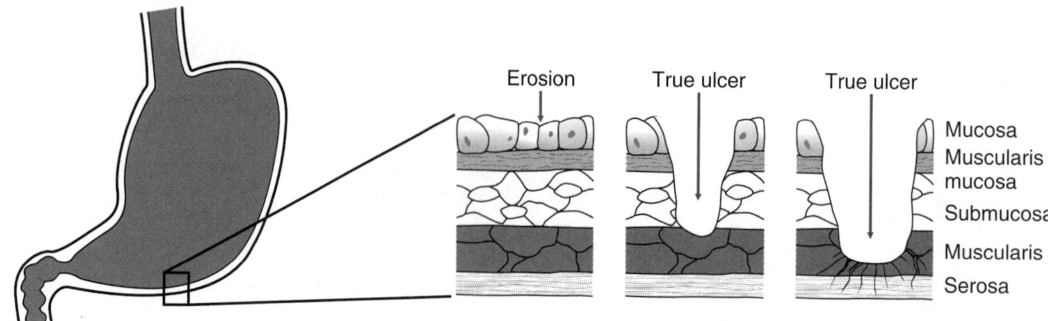

Figure **13–5.** Lesions caused by peptic ulcer disease.

Aspirin-containing compounds should be avoided unless specifically recommended by the physician. See also Special Implications for the Therapist: Signs and Symptoms of Gastrointestinal Disease (13–1) and Anemias (11–3).

Peptic Ulcer Disease

Definition and Overview. An ulcer is a break in the protective mucosal lining exposing submucosal areas to gastric secretions. The word *peptic* refers to pepsin, a proteolytic enzyme, the principal digestive component of gastric juice, which acts as a catalyst in the chemical breakdown of protein. Acute lesions of the mucosa that do not extend through the muscularis mucosae are referred to as *erosions*. Chronic ulcers involve the muscular coat, destroying the musculature and replacing it with permanent scar tissue at the site of healing. Ulcers extending to the muscularis mucosae damage blood vessels, causing hemorrhage (Fig. 13–5).

There are two kinds of peptic ulcer: the *gastric ulcer* (GU), which affects the lining of the stomach and the *duodenal ulcer* (DU), which occurs in the duodenum. DUs are two to three times more common than GUs. About 95% of DUs occur in the duodenal bulb or cap. About 60% of benign GUs are located at or near the lesser curvature and most frequently on the posterior wall (Fig. 13–6).

Stress ulcers, or secondary ulcers, occur in response to prolonged psychological or physiologic stress (e.g., severe trauma, surgery, extensive burns, brain injury) causing an upset in the aggressive-defensive balance (see Pathogenesis, this section). For example, gastric mucosal changes develop within 72 hours in 80% of clients with greater than 35% burns. The mechanism causing stress ulcers is unknown but probably involves ischemia of the gastric mucosa, which has large oxygen requirements and low gastric pH (high acidity). These ulcers differ pathologically and clinically from peptic ulcer with very few symptoms and are painless until perforation and hemorrhage occur (Ruder, 1993a).

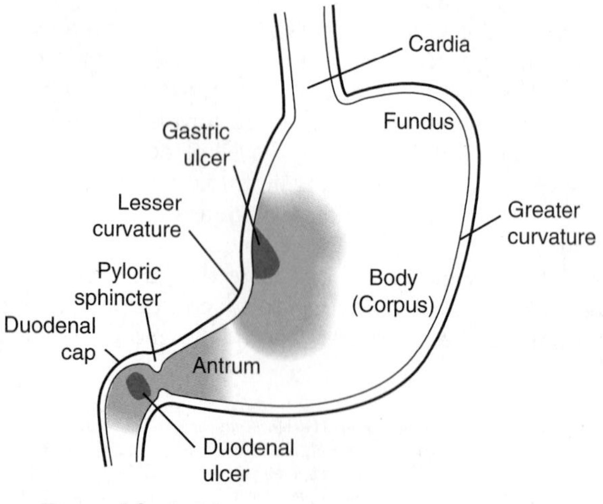

Figure **13–6.** Most common sites of peptic ulcers.

Incidence. In the United States, there are about 500,000 new cases per year of peptic ulcer and 4 million ulcer recurrences. Up to 10% of the American population will develop an ulcer at some time in their life (Harruff, 1994; McQuaid and Knauer, 1994). Older age groups, especially middle-aged and elderly people, are more likely to develop GUs; the peak incidence for GUs is in the sixth decade. Ten percent to 20% of people with GUs also have DUs.

DUs are the most common with an average age at onset in the mid-30s, although DUs can occur at any time from infancy on. In the past, men were more likely than women to develop gastric and duodenal ulcers, but now there is equal distribution between the sexes and the overall frequency of DU has been decreasing in the United States, especially in males.

Etiology and Risk Factors. There is no single cause of peptic ulcers. Rather the process is multifactorial, reflecting a few common and a few uncommon causes (Table 13–7). There are many genetic and environmental theories as to the causes of peptic ulcers. Both gastric and duodenal ulcers tend to occur in families; relatives of persons with DUs have three times the expected number of these same ulcers. There is a positive relationship between DUs and people with O blood type (Boren et al., 1993).

The most common risk factors responsible for GUs are smoking,[7] alcohol abuse, and chronic use of NSAIDs (see Table 4–4 for a listing of commonly prescribed NSAIDs).

[7] The exact mechanism of cigarette smoking in the development of peptic ulcers (most commonly, DU) is unknown. It does not increase gastric acid secretion but may be due to inhibition of pancreatic bicarbonate secretion (which neutralizes gastric acid) by nicotine or smoke or by accelerating gastric acid emptying into the duodenum or a combination of these. There is a positive correlation between the quantity of cigarettes smoked and the prevalence of ulcer disease; death due to peptic ulcer disease is more likely in people who smoke than in those who do not.

TABLE 13-7 CAUSES OF PEPTIC ULCER

Common forms of peptic ulcer
- *Helicobacter pylori*–associated
- NSAID-associated
- Stress ulcer

Uncommon forms of peptic ulcer
- Acid hypersecretion (e.g., gastrinoma, basophilic leukemias)
- Other infections (e.g., herpes simplex, CMV)
- Duodenal obstruction (e.g., congenital bands)
- Vascular insufficiency (e.g., crack cocaine–associated perforations)
- Radiation-induced
- Chemotherapy-induced (hepatic artery infusions)
- Rare genetic subtypes (e.g., amyloidosis)

NSAID, nonsteroidal anti-inflammatory drug; CMV, cytomegalovirus.
Adapted from Soll AH: Gastric, duodenal, and stress ulcer. *In* Sleisenger MH, Fordtran JS (eds): Gastrointestinal Disease, ed 5. Philadelphia, WB Saunders, 1993, p 582.

NSAIDs have deleterious effects on the entire GI tract, from the esophagus to the colon, although the most obvious clinical effect is on the gastroduodenal mucosa. The exact mechanism remains unknown but theoretically these drugs break down the mucous membrane which protects the GI tract by inhibiting the synthesis of gastric mucosal prostaglandins.[8] This interference with normal mucosal protective mechanisms leads to local injury by allowing stomach acids to dissolve the intestine (Soll, 1992; Babb, 1992) (for further discussion of the systemic effects of NSAIDs, see Chapter 4).

Psychological stress as a risk factor has not been conclusively proved. Individuals with multiple stressors, poor coping skills, and persistent anxiety and depression in the presence of recurrent ulcers lend support to the hypothesis that physiologic changes leading to ulcer occur secondary to psychological stress (Schineller and Ramchandani, 1991). In the case of emotional stress, an increase in gastric secretion, blood supply, and gastric motility by irritation of the vagal nerve stimulates the thalamus. The sympathetic nervous system then causes the blood vessels in the duodenum to constrict, making the mucosa more vulnerable to trauma from gastric acid and pepsin secretion (Ruder, 1993a).

Pathogenesis. Peptic ulcer develops when there is an unfavorable balance between gastric acid and pepsin secretion (aggressive factors) and factors that compromise mucosal defense or mucosal resistance to injury or ulceration. Multiple chemical, neural, and hormonal factors participate in regulation of gastric acid secretion, making ulcer development a multifactorial process (McGuigan, 1994). In the pathogenesis of GUs, defective mucosal defense appears to be the major contributing factor, either defective gastric mucosal resistance or direct gastric mucosal injury. In contrast, for DUs evidence favors the importance of relative gastric hypersecretion.

Helicobacter pylori, which inhabits the gastric mucosa of 95% of people with DU, has been proposed as an important factor in the pathogenesis of DU. It remains unclear whether this bacterium is a contributing factor, modifying factor, or if its presence just reflects a commensal association (i.e., an association in which one species derives benefit and the other is unharmed). Its eradication is shown to dramatically improve the rate at which ulcers relapse (Reilly and Walt, 1994; Bourke et al., 1994).

[8] Prostaglandins have two types of actions: inhibition of acid secretion and enhancement of mucosal resistance to injury by mechanisms independent of acid secretory inhibition, the latter phenomenon being called *cytoprotection* (Soll, 1993).

Clinical Manifestations. The classic symptom of peptic ulcer is epigastric pain described as burning, gnawing, cramping, or aching near the xiphoid, coming in waves that last several minutes. Distention of the duodenal bulb produces epigastric pain, which may radiate to the back (Ruder, 1993a). Perforation of the posterior duodenal wall causes steady midline pain in the thoracic spine from T6 to T10 with radiation to the right upper quadrant. The daily pattern of pain is related to the secretion of acid and the presence of food in the stomach (e.g., the presence of food may cause GU pain whereas pain occurs 1 to 3 hours after meals with DUs). Other symptoms include nausea, loss of appetite, and sometimes weight loss. Symptoms may occur for 3 or 4 days or weeks, subsiding only to reappear weeks or months later (O'Toole, 1992).

Many people report symptoms outside the "classic" presentation of DU. Some people are asymptomatic until complications occur, including hemorrhage, perforation, and obstruction accompanied by unremitting pain. Symptoms depend on the severity of the hemorrhage. In mild bleeding (less than 500 mL), slight weakness and diaphoresis may be the only symptoms. Signs of bleeding include bright-red blood in the vomitus, coffee-ground vomitus, and melena (black, tarry stools).

Medical Management

Diagnosis. Ulcers are diagnosed on the basis of symptoms and history, although the history is not as characteristic for GU as it is for DU. Decreased hematocrit and hemoglobin values on a complete blood count, and the presence of occult blood (blood present in feces, urine, or gastric juice not otherwise detectable) on stool analysis may be diagnostic. Specific tests may include barium radiographic examination and gastroscopy (endoscope passed into the stomach) used to determine the site of bleeding and to differentiate between benign and malignant ulcerations. Appropriate use of one of the many new tests (e.g., serology, urease breath testing, saliva test, biopsy, and culture) to diagnose *H. pylori* can identify those individuals likely to benefit from antimicrobial treatment (Peura, 1993; Patel et al., 1994).

Treatment. The primary goals of medical treatment of peptic ulcers are (1) relief of symptoms, (2) promotion of healing, (3) prevention of complications, and (4) prevention of recurrences. Each person responds differently to different treatment modalities, requiring individual treatment planning. In general, GUs tend to heal more slowly than DUs.

The medical management of ulcers requires a balance of antacids and histamine H_2 blocking agents (see discussion of GERD), use of antimicrobials (e.g. doxycycline, metronidazole) in the presence of *H. pylori*, elimination or at least reduction of alcohol and tobacco use, avoidance of aspirin or any over-the-counter drug containing acetylsalicylic acid, and stress reduction. NSAID-associated peptic ulcers respond well to medical therapy and discontinuation of the NSAIDs. Coffee, caffeinated or not, stimulates gastric acid secretion and should be avoided.

There is no substantial evidence to support dietary modifications as a treatment approach to peptic ulcers. Bland diets, soft diets, milk and cream diets, diets free of spices or fruit juices have no known effect in reducing gastric acid secretion, relieving symptoms, or promoting ulcer healing. It is reasonable to suggest that foods that seem to aggravate a person's symptoms should be avoided (McGuigan, 1994).

Surgical intervention is required for perforation because gastric and intestinal contents spilling into the peritoneal cavity can cause chemical peritonitis, bacterial septicemia, and hypovolemic shock. Peristalsis diminishes and paralytic ileus develops.

Prognosis. Prognosis is usually good and ulcers can be adequately controlled by medical management unless massive hemorrhage or perforation occurs, which carries a high mortality. Both duodenal and gastric ulcers tend to have a chronic course with remissions and exacerbations. Benign GUs should heal completely within 3 months of treatment. In the past 4 years, at least five well-controlled, double-blind studies have shown that curing *H. pylori* usually results in curing DU disease (Marshall, 1993).

Special Implications for the Therapist **13-7**

PEPTIC ULCER DISEASE

Ulcer presentation without pain occurs more frequently in elderly people and in persons taking NSAIDs for painful musculoskeletal conditions (Clinch et al., 1984; Pounder, 1989). Any client complaining of GI symptoms should be encouraged to report these findings to his or her physician. Musculoskeletal symptoms may recur after discontinuing the NSAIDs owing to the masking effects of these drugs. Once the drug is discontinued, painful symptoms may return in the presence of continued underlying ulcer disease. Medical follow-up is required in such situations.

Peptic ulcers located on the posterior wall of the stomach or duodenum can perforate and hemorrhage, causing back pain as the only presenting symptom. Occasionally ulcer pain radiates to the midthoracic back and right upper quadrant, including the right shoulder. Right shoulder pain alone may occur as a result of blood in the peritoneal cavity from perforation and hemorrhage. Back pain may be the only presenting symptom, but this is usually accompanied by vomiting of bright-red blood or coffee-ground vomitus. Back pain relieved by antacids is an indication of GI involvement and must be reported to the physician.

For the competitive athlete, during the acute episode, anxiety and nervousness may increase gastric secretions. This effect in combination with poor nutrition (often the athlete has not eaten at all) requires careful monitoring and maximizing the use of medications and food intake with the performance schedule. For the average adult uninvolved in competitive sports, regular exercise as part of stress reduction is essential during remission.

National Institute on Aging (NIA) researchers have reported that exercise at least three times a week greatly reduces the risk of GI bleeding. More strenuous forms of exercise such as swimming and bicycling do not provide greater protection from GI bleeding than do more moderate exercises such as walking (Pahor et al., 1994b).

Gastric Cancer

Primary Gastric Lymphoma

Primary lymphoma of the stomach is relatively uncommon, but is the most common extranodal location for lymphoma. Clinically, primary gastric lymphoma does not differ significantly in its clinical presentation from adenocarcinoma. The incidence is most often during the sixth decade of life characterized by epigastric pain, early satiety, and fatigue.

Gastric Adenocarcinoma

Definition and Incidence. Adenocarcinoma, a malignant neoplasm arising from the gastric mucosa, constitutes more than 90% of the malignant tumors of the stomach. In 1997, 22,400 new cases of stomach cancer were diagnosed in the United States and 14,000 Americans died from this disease (ACS, 1997). The incidence is decreasing for unknown reasons. The overall rate has decreased from 28 to 5.3 per 100,000 (men) and from 27 to 2.3 per 100,000 (women) (Mayer, 1994). Men over the age of 40 years are most likely to develop this disease, with a sharp increase in incidence after 50 years.

Etiology and Risk Factors. Chronic gastritis with intestinal metaplasia, possibly secondary to chronic *H. pylori* infection, is a strong risk factor for gastric cancer (Sipponen, 1994). Other nonenvironmental risk factors include pernicious anemia, which causes atrophy of the gastric mucosa in the same locations where gastric tumors arise, type A blood, gastrectomy, gastric polyps, dietary factors such as smoked fish and meat containing benzopyrene, and nitrosamines produced endogenously in chronic gastritis.

There is a very high incidence of gastric cancer in Japan, parts of South America, and in eastern Europe which drops when population groups emigrate from areas of high incidence to areas of low incidence. This phenomenon leads epidemiologists to consider geographic differences such as salt[9] added to food, food additives such as nitrates in pickled or salted foods (e.g., bacon), and protective food factors in water and vegetables, such as vitamin C, as environmental risk factors.

Pathogenesis. The most common site for adenocarcinomas appear to be the glands of the stomach mucosa located in the distal portion of the stomach on the lesser curvature of the prepyloric antrum (see Fig. 13–6). Duodenal reflux and insufficient acid secretion may contribute to intestinal metaplasia. The reflux contains caustic bile salts which destroy the normally protective mucosal barrier in the stomach. Insufficient acid secretion by the atrophic mucosa creates an alkaline environment that permits bacteria to multiply and act

[9] Dietary salt enhances the conversion of nitrates to carcinogenic nitrosamines. It is caustic to the stomach and can cause chronic atrophic gastritis. Salt solutions also delay gastric emptying, increasing the time during which nitrosamines exert an effect on the stomach mucosa (Huether and McCance, 1994).

on nitrates. The resulting increase in nitrosamines damages the DNA of mucosal cells further, promoting metaplasia and neoplasia (Huether and McCance, 1994).

Clinical Manifestations. The clinical presentation of gastric carcinoma depends on a variety of factors, including the morphologic characteristics of the tumor (e.g., infiltrating vs. ulcerating), size of the tumor, presence of gastric outlet obstruction, and metastatic vs. nonmetastatic disease (Andreoli et al., 1993). Early stages of gastric cancer may be asymptomatic or present with vague symptoms of indigestion, anorexia, and weight loss.

Medical Management

Diagnosis. Diagnosis may be delayed by the fact that symptomatic relief can be obtained from early GI symptoms using over-the-counter medications. The choice of diagnostic tests depends on the clinical manifestation at the time of presentation. Endoscopy with cytologic brushings and biopsies of suspicious lesions are highly sensitive for detecting gastric carcinoma. In areas of high incidence, screening upper endoscopy is performed to detect early gastric carcinoma.

Once the diagnosis has been made, staging to determine the local extent of disease and the presence of nodal or distant metastases must be done. Staging is accomplished through the use of liver chemistry tests, abdominal imaging studies (e.g., CT scan), and biopsy of suspected lymph nodes.

Treatment. Surgical therapy is still the treatment of choice for primary gastric adenocarcinoma. Despite many attempts, the postoperative strategies of adjuvant chemotherapy have been ineffective. Radiotherapy and chemotherapy have been considered palliative (symptomatic relief) with minimal success and no cures (Ajani et al, 1991). Multimodality treatment consisting of preoperative chemotherapy and surgery may provide improved results if endoscopic ultrasonography and staging laparoscopy provide early identification of locally advanced tumors (Meyer et al., 1994). At present, there is no role for *H. pylori* eradication in the prevention of gastric cancer, although this concept is being investigated (Fennerty, 1994).

Prognosis. Prognosis depends on the degree of gastric wall penetration, the presence of lymph node metastases, and the location of the primary site. Screening programs in other countries detect approximately 40% of tumors early with a 5-year survival rate of over 60%. Without screening, the prognosis is poor because symptoms do not occur until the tumor has penetrated muscle layers of the stomach, spread to local tissue by direct extension in the abdominal cavity, metastasized via the lymphatic system, or created a paraneoplastic manifestation (e.g., Trousseau's syndrome,[10] dermatomyositis, and acanthosis nigricans[11]). Metastatic gastric carcinoma is currently incurable. Surgical resection is only possible in one third of gastric cancers. Of those people in whom surgical resection is a possibility, 20% survive 10 years.

[10] Spontaneous peripheral venous thrombosis of the upper and lower extremities occurring in association with visceral carcinoma (O'Toole, 1992).

[11] A skin condition associated with an internal carcinoma characterized by diffuse thickening of the skin with gray, brown, or black pigmentation, usually in body folds such as the axillae.

Special Implications for the Therapist **13-8**

GASTRIC ADENOCARCINOMA

Epigastric or back pain, possibly relieved by antacids, is a frequent complaint that the physician must differentiate from peptic ulcer disease. Generally the first manifestations of carcinoma are caused by distant metastasis when the condition is quite advanced. The therapist may palpate the left supraclavicular (Virchow's) lymph node or the client may point out an umbilical nodule.

After surgery, position changes every 2 hours, deep breathing, coughing, and incentive spirometry (handheld device used to provide visual feedback for voluntary maximal inspiration) may be used to prevent pulmonary complications. The semi-Fowler position (head of the bed raised 6 to 12 in. with knees slightly flexed) facilitates breathing and drainage following any type of gastrectomy.

Congenital

Pyloric Stenosis

Definition and Overview. Pyloric stenosis (PS) is an obstruction at the pyloric sphincter (the sphincter at the distal opening of the stomach into the duodenum). The pyloric sphincter is a ring of muscles that serve to close the opening from the stomach into the intestine (Fig. 13–7). Obstruction occurs as a congenital condition or in adults as a result of scarring from peptic ulcer, pyloric spasm secondary to an ulcer, cancer, or gastritis. When present as a congenital condition, it is known as hypertrophic PS caused by hypertrophy of the sphincter and is one of the most common surgical disorders of early infancy.

Incidence and Etiology. The cause of congenital hypertrophy of the pyloric sphincter is unknown. White males are affected more commonly than females in a 4:1 ratio. It is more likely to occur in a full-term infant than in a premature infant, especially the first-born child. Siblings, offspring of affected persons, and fathers and sons are at increased risk of developing PS (genetic predisposition).

Increased third-trimester maternal gastric secretion associated with maternal stress-related factors increases the likelihood of PS in the infant. PS may also be associated with other congenital conditions such as Turner's syndrome, trisomy 18, intestinal malrotation, esophageal and duodenal atresia, and anorectal anomalies (Danek et al., 1994).

The incidence of adult PS is unknown. Although many physicians believe this condition is secondary to local disease, others think the condition in adults is the same entity as that observed in infants and children, but in a milder form and later in appearance (McGuigan and Ament, 1994).

Pathogenesis. The histologic and anatomic abnormalities in adult PS are indistinguishable from those in the infantile form (McGuigan and Ament, 1994). Individual fibers of the pyloric sphincter thicken or hypertrophy so that the entire sphincter is grossly enlarged and inelastic. Hyperplasia of the pyloric muscle occurs because of the extra peristaltic effort required to force the gastric contents through the narrow opening into the duodenum. This hypertrophy and hyperpla-

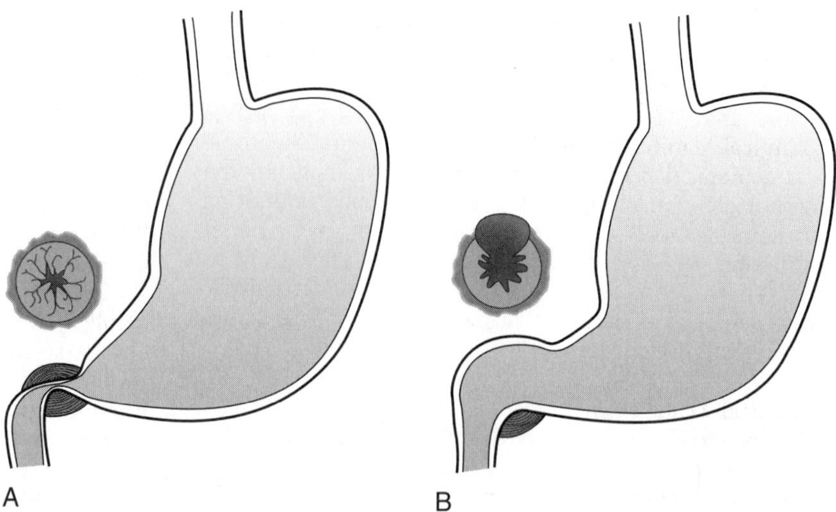

Figure **13–7.** Hypertrophic pyloric stenosis. *A*, Enlarged muscular area nearly obliterates the pyloric channel. *B*, Longitudinal surgical division of muscle down to the submucosa establishes an adequate passageway.

sia form a palpable "tumor" severely narrowing the pyloric canal between the stomach and the duodenum, causing partial obstruction. Over time, inflammation and edema further reduce the size of the lumen, progressing to complete obstruction. Progressive obstruction results in complications of malnutrition and fluid and electrolyte abnormalities (Danek et al., 1994).

Clinical Manifestations. Projectile vomiting[12] is the most common and dramatic early symptom and may occur at birth. Overall, the age of onset and pattern of vomiting varies, but usually regurgitation or occasional projectile vomiting develops around the second to fourth week after birth. Projectile vomiting quickly leads to dehydration and lethargy with rapid progression to complete obstruction and the accompanying complications of malnutrition, weakness, wasting, weight loss, and fluid and electrolyte imbalances. The palpable tumor is firm, movable, about the size of an olive, and felt in the right upper quadrant in approximately 80% of all infants with PS.

Persistent or episodic symptoms in some adults may extend from infancy with nausea and vomiting, epigastric pain, weight loss, and anorexia most commonly present. In contrast to congenital PS in the infant, there is no palpable abdominal mass in adult PS because the mass is small (McGuigan and Ament, 1994).

Medical Management

Diagnosis, Treatment, and Prognosis. In infancy, diagnosis is usually by history and recognition of the clinical presentation but radiographs with contrast media show the stenosis and obstruction. Ultrasonography is a noninvasive method of detection and usually the method of choice for screening adults with this condition; an upper GI series may also demonstrate the lesion.

Some infants are treated with antispasmodic drugs to relax the pylorospasm and nutritional management, including refeeding the infant after vomiting, hoping that the pylorus will spontaneously open by 6 to 8 months of age (Danek et al., 1994).

[12] Projectile vomiting describes forcible vomiting that ejects vomitus 1 ft or more when in a supine position and 3 to 4 ft when in an upright or side-lying position.

Surgical pyloromyotomy (local resection of the involved region of the pylorus) is the standard medical treatment with a very high success rate for the infant as well as the adult (see Fig. 13–7). Infants receive preoperative care to correct fluid and electrolyte imbalances (Bissonnette and Sullivan, 1991). Postoperative vomiting is not uncommon in the pediatric population, especially during the first 24 to 48 hours. Complications include surgical diagnosis of localized carcinoma in the adult, and, in both the adult and pediatric populations, persistent pyloric obstruction and partial, superficial, or total wound separation (dehiscence).

THE INTESTINES

Malabsorption Syndrome

Definition and Overview. Malabsorption syndrome is a group of disorders (celiac disease, cystic fibrosis, Crohn's disease, chronic pancreatitis, pancreatic carcinoma, pernicious anemia) characterized by reduced intestinal absorption of dietary components and excessive loss of nutrients in the stool. Traditionally, malabsorption disorders have been classified as *maldigestion* (failure of the chemical processes of digestion) or *malabsorption* (failure of the intestinal mucosa to absorb the digested nutrients). Nutrients most commonly malabsorbed include fat, fatty acids or bile salts, calories (fat, protein, carbohydrates), iron, vitamin B_{12}, folic acid, calcium, vitamin D, magnesium, potassium, vitamin K, water, and lactose (sugar in milk).

Both conditions can occur separately or together simultaneously. *Digestive defects* include cystic fibrosis, in which pancreatic enzymes are absent, biliary or liver diseases with altered bile flow, and lactase deficiency, in which there is a congenital or secondary lactose intolerance. *Absorptive defects* may be primary such as celiac disease or secondary to inflammatory disease of the bowel with the concomitant accelerated bowel motility and impaired absorption (e.g., ulcerative colitis, Crohn's disease).

Etiology. Clients in a therapy practice affected by malabsorption most often include people who develop gastroenteritis secondary to NSAID use, fibrosis caused by progressive systemic sclerosis or radiation injury, drug-induced malabsorption, and exocrine deficiency of the pancreas caused by diabetes mellitus. Hyperabsorption of substances such as vitamin D and the accompanying excessive absorption of calcium can also occur by intake of excessive amounts of calcium carbonate (Tums) for acid indigestion.

Pathogenesis. Generally, maldigestion is caused by deficiencies of enzymes (e.g., pancreatic lipase) and specific defects (e.g., poor digestion, lactose intolerance). Inadequate secretion of bile salts (e.g., advanced liver disease, obstruction of the common bile duct) and inadequate reabsorption of bile in the ileum also contribute to maldigestion (Andreoli et al., 1993).

In the case of inadequate absorption, food is fully digested, but not adequately absorbed. This situation occurs when the absorptive surface is normal but inadequate, or adequate but not functioning normally. This problem occurs within the mucosal cell and may be highly specific owing to a gene defect. Malabsorption syndrome can also be caused by a digestive defect, a mucosal abnormality, or lymphatic obstruction and can be a generalized malabsorption or an isolated malabsorption of a particular nutrient.

Clinical Manifestations. Early manifestations of malabsorption are progressive and not easily noticed by the person affected. Weight loss, fatigue, depression, and bloating are early symptoms. A change in bowel habits may occur with production of bulky, malodorous oil-covered stools (steatorrhea) that are difficult to flush. Excessive nocturnal reabsorption of intestinal fluids may cause nocturia. A gluten-related skin disorder, dermatitis herpetiformis, may also be present.

Other common signs and symptoms include explosive diarrhea, chronic diarrhea, abdominal cramps and bloating, indigestion, and flatulence. Late manifestations caused by nutritional deficiencies secondary to the malabsorption may include muscle wasting owing to diminished muscle mass, low blood pressure, and abdominal distention with active bowel sounds.

Any cause of decreased intrinsic factor can result in decreased absorption of vitamin B_{12} resulting in pernicious anemia. Other clinical findings are dependent on the particular condition or specific nutrient involved. The therapist is most likely to see the symptoms listed in Table 13–8.

TABLE 13-8 Symptoms Associated with Malabsorption

Symptoms	Malabsorbed Nutrients
Muscle weakness, muscle wasting, paresthesias	Generalized malnutrition; fat, protein, carbohydrates
Osteomalacia	Fat, protein, carbohydrates, iron, water; vitamins A, D, K
Tetany, paresthesias, Trousseau's sign, Chvostek's sign	Calcium, vitamin D, magnesium, potassium
Numbness and tingling; neurologic damage	Vitamin B_{12}, vitamin B
Bone pain, fractures, skeletal deformities	Calcium, vitamin D, protein
Muscle spasms	Electrolyte imbalance, calcium, pregnancy
Easy bleeding or bruising	Vitamin K
Generalized swelling	Protein

Medical Management

Diagnosis. It is important to differentiate between the various causes of malabsorption to determine the specific treatment. There are a large number of diagnostic tests (e.g., fecal fat analysis for fat malabsorption, oral tolerance tests and measurement of breath hydrogen for lactose intolerance, other breath tests to detect the presence of compounds produced by intraluminal bacteria). Specific tests are also available to assess pancreatic insufficiency. Biopsy of the small intestinal mucosa may be necessary. Sometimes clinical trials for treatable conditions are diagnostic (e.g., gluten-free diet for celiac disease, antibiotics for bacterial overgrowth, use of over-the-counter preparations of lactase enzyme [LactAid] for lactose intolerance).

Treatment and Prognosis. Therapy depends on the underlying condition such as avoidance of gluten for celiac disease or replacement of pancreatic enzymes for pancreatic insufficiency (cystic fibrosis). Muscular twitching and tetany are treated with calcium phosphate or gluconate administered orally or intravenously. Total parenteral nutrition (TPN)[13] may be the only treatment option, as in the case of reduced absorptive surface (e.g., short-bowel syndrome secondary to resection of the small intestine).

The prognosis is good for any of these conditions if the underlying defect can be corrected. There may be a slightly higher incidence of non-Hodgkin's lymphoma in adult life with gluten-sensitive enteropathy. Anyone who develops GI symptoms while in remission on a gluten-free diet should be evaluated for cancer (McQuaid and Knauer, 1994).

People with celiac disease have a greater risk of developing other related immune system disorders. Genes that make a person more susceptible to celiac disease are also known to be connected with autoimmune disorders, including insulin-dependent diabetes mellitus (IDDM, formerly called type I), systemic lupus erythematosus, Sjögren's syndrome, scleroderma, autoimmune chronic active hepatitis, Graves' disease, Addison's disease, and myasthenia gravis.

Special Implications for the Therapist **13-9**

MALABSORPTION SYNDROME

In the rehabilitation setting or for the acute care client who has not been eating solid foods, diarrhea may develop when the person begins to reestablish a normal diet. Prolonged viral conditions can wash out the enzymes normally present in the columnar epithelial cells. Reestablishing normal eating may require additional time to restore the enzymatic homeostasis in the intestines.

[13] Parenteral nutrition (sometimes called hyperalimentation) is a technique for meeting a person's nutritional needs by means of intravenous feedings, allowing bowel rest. Nutrition by intravenous feeding is administered via a central venous catheter, usually inserted into the superior vena cava and may be TPN or supplemental. TPN may also be given peripherally for short periods of time.

Paresthesias, muscle weakness, and muscle wasting accompanied by fatigue and weight loss can be signs of malnutrition (e.g., eating disorders) or malabsorbed fat, protein, or carbohydrates. Malabsorption of calcium, vitamin D, magnesium, and potassium can cause paresthesias, tetany, and positive Trousseau's and Chvostek's signs* (see Figs. 4–4 and 4–5).

Malabsorption of calcium, vitamin D, and protein can cause bone pain with pathologic (compression) fractures and skeletal deformities. In fact, 20% of osteoporosis is osteomalacia secondary to decreased absorption of vitamin D (see discussions of osteomalacia and osteoporosis in Chapter 20). On the other hand, excessive absorption of vitamin D and calcium through the use of calcium carbonate for acid indigestion should be evaluated by a physician; these antacids may be used by women to obtain the daily 1500 mg calcium requirement as protection against osteoporosis.

Other effects of malabsorption syndrome possibly seen in a therapy setting include muscle spasms caused by electrolyte imbalance (especially low calcium) and pregnancy, easy bleeding or bruising as a result of a vitamin K deficiency, and generalized swelling caused by protein depletion (see Table 13–8).

Physicians may recommend vitamin B_{12} or other B vitamin supplements for people with carpal tunnel syndrome. Malabsorption of these essential vitamins alters the structure and disrupts the function of the peripheral nerves, spinal cord, and brain and can cause numbness and tingling as well as permanent neurologic damage unresponsive to vitamin B_{12} therapy in extreme cases.

* Trousseau's sign is an indication of tetany seen as carpal spasm elicited by compressing the upper arm (as occurs when taking a blood pressure measurement). Chvostek's sign is a spasm of the facial muscles elicited by tapping the facial nerve in the region of the parotid gland; it is seen in tetany.

Celiac Disease

Celiac disease (CD), also known as gluten-induced enteropathy, gluten-sensitive enteropathy (GSE), and celiac sprue, is second only to cystic fibrosis as a cause of malabsorption in children. The term *celiac disease* is often used to describe a symptom complex that has four characteristics in common: (1) steatorrhea (fat in feces), (2) general malnutrition, (3) abdominal distention, and (4) secondary vitamin deficiencies.

The disease is defined by an inability to digest gluten, one of the proteins found in wheat, barley, rye, and oats. Gluten consists of two fractions: glutenin and gliadin. The exact pathologic process is unknown but susceptible people are unable to digest the gliadin fraction, resulting in an accumulation of a toxic substance that is damaging to the absorptive surface of the small intestine.

Symptoms of CD are first observed 3 to 6 months after the introduction of gluten-containing grains into the diet. Early symptoms are failure to thrive and diarrhea. Other symptoms include impaired fat absorption, impaired absorption of nutrients (malnutrition; muscle wasting, especially prominent in the legs and buttocks; anemia; abdominal distention), and behavioral changes (irritability, uncooperativeness, apathy). Musculoskeletal and neurologic manifestations may bring the child to the therapist's attention. Muscle twitching, tetany, and bone pain (especially in the lower back, rib cage, and pelvis) are musculoskeletal effects of calcium loss and vitamin D deficiency. Peripheral neuropathy or paresthesias may also develop.

Diagnosis is by jejunal biopsy performed by passing an endoscope through the mouth along the alimentary tract to the jejunum. Atrophic changes in the mucosa of the small intestine establish the diagnosis. Dramatic clinical improvement after a gluten-free diet with weight gain, improved appetite, elimination of diarrhea, and personality change confirms the diagnosis. Treatment and prognosis is as reported for malabsorption syndrome. CD is considered a chronic disease and strict permanent dietary avoidance of gluten to prevent symptoms may also minimize the risk of developing lymphoma, the most serious complication of this disease (Wong, 1993).

Vascular Diseases

Blood is supplied to the bowel by the celiac and superior and inferior mesenteric arteries. These arteries have anastomotic intercommunications at the head of the pancreas and along the transverse bowel. Obstruction of blood flow can occur as a result of atherosclerotic occlusive lesions or embolism (Ruder and Matassarin-Jacobs, 1993).

Intestinal Ischemia (*Tierney, 1994*)

Acute intestinal ischemia results from embolic occlusions of the visceral branches of the abdominal aorta, generally in people with valvular heart disease, atrial fibrillation, or left ventricular thrombus. Other causes include thrombosis of one or more visceral vessels involved with arteriosclerotic occlusive changes or nonocclusive mesenteric vascular insufficiency in people with congestive heart failure receiving recently instituted digitalis.

Symptoms of acute intestinal ischemia include acute onset of crampy or steady epigastric or periumbilical abdominal pain combined with minimal or no findings on abdominal examination and a high leukocyte count. Angiography of the superior mesenteric artery is essential to early diagnosis. If occlusion is present, laparotomy is performed to reestablish blood flow to the intestine if possible and remove necrotic bowel if some viable bowel exists.

Atherosclerotic plaque of the superior mesenteric, celiac, and inferior mesenteric arteries causes a significant decrease in blood flow to the intestines resulting in *chronic intestinal ischemia*. Symptoms of epigastric or periumbilical pains lasting for 1 to 3 hours in a person over 45 years of age who has peripheral vascular disease points to a diagnosis of intestinal ischemia. Arteriography may be performed if the person is a good candidate for surgery.

Special Implications for the Therapist **13–10**

INTESTINAL ISCHEMIA

Intestinal angina as a result of atherosclerotic plaque–induced ischemia can result in intermittent back pain (usually at the thoracolumbar junction) with exertion. Clinical presentation combined with past medical history, the presence of coronary artery disease risk factors (see Table 10–2), and the presence of peripheral vascular disease may alert the therapist to the need for a medical referral if the client has not been medically diagnosed.

Bacterial Infections

Botulism (*Abrutyn, 1994*)

Botulism is a rare paralytic disease that has a predilection for the cranial nerves and then progresses caudad and symmetrically to the trunk and extremities. Only foodborne botulism is discussed here; see Chapter 34 for a complete discussion of botulism.

In the case of foodborne botulism, ingested neurotoxins resist gastric digestion and proteolytic enzymes and are readily absorbed into the blood from the proximal small intestine. Minute amounts of circulating toxin reach the cholinergic nerve endings at the myoneural junction and bind to gangliosides of the presynaptic nerve terminals. Flaccid paralysis is caused by inhibition of acetylcholine release from cholinergic terminals at the motor end plate (Rubin and Farber, 1994).

Early symptoms of botulism are usually related to involvement of the cranial nerves producing weakness, visual changes (double vision or diplopia, and intolerance to light, or photophobia), ptosis, dysarthria or dysphagia, difficulty breathing, and impaired swallowing. There are no sensory changes. Motor weakness of the face and neck muscles can progress to involve the diaphragm, accessory muscles of breathing, and extremities. Vomiting, abdominal pain, headache, and constipation may occur before or after the onset of paralysis. The usual secondary effects of flaccid motor paralysis can occur, such as severe muscle wasting, pressure sores, and aspiration pneumonia.

Toxin identification is made by stool or serum analysis or cultures of the organism. Electromyography is confirmatory[14] and necessary to differentiate this condition from myasthenia gravis or Guillain-Barré syndrome. Immediate administration of antitoxin prevents further binding of free botulism to the presynaptic endings. Untreated food botulism can be fatal within 24 hours of toxin ingestion. Respiratory failure caused by rapid onset of respiratory muscle weakness is a complication that is often fatal.

Special Implications for the Therapist **13–11**

BOTULISM

The sudden onset of rapidly progressive symptoms associated with botulism is most likely to be reported to a physician rather than to a therapist. However, presentation of acute symmetrical cranial nerve impairment (ptosis, diplopia, dysarthria), followed by descending weakness or paralysis of the muscles in the extremities or trunk, and dyspnea from respiratory muscle paralysis, requires immediate medical referral. After the acute onset and initiation of medical treatment, treatment is as for cranial nerve palsy. In mild to moderate cases, there is a gradual recovery of muscle strength which can take as long as a year after disease onset; in severe cases, there is a 40% mortality.

Inflammatory Bowel Disease

Overview and Definition. Inflammatory bowel disease (IBD) refers to two inflammatory conditions: Crohn's disease (CD) and ulcerative colitis (UC) (Table 13–9). *Crohn's disease* is a chronic lifelong inflammatory disorder that can affect any segment of the intestinal tract and even tissues in other organs. It is characterized by exacerbations and periods of remission. CD is also referred to as regional enteritis, regional ileitis, terminal ileitis, or granulomatous colitis, depending on the location of the inflammation.

Ulcerative colitis is a chronic inflammatory disorder characterized by chronic diarrhea and rectal bleeding with ulceration, primarily just of the mucosa and submucosa in the colon. It may be referred to as ulcerative proctitis (involving the rectum only) or pancolitis (involving the entire colon).

Incidence and Etiology. Both CD and UC are disorders of unknown cause involving genetic and immunologic influences on the GI tract's ability to distinguish foreign from self-antigens. No single genetic marker (i.e., histocompatibility antigen) has been identified yet in clients with IBD, preventing early identification of susceptible individuals.

Inflammatory bowel conditions are considered to be autoimmune diseases in which either the antibodies or other defense mechanisms are directed against the body. A possible correlation between the onset of disease with life stresses and poor adaptation to those stresses is cited in the majority of literature regarding IBD, but this has not been proved conclusively. More likely, these factors exacerbate the illness but are not a cause of the condition. Autoimmune disorders such as systemic lupus erythematosus and fibromyalgia often accompany IBD.

These two conditions can occur in all age groups but have a peak incidence between the ages of 15 and 35. UC appears to be more common, but the incidence of CD has risen over the past 20 years; the combined prevalence of the two diseases is approximately 100 per 100,000 population (Hanauer, 1992).

Pathogenesis. There are two features that distinguish CD from UC. In CD, inflammation usually involves all layers of the bowel wall, referred to as *transmural inflammatory disease*, and the inflammatory process is discontinuous so that segments of inflamed areas are separated by normal tissue in a "skip" pattern. The transverse colon is affected in half of all cases; other more common sites include the small bowel, colon, and anorectal region. In UC, involvement extends uniformly and continuously, usually starting from the distal part of the rectum.

Inflammation accompanying CD produces thickened, edematous tissue and chronic inflammation leads to ulcerations which produce fissures that extend the inflammation into lymphoid tissue. Mesenteric[15] lymph nodes are often

[14] Nerve conduction velocities are normal but action potentials are decreased with a supramaximal stimulus. Facilitation is found after repetitive stimulation at high frequency.

[15] The mesentery is a membranous peritoneal fold attaching the small intestine to the dorsal abdominal wall.

TABLE 13-9 COMPARISON OF THE CHARACTERISTICS OF CROHN'S DISEASE AND ULCERATIVE COLITIS

CHARACTERISTICS	CROHN'S DISEASE	ULCERATIVE COLITIS
Incidence		
Age at onset	Any age; 10–30 yr most common	Any age; 10–40 yr most common
Family history	More common	Less common
Sex (prevalence)	About equal in women and men	Equal in women and men
Cancer risk	Increased; early detection best means of prevention	Increased; preventable with bowel resection
Pathogenesis		
Location of lesions	Any segment; usually small or large intestine	Large intestine; rectum
Skip lesions	Common	Absent
Inflammation and ulceration	Entire intestinal wall involved	Mucosal/submucosal layers involved
Granulomas	Typical	Uncommon
Thickened bowel wall	Typical	Uncommon
Narrowed lumen and obstruction	Typical	Uncommon
Fissures and fistulas	Common	Absent
Clinical Manifestations		
Abdominal pain	Mild to severe; common	Mild to severe; less frequent
Diarrhea	May be absent; moderate	Typical; often severe; chronic
Bloody stools	Uncommon	Typical
Abdominal mass	Common; right lower quadrant	Uncommon
Anorexia	Can be severe	Mild or moderate
Weight loss	Can be severe	Mild to moderate
Skin rashes	Common, mild	Common, mild
Joint pain	Common, mild to moderate	Common, mild to moderate
Growth retardation (pediatric)	Often marked	Usually mild
Clinical course	Remissions and exacerbations	Remissions and exacerbations

Adapted from Huether SE, McCance KL: Alterations in digestive function. *In* McCance KL, Huether SE (eds): Pathophysiology: The Biologic Basis for Disease in Adults and Children. St Louis, Mosby–Year Book, 1994, p 1341.

enlarged, firm, and matted together. The lesions are granulomatous (epithelioid cells rimmed by lymphocytes) with projections of inflamed tissue surrounded by fibrous scarring narrowing the intestinal lumen. A combination of the granulomas (nodular swelling), ulceration, and fibrosis results in a "cobblestone" appearance of the mucosal surface of the colon (Fig. 13–8).

Inflammation of the mucosa associated with UC results in small erosions and subsequent ulcerations with eventual abscess formation and necrosis (Fig. 13–9). Destruction of the mucosa causes bleeding, cramping pain, bowel frequency, and large volumes of watery diarrhea owing to decreased absorption and decreased transit time of intestinal contents through the colon.

Clinical Manifestations. Clinically, these disorders are characterized by recurrent inflammatory involvement of intestinal segments with diverse clinical manifestations often resulting in a chronic, unpredictable course (Glickman, 1994). For comparison of specific signs and symptoms, see Table 13–9.

Arthritis and Inflammatory Intestinal Diseases. The theory that an immune mechanism may be involved in the development of IBD is based in part on the presence of extraintestinal manifestations including inflammation of the eye (uveitis), mono- or polyarthritis, migratory arthralgias, and redness of the skin (erythema nodosum) (Mahoney, 1993; Musio et al., 1993). Ankylosing spondylitis (AS) may accompany IBD but is indistinguishable from idiopathic AS.

Joint involvement ranging from arthralgia only to acute arthritis is a common finding (25%) in IBD. Intestinal arthritis is usually asymmetrical, affects the knees, ankles, and

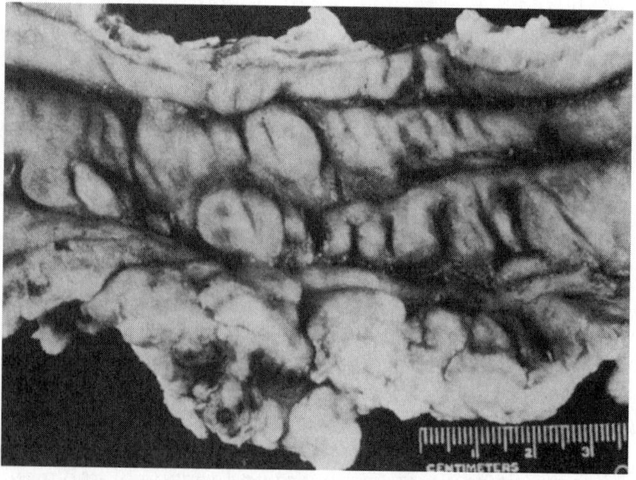

Figure 13-8. Crohn's disease. The mucosal surface of the colon displays a "cobblestone" appearance owing to the presence of linear ulcerations and edema and inflammation of the intervening tissue. (*From Marshak R, Lindner A: Radiology of the Small Intestine. Philadelphia, WB Saunders, 1976.*)

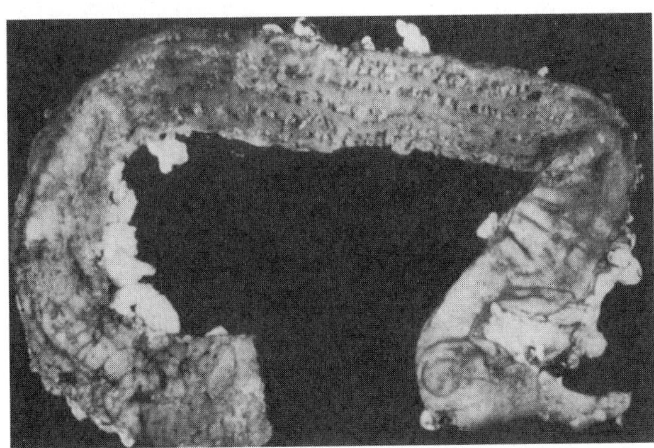

Figure 13–9. Ulcerative colitis. Prominent erythema and ulceration affecting the whole colon. (*From Sleisenger MH, Fordtran JS (eds): Gastrointestinal Disease, ed 5. Philadelphia, WB Saunders, 1993, p 1310.*)

wrists, but can affect any joint. Arthritis associated with chronic IBD comes and goes, occurring during the course of the bowel disease or preceding repeat episodes of bowel symptoms by 1 to 2 weeks. With proper medical treatment, there are no permanent sequelae or joint deformities.

Pathologically, the synovitis is nonspecific without crystals or evidence of infection. Tests for specific forms of arthritis (e.g., rheumatoid factor and antinuclear antibody) are usually negative; HLA-B27 (*h*uman *l*eukocyte *a*ntigen) is positive[16] (see explanation of HLA, Chapter 5; see also Table 35–17). Treatment of intestinal arthritis is toward control of the underlying intestinal inflammation; treatment of AS associated with IBD is the same as for idiopathic AS.

Medical Management

Diagnosis and Treatment. Since there are no specifically distinctive characteristic features or specific diagnostic tests, the diagnosis of CD and UC remains one of exclusion based on medical history and clinical presentation. Diagnostic procedures may include radiographic findings, upper GI series, barium enema, or colonoscopy with biopsy to evaluate the colon. Microscopically, granulomas present in CD (but not present in UC) distinguish CD from UC (Glickman, 1994).

Current treatment is directed toward symptomatic relief and control of the disease process on an individual basis. Some treatment measures may include diet and nutrition, symptomatic medications such as antidiarrheals or antispasmodics, or specific drug therapy to suppress inflammation and alleviate painful cramping (O'Brien et al., 1991; Prantera et al., 1992). Hospitalization may be required in the case of severe, unremitting disease with complications. Surgical resection of the colon, colostomy, or ileostomy may be performed for toxic megacolon or if medical intervention is unsuccessful with complications such as fistula, abscess, or for relief of obstruction (Hastings and Weber, 1993; Fazio, 1990).

Prognosis. CD is an incurable, chronic and sometimes debilitating disease with a known increased risk of intestinal cancer in people who develop this condition at a young age of onset (less than 30 years of age) (Gillen et al., 1994; Connell et al., 1994). Surgical removal of the diseased bowel does not prevent bowel cancer in CD so screening of stool specimens and periodic colonoscopic examination and biopsy are required for early detection. With proper medical and surgical treatment, the majority of people are able to cope with this disease and its complications. Few people die as a direct consequence of CD. The mortality rate (5% to 10%) increases with the duration of the disease (McQuaid and Knauer, 1994).

Like CD, UC is a chronic, occasionally debilitating disease for which there is no cure. The clinical course is variable but recurrent with long periods of remission possible. Approximately 85% of clients with UC will have mild to moderate intermittent disease managed without hospitalization. The remaining 15% demonstrate a full-blown course involving the entire colon, severe diarrhea, and systemic signs and symptoms (Glickman, 1994). There is a 20% mortality rate during the first 10 years of UC when complications occur. Also like CD, 10 years of chronic attacks of UC can predispose the colon to metaplastic changes leading to colon cancer, but unlike CD, in UC, removal of the affected bowel can prevent bowel cancer.

Special Implications for the Therapist **13–12**

INFLAMMATORY BOWEL DISEASE

When terminal ileum involvement in CD produces periumbilical pain, referred pain to the corresponding low back is possible. Pain of the ileum is intermittent and perceived in the lower right quadrant with possible associated iliopsoas abscess or ureteral obstruction from an inflammatory mass causing hip, thigh, or knee pain, often with an antalgic gait. Specific objective tests are available to rule out systemic origin of hip, thigh, or knee pain (Figs. 13–10 and 13–11; see also Fig. 13–17).

Twenty-five percent of all clients with IBD may present with migratory arthralgias, monarthritis, polyarthritis, or sacroiliitis. It is essential that any time a client presents with low back, hip, or sacroiliac pain of unknown origin, the therapist screen for medical disease by asking a few simple questions about the presence of accompanying intestinal symptoms, known personal history, or family history for IBD, and possible relief of symptoms after passing stool or gas (Goodman and Snyder, 1995). Articular symptoms may be the primary clinical manifestation of IBD; intestinal symptoms are usually present but disregarded as part of the whole picture by the client. Treatment of the musculoskeletal involvement follows the usual protocols for each area affected.

Sulfasalazine used in mild cases of IBD interferes with the absorption and utilization of folic acid, requiring supplemental folic acid. Clients taking sulfasalazine may complain of headache, nausea, and vomiting. Corticosteroids are an important and effective drug for treating moderate and severe IBD but carry with them all of the complications of prolonged high-dose steroid therapy (see Table 4–7).

[16] A statistical association has been shown between HLA-B27 and the development of AS (O'Toole, 1992).

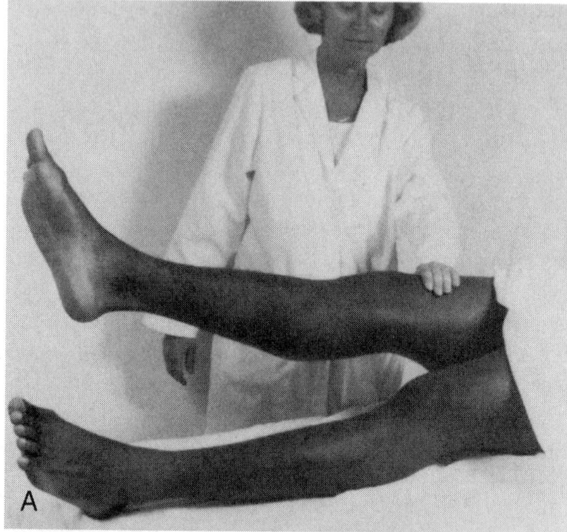

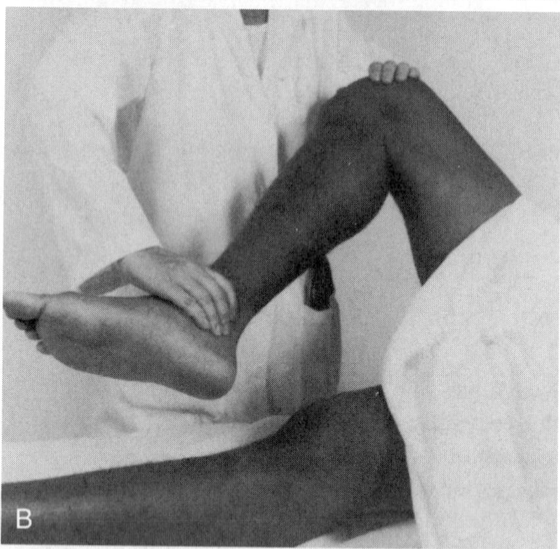

Figure **13-10.** *A*, Iliopsoas muscle test. With the client supine, instruct the client to lift the right leg straight up; apply resistance to the distal thigh as the client tries to hold the leg up. When the test is negative, the client feels no change; when the test is positive (i.e., the iliopsoas muscle is inflamed), pain is felt in the right lower quadrant. *B*, Obturator muscle test. With the client supine, perform active assisted motion, flexing at the hip and knee; hold the ankle and rotate the leg internally and externally. A negative or normal response is no pain; a positive test for inflamed obturator muscle is right lower quadrant pain. (*From Jarvis C: Physical Examination and Health Assessment. Philadelphia, WB Saunders, 1992, p 614.*)

People with IBD are known to have low bone mineral content. Low bone mineral density (BMD) may be more characteristic of CD than of UC, but no consistent differentiation has been made between CD and UC in this regard (Ghosh et al., 1994). It is always important for the therapist to know what medications clients are taking so that the first sign of possible side effects will be recognized and the physician alerted.

Hydration and nutrition are always long-term concerns with clients who have UC or CD. The client must be observed for any signs of dehydration (e.g., dry lips, hands, headache, brittle hair, incoordination, disorientation; see Box 4–7), as well as for any increase or pathologic change in symptoms. Any increase in painful symptoms or increased stool output or stool frequency must be reported to the physician.

People with IBD may have a characteristic personality susceptible to emotional stresses which precipitate or exacerbate their symptoms. No direct evidence proves the relationship between emotional factors and IBD. However, the chronic nature of IBD affecting persons in the prime of life often results in feelings of anger, anxiety, and possible depression. These emotions are important factors in the client's response to treatment and in modifying the overall course of the disease (Glickman, 1994). See also Chapter 2.

Antibiotic-Associated Colitis

Antibiotics can suppress normal GI flora, the bacteria usually residing within the lumen of the intestine, thus allowing yeasts and molds to flourish. Other kinds of microorganisms can replace normal GI flora suppressed by antibiotic therapy such as *Clostridium difficile*, the major cause of colitis in people with antibiotic-associated diarrhea. Although nearly all antibiotics have been associated with this syndrome, drugs such as clindamycin, ampicillin, and the cephalosporins are commonly implicated.

Clostridium difficile is not invasive, but replaces normal GI flora by producing toxins that damage the colonic mucosa. The mechanism by which C. *difficile* becomes pathogenic is not completely understood. The overgrowth of C. *difficile* causes lesions described as raised, exudative, necrotic, and inflammatory plaques. These plaques attach to the mucosal surface of the small intestine or colon, or both, giving this condition the name *pseudomembranous enterocolitis* (PMC). When the lesions are restricted to the small intestine, the term *pseudomembranous enteritis* is applied.

Onset of symptoms (primarily voluminous, watery diarrhea but also abdominal cramps and tenderness, and fever) occurs during early administration or within 4 weeks after the drug has been discontinued. Complications of untreated illness include dehydration with electrolyte imbalance, perforation, toxic megacolon, and death.

Reports of reactive arthritis occurring after C. *difficile* infection are most common with colitis associated with antibiotic therapy (Putterman and Rubinow, 1993). *Reactive arthritis* is defined as the occurrence of an acute, aseptic, inflammatory arthropathy arising after an infectious process, but at a site remote from the primary infection. The arthritis typically involves the large and medium joints of the lower extremities and first manifests 1 to 4 weeks after the infectious insult. Reactive arthritis may include some, but not all, of the three features associated with Reiter's syndrome (see discussion in Chapter 23) and is often designated incomplete Reiter's syndrome (Keating and Vyas, 1995).

Diagnosis is made on the basis of the history and if no other identifiable cause of diarrhea can be determined. Endoscopic procedures such as flexible sigmoidoscopy may be used in the diagnosis. Discontinuation of the antibiotics is usually enough to relieve symptoms, but antimicrobial agents such as metro-

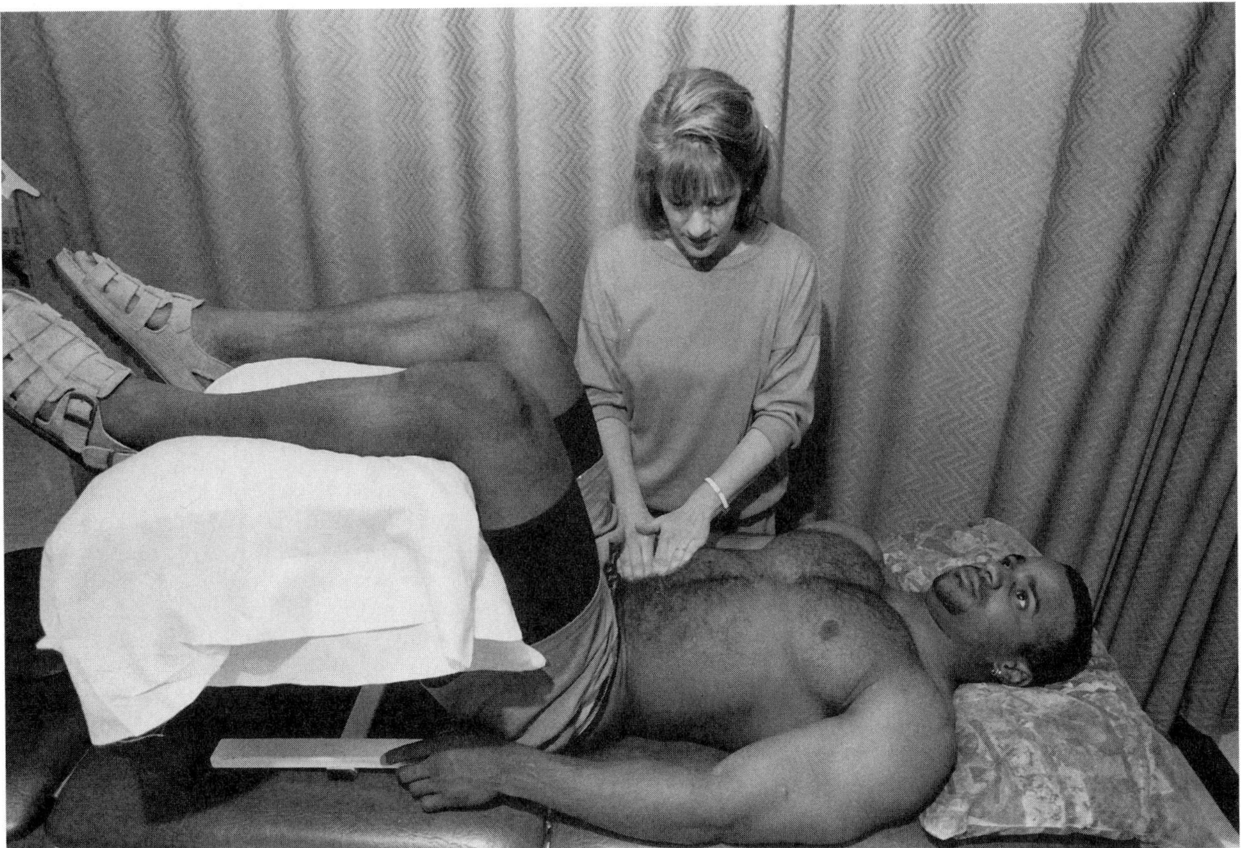

Figure **13-11.** Palpating the iliopsoas muscle. In addition to assessing McBurney's point, the examiner may also palpate the iliopsoas muscle by placing the client in a supine position with the hips and knees both flexed 90 degrees, and with the lower legs resting on a firm surface (a traction table stool works well for this; pillows under the lower legs may be necessary to obtain the full position). Palpate approximately one-third the distance from the anterior superior iliac spine toward the umbilicus; it may be necessary to ask the client to initiate hip flexion on that side to help isolate the muscle and avoid palpating the bowel. A positive test for iliopsoas abscess will produce right lower quadrant pain; alternatively, palpation may produce back pain or local muscular pain from a shortened or "tight" muscle indicating the need for soft tissue mobilization (STM) and stretching of the iliopsoas muscle. STM in this area would be contraindicated in the presence of any abdominal or pelvic inflammatory process involving the iliopsoas muscle until the infection has been treated with complete resolution.

nidazole or the more expensive vancomycin may be administered orally; supportive measures may include administration of intravenous fluids to correct fluid losses, electrolyte imbalance, and hypoalbuminemia. Recurrence of symptoms is common when treatment is discontinued, requiring retreatment, or in some cases, careful medical observation (Bartlett, 1993). In severe disease, mortality rates can be as high as 30% (Kasper and Zaleznik, 1994).

Special Implications for the Therapist **13-13**

ANTIBIOTIC-ASSOCIATED COLITIS

The primary concern with any client experiencing excessive watery diarrhea is fluid and electrolyte imbalance. See the implications previously discussed, as well as the discussion in Chapter 4. Since the onset of this condition may occur up to 1 month after the antibiotic has been discontinued, the client may not recognize the association between current GI symptoms and previous medications. Anytime someone taking antibiotics or recently completing a course of antibiotics develops GI symptoms, encourage physician notification.

Irritable Bowel Syndrome

Definition and Incidence. Irritable bowel syndrome (IBS) is a group of symptoms that represent the most common disorder of the GI system. IBS has been referred to as nervous indigestion, functional dyspepsia, spastic colon, nervous colon, and irritable colon, but because of the absence of inflammation, it should not be confused with colitis or other inflammatory diseases of the intestinal tract.

IBS is a chronic condition and is not limited to the colon, but can occur anywhere in the small and large intestines. Women are more often affected than men, especially in early adulthood, but IBS can occur in either sex at any age.

Etiology and Pathogenesis. IBS is a functional disorder of motility of the intestines as a result of the digestive tract's reaction to stress and diet. Episodes of emotional stress, fatigue, smoking, alcohol intake, or eating (especially a large meal with high fat content, roughage, or fruit) aggravate or precipitate symptoms (Snape, 1992). Intolerance of lactose and other sugars may account for IBS in some people.

There are no anatomic abnormalities or underlying organic disease. Colonic motor activity is abnormally increased and altered small bowel motility may also occur, which is especially associated with emotional tension. Rapid alterations in the speed of bowel movement create an obstruction to the natural flow of stool and gas. The resultant pressure buildup in the bowel produces the pain and spasm reported (Schuster, 1993).

Clinical Manifestations. Symptoms of IBS occur in up to 25% of otherwise healthy persons and are intermittent with variable periods of remission. The primary symptoms of IBS are altered bowel habits with diarrhea, constipation, and abdominal cramps and pain, or alternating diarrhea and constipation.

Pain may be steady or intermittent, and there may be a dull deep discomfort with sharp cramps in the morning or after eating. The typical pain pattern consists of lower left quadrant abdominal pain, constipation, and diarrhea (Ruder and Matassarin-Jacobs, 1993). Pain is relieved by defecation or associated with bowel habit change. Other symptoms may include nausea and vomiting, anorexia, foul breath, sour stomach, and flatus.

Medical Management

Diagnosis, Treatment, and Prognosis. Diagnosis is based on a classic history. Sigmoidoscopy often reveals marked spasm and mucus in the colonic lumen and will frequently provoke a spontaneous exacerbation of symptoms. Laboratory studies include a complete blood count and stool examination to rule out the presence of occult blood, parasites, and pathogenic bacteria. GI films may show altered motility without other evidence of abnormalities (McQuaid and Knauer, 1994).

General treatment may include a stress reduction program with a regular program of relaxation techniques and exercise. Psychotherapy, biofeedback training, and pharmacologic treatment may be suggested. Medications may include antianxiety or antidepressant drugs, and anticholinergic agents before meals to help control symptoms. Dietary exclusion of milk and milk products may be helpful for those people with lactose intolerance. Increased dietary fiber, use of bulking agents such as psyllium preparations, and avoidance of alcohol, tobacco, and GI stimulants such as caffeine-containing beverages are often recommended.

IBS is not a life-threatening disorder, and prognosis is good for controlling symptoms through diet, medication, regular physical activity, and stress management. There is no known relationship between IBS and malignancy of the bowel.

Special Implications for the Therapist **13-14**

IRRITABLE BOWEL SYNDROME

Regular physical activity helps relieve stress and assists in bowel function, particularly in people who experience constipation. The therapist should encourage anyone with IBS to continue with the prescribed therapy program during symptomatic periods. Therapists must be alert to the person with IBS who has developed breath-holding patterns or hyperventilation in response to stress. Teaching proper breathing is important for all daily activities, especially during exercise and relaxation techniques. See also Chapter 2.

Diverticular Disease

Definition and Incidence. *Diverticular disease* is the term used to describe diverticulosis (uncomplicated disease) and diverticulitis (disease complicated by inflammation). Diverticulosis refers to the presence of outpouchings (diverticula) in the wall of the colon or small intestine, a condition in which the mucosa and submucosa herniate through the muscular layers of the colon (Fig. 13–12) to form outpouchings containing feces (Fig. 13–13). This acquired deformity of the colon is rarely reversible and usually asymptomatic. The most common site is the sigmoid colon (95% of cases) because of the high pressures in this area required to move stool into the rectum, but any segment of the colon may be involved.

Diverticular disease is common, present in approximately 10% of people in the United States (Naitove and Smith, 1993). There is an increased incidence after age 50, the disease being present in as many as half of all elderly persons in the United States. Incidence is increased among the obese.

Etiology and Risk Factors. Causes of diverticular disease include atrophy or weakness of the bowel muscle, increased intraluminal pressure, obesity, and chronic constipation. Some people are born with diverticula, probably due to an inherited defect in the muscular wall of the intestines, but the majority of people who have diverticulosis develop it with age, indicating that both heredity and lifestyle play a role. The current hypothesis as to the primary cause (and major risk factor) of diverticular disease is a low fiber diet, which decreases stool bulk and predisposes individuals to constipation. The subsequent increased intraluminal pressure pushes the mucosa through connective tissue, weakening bowel muscle.

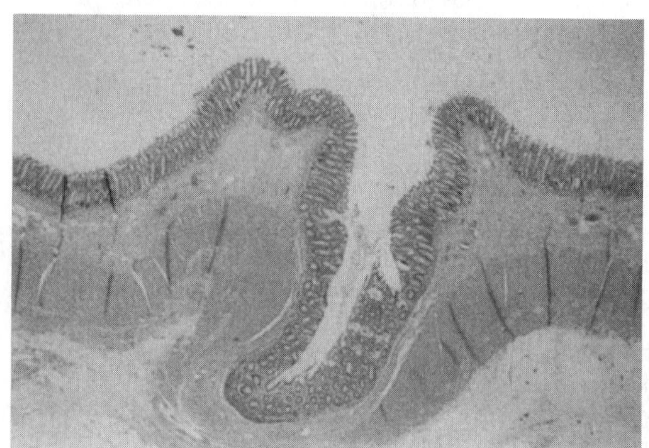

Figure **13–12.** Diverticulosis of the colon. A low-power photomicrograph shows a diverticulum, which extends through the muscle layers. (*From Rubin E, Farber JL (eds): Pathology, ed 2. Philadelphia, JB Lippincott, 1994, p 675.*)

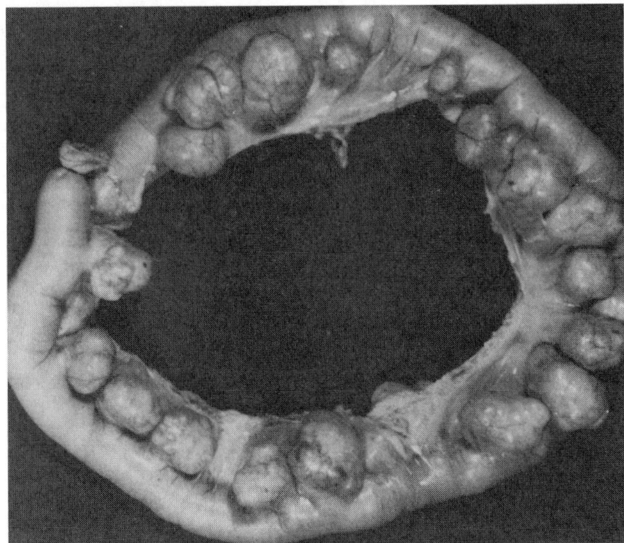

Figure 13–13. Multiple diverticula in resected section of the colon. Weak spots in the muscle layers of the intestinal wall permit the mucosa to bulge outward (herniate) into the pelvic cavity. (*From Rosai J: Ackerman's Surgical Pathology, 7th ed. St Louis, Mosby–Year Book, 1989.*)

In addition to a low fiber diet as a major risk factor, ingestion of poorly digested foods that can block the opening of the diverticulum and cause inflammation may also contribute to the development of diverticular disease. Such foods as corn, popcorn, and foods with tiny seeds (e.g. cucumbers, tomatoes, berries) have been implicated, but this remains a controversial issue.

Pathogenesis. Diverticula form at weak points in the colon wall, usually where arteries penetrate the muscularis to nourish the mucosal layer. Changes in the connective tissue of the gut wall contribute to the diminished resistance of the intestinal wall. The circular and longitudinal muscles (taeniae coli) surrounding the diverticula become thickened and hypertrophy as a result of age-related changes in collagen and progressive deposition of elastin in longitudinal muscle (Bornstein, 1976; Whiteway and Morson, 1985). Increased contraction of these muscles is required when hard, compact stools form in the absence of adequate fiber. Increased intraluminal pressure then increases the herniation. Over a person's lifetime, diverticula may increase in number and size, but only rarely extend to other portions of the colon.

Diverticulitis occurs when undigested food blocks the diverticulum (blind outpouchings), decreasing blood supply to the blood vessels penetrating the internal circular layer of bowel muscularis. This phenomenon leaves the bowel at risk for invasion by bacteria into the diverticulum and subsequent inflammation. The inflamed area becomes congested with blood and may bleed. Diverticulitis can lead to perforation when the trapped mass in the diverticula erodes the bowel wall. Chronic diverticulitis can result in increased scarring and narrowing of the bowel lumen, potentially leading to obstruction (Ruder and Matassarin-Jacobs, 1993).

Clinical Manifestations. Diverticular disease is asymptomatic in 80% of people affected. When diverticula become inflamed, diverticulitis develops, and the person experiences episodic or constant, severe abdominal pain located in the left quadrant or midabdominal region, often with extension into the back. The mechanism of pain is probably increased tension in the colonic wall with an associated rise in intraluminal pressure (Naitove and Smith, 1993).

Other symptoms may include constipation alternating with diarrhea, increased flatus, fever, sudden onset of painless rectal bleeding, and anemia in the presence of chronic blood loss. Eating and increased intra-abdominal pressure increase pain (see Box 13–1), whereas temporary partial or complete relief may follow a bowel movement or passage of flatus.

Medical Management

Diagnosis, Treatment, and Prognosis. Barium enema studies show the characteristic diverticula; colonoscopy and sigmoidoscopy may also provide diagnostic information and a CT scan may sometimes reveal the inflamed colon segment. There are no specific laboratory tests, but fecal examination for occult blood may be positive and anemia may be identified. Stool cultures may be used to exclude bacterial or parasitic infections.

Treatment directed at relieving symptoms and preventing diverticulitis is primarily dietary with adherence to a high fiber diet, prevention of constipation with bran and bulk laxatives, and exercise during periods of remission. Acute diverticulitis may require complete rest of the colon accomplished by nasogastric tube feedings and parenteral fluids until the inflammatory process has been resolved. Antibiotics are used for diverticulitis and surgery may be required for severely involved segments, with possible temporary colostomy.

Prognosis is good for the person with known diverticular disease, especially when prevention of diverticulitis is possible by consuming a high fiber diet and avoiding indigestible foods. If the diverticulum is not blocked and infected or inflamed (diverticulitis), the person may be asymptomatic. If the trapped fecal material (fecaliths) do not liquefy and drain from the diverticulum, diverticulitis develops. Only a small minority develop serious or life-threatening complications (Almy and Howell, 1980).

Special Implications for the Therapist **13–15**

DIVERTICULAR DISEASE

Exercise is an important treatment component during periods of remission. The therapist is instrumental in helping establish an appropriate exercise program. Throughout all activity and exercise, clients with diverticular disease must be careful to avoid activities that increase intra-abdominal pressure (see Box 13–1) to avoid further herniation. The therapist can provide valuable information regarding appropriate body mechanics and techniques to reduce intra-abdominal pressure for all activities.

Back pain can occur as a symptom of this disease. Anyone with back pain of nontraumatic or unknown origin must be screened for medical disease, including possible GI involvement. If infection occurs and penetrates the pelvic floor or retroperitoneal tissues, abscesses may result causing isolated referred hip or thigh pain. A variety of objective test procedures may be employed by the therapist to assess for iliopsoas abscess formation, including palpation of McBurney's point (see Fig. 13–17), the iliopsoas muscle test, the obturator test, and palpation of the iliopsoas muscle (see Figs. 13–10 and 13–11).

Neoplasms

Intestinal Polyps

A growth or mass protruding into the intestinal lumen from any area of mucous membrane can be termed a *polyp*. Polyps are either *neoplastic* or *non-neoplastic*. Adenomatous (benign neoplastic) polyps of the intestine usually develop during middle age and more than two thirds of the population over 65 years old have at least one polyp. Until a polyp becomes large enough to obstruct the intestine, there are no discernible symptoms. Early symptoms may be lower abdominal cramping pain, diarrhea with rectal bleeding, and passage of mucus.

Non-neoplastic polyps include are usually asymptomatic although inflammatory polyps may present with symptoms of the underlying inflammatory bowel disease usually present (e.g., UC or CD). Treatment is not required, but, polyps associated with rectal bleeding may be removed through a proctoscope. Polyps may be a risk factor for the development of adenocarcinomas (colorectal cancer) (Winawer et al., 1993). For this reason, regardless of the clinical manifestations, adenomatous polyps should be removed (by polypectomy, usually performed through a sigmoidoscope or colonoscope; large polyps may require removal by laparotomy).

Benign Tumors

Technically, benign tumors are non-neoplastic tumors. The most common benign tumors of the small intestine are adenomas, leiomyomas, and lipomas. Benign tumors of the small intestine rarely become malignant, may be symptomatic, or may be incidental findings at operation or autopsy. *Adenomas* account for 25% of all benign bowel tumors and are usually asymptomatic, although bleeding and intussusception (see discussion under Mechanical Obstruction) are occasional complications. *Leiomyomas* are smooth muscle tumors that can occur at any location in the intestine but are most common in the jejunum. They are usually associated with bleeding when they protrude into the lumen where necrosis of tumor tissue and ulceration of the mucosa occur. Obstruction is uncommon, but intussusception or volvulus may occur. Surgical removal of large leiomyomas is recommended because of the bleeding and the increased risk of malignancy with increasing size. *Lipomas* are fatty tumors that occur throughout the length of the small intestine but occur most frequently in the distal ileum. When symptomatic, the presenting symptom is obstruction due to tumor size causing intussusception. Other complications may include ulceration and bleeding of the overlying mucosa and subsequent sequelae.

Malignant Tumors

The most common malignant tumors of the small intestine are metastatic through direct extension from adjacent organs (e.g., stomach, pancreas, colon). Adenocarcinoma and primary lymphoma account for the majority of bowel malignancy. Other types of colorectal cancer, including melanoma and fibrosarcoma, and other types of sarcoma are rare and are not discussed further in this book.

TABLE 13–10 DUKES' STAGING OF COLORECTAL TUMORS

Stage	Description
Stage A	Cancer limited to the bowel wall; mucosal involvement only
Stage B	Cancer extending through the bowel wall; local invasion without penetration of the serous membrane
Stage C	Involvement of regional lymph nodes, with or without extension into the bowel wall
Stage D	Distant metastases regardless of primary tumor size

Adenocarcinoma

Overview and Incidence. Adenocarcinoma of the colon and rectum is the most common colorectal malignancy, occurring in approximately 150,000 people each year in the United States. Colorectal cancer accounts for 15% of cancer deaths, second in men only to cancer of the lung and third in women after lung and breast cancer. Incidence increases with age, starting at 40 years, and occurs more commonly in populations of high socioeconomic status, possibly owing to dietary factors. Colorectal tumors are staged using the Dukes' classification (Table 13–10).

Etiology and Risk Factors. The cause of colon cancer is unknown, although a number of environmental and familial factors have been considered. Known risk factors associated with increased risk of colonic cancer include increasing age, adenomatous polyps, ulcerative colitis, Crohn's disease, cancer elsewhere in the body, familial history of colon cancer, and immunodeficiency disease. Geographic distributions of highest incidence coincide with regional diet low in fiber and high in animal fat and protein; people who emigrate tend to acquire the risk characteristic of their new environment.

Genetic factors associated with colonic cancer such as the allelic deletion on chromosomes 5, 17, and 18 appear to promote transition from normal to malignant colon mucosa. Excess fats and colonic bacteria have been postulated to interact in some way to produce metabolites such as toxic bile acids or to cause somatic mutations. The recent identification of the adenomatous polyposis coli (APC) gene, which, when mutated, predisposes people to the development of colorectal tumors supports a genetic model (Fearon, 1991, 1992; Powell et al., 1992; Jen et al., 1994).

Two factors have been associated with a reduced risk of colon cancer. Taking aspirin daily for 20 years can reduce the risk of colon cancer by nearly one half (Paganini-Hill et al., 1991; Thun et al., 1991). Women who take estrogen replacement therapy, even for as little as 1 year, are less likely to die of colon cancer than those who have never used estrogen (Calle et al., 1995).[17] Researchers have found that the longer a woman takes estrogen, the less chance of death from colon cancer. It is not clear how estrogen acts to reduce

[17] This study looked only at the risk of dying from colon cancer; it did not examine whether taking estrogen reduced a woman's risk of developing colon cancer. It is possible that the women who took estrogen had higher survival rates simply because they had healthier lifestyles than those who did not take estrogen. Other studies have shown that, in general, estrogen users are better educated, exercise more, smoke less, and seek preventive care more often than women who do not use estrogen (Calle et al., 1995).

fatal colon cancer risk. One theory is that it lowers the concentration of bile acids, perhaps creating an environment that is hostile to the growth of cancer cells in the colon; another is that estrogen acts directly on the lining of the colon to suppress tumor growth.

Pathogenesis. Most colorectal cancers have a long preinvasive phase, growing slowly during invasion. Colorectal carcinoma starts in the glands of the mucosal lining. The lymphatic channels are located underneath the muscularis mucosae so that the lesions must extend across this layer before metastasis can occur. Such is the case with colorectal polyps that become invasive and malignant once the adenoma traverses the muscularis mucosae (Huether and McCance, 1994).

Clinical Manifestations. Colon carcinoma has very few early warning signs, as is the case with esophageal and stomach cancer. When symptoms do present, they present according to whether the lesion is in the right or left side of the colon. A persistent change in bowel habits is the single most consistent symptom for either side. Bright-red blood from the rectum is a cardinal sign of colon cancer, but must be differentiated from diverticulosis which is also a common cause of painless bright-red blood. Complications include intestinal obstruction, bleeding, perforation, anemia, ascites, distant metastases, to the liver most commonly, but also to the lungs, bone, and brain.

Medical Management

Diagnosis. Carcinoma of the colon should be suspected in anyone over the age of 40 who presents with occult blood in the stool, iron deficiency anemia, overt rectal bleeding, or alteration in bowel habits, especially if associated with abdominal discomfort or any of the risk factors mentioned earlier (Andreoli et al., 1993). Physical examination of the abdomen to detect liver enlargement and ascites is followed by palpation of appropriate lymph nodes. Diagnostic procedures include rectal examination, sigmoidoscopy, proctoscopy, colonoscopy with biopsy of lesion, CT scan, and barium enema studies. Laboratory diagnostic tests may include a screening test for occult fecal blood and a blood test for carcinoembryonic antigen (CEA), detected in some individuals with colorectal carcinoma. These are poor diagnostic tests with poor sensitivity; the client must be followed by the physician when these tests are negative.

Treatment. Surgical removal of the tumor is the mainstay of colorectal cancer treatment. Adjuvant chemotherapy may be administered, depending on the results of the staging process, to treat metastatic disease; radiation therapy is helpful for rectal carcinoma. Radiation therapy may be given before surgery to reduce the tumor size or alter the malignant cells to prevent tumor survival after surgery. Tumors in the distal rectum may require resection of the entire rectum with subsequent permanent colostomy. Given the link between adenomatous polyps and cancer, emphasis is on prevention through screening for colonic polyps and carcinomas.

Prognosis. Over 90% of clients with colorectal carcinoma can benefit from curative or palliative surgical resection with a low operative mortality rate, even among elderly clients. Prognosis can be predicted through the staging process for 5-year survival rates (after treatment): stage A—95%; stage B—60%; stage C—35%; stage D—poor. Local recurrence can occur if special operative precautions to prevent implantation of malignant cells are not followed. CEA is a marker for recurrent tumor and should be monitored every 6 months to improve survival. Routine follow-up colonoscopy is also recommended.

Special Implications for the Therapist **13-16**

ADENOCARCINOMA OF THE COLON AND RECTUM

Tumors of the rectum can spread through the rectal wall to the prostate in men and the vagina in women. Prostate involvement can cause dull, vague, aching pain in the sacral or lumbar spine regions. See Special Implications for the Therapist: Prostate Cancer, 16-3. Pelvic, hip, or low back pain may occur with extension to the vagina in women.

Systemic and pulmonary metastases occur through the hemorrhoidal plexus, which drains into the vena cava. Subsequent chest, shoulder, arm, or back pain can occur, usually accompanied by pulmonary symptoms; see also Special Implications for the Therapist: Lung Cancer, 12-20. Liver metastasis occurs following invasion of the mesenteric veins from the left colon or the superior veins from the right colon, which empty into the portal circulation; see also Hepatic Encephalopathy, Chapter 14 (Huether and McCance, 1994). Anytime a person with low back pain reports simultaneous or alternating abdominal pain at the same level as the back pain, or GI symptoms associated with back pain, a medical referral is required.

Anemia caused by intestinal bleeding associated with colon cancer requires special consideration. See Special Implications for the Therapist: Anemias, 11-3.

Primary Lymphoma

Primary lymphoma originates in nodules of lymphoid tissue within the bowel wall and accounts for 15% of small bowel cancers in the United States and two thirds of such cancers in undeveloped countries. The epidemiologic, clinical, and pathologic features of primary lymphoma in these geographic areas differ so the disease is labeled separately as Western type and Mediterranean type. Only the Western type which occurs most often in adults over 40 years and children under 10, is discussed here. The most common site of the Western type is the ileum.

The cause of primary lymphoma is unknown, although there appears to be a causal relationship between lymphoma and chronic inflammatory intestinal conditions such as celiac disease, possibly because of the persistent activation of lymphocytes in the bowel. The risk of intestinal lymphoma is also increased in conditions of immunodeficiency following treatment with immunosuppressive drugs.

Pathogenesis of this tumor may present as a fungating (rapidly growing fungus-like growth) mass projecting into the lumen, with or without ulceration; an elevated ulcerated lesion; or a diffuse, segmental thickening of the bowel wall. Any type of non-Hodgkin's malignant lymphoma may be seen (large or small cell, nodular or diffuse).

Signs and symptoms may include chronic abdominal pain, diarrhea, clubbing of the fingers, weight loss, and occult bleeding. Intestinal obstruction, intussusception, and perforation with massive hemorrhage and peritonitis are possible complications.

Clinical diagnosis is by radiographic studies of the small intestine, CT or magnetic resonance imaging (MRI) scans, and often laparoscopy. Chemotherapy and sometimes radiation therapy are the primary forms of therapy. Surgical resection for small, local involvement is possible. The overall prognosis is poor, especially when extraintestinal spread occurs (5-year survival rate is less than 10%). When the disease is localized and confined to the small intestine, it does not recur after surgical removal in over half the cases, but the disease is usually too diffuse to permit surgery.

Special Implications for the Therapist **13-17**

PRIMARY LYMPHOMA

Special considerations relate to any complications present with this condition such as anemia from intestinal bleeding or complications associated with radiation therapy. See also general guidelines for oncologic clients, Chapter 7.

Obstructive Disease

Anything that reduces the size of the gastric outlet, preventing the normal flow of chyme and delaying gastric emptying, can cause an obstruction of the bowel. Delayed gastric emptying may be secondary to obstruction of the stomach or secondary to an inability to generate effective propulsive forces (peristalsis). Obstruction of the intestines can occur as a result of (1) organic disease, (2) mechanical obstruction, or (3) functional obstruction (Table 13–11).

TABLE 13-11 CAUSES OF INTESTINAL OBSTRUCTION

ORGANIC DISEASE	MECHANICAL	FUNCTIONAL
Ulcers	Postoperative adhesions	Postoperative
Strictures	Intussusception	Drugs
Gallstones	Volvulus	Anticholinergics
Neoplasms	External hernia	β-Adrenergics
Granulomatous processes		Opiates
Viral infections		Electrolyte imbalance
Scleroderma		Metabolic disorders
Polymyositis		Diabetes mellitus
Brainstem tumors		Hypoparathyroidism
Gastroesophageal reflux		Pregnancy
Vascular occlusion		Vagotomy
Mesenteric infarction		Anorexia nervosa
Abdominal angina		Spinal cord injury
		Vertebral fracture
		Pneumonitis

Organic Disease

Clinical Manifestations. Distention develops accompanied by colicky, cramping pain and tenderness in the periumbilical area which progressively becomes constant. Vomiting occurs as a reflex associated with the waves of pain. Constipation develops into obstipation (intractable constipation) as fecal obstruction builds up in the distal bowel. Propulsion of gas through the intestines causes a rumbling noise called borborygmus and the person is aware of intestinal movement. Constitutional symptoms such as low-grade fever, perspiration, tachycardia, and dehydration may accompany this condition. The affected individual is restless, changing position frequently owing to the constant pain.

Signs of dehydration, hypovolemia, and metabolic acidosis may be seen within 24 hours of complete obstruction. Impaired blood supply to the bowel results in necrosis and strangulation. Strangulation is characterized by fever, leukocytosis, peritoneal signs, or blood in the feces. Further complications may develop such as perforation, peritonitis, and sepsis. In debilitated persons, distention of the abdomen can be severe enough to compress the diaphragm, decreasing lung compliance and resulting in atelectasis and pneumonia.

Pathogenesis. Gases and fluids accumulate proximal to the obstruction causing abdominal distention. The body's response to distention is temporarily increased peristalsis as the bowel attempts to force the material through the obstructed area. The distention also decreases the intestine's ability to absorb water and electrolytes, which are further imbalanced by vomiting. If the obstruction is at the pylorus or high in the small intestine, metabolic alkalosis develops as a result of vomiting and excessive loss of hydrogen ions. With prolonged obstruction or obstruction lower in the intestine, metabolic acidosis is more likely to occur because bicarbonate from pancreatic secretions and bile cannot be reabsorbed (Huether and McCance, 1994).

Medical Management

Diagnosis, Treatment, and Prognosis. Diagnosis requires differentiation of obstruction from other acute abdominal conditions such as inflammation and perforation of a viscus, renal or gallbladder colic, obstruction from other causes, vascular disease, and torsion of an organ, as occurs with an ovarian cyst. Abdominal radiography is the most useful diagnostic tool and laboratory findings may reveal electrolyte disturbances associated with vomiting and dehydration.

Supportive care to alleviate pain and symptoms and to facilitate passage of flatus and feces is instituted toward the goals of restoration of bowel function and prevention of surgical intervention. Intestinal intubation (insertion of a tube into the intestinal lumen to decompress the lumen and break up the obstruction) may relieve obstruction without surgery. Complete obstruction of the intestine is surgically resected; immediate surgery is required in the case of strangulation. Prognosis varies with the underlying cause; strangulation increases the mortality rate to 25%.

Special Implications for the Therapist **13-18**

ORGANIC OBSTRUCTIVE DISEASE

The therapist may see this client in an acute care setting for ambulation after the obstructive incident has been treated. Dehydration is the primary concern, requiring monitoring of symptoms (e.g., dry lips, hands, headache, brittle hair, incoordination, disorientation; see Box 4–7) and vital signs and encouragement of fluid intake throughout therapy. Movement and activity, along with deep-breathing exercises, will aid in promoting abdominal relaxation and restoring bowel function.

Mechanical Obstruction *(Rubin and Farber, 1994)*

Adhesions

Adhesions are the most common cause of small and large intestine obstruction caused by fibrous scars formed after abdominal surgery. These fibrous bands of scar tissue can loop over the bowel, either mechanically obstructing the bowel by constricting it or the fibrous band can become the axis around which the bowel can twist (volvulus) Peritonitis may cause obstruction by kinking or angulating the bowel or by directly compressing the lumen.

Intussusception

Intussusception is a telescoping of the bowel on itself, that is, one part of the intestine prolapses into the lumen of an immediately adjacent section (Fig. 13–14). In adults the leading point of an intussusception is often a lesion in the bowel wall, such as Meckel's diverticulum or a polypoid tumor. Once the leading point is entrapped, peristalsis drives it forward, dragging the mesentery into the enveloping lumen. As the two walls of the intestine press against each other, inflammation, edema, and decreased venous return and venous stasis occur. Untreated, necrosis and gangrene develop.

Clinical manifestations in adults are as listed for obstruction; complications in children include prolonged ischemia and subsequent necrosis with eventual perforation, peritonitis, and sepsis. Usually, diagnostic testing includes rectal examination, abdominal radiograph, and barium enema. The barium enema may be part of the diagnosis and treatment as the force of the flowing barium is usually enough to push the invaginated bowel into its normal position (Barr et al., 1990; Skipper et al., 1990). If the hydrostatic reduction is unsuccessful (in 30% to 40% of cases), surgical reduction of the intussusception and resection of any nonviable intestine is performed. The prognosis for children and adults with this condition is good if treated.

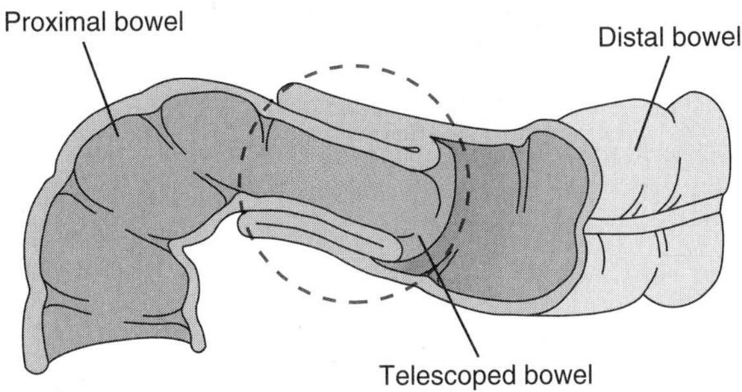

Figure **13–14.** Intussusception. A portion of the bowel telescopes into adjacent (usually distal) bowel.

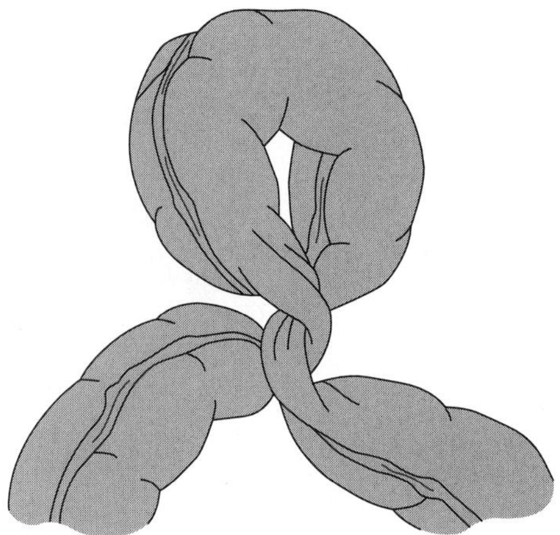

Figure **13–15.** Volvulus. The intestine twists, causing obstruction and ischemia.

Volvulus

Volvulus is a torsion of a loop of intestine twisted on its mesentery, kinking the bowel and interrupting the blood supply (Fig. 13–15). The cause of this phenomenon is usually a congenital abnormality such as a malrotation of the bowel that allows excess mobility of the bowel loops and predisposes the intestine to volvulus. Other focal points for a stationary object about which the bowel twists are tumors or Meckel's diverticulum. Treatment to decompress the bowel by inserting a long tube to release the pressure against the proximal end of the loop is tried first. If successful, the bowel volvulus relaxes. If unsuccessful, surgical intervention is sometimes required.

Hernia *(Nyhus and Condon, 1995)*

Definition and Incidence. A hernia is an acquired or congenital abnormal protrusion of part of an organ or tissue through the structure normally containing it. Half a million Americans each year have repair of a groin hernia. Hernias can occur at any age in men or women and most frequently occur in the abdominal cavity as a result of a congenital or acquired weakness of abdominal musculature. Weakness can occur as part of the aging process contributing to acquired hernias. As people age, muscular tissues become infiltrated by adipose and connective tissues, resulting in weakness. The most common types of hernias are *inguinal* (direct and indirect), *femoral*, *umbilical*, and *incisional* or *ventral* (Fig. 13–16) (Ruder and Matassarin-Jacobs, 1993). Hiatal hernia is discussed earlier in this chapter.

Etiology and Risk Factors. When muscular weakness (congenital or acquired) is accompanied by obesity, pregnancy, heavy lifting, coughing, or traumatic injuries from blunt pressure, the risk of developing a hernia increases. Often, herniation is the result of a multifactorial process involving one or more of these factors. For example, when increased abdominal pressure in a postoperative or posttraumatic injury is aggravated by nutritional or metabolic factors that result in poor wound healing and defective or poor collagen synthesis, herniation can occur. There are many other possible combinations of risk factors (Table 13–12).

Structural abnormalities account for most congenital her-

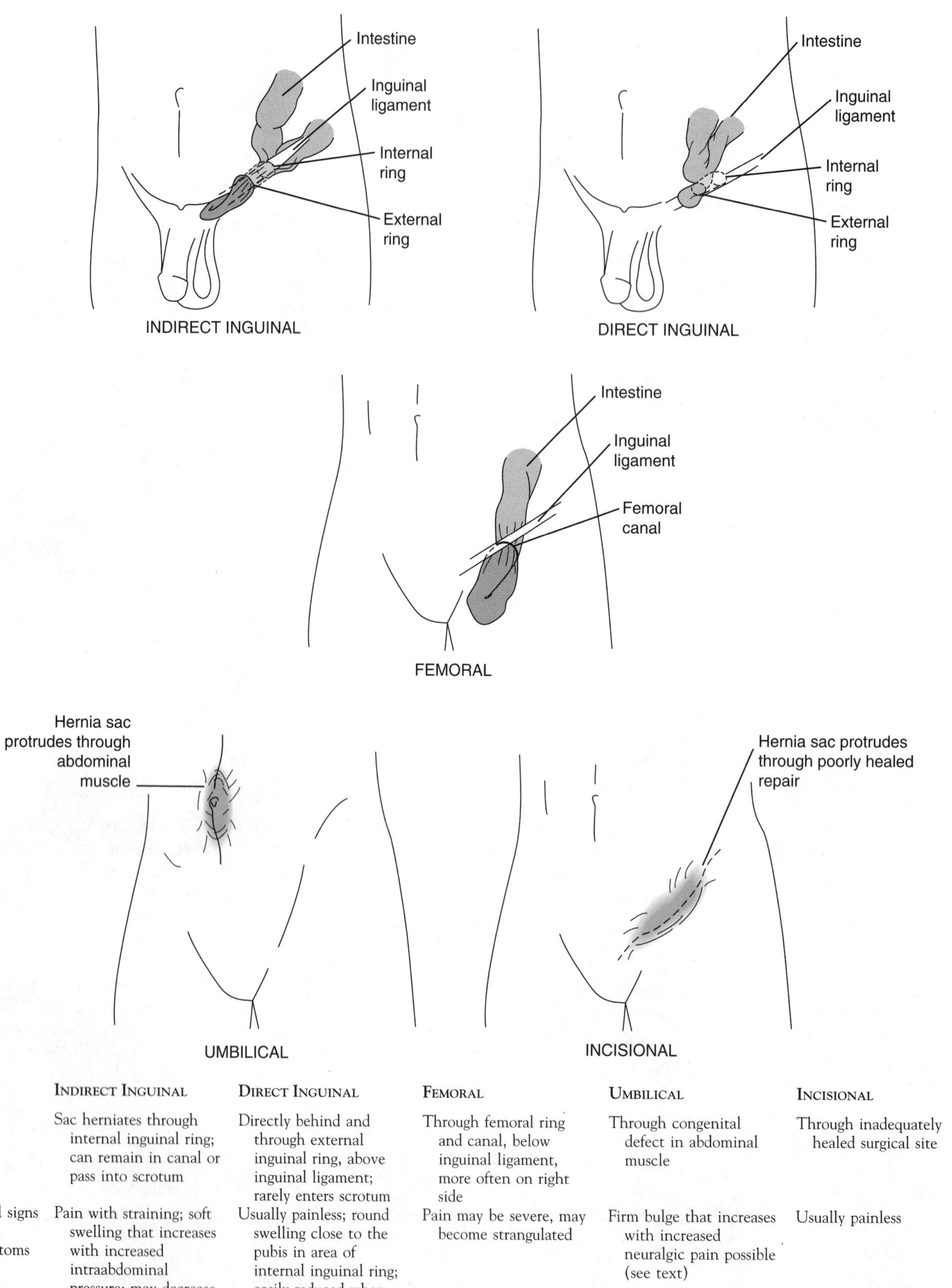

	Indirect Inguinal	Direct Inguinal	Femoral	Umbilical	Incisional
Course	Sac herniates through internal inguinal ring; can remain in canal or pass into scrotum	Directly behind and through external inguinal ring, above inguinal ligament; rarely enters scrotum	Through femoral ring and canal, below inguinal ligament, more often on right side	Through congenital defect in abdominal muscle	Through inadequately healed surgical site
Clinical signs and symptoms	Pain with straining; soft swelling that increases with increased intraabdominal pressure; may decrease when lying down	Usually painless; round swelling close to the pubis in area of internal inguinal ring; easily reduced when supine	Pain may be severe, may become strangulated	Firm bulge that increases with increased neuralgic pain possible (see text)	Usually painless

Figure 13–16. Hernias. (*Adapted from Jarvis C: Physical Examination and Health Assessment. Philadelphia, WB Saunders, 1992, p 827.*)

Illustration continued on facing page

TABLE 13-12 Risk Factors for Hernias

Inguinal	Femoral	Umbilical	Incisional
Advanced age	Pregnancy (multiparous)	Infants	Poor wound healing
Prematurity		Low birth weight	Infection
Positive family history		Black race	Inadequate nutrition
Abdominal wall defects		Congenital hypothyroidism	Abdominal distention
Undescended testis		Mucopolysaccharidoses	Obesity
Connective tissue disorders		Down syndrome	Prolonged use of steroids
Cystic fibrosis		Obesity	Advanced age
Shunt for hydrocephalus		Pregnancy	Immunosuppression
Ascites		Ascites	Postoperative pulmonary complications (coughing, straining)
			Type of incision (vertical)

Data from Nyhus LM, Condon RE: Hernia, ed 4. New York, Lippincott-Raven, 1995.

nias, but congenital factors alone do not explain the increased incidence of hernias (e.g., the direct inguinal type) in advancing age groups. Predisposing factors are equally important such as situational stress (e.g., repetitive local trauma, strenuous physical activities); degenerative changes associated with increased abdominal pressure; the wear and tear of living; multiparity; and altered collagen synthesis in middle age (Read, 1970, 1984). Sudden stress, as occurs in abdominal trauma or industrial accidents, may also contribute to the development of a hernia with or without an underlying congenital defect.

Pathogenesis. Structural and biochemical abnormalities and abnormalities of local collagen metabolism have all been proposed as factors in the eventual appearance of a hernia. Other biologic factors can affect the balance between collagen synthesis and lysis, eventually leading to the development of herniation. For example, any condition such as renal failure, diabetes mellitus, malnutrition, vitamin or mineral deficiencies, underlying systemic disease, altered immunity, or resistance to infection that can impair a person's ability to generate the proteinaceous constituents of collagen can alter collagen metabolism.

Inguinal hernias account for about 75% of all hernias and occur in the groin when a sac formed from the peritoneum and containing a portion of the intestine pushes either directly outward through the weakest point in the abdominal wall (direct hernia) or downward into the inguinal canal (indirect hernia). The direct hernias occur most often as a result of a deficient number of transversus abdominis aponeurotic fibers at a site called Hesselbach's triangle, the area between the pubic ramus and the musculofascial components in the lower abdominal wall. The direct inguinal hernia is more common in the elderly, especially in an area that is congenitally weak because of a deficient number of muscle fibers.

The indirect inguinal hernia pushes at an angle through the inguinal ring (the opening in the transverse fascia) into the inguinal canal (the oblique passage in the lower anterior abdominal wall through which passes the round ligament in the female and the spermatic cord in the male). The indirect inguinal hernia is most common in infants, young people, and males, the last because it follows the tract that develops when the testes descend into the scrotum before birth. A wide space at the inguinal ligament can also contribute to the development of an inguinal hernia.

Femoral hernia is a protrusion of a loop of intestine into the femoral canal, a tubular passageway into the thigh that carries nerves and blood vessels. The pathologic anatomy present is an enlarged femoral ring with a correspondingly narrowed transversus abdominis aponeurosis. This type occurs more often in multiparous women, acquired as a result of increased intra-abdominal pressure gradually forcing more and more preperitoneal fat into the femoral canal, enlarging the femoral ring.

The pathology of *umbilical hernias* is caused by increased

Figure **13-16.** *Continued*

	Indirect Inguinal	Direct Inguinal	Femoral	Umbilical	Incisional
Frequency	Most common; 60% of all hernias; more common in infants <1 yr and in males age 16 to 20 yr	Less common, occurs most often in men >40 yr, rare in women	Least common, 4% of all hernias; more common in women	More common in women	Affects men and women
Cause	Congenital or acquired	Acquired weakness; brought on by heavy lifting, muscle atrophy, obesity, chronic cough, or ascites	Acquired; due to increased abdominal pressure, muscle weakness, or frequent stooping	Increased abdominal pressure; obesity; multiparous women	Postoperative complications such as infection, inadequate nutrition, extreme distention, or obesity

abdominal pressure (see discussion of risk factors) exerted against a thinning of the umbilical ring and fascia. *Incisional hernia* occurs postoperatively (see discussion of risk factors) when the transected fibers are unable to form collagen links strong enough to hold the edges of the wound together (Grace and Cox, 1973).

Clinical Manifestations. The most common manifestation of a hernia of any type is a persistent or intermittent bulge, accompanied by persistent or intermittent pain. Inguinal hernia usually begins as a small, marble-sized soft lump under the skin. At first it is painless and can be reduced by pushing it back in place. As pressure from the abdominal contents pushes against the weak abdominal wall, the size of the lump formed by the hernia increases, requiring surgical repair (herniorrhaphy).

The pain associated with simple hernias depends on the involved structures and whether these are compressed or irritated. The pain is usually localized and sharp, aggravated by changes in position, by physical exertion, or by any activity causing the Valsalva maneuver (bearing down with increased intra-abdominal pressure), and relieved by cessation of the physical activity that precipitated it. It may radiate from the groin to the ipsilateral thigh, flank, or hypogastrium (lowest middle abdominal region). In the female, painful symptoms may be aggravated by the onset of menstruation.

The ilioinguinal nerve penetrates the abdominal wall cranially and somewhat laterally to the deep inguinal ring, passing the transverse and internal oblique muscles stepwise. Neuralgic pain may occur when the dull inguinal hernial pain causes a local reflex increase of tone in the internal oblique and transverse muscles of the abdomen. As the nerve passes these muscles in steps, it may be exposed to pressure, giving rise to pain of the neuralgic type. Ilioinguinal or femoral neuritis caused by nerve entrapment from sutures, adhesions, or the actual formation of a symptomatic neuroma after section of a nerve in this region can occur. These conditions usually resolve spontaneously without specific treatment, but therapy in conjunction with local nerve blocks may be indicated if symptoms persist after the first postoperative month.

Genitofemoral neuralgia (causalgia) occurs less commonly, but results in severe pain and paresthesia (or hyperesthesia) in the distribution of the genitofemoral nerve. Radiation of pain to the genitalia and upper thigh may occur and pain is aggravated by walking, stooping, or hyperextension of the hip. Recumbency and flexion of the thigh may relieve painful symptoms. This condition requires neurectomy for pain relief.

When the contents of the hernial sac can be replaced into the abdominal cavity by manipulation, the hernia is said to be reducible. Hernias that cannot be reduced or replaced by manipulation are referred to as irreducible and incarcerated. Complications occur when the protruding organ is constricted to the extent that circulation is impaired (strangulated hernia) or when the protruding organs encroach on and impair the function of other structures. When a hernia contains incarcerated or strangulated structures, the pain becomes persistent and is often associated with systemic signs or symptoms such as elevated temperature, tachycardia, vomiting, and abdominal distention.

Medical Management

Diagnosis, Treatment, and Prognosis. History and physical examination remain the most important aspects of diagnosis for all types of hernia; there may be a past history of hernia. The diagnosis of umbilical hernia is usually obvious because of protrusion of the umbilicus confirmed by palpation of the involved structures.

Various supports and trusses are available to contain hernias, but surgical repair is the only curative treatment. The use of strapping techniques is not recommended as the tape used may lead to ulceration of the thin skin covering the hernia and eventual rupture.

Prognosis varies with the type of hernia and accompanying complications. The incidence of incarceration is about 10% in indirect inguinal hernia and 20% in femoral hernia. Umbilical hernia in adults have a high morbidity and mortality associated with incarceration (Morgan et al., 1970).

Special Implications for the Therapist **13–19**

HERNIA

Early diagnosis is important in preventing incarceration and strangulation. Any client experiencing chronic cough, pregnancy, or back, hip, groin, or sacroiliac pain should be asked, Have you ever been told you have a hernia, or do you think you have a hernia now? For the client recovering from surgical repair of a hernia, heavy lifting and straining should be avoided for 4 to 6 weeks after surgery. Transient anesthesia of the skin beneath the hernial incision is a possible postoperative phenomenon. Whether in the presence of an uncorrected hernia or postoperatively, the client should avoid activities and positions that produce painful symptoms associated with the hernia.

The therapist should be aware of two complications that may occur in clients wearing a truss. In the client with a small hernia the pressure of the overlying truss on a protruding hernial mass enhances the chances of strangulation by obstructing lymphatic and venous drainage. In a person with a large direct inguinal hernia, the constant overlying pressure of the truss pad on the margins of the hernial defect eventually leads to atrophy of the fascial aponeurotic structures, enlarging the hernial opening and promoting growth of the hernia, thus making subsequent surgical repair more difficult. Anytime a person chooses to wear a truss without prior physician evaluation, the therapist is advised to encourage that client to seek medical advice.

Although uncommon, psoas abscess can still be confused with a hernia. The therapist may perform evaluative tests to rule out a psoas abscess (see the iliopsoas and obturator muscle tests (Fig. 13–10), iliopsoas palpation (Fig. 13–11), and McBurney's point (see Fig. 13–17), but the physician must differentiate between an abscess and a hernia. Psoas abscess isoften softer than a femoral hernia and has ill-defined borders, in contrast to the more sharply defined margins of the hernia. The major differentiating feature is the fact that a psoas abscess lies lateral to the femoral artery, not medial to it as is the case for the femoral hernia.

Whereas most people do well after surgical repair, some have persistent postoperative pain or discomfort.

If a person has had a previous inguinal hernial repair and now presents with painful groin or thigh pain, the physician must differentiate between ilioinguinal nerve entrapment or neuroma of a branch of the nerve severed previously. Any person (especially an older client) with a known hernia complaining of pain, nausea, vomiting, or other new symptom in the anatomic vicinity of the hernia should report these symptoms to the physician to rule out a systemic condition unrelated to the herniation.

Congenital muscle weakness complicated by the additional risk factors of obesity and increased intra-abdominal pressure should be identified and treated. Educate clients in proper lifting techniques and precautions to avoid heavy lifting and straining which reduce intra-abdominal pressure as an additional risk factor for the development of hernias and aids in preventing worsening of an already existing hernia. The mouth-open position as a reminder to breathe properly and to prevent increased intra-abdominal pressure is essential during all lifting procedures. Obesity as a cause of increased intra-abdominal pressure can be prevented by weight control through exercise (see Special Implications for the Therapist: Obesity, 2–5).

Special care must be taken when treating the client who has a vertical incision. When a vertical incision transects fascial aponeurotic fibers, the incision is made perpendicular to the direction of those fibers. Simple muscle contraction, as in coughing, straining, or turning over in bed, tends to distract the wound edges.

For a detailed treatise on hernia, see Nyhus and Condon, 1995.

Functional Obstruction

Adynamic or Paralytic Ileus

Adynamic or paralytic ileus is a neurogenic or muscular impairment of peristalsis that can cause functional intestinal obstruction. There are a variety of causes of this condition (see Table 13–11), most commonly occurring after abdominal surgery when the bowel ceases to function for a limited period of time (several hours to several days). Paralytic ileus is a common sequela of spinal cord injury. Neurogenic impairment may also occur following abdominal procedures in which the surgeon handles the bowel extensively or after surgery involving the retroperitoneal area.

Clinical manifestations include mild to moderate abdominal pain which tends to be continuous rather than colicky, as with mechanical obstruction. Borborygmus and bowel sounds are absent. Dehydration with prolonged vomiting and massive generalized abdominal distention may occur.

The diagnosis is suspected in the presence of a precipitating condition and signs and symptoms of obstruction in the absence of bowel sounds. Diagnosis is confirmed by radiography of the abdomen and barium enema to rule out organic obstruction.

Most cases of adynamic ileus respond to restricted oral intake with gradual reintroduction of foods as bowel function returns. Severe and prolonged ileus may require complete elimination of food and fluids and aspiration of gastric secretions by suctioning until the bowel begins to function again. In such cases, parenteral nutrition is utilized to reintroduce fluids and electrolytes.

Prognosis depends on the underlying cause of adynamic ileus. Removal of the cause may result in resolution of the ileus. Intubation with a rectal tube or colonoscope to decompress a dilated colon may be successful in returning bowel function, but is not a commonly performed procedure.

Special Implications for the Therapist **13–20**

ADYNAMIC OR PARALYTIC ILEUS

Anterior lumbar fusion procedures may indirectly cause a functional ileus when the client is unable to ambulate early or remains immobile and inactive for any reason. The short-term use of transcutaneous electrical nerve stimulation (TENS) in the acute care setting may be employed by the therapist to assist in pain control and to encourage mobility. Increased activity stimulates movement of air out of the bowel and helps prevent constipation and the subsequent development of a functional ileus.

Congenital *(Rubin and Farber, 1994)*

Intestinal atresia and stenosis, although rare, are the most frequent causes of neonatal intestinal obstruction. Either condition is diagnosed on the basis of persistent vomiting of bile-containing fluid during the first 24 hours after birth. Surgical correction is usually successful, but coexistent anomalies often exist and complicate treatment.

Stenosis and Atresia

Stenosis is a narrowing of a canal, in this case the small intestine. Intestinal *atresia* refers to defects caused by the incomplete formation of a lumen, in this case the tubular portion of the intestine. Many hollow organs originate as strands and cords of cells, the centers of which are programmed to die, thus forming a central cavity or lumen.

Most cases of intestinal atresia are characterized by complete occlusion of the lumen, which was not fully established in embryogenesis. Meconium ileus (accumulation of meconium in the small intestine causing neonatal intestinal obstruction) accounts for 25% of all cases and cystic fibrosis accounts for another 10%.

Intestinal atresia may have several forms: multiple intestinal occlusions giving the appearance of a string of sausages, disconnected blind ends, blind proximal and distal sacs joined by a cord, or a thin transluminal diaphragm across the opening. All forms require surgical intervention with good prognosis for recovery.

Meckel's Diverticulum

Meckel's diverticulum is an outpouching of the bowel located at the ileum of the small intestine, near the ileocecal valve. It occurs because of failure of destruction of the vitelline duct, an embryonic communication between the midgut and the yolk sac. Meckel's diverticulum is the most common congenital malformation of the GI tract, present in 1% to 3% of the population. Males are affected more often than females in a 2:1 ratio with accompanying complications in the same ratio.

Meckel's diverticulum may be asymptomatic or symptoms may include abdominal pain similar to appendicitis with nausea and vomiting, melena, and GI bleeding.[18] Common complications associated with Meckel's diverticulum include bleeding or hemorrhage from peptic ulceration of the ileum adjacent to the ectopic gastric mucosa; intestinal obstruction; diverticulitis that mimics appendicitis; and perforation caused by peptic ulceration in the diverticulum or in the ileum.

Diagnosis is usually made during the first 2 years, but may go undetected into adulthood when it is discovered on autopsy or during laparotomy for an unrelated condition. The diagnosis is usually made based on history, physical examination, and radionuclide scan. Prognosis is good with surgical resection to remove the diverticulum. Severe hemorrhage must be treated prior to surgery to correct hypovolemic shock through the administration of blood transfusion, intravenous fluids, and oxygen. Antibiotics may be used preoperatively to control infection.

THE APPENDIX

Appendicitis

Definition and Incidence. Appendicitis is an inflammation of the vermiform appendix that often results in necrosis and perforation with subsequent localized or generalized peritonitis. On the basis of operative findings and histologic appearance, acute appendicitis is classified as simple, gangrenous, or perforated. It is the most common disease of the appendix, occurring at any age, with the peak incidence among men in their second and third decades. The overall incidence is declining for unknown reasons, possibly as a result of increased dietary fiber intake in recent years (Walker and Segal, 1990) or improved hygiene and fewer intestinal infections associated with indoor plumbing (Barker et al., 1988).

Etiology. Approximately half of all cases of acute appendicitis have no known cause. At least one third are caused by obstruction preventing normal drainage. Obstruction may occur as a result of tumor, foreign body such as fecal material (fecalith) lodged in the lumen of the appendix, parasites (e.g., intestinal worms), or lymphoid hyperplasia. Because the appendix is chiefly lymphatic tissue, an infection that produces enlarged lymph nodes elsewhere in the body can also increase the glandular tissue in the appendix and obstruct its lumen (O'Toole, 1992). Other causes include Crohn's disease of the terminal ileum, ulcerative colitis when it spreads to the mucosa of the appendix, and tuberculous enteritis.

Pathogenesis. Classically, appendicitis is believed to develop primarily from obstruction of the lumen and secondarily from bacterial infection (Schrock, 1993). When the long, narrow appendiceal lumen becomes obstructed, inflammation begins in the mucosa, with swelling and hyperemia of the vermiform appendix. As secretions distend the obstructed appendix, the intraluminal pressure rises and eventually exceeds the venous pressure, causing venous stasis and ischemia. The accumulation of neutrophils produces microabscesses, and arterial thromboses aggravate the ischemia. The infected necrotic wall becomes gangrenous and may perforate, often in 24 to 48 hours (Rubin and Farber, 1994). The mucosa ulcerates and permits invasion by intestinal bacteria. *Escherichia coli* and other bacteria multiply and cause inflammation and infection that spread to the peritoneal cavity unless the body's defenses are able to overcome the infection or the appendix is removed before it ruptures (O'Toole, 1992).

Clinical Manifestations. The presenting symptoms of acute appendicitis occur in a classic sequence of abdominal (epigastric or periumbilical) pain, anorexia, nausea, vomiting, and low-grade fever in adults (children tend to have higher fevers). Pain is constant and may shift within 12 hours of symptom onset to the right lower quadrant with point tenderness over the site of the appendix at McBurney's point, a point between 1½ and 2 in. superomedial to the anterior superior iliac spine, on a line joining that process and the umbilicus (Fig. 13–17).

Aggravating factors include anything that increases intra-abdominal pressure (see Box 13–1) such as coughing, walking, laughing, and bending over. Elderly clients frequently have few or no symptoms with minimal fever and only slight tenderness until perforation occurs.

Atypical Appendicitis. Many cases of appendicitis are atypical because of the position of the appendix, the person's age, or the presence of associated conditions, such as pregnancy (Schrock, 1993). The person may not recognize the need for medical attention but will report symptoms to the

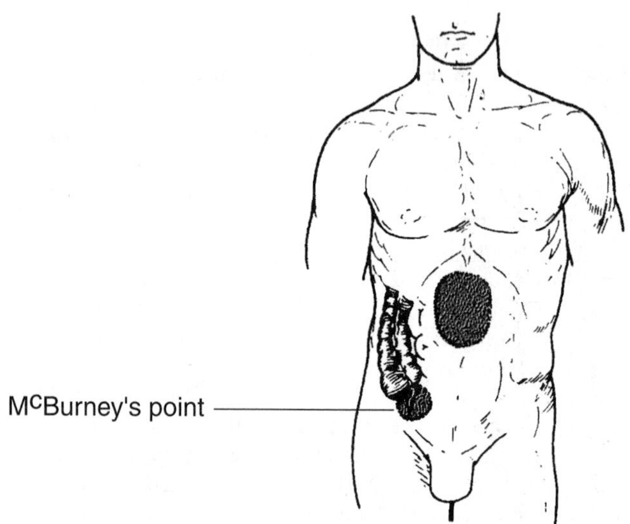

Figure **13–17.** Pain areas associated with appendicitis, including McBurney's point. Tenderness upon palpation of this point is indicative of appendicitis. With the client supine and legs extended, isolate the anterior superior iliac spine and the umbilicus, then gently palpate approximately one-half the distance between those two points. A positive test will produce painful symptoms in the right lower quadrant. (*Adapted from O'Toole M (ed): Miller-Keane Encyclopedia and Dictionary of Medicine, Nursing, and Allied Health, ed 5. Philadelphia, WB Saunders, 1992, p 111.*)

[18] GI bleeding in the pediatric population appears as dark red with mucus or "currant jelly–like" stools.

therapist. Early recognition of the need for medical evaluation is imperative.

Retrocecal appendicitis and *retroilieal appendicitis* may occur when the inflamed appendix is shielded from the anterior abdominal wall by the overlying cecum and ileum. The pain seems less intense, less localized, and there is less discomfort on walking or coughing. The pain may not shift as expected from the epigastrium to the right lower quadrant.

Pelvic appendicitis may begin with pain in the epigastrium, but quickly settles in the lower abdomen, commonly localized to the left side for an unknown reason. The absence of abdominal tenderness may be deceptive, but the physician will elicit this symptom on pelvic examination. *Appendicitis in the immunosuppressed* presents as abdominal pain and fever without leukocytosis, but concern about other causes usually delays recognition.

Appendicitis in the elderly is usually vague with minimal pain and only slight temperature elevation. Abdominal tenderness is present and localized to the right lower quadrant, but is deceptively mild. *Appendicitis in pregnancy* does not present a diagnostic problem in the first trimester, but later in gestation may be confused as an obstetric condition. Displacement of the appendix by the enlarged uterus may result in tenderness in the right subcostal area or adjacent to the umbilicus.

Medical Management

Diagnosis. Acute appendicitis must be differentiated from acute gastroenteritis, gallbladder disease, right kidney infection, mesenteric lymphadenitis, Meckel's diverticulitis, and gynecologic conditions such as ectopic pregnancy, twisted ovarian cyst, ovarian follicle rupture in the midmenstrual cycle, and acute salpingitis (inflammation of fallopian tube). The onset of right lower lobe pneumonia, rheumatic fever, or diabetic ketoacidosis can mimic appendicitis.

A careful history and thorough physical examination are the primary diagnostic tools. An elevated white blood cell count (leukocytosis), that is, higher than 20,000/mm^3, suggests ruptured appendix and peritonitis. Barium enema allowing visualization of the entire appendix and high-resolution sonography have reduced the incidence of negative laparotomy. Histologic examination of the resected appendix is used to confirm the diagnosis and at least 10% of appendices resected are normal (Harruff, 1994).

Treatment and Prognosis. Appendectomy, or surgical removal of the vermiform appendix, is performed as soon as possible. Antibiotics are administered preoperatively in the presence of systemic symptoms or when surgery is unavailable. With accurate diagnosis and early surgical removal, mortality and morbidity rates are less than 1%. Prognosis is good unless diagnosis is delayed and perforation occurs (rarely during the first 8 hours of symptomatic presentation). Perforation with complications such as peritonitis, hypovolemia, and septic shock have a poor prognosis. Perforation is more likely in infants under 2 years of age and in adults over 60 years.

Special Implications for the Therapist **13-21**

APPENDICITIS

When appendicitis is atypical the client may not recognize the need for medical attention but will report the symptoms to the therapist. Early recognition of the need for medical referral is important. In an athletic training or physical therapy setting, appendicitis may present with symptoms of right thigh, groin (testicular) pain, pelvic pain, or referred pain to the hip.

In addition to screening for the presence of constitutional symptoms, a variety of objective test procedures may be employed by the therapist including the iliopsoas muscle test and the obturator muscle test (see Fig. 13–10), palpation of the iliopsoas muscle (see Fig. 13–11), and palpation of McBurney's point (see Fig. 13–17). Ask the client to cough: localization of painful symptoms to the site of the appendix is typical.

If any of these tests is positive for reproduction of symptoms in the right lower quadrant, a medical referral is necessary. If appendicitis is suspected, medical attention must be immediate. The client should be instructed to lie down and remain as quiet as possible, taking nothing by mouth (including water); heat is contraindicated.

The physician will also assess for rebound tenderness by pressing down slowly and deeply at an abdominal site away from the painful area. Quickly lifting the examiner's hand allows the indented structures to rebound suddenly. Pain on release of pressure confirms rebound tenderness, a reliable sign of peritoneal inflammation.

THE PERITONEUM

Peritonitis

Overview. Peritonitis, or inflammation of the serous membrane lining the walls of the abdominal cavity, is caused by a number of situations that introduce microorganisms into the peritoneal cavity. Peritonitis that occurs spontaneously is called *primary peritonitis*. Peritonitis as a consequence of trauma, surgery, or peritoneal contamination by bowel contents (e.g., perforated duodenal ulcer or appendix) is referred to as *secondary peritonitis*.

Etiology. Specific causes of peritonitis are listed in Box 13–2. Primary peritonitis is associated with ascites and chronic liver disease or the nephrotic syndrome. Secondary peritonitis occurs as a result of inflammation of abdominal organs, irritating substances from a perforated gallbladder or gastric ulcer, rupture of a cyst, or irritation from blood, as in cases of internal bleeding (O'Toole, 1992).

Secondary peritonitis may be classified as bacterial, chemical, or metastatic. *Bacterial peritonitis* is caused by bacterial infection (*E. coli*, bacteroides, staphylococcus, streptococcus, pneumococcus, gonococcus) introduced most commonly by perforation of a viscus. Such perforation can occur in the case of appendicitis, an ulcer, a bowel infarct, colonic diverticulum, chronic peritoneal dialysis owing to instrument contamination or dialysate,[19] and urinary infection.

[19] Dialysate is the part of the mixture that passes through the dialyzing membrane. Peritonitis associated with chronic dialysis is probably caused by a chemical in the dialysate to which the peritoneum is sensitive. Approximately 25% of peritonitis associated with chronic dialysis is aseptic.

BOX **13-2**
Causes of Peritonitis

Gangrenous cholecystitis
Ruptured gallbladder
Perforated carcinoma of the stomach
Perforated gastric or duodenal ulcer
Ruptured spleen
Acute pancreatitis
Penetrating wound of the gastrointestinal tract
Ulcerative colitis
Gangrenous obstruction of the small bowel due to:
  Adhesions
  Carcinoma
  Volvulus or intussusception
Perforation of Meckel's diverticulum
Mesenteric thrombosis
Perforation of a diverticulum
Regional ileitis
Appendicitis with perforation
Ruptured retroperitoneal abscess
Strangulated hernia
Puerperal infection
Salpingitis
Septic abortion
Ruptured bladder
Iatrogenic perforation

Adapted from Ruder SM, Matassarin-Jacobs E: Nursing care of clients with intestinal disorders. *In* Black JM, Matassarin-Jacobs E: Luckmann and Sorensen's Medical-Surgical Nursing, ed 4. Philadelphia, WB Saunders, 1993, p 1638.

Chemical peritonitis is a noninfectious inflammation caused by bile leakage, usually from a perforated gallbladder, but sometimes from a needle biopsy of the liver. Other causes include substances such as gastric acid, blood, or foreign material introduced by surgery (e.g., talc), and acute pancreatitis, which releases and activates lipolytic and proteolytic enzymes. *Metastatic peritonitis* occurs when neoplasm perforates the viscus of the stomach and tumor cells infiltrate the peritoneum.

Pathogenesis. Once the inflammatory process has begun, a fibrinopurulent exudate covers the peritoneal surface. The exudate becomes organized and fibrotic, forming adhesions and causing obstruction. When a perforation drains contaminants into the peritoneal cavity, the ability of the peritoneum to combat the inflammatory process will be overpowered. The entire surface of the peritoneum may be involved (generalized peritonitis) or only specific sites (localized). When the pelvic peritoneum is involved, pelvic peritonitis (also called pelvic inflammatory disease) occurs.

Peritonitis creates severe systemic effects. Circulatory alterations, fluid shifts, and respiratory problems can cause critical fluid and electrolyte imbalances. The circulatory system undergoes great stress from several sources. The inflammatory response shunts extra blood to the inflamed area of the bowel to combat the infection. Peristaltic activity of the bowel ceases. Fluids and air are retained within its lumen, raising pressure and increasing fluid secretion into the bowel; circulating volume diminishes (Ruder and Matassarin-Jacobs, 1993).

Clinical Manifestations. Peritonitis presents as an acute abdomen with severe abdominal pain; the abdomen becomes rigid (involuntary guarding) and sensitive to the touch. Nausea, vomiting, and high fever follow. Complications may include paralytic ileus (diminished to absent peristalsis) and septic shock. A peritoneal abscess develops if the perforation becomes self-encased or walled off. Antibiotic therapy may mask or delay the recognition of signs of abscess.

In persons with underlying ascites, the signs and symptoms of peritonitis may be more subtle, with fever as the only manifestation of infection, or possibly nausea, vomiting, nonspecific abdominal pain, or altered mental status (Andreoli et al., 1993).

Medical Management

Diagnosis, Treatment, and Prognosis. Abdominal films, barium enema, and an abdominal tap may be used in the differential diagnosis of peritonitis. Peritonitis should be treated immediately to control infection, minimize the effects of paralytic ileus, and correct fluid, electrolyte, and nutritional disorders.

If peritonitis is advanced and surgery is contraindicated because of shock and circulatory failure, oral fluids are prohibited and intravenous fluids are necessary for replacement of electrolyte and protein losses. A long intestinal tube is inserted through the nose into the intestine to reduce pressure within the bowel. Once the infection has become walled off and the client's condition improves, surgical drainage and repair can be attempted (Ruder and Matassarin-Jacobs, 1993).

Despite treatment with antibiotics, surgical drainage and debridement, and supportive measures, generalized peritonitis is still associated with a mortality of 50% and is especially dangerous in the elderly client (Rubin and Farber, 1994).

Special Implications for the Therapist **13-22**

PERITONITIS

Special considerations associated with peritonitis are related to the underlying cause (e.g., liver or kidney disease, postoperative, cancer) and resultant complications (e.g., fluid and electrolyte imbalance, pulmonary compromise). The client with peritonitis is usually hospitalized and undergoing medical treatment. The therapist should be familiar with implications associated with the underlying cause and any complications present.

Vital signs should be regularly monitored (see Appendix B) and a semi-Fowler's position used to help the client breathe deeply with less pain to prevent pulmonary complications. Position changes must be accomplished with extreme caution as the slightest movement will intensify the pain. Watch for signs of dehiscence (separation of layers of a surgical wound) such as the person reporting that "something broke loose" or "gave way" inside. Follow all safety measures such as keeping the side rails up on the bed if fever and pain disorient the client.

THE RECTUM

Rectal Fissure

A rectal fissure is an ulceration or tear of the lining of the anal canal, usually on the posterior wall. An acute fissure occurs as a result of excessive tissue stretching such as childbirth or passage of a large, hard bowel movement through the area. The skin tear is very fragile and tends to reopen easily with the next bowel movement.

Chronic fissures are usually secondary to a tight rectal sphincter or infectious material retained in the anal sinuses. Sharp pain, followed by burning, accompanies defecation. Therapists may be involved with clients with chronic conditions who experience severe muscle spasm of the sphincter resulting in groin or pelvic pain and gluteal muscle trigger points.

Hemorrhoids

Hemorrhoids, or piles, are varicose veins in the perianal region and may be internal or external. Internal hemorrhoids are frequently first noticed when a small amount of bleeding occurs during passage of stool. Internal hemorrhoids are asymptomatic except in the presence of an anal fissure, thrombosis, or strangulation of the varicose vein. External hemorrhoids bleed (bright-red blood) if the hemorrhoid is injured or ulcerated and accompanying symptoms include pain, pressure, rectal itching, irritation, and a palpable mass.

Hemorrhoids are fairly common, affecting as many as half of all adults over 50 years of age. This condition is especially associated with anything that increases intra-abdominal pressure (see Box 13–1) such as pregnancy, congestive heart failure, prolonged sitting or standing, low fiber diet, constipation (hard, dry stool can cause prolonged sitting and straining during defecation), and delaying a bowel movement when the urge presents itself.

Severe bleeding or mild bleeding repeatedly from prolonged trauma to the vein during defecation can cause iron deficiency anemia. Strangulated hemorrhoids (prolapsed hemorrhoids in which the blood supply is cut off by the anal sphincter) can result in thrombosis when blood within the hemorrhoid clots (Ruder and Matassarin-Jacobs, 1993).

External hemorrhoids can be treated with local application of cold, astringent cream, sitz baths, high fiber diet, and avoidance of constipation and other causes of increased intra-abdominal pressure. A stool softener or psyllium preparation may be used when a modified diet is unsuccessful in eliminating constipation. Local topical preparations for hemorrhoids are used to reduce pain or itching. *Internal hemorrhoids* may require ligation, sclerosing, laser surgery, or cryosurgery to destroy the affected tissue. In the case of advanced chronic hemorrhoids, the client may be predisposed to carcinoma of the anus so surgical removal (hemorrhoidectomy) may be required.

Special Implications for the Therapist **13–23**

HEMORRHOIDS

Clients involved in any activity requiring increased abdominal support or causing increased intra-abdominal pressure should be questioned as to the presence of hemorrhoids. For clients with hemorrhoids postoperatively, prone positioning or side-lying supported with pillows between the knees and ankles is preferred. Supine positioning and sitting for brief periods can be accomplished with a rubber air ring under the buttocks for support. Fluid replacement during exercise is important in the prevention of constipation. Movement and exercise are also extremely helpful in preventing constipation.

References

Abrams WB, Beers MH, Berkow R: The Merck Manual of Geriatrics, ed 2. Rahway, NJ, Merck, 1995.

Abrutyn E: Botulism. *In* Isselbacher KJ, Braunwald E, Wilson JD, et al (eds): Harrison's Principles of Internal Medicine, ed 13. New York, McGraw-Hill, 1994, p 635.

ACS (American Cancer Society): Cancer statistics, 1997. CA Cancer J Clin 47:5–27, 1997.

Ajani JA, Ota DM, Jackson DE: Current strategies in the management of locoregional and metastatic gastric carcinoma. Cancer 67(suppl 1): 260–265, 1991.

Almy TP, Howell DA: Diverticular disease of the colon. N Engl J Med 302:324, 1980.

Andreoli TE, Bennett JC, Carpenter CC, et al (eds): Cecil Essentials of Medicine, ed 3. Philadelphia, WB Saunders, 1993.

Auch RD: Abdominal pain. *In* Blacklow RS: Signs and Symptoms, ed 6. Philadelphia, JB Lippincott, 1983, pp 165–180.

Babb RR: Gastrointestinal complications of nonsteroidal anti-inflammatory drugs. West J Med 157:444–447, 1992.

Barker DJP, Osmond C, Golding J, et al: Acute appendicitis and bathrooms in three samples of British children. Br Med J 296:956, 1988.

Barr LL, Stansberry SD, Swischuk LE: Significance of age, duration, obstruction, and the dissection sign in intussusception. Pediatr Radiol 20:454–456, 1990.

Bartlett JG: Pseudomembranous enterocolitis and antibiotic-associated colitis. *In* Sleisenger MH, Fordtran JS (eds): Gastrointestinal Disease, ed 5. Philadelphia, WB Saunders, 1993, pp 1174–1189.

Bissonnette B, Sullivan PJ: Pyloric stenosis. Can J Anaesthesiol 38:668–676, 1991.

Blaser MJ: *Helicobacter pylori*: Microbiolgoy of a "slow" bacterial infection. Trends Microbiol 1:255–260, 1993.

Boren T, Falk P, Roth KA, et al: Attachment of *Helicobacter pylori* to human gastric epithelium mediated by blood group antigens. Science 262:1892–1895, 1993.

Bornstein P: Disorders of connective tissue function and the aging process: A synthesis and review of current concepts and findings. Mech Aging Dev 5:305, 1976.

Bourke B, Sherman P, Drumm B: Peptic ulcer disease: What is the role for *Helicobacter pylori?* Semin Gastrointest Dis 5:24–31, 1994.

Calle EE, Miracle-McMahill HL, Thun MJ, et al: Estrogen replacement therapy and risk of fatal colon cancer in a prospective cohort of postmenopausal women. J Natl Cancer Inst 87:517–523, 1995.

Cappell MS: Gastritis: Making the differential diagnosis. Hosp Med 30:45–50, 1994.

Castell DO: Medical therapy for reflux esophagitis: 1986 and beyond. Ann Intern Med 104:112–114, 1986.

Clinch D, Banerjee AK, Ostick G: Absence of abdominal pain in elderly patients with peptic ulcer. Age Ageing 13:120, 1984.

Connell WR, Sheffield JP, Kamm MA, et al: Lower gastrointestinal malignancy in Crohn's disease. Gut 35:347–352, 1994.

Danek GD, Huether SE, Andrews MM: Alterations of digestive function in children. *In* McCance KL, Huether SE (eds.): Pathophysiology: The Biologic Basis for Disease in Adults and Children, ed 2. St Louis, Mosby–Year Book, 1994, pp 1376–1401.

Fazio VW: Crohn's disease. *In* Moody FG, Carey LC, Jones SR, et al (eds): Surgical Treatment of Digestive Diseases, ed 2. St Louis: Mosby–Year Book, 1990, pp 655–683.

Fearon ER: Genetic alterations underlying colorectal tumorigenesis. Cancer Surv 12:119–136, 1992.

Fearon ER: A genetic basis for the multi-step pathway of colorectal tumorigenesis. Princess Takamatsu Symp 22:37–48, 1991.

Fennerty MB: *Helicobacter pylori*. Arch Intern Med 154:721–727, 1994.

Fields HL, Martin JB: Pain. *In* Isselbacher KJ, Braunwald E, Wilson JD, et al (eds): Harrison's Principles of Internal Medicine, ed 13. New York, McGraw-Hill, 1994, pp 49–54.

Ghosh S, Cowen S, Hannan WJ, et al: Low bone mineral density in Crohn's disease, but not in ulcerative colitis, at diagnosis. Gastroenterology 107:1031–1039, 1994.

Gillen CD, Andrews HA, Prior P, Allan RN: Crohn's disease and colorectal cancer. Gut 35:651–655, 1994.

Glickman RM: Inflammatory bowel disease: Ulcerative colitis and Crohn's disease. *In* Isselbacher KJ, Braunwald E, Wilson JD, et al (eds): Harrison's Principles of Internal Medicine, ed 13. New York, McGraw-Hill, 1994, pp 1403–1416.

Goodman CC, Snyder TE: Differential Diagnosis in Physical Therapy, ed 2. Philadelphia, WB Saunders, 1995.

Goyal RK: Diseases of the esophagus. *In* Isselbacher KJ, Braunwald E, Wilson JD, et al (eds): Harrison's Principles of Internal Medicine, ed 13. New York, McGraw-Hill, 1994, pp 1355–1362.

Grace RH, Cox SJ: Incidence of incisional hernia following dehiscence of the abdominal wound. Proc Soc Med 66:1091, 1973.

Hanauer SB: Inflammatory bowel disease. *In* Wyngaarden JB, Smith LH, Bennett JC (eds): Cecil Textbook of Medicine, ed 19. Philadelphia, WB Saunders, 1992, pp 699–708.

Harford WV, McArthur KE: Diverticula, hernias, volvulus, and rupture. *In* Sleisenger MH, Fordtran JS (eds): Gastrointestinal Disease, ed 5. Philadelphia, WB Saunders, 1993, pp 478–485.

Harruff RC: Pathology Facts. Philadelphia, JB Lippincott, 1994.

Hastings GE, Weber RJ: Inflammatory bowel disease: Part II. Medical and surgical management. Am Fam Physician 47:811–818, 1993.

Herskovic A, Martz K, al-Sarraf M, et al: Combined chemotherapy and radiotherapy compared with radiotherapy alone in patients with cancer of the esophagus. N Engl J Med 326:1593–1598, 1992.

Huether SE: Structure and function of the digestive system. *In* McCance KL, Huether SE (eds): Pathophysiology: The Biologic Basis for Disease in Adults and Children, ed 2. St Louis, Mosby–Year Book, 1994, pp 1282–1319.

Huether SE, McCance KL: Alterations of digestive function. *In* McCance KL, Huether SE (eds): Pathophysiology: The Biologic Basis for Disease in Adults and Children, ed 2. St Louis, Mosby–Year Book, 1994, pp 1320–1375.

Jen J, Kim H, Piantadosi S, et al: Allelic loss of chromosome 18q and prognosis in colorectal cancer. N Engl J Med 331:213–221, 1994.

Kasper DL, Zaleznik DF: Gas gangrene and other clostridial infections. *In* Isselbacher, KJ, Braunwald E, Wilson JD, et al (eds): Harrison's Principles of Internal Medicine, ed 13. New York, McGraw-Hill, 1994, pp 636–640.

Keating RM, Vyas AS: Reactive arthritis following *Clostridium difficile* colitis. West J Med 62:61–63, 1995.

Kovacs TO, Jensen DM: Endoscopic diagnosis and treatment of bleeding Mallory-Weiss tears. Gastroenterol Clin North Am 1:387, 1991.

Lichtenstein DR, Syngal S, Wolfe MM: Nonsteroidal antiinflammatory drugs and the gastrointestinal tract: The double-edged sword. Arthritis Rheum 38:5–18, 1995.

Luk G: Cancer surveillance strategies. *In* Sleisenger MH, Fordtran JS (eds): Gastrointestinal Disease, ed 5. Philadelphia, WB Saunders, 1993, pp 115–126.

Mahoney BP: Rheumatologic disease and associated ocular manifestations. J Am Optom Assoc 64:403–415, 1993.

Marshall BJ: *Helicobacter pylori:* A primer for 1994. Gastroenterologist 1:241–247, 1993.

Mayer RJ: Neoplasms of the esophagus and stomach. *In* Isselbacher KJ, Braunwald E, Wilson JD, et al (eds): Harrison's Principles of Internal Medicine, ed 13. New York, McGraw-Hill, 1994, pp 1382–1385.

McGuigan JE: Peptic ulcer and gastritis. *In* Isselbacher KJ, Braunwald E, Wilson JD, et al (eds): Harrison's Principles of Internal Medicine, ed 13. New York, McGraw-Hill, 1994, pp 1363–1381.

McGuigan JE, Ament ME: Anatomy and developmental anomalies. *In* Isselbacher KJ, Braunwald E, Wilson JD, et al (eds): Harrison's Principles of Internal Medicine, ed 13. New York, McGraw-Hill, 1994, pp 459–477.

McQuaid KR, Knauer M: Alimentary tract. *In* Tierney LM, McPhee SJ, and Papadakis MA: Current Medical Diagnosis and Treatment, 33rd ed. Norwalk, Appleton & Lange, 1994, pp 467–527.

Meyer HJ, Jahne J, Pichlmayr R: Strategies in the surgical treatment of gastric carcinoma. Ann Oncol 5(suppl 3):33–36, 1994.

Morgan WW, White JJ, Stumbaugh S, Haller JA: Prophylactic umbilical hernia repair in childhood to prevent adult incarceration. Surg Clin North Am 50;839, 1970.

Musio F, Older SA, Jenkings T, Gregorie EM: Case report: Cerebral venous thrombosis as a manifestation of acute ulcerative colitis. Am J Med Sci 305:28–35, 1993.

Naitove A, Smith RE: Diverticular disease of the colon. *In* Sleisenger MH, Fordtran JS (eds): Gastrointestinal Disease, ed 5. Philadelphia, WB Saunders, 1993, pp 1347–1362.

Nyhus LM, Condon RE: Hernia, ed 3. New York, Lippincott-Raven, 1995.

O'Brien JJ, Bayless TM, Bayless JA: Use of azathioprine or 6-mercaptopurine in the treatment of Crohn's disease. Gastroenterology 101:39–46, 1991.

O'Toole M (ed): Miller-Keane Encyclopedia and Dictionary of Medicine, Nursing, and Allied Health, ed 5. Philadelphia, WB Saunders, 1992.

Paganini-Hill A, Hsu G, Ross RK, et al: Aspirin use and incidence of large-bowel cancer in a California retirement community. J Natl Cancer Inst. 83:1182–1183, 1991.

Pahor M, Guralnik JM, Salive ME, et al: Disability and severe gastrointestinal hemorrhage. A prospective study of community-dwelling older persons. J Am Geriatr Soc 42:816–825, 1994a.

Pahor M, Guralnik JM, Salive ME, et al: Physical activity and risk of severe gastrointestinal hemorrhage in older persons. JAMA 272:595–599, 1994b.

Patel P, Mendall MA, Khulusi S, et al: Salivary antibodies to *Helicobacter pylori:* Screening dyspeptic patients before endoscopy. Lancet 344:511–512, 1994.

Peura DA: *Helicobacter pylori:* Practical guidelines for diagnosis and treatment. Gastroenterologist 1:291–295, 1993.

Podolsky DK, Isselbacher KJ: Alcohol-related liver disease and cirrhosis. *In* Isselbacher KJ, Braunwald E, Wilson JD, et al (eds): Harrison's Principles of Internal Medicine, ed 13. New York, McGraw-Hill, 1994, pp 1483–1494.

Pounder R: Silent peptic ulceration: Deadly silence or golden silence? Gastroenterology 96:626, 1989.

Powell SM, Zilz N, Beazer-Barclay Y, et al: APC mutations occur early during colorectal tumorigenesis. Nature 359:235–237, 1992.

Prantera C, Pallone F, Brunetti G, et al: Oral 5-aminosalicylic acid (Asacol) in the maintenance treatment of Crohn's disease. Gastroenterology 103:363–368, 1992.

Putterman C, Rubinow A: Reactive arthritis associated with *Clostridium difficile* pseudomembranous colitis. Semin Arthritis Rheum 22:420–426, 1993.

Read RC: Attenuation of rectus sheath in inguinal herniation. Am J Surg 120:610, 1970.

Read RC: The development of inguinal herniorrhaphy. Surg Clin North Am 64:185, 1984.

Reilly TG, Walt RP: Duodenal ulcer treatment: Progress from pH to HP. J Clin Pharm Ther 19:73–80, 1994.

Rose SJ, Rothstein JM: Muscle mutability: General concepts and adaptations to altered patterns of use. Phys Ther 62:1773, 1982.

Rubin E, Farber JL: The gastrointestinal tract. *In* Rubin E, Farber JL (eds): Pathology, ed 2. Philadelphia, JB Lippincott, 1994, pp 618–703.

Ruder SM: Nursing care of clients with gastric disorders. *In* Black JM, Matassarin-Jacobs E (eds): Luckmann and Sorensen's Medical-Surgical Nursing, ed 4. Philadelphia, WB Saunders, 1993a, pp 1599–1626.

Ruder SM: Nursing care of clients with ingestive disorders. *In* Black JM, Matassarin-Jacobs E (eds): Luckmann and Sorensen's Medical-Surgical Nursing, ed 4. Philadelphia, WB Saunders, 1993b, pp 1571–1598.

Ruder SM, Matassarin-Jacobs E: Nursing care of clients with intestinal disorders. *In* Black JM, Matassarin-Jacobs E (eds): Luckmann and Sorensen's Medical-Surgical Nursing, ed 4. Philadelphia, WB Saunders, 1993, pp 1627–1674.

Schineller BA, Ramchandani D: Psychologic factors associated with peptic ulcer disease. Med Clin North Am 75:865–875, 1991.

Schrock TR: Acute appendicitis. *In* Sleisenger MH, Fordtran JS (eds): Gastrointestinal Disease, ed 5. Philadelphia, WB Saunders, 1993, pp 1339–1346.

Schuster MM: Irritable bowel syndrome. *In* Sleisenger MH, Fordtran JS (eds): Gastrointestinal Disease, ed 5. Philadelphia, WB Saunders, 1993, pp 917–929.

Shamburek RD, Farrar JT: Disorders of the digestive system in the elderly. N Engl J Med 322:438–443, 1990.

Silen W: Abdominal pain. *In* Isselbacher KJ, Braunwald E, Wilson JD, et al (eds): Harrison's Principles of Internal Medicine, ed 13. New York, McGraw-Hill, 1994, pp 61–65.

Sipponen P: Gastric cancer—A long term consequence of *Helicobacter pylori* infection? Scand J Gastroenterol Suppl 201:24–27, 1994.

Skipper RP, Boeckman CR, Klein RL: Childhood intussusception. Surg Gynecol Obstet 171:151–153, 1990.

Soll AH: Gastric, duodenal, and stress ulcer. *In* Sleisenger MH, Fordtran JS (eds): Gastrointestinal Disease, ed 5. Philadelphia, WB Saunders, 1993, pp 580–678.

Soll AH: Nonsteroidal anti-inflammatory drugs and ulcers (editorial). West J Med 157:465–468, 1992.

Snape WJ: Disorders of gastrointestinal motility. *In* Wyngaarden JB, Smith LH, Bennett JC (eds): Cecil Textbook of Medicine, ed 19. Philadelphia, WB Saunders, 1992, pp 671–680.

Thun MJ, Namboodiri MM, Heath CW: Aspirin use and reduced risk of fatal colon cancer. N Engl J Med 325:1593–1596, 1991.

Tierney LM: Blood vessels and lymphatics. *In* Tierney LM, McPhee SJ, Papadakis MA: Current Medical Diagnosis and Treatment, ed 33. Norwalk, Conn, Appleton & Lange, 1994, pp 385–414.

Walker AR, Segal I: What causes appendicitis? J Clin Gastroenterol 12:127, 1990.

Whiteway J, Morson BC: Elastosis in diverticular disease of the sigmoid colon. Gut 26:258, 1985.

Winawer SJ, Zauber AG, Ho MN, et al: Prevention of colorectal cancer by colonoscopic polypectomy. N Engl J Med 329:1977–1981, 1993.

Wong DL: Whaley and Wong's Essentials of Pediatric Nursing, ed 4. St Louis, Mosby–Year Book, 1993.

Wright V: The esophagus: Congenital anomalies. *In* Walker W (ed): Pediatric Gastrointestinal Disease. Philadelphia, BC Decker, 1991.

SECTION 2

chapter 14

The Hepatic, Pancreatic, and Biliary Systems

Catherine C. Goodman

The *liver* more than 500 separate functions, including the conversion of bilirubin (red bile pigment, an end-product of heme from hemoglobin in red blood cells [RBCs]) into bile. The liver is the sole source of albumin and other plasma proteins and also produces 500 to 1500 mL of bile each day. Other important functions of the liver include production of clotting factors, storage of vitamins, and metabolism of drugs, steroid hormones, toxins, carbohydrates, fats, and proteins.

The *pancreas* is both an exocrine and an endocrine gland. Its primary function in digestion is exocrine secretion of digestive enzymes and pancreatic juices, transported through the hepatic duct to the duodenum. Proteins, carbohydrates, and fats are broken down in the duodenum, aided by pancreatic and other secretions, which also help to neutralize the acidic chyme passed from the stomach to the duodenum.

The *gallbladder*, acting as a reservoir for bile, stores and concentrates the bile during fasting periods and then contracts to expel the bile into the duodenum in response to the arrival of food. Bile helps in alkalinizing the intestinal contents and plays a role in the emulsification, absorption, and digestion of fat. The signal for the gallbladder to contract comes from the release of cholecystokinin, a hormone released into the bloodstream from the wall of the duodenum and upper small intestine (Johnson and Triger, 1992).

SIGNS AND SYMPTOMS OF HEPATIC DISEASE

Primary signs and symptoms of liver diseases vary and can include gastrointestinal (GI) symptoms, edema/ascites, dark urine, light-colored or clay-colored feces, and right upper abdominal pain (Box 14–1). Impairment of the liver can result in *hepatic failure* when either the mass of liver cells is sufficiently diminished or their function is impaired as a result of cirrhosis, liver cancer, or infection and/or inflammation. Hepatic failure does not refer to one specific morphologic change but rather to a clinical syndrome that includes hepatic encephalopathy, renal failure (hepatorenal syndrome), endocrine changes, and jaundice (Goodman and Snyder, 1995).

Dark urine and *light stools* occur in association with jaundice (yellow pigmentation of skin, sclerae, and mucous membranes) (see Jaundice, later in the chapter) when the serum bilirubin level increases from normal (0.1 to 1.0 mg/dL) to a value of 2 or 3 mg/dL. Any damage to the liver impairs bilirubin metabolism from the blood. Normally, bile converted from bilirubin causes brown coloration of the stool. Light-colored (almost white) stools and urine the color of tea or cola indicate an inability of the liver or biliary system to excrete bilirubin properly.

Skin changes associated with the hepatic system include jaundice, pallor, and orange or green skin. When bilirubin reaches levels of 2 to 3 mg/dL, the sclera of the eye takes on a yellow hue. When bilirubin level reaches 5 to 6 mg/dL, the skin becomes yellow. The changes described here in urine, stool, or skin color may be caused by hepatitis, gallbladder disease, and/or pancreatic cancer blocking the bile duct, hepatotoxic medications, or cirrhosis. Other skin changes may include bruising, spider angiomas, and palmar erythema.

Spider angiomas (arterial spider, spider telangiectasis, vascular spider) are branched dilations of the superficial capillaries, which may be vascular manifestations of increased estrogen levels (hyperestrogenism) (see Fig. 8–2). Spider angiomas and palmar erythema both occur in the presence of liver impairment as a result of increased estrogen levels normally detoxified by the liver. *Palmar erythema* (warm redness of the skin over the palms, also called *liver palms*) especially affect the hypothenar and thenar eminences and pulps of the finger. The soles of the feet may be similarly affected. The person may complain of throbbing, tingling palms.

Neurologic symptoms such as confusion, sleep disturbances, muscle tremors, hyperreactive reflexes, and asterixis (see following discussion) may occur. When liver dysfunction results in increased serum ammonia and urea levels, peripheral nerve function can be impaired. Ammonia from the intestine (produced by protein breakdown) is normally transformed by the liver to urea, glutamine, and asparagine, which are then excreted by the renal system. When the liver does not detoxify ammonia, ammonia is transported to the brain, where it reacts with glutamate (excitatory neurotransmitter) to produce glutamine. The reduction of brain glutamate impairs neurotransmission, leading to altered CNS metabolism and function. Asterixis and numbness or tingling (misinterpreted as carpal tunnel syndrome) can occur as a result of this ammonia abnormality, causing intrinsic nerve pathology.

Asterixis, also called flapping tremors or liver flap, is a motor disturbance; specifically, it is the inability to maintain wrist extension with forward flexion of the upper extremities. Asterixis can be tested for by asking the client to dorsiflex the hand with the rest of the arm supported on a firm surface or with the arms held out in front of the body. Observe for quick, irregular extensions and flexions of the wrist and fingers (Fig. 14–1). Altered neurotransmission, in the form of impaired inflow of joint and other afferent information to the brainstem reticular formation, causes the movement dysfunction (Sherlock and Dooley, 1993).

BOX **14–1**
Most Common Signs and Symptoms of Hepatic Disease

- Gastrointestinal symptoms (see Table 13–1)
- Edema/ascites
- Dark urine
- Light- or clay-colored stools
- Right upper quadrant abdominal pain
- Skin changes
  - Jaundice
  - Bruising
  - Spider angioma
  - Palmar erythema
- Neurologic involvement
  - Confusion
  - Sleep disturbances
  - Muscle tremors
  - Hyperreactive reflexes
  - Asterixis
- Musculoskeletal pain (see text for sites)
- Hepatic osteodystrophy
- Hepatic failure
  - Hepatic encephalopathy
  - Renal failure (hepatorenal syndrome)
  - Endocrine changes
  - Jaundice
- Portal hypertension

Musculoskeletal locations of pain associated with the hepatic and biliary systems include thoracic pain between scapulae, right shoulder, right upper trapezius, right interscapular, or right subscapular areas. Sympathetic fibers from the biliary system are connected through the celiac and splanchnic (visceral) plexuses to the hepatic fibers in the region of the dorsal spine. These connections account for the intercostal and radiating interscapular pain that accompanies gallbladder disease. Although the innervation is bilateral, most of the biliary fibers reach the cord through the right splanchnic nerves, producing pain in the right shoulder (Ridge and Way, 1993).

Hepatic osteodystrophy, abnormal development of bone, can occur in all forms of cholestasis (bile flow suppression) and hepatocellular disease, especially in the alcoholic. Bone pain is frequently accompanied by either osteomalacia or, more often, osteoporosis. Hepatic osteoporosis is secondary to osteoblastic dysfunction rather than to excessive bone resorption.[1] Vertebral wedging, vertebral crush fractures, and kyphosis can be severe; decalcification of the rib cage and pseudofractures[2] occur frequently. Osteoporosis associated with primary biliary cirrhosis and primary sclerosing cholangitis (see text) parallels the severity of liver disease rather than the duration. Painful osteoarthropathy may develop in the wrists and ankles as a nonspecific complication of chronic liver disease (Sherlock and Dooley, 1993).

Portal hypertension, ascites, and hepatic encephalopathy are three other major symptoms of liver disease that are discussed in greater depth in this chapter as distinct clinical conditions.

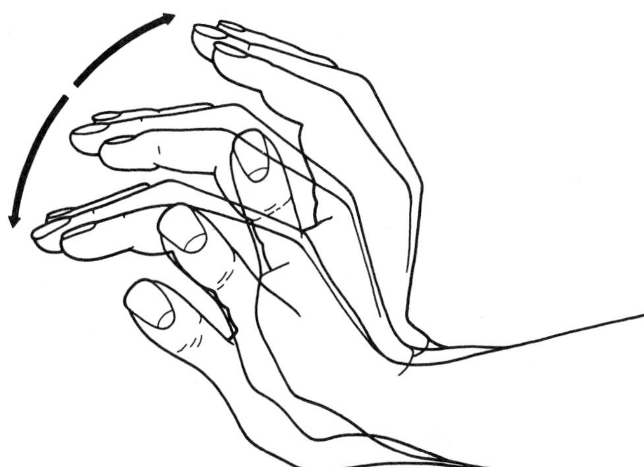

Figure **14–1.** "Flapping" tremor elicited by attempted dorsiflexion of the wrist while the forearm is fixed is the most common neurologic abnormality associated with liver failure. It can also be observed in uremia, respiratory failure, and severe heart failure. The tremor is absent at rest, decreased by intentional movement, and maximal on sustained posture. It is usually bilateral, although one side may be affected more than the other. (*From Sherlock S, Dooley J: Diseases of the Liver and Biliary System, ed 9. Oxford, Blackwell Scientific Publications, 1993, p 89.*)

Special Implications for the Therapist **14–1**

SIGNS AND SYMPTOMS OF HEPATIC DISEASE

Any client presenting with undiagnosed or untreated jaundice must be referred to the physician for follow-up. Active, intense exercise should be avoided when the liver is compromised (i.e., during jaundice or any other active disease), because the cornerstone of medical treatment and promotion of healing of the liver is rest. (See also Special Implications for the Therapist: Jaundice, Portal Hypertension, Ascites, and Hepatic Encephalopathy.)

An increased risk of coagulopathy (decreased clotting ability) also occurs with liver disease, necessitating precautions. Bleeding under the skin and easy bruising in response to the slightest trauma often occur when platelet production is altered (thrombocytopenia). This condition necessitates extreme care in the therapy setting, especially with any treatment requiring manual therapy or the use of any equipment, including modalities and weight-training devices (see also Special Implications for the Therapist: Thrombocytopenia, 11–11).

The most common neurologic abnormality associated with liver failure (called liver flap or asterixis) (see Fig. 14–1) can also be observed in uremia, respiratory failure, and severe heart failure. The rapid flexion-extension movements at the metacarpophalangeal and

---

[1] The pathogenesis is probably complex, and factors include calcium malabsorption, alcohol, corticosteroid therapy, estrogen deficiency in the postmenopausal woman, and vitamin D deficiency with secondary hyperparathyroidism (Sherlock and Dooley, 1993).

[2] Pseudofractures or Looser's zones are narrow lines of radiolucency (areas of darkness on x-ray film) usually oriented perpendicular to the bone surface. This may represent a stress fracture that has been repaired by the laying down of inadequately mineralized osteoid, or these sites may occur as a result of mechanical erosion caused by arterial pulsations, as arteries frequently overlie sites of pseudofractures (Key and Bell, 1994).

wrist joints are often accompanied by lateral movements of the digits. Sometimes movement of arms, neck, and jaws; protruding tongue; retracted mouth; and tightly closed eyelids are involved, and the gait is ataxic.

The tremor is absent at rest, decreased by intentional movement, and maximal on sustained posture. It is usually bilateral, although not bilaterally synchronous, and one side may be affected more than the other. It may be observed by gentle elevation of a limb or by the client's gripping the therapist's hand. In coma, the tremor disappears (Sherlock and Dooley, 1993).

AGING AND THE HEPATIC SYSTEM

The *liver* decreases in size and weight with advancing age, but liver function test results, such as levels of aspartate transaminase (AST), alanine transaminase (ALT), γ-glutamyl transpeptidase (GGTP), alkaline phosphatase, and total serum bilirubin (see Chapter 35) remain unchanged and within normal limits established for the adult (Abrams et al., 1995). However, these tests often measure hepatic damage rather than overall function; abnormal values for these tests in elderly people reflect disease rather than the effects of aging. The decreased liver weight is accompanied by diminished blood flow; this combination of decreased liver mass and blood flow may account for some changes in drug elimination observed in elderly persons.[3] Although age-related changes in renal function may require downward dosage adjustments, dosing changes based on hepatic function related to aging are not usually needed.

The liver itself becomes more fibrotic, but this change is not synonymous with pathologic cirrhotic changes. On autopsy, a buildup of brown pigment is seen, which is a result of accumulated unexcretable metabolic residue (end-stage metabolic products of lipids and proteins) acquired over a lifetime; no apparent physiologic significance has been identified with this pigment.

The *pancreas* undergoes structural changes, such as fibrosis, fatty acid deposits, and atrophy. Pancreatic secretion decreases, but there is usually no observable dysfunction. Much remains unknown about the *gallbladder* in the aging process, but aging apparently has little effect on gallbladder size, contractility, or function. No obvious change in secretion of bile acid is seen but lipid secretion may increase. This biliary lipid composition may explain the increased prevalence of gallstones in the aged.

HEALING IN THE HEPATIC SYSTEM

In general, older organs may not adapt to injury as well as younger organs, so severe hepatic illnesses (e.g., severe hepatitis) may not be tolerated as well by the older person. Delayed or impaired tissue repair may require longer time for recovery of homeostasis.

Liver injury is followed by complete parenchymal regeneration, the formation of scars, or a combination of both. The outcome depends on the extent and chronicity of the insult. Chronic hepatic injury, such as chronic viral hepatitis or alcoholic liver injury, destroys the extracellular matrix framework. This type of destruction results in a combination of regenerated nodules separated by bands of fibrous connective tissue (fibrosis), which is termed *cirrhosis* (Rubin and Farber, 1994).

LIVER

Jaundice (Icterus)

Overview and Incidence. Jaundice or icterus is not a disease but is rather a common symptom of many different diseases and disorders. It is characterized by yellow discoloration of the skin, sclerae, mucous membranes, and excretions owing to staining of tissues by the bile pigment bilirubin (hyperbilirubinemia).

Jaundice can occur at any age in any person with no predilection for sex. The probability of jaundice associated with cancerous biliary obstruction increases with age, but at no age is a person immune from hepatitis B and C. The incidence of hepatitis A decreases with age, and jaundice associated with this type of hepatitis is most commonly seen in children.

Risk Factors. Risk factors for the development of jaundice are listed in Box 14–2. Jaundice in the postoperative client is not uncommon and may be a potentially serious complication of surgery and anesthesia. Clinical management of jaundice is complicated by anything that can damage the liver, including stress, hypoxemia, blood loss, infection, and administration of multiple drugs. Drug-induced liver disease is a common cause of jaundice in older persons (see Tables 14–3 and 14–4). In most cases, drug toxicity stops when the agent is withdrawn.

Etiology and Pathogenesis. Jaundice may be classified according to the location of the pathologic change as *prehepatic*, *hepatic*, or *posthepatic*; causes of each state are listed in Table 14–1. In the prehepatic state, bilirubin increases before it

BOX **14–2**
Risk Factors for Jaundice

- Occupation or employment involving alcohol consumption
- History of jaundice, hepatitis, anemia, splenectomy, or cholecystectomy
- Place of origin: Mediterranean, Africa, Far East
- Contact with jaundiced persons (see Transmission, Table 14–2): persons on dialysis, drug abusers, homosexuals, or prostitutes
- Injections within the last 6 months for blood tests, drug abuse, tattoo (inscription or removal), blood or plasma transfusion
- Consumption of raw shellfish
- Recent travel to areas where hepatitis is present at all times (endemic)

[3] Many factors may influence drug metabolism in the elderly, including changes in body composition, decline in renal function, alterations in serum albumin levels (drugs such as sulfonamides and salicylates compete with bilirubin for binding sites on albumin, a transport plasma protein), individual variability, poor compliance, lack of understanding of drug therapy, presence of other systemic illnesses, and taking multiple drugs simultaneously (drug-drug interaction).

TABLE 14–1 Classification of Jaundice

Prehepatic	Hepatic	Posthepatic
Hemolytic blood transfusion reaction	Hepatitis	Bile duct strictures
Blood incompatibility (mother and infant)	Liver congestion	Gallstones
Autoimmune hemolytic anemia	Cirrhosis	Pancreatic stones
Severe burns	Metastatic cancer	Pancreatitis
Bacterial toxins	Prolonged use of medications metabolized by the liver	Tumors of the ducts or adjacent structures
Defective albumin binding	Anorexia	
Sickle cell disease	Physiologic jaundice of the newborn	
Hemolytic drugs	Primary biliary cirrhosis	

reaches the liver as a result of its overrelease, usually secondary to hemolysis (destruction) of RBCs. Hepatic jaundice results in bilirubin increase when pathology within the liver parenchyma impairs the liver's ability to adequately excrete bilirubin. Posthepatic (obstructive) jaundice occurs when bile duct obstruction impairs bilirubin transport after the bilirubin leaves the liver. Gallstones in the common bile duct are the most common cause of obstructive jaundice; cancer of the pancreas is also relatively common, particularly in older persons.

About 4 mg/kg of bilirubin is produced each day, 80% to 85% of which is derived from the catabolism of the heme of hemoglobin and subsequent conversion to bilirubin in worn out or defective RBCs. The remaining 15% to 20% of bilirubin is derived from the destruction of maturing but ineffective erythroid cells in the bone marrow. Normally, the liver cells absorb the bilirubin, but if the liver is diseased, flow of bile is obstructed, or destruction of erythrocytes is excessive, the bilirubin accumulates in the blood. The bilirubin binds with albumin, which transports it from the blood plasma to the liver, forming a complex known as *unconjugated bilirubin*. Unconjugated bilirubin cannot be excreted in the urine or bile, but it is easily taken up by fatty tissue and the brain. Bilirubin is easily bound to elastic tissue, such as the skin, blood vessels, sclerae, and synovium, which in turn become icteric (jaundiced or yellow).

Once the unconjugated bilirubin reaches the liver, it joins with glucuronic acid to form conjugated bilirubin. Conjugation transforms bilirubin from a lipid-soluble substance that can cross biologic membranes to a water-soluble substance that can be excreted in the bile or converted to urobilinogen, a yellow pigment that is subsequently excreted in the urine, giving normal urine its characteristic color. As a result of this pathologic process, jaundice may be categorized according to whether the bilirubin is primarily unconjugated or conjugated, which indicates whether the increase in bilirubin occurs before, at, or after it reaches the liver.

Clinical Manifestations. Jaundice is the predominant sign of hyperbilirubinemia, and it becomes obvious when bilirubin levels exceed 2.0 to 2.5 mg/dL, with yellowing of the sclerae of the eyes. When bilirubin level reaches 5 to 6 mg/dL, the skin becomes yellow. *Unconjugated hyperbilirubinemia* (indicating prehepatic pathology) may present as weakness or abdominal or back pain with acute hemolytic crisis. Stool and urine color are normal, but mild jaundice is observed in the skin, sclerae, or mucous membranes (Friedman and Knauer, 1994).

Conjugated hyperbilirubinemia (indicating hepatic or posthepatic pathology) may be asymptomatic when associated with factors that stop or suppress bile flow (cholestasis); in the case of intermittent cholestasis, symptoms may include light-colored stools, malaise, and pruritus (itching) from the deposition of bile salts in the skin. Conjugated hyperbilirubinemia associated with hepatocellular disease may be accompanied by malaise, anorexia, low-grade fever, and right upper quadrant discomfort. Dark urine, jaundice, vascular spiders, white nails, loss of sexual hair, palmar erythema, yellow plaque spots on eyelids (xanthelasma), asterixis, or fetor hepaticus (musty, sweet breath odor due to the liver's inability to metabolize the amino acid methionine) may be present, depending on the cause, severity, and chronicity of liver dysfunction (see Fig. 14–5).

Conjugated hyperbilirubinemia associated with biliary obstruction presents with right upper quadrant colicky pain, weight loss (carcinoma), jaundice, dark urine, and light-colored stools. Signs and symptoms may be intermittent when caused by stone or tumor.

Medical Management

Diagnosis. A careful history and physical examination are important in determining the nature and cause of jaundice. Past medical history of drug or alcohol use, exposure to persons with infectious hepatitis, recurrent abdominal pain and nausea (gallstones), and pre-existing liver disease are helpful clues as to the infectious cause of jaundice.

Specific urine and blood serum testing is used to determine the level of bilirubin and whether it is conjugated or unconjugated (see Overview earlier in this section) pointing to a prehepatic, hepatic, or posthepatic condition. Because bilirubin has to be conjugated to be excreted, and conjugation occurs in the liver, high levels of unconjugated bilirubin indicate a prehepatic problem (i.e., the bilirubin has not reached the liver to be conjugated) (see Table 14–1). High levels of conjugated bilirubin indicate that the bilirubin has passed through the liver, pointing to improper excretion of bilirubin from the liver or obstructed flow of bile outside the liver.

Other conditions may be demonstrated using ultrasonography, computed tomographic (CT) scan or magnetic resonance imaging (MRI). Percutaneous liver biopsy may also be used to determine the cause and extent of hepatocellular dysfunction; liver biopsy performed under ultrasound or CT may be performed when metastatic disease or hepatic mass is suspected.

Treatment and Prognosis. Treatment is determined by the underlying cause of the jaundice (e.g., surgery for obstructive jaundice, medical management [rest and supportive measures] for hepatitis, withdrawal of cholestatic drug). Likewise, prognosis depends on the underlying disease. The reader is referred to the Prognosis section for the individual disease or condition causing the jaundice. Once the underlying cause has been treated, jaundice fades slowly over 3 to 4 weeks, leaving the client looking particularly pale and washed out.

Special Implication Therapy **14–2**

JAUNDICE (ICTERUS)

With successful treatment of the underlying cause, jaundice usually begins to resolve within 4 to 6 weeks. Following this time, activity and exercise can be resumed or increased per individual tolerance, depending on the overall medical condition and presence of any complications. The return of normal stool and urine colors are an indication of resolution. (See also Special Implications: Signs and Symptoms of Hepatic Disease, 14–1.)

Hepatitis

Hepatitis is an acute or chronic inflammation of the liver caused by a virus, a chemical, a drug reaction, or alcohol abuse. Classifications of hepatitis discussed in this text are listed in Box 14–3. Five major viruses causing hepatitis have been identified and labeled as A, B, C, D, or E; there is evidence for at least one additional virus (HGV). Other viral causes of hepatitis include Epstein-Barr virus (mononucleosis), herpes simplex virus types I and II, varicella-zoster virus, measles, or cytomegalovirus (CMV). Hepatitis owing to any cause produces very similar symptoms and usually requires only a careful client history to establish the diagnosis.

Viral Hepatitis

Overview. Each of the five recognized hepatitis viruses belongs to a different virus family, and each has a unique epidemiology. Characteristics of these five strains of viruses are presented in Table 14–2. Personal contact with another person with hepatitis A is the primary source for infection among persons with hepatitis A; other potential sources account for fewer than 10% of all hepatitis A virus (HAV) cases. Drug use and contact with another person with hepatitis B are the two most frequent sources of hepatitis B virus (HBV). Parenteral drug use is the risk factor most commonly reported by clients with hepatitis C virus (HCV). Hepatitis D virus (HDV) has the same source as HBV, and HEV is transmitted by contaminated water.

BOX **14–3**
Hepatitis Classifications

Viral
Toxic
Chronic (active or persistent)
Autoimmune
Alcoholic

The identification of the specific virus is made difficult by the fact that a long incubation period often occurs between acquisition of the infection and development of the first symptoms. The incubation period for HAV is 2 to 7 weeks; it is 2 to 6 months for HBV and 1 to 2 weeks for HCV. Not all causative agents have been identified, and because hepatitis can be easily spread before symptoms appear, morbidity is high in terms of loss of time from school or work. More than half, and possibly as many as 90%, of all cases go unreported because symptoms are mild or even subclinical (Smelzer and Bare, 1992).

People with mild-to-moderate acute hepatitis rarely require hospitalization. The emphasis is on preventing the spread of infectious agents and avoiding further liver damage when the underlying cause is drug-induced or toxic hepatitis. Persons with fulminant hepatitis (of severe, sudden intensity; sometimes fatal) require special management because of the rapid progression of the disease and the potential need for urgent liver transplantation (Carithers, 1993). HBV, HCV, and HDV can result in chronic hepatitis and cirrhosis.

Incidence. Each year approximately 500,000 Americans are infected with some form of hepatitis virus; annually about 15,000 persons die from its complications. HAV is the predominant type of hepatitis among persons younger than 15 years; 70% of hepatitis B cases and 58% of hepatitis C cases are reported in the 20- to 39-year age group. Prevalence of HBV infection is more than four times higher among blacks than among whites (Centers for Disease Control and Prevention [CDC], 1992).

Pathogenesis. The pathology of hepatitis is similar to that of other viral infections. Hepatic cell necrosis, scarring, Kupffer cell hyperplasia, and infiltration by mononuclear phagocytes occur with varying severity in response to the virus. Cellular injury occurs via cytotoxic T cells and natural killer cells as part of the cell-mediated immune system response. The inflammatory process can damage and obstruct bile canaliculi, leading to cholestasis and obstructive jaundice. In milder cases, the liver parenchyma is not damaged. More severe liver damage tends to occur in cases of HBV and HCV. Regeneration of hepatic cells begins within 48 hours of injury (Heuther and McCance, 1994).

Clinical Manifestations. Hepatitis occurs in three stages: the initial or preicteric stage, the icteric or jaundice stage, and the recovery period (Table 14–3). During the *initial* or *preicteric* stage, which lasts for 1 to 3 weeks (sometimes also referred to as the *prodromal stage*), the urine darkens and the stool lightens as less bilirubin is conjugated and excreted.

The *icteric stage* is characterized by the appearance of jaundice, which peaks in 1 to 2 weeks and persists for 6 to 8 weeks. During this stage, the acuteness of the inflammation subsides. Persons who have been treated with human immune serum globulin (ISG) may not develop hepatitis. The *recovery stage* lasts for 3 to 4 months, during which time the person generally feels well but fatigues easily. Chronic hepatitis (covered more completely later in this section) may begin at this time.

TABLE 14–2 TYPES OF VIRAL HEPATITIS

	HEPATITIS A	HEPATITIS B	HEPATITIS C	HEPATITIS D	HEPATITIS E
Incidence	35,821 cases reported to CDC in 1995	CDC estimates 300,000 new acute cases in the US each year; 1 million carriers	CDC estimates 30,000 new cases each year in the US; 0.5% to 2.2% prevalence but transfusion-related cases decreasing with blood screening	Uncommon in US; most common in drug addicts, sexually active young adults, individuals receiving multiple transfusions	Epidemic in developing countries; rare in US; risk greatest to persons traveling to endemic regions
Morbidity	Results in acute infection only; does not progress to chronic hepatitis or cirrhosis; lifetime immunity	6%–10% of cases progress to chronic hepatitis; second major cause of cirrhosis in the US after alcohol abuse; responsible for 4,000 deaths due to cirrhosis and 800 deaths due to liver cancer in the US each year	50% of all cases progress to chronic hepatitis and 20% of chronic cases progress to cirrhosis; possibly associated with liver cancer	Most severe form of viral hepatitis; frequently progresses to chronic active hepatitis or death; mortality rate 2% to 20%	Causes acute self-limiting infection; does not progress to chronic hepatitis; high mortality in pregnant women, 10% mortality
Transmission	Spread by feces, saliva, and contaminated food and water	Exposure to blood and blood products, infected body fluids such as saliva, semen, and vaginal secretions through sexual contact; maternal-fetal; unidentified exposure	Exposure to blood or blood products, including transfusion, needlestick, and intravenous drug use; unidentified exposure	Same as B; requires co-infection with HBV to produce; transmission by sexual contact, contaminated blood and needles	Same as A; fecal contamination of water
Treatment	Supportive; most people recover within 6–10 wk	Interferon alfa-2b, recombinant, for chronic hepatitis B; HBIG for unvaccinated persons (see text)	Interferon alfa-2b, recombinant, for chronic hepatitis non-A, non B/C	Interferon alfa-2b can inhibit HDV replication but effect ends when therapy ends	None
Diagnosis	Blood test to identify antibody; anti-HAV; IgM	Blood test to identify antigen and antibodies; HBsAg; HBeAg; HbcAg	Blood test to identify antibody; does not distinguish between current and past infection; anti-HCV	Blood test to detect antigen and antibody; anti-HDV	No test available
Vaccine	Killed-virus vaccine now available	Recombinant vaccines available	None available	Immunization against hepatitis B can prevent hepatitis D infection	None available

From Hepatitis Fact Sheet, Schering Corporation, June 1992; and Gardner P, Schaffner W: Immunization of adults. N Engl J Med 328:1252–1258, 1993.

Medical Management

Diagnosis, Treatment, and Prognosis. In addition to the history and clinical examination, serodiagnosis may be helpful in detecting the presence of viral markers that indicate the cause of acute viral hepatitis (Herrera, 1994). Serial blood titers may be necessary, as the viral markers are only positive during certain periods of the disease process; a negative test result does not rule out viral hepatitis. A test for hepatitis E virus (HEV) has not been developed. Transaminases (enzymes normally present) are released from the acutely damaged hepatocytes, and serum transaminase levels rise, often to levels exceeding normal levels by 20-fold. Bilirubinuria and an elevated serum bilirubin level are usually found. Liver function tests (see Table 35–15) can indicate other viral liver diseases, drug toxicity, or alcoholic hepatitis (discussed further). None of the serodiagnostic tests are able to determine the current extent of liver damage; liver biopsy is required to identify the extent of liver disease.

TABLE 14-3 STAGES OF HEPATITIS

INITIAL/PREICTERIC (1–3 wk)	ICTERIC (6–8 wk)	RECOVERY (3–4 mo)
Dark urine Light stools Vague GI symptoms Constitutional symptoms Fatigue Malaise Weight loss Anorexia Nausea/vomiting Diarrhea Aversion to food, alcohol, cigarette smoke Enlarged and tender liver Intermittent pruritus (itching)	Jaundice GI symptoms subside Liver decreases in size and tenderness Enlarged spleen Enlarged postcervical lymph nodes	Easily fatigued

No specific treatment is available for acute viral hepatitis, and prognosis varies with each type (see Treatment and Prognosis sections for each individual type, see also Table 14–2). In the 1980s, plasma-derived and then recombinant hepatitis B vaccines were developed and introduced. A killed hepatitis A vaccine has been developed, and the virologic tools have been discovered that will ultimately provide a vaccine against hepatitis C (Katkov and Dienstag, 1995). A substantial proportion of hepatitis B morbidity and mortality that occurs in the health-care setting can be prevented by vaccinating health-care workers against HBV.[4] In addition, health-care workers must practice infection control measures (see Appendix A). Other prophylactic strategies are based on avoidance of high-risk behavior and use of immune globin.

Hepatitis A

Overview. HAV, formerly known as infectious hepatitis, most commonly affects children and young adults, although persons of any age are susceptible. A second peak incidence occurs in older persons who travel to parts of the world where the risk of HAV is increased. HAV is often spread in environments characterized by poor sanitation and overcrowding, such as day care centers, prisons, military training sites, and schools. The primary mode of transmission is the oral-fecal route;[5] major outbreaks of HAV occur when people consume water or shellfish from sewage-contaminated waters. HAV is rarely transmitted through transfused blood, and little placental transmission occurs, although the antibody is often detected in infants of infected mothers.

HAV is highly contagious, with the peak time of yiral excretion and contamination occurring during the 1-week period *before* the onset of symptoms of jaundice. Thus, the greatest danger of infection is during the incubation period, when a person is unaware that the virus is present. The illness can last from 4 to 8 weeks; it generally lasts longer and is more severe in persons older than 40 years (Smeltzer and Bare, 1992).

Medical Management

Treatment. Preventive measures include HAV vaccine (MMWR, 1995; Brewer et al., 1995), universal precautions, and the administration of ISG therapy, also referred to as gamma-globulin therapy, during the period of incubation. Gamma-globulin is a normal constituent of blood plasma that contains antibodies. When an infection begins, the body produces gamma-globulin that includes antibodies to fight the infection. In some cases, after the infection has been eliminated, enough gamma-globulin remains in the body to prevent a recurrence of that particular infection, providing lifetime immunity. If the ISG therapy is administered within 2 weeks of exposure to the HAV infection, it bolsters the person's own antibody production and provides 6 to 8 weeks of passive (temporary) immunity. ISG is also recommended for household members and sexual partners of persons with HAV.

HAV vaccine is recommended for anyone traveling to areas with intermediate to high rates of endemic hepatitis A, persons living in communities with high endemic rates or periodic outbreaks of HAV infection, and clients with chronic liver disease (American Academy of Pediatrics, 1996). Health care workers in high-risk areas (e.g., neonatal ICU, providing wound care) without serologic evidence of previous HAV infection should also be immunized (see Table 6–5).

Treatment is primarily symptomatic, and bed rest is recommended for persons who are jaundiced to avoid complications from liver damage. Hospitalization may be required for excessive vomiting and subsequent fluid and electrolyte imbalance. During the anorexic period, the client may receive nutritional supplements and, possibly, intravenous glucose infusions. Any hepatic irritants such as alcohol or chemicals (e.g., occupational exposure to carbon tetrachloride) must be avoided in all types of hepatitis.

Prognosis. HAV is rarely fatal and does not lead to chronic hepatitis or cirrhosis. Most people recover fully and become immune to HAV. Relapse may occur, characterized by arthralgia with positive rheumatoid factor (RF) as a common laboratory finding (Gilkson et al., 1992). Fulminant hepatitis resulting in death develops in a very small percentage of people with HAV (0.1%).

Hepatitis B

Overview. HBV, formerly called serum hepatitis, is transmitted through needle sticks, sexual relations, intravenous drug use, sharing needles, blood transfusions, dialysis, and perinatal transmission from mother to child. The major source of this infection is blood serum, but body secretions (nasopharyngeal washings, saliva, sweat, cerebrospinal fluid, synovial fluid, bile, urine, feces, semen, vaginal secretions [including menstrual blood] and breast milk) of an infected person can also transmit the virus (Ellis, 1993).

Incidence. Whereas HAV is usually eliminated from the body by the time jaundice appears, the body is not always

[4] According to the Occupational Safety and Health Administration (OSHA) Bloodborne Pathogen Standard (1991), hepatitis B vaccination must be offered to all potentially exposed employees within 10 days of employment. Records related to this vaccination must be maintained. Employees who decline vaccination must sign a standardized declination form.

[5] The oral-fecal route of transmission is primarily from poor or improper handwashing and personal hygiene, particularly after using the bathroom and then handling food for public consumption. This route of transmission may also occur through the shared used of oral utensils, such as straws, silverware, and toothbrushes.

able to rid itself of HBV, and the virus can persist in body fluids indefinitely. The carrier state occurs in 90% to 95% of infected neonates, 20% of older children, and 1% to 10% of adults; approximately 1 to 1.25 million persons are chronic carriers of HBV. Men are more likely than women to develop the carrier state; immunosuppressed individuals are also at increased risk (Meyers and Jones, 1990). See Table 14–2 for specific annual incidence rates.

Risk Factors. HBV is considered one of the most underreported diseases in this country. Persons at high risk for contact with HBV are listed in Box 14–4. Transfusion as a source for HBV is now ranked last among known sources for HBV infection since the initiation of donor screening for hepatitis B core antibody (anti-HBc) started in 1987 (Marx, 1993).

HBV can survive on environmental surfaces, such as countertops, for at least a week, making indirect inoculation of HBV onto mucous membranes, cutaneous scratches, abrasions, burns, or other lesions possible via inanimate objects (Ellis, 1993). This factor also makes it difficult to determine the source of viral transmission. Because this virus can be transmitted through heterosexual or homosexual intercourse, it is considered a sexually transmitted disease.

Medical Management

Diagnosis. Testing for hepatitis B surface antigen (HBsAg) permits detection of many, but not all, acutely infected people. Diagnosis of acute infection rests on the identification of the IgM antibodies to hepatitis B core antigen. Antibody to HBsAg appears in serum during the convalescent phase of HBV infection. It is the neutralizing, protective antibody largely responsible for immunity to reinfection (Koff, 1993).

Treatment. In the unvaccinated person, hepatitis B immune globulin (HBIG) should be administered within 24 hours of the exposure, followed by the HBV series at 0, 1, and 6 months. For vaccinated persons, anti-HBs level is measured and treated accordingly (e.g., anti-HBs level ≥10 mIU/mL needs no prophylaxis, but an additional dose of the HBV vaccine is recommended for a level <10 mIU/mL) (Diekema and Doebbeling, 1995). Current data indicate that approximately 50% of adults who have chronic infection achieve virologic, biochemical, and histologic remission from treatment with a new drug, interferon alfa-2b (Intron A) (Ching et al., 1996). Interferon is a recombinant DNA, a genetically engineered copy of a naturally occurring protein that acts as an antiviral agent. It has multiple biologic effects on cells of diverse origin including antiviral, immunomodulatory, and antiproliferative activities (Swartz, 1991; Trotta, 1991). Relapse on cessation of treatment is common, and significant side effects of this medication may include headache, fever, and other flu-like symptoms (Koff, 1993).

Hepatitis B vaccine (active immunization) obtained from inactivated HBsAg from the serum of chronic carriers of the B virus, as well as recombinant DNA vaccine, may provide permanent immunity to HBV when administered *prior to exposure*.

The World Health Organization (WHO) has recommended that all countries integrate HBV vaccination into their national immunization programs, but not all countries agree that the expense of universal vaccination is warranted (Van Damme et al., 1997). In the United States, this vaccine is recommended for persons in the high-risk category for HBV. Universal vaccination of health care workers against HBV is recommended (Diekema and Doebbeling, 1995).

Once individuals begin to engage in behaviors associated with the high-risk groups, they may become infected before vaccine can be given. A major obstacle in eliminating HBV is identifying persons and vaccinating them before they become infected. For this reason, it is now recommended that all infants receive the HBV vaccine. There is a high risk that children younger than 5 years of age, if infected, will become HBV carriers (MMWR, 1991).

Testing to identify pregnant women who are HBsAg-positive[6] and providing their infants with immunoprophylaxis effectively prevents HBV transmission during the perinatal period (MMWR, 1991).

The high cost of hepatitis B vaccine, along with recent recommendations for its expanded use, has stimulated increasing interest in the effectiveness and cost-saving potential of intradermal (ID) or intramuscular (IM) administration of reduced doses of vaccine (CDC, 1992).

Prognosis. HBV has a high mortality rate and is a very serious, potentially fatal illness. It can progress to cirrhosis, chronic hepatitis (5% to 10% of cases), hepatocellular carcinoma,[7] and death. Persistent infection leads to an asymptomatic carrier state; approximately 10% of infected persons become lifetime carriers of HBV. Orthotopic liver transplantation for cirrhosis caused by HBV is a possible treatment but has a poor prognosis because of almost universal reinfection.

Hepatitis C

Overview and Incidence. HCV, formerly post-transfusion non-A, non-B hepatitis, is another prevalent and underreported disease in the United States. HCV accounts for 25% of acute viral hepatitis and 90% of cases of post-transfusion hepatitis. A recently developed blood-screening test for HCV has reduced the numbers of blood transfusion-related cases of this virus by 50% in the United States. HCV also occurs among users of illicit drugs and their sexual partners, individuals with hemophilia receiving blood-derived factor replace-

BOX **14–4**
HBV Risk Factors

Dialysis
Occupational risk: morticians
Tattoo inscription or removal
Homosexual/bisexual activity
Health-care work in high-risk areas (i.e., areas of work in which contact with body fluid or blood is likely)
Multiple blood transfusions
Receipt of liver transplant
Certain ethnic groups (e.g., Hmong, Haitian)

---

[6] The HBsAg is a core protein antigen of the HBV present in the nuclei of infected cells. Presence of HBsAg in the blood usually indicates the individual is infectious. HBc antibodies appear during the acute infection but do not protect against reinfection.

[7] Hepatitis B is the most common cause of liver cancer worldwide (U.S. Department of Health and Human Services, 1992).

ment,[8] dialysis users, recipients of liver transplantation, infants born to HCV-infected mothers, and health-care personnel. The method by which millions without parenteral risk factors acquire HCV remains uncertain, so that control of community-acquired HCV remains a challenge (Alter, 1994; Purcell, 1994a; Purcell, 1994b). Vertical transmission and sexual and family spread occur only rarely (Sherlock, 1994a).

Clinical Manifestations. As with HAV, the period of infectivity begins before onset of symptoms, and the person may become a lifetime carrier of this virus. Clinically, HCV is very similar to HBV and often is asymptomatic; the acute HCV infection is usually mild. Significant symptoms include malaise, fever, headache, general muscle fatigue, loss of appetite, nausea, abdominal and joint pain, jaundice, and dark urine. Extrahepatic manifestations such as Hashimoto's thyroid disease, diabetes mellitus, corneal ulceration, and idiopathic thrombocytopenia appear to be more frequent in chronic HCV than in B or D.

Medical Management

Diagnosis. Formerly, the diagnosis of HVC was made by the exclusion of other causes. However, in 1989 cloning of an antigenic component of the hepatitis C virus was reported. It is now possible to detect an antibody to HCV (anti-HCV) in client serum 2 to 6 months after exposure to hepatitis C virus (Sherlock, 1994a). Appearance of this antibody indicates past infection with HCV, but it may not appear until over 1 year after infection and may persist up to 12 years after recovery (Kuo et al., 1989). Serum and liver tissue can be tested for viral RNA, which is evidence of ongoing viral replication.

Chronic HCV infection must be differentiated from autoimmune chronic active hepatitis. The most important difference is the response to corticosteroid therapy, which is good in autoimmune hepatitis and poor in HCV-related disease (Sherlock, 1994a).

Treatment. Currently, no vaccine is available to prevent this virus, and no immunoglobulin is effective in treating exposure. Interferon alfa-2b, used in the treatment of HBV, also reduces the inflammation and liver damage caused by HCV in 70% to 90% of cases (Douglas et al., 1993) but only 20% to 40% have a sustained benefit from therapy. It may be that HCV fails to induce an effective neutralizing antibody response, making the development of effective passive or active immunoprophylaxis against hepatitis C difficult (Alter, 1994). Universal precautions are indicated as a preventive measure.

Prognosis. The person with HCV can become a chronic carrier. When HCV continues to attack liver cells beyond a 6-month period, causing liver inflammation and scarring (cirrhosis), liver failure can occur; 60% to 80% of all cases progress to cirrhosis. An association has been suggested between the presence of long-standing chronic HCV and the development of hepatocellular cancer (Dana et al., 1994; Rubin et al., 1994). Chronic HCV necessitates most liver transplants among adults in the United States. The progression of HCV may be accelerated if a person is also infected with the acquired immunodeficiency syndrome (AIDS) virus (Ewenstein, 1994).

[8] Ninety percent of people with hemophilia who received clotting factor before the mid-1980s test positive for HCV (Ewenstein, 1994).

Hepatitis D

Hepatitis D (δ virus) is a defective single-stranded RNA that presents as a coinfection or superinfection of hepatitis B (Najm, 1997). This virus requires HBsAg for its replication, so only individuals with hepatitis B are at risk for hepatitis D. Risk factors and transmission mode are the same as for HBV; parenteral drug users have a high incidence of HDV. The symptoms of HDV are similar to those of HBV except that clients are more likely to have fulminant hepatitis and to develop chronic active hepatitis and cirrhosis (Smeltzer and Bare, 1992).

A short-lived anti-HDV antibody develops after symptoms occur, indicating past or present infection with hepatitis D. Universal precautions are indicated for prevention of this infection. Immunity to hepatitis B also confers immunity to hepatitis D; therefore, hepatitis B vaccination is recommended for preexposure immunization prophylaxis. Hepatitis D by itself appears to be relatively harmless, but it has a high mortality when it accompanies hepatitis B.

Hepatitis E

Hepatitis E, also called enteric non-A, non-B hepatitis, is transmitted by contaminated water and clinically resembles HAV. It is believed to be nonfatal except in pregnant women (10% to 20% mortality rate). This virus primarily occurs in developing countries and is rare in the United States. No blood serum test, vaccine, or prophylaxis exists for HEV.

Fulminant Hepatitis

Fulminant hepatitis is defined as hepatic failure with stage III or IV encephalopathy (confusion, stupor, and coma) as a result of massive hepatic necrosis. This type of hepatitis occurs in less than 1% of persons with acute viral hepatitis and can be fatal. Other causes can include exposure to hepatotoxins, such as acetaminophen (analgesic), isoniazid (antitubercular drug), halothane (anesthetic), valproic acid (anticonvulsant), mushroom toxins, or carbon tetrachloride. In addition to liver failure, numerous complications can occur, including additional infection, cerebral edema, hypoglycemia, GI hemorrhage, cardiorespiratory insufficiency, and renal insufficiency.

Diagnosis is made in the presence of a combination of hepatic encephalopathy, acute liver disease (elevated serum bilirubin and transaminase levels), and liver failure. Treatment is supportive, as the underlying etiology of liver failure is rarely treatable short of liver transplantation. Prognosis is determined in part by the cause of the condition. Persons with fulminant hepatitis from HAV or acetaminophen overdose are more likely to recover spontaneously than are those with idiosyncratic drug-induced liver failure (Table 14–4), HBV, or idiopathic fulminant liver failure without liver transplantation. Short-term prognosis without liver transplantation is very poor, and the mortality rate is high (20% survival) (Andreoli et al., 1993). Despite the poor prognosis, complete recovery can occur owing to liver cell regeneration with recovery of liver function.

TABLE 14-4 CAUSES OF DRUG-INDUCED HEPATITIS

DOSE-RELATED	IDIOSYNCRATIC
Acetaminophen* (Tylenol) (analgesic; suicide attempt)	α-Methyldopa (antihypertensive)
Amanita phalloides (poisonous mushroom)	Halothane (anesthetic)
Anabolic steroids	Isoniazid (antitubercular)
Aspirin	Monoamine oxidase inhibitors (antidepressant)
Benzene	Nitrofurantoin
Carbon tetrachloride	Phenytoin (Dilantin) (anticonvulsant)
Chloroform (anesthetic)	Rifampin (antitubercular)
Methotrexate (antineoplastic agent)	Quinidine (antiarrhythmic)
Oral contraceptives	Sulfasalazine (antibiotic)
Penicillin	
Tetracyclines (antibiotic)	

* Acetaminophen is Tylenol and is not an NSAID. It has no antiinflammatory properties, only analgesic and antipyretic uses. It has no relationship to ibuprofen.

Adapted from Matassarin-Jacobs E, Strasburg K: Nursing care of clients with hepatic disorders. *In* Black J, Matassarin-Jacobs E (eds): Luckmann and Sorensen's Medical-Surgical Nursing: A Pathophysiologic Approach, ed 4. Philadelphia, WB Saunders, 1993, p 1707.

Special Implications for Therapy **14-3**

HEPATITIS

Any direct contact with blood or body fluids of clients with hepatitis B or C requires the administration of immune globulin in the early incubation period. Therapists at risk for contact with HBV owing to their close contact with the blood or body fluids of carriers should receive active immunization against HBV. All therapists should follow universal precautions at all times to protect themselves; enteric precautions are required when caring for individuals with type A or E hepatitis.

Studies dealing with the natural history of acute hepatitis have provided perspective on the frequency of skin and joint manifestations (Gocke, 1982; Stewart et al., 1978). More than a third of the adults studied had joint pains during the course of the illness. The frequency of arthralgia as a symptom associated with hepatitis increases with age. Joint pains affected only 18% of children, compared with 45% of adults older than 30 years. No known studies have been published regarding the benefit of physical therapy in providing symptomatic joint relief until these symptoms resolve as the person recovers from the underlying pathology. In the case of a client with undiagnosed hepatitis presenting with joint symptoms, the systemically derived arthralgia will not respond to therapy. Any time treatment fails to provide symptomatic relief or resolution of symptoms, the results must be reported to the physician for further follow-up evaluation.

Overall, in the recovery process, adequate rest to conserve energy is important. The affected individual is encouraged to gradually return to preillness levels of activity. Fatigue associated with the anicteric phase of hepatitis may interfere with activities of daily living and may persist even after the jaundice resolves. A careful balance of activity is important to avoid weakness secondary to prolonged bed rest; a reasonable activity level is more conducive to recovery than is enforced bed rest. Whenever possible, therapy or increased activity should not be scheduled right after meals.

Watch for signs of fluid shift, such as weight gain and orthostasis; dehydration; pneumonia; vascular problems; pressure ulcers; and any signs of recurrence. After the diagnosis of viral hepatitis has been established, the affected individual should have regular medical checkups for at least 1 year and should avoid using any alcohol or over-the-counter drugs during this period.

HBV and the Athlete

No evidence has been reported that intense, highly competitive training is harmful for the asymptomatic HBV-infected person, whether the disease is acute or chronic. Therefore the presence of HBV infection does not contraindicate participation in sports or athletic activities; decisions regarding play are made according to clinical signs and symptoms such as fatigue, fever, or organomegaly. Chronic HBV infection with evidence of organ impairment requires reduction in intensity and duration of activity (McGrew, 1995).

Although risk of bloodborne pathogen infection during sports is exceedingly small, good hygiene practices concerning blood are still important. The American Medical Society for Sports Medicine (AMSSM) has made recommendations to minimize the risk of bloodborne pathogen transmission in the context of athletic events and has provided treatment guidelines for caregivers. The therapist in this type of setting is encouraged to read these proposed guidelines (AMSSM, 1995).

Toxic Hepatitis

Overview and Etiology. Toxic hepatitis is a form of nonviral liver inflammation that occurs secondary to exposure to certain chemicals or drugs. Despite safety precautions, occupational hepatotoxicity is on the rise, as a result of the modern development of many new chemicals. Specific chemical hepatotoxins may include alcohol, acetaminophen (Tylenol), carbon tetrachloride,[9] trichloroethylene, derivatives of benzene and toluene, organic pesticides, poisonous mushrooms (*Amanita phalloides* and related species, rare in the United States but more common in Europe), and vinyl chloride. Industrial toxins require rigorous safety precautions and ongoing monitoring to minimize the risk to industrial workers.

Drug-induced hepatitis occurs after the administration of one of various drugs. Substances that act as hepatotoxins may be categorized according to whether the hepatotoxic reaction is dose-related and predictable or idiosyncratic (i.e., unpredictable hypersensitivity reaction) (see Table 14–4). Some

[9] Carbon tetrachloride was the most common occupational inhalation poison until it was banned in most countries.

drugs, such as oral contraceptives, may impair liver function and produce jaundice without causing necrosis, fatty infiltration of liver cells, or a hypersensitivity reaction. By far the most common drug-induced liver failure is acetaminophen because of its availability, which makes possible the chronic ingestion of therapeutic dosages or overdose as a means of suicide.

Pathogenesis. Hepatic necrosis occurs when depletion of glutathione stores (nonessential amino acid occurring in proteins) in the liver allows the metabolized drug to bind with the liver rather than with the amino acid. Sensitive persons may be predisposed to idiosyncratic reactions either because they possess different metabolic pathways from those of the general population or because they are unusually sensitive to a uniform pharmacologic effect of the drug other than the desired therapeutic response (Rubin and Farber, 1994).

Clinical Manifestation. Toxic reactions are often difficult to identify, because the majority occur in acutely ill people who may be receiving a number of different drugs over a short period of time. Liver necrosis occurs within 2 or 3 days after acute exposure to a dose-related hepatotoxin. Several weeks may pass before manifestations of a reaction occurs. Clinical manifestations vary with the severity of liver damage and the causative agent. Some compounds can produce mild, subtle damage without any acute illness. In most individuals, symptoms resemble those of acute viral hepatitis and may include anorexia, nausea, and vomiting; fatigue and malaise; jaundice; dark urine; clay-colored stools; headache, dizziness, and drowsiness (carbon tetrachloride poisoning); and fever, rash, arthralgias, and epigastric or right upper quadrant pain (halothane anesthetic). Complications of unrecognized or untreated toxic hepatitis may include cirrhosis or renal failure.

Medical Management

Treatment and Prognosis. Treatment consists of removal of causative agent, rest, and alleviation of side effects. Gastric-emptying is used to eliminate acetaminophen intoxication. Once a drug has caused liver damage, this drug (as well as chemically similar compounds) must be avoided for life. Re-exposure to this drug is likely to cause the same symptoms with an increased risk of more severe liver damage on the second or third exposure. Industrial workers exposed to chemicals are encouraged to have regular medical examinations and blood tests, even if they are asymptomatic.

Special Implications for the Therapist **14-4**

TOXIC HEPATITIS

Therapists should be alert to the possibility of drug toxicity or drug reactions in clients taking multiple medications. Many people do not consider over-the-counter drugs as medications and may take the same drug with different names or combine over-the-counter drugs with prescription medications. People with memory loss or short-term memory deficits may take multiple doses in a short amount of time because they cannot remember when or whether they took their medication. Other guiding principles for the recovery process are as mentioned for viral hepatitis.

Chronic Hepatitis

Chronic hepatitis is the term used to describe an illness associated with prolonged inflammation of the liver (6 months or more). It is divided by findings on liver biopsy into *chronic active hepatitis* (CAH) and *chronic persistent hepatitis* (CPH). CAH occurs more often in females and is more serious, requiring careful differential diagnosis; CPH is usually benign and is seldom progressive, occurring more often in men.

Chronic Active Hepatitis

CAH is a seriously destructive liver disease with hepatic inflammation and hepatic necrosis that can result in progressive fibrosis and cirrhosis. It is uncertain why chronic hepatitis develops, although in the case of viral infection (CMV, HBV[10], HCV, and HDV), it is likely related to the persistence of the virus in the liver. However, this type of chronic hepatitis can also occur secondary to drug sensitivity. Drugs most commonly involved include methyldopa (Aldomet), an antihypertensive medication, and isoniazid (INH), an antituberculosis drug.

The onset of CAH is slow, and symptoms of acute viral hepatitis, cirrhosis, or extrahepatic problems (e.g., thyroiditis, hemolytic anemia, amenorrhea, arthritis, urticaria, or glomerulonephritis) may develop as the initial presentation (Fig. 14–2).

Steroids may be used to treat CAH; they can be prescribed for a period of 3 to 5 years. With steroid therapy, fatigue and anorexia resolve in a few days or weeks. Recombinant interferon alfa-2b injections in low doses over a 3- to 6-month period have been shown to improve hepatic function in this condition. This drug is expensive and may cause a number of side effects, necessitating careful medical supervision (Marx, 1993).

Other new drugs are being developed, and it is likely that the treatment for chronic viral hepatitis will improve substantially in the next few years. Nucleoside analogues (synthetic nucleic acids, the building blocks of DNA) appear to be extremely promising for the treatment of chronic hepatitis B. For chronic hepatitis C, prolonged therapy with interferon and combined therapy with multiple agents such as ribavirin are being tried toward an improved therapeutic response (Fried, 1996).

Left untreated, the course of CAH is unpredictable and may range from progressive deterioration of liver function to spontaneous remissions and exacerbations (Wilson and Lester, 1992). Death results from hepatic failure, bleeding varices, hepatic encephalopathy, or primary hepatocellular carcinoma. Liver transplantation is a consideration in the case of end-stage liver disease that cannot be managed medically.

Chronic Persistent Hepatitis

CPH may follow a viral infection (usually HBV, HCV, or HDV) representing a prolonged course of the acute illness. The person with CPH may present with symptoms of acute

[10] CAH is infectious if derived from HBV, requiring the same precautions as for HBV.

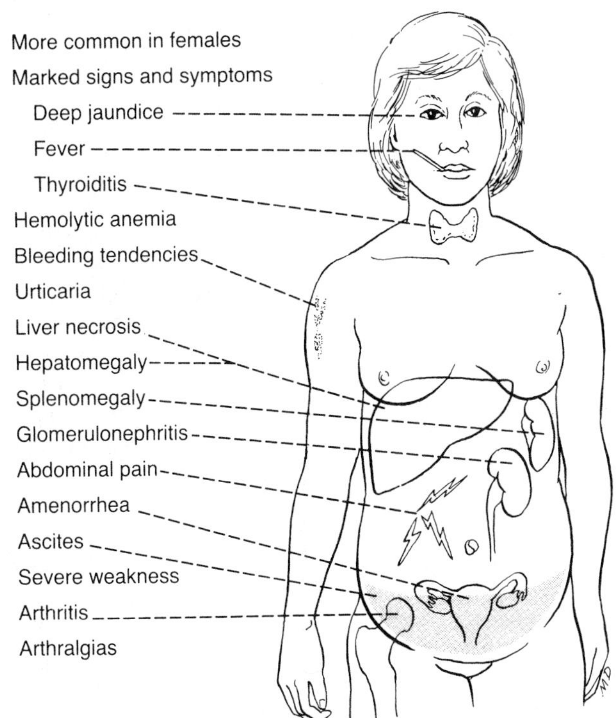

Figure **14–2.** Chronic active hepatitis (CAH). Clinical presentation associated with CAH. (*From Black JM, Matassarin-Jacobs E (eds): Luckmann and Sorensen's Medical-Surgical Nursing, ed 4. Philadelphia, WB Saunders, 1993, p 1709.*)

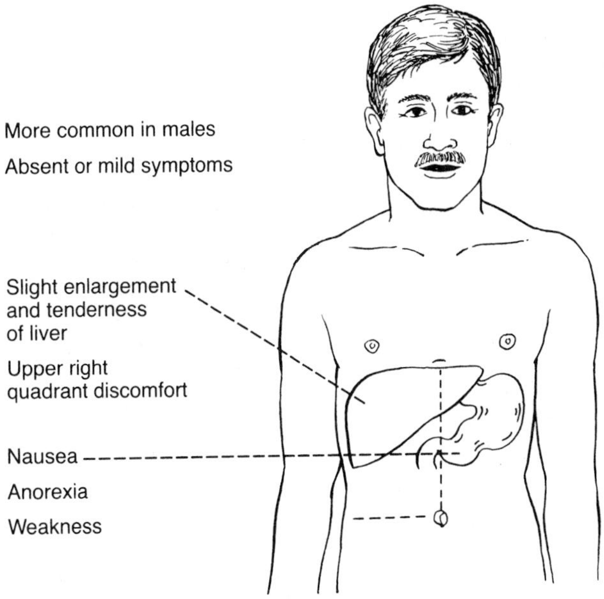

PHYSICAL ASSESSMENT

More common in males
Absent or mild symptoms

Slight enlargement and tenderness of liver
Upper right quadrant discomfort

Nausea
Anorexia
Weakness

Figure **14–3.** Chronic persistent hepatitis (CPH). Clinical presentation associated with CPH. (*From Black JM, Matassarin-Jacobs E (eds): Luckmann and Sorensen's Medical-Surgical Nursing, ed 4. Philadelphia, WB Saunders, 1993, p 1708.*)

viral hepatitis or may be asymptomatic and appear to be healthy or have only minor complaints (Fig. 14–3). No treatment is necessary, as the condition slowly resolves on its own. Typically, the prognosis for recovery is good, without extrahepatic involvement, jaundice, fibrosis or cirrhosis.

Autoimmune Hepatitis

Overview and Incidence. The association of hepatitis with systemic lupus erythematosus was first established in 1956 (Mackay et al., 1956). The availability of sensitive and specific immunoassays has made it possible to recognize hepatitis as a distinct autoimmune process. Type 1 autoimmune hepatitis (formerly referred to as *lupoid hepatitis*) is the most common form of autoimmune hepatitis in the United States, constituting at least 80% of cases in adults. Typically it appears in women (70% of all clients) and half of all cases are in persons 40 years old or younger; teenage girls are commonly affected (Czaja, 1994).

Etiology and Pathogenesis. This self-perpetuating inflammatory process within the liver is mediated by immunologic mechanisms rather than toxins, medications, or viruses. It is self-perpetuated by inadequate immunoregulation and untempered antibody production against itself. The pathogenesis is antibody-dependent as a cell-mediated cytotoxic reaction. A genetic predisposition in some people may heighten their immunoreactivity to auto- or extrinsic antigens and result in more active disease at an earlier age (Page et al., 1975).

Clinical Manifestations. Autoimmune hepatitis is characterized by hypergammaglobulinemia, periportal hepatitis ("piecemeal necrosis" on histologic examination), and frequent concurrence of extrahepatic immunologic disorders (Czaja et al., 1983). Systemic manifestations include arthralgia, acne, and amenorrhea. Other symptoms may include fever, malaise, recurrent or persistent jaundice, rash, or gynecomastia (breast development in the male). Pleurisy, pericarditis, or ulcerative colitis may be part of the client's history. Signs of chronic liver disease may be present, such as spider angiomas, palmar erythema, digital clubbing, and hepatosplenomegaly.

Medical Management

Diagnosis. Laboratory and histologic findings help determine the diagnosis. The demonstration of the lupus erythematosus cell is no longer required for the diagnosis of this autoimmune hepatitis. The presence of smooth muscle antibodies (SMA) and antinuclear antibodies (ANA) in the absence of epidemiologic and serologic evidence of viral infection or other explanations for the chronic disease is sufficient for the diagnosis.

Treatment. This disease responds to corticosteroid therapy. Prednisone alone or in combination with azathioprine (Imuran), an immunosuppressant drug that has a direct, anti-inflammatory effect, induces clinical, biochemical, and histologic remission in 75% of people within 1 to 2 years of treatment (Czaja, 1984). Treatment is continued until remission, deterioration despite compliance with treatment, drug toxicity, or lack of remission after protracted therapy (Czaja,

1992). Relapses occur in 40% to 50% of cases after cessation of therapy; repeat treatment is required, and remission usually follows.

Prognosis. Untreated disease that continues for months to years eventually results in postnecrotic cirrhosis. Persistent malaise, fatigue, and anorexia are present; bleeding from esophageal varices (see Chapter 13) and the development of ascites result in hepatic failure (Silverman and Sokol, 1993). Ninety percent of clients without cirrhosis at the time of diagnosis have life expectancies of 5 to 10 years; presentation with cirrhosis is associated with a 5-year life expectancy of 80% and a 10-year life expectancy of 65% (Czaja, 1984).

Special Implications for the Therapist **14-5**

AUTOIMMUNE HEPATITIS

Management of a client who has an autoimmune disease with liver involvement is a challenge. Energy conservation and maintaining quiet body functions during active liver disease must be balanced by activities to prevent musculoskeletal deconditioning with accompanying loss of strength, flexibility, and/or mobility.

Alcoholic Liver Disease

Alcohol abuse is the most common cause of liver disease in the Western world, resulting in alcoholic hepatitis and cirrhosis. Alcoholic hepatitis is potentially reversible but is also the most frequent cause of cirrhosis, which is not reversible and is potentially fatal. Although intake of alcohol causes the majority of cases of cirrhosis, it is important to note that the disease has other causes (see Cirrhosis, later in this chapter).

Alcoholic Hepatitis

Alcoholic hepatitis can be an acute or chronic inflammation of the liver caused by parenchymal necrosis as a result of heavy alcohol ingestion. The specific mechanism by which liver damage is sustained has not been fully determined. Immune-mediated hepatic damage is suspected in the pathogenesis of alcoholic hepatitis.

Unfortunately, many people with progressive liver damage have few symptoms until the disease is advanced; initial symptoms are those of the complications of cirrhosis (e.g., ascites, esophageal varices, and encephalopathy). If such is the case, irreversible liver damage has already occurred. Anorexia, nausea, vomiting, weight loss, jaundice, and abdominal pain are common presenting symptoms. Liver pain is rare despite the inflammation and parenchymal damage, because the liver parenchyma is relatively free of nerve fibers. Mild pain and tenderness may occur over the abdomen, sometimes mistaken for indigestion.

Fever is common, but persons with alcoholic liver disease are also prone to development of infections (e.g., pneumonia, urinary tract infection, infection of the peritoneal cavity) which could account for the fever. Cutaneous signs of chronic liver disease may be present, including spider angiomas, palmar erythema, loss of body hair, and gynecomastia.

Diagnosis includes a history of excessive, prolonged alcohol intake, but this information may not be available. Liver biopsy reveals a typical fatty-appearing liver associated with cirrhosis, and laboratory studies may show anemia, elevated WBC count, leukocytosis, elevated serum bilirubin, and prolonged prothrombin time. Treatment of acute alcoholic hepatitis is supportive, with high-carbohydrate diet, vitamin supplementation, parenteral fluids, and steroids in select cases.

Alcoholic hepatitis carries a poor prognosis if the person continues to drink alcohol. Frequently, the disease will stabilize if the person stops drinking. The person's condition can revert to normal, but it more commonly either progresses to cirrhosis or runs a rapid course to hepatic failure and death. Cirrhosis is often already present at the time of diagnosis, complicated by the development of ascites, encephalopathy, GI bleeding from varices, and deteriorating renal function (Andreoli et al., 1993).

Special Implications for the Therapist **14-6**

ALCOHOLIC HEPATITIS

Follow the same guidelines regarding liver protection as are discussed in Special Implications for the Therapist: Viral Hepatitis, 14–3. Increased susceptibility to infections requires careful handwashing *before* treating this client. (See also Special Implications for the Therapist: Cirrhosis, 14–7).

Alcoholic Cirrhosis

Alcoholic cirrhosis (Laënnec's cirrhosis) is only one cause of cirrhosis and is the primary form of cirrhosis discussed here.

Overview and Etiology. Cirrhosis of the liver is actually a group of chronic end-stage diseases of the liver resulting from a variety of chronic inflammatory, toxic, metabolic, or congestive damage. There are many potential causes of cirrhosis (e.g., drugs, autoimmune CAH, hereditary metabolic diseases, primary biliary cirrhosis) but alcohol abuse and hepatitis C are the most common causes in the Western world. Only 10% to 15% of clients with chronic alcoholism develop cirrhosis; however, more than 65% of all cases of cirrhosis are related to alcohol. In other words, not all alcoholism results in cirrhosis, but most cirrhosis is caused by alcohol. Men are more likely to develop Laënnec's cirrhosis. Cirrhosis is the fourth leading cause of death in persons between 35 and 54 years of age. It is the ninth leading cause of death overall in the United States (Matassarin-Jacobs and Strasburg, 1993).

Pathogenesis and Clinical Manifestations. Cirrhosis is characterized pathologically by the loss of the normal microscopic lobular architecture of the liver. Inflammation results in necrosis of parenchymal tissue, which is replaced with fibrous bands of connective tissue (Fig. 14–4). These fibrous bands eventually constrict and partition the organ into irregular nodules. Fibrous scarring distorts the liver, and biliary channels may be altered or obstructed, producing jaundice.

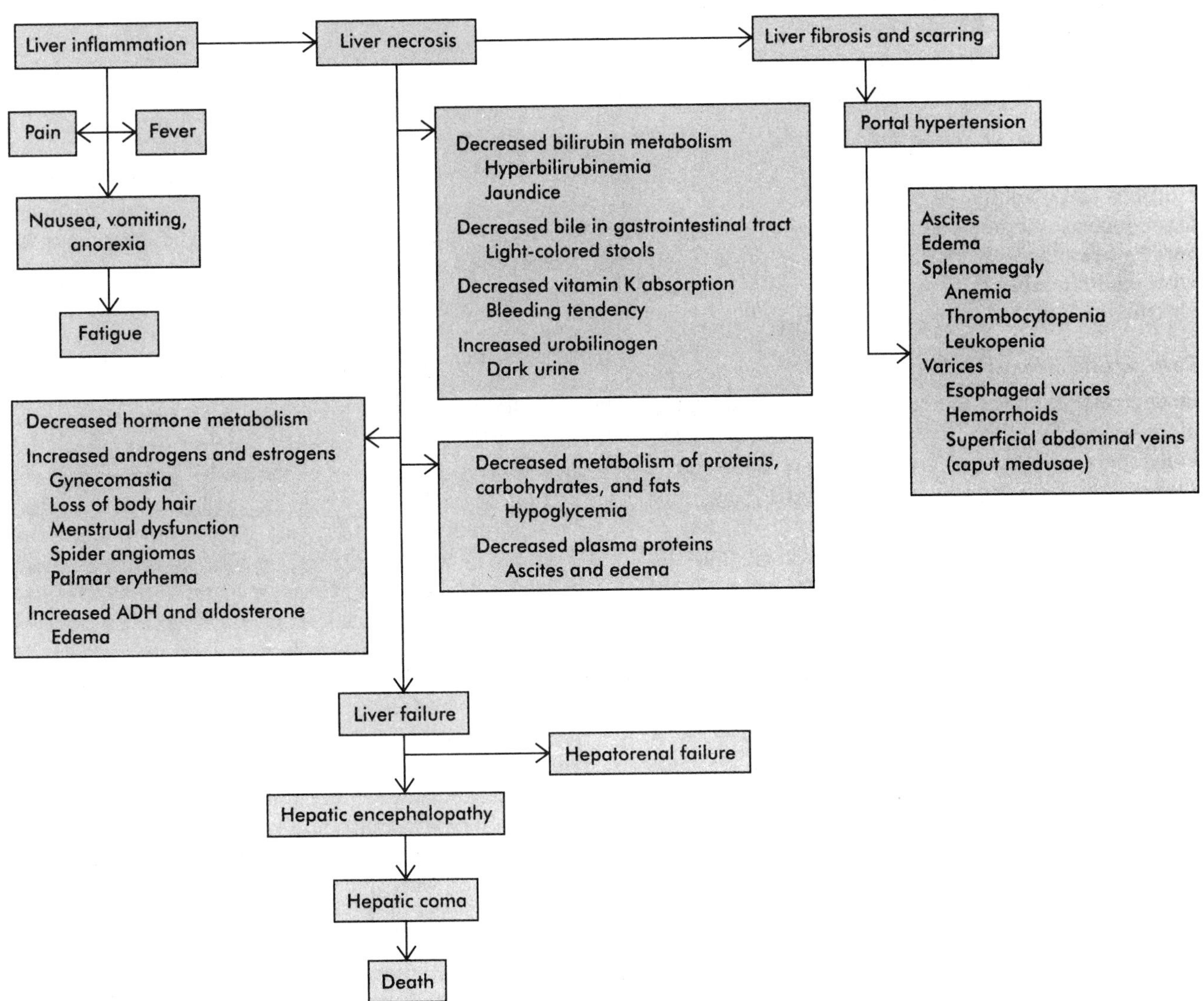

Figure **14–4.** Pathogenesis and resultant clinical manifestations associated with cirrhosis of the liver. (*From McCance KL, Huether SE (eds): Pathophysiology: The Biologic Basis for Disease in Adults and Children, ed 2. St Louis, Mosby–Year Book, 1993, p 1359.*)

Scarring may also distort the vascular bed, leading to portal hypertension and intrahepatic shunting. Portal hypertension causes a reverse flow of blood and enlargement of the esophageal, umbilical, and superior rectus veins. Subsequent bleeding varices, ascites, and incomplete clearing of metabolic wastes such as ammonia can lead to encephalopathy (see text for individual discussion).

The signs and symptoms of hepatic cirrhosis (Table 14–5; Fig. 14–5) are multiple and varied, representing interference with four major functions of the liver: (1) storage and release of blood to maintain adequate circulating volume, (2) metabolism of nutrients and detoxification of poisons absorbed from the intestines, (3) regulation of fluid and electrolyte balance, and (4) production of clotting factors. Individuals with cirrhosis who are asymptomatic and show little clinical evidence of hepatocellular dysfunction are said to have *well-compensated cirrhosis*. As evidence of complications develops, the clinical condition is referred to as *decompensated cirrhosis* (Andreoli et al., 1993).

Medical Management

Diagnosis. The presence of cirrhosis may remain undetected until autopsy. Laboratory results are used to evaluate liver function (see Table 35–15). Impaired hepatocellular function is revealed by elevated liver serum enzymes, reduced dye excretion, hypoalbuminemia, and elevated prothrombin time. Liver biopsy is the most specific diagnostic test and provides information as to the extent of the disease.

Treatment. Cirrhosis has no cure. Medical management of the client with any type of cirrhosis is supportive, with a view toward maximization of liver function, prevention of infection, and control of complications. Whenever possible, the primary causative agent for the cirrhosis is removed (e.g., abstinence from alcohol). A nutritious diet and adequate rest are essential to minimize trauma risk and to maximize regeneration in this progressive, degenerative disorder. Corticosteroids may be prescribed in the case of postnecrotic or posthepatic cirrhosis to reduce manifestations of cirrhosis and

TABLE 14-5 CLINICAL MANIFESTATIONS OF CIRRHOSIS

SIGNS AND SYMPTOMS	PATHOPHYSIOLOGIC BASES
Emaciation, ascites	Malnutrition, portal hypertension, hypoalbuminemia, and hyperaldosteronism
Splenomegaly	Portal hypertension
Lower extremity edema	Hypoalbuminemia, hyperaldosteronism, and pressure of massive ascites obstructing venous return from legs
Prominent abdominal wall veins (caput medusae)	Collateral vessels bypass scarred liver to carry portal blood to superior vena cava; portal hypertension causes dilation
Internal hemorrhoids	Superior rectal veins dilate with pressure of portal hypertension
Palmar erythema, spider nevi, altered hair distribution; amenorrhea, atrophy of testicles, gynecomastia	Decreased hormone metabolism in liver, resulting in estrogen excess
Bleeding tendency, especially gastrointestinal	Hypoprothrombinemia, thrombocytopenia; portal hypertension and esophageal varices; peptic ulcers common in alcoholism
Anemia	GI blood losses; erythrocyte destruction in enlarged spleen; folic acid deficiency due to inadequate diet
Renal failure	Rapidly falling hepatic function; occasionally precipitated by volume depletion; hepatorenal syndrome

From Matassarin-Jacobs E, Strasburg K: Nursing care of clients with hepatic disorders. *In* Black JM, Matassarin-Jacobs E (eds): Luckmann and Sorensen's Medical-Surgical Nursing, ed 4. Philadelphia, WB Saunders, 1993, p 1712.

to improve liver function. Complications are treated individually (see Portal Hypertension, Ascites, and Hepatic Encephalopathy following this section).

Prognosis. Cirrhosis develops slowly over a period of years. Its severity and rate of progression depend on the cause. In established cases with severe hepatic dysfunction, only 50% survive 2 years and 35% survive 5 years. Hematemesis, jaundice, and ascites are unfavorable signs (Friedman and Knauer, 1994). Liver failure and cirrhosis are indications for liver transplantation. A 6-month period of abstinence may be required for the person with alcoholic cirrhosis before trans-

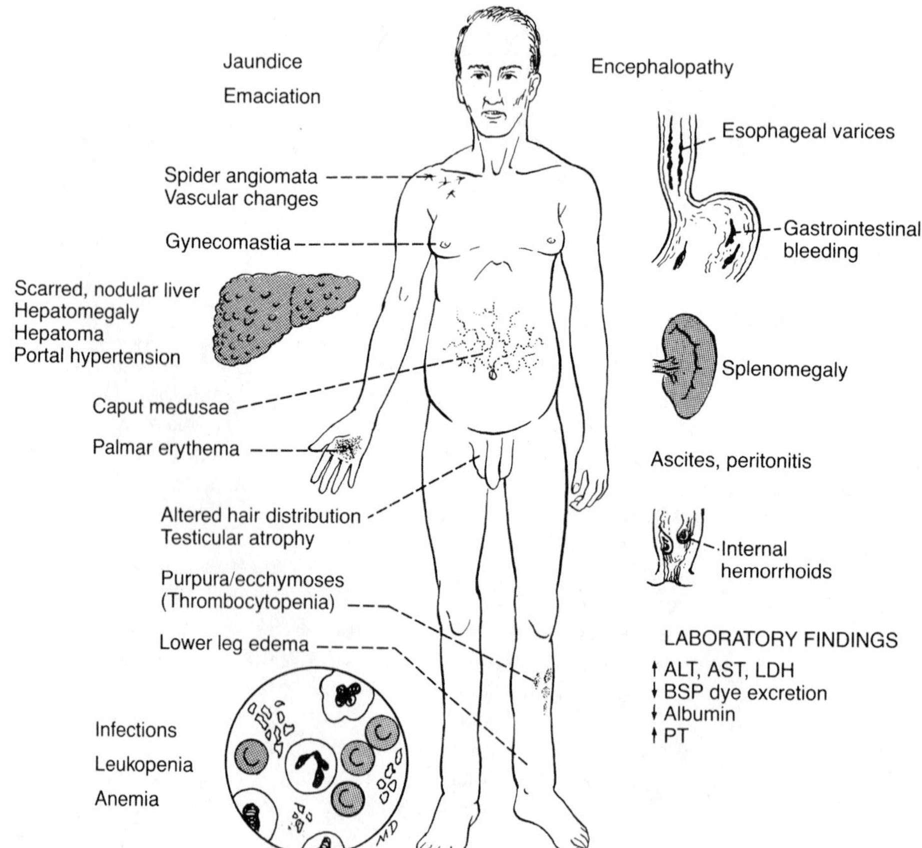

Figure **14-5.** Liver cirrhosis. Clinical presentation and laboratory findings associated with liver cirrhosis. ALT, alanine aminotransferase; AST, aspartate aminotransferase; LDH, lactate dehydrogenase; BSP, sulfobromophthalein; PT, prothrombin time. (*From Black JM, Matassarin-Jacobs E (eds): Luckmann and Sorensen's Medical-Surgical Nursing, ed 4. Philadelphia, WB Saunders, 1993, p 1713.*)

plantation. Without transplantation, prognosis is poor, although survival may be prolonged.

Special Implications for the Therapist **14-7**

CIRRHOSIS

One of the most common symptoms associated with cirrhosis is ascites, an accumulation of fluid in the peritoneal cavity surrounding the intestines. The distention often occurs very slowly over a number of weeks or months and may be seen as bilateral edema of the feet and ankles. The client may be unable to put on a pair of shoes, preferring to leave the shoes unlaced or to wear slippers. In a home health or inpatient hospital setting, this change in dress may not be as noticeable as in a private practice or outpatient clinic. It is always important to remain alert to these potential signs of fluid retention and to ask about any changes in health status or weight gain.

Detection of blood loss in the form of hematemesis, tarry stools, bleeding gums, frequent and heavy nosebleeds, or excessive bruising must be reported to the physician. Preventing increased intra-abdominal pressure (see Box 13–1) and preventing injury owing to falls requires client education regarding safety precautions.

Rest to reduce metabolic demands on the liver and to increase circulation is often recommended for clients with cirrhosis. Frequent rests during therapy and avoiding unnecessary fatigue are also important. The therapist must remain alert to any potential medicalcomplications in any client regardless of the physical therapy diagnosis. (See also Special Implications for Ascites, Hepatitis, Encephalopathy, Anemia, Splenomegaly, Esophageal Varices, or Renal Failure according to the client's condition.)

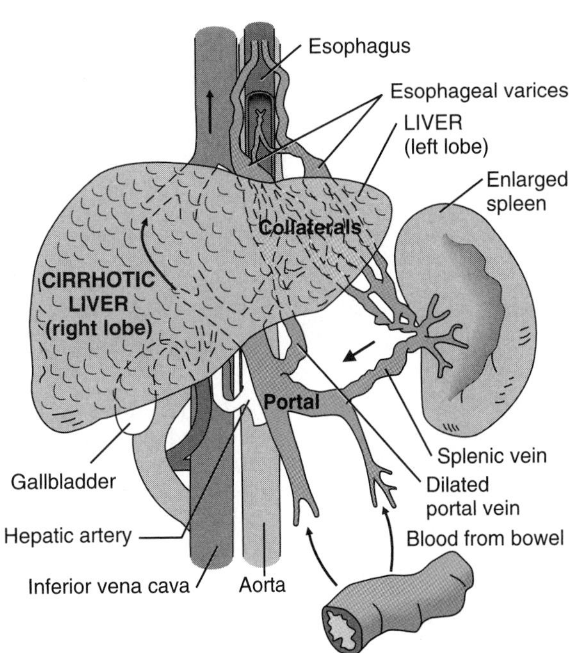

Figure **14-6.** Portal hypertension. Normally, in the portal venous system (consisting of the portal veins, sinusoids, and hepatic veins), the portal veins carry blood from the GI tract, pancreas, and spleen to the liver. In the liver, the blood flows through the sinusoids and empties into the hepatic veins, which carry it into the inferior vena cava. The inferior vena cava delivers blood to the right atrium of the heart. Normally, the spleen is small, but when the liver is cirrhotic and portal hypertension develops, the spleen becomes enlarged. As portal pressure rises, blood backs up into the spleen and flows through collateral channels to the venous system, bypassing the liver and causing large, tortuous veins, especially in the esophagus; these are called *esophageal varices*.

Portal Hypertension

Definition and Overview. Portal hypertension is abnormally high blood pressure in the portal venous system (Fig. 14–6); it occurs commonly, especially with cirrhosis, as a result of obstruction of the portal blood flow. This obstruction may be located in the portal vein (prehepatic), within the hepatic lobule (intrahepatic), or in the hepatic vein (posthepatic). Normal blood pressure in this system is 3 to 5 mm Hg; portal hypertension is characterized by pressure greater than 25 mm Hg.

Incidence and Etiology. Portal hypertension can occur at any age, depending on the cause. Most cases affect adults and are caused by alcoholic cirrhosis. Other causes include portal vein obstruction by a thrombus, tumor, or sarcoidosis; infection; Budd-Chiari syndrome (see footnote 13 on p. 517) and other veno-occlusive disease; splenomegaly; surgical trauma; pancreatitis; and inadequate decompression via varices (esophageal, retroperitoneal, periumbilical, or hemorrhoidal).

Pathogenesis and Clinical Manifestations *(Huether and McCance, 1994)*. As described, any condition or cause of obstruction to the blood flow through the portal system or vena cava results in portal hypertension. High pressure in the portal veins causes collateral vessels to enlarge between the portal veins and the systemic veins, where blood pressure is considerably lower. Collateral veins in the esophagus, anterior abdominal wall, and rectum enable blood to bypass the obstructed portal vessels. High pressure and increased flow volume through these collateral veins result in further problems, such as varices, splenomegaly, ascites, and hepatic encephalopathy.

Varices are distended, tortuous, collateral veins produced by the prolonged elevation of pressure in these collateral veins (see Fig. 14–6). The vomiting of blood from bleeding esophageal varices is the most common clinical manifestation of portal hypertension. Anemia may develop from the prolonged slow bleeding[11] associated with varices or rupture. Distended collateral veins may radiate over the abdomen, giving rise to the description *caput medusae* (Medusa's head) (Fig. 14–7). Hepatic vein thrombosis presents acutely with abdominal pain, liver enlargement, ascites, and jaundice.

Splenomegaly (enlargement of the spleen) is caused by in-

[11] In addition to anemia, the prolonged bleeding can also lead to increased toxic wastes (such as ammonia, since blood is a protein) and subsequent sequelae (e.g., hepatic encephalopathy, altered peripheral nervous system function).

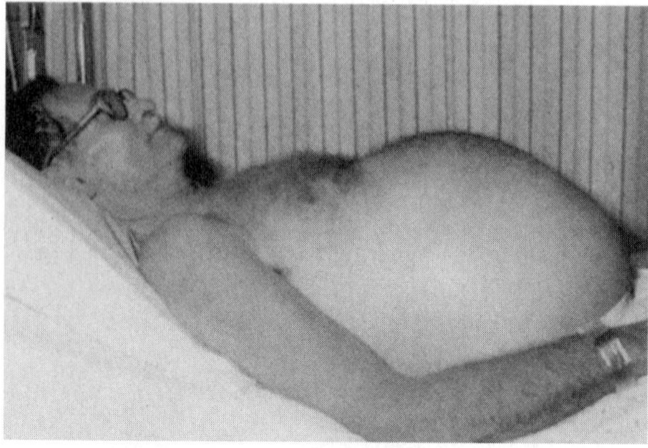

Figure **14-7.** Ascites in an individual with cirrhosis. Distended abdomen, dilated upper abdominal veins, and inverted umbilicus are classic manifestations. Peripheral edema associated with developing ascites may be observed first by the therapist. (*From Swartz MH: Textbook of Physical Diagnosis. Philadelphia, WB Saunders, 1989, plate XII.*)

creased pressure in the splenic vein, which branches from the portal vein. *Ascites* is caused by increased pressure forcing water and solids out of the tributaries of the portal vein into the peritoneal cavity. *Hepatic encephalopathy* occurs when blood that is shunted through collateral vessels to the systemic veins bypasses the liver, where toxins, hormones, and other harmful substances are normally removed. The presence of toxic substances (e.g., ammonia) in the blood reaching the brain results in hepatic encephalopathy.

Medical Management

Diagnosis, Treatment, and Prognosis. Diagnosis of portal hypertension is often made at the time of variceal bleeding and is confirmed by endoscopy and evaluation of portal venous pressure. The individual usually has a history of jaundice, hepatitis, or alcoholism. Liver function tests may be abnormal, and liver biopsy may determine the etiology.

Treatment usually addresses complications, especially emergency management of bleeding varices (see also Chapter 13), including administration of vasopressin (Pitressin), balloon tamponade, injection sclerotherapy, direct ligation of the bleeding varices, or, occasionally, emergency surgery to perform a portacaval shunt (from portal vein to the vena cava). Administration of vasopressin achieves temporary lowering of portal pressure by constricting afferent arterioles. Other pharmacologic measures may include administration of propranolol (Inderal), which also reduces portal pressure (Resnick, 1993).

Ruptured varices are associated with a high mortality rate (30% to 60%). Recurrent bleeding esophageal varices are a poor prognostic indicator. Most clients die within 1 to 2 years from complications of bleeding varices or hepatic failure.

Special Implications for the Therapist **14-8**

PORTAL HYPERTENSION

Various factors contribute to rupture of varices, especially anything that increases intra-abdominal pressure (see Box 13–1) such as coughing, straining at stool, or improper lifting. Any therapy program for a client with known varices must take this factor into account when presenting active or active-assisted exercises, or unsupported gait training. (See also Esophageal Varices and Anemia.)

Ascites

Definition and Overview. Ascites is the abnormal accumulation of serous (edematous) fluid within the peritoneal cavity, the potential space between the lining of the liver and the lining of the abdominal cavity. Ascites is most often caused by cirrhosis, but other diseases associated with ascites include heart failure, constrictive pericarditis, abdominal malignancies, nephrotic syndrome, and malnutrition.

Pathogenesis. The mechanisms of ascites caused by cirrhosis are complex, and several factors contribute to the development of ascites: (1) portal hypertension, resulting in increased plasma and lymphatic hydrostatic pressures; (2) hypoalbuminemia, resulting in decreased colloid osmotic pressure; and (3) hyperaldosteronism, resulting in sodium and water retention (Huether and McCance, 1994).

Portal hypertension and reduced serum albumin levels cause capillary hydrostatic pressure to exceed capillary osmotic pressure. This imbalance tends to push water into the peritoneal cavity. Portal hypertension also increases the production of hepatic lymph, which "weeps" into the peritoneal cavity. Decreased metabolic function of the liver results in the reduced albumin synthesis mentioned as well as in an accumulation of hormones that regulate sodium and water balance. As ascites sequesters more and more bodily fluid, the kidneys respond by retaining sodium and water, which expands plasma volume and thereby accelerates portal hypertension and further formation of ascites.

Clinical Manifestations. Ascites becomes clinically detectable when more than 500 mL has accumulated, causing weight gain, abdominal distention (with a downward protruding umbilicus), increased abdominal girth, and, eventually, peripheral edema (see Fig. 14–7). Dyspnea with increased respiratory rate occurs when the fluid displaces the diaphragm or when defects in the diaphragm allow ascites to pass into the pleural cavity, decreasing lung capacity. Complications include hepatorenal syndrome and bacterial peritonitis. Hepatorenal syndrome, a form of functional renal failure, occurs when liver function is compromised, which is usually progressive and fatal. Bacterial peritonitis (infection of the ascitic fluid) can be asymptomatic or accompanied by fever, chills, abdominal pain, and tenderness.

Medical Management

Diagnosis. Diagnosis of ascites is usually based on clinical manifestations in the presence of liver disease. Paracentesis may be used to aspirate ascitic fluid for bacterial culture, biochemical analysis, and microscopic examination, but this procedure may cause peritonitis and is not used as much as in the past. Abdominal x-rays, ultrasonography, and CT scan may locate fluid in the peritoneal cavity.

Treatment. Nonsurgical medical management of ascites includes restriction of fluids and sodium intake, and administration of diuretics. Electrolytes must be monitored carefully with supplementation of potassium and chloride if necessary (see Chapter 4). Review of current medications is required with withdrawal of any that inhibit prostaglandin synthesis and thus impair renal sodium excretion (e.g., aspirin and other NSAIDs).

Surgical intervention may be the insertion of a peritoneovenous shunt (LeVeen or Denver shunt) to move fluid from the peritoneal cavity into the venous blood of the superior vena cava. Complications of this procedure include infection, disseminated intravascular coagulation, congestive heart failure, and shunt clotting.

Prognosis. Resolution of ascites may be dramatic after implantation of a peritoneovenous shunt, but 25% of persons with cirrhosis-associated ascites still die within 1 year owing to continued heavy drinking and the difficulty of controlling the ascites.

Special Implications for the Therapist **14-9**

ASCITES

Most people with ascites are more comfortable in a high Fowler's position (head of the bed raised 18 to 20 in. above the level with the knees elevated). Breathing techniques are important to maintain adequate respiratory function and to prevent the development of atelectasis or pneumonia. The homebound person who has ascites should be monitored for the possible development of bacterial peritonitis. Onset of fever, chills, abdominal pain, and tenderness should be reported to the physician.

Decreases in serum albumin* associated with the development of ascites is accompanied by a parallel decrease in oncotic pressure in blood vessels causing peripheral edema. This edema may mask muscle wasting that occurs when the body does not have an adequate intake of protein to maintain structure and facilitate wound healing. The client must be encouraged to change position to maintain integrity of the skin and promote circulation. Small pillows or folded towels can be used to support the rib cage and the bulging flank while the client is lying on his or her side.

The abdominal distention associated with ascites may develop very slowly over a number of weeks or months and may be accompanied by bilateral edema of the feet and ankles. The client may be unable to put on a pair of shoes, preferring to leave the shoes unlaced or to wear slippers. In a home health, inpatient hospital, or nursing home setting, this change in dress may not be as noticeable as in a private practice an outpatient clinic. It is always important to remain alert to these potential signs of fluid retention and to ask about any changes in health status or weight gain.

Fluid intake and output are usually carefully measured and restricted, so in any setting the therapist is encouraged to know the individual's limits and to participate in reporting measurements as well. This is especially important because clients frequently ask the therapist for fluids in response to perceived exertion or increased exertion after exercise or ambulation. The client who is noncompliant or in denial requests fluids because of the false belief that fluids provided but not recorded do not "count." For the homebound client, who is receiving diuretics, the bedroom should be close to the bathroom.

* Persons with serum albumin levels between 2.5 and 3.5 g/dL are at moderate risk of malnutrition, and those whose levels are 2.5 g/dL or less are at great risk. Because albumin binds to calcium, serum albumin levels drop when serum calcium levels are low.

Hepatic Encephalopathy

Definition and Overview. Hepatic encephalopathy or hepatic coma refers to a variety of neurologic signs and symptoms in persons with chronic liver failure or in whom portal circulation is impaired. This neuropsychiatric syndrome can occur secondary to acute or chronic liver disease. *Acute hepatic encephalopathy* occurs as a result of fulminant hepatic failure; cerebral edema resulting in coma is common with high mortality. *Chronic hepatic encephalopathy* usually occurs with chronic liver disease and is often reversible.

Risk Factors. Any disease or condition of the liver that destroys liver parenchyma or causes abnormal shunting of blood around the liver tissue may predispose the client to hepatic encephalopathy. When cirrhosis progresses, portal hypertension may occur (see text for discussion of cirrhosis and portal hypertension) with possible subsequent hemorrhage. In addition to GI bleeding, other factors that may precipitate or severely aggravate hepatic encephalopathy in clients with severe liver disease include constipation, diuretics, infection, increased dietary protein, and CNS-depressant drugs, such as alcohol, benzodiazepines (e.g., Librium, Valium, Dalmane, Tranxene) and opiates.

Pathogenesis. The known etiology of this disorder is the liver's inability to metabolize ammonia, but the exact pathogenesis of hepatic encephalopathy remains unclear. Protein (food)- and gut-derived (GI bleed) toxins are normally taken up and detoxified by the liver. When these toxins are no longer absorbed into the portal vein and removed from the blood by the liver because of hepatocyte dysfunction, they pass directly to the brain, where they have direct harmful effects on the nervous system. Reduced hepatic function or bypass of blood around the liver results in rising ammonia levels that are toxic to central and peripheral nervous system function. Additionally, as blood ammonia levels rise, many unusual compounds, such as octopamine, begin to form and serve as false neurotransmitters in the CNS.

It is possible that specific causes of hepatic encephalopathy do not exist at all, but rather that brain function is affected to a certain degree by the *various* consequences of liver failure (e.g., accumulation of neuroactive compounds and neurotoxins, changes in the metabolism of amino acids, decreased availability of energy fuels and circulatory changes) finally precipitating the syndrome of hepatic encephalopathy (Ferenci, 1991).

Clinical Manifestations. Clinical manifestations of hepatic encephalopathy vary depending on the severity of neurologic involvement. Four stages of development occur as the ammonia level increases in the blood with the clinical features listed in Table 14–6.

Flapping tremors (asterixis) and numbness/tingling (mimicking carpal tunnel syndrome) are common early (stage I) symptoms of the ammonia abnormality associated with this condition. Subtle personality changes listed in stage I may include disorientation or confusion, euphoria or depression, forgetfulness, and slurred speech. Minor lapses in memory and inability to concentrate, slurred speech, and confusional episodes may be transient or permanent and are usually more noticeable to the affected person than to the outside observer. As this condition progresses, the person develops a sleep disorder or may become unconscious. This sequence may occur over a period of many months (chronic encephalopathy) or may develop rapidly in days or weeks as in the case of fulminant hepatic failure (acute encephalopathy).

The motor apraxia in stage II can be best observed by keeping a record of the client's handwriting and drawings of simple shapes, such as a circle, square, triangle, and rectangle. Progressive deterioration will be apparent in these handwriting samples. In stage III, the person will most likely be hospitalized or homebound with hospice care, and can still be aroused.

Stage IV is a comatose state from which the person cannot be aroused and can only respond to painful stimulus. Hepatic fetor is a musty, sweet odor of the breath caused by the liver's inability to metabolize the amino acid methionine.

Medical Management

Diagnosis, Treatment, and Prognosis. Diagnosis of hepatic encephalopathy is based on history of liver disease and clinical manifestations. No specific diagnostic test is available, but electroencephalography (EEG) and blood chemistry tests are used to confirm the diagnosis.

Because protein is the source of the toxins, many of the symptoms can be improved by restricting dietary protein. Pharmacologic treatment may include antibiotics (neomycin) to reduce bacterial production of ammonia. Lactulose, a bowel cathartic (causes evacuation) may also be used to increase gastric acid, another means of effectively killing the naturally occurring bacteria that survive in the intestines and produce ammonia.

More extreme measures may include peritoneal dialysis and exchange transfusions to remove and replace most of the person's blood. Liver transplantation may be performed for cases of fulminant liver failure. Without intervention, mortality is high, as the person's condition progresses into coma with hepatic failure.

Special Implications for the Therapist **14-10**

HEPATIC ENCEPHALOPATHY

The inpatient or homebound client with impending hepatic coma has difficulty ambulating and is extremely unsteady. Protective measures must be taken against falls and seizures. The home health therapist must be alert for any report of GI bleeding that will result in protein accumulation in the GI tract, exacerbating this condition (e.g., blood in stools or black, tarry stools). The client should be following a low-protein diet.

The physician may prescribe lactulose to decrease ammonia in the bowel, but diarrhea may be a side effect. The client experiencing prolonged diarrhea should be encouraged to report this information to the physician for possible follow-up. A reduced dosage may be required to prevent further electrolyte imbalance. (See also Electrolyte Imbalance, Chapter 4.)

The immobile client who lacks reflexes is vulnerable to numerous complications requiring attention to the prevention of pneumonia and skin breakdown. Skin breakdown in a client who is malnourished from liver disease and is immobile, jaundiced, and edematous can occur in less than 24 hours. Careful attention to skin care, passive exercise, and frequent changes in position are required.

Rest between activities is advocated, and strenuous exercise is to be avoided. The therapist should watch for (and immediately report) signs of anemia (e.g., reduced hemoglobin, weakness, dyspnea on exertion, easy fatigability, skin pallor, tachycardia; see also Anemia, Chapter 11), infection (see Table 6–1), and GI bleeding (e.g., melena, hematemesis, easy bruising).

Primary Biliary Cirrhosis

Definition and Overview. Primary biliary cirrhosis (PBC) is one type of cirrhosis characterized by chronic, progressive, inflammatory liver disease. Women between 30 and 65 years are most commonly affected. Secondary biliary cirrhosis can occur with prolonged partial or complete obstruction of the

TABLE 14-6 STAGES OF HEPATIC ENCEPHALOPATHY

STAGE I (PRODROMAL)	STAGE II (IMPENDING)	STAGE III (AROUSAL)	STAGE IV (COMATOSE)
Slight personality changes	Tremor progresses to asterixis	Hyperventilation	No asterixis
Slight tremor	Resistance to passive movement	Marked confusion	Positive Babinski's reflex
Bilateral numbness/tingling	Myoclonus	Abusive and violent	Hepatic fetor
Muscular incoordination	Lethargy	Noisy, incoherent speech	
Impaired handwriting	Unusual behavior	Asterixis (liver flap)	
Sleep disturbances	Apraxia	Muscle rigidity	
	Ataxia	Positive Babinski's reflex	
		Hyperactive deep tendon reflexes	

Adapted from Goodman CC, Snyder TE: Differential Diagnosis in Physical Therapy, ed 2. Philadelphia, WB Saunders, 1995, pp 307–308.

common bile duct or its branches. The obstruction may be caused by gallstones, tumors, fibrotic strictures, chronic pancreatitis, or in children, as a result of biliary atresia or cystic fibrosis. Clinical manifestations remain the same as for PBC, but treatment is centered on alleviating the underlying cause of obstruction. Persistent obstruction leads to advanced cirrhosis and liver failure.

Etiology and Pathogenesis. PBC is presumed to be an autoimmune disease as its presence is correlated with one of many autoimmune diseases in 85% of all cases. Some of the autoimmune diseases present include chronic thyroiditis, rheumatoid arthritis, scleroderma, Sjögren's syndrome, and systemic lupus erythematosus.

The initial lesion involves attack on bile duct epithelium by cytotoxic T cells; autoantibodies are present, which supports a suspected autoimmune basis. Antigenic alterations occur in the membranes of the bile duct epithelial cells, which appear to be an inviting target for sensitized cytotoxic T lymphocytes, but the reasons for this sensitization and the mechanism of T lymphocyte activation remain unknown.

Three pathologic steps are recognized in PBC; these are referred to as stages I to III and are characterized by ductal lesions, scarring, and cirrhosis, respectively. In stage I the lobular parenchyma remains normal but segmental bile duct injury occurs, with irregular, hyperplastic changes in the bile duct epithelium. Necrosis and ulceration of the epithelium commonly occur at this stage. As a result of the destructive inflammatory process that is characteristic of stage I, small bile ducts are obliterated and scarring occurs in the medium-sized ducts with chronic inflammation of the portal tracts (stage II). The disease terminates as end-stage liver disease (i.e., cirrhosis) in stage III, as the liver tissue is replaced by fibrotic nodules.

Clinical Manifestations. Fatigue and pruritus, with or without jaundice, are often initial symptoms. Other symptoms may include burning, pins-and-needles sensations, or prickling of the eyes; GI bleeding; right upper quadrant pain (posterior); and muscle cramping. Many women with PBC remain asymptomatic for years during the early stages of the disease, whereas others present with advanced disease and its complications. Complications include cirrhosis (and its complications, especially ascites and portal hypertension), malabsorption with steatorrhea (impairment of excretion of bile into the intestine), osteoporosis, and osteomalacia owing to malabsorption of vitamin D and calcium.

Medical Management

Diagnosis. Diagnosis is often sought by the client because of fatigue or pruritus. Liver function tests and blood serum analysis reflect cholestasis with elevation of bilirubin, alkaline phosphatase, γ-globulins, lipids, bile salts, aminotransferase, and presence of lipoprotein X, characteristic antibodies (antimitochondrial), and other autoantibodies.

Treatment. Treatment is symptomatic. Cholestyramine or colestipol is helpful to control pruritus by binding with bile salts in the intestine. Replacement of vitamins A, K, and D may be required in cases in which steatorrhea is present, especially if it is aggravated by drugs for the pruritus. Calcium supplementation may be helpful to prevent osteomalacia, but it is of uncertain benefit in osteoporosis associated with PBC (Friedman and Knauer, 1994). Liver transplantation is the only proven therapy for advanced primary biliary cirrhosis and should be considered sooner rather than later, but the disease probably recurs in the transplanted liver (Fennerty, 1993; Sherlock, 1994b).

Prognosis. PBC usually follows a progressive, indolent (painless, slow growing) course, with life expectancy being approximately 10 to 15 years after diagnosis. Death is usually a result of hepatic failure or complications of portal hypertension associated with cirrhosis. With liver transplantation, 1-year survival is 75%, with a projected 5-year survival of over 65%.

Special Implications for the Therapist **14-11**

PRIMARY BILIARY CIRRHOSIS

The most significant clinical problem for PBC clients is bone disease characterized by impaired osteoblastic activity and accelerated osteoclastic activity. Calcium and vitamin D should be carefully monitored and appropriate replacement instituted. Physical activity following an osteoporosis protocol should be encouraged (Carithers, 1993). (See also Special Implications for the Therapist: Signs and Symptoms of Hepatic Disease (14–1) and Liver Transplantation (14–2) and Osteoporosis and Osteomalacia [Chapter 20]).

Occasionally, sensory neuropathy (*xanthomatous neuropathy*) of the hands and/or feet may occur as a result of increased serum cholesterol levels and an abnormal lipoprotein X. Cholesterol-laden macrophages accumulate in the subcutaneous tissues and create local lesions, termed *xanthomas,* around the eyelids and over skin, tendons, nerves, joints, and other locations. Treatment and precautions are as listed for this condition associated with diabetes mellitus or other etiologics (see Special Implications for the Therapist: Diabetes Mellitus, 9–15).

Intrahepatic Cholestasis of Pregnancy

Intrahepatic cholestasis (suppression of bile flow) of pregnancy is a familial disorder characterized by pruritus and cholestatic jaundice; it usually occurs in the last trimester of each pregnancy and promptly resolves after delivery. A variant of this condition, without jaundice, is referred to as *pruritus gravidarum.* Of the women who develop pregnancy-induced intrahepatic cholestasis, 50% have other family members who have experienced jaundice during pregnancy or after the use of oral contraceptives. Women who have experienced cholestatic jaundice of pregnancy should avoid all contraceptives because of a high risk of disease recurrence (Lindberg, 1992).

The increase in gonadal and placental hormones during pregnancy is most likely responsible for the cholestasis in susceptible women. Maternal health is unaffected by this condition, but the effects on the unborn child can be serious, including fetal distress, stillbirth, prematurity, and an increased risk of intracranial hemorrhage during delivery. There are no apparent effects on the liver of the mother other than centrilobular cholestasis at the time of the pregnancy (Rubin and Farber, 1994).

Liver Transplantation

Overview. The first liver transplant in a human was performed in 1963. Since that time, the success of this procedure has improved so much that 1600 liver transplant operations were completed in the United States in 1990. Transplantation of the liver differs from renal, lung, or heart transplantation because there is no intervening assistance from an artificial liver, and the technical aspects of liver transplantation require precise connection of the hepatic artery, hepatic and portal veins, and the bile duct (Johnson and Triger, 1992).

Transplant Candidates. Theoretically, anyone with advanced, irreversible liver disease with certain mortality may be considered for a liver transplant (Table 14–7). Also, the disease must be correctable by liver transplantation. The decision to perform a transplant may be determined by how long the procedure will extend the recipient's life. Recipients are selected on the basis of ABO (blood type) matching and organ size. At present, the most common indications for liver transplantation are nonalcoholic cirrhosis and hepatic or biliary malignancy, although liver transplantation for hepatic malignancy has decreased significantly because of the poor long-term results. Some carefully selected clients with cancer remain good candidates, especially those with resectable hepatocellular carcinoma (Meyers and Jones, 1990).

Some metabolic disorders (e.g., familial hypercholesterolemia) that arise in the liver but produce damage elsewhere in the body can be cured if the liver is replaced with a liver from a normal individual. Many inborn errors of liver metabolism are benign and are not associated with end-stage liver disease. Acute fulminant liver failure secondary to severe hepatitis owing to a virus, toxin, or poison can be life-threatening and require liver transplantation to prevent death.

With the exception of metastatic malignancy and hepatic lymphoma, there are few absolute contraindications to liver transplantation (Woolf et al., 1994; Zetterman, 1994). In general persons with nonmalignant, nonalcoholic liver disease between ages 2 and 60 years are considered most suitable. Elderly people may be unable to survive the procedure, and clients with considerable damage to other major organs (e.g., heart or lungs) cannot handle the stress of the surgery.

Clients with alcoholic cirrhosis may be required to remain abstinent 6 months prior to the transplant, although it has been suggested that liver transplantation itself contributes to recovery from alcoholism. Only 10% to 15% of alcoholic persons return to drinking after transplantation, and most do so only transiently (Keefe and Esquivel, 1993).

Hepatitis B is not eliminated by transplantation, but its recurrence and the damage it can cause may be substantially reduced by giving the client hepatitis B globulin. Hepatitis recurs in the transplanted liver in 80% to 90% of cases, but the damage to the new liver is slow so that many years of symptom-free living can occur. At present long-term survival after reinfection of the allograft is 45% to 50%.

TABLE 14–7 Liver Transplantation

Indications	Possible Contraindications
Primary biliary cirrhosis	Sepsis
Neoplasm (selected cases)	Hepatic lymphoma
Acute fulminant liver failure	AIDS
Inborn errors of metabolism	Poor client understanding
Alcoholic cirrhosis after documented treatment and recovery	Alcoholic cirrhosis (documented continued abuse)
Drug-induced liver disease	Cirrhosis secondary to drug abuse
Chronic active hepatitis (see text)	Chronic active (type B) hepatitis
Neonatal cholestasis (bile suppression)	Advanced cardiopulmonary disease
Biliary atresia	Inability to follow-up with treatment
Sclerosing cholangitis	
Budd-Chiari syndrome	
Congenital hepatic fibrosis	
Cystic fibrosis	

Risk Factors. Besides having an end-stage liver disease that is correctable by a liver transplant, the client must be a good operative candidate. Many potential risk factors have been reported to increase the risk of transplantation (Table 14–8). A definite age cutoff has not been determined, although many transplant centers do not accept most people as candidates if they are older than 60 years. However, recent data demonstrate that this group has excellent survival and good quality of life after transplantation (Keefe and Esquivel, 1993). For technical reasons, with small-birth-weight infants, most surgeons prefer to wait until significant growth has occurred.

Complications. Mechanical postoperative complications include biliary strictures, nonfunction of the graft (i.e., the transplanted liver does not function), hemorrhage, and vascular thrombosis of the hepatic artery, portal vein, or hepatic veins. Rejection is the most common cause of liver dysfunction after transplantation, most likely after the first week and during the first 3 postoperative months.

As with all organ transplantation procedures, the chances of organ rejection require the use of immunosuppressants such as corticosteroids, azathioprine, cyclosporine, and a new, more potent drug tacrolimus.[12] Unfortunately these drugs also suppress the body's natural defenses, making infections a common complication; each person is also maintained on prophylactic medications to decrease the risk of opportunistic infection. Cytomegalovirus (CMV), a common infectious process, occurs early after transplantation. CMV remains a major cause of morbidity but is no longer a major cause of mortality after liver transplantation (Stratta et al., 1992).

Clinical manifestations of rejection may be minimal; the client may be asymptomatic or may present with malaise, anorexia, a vague feeling of illness, abdominal pain, fever,

[12] At present, tacrolimus is used in liver grafts that fail cyclosporine-based immunosuppression and provides a valuable therapeutic alternative to retransplantation. Trials comparing tacrolimus with cyclosporine report fewer acute rejections with tacrolimus (High and Washburn, 1997; Mirza et al., 1997). Direct comparisons between tacrolimus and cyclosporine will determine the role of tacrolimus as a primary transplant therapy. Paraplegia can result as a nonreversible side effect from this drug in approximately 4 out of 1,000 cases (Sineath, 1995).

TABLE 14-8 LIVER TRANSPLANT RISK FACTORS

LOW	INTERMEDIATE	HIGH
Increasing age	Active extrahepatic infection	More than one other failing organ
Severity of liver dysfunction in otherwise stable person without encephalopathy	Hepatobiliary sepsis	Prolonged, severe coma
Previous abdominal surgery	Hepatorenal syndrome	Preoperative hemodynamic instability
Preexisting thrombotic disorder	Small-sized infant	Extrahepatic malignancy
	Short-duration coma	Immunosuppressive disorders
	Transplantation across ABO barrier	
	Previous portosystemic shunt	
	Portal vein thrombosis	
	Operative variable	

From Meyers WC, Jones RS: Textbook of Liver and Biliary Surgery. Philadelphia, JB Lippincott, 1990, p 406.

tenderness, or a palpable liver. Other causes of graft dysfunction may include infection, hemolysis, and drug injury from immunosuppressants and antibiotics. Extrahepatic complications may include renal failure, neurologic disorders, and pulmonary involvement (e.g., pneumonia, atelectasis, respiratory distress syndrome, or pleural effusion). Hepatocellular carcinoma, hepatitis B, and Budd-Chiari syndrome[13] may recur in the transplanted liver, but other chronic liver diseases do not recur.

Clinically significant neurologic events may occur in 27% to 90% of adult liver transplant recipients (Boon et al., 1991; Power et al., 1990; Vogt et al., 1988). CNS complications after liver transplantation may be a consequence of liver disease itself or may result from a wide array of metabolic abnormalities or vascular insults occurring in the early postoperative period (range, 1 to 47 days; median, 5 days) (Singh et al., 1994). The most common CNS lesions are listed in Box 14–5 (see also Box 4–3). The therapist is likely to be familiar with most of these terms, with the possible exception of central pontine myelinosis, which is demyelination of the central pons that causes a "locked-in" syndrome that is characterized by paralysis of the limbs and lower cranial nerves with intact consciousness.

Medical Management

Diagnosis. In many cases, end-stage liver disease must be confirmed by percutaneous, or occasionally by open, liver biopsy. Pathologic confirmation via biopsy may not be necessary in the case of previously diagnosed fulminant hepatic failure or Budd-Chiari syndrome. In the case of suspected liver transplant rejection, the most common chemical abnormalities are elevated transaminase (normally present enzymes that are released in greater amounts from damaged hepatocytes) and bilirubin levels (see Table 35–15). A liver biopsy is necessary.

Prognosis. Factors determining survival include the underlying cause of liver failure (e.g., poorer prognosis for advanced cirrhosis), the person's ability to stop the intake of alcohol in the case of alcoholic cirrhosis, and the presence of complications or symptoms of hematemesis, jaundice, and ascites. The use of cyclosporine-steroid combinations has increased survival rates through effective immunosuppression with minimal toxicity.

One-year survival rates range between 70% and 85%; 5-year survival rates can be as high as 70%. The survival after emergency liver transplantation for acute liver failure is less than 70%, because such clients are seriously ill at the time of the operation.

The expected 1-year survival rate after a second or subsequent liver transplantation is about 50%. Two groups of people qualify for retransplantation: those with serious postoperative complications due to mechanical failure or rejection and those who have a slow progressive course of chronic hepatic dysfunction, usually caused by rejection.

Special Implications for the Therapist **14-12**

LIVER TRANSPLANTATION

The majority of transplanted livers begin to function well within minutes to hours after the vascular clamps are released. The client must be closely monitored for signs of respiratory compromise, bleeding, infection,

BOX 14-5
Central Nervous System Complications: Liver Transplantation

- Focal seizures
- Encephalopathy
- Central pontine myelinolysis
- Hemorrhages, infarcts, or both (intracranial, intracerebral, subarachnoid)
- Confusion
- Coma
- Psychosis
- Cortical blindness
- Quadriplegia
- Tremors
- Alzheimer type II astrocytosis
- CNS aspergillosis (fungal infection)
- Cytomegalovirus (viral infection)

[13] In the *Budd-Chiari syndrome*, occlusion of the hepatic veins impairs blood flow out of the liver, producing massive ascites and hepatomegaly. It is associated with any condition that obstructs the hepatic vein (e.g., abdominal trauma, use of oral contraceptives, polycythemia vera, paroxysmal nocturnal hemoglobinuria, other hypercoagulable states, and congenital webs of the vena cava).

rejection, and fluid or electrolyte imbalance (see Chapter 4). Vital signs must be monitored as activities are slowly resumed with physician approval and according to the client's tolerance levels. (See Appendix B.)

Postoperatively, the client will have multiple intravenous lines, drains, and a Foley catheter, as well as a painful abdomen with a large abdominal incision and a 4 to 5-in. left axillary incision (bypass procedure) restricted by staples and dressings. Standing postoperative orders are usually followed in the ICU. The large incisions are contraindications for resistive exercises; gradual low-resistance training can be introduced according to the physician's protocol. Upper extremity range of motion exercises and client education for prevention of adhesive capsulitis (i.e., "frozen shoulder") are important concerns. Staples are removed in approximately 7 to 10 days.

Often postoperative ascites is a significant problem, making functional training (e.g., bed mobility training, transfers) more difficult in the presence of an altered center of gravity. Hand and pedal edema from dependent positioning frequently develop, requiring active range of motion and bed mobility training as soon as possible. Assisted ambulation should occur as soon as the client is stable in the upright position; once the telemetry is removed, rehabilitation can progress rapidly. Ascites and associated edema usually resolve within 3 to 4 weeks.

Outpatient therapy continues approximately 8 weeks postoperatively. The liver transplant recipient with healthy heart and lungs can usually function well at home and resume independent activities of daily living. Rest and energy conservation balanced with nutrition, exercise, and correct, consistent, life-long drug-self administration are all important features of the rehabilitation process.

The therapist must be alert to any self-medicating or use of over-the-counter drugs by the client; the client should be encouraged to check with the physician before continuing unmonitored drug use. Steroid usage in older women can cause posttransplant confusion; the woman may become uncooperative, disoriented to time and place, and experience hallucinations (Sineath, 1995).

Vascular Disease of the Liver

Congestive Heart Failure

Congestive heart failure is the major cause of liver congestion, especially in the Western world, where ischemic heart disease is so prevalent. Backward congestion of the liver as well as the decreased perfusion of the liver secondary to decline in cardiac output result in abnormal liver function tests. Hepatic encephalopathy may contribute to the altered mentation seen with severe congestive heart failure. Decreased cerebral perfusion, hypoxemia, and electrolyte imbalance are usually the major contributors to the confused state that can be seen in people with severe congestive heart failure (Gibbons and Levy, 1989).

Shock

Shock from any cause results in decreased perfusion of the liver and often leads to ischemic necrosis of the centrilobular hepatocytes.

Infarction

Owing to its dual blood supply and the anastomotic structure of the hepatic sinusoids, infarcts of the liver are uncommon. Occlusion of the portal vein or the hepatic artery or its branches can occur as a result of embolism, polyarteritis nodosum, unknown cause, or accidental surgical ligation. Thrombosis interrupts the portal blood flow through the sinusoids, which allows a backflow of venous blood into the sinusoids that results in liver congestion (Rubin and Farber, 1994). (See also Portal Hypertension, this chapter.)

Liver Neoplasms

Hepatic neoplasms can be divided into three groups: benign neoplasms, primary malignant neoplasms, and metastatic malignant neoplasms. Cancer arising from the liver itself is called *primary;* liver cancer that has spread from somewhere else is labeled *secondary*. Primary liver tumors may arise from hepatocytes, connective tissue, blood vessels, or bile ducts and are either benign or malignant (Table 14–9). Primary liver cancer is commonly found in Africa and East Asia but is much rarer in the Western world, accounting for 2% of all cancer deaths in the United States (American Cancer Society, 1997). Primary malignant cancer is almost always found in a cirrhotic liver and is considered a late complication of cirrhosis. Benign and malignant neoplasms occur in women taking oral contraceptives.

A few rare tumors arise from the bile ducts within the liver and are associated with certain hormonal drugs and cancers. These *cholangiocarcinomas* are discussed later in the chapter (see Biliary section).

Benign Neoplasms

Hemangioma *(Meyers and Jones, 1990)*

About 2% of autopsied livers contain hemangiomas, making this lesion the most common benign liver tumor. It is of unknown etiology and occurs in all age groups, more commonly among women. The pathology is similar to that of hemangiomas anywhere in the body; it is a solitary, blood-filled mass of variable size and can be located anywhere in the liver. Areas of thrombosis are common, and older lesions may begin to calcify. The end-stage is a fibrous scar.

TABLE 14-9 CLASSIFICATION OF PRIMARY LIVER NEOPLASMS

ORIGIN	BENIGN	MALIGNANT
Hepatocytes	Adenoma	Hepatocellular carcinoma
Connective tissue	Fibroma	Sarcoma
Blood vessels	Hemangioma	Hemangioendothelioma
Bile ducts	Cholangioma	Carcinoma

From Matassarin-Jacobs E, Strasburg K: Nursing care of clients with hepatic disorders. *In* Black JM, Matassarin-Jacobs E (eds): Luckmann and Sorensen's Medical-Surgical Nursing, ed 4. Philadelphia, WB Saunders, 1993, p 1725.

Most hepatic hemangiomas are asymptomatic until they become large enough to cause a sense of fullness or upper abdominal pain. Hepatomegaly or an abdominal mass is the most common physical finding. About 10% of clients with clinically detectable lesions are febrile. Hepatic hemangiomas are often discovered coincidentally on CT scan, by MRI, or during laparotomy; otherwise radiographic arteriography or dynamic radionuclide scanning is used to make the diagnosis. Needle aspiration or biopsy is avoided because of the risk of hemorrhage.

Treatment is not usually recommended, because most hepatic hemangiomas have a benign course with negligible risk of malignancy and minimal chance of spontaneous hemorrhage. Surgical resection may be performed if the hemangioma is consistently symptomatic, producing pain or fever, or if the tumor is large enough for traumatic rupture to be considered a risk (e.g., a palpable lesion in an athlete).

Special Implications for the Therapist **14-13**

LIVER HEMANGIOMA

In the case of a known liver hemangioma, the client must be cautioned to avoid activities and positions that will increase intra-abdominal pressure to avoid risk of rupture (see Box 13-1). For the same reason, throughout therapy and especially during exercise, the client must be instructed in proper breathing techniques.

Adenomas

Liver cell adenomas occur most commonly in the third and fourth decades, almost exclusively in women. The incidence of benign hepatic cell tumors, called *adenomas*, is increasing, possibly in association with environmental estrogens, estrogens in oral contraceptives used by women, or the use of androgens in the case of liver adenomas in men. Although classified as benign tumors, they are highly vascular and carry a risk for rupture and subsequent hemorrhage. The clinical presentation is often one of acute abdominal disease due to necrosis of the tumor with hemorrhage (Friedman and Knauer, 1994). Pain, fever, and circulatory collapse occur in the presence of hemorrhage.

Hepatic arteriography is an early diagnostic test used for this condition, and liver biopsy may be employed, but the risk of hemorrhage is present. Liver function test results are usually within normal limits. The treatment for benign adenomas is dependent on the underlying cause. Hormone-dependent tumors may resolve with cessation of the oral contraceptives or androgens. Surgical excision (or hepatic lobectomy in the case of acute hemorrhage) of the involved liver segment is indicated in the absence of hormonally induced tumor. Prognosis is excellent; although malignant transformation can occur, it is a rare phenomenon (Foster and Berman, 1994).

Special Implications for the Therapist **14-14**

LIVER ADENOMA

The therapist is most likely to see this client postoperatively after the danger of rupture and hemorrhage have passed. Standard postoperative protocols are usually sufficient.

Malignant Neoplasms

Primary Hepatocellular Carcinoma

Overview and Incidence. Hepatocellular carcinoma, also referred to as *hepatoma*, constitutes about 90% to 95% of primary liver cancers in adults and appears to be on the rise in the United States, based on findings of autopsy studies. Although hepatocellular carcinoma can develop at any age, in the Western world, incidence increases at age 60 years, occurs more frequently in men, and appears to be closely associated with cirrhosis. Geographic variations exist in the United States with significantly higher death rates reported in western, southern, and central states (Meyers and Jones, 1990).

Staging and prognosis are based on histopathologic criteria that includes the size of the primary tumor, the number and lobar distribution of the tumors, the presence of vascular invasion, lymph node involvement, and distant metastases (Beahrs et al., 1992). Primary metastasis is to the heart and lungs via the hepatic and portal veins, but other sites of metastases include the brain, kidney, and spleen.

Etiology and Risk Factors. Epidemiologic and laboratory studies have firmly established a strong and specific association between HBV (chronic persistent form) and hepatocellular carcinoma. The presence of serum markers for hepatitis virus (HBsAg, anti-HBc, and anti-HCV), particularly in conjunction with cirrhosis, has a significant association with the risk of liver cancer (Tsukuma et al., 1993; Yu et al., 1990). These markers act either as a carcinogen or as a co-carcinogen in chronically infected hepatocytes (Huether and McCance, 1994).

Evidence also points to a link between ethanol abuse and hepatocellular carcinoma, probably mediated by its capacity to induce cirrhosis (Adami et al., 1992; Naccarato and Farinati, 1991). Other risk factors include gender (men have 3 to 8 times greater risk), increasing age (over 60 years), certain mycotoxins,[14] anabolic steroids, long-term oral contraceptive use,[15] polyvinylchloride, and nitrosamines. In addition, metabolic conditions such as hemochromatosis, α_1-antitrypsin deficiency, Wilson's disease, and glycogen storage diseases (see Chapter 9) have been linked by epidemiologic study more than by a direct causal relationship (Farmer et al., 1994). Rarely, hepatobiliary complications occur in women using oral contraceptive agents. Women with current or previous benign or malignant hepatic tumors should not take oral contraceptives (Lindberg, 1992).

Pathogenesis. The exact events leading to malignant transformation of the hepatic cell remains unknown. HBV appears to be an oncogenic virus that can integrate its viral DNA sequences into the cellular genome. This integration appears to be a necessary step for the mentioned transforma-

[14] The most significant mycotoxins are the aflatoxins, particularly those produced by *Aspergillus flavus*, a fungus from mold found in wheat, soybeans, corn, rice, oats, peanuts, milk, and cheese.

[15] This risk factor increases with higher dosage, longer duration of use, and older age (MacKay and Evans, 1994).

tion. Histologically, hepatocellular carcinoma is made up of cords or sheets of cells that resemble the hepatic parenchyma. Blood vessels such as portal or hepatic veins are commonly involved by tumor (Friedman and Knauer, 1994).

Clinical Manifestations. Clients with primary (benign and malignant) and secondary (metastatic) tumors often present with a similar clinical picture. Symptoms may be vague initially with minor temperature elevation and GI symptoms. Common clinical manifestations include jaundice, right upper quadrant pain, right shoulder pain, abdominal mass or distention, weight loss, diarrhea or constipation, and nausea (Matassarin-Jacobs and Strasburg, 1993).

Complications may include cachexia (see discussion, Chapter 13), tumor rupture, thrombosis of portal or hepatic vein, tumor embolism, portal hypertension with esophageal varices, ascites, hepatic failure, and widespread metastases (Harruff, 1994).

Medical Management

Diagnosis. Serum levels of α-fetoprotein are high in up to 60% of cases (400 ng/mL compared to the normal adult level of 10 ng/mL) but are not absolutely diagnostic (Columbo, 1992). Tumors detected or suspected at the time of α-fetoprotein measurement or ultrasonography are further examined. HBsAg is present in a majority of cases in endemic areas, whereas in the United States anti-HCV is found in up to 40% of cases (Friedman and Knauer, 1994).

Liver biopsy is diagnostic and real-time ultrasonography can detect hepatocellular carcinomas of 1 cm, offering the advantage of allowing guided percutaneous biopsy or aspiration cytology. Dynamic CT scanning with intravenous contrast material may also demonstrate lesions as small as 1 cm (Baron, 1994). Final diagnosis is based on histologic findings in resected hepatic tumors, biopsy specimens, or on the radiologic findings of hepatic arteriography.

Treatment. The use of vaccination to prevent infection with hepatitis B is expected to reduce the incidence of hepatocellular carcinoma associated with HBV. This is the only malignancy for which effective immunization is available. In the meantime, early screening of high-risk populations and detection remains the key to successful treatment of this malignancy (Smith and Paauw, 1993). Surgical resection (partial or total hepatectomy) has been the primary treatment if no nodal involvement or distant spread is present.

Newer treatment techniques for unresectable hepatocellular carcinoma to reduce tumor size now include transarterial chemoembolization (angiography to embolize the tumor arterial supply) and percutaneous ethanol injection (alcohol injection into the tumor) (Farmer et al., 1994; Matsui et al., 1993; Yamada, et al., 1990). Radioimmunotherapy is an experimental form of treatment used for some types of liver cancer. A radioactive isotope is attached to a radiolabeled antibody against ferritin, a specific protein found in human liver tumors. The isotope is given intravenously and concentrates in the liver, where it irradiates the tumor internally (Alkire, 1991).

Liver transplantation is a possible treatment option for clients with decompensating cirrhosis (see discussion Cirrhosis: Pathogenesis) and a small hepatocellular carcinoma confined to the liver; but even with transplantation, recurrence rates are as high as 65% (Farmer et al., 1994). The survival rate may be better for those in whom the tumor is incidental to another disorder (e.g., biliary atresia, cirrhosis). Clients with portal vein thrombosis secondary to tumor invasion are not candidates for a liver transplantation.

Prognosis. Untreated hepatocellular carcinoma has a very poor prognosis, especially in clients with multiple tumor nodules. Factors affecting the prognosis favorably include early detection, tumor size (less than 5 cm), tumor location, presence of a tumor capsule, well-differentiated tumor, lack of vascular invasion, and absence of cirrhosis (Farmer et al., 1994). Even so, with treatment the 5-year survival rate is only 15% to 30%. If treatment fails to eradicate the tumor process, the expected survival is no more than 4 to 6 months. Five-year survival rates can be as high as 45% with treatment of small, well-differentiated tumors in the absence of cirrhosis. Tumor resection in the presence of cirrhosis is accompanied by risk of tumor recurrence or death from the remaining underlying liver dysfunction.

Special Implications for the Therapist **14-15**

LIVER MALIGNANT NEOPLASMS

Liver tumors that cause elevation of the diaphragm can cause right shoulder pain or symptoms of respiratory involvement. Peripheral edema associated with developing ascites may be observed first by the therapist (see Ascites, this chapter). As the tumor grows, pain may radiate to the back (mid-thoracic region). Paraneoplastic syndromes (Chapter 7) due to ectopic hormone may occur including polycythemia, hypoglycemia, and hypercalcemia. (See general principles related to the oncology client, Chapter 7).

Metastatic Malignant Tumors

The liver is one of the most common sites of metastasis from other primary cancers (e.g., colorectal, stomach, pancreas, esophagus, lung, breast, melanoma, Hodgkin's disease, and non-Hodgkin's lymphoma). Metastatic tumors occur 20 times more often than primary liver tumors and constitute the bulk of hepatic malignancy. As with other types of cancers, secondary liver cancer can occur as a result of local invasion from neighboring organs, lymphatic spread, spread across body cavities, and spread via the vascular system. The liver filters blood from anywhere else in the body, but since all blood from the digestive organs pass through the liver before joining the general circulation, the liver is the first organ to filter cancer cells released from the stomach, intestine, or pancreas.

Metastatic tumors to the liver originating in some organs (e.g., stomach, lung) never give rise to hepatic symptoms, whereas others produce hepatic symptoms or jaundice with less than 60% replacement of the liver. Certain tumors (colon, breast, melanoma) typically replace 90% of the liver before jaundice develops. Melanomas are associated with such minimal tissue reaction that almost complete hepatic replacement occurs before hepatic symptoms develop. Clinical manifestations, diagnosis, and treatment are as for primary liver neoplasm.

Liver Abscess

Liver abscess most often occurs among individuals with other underlying disorders. Most common underlying causes include *bacterial cholangitis* secondary to obstruction of the bile ducts by stone or stricture; *portal vein bacteremia* secondary to bacterial seeding via the portal vein from infected viscera following bowel inflammation or organ perforation; *liver flukes*, a parasitic infestation, or *amebiasis*, an infestation with amebae from tropical or subtropical areas. Other predisposing factors are diabetes mellitus, infected hepatic cysts, metastatic liver tumors with secondary infection, and diverticulitis. Pyogenic (pus-filled) abscesses may be single or multiple; multiple abscesses often arise from a biliary source of infection.

Clinical manifestations are commonly right-sided abdominal and right shoulder pain, nausea, vomiting, rapid weight loss, high fever, and diaphoresis. The liver's close proximity to the base of the right lung may contribute to the development of right pleural effusion. Complications of hepatic abscess relate to rupture and direct spread of infection. Pleuropulmonary involvement from the rupture of an abscess through the diaphragm, and peritonitis from leakage into the abdominal cavity can occur.

Diagnosis is accomplished by a variety of possible tests including liver function tests, chest roentgenograms, contrast-enhanced CT scan of the abdomen, ultrasonography of the right upper quadrant, liver scan, or arteriography. Treatment may consist of antimicrobial therapy alone or percutaneous drainage of the abscess with antimicrobial therapy. Surgery may be required to relieve biliary tract obstruction and to drain abscesses that do not respond to percutaneous drainage and antibiotics.

Unrecognized and untreated, pyogenic liver abscess is universally fatal. The mortality from hepatic abscess in treated cases remains high, ranging from 40% to 80%. Amebic abscesses are an exception; when treated, the mortality rate is less than 3%). Early diagnosis and aggressive treatment can significantly reduce the mortality in some cases (Rubin and Farber, 1994). Specific antibiotics are required whenever abscess is caused by amebic infestation.

Special Implications for the Therapist **14-16**

LIVER ABSCESS

Clients with liver abscess are very ill and are usually only seen by the therapist assigned to an intensive care unit team. In such situations, vital signs are assessed regularly to detect high fever and rapid pulse, which are early signs of sepsis (a common complication). Movement, coughing, and deep breathing are important to prevent or limit pulmonary complications related to hepatic abscess, and skin care in the presence of high fever is essential. Careful disposal of feces and careful handwashing to avoid transmission are required when abscess is caused by amebic infestation.

Liver Injuries

Toxic Liver Injury

Toxic liver injury can occur as a result of drugs or from occupational exposure to chemicals and toxins. Hepatotoxic chemicals produce liver cell necrosis, a consequence of the metabolism of the compound by the oxidase system of the liver. Agents responsible for toxic liver injury include yellow phosphorus, carbon tetrachloride, phalloidin (mushroom toxin), and acetaminophen (analgesic). Reye's syndrome in children may be related to aspirin toxicity.

In addition to jaundice, other symptoms of liver toxicity may occur (e.g., cholestasis, chronic hepatitis). Toxic liver injury produces toxic hepatitis (discussed earlier in the chapter). The prognosis is usually good if the toxin is withdrawn and never reintroduced. Whatever drug is responsible, it is well documented that liver toxicity becomes more severe with advancing age (Gilliam, 1990).

Liver Trauma

Liver injury by trauma may be either penetrating or blunt, leading to laceration and hemorrhage. Penetrating injuries are usually knife or missile wounds (gunshot). A knife wound leaves a sharp clear incision, whereas gunshot wounds enter and exit with greater damage. Blunt trauma from a fall or from hitting a steering wheel have varying effects, from small hematomas to large lacerations as a result of severe impact forces.

Special Implications for the Therapist **14-17**

LIVER INJURIES

The therapist will likely be treating clients with liver injury secondary to trauma postoperatively in the trauma unit. The common postoperative problems include pulmonary infections and abscess formation. Clients are assessed postoperatively for manifestations of infection (e.g., fever, chills, difficulty breathing). Physical therapy intervention is focused on prevention of respiratory complications, especially pneumonia and provision of skin care and extremity movement, until the client can begin progressive transfer and mobility skills.

PANCREAS

Diabetes Mellitus

The pancreas has dual functions, acting as both an endocrine gland in secreting hormones insulin and glucagon and as an exocrine gland in producing digestive enzymes. The cells of the pancreas that function in the endocrine capacity are the islets of Langerhans, constituting 1% to 2% of the pancreatic mass. Defective endocrine function of the pancreas resulting in ineffective insulin (whether deficient or defective in action within the body) characterizes diabetes mellitus (see Chapter 9).

Pancreatitis

Definition and Overview. Pancreatitis is a potentially serious inflammation of the pancreas that may result in autodigestion of the pancreas by its own enzymes. Pancreatitis may be acute or chronic; the acute form is brief, usually mild, and reversible, whereas the chronic form is recurrent or persisting.

BOX 14–6
Conditions Associated with Acute Pancreatitis

- Alcoholism
- Cystic fibrosis
- Hereditary (familial) pancreatitis
- Hypercalcemia
- Hyperlipidemia
- Medications
- Gallstones
- Peptic ulcers
- Postoperative inflammation
- Trauma (including surgery)
- Vasculitis
- Viral infections

Acute Pancreatitis

Incidence and Etiology. Acute pancreatitis can arise from a variety of etiologic factors; it can occur in association with one of several other clinical conditions (Box 14–6) or as the result of an unknown cause (10% to 20%). The incidence varies with the circumstances and age of the affected person; incidence increases after age 55 years (Abrams et al., 1995). In metropolitan areas, affected people tend to be younger, and alcoholism is the most common etiology. In rural areas and in geriatric clients, gallstones predominate as a cause.

Pathogenesis. Acute pancreatitis is thought to result from "escape" of activated pancreatic enzymes from acinar cells[16] into surrounding tissues. The exact pathogenesis is unknown, but it may include edema or obstruction (e.g., stone) of the ampulla of Vater (Fig. 14–8) with resultant reflux of bile into pancreatic ducts or direct injury to the acinar cells, which allows leakage of pancreatic enzymes into pancreatic tissue.

Enzyme activation breaks down tissue and cell membranes, causing pathologic changes varying from acute connective tissue edema and cellular infiltration with subsequent scarring to necrosis of the acinar cells, hemorrhage from necrotic blood vessels, and intrahepatic and extrahepatic fat necrosis. Autodigestion and inflammation of all or part of the pancreas may occur, resulting in the formation of a soap-like substance that binds with calcium. Other organs, such as the lungs and kidneys, can be affected by toxic enzymes released into the bloodstream. These systemic effects are major causes of morbidity and mortality.

Clinical Manifestations. Symptoms in clients presenting with acute pancreatitis can vary from mild, nonspecific abdominal pain to profound shock with coma and, ultimately, death. Abdominal pain begins abruptly in the mid-epigastrium, increases in intensity for several hours, and can last from days to more than a week (Kallsen, 1993; Steinberg, 1992). The pain is caused by edema, which distends the pancreatic ducts and capsule; chemical irritation and inflammation of the peritoneum; and irritation or obstruction of the biliary tract. Pancreatic pain has a penetrating quality and radiates to the upper back because of the retroperitoneal location of the pancreas. Pain is made worse by walking and lying supine and is relieved by sitting and leaning forward.

Other common symptoms include nausea and vomiting, fever and sweating, tachycardia, malaise and weakness, and mild jaundice from impingement on the common bile duct. Tetany may develop as a result of calcium deposition in areas of fat necrosis, leading to reduced calcium levels or as a decreased response to parathormone (parathyroid hormone). Symptoms are often preceded by a heavy meal or excessive alcohol consumption. Complications may include shock, adult respiratory distress syndrome (ARDS), acute renal failure, hypercalcemia, pancreatic pseudocysts,[17] abscess, or chemical or septic peritonitis.

Medical Management

Diagnosis. Diagnosis is based on clinical presentation and clinical studies, including abdominal x-ray, ultrasound for the diagnosis of gallstones, CT scan to evaluate the pancreas (possibly serial examinations if symptoms fail to resolve with treatment), and laboratory studies. Early in the disease (within 24 to 72 hours), pancreatic digestive enzymes released from injured acinar cells into the blood result in elevated serum amylase and lipase levels, which are diagnostic for acute pancreatitis. Urine amylase level is also elevated, which is significant in the diagnosis. The ratio of amylase clearance to creatinine clearance by the kidney increases significantly in cases of pancreatitis. Acute pancreatitis must be differentiated from perforating duodenal ulcer, leaking aortic aneurysm, acute cholecystitis, small bowel obstruction, mesenteric thrombosis or embolism, and kidney stones, which can cause similar clinical and laboratory findings.

Treatment. For most persons, acute pancreatitis is a mild disease that subsides spontaneously within several days. The pathogenesis of pancreatitis is not understood well enough to develop a specific therapy to stop the inflammatory cascade. Treatment for pancreatitis is largely symptomatic and is designed to provide rest for the pancreas by stopping the process of autodigestion. Oral foods and fluids may be withheld to decrease pancreatic secretions, with gradual reintroduction of clear liquids and progression to a regular low-fat diet per tolerance. Nasogastric suction may be required to relieve pain and prevent paralytic ileus in individuals with nausea and vomiting. Analgesics, fluid management, and cessation of alcohol intake are essential components of medical treatment. Calcium gluconate is given intravenously in the presence of hypocalcemia with tetany. Long-term parenteral feeding may be required for protracted cases. Surgical intervention is indicated in the presence of cholelithiasis (removal of gallstones) or pancreatic necrosis.

Prognosis. Prognosis depends on the severity of the condition; treatment produces varying results, but the clinical course follows a self-limited pattern, resolving within 2 weeks in up to 90% of cases. Many people, especially those with gallstone pancreatitis, improve rapidly, but recurrences are

---

[16] *Acinus* is the smallest functional unit of the liver; the term is also used to refer to a terminal respiratory unit (*pulmonary acinus*).

[17] A pseudocyst is a liquefied collection of necrotic debris and pancreatic enzymes surrounded by a rim of pancreatic tissue or adjacent tissues; it contains no true epithelial lining. Complications of pseudocysts include infection, bleeding, and rupture into the peritoneum (Andreoli et al., 1993).

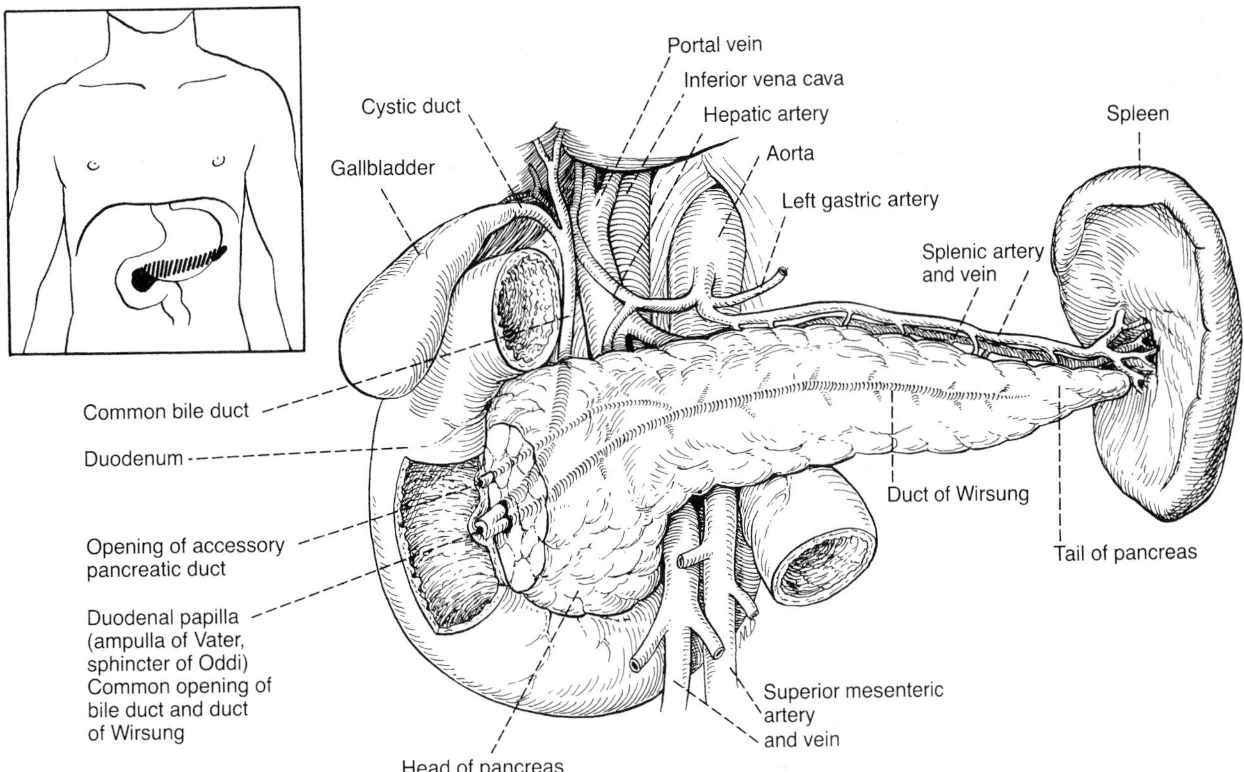

Figure 14–8. The pancreas (located behind the stomach) and gallbladder. Obstruction of either the hepatic or common bile duct by stone or spasm blocks the exit of bile from the liver, where it is formed, and prevents bile from ejecting into the duodenum. (*From Black JM, Matassarin-Jacobs E (eds): Luckmann and Sorensen's Medical-Surgical Nursing, ed 4. Philadelphia, WB Saunders, 1993, p 1681.*)

common in alcoholic pancreatitis. Complications of shock and ARDS develop in approximately 10% of cases, resulting in lengthy hospitalizations and high mortality. Chronic pancreatitis develops in about 10% of cases.

Chronic Pancreatitis

Incidence. The distribution of idiopathic chronic pancreatitis is bimodal, with a juvenile form of the disease occurring in young persons (mean age, 25 years) and a second distribution peak at age 60 years. Chronic pancreatitis is caused by long-standing alcohol abuse in more than 90% of adult cases; cases in children are related to cystic fibrosis (Holt, 1993).

Pathogenesis. Structural or functional impairment of the pancreas leads to chronic pancreatitis. Progressive destruction of the pancreas occurs with resulting irregular fibrosis and chronic inflammation (Scarpelli, 1994). Functional obstruction of the pancreatic duct may be caused by mechanical obstruction (e.g., cancer, cystic fibrosis mucus).

Although the etiologic role of alcohol is well established, the mechanism by which it causes pancreatitis is unclear. Alcohol stimulates precipitation of protein plugs in the ducts, which serve as the point of origin (nidus) for subsequent calculi. These stones obstruct the ductal system, leading to progressive necrosis and scarring.

The fact that chronic pancreatitis is often characterized by intermittent "acute" attacks followed by periods of quiescence suggests that in many persons the pathogenesis involves repeated bouts of acute pancreatitis followed by scarring. In persons without a history of acute episodes, the pathogenesis of chronic pancreatitis may relate to persistent necrosis and insidious scarring, similar to the progression of cirrhosis of the liver (Scarpelli, 1994).

Clinical Manifestations. In clients with alcohol-associated pancreatitis, epigastric and left upper quadrant pain often begin 12 to 48 hours after an episode of excessive alcohol consumption. Pain may eventually become almost continuous, and referred upper left lumbar pain with muscle guarding may occur.

Gallstone-associated pancreatitis typically produces symptoms after a large meal. Attacks may last only a few hours or as long as 2 weeks, and symptoms are similar to those of acute pancreatitis with additional symptoms of weight loss, flatulence, diarrhea owing to loss of enzymes, or constipation. When greater than 90% destruction of the pancreas occurs, malabsorption syndrome with steatorrhea and long-term pancreatic enzyme deficiency and loss of islet cell function with diabetes mellitus may result.

Complications may include narcotics addiction (used for pain control in severe form, called *pancreatolithiasis*), diabetes mellitus, pancreatic pseudocyst or abscess, cholestatic liver disease (with or without jaundice) common bile duct stricture, fat malabsorption (steatorrhea, malnutrition), and peptic ulcer.

Medical Management. Clinical history in the presence of typical findings on examination are correlated with laboratory studies and imaging (e.g., abdominal films, ultrasound, upper GI tract series, endoscopy) to make the diagnosis. In contrast to acute pancreatitis, chronic pancreatitis does not usually produce an elevated amylase level unless associated with a distinct attack (Andreoli et al., 1993). Calcium levels may be decreased, but unlike the case with acute pancreatitis, this does not lead to tetany.

The treatment of chronic pancreatitis is directed toward prevention of further pancreatic injury, pain relief, and replacement of lost endocrine/exocrine function. In the case of cystic fibrosis and for selected individuals with alcoholic pancreatitis, oral enzyme replacements are taken before and during meals to correct enzyme deficiencies and to prevent malabsorption. Cessation of alcohol intake is essential in the management of chronic pancreatitis; insulin may be required in the case of islet cell dysfunction. Surgical drainage for persistent pseudocysts as well as surgical intervention to eliminate obstruction of the bile ducts may be indicated.

Chronic pancreatitis is a serious disease, often leading to chronic disability. Chronic pancreatitis associated with cystic fibrosis may produce death secondary to lung infection. For those persons who cannot be helped by treatment, addiction to narcotics is a frequent result.

Special Implications for the Therapist **14-18**

ACUTE PANCREATITIS

The therapist is most likely to see acute pancreatitis either when the early presentation is back pain (undiagnosed) or when ARDS develops as a complication, necessitating assisted respiration and pulmonary care. Pancreatic inflammation and scarring occurring as part of the acute pancreatic process can result in decreased spinal extension, especially of the thoracolumbar junction (see Pathogenesis). This problem is difficult to treat and requires the therapist to make reasonable goals (e.g., maintain function and current range of motion), especially when the pancreatitis is in an active, ongoing phase. Even with client compliance with treatment and subsiding of inflammation, the residual scarring is difficult to reach or affect with mobilization techniques and continues to reduce mechanical motion.

Back pain associated with acute pancreatitis may be accompanied by GI symptoms such as diarrhea, pain after a meal, anorexia, and unexplained weight loss. The client may not see any connection between GI symptoms and back pain and may not report the additional symptoms. The pain may be relieved by heat initially (decreases muscular tension); preferred positions include leaning forward, sitting up, or lying motionless.

Promoting comfort and rest as part of the medical rehabilitation process may necessitate teaching the client positioning (side-lying, knee-chest position with a pillow pressed against the abdomen, or sitting with the trunk flexed may be helpful) and relaxation techniques.

For the client who is restricted from eating or drinking anything to rest the GI tract and decrease pancreatic stimulation, even ice chips can stimulate enzymes and increase pain. In such cases, the therapist must be careful not to give in to the client's repeated requests for water or ice chips unless approved by nursing or medical staff. Clients with acute pancreatitis are allowed to resume oral intake when all abdominal pain and tenderness have resolved. (See also Chapter 4 for care of the client with fluid or electrolyte imbalance.)

Pancreatic Cancer

Overview and Incidence. Pancreatic cancer represents the fourth and fifth most common cause of cancer-related death in men and women, respectively; 27,600 new cases will be diagnosed in the United States during 1997 (ACS, 1997). Most pancreatic neoplasms are adenocarcinoma of ductal origin (90%), which are discussed here (Murr et al., 1994). From 1930 until 1980, the incidence of pancreatic cancer doubled and then peaked in the 1980s. The reason(s) for this remain unknown. Pancreatic cancer is more common in black men than in whites and has a peak incidence in the seventh and eighth decades

Etiology and Risk Factors. Clear evidence of increased risk of pancreatic cancer with smoking, diabetes mellitus (especially in women), and prior gastrectomy has been shown. There is no support for any direct effect from alcohol intake or coffee consumption, but these risk factors are in question (Boyle et al., 1989; Fontham and Correa, 1989). Although unusual, a genetic predisposition to pancreatic cancer has been documented (Lynch et al., 1992). Gene mutations and other acquired chromosomal abnormalities are being recognized with increasing frequency. How mutations or abnormalities in gene expression relate to the pathogenesis of pancreatic cancer remains unknown.

Pathogenesis. Most pancreatic tumors arise from exocrine cells in the ducts and are called *ductal adenocarcinomas*. About 75% of the ductal pancreatic neoplasms are located in the head of the pancreas and 25% are located in the body and tail of the organ. Obstructive jaundice caused by pancreatic carcinoma occurs when the lower end of the bile duct is enveloped by the cancer as it passes through the pancreas.

A number of physiologic changes occur as a consequence of biliary obstruction and vary according to the extent and duration of obstruction. One of the more important physiologic responses to bile duct obstruction is the production of pain. Intrinsic nerve plexuses are found throughout the extrahepatic biliary system that are composed of parasympathetic and sympathetic fibers. The precise mechanism of biliary pain stimulated by obstruction remains unexplained (Meyers and Jones, 1990).

Clinical Manifestations. The clinical features of pancreatic cancer are initially nonspecific and vague, which contribute to the delay in diagnosis. The most common symptoms include weight loss, epigastric pain radiating to the back (thoracic) or back pain alone, and jaundice with pruritus. Radiating pain associated with carcinoma of the body and tail of the pancreas localizes in the left lumbar region. The pain associated with pancreatic cancer, especially with an advanced lesion, that radiates to the back may be incapacitating. Sitting up and leaning forward may provide some relief initially and usually indicates that the lesion has spread beyond the pancreas and is inoperable. Less commonly, the client may experience nausea, vomiting, diarrhea, and anorexia.

Medical Management

Diagnosis. With the expanding knowledge of cell biology and nuclear control of cellular proliferation, strategies for screening (or directed treatment) are not far off (Murr et al., 1994). At the present time, there is no single diagnostic test, but rather a range of serologic and radiologic studies are available for evaluation and staging of this disease. However, invasive studies, including laparotomy, are often necessary to establish the diagnosis and resectability of the tumor. CT scan is usually the diagnostic procedure of choice for the jaundiced client with a suspected malignancy.

The TNM staging system (for *t*umor, *n*ode, *m*etastases) (see Chapter 7) classifies pancreatic carcinoma according to tumor size, extent of local invasion, presence or absence of regional lymph node metastases, and presence or absence of distant non-nodal metastatic disease. Staging provides information required for determining resectability and prognosis.

Treatment. Management of symptoms such as obstructive jaundice, duodenal obstruction, and back pain is often difficult. Palliative therapy may be operative or nonoperative to provide significant relief of symptoms. Pancreatic resection currently provides the only opportunity for cure. Despite sophisticated preoperative staging methods, 60% to 70% of clients with adenocarcinoma of the pancreatic head that appears to be resectable preoperatively are found to have metastatic or locally invasive disease at laparotomy, precluding resection. Combined-modality treatment with chemotherapy and radiation therapy prolongs survival minimally following curative resection, but it provides symptomatic relief. When tumors of the pancreas cannot be removed, a bypass operation (cholecystojejunostomy or choledochoduodenostomy) to relieve jaundice without removing the tumor is recommended.

Pharmacology for pain control may include non-narcotic analgesics (e.g., NSAIDs, Tylenol) initially, with later introduction of narcotics and other adjuvant drugs (e.g., tricyclic antidepressants). Percutaneous chemical splanchnicectomy (destruction of the splanchnic nerve) is routinely used for the nonoperative treatment of pain, to reduce the need for oral narcotics (Lee et al., 1993).

Prognosis. The overall prognosis for pancreatic carcinoma is very poor with a mortality rate of nearly 100%. Despite advances in diagnostic technology that have shortened the interval between onset of symptoms and definitive treatment, no appreciable impact on survival has occurred. Operative resection offers the only hope for cure, but fewer than 15% of clients have resectable disease at the time of diagnosis, and 5-year survival after curative resection remains around 5% to 10% (Livingston et al., 1991; Spencer et al., 1990).

Return of hepatic function following relief of obstruction is variable. Bile secretion may return to normal within hours; immunologic dysfunction may take weeks to normalize; jaundice characteristically improves dramatically within the first several days but may not disappear for weeks, and some of the other symptoms such as pruritus, loss of appetite, and malaise correct within hours or days following relief of the obstruction (Meyers and Jones, 1990).

Special Implications for the Therapist **14-19**

PANCREATIC CANCER

Vague back pain may be the first symptomatic presentation, and cervical lymphadenopathy (called *Virchow's node*) may be the first sign of distant metastases. The therapist is most likely to palpate an enlarged supraclavicular lymph node (usually left-sided), a finding that should always alert the therapist to the need to screen for medical disease. Paraneoplastic syndrome (see Chapter 7) associated with pancreatic carcinoma may present as neuromyopathy, dermatomyositis, or thrombophlebitis associated with abnormalities in blood coagulation (coagulopathy) (Rugo, 1994).

The therapist is most likely to be involved with the client with diagnosed pancreatic cancer who experiences intractable back pain. Referral to chronic pain clinics or hospice centers will likely include physical therapy services. Repeated nerve blocks may be performed after a reasonable effort to manage pain through the use of transcutaneous electrical nerve stimulation (TENS), biofeedback, analgesics, or other pain control techniques. Indwelling infusion pumps implanted to deliver analgesics directly to the site of visceral afferent nerves in the epidural or intrathecal spaces may be used for short periods (i.e., 1 to 3 months).

Cystic Fibrosis

Cystic fibrosis is a disease of the exocrine glands that results in the production of excessive, thick mucus that obstructs the digestive and respiratory systems. When the disease was first being differentiated from other conditions, it was given the name cystic fibrosis of the pancreas, because cysts and scar tissue on the pancreas were observed during autopsy. This term describes a secondary rather than primary characteristic (in-depth discussion of this disorder is found in Chapter 12).

BILIARY *(Table 14-10)*

Cholelithiasis (Gallstones)

Definition and Overview. Cholelithiasis is the formation or presence of gallstones that remain in the lumen of the gallbladder or are ejected with bile into the cystic duct. Gallstones are stonelike masses called *calculi* (singular: calculus) that form in the gallbladder as a result of changes in the normal components of bile. There are two types classified according to composition: 75% consist primarily of cholesterol (*cholesterol stones*), whereas 25% are composed of bilirubin salts (e.g., calcium bilirubinate and other calcium salts), called *pigment stones*. Chronic cholecystitis (gallbladder or cystic duct inflammation) usually accompanies cholelithiasis

TABLE 14–10 Biliary Tract Terminology

Term	Definition
Chole-	Pertaining to bile
Cholang-	Pertaining to bile ducts
Cholangiography	X-ray study of bile ducts
Cholangitis	Inflammation of bile duct
Cholecyst-	Pertaining to the gallbladder
Cholecystectomy	Removal of gallbladder
Cholecystitis	Inflammation of gallbladder
Cholecystography	X-ray study of gallbladder
Cholecystostomy	Incision and drainage of gallbladder
Choledocho-	Pertaining to common bile duct
Choledocholithiasis	Stones in common bile duct
Choledochostomy	Exploration of common bile duct
Cholelith-	Gallstones
Cholelithiasis	Presence of gallstones
Cholescintigraphy	Radionuclide imaging of biliary system
Cholestasis	Stoppage or suppression of bile flow

Adapted from Kallsen C: Nursing care of clients with biliary and exocrine pancreatic disorders. *In* Black JM, Matassarin-Jacobs E (eds): Luckmann and Sorensen's Medical-Surgical Nursing, ed 4. Philadelphia, WB Saunders, 1993, p 1732.

when gallstones become lodged in the cystic duct and obstruct the flow of bile in and out of the gallbladder.

Incidence. Gallstones, the most common cause of biliary tract disease in the United States, occur increasingly with advancing age, so that gallstones are present in 20% of men and 35% of women by age 75 years. In the United States, an estimated 15 million people have gallstones. Twenty-five years ago, the typical person with gallstones was described as a "fat, fair, fertile, flatulent, forty, female." As the incidence of gallstones continues to increase, this descriptor no longer strictly applies. For example, very elderly people with associated conditions such as heart and lung disease develop gallstones as a complication.

Risk Factors. Specific risk factors for the development of gallstones are listed in Box 14–7. Fasting overnight for 14 hours or more (presumably skipping breakfast) has been associated with a higher rate of gallstones. Without the stimulation of food, the gallbladder does not put out enough "solubilizing" bile acids that keep cholesterol dissolved and unable to form stones. (Sichieri et al., 1991). Elevated estrogen levels associated with gallstones may occur during the last trimester of pregnancy, when gallbladder stasis reduces precipitation of cholesterol from the gallbladder and/or possibly some chemical alteration of bile. Other estrogen-associated causes of gallstones include use of oral contraceptives, postmenopausal therapy, or multiparity (two or more pregnancies resulting in viable offspring).

The formation of gallstones does not appear to be related to smoking or alcohol intake. Genetic predisposition is difficult to establish, because the disease is very common in the general population. Two known familial-related causes of gallstones are American Indian ancestry (specifically Pima Indian) and hemolytic anemia (e.g., congenital spherocytosis and sickle cell anemia), which can cause pigment stones.

BOX 14–7
Risk Factors Associated with Gallstones

- Age (increasing incidence with increasing age)
- Sex (female-male ratio = 3 : 1)
- Elevated estrogen levels
  - Pregnancy
  - Use of oral contraceptives
  - Estrogen replacement therapy (ERT)
- High bile cholesterol
  - Obesity
  - Diabetes mellitus
  - Hyperlipidemia
- Low levels of bile salts
  - Hydroxylase deficiency
  - Malabsorption
- Diet
- Liver disease
- American Indian ancestry (Pima indian)
- Hemolytic anemia (pigment stones)

Pathogenesis. Lifestyle and diet alone do not account for the variation within high incidence areas, and even excessive cholesterol in the bile probably requires another particle or substance to trigger gallstone formation. Cholesterol, which is insoluble in water, is carried in bile solubilized by bile acids and phospholipids. In most persons, many of whom do not develop gallstones, bile contains more cholesterol than can be maintained in stable solution; in other words, it is supersaturated with cholesterol. In this supersaturated bile, microscopic cholesterol crystals form. Gradual deposition of additional layers of cholesterol leads to the appearance of macroscopic cholesterol gallstones (Andreoli et al., 1993). Although the chemical imbalance causing cholesterol stones to form has been identified, the cause of the imbalance remains undetermined. In obese individuals, the mechanism appears to involve cholesterol synthesis, whereas in people who are not obese, decreased secretion of bile acids seems to be the key.

Pigmented gallstones are formed by supersaturation of bile with calcium hydrogen bilirubinate, the acid calcium salt of unconjugated bilirubin (see Jaundice, this chapter). The formation of pigmented stones is associated with biliary infection and increased amounts of unconjugated bilirubin in bile rather than gallbladder hypomotility present with cholesterol stones. The unconjugated bilirubin precipitates in the gallbladder or bile ducts to form stones (Carey, 1993).

Clinical Manifestations. Most gallstones are asymptomatic; approximately 30% cause symptoms of biliary colic or chronic cholecystitis with right upper quadrant pain. Obstruction of the cystic duct (see Fig. 14–8) distends the gallbladder and produces this abdominal pain, called *biliary colic*. The pain of biliary colic may be intermittent or steady; it is usually severe and is located in the right upper quadrant with abdominal tenderness, muscle guarding, and rebound pain. Painful symptoms often radiate to the mid-upper back, below or between the scapulae.[18]

[18] Radiating pain to the mid-back and scapula occur owing to splanchnic (visceral) fibers synapsing with adjacent phrenic nerve fibers (major branch of the cervical plexus innervating the diaphragm).

Other symptoms are vague, including heartburn, belching, flatulence, epigastric discomfort, and food intolerance (especially for fats and cabbage). Gallstones in the elderly may not cause pain, fever, or jaundice. Mental confusion and shakiness may be the only manifestations of gallstones in the elderly. Serious complications occur in 20% of cases when a stone becomes lodged in the lower end of the common bile duct, causing inflammation (cholecystitis) leading to bacterial infection and jaundice (indicating the stone is in the common bile duct). Sometimes acute pancreatitis develops when the duct from the pancreas that joins the common bile duct also becomes blocked (see Fig. 14–8). About 15% of clients with gallstones also have stones in the common bile duct (choledocholithiasis).

Medical Management

Diagnosis. Diagnosis is based on the history, physical examination, and radiographic evaluation (stones containing calcium show up on plain x-ray). In the past, oral cholecystogram was used for imaging of the stones, but this has been replaced by ultrasonography. Ultrasonography demonstrates gallstones in more than 95% of cases. Other more specialized radiography may be required, such as intravenous cholangiography (to differentiate cholelithiasis from other causes of extrahepatic biliary obstruction) and endoscopic or percutaneous cholangiography.

Treatment. No treatment is recommended for the person with asymptomatic gallstones, and there is no indication for prophylactic cholecystectomy in such a case. A low-fat diet that reduces stimulation of the gallbladder can often relieve mild or moderate symptoms. Laparoscopic cholecystectomy has replaced open cholecystectomy as the treatment of choice for symptomatic gallbladder disease. Lithotripsy using focused shock waves from outside the body can crush stones into fine gravel, which can be easily dissolved by bile salts. In the past, a variety of conditions precluded the safe use of lithotripsy, but currently pregnancy is the only absolute contraindication to this treatment (Streem, 1997).

Prognosis. Cholelithiasis is the fifth leading cause of hospitalization among adults and accounts for 90% of all gallbladder and duct diseases. However the prognosis with medical treatment is usually good, depending on the severity of disease, presence of complications (especially infection), and response to antibiotics. Cholecystectomy in the older population has a higher risk for injury related to anesthesia, pain medications, and, sometimes, the response to the trauma of surgery. Gallstones recur within 3 to 5 years after cessation of treatment in 50% of cases. Gallstones may be a risk factor for gallbladder cancer, but this is a rare tumor that is easily detected by x-ray or ultrasound.

Special Implications for the Therapist **14–20**

CHOLELITHIASIS (GALLSTONES)

When the gallbladder has been removed (or is blocked by a stone) a small amount of less concentrated bile is still secreted into the intestine. The loss of a gallbladder itself does not appear to have an impact on physical activity and exercise. In the past, gallbladder removal required a significant incision with muscle disruption, scarring, and, frequently, postoperative back pain associated with the formation of deep scar tissue. Now the closed procedure (laparoscopic cholecystectomy) can be performed as outpatient (day) surgery without these complications.

The usual postoperative exercises (e.g., breathing, turning, coughing, wound splinting, compressive stockings, leg exercises) for any surgical procedure apply, especially in case of complications. Early activity helps to prevent pooling of blood in the lower extremities and subsequent development of thrombosis. Early activity also assists the return of intestinal motility, so the client is encouraged to begin progressive movement and ambulation as soon as possible.

Choledocholithiasis

Defined as calculi in the common bile duct, choledocholithiasis occurs in 15% of persons with gallstones and has the same etiology and pathogenesis. The percentage rises with age and the incidence in elderly people may be as high as 50%. Common duct stones usually originate in the gallbladder, but they may also form spontaneously in the common duct and can therefore occur after a person has had a cholecystectomy. Stones that occur in the absence of a gallbladder are referred to as *primary common duct stones*.

Approximately 30% to 40% of duct stones are asymptomatic when there is no obstruction. When symptomatic, duct stones may produce severe and persistent biliary colic (see Cholelithiasis: Clinical Manifestations, this chapter) accompanied by chills and fever, obstructive jaundice, cholangitis (bile duct inflammation[19]), pancreatitis, or a combination of these.

Diagnosis is based on clinical picture and radiologic or endoscopic evidence of dilated bile ducts, ductal stones, or impaired bile flow. Percutaneous transhepatic cholangiography[20] or endoscopic retrograde cholangiopancreatography (ERCP)[21] provides the most direct and accurate means of determining the cause, location, and extent of obstruction in the symptomatic client. If the obstruction is thought to be due to a stone, ERCP is the procedure of choice, because it permits endoscopic sphincterotomy, which opens the sphincter of Oddi (see Fig. 14–8) and allows passage of gallstones up to 1 cm in size. Alternately, endoscopic sphincterotomy and stone extraction may be combined with laparoscopic cholecystectomy. Shock wave lithotripsy is used when stones are too large to extract via the endoscopic approach. Medical management includes antibiotic therapy when cholangitis is present.

A high mortality (50%), caused by rapidly developing and fatal sepsis, occurs when common bile duct stones (choledocholithiasis) are accompanied by inflammation of the bile duct (cholangitis).

[19] The combination of pain, fever and chills, and jaundice is referred to as *Charcot's triad*, the classic picture of cholangitis.

[20] ERCP consists of introduction of radiopaque medium into the biliary system by percutaneous puncture of a bile duct to provide x-ray examination of the bile ducts.

[21] The endoscope is advanced into the duodenum, a tube is inserted into the lumen of the biliary tract, and contrast medium is injected to visualize all portions of the biliary tree.

Special Implications for the Therapist **14-21**

CHOLEDOCHOLITHIASIS

Special considerations for the therapist are the same as for the client with cholelithiasis. When choledocholithiasis occurs in the absence of a gallbladder (primary common duct stones), the presenting symptom can be shoulder pain. The therapist must be alert to this possibility in anyone who has had a cholecystectomy. (See also Obstructive Jaundice, this chapter.)

Cholecystitis

Cholecystitis, or inflammation of the gallbladder, may be acute or chronic and occurs as a result of impaction of gallstones in the cystic duct (see Fig. 14–8) causing painful distention of the gallbladder. The acute form is most common during middle age, whereas the chronic form is most common among the elderly.

Painful symptoms are similar to those caused by gallstones (see Cholelithiasis, earlier), with biliary colic (described as severe) and steady right upper quadrant abdominal pain with abdominal tenderness, muscle guarding, and rebound pain. Upper quadrant pain often radiates to the upper back (between the scapulae) and into the right scapula or right shoulder. Accompanying GI symptoms usually include nausea, anorexia, and vomiting. Gallbladder "attacks" are usually precipitated by a large or fatty meal, because decreased bile production results in decreased fat digestion.

Diagnosis is made on the basis of clinical history, examination, laboratory findings, and imaging. The WBC count is usually elevated (12,000 to 15,000/μL). Total serum bilirubin, serum aminotransferase, and alkaline phosphatase levels are often elevated in the acute disease, but they are normal or minimally elevated in the chronic form. X-ray films of the abdomen show radiopaque gallstones in 15% of cases. Right upper quadrant abdominal ultrasound may show the presence of gallstones, but it is not specific for acute cholecystitis (much higher sensitivity for cholelithiasis). Radionuclide scanning (hepatobiliary imaging, also known as hepatoiminodiacetic acid [HIDA] scan) is useful in demonstrating an obstructed cystic duct; if the gallbladder fills with the isotope, acute cholecystitis is unlikely, but filling of the bile duct strongly suggests a positive diagnosis.

Acute cholecystitis usually subsides within 1 to 7 days on a conservative plan of medical treatment including analgesic, antibiotics, withholding of oral feedings, and intravenous alimentation. Cholecystectomy (gallbladder resection) is required when symptoms do not resolve, or it may be indicated in the case of chronic cholecystitis.

Prognosis for both acute and chronic cholecystitis is good with medical intervention. Acute attacks may resolve spontaneously, but recurrences are common. Complications are often quite serious and are usually associated with infection and sepsis. The mortality of acute cholecystitis is 5% to 10% for clients older than 60 years with serious associated diseases.

Special Implications for Therapy **14-22**

CHOLECYSTITIS

Special considerations for the therapist are the same as for the client with Cholelithiasis (see also Obstructive Jaundice, this chapter). It is possible for a person to develop acholelithiasis cholecystitis, or inflammation of the gallbladder without gallstones. The therapist may see a clinical picture typical of gallbladder disease, including mid-upper back or scapular pain (below or between the scapulae) or right shoulder pain associated with right upper quadrant abdominal pain. Close questioning may reveal accompanying associated GI signs and symptoms.

The person may have been evaluated for gallbladder disease, but ultrasonography does not always show small stones. Unless further and more elaborate testing has been performed to examine gallbladder function, the individual may end up in therapy for treatment of the affected musculoskeletal areas. Lack of results from therapy and/or progression of symptoms corresponding to progression of disease require further medical follow-up.

Primary Biliary Cirrhosis

(See Primary Biliary Cirrhosis, earlier in this chapter, in the Cirrhosis section.)

Sclerosing Cholangitis

Sclerosing cholangitis is an inflammatory disease of the bile ducts that has been linked to altered immunity, toxins, and infectious agents, and is thought to have a possible genetic etiology. Approximately two-thirds of cases occur in clients 20 to 40 years of age; it has a higher incidence in men and is often seen in association with ulcerative colitis.

The inflammatory process associated with this disease results in fibrosis and thickening of the ductal walls and multiple concentric strictures. This fibrosing process narrows and eventually obstructs the intrahepatic and extrahepatic bile ducts. Symptomatic presentation usually includes pruritus and jaundice accompanied by fatigue, anorexia, and weight loss. Vague upper abdominal pain may be present.

Diagnosis is made on the basis of clinical findings confirmed by ERCP or liver biopsy. Medical management may include corticosteroids and long-term antibiotic therapy for recurrent cholangitis (see earlier section, Choledocholithiasis). Liver transplantation is the only medical treatment that offers a cure for this condition.

The prognosis is poor owing to the progressive nature of this disease, with gradual development of cirrhosis, portal hypertension, and death from hepatic failure. Death occurs within 2 to 3 years after the appearance of symptoms. Clients with this condition may also be predisposed to the development of cholangiocarcinoma. Survival rates with liver transplantation are 71% at 1 year and 57% at 3 years (LaRusso, 1991).

Special Implications for the Therapist **14-23**

SCLEROSING CHOLANGITIS

Special considerations for the therapist are the same as for the client with Cholelithiasis (see also Obstructive Jaundice, this chapter).

Neoplasms of the Gallbladder and Biliary Tract

Benign Neoplasms

Biliary neoplasms, whether benign or malignant, are rare. *Papillomas* are the most common benign tumors affecting the gallbladder or common bile duct; they may be single or multiple and are often associated with gallstones. Benign tumors of the common bile duct are more clinically significant because they can obstruct biliary flow and cause obstructive jaundice. *Adenomas*, benign epithelial tumors, may be premalignant based on the observation that adenocarcinoma occurs in as many as 50% to 80% of persons with adenoma. Treatment is usually removal by cholecystectomy as most lesions that are found cause symptoms and are possibly premalignant.

Malignant Neoplasms

Adenocarcinoma of the gallbladder is the most common malignant lesion of the biliary tract (90% of cases), but it only accounts for 5% of all cancers at the time of autopsy. Predisposing factors include age over 60 years, female sex, gallstones, ulcerative colitis, and membership in certain racial or ethnic groups (Japanese, Japanese-American, Mexicans, Mexican-American, certain American Indian tribes, native Alaskan, and Bolivian). Workers in the textile, rubber, and metal-fabricating industries may have an increased incidence (Meyers and Jones, 1990).

Bile duct cancer is the second most common biliary tract malignancy; it occurs predominantly in men. Gallstones are also present in 70% of all cases. Spread of cancer, whether originating in the gallbladder or bile duct, occurs by direct extension into the liver or to the peritoneal surface, and it may do so before symptoms develop. Other metastatic sites include the lymph nodes, lung, bone, and adrenal glands.

Clinical presentation of malignant gallbladder diseases depends on the stage of disease and the location and extent of the lesion, but it is often insidious. By the time the tumor becomes symptomatic, it is almost invariably incurable. Symptoms most often mimic gallstone disease (acute and chronic cholecystitis). Right upper quadrant pain radiating to the upper back is the most common symptom (75% of cases), with weight loss, progressive (obstructive) jaundice, anorexia, and right upper quadrant mass occurring in 40% to 50% of cases. Pruritus and skin excoriations are commonly associated with the presence of jaundice.

Diagnosis is often made unexpectedly during surgery. Most gallbladder cancers have caused significant clinical problems at the time of diagnosis (laparotomy). The most helpful diagnostic studies before surgery are either percutaneous transhepatic cholangiography or ERCP with biopsy.

Treatment varies; it may include radical resection if the tumor is well localized without metastases, palliative relief of duct obstruction (obstructive jaundice) for unresectable tumor, and chemotherapy or radiation for local control and pain relief. Prognosis is poor even with treatment, and few people survive more than 6 months after diagnosis; the 5 year survival rate is 5% (Chao and Greager, 1991).

Special Implications for the Therapist **14-24**

GALLBLADDER AND BILIARY TRACT NEOPLASM

Special considerations for the therapist are the same as for the client with cholelithiasis (See also Obstructive Jaundice, this chapter.) See also general principles related to the oncology client (Chapter 7).

References

Abrams WB, Beers MH, Berkow R: The Merck Manual of Geriatrics, ed 2. Rahway, NJ, Merck & Co, 1995.
Adami H-O, Hsing AW, McLaughlin JK, et al: Alcoholism and liver cirrhosis in the etiology of primary liver cancer. Int J Cancer 51:898–902, 1992.
Alkire KT: Cancers of the pancreas, hepatobiliary, and endocrine systems. *In* Baird SB (ed): A Cancer Source Book for Nurses, ed 6. Atlanta, American Cancer Society, 1991, pp 200–208.
Alter MJ: Review of serologic testing for hepatitis C virus infection and risk of posttransfusion hepatitis C. Arch Pathol Lab Med 118:342–345, 1994.
American Academy of Pediatrics: Prevention of hepatitis A infections: Guidelines for use of hepatitis A vaccine and immune globulin. Pediatrics 98(6 pt 1):1207–1215, 1996.
American Cancer Society: Cancer statistics 1997. CA Cancer J Clin 47:5–27, 1997.
American Medical Society for Sports Medicine and American Orthopaedic Society for Sports Medicine: Position statement on HIV and other blood-borne pathogens in sports. American J of Sports Medicine 23(4):510–516, 1995.
Andreoli TE, Bennett JC, Carpenter CCJ, et al (eds): Cecil Essentials of Medicine, ed 3. Philadelphia, WB Saunders, 1993.
Baron RL: Understanding and optimizing use of contrast material for CT of the liver. AJR 163:323–331, 1994.
Beahrs OH, Henson DE, Hutter RVP, et al (eds): American Joint Committee on Cancer (AJCC) Manual for Staging of Cancer. Philadelphia, JB Lippincott, 1992, pp 89–90.
Boon AP, Adams DH, Buckels JAC, et al: Neuropathological findings in autopsies after liver transplantation. Transplant Proc 23:1471–1472, 1991.
Boyle P, Hsieh CC, Maisonneuve P, et al: Epidemiology of pancreas cancer. Int J Pancreatol 5:327–346, 1989.
Brewer MA, Edwards KM, Decker MS: Who should receive hepatitis A vaccine? Pediatr Infect Dis J 14:258–260, 1995.
Carey MC: Pathogenesis of gallstones. Am J Surg 165:410–419, 1993.
Carithers RL: Liver diseases. *In* Ramsey PG, Larson EB: Medical Therapeutics, ed 2. Philadelphia, WB Saunders, 1993, pp 330–373.
Centers for Disease Control and Prevention (CDC): Intradermal Administration of Hepatitis B Vaccine: An update. Hepatitis Surveillance report No. 54. Atlanta, CDC, 1992.
CDC: Why does my baby need hepatitis B vaccine? Atlanta, US Dept of Health and Human Services, 1994.
Chao TC, Greager JA: Primary carcinoma of the gallbladder. J Surg Oncol 46:215, 1991.
Ching N, Lumeng J, Pang R, et al: Long-term low dose interferon alpha-2b in the treatment of chronic hepatitis B in multi-ethnic patients in Hawaii. Hawaii Med 55:201–203, 1996.
Columbo M: Hepatocellular carcinoma. J Hepatol 15:225–236, 1992.
Czaja AJ: Chronic active hepatitis. *In* Lichtenstein LM, Dauci AS (eds): Current Therapy in Allergy, Immunology, and Rheumatology. St Louis, Mosby–Year Book, 1992, pp 273–278.
Czaja AJ, Davis GL, Ludwig J, et al: Autoimmune features as determinants of prognosis in steroid-treated chronic active hepatitis of uncertain etiology. Gastroenterology 85:713–717, 1983.
Czaja AJ: Natural history, clinical features, and treatment of autoimmune hepatitis. Semin Liver Dis 4:1–12, 1984.
Czaja AJ: Type 1 autoimmune hepatitis new term for lupoid hepatitis. Musculoskel Med 11:11–15, 1994.
Dana F, Becherer PR, Bacon BR: Hepatitis C virus: What recent studies can tell us. Postgrad Med 95:121–130, 1994.
Danek GD, Huether SE: Alterations of digestive function in children. *In* McCance KL, Huether SE (eds): Pathophysiology: The Biologic Basis for Disease in Adults and Children, ed 2. St Louis, Mosby–Year Book, 1994, pp 1376–1403.
Diekema DJ, Doebbeling BN: Employee health and infection control. Infect Control Hosp Epidemiol 16:292–301, 1995.
Douglas DD, Rakela J, Hin HJ, et al: Randomized controlled trial of recombinant alpha-2a-interferon for chronic hepatitis C. Dig Dis Sci 38:601–607, 1993.

Ellis RW: Hepatitis B vaccines in clinical practice. New York, Marcel Dekker, 1993.

Ewenstein B: Hepatitis C: New understanding about an old viral enemy. Natl Hemophilia Foundation Community Alert Publ 1:1–2, May 1994.

Farmer DG, Rosove MH, Shaked A, et al: Current treatment modalities for hepatocellular carcinoma. Ann Surg 219:236–247, 1994.

Fennerty MB: Primary sclerosing cholangitis and primary biliary cirrhosis: How effective is medical therapy? Postgrad Med 94:81–88, 92, 1993.

Ferenci P: Pathophysiology of hepatic encephalopathy. Hepatogastroenterology 38:371–376, 1991.

Fontham ET, Correa P: Epidemiology of pancreatic cancer. Surg Clin North Am 69:551–567, 1989.

Foster JH, Berman MM: The malignant transformation of liver cell adenomas. Arch Surg 129:712–717, 1994.

Fried MW: Therapy of chronic viral hepatitis. Med Clin North Am 80:957–972, 1996.

Friedman LS, Knauer CM: Liver, biliary tract, and pancreas. *In* Tierney LM, McPhee SJ, Papadakis MA: Current Medical Diagnosis and Treatment, ed 33. Norwalk, Conn, Appleton & Lange, 1994, pp 528–562.

Gibbons JC, Levy SM: Gastrointestinal diseases in the aged. *In* Reichel W (ed): Clinical Aspects of Aging, ed 3. Baltimore, Williams & Wilkins, 1989, pp 188–198.

Gilkson M, Galun E, Oren R, et al: Relapsing hepatitis A. Medicine 71:14–23, 1992.

Gilliam JH: Hepatobiliary disorders. *In* Hazzard WR, Andres R, Bierman EL, et al (eds): Principles of Geriatric Medicine and Gerontology. New York, McGraw-Hill, 1990, pp 631–639.

Gocke DJ: Systemic manifestations of viral liver disease. *In* Gitnick GL (ed): Current Hepatology, vol 2. New York, John Wiley & Sons, 1982, pp 273–288.

Goodman CC, Synder TE: Differential Diagnosis in Physical Therapy, ed 2. Philadelphia, WB Saunders, 1995.

Harruff RC: Pathology Facts. Philadelphia, JB Lippincott, 1994.

Herrera JL: Serologic diagnosis of viral hepatitis. South Med J 87:677–684, 1994.

High KP, Washburn RG: Invasive aspergillosis in mice immunosuppressed with cyclosporin A, tacrolimus (FK506), or sirolimus (rapamycin). J Infect Dis 175:222–225, 1997.

Holt S: Chronic pancreatitis. South Med J 86:201–207, 1993.

Huether SE, McCance KL: Alterations of digestive function. *In* McCance KL, Huether SE: Pathophysiology: The Biologic Basis for Disease in Adults and Children, ed 2. St Louis, Mosby–Year Book, 1994, pp 1320–1375.

Johnson AG, Triger DR: Liver Disease and Gallstones: The Facts, ed 2. Oxford, Oxford University Press, 1992.

Kallsen C: Nursing care of clients with biliary and exocrine pancreatic disorders. *In* Black J, Matassarin-Jacobs E (eds): Luckmann and Sorensen's Medical-Surgical Nursing: A Psychophysiologic Approach, ed 4. Philadelphia, WB Saunders, 1993, pp 1731–1754.

Katkov WN, Dienstag JL: Hepatitis vaccines. Gastroenterol Clin North Am 24:147–159, 1995.

Keefe EB, Esquivel CO: Controversies in patient selection for liver transplantation. West J Med 159:586–593, 1993.

Key LL, Bell NH: Osteomalacia and disorders of vitamin D metabolism. *In* Stein JH (ed): Internal Medicine, ed 4. St Louis, Mosby–Year Book, 1994, pp 1520–1528.

Koff RS: Hepatitis B today: Clinical and diagnostic overview. Pediatr Infect Dis J 12:428–432, 1993.

Kuo, G, Choo QL, Alter HJ: An assay for circulating antibodies to a major etiologic virus of human non-A, non-B hepatitis. Science 244:362–364, 1989.

LaRusso NF: Primary sclerosing cholangitis. Semin Liver Dis 11:1, 1991.

Lee MJ, Mueller PR, vanSonnenberg E, et al: CT-Guided celiac ganglion block with alcohol. AJR 161:633–636, 1993.

Lindberg MC: Hepatobiliary complications of oral contraceptives. J Gen Intern Med 7:199–209, 1992.

Livingston EH, Welton ML, Reber HA: Surgical treatment of pancreatic cancer: The United States experience. Int J Pancreatol 9:153–157, 1991.

Lynch HT, Fusaro L, Lynch JG: Familial pancreatic cancer: A family study. Pancreas 7:511–515, 1992.

MacKay HT, Evans AT: Gynecology and obstetrics. *In* Tierney LM, McPhee SJ, Papadakis MA: Current Medical Diagnosis and Treatment, ed 33. Norwalk, Conn, Appleton & Lange, 1994, pp 587–639.

Mackay JR, Taft LI, Cowling DD: Lucoid hepatitis. Lancet 2:1323–1326, 1956.

Marx J: Viral hepatitis: Unscrambling the alphabet. Nursing 93 23:34–41, 1993.

Matassarin-Jacobs E, Strasburg K: Nursing care of clients with hepatic disorders. *In* Black JM, Matassarin-Jacobs E (eds): Luckmann and Sorensen's Medical-Surgical Nursing, ed 4. Philadelphia, WB Saunders, 1993, pp 1697–1730.

Matsui O, Kadoya M, Yoshikawa J, et al: Small hepatocellular carcinoma: Treatment with subsegmental transcatheter arterial embolization. Radiology 188:79–83, 1993.

Meyers WC, Jones RS: Textbook of Liver and Biliary Surgery. Philadelphia, JB Lippincott, 1990.

Mirza DF, Gunson BK, Soonawalla Z: Reduced acute rejection after liver transplantation with Neoral-based triple immunosuppression. Lancet 349:701–702, 1997.

MMWR: Immunization Practices Advisory Committee: Hepatitis B virus: A comprehensive strategy for eliminating transmission in the United States through universal childhood vaccination. MMWR 40(No. RR-13):1–25, 1991.

MMWR: Licensure of inactivated hepatitis A vaccine and recommendations for use among international travelers. MMWR 44:559–560, 1995.

Murr MM, Sarr MG, Oishi AJ, et al: Pancreatic cancer. CA Cancer J Clin 44:304–318, 1994.

Naccarato R, Farinati F: Hepatocellular carcinoma, alcohol, and cirrhosis: Facts and hypotheses. Dig Dis Sci 36:1137–1142, 1991.

Najm W: Viral hepatitis: How to manage type C and D infections. Geriatrics 52:28–30, 33–34, 37, 1997.

OSHA/US Department of Labor: Occupational exposure to bloodborne pathogens: Final rule. Federal Register 56:64004, 1991.

Page AR, Sharp HL, Greenberg LJ: Genetic analysis of patients with chronic active hepatitis. J Clin Invest 56:530–535, 1975.

Power C, Poland SD, Kassim KH, et al: Encephalopathy in liver transplantation: Neuropathology and CMV infection. Can J Neurol Sci 17:378–381, 1990.

Purcell RH: Hepatitis viruses: Changing patterns of human disease. Proc Natl Acad Sci USA 91:2401–2406, 1994a.

Purcell RH: Hepatitis C virus: Historical perspective and current concepts. FEMS Microbiol Rev 14:181–191, 1994b.

Resnick RH: Management of varices in cirrhosis. Hosp Pract 28:123–130, 1993.

Ridge JA, Way LW: Abdominal pain. *In* Sleisenger MH (ed): Gastrointestinal Disease, ed 5. Philadelphia, JB Lippincott, 1993, pp 150–161.

Rubin E, Farber JL: The liver and biliary system. *In* Rubin E, Farber JL (eds): Pathology, ed 2. Philadelphia, JB Lippincott, 1994, pp 705–784.

Rubin RA, Falestiny M, Malet PF: Chronic hepatitis C: Advances in diagnostic testing and therapy. Arch Intern Med 154:387–392, 1994.

Rugo HS: Cancer. *In* Tierney LM, McPhee SJ, Papadakis MA: Current Medical Diagnosis and Treatment, ed 33. Norwalk, Conn, Appleton & Lange, 1994, pp 61–88.

Scarpelli DG: The pancreas. *In* Rubin E, Farber JL (eds): Pathology, ed 2. Philadelphia, JB Lippincott, 1994, pp 787–803.

Sherlock DS: Chronic hepatitis C. Dis Month 40:117–126, 1994a.

Sherlock DS: Primary biliary cirrhosis: Clarifying the issues. Am J Med 96:27S–33S, 1994b.

Sherlock S, Dooley J: Diseases of the Liver and Biliary System, ed 9. Oxford, Blackwell Scientific Publications, 1993.

Sichieri R, Everhart JE, Roth H: A prospective study of hospitalization with gallstone disease among women: Role of dietary factors, fasting period, and dieting. Am J Public Health 81:880–884, 1991.

Silverman A, Sokol RJ: Liver and pancreas. *In* Hathaway WE, Hay WW, Groothuis JR, et al (eds): Current Pediatric Diagnosis and Treatment, ed 11. Norwalk, Conn, Appleton & Lange, 1993, pp 611–647.

Sineath L: Unpublished data (personal communication), 1995.

Singh N, Yu VL, Gayowski T: Central nervous system lesions in adult liver transplant recipients: Clinical review with implications for management. Medicine 73:110–118, 1994.

Smeltzer S, Bare B: Brunner and Suddarth's Medical-Surgical Nursing, ed 7. New York, JB Lippincott, 1992, pp 971–1021.

Smith CS, Paauw DS: Hepatocellular carcinoma: Identifying and screening populations at increased risk. Postgrad Med 94:71–74, 1993.

Spencer MP, Sarr MG, Nagomey DM: Radical pancreatectomy for

pancreatic cancer in the elderly: Is it safe and justified? Ann Surg 212:140–143, 1990.

Steinberg WM: Pancreatitis. *In* Wyngaarden JB, Smith LH, Bennett JC (eds): Cecil Textbook of Medicine, ed 19. Philadelphia, WB Saunders, 1992, pp 721–727.

Stewart JS, Farrow JL, Clifford RE, et al: A three-year survey of viral hepatitis in West London. Q J Med 187:365, 1978.

Stratta RJ, Shaeffer MS, Markin RS, et al: Cytomegalovirus infection and disease after liver transplantation: An overview. Dig Dis Sci 37:673–688, 1992.

Streem SB: Contemporary clinical practice of shock wave lithotripsy: A reevaluation of contraindications. J Urol 157:1197–2203, 1997.

Swartz ML: Intron A (interferon-alpha-2b recombinant) for injection. Gastroenterol Nursing 14:40–43, 1991.

Trotta PP: The clinical potential of recombinant human interleukin 4 and alfa-2b interferon. Am J Reprod Immunol 25:124–128, 1991.

Tsukuma H, Hiyama T, Tanaka S, et al: Risk factors for hepatocellular carcinoma among patients with chronic liver disease. N Engl J Med 328:1797–1801, 1993.

US Department of Health and Human Services, Division of Viral and Rickettsial Diseases: Hepatitis B Prevention. Atlanta, CDC, October 1992.

Van Damme P, Kane M, Meheus A: Integration of hepatitis B vaccination into national immunization programs. BMJ 314:1033–1036, 1997.

Vogt DP, Lederman RJ, Carey WD, et al: Neurologic complications of liver transplantation. Transplantation 6:1057–1061, 1988.

Wilson L, Lester L: Liver, biliary tract and pancreas. *In* Price S, Wilson L (eds): Pathophysiology: Clinical Concepts of Disease Processes, ed 4. St Louis, Mosby-Year Book, 1992, pp 337–368.

Wong DL: Whaley & Wong's Essentials of Pediatric Nursing, ed 4. St Louis, Mosby–Year Book, 1993.

Woolf GM, Petrovic LM, Rojter SE, et al: Acute liver failure due to lymphoma: A diagnostic concern when considering liver transplantation. Dig Dis Sci 39:1351–1358, 1994.

Yamada R, Kishi K, Sonomura T, et al: Transcatheter arterial embolization in unresectable hepatocellular carcinoma. Cardiovasc Int Radiol 13:135–139, 1990.

Yu MC, Tong MJ, Coursaget P, et al: Prevalence of hepatitis B and C viral markers in black and white patients with hepatocellular carcinoma in the United States. J Natl Cancer Inst 82:1038–1041, 1990.

Zetterman RK: Primary care management of the liver transplant patient. Am J Med 96:10S–17S, 1994.

SECTION 2

chapter 15

Urinary Tract Disorders

William G. Boissonnault

The structures associated with the excretion of urine are the kidneys, ureters, bladder, and urethra (Fig. 15–1). The process of excretion involves filtration (kidney) and storage (bladder). These functions expose the kidney and bladder to carcinogens for extended periods, increasing the risk of cancer developing in these organs compared to the other urinary tract structures. In addition, the urethra of females lies close to the vaginal and rectal openings, allowing for relative ease of bacterial transport and increased risk of infection. The fact that the urethra is shorter in females is one reason why urinary tract infections (UTIs) are more common in females.

UTIs and urinary incontinence are extremely common. UTIs rank second only to upper respiratory tract infections in incidence of bacterial infections. Urinary incontinence afflicts a significant percentage of the geriatric population. Therapists encounter these two disorders frequently in the clinical arena.

Although specific age-related anatomic changes have not been associated with urinary tract disease, certain age groups, such as the elderly, are at significant risk of developing a variety of disorders. The effect of multiple medications, conditions such as benign prostatic hyperplasia (BPH), and pelvic floor disorders, and the incidence of pelvic surgeries and catheterization in this population all increase the risk of developing urinary tract disease. Considering the percentage of the rehabilitation population made up by the elderly, therapists are frequently confronted by disorders of the system.

Therapists have an important role on the medical team for treatment of a number of urinary tract diseases. For example, rehabilitation for those on dialysis or postrenal transplant is vital. Therapists also have a key role in the conservative management of urinary incontinence. Other conditions, such as infections, are common comorbidities confronting the therapist. The presence of UTI increases the risk of infection developing elsewhere. This could occur while the therapist is treating someone for a knee injury or postcerebral vascular accident. Understanding how these diseases and the prescribed medical treatment can influence rehabilitative efforts is essential to help ensure a positive functional outcome.

INFECTIONS

Lower Urinary Tract Infections

Cystitis is an example of a lower UTI. Pyelonephritis is an example of an upper UTI. This section covers lower UTIs. Pyelonephritis is discussed separately. Geriatric and pediatric concerns are discussed first.

UTIs are very common in the geriatric population. Approximately 20% of women and 10% of men living at home have bacteriuria. For those living in nursing homes or extended care facilities the prevalence of infection is even higher: 25% for women and 20% for men (Baldassare and Kaye, 1991). The elderly are at higher risk for this disease for several reasons: general immobility or inactivity, which causes impaired bladder emptying; bladder ischemia resulting from urine retention; urinary outflow obstruction from renal calculi and prostatic hyperplasia; senile vaginitis; constipation; and diminished bactericidal activity of prostatic secretions (Zweig, 1987). The clinical manifestations in this population can be varied and somewhat surprising. The expected complaints of fever, chills, and sweats may be absent. Flank pain, urgency, frequency, and incontinence are potential symptoms, but may not be present until the infection is well advanced (Baldassare and Kaye, 1991). Lastly, the communication difficulties that occur with this population can delay detection of this disease.

Up to 5% of female and 1% to 2% of male children experience UTIs. In addition, recurrent UTIs can occur in up to 80% of children who experience uncomplicated infection. Risk factors for this condition include premature birth; the presence of urinary tract abnormalities such as neurogenic bladder and systemic or immunologic disease; and a family history of UTI (Zelikovic et al., 1992). The classic features of UTIs—enuresis, frequency, dysuria, suprapubic pain—become evident in older children (Mattson Porth, 1994).

Risk Factors. Urinary tract instrumentation and urinary catheterization are the most common predisposing factors related to the development of UTIs (Kunin, 1984). A history of urinary obstruction and reflux also increases the risk of UTI. The obstruction results in urinary stasis and the reflux may cause bacteria to be drawn up into the bladder or ureters. Urinary tract calculi, prostatic hyperplasia, and pregnancy can all cause urinary obstruction.

Adult women are at greater risk of developing UTI than men for several reasons. As mentioned, the urethra in females is shorter and also close to the entrances to the vagina and rectum. The bacteria that result in most UTIs are acquired from the large bowel. The urethral meatus is close to the fecal reservoir and rectum. Sexually active women are at higher risk of developing UTIs because it is thought that sexual intercourse can influence the movement of bacteria in the direction of the bladder. This again is due to the proximity of the urethral meatus and vagina. UTIs are more common during pregnancy. The increased risk is due to dilation of the upper urinary system, reduction of the peristaltic activity of the ureters, and displacement of the urinary bladder, which moves to a more abdominal position, thus further affecting the ureteral position (Mattson Porth, 1994).

Clinical Manifestations. Adults with UTI may present with urinary irritative symptoms including frequency, ur-

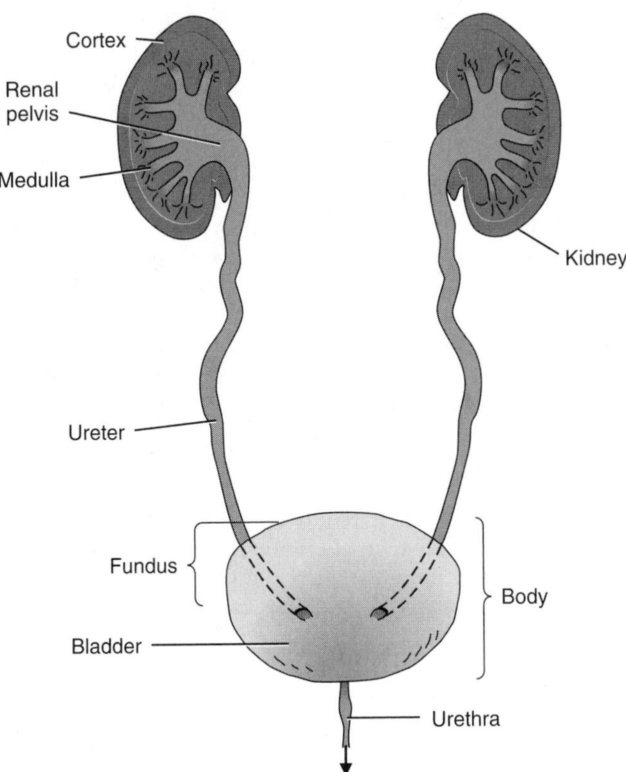

Figure **15-1.** Urinary tract structures.

gency, and dysuria. Pain may be noted in the suprapubic, lower abdominal, or flank areas depending on the location of the infection. Fever, chills, and malaise may also be present.

Medical Management

Diagnosis. The diagnosis of UTI is typically made following urinalysis. A bacterial count of greater than 100,000 organisms per milliliter of urine is a commonly accepted criterion for diagnosis. Besides the bacterial count the urine leukocyte count is also used. Ultrasound, radiographs, computed tomography (CT), and renal scans may be used to identify contributing factors such as obstruction.

Treatment. Antibiotic agents are typically used to treat acute infections. Increased fluid intake may also help relieve symptoms and signs and is often used as an adjunct to pharmacologic treatment. (See Special Implications for the Therapist: Pyelonephritis).

Pyelonephritis

Overview. Pyelonephritis is an infectious, inflammatory disease involving the kidney parenchyma and renal pelvis. The disease can be acute or chronic. Acute pyelonephritis is typically related to a bacterial infection. Chronic pyelonephritis is a tubulointerstitial disorder marked by progressive, gross, and irregular scarring and deformation of the calices and overlying parenchyma (Spargo and Haas, 1994). The anatomic changes can lead to insufficient renal function. Chronic pyelonephritis may be responsible for up to 25% of the population with endstage renal disease (Mattson Porth, 1994).

Etiology. Gram-negative bacteria such as *Escherichia coli*, and *Proteus*, *Klebsiella*, *Enterobacter*, and *Pseudomonas* species are the most common agents associated with acute pyelonephritis (Presti et al., 1995). Infection may also be associated with chronic disease, but when present is superimposed on either obstruction or vesicoureteral reflux[1] or both.

Risk Factors. The majority of cases of acute pyelonephritis are associated with ascending UTIs. Catheterization, urinary tract instrumentation, vesicoureteral reflux, pregnancy, diabetes, and neurogenic bladder increase susceptibility to UTI. Catheterization and urinary tract instrumentation may transfer bacterial organisms that lie at the distal end of the urethra into the bladder. Females are more prone to ascending UTI because of the absence of prostatic secretions, which have an antibacterial action, and the fact that they have a shorter urethra. People with diabetes are more prone to infection because of the associated glycosuria which provides a fertile medium for bacterial growth. The increased risk of infection during pregnancy is associated with a decreased tone of bladder musculature. This does not allow for urine to be expelled with the usual efficiency. Other conditions that can result in this increased residual urine volume are prostatic obstruction and atonic bladder associated with paraplegia or diabetic neuropathy.

In other cases pyelonephritis can stem from bloodborne pathogens associated with infection elsewhere. People with bacterial endocarditis and miliary tuberculosis are susceptible to kidney involvement. In addition, immunocompromised persons are at risk for fungi seeding the kidney.

Pathogenesis. While urine is typically sterile, the distal end of the urethra is commonly colonized by bacterial flora. As described under Risk Factors there are many ways in which bacteria can be transported to the urinary bladder. After urination, the subsequent passage of sterile urine from the kidneys to the bladder dilutes any bacteria that may have entered the bladder. If the residual urine volume is increased, as with an atonic bladder, an accumulation of insufficiently diluted bacteria can occur. Bacteria in the bladder urine typically does not gain access to the ureters for a variety of anatomic reasons. But people with an abnormally short passage of the ureter within the bladder muscle wall and an angle of ureter insertion into the bladder wall that is more perpendicular are at risk for reflux of urine into the ureter itself. This reflux can be of sufficient force to carry the urine and the accompanying bacteria into the renal pelvis and calices. The bacteria will not necessarily enter the renal parenchyma unless the reflux pressure is prolonged.

Clinical Manifestations. The onset of symptoms and signs associated with acute pyelonephritis is usually abrupt. The complaints may include fever, chills, malaise, headache, and back pain. The person may also complain of tenderness over the costovertebral angle. Also, often present are symptoms of bladder irritation, including dysuria, urinary frequency, and urgency.

---

[1] Urine forced from the urinary bladder into the ureters and kidneys.

Medical Management

Diagnosis. The presence of the above symptoms calls for laboratory testing. Urinalysis will reveal pyuria, bacteriuria, and varying degrees of hematuria. A urine culture will demonstrate heavy growth of the bacterial agent. In addition, the blood count may show leukocytosis.

Treatment. If the infection is severe enough or if complicating factors are present, hospital admission may be required for treatment. Typically, however, the condition is treated with an appropriate antibiotic medication. Symptoms typically begin disappearing within several days. If the person does not show improvement within 48 to 72 hours, contact with their physician is warranted.

Special Implications for the Therapist **15-1**

URINARY TRACT INFECTIONS

Depending on the severity of the infection the patient may not be able to participate fully in a rehabilitation program until the disease is brought under control. If the client begins to complain of nausea or vomiting, has a fever greater than 102° F, or the therapist notes a change in mental status, immediate contact with the client's physician is warranted. These may be indications for hospital admission. Lastly, being aware of the symptoms and signs associated with this disease may allow the therapist to recognize the onset of pyelonephritis in its early stages. The initial symptoms may be subtle enough that the client is not alarmed to the point that he or she visits a physician. Early detection and treatment of this disorder is important to prevent possible permanent structural damage. UTIs also increase the risk of development of infection elsewhere in the body, including osteomyelitis, pleurisy, and pericarditis. See Chapters 21, 12, and 10, respectively, for a description of these disorders.

RENAL DISORDERS

Cancer

Renal Cell Carcinoma

Overview. Renal cell carcinoma is the most common adult renal neoplasm accounting for approximately 80% to 90% of renal tumors (Spargo and Haas, 1994; Mattson Porth, 1994). The term *renal cell carcinoma* is based on the cell of origin, the nephron, consisting of the renal corpuscle, the proximal convoluted tubule, the nephronic loop, and the distal convoluted tubule (Tannenbaum, 1971).

Etiology. Although a genetic basis is strongly suggested, no specific etiologic agent has been identified (Robertson, 1994). Renal cell carcinoma has been linked with von Hippel-Lindau disease, which is an autosomal dominant hereditary disorder. This disease is linked to a defect of a gene on chromosome 3. Defects of this chromosome have also been demonstrated in people with renal cell carcinoma (Spargo and Haas, 1994).

Incidence. Adult kidney neoplasms account for approximately 2% of all cancers. An estimated 28,800 new cases are expected to be diagnosed and approximately 11,300 deaths related to kidney cancer are estimated to occur in 1997 (Parker et al., 1997). Renal cell carcinoma is the most commonly diagnosed kidney neoplasm in adults, but this disease can also occur in children and young adults.

Risk Factors. Renal cell carcinoma occurs twice as frequently in males as in females. The age range of peak incidence is 60 to 70 years. Cigarette smoking is linked to this condition with an estimated 25% to 33% of these cancers being directly caused by smoking (Spargo and Haas, 1994; Frank et al., 1991). Obesity has also been linked to an increased risk of renal cell carcinoma, especially in women.

Pathogenesis. Renal cell carcinomas are of four histologic subtypes: (1) clear cell, (2) granular cell, (3) papillary adenocarcinoma, and (4) the sarcomatoid variant. The tumors are typically yellow-orange in color and often demonstrate focal hemorrhage and necrosis. The lesions are solid or focally cystic. Metastasis most frequently occurs to the lungs and the skeletal system (Spargo and Haas, 1994).

Clinical Manifestations. Kidney cancers are generally silent during the early stages. Symptoms associated with metastasis are often the initial manifestations. The client may develop a cough or convulsions secondary to metastasis to the lungs or brain or an onset of back pain may occur secondary to a pathologic fracture.

The classic triad associated with renal cancers consists of hematuria, abdominal or flank pain, and a palpable abdominal mass. This combination of findings, however, occurs only in approximately 10% of cases. When it does occur, it carries a poor prognosis (Robertson, 1994). Hematuria is the single most common presenting finding, occurring in up to 50% of cases (Robertson, 1994). In the early stages of this disease the hematuria may be intermittent and microscopic. Other findings include flank pain, weight loss, anemia, abdominal mass, and fever.

Potentially confusing the clinical presentation of this condition is the fact that renal cell carcinomas are a source of ectopic hormone production. Hypertension, hyperparathyroidism, and erythrocytosis can result via this mechanism (Spargo and Haas, 1994; Robertson, 1994).

Medical Management

Diagnosis. The primary feature of renal cell carcinoma is the renal parenchymal mass which can be detected by a variety of imaging modalities. Examples are CT scanning, ultrasonography, excretory urography, and renal angiography. Determining whether the mass is benign or malignant is often difficult, requiring surgical removal before a definitive diagnosis can be made (Robertson, 1994). If hematuria is present, intravenous pyelography (IVP)[2] may be the initial procedure to identify renal abnormalities. Ultrasonography can be used to further evaluate the renal parenchyma, detecting small tumors (less than 1 cm). The advantage of the CT

---

[2] A radiographic test which allows for evaluation of the kidneys, ureters, and bladder. A dye injected into the bloodstream is filtered and secreted by the renal tubules. The IVP provides information including renal size, function, position, the presence of calculi, masses, and congenital variants.

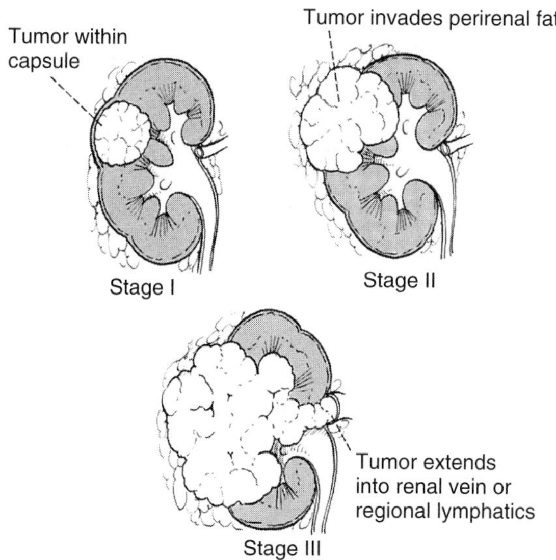

Figure **15–2.** Renal cell carcinoma stages.

scan is that the greatest renal anatomic detail is obtained and in addition details of neighboring organs such as liver, colon, spleen, and lymphatics will also be available.

Staging. The TNM system for staging of this disease was recently updated by the American Joint Committee on Cancer (Beahrs et al., 1992). Organ-confined lesions are associated with a 90% five-year survival rate. If the disease has penetrated the renal capsule and invaded Gerota's fascia[3] or has spread into the regional lymph nodes, the prognosis is poor (Fig. 15–2).

Treatment. Surgery, including radical nephrectomy and regional lymph node dissection, is the treatment of choice for all resectable tumors. For clients with a solitary kidney or abnormal renal function, partial nephrectomy may be performed. No single chemotherapeutic agent has been identified to have significant results with this disease (Pouillson and deVere White, 1993).

Special Implications for the Therapist **15–2**

RENAL CELL CARCINOMA

Therapists working primarily with the geriatric population need to be aware of the symptoms and signs of this disease. Questions related to hematuria, unexplained weight loss, fatigue, fever, and malaise in the history when examining this population is important regardless of the reason for the physical therapy care. Awareness of new onset of unexplained abdominal, flank, or back pain; cough; or other signs of pulmonary involvement should raise concern on the therapist's part and warrants communication with a physician. In addition, renal cell carcinoma is the most common metastatic tumor to the sternum. An onset of sternal pain or a mass in someone with a history of renal cell carcinoma should be brought to the physician's attention.

The extensive abdominal and thoracic surgical sites may produce scarring that affects the client's posture and ability to move, increasing mechanical stress on the musculoskeletal system. Myofascial and soft tissue mobilization treatment of the abdominal and thoracic regions may be of benefit to these people. If there is a history of abnormal renal function in addition to the cancer, additional precautions may need to be taken by the therapist. See Chronic Renal Failure later in this chapter.

[3] A fibroareolar tissue surrounding the kidney and perirenal fat.

Wilms' Tumor

Overview. Wilms' tumor, or nephroblastoma, is the most common malignant neoplasm in children. Grossly, the tumor appears to be fleshy but may have areas of necrosis that lead to cavity formation. There is often a unique mixture of primitive cells, as well as highly differentiated tubular cells resembling embryonic glomeruli and tubules. The tumor can occur bilaterally.

Incidence. Approximately 500 new cases are reported annually in the United States.

Risk Factors. Age is the primary risk factor. The disease most commonly occurs during the first 7 years of life with approximately 75% of cases occurring in children under the age of 5. The peak incidence occurs between the ages of 3 and 4 and the tumor occurs equally in boys and girls.

Clinical Manifestations. The most common presenting feature is a large abdominal mass. Up to 30% of children may complain of abdominal pain, while hematuria may occur in up to 15% to 20% of cases. Symptoms associated with hypertension may occur in up to 50% of children. Lastly, fever, anorexia, and nausea and vomiting may be part of the presentation.

Medical Management

Diagnosis. Abdominal ultrasonography helps define the cystic or solid nature of the mass and helps determine whether the renal vein or vena cava is involved. Excretory urography is also diagnostic. Chest films are indicated to determine whether metastasis has occurred to the pulmonary system. CT scan of the abdomen is helpful in determining the extent of the tumor, but can be difficult to perform with small children.

Treatment. Surgical resection of the tumor is the primary treatment regardless of the stage of the disease. An abdominal surgical approach is generally utilized to allow for bilateral exploration and confirmation of the extent of the disease. Regional lymphadenectomy is carried out, as lymph node involvement strongly affects the prognosis. Chemotherapy is also utilized for all stages of the disease with radiation therapy being added to the treatment regimen for stage III and IV disease. (See Chapter 7 for a discussion of the side effects associated with chemotherapy and radiation therapy.) Wilms' tumor may recur after 9 to 11 years.

Prognosis. Prognosis depends on the histologic appearance of the lesion, stage of the disease, and age of the child. A poor prognosis is indicated by invasion of the mass beyond the renal capsule and by anaplasia of the tumor, which is manifested by nuclear enlargement and hyperchromasia with atypical mitotic figures. Children younger than 2 years of age tend to have a better prognosis with a 2-year survival rate of up to 73%.

Renal Cystic Disease

A renal cyst is a cavity filled with fluid or renal tubular elements making up a semisolid material. The cyst may also be a segment of a dilated nephron. The presence of these cysts can lead to degeneration of renal tissue and obstruction of tubular flow. Renal cysts vary in size considerably, ranging from microscopic to several centimeters in diameter, and can be single or multiple, unilateral or bilateral.

There are four types of renal cystic disease: (1) polycystic kidney disease, (2) medullary sponge kidney, (3) acquired cystic disease, and (4) single or multiple cysts (Bennett et al., 1992). Simple renal cysts are the most common. They are usually less than 1 cm in diameter and do not often produce symptoms or compromise renal function.

Polycystic kidney disease is one of the most common hereditary disorders in the United States (Grantham, 1992). Polycystic kidney disease with the onset in infancy is usually associated with autosomal recessive inheritance and with the onset in adults, is usually associated with autosomal dominant inheritance.

Etiology. In general, renal cystic disease is thought to develop from either tubular obstructions which increase intratubular pressure or from renal tubule basement membrane changes that would allow dilation. The autosomal dominant disease results from a defect on the short arm of chromosome 16. Persons who inherit this gene defect are likely to develop the disorder.

Incidence. Polycystic kidney disease affects more than 500,000 Americans (Grantham, 1992). Approximately 10% of people who develop endstage renal disease have autosomal dominant polycystic kidney disease (Mattson Porth, 1994).

Risk Factors. Regarding autosomal dominant polycystic kidney disease, a positive family history is noted in approximately 75% of cases (Morrison, 1995). A history of UTIs and kidney stones is also a frequent finding.

Pathogenesis. Renal cysts can occur at any point along the nephron. Once the dilation of the tubule occurs forming the cyst, local fluid accumulation results in gradual, but continued growth of the lesion. The tubular dilation can occur from tubular obstruction which elevates luminar pressure or from a defective and highly compliant basement membrane. The expanding cysts can eventually compromise the intrinsic renal vascular system which can obstruct tubular flow and result in degeneration of the renal parenchyma (Spargo and Haas, 1994).

Clinical Manifestations. The simple or solitary cysts are usually asymptomatic and found incidentally on routine urographic examination. Symptoms associated with autosomal dominant disease may include pain, hematuria, fever, and hypertension. Abdominal or flank pain is associated with bleeding into the cyst or growth of the cyst. Most of these clients will have enlarged kidneys, palpable abdominally. The hematuria can be gross or microscopic. Rupture of a cyst usually accounts for the gross hematuria. Fever can be related to an infected cyst secondary to an ascending UTI. The hypertension is caused by compression of the intrarenal blood vessels and the resultant activation of the renin-angiotensin system (Mattson Porth, 1994).

Medical Management

Diagnosis. Most simple cysts are discovered on routine urographic examination. Often urinalysis will detect hematuria and proteinuria or the clinical examination may reveal enlarged, palpable kidneys. The primary concern is to determine if a malignancy is present. Ultrasonography and CT scanning help determine this. At times tissue biopsy or surgical exploration is necessary to make the definitive diagnosis (Presti et al., 1995).

Treatment. If a simple or solitary cyst is found, observation and periodic reassessment is standard procedure. If polycystic kidney disease is present, treatment is primarily supportive. Treating the hypertension and implementing a low protein diet may slow the development of renal failure, but will not prevent it from occurring.

Special Implications for the Therapist **15-4**

RENAL CYSTIC DISEASE

When treating a client with a history of renal cystic disease, therapists should be aware of symptoms and signs suggesting that the condition is worsening. The presence of any of these clinical findings warrants a referral to a physician. An awareness of what this population is at risk for is also necessary. Besides hypertension (see Chapter 10) and UTIs (described earlier) these clients are at increased risk of developing cerebral and aortic aneurysms and mitral valve problems (see Chapter 10). The presentation of any symptoms or signs suggestive of the presence of these conditions again warrants referral to a physician. Lastly, the fact the kidneys may be enlarged can account for atypical findings on palpation.

Renal Calculi

Overview. Urinary stone disease is the third most common urinary tract disorder, exceeded only by infections and prostate disease. A majority of the stones develop in the kidneys and are designated by the term *nephrolithiasis*. The calculi are crystalline and when 1 to 5 mm in diameter can cause urinary obstruction (Mattson Porth, 1994). Urinary obstruction typically occurs at one of the following three sites: (1) the ureteropelvic junction, (2) where the ureter crosses over the iliac vessels, and (3) at the ureterovesical junction (Fig. 15–3) (Presti et al., 1995). There are four basic types of stones: calcium, magnesium ammonium phosphate, uric acid, and cystine. Eighty percent to 90% of kidney stones are composed of calcium (Mattson Porth, 1994; Spargo and Haas, 1994).

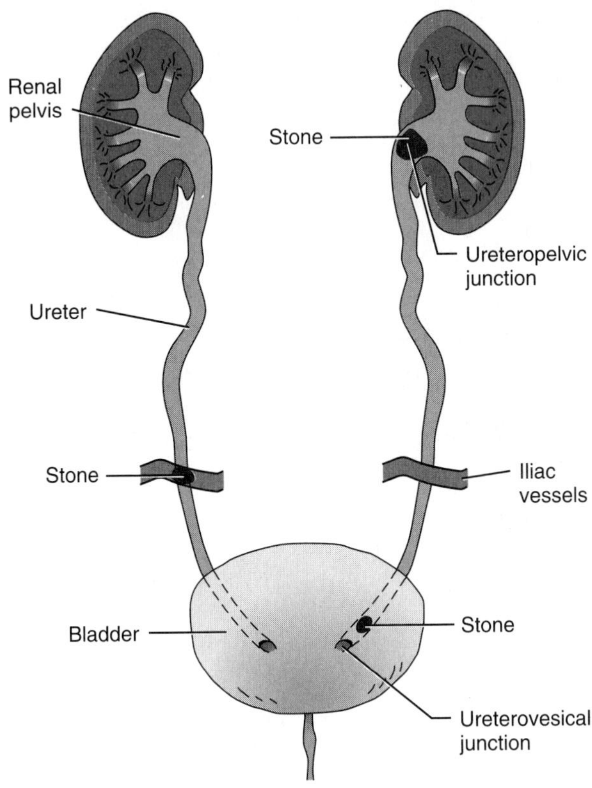

Figure **15-3.** The three common sites of urinary obstruction secondary to renal calculi.

Etiology. In most instances, the presence of a renal stone is associated with an increased blood level and urinary excretion of the principle component. An example of how this occurs is increased intestinal absorption of calcium and a decrease in its reabsorption in the proximal tubules of the kidney.

Risk Factors. A wide variety of risk factors are associated with urinary calculi, including sex, age, geography, climate, diet, genetics, and environment. The primary age span for the initial presentation of the disease is 30 to 50 years of age. Men are more frequently afflicted than women by a ratio of 4:1 until the sixth or seventh decade when the incidence increases in women. There is a higher incidence of renal calculi in industrialized countries and areas noted for high temperatures and humidity. The incidence of this disease is highest in the hot summer months. Excess intake of calcium, oxalate, and purines can increase the incidence of stones while adequate fluid intake and bran ingestion can help prevent calculi formation (Presti et al., 1995).

Pathogenesis. There are three primary theories related to calculi formation: the saturation theory, the inhibitor deficiency theory, and the matrix theory (Abraham and Smith, 1984). Regarding the saturation theory, there is increased risk of stone formation due to the urine being supersaturated with calculi components such as calcium salts, uric acid, magnesium ammonium phosphate, or cystine. The inhibitor theory states that people with a reduced urinary level of endogenous compounds that inhibit stone formation are at increased risk for this condition. One such endogenous compound is nephrocalcin (Coe et al., 1992). The matrix theory suggests that organic materials become a nidus for calculi formation. An example is the mucopolysaccharides that line the kidney tubules. Whether the organic matrix actually helps initiate stone formation or the material is simply entrapped during stone formation is unclear. Most likely, a combination of the three mechanisms leads to development of calculi.

Clinical Manifestations. *Renal colic* is the term used to describe the pain associated with urinary tract obstruction. Acute, excruciating flank and upper outer abdominal quadrant pain is the classic complaint. The pain may also radiate into the lower abdominal, bladder, and perineal areas, including the scrotum in males and labia in females. Nausea and vomiting, urinary urgency and frequency, and a cool and clammy skin may also be present (Mattson Porth, 1994; Presti et al., 1995).

Medical Management

Diagnosis. A variety of tests are used to diagnose this disease. Approximately 90% of calculi are radiopaque, making them visible on an abdominal radiograph. Ultrasonography, CT scanning, and magnetic resonance imaging (MRI) may be used. Hematuria, infection, the presence of stone-forming crystals, and urine pH can be determined on urinalysis. Excretory urography allows for visualization of the urinary collecting and drainage system by the use of a contrast medium prior to the abdominal film.

Treatment. A majority of stones 5 to 6 mm in diameter will pass spontaneously. Pain medication and antibiotic therapy (if infection is present) are commonly administered during the initial 6-week period. Onset of a fever during this period is a medical emergency, requiring prompt drainage by catheterization or a percutaneous nephrostomy tube. If spontaneous passage does not occur, more aggressive intervention is utilized.

Distal ureteral stones are managed by ureteroscopic stone extraction (USE) or in situ extracorporeal shock wave lithotripsy (ESWL). The USE method involves placing an endoscope through the urethra. Then basket extraction or fragmentation followed by extraction is performed. In situ ESWL utilizes the transmission of shock waves to break the calculi into fragments. Since the soft tissues of the body have similar densities the shock waves pass through these structures with low attenuation. When the shock wave encounters a boundary between substances of differing acoustic density (i.e., a calculus in the ureter), high compressive forces are generated causing a breakdown of the stone. The goal is to reduce the diameter to the point where spontaneous passage of the stone occurs (Preminger, 1994).

Recurrence of calculi is common if appropriate steps are not taken. Otherwise calculi may recur in up to 50% of people within 5 years (Presti et al., 1995). Appropriate preventive measures are determined by the cause of the stone formation. Adequate fluid intake is essential to the prevention of recurrences by reducing the saturation of stone-forming crystals. Clients with calcium oxalate calculi are required to reduce their intake of foods high in oxalate, including spinach, cocoa, chocolate, pecans, and peanuts. If the stones are associated with underlying disease such as hyperparathyroidism, the comorbidity must be effectively treated.

Special Implications for the Therapist **15-5**

RENAL CALCULI

If the classic symptoms are present, the renal colic associated with the calculi will not be confused with pain from mechanical dysfunction. The condition, however, may be manifested by symptoms that are intermittent and not severe. Depending on where the urinary collecting system is obstructed, the condition may be manifested solely by unilateral back pain ranging from the thoracolumbar junction to the iliac crest. The therapist needs to be vigilant for complaints of urinary dysfunction, as well as the risk factors associated with this disease.

If working with someone who is concurrently being treated conservatively for renal calculi, the therapist must be vigilant for complaints of fever, chills, or sweats. An onset of these symptoms warrants immediate communication with the patient's physician.

Chronic Renal Failure

Overview. Chronic renal failure can be attributed to a variety of conditions that result in permanent loss of nephrons. The loss of nephrons results in progressive deterioration of glomerular filtration, tubular reabsorption, and endocrine functions of the kidneys. The progressive inability of the kidneys to function has significant systemic effects, influencing all the other body systems.

Etiology and Risk Factors. The presence of a number of diseases can account for destruction of nephrons. The most common of these disorders includes uncontrolled hypertension, urinary tract obstruction and infection, hereditary defects of the kidneys, glomerular disorders, diabetes mellitus, and systemic lupus erythematosus. An increased risk of kidney failure is also associated with over-the-counter analgesic drug use. Heavy average intake (more than one pill per day) and medium to high cumulative intake (1000 or more pills in a lifetime) of acetaminophen doubled the odds of developing endstage renal disease. In addition, high cumulative intake of nonsteroidal anti-inflammatory drugs (5000 or more pills in a lifetime) increased the risk of developing the disease (Perneger et al., 1994).

Age is also a factor as adults 65 and older account for a large percentage of newly diagnosed conditions. This is linked with the age-related reduced glomerular filtration rate (GFR) and the often-present concurrent medical diseases in the elderly (Harum, 1984). The reduced GFR also increases the susceptibility of older people to the harmful effects of nephrotoxic drugs.

Incidence. Physical therapy care of patients with chronic renal failure has increased significantly in the past 20 years. In the early 1970s federal government support for dialysis and transplantation began. The technologic advances in dialysis and transplantation have resulted in improved outcomes for those with renal disease. Prior to this, there was a very high mortality rate for these clients as well as a tremendous cost of treatment.

Pathogenesis. Owing to the loss of nephrons, renal failure is marked by the kidneys' inability to adequately remove metabolic waste products from the blood and regulate fluid, electrolyte, and pH balance of extracellular fluids. The rate of nephron destruction can vary considerably, occurring over a period of several months to many years. There are typically four stages that mark the progression of chronic renal failure: (1) diminished renal reserve, (2) renal insufficiency, (3) renal failure, and (4) endstage renal disease. In the first stage, diminished renal reserve, the GFR is approximately 50% of normal. During this stage no overt symptoms of impaired renal function are evident. Depending on the health of the person, the kidneys have tremendous adaptive and compensatory capabilities, accounting for the delay in symptoms. The unaffected nephrons undergo structural and physiologic hypertrophy in an attempt to make up for those nephrons that are no longer functioning. In addition, blood urea nitrogen (BUN) and creatinine levels are normal. The second stage, renal insufficiency, is manifested by a reduction in GFR to approximately 20% to 35% of normal. It is during this stage that azotemia (abnormally high level of nitrogenous waste in the blood), anemia, and hypertension can appear. The third stage is renal failure. This occurs when the GFR is less than 20% to 25% of normal. At these levels the kidneys cannot regulate volume and solute composition. This inability leads to edema, metabolic acidosis, and hypercalcemia. Neurologic, gastrointestinal, and cardiovascular complications now become a part of the clinical manifestations of this disease. Endstage renal disease, the fourth stage, occurs when the GFR is less than 5% of normal. The complications noted in the first three stages are magnified by the continued progressive loss of kidney function. *Uremia* (urine in the blood) is the term used to describe the clinical manifestations of this stage. Virtually all body systems are involved, with a multitude of symptoms and signs being present. Besides the physiologic changes that are occurring, anatomic changes are also evident. The mass of the kidneys is generally reduced and histologic investigation reveals a reduction in renal capillaries and scarring of the glomeruli. In addition, atrophy and fibrosis are evident in the kidney tubules. During this final stage, survival is dependent upon dialysis or transplantation.

Clinical Manifestations. Chronic renal failure is marked by a multitude of symptoms and signs. The onset of these findings is typically very gradual and subtle, often resulting in a delay in diagnosis. Table 15–1 summarizes the systemic effects associated with chronic renal failure.

Anemia is the most significant hematologic problem associated with chronic renal failure. Controlling the production of red blood cells is the hormone erythropoietin which is primarily produced by the kidneys. Renal failure leads to decreased erythropoietin production which results in subsequent decrease in red blood cell numbers. In addition, the red blood cells that are produced have a shortened life span. (See Chapter 11 for additional information regarding anemia.) The tendency to bleed and bruise easily is related to impaired platelet function. Up to 20% of those with chronic renal failure have a tendency to bleed easily (Lancaster, 1990).

Cardiovascular diseases occur frequently in those with chronic renal failure. Hypertension often appears early in the course of this disease because of increased renin production and excess extracellular fluid volume (Brenner and Lazarus, 1991). Retrosternal pain can be a result of pericarditis. Owing

TABLE 15-1 CHRONIC RENAL FAILURE: SUMMARY OF CLINICAL MANIFESTATIONS

SYSTEM	MANIFESTATIONS
General	Fatigue, weakness, decreased alertness, inability to concentrate
Skin	Pallor, ecchymosis, pruritus, dry skin and mucous membranes, thin/brittle fingernails, urine odor on skin
Hematologic	Anemia, tendency to bleed easily
Body fluids	Polyuria, nocturia, dehydration, hyperkalemia, metabolic acidosis, hypocalcemia, hyperphosphatemia
Eye, ear, nose, throat	Metallic taste in mouth, nosebleeds, urinous breath, pale conjunctiva
Pulmonary	Dyspnea, rales, pleural effusion
Cardiovascular	Dyspnea on exertion, hypertension, friction rub, retrosternal pain on inspiration
Gastrointestinal (GI)	Anorexia, nausea, vomiting, hiccups, GI bleeding
Genitourinary	Impotence, amenorrhea, loss of libido
Skeletal	Osteomalacia, osteoporosis, bone pain, fracture, metastatic calcification of soft tissues
Neurologic	Recent memory loss, coma, seizures, muscle tremors, paresthesias, muscle weakness, restless legs, cramping

to the immunologic complications associated with chronic renal failure, infections can more easily occur, potentially leading to pericarditis.

Gastrointestinal system complaints occur frequently in uremia. High concentrations of ammonia and increased gastric acid secretion can contribute to the nausea and vomiting and the metallic taste in the mouth. The resultant depressed appetite contributes to fatigue, weakness, and malaise.

The skeletal changes associated with chronic renal failure occur early in the disease secondary to abnormalities in calcium, phosphate, and vitamin D metabolism. A drop in serum calcium stimulates the release of parathyroid hormone which results in increased calcium resorption from bone. The hyperparathyroid function is related to the impaired ability of the individual to convert vitamin D to its active form. The reduced calcium and phosphate levels in bone lead to osteomalacia and osteoporosis (see Chapter 20). After dialysis is initiated, a rapid rise in calcium levels occurs, preceding a fall in phosphate levels. Metastatic calcification is the result, affecting the eyes (conjunctivitis), muscle, arteries, and skin (pruritus—intense itching).

Alteration of central (CNS) and peripheral nervous system (PNS) function often occurs with chronic renal failure. CNS involvement is manifested by recent memory loss, inability to concentrate, perceptual errors, and decreased alertness. The lower extremities are much more commonly affected than the upper extremities with PNS involvement. The atrophy and demyelination of both sensory and motor nerves is possibly caused by uremic toxins. The neurologic changes are typically symmetrical and can also be manifested as the restless legs syndrome, which is more pronounced at rest (Van Stone, 1983).

Medical Management

Diagnosis. In addition to the symptoms and signs associated with this disease, documentation of elevated BUN and serum creatinine valves lead to the diagnosis of renal failure. Imaging modalities are also utilized to support a diagnosis of chronic renal failure. These include ultrasonography, where the finding of bilateral small kidneys (less than 10 cm) is supportive of the diagnosis. This disease is also marked by subperiosteal reabsorption along the radial borders of the digits of the hand. This finding confirms hyperparathyroidism, which would have to have been present for at least 1 year to be demonstrable.

Treatment. The treatment of chronic renal failure falls under two categories: conservative management and renal replacement therapy. The goals of conservative care are to slow the deterioration of the remaining renal function and to assist the body in its fight to compensate for the existing condition. Renal replacement therapy consists of dialysis or renal transplantation. The stage of the disease will determine which of the treatment approaches will be instituted.

Conservative management consists of a wide variety of interventions. Treating hypertension and restricting dietary protein can significantly retard disease progression (Zeller, 1991). Proteins are broken down to form nitrogenous wastes which adds to the problem of azotemia. A carefully controlled diet regarding potassium, sodium, carbohydrate, fat, and caloric and fluid intake is vital for these clients. The development of recombinant human erythropoietin for treatment of anemia in clients with renal disease has increased hematocrit levels and improved appetite, energy levels, sexual function, and skin characteristics (Lundin, 1991). Early and aggressive treatment of hypocalcemia and hyperphosphatemia is vital to slowing the concurrent osteodystrophy. Phosphate-binding antacids and calcium supplements are frequently prescribed.

The treatment of endstage renal disease is dialysis or transplantation. The choice is based on the client's age, general health, donor availability, and personal preference. Dialysis can take the form of hemodialysis or peritoneal dialysis. Hemodialysis typically requires three sessions per week for 3 to 4 hours per session. The blood flows from an artery, through the dialysis machine chambers, then back to the body's venous system, with the waste products and excess electrolytes diffusing into the dialyzing solution.

Peritoneal dialysis relies on the same principles as hemodialysis. A catheter is implanted in the peritoneal cavity and sterile dialyzing solution is instilled and then drained over a specific period of time. This process is completed four times daily. The advantages of this continuous exchange are fewer dietary restrictions and fewer of the often dramatic symptom swings associated with hemodialysis (Morrison, 1995; Gallagher-Lepak, 1994). Potential complications of peritoneal dialysis include infection, catheter malfunction, dehydration, hyperglycemia, and hernia. Peritonitis is the most serious potential complication.

The steady improvement in the outcome of renal allografts has made kidney transplantation the treatment of choice for many people with chronic renal failure (Morris, 1991). Donor availability limits the number of transplants performed. In adults, the renal graft is placed extraperitoneally in the iliac fossa through an oblique lower abdominal incision. In small children, the graft is located retroperitoneally with a midline abdominal incision. Complications of the procedures include renal artery thrombosis, urinary leak, and lymphocele (Suthanthiran and Strom, 1994). Post-transplant immunosuppression with corticosteroids, azathioprine, or cyclosporin is regularly utilized with cadaveric kidney transplantation and generally in living related donor transplants (Morrison, 1995). Successful graft rates at 1 year are approximately 80% after cadaveric transplantation and 90% after living-related-donor transplantation (Morris, 1991).

Special Implications for the Therapist **15-6**

CHRONIC RENAL FAILURE

Treating people with a diagnosis of chronic renal failure can be extremely challenging because of the number of body systems involved. The decreased alertness, inability to concentrate, and short-term memory deficits will interfere with following instructions, including transfers, exercises, body mechanics, and so on. Reliance on the assistance of family and other health care providers is often necessary. The fatigue and general weakness may dictate that the therapist provide rest periods during a rehabilitation session. The potential osteodystrophy will require modification of evaluation and treatment techniques (see Implications for the Therapist: Osteoporosis, in Chapter 20).

There are a number of potential renal transplantation complications the therapist should be aware of. Hypertension, lipid disorders, hepatitis, cancer, and osteopenia occur with increased frequency in graft recipients (Suthanthiran and Strom, 1994). Hypertension occurs in 60% to 80% of renal graft recipients. (See Chapter 10 for the clinical implications associated with hypertension.) Approximately 15% of graft recipients develop chronic hepatitis (Parfrey et al., 1985; Rao et al., 1993) (see Chapter 14 for the clinical implications associated with hepatitis). Basal cell and squamous cell carcinoma (Chapter 8) and lymphomas (Chapter 7) are more frequent in this population, whereas the more common cancers of breast, lung, prostate, and colon are not (Penn, 1991). Lastly, corticosteroids appear to be the primary factor in the impaired bone formation associated with graft recipients (see Chapter 4).

Inflammatory Glomerular Lesions

Overview. The glomeruli are tufts of capillaries connecting the afferent and efferent arterioles of the nephron (Fig. 15–4). The capillaries are supported by a stalk made up of mesangial cells and a basement membrane and are arranged in lobules. The circulating blood is filtered in the glomeruli, with the urine filtrate being an end product. Glomerulonephritis is the leading cause of chronic renal failure in the United States. It accounts for approximately 50% of those who require dialysis. Glomerular disease can occur independently of other diseases or secondarily to diseases such as vasculitis or systemic lupus erythematosus (Mattson Porth, 1994). There exist two categories of glomerular disease: the nephrotic and nephritic syndromes. Nephrotic syndrome affects the integrity of the glomerular capillary membrane; the nephritic syndrome results in an inflammatory response within the glomeruli.

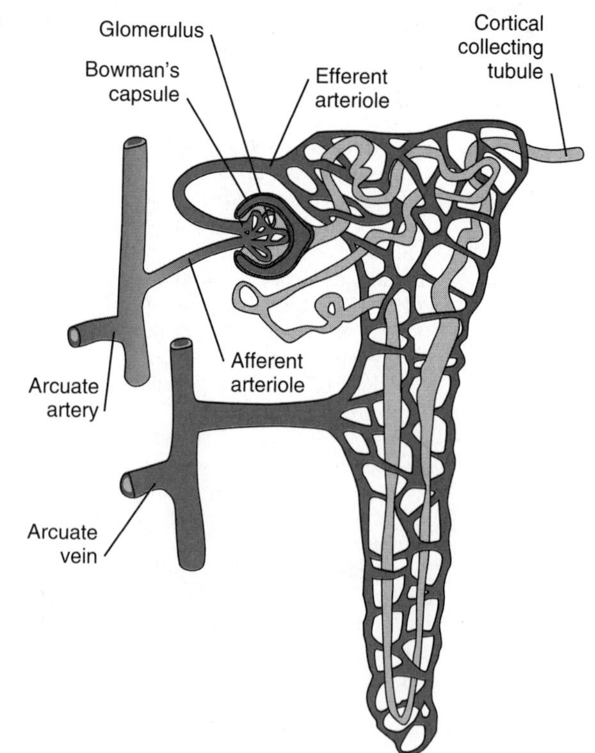

Figure **15-4.** The glomerulus.

Etiology. Most cases of primary glomerular disease and many cases of secondary disease have an immune origin (Harum, 1984; Cogan et al., 1981). Two different immune mechanisms have been suggested: (1) injury secondary to deposition of soluble circulating antigen-antibody complexes in the gomeruli and (2) injury secondary to antibodies reacting with insoluble fixed glomerular antigens. The antigen of the immune complexes can be endogenous, for example, DNA in systemic lupus erythematosus. The antigen can also be exogenous, for example, streptococcal membrane antigens in poststreptococcal glomerulonephritis (Mattson Porth, 1994).

Risk Factors. The presence of a variety of common disorders can significantly increase the risk of glomerular damage. Approximately 55% of those with (type I) insulin-dependent diabetes and 30% of those with (type II) non–insulin-dependent diabetes develop endstage kidney disease. The glomerulus is the primary component of the kidney affected by diabetic neuropathy. Besides diabetes and systemic lupus erythematosus, hypertension is also associated with glomerular disease.

The nephrotic syndrome can occur at any age. In children the disease is most prevalent between 1½ and 4 years of age. Boys are more commonly involved than girls, but the sex distribution is roughly equal in the adult population.

Pathogenesis. Whether the antigens are endogenous or exogenous, the antigen-antibody complex is formed in the circulation and becomes trapped in the glomerular membrane as the blood is being filtered. Injury to the glomerular membrane can occur through cell lysis or chemotaxis. Leukocytes are then drawn into the area (Michael, 1985). If the inciting antigen is short-lived, the inflammatory process is acute, but then subsides. If the antigen is being chronically produced, the recurrent inflammatory reactions lead to chronic glomerulonephritis.

The histologic changes associated with glomerular disease include proliferative, sclerotic, and membranous changes. There is a local increase in both the cellular (proliferative) and noncellular (sclerotic) components of the glomerulus. In addition, an increase in the thickness of the glomerular capillary wall (membranous) occurs. These changes adversely affect the glomerular filtration mechanism and alter capillary permeability. Increased glomerular capillary permeability results in proteinuria, hematuria, pyuria, oliguria, edema, hypertension, and azotemia (Mattson Porth, 1994).

Clinical Manifestations. Typically, the earlier stages of glomerular disease are marked by the absence of overt symptoms. The usual initial manifestation of the nephrotic syndrome is generalized edema. The edema can be severe enough to be disabling. The nephritic syndrome is typically marked by hematuria. The damaged capillary walls allow red blood cells to become part of the urine filtrate. In addition, pyuria, oliguria, and hypertension are associated with this condition.

Medical Management

Diagnosis. Owing to the lack of symptoms in the early stages of glomerulonephritis the disease is often found incidently by urinalysis or elevated blood pressure readings. Urinalysis may reveal proteinuria, hematuria, and pyuria, while blood analysis will reveal azotemia. Renal ultrasound and renal biopsy may be utilized depending on the initial presenting symptoms and signs.

Treatment. The management of this condition is multifaceted. To prevent protein malnutrition, additional dietary protein intake, equivalent to the daily protein loss, may be necessary. Restricted dietary salt intake is vital in the management of edema. Diuretics are also typically needed by these clients. A low fat diet with a general weight control and exercise program are essential if hypercholesterolemia and hypertriglyceridemia are present (Morrison, 1995). Lastly, dialysis and transplantation may be necessary for those in the late stages of glomerulonephritis (see Chronic Renal Failure).

Special Implications for the Therapist **15-7**

INFLAMMATORY GLOMERULAR LESIONS

Therapists working with clients with a diagnosis of diabetes, systemic lupus erythematosus vasculitis, and hypertension need to be aware of the association of glomerulonephritis and these disorders. Being vigilant for the clinical manifestations of glomerulonephritis (edema, hypertension, hematuria, oliguria) is important and their presence warrants referral of the client to a physician. An awareness of the side effects associated with diuretics is also important. Potential side effects include muscle weakness, fatigue, muscle cramps, headaches, and depression, all of which can interfere with the rehabilitation program. (See Chapter 4 for additional information regarding diuretics.) The onset of any of these complaints also warrants communication with a physician. Finally, many clients with glomerulonephritis progress to chronic renal failure.

DISORDERS OF THE BLADDER AND URETHRA

Bladder Cancer

Overview. Approximately 95% of urinary tract cancers occur in the bladder. The other 5% occur in the renal pelvis and ureter. A majority of primary bladder cancers involve the epithelium.

Incidence. Approximately 54,500 new cases of bladder cancer and 11,700 associated deaths are projected for 1997 in the United States (Parker et al., 1997). These tumors are the most common urinary tract cancer in females.

Etiology. The cause of bladder cancer is unknown, but the carcinogens that are stored in the bladder and excreted in the urine have been linked to environmental factors.

Risk Factors. See Box 15–1 for a list of risk factors related to bladder cancer. Transitional cell carcinoma of the bladder was one of the earliest cancers to be linked with environmental hazards. In 1895 a markedly higher incidence of bladder cancer was noted in German workers in the aniline dye industry. Since then, an increased incidence of bladder cancer has been associated with other industries, such as leather, rubber, and paint manufacturing (Murphy, 1989; Peterson, 1986). Males are affected two to four times more often than females, and 80% of the population is 50 years of age and older (Frank et al., 1991; Murphy, 1989; Ross et al., 1988).

Cigarette smoking has also been associated with a significant risk of developing cancer. One of the first noted bladder carcinogens, 2-naphthylamine, is absorbed from unfiltered cigarette smoke (Murphy, 1989). Cigarette smoking may be responsible for as many as 50% of male cases and 33% of female cases (Mattson Porth, 1994). The highest incidence of bladder cancer is noted in urban whites living in the United States and western Europe. A lower incidence is noted in Japan and in American blacks. Chronic use of cyclophosphamide (Cytoxan: antineoplastic agents) or analgesics containing phenacetin can also predispose to the development of bladder cancer (Wall and Clausen, 1975). Lastly, a history

BOX **15-1**

Risk Factors for Bladder Cancer

Male sex
Fifty years and older
Cigarette smoking
Environmental hazards
White race
Western industrialized nation
History of chronic bladder infections and bladder stones

of chronic bladder infections and bladder stones increases the risk of bladder cancer (Mattson Porth, 1994).

Pathogenesis. Tumors of the urinary collecting system can arise from epithelial, mesenchymal, or hematopoietic tissues, but the majority of bladder cancers arise from the epithelium. Approximately 90% to 98% of these cancers are transitional cell carcinomas with squamous cell carcinomas and adenocarcinomas making up the remainder (Peterson, 1994; See et al., 1994). The systemic absorption of environmental carcinogens, including cigarette smoke, followed by urinary excretion exposes the urinary epithelium to concentrated levels of the agents for prolonged periods of time. This interaction of the urine-soluble carcinogens with the epithelium is known as contact chemical carcinogenesis. The precise molecular events leading to the formation of bladder cancer are not known (See et al., 1994).

Clinical Manifestations. Hematuria is the most common sign of bladder cancer. Gross hematuria is present in up to 75% to 80% of persons with this condition and microscopic hematuria is present in a majority of the remainder (Frank et al., 1991; Raghavan et al., 1990; McCarron et al., 1983). The onset of hematuria is often sudden and frequently intermittent. The intermittent pattern can result in a delay in diagnosis. Other signs of voiding dysfunction may also be present including frequency, urgency, and dysuria (See et al., 1994; Mattson Porth, 1994).

In the presence of metastatic disease, back pain secondary to bony invasion or involvement of the periaortic lymph nodes may occur. Supraclavicular lymphadenopathy may also occur, as well as hepatomegaly. Lymphedema of the lower extremities may occur secondary to locally advanced masses or pelvic lymph node involvement (Presti et al., 1995).

Medical Management

Diagnosis. Diagnostic methods utilized to detect bladder cancer include ultrasound, excretory urography, cytologic studies, CT, and MRI. Confirmation is obtained with cystoscopy and transurethral resection. An abdominal CT scan, bone scan, and chest film can be used to investigate potential spread of the disease (Presti et al., 1995).

Staging. Tumors that are limited to the mucosal lining are classified as stage 0. The overall 3-year survival rate with stage 0 disease is approximately 90%. Stage A disease includes invasion of the lamina propria. Stage B disease is marked by invasion of the bladder smooth muscle wall. The 5-year survival rate of patients with stage B disease is 35% to 40%. Perivesical tumor invasion extending to the prostate and seminal vesicles marks stage C (Fig. 15–5). The invasion of the bladder wall may obstruct the ureter, causing hydroureter. Stage D includes metastasis, regional or distant. Distant sites of metastasis include the liver, lung, and bone (Peterson, 1994).

Treatment. Treatment of bladder cancer depends on the extent of the lesion and the person's general health. Endoscopic resection of superficial lesions is performed, as is electrocautery. Segmental surgical resection is done to remove large solitary lesions. Radical cystectomy is performed in the presence of stage B disease, including resection of the pelvic lymph nodes. In males, the prostate and seminal vesicles may also be removed.

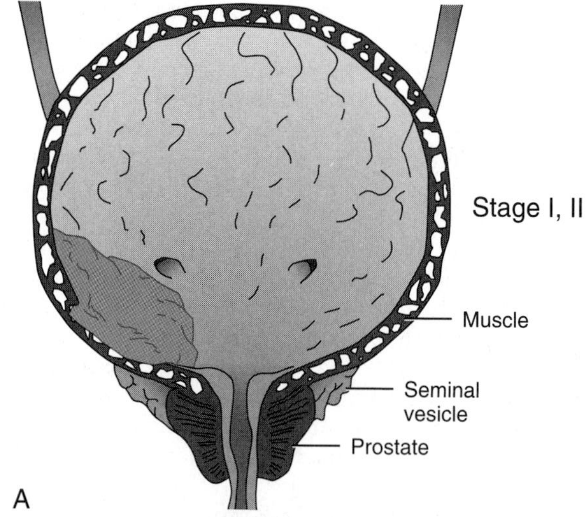

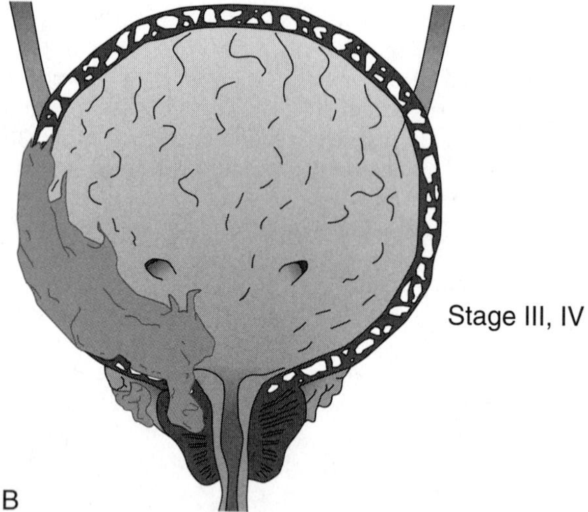

Figure **15–5.** Bladder cancer staging. *A*, Stages I and II. *B*, Stage III.

Metastatic bladder cancer appears to develop resistance to chemotherapy. The use of intravesicular chemotherapy, wherein the cytotoxic drug is administered directly into the bladder, is increasing (Mattson Porth, 1994; See et al., 1994). Chemotherapy is being combined with radiation therapy in an effort to lower local and distant relapse rates (Presti et al., 1995).

Special Implications for the Therapist **15-8**

BLADDER CANCER

Approximately 15% of those with newly diagnosed bladder cancer and 40% of those considered to have local disease only at the time of diagnosis will develop metastases within 2 years (Presti et al., 1995). Therapists working with people diagnosed with this condition must be vigilant for the onset or return of symptoms and signs suggestive of urogenital system disease or metastatic spread.

Neurogenic Bladder Disorders

Overview. The sensorimotor innervation of the urinary bladder can be interrupted at multiple levels, resulting in urinary dysfunction. Neurologic lesions above the sacral micturition reflex center level typically result in spastic bladder dysfunction. "Reflex neurogenic bladder," "spastic neurogenic bladder," "cord bladder," and "uninhibited bladder" are terms used to describe neurogenic disorders that result in spastic bladder dysfunction. Neurogenic lesions at the level of the sacral micturition reflex center or affecting the peripheral innervation of the bladder typically result in flaccid bladder dysfunction.

Neurogenic bladder disorders can result in a variety of bladder abnormalities. These include diminished bladder capacity, a constricted external bladder sphincter, an atonic bladder that is unable to contract, a hyperactive detrusor (bladder) muscle, and loss of perception of bladder fullness. The inability of the bladder to function normally can lead to serious complications such as ascending urinary tract infections; vesicoureteral reflux, which can seriously impair kidney function; and urinary calculi.

Etiology. The common disorders that can result in spastic bladder dysfunction include cerebrovascular accident, dementia, multiple sclerosis, and brain tumors. Spastic bladder dysfunction can also occur secondary to spinal cord lesions such as spinal cord injury, herniated intervertebral disk, vascular lesions, spinal cord tumors, and myelitis. Local pelvic irritation can result in spasm of the external bladder sphincter, impairing urinary function. The local irritation can occur in the presence of vaginitis, perineal inflammation, urethral inflammation, and chronic prostatitis (Thon and Altwein, 1984). Flaccid bladder dysfunction can be secondary to meningomyelocele, spina bifida, diabetes mellitus, and anxiety or depression (Mattson Porth, 1994).

Pathogenesis. The type of bladder disorder that occurs is dependent upon the underlying cause. Following a stroke or in the early stages of multiple sclerosis an uninhibited bladder can develop. The sacral reflex arc and sensation are retained, the urine stream is normal, but the bladder capacity is diminished secondary to increased detrusor muscle tone and spasticity.

Conditions that affect the micturition center in the brainstem or impair reflex activity between the micturition center and the spinal cord can affect the coordinated activity of the detrusor muscle and the external bladder sphincter. This event is termed *detrusor-sphincter dyssynergia*. The external sphincter tightens during micturition as the detrusor muscle is contracting, resulting in increased intravesicular pressure and vesicoureteral reflux.

Immediately following a spinal cord injury all reflexes are depressed. During this phase the urinary bladder is atonic. Catheterization is essential to prevent overdistention of the bladder. One to 2 months following injury the reflexes become hyperactive. Frequent, spontaneous detrusor muscle contractions result in a small, hyperactive bladder. The act of voiding is interrupted, involuntary, or incomplete. In addition, trigone hypertrophy occurs, which can cause vesicoureteral reflux and renal damage.

Diabetic bladder neuropathy occurs in 43% to 87% of persons with insulin-dependent diabetes (Frimodt-Miller, 1980). Initially, the sensory supply of the bladder is affected, resulting in decreased urinary frequency. Then urinary hesitancy, weakness of stream, dribbling, and a sensation of the bladder not being fully emptied occurs. Vesicoureteral reflux and ascending UTIs are potential complications (Mattson Porth, 1994).

Clinical Manifestations. Neurogenic bladder dysfunction is manifested by partial or complete urinary retention, incontinence, or frequent urination.

Medical Management

Diagnosis. Numerous urologic tests are utilized to assess the anatomic and physiologic status of the bladder and associated structures. Serial cystometrograms provide an index of detrusor functional capacity and cystourethroscopic evaluation determines the degree of bladder outlet obstruction. Intravenous urography, ultrasonography, and cystosonography help assess the anatomic status of the bladder. Urodynamic evaluation to assess bladder function includes voiding flow rates, sphincter electromyograms (EMGs), and urethral pressure profile studies.

Treatment. The primary goals of treatment include preventing bladder overdistention, UTIs, and renal damage. Treatment modalities include catheterization, bladder training, surgery, and pharmacologic bladder manipulation.

Catheterization is a commonly employed intervention. Permanent indwelling catheters are utilized in people who are debilitated and have urinary retention or incontinence. In addition, if conservative or surgical options for treatment of incontinence are not feasible, permanent indwelling catheters may be utilized. Although a medical necessity in certain situations, permanent indwelling catheters also carry a risk. UTIs, urethral irritation, epididymo-orchitis, pyelonephritis, and renal calculi have all been associated with the use of permanent indwelling catheters in people with spinal cord injury (Jacobs and Kaufman, 1978).

Intermittent catheterization is utilized to treat urinary retention, and prevents bladder overdistention when performed at 3- to 4-hour intervals. Advantages of intermittent vs. permanent catheterization include decreased urethral irritation and periodic bladder distention, which maintains some degree of muscle tone. Intermittent catheterization is often used in conjunction with pharmacologic intervention.

Medications are utilized to relax the external sphincter, decrease the outflow resistance of the internal sphincter, and alter the muscle tone of the bladder. Muscle relaxers such as diazepam (Valium) and baclofen (Lioresal) are used to decrease external sphincter tone. Parasympathomimetic drugs (except bethanechol chloride [Urecholine]) can increase bladder muscle tone, while anticholinergic drugs (except propantheline bromide [Pro-Banthine]) will decrease detrusor muscle tone and increase bladder capacity.

A variety of surgical interventions for neurogenic bladder exist. Sphincterectomy or transurethral resection of the bladder neck are performed in men with prostatic hyperplasia. Reconstruction of the sphincter, nerve resection, and urinary diversion are also surgical options. Resection of the sacral reflex nerves and of the pudendal nerve that controls the external sphincter can be done when spasticity is present. An example of urinary diversion is the attachment of the ureters to the sigmoid colon with the rectum serving as the urinary receptacle (Mattson Porth, 1994).

Lastly, bladder training methods are designed to enhance bladder function and prevent complications. Adequate fluid intake is essential for the prevention of infection and overconcentrated urine. With a hyperreflexive bladder or detrusor-sphincter dyssynergia the abnormally concentrated urine can stimulate afferent nerve endings, exacerbating the bladder disorder. This could increase vesicular pressures, vesicoureteral reflux, and overflow incontinence. Fluid intake must be controlled and monitored to prevent bladder distention. Biofeedback techniques utilizing EMG or cystometry help the person control external sphincter function or increase intravesicular pressure sufficiently to overcome outflow resistance.

Special Implications for the Therapist **15-9**

NEUROGENIC BLADDER DISORDERS

Therapists provide care for many people who have sustained spinal cord injuries and cerebrovascular accidents. Also, clients with multiple sclerosis and brain tumors make up a significant portion of the population in rehabilitation centers. Neurogenic bladder disorders are usually only one of the complications associated with these conditions, but familiarity with this complication is important. The potential for UTIs, renal calculi, and renal damage is high in those with neurogenic bladder disorders. Familiarity with the signs and symptoms associated with these potential diseases is a necessity. The development of any of these comorbidities can interfere with the rehabilitation process. Detection of any of these symptoms warrants immediate communication with a physician.

Urinary Incontinence

Overview. *Urinary incontinence* may be defined as an involuntary loss of urine that is sufficient to be a problem (Urinary Incontinence Guideline Panel, 1992). Four categories are utilized to classify urinary incontinence: (1) *total incontinence* includes people who lose urine at all times regardless of body position; (2) *stress incontinence* is the loss of urine during activities that increase intra-abdominal pressure such as coughing, lifting, or laughing; (3) *urge incontinence* is the uncontrolled loss of urine, which is preceded by an unexpected, strong urge to void; (4) *overflow incontinence* is the uncontrolled loss of urine when intravesicular pressure exceeds outlet resistance. The last three categories are the ones most commonly found and are the focus of this discussion.

Urinary incontinence is common, yet the condition is poorly understood, underdiagnosed, and often inadequately treated. Many people are embarrassed to acknowledge that they are incontinent. It is estimated that only 20% to 50% of incontinent adults seek medical care (Weinberger, 1995). Others regard incontinence as part of the normal aging process. The economic price tag associated with urinary incontinence is estimated to be greater than $8 billion per year in the United States. Incontinence can be a significant contributory factor related to pressure sores, UTIs, institutionalization, depression, and isolation (Abrams and Berkow, 1990).

Although there is no evidence that the normal aging process directly causes incontinence, the incidence of urinary incontinence in the elderly population is quite high. Depending upon the individual's setting, the incidence of incontinence in the elderly ranges from 11% to 43% (Palmer, 1988). A variety of factors may contribute to numbers such as these. Pelvic relaxation disorders in elderly women and BPH in elderly men are common and can contribute to the development of incontinence. Medications commonly prescribed for this age group can also increase the risk of incontinence. Certain diuretics can cause urge incontinence, especially in those with reduced bladder capacity. Tranquilizers and sedatives may impair awareness of the usual cues related to urinary urgency and may also depress the cerebral corticoregulatory tract affecting detrusor muscle activity. Drugs producing anticholinergic side effects can induce urinary retention and overflow incontinence. These medications include major tranquilizers and antiparkisonian agents. Also, certain hypertensive medications such as prazosin can reduce urethral resistance and induce stress incontinence.

Inadequate fluid intake can also contribute to the development of urinary incontinence. Constipation may cause urethral obstruction and overflow incontinence. These clients will also be at risk for UTIs resulting in bladder irritability and an increased risk of incontinence. Lastly, as the elderly lose their mobility and manual dexterity secondary to a multitude of ailments, including arthritis, getting to the bathroom or commode in a timely fashion and manipulating clothing become increasingly difficult (Mattson Porth, 1994; Abrams and Berkow, 1990).

Incidence. Urinary incontinence is more prevalent in women than men and in the elderly vs. the young. An estimated 10 million adults in the United States experience incontinence, including 15% to 30% of the community-dwelling elderly and more than 50% of nursing home residents (Consensus Conference, 1989). The condition is not rare in younger populations, as up to 30% of healthy middle-aged women experience urinary incontinence (Weinberger, 1995). Lastly, 28% of nulliparous "elite" college athletes reported urine loss while participating in their sport (Nygaard et al., 1994).

Risk Factors. A wide range of factors can contribute to the increased risk of developing urinary incontinence (Box 15–2): altered local anatomy and physiology, medications,

BOX **15-2**
Risk Factors for Urinary Incontinence

Pelvic floor muscle weakness
History of myelomeningocele
History of benign prostatic hyperplasia
Fecal impaction
Medication use, including diuretics, tranquilizers, and decongestants
Pelvic surgery
Bladder irritation

preexisting disease, decreased mentation, impaired mobility, radiation therapy, and surgery. In women, weakness of the pelvic floor musculature secondary to normal aging, childbirth, or pelvic surgery changes the important posterior ureterovesical angle. With the loss of this angle, any activity that places caudal pressure on the bladder will result in involuntary flow of urine. These activities include coughing, laughing, sneezing, and lifting, all of which increase intra-abdominal pressure. Congenital sphincter weakness also results in the involuntary flow of urine. Myelomeningocele is such a condition. The presence of conditions that cause urethral or bladder neck obstruction, such as BPH (see Chapter 16) or fecal impaction can result in overflow incontinence. In this situation intravascular pressure will exceed the maximal urethral pressure as the bladder distends.

The use of a variety of medications increases the risk of becoming incontinent. Diuretics, tranquilizers, sedatives, antiparkinsonian agents, decongestants, and α-adrenergic blockers can induce involuntary loss of urine. These pharmacologic agents can interfere with conscious inhibition of voiding, induce a quick diuresis, induce urinary retention to the point of overflow incontinence, and reduce urethral resistance to the point of stress incontinence. Incontinence can also be a side effect of pelvic surgery. One of the most commonly employed procedures in treating this side effect is transurethral prostatic resection (Mattson Porth, 1994; Abrams and Berkow, 1990; Riehmann and Bruskewitz, 1994). Lastly, bladder irritation can contribute to the events leading to urinary incontinence. UTIs, caffeine, alcohol, and citrus fruits are all potential bladder irritants.

Medical Management

Diagnosis. Since urinary incontinence is related to a wide variety of disorders and factors, a detailed investigation is necessary to determine the cause(s). An important part of this investigation is a voiding diary to determine the frequency, timing, amount of voiding, and to assess the numerous other factors potentially associated with incontinence (Urinary Incontinence Guideline Panel, 1992). A careful history will investigate medication usage (prescribed and over-the-counter), past and current illnesses and surgical history. Urinalysis and urodynamic evaluation are important to rule out the presence of diseases such as UTI and to assess bladder and sphincter function, respectively. Cystometry is utilized to assess bladder capacity, sensation, voluntary control, and contractility. Cystometry consists of filling the bladder with water or carbon dioxide and recording changes in intravesicular pressure (Presti et al., 1995; Tucker, 1994). When stress incontinence is suspected, provocative stress testing is carried out. The client is asked to cough vigorously while the examiner observes for urine loss. The test is initially done in the lithotomy position, but if negative is repeated in a standing position (Urinary Incontinence Guideline Panel, 1992).

Treatment. Management of urinary incontinence depends on the type of incontinence and the person's age and general health. Stress incontinence can be treated by physiotherapeutic, surgical, and pharmacologic interventions, singly or in combination. Exercises can be performed to retrain and strengthen the pelvic floor musculature. This type of exercise has been advocated for decades (Kegel, 1948). Reported cure rates utilizing pelvic floor exercises range from 30% to 75% (Wells, 1990). With verbal and manual cues, biofeedback, and EMG, the client can be taught to disassociate pelvic floor muscle activity from other hip and pelvic muscle activity and to maintain pelvic floor muscle tone while avoiding a Valsalva maneuver. Weighted vaginal cones and electrical stimulation can also be utilized to rehabilitate the pelvic floor.

Drugs are also prescribed for stress incontinence. Estrogens with phenylpropanolamine have been shown to be more effective than the use of either agent alone (Ahkstrom et al., 1990). Surgery may be used to correct a cystocele or alter the position of the bladder neck. A bladder neck suspension procedure is utilized to prevent the bladder neck from displacing caudally when straining (Tucker, 1994).

Various interventions are utilized to treat urge incontinence, with the primary focus being behavioral modification and pharmacologic therapy. Urge incontinence is related to detrusor instability. Continence requires the ability to inhibit automatic detrusor contractions. The bladder needs to be trained to respond to a specific voiding schedule. Clients void at scheduled intervals to suppress the micturition reflux, increase bladder capacity, and decrease urinary frequency. The initial retraining interval is usually 60 minutes. The voiding intervals are increased by 15- to 60-minute extensions. Success is marked by voiding at 3- to 4-hour intervals, continence, and minimal sensory symptoms. Success occurs in 50% to 90% of clients (Hadley, 1986). Biofeedback can also be utilized with cystometry to train the client to inhibit bladder contractions and reduce detrusor pressure (Weinberger, 1995). Recommended medications for urge incontinence include antispasmodics (oxybutynin), anticholinergics, and tricyclic antidepressants (Presti et al., 1995).

Other forms of treatment include catheterization, penile clamps, intravaginal urethral compression devices, urine collection devices, and surgically implanted artificial sphincters. Careful diagnosis to determine the type of incontinence and the underlying cause will allow for the proper choice of interventions.

Special Implications for the Therapist **15-10**

URINARY INCONTINENCE

Therapists have an important direct role in the treatment of urinary incontinence. A valuable reference for these treatment approaches is *Obstetric and Gynecologic Care in Physical Therapy* by O'Connor and Gourley (1990). For most clients seen by therapists, though, urinary incontinence will be a comorbidity or a condition which has yet to be evaluated. The generally positive rapport that develops between client and therapist may facilitate the acknowledgment that this condition exists. The therapist may be in a position to direct the person to the appropriate physician for evaluation. Successful treatment of urinary incontinence may enhance rehabilitation efforts geared to improve the client's physical and social activity level.

References

Abraham PA, Smith CL: Medical evaluation and management of calcium nephrolithiasis. Med Clin North Am 68:1984, 281.

Abrams WB, Berkow R (eds): The Merck Manual of Geriatrics. Rahway, NJ, Merck, 1990, pp 88–104.

Ahkstrom K, Sandahl B, Sjoberg B, et al: Effect of combined treatment with phenylpropanolamine and estriol, compared with estriol treatment alone in postmenopausal women with stress incontinence. Gynecol Obstet Invest 30:37–43, 1990.

Baldassare JS, Kaye D: Special problems of urinary tract infection in the elderly. Med Clin North Am 75:375–390, 1991.

Beahrs OH, Henson DE, Hutler RUP, Kennedy BJ: Manual for Staging Cancer, 4th ed. Philadelphia, JB Lippincott, 1992, p 201.

Bennett WM, Elzinga LW, Barry JM: Polycystic kidney disease: II. Diagnosis and management. Hosp Pract 23 (4):165, 1992.

Brenner BM, Lazarus JM: Chronic renal failure. *In* Wilson JD, Braunwald E, Isselbacher KJ, et al. (eds). Harrison's Principles of Internal Medicine, ed 12. New York, McGraw-Hill, 1991, pp 1150–1156.

Coe FL, Parks JH, Asplin JR: The pathologenosis and treatment of kidney stones. N Engl J Med 327:1141–1152, 1992.

Cogan MG, Sargent JA, Yarbrough SG, et al: Prevention of prednisone-induced negative nitrogen balance. Ann Intern Med 95:160, 1981.

Consensus Conference: Urinary incontinence in adults. JAMA 261:2685–2690, 1989.

Frank IN, Graham SO, Nabors WL: Urologic and male genital cancers. *In* Hollies AI, Fink OJ, Murphy GP (eds): Clinical Oncology. American Cancer Society, Atlanta 1991, pp 276–280.

Frimodt-Miller C: Diabetic cystopathy: Epidemiology and related disorders. Ann Intern Med 92:318, 1980.

Gallagher-Lepak S: Renal failure. In Mattson Porth C (ed): Pathophysiology, ed 4. Philadelphia, JB Lippincott, 1994, pp 684–696.

Grantham JJ: Polycystic kidney disease: I. Etiology and pathogenesis. Hosp Pract 27(3A):51–59, 1992.

Hadley EC: Bladder training and related therapies for urinary incontinence in older people. JAMA 256:372, 1986.

Harum P: Renal nutrition for the renal nurse. Am Nephrol Nurses Assoc J 8:39, 1984.

Jacobs SC, Kaufman JM: Complications of permanent bladder catheter drainage in spinal cord injury patients. J Urol 119:740, 1978.

Kegel AH: Progressive resistance exercises in the functional restoration of the perineal muscles. Am J Obstet Gynecol 56:238, 1948.

Kunin CM: Genitourinary infections in the patient at risk: Extrinsic risk factors. Am J Med 76:141, 1984.

Lancaster L: Renal response to shock. Critic Care Clin North Am 2:221–233, 1990.

Lundin AP: Recombinant erythropoietin and chronic renal failure. Hosp Pract 26:62, 1991.

Mattson Porth C: Alterations in renal function. *In* Mattson Porth C (ed): Pathophysiology, ed 4. Philadelphia, JB Lippincott, 1994, pp 665–667, 706–710.

McCarron JP, Mills C, Vaughn ED Jr: Tumors of the renal pelvis and ureter: Current concepts and management. Semin Urol 1:75, 1983.

Michael AF: Immunologic mechanisms in immune complex disease. Kidney Int 28:569, 1985.

Morris PJ: Kidney transplantation, 1960–1990. Adv Nephrol 20:14, 1991.

Morrison G: Kidney. *In* Tierney LM, McPhee SJ, Papadakis MA (eds): Current Medical Diagnosis and Treatment, ed 34. Norwalk, Conn, Appleton & Lange, 1995, pp 773–780.

Murphy WM: Diseases of the urinary bladder, urethra, ureters and renal pelves. *In* Murphy WM (ed): Urologic Pathology. Philadelphia, WB Saunders, 1989.

Nygaard IE, Thompson FL, Svengalis SL, Albright JP: Urinary incontinence in elite nulliparous athletes. Obstet Gynecol 84:183–187, 1994.

O'Connor LJ, Gourley RJ: Obstetric and Gynecologic Care in Physical Therapy. Thorofare, NJ, Slack, 1990.

Palmer MH: Incontinence: The magnitude of the problem. Nurs Clin North Am 23:139, 1988.

Parfrey PS, Farge O, Forbes ROC, et al: Chronic hepatitis in end-stage renal disease: Comparison of HbsAg-negative and HBsAg-positive patients. Kidney Int 28:959–967, 1985.

Parker SL, Tong T, Bolden S, Wingo PA: Cancer statistics, 1997. CA Cancer J Clin 47(1):5–27, 1997.

Penn I: Cancer in the immunosuppressed organ recipient. Transplant Proc 23:1771–1772, 1991.

Perneger TV, Whelton PK, Klag MJ: Risk of kidney failure associated with the use of acetaminophen, aspirin and nonsteroidal anti-inflammatory drugs. N Engl J Med 331:1675–1679, 1994.

Peterson RO: Urinary bladder. *In* Peterson RO (ed): Urologic Pathology. Philadelphia, JB Lippincott, 1986.

Peterson RO: The urinary tract and male reproductive system. *In* Rubin E, Farber JL (eds): Pathology, 2nd ed. Philadelphia, JB Lippincott, 1994, pp 867–907.

Pouillson DR, deVere White R: Surgery of renal cell carcinoma. Urol Clin North Am 20:263, 1993.

Preminger GM: Surgical management of calculus disease. *In* Bahnson RR (ed): Management of Urologic Disorders. London, Wolfe, 1994, pp 14.1–14.9.

Presti JC, Stoller ML, Carroll PR: Urology. *In* Tierney LM, McPhee SJ, Papadakis MA (eds): Current Medical Diagnosis and Treatment, ed 34. Norwalk, Conn, Appleton & Lange, 1995, pp 797–799, 802–806.

Raghavan D, Shipley WU, Garnick MB, et al: Biology and management of bladder cancer. N Engl J Med 322:1129, 1990.

Rao KV, Anderson WR, Kasiske BL, Dahl DC: Value of liver biopsy in the evaluation and management of chronic liver disease in renal transplant recipients. Am J Med 94:241–250, 1993.

Riehmann M, Bruskewitz R: Treatment of benign prostatic hyperplasia. *In* Bahnson RR (ed): Management of Urologic Disorders. London, Wolfe, 1994, pp 2.1–2.14.

Robertson CN: Renal tumors. *In* Bahnson RR (ed): Management of Urologic Disorders. London, Wolfe, 1994, pp 3.1–3.26.

Ross RK, Paganini-Hill A, Henderson BE: Epidemiology of bladder cancer. *In* Skinner DG, Lieskovsky G (eds): Genitourinary Cancer. Philadelphia, WB Saunders, 1988.

See WA, Dreicer R, Cohen MB: Adult tumors of the ureter and bladder. *In* Bahnson RR (ed): Management of Urologic Disorders. London, Wolfe, 1994, pp 4.2–4.25.

Spargo BH, Haas M: The Kidney. *In* Rubin E, Farber JL (eds): Pathology, ed 2. Philadelphia, JB Lippincott, 1994, pp 810–812, 842–844, 859–860.

Suthanthiran M, Strom TB: Renal transplantation. N Engl J Med 331:365–376, 1994.

Tannenbaum M: Ultrastructural pathology of human renal cell tumors. Pathol Annu 6:259, 1971.

Thon W, Altwein JE: Voiding dysfunction. Urology 23:323, 1984.

Tucker MS: Diagnosis and management of urinary incontinence. *In* Bahnson RR (ed): Management of Urologic Disorders. London, Wolfe, 1994, pp 10.1–10.28.

Urinary Incontinence Guideline Panel: Urinary incontinence in adults: Clinical practice guidelines. US Department of Health and Human Services. APCPR Publication (PHS) No. 92-0038. Rockville, Md, Agency for Health Care Policy and Research, 1992.

Van Stone JC: Dialysis and the Treatment of Renal Insufficiency. New York, Grune & Stratton, 1983, pp 1–31.

Wall RL, Clausen KP: Carcinoma of the urinary bladder in patients receiving cyclophosphamide. N Engl J Med 293:271, 1975.

Weinberger MW: Conservative treatment of urinary incontinence. Clin Obstet Gynecol 38:175–188, 1995.

Wells TJ: Pelvic (floor) muscle exercise. J Am Geriatr Soc 38:333–337, 1990.

Zelikovic I, Adelman RD, Nancarrow RA: Urinary tract infections in children—An update. West J Med 157:554–556, 1992.

Zeller KR: Low protein diets in renal disease. Diabetes Care 14:859–861, 1991.

Zweig S: Urinary tract infections in the elderly. Am Fam Pract 35:123–130, 1987.

SECTION 2

chapter 16

The Male Genital/ Reproductive System

William G. Boissonnault

The male genital or reproductive system is made up of the testes, epididymis, vas deferens, seminal vesicles, prostate gland, and penis (Fig. 16–1). These structures are susceptible to inflammatory disorders, neoplasms, and structural defects. The reproductive system also undergoes degenerative changes associated with aging that can affect sexual function. The testes become smaller, with thickening of the seminiferous tubules impeding sperm production; the prostate gland enlarges, potentially affecting urine outflow; and sclerotic changes occur in the local blood vessels possibly resulting in sexual dysfunction. The age-related decrease in male sex hormone levels also has significant local and systemic effects. Protein synthesis, salt and water balance, bone growth, and homeostasis and cardiovascular function are all under the influence of these hormones.

Unless treating patients with urinary incontinence, therapists do not typically treat patients for primary reproductive system disease, but because of the incidence and nature of these disorders an understanding of their clinical presentation is essential. Prostate cancer is the most common cancer in males in the United States and testicular cancer, although relatively rare, is the most common cancer in males aged 15 to 35 years. Benign prostatic hyperplasia (BPH) is one of the most common disorders of the elderly male population. Owing to the high incidence of these diseases, therapists will see clients with such a history and the disorder or prescribed medical treatment could have a profound effect on the client's clinical presentation and response to treatment. The initial presenting symptom for some of these disorders could be back pain, a condition for which physical therapy care is frequently sought. An awareness of other symptoms, besides pain, and signs associated with urogenital system diseases may alert the therapist to other origins of the back pain. The presence of such symptoms warrants communication with a physician regarding the client's status. Therapists have long been taught to ask clients with back pain questions regarding sexual function, the concern being the possible presence of cauda equina syndrome. An awareness of the more probable causes of sexual dysfunction will help the therapist determine the relevance and potentially urgent nature of a client's complaints. The disorders discussed in this chapter are those of the highest incidence or of greatest implications for therapists.

DISORDERS OF THE PROSTATE

Prostatitis

Overview. Inflammation of the prostate gland can be acute or chronic and bacterial or nonbacterial. These conditions are typically preceded by lower urinary tract infections (UTIs) (see Chapter 15). Therapists are least likely to encounter problems associated with acute prostatitis as the symptoms are usually severe enough that physician contact is initiated by the client and family and rehabilitation is typically placed on hold until the antibiotic therapy is successful. On the other hand, therapists are likely to encounter chronic bacterial prostatitis, which is a much more subtle disorder, and complete resolution with treatment is often difficult to obtain.

Incidence and Risk Factors. Although generally occurring with much higher frequency in women than men, UTIs are among the more common infections afflicting the male population. Elderly men are especially prone to develop UTI secondary to bladder outlet obstruction associated with BPH. As the infection ascends through the urogenital system the prostate can become involved (Norrby, 1990). Besides a history of UTI and BPH, recent urethral catheterization or instrumentation and multiple sexual partners increase the risk of developing prostatitis (Stewart, 1994). Lastly, poorly controlled diabetes mellitus increases the risk of UTI and prostatitis developing because the increased urine glucose provides the substrate for bacterial growth (Norrby, 1990; Stewart, 1994).

Pathogenesis. The most common form of prostate inflammation is nonbacterial prostatitis (Moldwin, 1994b). The cause is unknown, but a possible cause is intraprostatic urine reflux (Kirby, 1982). The urine reflux is theorized to cause a chemical prostatitis or to initiate an immunologic response to the urine (Meares, 1992). Although controversial, infectious agents such as gonococci, *Ureaplasma* species, chlamydiae, and mycoplasmata are thought to possibly play a role in the development of this disease.

The most commonly found pathogens associated with chronic bacterial infections are the gram-negative enterobacteria such as *Escherichia coli*, *Proteus mirabilis*, *Klebsiella pneumoniae*, and *Pseudomonas aeruginosa*. The pathogens associated with acute bacterial prostatitis include *E. coli*, pseudomonads, staphylococci, and streptococci (Stewart, 1994; Moldwin, 1994b).

Clinical Manifestations. See Table 16–1 for a summary of symptoms associated with nonbacterial prostatitis, chronic bacterial prostatitis, and acute bacterial prostatitis (Stewart, 1994; Moldwin, 1994b).

Medical Management

Diagnosis. Urinalysis, analysis of an expressed prostatic specimen, and a digital rectal examination (DRE) are used

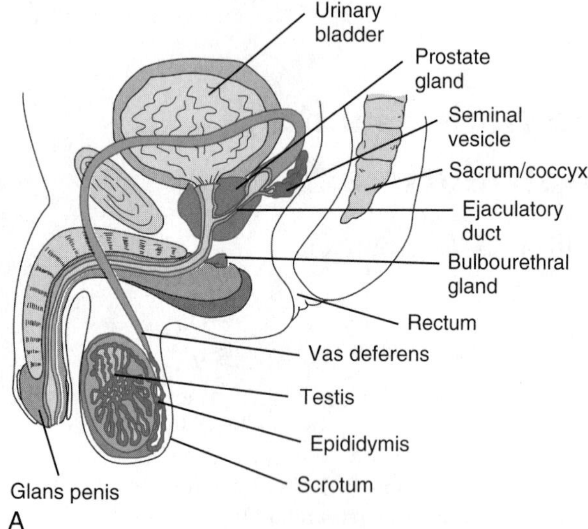

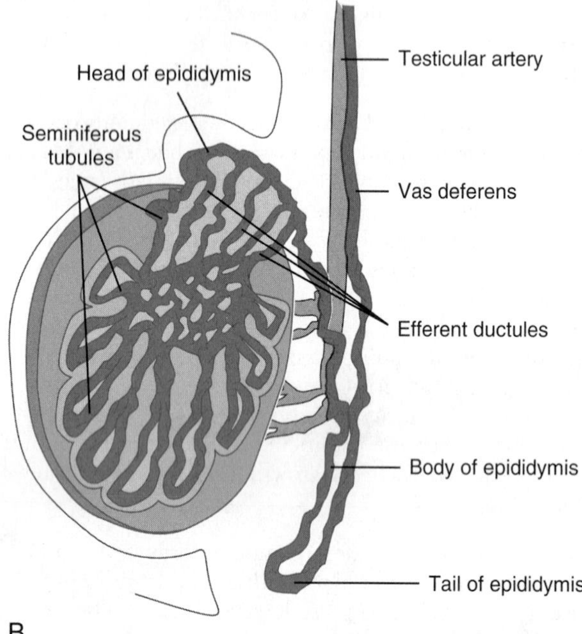

Figure **16–1.** *A*, The male reproductive system. *B*, Internal structure of the testis and relationship of the testis to the epididymis. (*From Guyton AC: Anatomy and Physiology. Philadelphia, WB Saunders, 1985.*)

to establish a diagnosis of prostatitis. The DRE may reveal a swollen, tender, and warm prostate. Computed tomography (CT) and transrectal ultrasound are utilized if a prostatic abscess is suspected (Stewart, 1994; Moldwin, 1994b).

Treatment. Because the cause of nonbacterial prostatitis is unknown, treatment is often given to simply provide symptom control and relief. Anti-inflammatory medications are administered. Tetracycline, erythromycin, and antifungal agents may also be given.

Treatment of chronic bacterial prostatitis can be equally as difficult, as the antibiotic agents have difficulty penetrating the chronically inflamed prostate. Drug therapy of 4 to 6 months' duration may be used in an attempt to treat this infection. Transurethral prostatectomy (TURP) may be indicated if the disease is not cured with medications.

Unlike chronic bacterial prostatitis, acute bacterial infections typically respond to antibiotic therapy. If the symptoms are severe, bed rest, antipyretics, analgesics, and stool softeners may be indicated. Hospitalization may be necessary and a suprapubic catheter may be indicated if urination is difficult (Moldwin, 1994b).

TABLE 16–1 CLINICAL MANIFESTATIONS OF PROSTATITIS

ACUTE	NONBACTERIAL	CHRONIC BACTERIAL
Urinary Frequency Urgency	Urinary Frequency Urgency	Urinary Frequency Urgency
Dysuria	Dysuria	Dysuria
Urethral discharge	Impotence	Myalgia
High fever	Decreased libido	Arthralgia
Chills	Pain Low back Rectal Scrotal	Pain Low back Rectal
Malaise		
Myalgia		
Arthralgia		
Pain Rectal Sacral		

Special Implications for the Therapist **16–1**

PROSTATITIS

When treating persons at risk of developing prostatitis, therapists need to be vigilant for the onset of symptoms listed in Table 16–1. The symptoms may be subtle initially or difficult to ascertain because of communication difficulties common in the elderly population. The fact that therapy may extend over a number of weeks may allow the therapist to detect the subtle changes and initiate contact with the primary physician.

In young people with back pain, the thought of visceral disease accounting for the back pain is not always at the forefront. Prostatitis can be the cause of back pain of unknown cause in young males. The presence of any of the symptoms listed in Table 16–1, along with the onset of back pain, should raise concern.

Lastly, when rehabilitating someone with a history of chronic bacterial prostatitis, therapists need to be aware of symptoms associated with UTIs. Many of these men will suffer recurrent UTIs as the prostatic bacteria continue to invade the bladder. The waxing and waning of symptoms may interfere with the client's compliance with a rehabilitation program.

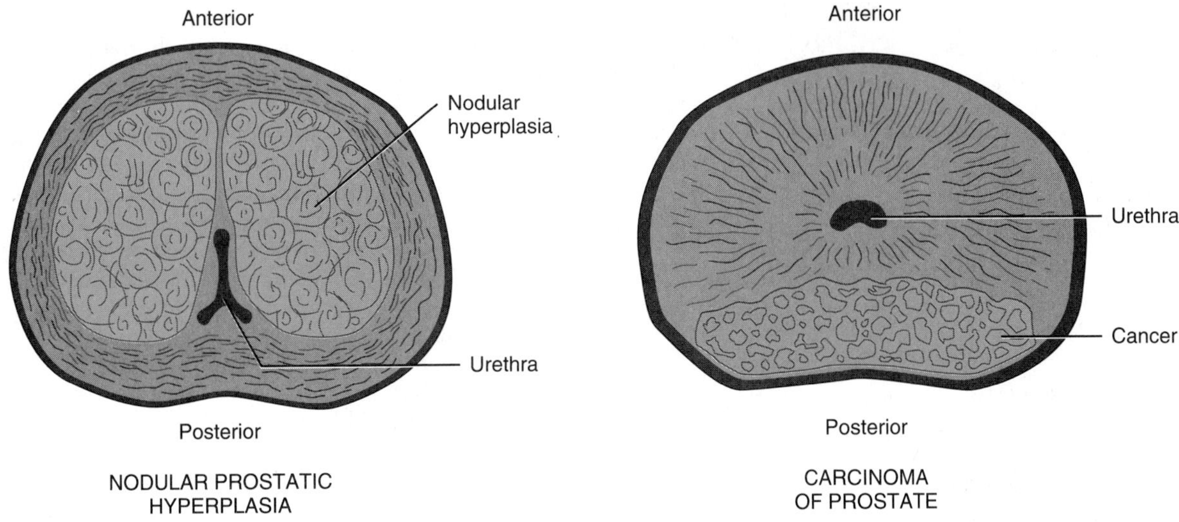

Figure **16–2.** In benign prostatic hyperplasia the nodules initially develop in the periurethral region, compressing the urethra. Cancer of the prostate typically develops initially in the periphery of the gland.

Benign Prostatic Hyperplasia

Overview. Benign prostatic hyperplasia is an age-related nonmalignant enlargement of the prostate gland.

Incidence and Risk Factors. Of men 50 years of age and older, 75% experience symptoms of prostate enlargement (Smith et al., 1988). Twenty-five percent of the subjects had symptoms severe enough that surgery was required. The disease is rarely noted in men below the age of 40 (Peterson, 1994).

Besides age, geography and race are important factors in the incidence of this disease. BPH is found most frequently in the United States and western Europe and least frequently in the Orient. The incidence of BPH is also higher in blacks than in whites (Peterson, 1994).

Pathogenesis. Although the cause is unknown, it is postulated that changes in hormone balance associated with aging are responsible for the development of BPH. Although commonly referred to as benign prostatic hypertrophy, the pathologic changes are marked by *hyperplasia*, not hypertrophy. Multiple prostatic nodules develop, resulting from the proliferation of epithelial cells, smooth muscle cells, and stromal fibroblasts of the gland. These nodules initially develop in the periurethral region of the prostate as opposed to the periphery of the gland (Fig. 16–2). The lumen of the urethra becomes progressively narrowed.

Regarding hormonal balance and aging, it appears that both androgens and estrogens contribute to the hyperplasia. Dihydrotestosterone (the biologically active metabolite of testosterone) is thought to be the primary mediator of hyperplasia, while estrogens sensitize the prostatic tissue to the growth-producing effects of dihydrotestosterone (Stewart, 1994; Robertson, 1994). The increased levels of estrogen that occur with aging may enhance the action of androgens at this point in the life cycle (Gillenwater et al., 1991).

Clinical Manifestations. The clinical presentation of BPH is related to secondary involvement of the urethra. The nodular hyperplasia results in a narrowing of the urethra, producing urinary outflow obstruction. The client may note a decreased caliber and force of the urine stream and difficulty initiating the urine stream. In addition, residual urine in the bladder results in urinary frequency, which is particularly troublesome at night (nocturia). As the urethral obstruction progresses, the risk of developing UTIs, marked bladder distention with destructive bladder wall changes, hydroureter,[1] and hydronephrosis[2] increases (Fig. 16–3). Ultimately, renal failure and death may occur if treatment is not initiated. Other urinary symptoms associated with the later stages of the disease include urge incontinence, terminal urinary dribbling, urgency, hematuria, and dysuria (Stewart, 1994; Peterson, 1994).

Medical Management

Diagnosis. Correlation of the history, palpation findings, and urodynamic test results (flow rate and force of stream) typically give rise to the diagnosis of BPH and indicate the choice of treatment. Regarding palpation, the bladder may be palpable as urinary retention progresses. In addition, a smooth, rubbery enlargement of the prostate may be noted during DRE, although the perceived size of the prostate does not always correlate with the degree of urethral compression (Riehmann and Bruskewitz, 1994).

The most commonly employed urodynamic test for the assessment of BPH is uroflowmetry.[3] The urine flow rate and the force of the urine stream are measured. Uroflowmetry by itself is a screening modality, not diagnostic, because the urinary obstruction could be occurring at sites other than at the prostate gland (Stewart, 1994; Riehmann and Bruskewitz, 1994).

---

[1] The ureteral wall becomes severely stretched secondary to the bladder outflow obstruction which increases the pressure in a retrograde direction. The ureteral wall can become stretched to the point where it loses the ability to undergo peristaltic contractions.

[2] Urine-filled dilation of the renal pelvis and calices. Destruction of renal tissue may occur.

[3] It is generally agreed that a peak urine flow rate of less than 10 mL/second is suggestive of obstruction.

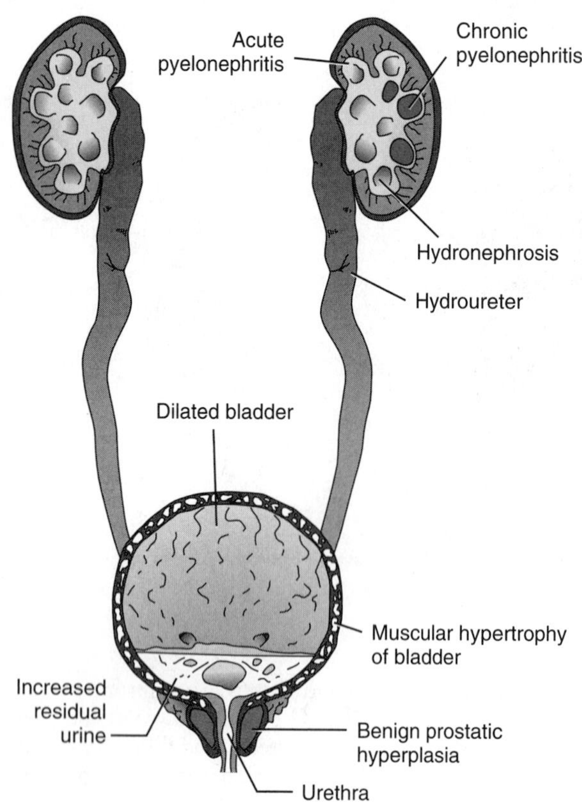

Figure **16–3.** A cascade of destructive events potentially associated with advanced benign prostatic hyperplasia.

In addition, diagnostic ultrasound and abdominal radiographs may be used to evaluate the size and length of the urethra, the size and configuration of the prostate, and the bladder capacity (Presti et al., 1995).

Treatment. If symptoms related to BPH are mild, the condition is often just monitored because the clinical status of the disorder may stabilize or even improve. Aggressive treatment is indicated, however, if the more severe symptoms of obstruction develop. Symptoms suggesting advanced disease include urine retention, incontinence, hematuria, and chronic UTIs. The goals of treatment include providing client comfort and avoiding serious renal damage (Christensen and Bruskewitz, 1990). For those with moderate to severe symptoms the two medical treatment approaches for BPH are surgical and pharmacologic.

The goal of surgical intervention is to alleviate the obstruction to urine flow. Transurethral resection of the prostate (TURP) has been the most commonly employed procedure, with approximately 400,000 surgeries done annually. An alternative technique is transurethral incision of the prostate (TUIP).[4] TURP is preferable in patients with a large gland, severe and recurrent gross hematuria, and prostatitis, where the goal is to remove infected tissue and calculi (Riehmann and Bruskewitz, 1994; Tafelski and Navarre, 1992).

Laser surgery to remove prostatic tissue is also being studied. The potential advantages of this procedure over TURP and TUIP are shorter hospitalization, shorter operative time, minimal bleeding, and decreased incidence of postoperative retrograde ejaculation and bladder neck contracture. Potential disadvantages include postoperative urinary retention, no tissue being available for histologic study, and less than optimal prospects for treating large lesions. The larger the lesion, the more passes required, increasing the risks associated with using a free-beam laser (Riehmann and Bruskewitz, 1994).

An alternative treatment to prostatectomy for patients with moderate symptoms and a small to moderate-sized gland (less than 40 g) is balloon dilation. Balloon dilation is less expensive, can be an outpatient procedure, and has fewer side effects, but its efficacy has not reached the levels of TURP (Stewart, 1994; Riehmann and Bruskewitz, 1994; Willis, 1992).

Pharmacologic agents can also be used to treat BPH. Three selective α-adrenergic blocking drugs have been utilized to decrease urethral obstruction. Prazosin, doxazosin, and terazosin cause smooth muscle relaxation. The α-adrenergic receptors are located in the muscle fibers of the adenoma and prostate capsule. The resultant smooth muscle relaxation decreases pressure on the urethra, enhancing urinary flow (Stewart, 1994; Riehmann and Bruskewitz, 1994).

Androgen suppression drug therapy can also be utilized to block the synthesis and action of testosterone, including dihydrotestosterone (DHT). A 20% to 30% reduction in prostate volume can be noted. This can result in a lessening of the severity of symptoms and improvement in the objective criteria related to urinary obstruction. Despite this, the efficacy of this treatment approach does not yet match that of the surgical approaches (Riehmann and Bruskewitz, 1994).

Special Implications for the Therapist **16–2**

BENIGN PROSTATIC HYPERPLASIA

Surgical procedures for BPH carry the risk of complications. The perineal prostatectomy approach has the highest risk of causing impotence, which occurs in approximately two thirds of cases. The risk of impotence is also substantial with TURP and TUIP. Retrograde ejaculation is also a risk with all three surgical approaches, although it is less frequently noted with TUIP. Unexplained patient complaints of sexual dysfunction warrant communication with a physician. If the patient notes sexual dysfunction and has a history of the above procedures, then ask the patient periodically about changes in sexual function. If there appears to be a worsening, communication with a physician would again be warranted.

Pharmacologic agents used to treat BPH are associated with numerous side effects. These include impotence, loss of libido, gynecomastia, drowsiness, dizziness, tachycardia, and postural hypotension. Monitoring pre–drug therapy side effects is important because a change or new onset of symptoms may necessitate communication with a physician.

Prostate Cancer

Overview. Adenocarcinoma of the prostate accounts for 98% of primary prostatic tumors (Peterson, 1994). Ductal

[4] The incisions in the muscle wall of the prostate and bladder neck allow for an outward expansion of the gland, relieving some of the pressure on the urethra.

and transitional cell carcinomas make up the remainder of the tumors (Whitmore, 1984). Bony metastasis is common, especially to the spine, ribs, and pelvis (Peterson, 1994; Presti et al., 1995). Of the primary tumors that metastasize to the spine, prostate lesions rank fourth behind breast, lung, and myeloma (McLain and Weinstein, 1990). Prostate cancer can also metastasize to the lungs and liver.

Incidence. Prostate cancer, the most common cancer in American men, is the second most common cause of male death from cancer (National Cancer Institute, 1988). In 1997 it is estimated that prostrate cancer will account for approximately 43% (334,500) of the new male cancer cases and for 14% of male cancer deaths. The number of new cases of prostate cancer in 1997 represents an increase of 200% compared to 1990 figures (Parker et al., 1997). Autopsy studies indicate the actual incidence of this disease is much higher than these figures indicate (Peterson, 1994).

Risk Factors. Box 16–1 lists risk factors related to prostate cancer. Prostate cancer is a disease of the elderly male (Meikle and Smith, 1990). Autopsy studies indicate that occult prostate cancer is present in 25% of men aged 60 to 69, in 40% of men aged 70 to 79, and in over 50% of men 80 years of age and older (Scardino, 1989). Men less than 50 years old make up less than 1% of those with prostate cancer (Peterson, 1994). The other known risk factor besides age is race. Blacks are twice as likely as whites to develop the disease (Paulson, 1989; Peterson, 1994).

Other risk factors have been suggested. Geographically, the highest frequencies of prostate cancer are found in the United States and Scandinavian countries, while the lowest are found in Mexico, Greece, and Japan (Peterson, 1994; Hanchette and Schwartz, 1992). Although no genetic marker has been found, a familial history of prostate cancer is a risk factor. An eightfold increase in risk has been estimated for men who have both a first- and second-degree relative with the disease (Steinber et al., 1990). In addition, mortality from prostate cancer is believed to be three times greater in relatives of men with prostate cancer compared with those without such a family history (Stewart, 1994). Exposure to cadmium through welding, electroplating, alkaline battery production, farming, typesetting, and ship fitting places men at higher risk of prostate cancer (Stewart, 1994; Hanchette and Schwartz, 1992). Lastly, high dietary fat intake has been correlated with prostate cancer (Chamberlain et al., 1993; Giovannucci, 1994).

Etiology and Pathogenesis. Although the precise cause of prostate cancer is unknown, a strong endocrine system link is theorized. Androgens in particular have been implicated based on the androgenic control of normal growth and development of the prostate and the fact that males castrated before puberty do not develop prostate cancer or BPH. In addition, the responsiveness of prostate cancer to surgical castration and estrogen therapy supports this theory. Lastly, the higher incidence of cancer in blacks is correlated with a 15% higher serum testosterone level in blacks (Edelstein and Babayan, 1993).

Most prostatic adenocarcinomas are characterized by small to moderate-sized disorganized glands that infiltrate the stroma of the prostate. The tumors are more likely to develop initially in the periphery of the prostate, unlike BPH where the pathologic changes typically originate close to the urethra (see Fig. 16–2). The cancer invades adjacent local structures such as the seminal vesicles and urinary bladder, and spreads to the musculoskeletal system, particularly the axial skeleton, and lungs. Lymphatic metastasis may involve the obturator, iliac, and periaortic lymph nodes, extending up through the thoracic duct.

BOX 16–1
Risk Factors for Prostate Cancer

- Age >50 yr
- Black race
- Geography (United States and Scandinavian countries)
- Family history
- Environmental exposure to cadmium
- Diet—high fat intake

Clinical Manifestations. The clinical presentation of prostate cancer is extremely variable. In many patients the disease is noted incidentally on DRE or discovered in fragments of prostatic tissue removed via TURP for BPH. Depending on the size and location of the lesion, the initial presenting symptom could be related to urinary obstruction, onset of pain, or constitutional symptoms such as fatigue and weight loss.

The urinary obstruction symptoms associated with cancer are similar to those associated with BPH, but typically present in later stages of the disease compared to BPH. Cancer originating in the subcapsular region of the prostate as opposed to the periurethral area would account for this difference. The obstructive symptoms include urinary urgency, frequency, hesitancy, dysuria, hematuria, difficulty initiating the urine stream, and decreased urine stream. Blood in the ejaculate may also be noted.

Pain complaints associated with prostate cancer can vary tremendously. A dull, vague ache may be noted in the rectal, sacral, or lumbar spine region. The sacral and lumbar pain is typically associated with bony metastasis. Pain may be noted in the thoracic and shoulder girdle areas secondary to lymphatic spread of the disease or again secondary to bony metastasis. Lastly, symptoms such as fatigue, weight loss, anemia, and dyspnea have all been attributed to metastatic spread of the disease (Stewart, 1994; Robertson, 1994; McGinnis and Gomella, 1994).

Medical Management

Diagnosis. The diagnosis of prostate cancer is made by a variety of tests, including DRE, transrectal ultrasound, serum prostate-specific antigen (PSA) assay, and radiographic imaging modalities. Ultimately, tissue biopsy is performed to confirm the diagnosis.

The DRE may reveal a hardened, fixed structure or a diffusely undulated gland. A limitation to this procedure is that typically only the posterior and lateral aspects of the prostate can be palpated (Canter et al., 1990). Transrectal ultrasound is being used less as a first-line screening tool because of its poor specificity, expense, and because its detection rate of cancer varies little compared with the combined use of DRE and PSA testing. The modality is useful, though, in directing the biopsy procedure and staging of the disease.

The PSA assay is now an important part of the screening process. PSA is a glycoprotein produced exclusively in the cytoplasm of benign and malignant prostatic cells. The average prostatic cancer produces approximately 10 times the PSA a normal prostate gland does (Gittes, 1991). An elevated PSA assay, however, may also be related to prostatitis, BPH, prostatic infarcts, and prostatic biopsy and surgery. Therefore, an elevated PSA is organ-specific but is not diagnostic by itself. Lastly, the PSA may be false-negative in up to 30% of patients with localized prostate cancer (Small, 1993).

Recent research has focused on PSA velocity and density, hoping to enhance the diagnostic capabilities of this test. There are indications that higher PSA velocities and densities are found in prostate cancer (Carter et al., 1992; Oesterling, 1993).

Radiographic imaging modalities are also utilized for staging of the disease. Magnetic resonance imaging (MRI) allows for evaluation of the prostate gland and regional lymph nodes. Lymph node involvement must typically be advanced (nodes larger than 1 cm) to be for demonstrable. Radiographs may detect metastatic lesions, but the radionuclide bone scan, although not diagnostic, is a more sensitive modality for detection of a metabolically active lesion (Presti et al., 1995; McGinnis and Gomella, 1994; Stewart, 1994).

Staging. The Whitmore-Jewett staging system is the one most commonly used. The spread of prostate cancer has been divided into four stages, A through D (Fig. 16–4). The stage of the disease at the time of the diagnosis helps dictate the course of treatment (Peterson, 1994; McGinnis and Gomella, 1994).

Treatment. The medical treatment of prostate cancer depends on the patient's age, health, and the stage of the disease. The disease is treated by surgery, radiation therapy, and hormone manipulation.

Unless relatively young, men with early stage A disease are simply monitored because prostate cancer can be an indolent disease. These cancers rarely progress during the initial 5 years after diagnosis, but do progress in 10% to 25% of clients 10 years after diagnosis (Blute et al., 1986; Epstein et al., 1986). Generally, though, men with a life expectancy of 10 years or more and with disease diagnosed in later stage A or B undergo radical prostatectomy and possibly radiation therapy (Catalona, 1994). Radical prostatectomy involves removal of the prostate, seminal vesicles, and a portion of the bladder neck. The surgical approach can be retropubic or perineal. The retropubic approach involves an incision from the pubic symphysis to the umbilicus and allows for staging pelvic lymphadenectomy. The primary postoperative complications are infection, incontinence, impotence, excessive bleeding, and rectal injury. Potency may return gradually over the course of a year (McGinnis and Gomella, 1994).

Radiation therapy may be utilized to treat localized prostatic lesions, be an adjunctive treatment after radical prostatectomy, or be used for palliative effects in the presence of widespread disease. Relief of pain and improvement in symptoms associated with urethral obstruction are possible benefits of this treatment modality. Radiation therapy is most

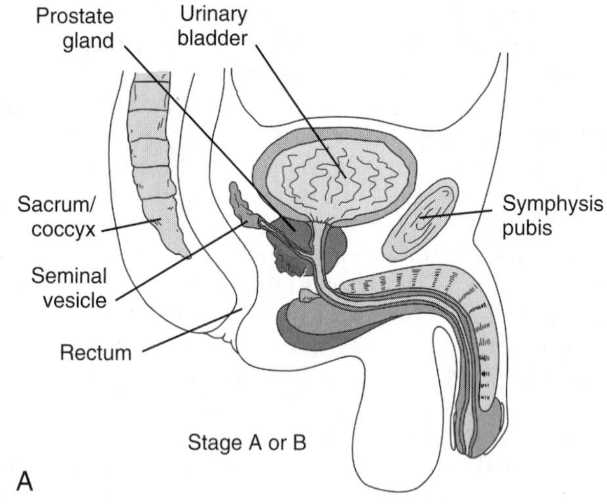

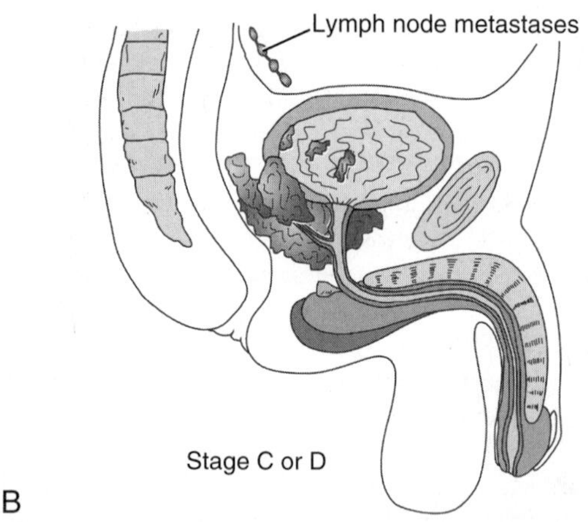

Figure 16–4. Prostate cancer: clinical staging. A, The tumor has not spread beyond the gland's capsule in stages A and B. B, In stage C the tumor has spread into adjacent tissues; in stage D the disease has spread into the lymphatic system and beyond.

often used with stage C disease because many of the patients have occult pelvic lymph node metastases. The radiation therapy can be administered by external beam radiation or by seed implantation (McGinnis and Gomella, 1994; Catalona, 1994).

Hormone therapy is the treatment of choice in the presence of stage D disease, the goal being androgen deprivation. Since the testes produce 95% of the circulating testosterone, orchiectomy is the primary method of manipulating hormone levels. A second option is estrogen therapy, but because of its side effects it is utilized less frequently. The adverse effects include impotence, gynecomastia, loss of libido, bloating, and pedal edema. Also, serious cardiovascular disease, including stroke, heart attack, and deep venous thrombosis, can be associated with estrogen therapy in those patients at high risk. Luteinizing hormone–releasing hormone (LH-RH) agonists and androgen blockers are also used, but their use is limited.

Lastly, total androgen block is a new concept designed to shut down the production of androgens taking place in the testes and adrenal glands. This can be achieved by either orchiectomy or LH-RH agonists in combination with an androgen blocker (McGinnis and Gomella, 1994; Catalona, 1994).

Once the cancer treatment has begun, most clients are reevaluated every 3 to 6 months. At follow-up visits symptoms of urinary obstruction and pain are investigated. DRE and a PSA assay are carried out and prostatic acid phosphatase levels are measured. Other tests may be routinely ordered depending on the patient's status.

Special Implications for the Therapist **16-3**

PROSTATE CANCER

Considering the number of elderly clients that physical therapists work with and the incidence of prostate disease, therapists are seeing a number of clients with preexisting prostate conditions. Investigating the symptoms or signs associated with the condition provides the therapist with the baseline information needed to monitor the client's status. For example, if the client experiences difficulty with initiating the urine stream and with urinary frequency, the therapist should periodically ask if there has been a change regarding the urinary dysfunction. If there has been a worsening, the client should be referred to the physician who is managing the prostate condition. Knowledge of other potential symptoms associated with prostate conditions provide the basis for a screening checklist the therapist could utilize periodically while treating the patient. Once again, if an onset of new symptoms is noted, referral to the physician is warranted.

Pain is often the primary or only symptom associated with prostate disease. If the pain is located in the thoracic, lumbar, or sacral area the client may seek care from a therapist, thinking the pain is of mechanical origin. Metastatic spread of the disease to the axial skeleton or the periaortic lymph nodes may account for these complaints. If the patient's back pain does not present in a mechanical fashion (based on history and physical examination findings) or the patient notes urologic dysfunction, referral to a physician is warranted.

Important implications exist related to the commonly employed treatment approaches to the various prostate conditions. Complications associated with radical prostatectomy procedures include infection, incontinence, and impotence. If the therapist is seeing a patient who has undergone such a procedure, being vigilant for symptoms associated with infection is necessary for months after the surgery. If the patient notes malaise, fever, chills, sweats, or sudden worsening of symptoms, communication with the physician is warranted. The surgery may account for the patient's complaints of incontinence and impotence. The average time to achieve continence is 3 weeks with virtually all patients being continent within 6 months. Postoperative impotence occurs in 70% of patients who undergo retropubic prostatectomy. Potency can gradually return over the course of a year (McGinnis and Gomella, 1994).

Although reduced in recent years, complications of radiation therapy can occur. Diarrhea, gastrointestinal or urinary bleeding, irritative voiding symptoms, and tenesmus (painful spasm of the anal sphincter with straining) are all possible complications. The presence of these problems could interfere with a rehabilitation program, slowing progress. A recent onset or worsening of any of these complications should be brought to the physician's attention.

Multiple potential side effects are associated with endrocine or hormonal manipulation (Box 16–2). As with the complications associated with surgical procedures and radiation therapy, these problems may interfere with rehabilitation of the patient, altering the prognosis. Knowing the patient is being treated with endocrine manipulative therapy and being familiar with the side effects can lessen alarm on the therapist's part if the client reports any of these symptoms. If symptoms or signs of myocardial infarct, cerebral vascular accident, or deep venous thrombosis develop, immediate referral to a physician is warranted (see Chapter 10).

DISORDERS OF THE TESTES

Orchitis

Description and Etiology. Orchitis is inflammation of the testis and can be acute or chronic. It is often associated with epididymitis. Gram-negative bacteria and *Chlamydia trachomatis* are the usual infectious agents.

Incidence and Risk Factors. Patients with primary infections of the genitourinary tract or infections in other body regions (e.g., pneumonia, scarlet fever) are at risk of developing orchitis. Sexually active males with multiple partners are at higher risk of developing genitourinary infections. Males 10 years of age and older who have parotitis (mumps), are also at risk of developing orchitis (Stewart, 1994). The incidence of orchitis in this group can be as high as 25% to 33% (Gillenwater et al., 1991). Catheterized (indwelling) males are also at higher risk of developing orchitis secondary to genitourinary tract infection.

Pathogenesis. Orchitis is often secondary to UTIs. The bloodstream and lymphatics are then the route of spread from other body areas to the testes. Systemic infections, such as

BOX **16-2**
Side Effects of Hormonal Manipulation

- Loss of libido
- Impotence
- Hot flashes
- Gynecomastia
- Bloating and pedal edema
- Nausea and vomiting
- Diarrhea
- Myocardial infarction, cerebrovascular accident, deep venous thrombosis

pneumonia, scarlet fever, and parotitis, utilize the same routes to spread to the testes (Stewart, 1994; Peterson, 1994).

Clinical Manifestations. Orchitis is marked by testicular pain and swelling. Pain may also be noted in the lower abdominal area. Fever and malaise can be present, but symptoms of urinary dysfunction are usually absent.

Medical Management

Diagnosis. Physical examination reveals a tender and swollen testicle. Laboratory tests revealing an elevated white blood cell count and urinalysis is an important component of the diagnostic process.

Treatment. See under Epididymitis and Special Implications for the Therapist.

See Special Implications for the Therapist: Testicular Torsion.

Epididymitis

Description and Risk Factors. Epididymitis is an inflammation of the epididymis. There are two primary types of epididymitis: sexually and nonsexually transmitted infections. Males, typically under the age of 40, sexually active with multiple partners, are at higher risk of developing genitourinary disease which can lead to epididymitis. Iatrogenic sources of infection include cystoscopy and indwelling catheters. In the older male population this condition can be precipitated by prostatitis and UTIs.

Pathogenesis and Etiology. Epididymitis is typically caused by bacterial pathogens. The sexually transmitted infections leading to epididymitis are associated with urethritis. In the nonsexually transmitted infections, urine-containing pathogens may be forced up the ejaculatory ducts, through the vas deferens, and into the epididymis. Pressure associated with voiding and physical strain can force the urine from the urethra. Infection originating elsewhere in the body can spread to the epididymis via the lymphatics of the spermatic cord. Congenital urinary tract abnormalities can lead to epididymitis in children (Stewart, 1994; Moldwin, 1994a).

Clinical Manifestations. Epididymitis may be associated with pain, urinary dysfunction, fever, and urethral discharge. Unilateral scrotal pain is common, but pain may also be noted in the lower abdominal, groin, or hip adductor muscle areas. When bacteriuria is present, urinary frequency and urgency and dysuria can occur. When the epididymitis is related to sexually transmitted disease, urethritis and urethral discharge are present concurrently (Berger et al., 1979). Lastly, local scrotal erythema and swelling are associated with epididymitis (Stewart, 1994; Moldwin, 1994).

Medical Management

Diagnosis. In addition to the findings noted under Clinical Manifestations, urinalysis, urethral smear, and urine culture are important for the diagnosis of epididymitis. An elevated white blood cell count is also usually present (Stewart, 1994; Moldwin, 1994a).

Treatment. During the acute phase, treatment includes bed rest, scrotal elevation and support, nonsteroidal anti-inflammatory medication, or antibiotics. Hospitalization may be necessary if signs of sepsis or abscess formation are present or if the pain is severe. Once treatment has been initiated, a significant decrease in pain should be noted within a week, but the scrotal edema may be present for 2 to 3 months (Moldwin, 1994a; Stewart 1994). (See discussions on epididymitis and testicular torsion.)

Testicular Torsion

Overview. Testicular torsion is an abnormal twisting of the spermatic cord as the testis rotates within the tunica vaginalis. The torsion can occur intra- or extravaginally, but intravaginal torsion is the more common. This condition is a surgical emergency. Early diagnosis and treatment is imperative to save the testis (Stewart, 1994).

Etiology. Torsion of the spermatic cord is often associated with congenital abnormalities. These include absence of the scrotal ligaments, incomplete descent of the testis, and a high attachment of the tunica vaginalis. Increased mobility of the testis and epididymis within the tunica vaginalis, facilitate twisting of the spermatic cord. Testicular torsion can also occur after heavy physical activity (Peterson, 1994).

Incidence and Risk Factors. Intravaginal torsion most frequently occurs in males 8 to 18 years of age. The condition is rarely seen after age 30. The extravaginal torsions occur primarily in neonates. A firm, painless scrotal mass is discovered shortly after birth (Stewart, 1994).

Pathogenesis. The spermatic cord contains the vas deferens and the nerve and blood supply for the scrotal contents. If the torsion is severe enough to occlude the arterial supply, infarction of testicular germ cells can quickly occur. Intravaginal torsions are often precipitated by congenital abnormalities. These anomalies allow for rotation of the testis around the spermatic cord or the torsion may occur between the testis and epididymis. Extravaginal torsion occurs most often during the fetal descent of the testes, before the tunica adheres to the scrotal wall. This allows the testis and fascial tunica to rotate around the spermatic cord above the level of the tunica vaginalis (Stewart, 1994).

Clinical Manifestations. An abrupt onset of scrotal pain and then swelling suggests testicular torsion. The pain may extend up into the inguinal area. Nausea, vomiting, and tachycardia may be present.

Medical Management

Diagnosis. Physical examination reveals a firm, tender testis that is often positioned high in the scrotum. Erythema and scrotal edema may be present. The cremasteric reflex is often absent. Doppler ultrasound and radionuclide scanning may aid in the diagnosis. A urinalysis is performed to help rule out infection (Stewart, 1994).

Treatment. Once the diagnosis of testicular torsion is made, emergency surgery is performed. The procedure includes detorsion and if the testis is deemed nonviable, then an orchiectomy is performed. The duration of the torsion is critical regarding salvage of the testis. If the surgery is performed within 3 hours of onset, a greater than 80% salvage rate occurs. The salvage rate drops to 20% if more than 12 hours passes before the surgery (Stewart, 1994).

Special Implications for the Therapist **16–4**

TESTICULAR TORSION

Pain extending into the groin and scrotum can occasionally be referred from muscle or joint structures, but if a client notes the onset of scrotal pain, immediate communication with a physician is warranted. Ask the client if he has noted scrotal swelling or tenderness, if he feels feverish or nauseated, if he has any difficulties with urination, including urgency, frequency, or dysuria, or if he has noted any urethral discharge. If the scrotal or groin pain is associated with musculoskeletal dysfunction one would expect that the therapist could alter the symptoms by mechanically stressing a component of the musculoskeletal system.

Testicular Cancer

Overview. Testicular tumors are divided into two primary histogenetic categories. Germ cell tumors make up more than 90% of testicular tumors, while tumors of stromal or sex cord origin make up a majority of the remaining neoplasms.

Incidence. Approximately 7200 new cases of testicular cancer were estimated to occur in the United States in 1997 (Parker et al., 1997). Testicular cancer accounts for approximately 3% of male urogenital cancers (Stewart, 1994). Although relatively rare, testicular cancer is the most common cancer in the 15- to 35-year-old male age group.

Etiology and Risk Factors. Although the cause is unknown, congenital and acquired factors have been associated with the development of testicular cancer. The most significant factor is the association of cryptorchidism (the testes not descending into the scrotum) and testicular cancer. The incidence of testicular cancer is 35 times higher in males with a cryptoid testis (Lasater, 1990). Other risk factors include a 2% to 6% higher incidence in males whose mothers took exogenous estrogen during pregnancy (Presti and Herr, 1992). Lastly, a history of infertility, scrotal trauma, or infection has been associated with an increased risk of developing testicular cancer, though a causal relationship has not been established (Stewart, 1994; Foster and Donohue, 1994).

Pathogenesis. Since germ cell tumors make up the vast majority of testicular cancers, the following discussion focuses solely on such tumors. The neoplastic transformation of a germ cell results in either a seminoma, an undifferentiated tumor, or an embryonal carcinoma. Seminomas are the most common testicular cancers, accounting for approximately 40% to 50% of germ cell tumors (Peterson, 1994; Stewart, 1994). Seminomas appear as a solid, gray-white growth. The entire testis can be replaced by the tumor. As opposed to embryonal carcinomas, hemorrhage, necrosis, or cystic changes are uncommon in seminomas.

Yolk cell tumors are the most common germ cell tumors of infants. These tumors result in enlarged testes which appear grossly as poorly defined lobulated masses. Focal areas of hemorrhage are common (Peterson, 1994; Stewart, 1994).

Clinical Manifestations. The most common initial sign of testicular cancer is enlargement of the testis. This sign may go undetected if the male is not periodically performing testicular self-examination. The enlargement may be accompanied by an ache in the abdomen or scrotum, or a sensation of heaviness in the scrotum. There may be metastasis though with little or no local change noted in the scrotum.

Metastatic testicular cancer can present as back pain (may be the primary presenting complaint), abdominal mass, hemoptysis, or neck or supraclavicular adenopathy. Pain may be the sole presenting symptom in metastasis to the retroperitoneal, cervical, and supraclavicular lymphatic chains. Twenty-one percent of men with testicular germ cell cancer had back pain as the primary presenting symptoms in the study of Cantwell et al. (1987). There was a significant delay in diagnosis of testicular cancer in these patients compared to patients who also had symptomatic unilateral testicular enlargement.

Medical Management

Diagnosis. A thorough urologic history and physical examination are the basis for making a diagnosis of testicular cancer. A painless testicular mass is highly suggestive of testicular cancer. Transillumination of the scrotum may also reveal a testicular mass. Testicular ultrasound is used to differentiate a variety of scrotal disorders besides cancer (e.g., epididymitis, orchitis, hydrocele, or hematocele). The modalities utilized to assess metastatic spread include computed tomography (CT) scans and MRI.

Staging. Clinical staging is based on the TNM classification system: stage I—tumor confined to the testis; stage II—spread to the retroperitoneal lymph nodes; stage III—distant metastasis.

Generally, the prognosis with testicular cancer is excellent. The prognosis, though, is contingent upon prompt diagnosis. One confounding factor related to the diagnosis being delayed is the potential lack of perceptible testicular changes while the disease spreads.

Treatment. Once diagnosed, treatment of testicular cancer includes orchiectomy. Additional therapies that may be utilized include chemotherapy, radiation therapy, and peritoneal lymphatic dissection. The recommendation of which therapies to include is based on pathologic findings from the orchiectomy and results of the CT and MRI procedures. Radiation therapy is included in the treatment of stage I or II seminomas with irradiation of the retroperitoneal and homolateral lymph nodes to the level of the diaphragm. Retroperitoneal lymph node dissection is often utilized to treat stage II seminomas and nonseminoma germ cell tumors. Chemotherapy is used in patients with extensive metastasis (Stewart, 1994; Foster and Donohue, 1994).

Special Implications for the Therapist **16-5**

TESTICULAR CANCER

Therapists need to be aware of the potential symptoms and signs related to this disease because clients may be seen by the therapist for other conditions before the cancer is diagnosed. The most likely scenario is someone with thoracic or lumbar pain secondary to undiagnosed lymph node adenopathy or with low lumbar pain that seems to spread around the iliac crest to the groin. Low lumbar and iliac crest pain may be secondary to dysfunction while the groin pain could be secondary to the cancer. Correlation of findings from the history and physical examination and the client's response to treatment may raise suspicion, warranting communication with a physician.

An awareness of the location of superficial lymph nodes is also important for the therapist (Fig. 16-5). Observation of a mass or even a "filling in" of the concavity normally found in the left supraclavicular region should alert the therapist to palpate this area. Palpation of a nodule warrants a referral to a physician.

Treatment of testicular cancer also holds implications for the therapist. The surgical scars related to orchiectomy and retroperitoneal lymph node dissection may affect the patient's posture or movement mechanics of the trunk, pelvis, and hip regions. Other potential adverse effects of the surgery include sexual dysfunction, such as retrograde ejaculation or failure to ejaculate. See Treatment and Special Implications for the Therapist: Prostate Cancer for a description of side effects of radiation and chemotherapy.

IMPOTENCE

Overview. Impotence is a general term which expresses a problem with libido, penile erection, ejaculation, or orgasm.

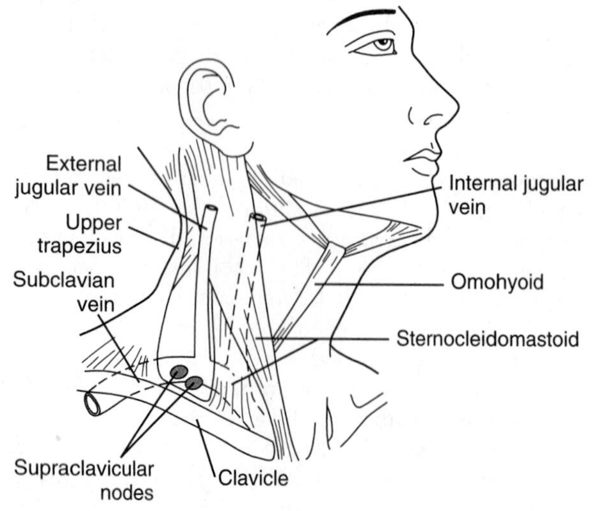

Figure **16-5.** Anatomic location of supraclavicular nodes.

The contemporary diagnostic term is erectile dysfunction (Broderick, 1994).

Incidence and Risk Factors. The Massachusetts Male Aging Study revealed that 51% of 1290 men aged from 40 to 70 had a complaint of impotence. The complaints ranged from minimally impotent (16%), to moderately impotent (25%), to completely impotent (10%) (Feldman et al., 1992). See Box 16-3 for a list of medications, diseases, and surgeries associated with sexual dysfunction.

Etiology. Impotence may be organic or psychogenic. Approximately 50% to 80% of men seeking treatment for sexual dysfunction have an organic lesion (Jünemann et al., 1990). The ratio of organic to psychogenic lesions is directly proportional to age. In 70% of men less than 35 years old the cause is psychogenic. In 85% of men over the age of 50 the cause is organic (Masters, 1986; Mellinger and Weiss, 1992). The psychogenic factors include anxiety, fear, depression, stress, fatigue, and so forth. The organic causes may be neurogenic, vascular, or endocrine factors.

Pathogenesis. Numerous factors and structures can influence the process of sexual function and dysfunction. Coordinated interaction between regulatory centers in the diencephalon, brainstem, and spinal cord are required for sexual function. In addition, the end organs of the vascular and nerve tree of the penis, the smooth muscle of the corpora cavernosa, the skeletal muscle of the penis, and the accessory sex glands all have important roles in sexual function. It is beyond the scope of this textbook to cover all of the possible mechanisms leading to sexual dysfunction, but some examples follow.

Neurogenic erectile dysfunction can result from surgical or traumatic injury to the autonomic or somatic penile innervation. The other possible neurologic mechanism is microscopic neuropathy with breakdown of cholinergic, adrenergic, noncholinergic, or nonadrenergic neurotransmis-

BOX **16-3**
Risk Factors for Impotence

Medical History
- Diabetes
- Coronary heart disease
- Hypothyroidism
- Hypopituitarism
- Hypertension
- Chronic uremia
- Neuromuscular disease
- Psychiatric disorders
- Multiple sclerosis
- Chronic alcoholism

Surgical History
- Transurethral procedures
- Aortoiliac procedures
- Proctocolectomy
- Abdominoperineal resection

Medications
- Antihypertensives
- Tranquilizers
- Amphetamines

sion. Patients with diabetes mellitus experience change in the ultrastructure of the cavernous nerves arising from the S2–S4 spinal nerves. These changes include diffuse thickening of the Schwann cells and perineural basement membranes.

Conditions resulting in arterial insufficiency can also result in local penile changes. Changes in smooth muscle cells can occur with vascular insufficiency, including irregular contour, fragmentation, loss of basement lamina, and the cytoplasm showing deficits of contractile myofilaments (Khawand et al., 1987).

Clinical Manifestations. Manifestations of sexual dysfunction include inability to have or maintain penile erection, inability to achieve orgasm, infertility, and dyspareunia.

Medical Management

Diagnosis. Owing to the sheer number of possible etiologic factors, a definitive diagnosis related to impotence can be difficult. Differentiating between an organic vs. psychogenic cause is the initial challenge. The nocturnal penile tumescence test, which monitors the incidence of nocturnal erections, helps with this distinction. Men with psychogenic impotence will have nocturnal erections, whereas those with an organic lesion will not (Presti et al., 1995). Arteriography is the standard test for vascular diagnostic testing, but ultrasonography is also utilized to assess the vascular integrity of the genital area.

Treatment. Medical treatment for impotence varies depending on the cause. Testosterone injections are an option for men with documented androgen deficiency. Injection of vasoactive substances directly into the penis is also utilized. Penile prosthetic devices can be implanted surgically and men with arterial and venous deficiencies are candidates for vascular reconstruction procedures. Lastly, psychological counseling is indicated for those with a psychogenic basis for the impotence (Presti et al., 1995).

Special Implications for the Therapist **16-6**

IMPOTENCE

Therapists ask patients with back pain about the presence of sexual dysfunction as part of the screening for cauda equina syndrome. Many patients who answer yes to these questions may have a preexisting condition that accounts for the impotence. Sexual dysfunction may be a postoperative complication related to some of the procedures described earlier in this chapter. If the patient notes a sudden change in sexual function, communication with a physician is warranted.

References

Berger RE, Alexander ER, Harnisch JP, et al: Etiology, manifestations and therapy of acute epididymitis: Prospective study of 50 cases. J Urol 121:750–754, 1979.

Blute ML, Zincke H, Farrow GM: Long term follow-up of young patients with stage A adenocarcinoma of the prostate. J Urol 136:840–843, 1986.

Broderick GA: Impotence. *In* Bahnson RR (ed): Management of Urologic Disorders. London, Wolfe, 1994 pp 11.2–11.31.

Canter H, Piantadosis S, Isaccs J: Clinical evidence for and implications of the multistep development of prostate cancer. J Urol 143:742–748, 1990.

Cantwell B, Mannix KA, Harris AL: Back pain—A presentation of metastatic testicular germ cell tumors. Lancet 1:262–264, 1987.

Carter HB, Pearson TD, Metter EJ, et al: Longitudinal evaluation of prostate-specific antigen levels in men with and without prostate disease. JAMA 267:2215–2220, 1992.

Catalona WJ: Management of cancer of the prostate. N Engl J Med 331:996–1004, 1994.

Chamberlain J, Melia J, Shearer RJ, et al: Prostate cancer—Grand rounds. Lancet 342:901–905, 1993.

Christensen MM, Bruskewitz RC: Clinical manifestations of benign prostatic hyperplasia and indications for therapeutic interventions. Urol Clin North Am 17:509–515, 1990.

Edelstein R, Babayan R: Managing prostate cancer. Part I: Localized disease. Hosp Pract 28(4):61–78, 1993.

Epstein JI, Paull G, Eggleston JC, Walsh PC: Prognosis of untreated stage A1 prostatic carcinoma: A study of 94 cases with extended follow-up. J Urol 136:837–839, 1986.

Feldman H, Goldstein I, Hatzichristou DG, et al.: Impotence and its medical and psychological correlates: Results of the Massachusetts male aging study. Int J Impot Res 4(suppl 2):A17, 1992.

Foster RS, Donohue JP: Management of testis cancer. *In* Bahnson RR (ed): Management of Urologic Disorders. London, Wolfe, 1994, pp 6.2–6.12.

Gillenwater JY, Grayhoch JT, Howards SS, et al: Adult and Pediatric Urology, ed 2. St Louis, Mosby–Year Book, 1991.

Giovannucci E: A prospective study of dietary fat and risk of prostate cancer. J Natl Cancer Inst 271:498, 1994.

Gittes RF: Carcinoma of the prostate. N Engl J Med 324:236–245, 1991.

Hanchette C, Schwartz G: Geographic patterns of prostate cancer mortality: Evidence for a protective effect of ultraviolet radiation. Cancer 70:2861–2869, 1992.

Jünemann KP, Personn-Jünemann C, Alken P: Pathophysiology of erectile dysfunction. Semin Urol 8:80–93, 1990.

Khawand N, Vidic B, Jeutich MJ: Clinical application of electron microscopy of the corpora cavernosa in normal and impotent men. J Urol 519:137 (pt 2):233A.

Kirby RS, Lowe D, Bultitude MI, et al: Intra-prostatic urinary reflux: An aetiological factor in abacterial prostatitis. Br J Urol 54:729–731, 1982.

Lasater SJ: Testicular cancer: A perioperative challenge. AORN J 51:513–523, 1990.

Masters WH: Sex and aging: Expectations and reality. Hosp Pract 175–198, 1986.

McGinnis DE, Gomella LG: Tumors of the prostate. *In* Bahnson RR (ed): Management of Urologic Disorders. London, Wolfe, 1994, pp 5.2–5.31.

McLain RF, Weinstein JN: Tumors of the spine. Semin Spine Surg 2:157–180, 1990.

Meares EM Jr: Nonspecific infections of the genitourinary tract. *In* Tanagho EA, McAninch JW (eds): Smith's General Urology, ed 13. Norwalk, Conn, Appleton and Lange. 1992, pp 231–232.

Meikle A, Smith J: Epidemiology of prostate cancer. Urol Clin North Am 17:709–718, 1990.

Mellinger BC, Weiss J: Sexual dysfunction in the elderly male. Am Urol Assoc Update Ser 11:146–152, 1992.

Moldwin R: Epididymitis. *In* Bahnson RR (ed): Management of Urologic Disorders. London, Wolfe, 1994a, pp 16.2–16.4.

Moldwin R: Prostatitis. *In* Bahnson RR (ed): Management of Urologic Disorders. London, Wolfe, 1994b, pp 17.2–17.8.

National Cancer Institute: 1987 Annual cancer statistics review. Bethesda Md, National Cancer Institute, NIH Publication No. 8802789, 1988.

Norrby SR: Urinary tract infection. *In* Abrams WB, Berkow R (eds): The Merck Manual of Geriatrics. Rahway, NJ, Merck, 1990, pp 615–616.

Oesterling JE: PSA leads the way for detecting and following prostate cancer. Contemp Urol 5:60–91, 1993.

Parker SL, Tong T, Bolden S, et al: Cancer statistics, 1997. CA Cancer J Clin 47(1):5–27, 1997.

Paulson D: Diseases of the prostate. Clin Symp 41:17–32, 1989.

Peterson RO: The urinary tract and male reproductive system. *In* Rubin E, Farber JL (eds): Pathology, ed 2. Philadelphia, JB Lippincott, 1994, pp 867–907.

Presti JC, Herr HW: Genital tumors. *In* Tanagho EA, McAninch JW (eds): Smith's General Urology, ed 13. Norwalk, Conn, Appleton & Lange, 1992, pp 413–425.

Presti JC, Stoller ML, Carroll PR: Genitourinary tract. *In* Tierney LM, McPhee SJ, Papadakis MA (eds): Current Medical Diagnosis and Treatment, ed 33. Norwalk, Conn, Appleton & Lange, 1995, pp 736–778.

Riehmann M, Bruskewitz R: Evaluation of benign prostatic hyperplasia. *In* Bahnson RR (ed): Management of Urologic Disorders. London, Wolfe, 1994, pp 1.2–2.14.

Scardino PT: Early detection of prostate cancer. Urol Clin North Am 16:635–655, 1989.

Small EJ: Prostate cancer: Who to screen, and what the results mean. Geriatrics 48:28–38, 1993.

Smith RH, Wake R, Soloway MS: Benign prostatic hyperplasia: A universal problem among aging men. Postgrad Med 83(6):79, 1988.

Steinber GD, Carter BS, Beaty TL, et al: The familial aggregation of prostate cancer. A case control study (abstract). J Urol 143:131A, 1990.

Stewart SM: Alterations in structure and function of the male genitourinary system. *In* Mattson Porth C (ed): Pathophysiology: Concepts of Altered Health States, ed 4. Philadelphia, JB Lippincott, 1994, pp 727–744.

Tafelski TJ, Navarre R: Prostate gland enlargement. Mayo Clinic Health Lett 10:4–5, 1992.

Whitmore W: Natural history and staging of prostate cancer. Urol Clin North Am 11:205–220, 1984.

Willis D: Taming the overgrown prostate. Am J Nurs 92:35–39, 1992.

SECTION 2

chapter 17

The Female Genital/ Reproductive System

William G. Boissonnault

The female genital or reproductive system is made up of the ovaries, fallopian tubes, uterus, vagina, and external genitalia (Figs. 17–1 and 17–2). The primary functions of this system are related to preparing the woman for conception and gestation and for gestation itself. The female hormonal system, including the ovarian hormones, estrogen and progesterone, plays a key role in these functions (Guyton, 1991). Malfunctioning of this system can result in a multitude of local disorders, some benign and others life-threatening, as well as widespread systemic changes via the hormonal influences. The incidence of some of the disorders discussed in this chapter is quite high. For example, endometriosis is present in approximately 50% of women receiving treatment for infertility and in 10% to 15% of all premenopausal women. Furthermore, breast cancer accounts for approximately one third of all female cancers. Therefore, disorders of this system are frequently encountered by therapists.

The most significant age-related change associated with the female reproductive system is menopause, which is the permanent cessation of menses. The average age at which this event occurs is 45 to 50 years (McCowen-Mehring, 1994). Menopause is caused by the gradual cessation of ovarian function with the resultant reduced estrogen levels. During the reproductive years the primordial ovarian follicles, from which ova are expelled, steadily decrease in number. Ovarian production of estrogens decreases significantly when the number of these follicles approaches zero. The reduced level of estrogens results in a cascade of events resulting in altered physiology of multiple systems (Guyton, 1991). Symptomatically, women may experience hot flashes, fatigue, anxiety, and irritability. Physiologic changes include decreased thyroid function, hyperparathyroidism, and decreased renal function, insulin release, and response to catecholamines. In addition, if not receiving hormonal replacement therapy, postmenopausal women are at greater risk of developing arteriovascular disease including heart disease, hypertension, and cerebrovascular accidents, as well as osteoporosis and depression. Any of these conditions may account for the need for rehabilitation or complicate rehabilitative efforts if present as comorbidities.

Local changes of the reproductive organs also occur secondary to the decreased estrogen levels. The myometrium, endometrium, cervix, vagina, and labia all become atrophic to some degree. In addition, the pelvic floor musculature loses strength and tone, which can contribute to the development of cystocele, rectocele, uterine prolapse, and stress urinary incontinence (O'Connor and Gourley, 1990).

The diseases discussed in this chapter have several implication for therapists. Some conditions, for example, pelvic floor disorders or postsurgical rehabilitation following radical mastectomy, may be the primary reason the woman is seeing the therapist. Other conditions, such as endometriosis, may be manifested solely by pain, and the woman presents to the therapist with back or pelvic pain of unknown cause. Lastly, the presence of some of these conditions places the woman at higher risk of developing other diseases. For example, a history of endometriosis increases the risk of ectopic pregnancy which is a potentially life-threatening disorder.

DISORDERS OF THE UTERUS AND FALLOPIAN TUBES

Endometriosis

Overview. Endometriosis is marked by functioning endometrial tissue found outside the uterus. The most common sites of ectopic implantation include the ovaries, broad ligaments, pouch of Douglas, bladder, pelvic musculature, perineum, vulva, vagina, or intestines. Although less common, endometrial tissue can also be found in the abdominal cavity, implanted on the kidneys, small bowel, pleura, and bony elements of the spine (Fig. 17–3).

Etiology. The cause of endometriosis is unknown.

Incidence. The incidence of endometriosis has increased in the past 40 to 50 years in western countries. Approximately 10% to 15% of premenopausal women have endometriosis (McCowen-Mehring, 1994). In addition, the condition has been found in up to 50% of women undergoing diagnostic laparoscopy for infertility (Malinak and Wheeler, 1985).

Risk Factors. Any woman of childbearing age is at risk of developing endometriosis, but it is more common in those who have postponed pregnancy. In addition, other risk factors include early menarche; regular menstruation, but of cycles 27 days or less; and menstrual periods lasting 7 days or longer (Cramer et al., 1986).

Pathogenesis. Several theories exist regarding the pathogenesis of endometriosis. The most widely espoused theory suggests that foci of menstrual endometrium regurgitate from the uterus, through the fallopian tubes, and into the pelvis and peritoneal cavity. This retrograde menstruation has been shown to occur in up to 90% of women, but it is unclear

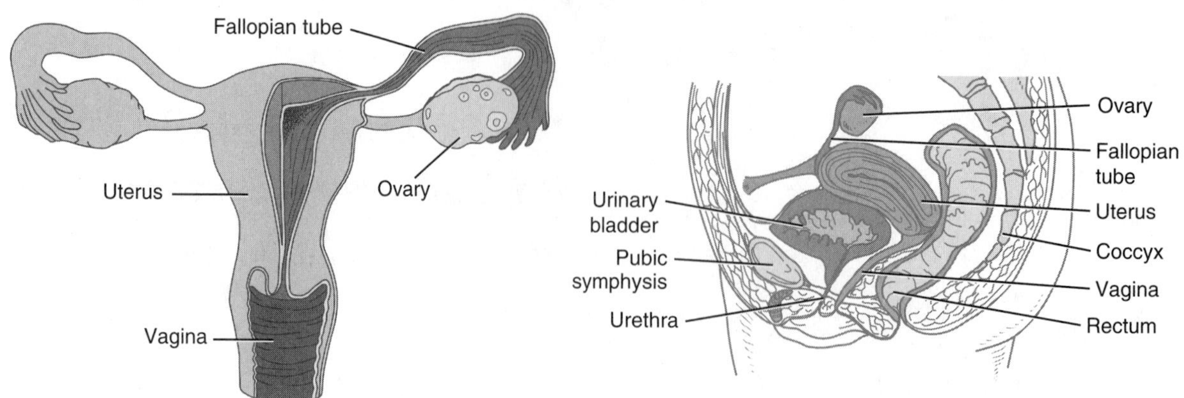

Figure **17–1.** Female reproductive organs.

why endometrial cells implant in some women and not in others (Robboy et al., 1994). Since the fimbrial openings of the fallopian tubes are in the posterior aspect of the pelvis, more of the endometrial implants are found on posterior structures.

Other theories include intraoperative implantation, lymphatic and hematogenous metastasis, and celomic metaplasia. The implantation of endometrial tissue has been associated with procedures such as hysterectomy and episiotomy. The observation of endometrial implants in the lungs and kidneys has been attributed to hematogenous spread. Endometrial tissue has also been found in lymph nodes. Lastly, another theory suggests that during embryonic development dormant, immature cells spread over a wide area. Then, during adult life, metaplasia occurs resulting in ectopic endometrial tissue (Robboy et al., 1994).

Pathologic changes associated with endometriosis include the formation of cysts (ovarian) that are filled with old blood that resembles chocolate syrup (chocolate cysts). Peritonitis and adhesions can occur if these cysts rupture. The ectopic implants found elsewhere in the pelvis respond to hormonal stimulation the same way normal endometrium does. Proliferation occurs initially, followed by a secretory phase and then menstrual breakdown. Bleeding into the area can cause pain and the development of significant adhesions.

Clinical Manifestations. The symptoms and signs associated with endometriosis depend upon the location of the implants. Dysmenorrhea will be the chief complaint if the implants are on the uterosacral ligaments. These lesions swell immediately before or during menstruation, resulting in pelvic pain. Dyspareunia (painful intercourse) is also associated with this condition as penile penetration during intercourse can aggravate the local adhesions. Pain during defecation can occur when there are adhesions on the large bowel. The fecal material moves through the intestine, stretching and aggravating the scar tissue. Surprisingly, the extent of the disease does not always correlate with the intensity of the

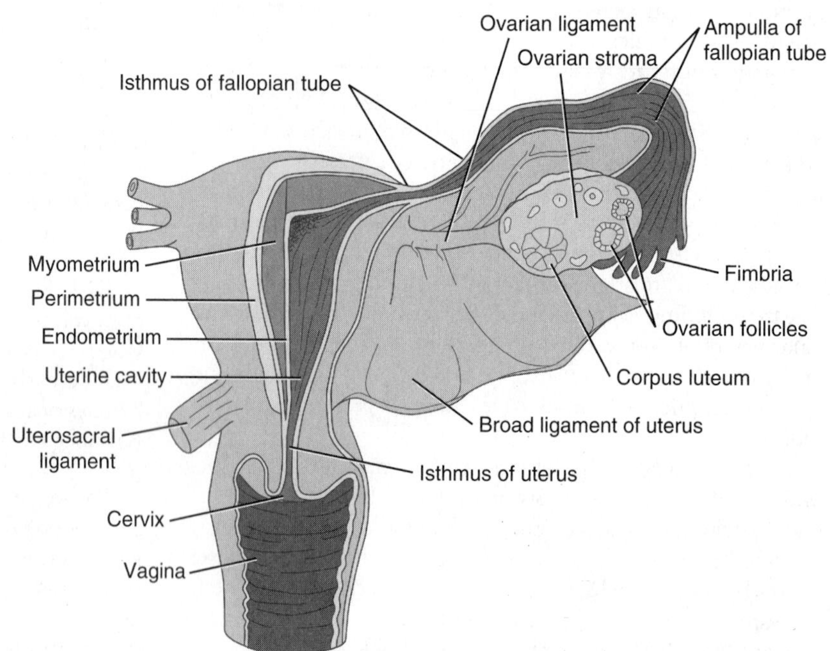

Figure **17–2.** Expanded view of female reproductive organs.

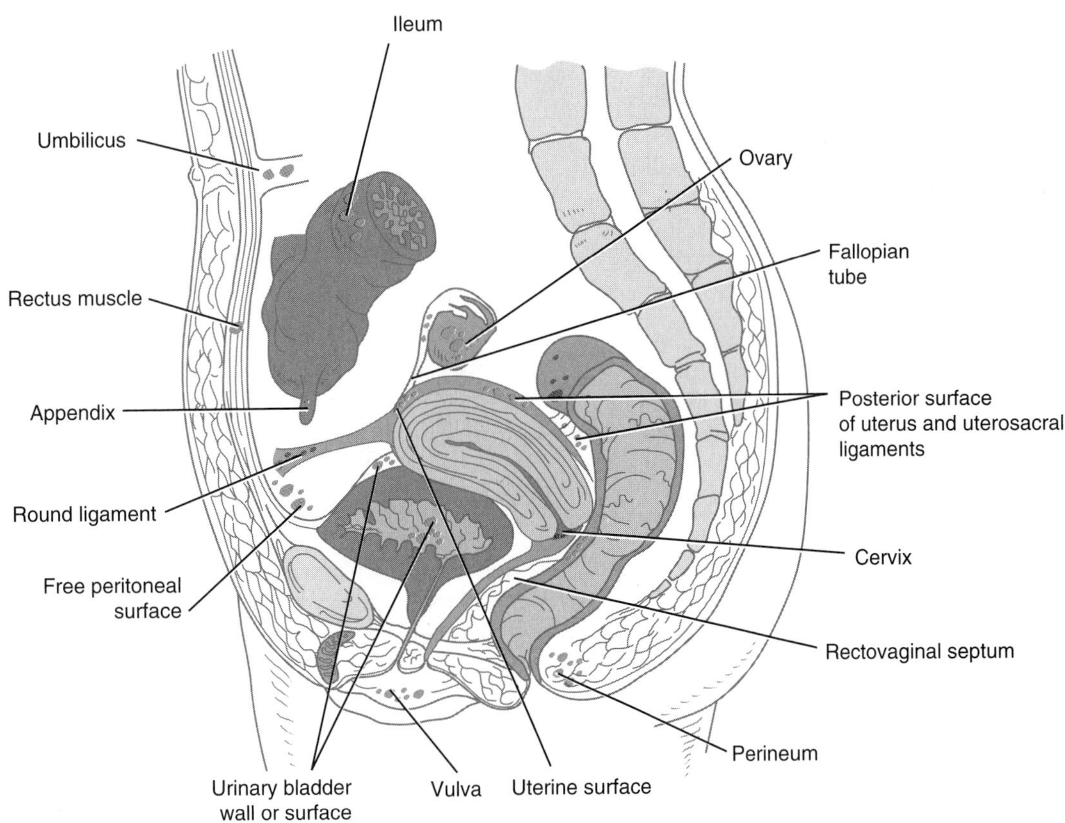

Figure **17–3.** Potential sites of endometrial implantation.

symptoms. A woman with widespread lesions may be asymptomatic, while a woman with few implants may have considerable pain.

Medical Management

Diagnosis. Although the classic triad of dysmenorrhea, dyspareunia, and infertility strongly suggests the presence of endometriosis, accurate diagnosis can be made only with laparoscopy or laparotomy. The other advantage of laparoscopy is that the technique is also therapeutic in that lesions can be removed immediately. Ultrasound and magnetic resonance imaging (MRI) are generally utilized to examine the pelvis, but MRI is more sensitive in detecting the implants (MacKay and Evans, 1995; McCowen-Mehring, 1994).

Treatment. The goal of medical treatment is to preserve fertility (if fertility is an issue) and pain relief. Nonsteroidal anti-inflammatory drugs may sufficiently relieve the pain or other analgesics can be administered before or during menstruation. Other medications are used to inhibit ovulation and lower hormone levels to prevent the cyclic stimulation of the endometrial implants. Eventually, the implants will decrease in size. These medications include danazol,[1] a combination estrogen–progesterone acetate, and nafarelin nasal spray, a gonadotropin-releasing hormone.

Surgical intervention is another commonly utilized approach. If the endometriosis is mild without extensive adhesions, laparoscopic cauterization or laser surgery is indicated. If the woman is over 35 to 40 years of age, disabled by the pain, and childbearing is completed, a total hysterectomy, bilateral salpingo-oophorectomy, and implant removal is considered.

Special Implications for the Therapist **17–1**

ENDOMETRIOSIS

As common as this disease is, therapists encounter endometriosis either as a comorbidity or an undiagnosed condition. Many women note that their back or pelvic pain is cyclic. Therapists often justify this observation with an explanation that the hormonal changes associated with menstruation can result in ligamentous laxity, thereby stressing the joints of the pelvis. This is only one possible scenario. Therapists need to consider all possibilities, including pelvic disease. Dyspareunia is a common complaint associated with sacroiliac, lumbar, or hip dysfunction. If the painful intercourse is related to endometriosis, the pain will be present regardless of position. If the pain is related to joint dysfunction, typically certain intercourse positions will be comfortable and others painful.

Endometriosis may account for false-positive findings during the therapist's physical examination. For example, if there are endometrial implants on the psoas

[1] The primary adverse side effects include weight gain, edema, decreased breast size, acne, oily skin, headache, muscle cramps, and deepening of the voice.

major muscle, local palpation and length or strength testing of the psoas may be provocative. The therapist may be led to believe the psoas is the culprit regarding the origin of the pain complaints. Endometrial implants on pelvic floor muscles and ligaments, sacroiliac ligaments, and abdominal wall muscle may lead to similar false-positive findings.

The medications commonly given to treat endometriosis can result in a variety of side effects which may account for a woman's complaints. Gastrointestinal system complaints (dyspepsia, nausea, etc.) may be related to the pain or the anti-inflammatory medication being taken. The gonadotropin-releasing hormone medications can result in hot flashes and vaginal dryness. Danazol can cause weight gain, acne, decreased breast size, and hirsutism (MacKay and Evans, 1995).

Ectopic Pregnancy

Overview. Ectopic pregnancy is marked by the implantation of a fertilized ovum outside the uterine cavity (Fig. 17–4). The fallopian tube is the most common site of ectopic pregnancy with approximately 95% implanting there. Ectopic pregnancy is a true gynecologic emergency as accompanying complications are one of two primary causes of maternal death in the United States.

Etiology. Ectopic pregnancy is caused by delayed ovum transport secondary to decreased fallopian tube motility or distorted tubule anatomy.

Incidence. The incidence of ectopic pregnancy has risen to approximately 1.5% of reported pregnancies. Between 1970 and 1987 the annual number of ectopic pregnancies rose from 17,800 to 88,000. This is in part due to new testing procedures which detect pregnancy earlier in the gestation process. Despite this increase, the death rate has steadily declined to the rate of 3.4 deaths per 10,000 ectopic pregnancies (Centers for Disease Control, 1990).

Risk Factors. Any condition that impedes the migration of the fertilized ovum to the uterus increases the risk of ectopic pregnancy. A previous history of pelvic inflammatory disease, prior tubal surgery, ruptured appendix, endometriosis, and previous ectopic pregnancy could account for potential damage to the fallopian tubes. This damage could impair transport of the ovum. In addition, a history of infertility and the use of clomiphene citrate to induce ovulation are associated with an increased risk of this condition.

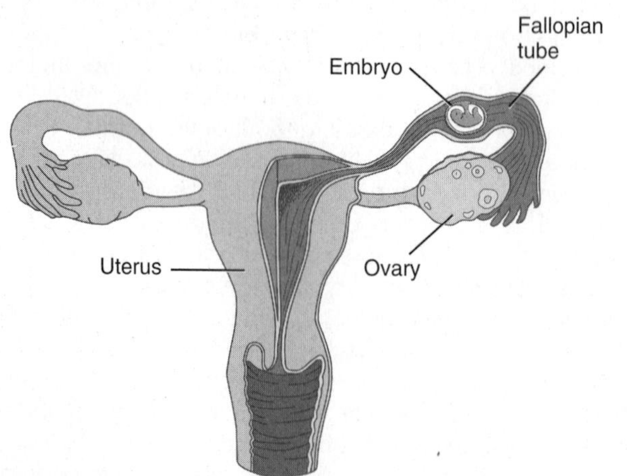

Figure **17–4.** Ectopic pregnancy with implantation occurring in the fallopian tube.

Pathogenesis. Fertilization does not occur in the uterus. The sperm fertilizes the ovum soon after the ovum enters the ampulla of the fallopian tube. Three to four days is typically required for the ovum to travel through the fallopian tube to the uterus. The ovum is rapidly dividing and growing throughout the journey. If the journey is slowed sufficiently (tubule motility), the ovum becomes too large to complete the passage through the tubule. If the tubule anatomy has been affected by recurrent infection or endometriosis the same problem occurs. The trophoblasts that cover the surface of the ovum easily penetrate the mucosa and wall of the tubule and implantation occurs.

Bleeding occurs during implantation with leakage into the pelvis and abdominal cavity. Vaginal bleeding that may be perceived as menstruation may occur. The pregnancy will typically outgrow its blood supply, terminating the pregnancy. If the pregnancy does not terminate, the thin-walled tubule will no longer support the growing fetus, and rupture can occur by the 12th week of gestation. Tubal rupture is life-threatening because rapid exsanguinating intra-abdominal hemorrhage can occur.

Clinical Manifestations. The classic presentation of ectopic pregnancy is marked by amenorrhea or irregular bleeding and spotting, lower abdominal quadrant or back pain, and a pelvic mass. The woman may believe she had a menstrual period, but when questioned will report the period was atypical for her. The pain reported can be diffuse and aching or localized and will progress to a sharper, lancinating type of pain. The pain can be sudden in onset and intermittent. The pain is thought to be primarily due to the leakage of blood into the pelvic and abdominal cavity. Pain referred to the shoulder area can occur if the blood comes in contact with structures found high (cranially) enough in the abdominal cavity.

Since the woman is pregnant, symptoms and signs associated with normal pregnancy may also be present. These findings include fatigue, nausea, breast tenderness, and urinary frequency.

Medical Management

Diagnosis. Physical examination reveals a pelvic mass in approximately 50% of the cases (McCowen-Mehring, 1994). Pelvic ultrasound studies can reliably reveal a gestational sac by 5 to 6 weeks into the pregnancy. An empty uterine cavity with elevated (slight) human chorionic gonadotropin β subunit (HCG-β) and symptoms strongly implies an extrauterine pregnancy. Blood studies may show anemia while serum pregnancy tests (HCG-β hormonal levels) will be positive but show levels lower than expected in the presence of a normal pregnancy (lack of doubling over 2 days). Definitive diagnosis requires laparoscopy.

Treatment. Surgical intervention consisting of a laparoscopic salpingostomy to remove the ectopic pregnancy is performed if the fallopian tube has not ruptured. Laparotomy is indicated if there is internal bleeding or if the ectopic site cannot be adequately visualized with the laparoscope (Catlin and Wetzel, 1991).

A chemotherapeutic-agent, methotrexate, can be administered to remove residual ectopic tissue following laparoscopy. The drug is also used when the pregnancy is intact and surgery is contraindicated or the diagnosis is made early enough that the condition is not life-threatening and preserving fertility is desirable.

Special Implications for the Therapist **17-2**

ECTOPIC PREGNANCY

An awareness of this potentially life-threatening condition is important for the therapist. This awareness should include knowledge of the preexisting conditions that increase the risk of ectopic pregnancy and of the symptoms associated with pregnancy. If a woman of childbearing age complains of an onset of lower abdominal, ipsilateral shoulder or back pain, the therapist should ask questions regarding her menstrual cycle and if any of the symptoms of pregnancy are present. If the therapist suspects ectopic pregnancy, an immediate telephone call to the physician is warranted.

DISORDERS OF THE OVARIES

Ovarian Cystic Disease

Overview. Ovarian cysts, most of which are benign, are the most common form of ovarian tumor. The different types of cysts include follicular cysts, luteal cysts, functional cysts, and a disorder marked by the presence of multiple cysts called polycystic ovary syndrome. This polycystic disorder is one of the most common causes of infertility. These disorders can also cause menstrual problems. Most of the following discussion focuses on polycystic ovary syndrome.

Incidence. The polycystic ovary syndrome affects 3% to 7% of women of childbearing age. This level of incidence makes this disorder one of the most common endocrine disorders (Robboy et al., 1994).

Risk Factors. Women of childbearing years, especially those in their 20s, are at risk of developing polycystic ovary syndrome.

Etiology. Excess androgen production from any source can initiate a self-perpetuating cycle that can lead to polycystic ovary syndrome.

Pathogenesis. Excess circulating androgens are converted to estrone in the peripheral adipose tissue. The elevated levels of circulating estrogens stimulate the release of gonadotropin-releasing hormone (Gn-RH) by the hypothalamus and inhibit the secretion of follicle-stimulating hormone (FSH) by the pituitary. Gn-RH stimulates the pituitary which produces lutenizing hormone (LH). The increased secretion of LH stimulates the ovary to produce and secrete more androgens. This self-perpetuating cycle results in abnormal maturation of the ovarian follicles, the development of multiple follicular cysts, and a persistent anovulatory state (Robboy et al., 1994).

Clinical Manifestations. Polycystic ovarian syndrome is characterized by obesity, hirsutism, infertility, and menstrual problems. Fifty percent of these women have amenorrhea and another 30% have abnormal uterine bleeding.

Pain can be a manifestation of other types of cysts. A dull, aching sensation experienced in the lower abdominal, groin, or buttock areas can occur. The sensation may also be described as a heaviness. This pain is associated with bleeding into the cyst or with quick enlargement of the cyst. Sudden or sharp pain can indicate a cyst rupturing or hemorrhaging or a torsion occurring.

Medical Management

Diagnosis. The history and pelvic examination lead to suspicion of cystic disease. Confirmation is made by ultrasonography or laparoscopy.

Treatment. The treatment of polycystic ovary syndrome is primarily hormonal with the goal being an interruption of the persistent elevated levels of androgens. Clomiphene citrate (Clomid) is often administered to induce ovulation. If medication is not effective, laser surgery can be instituted to puncture the multiple follicles. Weight reduction can be helpful, resulting in a lowering of the level of androgens being converted to estrone (McCowen-Mehring, 1994; MacKay and Evans, 1995).

Special Implications for the Therapist **17-3**

POLYCYSTIC OVARY SYNDROME

Considering how common polycystic ovary syndrome is, therapists need to be aware of the potential side effects of clomiphene citrate. These include insomnia, blurred vision, nausea, vomiting, urinary frequency, and polyuria (Baer and Williams, 1992). The onset of any of these symptoms warrants communication with the physician.

Therapists ask women if menstrual dysfunction is present. A history of ovarian cystic disease could account for a woman's complaints.

Ovarian Cancer

Overview. Ovarian cancer is estimated to be the second most common female urogenital cancer and the most lethal of these cancers (Parker et al., 1997). The poor outcome is based on the difficulty of diagnosing the disease, which results in 60% to 70% of the women having metastatic disease at the time of diagnosis. Although there are a number of types of ovarian cancers, epithelial tumors make up approximately 90% of the cases (Saigo, 1993).

Incidence. An estimated 26,800 women in the United States were projected to develop ovarian cancer in 1997 with 14,200 deaths from ovarian cancer (Parker et al., 1997).

Risk Factors. Numerous factors increase the risk of developing ovarian cancer, including age, geographic location, race, nulliparity, family history, and a history of infertility, or endometrial or breast cancer (Box 17–1). On the other hand, a history of one or more full-term pregnancies, a history of breast-feeding, and the use of oral contraceptives reduces the risk of ovarian cancer (Tortolero-Luna et al., 1994). Since epithelial tumors make up approximately 90% of ovarian cancers, most of the risk factors described relate to this entity.

While epithelial tumors are rare before puberty, the incidence peaks in a women's 50s and 60s. The most common type of epithelial tumor, serous carcinoma, has a peak incidence between the ages of 40 and 60 years. The highest rates of ovarian cancer are found in northwestern Europe, the United States, and Canada, while the lowest rates occur in Asia, Africa, and Latin America (Muir et al., 1987; Parkin et al., 1988). In the United States white and Hawaiian women have the highest incidence of ovarian cancer, while Native American women have the lowest incidence. Nulliparous women are at increased risk of developing ovarian cancer. This factor is thought to be related to the repeated epithelial surface disruption that occurs with cyclic ovulation. A history of breast-feeding also is important as women who breast-feed are at decreased risk of developing this condition compared to nulliparous women and parous women who have not breast-fed. Finally, a family history of ovarian cancer is an important factor. Women with two or more first-degree relatives with ovarian cancer carry a lifetime risk of approximately 50% compared with women with no family history who have only 1.4% lifetime risk (Tortolero-Luna et al., 1994).

Etiology. The cause of ovarian cancer is unclear, but three hypotheses have been proposed: (1) the incessant ovulation, (2) the gonadotropin, and (3) the pelvic contamination theories. The incessant ovulation hypothesis theorizes that repetitive microtrauma to the epithelial surface of the ovary secondary to continuous ovulation initiates the process (Fathalla, 1971). The gonadotropin hypothesis states that the exposure of the ovary to continuous, high circulating pituitary gonadotropin levels increases the risk of cancer (Stadel, 1975). Lastly, the pelvic contamination theory suggests that carcinogens come in contact with the ovaries (Heintz et al., 1985).

Pathogenesis. The classification of ovarian tumors is based on the tissue of origin. The most common tumors arise from the surface epithelium or serosa of the ovary. As the ovary develops the epithelium extends into the stroma of the ovary forming glands and cysts. In certain cases these inclusions become neoplastic (Robboy et al., 1994). Other categories of tumor include germ cell tumors, sex cord and stromal tumors, and steroid cell tumors. Once present, ovarian cancer spreads to the pelvis, abdominal cavity, and bladder, while lymphatic metastasis carries the disease to the para-aortic lymph nodes and to a lesser extent the inguinal or external iliac lymph nodes. Hematogenous spread of the cancer can result in liver and lung involvement.

BOX **17–1**
Risk Factors for Ovarian Cancer

- Forty years of age and older
- Nulliparity
- Positive family history
- White race
- Industrialized western nation
- History of breast or endometrial cancer

Clinical Manifestations. Most ovarian cancers are asymptomatic or present with symptoms so vague that the disease is advanced in many cases by the time the woman seeks care. The vague complaints include abdominal bloating, flatulence, or general abdominal discomfort. Abnormal vaginal bleeding can occur, but is not common. Local pelvic pain also occurs late in the disease. Symptoms associated with metastatic spread of the disease include unexplained weight loss, weakness, ascites,[2] and cachexia (general feebleness and wasting).

Medical Management

Diagnosis. A pelvic mass with ascites is usually indicative of ovarian cancer. A cervical smear may reveal malignant cells. Ultimately biopsy will reveal whether the mass is benign or cancerous.

Staging. Staging of the disease is as follows: stage I—disease limited to the ovaries; stage II—extension to the pelvis; stage III—intraperitoneal metastasis; and stage IV—distant metastasis.

Treatment. Surgery is the primary treatment for removal of the primary tumor. If the woman is young and the disease localized, a cystectomy is performed. Otherwise the ovary is removed and the abdominal cavity is examined to determine the extent of the disease. As much of the metastatic disease is removed as possible. Chemotherapy is also utilized in the presence of widespread (stage IV) cancer. For patients with common epithelial tumors, the 5-year survival rate without evidence of recurrence is only 15% to 45%.

Special Implications for the Therapist **17–4**
OVARIAN CANCER

Therapists treating women with a history of ovarian cancer need to be cognizant of the moderate to high risk of recurrence of the disease. Symptoms associated with spread may include thoracic or shoulder girdle pain secondary to lymphadenopathy; symptoms associated with lung (see Chapter 12) or liver (see Chapter 14) disease; and weight loss and fatigue. Onset of any of these complaints warrants communication with the physician. Oophorectomy induces menopause in women. Therefore an onset of the symptoms described in the beginning of this chapter may occur in addition to headaches, depression, and insomnia.

PELVIC FLOOR DISORDERS

Cystocele, Rectocele, and Uterine Prolapse

Overview. Three types of pelvic floor disorders are discussed here: cystocele, rectocele and uterine prolapse. A cys-

[2] Ascites is an accumulation of fluid within the peritoneal cavity. This can occur when there is marked increased pressure within the liver sinusoids or portal hypertension which results in serum exuding through the superficial capillaries into the peritoneal cavity.

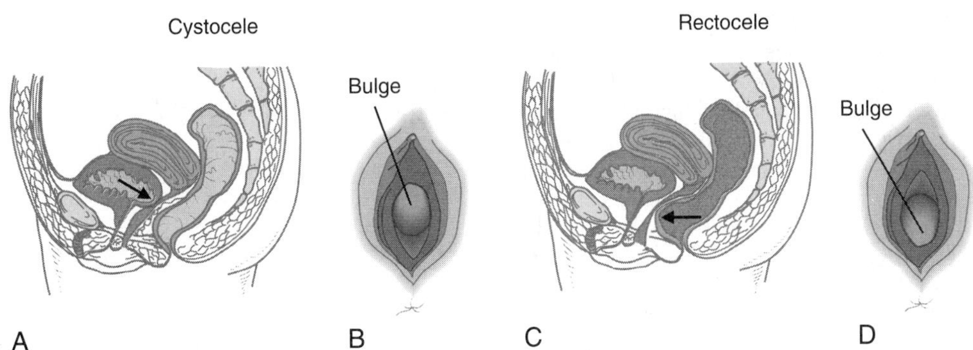

Figure 17–5. *A*, Cystocele. Note the bulging of the anterior vaginal wall. The urinary bladder is displaced downward. *B*, The bladder pushes the anterior vaginal wall downward into the vagina. *C*, Rectocele. *D*, Note the bulging of the posterior vaginal wall associated with rectocele.

tocele is a herniation of the urinary bladder into the vagina (Fig. 17–5*A* and *B*). A rectocele is a herniation of the rectum into the vagina (Fig. 17–5*C* and *D*). A uterine prolapse is the bulging of the uterus into the vagina (Fig. 17–6).

Etiology. Cystocele, rectocele, and uterine prolapse are a result of pelvic floor relaxation or structural overstretching of the pelvic musculature or ligamentous structures.

Risk Factors. Multiple pregnancies and deliveries increase the risk of these disorders developing. In addition, pelvic tumors and neurologic conditions such as spina bifida and diabetic neuropathy, which interrupt the innervation of pelvic muscles, can also increase the risk.

Incidence. Pelvic floor disorders are common in multiparous women (MacKay and Evans, 1995).

Pathogenesis. The uterus and other pelvic structures are maintained in their proper position by the uterosacral, round, broad, and cardinal ligaments. The pelvic floor musculature forms a slinglike structure that supports the uterus, vagina, urinary bladder, and rectum. Multiple pregnancies and deliveries progressively stretch and potentially weaken these important structures.

Cystocele occurs when the muscle support for the bladder is impaired. This allows the bladder to drop below the uterus. Over a period of time the vaginal wall will stretch and bulge downward. Eventually the bladder can herniate through the anterior vaginal wall and form a cystocele. A rectocele occurs when the posterior vaginal wall and underlying rectum bulge forward. Eventually protrusion occurs through the introitus as the supporting structures continue to weaken. Uterine prolapse occurs when the supporting ligaments become overstretched (McCowen-Mehring, 1994).

Clinical Manifestations. The symptoms associated with a cystocele include urinary frequency and urgency, difficulty in emptying the bladder, cystitis, and a painful bearing-down sensation in the perineal area. Urinary stress incontinence may also be associated with the presence of a cystocele.

The symptoms associated with a rectocele include perineal pain and difficulty with defecation. Lastly, the primary symptoms resulting from uterine prolapse are backache, perineal pain, and irritation of the exposed mucous membranes of the cervix and vagina.

Medical Management

Diagnosis. The diagnosis of these disorders is primarily derived from observation and the pelvic examination. A uterine prolapse is graded as first, second, or third degree, depending on how far the uterus protrudes through the introitus. A first-degree prolapse is marked by some descent, but the cervix has not reached the introitus. A second-degree prolapse is marked by the cervix as part of the uterus having descended through the introitus. A third-degree prolapse is manifested by the entire uterus protruding through the vaginal opening (McCowen-Mehring, 1994).

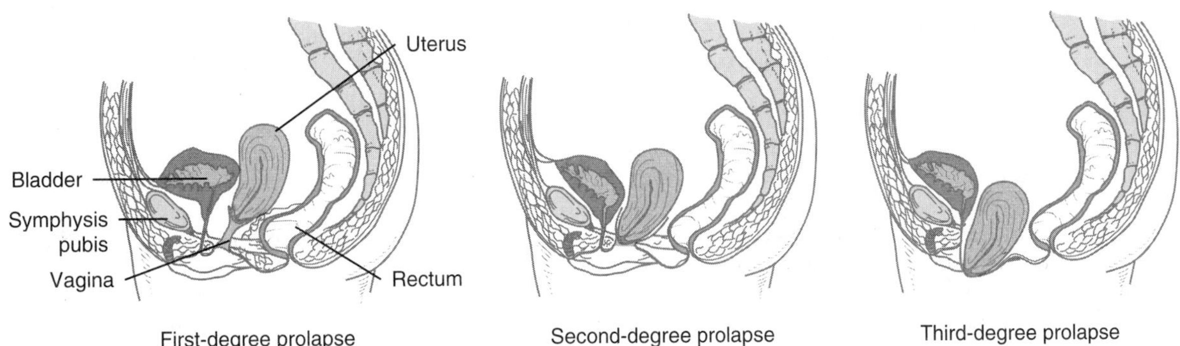

Figure 17–6. Stages of uterine prolapse.

Treatment. Although physical therapy intervention can play an important role in the management of these disorders, surgery is often required. This is especially the case with second- and third-degree uterine prolapse. Vaginal hysterectomy, vesicourethral suspension, and abdominal hysterectomy are possible surgical approaches depending upon the diagnosis. Strengthening of the pelvic floor should be incorporated into the postoperative rehabilitation program. In addition, pelvic floor rehabilitation, including biofeedback, pelvic floor strengthening exercises, and electrical stimulation, is the primary treatment approach for first-degree uterine prolapse.

Special Implications for the Therapist **17–5**

PELVIC FLOOR DISORDERS

As with urinary incontinence, physical therapists may have a primary role in the treatment of pelvic floor disorders. See O'Connor and Ghorley (1990) for details regarding these treatment approaches. Therapists will also see patients with pelvic floor disorders as a comorbidity. In these cases, therapists must be vigilant that the woman does not hold her breath or perform a Valsalva maneuver because these could exacerbate the pelvic floor condition. In addition, a woman with a second- or third-degree uterine prolapse will have difficulty tolerating extended periods of weight-bearing activities. Alternative positions for exercise will need to be incorporated into the rehabilitation program.

BREAST DISEASE

Breast Cancer

Overview. Breast cancer is the most common malignancy of females in the United States. Most breast carcinomas are adenocarcinomas, derived from the glandular epithelium of the terminal duct lobular unit. The evolution of this disease consists of a series of functional and structural changes.

Incidence. Breast carcinomas account for approximately 30% of all the female cancers in the United States. In addition, breast cancer is the number two cause of female cancer deaths in the United States, second only to lung cancer. Approximately 17% of the deaths are from breast cancer and 25% from lung cancer (Parker et al., 1997).

Etiology. The cause of breast cancer is unknown although a number of risk factors have been associated with the disease.

Risk Factors. Gender, age, race, family history, medical history, menstrual history, pregnancy, and geography are all factors linked to breast cancer (Box 17–2). Gender is the most significant risk factor associated with this disease; less than 1% of breast cancers occur in males (Parker et al., 1997). Age is the second most significant factor; the incidence increases with advancing age. The median and mean age of women with breast cancer is between 60 and 61 years (Giuliano, 1995). White women in western industrial nations are also at higher risk. A history of breast cancer among first-degree relatives is also a factor. Increased risk is noted if two or more first-degree relatives have the disease or if the cancer occurred before menopause or was bilateral (Bartow, 1994; Giuliano, 1995). A history of breast, ovarian, and uterine cancer carries an increased risk of developing breast cancer. Women with a history of breast cancer have a two to four times higher risk of recurrence of the disease than women without this history (Stenbeck, 1995). In addition, a history of fibrocystic breast disease, when accompanied by proliferative changes, papillomatosis, or atypical epithelial hyperplasia, increases the risk of cancer. An association between hormonal status and breast cancer is also present. Early menarche, under the age of 12, and late natural menopause, after the age of 50, have been related to an increased risk of developing breast cancer. Also, nulliparous women and those whose initial full-term pregnancy occurred after the age of 35 are at increased risk (Giuliano, 1995).

BOX **17–2**
Risk Factors for Breast Cancer

- Female sex
- Age ≥60 yr
- Positive family history
- History of breast cancer, fibrocystic breast disease
- White race
- Early menarche
- Late menopause
- Nulliparity

Pathogenesis. The pathogenesis of breast cancer is unknown, but most carcinomas develop in the glandular epithelium of the terminal duct lobular unit. A stromal invasion by malignant cells usually results in fibroblastic proliferation. A palpable mass within the breast tissue will typically develop. If not diagnosed and treated early the cancer will spread to the regional lymph nodes, including the axillary, internal mammary, and supraclavicular nodes (Fig. 17–7). Lesions can develop anywhere in the breast, but most commonly occur in the upper, outer quadrant of the breast (Giuliano, 1995; Bartow, 1994). As the disease progresses the cancer commonly spreads to the lungs, liver, bone, adrenals, skin, and brain (Bartow, 1994).

Clinical Manifestations. The most common initial presenting sign of breast cancer is a palpable mass. Approximately 90% of breast masses are discovered by the woman herself. The mass tends to be firm and irregular if it is a carcinoma vs. smooth and rubbery if it is benign. The mass is typically not painful if it is cancer. Other manifestations include a change in breast contour, nipple discharge and retraction, local skin dimpling, erythema, and a local rash. Lymphadenopathy may also be the initial presentation of this disease. Symptoms associated with metastases can include upper extremity edema, bone pain, jaundice, or weight loss. These findings are rarely the initial complaint though.

Medical Management

Diagnosis. Clinical examination, mammography, and ultrasonography are all utilized to detect breast abnormalities. Tissue biopsy is the standard for a definitive diagnosis. Ultra-

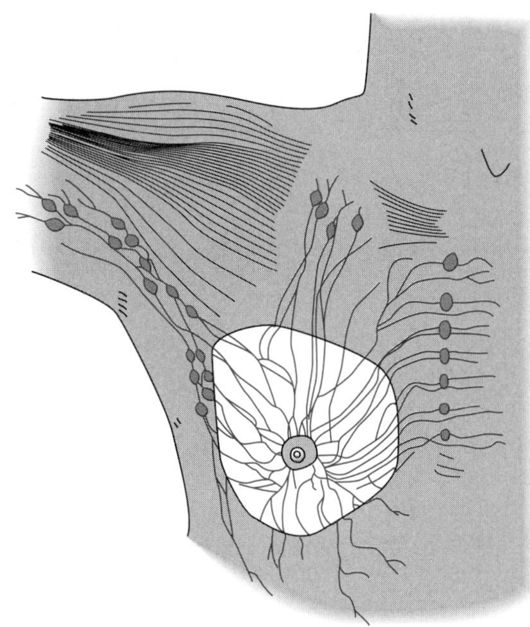

Figure **17-7.** Regional lymph nodes associated with breast cancer.

sonography is primarily used to differentiate a cystic from a solid lesion. Mammography is an important tool for the detection of a lesion before the mass (cancerous or benign) is large enough to be palpable, but is not a substitute for biopsy because by itself it is not diagnostic and it may not detect cancer in very dense breast tissue.

Staging. Once the diagnosis is established the clinical stage is determined. Stage I disease is marked by a tumor 2 cm in size or smaller. Stage II disease is marked by a tumor between 2 and 5 cm in size without nodal metastases or a tumor less than 5 cm with homolateral axillary lymphatic metastases (the nodes are movable). A tumor larger than 5 cm is classified as Stage III, as is a tumor fixed to the pectoral muscle or fascia or if the diseased axillary lymph nodes are fixed to adjacent tissues. Stage IV disease is a tumor fixed to the chest wall or skin and any tumor with metastases to the homolateral infraclavicular or supraclavicular nodes, with upper extremity edema or with any distant metastasis (Bartow, 1994).

Treatment. The hallmark of effective treatment of breast cancer is early detection. The American Cancer Society makes the following screening recommendations for asymptomatic women at average risk: for women aged 20 to 40 years, a monthly breast self-examination and a clinical breast examination every 3 years; for women aged 40 to 49 years, a monthly breast self-examination, annual clinical breast examination, and mammography every 1 to 2 years; and for women aged 50 years old and older, a monthly breast self-examination, annual mammography, and clinical breast examination (Mettlin and Smart, 1994).

Once the diagnosis of breast cancer is made the treatment options include surgery, chemotherapy, radiation therapy, and hormonal manipulation. Radical mastectomy was the most commonly employed procedure until the 1970s. This technique included removal of the entire breast, pectoral muscles, axillary lymph nodes, and some additional skin. Postsurgical problems included lymphedema, restricted shoulder mobility, impaired muscle function, and paresthesia. More recent treatment recommendations for women with stage I or II breast cancer include breast-conserving surgery and radiation therapy. Modified radical mastectomy, which spares the pectoralis major muscle, is also a commonly utilized procedure with the primary advantage being avoidance of radiation therapy. The major disadvantage is the comparative psychological and cosmetic trauma associated with this procedure (Giuliano, 1995).

Following surgery and radiation therapy, chemotherapy or hormone therapy, or both, are often employed. The primary objective of these treatments is to reduce the odds of occult metastases developing into disease. The most widely studied chemotherapy is the CMF regimen (cyclophosphamide, methotrexate, and fluorouracil). Increased disease-free survival times following chemotherapy have been noted consistently in premenopausal women with metastases to the axillary lymph nodes. The addition of hormone therapy (i.e., tamoxifen) may enhance the effects of chemotherapy in postmenopausal women whose tumors contain estrogen receptors. Survival rates reflect the importance of early detection. The 5-year survival rate for localized tumors is 92%. If there is nodal involvement the rate is approximately 71% (McCowen-Mehring, 1994). Women with stage III or IV disease have little hope of cure and the goal of treatment is palliative (Bartow, 1994).

Special Implications for the Therapist **17-6**

BREAST CANCER

Therapists examining the shoulder and shoulder girdle region need to be aware of the nonmusculature structures located in these areas. These structures include breast tissue and regional lymph nodes. The upper, outer quadrant of the breast can extend up toward the glenohumeral joint and more cancerous masses occur in this area than in any other part of the breast. In addition, approximately 50% of women with breast cancer have metastasis to the axillary nodes at the time the diagnosis is made (Bartow, 1994). Palpation of a lump or mass in these areas should raise concern on the therapist's part and lead to questioning of the patient regarding the clinical findings. If the mass lies in the pectoralis major muscle, the mass should change during palpation when the muscle is actively contracting. If the therapist is in doubt, the patient should be evaluated by a physician (see discussion of lymphedema in Chapter 10).

When treating a woman with a history of breast cancer, an awareness of the symptoms and signs associated with breast cancer is important. Approximately 10% of these women will develop cancer in the opposite breast. Local and distant metastases occur most frequently within 3 years of the initial diagnosis (Giuliano, 1995).

Women receiving adjuvant therapy (chemotherapy or hormonal therapy) may experience numerous side effects that could interfere with rehabilitation (see

Chapter 4). Women receiving chemotherapy will likely be fatigued and experience flulike symptoms. Therefore, the timing of scheduled therapy visits is important to maximize productivity during the session. Exercises and functional activities may have to be paced or therapy visits shortened to accommodate the woman's energy level. Potential side effects of hormone therapy include hot flashes, genital itching and bleeding, nausea, vomiting, diarrhea, and urinary frequency. Women who have undergone mastectomy should be instructed postoperatively and assisted with breathing and coughing exercises to prevent pulmonary complications. In addition, lower extremity exercises are also important to prevent thromboemboli. Lastly, phantom breast pain may be noted by the woman postoperatively.

Fibrocystic Disease and Fibroadenoma

Overview. *Fibrocystic breast disease* or *mammary dysplasia* is a term used to describe a number of benign breast irregularities. The constellation of morphologic changes can include cystic dilation of terminal ducts, a relative increase in the fibrous stroma, and proliferation of the terminal duct epithelial elements. Fibroadenoma is the most common benign neoplasm of the breast. Epithelial and stromal elements that arise from the terminal duct lobular unit make up the tumor.

Incidence and Risk Factors. Fibrocystic breast disease is the single most common breast disorder and accounts for approximately 50% to 75% of surgical procedures on the female breast (McCowen-Mehring, 1994).

The risk factors for developing breast cancer (see earlier discussion) also apply to the development of this condition. Fibroadenomas occur most commonly in premenopausal women, especially women between the ages of 20 to 35 years (Bartow, 1994).

Etiology. The cause of fibrocystic breast disease and fibroadenoma is unknown.

Pathogenesis. The fibrocystic changes typically involve the terminal ducts and surrounding stroma and can be proliferative or nonproliferative. Nonproliferative fibrocystic changes are generalized, occurring in multiple areas of both breasts. A majority of the time these cystic changes are minimal and do not result in a discrete mass. Cysts up to 5 cm can develop though.

Fibroadenomas are typically solitary lesions and are 2 to 4 cm in size when first detected. This round and rubbery lesion is sharply demarcated from surrounding breast tissue and as a result moves freely within the surrounding tissue.

Clinical Manifestations. A fibrocystic breast mass may or may not be painful. The tenderness may become evident during the premenstural phase of the cycle when the cysts tend to enlarge. These cysts can fluctuate in size with rapid appearance or disappearance. A typical fibroadenoma is a nontender, round, firm, and discrete mass (Giuliano, 1995; McCowen-Mehring, 1994).

Medical Management

Diagnosis. Diagnosis of these benign lesions is based on physical examination, mammography, and biopsy. Because fibrocystic disease and fibroadenoma are often indistinguishable from carcinomas, biopsy is often utilized to confirm the diagnosis.

Treatment. Treatment for these conditions is often palliative and includes aspirin, mild analgesics, and local heat or cold. Dietary changes are often recommended such as avoiding coffee, colas, chocolate, and tea (foods that contain xanthines). Women are encouraged to wear a brassiere that provides adequate support. For women in severe pain, danazol may be given. Surgery is performed if a suspicious mass that is deemed not to be malignant upon cytologic examination does not resolve over several months (Giuliano, 1995; McCowen-Mehring, 1994).

References

Baer CL, Williams BR (eds): Clinical Pharmacology and Nursing, ed 2. Springhouse, Pa, Springhouse, 1992, pp 1197, 1272.

Bartow S: The breast. *In* Rubin E, Farber JL (eds): Pathology, ed 2. Philadelphia, JB Lippincott, 1994, pp 973–992.

Catlin AJ, Wetzel WS: Ectopic pregnancy—Clinical evaluation, diagnostic measures and prevention. Nurse Pract 16:38, 43, 1991.

Centers for Disease Control: Ectopic pregnancy mortality, 1970–1987. MMWR 39:1990.

Cramer DW, Wilson E, Stillman RJ, et al: The relationship of endometriosis to menstrual characteristics, smoking and exercise. JAMA, 155:1904, 1986.

Fathalla MF: Incessant ovulation—A factor in ovarian neoplasia? Lancet 2:163, 1971.

Giuliano AE: Breast. *In* Tierney LM, McPhee SJ, Papadakis MA (eds): Current Medical Diagnosis and Treatment, ed 34. Norwalk, Conn, Appleton & Lange, 1995, pp 593–599.

Guyton AC: Textbook of Medical Physiology, ed 8. Philadelphia, WB Saunders, 1991, pp 899–905.

Heintz APM, Hacker NF, Lagasse LD: Epidemiology and etiology of ovarian cancer: A review. Obstet Gynecol 66:127–135, 1985.

MacKay HT, Evans AT: Gynecology and obstetrics. *In* Tierney LM, McPhee, SJ, Papadakis MA (eds): Current Medical Diagnosis and Treatment, ed 34. Norwalk, Conn, Appleton & Lange, 1995, pp 628–629.

Malinak LR, Wheeler JM: A practical approach to endometriosis—Part 1: Diagnosis. Female Patient 10:39, 1985.

McCowen-Mehring P: Alterations in structure and function of the female reproductive system. *In* Mattson Porth C (ed): Pathophysiology: Concepts of Altered Health States, ed 4. Philadelphia, JB Lippincott, 1994, pp 765–766.

Mettlin C, Smart CR: Breast cancer detection guidelines for women aged 40 to 49 years: Rationale for the American Cancer Society reaffirmative of recommendations. CA Cancer Journal for Clinicians. 44(4):248–255, 1994.

Muir C, Waterhouse J, Mack T, et al: Cancer Incidence in Five Continents. Publication No. 88. Lyon, France, International Agency for Research on Cancer, 1987, pp 892–893.

O'Connor LJ, Gourley RJ: Obstetric and Gynecologic Care in Physical Therapy. Thorofare, NJ, Slack, 1990, pp 248–253.

Parker SL, Tong T, Bolden S, et al: Cancer statistics, 1997. CA Cancer J Clin 47(1):5–27, 1997.

Parkin DM, Laara E, Muir CS: Estimates of the worldwide frequency of sixteen major cancers in 1980. Intl J Cancer 41:184–197, 1988.

Robboy SJ, Duggan MA, Kurman RJ: The female reproductive system. *In* Rubin E, Farber JL (eds): Pathology, ed 2. Philadelphia, JB Lippincott, 1994, pp 936–938.

Saigo PE: The histology of malignant ovarian tumors. *In* Markman M, Hoskin WJ (eds): Cancer of the Ovary. New York, Raven Press, 1993, pp 21–46.

Stadel BV: The etiology and prevention of ovarian cancer. Am J Obstet Gynecol 123:772–774, 1975.

Stenbeck M: Breast. Acta Oncol 34:49–51, 1995.

Tortolero-Luna G, Mitchell MF, Rhodes-Morris HE: Epidemiology and screening of ovarian cancer. Obstet Gynecol Clin North Am 21:1–23, 1994.

section 3

Pathology of the Musculoskeletal System

SECTION 3

chapter 18

Introduction to Pathology of the Musculoskeletal System

William G. Boissonnault

Primary musculoskeletal system disease is extremely common in our society. The fact that the skeletal system with its associated soft tissues provides a protective covering for important structures like the brain and heart and essentially makes up the limbs puts this system at risk for traumatic and repetitive insults and injuries (See Box 18–1). In addition, the musculoskeletal system is often confronted with immobilization secondary to bed rest or casting or splinting of a specific body region. The musculoskeletal system reacts quickly to the lack of mechanical stress (immobilization) in ways that may adversely affect recovery and rehabilitation.

Like all other body systems the musculoskeletal system does not function in isolation. Therefore, primary disease of the musculoskeletal system can significantly affect other body systems and vice versa. In addition, certain diseases are systemic, meaning that all body systems, including the musculoskeletal system, can be involved to some degree. The challenge to develop an effective rehabilitation program is heightened when one is faced with complex, multisystem disorders (see Chapter 4). The purpose of this chapter is to describe the common types of injuries and disorders sustained by the musculoskeletal system, including a generalized response to trauma and immobilization. In addition, examples of how primary diseases in other organs affect the musculoskeletal system are described. The remainder of the chapters in Section 3 describe a variety of specific musculoskeletal conditions.

BIOLOGIC RESPONSE TO TRAUMA

The immediate biologic response to trauma is a generalized inflammatory reaction regardless of what tissue is damaged or the nature of the injury. The response is marked by vascular, chemical, and cellular events with the ultimate purpose being to prepare the area for repair. The primary objective of the vascular response to injury is to mobilize and transport the body's defenses (white blood cells). Vasoconstriction occurs initially and can last up to 5 to 10 minutes (Zarins, 1982). This, along with reduced fluid flow through the injured area, due to development of fibrinogen clots in the tissue spaces and lymphatic channels (which prevents the spread of bacteria and toxins), allows for the white blood cells to migrate to the periphery of the vessel in a process called margination. These white blood cells will eventually adhere to the walls of the damaged capillary, a process called pavementing.

Shortly after the injury and vasoconstriction, vasodilation of the local blood vessels occurs. The increased blood flow is accompanied by increased permeability of the small blood vessels. The permeability changes occur secondary to direct trauma to the vessels and to the presence of chemical mediators such as histamines, serotonin, and bradykinins. The increased permeability allows for the white blood cells to squeeze through the blood vessel wall. This process is called diapedesis. The increased blood volume and vessel permeability also result in a significant transfer of fluid into the injured area. The fluid shift occurs because of the heightened intravascular hydrostatic pressure and the altered osmotic pressure gradient (as larger molecules escape into the tissues).

Once beyond the blood vessel walls the white blood cells are guided to the site of injury by a process called chemotaxis (Fig. 18–1). Numerous elements of the damaged tissue (i.e., bacterial toxins and tissue polysaccharides) draw the white blood cells to the area of highest concentration of these elements. Upon arriving at the site of damage, the white blood cells begin to clean up the area by the process of phagocytosis. The neutrophils, monocytes, and macrophages recognize, engulf, and digest debris, necrotic tissue, red blood cells, proteins, and so forth to prepare the area for repair and growth of new tissue (Guyton, 1991).

Clinical Manifestations. The cardinal signs of acute inflammation are listed in Table 18–1. Accompanying clinical findings include increased muscle tone or spasm and loss of function. Movements of the involved area are generally slow and guarded. Cyriax describes two components of passive movement testing that also suggest acute inflammation: a spasm end feel and pain reported before resistance is noted by the practitioner as the limb is moved passively (Cyriax, 1982).

Medical Management

Treatment. If surgery is not indicated, the most common medical intervention for acute inflammation is pharmacotherapy. Salicylates (except aspirin) and nonsteroidal anti-inflammatory drugs (NSAIDs)[1] are the most commonly administered medications for pain and inflammation. The anti-inflammatory affect is chiefly attained by inhibition of the biosynthesis of prostaglandins. Other anti-inflammatory mechanisms include decreasing the release of chemical mediators from granulocytes, basophils, and mast cells, decreasing the sensitivity of vessels to bradykinin and histamine, and reversing or controlling the degree of vasodilation (Payan, 1992; MacDermott, 1992).

[1] Examples of commonly prescribed NSAIDs are ibuprofen, ketoprofen, nabumetone, naproxen, piroxicam, diclofenac sodium, and sulindac.

BOX 18-1
Common Musculoskeletal Disorders

Fracture
Dislocation
Subluxation
Contusion
Hematoma
Repetitive overuse, microtrauma
Sprain
Degenerative disease

TABLE 18-1 Cardinal Signs of Inflammation

Sign	Precipitating Events
Heat	Vasodilation and increased blood flow
Erythema	Vasodilation and increased blood flow
Edema	Fluid leaking from local blood vessels
Pain	Chemical mediation by bradykinins, histamines, serotonin, etc. Mechanical mediation by direct trauma or by internal pressure secondary to edema

Special Implications for the Therapist **18-1**

BIOLOGIC RESPONSE TO TRAUMA

Therapists have an important role in the rehabilitation of acute injuries. The specific goals of treatment are to facilitate wound healing and maintain the normal function of noninjured tissue and body regions. The overall goal of the rehabilitation program is to return the person to normal activity as soon as possible, yet not so fast that irritation and further inflammation of the injured area occur. There is often a fine line between maximizing activity and overdoing the activity to the point of injury aggravation. Client education is essential regarding their role in facilitating wound healing. Adherence to weight-bearing guidelines, avoiding prolonged sitting or flexion of the trunk, applying ice appropriately, and doing the prescribed exercises are key to the recovery process. Careful monitoring of the presenting symptoms and signs will guide the therapist in deciding when and how to progress therapy and activity level. This monitoring can also be taught so the client understands the limits of his or her condition. This process is somewhat more difficult with acute back or neck injuries than with peripheral injuries. Owing to the depth of the tissues of the spine, increased temperature and erythema are not always present. The therapist must rely more on muscle tone and the degree of pain with movement changes in deciding when the program can be progressed.

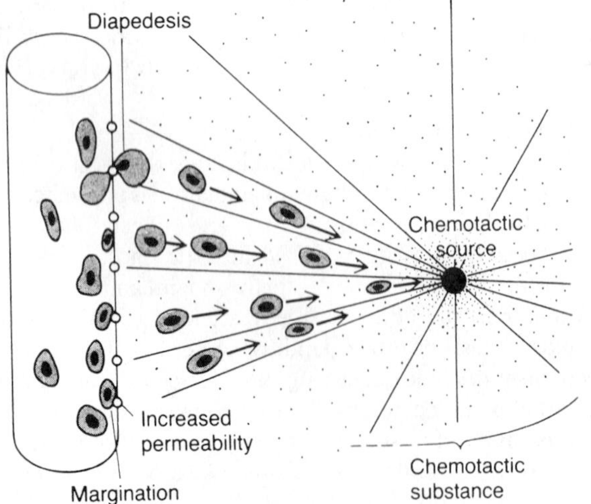

Figure 18-1. Movement of neutrophils by the process of chemotaxis toward an area of tissue damage. (*From Guyton AC: Textbook of Medical Physiology, ed 8. Philadelphia, WB Saunders, 1991, p 367.*)

Certain components of the inflammatory process must be controlled quickly for recovery to proceed. For example, if edema is a component of a joint injury it must be controlled as quickly as possible. Studies have demonstrated that joint edema can inhibit or hinder local muscle activity, which could result in altered joint mechanics and further irritation (Spencer et al., 1984; deAndrade et al., 1965).

A significant percentage of those coming to outpatient physical therapy clinics are taking salicylates or NSAIDs (Boissonnault and Koopmeiners, 1994). These medications can play a key role in recovery from an acute injury, facilitating the therapist's role and clinical decision making. Individuals respond very differently to NSAIDs so what works for one person may not work for another who presents with similar manifestations. If an acute injury is not responding to therapy by 2 weeks, communicating with a physician regarding possibly trying a different anti-inflammatory medication is warranted. This is based on the assumption that no other factors exist that could delay recovery.

Considering the widespread use of salicylates and NSAIDs, therapists must also be aware of potential side effects that would warrant communication with a physician. Box 18–2 summarizes potential adverse reactions to NSAIDs. Irritation of the gastrointestinal system is the most common potential side effect. The risk of developing peptic ulcer disease increases significantly if someone is taking more than one of these types of drugs. This pattern of drug use exists in the physical therapy population, in which significant numbers of subjects are taking an over-the-counter anti-inflammatory agent along with a prescribed NSAID (Boissonnault and Koopmeiners, 1994). See Chapter 13 for a description of peptic ulcer disease.

Besides ineffective medications, numerous other factors may delay or inhibit wound healing. Box 18–3 lists factors that could delay recovery from an injury. Since local blood supply is vital to the delivery of the

BOX **18–2**
Potential Adverse Reactions to Nonsteroidal Anti-inflammatory Drugs

- Central nervous system
  - Drowsiness
  - Headache
  - Dizziness
  - Confusion
  - Tinnitus
  - Vertigo
  - Depression
- Gastrointestinal system
  - Abdominal pain
  - Bleeding
  - Anemia
  - Diarrhea
  - Nausea
  - Ulcerations
  - Perforation
  - Hepatotoxicity
- Renal system
  - Cystitis
  - Hematuria
  - Kidney necrosis
  - Nephrotic syndrome (rare)
- Eyes
  - Blurred vision
  - Decreased acuity
  - Corneal deposits

From MacDermott BL: Non-narcotic analgesic, antipyretic and nonsteroidal anti-inflammatory agents. *In* Baer CL, Williams BR (eds): Clinical Pharmacology and Nursing, ed 2. Springhouse, Pa, Springhouse, 1992, p 341.

materials necessary for wound healing, factors that impede local circulation or a depletion of the necessary materials could delay rehabilitation. Certain tissues (e.g., tendons) have a decreased blood supply, and thus the healing process may require additional time. Therapists should screen a patient's medical history for the presence of conditions such as diabetes, chemical dependency (alcoholism), cigarette smoking, and so on to identify factors that could delay recovery. Lastly, local infection delays healing. If an abscess is present, the expected fever, chills, and sweats associated with infection will not be present. A sudden worsening of symptoms, the presence of a hot, acutely inflamed joint, or the onset of fever should warn the therapist that something more serious may exist (see Chapter 21). In general, the more compromised the host, the greater the chance of a slow or incomplete recovery.

BOX **18–3**
Factors Delaying Wound Healing

- Age
- General health of the host
- Presence of comorbidities (diabetes, peripheral vascular disease)
- Tobacco, alcohol
- Protein, vitamins, heavy metals depletion
- Local infection
- Type of tissue

TABLE **18–2** Synovial Joint Changes Observed After Prolonged Immobilization

Tissue	Results of Immobilization
Synovium	Proliferation of fibrofatty connective tissue into joint space
Cartilage	Adherence of fibrofatty connective tissue to cartilage surfaces Loss of cartilage thickness Pressure necrosis at points of contact where compression has been applied
Ligament	Disorganization of parallel arrays of fibrils and cells
Ligament insertion site	Destruction of ligament fibers attaching to bone
Bone	Generalized osteoporosis of cancellous and cortical bone

From Engles M: Tissue response. *In* Donatelli R, Wooden MJ (eds): Orthopaedic Physical Therapy, ed 2. New York, Churchill Livingstone, 1994 p 24.

Tissue Response to Immobilization

In addition to having an important role in the rehabilitation of acute injuries, therapists frequently deal with clinical problems secondary to the effects of immobilization. Although not traumatic in the classic sense, immobilization of a limb or joint can result in significant impairment and functional limitations. Immobilization takes a variety of forms, including bed rest, casting or splinting of a body part, or non–weight-bearing status of a lower extremity. On a tissue level, significant changes can occur with immobilization (Tables 18–2 and 18–3). Besides the inert joint structures, changes also occur in muscle, particularly a loss of strength. Such changes can occur without injury,

TABLE **18–3** Changes Associated with Joints Immobilized for 12 Weeks

Tissue	Results of Immobilization
Joint composite	Range of motion on an arthrograph indicates that the force required for the first flexion-extension cycle is increased more than 12-fold
Ligament	Stress-strain diagrams of collateral ligaments show increased deformation with a standard load (i.e., greater compliance) Tensile failure tests of collateral and cruciate ligaments show failure at lower load as well as lower energy-absorbing capacity of the immobilized bone-ligament complex (to about one-third of controls)

Modified from Engle M: Tissue response. *In* Donatelli R, Wodden MJ (eds): Orthopaedic Physical Therapy, ed 2. New York, Churchill Livingstone, 1994, p 24.

which magnifies the importance of maintaining function in noninjured tissue and body areas. A rehabilitation program should be designed to address the needs of each of the tissues.

While initiating rehabilitation after immobilization, the therapist must remain vigilant for the possible presence of deep vein thrombosis (DVT). A potential complication of DVT is pulmonary embolus, which represents one of the leading causes of morbidity and mortality after orthopedic surgical procedures (Ferree et al., 1993). Although a large percentage of clients with DVT are asymptomatic, severe local pain and edema, fever, chills, and malaise are all possible manifestations. The types of immobilization that carry the risk of DVT include bed rest, the limb's being placed in a cast or splint, and non–weight bearing status following a lower extremity injury or procedure or a long car or plane ride. (See Chapter 10 for more information about DVT.)

SPECIFIC TISSUE INJURY

Fracture

Description. A fracture is any defect in the continuity of a bone, ranging from a small crack to a complex fracture with multiple segments. Fractures can be classified into three general categories: (1) fracture by sudden impact; (2) stress or fatigue fracture; and (3) pathologic fracture (Gunta, 1994). By far the most common of these fractures are those associated with sudden impact. Fractures can also be classified as open (also called compound) or closed depending upon whether the skin is breached or not. Figure 18–2 shows the different types of fractures.

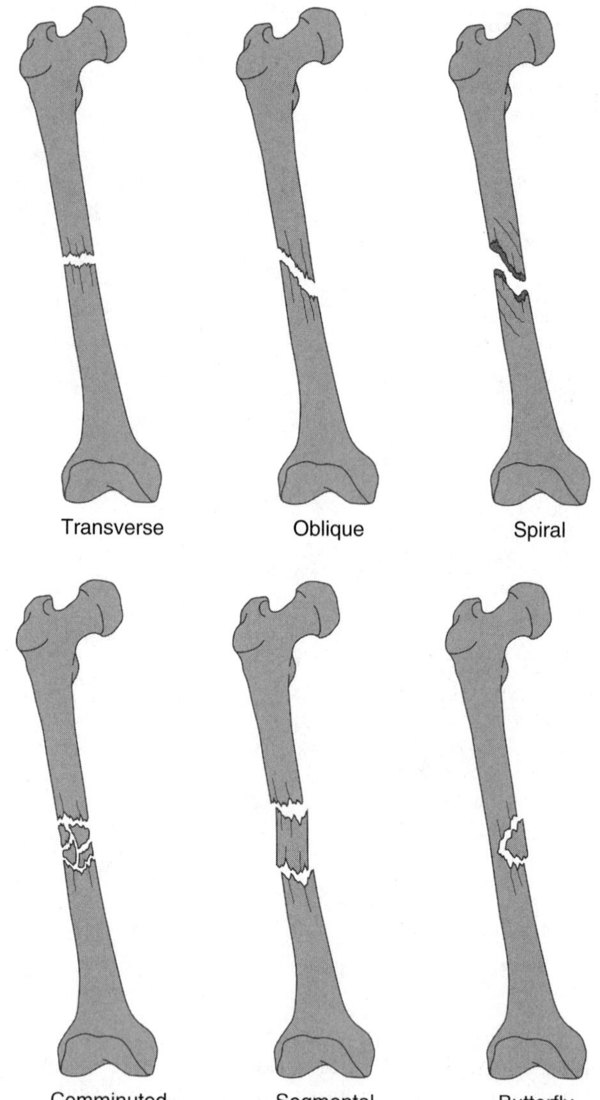

Figure **18–2.** Classification of fractures.

Clinical Manifestations. The primary manifestations of fracture are listed in Box 18–4. Point tenderness over the site of the fracture will be present. With many fractures, attempts to move the injured limb will provoke severe pain, but in the presence of a fatigue (stress) fracture active movement is typically painless.[2] Repetitive weight bearing will cause pain, and local palpation will be exquisitely tender. In the presence of a compression fracture of a thoracic vertebra, the initial pain may be sharp and severe, but after a few days may become dull and achy. The deformity associated with an extremity fracture is often obvious, but the deformity of a spinal fracture is not always so. For example, a compression fracture of a thoracic vertebral body may result in an anterior wedging of the body, but only a mildly accentuated thoracic kyphosis. In the long bones of the extremities three types of deformities are possible: (1) angulation, (2) shortening, and (3) rotational (Gunta, 1994).

Fracture Healing

The complex process of fracture healing can be broken down into five stages: (1) hematoma formation, (2) cellular proliferation, (3) callus formation, (4) ossification, and (5) consolidation and remodeling. During the initial 48 to 72 hours post fracture, hematoma formation occurs. Clotting factors from the blood initiate the formation of a fibrin meshwork. This meshwork is the framework for the ingrowth of fibroblasts and capillary buds around and between the bony ends. During the cellular proliferation phase, osteogenic cells proliferate and eventually form a fibrocartilage collar around the fracture site. Eventually the collars and the ends of the bones unite. The cartilage is eventually replaced by bone as osteoblasts continue to move into the site (callus formation and ossifica-

BOX **18–4**
Signs and Symptoms of Fractures

- Pain and tenderness
- Deformity
- Edema
- Ecchymosis
- Loss of general function
- Loss of mobility

[2] In addition, initial radiographs are also frequently normal because of the subtle nature of stress fractures. A repeat radiograph a few weeks after the initial radiograph, or a bone scan, will reveal the lesion.

tion). Lastly, the excessive bony callus is resorbed and the bone remodels in response to the mechanical stresses placed upon it. In general, fractures in children heal in 4 to 6 weeks; in adolescents in 6 to 8 weeks; and in adults in 10 to 18 weeks (Gunta, 1994).

Special Implications for the Therapist **18–2**

FRACTURES

Complications of fractures require vigilance on the therapist's part and possibly quick action. Significant swelling can occur around the fracture site, and if the swelling is contained within a closed soft tissue compartment, compartmental syndrome may occur. Because of the progressively increased intracompartmental pressure, nerve and circulatory compromise can occur. This condition may be acute or chronic. The compartment becomes exquisitely painful. If the therapist notes decreased motor function, burning, paresthesia, or diminished reflexes, physician contact is warranted. Permanent damage and loss of function may result if this condition is not treated.

Another complication, fat embolism, is potentially fatal. The risk of developing this condition is related to fracture of long bones and the bony pelvis, which contain the most marrow. The fat globules from the bone marrow (or from the subcutaneous tissue at the fracture site) migrate to the lung parenchyma and can block pulmonary vessels, decreasing alveolar diffusion of oxygen. The initial symptoms typically appear within 1 week post injury. Subtle changes in behavior and orientation occur if there are emboli in the cerebral circulation. There may also be complaints of dyspnea and chest pain, diaphoresis, pallor, or cyanosis. A rash on the anterior chest wall, neck, axillae, and shoulders may develop. The onset of any of these symptoms warrants immediate physician contact (Gunta, 1994).

Soft Tissue Injuries

Sprains, dislocations, and subluxations are described in this section. A sprain is an injury of the ligamentous structures around a joint caused by abnormal or excessive joint motion. Sprains can be classified as injuries of first, second, or third degree, ranging from injury of a few fibers without loss of ligamentous integrity (first degree) to complete loss of structural or biomechanical integrity (third degree). Common sites for this type of injury include the ankle, knee, and fingers. The clinical manifestations of sprains are local pain, edema, increased local tissue temperature, ecchymosis, hypermobility or instability, and loss of function. If, after an injury, the therapist notes quick onset of joint effusion and the joint feels hot to the touch and movement is extremely painful and limited, the joint needs to be examined by a physician to rule out hemarthrosis.

The terms *dislocation* and *subluxation* relate to joint integrity. Dislocation implies complete loss of joint integrity with loss of anatomic relationship. Often significant ligamentous damage occurs with this type of injury. Dislocations most often occur at the glenohumeral joint. Congenital dislocations are most frequently seen at the hip joints. Joint dislocation can also be a late manifestation of chronic disease such as rheumatoid arthritis, paralysis, and neuromuscular disease. In the presence of a joint dislocation, the integrity of nerve and vascular tissue must be assessed. If compromise is suspected, timely reduction is essential to prevent serious complications.

Lastly, subluxation is partial disruption of the anatomic relationship within a joint. Mobile joints are at risk of subluxation. These include the glenohumeral, acromioclavicular, sacroiliac, and atlantoaxial joints. Once the joint condition has stabilized, rehabilitation should address local muscle imbalances and adjacent joint hypomobility, which could increase mechanical stresses at the joint.

MUSCULOSKELETAL SYSTEM DISEASE

Although not nearly as common as traumatic and repetitive or overuse injuries, musculoskeletal system diseases are significant from the standpoint of disability, mortality, and cost in terms of health-care dollars. The most serious of these diseases are cancer and infection. The pathogenesis of these two types of diseases illustrates the intricate interrelationships between the musculoskeletal system and other body systems. The primary highways or communication networks connecting the musculoskeletal and other body systems are the circulatory and lymphatic systems. These pathways are the routes utilized by disease to travel from one system to another. In addition, these highways deliver the nutrients and other supplies needed by the musculoskeletal system.

Cancer

While primary malignant bone and soft tissue tumors are rare, metastatic disease of the musculoskeletal system is relatively common. Although a wide variety of primary cancers can spread to the musculoskeletal system, the four most common primary lesions are breast, lungs, myeloma, and prostate (McLain and Weinstein, 1990). Cancer cells typically invade the thin-walled lymphatic channels, capillaries, and venules as opposed to the thicker-walled arterioles and arteries. Once the cancer cells enter the bloodstream, they must lodge in the vascular network of the host tissue before the secondary cancer can develop. Organs with extensive circulatory or lymphatic systems, like the lungs and liver, are the most common sites of metastasis. Of the other potential sites of metastasis, the axial skeleton is among the most common (Rubin and Farber 1994). The blood supply to the axial skeleton is extensive compared to that to the distal components of the extremities, and the spinal blood flow through the thin-walled, valveless veins is slow and sluggish. This gives the circulating cancer cells ample opportunity to attach to the vessels' endothelium. The bony thorax, lumbar spine, and pelvis are the most common components of the axial skeleton for seeding of cancer to occur, and the vertebral bodies, because of the extensive venous plexus, appear to be the initial site for development of disease (Asdourian et al., 1990).

As with primary bone tumors, the major manifestation of metastatic bone cancer is pain. The pain can be caused by stretching of the periosteum, irritation of a nerve root or spinal cord, or be secondary to bone collapse (pathologic fracture). Once the cancer begins to spread, clients complain

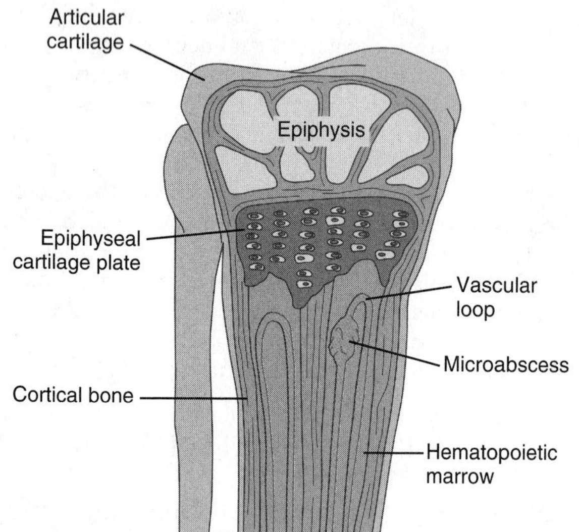

Figure 18–3. The vascular loop in growing bone is a common initial site of bacterial seeding.

of fatigue, malaise, fever, nausea, and so forth. Therapists working with clients diagnosed with cancer must be vigilant for symptoms or signs suggestive of systemic compromise and be aware of common sites of metastasis for the particular primary tumor. An awareness of complaints associated with the potential target organs is important and any suspicious findings should be reported to the physician. Unfortunately, often the initial presenting complaint associated with the disease is pain from the bone metastasis (back pain), which can result in a delay in the diagnosis. See Chapters 7 and 22 for extensive information related to cancer.

Infection

As with cancer, infection can originate in the musculoskeletal system or it can spread to the musculoskeletal system from elsewhere in the body. The most common cause of osteomyelitis is direct extension of bacterial organisms by penetrating wounds, fractures, or surgical intervention (Schiller, 1994). Staphylococci and streptococci are the most common infecting agents. The other common mechanism by which bacterial organisms reach the musculoskeletal system is via the hematogenous route. The original infection could be of the urinary tract (adults) or skin or teeth (children). In adults, the most common site of osteomyelitis is the vertebral body or intervertebral disk. The sluggish blood flow through the valveless veins facilitates bacterial seeding. Cases have been described illustrating the lengthy delay in diagnosis of vertebral osteomyelitis when back pain is the primary complaint (Heggeness et al., 1993; Schofferman et al., 1989).

In children, the ends of the long bones are the most frequently involved areas in hematogenous osteomyelitis. The infection typically begins in the metaphyseal region adjacent to the growth plate. Blood flow is sluggish and relatively slow because the arterioles form a loop (Fig. 18–3), then drain into the medullary cavity without establishing a capillary bed (Schiller, 1994; Almekinders, 1994).

The primary manifestations of osteomyelitis vary between adults and children. Back pain is typically the chief complaint in adults, but once the infection becomes systemic (as opposed to an abscess) a low-grade fever may be present. Children are more likely to present with acute, severe complaints such as high fever and intense pain, but in some cases local manifestations will predominate, such as edema, erythema, and tenderness. These signs are easier to detect in the extremities, unlike vertebral osteomyelitis where the infected structures lie much deeper. Therapists working with clients with a recent history of infection or of trauma or surgery (within the previous 12 months) need to be vigilant for manifestations of infection.

References

Almekinders LC: Osteomyelitis: Essentials of diagnosis and treatment. J Musculoskel Med, pp 31–40, Nov 1994.
Asdourian PL, Weidenberg M, DeWald RL, et al.: The pattern of involvement in metastatic vertebral breast cancer. Clin Orthop 250:164–170, 1990.
Boissonnault WG, Koopmeiners MB: Medical history profile: Orthopaedic physical therapy outpatients. J Orthop Sports Phys Ther 20:2–10, 1994.
Cyriax J: Textbook of Orthopaedic Medicine: Diagnosis of Soft Tissue Lesions, ed 8, vol 1. London, Bailliere-Tindall, 1982.
deAndrade JR, Grant C, Dixon AS: Joint distention and reflex muscle inhibition in the knee. J Bone Joint Surg [Am] 47:313–322, 1965.
Ferree BA, Stern PJ, Jolson RS, Roberts JM, Kahn A: Deep venous thrombosis after spinal surgery. Spine 18:315–319, 1993.
Gunta K: Alterations in skeletal function: Trauma and infection. *In* Mattson-Porth C (ed): Pathophysiology: Concepts of Altered Health States, ed 4. Philadelphia, JB Lippincott, 1994, pp 1203–1209.
Guyton AC: Textbook of Medical Physiology, ed 8. Philadelphia, WB Saunders, 1991.
Heggeness MH, Esses SI, Errico T, Yuam HA: Late infection of spinal instrumentation by hematogenous seeding. Spine 18:492–496, 1993.
MacDermott BL: Non-narcotic analgesic, antipyretic and nonsteroidal anti-inflammatory agents. *In* Baer CL, Williams BR (eds): Clinical Pharmacology and Nursing, ed 2. Springhouse, Pa, Springhouse, 1992, p 341.
McLain RF, Weinstein JN: Tumors of the spine. Semin Spine Surg 2:157–180, 1990.
Payan DG: Nonsteroidal anti-inflammatory drugs: Nonopioid analgesics; drugs used in gout. *In* Katzung BG (ed): Basic and Clinical Pharmacology, ed 5. Norwalk, Conn, Appleton & Lange, 1992, pp 491–501.
Rubin E, Farber JL: Neoplasia. *In* Rubin E, Farber JL (eds): Pathology, ed 2. Philadelphia, JB Lippincott, 1994, pp 152–156.
Schiller AL: Bones and joints. *In* Rubin E, Farber JL (eds): Pathology, ed 2. Philadelphia, JB Lippincott, 1994, pp 1294–1297.
Schofferman L, Schofferman J, Zucherman J, et al: Occult infections causing persistent low back pain. Spine 14:417–419, 1989.
Spencer JD, Hayes KC, Alexander IJ: Knee joint effusion and quadriceps reflex inhibition in man. Arch Phys Med Rehabil 65:171–177, 1984.
Zarins B: Soft tissue injury and repair: Biomechanical aspects. Int J Sports Med 3:9–11, 1982.

SECTION 3

chapter 19

Genetic and Developmental Disorders

Catherine C. Goodman
and Jim Miedaner

TERMINOLOGY FOR NEURAL TUBE DEFECTS

Anencephaly The most severe form of neural tube defect in which there is no development above the brainstem; absence of the brain

Bifid Split in two

Cele Sac

Encephalocele Hernial protrusion of brain substance and meninges through a congenital or traumatic opening in the skull

Encephalocystocele Hernial protrusion of the brain distended by fluid

Lipo(myelo)meningocele A variation in which a lipomatous tumor is embedded within the lumbar spinal cord and replaces the overlying dura; the lipoma typically causes minimal (if any) early impairment but can produce progressive myelopathy as the child grows

Meninges The three membranes covering the brain and spinal cord: the dura mater, arachnoid, and pia mater

Meningocele Hernial protrusion of the meninges through a defect in the vertebral column; a form of spina bifida cystica consisting of a saclike cyst of meninges filled with spinal fluid

Meningomyelocele (myelomeningocele or MM) Hernial protrusion of a saclike cyst of meninges, spinal fluid, and a portion of the spinal cord with its nerves through a defect in the vertebral column

Myelo The spinal cord and medulla oblongata

Myelodysplasia A general term used to describe defective development of any part of the spinal cord but especially of the lower spinal cord levels

Myelomeningocele See Meningomyelocele

Rachischisis Congenital fissure of the vertebral column; *right posterior*, spina bifida

Spina bifida A term used to describe various forms of myelodysplasia. A defective closure of the bony encasement of the spinal cord, that is, the bony vertebral column is divided into two parts through which the spinal cord and meninges may or may not protrude. If the anomaly is not visible, the condition is called *spina bifida occulta*. If there is an external protrusion of the saclike structure, it is called *spina bifida cystica*, which is then further classified according to the extent of involvement (e.g., meningocele, meningomyelocele, or myelomenigocele)

Spina bifida cystica Spina bifida in which there is protrusion through the defect of a saclike cyst that contains the meninges (meningocele), or the meninges and spinal cord (meningomyelocele)

Spina bifida occulta Spina bifida in which there is incomplete closure of one or more vertebrae (failure of the vertebral arch to fuse posteriorly) without protrusion of the cord or meninges (*occulta* means hidden or not visible). These defects are skin-covered but may be marked by a patch of dark hair at the level of the lesion

Pediatric diseases and disorders comprise a large number of conditions, so many that entire volumes have been devoted just to pediatric pathologies. Given the format of this book and space limitations, in this chapter we have included as many of the more commonly encountered genetic and developmental disorders as possible.

A brief discussion of several other rare but important diagnoses is also included. Since physical and occupational therapy treatment is not the focus here, the reader is referred to other, more appropriate resources for specific and thorough treatment guidelines for these conditions (Campbell, 1995; Dunn, 1991; Gilfoyle et al., 1993; Kurtz and Scull, 1993).

CEREBRAL PALSY

Overview. Cerebral palsy (CP) is a nonhereditary and nonprogressive lesion of the cerebral cortex resulting in a group of neuromuscular disorders of posture and voluntary movement. Patterns of abnormal movement develop to compensate for the lack of voluntary control. CP may be accompanied by impairment of speech, vision, hearing, and perceptual functions, a seizure disorder, hydrocephalus, microcephalus, or mental retardation.

CP is often classified by the type of muscle tone and limb involvement. The types of muscle tone include hypotonia (low tone), hypertonia (high tone, spasticity), or a mixture of these two types. Muscle tone is graded on a scale of mild, to moderate, to severe. The patterns of motor involvement are described in Table 19–1. Spastic CP accounts for the majority of cases, often with a clinical picture of spastic hemiplegia. Spastic diplegia is seen in approximately one third of

TABLE 19–1 CLASSIFICATION OF CEREBRAL PALSY

TYPE	DESCRIPTION	INCIDENCE
Spastic		75%
Monoplegia	Only one limb affected	
Diplegia	Involves trunk and lower extremities; upper extremities to a lesser degree	
Hemiplegia	Primarily one total side involved; upper extremity usually more than the lower extremity	
Quadriplegia (tetraplegia)	Involvement of all four limbs, head, and trunk	
Ataxia	Irregularity of muscular action; may be pure or combined with other forms	15%
Dyskinesia (choreoathetosis)	Impairment of the power of voluntary movement; ceaseless rapid, jerky involuntary movements (chorea) alternating with repetitive, involuntary, slow, writhing movements (athetosis); movements increase with emotional stress and around adolescence; often associated with rigidity or spastic quadriplegia or diplegia	5%
Hypotonia	Abnormally reduced tension or muscle tone; accompanied by variable degrees of weakness	<1%

all cases. Quadriplegia, ataxia, and athetoid CP affect a small number of children.[1]

Incidence, Etiology, and Risk Factors. The reported incidence of CP ranges from 2.5 to 4.2 cases per 1000 births in the United States with an estimated 7000 to 12,000 children per year affected. The cause of CP can remain unknown but is often multifactorial. Any prenatal, perinatal, or postnatal condition that results in cerebral anoxia, hemorrhage, or damage to the cerebral cortex can cause CP (Table 19–2).

Pathogenesis. There is no consistent or uniform pathology associated with CP. Several types of neuropathic lesions have been identified on the basis of autopsy: (1) hemorrhage below the lining of the ventricles (subependymal) or (2) malformations of the central nervous system (CNS) resulting in neuropathy and anoxia or (3) hypoxia causing encephalopathy (brain degeneration) (Weinstein and Tharp, 1989).

The most common cause (prenatal cerebral hypoxia) can be responsible for systemic degeneration of immature areas of the brain and can interfere with cell maturation. Hypoxia and asphyxia are known to cause edema in the brain. The accumulation of carbon dioxide and lactic acid contributes to the development of acidosis, causing osmotic pressure changes and generalized cerebral swelling with subsequent brain damage. The severity of the damage depends on the gestational age at the time of the injury and the degree of injury sustained (Farley and Mooney, 1994).

Clinical Manifestations. Clinical manifestations of CP may include alterations of muscle tone, abnormal postures, reflex abnormalities, delayed motor development, and abnormal motor performance.[2] Associated disabilities may include mental retardation, learning disabilities, seizure disorders, sensory impairment (vision, hearing), bowel and bladder incontinence as a result of spasticity or flaccidity with increased risk of urinary tract infection, and orthopedic disabilities. Abnormal head circumference usually accompanies microcephalus or hydrocephalus. Behavioral signs may include extreme irritability or crying or failure to smile by 3 months.

Although this condition is considered nonprogressive, clinical manifestations change with growth and maturation and may become more apparent as the affected child grows. Musculoskeletal problems of altered muscle tone, muscle weakness, and joint restrictions are common. Joint restrictions are often due to atrophy of muscle fibers resulting in an increase in fibrous tissue in the periarticular structures. In this process, bone will grow faster than muscle, resulting in a disadvantageous length-tension relationship and an increased risk of subsequent contracture (Tardieu, 1988). A characteristic decreased muscle mass also results in decreased muscle power and endurance.

Changes in muscle tone affect a person's ability to control movement, resulting in poor selective control of muscles, poor regulation of activity and muscle groups, decreased ability to learn unique movements, inappropriate sequencing of movements, and poor anticipatory response (Table 19–3). Most often the timing and sequence of muscle activity are also affected. Each type of CP is characterized by its own clinical picture based on the presence and extent of these clinical manifestations.[3]

Medical Management

Diagnosis. Observation, a good history, and a neurologic examination will provide the physician with the information necessary to make an accurate and early diagnosis. The diagnostic studies performed depend on clinical findings. For example, electroencephalography (EEG) is indicated when sei-

[1] New cases of athetoid CP (characterized by an ongoing fluctuating movement pattern) have become almost nonexistent in the United States and Canada as a result of improved prenatal care in the prevention of Rh incompatibility and hyperbilirubinemia. It remains a problem in developing countries.

[2] Impaired motor function affects the head, neck, trunk, and extremities but also impairs sucking and swallowing resulting in feeding difficulties, a major focus of the occupational therapist.

[3] The progression of motor development associated with each type of CP is beyond the scope of this book. The reader is referred to other texts for a more detailed discussion (Campbell, 1995; Kottke and Lehmann, 1990).

TABLE 19-2 Risk Factors for Cerebral Palsy

Prenatal	Perinatal	Postnatal
Maternal infection	Prematurity	Neonatal infection (meningitis, encephalitis)
Rubella	Obstetric complications	Environmental toxins
Cytomegalovirus	Mechanical birth trauma	Trauma
Herpes simplex	Breech delivery	Kernicterus
Toxoplasmosis	Forceps delivery	Brain tumor
Maternal diabetes	Twin or multiple births	Anoxia (e.g., near drowning, assault)
Rh incompatibility	Prolapsed umbilical cord	Cerebrovascular accident
Toxemia (undiagnosed or untreated)	Low birth weight (<1750 g)	Neonatal hypoglycemia
Maternal malnutrition	Small for gestational age (SGA)	Acidosis
Maternal seizures	Low Apgar scores (≤4 at 5 min)	
Maternal radiation	Placenta previa (intrauterine bleeding)	
Abnormal placental attachment	Abruptio placentae	
Congenital anomalies of the brain		

zures are present or suspected; hip radiographic films may be indicated to rule out hip dislocations, particularly in the presence of spasticity; blood or urine screening tests may be utilized to rule out certain metabolic causes of CP. The computed tomography (CT) scan can provide definitive confirmation of a diagnosis of CP, but these are usually in the more severe cases which also tend to be easier to recognize clinically.

Treatment. Comprehensive and cooperative planning involving physicians, therapists, nurses, special educators, psychologists, and family members is essential.

Some of the most common medical management strategies include pharmaceuticals, neurosurgical intervention, and orthopedic surgery. Skeletal muscle relaxants (e.g., baclofen, diazepam, dantrolene) can be used to assist in controlling increased spasticity and can be administered orally or intrathecally.[4]

Motor point blocks can also be used to control spasticity. Muscles such as the gastrocnemius, hip adductors, or hamstrings are injected with a botulinum toxin to temporarily decrease tone and increase movement[5] (Epperson, 1995–1996; Lu et al., 1995). The effects of these injections will wear off anywhere from several weeks to several months later (Koman, 1993).

Dorsal rhizotomy (surgically identifying the posterior roots of the spinal cord and selectively resecting some or all of them) to reduce spasticity has been used with increasing frequency over the past 5 to 10 years. This is usually performed at the L2–5 spinal levels for clients with spastic diplegia or mild increased tone who are independent ambulators but who have abnormalities of posture and gait. A rhizotomy may also be used effectively for clients with severe positioning difficulties such as severe quadriplegia. This procedure may reduce muscle tone enough to facilitate personal hygiene and provide improved sitting and comfort.

Orthopedic surgery may include muscle lengthening or releases (e.g., adductors, iliopsoas, hamstrings), muscle transfers to increase control or decrease excessive muscle pull,[6] or bone procedures (e.g., femoral derotational osteotomy [see Fig. 19–14], triple arthrodesis, spinal fusions). Orthoses to support or stabilize a joint, extremity, or the torso may also be prescribed.

Prognosis. Individuals with mild cases of CP may experience resolution of motor impairment with maturation of the CNS. Most children with mild to moderate CP have normal life spans, although motor impairment may limit mobility, especially ambulation. Severe CP (spastic type with profound retardation and seizures difficult to control) has a poor prognosis. Nearly half die by 10 years of age, often as a result of infections.

Ambulation potential may be predicted based on motor milestones (Table 19–4). Independent sitting prior to age 2 years and seat-scooting along the floor on the buttocks are positive indicators of future ambulation. If it is going to occur, ambulation usually takes place by 8 years of age.

Special Implications for the Therapist **19-1**

CEREBRAL PALSY

Early Intervention

An assessment of current management practices with guidelines for the management of clients with CP is available (Campbell, 1990). A general review of intervention studies shows that children with CP involved with handling and direct intervention services benefit compared with those children not involved in specific programming activities. The potential for improvement is better for children less than 9 months old and no

[4] Intrathecal administration (through the sheath of the spinal cord into the subarachnoid space) uses an implantable intrathecal infusion pump to allow a more direct effect and may be more effective in controlling spasticity with subsequent improved movement. Any attempts to control excess muscle tone (pharmaceutically or otherwise) should always be paired with activities to take advantage of the modulated tone.

[5] The type A toxin (Botox) is injected directly into the muscle and is used to blockade the neuromuscular junction by acting presynaptically to reduce the release of acetylcholine. Muscle weakness and decrease in muscle spasm occur in 3 to 7 days.

[6] Transfer of the tibialis posterior to improve neutral ankle position and foot clearance during gait is probably the most common transfer in this population.

TABLE 19-3 EFFECTS OF CHANGES IN MUSCLE TONE

EFFECTS OF MODERATE HYPERTONIA	EFFECTS OF MODERATE HYPOTONIA
Decreased movement: gross motor delays	Decreased movement: gross motor delays
Tightness/contractures of hip and knee flexors, lower extremity adductors, gastrocnemius and soleus (heel cords)	Possible lower extremity external rotation tightness
Weak trunk; unstable kyphotic sitting	Truncal kyphosis
Flexed, adducted, pronated upper extremity (severe cases)	Compensatory widened lower extremity base of support in prone position, creeping, sitting, standing, and walking
Significant upper extremity compensations (pulling up with arms, using arms for sitting balance)	Delayed ambulation (at least 6–12 mo)
Standing and ambulation usually require assistance (splinting, walking aids)	Unstable (pronated) feet
Usually at least one orthopedic (surgical) intervention required by age 5 yr	Future difficulties with hopping, jumping, skipping
Adaptive equipment required by age 5 yr (e.g., stander, wheelchair or stroller, adaptive chair)	

greater than 2 years of age at a minimum frequency of intervention of two times per week (Binder, 1989).

A significant number of children with a diagnosis of spastic CP begin with low muscle tone. As a result they have insufficient support to position themselves against gravity for activities such as lifting the head, reaching, or kicking. The child will attempt to develop alternative strategies to complete the tasks. If control is not available, these strategies will result in postures that allow a particular sequence but do not allow for subsequent movement and transitions.

Examples of such situations are a wide-based sitting posture which allows the child to maintain sitting but decreases the ability to turn and rotate in and out of the position. Pulling with the arms only (without using the lower extremities) to stand is another example of an alternative strategy used by the child. If practiced and repeated over time, these abnormal movements become habitual and are difficult to change.

TABLE 19-4 PREDICTORS OF AMBULATION FOR CEREBRAL PALSY

PREDICTORS	AMBULATION POTENTIAL
By diagnosis:	
Monoplegia	100%
Hemiplegia	100%
Ataxia	100%
Diplegia	85%–90%
Spastic quadriplegia	0%–70%
By motor function:	
Sits independently by 2 yr	100%
Sits independently by 3–4 yr	50% community ambulation
Presence of primitive reactions beyond 2 yr	Poor
Absence of postural reactions beyond 2 yr	Poor
Independently crawled symmetrically or reciprocally by 2½–3 yr	100%

Early and accurate identification of CP provides the most likely opportunity for significant change and facilitation of more normal motor performance (Sharkey, 1990). There are many motor milestone checklists available from which a comparison with the normal can be made.

Postoperative Concerns

After orthopedic surgery, the therapist can assist in reducing muscle spasms that increase postoperative pain by moving and turning the child carefully and slowly. In the case of postoperative casting, the therapist can instruct the family to wash and dry the skin at the edge of the cast frequently, inspecting often for signs of skin breakdown. Repositioning and ventilation under the cast with a cool-air blow dryer can also assist in preventing skin breakdown. A flashlight can be used daily to inspect beneath the cast.

Surgical procedures (orthopedic or neurosurgical) may expose areas of underlying muscle weakness and instability. It is critical that an inpatient program begin following surgery to assist with strengthening and improving functional performance.

Adaptive Equipment

The selection and use of adaptive equipment is a critical part of the overall management of CP. Carefully adapted equipment can improve speech intelligibility and vocalization, increase head and trunk control, improve self-feeding and drinking skills, increase upper extremity function, and improve mobility.

Appropriately selected equipment and postioning have been shown to encourage smoother and faster reach, decrease extensor tone, increase vital capacity, and improve performance on cognitive testing (Myhr, 1995). Children as young as 2 years of age with comparable cognitive skills have been shown to be capable of controlling powered mobility.

A wide variety of technical aids are also available to improve the functioning of children with CP. These include communication boards, electromechanical toys that are manipulated by correct movement of the head and trunk or other body parts, and microcomputers

TABLE 19-5 General Foot and Ankle Splinting Guidelines

Splints	Status	Application
Solid AFO neutral to +5 degrees DF	Nonambulators, beginning standers/ambulators	1. Less than antigravity DF in standing 2. Genu recurvatum associated with decreased ankle DF 3. Need for medial-lateral stability 4. Nighttime/positional stretching
AFO with 90 degrees posterior stop and free DF (adjustable angle) (hinged AFO)	Clients with some, but limited, functional mobility	Applications 1–4 above, but need more passive DF during movement, such as ambulation, squatting, steps, and sit to stand
Floor reaction AFO	Crouch Gait Standers Full passive knee extension in standing	For clients with decreased ability to maintain knee extension during standing/ambulation
SMO	Standers/ambulators with unstable ankles	1. Need medial-lateral ankle stability 2. Would like opportunity to use active plantar flexion 3. Decreased DF not a problem during gait

AFO, ankle-foot orthosis; DF, dorsiflexion; SMO, supramalleolar orthosis.

combined with voice synthesizers to aid speech and communication.

Manual Passive Range-of-Motion Exercise

It is generally accepted that manual straight-plane passive range-of-motion (ROM) exercise for children with a chronic neurologic disorder such as CP is of limited use as it does not meet the physiologic requirements necessary to stretch a muscle.* Instead, splinting or positioning that offers a low-load prolonged stretch greater than 30 minutes and that is utilized throughout the day is recommended. For example, splints such as lower extremity ankle-foot orthoses (AFOs) to maintain ankle ROM or supported standing to control lower extremity flexion contractures and assist with hip development and stability may be implemented.

Manual passive ROM exercise is, however, not without its application. It is very useful for maintaining or increasing lower or upper extremity ROM for children less than 2 years of age, particularly for those with an isolated ROM limitation.

Other treatment options used by therapists to improve ROM and facilitate motor development or improve function include relaxation techniques such as neutral warmth or acupressure points, serial or tone casts, therapy ball activities, aquatic programs, and manual therapy techniques.

Orthoses

AFOs are probably the most commonly used orthoses for children with CP. A rigid polypropylene AFO is used to provide medial-lateral stability to the foot and ankle while at the same time assisting with foot clearance during gait. The AFO can be set at +3 to +5 degrees of dorsiflexion to facilitate the increased ankle dorsiflexion necessary for the swing phase of gait or to decrease genu recurvatum (hyperextensibility at the knee). Hinged AFOs may be recommended once a child is moving in the upright position, especially when the child is beginning to squat or move up- and downstairs.

A supramalleolar orthosis (SMO) provides medial-lateral stability for the foot and ankle while allowing free plantar flexion† and dorsiflexion. The SMO can be used when decreased ankle dorsiflexion or excessive genu recurvatum are not problems. Extending the SMO proximally to the malleoli provides important support whereas support distal to the malleoli usually shifts the deformity in a proximal direction. General guidelines and recommendations for foot and ankle splinting can be found in Table 19–5.

Adults with Cerebral Palsy

Therapists must also recognize and address the ongoing and unique needs of adults with CP. Group homes, independent living centers, and sheltered workshops are now making it possible for many nonambulatory adults with disabilities to function independently or semi-independently. Regular daily living assistance is required by adults with spastic quadriplegia, especially in the area of lifts and transfers. Degenerative arthritis, severe joint contractures, and other orthopedic deformities present the most common and challenging problems within this population.

Management strategies for older children and adults with CP are just evolving. Isokinetic strengthening three times per week for 8 weeks can improve gross motor skills such as running and walking for those persons who remain ambulatory into adulthood (Macphail, 1995). A traditional upper extremity strengthening program of 6 to 10 repetitions three times per week for 8 weeks has been useful in improving speed and endurance with independent wheelchair propulsion.

* Passive trunk *rotation* has been found to be useful in assisting with general flexibility and modulation of increased tone for persons with spastic quadriplegia.
† It is always helpful to have whatever plantar flexion is available since this motion helps decelerate the limb during mid and late stances and facilitates the initial progression of the limb during late stance and early swing.

DOWN SYNDROME

Definition and Incidence. Down syndrome was the first genetic disorder attributed to a chromosomal aberration referred to as trisomy 21.[7] Down syndrome is characterized by muscle hypotonia, cognitive delay, abnormal facial features, and other distinctive physical abnormalities.

The overall prevalence of Down syndrome is 1 in 650 to 800 live births. The incidence rises with age. Before maternal age 30 the incidence is 1 in 2000 births; it is 1 in 50 for mothers aged 35 to 39, and 1 in 20 in mothers over 40 years. There is a 2% risk of recurrence for a couple[8] who have had a child with Down syndrome.

Etiology and Pathogenesis. The actual cause of Down syndrome is not yet known but evidence from cytogenetic and epidemiologic studies supports multiple causality. Trisomy 21 produces three copies of chromosome 21 instead of the normal two because of faulty meiosis (cell division by which reproductive cells are formed) of the ovum or, sometimes, the sperm. This results in a karyotype (chromosomal constitution of the cell nucleus) of 47 chromosomes instead of the normal 46.

In a small number of cases (3% to 4%) Down syndrome occurs as a result of a translocation of chromosome 15, 21, or 22 (i.e., the long arm of the chromosome breaks off and attaches to another chromosome). This type of genetic aberration is usually hereditary and is not associated with advanced parental age.

Because of the positive correlation between increasing age and Down syndrome, it is hypothesized that deterioration of the oocyte (immature ovum) or environmental factors such as radiation and viruses may cause the chromosomal abnormality. Persons with Down syndrome have an overall reduced brain weight especially affecting the brainstem and cerebellum. It is this factor that likely accounts for the muscle hypotonia.

Additional abnormal findings may include smaller convolutions within the brain, structural abnormalities in the dendritic spines of the pyramidal neurons of the motor cortex, and abnormality of the pyramidal system as a whole, including decreased pyramidal neurons in the hippocampus. This last finding has particular significance as it relates to the increased incidence of Alzheimer's symptoms in older persons with Down syndrome.

[7] Trisomy is the presence of an extra chromosome instead of the normal pair of homologous chromosomes. In trisomy 21 there is an extra, shorter chromosome 21.

[8] Although Down syndrome is usually attributed to the aging woman, recent evidence supports the notion that paternal age is also a factor though in a smaller percentage of cases and these are associated with chromosomal translocation (Cooley and Graham, 1991).

TABLE 19-6 DOWN SYNDROME: CLINICAL CHARACTERISTICS

Most Frequently Observed Manifestations	Associated Manifestations

Flat faces and nasal bridge (90%)
Flat occiput
Muscle hypotonia and joint hyperextensibility
Congenital heart disease
Language and cognitive delay
Short limbs, short broad hands and feet
Epicanthal folds
High arched palate; protruding, fissured tongue
Delayed acquisition of gross motor skills
Simian line (transverse palmar crease)
	Other congenital anomalies
	  Absence of kidney
	  Duodenal atresia
	  Tracheoesophageal fistula
	Feeding difficulties
	Atlantoaxial instability
	Sensory impairment
	  Hearing loss (conductive)
	  Visual impairment
	    Strabismus
	    Myopia
	    Nystagmus
	    Cataracts
	    Conjunctivitis
	Delayed growth and sexual development
	Obesity

Clinical Manifestations. Children with Down syndrome are readily identified by their flat faces, nasal bridges, short limbs, and mild to moderate hypotonia. The most frequently observed clinical characteristics are listed in Table 19–6. Many other associated clinical manifestations may also be present.

For example, these persons tend to exhibit increased susceptibility to infections such as otitis media (ear infection). They are frequently hepatitis B carriers, have an increased incidence of thyroid dysfunction with age, experience constipation associated with gastrointestinal tract anomalies, develop acute leukemia, and present with congenital cardiac anomalies such as atrioventricular and ventricular septal defects.

These children frequently present with a variety of musculoskeletal or orthopedic problems believed to be acquired secondary to soft tissue laxity and muscle hypotonia. Some of the more common findings include recurrent patellar dislocation, flatfeet, scoliosis, slipped capital femoral epiphyses (secondary to persistent hip abduction associated with hypotonia), and hip dislocation.

Atlantoaxial instability (AAI) (subluxation between C1 and C2) is a much written about characteristic of children with Down syndrome and is present in 10% to 40% of all cases (Litman et al., 1995; Morton et al., 1995; Rizzolo et al., 1995). This instability is thought to be secondary to ligamentous laxity or odontoid maldevelopment or possibly abnormal syringomyelia[9] in the area of the odontoid process. No significant correlation has been made between the general laxity associated with Down syndrome and AAI (Cremers and Beijer, 1993). Clinical changes indicative of AAI include hyperreflexia, clonus, positive Babinski's sign, torticollis, increased loss of strength, changes in sensation, loss of established bladder and bowel control, and a decrease in motor skills.

[9] A slowly progressive syndrome in which cavitation (the formation of a cavity from destruction of tissue) occurs in the central segments of the spinal cord.

Children with Down syndrome predictably present with feeding difficulties and delayed acquisition of motor skills. These skills, however improve with age. Because of the hypotonia and decreased strength, midline upper extremity movement is difficult and gait is usually characterized by smaller step lengths, increased knee flexion at contact, decreased single limb support, and an increased hip flexion posture. These children present with slower reaction times and slower postural reactions.

Medical Management

Diagnosis. Prenatal diagnosis may be made by amniocentesis. Postnatal diagnosis usually begins with suspected physical findings at birth. Genetic studies showing the chromosomal abnormality can confirm the diagnosis. Specific diagnostic testing varies depending on the organ system suspected of dysfunction.

Treatment. Since there is no known cure for Down syndrome, treatment is directed toward specific medical problems (e.g., antibiotics for infection, cardiac surgery, monitoring thyroid function, and development of Alzheimer's disease). Larger medical centers are pursuing plastic surgery to eliminate the hypoplastic facial features (see Table 19–6) based on the premise that this type of surgery has a positive influence on rehabilitation. The overall goal of treatment is to help affected children develop to their full potential. This involves a team of experts, including therapists.

Prognosis. Life expectancy has improved with more sophisticated medical care but remains lower than that for the general population. Over 80% of these persons survive to age 30 years and beyond. The presence of heart defects is a major factor in outcome; respiratory tract infections are very common secondary to hypotonicity of chest and abdominal muscles and immune system dysfunction. This combination can prove fatal, particularly in the first year of life.

Special Implications for the Therapist **19-2**

DOWN SYNDROME

Precautions

Since AAI is a potential problem, radiographs are recommended before any type of event that could result in a direct downward force on the cervical area (e.g., surgery, especially head and neck surgery; manual therapy; tumbling; diving; horseback riding; and so forth).* Subluxation of the cervical vertebrae greater than 4.5 mm (occurs in 1% to 2% of cases) with or without neurologic symptoms is considered to be an indicator for intervention (e.g., cervical fusion). The therapist is an important source of information for increasing family and community awareness regarding the potential precautions and contraindications associated with AAI (Wong, 1993).

The presence of cardiac defects may affect the client's overall level of activity, especially in the school setting, regarding fitness and endurance training. Similarly, for any client with Down syndrome interested in participating in the Special Olympics, the therapist and support staff must work closely with the physician to establish guidelines for safety.

Decreased muscle tone compromises respiratory expansion. In addition, the underdeveloped nasal bone causes a chronic problem of inadequate drainage of mucus. The constant stuffy nose forces the child to breathe by mouth, which dries the oropharyngeal membranes, increasing susceptibility to upper respiratory tract infections.

The parents should be instructed in taking measures to lessen these problems such as clearing the nose with a bulb-type syringe, rinsing the mouth with water after feedings, changing the child's position frequently, practicing good handwashing, and performing postural drainage and percussion if necessary (Wong, 1993).

Feeding

The protruding tongue interferes with feeding, especially solid foods. Inadequate drainage with pooling of mucus in the nose also interferes with breathing. Because the child breathes by mouth, sucking for any length of time is difficult. When eating solids, the child may gag on food because of mucus in the oropharynx. The nose must be cleared before each feeding and the child should be given small, frequent feedings with opportunities for rest (Wong, 1993).

* Transportation in a car, bus, or on a bicycle alone or with an adult may be considered a potentially risky activity requiring specific head support. Likewise, riding carnival-type rides such as fast-moving carousels, roller coasters, and so on must be discussed with the family. To the contrary, at least one study (Cremers et al., 1993) suggests that there is no reason to stop children with Down syndrome from playing certain sports and no need to screen them by radiography before participating in such sports.

SCOLIOSIS

Definition. Scoliosis is an abnormal lateral curvature of the spine. The curvature may be toward the right (more common in thoracic curves) or the left (more common in lumbar curves). Rotation of the vertebral column around its axis occurs and may cause rib cage deformity. Scoliosis is often associated with kyphosis and lordosis.

Overview. Scoliosis is classified as *idiopathic* (unknown cause; 80% of all cases), *osteopathic* (due to spinal disease or bony abnormality), *myopathic* (due to muscle weakness), or associated with various *neurologic* disorders. Age of onset can vary from birth onward and is referred to as *infantile* (0 to 3 years), *juvenile* (skeletal age of 4 to puberty), or *adolescent* (skeletal age of 12 in girls and 14 in boys).

Infantile idiopathic scoliosis (rare in the United States) is characterized by curvatures that are most often thoracic and toward the left and affect males. Juvenile idiopathic scoliosis is most often characterized by a right thoracic curvature and can be rapidly progressive. Adolescent idiopathic scoliosis is seen mostly in females in a 10 : 1 ratio.[10]

Incidence and Etiology. As many as 1 in 10 children may present with some type of scoliosis with 1 in 4 of those requiring some type of treatment. Scoliosis may be functional

[10] In its milder forms, scoliosis affects boys and girls equally, but girls are more likely to develop more severe curvatures requiring treatment.

or structural. Functional (postural) scoliosis may be caused by factors other than vertebral such as pain, poor posture, leg length discrepancy, or muscle spasm induced by a herniated disk or spondylolisthesis. Functional scoliosis can become structural if untreated.

Structural scoliosis is a fixed curvature of the spine associated with vertebral rotation and asymmetry of the ligamentous supporting structures. It can be caused by deformity of the vertebral bodies and may be *congenital* (e.g., wedge vertebrae, fused ribs or vertebrae, hemivertebrae), *musculoskeletal* (e.g., osteoporosis, spinal tuberculosis, rheumatoid arthritis), *neuromuscular* (e.g., cerebral palsy, polio, myelomeningocele, muscular dystrophy), or, most commonly, *idiopathic*, but possibly transmitted as an autosomal dominant trait.

Suggestions as to the causes of idiopathic scoliosis include negative fetal environmental factors during the first trimester of pregnancy, abnormalities of collagen fibers, paraspinal weakness and subsequent asymmetry, insufficiency of the costovertebral ligaments, decreased muscle strength, decreased proprioception, and decreased spinal stability.

Pathogenesis. The pathogenesis of scoliosis remains unclear but may be better understood in relation to the underlying cause. Abnormal embryonic formation and segmentation of the spinal column are possible pathologic pathways in congenital scoliosis. Neuromuscular scoliosis is often the result of an imbalance or asymmetry of muscle activity through the trunk and spine. Adolescent scoliosis may be the result of an abnormality of the CNS involving the balance mechanism in the midbrain. Postural and equilibrium dysfunction, alterations in vibratory sensation, vestibular dysfunction, growth hormone levels, and genetic factors play a role as well (Weinstein, 1991).

Additionally, adolescent idiopathic scoliosis may be associated with abnormal function of the posterior columns of the spinal cord. This results in abnormal or decreased proprioception but it remains unclear whether these findings are causative or secondary to the scoliosis (Barrack et al., 1988; Byrd, 1988).

The earliest pathologic changes associated with idiopathic scoliosis occur in the soft tissues as the muscles, ligaments, and other tissues become shortened on the concave side of the curve. In time bone deformities occur as compression on one side of the vertebral bodies applies asymmetrical forces to the epiphyseal ossification center. The compressive force is greatest on the vertebrae in the apex of the concavity so that the apical vertebrae become most deformed (McCullough, 1994) (Fig. 19–1).

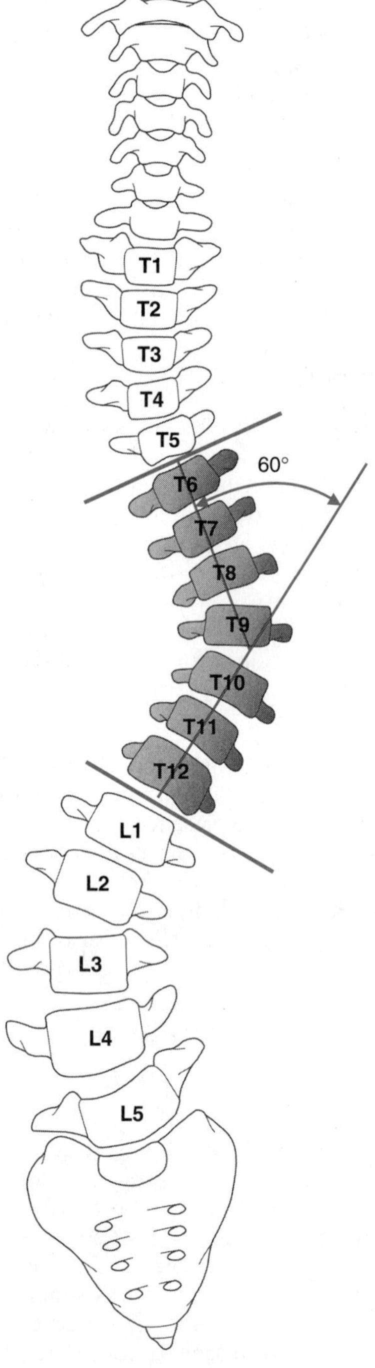

Figure **19–1.** Cobb's method of measuring scoliosis is the method most commonly used, since it is readily reproduced. The top vertebra used in the measurement is identified as the uppermost vertebra whose upper surface tilts toward the curvature's concave side. (The superior surface of the vertebra above it usually tilts in the opposite direction or may be parallel to it.) The bottom vertebra is the lowest vertebra whose inferior surface tilts toward the curvature's concave side. (Likewise, the inferior surface of the vertebra below it usually tilts in the opposite direction or may be parallel to it.) A line is drawn parallel to each of these vertebrae. The angle formed by perpendicular lines drawn to each of the parallel lines is the angle of the curvature.

Clinical Manifestations. Curvatures of less than 20 degrees (mild scoliosis) rarely cause significant problems. Severe untreated scoliosis (curvatures greater than 60 degrees) may produce pulmonary insufficiency and reduced lung capacity, back pain, degenerative spinal arthritis, disk disease, vertebral subluxation, or sciatica. Back pain is not typical in children or adolescents with mild scoliosis; back pain in this population should be evaluated by a physician who will rule out possible tumor, infection, or occult trauma.

Common characteristics of scoliosis are asymmetrical shoulders and pelvis, often identified when clothes do not hang evenly. Curves are designated as right or left depending on the convexity (e.g., right thoracic scoliosis describes a curve with convexity to the right). Usually there is one primary curvature with a secondary or compensatory curvature that develops to balance the body. There may be two primary curvatures (usually right thoracic and left lumbar). If the curvatures of the spine are balanced (compensated), the head is centered over the center of the pelvis; if the spinal alignment is uncompensated, the head will be displaced to one side.

Paraspinal muscles become asymmetrical as the muscles on the convex side of the curve become rounded, appearing prominent or bulging, while the muscles on the concave side flatten. Rotational deformity on the convex side is observed as a rib hump (gibbus) sometimes seen in the upright position but always apparent in the forward bend position.

Medical Management

Diagnosis. Diagnosis by clinical examination requires the client to bend forward 90 degrees with the hands joined in the midline as if taking a dive into a swimming pool. An abnormal finding includes asymmetry of the height of the ribs or paravertebral muscles on one side. The examiner also checks for leg length discrepancy and other asymmetries and for the presence of hair patches, nevi, pits, or areas of abnormal skin pigmentation in the midline indicating possible underlying spinal abnormality.

Differential diagnosis is important in determining whether the scoliosis is structural or functional. Structural curvatures maintain their position irrespective of whether the spine is in an upright or forward bending position. Functional curvatures straighten when placed in a forward bend position. This is especially easy to see when the client is sitting, thereby eliminating weight bearing through the feet. The physician also performs a neurologic examination to rule out an underlying neurologic disorder, especially in the presence of left thoracic curvature.

Full-length radiographs of the spine using the Cobb method (see Fig. 19–1) measure the angle of curvatures. A scoliometer can also be used to measure the angle of trunk rotation (ATR) (Fig. 19–2). Bone scan may be used to rule out neoplasms, infections, spondylolysis, or compression fractures as the underlying cause. Magnetic resonance imaging (MRI) is also used to differentiate cord lesions, disk herniations, neoplasms, infections, spondylolysis, and compression fractures.

Treatment. Prevention of postural or idiopathic structural scoliosis is the key to management of the majority of scoliosis cases. Early detection allows for early treatment without surgical intervention and with good long-term results.

Overall goals of management are to prevent severe and progressive deformities that might lead to decreased cardiorespiratory function. Conservative care may include exercise, electrical stimulation, observation, and monitoring every 4 to 6 months for curvatures less than 25 degrees, spinal orthoses for curvatures 25 to 40 or 45 degrees (Table 19–7), or surgery for curvatures greater than 45 degrees (Krengel and King, 1995).

The goal of the use of spinal orthoses is to serve as a passive restraint system to maintain curvatures within 5 degrees of the curvature measurement at the time of initial application. This is accomplished successfully in 85% to 88% of cases (Willers, 1993). Curvatures with an apex between T8 and L2 respond the most favorably to bracing, whereas curvatures with an apex at T6 or above have the poorest outcome.

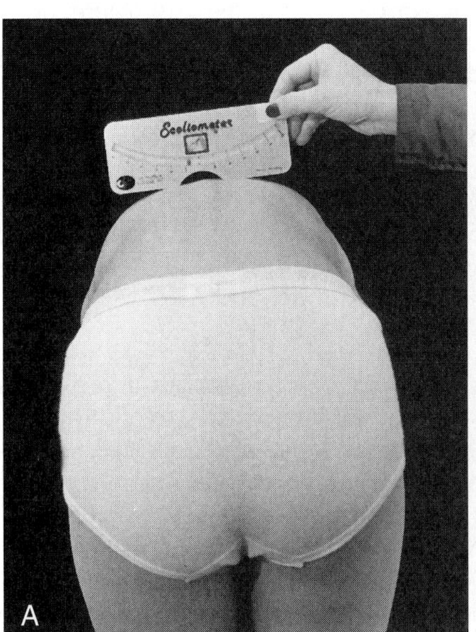

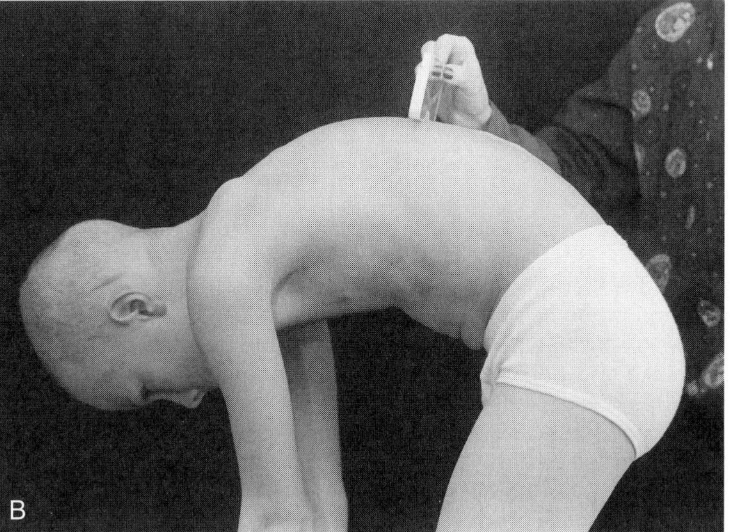

Figure 19–2. A and B, The scoliometer can be used by any health-care worker trained to screen for scoliosis. Some medical personnel also use this device to monitor curvatures over time, thereby avoiding unnecessary radiographs. Ask the client to bend forward slowly, stopping when the shoulders are level with the hips. View the client from both the front and back, keeping your eyes at the same level as the back. Before measuring with the scoliometer, adjust the height of the person's bending position to the level where the deformity of the spine is most pronounced. This position will vary from one person to another depending upon the location of the curvature (e.g., a low lumber curvature requires further bending than an upper thoracic curvature). Lay the scoliometer across the deformity with the 0 mark over the top of the spinous process. A measurement 5 degrees or more in the screening test is considered positive and requires medical follow-up. (*Courtesy of Todd Goodrich, University of Montana, Missoula.*)

TABLE 19-7 Scoliosis: Bracing Options

Brace	Use
Milwaukee (CTLSO)	Best with curvature at T8 or above
Boston (TLSO)	Best with curvature apex lower than T9 or T10
Lyon	For idiopathic scoliosis with thoracic hypokyphosis
Charleston	For idiopathic curves fabricated in maximum side-bend correction

CTLSO, cervicothoracolumbosacral orthosis; TLSO, thoracolumbosacral orthosis.

Surgical intervention (e.g., fusion with spinal rods for stability) may be necessary for curvatures greater than 45 degrees, in the presence of chronic pain, or when the curvature appears to be causing neurologic changes. Surgical goals are to halt progression of the curvature and improve alignment, decrease deformity, prevent pulmonary problems, and eliminate pain.

The surgical options include Luque rod instrumentation or a Harrington rod procedure (posterior fusion procedures), or a Dwyer procedure (anterior fusion), which is usually reserved for more severe curvatures. Whenever possible, the fusions are stabilized at L3 or L4 and above as back pain with fusions below these levels can occur.

Prognosis. Postural curvatures resolve as the primary problem is treated. Structural curvatures are not eliminated but rather increase during periods of rapid skeletal growth. If the curvature is less than 40 degrees at skeletal maturity, the risk of progression is small. In curvatures greater than 60 degrees, the spine is biomechanically unstable and the curvature will likely continue to progress at a rate of 1 degree per year throughout life. In severe kyphoscoliosis, pulmonary compromise can lead to death.

Special Implications for the Therapist **19-3**

SCOLIOSIS

Intervention

Key roles of the therapist are screening for scoliosis and the education of the public about scoliosis. Consumer education must include recommendations for adequate calcium intake and participation in weight-bearing activities. This is especially important for girls; studies show a higher risk of developing osteoporosis in this population (Lonstein and Winter, 1988; Notelovitz, 1993).

Exercise programs continue to be employed, but have not been found to halt or improve scoliosis even when used in conjunction with orthoses (Krengel and King, 1995). When utilized, the focus of strengthening programs is on trunk extensors, abdominals, and gluteals (especially hip extensors). Stretching activities focus on the iliopsoas and low back extensors and lateral trunk flexors on the concave side of the curvature.

Electrical stimulation (ES) has been used for the management of scoliosis with success in halting the progression of the curvature (Anciaux et al., 1991; Lonstein and Winter, 1988) but has lost favor in the past few years. Theoretically this treatment strengthens the muscles on the convex side of the curvature and pulls the spine into alignment.

Postoperative

During the hospital stay following surgery the therapy and nursing staff must check sensation, color, and blood supply in all extremities to detect neurovascular deficit, a serious complication following spinal surgery. Logroll the client often and encourage deep-breathing exercises to avoid pulmonary complications. Promote activities of daily living (even brushing the hair or teeth can be beneficial) and active ROM exercises of the extremities to help maintain circulation and muscle strength. Clients should be instructed in quadriceps setting, calf pumping, and other ROM exercises to perform frequently on their own throughout the day.

Cast syndrome is a serious complication that sometimes follows spinal surgery and application of a body cast. Characterized by nausea, abdominal pressure, vomiting, and vague abdominal pain, cast syndrome probably results from hyperextension of the spine. This hyperextension accentuates lumbar lordosis with compression of the third portion of the duodenum between the superior mesenteric artery and the aorta and vertebral column posteriorly (Norris, 1995).

The therapist encountering anyone in a body jacket, localizer cast, or high hip spica cast must be aware of this condition as it can develop as late as several weeks to months after application of the cast. Medical treatment is necessary for this condition.

The incidence of other postsurgical complications is low but may include infection at the surgical site, dislodgment of instrumentation, failure of fusion, and urinary tract infection, among other common postoperative complications. Osteophytes and foraminal narrowing in the concavity of the lumbar curvature may develop in older clients causing nerve root impingement and radicular pain (Krengel and King, 1995).

Precautions

Precautions following spinal fusion include avoiding excessive bending, squatting, trunk rotation, or hyperextension. These precautions are to help prevent loosening or dislodging hardware while promoting bony union in the corrected position.

Lifting limitations are imposed completely the first month and gradually increased (beginning with 1 lb at the end of the first month and gradually increasing to 10 lb by the end of the first year). The therapist can provide necessary instructions for safe lifting. Following physician clearance, unrestricted lifting can be reinitiated.

Functional mobility is severely limited for the first 4 weeks following surgery. After 3 months any type of noncontact sport is acceptable, including aerobic exercise such as walking or stationary bicycling;

swimming is especially encouraged but diving is contraindicated. By 1 year, other noncontact activities such as horseback riding, skating, or skiing may be reinitiated. Vigorous activities and contact sports are usually avoided unless directed otherwise by the physician. These same guidelines are usually followed for the child or adolescent who is wearing a brace but has not had surgery.

Skin care and prevention of breakdown is essential for anyone wearing a cast or spinal orthosis or brace. The client should be taught good skin care and how to recognize signs of irritation that can lead to lesions.

KYPHOSCOLIOSIS

Overview and Etiology. *Scheuermann's disease* (juvenile kyphosis, vertebral epiphysitis) is a condition of kyphoscoliosis (anteroposterior curvature of the spine) affecting adolescents between the ages of 12 and 16. The cause and pathogenesis of this excessive kyphosis remain unknown. Growth retardation or vascular disturbance in the vertebral epiphyses (usually at the thoracic level) during periods of rapid growth are the two most common hypotheses. Other proposed causes are poor posture, congenital deficiency in the thickness of the vertebral end plates, infection, inflammation, aseptic necrosis (osteochondritis), and disk degeneration.

In the aging population, kyphoscoliosis (adult round back) is more likely to develop as a result of poor posture, aging, degeneration of the intervertebral disks, vertebral compression fractures or osteoporotic collapse of the vertebrae, endocrine disorders (e.g., hyperparathyroidism, Cushing's disease), arthritis, Paget's disease, metastatic tumor, or tuberculosis.

Clinical Manifestations. Adolescent kyphosis is usually asymptomatic, although some adolescents experience mild pain at the apex of the curvature, fatigue, prominent vertebral spinous processes, and tenderness or stiffness in the involved area or along the entire spine. The pectoral, hamstring, and hip flexor muscles are often tight producing a crouched posture with anterior pelvic tilt and lumbar lordosis. Signs and symptoms associated with adult kyphosis are similar to the adolescent form but rarely produce local tenderness unless caused by vertebral compression fractures.

In both adolescent kyphoscoliosis (Scheuermann's) and adult kyphosis, the vertebrae are wedged anteriorly and disk lesions called Schmorl's nodes develop. Schmorl's nodes are localized extrusions of the nuclear material through the cartilage plates and into the spongy bone of the vertebral bodies. The cancellous bone reacts by encapsulating the herniated tissue within a wall of fibrous tissue and bone producing the Schmorl's node.

Medical Management

Treatment. Treatment is determined by the underlying cause and may include therapeutic exercises (e.g., postural exercises, stretching, thoracic hyperextension, exercises to strengthen abdominal and gluteal muscles), soft tissue and joint mobilization, traction, bracing, and rarely (in skeletally mature adults only), surgery when the curvature causes neurologic damage or intractable pain.

BOX 19–1
Clinical Features of Myelomeningocele

Thoracic (25%)
Low- to midthoracic region
- Increasing neurologic deficit

Upper thoracocervical region
- Minimal neurologic deficit
- Hydrocephalus rare

Lumbosacral (75%)
Low sacral
- Bowel and bladder incontinence
- Anesthesia in the perineal area
- No impairment of motor function

Midlumbar
- Constant urinary dribbling with relaxed anal sphincter
- Lower motor neuron signs:
  - Flaccid paralysis of the lower limbs
  - Absence of deep tendon reflexes
  - Lack of response to pain and touch
- High incidence of postural abnormalities
  - Clubfoot (talipes equinovarus), hip subluxation
- Trophic ulcers of the lower limbs

SPINA BIFIDA OCCULTA, MENINGOCELE, MYELOMENINGOCELE

Definition. Congenital neural tube defects (NTDs) encompass a variety of abnormalities as defined in Box 19–1. The term *spina bifida* is the one most often used to describe the more common congenital defects of neural tube closure. Normally, the spinal cord and cauda equina are encased in a protective sheath of bone and meninges (Fig. 19–3). Failure of neural tube closure produces defects that may involve the entire length of the neural tube or may be restricted to a small area.

The three most common NTDs presented here are *spina bifida occulta* (incomplete fusion of the posterior vertebral arch), *meningocele* (external protrusion of the meninges), and *myelomeningocele* (protrusion of the meninges and spinal cord). Generally these defects occur in the lumbosacral area but may be found in the sacral, thoracic, and cervical areas as well.

Incidence and Etiology. NTDs occur in 1 to 2 cases per 1000 live births with an estimated 6000 to 10,000 children born with some form of spina bifida each year in the United States. The incidence of spina bifida appears to be declining; the reason for this remains unclear[11] (Edmonds and James, 1990).

Evidence supports the hypothesis that NTDs may be caused by the interaction of a genetic predisposition with an essential nutrient deficiency (folic acid, a B vitamin found

[11] Termination of pregnancies as a result of the wider availability of maternal serum screening and better nutrition may contribute to this decline.

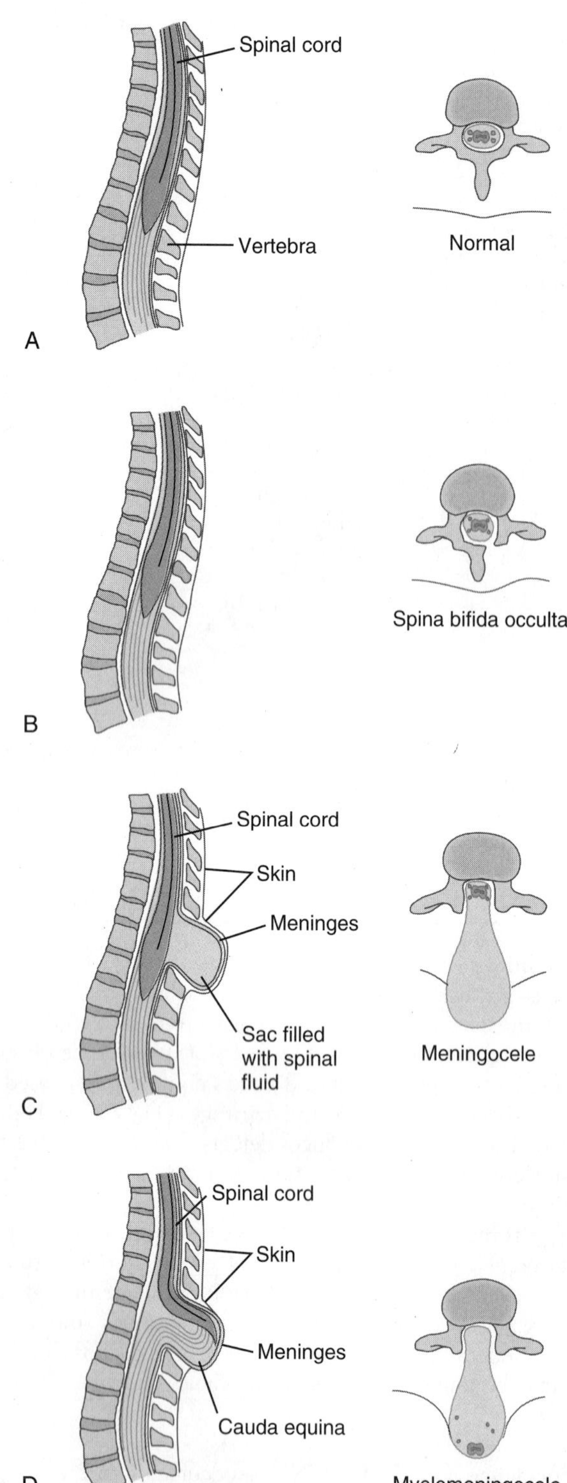

Figure **19–3.** Various degrees of spina bifida. *A*, Normal anatomic structure. *B*, Spina bifida occulta results in only a bony defect with the spinal cord, meninges, and spinal fluid intact. *C*, Meningocele involves the bifid vertebra with only a cerebrospinal fluid (CSF)–filled sac protruding; the spinal cord or cauda equina (depending on the level of the lesion) remains intact. *D*, Myelomenigocele is the most severe form because not only is the spine open but the protruding sac contains CSF, the meninges, and the spinal cord or cauda equina.

chiefly in yeast, orange juice, and green leafy vegetables). Multivitamins containing folic acid taken when planning a pregnancy and especially during the first 6 weeks of pregnancy will prevent (by up to 86%) NTDs (Daly et al., 1995; Locke and Sarwark, 1996).

Genetic factors are considered important since couples who have had one child with spina bifida have a recurrence rate approximately 50 times higher than the general population. Radiation, environmental influences, maternal alcohol intake, maternal treatment with antiepileptic drugs, and viral causes continue to be investigated.

Pathogenesis. Normally, about 20 days after conception, the embryo develops a neural groove in the dorsal ectoderm which deepens as the two edges fuse to form the neural tube. By about day 23 this tube is completely closed except for an opening at each end. The upper end will continue to fold and develop forming the brain while the bottom end will form the spinal cord.

Exposure to a risk factor may alter hyaluronate metabolism which results in failure of vertebral architecture to develop normally. When the posterior portion of the neural tube fails to close by the fourth week of gestation, or if it closes but then splits open from a cause such as an abnormal increase in cerebrospinal fluid (CSF), the meninges or the spinal cord, or both, bulge out of the normal confines of the spine. The degree of subsequent dysfunction is related to the anatomic level of the defect, with loss of neurologic function (sensory and motor) below the level of the lesion.

Clinical Manifestations. Approximately 75% of these vertebral defects are located in the lumbrosacral region, most commonly at the L5–S1 level (see Box 19–1). Motor dysfunction depends on the level of involvement and sparing of muscle sensory and motor innervation (Fig. 19–4 and Table 19–8). The loss of motor function is not evenly distributed over the limbs and spine, resulting in muscle imbalance contributing to the development of scoliosis and various musculoskeletal deformities. Other associated characteristics are listed in Box 19–2.

Spina bifida occulta does not protrude visibly but is often accompanied by a depression or dimple in the skin, a tuft of dark hair, soft fatty deposits (subcutaneous lipomas or dermoid cyst), port wine nevi, or a combination of these abnormalities on the skin at the level of the underlying lesion. Spina bifida

BOX **19–2**
Myelomeningocele: Associated Characteristics

0–2 years: truncal hypotonia
Delayed automatic reactions
90% have normal intelligence (IQ > 80)
Increased incidence of learning disabilities
90% present with hydrocephalus
10%–30% risk of seizures
Obesity
Late childhood and early adolescence: kyphoscoliosis
30% demonstrate decreased ambulatory status by age 12 years
Increased risk for strabismus (deviation of the eye)
Vasomotor insufficiency

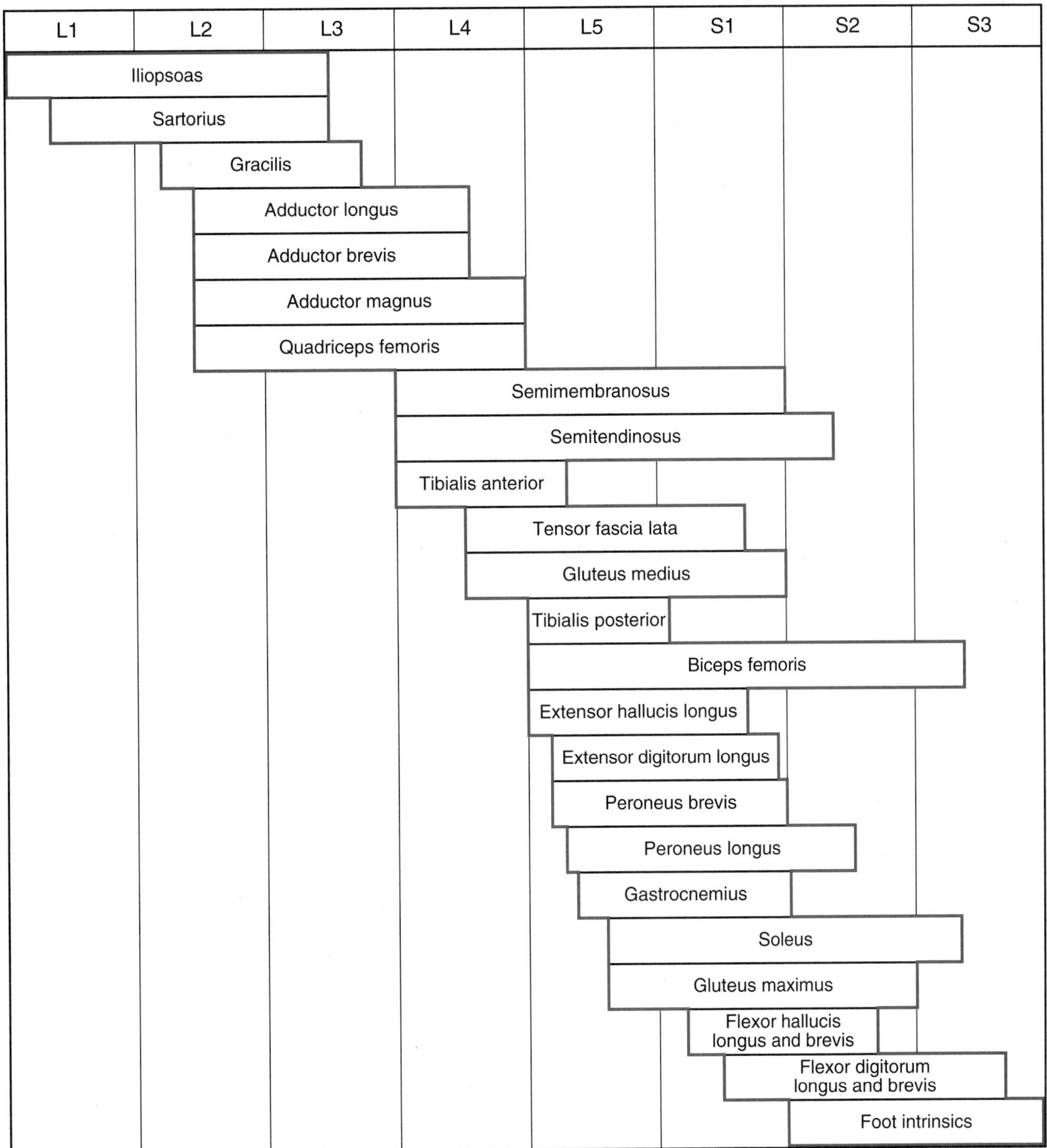

Figure **19–4.** Normal lumbar and sacral segmental innervation. For the child with myelomenigocele, once the level of the lesion has been identified, the therapist can begin to assess muscle involvement above and below that level. (*From Sharrard WJ: The segmental innervation of the lower limb muscles in man. Ann R Coll Surg Eng 35:106–122, 1964.*)

occulta usually does not cause neurologic dysfunction but occasionally bowel and bladder disturbances or foot weakness occurs.

In *spina bifida cystica* (meningocele and myelomeningocele), a saclike cyst protrudes outside the spine. Like spina bifida occulta, meningocele rarely causes neurologic deficits whereas myelomeningocele causes permanent neurologic impairment depending on the level of involvement. During the first 2 years of life, children with myelomeningocele often present with various degrees of truncal hypotonia and delayed autonomic postural reactions, even those children with sacral level lesions.

TABLE 19-8 Myelomeningocele: Functional Mobility

LE Spasticity	Motor Level Spinal Cord Segment	Critical Motor Function Present	Bracing/External Support for Ambulation	Typical Functional Activity
Presence decreases ability to ambulate by 36%	≤T10 T12	No LE movement Strong trunk	Standing brace or equipment HKAFOs	Supported sitting* Sliding board transfers Good sitting balance*
		No LE movement	Sometimes with thoracic corset	Therapeutic ambulation Independent wheelchair mobility
Presence decreases ability to ambulate by 62%	L1–2	Unopposed hip flexion, some adduction	Standing brace or equipment HKAFOs or KAFOs RGOs after 2½–3 yr Crutches	Household ambulation*
	L3	Quadriceps‡	KAFOs Crutches	Household and short community ambulation*
	L4	Quadriceps‡	Floor reaction AFOs/twister cables Crutches	Household and short community ambulation*
	L5	Medial hamstrings Anterior tibia Weak toe activity	Floor reaction AFOs (yes and no) Crutches (yes and no)	Community ambulation§
Minimal effect	S1	Lateral hamstring Peroneals	Usually no AFOs or upper limb support	Community ambulation
	S2–3	Mild intrinsic foot weakness	Possible crutch or cane with increased age	Community ambulation Possible decreased endurance with increasing age

LE, lower extremity; HKAFO, hip-knee-ankle-foot orthosis; KAFO, knee-ankle-foot orthosis; RGO, reciprocating gait orthosis; AFO, ankle-foot orthosis.
* Do not usually walk as adults.
‡ Approximately 50% probability of long-distance ambulation with muscle grade 4/5.
§ Able to use ambulation as the primary means of locomotion outside the home.

Myelomeningocele may be accompanied by flaccid or spastic paralysis, various combinations of bowel and bladder incontinence, musculoskeletal deformities[12] (e.g., scoliosis, hip dysplasia, hip dislocation, clubfoot [talipes equivarus], hip and knee flexion contractures), hydrocephalus, and sometimes mental retardation.

Approximately 90% of children born with this condition have an associated hydrocephalus (Box 19–3). Hydrocephalus accompanying spina bifida is usually a result of the Arnold-Chiari malformation,[13] a defect in the formation of the brainstem. The hindbrain[14] is displaced through the foramen magnum (Fig. 19–5) leading to increased CSF pressure and actual splitting of the neural tube during fetal development.

Severe Arnold-Chiari malformations are rare but can lead to hindbrain dysfunction and cranial nerve involvement with feeding difficulties, choking, pooling of secretions, repeated aspirations, apnea (cessation of breathing), neck pains, vocal cord paralysis with subsequent stridor (noisy breathing), and upper extremity spasticity, weakness, motor incoordination, and immature hand function.

Sensory disturbances usually parallel motor dysfunction. Pressure ulcers at the ischial tuberosities, knees, and dorsum

BOX 19–3
Signs and Symptoms of Hydrocephalus

- Full, bulging, tense soft spot (fontanel) on top of the child's head
- Large prominent veins in the scalp
- Setting sun sign (child appears to only look downward; the whites of the eyes are obvious above the colored portion of the eyes)
- Behavioral changes (e.g., irritability, lethargy)
- High-pitched cry
- Seizures
- Vomiting or change in appetite

From McLone, DG: An introduction to spina bifida. Rockville, Md, Spina Bifida Association of America, 1986.

[12] For an in-depth discussion of the musculoskeletal deformities associated with myelomeningocele, see Campbell, 1995.

[13] There are different forms of Arnold-Chiari malformations, but most are either type I or type II. Generally speaking, all children with myelomingocele have some degree of type II malformation, regardless of the presence of hydrocephalus. Although it may be present radiographically, it may not be causing any symptoms and is not necessarily treated.

[14] The brainstem consists of the mesencephalon (midbrain), pons, and medulla oblongata. The hindbrain or rhombencephalon includes part of the brainstem (medulla, pons) and the cerebellum.

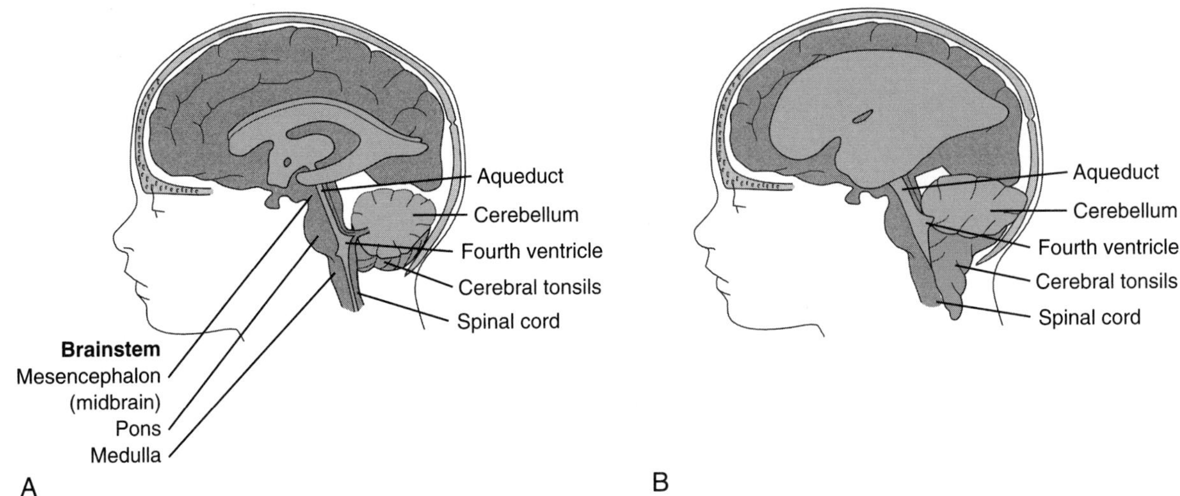

Figure **19–5.** *A*, Normal brain with patent cerebrospinal fluid (CSF) circulation. *B*, Arnold-Chiari type II malformation with enlarged ventricles, which predisposes a child with myelomenigocele to hydrocephalus. The brainstem, fourth ventricle, part of the cerebellum, and the cerebral tonsils are displaced downward through the foramen magnum, leading to blockage of CSF flow. Additionally, pressure on the brainstem housing the cranial nerves may result in nerve palsies.

of the feet occur with increasing frequency as the person ages, with an estimated incidence of 85% to 90% by adulthood (Shurtleff, 1986). Factors contributing to pressure ulcers in this population are listed in Box 19–4. Many of these same risk factors are present in other conditions prone to pressure ulcers (e.g., diabetic neuropathy) (see also Tables 8–13 and 8–14).

Bowel and bladder problems are present in virtually all children with myelomeningocele, since these functions are controlled at the S2–4 level. Even children with sacral lesions and normal leg movement often have bowel and bladder problems.

Problems with urinary incontinence and infection can occur if the bladder is small and spastic (bladder holds little urine) or large and hypotonic (incomplete emptying of the bladder and ureteral reflux). Bladder dyssynergy occurs with either a flaccid or spastic sphincter. Normally, when the bladder contracts, the sphincter relaxes, allowing urine to flow. In a dyssynergistic state, the bladder and sphincter contract together, predisposing the child to urethral reflux.

Medical Management

Diagnosis. Frequently, NTDs are detected prenatally with ultrasonic scanning and serum alpha-fetoprotein (AFP) testing.[15] Amniocentesis can detect only open NTDs and is recommended for pregnant women who have previously had children with NTDs. Prenatal diagnosis makes it possible for a planned cesarean section to avoid trauma to the neural sac during vaginal delivery (Luthy et al., 1991) or for a therapeutic abortion.

Postnatally, meningocele and myelomeningocele are obvious on examination. Transillumination of the protruding sac can usually distinguish between these two conditions.[16] Spinal films can be used to detect defects and the CT scan demonstrates the presence of hydrocephalus. Other laboratory tests may include urinalysis, urine cultures, and tests for renal function.

Treatment. Infection and drying of the nerve roots leading to further loss of function necessitates surgical closure within 48 hours of birth. Ventriculoperitoneal shunting (Figs. 19–6 and 19–7) is recommended in the presence of hydrocephalus; shunt revision is often required as the child grows or if the shunt becomes obstructed, infected, or separated.

A variety of orthopedic surgical interventions may be required throughout the child's growing years (e.g., hip varus or derotation osteotomies for hip dislocation [see Fig. 19–14]; spinal fusion for scoliosis; tendon transfers and muscle releases).

Medical management of the bowel and bladder is critical to prevent infection and to assist with independence and functional toileting. Complete bladder emptying using man-

BOX **19–4**
Factors Contributing to Pressure Ulcers in Myelomeningocele

- Ammonia from urine burns
- Friction burns (feet and knees of young active children)
- Pressure from casts or splints
- Bony prominences
- Vascular problems
- Poor transfer skills
- Obesity
- Asymmetrical weight bearing or posture (scoliosis, orthopedic deformities)

[15] Alpha-fetoprotein is a glycoprotein produced by the yolk sac and fetal liver. Elevated AFP usually occurs by 14 weeks' gestation in the presence of NTDs. This type of screening will not detect skin-covered (closed) neural defects such as spina bifida occulta or defects distal to the S2 vertebra. The potential for false-negative results with this test may result in unnecessary intervention. Additionally, as the incidence of this condition continues to decrease, the less reliable the test will become because the positive predictive value of the AFP test is dependent on the prevalence of the disease in a population. The less prevalent the disease, the less accurate laboratory results may be. See Chapter 35 for further explanation of the limitations of laboratory tests.

[16] In meningocele, the sac with its CSF contents is transilluminated (light shines through the sac); in myelomeningocele, the light does not shine through the neural bundle that is present.

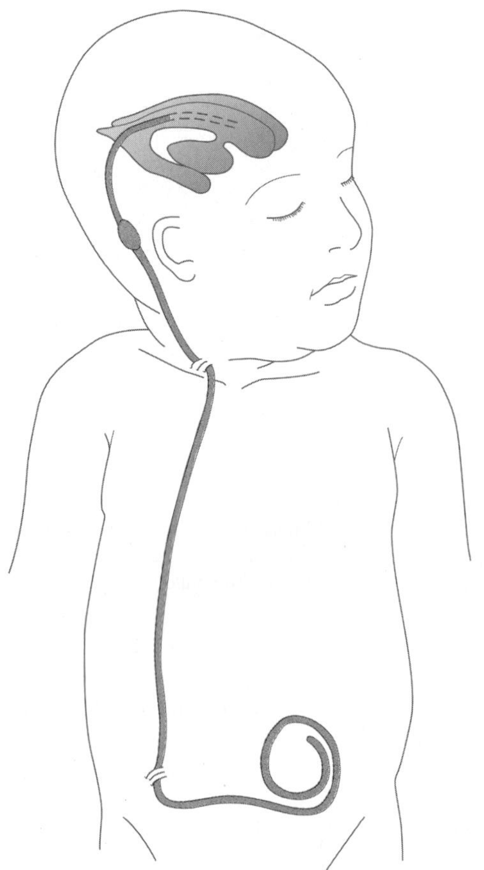

Figure 19–6. Ventriculoperitoneal (VP) shunt provides primary drainage of cerebrospinal fluid from the ventricles to an extracranial compartment (usually either the heart or the abdominal or peritoneal cavity, as shown here). Extra tubing is left in the extracranial site to uncoil as the child grows. A unidirectional valve designed to open at a predetermined intraventricular pressure and close when the pressure falls below that level prevents backflow of fluid.

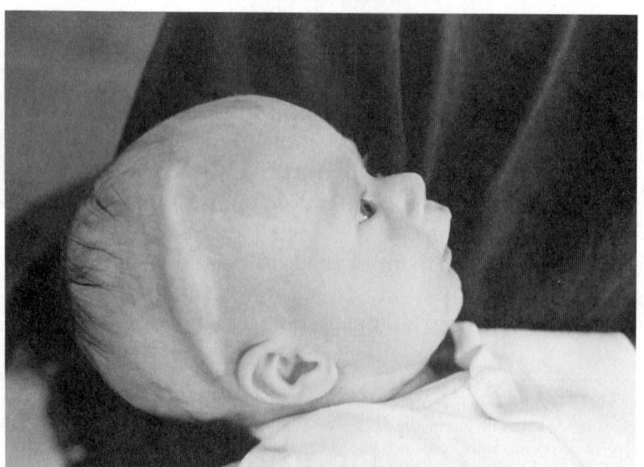

Figure 19–7. The shunt is placed very superficially, necessitating caution when handling the infant. The therapist must be careful to avoid placing pressure over the shunt, stretching the neck, or placing the child in the head-down position. (*Courtesy of Todd Goodrich, University of Montana, Missoula.*)

ual pressure on the bladder (Credé's method) or intermittent catheterization helps prevent urinary tract infections. High fluid intake is a critical part of the overall program. Implantation of an artificial urinary sphincter may be employed in the older child or adolescent.[17] Stool incontinence is managed by a program to regulate bowel movements using timed enemas or suppositories.

Prognosis. Early, aggressive care of NTDs has now improved the overall prognosis associated with this condition. Prognosis varies with the degree of accompanying neurologic deficit and is poorest for those children who have total paralysis below the lesion, kyphoscoliosis, hydrocephalus, and progressive loss of renal function secondary to chronic infection. Most deaths occur before age 4. At present, survival to adulthood is approximately 85%.

Approximately two thirds of children with myelomeningocele and shunted hydrocephalus have normal intelligence. The remaining one third have mental retardation, usually mild. Children who do not have mental retardation may still have difficulties in perceptual organizational abilities, attention, speed of motor response, memory, and hand function (Charney, 1990). Overall cognitive delays occur less often and with less severity now as an outcome of improved medical treatment for these children.

Adult outcome data are incomplete at this time. Most adults over 30 years of age survived the preshunt era of the 1950s and are without hydrocephalus, while adults now in their 20s include persons with more severe disabilities who benefited from the recent advances in medical and surgical management (Charney, 1990).

Adults with myelomeningocele continue to need therapy and medical management secondary to joint and spinal deformities, joint pain, pressure ulcers, neurologic deterioration, depression, and poor social interaction and adjustment.

Prognosis for Motor Function. The child's motor abilities vary according to the level of the lesion (see Box 19–1 and Table 19–8). A child's ability to walk outdoors and use a wheelchair by age 7 usually suggests a good ambulation prognosis (Dudgeon, 1991). If functional ambulation is not present by 7 to 9 years of age, it is unlikely to occur subsequently (Asher, 1983; Findley, 1987).

However, a third of all persons with myelomeningocele demonstrate a decline in ambulatory status with increasing age, usually around age 12. These losses in ambulatory status often correlate with a variety of adolescent changes including increasing body proportion and composition, loss of upper and lower extremity strength, or immobilization for varied periods of time secondary to musculoskeletal surgery or fracture healing (Liptak, 1992; McDonald, 1991).

Special Implications for the Therapist 19–4
SPINA BIFIDA, MENINGOCELE, MYELOMENINGOCELE

Neonatal Intensive Care Unit (NICU)

Before surgery to repair the meningocele, pressure of any kind against the sac must be avoided. Whenever

[17] In most of these devices, the opening and closing of the bladder outlet is accomplished by a cuff placed around the outlet. The cuff can be constricted to close the outlet or relaxed to open the outlet and allow urine to flow.

holding the (unrepaired) infant the spine must be maintained in good alignment without tension in the area of the defect. The infant must be kept in the prone position to minimize tension on the sac and to reduce the risk of trauma.

The prone position allows for optimal positioning of the legs, especially in cases of associated hip dysplasia. The infant is placed flat with the hips slightly flexed to reduce tension on the defect. The legs are maintained in abduction with a pad (a folded diaper or towel or small stuffed animal works well) between the knees and a small diaper roll is placed under the ankles to maintain a neutral foot position.

The prone position is maintained after operative closure, although many neurosurgeons allow a side-lying or partial side-lying position unless it aggravates a coexisting hip dysplasia (see Congenital Hip Dysplasia) or permits undesirable hip flexion. The side-lying positioning offers an opportunity for position changes, which reduces the risk of pressure sores and facilitates feeding. If permitted,* the infant can be held upright against the body. In all handling procedures, care must be taken to avoid pressure on the sac preoperatively or on the operative site postoperatively (Wong, 1993).

Skin Care

Areas of sensory and motor impairment are subject to skin breakdown and require meticulous care. The loss of skin sensation accompanied by lack of pain can lead to injury and pressure ulcers. Inadequate circulation increases the problem because the wounds do not heal properly.

Placing the infant on a soft foam or fleece pad reduces pressure on the knees and ankles. Periodic cleansing, application of lotion, and gentle massage aid circulation, which is often compromised. Bath water must be tested carefully because the child cannot feel the water temperature. The family should be advised to use sunscreen to prevent sunburn and to observe for tight-fitting shoes or braces. The skin should be checked daily for red areas that do not disappear readily when the pressure is removed.

Early and Ongoing Intervention

Precautions

An early role of the therapist in assessment is to assist in establishing baseline information regarding the level of initially available muscle function and sensation. Ongoing assessment includes an awareness of signs and symptoms associated with changes due to increased CSF pressure in the presence of hydrocephalus with or without a shunt† (Box 19–5) or a tethered cord‡ (Box 19–6). Before age 2 years, children do not show typical signs of increased intracranial pressure, since skull suture lines are not fully closed. In this age group, a bulging fontanel is the most obvious sign of pathology. Once the skull bones have fused, pressure can build inside the closed space, resulting in a variety of symptoms.

Likewise, children with spina bifida have been identified as having a greater risk of becoming allergic to latex (see Latex Rubber Allergy, Chapter 3). Typical symptoms include watery eyes, wheezing, hives, rash, swelling, and in severe cases, anaphylaxis, a life-threatening reaction. These responses occur when items containing latex touch the skin, mucous membranes (mouth, genitals, bladder, or rectum), or open areas. The therapist must avoid using toys, feeding utensils, or other items the infant or child may put in its mouth that are made of latex.

Passive ROM exercises must be performed slowly and cautiously given the tendency toward fracture in this population. When the hip joints are unstable, stretching against hip flexor or adductor muscles may aggravate a tendency toward subluxation. For this reason the prone hip extension test for measuring hip extension is the method of choice over the traditional Thomas test (Hinderer et al., 1995).

Controversies

The philosophy regarding surgical repair of myelomeningocele varies greatly. There are those who question whether operative procedures should be considered for children with overwhelming neurologic deficit or whether the disorder should be allowed to assume its natural course. Some people advocate criteria for selection or nonselection based on the

BOX 19–5
Signs and Symptoms of Shunt Malfunction

Congestion of scalp veins
Firm or tense soft spot on cranium (fontanel)
Listlessness, drowsiness, irritability
Vomiting, change in appetite
Marked depression of the anterior fontanel (overdrainage)
Disturbance in urinary and bowel patterns
Increasing head circumference
Swelling along the shunt
Seizures
Nuchal (nape of the neck) rigidity
Additional symptoms for older children and adults:
- Gradual personality change
- Headaches
- Blurring vision
- Memory loss
- Progressive coordination problems
- Declining school or work performance
- Decrease in sensory or motor functions

BOX 19–6
Signs and Symptoms of Tethered Cord Syndrome

Scoliosis
Increased spasticity
Increased asymmetrical postures or movement
Altered gait pattern
Decreased upper extremity coordination
Changes in muscle strength (at or below the lesion)
Back pain

prognosis for quality of life. Such controversies present serious ethical problems (Wong, 1993).

The timing of the operative repair of the lesion remains under heavy debate. Most authorities advocate early closure§ (within the first 24 to 48 hours) to prevent local infection, avoid trauma to the exposed tissues, and avoid stretching of other nerve roots, thus preventing further motor impairment. Other experts contend that surgical repair is best delayed until after further assessment of neurologic function, intellectual potential, and extent of complications. This delay increases the infant's ability to tolerate the surgical procedure, allows for better epithelialization of the sac (thereby reducing the risk of infection), and permits easier mobilization of skin for closure (Wong, 1993).

Philosophical differences exist regarding the extent and direction of management programs for children with myelomeningocele. At present, research results show that children whose program emphasizes upright activities and ambulation (compared with children whose program focuses primarily on wheelchair mobility) show better outcomes with transfer skills (even after they have stopped ambulating), greater bone density, fewer lower extremity fractures, and a smaller incidence of pressure ulcers (Mazur, 1989). High-level lesions do not preclude ambulation; many established programs for the child with myelomeningocele are ambulation-oriented, reserving wheelchair mobility for older or cognitively impaired children.

Controversy also exists as to the best choice of lower extremity bracing and ambulation method (e.g., the hip-knee-ankle-foot orthosis [HKAFO] for swing-through gait only vs. the reciprocating gait orthosis [RGO],¶ which allows the individual options of a swing-to, swing-through, or reciprocating gait). Given the many improvements and number of bracing options available, the overall key to maintaining ambulatory status is good lower extremity ROM and a level pelvis.

* For the infant with hydrocephalus, until the shunt is in place and draining well, elevation of the head above 25 degrees may be contraindicated. The baby must be kept level as much as possible to avoid any disruption of the CSF or increased pressure on the brain.

† A shunting mechanism is used for hydrocephalus associated with a variety of conditions other than myelomeningocele. Depending on the underlying condition, shunts can become obstructed or stop functioning for many reasons (e.g., occlusion due to blood clots or brain fragments, tumor cell aggregates, bacterial colonization or other debris; the tube itself can become kinked or blocked at the tip; or growth of the infant or child or physical activities can result in disconnection of the shunt components or withdrawal of a distal catheter from its intended drainage site). Shunt systems may also fail owing to mechanical malfunction, including fracture of the catheters, leading to underdrainage or overdrainage.

‡ Tethering of the spinal cord may develop with myelodysplasia. The cord becomes caught or tethered from scar tissue as it grows beyond the vertebral canal.

§ A variety of plastic surgical procedures can be used for skin closure. The goal is to place the sac and its contents back in the body with good skin coverage of the lesion and careful closure. Excision of the membranous covering or removal of any portion of the sac may damage functioning neural tissue and is avoided completely. Although this corrective procedure may prevent an infection of the spinal cord or brain, the surgery has little or no effect on the neurologic function of the infant.

¶ Contraindications to HKAFO or RGO include severe spinal deformity, spasticity, decreased upper extremity strength, moderate obesity, plantar flexion contractures greater than 15 to 20 degrees, and hip flexion contracture greater than 35 degrees.

CONGENITAL HIP DYSPLASIA

Overview. Congenital hip dysplasia (CHD), or developmental dysplasia of the hip (DDH), is a common hip disorder affecting children under age 3.[18] CHD can be unilateral or bilateral and occurs in three forms of varying severity: (1) *unstable hip dysplasia*, in which the hip is positioned normally but can be dislocated by manipulation; (2) *subluxation* or *incomplete dislocation*, in which the femoral head remains in contact with the acetabulum but the head of the femur is partially displaced or uncovered; and (3) *complete dislocation*, in which the femoral head is totally outside the acetabulum (Norris, 1995).

Incidence and Risk Factors. CHD occurs in approximately 1 in 1000 live births. About 85% of affected infants are females. The risk of hip dysplasia increases dramatically in the presence of certain obstetric conditions (e.g., breech delivery, large neonates, twin or multiple births) and other conditions such as idiopathic scoliosis, myelomeningocele (spina bifida), arthrogryposis, and CP. The presence of other musculoskeletal deformities such as torticollis, metatarsus adductus, and calcaneal valgus deformity should alert the medical practitioner to the need for further evaluation.

Other risk factors include family history, first pregnancies, and oligohydramnios (deficient volume of amniotic fluid limiting fetal movement). One fourth of all cases involve both hips; when only one hip is involved, the left hip is affected three times more often than the right.

Etiology. The cause varies depending on the associated condition but is usually the result of mechanical, physiologic, or environmental factors. Hormonally derived laxity of the ligaments about the joint, in utero positioning, spasticity, and spinal instability are all possible etiologic factors.

Cultural customs of how babies are carried or positioned may affect the formation of the acetabular cup and hip stability. For example, carrying the infant or young child with hips and lower extremities abducted, flexed, and externally rotated may increase stability of the femoral head in relationship to the acetabulum. Conversely, those cultures that swaddle infants with the hips in extension and adduction are at greater risk of causing hip dislocations.

Pathogenesis. The femur, acetabulum, and hip joint capsule are usually well developed by approximately 10 weeks' gestation. Most dislocations occur in the perinatal period, at which time there is maximal joint distention and elasticity. In the case of the breech position in utero, not only is movement limited but this presentation places the hips in a position of acute flexion and adduction with knees extended.

The subluxated hip maintains contact with the acetabulum but is not well seated within the hip joint. Often this occurs because the acetabulum is shallow or sloping with CHD rather than a normal cup shape (Fig. 19–8). The dislocated hip has no contact between the femoral head and the acetabulum and the ligamentum teres is elongated and taut.

If the dislocation is not diagnosed and treated early, sec-

[18] CHD can affect the acetabulum, femoral head, and the relationship of the femoral head to the acetabulum.

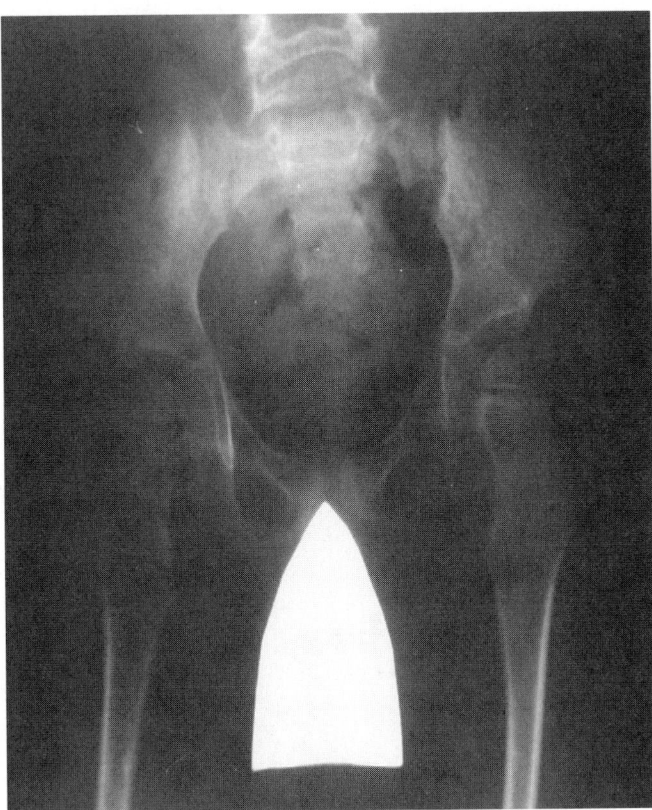

Figure **19–8.** Anteroposterior radiograph of a young child with spastic quadriplegia and subsequent hip dysplasia with subluxation on the left. Note that a line drawn vertically down from the outermost edge of the acetabulum would bisect the head of the femur. Failure of the acetabulum to become cup-shaped and subsequent (acquired) hip dysplasia and subluxation occur as a result of non–weight-bearing status and uneven muscular forces pulling on the bone. (*Courtesy of Rae Johnston, MD, Missoula, Montana.*)

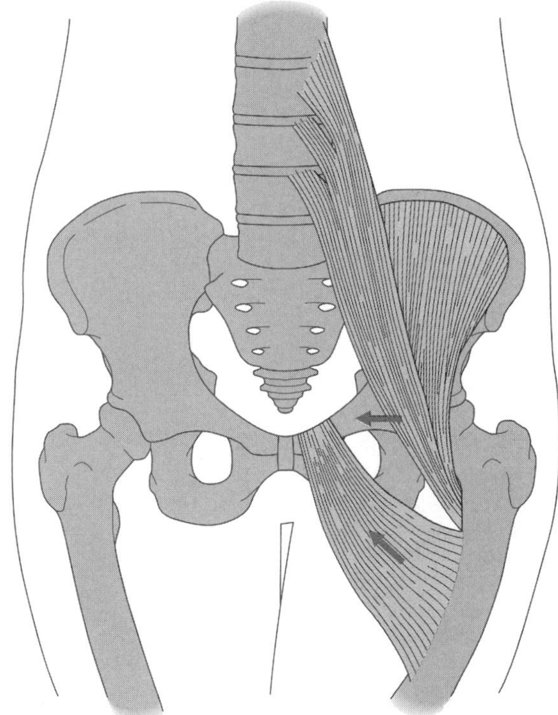

Figure **19–9.** Spastic iliopsoas and adductor muscles are the initiating deforming force in acquired hip dislocation.

ondary changes in both soft tissues and bony structures will occur. The longer the dislocation has been present, the greater the secondary changes that occur. These changes include stretching of the hip capsule, contracture and shortening of the structures of the hip joint, changes in the blood supply to the hip, flattening of the femoral head, and acetabular dysplasia,[19] sometimes with development of a false acetabulum (McCullough, 1994).

In the case of the child with spasticity, the abnormal pull of the iliopsoas and adductor muscles are the initiating deforming force in hip dislocations (Fig. 19–9). When overactivity and contracture of the iliopsoas occur, the medial joint capsule is compressed and the femoral head is pushed laterally. As lateral drift of the femoral head occurs, the iliopsoas insertion on the lesser trochanter becomes the center of rotation. Acetabular development ceases, and when the femoral head is completely displaced laterally, further hip flexion pushes the head posteriorly to complete the dislocation (Bleck, 1979).

Clinical Manifestations. Clinical manifestations of CHD vary with age. In the newborn and nonambulator up to 12 months, there may be one or more positive signs (Fig. 19–10).[20] Any observed physical asymmetries in ROM (even as little as 10 degrees is considered significant, especially limitation of hip abduction), asymmetry in the buttock or gluteal fold (higher on the affected side), extra thigh skin folds, or leg length discrepancy requires medical evaluation.

In the ambulating child, uncorrected bilateral dysplasia may cause a characteristic gait pattern known as a "duck waddle" as the child sways from side to side. Unilateral dysplasia is usually characterized by a limp with a positive Trendelenburg's sign during the stance phase of gait on the involved side (Fig. 19–11). A flexion contracture on the involved side(s) develops as a result of posterior displacement of the hips, which then contributes to marked lumbar lordosis.

Medical Management

Diagnosis. In the newborn period, clinical examination is the most important diagnostic tool. A positive Ortolani's, Barlow's, or Galeazzi's sign confirms CHD. There are cases in which dislocation is not diagnosed by these standard tests and the disorder may not be apparent at birth. Regular well-

[19] Lack of contact of the femoral head in the acetabulum is a known cause of acetabular dysplasia occurring in the older child (median age at the time of dislocation is 7 years). This phenomenon is the basis for standing programs for nonambulatory children (i.e., standing provides mechanical forces to assist in the development of the acetabular cup, thus preventing dislocation).

[20] As ligamentous structures become stronger or if the joints become stretched and worn, it is more difficult to elicit the characteristic popping in and out. These tests are considered significantly less diagnostic past 2 to 3 months by some experts. For a more in-depth description of these tests, see Magee, 1996.

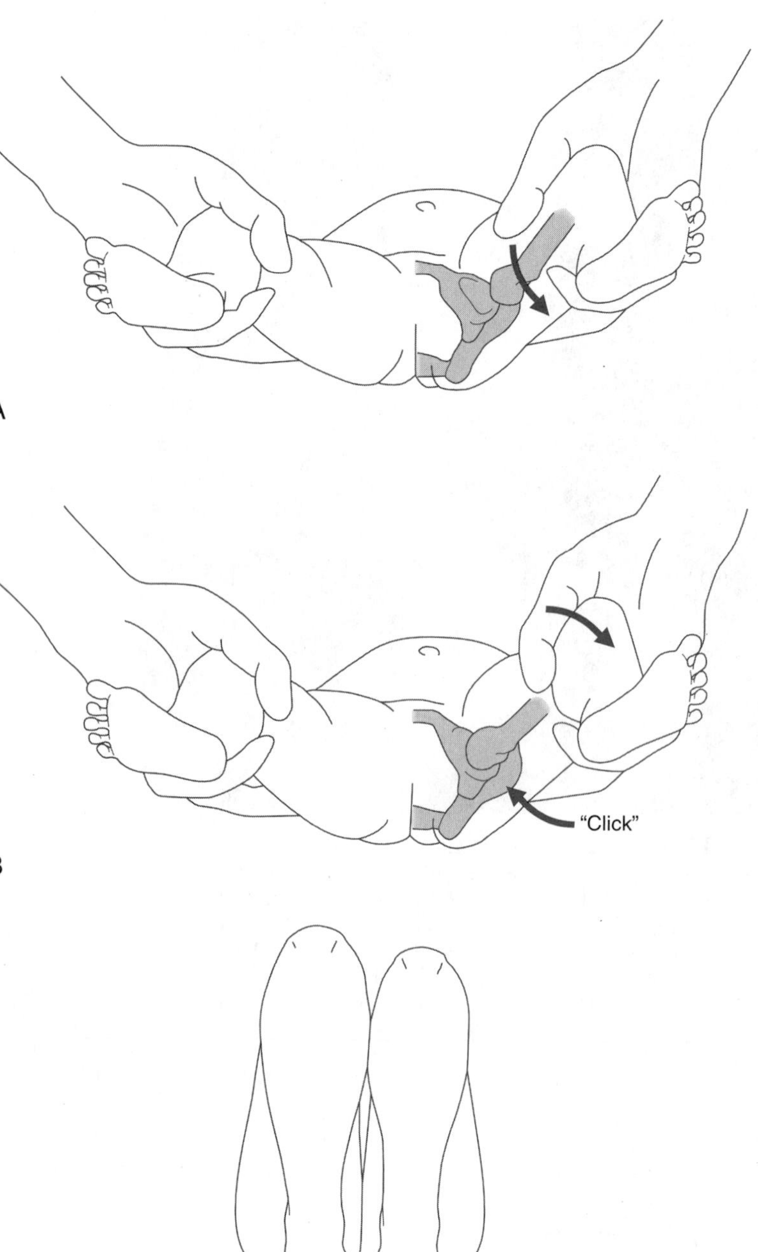

Figure **19–10.** Signs of congenital hip dislocation. A, Ortolani's maneuver No. 1 (also the second part of the Barlow test): Hip flexion and adduction with downward pressure dislocates the hip. B, Ortalani's maneuver No. 2: Gentle hip flexion, abduction, and slight traction reduce the hip with a discernible click or clunk and increased hip abduction is possible. This test is valid only for the first few weeks after birth. C, Galeazzi's test (Allis' sign): In the supine position, with hips and knees flexed and feet flat on the floor, the knee is lower on the dislocated side indicating the head of the femur is positioned posterior to the rim of the acetabulum. This test is used to assess unilateral hip dislocation but can be used in older children (from 3 months on).

baby check-ups should include hip examination until the child begins to walk with a normal gait pattern. Radiographic examination is unreliable until about 6 weeks of age and is used more commonly in older infants and children. Ultrasonography allows visualization of the cartilaginous structures of the hip and is especially accurate during the first 6 months of life.

Treatment. Treatment depends on the age of the child, and the severity and duration of the dysplasia. The most common treatment in the infant is placement of the hip in a position of flexion and abduction until the joint capsule tightens and the acetabulum is molded to assume a cup shape. This can be accomplished in some children simply by double diapering but in others requires the use of a hip harness such as the Pavlik harness (Fig. 19–12).

The infant must wear this apparatus continuously for 2 to 3 months and then use a night splint for another month to stabilize the hip in the correct alignment (Fig. 19–13). Criteria for discontinuation of the harness are not standard. Some physicians advocate complete removal of the harness 6 weeks after the hip can no longer be moved in and out of the acetabulum. Others recommend discontinuation when radiographic findings confirm hip stabilization.

Treatment in older children who have been walking and for children with spasticity-induced dysplasia is usually surgi-

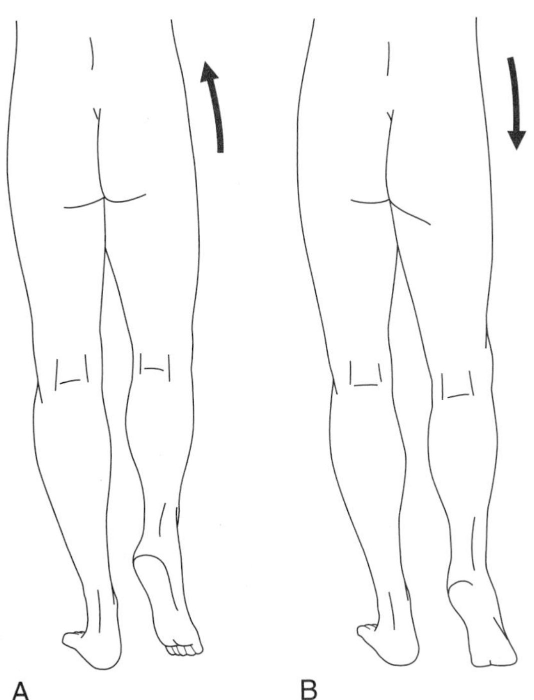

Figure 19–11. Trendelenburg's test. *A*, Negative: With the weight on one leg, the pelvis on the opposite side will be slightly elevated (observed from behind the client). *B*, Positive: With weight on one leg, the pelvis will drop on the opposite side because of muscle weakness or pain in the hip joint on that side. Trendelenburg's test measures weakness of the hip abductor muscles, especially the gluteus medius.

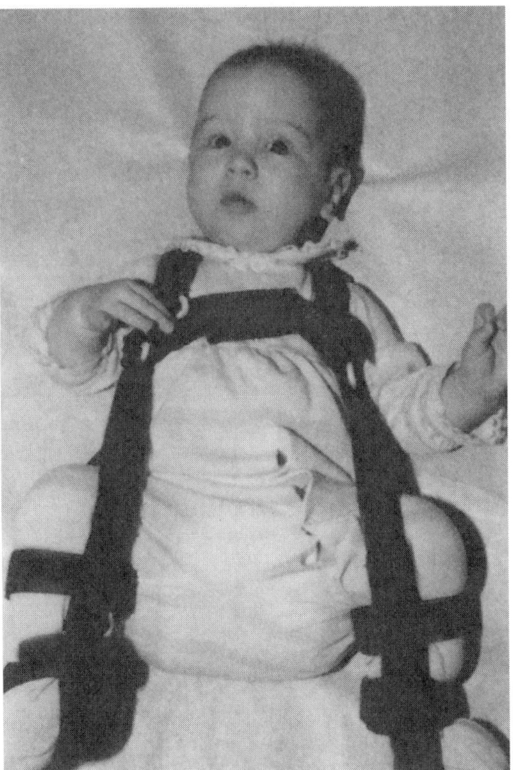

Figure 19–12. The Pavlik harness can be used to treat acetabular dysplasia, to stabilize a lax hip, or to reduce a dislocated hip. (*From Leach J: Orthopaedic conditions.* In *Campbell SK (ed): Physical Therapy for Children. Philadelphia, WB Saunders, 1995, p 364.*)

cal (e.g., skin or skeletal traction,[21] closed reduction, open reduction, tenotomy of contracted muscles, or osteotomy) (Fig. 19–14) depending on the clinical presentation.

Prognosis. If the dislocation is corrected in the first few days or weeks of life, the dysplasia is completely reversible and a normal hip will develop. As the child becomes older (prior to the developmental stage of walking) and the primary subluxation or dislocation persists, the deformity will worsen and become permanent.

When untreated, long-term problems can include degenerative joint disease, hip pain, antalgic gait, scoliosis, back pain, or the need for total hip replacement. In the case of hip dysplasia associated with other medical conditions such as CP, the long-term results are not nearly as good compared to the outcome of uncomplicated CHD.

Special Implications for the Therapist 19-5
CONGENITAL HIP DYSPLASIA

Often therapists are involved early and regularly in managing a child's program for some condition other than hip dysplasia and may be the first health-care workers to observe signs of hip pathology. An awareness of quick screening strategies for hip dysplasia is critical (Box 19–7).

Precautions

Positioning and splinting strategies focus on hip abduction and external rotation. Positions to avoid include lower extremity adduction and flexion as occurs in the side-lying position, especially with one lower extremity drifting across the midline (Campbell, 1995). Force should not be used in flexing and abducting the hip as the excessive pressure can cause avascular necrosis. Tests for hip subluxation or dislocation (see Fig. 19–10) should not be repeated too often as they can result in articular damage to the head of the femur and dislocation. Internal rotation is avoided because this movement tends to "wring out" the blood vessels in the capsule of the joint (Eilert and Georgopoulos, 1995).

When transferring a child immediately after casting, use the palms to avoid making dents in the cast. Any indentations in the cast can predispose the child to pressure ulcers. The cast will need 24 to 48 hours to completely air-dry; artificial heat sources such as lamps or blow dryers should not be used to hasten drying since heat also makes the cast more fragile. Check

[21] Skin traction (moleskin or some other type of adhesive wrap is used to cover the affected limb and traction is applied to the bandage) in infants and skeletal traction (force applied directly upon a bone by means of surgically installed pins and wires or tongs) in children who have started walking are used in an attempt to reduce the dislocation by gradually abducting the hips.

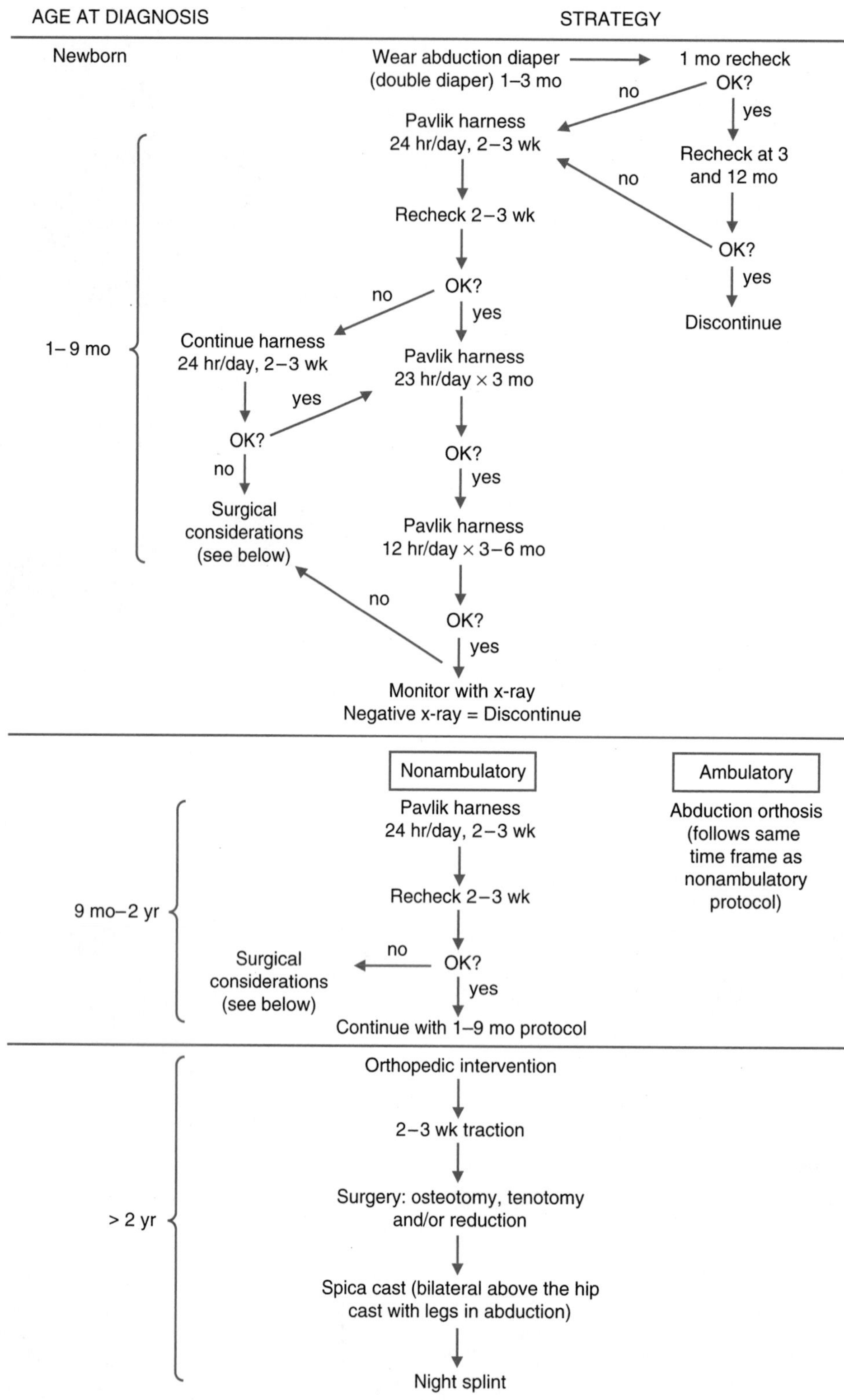

Figure **19–13.** Treatment of hip dysplasia. Management will vary for children with increased lower extremity muscle tone or chronic developmental disability.

color, sensation, and motion of the child's legs and feet and notify the physician immediately of dusky, cool, or numb toes. Observe for signs that the child is outgrowing the cast (e.g., cyanosis, cool extremities, pain).

Motor Development

The widely abducted position of the lower extremities limits opportunities to initiate or continue development of low back and hip extension, especially in the absence of the prone position. Likewise, the widely abducted

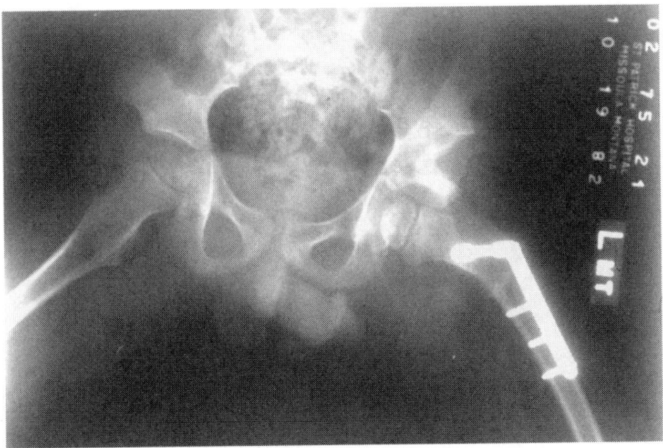

Figure **19–14.** Anteroposterior (AP) radiograph of left hip following derotational osteotomy for chronic hip dislocation. The femoral shaft is cut obliquely, then internally rotated to correct the femoral anteversion (derotation), and a portion of the iliac crest is removed and used as a wedge above the acetabulum to create an extended acetabular shelf (osteotomy). (*Courtesy of Rae Johnston, MD, Missoula, Montana.*)

base of support in sitting decreases opportunities for the use of trunk rotation necessary for transitioning in and out of positions such as sitting and lying prone. The therapist must closely monitor overall progression of motor development during this time and provide as many opportunities as possible for the development of these important skills.

MUSCULAR DYSTROPHY

Definition and Overview. Muscular dystrophy (MD) is the largest and most common group of progressive neuromuscular disorders of childhood, although signs of MD can occur at any point in the life span. It has a genetic origin and is characterized by ongoing symmetrical muscle wasting without neural or sensory deficits but with increasing deformity and disability. Paradoxically, the wasted muscles tend to hypertrophy because of connective tissue and fat deposits, giving the visual appearance of muscle strength.

There are four types of MD: (1) Duchenne's (pseudohypertrophic) muscular dystrophy (DMD, 50% of all cases), (2) Becker's (benign pseudohypertrophic) muscular dystrophy (BMD), (3) facioscapulohumeral (Landouzy-Dejerine) dystrophy (FSH), and (4) limb-girdle dystrophy (LGD). In all forms of MD there is a primary degeneration of muscle with a gradual loss of strength, but each type differs as to which muscle groups are affected (Fig. 19–15).

Incidence and Etiology. The overall incidence of MD is approximately 20 to 30 per 100,000 live births. DMD occurs in approximately 1 in 3500 live male births. BMD occurs in approximately 1 to 3 in 100,000 live male births.

All dystrophies are inherited disorders. DMD and BMD are X-linked recessive caused by mutations in the dystrophin gene (muscle protein) Xp21.[22] In these two forms of MD, males are affected clinically and females are the carriers. FSH is an autosomal dominant disorder with onset in early adolescence. The son or daughter of a person affected with FSH is at 50% risk of inheriting the defective gene.

LGD may be inherited in several ways but is usually an autosomal recessive disorder of late childhood or adolescence. This means the parents will not exhibit the disorder but there is a 1 in 4 chance of every pregnancy producing a child (son or daughter) with the disorder. These two types of MD (FSH, LGD) affect both sexes equally.

Pathogenesis. The affected gene encodes messenger RNA (mRNA) for a protein called dystrophin which is localized to the skeletal and cardiac muscle surface membrane, the sarcolemma. Dystrophin is the protein that links the muscle surface membrane (sarcolemma) with the contractile muscle protein (actin) (Matsumura et al., 1993).

Lack of normal dystrophin makes the sarcolemma susceptible to damage during contraction and relaxation cycles; thus muscle fiber necrosis is initiated by muscle contraction. Skeletal muscle fibers, especially during eccentric contraction, are susceptible to damage (Brown and Lucy, 1993; Ervasti and Campbell, 1993; Matsumura and Campbell, 1994). Males with low or undetectable levels of dystrophin have the Duchenne-type MD, whereas those with nearly normal levels but dystrophin of an abnormal size have the Becker-type MD. The levels of dystrophin seem to correlate with clinical prognosis.

The absence or altered state of dystrophin causes the slowing of muscle protein synthesis so that there is a failure of muscle growth maintenance and slowing of muscle turnover. This alteration in protein synthesis results in higher loads of calcium entering the muscle cells. Subsequently, muscle cells are destroyed and replaced by fatty and connective tissues, often producing contractures. Fat cells then continue to accu-

BOX **19–7**
Hip Dysplasia: Quick Screen

- History
  - Breech delivery
  - Family history
  - Female
- Lower extremity examination
  - Foot alignment
  - Hip range of motion (asymmetry, limited abduction)
  - Asymmetrical skin folds (thigh, gluteal)
  - Buttocks appear flattened
  - Leg length discrepancy
- Hip stability (only one positive test required)
  - Ortolani's sign
  - Barlow's sign
  - Galeazzi's sign
- Gait (if ambulating)
  - Abnormal (waddling gait, limp)
  - Positive Trendelenburg's sign
  - Pain
- Typical posture
  - Lower extremity hip flexion, abduction, adduction, internal and external rotation
  - Asymmetrical head and neck alignment when associated with torticollis

[22] The affected gene on the short arm of the X chromosome in band Sp21 is one of the largest genes in the human genome, which may explain its high rate of spontaneous mutation. About 60% to 65% of families affected by MD have a deletion in this gene.

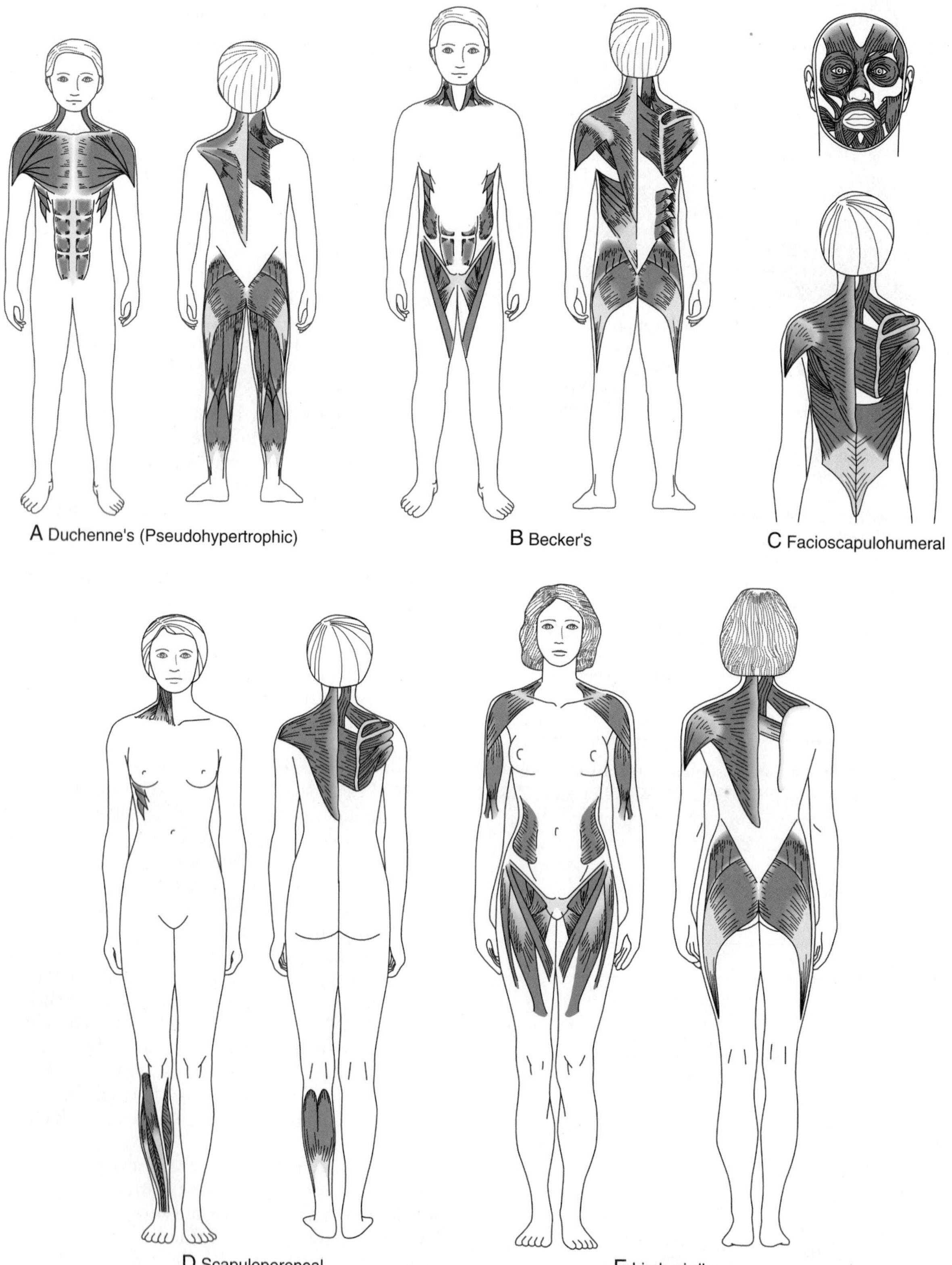

Figure **19–15.** Muscle groups involved in muscular dystrophies. *A*, Duchenne's: shoulder girdle (trapezius, levator scapulae, rhomboids, serratus anterior), pectoral muscles, deltoid, rectus abdominis, gluteals, hamstrings, calf muscles. *B*, Becker's: neck, trunk, pelvic and shoulder girdle. *C*, Facioscapulohumeral: muscles of the face and shoulder girdle. *D*, Scapuloperoneal: muscles of the legs below the knees (first), shoulder girdle (later). *E*, Limb-girdle: upper arm (biceps and deltoid) and pelvic girdle.

TABLE 19-9 NEUROMUSCULAR CLASSIFICATIONS

TYPE	ONSET	INHERITANCE	COURSE
Duchenne's (pseudohypertrophic)	1–4 yr	X-linked	Rapidly progressive; loss of walking by 9–10 yr; death in late teens
Becker's	5–10 yr	X-linked	Slowly progressive; walking maintained past early teens; life span into 20s
Facioscapulohumeral (Landouzy-Dejerine)	Any age; usually early adolescence	Autosomal dominant or recessive	Slowly progressive loss of walking in later life; variable life expectancy
Scapuloperoneal (variant of facioscapulohumeral)	Any age from early childhood to adult	Autosomal dominant or recessive	Normal life span
Limb-girdle	Late adolescence; early adulthood	Autosomal recessive	Slowly progressive; mild impairment
Werdnig-Hoffmann (acute) (SMA type I)	0–3 mo	Autosomal recessive	Rapidly progressive; severe hypotonia; death within first 3 yr
Werdnig-Hoffman (chronic) (SMA type II)	3 mo–4 yr	Autosomal recessive	Rapid progress that stabilizes; moderate to severe hypotonia; shortened life span
Kugelberg-Welander, juvenile onset (SMA type III)	5–10 yr	Autosomal recessive	Slowly progressive; mild impairment

SMA, spinal muscular atrophy.

mulate between damaged muscle fibers as a response to the ongoing muscle atrophy. Disorganization of tendinous insertions is also associated with fat accumulation.

The involved muscle fibers are randomly distributed with no distinct pattern. Although fibers regenerate in the younger child, they are abnormal in many ways and become nonfunctional.

Clinical Manifestations. Persons with MD have muscular weakness, wasting, and hypotonia. The degree of severity and age of onset vary with the type of MD present (Table 19–9). *Duchenne's* is usually identified when the child has difficulty getting up off the floor (Gower's sign; Fig. 19–16), falls frequently, has difficulty climbing stairs, and starts to walk with a waddling gait (proximal muscle weakness) and increased lumbar lordosis (compensation for hip extensor weakness). At the same time the child begins to walk on the toes because of weakness and contracture of the anterior tibial and peroneal muscles.

Hip abductor weakness produces a positive Trendelenburg's sign (see Fig. 19–11) which will eventually change to a compensated gluteus medius gait as hip abductor weakness progresses. Ambulation continues to deteriorate up to the ages of 10 to 12 years at which time the majority of persons with DMD are no longer able to walk (Smith, 1990).

Within 3 to 5 years, muscles of the shoulder girdle become involved with excessive scapular winging and muscle hypertrophy (especially the upper arms, calves, and thighs) (Fig. 19–17). One of the major problems in gait occurs when the affected person requires upper extremity support. Shoulder girdle weakness often prevents the use of crutches to support the body weight. Weakness of the shoulder girdle also causes difficulty in performing overhead activities related to hygiene and work. Bicipital tendinitis or other impingement disorders at the shoulder occur as muscle imbalances create biomechanical dysfunction.

Later, other complications develop such as altered mentation, depressed deep tendon reflexes, contractures, kyphosco-

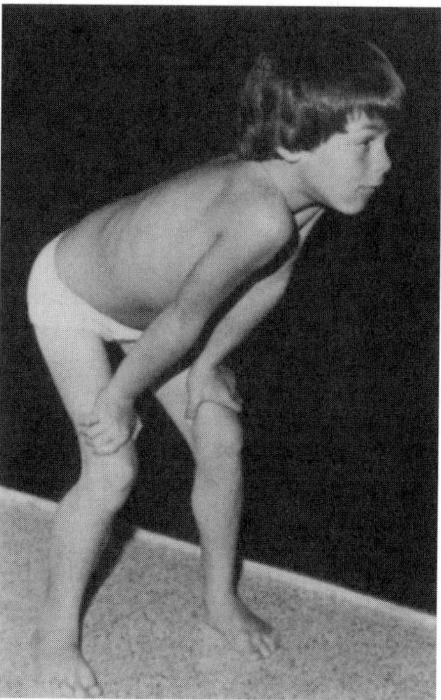

Figure **19–16.** This boy adopts the typical movement seen with proximal weakness, such as myopathies, when arising from the floor, a chair, or even when climbing stairs. During Gower's maneuver the client places the hands on the thighs and "walks" up the legs with the hands until the weight of the trunk can be placed posterior to the hip joint. This sign is characteristic of weakness of the lumbar and gluteal muscles. (*From Vinken PJ, Bruyn GW (eds): Handbook of Clinical Neurology. Diseases of Muscle. New York, Elsevier–North Holland, 1979, p 315.*)

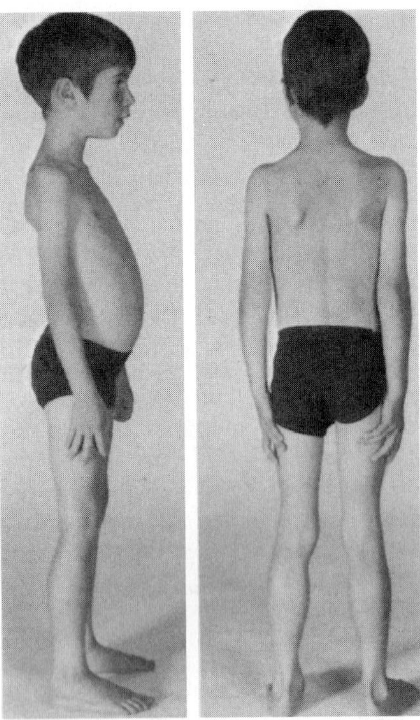

Figure **19–17.** Duchenne's muscular dystrophy with pseudohypertrophy of calves and lordotic posture that place the weight of the trunk behind the hip joint. Even though weakness occurs symmetrically, habitual standing postures may create asymmetries in flexibility. (*From Morgan-Hughes JA: Diseases of striated muscle. In Asbury AK, McKhann GM, McDonald WI (eds): Diseases of the Nervous System: Clinical Neurobiology, ed 2. Philadelphia, WB Saunders, 1992, p 167.*)

liosis, respiratory involvement, and chronic heart failure. These changes occur as a result of the loss of the protein dystrophin normally present in skeletal muscle as well as cardiac muscle and brain tissue.

Signs and symptoms of *Becker's* resemble Duchenne's but with a slower progression and later life expectancy. Ambulation is preserved into midadolescence or later but is often marked by the tiptoe pattern with bilateral calf muscle hypertrophy. Proximal muscles tend to be affected more and prior to the distal musculature, with primary involvement in the neck, trunk, pelvis, and shoulder girdle. Muscle cramps are a common complaint in late childhood and early adolescence. Scoliosis and contractures (elbow flexors, forearm pronators, and wrist flexors) are common when the child becomes wheelchair-dependent.

Facioscapulohumeral dystrophy is a mild form of MD beginning with weakness and atrophy of the facial muscles and shoulder girdle. Inability to close the eyes may be the earliest sign; the face is expressionless even when laughing or crying, forward shoulders and scapular winging develop, and the person has difficulty raising the arms overhead (Fig. 19–18).

Other changes in the face include diffuse facial flattening, a pouting lower lip, and inability to pucker the mouth to whistle, or for the infant, an inability to suckle. Weakness of the lower extremities may occur but is delayed for many years. Contractures, skeletal deformities, and hypertrophy of the muscles are uncommon. This form of MD responds well to steroid therapy and may be arrested for long periods of time.

A variation of FSH is *scapuloperoneal muscular dystrophy* with involvement of the distal muscles of the lower extremities instead of the face and proximal muscles of the shoulder girdle. Early symptoms may include footdrop with shoulder weakness developing later.

Limb-girdle dystrophy follows a slow course, often with only mild impairment. Early symptoms develop as a result of muscle weakness in the upper arm (biceps and deltoid muscles) and pelvic muscles, usually noticed in late adolescence or early adulthood but as late as the person's 40s. The lack of consistent clinical features make this type of MD more difficult to diagnose. Winging of the scapulae, lumbar lordosis, abdominal protrusion, waddling gait, poor balance, and inability to raise the arms may also develop.

Medical Management.

Diagnosis. Diagnosis is based on clinical presentation, family history, and diagnostic testing such as electromyography (EMG), serum enzymes, and muscle biopsy. EMG demonstrates short (decreased duration), weak bursts (decreased amplitude) of electrical activity in affected muscles. Muscle biopsy shows variation in the size of muscle fibers, and in later stages shows fat and connective tissue deposits. In DMD, muscle biopsy reveals an absence of dystrophin (Norris, 1995).

If the affected person marries and has children, all daughters will be carriers of this X-linked recessive disorder. Female carriers of and males affected by DMD and BMD usually

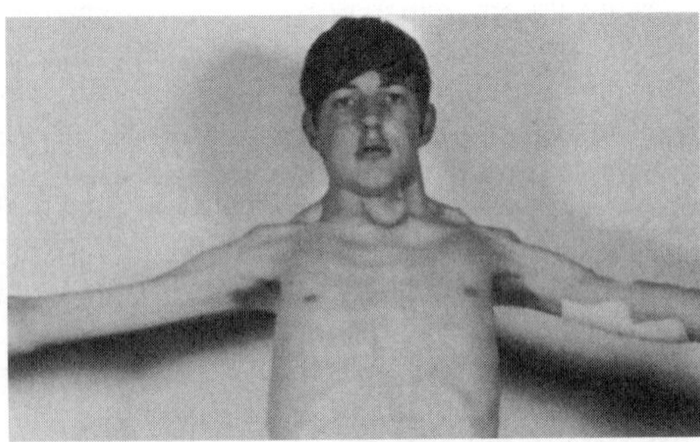

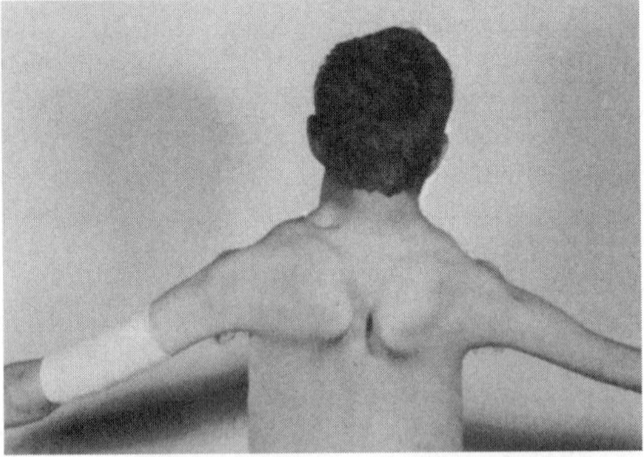

Figure **19–18.** Facioscapulohumeral dystrophy. Weakness of shoulder girdle musculature makes it difficult to perform overhead activities; wasting also causes the clavicles to jut forward and the shoulders to have a drooping appearance. During humeral movement, the scapulae "wing" and ride up over the thorax. (*From Morgan-Hughes JA: Diseases of striated muscle. In Asbury AK, McKhann GM, McDonald WI (eds): Diseases of the Nervous System: Clinical Neurobiology, ed 2. Philadelphia, WB Saunders, 1992, p 170.*)

present with creatinine kinase (CK) levels that are approximately 2 to 10 times normal (see Serum Enzymes, Chapter 35. Levels are extremely high in the first 2 years of life before the onset of clinical weakness, diminish with muscle deterioration, but do not return to normal levels until severe muscle wasting and disability occur.

Newer molecular techniques, including linkage studies, are now able to accurately diagnose DMD and BMD as well as predict carrier status. These tests will eventually replace muscle biopsy and serum enzyme testing.

Chorion biopsy is a prenatal diagnostic technique in which DNA is removed as early as 10 weeks' gestation to determine the presence or absence of the defective gene. Currently, laboratory testing can detect a deletion of the dystrophin gene in approximately 70% of fetuses with DMD.

Treatment. At present there is no known treatment to halt the progression of MD. Treatment is directed toward maintaining function in unaffected muscle groups for as long as possible, utilizing supportive measures such as physical and occupational therapy, orthopedic appliances, orthopedic surgery, and pharmaceuticals. Children who remain active as long as possible avoid complications (e.g., contractures, pressure ulcers, infections) and deconditioning that are common once they are wheelchair-bound.

The effective use of glucocorticoid therapy (e.g., prednisolone) to slow the progression of DMD and BMD has been reported. The addition of glucocorticoids to muscle increases myogenesis and enhances the expression of dystrophin, thereby improving muscle force and function and diminishing the deterioration of muscle function (Backman and Henriksson, 1995; Hardiman et al., 1993). The functional advantage of this treatment is the child's ability to maintain independent ambulation for longer periods of time.

Cell and gene therapy for MD are currently under investigation exploring a variety of treatment possibilities. Experiments in mice have investigated the use of viruses to implant normal muscle precursor cells into dystrophin-deficient muscles (Hauser and Chamberlain, 1996; Mateos, 1995).

In other research models, attempts have been made to inject skeletal muscles with donor cells (myoblast transfer). These myoblasts fuse with diseased muscle fibers and provide the missing gene to replace dystrophin. To date, there have been no reports of improved strength in persons with DMD with this procedure (Mendell et al., 1995).[23] Whether this procedure would allow a person to stabilize at current functional levels without necessarily increasing strength has not been evaluated.

Prognosis. All forms of MD are progressive, but the prognosis varies with the type of MD present. As a general rule, the earlier the clinical signs appear, the more rapid, progressive, and disabling the dystrophy. DMD generally occurs during early childhood with rapid progression of symptoms and results in death by age 20. Pulmonary complications due to respiratory muscle dysfunction or cardiac weakness are common sources of morbidity and mortality. People with BMD usually live into their 40s and death occurs secondary to respiratory dysfunction or heart failure. Those with FSH involvement may appear almost stable over a period of years; there is variable progression among those with LGD. Both FSH and LGD have a normal life span.

[23] Two factors may account for the failure of these trials: (1) human muscle appears to be a much less fertile bed for myoblast fusion compared with mice used in animal trials, and (2) immune responses directed against the injected myoblasts may have prevented the stable engraftment of myoblasts (Leiden, 1995).

Special Implications for the Therapist 19-6

MUSCULAR DYSTROPHY

Precautions

When persons become ill or injured and are on bed rest (at home or in hospital) even for a few days they may lose many of their functional abilities. For example, a child who develops chickenpox and is on bed rest may never regain the ability to ambulate. These children should be encouraged to stand, and if possible, ambulate for even a few minutes during the course of the illness.

Although activity helps the client maintain functional abilities, strenuous exercise may facilitate the breakdown of muscle fibers so that exercise must be approached cautiously. Low-repetition maximum weightlifting or strengthening is contraindicated. General guidelines for a strengthening program should include 8 to 12 repetitions (two to three sets) with only minimal fatigue noted after the second and third sets.

Respiratory involvement requires careful monitoring of breathing techniques, respiratory movements, and oxygen saturation levels. Monitoring oxygen during exercise and activity is highly recommended. See Appendix B. The client should be instructed in deep-breathing and diaphragmatic breathing exercises and encouraged to cough.

Investigators have shown that the inspiratory muscles are similar to other skeletal muscle groups in that they can be trained for both force and endurance in this population. These training-related improvements in inspiratory muscle performance are more likely to occur in those who are less severely affected by the disease. In those clients who have disease to the extent that they are already retaining carbon dioxide, there is little change in respiratory muscle force or endurance with training. In this group, the inspiratory muscles may already be working at a level of carbon dioxide sufficiently severe to provide a training stimulus with each breath (McCool and Tzelepis, 1995).

Therapy Interventions

The therapist can provide valuable information regarding the use of grab bars, overhead slings, wheelchairs, standing equipment, splints, active ROM exercises (passive ROM exercises are not effective), prolonged positioning, home environment assessment, lift equipment, and so on. Both children and adults can benefit from ambulation and pool therapy programs aimed at improving endurance. For a more in-depth discussion of the direct treatment protocols for this condition, the reader is referred to other resources (Campbell, 1995; Kurtz and Scull, 1993).

TORTICOLLIS

Definition and Overview. Torticollis (wry neck) means "twisted neck" and is a contracted state of the sternocleidomastoid muscle (SCM), producing bending of the head to the affected side with rotation of the chin to the opposite side.

This musculoskeletal condition usually develops in utero and is therefore considered congenital, but it can be acquired secondary to pressure on the accessory nerve, to inflammation of glands in the neck, or to muscle spasm. Torticollis, sometimes referred to as spasmodic torticollis, is often confused with cervical dystonia (also referred to as spasmodic torticollis). However, torticollis as presented here is a musculoskeletal phenomenon viewed as an orthopedic condition, whereas cervical dystonia is a movement disorder with an underlying CNS pathology (see discussion of dystonia, Chapter 27).

In the congenital form of torticollis, there is a 20% incidence of hip dysplasia, which most often presents on the same side as the shortened SCM. The reason for this relationship remains unknown.

Incidence. The incidence of congenital torticollis is highest after obstetric complications such as breech delivery, in first-born infants, and in girls. Acquired torticollis usually develops during the first 10 years of life or after age 40, with both sexes affected equally.

Etiology. There are a variety of possible causes of torticollis, both orthopedic and nonorthopedic. Orthopedic causes usually relate to tightness or contracture of the SCM or subluxation of the cervical spine. Nonorthopedic causes include pseudotumor or ocular problems.

Torticollis in children caused by atlantoaxial rotational subluxation (Grisel's syndrome) occurs spontaneously or secondary to minor trauma, upper respiratory tract infections (or infections anywhere in the head and neck region), juvenile rheumatoid arthritis, and surgical procedures in the oropharynx (Engelhardt et al., 1995; Samuel et al., 1995).

Pseudotumor of infancy presents as a discrete, firm mass in the distal SCM in infants 2 to 4 weeks of age, resulting in fibrosis and torticollis. Ocular causes include underaction of the superior oblique muscle, paresis of the lateral rectus muscle, or nystagmus (Williams et al., 1996).

Pathogenesis. Previously it was hypothesized that some types of birth trauma led to a tearing of the SCM at birth resulting in hematoma formation. The hematoma underwent fibrous changes resulting in muscle shortening or tightness which could not lengthen with the growing neck (Lawrence, 1989).

However, it now seems more likely that malposition of the head in utero is the probable cause of facial asymmetry associated with congenital torticollis. The malposition of the head potentially leads to a compartmental syndrome resulting in a venous occlusion. In this scenario, the SCM is not stretched or torn but rather kinked or crushed. With the head and neck in a position of forward flexion, lateral bend, and rotation, the ipsilateral SCM kinks, causing an ischemic injury and subsequent edema at the site of the kink (Davids, 1993).

TABLE 19-10 Torticollis Severity

Movement		Severity (Degrees) Mild	Moderate	Severe
Lateral flexion (opposite side)	Active	25–45	10–25	0–5
	Passive	90	20–80	0–10
Rotation (same side)	Active	70	45–60	0–20
	Passive	80	65–75	0–15

Clinical Manifestations. The first sign of *congenital torticollis* is often a firm, nontender, palpable enlargement of the SCM visible at birth and for several weeks afterward. Approximately half of all cases of torticollis demonstrate bulbous fibrotic tissue at the base or midportion of the involved SCM. This local lesion usually reaches its maximal size by 1 month and often slowly regresses within 2 to 6 months, although incomplete regression can cause permanent contracture.

If the deformity is severe (Table 19–10), the infant's face, ear, and head flatten from sleeping on the affected side; this asymmetry gradually worsens. The infant's chin turns away from the side of the shortened muscle, the head tilts to the shortened side, and the shoulder is elevated on the affected side, further limiting cervical movement (Norris, 1995).

The first sign of *acquired torticollis* is usually recurring unilateral stiffness of the neck muscles, followed by a drawing sensation and momentary twitching or contraction that pulls the head to the affected side. In the early stages, the affected person can voluntarily overcome the muscle spasm. The acquired type of torticollis often produces severe neuralgic pain throughout the head and neck.

Chronic, unresolved torticollis (whether congenital or acquired) results in muscle hypertrophy, SCM trigger point dysfunction, and subsequent significant myofascial component (Travell and Simons, 1983).

Medical Management

Diagnosis. Clinical observation combined with the history forms the basis of the initial diagnostic process. Radiographic studies of the spine are always indicated to rule out tumors, congenital deformities of the cervical spine, tuberculosis of the cervical spine, subdural hematoma, dislocations or fractures, scoliosis, or arthritic changes.

Treatment. Congenital torticollis is treated conservatively, utilizing active and passive ROM exercises, heat, positioning, and splinting[24] as necessary to stretch the shortened muscle (Fig. 19–19). Active movement in the opposite direction to the typical resting head position is by far the most useful treatment strategy. Particular emphasis is placed on active and passive lateral flexion in a direction opposite to the involved SCM (Emery, 1994).

Surgical intervention is rare (e.g., SCM tenotomy, plastic

[24] A cervical collar can be helpful in providing tactile cueing for movement in the direction opposite the lateral tilt. Usually these collars are the most effective from 4 to 12 months of age or at a time that is compatible with active head control.

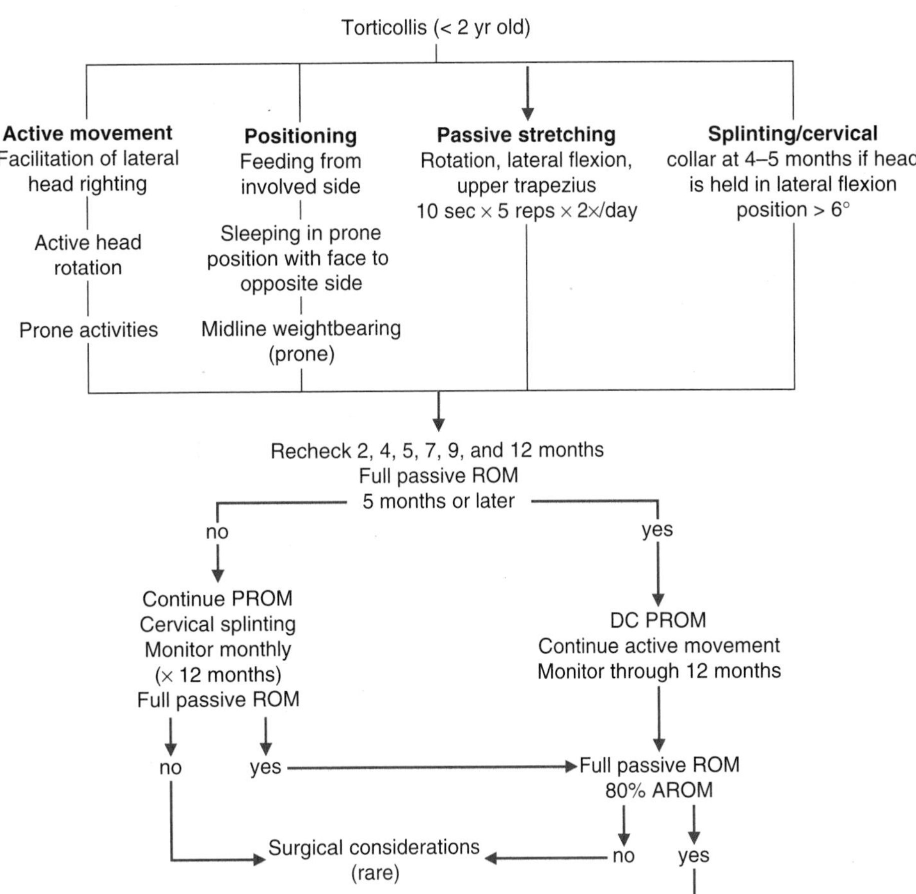

Figure **19-19.** Conservative treatment protocol for torticollis in children under 2 years old.

surgery for craniosacral asymmetry) and considered only if the individual continues to demonstrate significant motion restrictions (loss of more than 30 degrees of neck rotation) past 12 to 15 months of age.

Treatment of acquired torticollis is directed toward correction of the underlying cause. Physical therapy can be utilized to relieve pain and improve movement. Stretching exercises and a neck brace may be helpful. In the case of atlantoaxial rotational subluxation, treatment may be physical therapy or in some cases, surgical mobilization followed by halo cast fixation (2 to 4 days), then casting for 4 to 8 weeks.

Treatment of elderly clients with acquired torticollis may include administration of anticholinergics (e.g., carbidopa-levodopa, carbamazepine [Tegretol], benzodiazepines [Valium], baclofen, and haloperidol [Haldol]). Mixed results have been reported using these drugs and side effects such as blurred vision, dry mouth, voiding and sleeping difficulties, and personality changes can develop.

Prognosis. Torticollis in infancy is usually a self-limiting condition. Complete recovery, including full passive ROM, can be expected to take approximately 10 months with an associated treatment duration of approximately 5 to 7 months. Treatment of acquired torticollis is often unsatisfactory, with significant pain, loss of motion, and craniofacial asymmetry and postural deformity such as scoliosis. The majority of clients show steady progression and reach maximal disability after 5 years (Van Zandijcke, 1995).

Special Implications for the Therapist **19-7**

TORTICOLLIS

The prognostic information provided makes it possible for therapists to better predict treatment duration at the time of initial assessment. By providing parents with more precise information about the length of treatment, parents may be more willing to adhere to the exercise program (Emery, 1994).

The therapist must remain alert to recognize cervical subluxation in cases of congenital muscular torticollis. This may be observed as residual head-neck posturing problems, even after successful neck muscle therapy; usually there are no neurologic deficits present. In such cases, physical therapy is often prescribed, although some cases may require surgical intervention (Slate et al., 1993).

Likewise, torticollis that does not respond to physical therapy may have a nonorthopedic cause such as ocular torticollis, requiring further medical evaluation. Do not hesitate to ask for reevaluation if and when a child does not respond to therapy.

Postoperative

Following surgery for this condition, the client may be in traction 24 hours a day or at night only. Frequent monitoring of circulation, sensation, and color around the cast is important. Check the skin for any signs of irritation or pressure.

ERB'S PALSY

Definition and Overview. Erb's palsy is a paralysis of the upper limb resulting from a traction injury to the brachial plexus at birth. Erb's palsy actually comprises three distinct types of brachial plexus palsies: (1) *Erb-Duchenne palsy* affecting the C5–6 nerve roots (95% to 99% of all cases), (2) *whole-arm palsy* affecting C5–T1, and (3) *Klumpke's palsy* affecting the C8 and T1 (lower plexus) nerve roots.

Incidence. The incidence of brachial plexus injuries has decreased secondary to improved obstetric management of difficult labors. Traction injuries are most common in newborns, occurring in 0.1% of spontaneous, 1.2% of breech, 1.3% of forceps, and 0.25% of all deliveries.

Etiology and Risk Factors. The major contributing factor to these injuries is forced stretching of the brachial plexus, that is, a pulling away of the shoulder from the head secondary to a traction maneuver during the birth process. The lower plexus injury resulting in Klumpke's palsy is usually caused by manipulation during delivery resulting from hyperabduction of the arm at the shoulder, that is, the head and trunk remain relatively immobile in the pelvis while the upper extremity is stretched severely. Swinging a child by one arm or jerking the arm may also cause lower plexus injuries called "nursemaid's palsy."

Obstetric history associated with Erb's palsy is characterized by high birth weight, brow or face presentation,[25] with shoulder dystocia,[26] difficult breech delivery, or instrumental vaginal delivery (e.g., forceps delivery or misapplication of the vacuum extractor) (Moe and Seay, 1995). Other risk factors include idiopathic respiratory distress syndrome and gestational diabetes.

Pathogenesis. The palsies are usually caused by avulsion of the plexus with contusion, edema, and hemorrhage. A mild lesion involves stretching of the nerve fibers and is associated with perineural edema and possible hemorrhage. With a moderate injury some nerve fibers are stretched, some are actually torn, and internal and external bleeding occurs. Some permanent residual damage can be expected.

A severe injury is characterized by a complete rupture of the plexus trunks with avulsion of the roots from the spinal cord. The degree of residual stability will depend on the site of injury. If the upper roots are involved the injury is usually a rupture. If the lower roots are involved the injury is attributed to an avulsion. Most likely the disruption of the plexus occurs at the foramen or groove of the transverse processes.

[25] Brow or face presentation makes vaginal delivery impossible. Brow presentation rarely persists; in face presentation, the head is hyperextended and the chin presents.

[26] During delivery the baby's shoulder impinges on the mother's symphysis pubis.

Clinical Manifestations. Children with brachial plexus injuries are unlikely to demonstrate postural or placing responses with the involved upper extremity when tested. In Erb's palsy the arm is maintained in adduction and internal rotation at the shoulder with the lower arm pronated, assuming the "waiter's tip" position. Children with this type have difficulty with activities such as hand-to-mouth, hand-to-head, and hand-to-back of neck movements, but will usually have control of the wrist and fingers and normal sensation will be present.

In Klumpke's palsy, paralysis of the small muscles of the hand and wrist flexors causes a claw hand appearance. There is good proximal shoulder control but difficulty with voluntary forearm, wrist, and hand control. In severe forms of brachial palsy (whole-arm palsy), the entire arm is paralyzed and hangs limp and motionless at the side.

The clinical characteristics of brachial plexus injury are summarized in Table 19–11.

Medical Management

Diagnosis, Treatment, and Prognosis. Some injuries are readily recognizable at or soon after birth. Radiographs may be taken to rule out associated fractures of the clavicle. EMG and CT-myelography can delineate the extent of injury and aid in the prognosis, as well as identify those individuals for whom surgical repair may be attempted. In most instances, once the swelling decreases, full recovery can be expected, usually within a few days or weeks.

For more involved cases, recovery can take months. The long-term prognosis for recovery of motor control is poor beyond 18 months (Table 19–12). Recovery of shoulder external rotation is highly indicative of a good long-term outcome and a key movement for performing a variety of functional tasks. Almost half of the Erb-Duchenne–type injuries do not recover shoulder external rotation and contractures of the shoulder and elbow joint with atrophy of the affected muscles can occur.

Treatment is primarily with a therapist following the strategies outlined in Table 19–11. In the rare case, surgical correction may be applied following a lengthy trial of conservative care.

Special Implications for the Therapist **19-8**

ERB'S PALSY

Treatment should focus on activities that encourage active and active assistive movement. Presently there are no studies to clearly identify which individual technique or combination of techniques is most effective in the treatment of this condition. Some strategies used to encourage functional upper extremity position* and movement include therapeutic electrical stimulation or biofeedback, aquatic activities, ball therapy, craniosacral therapy, myofascial release techniques (sometimes referred to as soft tissue mobilization), and positioning using splints or serial casts.

Passive ROM exercises or joint mobilization performed three times a day for the first 9 to 12 months in the direction of limited movement may be useful but are considered inadvisable by some therapists because traction of the affected nerve roots may result in

TABLE 19-11 Brachial Plexus Injury: Clinical Characteristics

Type	Typical Posture	Strength Losses	Sensory Losses	Skeletal Changes	Treatment Strategies
Erb's (C5–6)	Shoulder IR, adduction (difficulty with hand to mouth, hand to head, and back of neck)	Deltoid, supraspinatus, infraspinatus, teres minor, biceps, brachialis, brachioradialis, supinator	Mild deficits	Flattening of glenoid fossa/humeral head Elongating deformity of coracoid process hooking down and lateral; interference with return of humeral head to socket Scapular winging secondary to abduction contracture of scapulohumeral joint; scapulothoracic instead of scapulohumeral movement	Active/active assistive exercise: shoulder abduction; elbow flexion; forearm supination and shoulder ER
Klumpke's (C8–T1)	Pronation, elbow flexion contractures; no grasp reflex	Wrist flexors, long finger flexors; hand intrinsics	Sensation normal	Hypertrophy of olecranon and coronoid process: elbow flexion contracture; posterior dislocation of radial head (25%)	Active/active assistive exercise: forearm supination, elbow extension, finger flexion Positional splint to assist with elbow extension; combined with UE weight bearing
Total plexus injury (whole arm)	Combinations of above	Combination of Erb's and Klumpke's types	Moderate losses	Posterior glenohumeral dislocation	Combination of above

IR, internal rotation; ER, external rotation; UE, upper extremity.

TABLE 19-12 KEY INDICATORS OF RECOVERY OF MOTOR CONTROL*

MUSCLE	TIME SINCE BIRTH (MO)
Triceps	1½
Deltoid, biceps	2
Shoulder external rotators	3
Finger extension	6
Wrist extension	10
Thumb extension, abduction	14

* There is a reasonable expectation of functional recovery if the child achieves a strength grade of 3 or better within the listed time frames.

increased protective muscle spasm. When splints are used, careful follow-up by the therapist is necessary to avoid contractures developing in the splinted position.

* A functional position is described as approximately 70 degrees shoulder abduction, 90 degrees shoulder flexion, 90 degrees shoulder external rotation, 50 to 60 degrees elbow flexion, and a forearm position in midpronation.

SPINAL MUSCULAR ATROPHY

Overview and Incidence. Spinal muscular atrophy (SMA), also known as Werdnig-Hoffmann disease, progressive infantile spinal muscular atrophy, and floppy infant syndrome, is a neuromuscular disease characterized by progressive weakness and wasting of skeletal muscles. SMA is the second most common fatal autosomal recessive disorder after cystic fibrosis.

Childhood SMAs are divided into severe (type I), intermediate (type II), and mild (type III). Types I (acute form) and II (chronic form) are referred to as Werdnig-Hoffmann disease. These more severe forms cause early death or increasing disability in childhood. Kugelberg-Welander disease, or type III SMA, is the mildest form with an onset at 3 to 15 years of age and slow progression (see Table 19–9).

SMA types I and II affect approximately 1 in 15,000 to 25,000 live births; SMA type III occurs in approximately 6 in 100,000 live births.

Etiology and Pathogenesis. The basis of this inherited pathologic condition (autosomal recessive trait) is gene deletions in the SMA critical region (long arm of chromosome 5q13.1). The extent of the deletions seems to correlate with disease severity (Spiegel et al., 1996). Progressive degeneration of anterior horn cells of the spinal cord and selective motor nuclei of the brainstem develop. Gliosis[27] of the spinal cord is usually associated with this degeneration and cell loss in the motor nuclei of the brainstem occurs along with associated thinning of motor roots.

Secondary to these degenerative changes, progressive paralysis with muscular atrophy occurs. EMG analysis of muscles shows prolongation of individual motor unit potentials and increased nerve conduction velocities.

[27] An excess of astroglia (neuroglia or glial tissue, the supporting structure of the nervous system, which is made up of astrocytes, as in the case of astroglia, as well as oligodendrocytes, and microglia) in damaged areas of the CNS.

Clinical Manifestations. The primary effect of SMA is atrophy of skeletal muscles with marked hypotonia and significant weakness. Static postures, significant developmental delays, and feeding problems (muscles to the tongue affected) and respiratory problems (involvement of the intercostals) are common. Cardiac involvement is often secondary to the chronic respiratory insufficiency typical of this disease. Fifty-five percent to 100% of persons with SMA type I or II will develop some type of scoliosis and usually much earlier than expected compared with the average population (Merlini et al., 1989) (Table 19–13).

SMA type III clients are most likely to ambulate, although about half of this group lose ambulatory skills by age 10 and fractures are common. Decrease in normal vital capacity values has been associated with decrease in ambulation skills in this population.

Medical Management

Diagnosis and Treatment. The diagnosis is suspected on the basis of clinical manifestations (see Table 19–13) but is established from EMG demonstrating a denervation pattern and confirmed by muscle biopsy. Treatment is symptomatic and preventive, primarily preventing infection and treating orthopedic problems, the most serious of which is scoliosis (Wong, 1993). Surgical intervention such as muscle releases and hip osteotomies may be necessary as a result of deforming forces from persistent frog-leg posturing.

Prognosis. Prognosis varies according to age of onset or

TABLE 19-13 CHARACTERISTICS OF SPINAL MUSCULAR ATROPHY (SMA)

Werdnig-Hoffmann (Types I and II)

- Disease acquired in utero or first 2 mo (SMA I); 2–12 mo (SMA II)
- LEs flexed, abducted, and externally rotated (frog position)
- UEs abducted, externally rotated, unable to move to midline against gravity
- Poor head control
- Significantly decreased muscle tone
- Decreased newborn movements, decreased diaphragmatic movements
- High risk of scoliosis
- Proximal muscle weakness greater than distal weakness
- Weak cry and cough
- Normal sensation and intellect
- Early death from respiratory failure or infection (usually by age 3 yr in SMA I, by age 7 yr in SMA II)

Kugelberg-Welander Disease (Type III)

- Onset of symptoms in second year of life
- Proximal LE weakness; greatest with hip, knee, trunk extension
- Trendelenburg's gait, especially with running
- Slow continued developmental progression
  - Sits independently by 1 yr
  - Walks independently by 3rd yr (lumbar lordosis, waddling gait, genu recurvatum, protuberant abdomen)
- Wheelchair-bound by early adulthood
- Good UE strength

LE, lower extremity; UE, upper extremity.

type of SMA (see Table 19–9). The earlier the disease occurs, the faster the progression of muscle weakness with secondary deformities, and the poorer the prognosis. The presence of respiratory distress also contributes to a poorer prognosis. SMA type I is the most severe and has a very poor prognosis with death likely in the first 6 months of life. Most children with this form of SMA do not survive past 3 years.

Special Implications for the Therapist **19-9**

SPINAL MUSCULAR ATROPHY

A variety of opinions exist regarding the usefulness or effectiveness of an active developmental program for children with SMA. However, often children with SMA type I or II outlive predictions and therapy intervention is very helpful in improving function and preventing musculoskeletal problems.

Precautions

The infant or child with SMA who is immobile requires frequent change of position to prevent physical injury and complications, especially pneumonia. The pharynx may require suctioning to remove secretions and feeding must be carried out slowly and carefully with good positioning to prevent aspiration. These children are intellectually normal so verbal, tactile, and auditory stimulation is an important aspect of treatment.

Respiratory weakness or diminished head control may prevent the child from benefiting from prone positioning. This is especially problematic when the child cannot lift the head to clear the airway. The use of prone positioning must be evaluated and monitored carefully by the therapist.

Monitoring oxygen saturation levels may be necessary in evaluating programming effectiveness. Observe how much work is required to breathe and whenever possible use a pulse oximeter (see Fig. B–1, Appendix B: Guidelines for Activity and Exercise) to measure arterial oxygen saturation noninvasively. Pulse oximetry can provide an outcome measure for documentation (see Appendix B).

Therapy Intervention

Specific treatment protocols for this condition are beyond the scope of this book. The therapist is referred to a more appropriate resource (Campbell, 1995). An overall management program should include positioning to encourage head and trunk control and to promote functional strengthening, as well as splinting, and mobility.

Facilitation and active assistive work toward standing and ambulation have been found to be effective in increasing forced vital capacity and in reducing the incidence of hip dislocation and contracture. More severely involved clients may benefit from instruction in standing to assist with or perform transfers independently (Stuberg, 1995).

Elastic chest binders similar to those used in spinal cord injury can be used to provide increased trunk, abdominal, and diaphragmatic stability, especially if there is evidence of decreased oxygen saturation with or without activity.

OSGOOD-SCHLATTER DISEASE

Definition and Overview. Osgood-Schlatter (OS) disease (osteochondrosis, Schlatter-Osgood disease) results from fibers of the patellar tendon pulling small bits of immature bone from the tibial tuberosity. In the past, OS was considered a form of osteochondritis (inflammation of bone and cartilage) but more recent thinking views the process as one part of the spectrum of mechanical problems related to the extensor mechanism. Rather than being an actual degenerative "disease," OS is considered a form of tendinitis of the patellar tendon (Hertling and Kessler, 1995).

OS is most commonly seen in active adolescent boys (10 to 15 years old) but can also affect adolescent girls (8 to 13). Overall, boys have an approximately three times higher incidence than girls.

Etiology and Pathogenesis. This condition is probably the result of indirect trauma (force produced by the sudden, powerful contraction of the quadriceps muscle during an activity) or repetitive stress (repeated knee flexion against a tight quadriceps muscle) before complete fusion of the epiphysis to the main bone has occurred. It is further aggravated by the longitudinal traction associated with bone growth in adolescents. Other causes include local deficient blood supply and genetic factors.

In young athletes, the tendon is attached to prebone, which is weaker than normal adult bone. With excessive stresses on the tendon from running and jumping, the structure becomes irritated and a tendinitis begins (Hertling and Kessler, 1995) (Fig. 19–20). Often fragments representing cartilage or bone formations are found on the surface of the patellar tendon and are a potential cause of pain. These

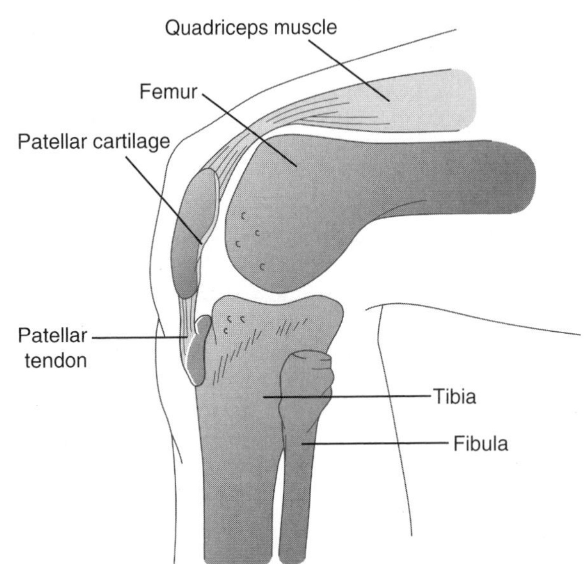

Figure 19–20. Osgood-Schlatter disease. Swelling below the knee and an enlarged tibial tuberosity may be observed clinically.

patellar tendon fibers can actually pull fragments away from the tibial epiphysis.

Clinical Manifestations. Clinically, clients report constant aching and pain at the site of the tibial tubercle (just below the kneecap) which is often enlarged on visual examination. Symptoms are aggravated by any activity that causes forceful contraction of the patellar tendon against the tubercle, such as active knee extension or resisted knee flexion (e.g., going up- or downstairs, running, jumping, biking, kneeling, squatting).

Besides the obvious soft tissue swelling, there may be localized heat and tenderness, the latter elicited with direct pressure over the tibial tubercle. Many clients with this condition also have significant tightness in the hamstrings, iliotibial band, triceps surae (bellies of the gastrocnemius and soleus), and quadriceps muscles. Tightness in these areas can potentially increase the flexion moment and subsequent stresses at the tibial tubercle.

Medical Management

Diagnosis. On physical examination, the examiner forces the tibia into internal rotation while slowly extending the client's knee from 90 degrees flexion; at about 30 degrees of knee flexion pain is reproduced which can be relieved by externally rotating the tibia. Clinical diagnosis may be confirmed by radiograph. Although the films may be normal, epiphyseal separation, soft tissue swelling, and bone fragmentation can be visualized in many cases.

Treatment and Prognosis. Immobilization is no longer advocated with this condition, although rest from aggravating activities is recommended until symptoms have subsided. This time frame ranges anywhere from 2 to 3 weeks in some individuals to 2 to 3 months in others. Enough time must be allowed for revascularization, healing, and ossification of the tibial tubercle before resuming unrestricted athletic participation. Nonsteroidal anti-inflammatory medication and ice are used regularly.

Treatment should include exercises to address the mechanical inefficiencies of the extensor mechanism, stretching for any areas of inflexibility, and strengthening areas of weakness (e.g., ankle dorsiflexion, pain-free quadriceps strengthening). Support may be provided through the use of a neoprene knee sleeve or narrow strap wrapped around the leg placing pressure over the tibial tubercle. This device is used to reduce the pulling stresses of the patellar tendon on the tubercle and subsequently reduce pain.

Conservative measures are usually sufficient to provide pain relief and resolution of local swelling. When conservative care fails to resolve painful symptoms, full-extension immobilization of the leg through reinforced elastic knee support, plaster cast, or splint may be prescribed for 6 to 8 weeks. Beyond that, surgery may be necessary to remove the epiphyseal ossicle that forms in the tendon. In extreme cases, the epiphysis may actually be removed or holes drilled into the tibial tubercle to facilitate revascularization of the area.

OSTEOGENESIS IMPERFECTA

Definition and Incidence. Osteogenesis imperfecta (OI), sometimes referred to as "brittle bones," is a rare congenital disorder of collagen synthesis affecting bones and connective tissue. There are four primary types of OI, each with specific symptoms and genetic characteristics (Table 19–14).

Type I OI is the most common form, affecting approximately 1 in 30,000 people. There are approximately 20,000 to 50,000 Americans with this type of OI. Type II is the most lethal, usually resulting in stillbirth or death soon after birth, although some survive into childhood. Type III is rarely seen and type IV is the most variable.

Etiology and Pathogenesis. OI can result from autosomal dominant (most common) or recessive (most lethal) inheritance. More than 90% of persons with OI have mutations in the type I collagen genes. The variable clinical expression could be the result of abnormalities in other connective tissue proteins or due to the differing genetic backgrounds of the individual (Dyne et al., 1996).

Clinical signs may result from defective osteoblastic activity and a defect of mesenchymal collagen (embryonic connective tissue) and its derivatives (sclerae, bones, and ligaments). The reticulum fails to differentiate into mature collagen or causes abnormal collagen development, leading to immature and coarse bone formation. Cortical bone thinning also occurs characterized by a reduced number of slender and delicate cancellous trabeculae (supporting structure of bone). Osteocytes (osteoblasts embedded in bone matrix, the intercellular substance of bone) are overcrowded with no intervening matrix. The result is decreased bone volume, brittle and unstable bones, and restriction of joint motion.

Clinical Manifestations. This disease has a wide range of clinical presentations ranging from a normal appearance with occasional fractures to very severe involvement with growth retardation and long bone deformities. In its severe forms, OI is evident at birth because of the fractures and deformity that have occurred in utero. The less severe forms may not become evident until the child begins to walk and fractures develop. The tendency to fracture disappears after puberty when the increased production of hormones helps strengthen bones, and increases later for women with type I OI following menopause. Some children with this form can be mistaken for battered children until the diagnosis is made.

Shortened statures are common in children with OI. This is due, at least in part, to the abnormal development of epiphyseal growth plates. Deformities following fractures, osteoporosis, and vertebral collapse contribute to loss of height with increasing age. Lower extremities tend to be more involved than upper extremities. These children often bruise very easily and ligaments tend to show increased laxity (Resnick, 1995).

Additional clinical features may include blue sclerae, thin skin, deformity of bony auditory structures, scoliosis, deformed teeth, a tendency toward recurrent epistaxis, excess diaphoresis, cardiovascular complications (e.g., aortic and mitral valve insufficiency, aortic dissection), and metabolic defects (e.g., elevated serum pyrophosphate, decreased platelet aggregation). Children with type III OI are born with a triangular-shaped face and a large skull, a feature that makes them easily identifiable.

Developmental motor skills are often delayed because of poorly developed muscles (atrophy), hypermobility of joints,

TABLE 19-14 Silence Classification of Osteogenesis Imperfecta (OI)

Type	Genetic Status	Description
I	Autosomal dominant	Mildest form of OI Mild to moderate bone fragility without deformity Associated with blue sclerae, early hearing loss, easy bruising May have mild to moderate short stature Type IA: dentinogenesis imperfecta absent Type IB: dentinogenesis imperfecta present
II	Autosomal dominant or recessive	Perinatal lethal (OI congenita) Extreme fragility of connective tissue Multiple in utero fractures Usually intrauterine growth retardation Soft, large cranium Micromelia: long bones crumpled and bowed; ribs beaded
III	Autosomal recessive	Triangular-shaped face, large skull Severe osteoporosis Severe fragility of bones; usually in utero fractures Fractures heal with deformity and bowing Associated with white sclerae and extreme short stature, scoliosis Usually wheelchair-bound by teenage years.
IV	Autosomal dominant	Mild to moderate skeletal fragility and osteoporosis (more severe than type I) Associated with bowing of long bones Some children improve at puberty Light or normal sclerae; may or may not have moderate short stature and joint hyperextensibility Type IVA: dentinogenesis imperfecta absent Type IVB: dentinogenesis imperfecta present

From Gerber L: Rehabilitation of children and infants with osteogenesis imperfecta. Clin Orthop 251:255, 1990.

and multiple fractures with subsequent immobilization. The majority of children with OI ambulate either as functional or household ambulators and approximately 50% walk without any type of assistive device (Gertner, 1990). For those children whose fractures occur after birth, the potential for ambulation is significantly better, with almost 85% ambulating and the rest relying on a wheelchair (Shapiro, 1985).

Medical Management

Diagnosis. Diagnosis of OI is based on clinical manifestations and serologic tests. Bone scans and x-ray films will show evidence of multiple old fractures and skeletal deformities. Skull radiographs show wide sutures with small, irregularly shaped islands of bone called *wormian* bones. Serum alkaline phosphatase is elevated in all forms of the disease. These findings can help exclude child abuse.

Treatment. There is no effective treatment for type II OI. Orthopedic management is central to the overall care. Fracture prevention and control is the primary focus; careful positioning and handling are required to prevent fractures in the neonate. Lightweight braces and splints may also be used to help support the limbs, prevent fractures, and aid in ambulation. Fracture immobilization is as minimal as possible with a maximum of 6 weeks for the lower extremities and 3 to 4 weeks for the upper extremities. Frequently no intervention takes place and the family is advised to maintain proper body alignment and handling techniques to support the affected body part.

The use of intermedullary rods is one way of managing recurring fractures. Indications for this procedure include more than two fractures in the same long bone within a 6-month period, lower extremity bone angles greater than 40 degrees, or very unstable lower extremities in a child ready to walk. These rods must be replaced every 2 to 4 years to accommodate for growth. Osteotomies are also performed to help control rotational deformities, with appropriate bracing to prolong the time period between potential surgeries.

Studies in cell cultures using mice with an antisense gene have raised the possibility that several strategies may be developed to treat OI by converting severe forms of the disease to milder forms (Prockop et al., 1994).

Prognosis. Delivery trauma may lead to intracranial hemorrhage and stillbirth because of the soft skull. Infants born alive may often die suddenly during the first few days or weeks of life, but many survive with normal intelligence. Incomplete and relatively painless fractures after birth that receive no treatment can produce deformities from bones healing in poor alignment. Short stature and deformities give some the appearance of being deformed dwarfs. Milder forms of this condition have fewer clinical problems and these children survive into adulthood.

Special Implications for the Therapist **19-10**

OSTEOGENESIS IMPERFECTA

Precautions

Infants and children with this disorder require careful handling to prevent fractures. They must be supported when they are being turned, positioned, moved, and cuddled or held. Diaper changing must be carried out gently, never lifting the legs by the ankles but rather by gently lifting the buttocks.

With the older child passive ROM exercises should not be used. The child must be encouraged to use full active ROM without force. Strengthening activities should avoid placing weight near joint lines and if manual resistance is applied, long lever arms should be avoided.

Family Education

Educational material and information can be obtained from the Osteoporosis Imperfecta Foundation.* The family must be instructed in handling and positioning techniques. Precautions should be given to avoid lifting the child under the arms or by the hands. The young child should not be tossed into the air or roughhoused in play.

At the same time, families should be encouraged to hold and play with their child appropriately and to develop interests that do not require strenuous physical activity. Fine motor skills are especially encouraged. Swimming is frequently recommended, but the child must be monitored carefully to avoid falls in the shower and pool area. Nonskid aquatic shoes can be worn to assist with this precaution.

Family members must also be instructed to assess for fractures daily. Symptoms to look for include crepitus (the crackling sound produced by the rubbing together of fractured bone fragments), which can be heard or felt, limited use of an extremity, malposition of an extremity, an asymmetrical Moro's reflex, focal swelling or tenderness, or crying when a body part is moved or when the child attempts to move.

Therapy Intervention

Therapy helps to prevent disuse osteoporosis and strengthens muscles to build bone density. Light resistance to exercise or movement can be used; aquatic programs are especially helpful in allowing exercise with light resistance. Strengthening programs emphasize hip extension, hip abduction, trunk extension, and abdominal muscles. A hip extension, hip abduction, and spinal muscular strengthening program complemented by a swimming program two times per week has been found to correlate with an increased ability to assume and maintain an upright position and subsequent ambulation (Bleck, 1981).

Positioning is a significant part of the overall management program for these children. Positioning emphasizes a neutral position of the head, trunk, and lower extremities, neutral hip rotation, and hip extension. In fragile cases, the prone position should be avoided except when fully supported or while being supported in the swimming pool.

The ability to stand is important and should be implemented at approximately 10 to 14 months' chronological age. Standing can be initiated in a standing frame for 30 minutes twice daily. Special care must be taken to avoid fractures when placing and securing the child in the stander. Hydrotherapy can also be used as a medium for initiating standing activities in more severe cases. Throughout any standing activity the therapist must continue to monitor for lower extremity bowing secondary to bone instability.

Mobility

The therapist may have to use a significant amount of creativity to adapt ambulating devices and to accommodate for various musculoskeletal deficiencies while fostering the skills necessary for independent mobility. If ambulation is unlikely, the therapist should not hesitate to move quickly toward a power wheelchair as the child's primary means of mobility. Children as young as 2 years old cognitively can use and benefit from powered mobility.

* Osteoporosis Imperfecta Foundation, Inc., 804 W. Diamond Avenue, Suite 210, Gaithersburg, MD 20878 (301-947-0083).

ARTHROGRYPOSIS MULTIPLEX CONGENITA

Definition and Overview. Arthrogryposis multiplex congenita (AMC) is the presence at birth of multiple congenital contractures in an intact skeleton. There may be contractures either in flexion or extension and the muscles may be nothing more than fibrous bands.

AMC is considered a nonprogressive neuromuscular syndrome. There are three different types of AMC: (1) contracture syndromes, (2) amyoplasia (lack of muscle formation or development), and (3) distal arthrogryposis, primarily affecting the hands and feet. Occasionally the child presents with associated abnormalities such as cleft palate, cardiac lesions, urinary tract malformations, and cryptorchidism (failure of testes to descend into the scrotum).

Incidence and Etiology. AMC affects 1 in 3000 to 4000 births. The absolute causes are unknown, but various investigations have attributed the basic defect to an abnormality of muscle or of the lower motor neuron. Previously there were no known genetic links or hereditary factors, but isolated cases of a new type of autosomal dominant arthrogryposis have been confirmed as a distinct type of AMC (Schrander-Stumpel et al., 1993). Several reports of recurrence within a family point to autosomal recessive inheritance as a possible cause in some cases (Vuopala et al., 1994)

The joint deformities appear to be secondary to a lack of active motion during intrauterine development. Failed terminations of pregnancy resulting in AMC have been reported.[28] Vascular compromise during the attempted termination with secondary loss of functional neurons leading to fetal akinesia

[28] These cases involved incomplete spontaneous miscarriage followed by dilation and curettage and subsequent ongoing pregnancy or medical abortion to end the pregnancy with continued fetal development.

and subsequent contractures is suspected (Hall, 1996). Other possible causes are prenatal viral infection, drugs, maternal hyperthermia, vascular compromise between mother and fetus, and decreased amniotic fluid in utero (oligohydramnios) limiting fetal movement.

Pathogenesis. In all likelihood, AMC is neurogenic as there is histologic and EMG evidence of nervous system involvement. Specifically, there may be a disturbance in the development of the anterior horn cells of motor neurons resulting in variable lesions throughout the spinal cord and variable muscle contractures. These persons usually have a normal muscle spindle with normal sensation but demonstrate fibrofatty changes in the muscle resulting in fibrous tissue and lack of muscle development. The joints are affected with decreased volume in the joint capsules, producing contractures.

Clinical Manifestations. The dominant features of AMC include joint contracture, articular rigidity, and muscle weakness. Arthrogryposis can affect all joints of the body, but tends to have a preference for the feet, hips, wrists, knees, elbows, and shoulders (in order of decreasing frequency). A typical clinical picture of a child with arthrogryposis is outlined in Box 19–8.

Because many of these children demonstrate average or above-average intelligence, they are able to accommodate for loss of motion with a variety of alternative mobility patterns such as seat-scooting or rolling. They usually do not choose (or are unable to assume or maintain) a four-point position.

The jackknife or frog posture will also affect the child's ability to accommodate for movement. Those children with knee flexion (frog-leg posture) are typically slower to roll but quicker to sit and scoot. Many of the children are unable to transition from sitting to standing, but can maintain a standing position once placed upright.

As adults, these persons commonly develop arthritis in a variety of different joints as a result of overuse. Many will eventually require some type of wheeled or powered mobility for long distances because of the wear and tear on malaligned joints and the amount of energy required to move in a malaligned position.

BOX **19–8**
Arthrogryposis: Clinical Picture

Speech, cognition usually within average limits
Facial asymmetry
Oral-motor: hypotonia, congenitally absent muscles, jaw stiffness contribute to oral-motor difficulties
Trunk: thoracolumbar scoliosis (20%), rigid movement, slow responses, minimal rotation, all affecting equilibrium and balance
Lower extremity jackknife posture (55%)
- Flexed dislocated hips with extended knees
- Clubfeet (talipes equinovarus)

Lower extremity frog posture (45%)
- Abducted, externally rotated hips
- Knee flexion
- Clubfeet (talipes equinovarus)

Upper extremity posture
- Shoulder adduction and internal rotation
- Extended elbow, wrist ulnar deviation
- Flexed wrists with stiff straight fingers; poor thumb control

Functional reach impaired requiring multiple muscle substitution, co-contraction of flexors and extensors, use of opposite arm or hand to assist
Delayed motor development
- Sitting independently: approximately 15 months
- Ambulation: approximately 2 to 3 years if musculoskeletal limitations allow

Medical Management

Diagnosis. Definitive diagnosis is made by clinical observation and radiographs, if needed. However, congenital joint contractures may be secondary to many conditions requiring differential diagnosis. The long-term prognosis is good in that this condition is nonprogressive and not life-threatening.[29] Distal arthrogryposis and amyoplastic types of AMC seem to respond best to intervention.

Treatment and Prognosis. Physical and occupational therapy are the mainstays of early treatment with passive mobilization of the joints, positioning, strengthening, and enhancement of functional adaptation skills (e.g., prevention of falls, mobility training, movement up- and downstairs or on uneven terrain).

Orthopedic surgery is often used to address the many musculoskeletal limitations associated with AMC. Some of the more common procedures include posterior spinal fusion for thoracolumbar scoliosis, quadriceps lengthening to increase knee flexion for functional movement, posterior capsulotomies to allow for increased functional knee extension, and distal femoral osteotomies to improve upright skeletal alignment for standing and ambulation.

Multiple operative hip procedures are contraindicated because increased stiffness may be produced with further impairment of motion. The hip dislocations associated with AMC are associated with severe dysplasia of the bones and do not respond to treatment. Affected children are often able to walk with bilateral dislocation of the hips, and in cases of severe rigidity it is better to leave the hips out of joint (Eilert and Georgopoulos, 1995).

Surgeries are timed to coincide with the acquisition of motor skills. For example, a posteromedial surgical release for talipes equinovarus (clubfoot) is considered when the child begins to stand or is already standing (usually before 2 years of age).

For the adult with AMC, the long-term prognosis for physical and vocational independence is poor. Despite normal intelligence, gainful employment is difficult to find.

Special Implications for the Therapist **20-11**

ARTHROGRYPOSIS MULTIPLEX CONGENITA

Precautions

Prolonged casting for correction of deformities is contraindicated in these children because further stiffness is often produced. For this reason, removable

[29] There is an extreme form of AMC called fetal akinesia deformation sequence (FADS) that is lethal pre- or postnatally. The reader is referred elsewhere (Porter, 1995) for further information.

TABLE 19–15 Stages of Legg-Calvé-Perthes Disease

Stage	Time Period	Pathogenesis
Avascular (stage I)	1–3 wk	Spontaneous vascular interruption causes necrosis of the femoral head with degenerative changes; hip synovium and joint capsule are swollen, edematous, and hyperemic; joint space widens
Revascularization (stage II) (fragmentation stage)	6 mo–1 yr	New blood supply causes bone resorption and deposition of new bone cells; deformity from pressure on weakened area occurs; the entire or anterior half of the epiphysis of the femoral head is necrotic; increased blood supply and decalcification of bone causes softening at the junction of the femoral neck and the capital epiphyseal plate is softened; granulation tissue and blood vessels invade the dead bone
Reparative (stage III) (residual stage)	2–3 yr	New bone replaces necrotic bone; the necrotic femoral head is replaced by new bone; collapse and flattening of the femoral head causes the femoral neck to become short and wide
Regenerative (intravascular)	Final months	Completion of healing or regeneration gradually re-forms the head of the femur into live spongy bone; restoration of the femoral head to a normal shape is more likely in younger children and only if the anterior epiphysis was involved

splints such as AFOs are recommended for positioning and stretching. These must be worn a minimum of 6 to 8 hours a day and preferably up to 22 hours per day.

Strengthening

The child will benefit maximally from therapy from 0 to 2 years of age during periodic growth spurts. Strengthening programs focus on weak muscles or movement in opposition to typical resting postures. A general strengthening protocol* would include three to five sets per day, three to five repetitions per set.

* Applying generally accepted and proven treatment principles regarding strengthening is suggested as a place to begin rather than as a definitive model. Research has not clarified the most beneficial exercise protocol for specific pathologic conditions such as this one.

LEGG-CALVÉ-PERTHES DISEASE

Definition and Overview. Legg-Calvé-Perthes disease, also known as coxa plana and osteochondritis deformans juvenilis, is avascular necrosis of the proximal femoral epiphysis. It is the most common of the osteochondroses[30] with flattening of the head of the femur caused by vascular interruption and ischemic necrosis.

This self-limiting condition lasts from 2 to 5 years but can have long-term effects such as premature osteoarthritis in adulthood as a result of misalignment of the acetabulum and flattened femoral head.

Incidence. Legg-Calvé-Perthes disease is usually a unilateral phenomenon affecting boys aged 3 to 12 years (most cases occur between 4 and 8) but it can occur bilaterally. The male-to-female ratio is 5 : 1 and white children are affected 10 times more often than black children.

Etiology and Pathogenesis. Although the pathogenesis of this condition is well understood, the cause or vascular obstructive changes that initiate Legg-Calvé-Perthes disease are not generally agreed upon. Some suspected factors are trauma, inflammation, coagulation defects, and a variety of other causes. This disease involves the replacement of necrotic tissue in a process that takes place in four stages (Table 19–15).

Clinical Manifestations. This condition is characterized by insidious onset, initially presenting as intermittent appearance of a limp on the involved side with hip pain described as soreness or aching with accompanying stiffness. The pain may be present in the groin and along the entire length of the thigh following the path of the obturator nerve or just in the area of the knee. There is usually point tenderness over the hip capsule.

Painful symptoms are aggravated by activity and fatigue and relieved by rest. Clinically, there are decreases in active and passive ROM as well as limited physiologic (accessory) motion. As the condition progresses, atrophy of thigh muscles, external hip rotation, and severely restricted hip abduction and internal rotation develop.

Medical Management

Diagnosis. Physical examination, clinical history, and x-ray examination confirm the diagnosis. MRI is widely accepted as the imaging method of choice; it not only allows early diagnosis but also yields exact staging information in advanced disease which is a requirement for adequate therapy. Aspiration and culture of synovial fluid rule out joint sepsis.

Treatment. The goals of all therapy are to preserve full hip ROM and prevent premature degenerative changes by maintaining a round, well-shaped femoral head that is contained by and congruous with the acetabulum (Hubbard and Dormans, 1995). Initial treatment consists of 1 to 2 weeks of bed rest to reduce inflammation, followed by a balanced approach to weight bearing to protect the joint.

In the past, weight bearing was minimized but more recently therapy allows the child to continue weight bearing with the femur in an abducted and internally rotated position.

[30] Osteochondrosis is a disease of the growth ossification centers in children known by various names depending on the bone involved (e.g., tarsal-navicular = Köhler's bone disease; calcaneus = Sever's disease; second metatarsal head = Freiberg's disease).

Keeping the head of the femur well seated in the acetabulum decreases focal areas of increased load and minimizes distortion, thereby maintaining ROM and preventing deformity. A variety of splints, braces, and positional devices may be used to maintain this position. Conservative treatment is usually continued for 2 to 4 years.

For a young child in the early stages of the disease, surgical correction (e.g., osteotomy and subtrochanteric osteotomy) may be used. With the surgical approach, a hip spica cast is used for 6 to 8 weeks and the child can return to normal activities in 3 to 4 months.

Prognosis. Although the disease is self-limiting, the final outcome is determined by how early the diagnosis is made, that is, the amount of deformity that develops during the time the hip structures are softened. In general, metaphyseal defects, older age, complete involvement of the femoral head, and noncompliance with treatment contribute to a poorer prognosis.

Special Implications for the Therapist **19-12**

LEGG-CALVÉ-PERTHES DISEASE

See Precautions in Special Implications for the Therapist: Congenital Hip Dysplasia, 19-5 regarding handling of the child in a spica cast.

References

Anciaux M, Lenaert A, Van Beneden ML, et al: Transcutaneous electrical stimulation (TCES) for the treatment of adolescent idiopathic scoliosis: Preliminary results. Acta Orthop Belg 57:399–405, 1991.

Asher M: Factors affecting the ambulatory status of patients with spina bifida cystica. J Bone Joint Surg Am 65:350–356, 1983.

Backman E, Hendriksson KG: Low-dose prednisolone treatment in Duchenne and Becker muscular dystrophy. Neuromuscul Disord 5:233–241, 1995.

Barrack R, Wyatt M, Whitecloud T, et al: Vibratory hypersensitivity in idiopathic scoliosis. J Pediatr Orthop 8:389–395, 1988.

Binder H: Rehabilitation management of children with spastic diplegic cerebral palsy. Arch Phys Med Rehabil 70:482–489, 1989.

Bleck EE: A non-operative treatment of osteogenesis imperfecta: Orthotic and mobility management. Clin Orthop 159:111–122, 1981.

Bleck EE: Orthopedic Management of Cerebral Palsy. Philadelphia, WB Saunders, 1979.

Brown SC, Lucy JA: Dystrophin as a mechanochemical transducer in skeletal muscle. Bioassays 15:413–419, 1993.

Byrd J: Current theories on the etiology of idiopathic scoliosis. Clin Orthop 299:114–119, 1988.

Campbell SK: Pediatric consensus statement. Phys Ther 2:121–122, 1990.

Campbell SK (ed): Physical Therapy for Children. Philadelphia, WB Saunders, 1995.

Charney EB: Myelomenigocele. *In* Schwartz MW, Charney EB, Curry TA, et al (eds): Pediatric Primary Care: A Problem-Oriented Approach, ed 2. St Louis, Mosby–Year Book, 1990, pp 660–671.

Cooley SC, Graham JM: Down syndrome—An update and review for the primary pediatrician. Clin Pediatr 30:233–253, 1991.

Cremers MJ, Beijer HJ: No relation between general laxity and atlantoaxial instability in children with Down syndrome. J Pediatr Orthop 13:318–321, 1993.

Cremers MJ, Bol E, de Roos F, et al: Risk of sports activities in children with Down syndrome and atlantoaxial instability. Lancet 342:511–514, 1993.

Daly LE, Kirke PN, Molloy A, et al: Folate levels and neural tube defects: Implications for prevention. JAMA 274:1698–1702, 1995.

Davids J: Congenital muscular torticollis: Sequelae of intrauterine or perinatal compartment syndrome. J Pediatr Orthop 13:141–147, 1993.

Dudgeon D: Variations in mid-lumbar myelodysplasia: Implications for ambulation. Pediat Phys Ther 3:57–62, 1991.

Dunn WW: Pediatric Occupational Therapy: Facilitating Effective Service Provision. Thorofare, NJ, Slack, 1991.

Dyne KM, Valli M, Forlino A, et al: Deficient expression of the small proteoglycan decorin in a case of severe lethal osteogenesis imperfecta. Am J Med Genet 63:161–166, 1996.

Edmonds LD, James LM: Temporal trends in the prevalence of congenital malformations at birth based on the Birth Defects Monitoring Program, United States, 1979–1987. MMWR 39(SS-4):19–23, 1990.

Eilert RE, Georgopoulos G: Orthopedics. *In* Hathaway WE, Hay WW, Groothuis JR, et al (eds): Current Pediatric Diagnosis and Treatment, ed 12. Norwalk, Conn, Appleton & Lange, 1995, pp 786–806.

Emery C: The determinants of treatment duration for congenital muscular torticollis. Phys Ther 74:921–929, 1994.

Engelhardt P, Frohlich D, Magerl F: Atlanto-axial rotational subluxation in children: Therapy in delayed diagnosis. Z Orthop Ihre Grenzgeb 133:196–201, 1995.

Epperson LW: Therapeutic uses of botulinum toxin (Botox). Ala Med 65(5–7):49–50, 1995–1996.

Ervasti JM, Campbell KP: Dystrophin-associated glycoproteins: Their possible roles in the pathogenesis of Duchenne muscular dystrophy. Mol Cell Biol Hum Dis Ser 3:139–166, 1993.

Farley JA, Mooney KH: Alterations of neurologic function in children. *In* McCance KL, Huether SE (eds): Pathophysiology: The Biologic Basis for Disease in Adults and Children, ed 2. St Louis, Mosby–Year Book, 1994, pp 587–625.

Findley T: Ambulation in adolescents with myelodysplasia: Early childhood predictors. Arch Phys Med Rehabil 68:518–522, 1987.

Gertner J: Osteogenesis imperfecta. Orthop Clin North Am 21:151–162, 1990.

Gilfoyle EM, Grady AP, Moore JC: Adapt: A Theory of Sensorimotor Development, ed 2. Thorofare, NJ, Slack, 1993.

Hall JG: Arthrogryposis associated with unsuccessful attempts at termination of pregnancy. Am J Med Genet 63:293–300, 1996.

Hardiman O, Sklar RM, Brown RH Jr: Methylprednisolone selectively affects dystrophin expression in human muscle cultures. Neurology 43:342–345, 1993.

Hauser MA, Chamberlain JS: Progress towards gene therapy for Duchenne muscular dystrophy. J Endocrinol 149:373–378, 1996.

Hertling D, Kessler RM: Management of Common Musculoskeletal Disorders: Physical Therapy Principles and Methods, ed 3. New York, Lippincott-Raven, 1995.

Hinderer KA, Hinderer SR, Shurtleff DB: Myelodysplasia. *In* Campbell SK (ed): Physical Therapy for Children. Philadelphia, WB Saunders, 1995.

Hubbard AM, Dormans JP: Evaluation of developmental dysplasia, Perthes disease, and neuromuscular dysplasia of the hip in children before and after surgery: An imaging update. AJR 164:1067–1073, 1995.

Koman O: Management of cerebral palsy with botulin toxin: Preliminary investigation. J Pediatr Orthop 13:489–495, 1993.

Kottke FJ, Lehmann JF: Krusen's Handbook of Physical Medicine and Rehabilitation, ed 4. Philadelphia, WB Saunders, 1990.

Krengel WF, King HA: Scoliosis: Diagnostic basics and therapeutic choices. J Musculoskel Med 12:54–69, 1995.

Kurtz LA, Scull SA: Rehabilitation for developmental disabilities. Pediatr Clin North Am 40:629–643, 1993.

Lawrence T: Congenital muscular torticollis: A spectrum of pathology. Ann Plast Surg 23:523–530, 1989.

Leiden JM: Gene therapy—Promise, pitfalls, and prognosis. N Engl J Med 333:871–873, 1995.

Liptak G: Mobility age for children with high level myelomeningocele: Parapodium versus wheelchair. Dev Med Child Neurol 34:787–796, 1992.

Litman RS, Zerngast BA, Perkins FM: Preoperative evaluation of the cervical spine in children with trisomy-21: Results of a questionnaire study. Paediatr Anaesth 5:355–361, 1995.

Locke MD, Sarwark JP: Orthopedic aspects of myelodysplasia in children. Curr Opin Pediatr 8:65–67, 1996.

Lonstein JE, Winter RB: Adolescent idiopathic scoliosis. Nonoperative treatment. Orthop Clin North Am 19:239–246, 1988.

Lu CS, Chen RS, Tsai CH: Double-blind, placebo-controlled study of botulinum toxin injections in the treatment of cervical dystonia. J Formos Med Assoc 94:189–192, 1995.

Luthy DA, Wardinsky T, Shurtleff DB, et al: Cesarean section before the onset of labor and subsequent motor function in infants with myelomingocele diagnosed internally. N Engl J Med 324:662–666, 1991.

Macphail H: The effect of isokinetic strength training on functional mobility and walking efficiency in adolescents with cerebral palsy. Dev Med Child Neurol 37:763–776, 1995.

Magee DJ: Orthopedic Physical Assessment, ed 3. Philadelphia, WB Saunders, 1996.

Mateos F: Duchenne muscular dystrophy: Clinical analysis and prospects of genetic therapy. Rev Neurol 23(suppl 3):S404–407, 1995.

Matsumura K, Campbell KP: Dystrophin-glycoprotein complex: Its role in the molecular pathogenesis of dystrophies. Muscle Nerve 17:2–15, 1994.

Matsumura L, Ohlendieck K, Ionasescu W, et al: The role of dystrophin-glycoprotein complex in the molecular pathogenetics of muscular dystrophies. Neuromuscul Disord 3:533–535, 1993.

Mazur J: Orthopedic management of high level spina bifida. J Bone Joint Surg [Am] 71:56–61, 1989.

McCool FD, Tzelepis GE: Inspiratory muscle training in the patient with neuromuscular disease. Phys Ther 75:1006–1014, 1995.

McCullough FL: Alterations in musculoskeletal function in children. *In* McCance KL, Huether SE (eds): Pathophysiology: The Biologic Basis for Disease in Adults and Children, ed 2. St Louis, Mosby–Year Book, 1994, pp 1482–1509.

McDonald C: Ambulatory outcome with myelodysplasia: Effect of lower extremity muscle strength. Dev Med Child Neurol 22:482–490, 1991.

Mendell JR, Kissel JT, Amato AA, et al: Myoblast transfer in the treatment of Duchenne's muscular dystrophy. N Engl J Med 333:832–838, 1995.

Merlini L, Granata C, Capelli T, et al: Natural history of infantile and childhood spinal muscular atrophy. *In* Merlini L, Granata C, Dubowitz V (eds.): Current Concepts in Childhood Spinal Muscular Atrophy. New York, Springer-Verlag, 1989, pp 95–100.

Moe PG, Seay AR: Neurologic and muscular disorders. *In* Hathaway WE, Hay WW, Groothuis JR, et al: Current Pediatric Diagnosis and Treatment, ed 12. Norwalk, Conn, Appleton & Lange, 1995, pp 710–785.

Morton RE, Khan MA, Murray-Leslie C, et al: Atlantoaxial instability in Down's syndrome: A five-year follow-up study. Arch Dis Child 72:115–118, 1995.

Myhr U: A five year follow up of functional sitting position in children with cerebral palsy. Dev Med Child Neurol 37:587–596, 1995.

Norris J (ed): Professional Guide to Diseases, ed 5. Springhouse, Pa, Springhouse, 1995.

Notelovitz M: Osteoporosis: Screening, prevention, and management. Fertil Steril 59:707–725, 1993.

Porter HJ: Lethal arthrogryposis multiplex congenital (fetal akinesia deformation sequence, FADS). Pediatr Pathol Lab Med 15:617–637, 1995.

Prockop DJ, Kulvaniemi H, Tromp G: Molecular basis of osteogenesis imperfecta and related disorders of bone. Clin Plast Surg 21:407–413, 1994.

Resnick F: Diagnosis of Bone and Joint Disorders. Philadelphia, WB Saunders, 1995.

Rizzolo S, Lemos MJ, Mason DE: Posterior spinal arthrodesis for atlantoaxial instability in Down syndrome. J Pediatr Orthop 15:543–548, 1995.

Samuel D, Thomas DM, Tierney PA, et al: Atlanto-axial subluxation (Grisel's syndrome) following otolaryngological diseases and procedures. J Laryngol Otol 109:1005–1009, 1995.

Schrander-Stumpel CT, Howeler CJ, Reekers AD, et al: Arthrogryposis, ophthalmoplegia, and retinopathy: Confirmation of a new type of arthrogryposis. J Med Genet 30:78–80, 1993.

Shapiro F: Consequences of osteogenesis imperfecta: Diagnosis for survival and ambulation. J Pediatr Orthop 5:456–462, 1985.

Sharkey M: The effects of early referral and intervention on the developmentally disabled infant: An evaluation at eighteen months of age. J Am Board Fam Pract 3:163–170, 1990.

Shurtleff D: Decubitus Formations and Skin Breakdown in Myelodysplasia: Significance, Prevalence, and Treatment. Orlando, Fla, Grune & Stratton, 1986.

Slate RK, Posnick JC, Armstrong DC, et al: Cervical spine subluxation associated with congenital muscular torticollis and craniofacial asymmetry. Plast Reconstr Surg 91:1187–1195, 1993.

Smith R: Early development of boys with Duchenne's muscular dystrophy. Dev Med Child Neurol 32:519–527, 1990.

Spiegel R, Hagmann A, Boltshauser E, et al: Molecular genetic diagnosis and deletion analysis in Type I–III spinal muscular atrophy. Schweiz Med Wochenschr 126:907–914, 1996.

Stuberg W: Muscular dystrophy and spinal muscular therapy. *In* Campbell SK (ed): Physical Therapy For Children. Philadelphia, WB Saunders, 1995, pp 295–324.

Tardieu C: For how long must the soleus muscle be stretched each day to prevent contracture? Dev Med Child Neurol 30:3–10, 1988.

Travell JG, Simons DG: Myofascial Pain and Dysfunction: The Trigger Point Manual, vol I. Baltimore, Williams & Wilkins, 1983.

Van Zandijcke M: Cervical dystonia (spasmodic torticollis). Some aspects of the natural history. Acta Neurol Belg 95:210–215, 1995.

Vuopala K, Leisti J, Herva R: Lethal arthrogryposis in Finland—A clinical-pathological study of 83 cases during thirteen years. Neuropediatrics 25:308–315, 1994.

Weinstein SL: Scoliosis. Semin Spine Surg 4:186–265, 1991.

Weinstein SL, Tharp BR: Etiology and timing of static encephalopathies of childhood (cerebral palsy). Dev Med Child Neurol 31:766–773, 1989.

Willers U: Long term results of Boston brace treatment on vertebral rotation. Spine 18:472–475, 1993.

Williams CR, O'Flynn E, Clarke NM, et al: Torticollis secondary to ocular pathology. J Bone Joint Surg [Br] 78:620–624, 1996.

Wong DL: Whaley and Wong's Essentials of Pediatric Nursing, ed 4. St Louis, Mosby–Year Book, 1993.

SECTION 3

chapter 20

Metabolic Disorders

William G. Boissonnault

Metabolic disorders can affect numerous body tissues. The disorders physical therapists are most likely to encounter clinically are those involving bony structures. Metabolic diseases of bone also tend to be the most disabling and costly to the client and society.

The skeletal system serves numerous functions in the human body. Bone is the primary storage depot for calcium, phosphate, sodium, and magnesium. Bones are the hosts for the hemopoietic bone marrow (growth and development of elements of blood; see Chapter 11). Bones also serve important mechanical functions such as protection of components of the nervous system and visceral organs; provision of rigid internal support for the trunk and extremities; and provision of attachment sites for numerous soft tissue structures. Bone is constantly remodeling throughout life. While osteoclasts resorb the existing bone, new bone is being formed by osteoblasts. There are three primary influences on this remodeling process: (1) mechanical stresses; (2) calcium and phosphate levels in the extracellular fluid; and (3) hormonal levels of parathyroid hormone, calcitonin, vitamin D, cortisol, growth hormone, thyroid hormone, and sex hormones (Gunta, 1994).

Metabolic bone disease is typically manifested by diffuse loss of bone density and bone strength, but there can be increased bone density yet decreased bone strength (e.g., in Paget's disease). Significant disability , marked by bone pain, postural deformity, and fracture, can occur secondary to these bony changes. The commonly observed accentuated thoracic spine kyphosis in clients with vertebral collapse secondary to osteoporosis can compromise cardiopulmonary function. This compromise could impair the patient's ability to participate in a rehabilitation program. The spine and extremity deformities associated with this group of diseases can result in increased mechanical stress on bony and soft tissue structures manifested by pain. Decreased bone strength can be present without postural deformity though and yet be sufficient to cause pain as the person attempts to participate in activities of daily living. The bone is now mechanically inadequate to withstand what once were normal stress levels.

The most serious, potentially life-threatening, and costly complication of metabolic bone disease is fracture. It is estimated that osteoporosis alone is responsible for more than 1.3 million fractures annually (National Osteoporosis Foundation, 1991). The monetary cost of these fractures is projected to reach an estimated $31 to $62 billion in the United States by the year 2020 (Cummings et al., 1990). Approximately 250,000 osteoporosis-related hip fractures occur annually in the United States (Raisz, 1989; Raisz and Rodan, 1990). Deaths related to hip fractures alone were estimated to reach 20,000 to 30,000 in 1993, making it the leading cause of orthopedic mortality (Robb, 1993).

Therapists have an important role in the primary prevention of disability secondary to the complications associated with metabolic bone disease. Client education regarding posture, body mechanics, and proper exercise is an important component of any prevention program. Physical therapy intervention is also a vital part of the rehabilitation of clients disabled by the resultant pain or postural deformities that can accompany these diseases. Therapists also treat many clients who have suffered traumatic injury precipitated by the presence of metabolic bone disease. Lastly, therapists treat clients with a primary diagnosis of low back, knee, or shoulder conditions and osteoporosis is present as a secondary diagnosis. The presence of such a secondary diagnosis may influence the therapist's choice of evaluation and treatment techniques. A thorough understanding of this group of diseases will enable the therapist to treat clients safely and effectively.

OSTEOPOROSIS

Definition. The term *osteoporosis* applies to a group of disorders which have as their common denominator a reduction of bone mass per unit of bone volume (Schiller, 1994). The disorders can be classified as primary or secondary osteoporosis. (Box 20–1.) Included in the *primary osteoporosis* category is idiopathic osteoporosis, which occurs in children and young adults with normal gonadal function. Postmenopausal osteoporosis (the most common type) and senile or involutional osteoporosis also fall under the heading of primary osteoporosis. Both are associated with the aging process. Osteoporosis is also associated with other disorders and when this occurs, the term *secondary osteoporosis* applies. Examples of these disorders are endocrine conditions such as hyperthyroidism, hyperparathyroidism, hypogonadism, Cushing's disease, and diabetes mellitus. Other relevant disorders are chronic renal failure, rheumatoid arthritis, malabsorption syndrome related to gastrointestinal and hepatic disease, chronic respiratory disease, malignancies, and chronic alcohol dependency (Gunta, 1994; Hahn, 1993; Schiller, 1994).

Incidence. Osteoporosis is by far the most common metabolic bone disease, affecting approximately 25 million people living in the United States (National Osteoporosis Foundation, 1991). The disease is much more common in females. The disease most commonly affects white women, and 30% to 45% of white women over the age of 45 will be affected (AAOS, 1988; Baran, 1994).

Risk Factors and Pathogenesis. Box 20–2 lists the risk factors associated with osteoporosis. Age, sex, heredity, and race are important risk factors. Between the ages of 25 and

BOX **20-1**
Classification of Osteoporosis

Primary
- Idiopathic
- Postmenopausal
- Senile

Secondary
- Endocrine disorders
  - Hyperthyroidism
  - Hyperparathyroidism
  - Type II diabetes
  - Cushing's disease
  - Hypogonadism
- Malabsorption syndrome
  - Gastrointestinal disease
  - Hepatic disease
- Chronic renal failure
- Rheumatoid arthritis
- Chronic respiratory disease
- Neoplasms
- Chemical dependency (alcohol)
- Amenorrhea

BOX **20-2**
Risk Factors Associated with Osteoporosis

- Age 50 yr and older
- Female sex
- White race
- Post menopause
- Northern European ancestry
- Thin, small, bony body frame
- Familial history of osteoporosis
- Long periods of inactivity, immobilization
- Long-term intake of
  - Alcohol
  - Tobacco
  - Caffeine
- Long-term use of
  - Corticosteroids
  - Heparin
  - Antacids
  - Laxatives
  - Anticonvulsants
- Diet deficiencies of
  - Calcium
  - Vitamin D
- Medical history of
  - Malabsorption secondary to gastrointestinal and hepatic disease
  - Hyperthyroidism
  - Hyperparathyroidism
  - Hypogonadism
  - Chronic pulmonary disease
  - Cancer
  - Rheumatoid arthritis
  - Diabetes mellitus

35 years, bone mass peaks and the rate of bone resorption begins to exceed the rate of bone formation (Schiller, 1994). This physiologic mismatch can progress to a point at which osteopenia (decreased bone density) may be noted radiographically and a diagnosis of osteoporosis made. Postmenopausal females are at higher risk to develop the disease. Diagnosis of primary postmenopausal osteoporosis occurs with increasing frequency from age 51 to 75 years (Rauscher, 1993). The increased risk of osteoporosis related to menopause is due primarily to the decreased production of estrogen. Decreased intestinal calcium absorption, increased bone resorption to compensate for low calcium levels, and impaired osteoblastic activity have all been associated with estrogen deficiency (Baran, 1994). An estimated 11% of bone loss occurs during the first 5 years after menopause, and an additional 5% loss occurs during the next 20 years (Nordin et al., 1990).

Race is also a factor because bone mass correlates positively with skin pigmentation. Whites have the least amount of bone mass, whereas blacks have the greatest amount (Gordon and Vaughn, 1980). Peak bone mass is also generally higher in males. Therefore, black men are at lowest risk of developing osteoporosis. Because white women generally have lower peak bone mass, the complications of the bone loss associated with aging can affect them earlier in life.

Body build is related to bone fragility. Thin women have less cortical bone (Daniell, 1976; Tylavsky et al., 1989) and are therefore at greater risk of fractures (Kleerekoper et al., 1989). Obesity, by increasing the mechanical strain on bone, may result in increased peak bone mass, reducing bone fragility. In addition, obesity increases the amount of biologically available estrogen, protecting against fracture (Cummings et al., 1985). Women with a family history of osteoporosis are at high risk of developing osteoporotic fractures (Bouillon et al., 1991).

Inactivity and immobilization have been associated with decreased bone formation. The prolonged inactivity results in reduced gravitational and muscular forces acting on the skeletal system. The decreased mechanical stress on bony structures alters bone physiology, resulting in decreased bone mass (Baran, 1994; Deitrich et al., 1948; Donaldson et al., 1970; Whedon, 1984).

Cigarette smoking has been reported as a risk factor for spinal and hip fractures (Seeman et al., 1983; Wickham et al., 1989). Smoking was associated with a 5% to 10% reduction of bone mass in women.[1] This reduction is sufficient to increase the risk of fracture (Hopper and Seeman, 1994). Chronic alcohol abuse has been linked to the development of osteoporosis by directly inhibiting osteoblastic activity and possibly inhibiting calcium resorption (Schapira, 1990).

Long-term use of medications, including corticosteroids, has been associated with the presence of osteoporosis. Corticosteroids impair osteoblastic activity and the maturation of preosteoblastic cells to osteoblasts, increase osteoclastic activity, and impair vitamin D–dependent intestinal calcium absorption, which can result in secondary hyperparathyroidism. The hyperparathyroidism increases bone resorption and

[1] Hypotheses for this association include a reduction in levels of circulating estrogens, calcitonin resistance, and interference with osteoblastic function.

decreases renal resorption of calcium, thereby increasing the amount of calcium excretion (Gunta, 1994; Schiller, 1994).

Clinical Manifestations. Back pain and fracture are the most common presenting features of osteoporosis (Gunta, 1994; Rauscher, 1993). These may or may not be associated with postural changes. Marked thoracic spine kyphosis and loss of overall body height are common findings following a vertebral compression fracture (Fig. 20–1). Similarly, bone loss in the mandible can contribute to changes in facial appearance.

Medical Management

Diagnosis. Most patients are unaware they have osteoporosis until a fracture occurs (Hahn, 1993; Rauscher, 1993; Schiller, 1994). The radiograph that demonstrates the fracture also reveals the osteopenia leading to the diagnosis of osteoporosis (Fig. 20–2). The vertebral bodies, ribs, radius, and femur are the most common fracture sites (Gunta, 1994; Hahn, 1993). Histologically, there is a thinning of cortical bone and a reduction in the number and size of the trabeculae of cancellous bone. Thirty percent or greater bone density loss must occur before such abnormalities can be noted on an x-ray film. A computed tomographic (CT) scan is a more accurate and sensitive indicator of bone loss, but it is more expensive and exposes the client to higher doses of radiation. Once osteopenia is noted, other causes of metabolic bone disease must be ruled out, including hyperthyroidism, hyperparathyroidism, osteomalacia, testicular failure, malignancies, and so forth. Once these conditions are ruled out, tests such as single and dual photon absorptiometry, dual energy x-ray absorptiometry, and quantitative CT are utilized to obtain baseline bone density levels.

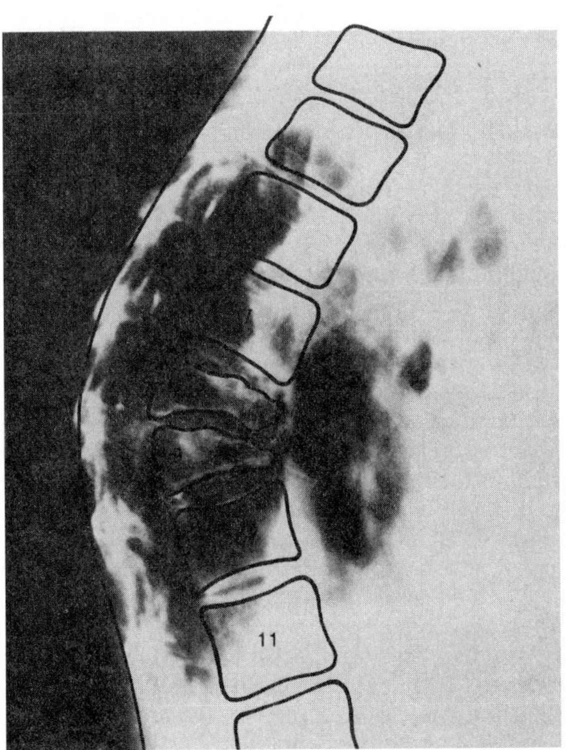

Figure 20–1. Increased thoracic kyphosis with vertebral collapse secondary to osteoporosis. (*From Richardson JK, Iglarsh ZA: Clinical Orthopaedic Physical Therapy. Philadelphia, WB Saunders, 1994.*)

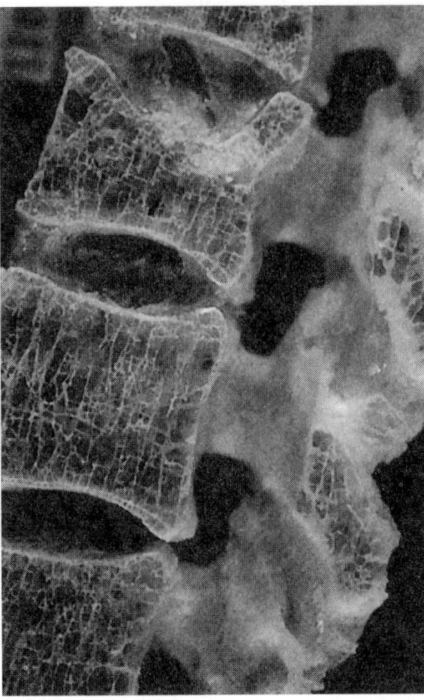

Figure 20–2. Decreased bone density of vertebrae with compression fracture. (*From Schiller AL: Bones and joints. In Rubin E, Farber JL (eds): Pathology, ed 2. Philadelphia, JB Lippincott, 1994, p 1302.*)

Single photon absorptiometry assesses bone mass by measuring the transmission of γ-rays through bone. A narrow pencil-width beam of radiation is passed across a long bone (usually the distal radius) and the absorption profile of the beam is recorded. The bone mass levels are directly related to the degree of beam absorption by the bone. The limitations of this modality are inability to differentiate cortical vs. trabecular bone and to measure the spine and femur.

Dual photon and dual energy x-ray absorptiometry assess bone mass by measuring the transmission of a narrow γ-ray and x-ray beam, respectively, through bone, most often the proximal femur or lumbar spine. Bone density is calculated by dividing the bone mineral content by the projected area of the scanned region. In dual photon absorptiometry, the energy source emits photons of two different energies. In dual energy x-ray absorptiometry, the x-ray tube is pulsed between high and low. The primary disadvantage of this modality is the inability to differentiate cortical from trabecular bone. Single and dual photon absorptiometry are used as inexpensive diagnostic tools in osteoporosis screening programs (Gunta, 1994).

Quantitative CT differentiates between cortical and trabecular bone. The disadvantages include increased radiation exposure and bone marrow fat content affecting measurement accuracy (Baran, 1994).

Treatment. Because there is no cure for osteoporosis, the best treatment is prevention. There is an overlap between the treatment modalities designed to prevent abnormal bone loss and those designed to retard the pathophysiologic process (inhibitory) once the disease is present.

Besides eliminating factors such as chronic alcohol abuse and cigarette smoking, a key to prevention is developing as great a peak bone mass as possible through adequate calcium intake and regular exercise. Reports suggest that premenopausal women need over 1000 mg and postmenopausal women need over 1500 mg of calcium daily. The average calcium intake of postmenopausal women is 400 to 500 mg/day, well below the recommended levels (Dawson-Hughes et al., 1990; Holbrook et al., 1988).

Exactly how much benefit can be gained from given levels or types of exercise remains unclear, but the consensus is that regular exercise has a positive effect on bone mass levels (Hahn, 1993; Orwall, 1994; Schiller, 1994). Weight-bearing exercises such as walking and jogging stress the skeletal system, resulting in larger bone mass. Swimmers also have higher mineral densities than those of control groups (Block et al., 1989; Orwall et al., 1989). The suggestion remains that weight-bearing exercises are associated with greater changes in bone remodeling and mass (Davee et al., 1990). Persons with sedentary lifestyles are at higher risk of bone loss and fracture.

Loss of ovarian function due to menopause or oophorectomy is associated with an increased rate of bone loss. Estrogen is commonly administered as a preventive measure. Androgens are used similarly in hypogonadal men. Other agents used to treat osteoporosis include calcium, vitamin D, calcitonin, biphosphonates (including etidronate disodium), and fluoride. Calcium is required for bone mineralization and also suppresses bone turnover, slowing the remodeling process. Vitamin D (800 units/day) is advocated to assist in maximal absorption of dietary calcium. Calcitonin acts directly on osteoclasts, suppressing activity. Biphosphates inhibit both bone generation and resorption with a greater effect on the resorption process. Unlike the above-described agents, fluoride can activate osteoblasts, increasing bone formation, but the quality of the bone is questioned because there is not a concurrent reduction in fracture rates (Riggs et al., 1990).

Special Implications for the Therapist **20–1**

OSTEOPOROSIS

The clinical implications of osteoporosis are varied, numerous, and significant. Considering the prevalence of primary osteoporosis, as well as the prevalence of diseases osteoporosis can be associated with, therapists will encounter this disease frequently.

Therapists have an important role in prevention. As mentioned, exercise is considered to have an important role in maintaining and possibly increasing peak bone mass and theoretically should be started early in life to minimize the risks of osteoporosis. The level of exercise must be maintained because the benefits are lost if exercise is discontinued (Hahn, 1993). To minimize the risk of development of musculoskeletal repetitive overuse syndromes, education regarding the proper use of exercise equipment, proper body mechanics, variety in the exercise program, and awareness of warning signs of overuse injuries is essential. Exercising excessively can have detrimental effects. For example, women who exercise to the point of amenorrhea may lose bone rapidly, enhancing the risk of developing osteoporosis (Fahy et al., 1994; Prior et al., 1990).

Therapists also have a role in the prevention of the most serious complication associated with osteoporosis: fracture. A rehabilitation program designed to improve flexibility, balance, and strength may help prevent falls. Choosing the appropriate gait assistive device and teaching the patient how to use the walker, cane, and other aids properly could also prevent injury. Educating the patient and family regarding home ambulatory hazards such as throw rugs, faulty footwear, and so on is important.

In patients with known osteoporosis or those at high risk of having the disease, caution should be taken with certain evaluation and treatment techniques. For example, utilizing a posteroanterior pressure technique at the thorax for provocation and mobility assessment with the patient positioned prone is risky. In the prone position the thorax is stabilized anteriorly by the table and with the therapist applying pressure over the posterior thorax significant stress levels could develop in the rib cage, possibly resulting in a fracture. The same risk applies if the therapist uses this technique for manipulation. Although it is important that provocation and mobility information be collected and joint dysfunction treated in these patients to improve their functional abilities, precautions must be taken, including using other techniques or altering the patient's position (side-lying or sitting, for example) so that the anterior thorax is not stabilized.

Therapists should be aware of the symptoms and signs associated with osteoporosis as they may be in a position to refer a patient to a physician for examination based on a change in the patient's status. For example, a 65-year-old woman being treated for a rotator cuff disorder may report the onset of sharp midthoracic pain associated with sneezing since her last visit, and she now notes a constant dull ache in the area. In addition, the client and therapist note an increase in the thoracic kyphosis. Communication with a physician regarding these clinical changes is warranted due to the concern about a possible fracture.

As with other metabolic bone diseases, delayed healing and poor retention of internal fixation devices following fracture can occur in clients with osteoporosis. Postoperatively, the response to rehabilitation may be slowed and adjustments may have to be made in the program to protect the injured area as recovery takes place. Close communication with the physician is called for to ensure patient safety.

The medical interventions for the prevention or treatment of osteoporosis also have implications for the therapist. Medication side effects may occur at any time and may warrant communication with the physician. Box 20–3 lists the side effects of estrogens. Estrogen therapy has been associated with blood clots, heart attack, and stroke (see Chapter 10) and breast and endometrial cancer (see Chapter 17). To reduce the risk of endometrial carcinoma, estrogen is taken with a progestin (Fitzgerald, 1994). Clients with a history of these conditions are at greater risk of developing side effects. Nevertheless, hormone replacement therapy has

BOX **20–3**
Side Effects of Estrogens*

Sudden onset of or change in headache, coordination, vision, breathing, speech, or extremity strength or sensation.*
Chest pain*
Groin or calf pain*
Change in vaginal bleeding
Urinary incontinence
Increased blood pressure
Breast discharge or lumps
Skin rash
Extremity edema
Jaundice
Abdominal pain
Tremors

* The above side effects warrant communication with a physician. Those marked with an asterisk call for *immediate* communication.

an important role in reducing the rate of bone mass loss as well as reducing the risk of developing cardiovascular disease (Barrett-Connor and Bush, 1991; Philosophe and Seibel, 1991). Calcium supplements are also commonly used. A side effect of these agents that warrants immediate communication with a physician is urinary dysfunction. Mild diarrhea or constipation or a chalky taste that does not resolve should be brought to a physician's attention. A major advantage of calcitonin is the lack of significant side effects. Nausea is the primary side effect and cost and route of administration (subcutaneous) are major disadvantages (Baran, 1994).

OSTEOMALACIA

Definition. In contrast to osteoporosis, which results in a loss of bone mass and brittle bones, osteomalacia results in a softening of bone without loss of bone matrix. Osteomalacia is a generalized bone condition in which insufficient mineralization of the bone matrix results from calcium and/or phosphate deficiency. The disease is sometimes referred to as the adult form of rickets.

Etiology. The two primary causes of osteomalacia are insufficient intestinal calcium absorption and increased renal phosphorus losses. The insufficient calcium absorption could occur because of either a lack of calcium or a resistance to the action of vitamin D. The increased renal phosphorus losses can occur secondary to renal tubular defects. In addition, the long-term use of antacids[2] and the presence of longstanding hyperparathyroidism can lead to phosphate deficiencies which can contribute to the development of osteomalacia.

Incidence and Risk Factors. Diseases of the small intestine, cholestatic disorders of the liver, biliary obstruction, and chronic pancreatic insufficiency increase the risk of developing osteomalacia. These conditions adversely affect the absorption of calcium and the action of vitamin D (Schiller, 1994). The incidence of osteomalacia is greater in the world's colder regions. This is related to decreased exposure to sunlight, affecting vitamin D levels. Osteomalacia is seen with greater frequency in cultures where the diet is vitamin D–deficient (e.g., northern China, Japan, and northern India). Osteomalacia is common in the elderly owing to calcium and vitamin D–deficient diets. This situation is worsened by the intestinal malabsorption problems associated with aging (Gunta, 1994). Long-term use of commonly prescribed medications also increases the risk of developing osteomalacia. Anticonvulsant medications such as phenobarbitol and phenytoin accelerate breakdown of the active forms of vitamin D by inducing hepatic hydroxylases. As mentioned, antacids can cause phosphate deficiency (Gunta, 1994). Box 20–4 summarizes the risk factors associated with osteomalacia.

Pathogenesis. Demineralization results in an exaggeration of the osteoid seams, including their thickness and the proportion of trabecular surface covered (Fig. 20–3). As the osteoid accumulates, bone strength declines. These exaggerated seams occur due to the excessive time lag between collagen deposition and the appearance of the calcium salt. Areas of abundant osteoid appear radiologically as radiolucent stripes. These so-called pseudofractures are characteristic of the Milkman syndrome (Schiller, 1994). The areas of pseudofracture, which most commonly occur on the concave side of long bones, the ischial and pubic rami, and the ribs and scapula, may function as mechanical stress points allowing true fractures to develop.

Clinical Manifestations. The diagnosis of osteomalacia is difficult and often delayed because many patients present initially with diffuse, generalized aching and fatigue. Proximal myopathy and sensory polyneuropathy may also be present, resulting in a confusing clinical presentation. Bone pain and

BOX **20–4**
Risk Factors Associated with Osteomalacia

Old age
Residence in cold geographic area
Vitamin D deficiency
Gastrectomy
Intestinal malabsorption associated with
- Diseases of the small intestine
- Cholangiolitic disorders of the liver
- Biliary obstruction
- Chronic pancreatic insufficiency

Long-term use of
- Anticonvulsants
- Tranquilizers
- Sedatives
- Muscle relaxants
- Diuretics
- Antacids containing aluminum hydroxide

History of
- Hyperparathyroidism
- Chronic renal failure
- Renal tubular defects

[2] Antacids containing aluminum hydroxide bind with dietary forms of phosphate to prevent gastrointestinal absorption.

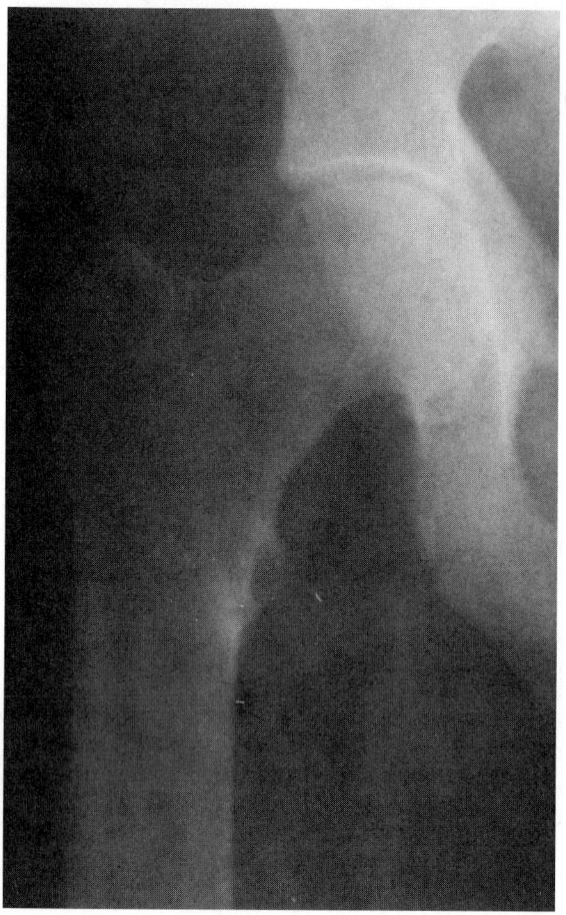

Figure **20–3.** Osteomalacia of the femur. Note the loss of the sharp interface between cortical bone and cancellous bone caused by demineralization of the cortex. (*From Richardson JK, Iglarsh ZA: Clinical Orthopaedic Physical Therapy. Philadelphia, WB Saunders, 1994.*)

periarticular tenderness can occur in the spine, ribs, pelvis, and proximal extremities.

The combination of muscle weakness and softening of bone contributes to postural deformities, including increased thoracic kyphosis, a heart-shaped pelvis, and marked bowing of the femora and tibiae. The muscular weakness may lead to a waddling gait and difficulties with transitional movements, such as rising from sitting to standing and moving into and out of bed (Gunta, 1994; Hahn, 1994).

Medical Management

Diagnosis. Numerous methods are used to diagnose osteomalacia, including radiographs, bone scan, bone biopsy, and a laboratory workup (blood tests and urinalysis). Radiologically, osteomalacia, like osteoporosis, may present as osteopenia. A bone biopsy may be done at the site of osteopenia to evaluate the bone matrix. Besides osteopenia, radiolucent bands in the bone cortex (Looser's zones) may be revealed radiographically (Gunta, 1994).

Although not occurring nearly as frequently as in osteoporosis, acute fracture may be what leads to the diagnosis of osteomalacia. The radius, femur, vertebral bodies, ribs, and pubic ramus are common sites of fracture.

Serum for levels of calcium, albumin, phosphate, alkaline phosphatase, and parathyroid hormone are also obtained. Lastly, urine is collected to assess calcium and phosphate excretion rates (Fitzgerald, 1994).

Treatment. The treatment of osteomalacia depends on the cause. If inadequate nutrition is the problem, strengthening the dietary regimen with calcium and vitamin D may be sufficient. If osteomalacia is a result of intestinal malabsorption, treatment is directed to correct the primary disease. (See Chapter 13 for a description of these diseases.) Phosphate supplementation can be prescribed in the presence of renal phosphate wasting. If utilized, vitamin D must be given to enhance calcium absorption impaired by the phosphate.

Special Implications for the Therapist **20–2**

OSTEOMALACIA

There is considerable overlap between osteomalacia and osteoporosis regarding implications for the therapist. The reader is directed to the section associated with osteoporosis for the discussion of prevention of fracture, patient injury during examination and treatment, recognition of possible fracture, postoperative care, and side effects of calcium agents.

PAGET'S DISEASE

Definition. Although not a true metabolic disease, Paget's disease, or osteitis deformans, is placed in this chapter because of the many similarities between it and metabolic bone diseases. Paget's disease is a progressive disorder of the adult skeletal system marked by abnormal bone remodeling. Initially, excessive bone resorption occurs followed by disorganized and excessive bone formation.

Etiology. The cause of Paget's disease is unknown. Sir James Paget, who described the disease over a century ago, thought it was likely a bone infection. A more recent theory proposes that a virus associated with osteoclasts that remains dormant for years may be responsible (Schiller, 1994; Wallach, 1982).

Incidence and Risk Factors. Paget's disease is a common disease of the elderly. Approximately 3% of the population over the age of 40 and 10% of those over 70 years may be affected (Daliuka et al., 1983). The disease is frequently familial and has an unusual geographic distribution. Populations of the British Isles and countries where migration occurred from Britain (the United States, Australia, New Zealand, and Canada) have a greater incidence. The disease is almost nonexistent in Asia and in the native African and South American populations (Schiller, 1994).

Pathogenesis. Paget's disease begins insidiously and progresses slowly. There is an initial osteoclastic, resorptive stage where abnormal osteoclasts proliferate. The bone resorption is so rapid that osteoblastic activity cannot keep up and fibrous tissue replaces bone. Radiologically, the resultant lytic areas are sharply defined and flame- or wedge-shaped. The initial resorption is followed by abnormal regeneration called the osteoblastic sclerotic phase. The normal cancellous architecture is replaced by coarse, thickened struts of trabecular bone, and the cortical bone is irregularly thickened, rough, and pitted. The abnormal arrangement of the lamellar bone, separated by so-called cement lines, gives the bone the look of a mosaic. Although heavily calcified, the bone is now enlarged but weakened. Involvement of the vertebral bodies presents with a picture frame appearance radiologically as the cortical shell and end plates become greatly exaggerated in comparison to the coarse, cancellous bone portion of the vertebral body (Fig. 20–4). The final stage of the disease is characterized by little cellular activity (Gunta, 1994; Schiller, 1994).

The progressive deossification that weakens the bony structure primarily affects the axial skeleton. The lesions occur at multiple sites, particularly the skull, spine, and pelvis. The proximal femur and tibia may also be involved. Pathologic fractures can occur, especially in the proximal femora, pelvis, and lumbar spine.

Clinical Manifestations. Approximately 20% of people with Paget's disease are asymptomatic (Wallach, 1982). The most common symptom is pain, which is described as a deep ache, accentuated at night. If the skull is involved, the client may complain of headaches, tinnitus, vertigo, and hearing loss. The pain is thought to be related to microfractures, hypervascularity, or to weakened bones being excessively stressed mechanically. The hearing loss may be related to involvement of the ossicles or bony foraminal encroachment of the eighth cranial nerve. Clients may also experience fatigue, lightheadedness, and general stiffness. New onset of pain may be related to pathologic fracture of the vertebral bodies, pelvis, or long bones.

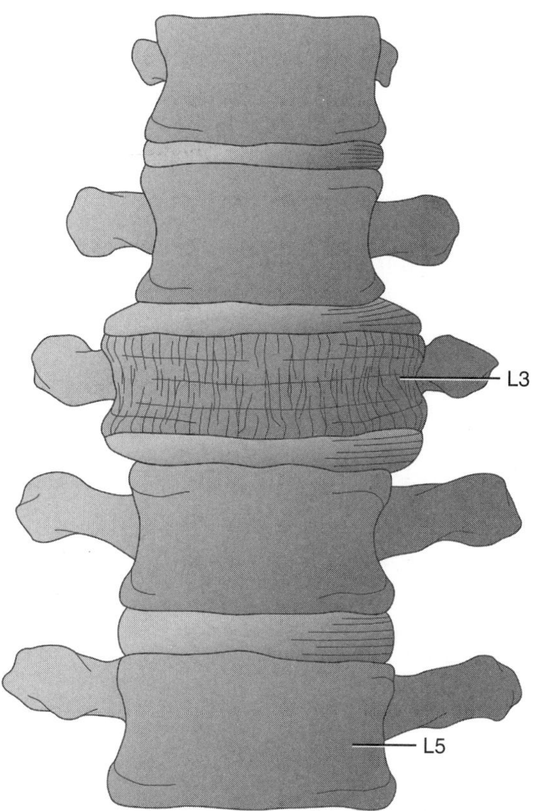

Figure **20–4.** Anterior view of lumbar spine in Paget's disease. L3 is compressed. This will be evident radiographically.

Clinical findings also include postural deformities such as increased thoracic kyphosis and bowing of the femora and tibiae. Bony softening of the femoral neck can cause coxa vara (reduced angle of the femoral neck) and may result in a waddling gait. These changes may produce increased local mechanical stresses resulting in pain.

Other manifestations include nerve palsy syndromes, mental deterioration, and cardiovascular disease. The nerve palsy syndromes can occur secondarily to compression entrapments. The cardiovascular disease is due to vasodilation of blood vessels in the bones and skin and subcutaneous tissues overlying the affected bones. When one third to one half of the skeleton is involved, an increase in cardiac output may be severe enough to cause heart failure. This is the most common cause of death in patients with advanced Paget's disease (Schiller, 1994; Wallach, 1982).

Sarcoma occurs in approximately 7% of those with Paget's disease (Schajowicz et al., 1983). Twenty percent of people 50 years or older diagnosed with osteogenic sarcomas have Paget's disease (Rubin, 1983). The bones most commonly affected, in order of frequency, are femur, pelvis, humerus, and tibia. The bones most commonly affected in Paget's disease, the skull and vertebrae, rarely undergo sarcomatous change (Schiller, 1994). See Chapter 22 for an overview of osteogenic sarcoma.

Medical Management

Diagnosis. Because Paget's disease progresses slowly and the severity of the disease varies considerably among individuals, it may be present years before a diagnosis is made. In fact, the diagnosis is often made incidentally on the basis of radiographs or laboratory tests done for other reasons (Berkow, 1992).

If the disease is advanced, the diagnosis is made based on the characteristic bone deformities and radiologic bony changes. Elevated levels of serum alkaline phosphatase and urinary hydroxyproline support the diagnosis. Bone scans are positive only if the disease is active, marked by rapid bone turnover. But the test is not diagnostic by itself as other conditions are also accompanied by a metabolically active lesion. A bone biopsy may occasionally be done to make a differential diagnosis. The differential diagnosis includes hyperparathyroidism, bone metastasis, multiple myeloma, and fibrous dysplasia (Berkow, 1992; Gunta, 1994; Schiller, 1994).

Treatment. Treatment of Paget's disease depends on the degree of pain and extent of the pathologic changes. Nonsteroidal and other anti-inflammatory agents are used to control the pain. Etidronate disodium and calcitonin inhibit osteoclast activity, but only calcitonin has the potential to heal the existing osteolytic lesions. The healing potential of calcitonin is limited because serum antibodies may form, resulting in resistance to the drug. If these drugs are successful in slowing down the disease, the patient may note a corresponding decrease in pain.

Surgical intervention may be indicated for reasons other than fracture repair. Interventions include occipital craniectomy to relieve basilar and nerve compression, tibial osteotomy if the deformity is severe, and total hip replacement if severe degenerative joint disease is present (Abrams and Berkow, 1990).

Special Implications for the Therapist **20-3**

PAGET'S DISEASE

The reader is directed to the section associated with osteoporosis as there is considerable overlap between Paget's disease and osteoporosis regarding implications for the therapist. The overlap includes the discussion of prevention of fracture, patient injury during examination and treatment, recognition of possible fracture, and postoperative care.

Other important considerations exist for the therapist. If working with an elderly population, therapists need to be aware of the symptoms and signs of Paget's disease. Because pain is often the initial symptom and is usually a vague diffuse ache, there can be difficulty in distinguishing this disease from degenerative joint disease of the lumbar spine, hips, or knees. Also, clients with diffuse headaches may present to the therapist with undiagnosed Paget's disease. These clients may complain of hearing loss, tinnitus, incontinence, diplopia, or swallowing difficulties. There may be slurring of speech or the onset of symptoms or signs associated with heart disease. The presentation of any of the above warrants communication with a physician. Awareness of the side effects of anti-inflammatory medications is also important. These side effects include indigestion, nausea, vomiting, melena, tinnitus, hearing loss, vertigo, and hyperpnea (Payan, 1992). Again, if any of the above are reported by the patient, communication with a physician is warranted.

References

AAOS (American Academy of Orthopaedic Surgeons): Osteoporosis. Park Ridge, Ill, Author, 1988.

Abrams WB, Berkow R (eds): The Merck Manual of Geriatrics. Rahway, NJ, Merck, 1990, pp 721–724.

Baran DT: Osteoporosis: Monitoring techniques and alternate therapies, calcitonin, fluoride, biophosphates, vitamin D. Obstet Gynecol Clin North Am 21:321–335, 1994.

Barrett-Connor E, Bush TL: Estrogen and coronary heart disease in women. JAMA 265:1861–1867, 1991.

Berkow R (ed): The Merck Manual of Diagnosis and Therapy, ed 16. Rahway, NJ, Merck, 1992, pp 1359–1360.

Block JE, Friedlander AL, Brooks GAD, et al: Determinants of bone density among athletes engaged in weight-bearing and non–weight-bearing activity. J Appl Physiol 67:1100–1105, 1989.

Bouillon R, Burckhard P, Christiansen C, et al: Consensus development conference: Prophylaxis and treatment of osteoporosis. Osteoporos Int 1:114–117, 1991.

Cummings S, Kelsey J, Nevitt M, O'Dowd K: Epidemiology of osteoporosis and osteoporotic fractures. Epidemiol Rev 7:178–208, 1985.

Cummings S, Rubin S, Black D: The future of hip fractures in the United States. Clin Orthop 252:163–166, 1990.

Dalinka MK, Aronchick JM, Haddad JG: Paget's disease. Orthop Clin North Am 14:3–19, 1983.

Daniell H: Osteoporosis of the slender smoker. Vertebral compression fractures and loss of metacarpal cortex in relation to postmenopausal cigarette smoking and lack of obesity. Arch Intern Med 136:298–304, 1976.

Davee AM, Rosen CJ, Adler RA: Exercise patterns and trabecular bone density in college women. J Bone Miner Res 5:245–250, 1990.

Dawson-Hughes B, Dallal GE, Krall EA, et al: A controlled trial of the effect of calcium supplementation on bone density in postmenopausal women. N Engl J Med 323:878–883, 1990.

Deitrick J, Whedon G, Schorr E: Effects of immobilization upon various metabolic and physiologic functions of normal men. Am J Med 4:3–36, 1948.

Donaldson C, Hulley S, Vogel J: Effect of prolonged bed rest on bone mineral. Metabolism 19:1071–1084, 1970.

Fahy UM, Cahill DJ, Wardle PG, Hull M: Osteoporotic fractures in young amenorrheic women. Acta Obstet Gynecol Scand 73:417–419, 1994.

Fitzgerald PA: Endocrine disorders. *In* Tierney LM, McPhee SJ, Papadakis MA (eds): Medical Diagnosis and Treatment, ed 33. Norwalk, Conn, Appleton & Lange, 1994, pp 949–952.

Gordon GS, Vaughn C: Osteoporosis: Early detection, prevention and treatment. Consultant 25:64, 1980.

Gunta KE: Alterations in skeletal function: Congenital disorders, metabolic bone disease, and neoplasms. *In* Porth C (ed): Pathophysiology: Concepts of Altered Health States, ed 4. Philadelphia, JB Lippincott, 1994, pp 1230–1235.

Hahn BH: Osteopenic bone diseases. *In* McCarty DJ, Koopman WJ (eds): Arthritis and Allied Conditions, ed 12, vol 2. Philadelphia, Lea & Febiger, 1993, pp 1935–1938.

Holbrook TL, Barrett-Conor E, Wingard DL, et al: Dietary calcium and the risk of hip fracture: 14 year prospective population study. Lancet 2:1046–1048, 1988.

Hopper JL, Seeman E: The bone density of female twins discordant for tobacco use. N Engl J Med 330:387–392, 1994.

Kleerekoper M, Peterson E, Nelson D, et al. Identification of women at risk for developing postmenopausal osteoporosis with vertebral fractures: Role of history and single photon absorptiometry. Bone Miner 7:171–186, 1989.

National Osteoporosis Foundation: The Older Person's Guide to Osteoporosis. Washington, DC, Author, 1991.

Nordin C, Need A, Chatterton B, et al: The relative contributions of age and years since menopause to postmenopausal bone loss. J Clin Endocrinol Metab 70:83–88, 1990.

Orwall ES, Ferar J, Oviatt SK, et al: The relationship of swimming exercise to bone mass in men and women. Arch Intern Med 149:2197–2200, 1989.

Orwall ES: The influence of exercise on osteoporosis and skeletal health. *In* Goldberg L, Elliot DL (eds): Exercise for Prevention and Treatment of Illness. Philadelphia, FA Davis, 1994, pp 228–243.

Payan DG: Nonsteroidal anti-inflammatory drugs; nonopioid analgesics; drugs used in gout. *In* Katzung BG (ed): Basic and Clinical Pharmacology, ed 5. Norwalk, Conn, Appleton & Lange, 1992, pp 491–512.

Philosophe R, Seibel MM: Menopause and cardiovascular disease. *In* McCormick A (ed): Clinical Issues in Perinatal and Women's Health Nursing. Philadelphia, JB Lippincott, 1991, pp 441–451.

Prior JC, Vigna YM, Schechter MT, Burgess AE: Spinal bone loss and ovulatory disturbances. N Engl J Med 323:1221–1227, 1990.

Raisz LG, Rodan GA: Cellular basis for bone turnover. *In* Avioli L, Krane S (eds): Metabolic Bone Disease and Clinically Related Disorders, ed 20. Philadelphia, WB Saunders, 1990.

Raisz L: Osteoporosis. Annu Rev Med 40:251–267, 1989.

Rauscher NA: Nursing care of clients with musculoskeletal disorders. *In* Black JM, Matassarin-Jacobs E (eds): Luckmann and Sorensen's Medical-Surgical Nursing, ed 4. Philadelphia, WB Saunders, 1993, pp 1901–1914.

Riggs BL, Hodgson SF, O'Fallon WM, et al: Effect of fluoride treatment on the fracture rate in postmenopausal women with osteoporosis. N Engl J Med 322:802–809, 1990.

Robb WJ: Hip fracture disease: Coping with a contemporary epidemic. J Musculoskel Med 10:12–24, 1993.

Rubin R (ed): Clinical Oncology: A Multi-disciplinary Approach. New York, American Cancer Society, 1983, pp 296–306.

Schajowicz F, Arauyo ES, Berenstein M: Sarcoma complicating Paget's disease of bone. J Bone Joint Surg [Br] 65:299, 1983.

Schapira D: Alcohol abuse and osteoporosis. Semin Arthritis Rheum 19:371–376, 1990.

Schiller AL: Bones and joints. *In* Rubin E, Farber JL (eds): Pathology, ed 2. Philadelphia, JB Lippincott, 1994, pp 1300–1304.

Seeman E, Melton LJ III, O'Fallon WM, Riggs BL: Risk factors for spinal osteoporosis in men. Am J Med 75:977–983, 1983.

Tylavsky F, Bortz A, Hancock R, Anderson J: Familial resemblance of radial bone mass between premenopausal mothers and their college-age daughters. Calcif Tissue Int 45:265–272, 1989.

Wallach S: Treatment of Paget's disease. Adv Intern Med 27:1–43, 1982.

Whedon G: Disuse osteoporosis: Physiological aspects. Calcif Tissue Int 36:S146–S150, 1984.

Wickham CAC, Walsh K, Cooper C, et al: Dietary calcium, physical activity, and risk of hip fracture: A prospective study. Br Med J 299:889–892, 1989.

SECTION 3

chapter 21

Infectious Diseases of the Musculoskeletal System

Terry Randall

Infectious diseases are common in the general population. Fortunately, most of the microorganisms that humans encounter do not produce disease. In fact, staphylococci can be found on the skin of many healthy adults. The interaction between host and organism is complex but is responsible for determining whether an infectious disease ensues. The method by which a microorganism attaches itself to a host cell is not well understood, but it is the important first step in establishing an infection (Gibbons, 1992). Once the methods of adhesion of the microorganism to the host are better understood, new methods of prevention with vaccines that block linkage to the host may offer better control of infectious diseases. The body has a number of defense systems in place to prevent an infection from becoming established. These are important in understanding musculoskeletal infections.

The skin serves as an effective barrier to invasion by microorganisms but can be broken down by trauma, invasive procedures, or insect bites. Even the best of defense systems can fail or be overwhelmed by the numbers of invading microorganisms. When bacteria become established in the host, the multiplication of the organism is what triggers the inflammatory response. The presence of the foreign microorganism also initiates the immune response. This includes the phagocytic system, which consists of neutrophils, monocytes, and macrophages, which attempt to ingest invading microorganisms (Berkow, 1992). This occurs as a general response to any invasion. A more specific response is delivered by lymphocytes and immunoglobulins (see Chapter 5). Depending on the location of the infection, the functioning of the hematologic, cardiopulmonary, gastrointestinal, endocrine, and genitourinary systems may be impaired.

The use of implants and prosthetic materials is now commonplace. Therapists frequently treat clients with biomaterial implants. Joint replacements, heart valves, vascular prostheses, dental implants, sutures, catheters, and allografts are but a few of the devices that can harbor infections. Musculoskeletal infections can require drastic measures to treat and to prevent morbidity. For example, infection following total joint replacement often requires removal of the hardware, and joint sepsis requires surgical debridement (Gristina et al., 1991).

Understanding the epidemiology, pathogenesis, and treatment of musculoskeletal infections will allow the clinician to play an active role in all phases of diagnosis and treatment. From early detection of signs and symptoms that reflect the need for further medical evaluation to rehabilitation of those clients who undergo surgical intervention for musculoskeletal infections, therapists can have an important impact on the outcome of treatment. Only the most common infectious diseases are covered in this chapter. Therapists will likely be involved with the diagnosis or rehabilitation of clients with osteomyelitis, tuberculosis, septic arthritis, and soft tissue infections.

OSTEOMYELITIS

Overview. Osteomyelitis is an inflammation of bone caused by an infectious organism. Osteomyelitis is usually caused by bacteria, but fungi, parasites, and viruses can also cause skeletal infections (see Chapter 6). Bacteria can enter the body through scratches on the skin or through the mucous membranes in the alveoli when an upper respiratory infection is present. In adults the source is usually by direct inoculation into the bone. In children the infection is spread hematogenously and usually develops in the metaphysis of the distal femur and proximal tibia, humerus, and radius and can then spread, causing a septic joint (Almekinders, 1994). Vertebral osteomyelitis is seen in adults and is also spread hematogenously, usually from pelvic or urinary tract infections. The lumbar spine is the most commonly involved area (Patzakis et al., 1991; Sapico and Montgomerie, 1990). Osteomyelitis is characterized as acute or chronic, although the separation between the two is vague. Acute osteomyelitis can develop into the chronic reaction when treatment is delayed or inadequate.

Acute osteomyelitis is a rapidly destructive pyogenic infection often seen in children, older adults, and intravenous (IV) drug abusers. The infection has the capability to spread quickly via the bloodstream, resulting in septicemia. While the initial presentation may be of joint pain with minimal impairment, increased joint pain, diminished function, and systemic signs such as fever and malaise may rapidly develop.

Chronic osteomyelitis can be the result of the acute disease being undiagnosed. Since chronic osteomyelitis is a recognized complication of treatment of open fractures, prevention of infection should always be stressed. The risks can be minimized if the wound is thoroughly debrided, irrigated, and left open for delayed primary closure. Delayed primary closure allows the wound bed to be inspected and further debridement can be carried out if necessary.

Incidence. Generally, osteomyelitis occurs more often in children than adults and affects boys more often than girls. Acute hematogenous osteomyelitis is the most common type and is usually seen in children. Chronic osteomyelitis is more common in adults and immunocompromised persons. With the use of antibiotics the incidence of osteomyelitis is gradually decreasing except in IV drug abusers.

Etiology. *Staphylococcus aureus* is the usual cause of osteomyelitis, but other organisms such as group B streptococcus, pneumococcus, *Pseudomonas aeruginosa*, *Haemophilus influenzae*, and *Escherichia coli* also produce bone infections. Among people with sickle cell anemia, salmonella infection is associated with osteomyelitis. Older adults and persons with impaired immunity may develop osteomyelitis as a result of gram-negative infections. Osteomyelitis can be acquired from exogenous or hematogenous sources. *Exogenous osteomyelitis* is acquired by invasion of the bone by direct extension from the outside as a result of inoculation, by a penetrating or puncture wound, extension from an overlying abscess or burn, or other trauma such as an open fracture. Surgical procedures and open fractures are common sources of acute osteomyelitis infection. These examples of osteomyelitis secondary to a contiguous area of infection are common in immunocompromised persons, and those with diabetes or severe vascular insufficiency.

Hematogenous osteomyelitis is acquired from spread of organisms from preexisting infections such as occurs in impetigo, furunculosis (persistent boils), infected lesions of varicella (chickenpox), and sinus, ear, dental, soft tissue, respiratory, and genitourinary infections. Vaginal, uterine, ovarian, bladder, and intestinal infections can lead to iliac or sacral osteomyelitis. Osteomyelitis of the arm and hand bones may occur in drug abusers. Hematogenous osteomyelitis is more common in children than adults.

Risk Factors. In general, anyone who is chronically ill, including diabetes or alcoholism, or receives large doses of steroids or immunosuppressive drugs is particularly susceptible to osteomyelitis (Table 21–1) (Mourad, 1994). Clients with these conditions should be aware of the increased risk of infection and be taught proper preventive measures and early warning signs. As mentioned, persons with biomaterial implants will have an increased risk of infection, especially in the immediate postoperative period. Although rare, late infections occurring 1 year postoperatively have been reported (Heggeness et al., 1993).

TABLE 21–1 States Associated with Musculoskeletal Infection

- Congenital
  - Chronic granulomatous disease
  - Hemophilia
  - Hypogammaglobulinemia
  - Sickle cell hemoglobinopathy
- Acquired
  - Diabetes mellitus
  - Hematologic malignancy
  - Human immunodeficiency virus infection
  - Pharmacologic immunosuppression
    - Organ transplantation
    - Collagen-vascular diseases
  - Uremia

From Brennan PJ, DeGirolamo MP: Musculoskeletal infections in immunocompromised hosts. Orthop Clin North Am 22:390, 1991.

Nutrition is often overlooked but can play a significant role in preventing infections. Anyone who has lost 10% of his or her body weight or weighs less than 90% of ideal weight is considered malnourished (Smith, 1991). These persons risk surgical complications such as infection, wound breakdown, and poor fracture healing (Brennan and DeGirolamo, 1991).

Pathogenesis. Acute osteomyelitis may develop in the metaphysis of long bones owing to the decreased amount of phagocytosis and/or slower rate of blood flow in the terminal arterioles (Green, 1988). Trauma, including microtrauma, may also increase susceptibility to infection by slowing the blood flow.

Regardless of the source of the pathogen, the pathogenesis of bone infection initially involves an inflammatory response. The metaphysis of long bones is very porous, allowing exudate from the infection to spread easily. As the organisms grow and form pus within the bone, tension builds within the rigid medullary cavity, forcing pus through the haversian canals.[1] This forms a subperiosteal abscess that deprives the bone of its blood supply and eventually may cause necrosis. Necrotic cells then become a fertile bed for the organisms to multiply. Because sensory nerve endings are absent in cancellous bone this process can progress without pain. Necrosis then stimulates the periosteum (osteoblasts) to create new bone. The sheath of new bone, called an *involucrum*, forms around the *sequestrum*, necrotic tissue that has become separated, which works its way out through an abscess or the sinuses (Fig. 21–1) (Norris, 1995).

By the time the sequestrum forms, the osteomyelitis is chronic. In adults this complication is rare because the periosteum is firmly attached to the cortex and resists displacement. Instead, infection disrupts and weakens the cortex, which predisposes the bone to pathologic fracture (Mourad, 1994).

In vertebral osteomyelitis the infection is first found in the metaphysis or cartilaginous end plates and quickly spreads to the intervertebral disk (Wood, 1992). *Staphylococcus aureus* is the most common organism found. Abscess formation is common via direct extension of the infection to adjacent tissues. The abscesses can advance posteriorly to involve the epidural area or anteriorly to produce a paravertebral abscess that can extend to the psoas muscle, producing hip pain.

Clinical Manifestations. In the initial phases of the infection pain may not be a factor because of the lack of pain fibers in cancellous bone. This is unfortunate because osteomyelitis can spread rapidly and antibiotics should be administered as soon as possible. When the infection extends into the periosteum, pain may become a factor (Cohen et al., 1990). The pain will likely be described as a deep, continuous pain, which may increase with weight bearing.

Once present, spinal osteomyelitis can produce intermittent or constant back pain. The pain is aggravated by motion and is throbbing at rest. It may radiate in a radicular distribution and is commonly accompanied by spinal tenderness and rigidity; accessory motions of the spine are often difficult to perform. Sacroiliac osteomyelitis is usually characterized by

[1] Haversian canals are anastomosing channels that constitute the basic inut of structure in compact bone. These canals contain blood, lymph vessels, and nerves. Once bacteria gain access to these channels, they are able to proliferate unimpeded.

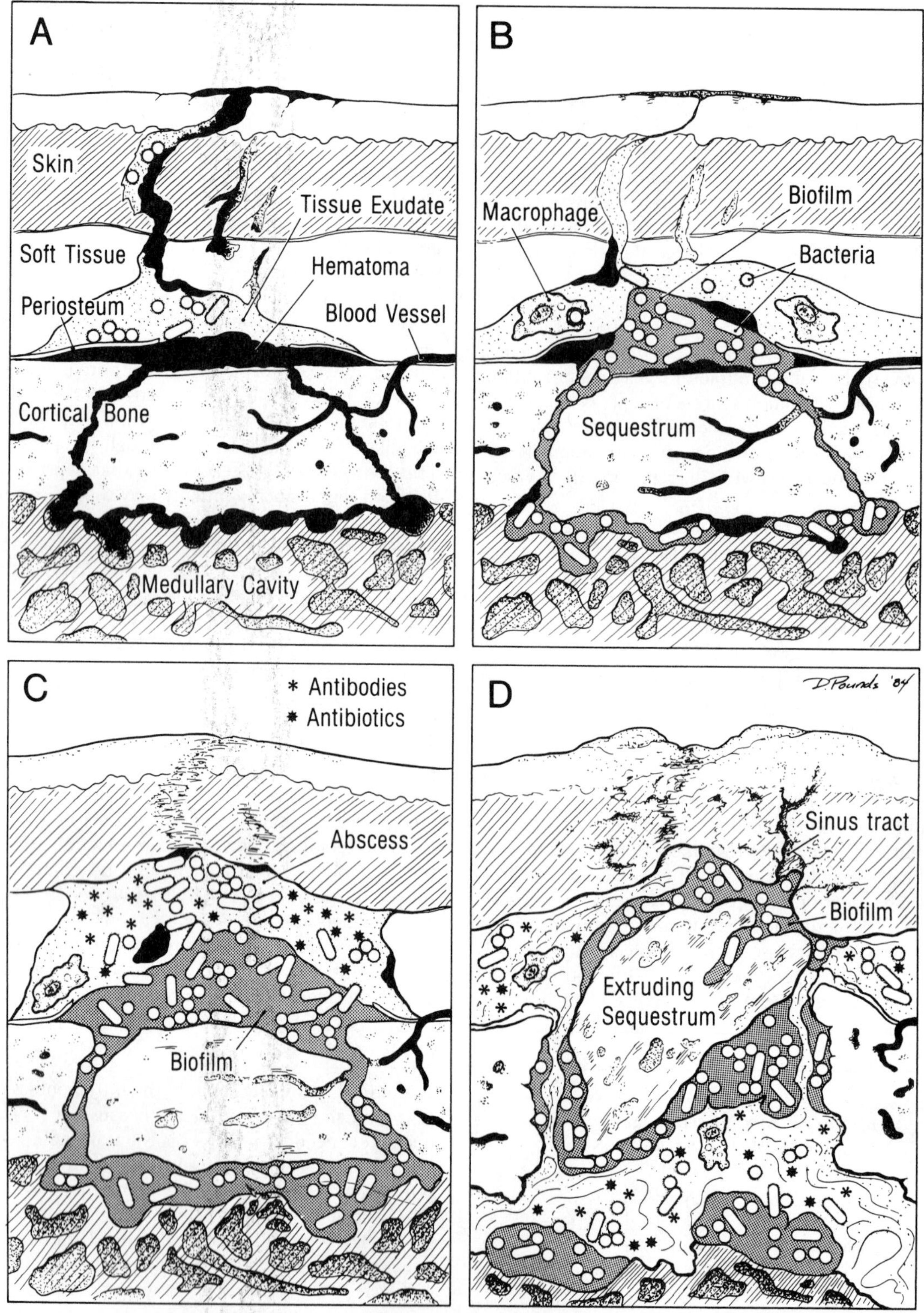

Figure 21–1. The sequence of pathogenesis in osteomyelitis. A, Initial trauma produces soft tissue destruction and bone fragmentation, as well as wound contamination by bacteria. In closed wounds, contamination may occur by hematogenous seeding. *B*, As the infection progresses, bacterial colonization occurs within a protective exopolysaccharide biofilm. The biofilm is particularly abundant on the devitalized bone fragment, which acts as a passive substratum for colonization. C, Host defenses are mobilized against the infection but are unable to penetrate or be effective in the presence of the biofilm. *D*, Progressive inflammation and abscess formation eventually result in the development of a sinus tract and, in some cases, ultimate extrusion of the sequestrum that is the focus of the resistant infection. (*From Gristina AG, Bath E, Web L: Microbial adhesion and the pathogenesis of biomaterial centered infections.* In *Gustilo RR, Gruninger RR, Tsukayama DA (eds): Orthopaedic Infection. Diagnosis and Treatment. Philadelphia, WB Saunders, 1989, p 8.*)

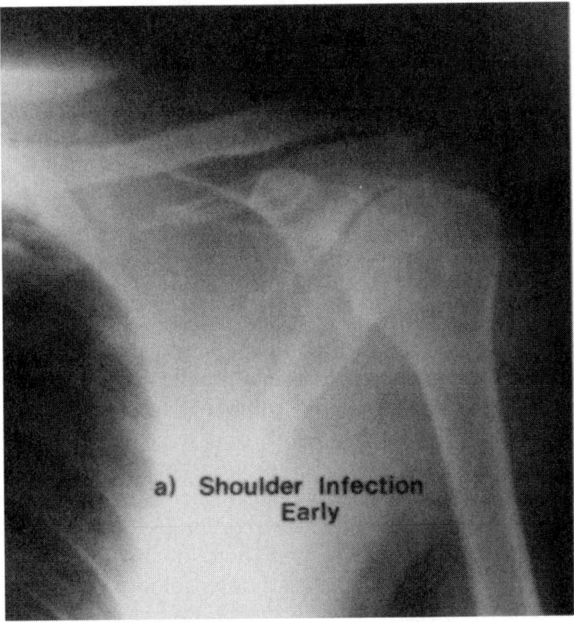

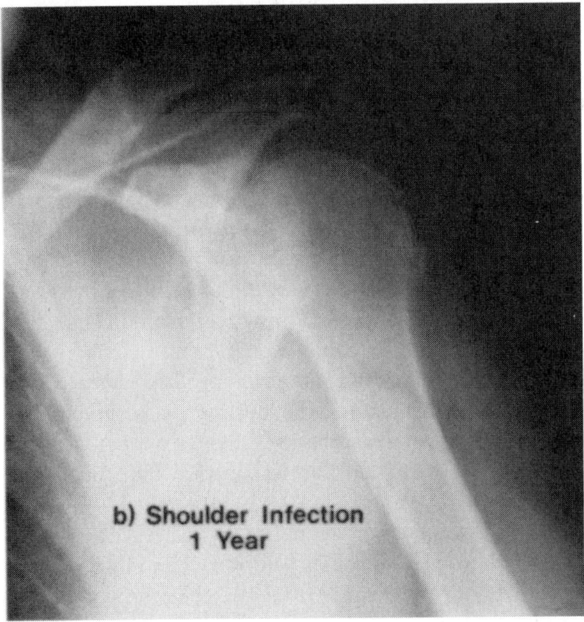

Figure 21–2. Hematogenous osteomyelitis secondary to intra-articular sepsis. *A*, Minimal lucency of proximal humerus at 2 weeks after probable onset of infection. *B*, After arthrotomy, antibiotic treatment, and resolution of infection, radiograph reveals periosteal new bone formation and joint contracture. Organism: *Staphylococcus aureus*. (*From Gristina A, Kammire G, Voytek A, Web L: Sepsis of the shoulder.* In *Rockwood C, Matsen F (eds): The Shoulder. Philadelphia, WB Saunders, 1990, p 933.*)

severe, local pain with tenderness and an antalgic gait. The pain may radiate to the buttocks or abdomen. The history will be that of recent onset of localized pain. Besides pain symptoms may include fever, local tenderness, and swelling.

Medical Management

Diagnosis. Although diagnosing infectious diseases is beyond the purview of the therapist, a thorough history and a review of systems can help to identify pathology that requires further medical evaluation (Boissonnault, 1995). Signs and symptoms of systemic disease can sometimes be easily detected. For screening purposes the presence of a fever, unexplained weight loss, history of cancer, and failure to respond to adequate treatment are good indicators of more serious pathology (Deyo et al., 1992). Sometimes the history alone is quite informative. Disturbances in the sleep pattern such as awakening with pain, requiring sleep medications, or inability to fall asleep, along with symptoms that increase with walking, have been found to be associated with serious back problems (Roach et al., 1995). In other areas of the body localized pain in the presence of other risk factors may raise suspicion. Laboratory studies showing an increase in white blood cells (WBCs) and elevation of the erythrocyte sedimentation rate (ESR) are added evidence for osteomyelitis.

Diagnosis is often delayed due to lack of specific signs and symptoms, especially in chronic osteomyelitis. Laboratory values and radiographs are negative in the early stages. Radiographs may not detect bony abnormality in infections of less than 10 days' duration (Fig. 21–2). Radionuclide bone scan can detect early stage disease and is helpful in detection and identifying multiple sites of involvement. Lytic lesions may be demonstrable on radiographs within 2 weeks of onset of the disease. A periosteal reaction develops later. Magnetic resonance imaging (MRI) and computed tomography scans have been used to plan surgical procedures but are not as commonly used for diagnosis. The use of MRI will probably increase as its value in differentiating bone from soft tissue involvement is better demonstrated. MRI can also help in the differentiation of cellulitis and arthritis from osteomyelitis (Tehranzadeh et al., 1992). The diagnosis is confirmed by cultures from the involved area.

Identification of the infectious pathogen is of utmost importance because the type of medication used often depends on the infecting microorganism. Specimens are obtained for culture or stains by aspiration, needle biopsy, or swab. Accurate identification is often difficult due to the technical problems of obtaining an acceptable sample (Neu, 1992). Image-enhanced needle biopsy can improve the specimen quality. Other factors to consider in choosing an antibiotic are the client's age and health status, site of infection, and previous antimicrobial therapy.

Treatment. Immediate treatment is called for, especially in *acute osteomyelitis*. Antibiotics can be given intravenously or delivered orally.[2] The choice of antibiotics is based on the culture results. Antibiotics are delivered intravenously to hasten their effect when faced with serious infection that can progress rapidly. Often 6 weeks of therapy is indicated before clinical signs of healing such as absence of drainage and diminished pain are noted. Surgery is indicated if the infection has spread to the joints. In fact, this is considered an

[2] Adverse effects of antibiotics include fever, rash, anaphylaxis, diarrhea, vomiting, impairment of renal and hepatic function, and depression.

orthopedic emergency. Articular cartilage can be damaged in a matter of hours. The goal of surgery is to drain exudate or pus from the bone or joint. Often extensive debridement of both bone and surrounding soft tissue is required. Various reconstructive procedures may be considered once the infection is eliminated. These include soft tissue procedures to provide coverage of defects, as well as bone grafting. In adults both surgery and antibiotics are often required.

The goals for treatment of *chronic osteomyelitis* are to eliminate the infection by use of antibiotics if possible or by surgically removing infected tissue. If surgery is indicated the current trend is toward more radical surgery rather than serial debridements. In general, chronic osteomyelitis is more difficult to treat than the acute type because it is difficult to eradicate completely. Exacerbations may respond well to treatment with rest and antibiotics only to flare up again months later.

In the spine, surgery may be necessary to treat the infection, as well as to address spinal deformity (Berchuck et al., 1991). Deformity of the spine from the infection or subsequent surgery may lead to pain or neurologic compromise. If surgery is not indicated the person may be treated with short-term bed rest or the use of a brace for immobilization.

The use of appropriate antibiotics prophylactically is standard for some procedures such as total joint replacements and in open wounds that are contaminated. The cephalosporins are commonly used because they are inexpensive, relatively nontoxic, and effective against the most common infecting organism, *S. aureus* (Warner, 1992a). Gentamicin-impregnated beads can be implanted in the infected area to achieve concentrated levels of antibiotics in the local tissue without raising serum levels to toxic ranges. Antibiotic bead chains can be an effective method of prophylaxis as well as treatment of established infections (Klemm, 1993).

Prognosis. Fifty years ago osteomyelitis carried a mortality risk of 20%. The risk of death is now negligible, but treatment remains a challenge to the orthopedic surgeon, radiologist, infectious disease specialist, and therapist. With current medical interventions an infection arrest rate of 90% can be expected, even in chronic cases (Patzakis and Mader, 1994). Still, complications such as growth arrest can occur when the diagnosis or treatment is delayed or treatment is not maintained for an adequate length of time. When osteomyelitis is diagnosed in the early clinical stages and treated with antibiotics, the prognosis is excellent. If the process is unattended for a week to 10 days, there is almost always some permanent loss of bone structure, as well as the possibility of growth abnormality in the pediatric population (Eilert and Georgopoulos, 1995).

When osteomyelitis persists for a long period of time, infected necrotic bone serves as a harbor for infection that will not respond well to systemic antibiotics. Reduced blood flow is responsible for increasing the chance of establishing an infection, as well as preventing the antibiotic from reaching the focus of infection.

Chronic osteomyelitis also has a poor prognosis, even when treated surgically. People with chronic osteomyelitis are often in great pain, require prolonged hospitalization or medical care, and may, although rarely, require amputation of an extremity.

Special Implications for the Therapist **21-1**

OSTEOMYELITIS

In cases in which prostheses or hardware for open reduction and internal fixation are inserted, signs of infection should be monitored (see Box 6–9). The increased chance of infection is thought to be due to the enhanced ability of the infectious organism to attach to the implant. Regular inspection will reveal drainage from the wound, pain with rehabilitation exercises or movement, low-grade fever, and swelling or redness.

Prevention of infection through hospital infection control policies is crucial and important for therapists to become familiar with (see Chapter 6). Person-to-person transmission can be limited by following standard handwashing recommendations. Isolation procedures should be followed when indicated. Most hospitals utilize universal precautions, which controls the contact and disposal of blood and bodily fluids and material such as contaminated dressings (see Appendix A).

Surgery

If surgery is indicated, current techniques are more likely to result in soft tissue and bony defects that may require secondary reconstruction with split-thickness skin grafting, pedicle muscle flaps, or bone grafting (Zinberg, 1992). If the infection has affected the articular cartilage weight bearing and controlling compressive forces with exercise should be a priority. For example weight bearing on the affected leg may be restricted, and crutches may not be advised when arm(s) and leg(s) are affected simultaneously until sufficient healing occurs to avoid pathologic fractures. The physician must make this determination.

Often surgery and initial management are performed without adequate consideration for adjacent joints. Prolonged immobilization or limited mobility and weight bearing with external fixators may lead to significant impairment of previously uninvolved joints and muscles. Attention must not be focused on the infection site to the exclusion of the rest of the limb. Important elements of a successful rehabilitation include minimizing the original effects of the trauma or disease process and preventing as many complications as possible (Nickel, 1992).

Preventing Complications

Preventing complications is best done by beginning rehabilitation early. Therapists should first recognize the possible side effects of medical treatment that may lead to complications such as contractures, atrophy, impaired joint mechanics, and loss of function. Treatment of osteomyelitis is complex and the rehabilitation sometimes perplexing under the best of circumstances. Sequelae of hip joint sepsis and treatment can include joint destruction, avascular necrosis, and fracture (Hicklin and DePretis, 1995). When complications such as these arise, a full recovery is jeopardized. In addition to the musculoskeletal problems, the therapist should consider other involved organ systems such as the cardiovascular system and what impact the co-morbidities may have on healing, rehabilitation, and return to a high level of function.

Strict aseptic technique must be used when changing dressings and performing *wound care*. Reconstructive surgery to cover bone or soft tissue defects require careful monitoring, dressing changes, and protection. If the client is in skeletal traction for fractures, the insertion points of pin tracks should be covered with small, dry dressings. Pins used in external fixators also deserve close inspection. Therapist and client must avoid touching the skin around the pins and wires. Assess vital signs, wound appearance, and any new pain daily for signs of secondary infection. During the acute phase of this illness, any movement of the affected limb will cause discomfort or pain. The affected limb should be firmly supported and kept level with the body. Active, active assisted, and passive range-of-motion exercise of adjacent joints are essential. Good skin care is essential with proper positioning, frequent (but careful and gentle) position changes (at least every 2 hours), and skin assessment for any signs of developing pressure ulcers. Massage or any technique that can possibly spread the infection through mechanical means is to be avoided.

Cast Care

Good cast care is important and in most settings the cast is already "petalled" (edges covered with adhesive tape or moleskin to smooth rough edges), but in some situations the therapist may be called upon to provide this service. Also, monitor sensation, circulation, and drainage and report any wet spots from drainage soaking through the cast or dressings. Palpating the cast over the incision may reveal softening of the plaster before the drainage is visible. Usually new spots are circled with a marking pen and the date and time recorded. The circled spot should be checked every 4 hours and any enlargement is reported immediately. Any sign of recurrent infection (increased temperature, redness, localized heat, swelling) or recurring sources of infection (e.g., boils, styes, impetigo, blisters) must be brought to the physician's attention.

DISCITIS

Overview and Incidence. Although spinal infections are rare, the disk is the most common site. Discitis can range from a self-limiting inflammatory process to a pyogenic infection. It may involve the intervertebral disk or vertebral end plates, or both. The infection rate in adults following disk surgery is less than 3%.

Etiology and Risk Factors. Children as young as 2 years old can develop discitis. The origin of the infection in children may be traumatic. A focus of infection, such as in the upper respiratory or urinary tract, may also precede the discitis.

Discitis may develop as a postoperative complication following discectomy. Other procedures capable of directly inoculating the disk, such as discography, also carry the risk of infection. Direct inoculation is the only method by which an infection can arise from within the disk (Wood, 1992).

Pathogenesis. A bacterial origin is usually the cause of the infection. *Staphylococcus aureus* is commonly found but in some cases no organism can be isolated. *Mycobacterium tuberculosis* is also detected in disk infections. A hematogenous spread of a bacterial infection is likely in children but in adults, in whom the disk is relatively avascular, the infection may involve the adjacent vertebrae and spread to the disk via the cartilaginous end plates. If the infection arises within the disk itself, formation of a peridural abscess is not common. However, an infection extending to the disk from the cartilaginous plate can spread to cause an epidural abscess posteriorly or a paravertebral abscess anteriorly.

Clinical Manifestations. Fever and spinal pain are classic symptoms in children. In the very young child a refusal to ambulate and pain with hip extension may be the first symptoms. Abdominal pain is also common, but the lumbar spine (low back pain) occurs more frequently.

In adults, disk infection following spinal procedures usually is noted within a few days while those developing from an infection at a distant site may not be evident for months. Spinal pain will be common and sometimes severe with radiation of the pain into the lower extremities. The lower extremity pain is not usually radicular; rather it may involve multiple nerve levels. Persons may present with unusual posture and movement patterns which could be erroneously labeled pain of psychogenic origin (Wood, 1992).

Medical Management

Diagnosis. In children routine radiographs are positive and often diagnostic but may not become so until 2 weeks have passed. Disk space narrowing, end plate irregularity, and a loss of lumbar lordosis are noted. Bone scans are also used for initial evaluation. The ESR and the WEC count may be elevated.

In adults the use of MRI in conjunction with bone scan using gadolinium enhancement has been found to be useful in differentiating normal postoperative disk space changes from those caused by infection (Boden et al., 1992). MRI is most useful in determining the extent of the infection but less valuable in demonstrating the type of infection. The sclerosis present later in the disease course may be confused with a benign degenerative process or even with metastatic disease. MRI and biopsy may be used to differentiate chronic cases (Pope et al., 1990).

Treatment. Treatment for the younger person may consist of bed rest, hip spica casting, and bracing. Antibiotics are used but do not appear to radically alter the natural course of the infection in children. In adults a removable body jacket can be used along with specific or empiric antibiotic therapy. The use of antibiotics prophylactically is common following spinal surgery in adults.

Prognosis. In both adults and children the prognosis is good, although pain may persist for several months. In children, long-term follow-up has shown a resolution of the pain in spite of persistent radiographic changes (Crawford et al., 1991). Late radiographic changes in adults include vertebral collapse, kyphosis, and, eventually, bony ankylosis, which can take up to 2 years to run its course. Adults can expect similar spontaneous healing to occur, especially in those individuals with a strong immune response. Complications can arise when the infection spreads or when an abscess forms. An epidural abscess can result in paralysis and is noted in older persons, in those who have involvement of the cervical region, and in those with associated medical problems, such as diabetes.

Special Implications for the Therapist **21-2**

DISCITIS

Because very young children can be affected, discitis must be considered a possible cause of spinal pain or refusal to bear weight or walk. Because the pain is usually related to activity, increasing with weight bearing, it is easy to mistakenly attribute the symptoms to musculoskeletal origins.

SEPTIC ARTHRITIS

Overview and Incidence. The incidence of septic arthritis may be increasing as a result of the greater number of people with immunocompromised conditions. Any person with an acute onset of joint pain and disability should be evaluated for possible sepsis.

Etiology and Risk Factors. Osteomyelitis is but one type of infection that is capable of extending into a joint and causing sepsis. Bacteria, viruses, and fungi are all capable of infecting a joint. *Staphylococcus aureus* and *Neisseria gonorrhoea* are the most common organisms responsible. Predisposing factors for development of septic arthritis are listed in Table 21–2 (Esterhai and Gelb, 1991). A history of alcohol abuse, IV drug abuse, human immunodeficiency virus (HIV) infection, joint prosthesis, rheumatoid arthritis, or other infectious disease increases the likelihood of having a septic joint (Dubost et al., 1993).

TABLE 21-2 PREDISPOSING FACTORS IN ADULT SEPTIC ARTHRITIS AND THEIR FREQUENCY*

Factor	Frequency
Systemic corticosteroid use	33%
Preexisting arthritis	24%
Arthrocentesis	23%
Distant infection	22%
Diabetes mellitus	13%
Trauma	12%
Other diseases	19%
None	8%

* More than one factor may exist in a patient.

From Esterhai J, Gelb I: Adult septic arthritis. Orthop Clin North Am 22:504, 1991.

TABLE 21-3 PATHOGENESIS OF BACTERIAL ARTHRITIS

Hematogenous spread

Direct inoculation and penetrating injury
- Trauma
- Arthrocentesis
- Arthroscopy
- Total joint arthroplasty

Contiguous soft tissue infection

Periarticular osteomyelitis

From Esterhai J, Gelb I: Adult septic arthritis. Orthop Clin North Am 22(3):504, 1991.

Pathogenesis. Microorganisms can be introduced into the joint by direct inoculation, direct extension, or via the circulatory system. Hematogenous spread is the most common. Other causes of septic arthritis are listed in Table 21–3 (Esterhai and Gelb, 1991). In animal models it has been established that within 24 hours of infection lysosomal enzymes are released and by day 7 cartilage softening is occurring. Pannus, an inflammatory exudate, forms over the synovial lining of the joint in 11 days with erosion of the joint capsule in 17 days (Esterhai and Gelb, 1991). This underscores the need for urgency in detection and treatment in septic arthritis.

Clinical Manifestations. Persons with septic arthritis can be of any age and present with an acute onset of joint pain, swelling, tenderness, and loss of motion. These symptoms may be accompanied by fever, chills, and other systemic symptoms depending on the stage of the illness. Physical examination may reveal the classic signs of infection such as increased temperature of the joint, swelling, redness, and loss of function. Only the severity and the nature of these signs will differentiate the septic joint from more mundane causes such as tendinitis and other noninfectious inflammatory diseases.

A child with a septic joint will often refuse to bear weight and be extremely tender to palpation at the joint and along the metaphysis. Destruction of the joints can proceed rapidly, and have long-lasting effects. In addition to the infection, the WBCs that enter the joint to combat the infection release enzymes that have a deleterious effect on articular cartilage (Sullivan, 1993). In a series of young children studied under the age of 2 years with septic knees, 24% had a varus or valgus deformity at long-term follow-up (Strong et al., 1994). In adults, *S. aureus* produces a monarticular sepsis, usually at the hip or knee. In children, the ankle and elbow are also common sites. Although not as common, polyarticular septic arthritis has been reported. Gonococcus affects mostly women and may produce skin lesions, tenosynovitis, and polyarthralgias, in addition to systemic symptoms (Simon, 1995). Prosthetic joints are also sites of infection, which is probably introduced at the time of surgery. *Staphylococcus epidermidis* is frequently the cause.

Medical Management

Diagnosis. Diagnosis is made by analysis of the joint fluid obtained by aspiration. The decision to aspirate the joint, however, is made on the basis of history and physical examination. Aspiration of the sacroiliac and hip joints is difficult, and fluoroscopy is sometimes used. Decisions on treatment and appropriate antibiotics are aided by the results of cultures, stains, and laboratory studies such as the WBC count and ESR.

Treatment. All joint infections are considered a medical emergency. Admission to the hospital for treatment with specific IV antibiotics such as penicillin, nafcillen, or gentamicin is required. Continued treatment with oral medication for an additional 2 to 3 weeks is standard (Korkis and Gantz, 1992). Open drainage is indicated for hip joint infections. In prosthetic joints the infection may require removal of the hardware and cement along with a more prolonged course of antibiotics. Early in the course of treatment the joint should be rested. This may be accomplished by splinting, traction, or casting. Care in application of the splint will preserve function and the splint should be removed periodically for range-of-motion exercise. More vigorous types of exercise are performed when signs of infection have resolved (Swezey, 1982).

The aggressiveness of treatment is dictated by the specific organism, the joint involved, duration of symptoms, and the health of the individual. Surgical drainage is often required to preserve function and prevent complications.

Prognosis. As for other infectious diseases prompt treatment is the key to a successful outcome. If treatment is initiated within 5 days of onset a good or excellent long-term result can be expected (Studahl et al., 1994). The more common complications include osteomyelitis, abscess formation, and permanent loss of joint motion.

Special Implications for the Therapist **21-3**

SEPTIC ARTHRITIS

Immediate referral of a client with a suspected septic joint to a specialist may save the joint from unnecessary destruction. Including joint infection in the differential diagnosis of some clients with joint pain may expedite appropriate treatment. This is important because the prognosis is related to the time between onset of symptoms and definitive treatment. Treatment of hip infections within 4 days of symptomatic presentation can result in preservation of the joint and complete resolution of the infection (Bennett and Namnyak, 1992). On the other hand, delayed treatment can result in serious complications leading to total hip replacement (Bennett and Namnyak, 1992).

The age of the client and the previous condition of the joint are also important factors. The elderly, who often have additional joint pathology such as degenerative joint disease, rheumatoid arthritis, or complications from diabetes, may not recover full function of the joint (Cooper and Cawley, 1986). The presence of associated joint pathology also tends to delay the diagnosis of sepsis, which further diminishes the chances of a favorable outcome and may result in a significant amount of residual impairment (e.g., contractures, fibrous ankylosis), especially among the elderly (Kelly et al., 1970).

INFECTIONS OF BURSAE AND TENDONS

Overview and Incidence. Acute infections affecting the bursae and tendons are not common but must be treated appropriately to avoid complications. The hand is very susceptible to scratches, bites, and subsequent infections. Hand infection can range from cellulitis to tenosynovitis. Hand infections are given special attention in the following paragraphs.

Etiology and Risk Factors. The bursae and tendons that lie close to the skin surface are most susceptible to infection from direct contact with microorganisms. Trauma to the elbow and knee is common, especially in sports such as wrestling. The infection is normally caused by *S. aureus* which enters the body through a local skin abrasion.

Hand infections often develop from untreated injuries. Up to 60% of hand infections are related to trauma, 25% are due to human bites, and 10% are due to animal bites (Brown and Young, 1993). As with all infections, persons with diabetes or who are immunocompromised have a greater risk of developing an infection in the hand.

Pathogenesis. Infection in the hand can spread along synovial sheaths, fascial planes, and via lymphatic channels. *S. aureus* is the most common organism isolated and may cause up to 80% of infections. Anaerobic bacteria are more commonly seen in wounds from bites and in persons with diabetes. Bursae are lined with a membrane similar to synovium and are therefore subject to the same pathologic processes, namely, inflammatory conditions due to acute or chronic infections.

Clinical Manifestations. The olecranon and prepatellar bursae can be sites of localized infection (Ho et al., 1978). An olecranon bursal infection will cause pain, loss of function, and swelling, which may be accompanied by cellulitis (Goldenberg, 1995). Infections of other bursae such as the prepatellar and subdeltoid bursae have similar presentations.

Tendon sheaths of the extremities can also become infected. As mentioned earlier, the hand is a common site because of its susceptibility to minor trauma. The anatomy of the hand determines the nature and presentation of the infection. For example, the tendon sheaths of the thumb and small finger extend proximally to the wrist, whereas the sheaths of the index, long, and ring fingers stop at the proximal pulley. An infection of the flexor tendon of the thumb could rapidly spread to the small finger (Brown and Young, 1993). Common signs associated with an infectious tenosynovitis include a finger maintained in slight flexion, fusiform (spindle-shaped) swelling, pain on extension (passive or active), and tenderness along the tendon sheath into the palm (Kanavel, 1939).

Medical Management

Diagnosis, Treatment, and Prognosis. In most joints, examination will identify a localized swelling, not a joint effusion. Aspiration of fluid for laboratory analysis is performed before treatment. The use of antibiotics is often adequate, but surgical incision and drainage is sometimes required; occasionally bursectomy is required (Phillips, 1992). Prompt treatment with drainage, irrigation, and antibiotics is crucial. The benefits of therapy have long been recognized.

Appropriate treatment of hand infections is based on an accurate identification by culture of the organism causing the infection. In addition to the appropriate antibiotic, the hand is immobilized, elevated, and often surgical drainage is necessary. Necrotic tissue is cautiously debrided and the wound is left open to drain. Kanavel (1939) long ago advocated earlier involvement of physical and occupational therapy to maximize function, and this is still advised.

Special Implications for the Therapist **21-4**

INFECTIONS OF BURSAE AND TENDONS

Treatment of hand injuries has developed into a subspecialty, and rightfully so, not only for the orthopedic surgeon but also for the therapist. Clients recovering from infection and surgery must be monitored carefully and their treatment adjusted often. Splinting of the hand is an important feature throughout the course of treatment. Early immobilization must be done with eventual recovery and function in mind. The wrist should be placed in 30 to 50 degrees of extension, the metacarpophalangeal joints in 75 to 90 degrees of flexion, and the interphalangeal joints in full extension. Active range-of-motion exercise is initiated early, as soon as the infection begins to subside and it is apparent that treatment will be successful, often within 48 hours. Prognosis is dependent on the extent of the infection and how soon treatment was initiated. Delayed treatment usually requires more extensive surgical debridement, an increased chance of scar tissue formation, the need for possible skin grafts, and a prolonged rehabilitation to maximize function.

EXTRAPULMONARY TUBERCULOSIS

Overview. Tuberculosis (TB) is an acute or chronic infection caused by *Mycobacterium tuberculosis* that can affect multiple organ systems via lymphatic and hematogenous spread during the initial pulmonary infection (see Chapter 12). Systems involved may include the pulmonary, genitourinary, musculoskeletal, and lymphatic systems. Of these the lymphatic system is most commonly involved. Disseminated or miliary TB involves not only the lungs but also most other organ systems. It is commonly seen in immunocompromised hosts. Extrapulmonary TB is more difficult to diagnose and treat than pulmonary TB. This is due in part to clinicians' lack of familiarity with the condition. In addition, extrapulmonary TB is often in inaccessible areas which makes aspiration or biopsy, and therefore diagnosis, more difficult. Also, smaller numbers of bacilli can cause extensive damage to joints but are harder to detect (Hopewell, 1995).

TB involving the bone is usually transferred hematogenously from some other organ, usually the lung. Only one fourth of persons with skeletal TB have a history of TB. Vertebral TB is called Pott's disease.

Skeletal Tuberculosis

Overview and Incidence. Because skeletal TB is relatively uncommon, delays in diagnosis are frequent. After years of decline the incidence of TB has increased over the past few years. The incidence rate was 9.5 per 100,000 person-years in 1989, 10.3 in 1990, and 10.4 in 1991 (Jereb et al., 1994). This increase is due in part to the presence of acquired immunodeficiency syndrome (AIDS). While TB is found in all 50 states, New York, California, and Hawaii have had the highest incidence.

Skeletal TB is uncommon but infection rates have held constant over the years. About 10% to 15% of TB is extrapulmonary and only 10% of extrapulmonary TB is skeletal. The spine is primarily affected, but other weight-bearing joints can also be affected (Rich and Kilner, 1994).

Pathogenesis and Clinical Manifestations. The tuberculin bacilli are transmitted hematogenously. In adults the onset of skeletal TB is insidious, developing 2 to 3 years after the primary infection. Early signs and symptoms include pain and stiffness. Pain may be localized or referred. Systemic signs such as fever, chills, weight loss, and fatigue are not common in the early phase. The lower thoracic and lumbar spine are commonly involved. Infection begins in the cancellous bone of the vertebral body and eventually spreads to the intervertebral disk and adjacent vertebrae. As the disease progresses nerve root irritation, pressure from abscess, and collapse of the vertebral body will cause a progressive increase in pain and protective spasm. The abscess may extend from the lumbar region to the psoas muscle, producing hip pain. TB is also found in other joints and is spread hematogenously from other organs.

Medical Management

Diagnosis. Early diagnosis is very helpful in preserving articular cartilage and the joint space, but is often delayed for several months to years after the initial presentation. This is because there are no symptoms pathognomonic of extrapulmonary TB. Chen reports a typical case where treatment may have been delayed because symptoms were consistent with chronic sciatica, in which the cause of the radiating pain was tuberculous sacroiliitis with an anterior synovial cyst (Chen, 1995). Conventional radiographs are important in the initial detection and CT and MRI can assist in further evaluation. Confirmation of skeletal TB requires microbiologic assessment with smear and culture (Talavera et al., 1994). In the spine this can be accomplished with fine-needle aspiration. Tissue biopsy is more often required for extrapulmonary disease.

Treatment and Prognosis. Treatment does not differ for pulmonary and extrapulmonary TB. Although surgical debridement is sometimes necessary, usually pharmacologic treatment is sufficient. Isoniazid, rifampin, and pyrazinamide are often used in combination. It should be noted, however, that strains of M. *tuberculosis* that are resistant to multiple antibiotics exist and are apparently increasing. Treatment continues for 6 to 9 months (Thijn and Steensma, 1990). See Chapter 12 for discussion of medical management of TB.

Rehabilitation after surgery for TB of the extremities follows standard orthopedic principles. Medical treatment and subsequent rehabilitation are individualized based on the extent of the infection. Surgical treatment of joint infection may include arthrotomy, synovectomy, and treatment of articular erosions. Extra-articular infections can sometimes be treated with curettage and bone grafting. For more advanced infections resection of bones and joints, arthrodesis, or amputation may be indicated. Factors to be considered include the affected bone, extent of surgical excision, and involvement of soft tissue, articular cartilage, or bone. Weight bearing is often limited but active range-of-movement exercise is often encouraged.

In the spine, surgery is more often needed to address nerve compression or deformity secondary to collapse of the vertebral body rather than the infection. The resultant deformity often includes a marked kyphotic curve with a gibbus formation (Fig. 21–3). Paralysis can be a serious complication of vertebral TB and can be a result of the disease process or a secondary spinal deformity.

If TB is diagnosed early when the infection is confined to the synovium, rest, medication, and joint protection may be adequate. In advanced disease with caseation, fibrosis, and scarring, the vascularity is reduced (Fig. 21–4). This makes the medications less effective and surgical excision or curettage of the affected areas may be necessary (Warner, 1992b). In joints the granulomatous tissue acts to separate the articular cartilage from the underlying bone (Bullough and Vigorita, 1984).

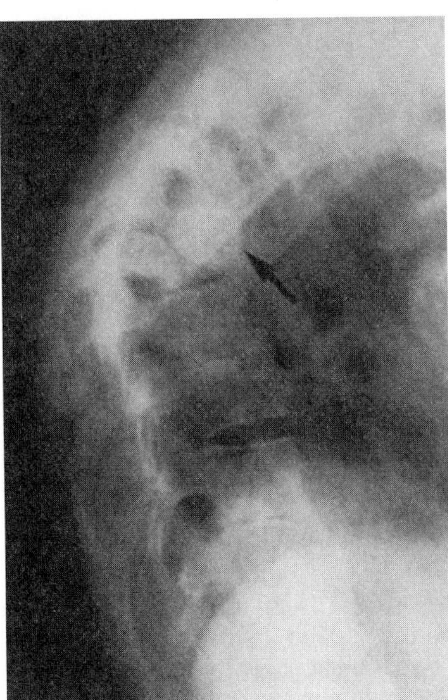

Figure **21–3.** Tuberculous spondylitis. Involvement at multiple levels. Gibbus deformity is seen in the upper thoracic region (*arrow*). (*From Yao D, Sartoris D: Musculoskeletal tuberculosis. Radiol Clin North Am 33;681, 1995.*)

Special Implications for the Therapist **21–5**

EXTRAPULMONARY AND SKELETAL TUBERCULOSIS

Therapists may provide treatment to clients with pulmonary TB that involves postural drainage and percussion to remove secretions from the lung (Starr, 1995). Care must be taken with clients' sputum. All health-care professionals must be aware of the risk of spreading the infection when working with people who have TB. This is equally important for extrapulmonary TB (see Table 12–15).

The risk of spreading the infection is also of primary importance in skeletal TB. Even though it is thought that once the client is started on appropriate medical therapy the risk of transmission decreases in as little as 2 weeks, there are types of drug-resistant TB that may be infectious for longer periods.

In addition to the obvious orthopedic concerns that will evolve during the treatment of skeletal TB, therapists should be aware of psychosocial issues that may develop. Clients undergoing long-term treatment for infectious diseases will undoubtedly have some difficulties in managing their disease. Chronic pain, repeated hospitalizations, frequent setbacks, fear of long-term disability, and loss of independence may all contribute to a number of abnormal, but expected, illness behaviors. A multidisciplinary team that includes occupational and physical therapists, psychologists, and community health nurses, among others, will be useful in achieving functional goals (Cheatle, 1991).

Summary of Special Implications for the Therapist

Rehabilitation following medical treatment for infectious diseases must proceed in a comprehensive and coordinated fashion. The pathology of each type of infectious disease process, as well as every medical decision made in treatment, will have some bearing on rehabilitation and outcome. When should range-of-motion exercise begin? Should it be active or passive? What is the client's weight-bearing status? What is the general health of the client? What are the client's goals and expectations? Many questions such as these must be addressed when planning the rehabilitation program.

The hip joint is commonly affected and has been alluded to in several chapters as a site of infectious processes of many origins and will be used here again to illustrate some factors that should be considered in planning rehabilitation. The client and therapist may be anxious for an exercise program to begin, but this must be done in concert with medical treatment and consideration of the stage of recovery. Early in the course of treatment, rest may be a predominant feature, but even this calls for therapy intervention. All health-care providers must be made aware of the potentially adverse effects of apparently simple movements. For example, using a bedpan and performing isometric

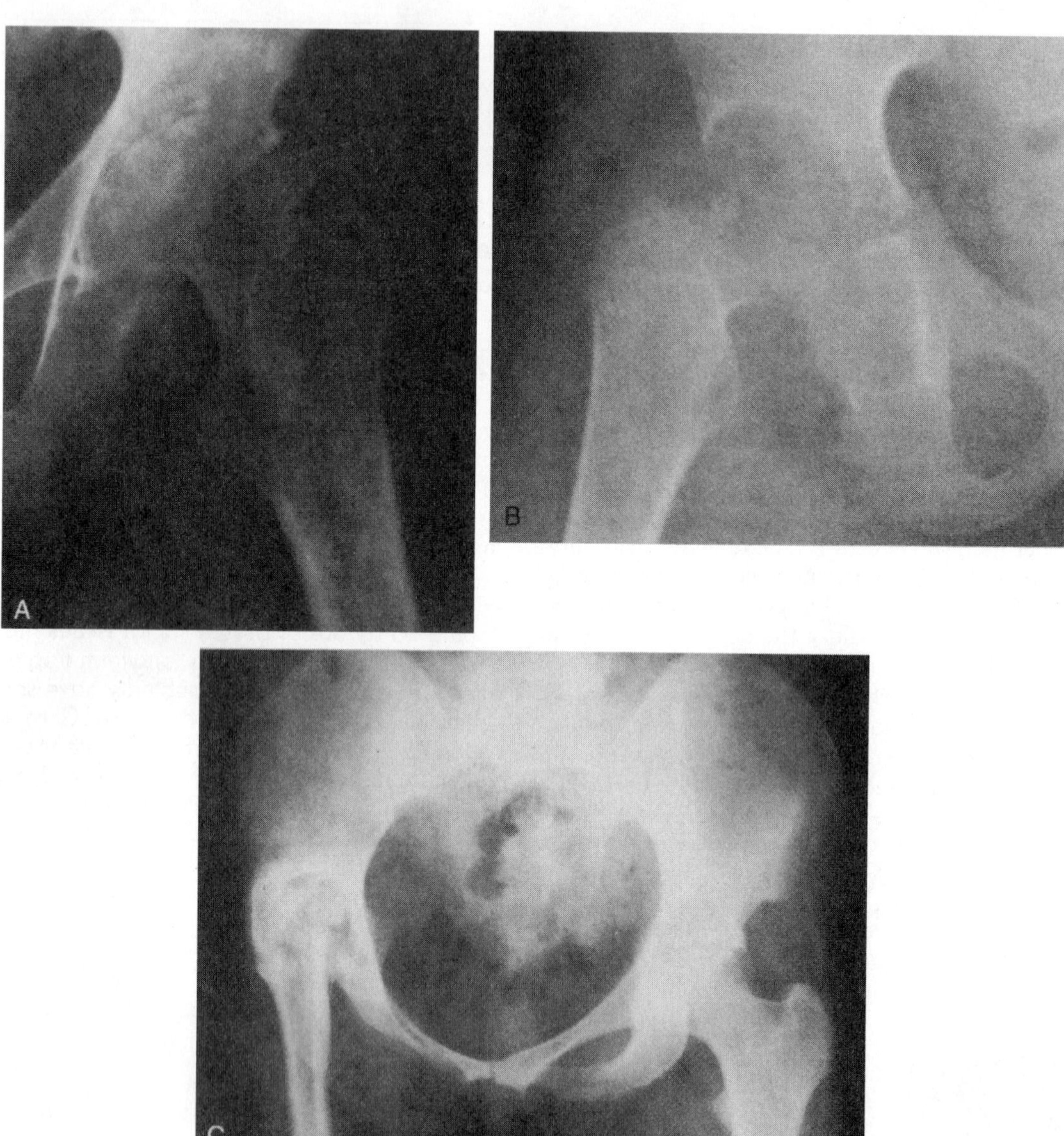

Figure **21–4.** Tuberculous arthritis. *A*, Bony erosion of acetabulum and femoral head with joint space loss. There also is evidence of periarticular osteopenia. *B*, Similar findings to *A* but with further destruction of the femoral head and acetabulum. C, Advanced tuberculosis of the hip with superior displacement and ankylosis of the right hip joint. (*From Yao D, Sartoris D: Musculoskeletal tuberculosis. Radiol Clin North Am 33;687, 1995.*)

exercises produce acetabular contact pressure close to that of walking (Hodge et al., 1989). Therefore, clinicians should not assume that a client who is on bed rest is not producing elevated joint compressive forces. Clients must be instructed in proper methods of moving, transferring, and positioning themselves.

Active range-of-motion exercise is often the first type of supervised exercise permitted. Even these innocuous movements must be done while noting limits set by pain, spasm, or apprehension. Active hip flexion has been found to increase acetabular contact pressure similar to that of full weight bearing (Strickland et al., 1992). However, passive range-of-motion exercise has been found to have a beneficial affect on healing joints (Salter et al., 1980; Gelberman et al., 1982). It may be worth remembering the motion requirements of certain positions so that functional goals can be set, for example, ascending stairs requires just over 65 degrees of hip flexion, whereas sitting in a chair requires about 105 degrees (Johnston and Schmidt, 1970). Restoring "normal" range of motion may not be as realistic or necessary as obtaining the range of motion required to restore normal function.

Once the client is ambulatory, his or her weight-bearing status must be determined. This again depends on the type of infection, surgical procedure, stage of recovery, and extent of joint destruction. Articular cartilage heals very slowly, and that portion on weight-bearing surfaces should be protected from undue compressive or shear forces. In addition, immobilization has deleterious effects on articular cartilage as well as on other periarticular tissue (Akeson et al., 1967;

Enneking and Horowitz, 1972). Exercise following prolonged immobilization should take these factors into consideration. Often a non–weight-bearing status is used with the intention of minimally loading the joint. In fact the compressive forces may actually increase when compared to those of a touch-down weight-bearing gait pattern (Radin et al., 1979). Other factors such as the weight of the limb and muscular contraction must be considered. Long-term use of an ambulatory aid may be indicated over a 2- to 3-year period (Givens-Heiss et al., 1992). The use of a cane in the contralateral hand can reduce weight-bearing forces by up to 15% (Ely and Schmidt, 1977).

References

Akeson W, Amiel D, La Violette D: The connective tissue response to immobility: A study of the chondroitin 4 and 6 sulfate; dermatan sulphate changes in periarticular connective tissue of control and immobilized knees of dogs. Clin Orthop 51:183–197, 1967.

Almekinders L: Osteomyelitis: Essentials of diagnosis and treatment. J Musculoskel Med 11:31–40, 1994.

Behrman R, Kliegman R, Nelson W, Vaughn V: Nelson Textbook of Pediatrics. Philadelphia, W.B. Saunders, 1992.

Bennett OM, Namnyak SS: Acute septic arthritis of the hip joint in infancy and childhood. Clin Orthop 281:123–132, 1992.

Berchuck M, Garfin S, Abitbol J, Wilber G: Vertebrectomy for tumors and infections in the lumbar spine. Operative Techniques Orthop 1:97–105, 1991.

Berkow R: Biology of infectious disease. *In* The Merck Manual of Diagnosis and Therapy, ed 16. Rahway NJ, Merck, 1992, pp 2399–2460.

Boden S, Davis D, Dina T, Sunner J: Postoperative diskitis: Distinguishing early MR imaging findings from normal postoperative disk space changes. Radiology 184:765–771, 1992.

Boissonnault W: Examination in Physical Therapy Practice, ed 2. New York, Churchill Livingstone, 1995, pp 1–30.

Brennan PJ, DeGirolamo MP: Musculoskeletal infections in immunocompromised hosts. Orthop Clin North Am 22:389–399, 1991.

Brown D, Young L: Hand infections. South Med J 86:56–66, 1993.

Bullough P, Vigorita V: Atlas of Orthopaedic Pathology. Baltimore, University Park Press, 1984.

Cheatle M: The effect of chronic orthopedic infection on quality of life. Orthop Clin North Am 22:539–547, 1991.

Chen, WS: Chronic sciatica caused by tuberculous sacroiliitis. Spine 20:1194–1196, 1995.

Cohen J, Bonfiglio M, Campbell C: Orthopedic Pathophysiology in Diagnosis and Treatment. New York, Churchill Livingstone, 1990.

Cooper C, Cawley M: Bacterial arthritis in the elderly. Gerontology 32:222–227, 1986.

Crawford A, Kucharzyk D, Ruda R, Smitherman H: Diskitis in children. Clin Orthop 266:70–79, 1991.

Deyo R, Rainville J, Kent D: What can the history and physical examination tell us about low back pain? JAMA 268:760–765, 1992.

Dubost JJ, Fis I, Denis P, et al: Polyarticular septic arthritis. Medicine (Baltimore) 72:296–310, 1993.

Eilert RE, Georgopoulos G: Orthopedics. *In* Hathaway WE, Hay WW, Groothuis JR, Paisley JW (eds): Current Pediatric Diagnosis and Treatment, ed 13. Norwalk, Conn, Appleton & Lange, 1995, pp 748–767.

Ely DD, Schmidt GI: Effect of cane on variables of gait for patients with hip disorders. Phys Ther 57:507–516, 1977.

Enneking WF, Horowitz M: The intraarticular effects of immobilization on the human knee. J Bone Joint Surg [Am] 54:973–985, 1972.

Esterhai J, Gelb I: Adult septic arthritis. Orthop Clin 22:503–514, 1991.

Gelberman RH, Woo SL, Lothringer K, et al: Effects of early intermittent passive mobilization on healing canine tendons. J Hand Surg 7:170–175, 1982.

Gibbons R: Bacterial attachment to host tissues. *In* Gorbach SL, Bartlett JG, Blacklow NR (eds): Infectious Diseases. Philadelphia, WB Saunders, 1992, pp 7–16.

Givens-Heiss D, Krebs D, O'Riley P, et al: In vivo acetabular contact pressures during rehabilitation, Part II: Postacute phase. Phys Ther 72:7007–710, 1992.

Goldenberg D: Septic arthritis. *In* Goroll A, May L, Mulley A (eds): Primary Care Medicine; Office Evaluation and Management of the Adult Patient, ed 3. Philadelphia, JB Lippincott, 1995, pp 821–829.

Green N: What to do when you suspect acute hematogenous osteomyelitis in children. J Musculoskel Med 5(8):62–74, 1988.

Gristina A, Naylor P, Myrvik Q: Mechanisms of musculoskeletal sepsis. Orthop Clin North Am 22:363–371 1991.

Heggeness M, Esses S, Errico T, Hansen A: Late infection of spinal instrumentation by hematogenous seeding. Spine 18:492–496, 1993.

Hicklin S, DePretis M: Lower Extremity: Hip. *In* Myers RS (ed): Saunders Manual of Physical Therapy Practice. Philadelphia, WB Saunders, 1995, pp 955–1000.

Ho G Jr, Tice AD, Kaplan SR: Septic bursitis in the prepatellar and olecranon bursae. Ann Intern Med 89:21–27, 1978.

Hodge WA, Carlson K, Figan R, et al: Contact pressure from an instrumented hip endoprosthesis. J Bone Joint Surg [Am] 71:1378–1386, 1989.

Hopewell PC: A clinical view of tuberculosis. Radiol Clin North Am 33;641–653, 1995.

Jereb J, Cauthen G, Kelly G, Geiter L: The epidemiology of tuberculosis. *In* Friedman L: Tuberculosis—Current Concepts and Treatment. Boca Raton, Fla, CRC Press, 1994, pp 2–26.

Johnston RC, Schmidt GL: Hip motion measurements for selected activities of daily living. Clin Orthop 72:205–215, 1970.

Kanavel AB: Infections of the Hand; A Guide to the Processes in the Fingers, Hand, and Forearm, ed 7. Philadelphia, Lea & Febiger, 1939.

Kelly PJ, Martin WJ, Coventry MB: Bacterial arthritis in the adult. J Bone Joint Surg [Am] 52:1595–1602, 1970.

Klemm K: Antibiotic bead chains. Clin Orthop 295:63–76, 1993.

Korkis A, Gantz N: Osteomyelitis and septic arthritis. *In* Steinberg G, Akins C, Baran D (eds): Ramamurti's Orthopaedics in Primary Care, ed 2. Baltimore, Williams & Wilkens, 1992, pp 346–353.

Mourad LA: Alterations of musculoskeletal function. *In* McCance KL, Huether SE (eds): Pathophysiology: The Biologic Basis for Disease in Adults and Children, ed 2. St Louis, Mosby–Year Book, 1994, pp 1434–1481.

Neu H: General Therapeutic Principles. *In* Gorbach SL, Bartlett JG, Blacklow, NR (eds): Infectious Diseases. Philadelphia, WB Saunders, 1992, pp 153–159.

Nickel V: General principles of orthopaedic rehabilitation. *In* Nickel V, Botte M (eds): Orthopaedic Rehabilitation, ed 2. New York, Churchill Livingstone, 1992, pp 3–10.

Norris J, (ed): Professional Guide to Diseases, ed 5. Springhouse, Pa, Springhouse, 1995.

Patzakis M, Mader J: Symposium: Current concepts in the management of osteomyelitis. Contemp Orthop 28:157–185, 1994.

Patzakis M, Rao W, Wilkins J, et al: Analysis of 61 cases of vertebral osteomyelitis. Clin Orthop 264:178–183, 1991.

Phillips B: Nontraumatic disorders. *In* Crenshaw AH (ed): Campbell's Operative Orthopaedics. St Louis, Mosby–Year Book, 1992, pp 1939–1955.

Pope T, Wang G, Whitehill R: Discogenic vertebral sclerosis: A potential mimic of disc space infection or metastatic disease. Orthopedics 13:1389–1397, 1990.

Radin EL, Simon SR, Rose RM, Paul IL: Practical Biomechanics for the Orthopedic Surgeon. New York, Wiley, 1979.

Rich E, Kilner J: Pathogenesis of tuberculosis. *In* Friedman L (ed): Tuberculosis—Current Concepts and Treatment. Boca Raton, Fla, CRC Press, 1994, pp 27–51.

Roach K, Brown M, Ricker E, et al: The use of patient symptoms to screen for serious back problems. J Orthop Sports Phys Ther 21:2–6, 1995.

Salter RB, Simmonds DF, Malcolm BW, et al: The biological effect of continuous passive motion on the healing of full thickness defects in articular cartilage. J Bone Joint Surg Am 62:1232–1251, 1980.

Sapico FL, Montgomerie JZ: Vertebral osteomyelitis. Infect Dis Clin North Am 4:539–550, 1990.

Simon H: Management of tuberculosis. *In* Goroll A, May L, Mulley A (eds): Primary Care Medicine: Office Evaluation and Management of the Adult Patient, ed 3. Philadelphia, JB Lippincott, 1995, pp 701–705.

Smith TK: Nutrition: Its relationship to orthopedic infections. Orthop Clin North Am 22:373–377, 1991.

Starr J: Pulmonary system. *In* Myers R (ed): Saunders Manual of Physical Therapy Practice. Philadelphia, WB Saunders, 1995, pp 253–321.

Strickland E, Fares M, Krebs D, et al: In vivo acetabular contact pressures during rehabilitation, Part I: Acute phase. Phys Ther 72:691–699, 1992.

Strong M, Lejman T, Michno P, Hayman M: Sequelae from septic arthritis of the knee during the first two years of life. J Pediatr Orthop 14:745–751, 1994.

Studahl M, Bergman B, Kalebo P, Lindberg J: Septic arthritis of the knee: A 10 year review and long-term follow-up using a new scoring system. Scand J Infect Dis 26:85–93, 1994.

Sullivan JA: Infectious and inflammatory processes of the knee. *In* Larson RL, Grana WA (eds): The Knee: Form, Function, Pathology, and Treatment. Philadelphia, WB Saunders, 1993 pp 258–272.

Swezey R: Rehabilitation in arthritis and allied conditions. *In* Kottke F, Stillwell K, Lehmann J (eds): Krusen's Handbook of Physical Medicine and Rehabilitation, ed 3. Philadelphia, WB Saunders 1982, pp 679–716.

Talavera W, Lessnau KD, Handwerger S: Extrapulmonary tuberculosis. *In* Friedman L (ed): Tuberculosis—Current Concepts and Treatment. Boca Raton, Fla, CRC Press, 1994, pp 113–151.

Tehranzadeh J, Wang F, Mesgarzadeh M: Magnetic resonance imaging of osteomyelitis. Crit Rev Diagn Imaging 33:495–534, 1992.

Thijn CJP, Steensma JT: Tuberculosis of the Skeleton. New York, Springer-Verlag, 1990.

Warner W: Osteomyelitis. *In* Crenshaw A (ed): Campbell's Operative Orthopaedics, ed 8. St Louis, Mosby–Year Book, 1992a, pp 119–130.

Warner W: Tuberculosis and other unusual infections. *In* Crenshaw A (ed): Campbell's Operative Orthopaedics, ed 8. St Louis, Mosby–Year Book, 1992b, pp 177–189.

Wood G: Infections of spine. *In* Crenshaw A (ed): Cambell's Operative Orthopaedics, ed 8. St Louis, Mosby–Year Book, 1992, pp 3791–3823.

Zinberg E: Chronic osteomyelitis. *In* Nickel V, Botte M (eds): Orthopaedic Rehabilitation, ed 2. New York, Churchill Livingstone, 1992, pp 659–677.

SECTION 3

chapter 22

Musculoskeletal Neoplasms

Terry Randall

Neoplasm is defined as a new or abnormal growth of cells. It is often used interchangeably with *tumor*, which means any swelling or mass. Neoplasms are divided into two broad categories: benign and malignant. Benign neoplasms are those which show no tendency to metastasize, are noninvasive, and usually slow-growing. A malignant neoplasm is one that can be invasive or metastasize (see Chapter 7).

Although neoplasms represent a small portion of the spectrum of pathology seen in clinics, their severity and potential for serious consequences necessitate an understanding of their detection and treatment. The purpose of this chapter is to review the characteristics of primary and secondary skeletal neoplasms. Those that may be encountered by therapists are highlighted. It is hoped that by increasing awareness of the clinical manifestations, earlier detection will be possible. Appropriate treatment interventions and explanations of the ramifications of treatment and the disease process are given.

To grasp the concepts of tumor formation one must understand that bone metabolism is a balancing act of bone formation and resorption. Cortical bone is most abundant in the outer walls of the shafts of long bones and is quite dense. The haversian canal system, which refers to the concentric rings of lamellae, is found in the cortical bone. The cortical bone surrounds the trabecular or cancellous bone, which is the honeycomb-like bone found in the ends of long bones. Trabeculae are aligned with applied stresses in the bone. The metabolic activity is higher in cancellous bone than cortical bone. This is why many disorders that create disturbances in metabolic activity are first noted in cancellous bone.

Bone remodeling is a structured process governed by highly specialized cells. Osteoblasts are derived from mesenchymal fibroblast-like cells and are responsible for bone formation. Bone formation is accomplished by synthesizing various collagens, alkaline phosphatase, and other chemicals. This is done in response to the resorption performed by the osteoclasts. The osteoclast is a multinucleated giant cell derived from granulocyte-macrophage precursors. The coupling of these two processes usually results in a balance of bone resorption and formation. When metabolic bone disease and neoplastic formations occur, this balance is upset.

PRIMARY TUMORS: OVERVIEW

Description. Primary tumors are those which have developed from or within tissue in a localized area. Hence a tumor may originate from bone, cartilage, nerve, collagen, adipose, or muscle. Primary tumors can be benign or malignant. Some benign bone tumors pose difficult evaluation and treatment decisions and can result in a significant level of impairment. Although rare, some benign lesions can develop into a malignancy. Benign lesions usually do not cause the constant, severe pain that is commonly associated with progressive malignant disease. Table 22–1 shows the major types of soft tissue sarcomas, their origin, and their usual sites.

Malignant primary tumors of bone by definition have the capacity to spread to other sites. Skeletal neoplasms often metastasize to the lungs via the bloodstream. Fortunately, malignant tumors are not as common as benign lesions. Their rarity has made it difficult to standardize treatment. For this reason most individuals with malignant primary tumors are referred to regional centers where valuable experience concerning evaluation and treatment can be gained and then applied to future cases.

Incidence. Primary tumors of the musculoskeletal system are rare. Excluding myeloma, as few as 2000 new cases of primary bone tumors and 6400 cases of soft tissue sarcomas are detected annually in the United States (Parker et al., 1996). This does not mean that they are unimportant. A great deal of time is devoted to research, reporting, and educating physicians in the proper management of people with primary tumors. These efforts are indicative of the serious nature of the problem rather than the frequency.

Etiology. The histogenesis of benign tumors is generally poorly understood.

Risk Factors. Although bone tumors may have a predilection for certain sites, age groups, and gender, risk factors have not been identified. Soft tissue tumors may be associated with high doses of radiation or exposure to toxic chemicals in the workplace (herbicides, preservatives, etc.).

Pathogenesis. Bone tumors are considered to be either osteoblastic or osteolytic, although most have characteristics of both processes. The osteoblastic process can be preceded by tumor cells or by normal cells in the host bone reacting to the tumor. Since the host bone continues with the normal process of resorption and bone formation, there will likely be a variety of cell types within the lesion. This makes histologic interpretation difficult.

Clinical Manifestations. It is the clinical features that must be well understood to ensure that the diagnostic evaluation proceeds expeditiously. Unfortunately, many tumors are not diagnosed on their initial presentation. This is due to the ambiguous presentation of most tumors in their early stages rather than to any degree of ineptness on the part of a health-care provider. In fact, rarely does one actually find the case that everyone describes as typical for a given lesion. This applies to benign and malignant tumors and to the

TABLE 22–1 Soft Tissue Sarcomas: Their Origin and Usual Sites

Origin	Type of Tumor	Usual Sites
Fibrous tissue	Fibrosarcoma	Arms, legs, trunk
	Malignant fibrous histiocytoma	Legs
Fat	Liposarcoma	Arms, legs, trunk
Muscle		
Striated	Rhabdomyosarcoma	Arms, legs
Smooth	Leiomyosarcoma	Uterus, gastrointestinal system
Blood vessels	Hemangiosarcoma	Arms, legs, trunk
	Kaposi's sarcoma	Legs, trunk
Lymph vessels	Lymphangiosarcoma	Legs
Synovial tissue	Synovial sarcoma	Legs
Peripheral nerves	Neurofibrosarcoma	Arms, legs, trunk
Cartilage	Chondrosarcoma	Legs

Modified from Pfalzer L: Oncology: Examination, diagnosis, and treatment; Medical and surgical considerations. *In* Myers RS (ed): Saunders Manual of Physical Therapy Practice. Philadelphia, WB Saunders, 1995, pp 65–147.

initial presentation, as well as to the appearance of the lesion (Cohen et al., 1990).

Pain is a hallmark of tumor development, especially with malignant lesions. Since pain is the overriding symptom in many persons who seek treatment, a great deal of information should be obtained concerning the pain. The onset, progression, nature, quality, intensity, and aggravating factors are just some of the factors that may be important in identifying a tumor in the early stages. Pain is not a measure of disease progression. Some tumors can progress to advanced stages without causing significant pain. Soft tissue tumors may progress with relatively little pain because the soft tissue allows the growth to occur without putting undue pressure on nerve endings.

Intense pain is more likely to occur with rapidly growing lesions. Constant pain is often present which is not dependent on position or activity. The presence of night pain is considered an important finding. When the client reports night pain, further questioning is required. Ensure that he or she is reporting true night pain, which awakens the person from sleep, rather than a pain that makes it difficult to fall asleep. The intensity of pain is again important. Often, persons with tumors will report a severe pain that awakens them consistently and prevents them from returning to sleep for some time. Roach et al. (1995) reported that a positive report of sleep disturbance and pain with walking had a sensitivity of .87. This means that 87% of clients with serious spinal pathology would report at least one of these symptoms.

It is also important to remember the common referral patterns for pain. These may give important clues to the origin of symptoms. The varied pain pattern is due to the nature, site, and rate of growth of the tumor. Other signs and symptoms that are frequently encountered include swelling, fever, and the presence of a mass.

Swelling surrounding a tumor may not be detectable in a bone tumor, but with soft tissue tumors close to the skin surface, swelling may be one of the first presenting signs. The nature of swelling, to include the location, amount, temperature, and tenderness, is somewhat dependent on the vascularity of the lesion.

Other factors that are useful in screening for serious pathology include unexplained weight loss, failure of rest to provide relief of pain, age, and history of cancer. Deyo found that the combination of these factors gave a sensitivity of 1.00, although the specificity was just .60 (Deyo et al., 1992). The history will often give more meaningful information regarding the possibility of skeletal neoplasms than the physical examination. A careful physical examination may reveal a mass or other signs of an inflammatory process.

The presence of a mass should raise questions concerning the location, mobility, tenderness, dimensions, and recent changes in any of these factors. As with pain, the size of the mass is not indicative of the severity of the lesion but is but one factor to consider. Any recent change in the mass is of great interest.

Medical Management

Diagnosis. Many tumors cannot be palpated but if a mass is present its characteristics must be noted. A tumor overlying bone and muscle can be evaluated by contracting the muscle and checking for movement or change in consistency of the tumor. Radiographs also help to differentiate between bone and soft tissue involvement.

Plain radiographs are a mainstay in detection and evaluation of many skeletal tumors. In many cases skeletal tumors are found incidentally on routine radiographs for associated injuries. The radiograph provides unique information concerning skeletal tumors. The location of the tumor will give many clues to the type of lesion (Fig. 22–1). Some tumors develop exclusively in the epiphysis whereas others develop in the diaphysis of long bones. The effect that the tumor has on bone is described as destructive or lytic if the normal bone pattern is disruptive.[1] This may be evident by an irregular, erosive border surrounding the lesion, loss of trabeculae, or disruption of the cortex. Table 22–2 summarizes the differential criteria for specific tumors.

The response of surrounding bone to the tumor is another important feature to note on plain radiographs. Sclerotic borders give an indication of the growth characteristics of the tumor. A well-defined border with definite sclerotic margins is seen with a slow-growing lesion. A tumor with a permeated or motheaten appearance (i.e., an area with multiple holes with irregular edges randomly distributed) with an expansive cortical shell indicates an aggressive malignant lesion (Fig. 22–2). Codman's triangle is formed when the lesion has an interrupted layer of bone that has expanded beyond the periosteum (Fig. 22–3). The tumor's location, its effect on bone, and the local bone response to the lesion are just some of the radiographic features to be noted and that will help in planning the rest of the evaluation. Radionuclide bone scans, computed tomography (CT), and magnetic resonance imaging (MRI) all have a place in the evaluation of bone lesions.

A biopsy is the definitive diagnostic procedure in both bone and soft tissue tumors. This procedure can take many

[1] Approximately 50% of the bone must be destroyed before the lesion can be detected.

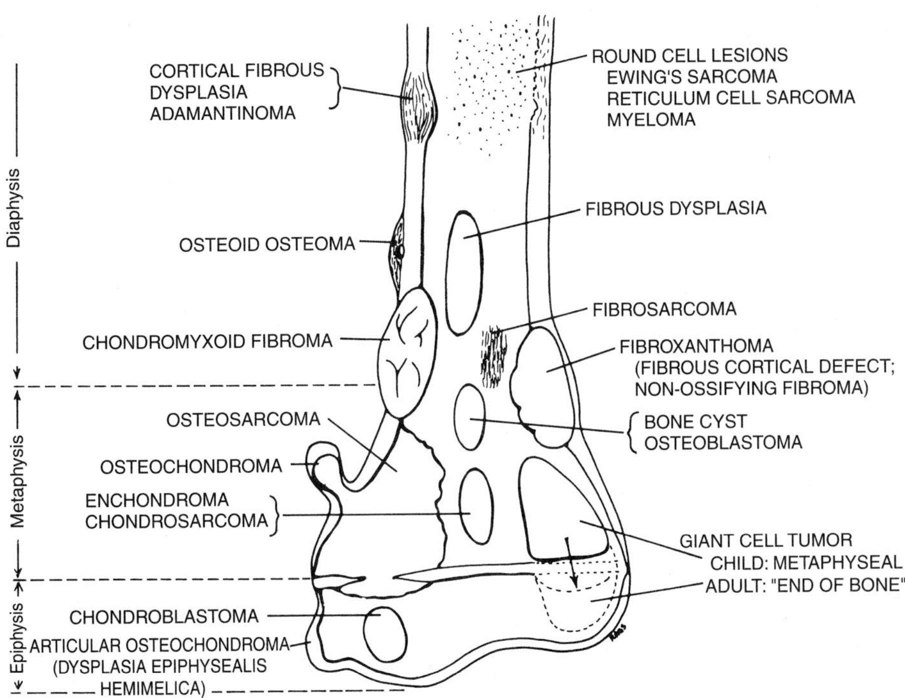

Figure 22-1. Composite diagram illustrating frequent sites of bone tumors. The diagram depicts the end of a long bone that has been divided into the epiphysis, metaphysis, and diaphysis. The typical sites of common primary bone tumors are labeled. Bone tumors tend to predominate in those ends of long bones that undergo the greatest growth and remodeling and hence have the greatest number of cells and amount of cell activity (shoulder and knee regions). When small tumors, presumably detected early, are analyzed, preferential sites of tumor origin become apparent within each bone, as shown in this illustration. This suggests a relationship between the type of tumor and the anatomic site affected. In general, a tumor of a given cell type arises in the field in which the homologous normal cells are most active. These regional variations suggest that the composition of the tumor is affected or may be determined by the metabolic field in which it arises. (*From Madewell JE, Ragsdale BD, Sweet DE: Radiologic and pathologic analysis of solitary bone lesions: I. Internal margins. Radiol Clin North Am 19:715, 1981.*)

forms. The decision to do an open, closed, incisional, or excisional biopsy is based on the location and type of tumor. The biopsy can result in significant morbidity and should be performed by the same persons involved with the definitive treatment (Mankin et al., 1982).

Various laboratory studies are used to detect, diagnose, and differentiate musculoskeletal neoplasms. Laboratory tests that may be of value include the complete blood count (CBC); urinalysis; erythrocyte sedimentation rate (ESR); serum calcium, phosphorus, alkaline phosphatase, and protein values; and serum protein electrophoresis.[2]

Pathologic fractures are rare in primary neoplasms, but if the lytic process affects a significant portion of the cortex (over 50%), or occupies 60% of the bone diameter, the risk of fracture increases (Levinson, 1993). A relatively small lytic lesion in the femoral neck that destroys the inferior cortex of the femoral neck also places the client at increased risk. In benign lesions there may be no other symptoms to warn of the impending fracture. Solitary bone cysts, fibrous dysplasia, nonossifying fibroma, and enchondromas may only be detected after presentation with a pathologic fracture. In addition to the tumor itself, other factors such as disuse, treatment (biopsy, radiation), and other health problems (osteoporosis) may increase the risk of pathologic fracture.

[2] For example, serum levels of alkaline phosphatase and calcium are frequently elevated with metastatic disease.

The purpose of much of the extensive workup once a tumor is identified is to determine the grade and stage of the tumor. Grading determines the extent of anaplasia, or differentiation, of the cells. Grade I signifies cells that are very differentiated and grade IV, those which are undifferentiated. Staging of a tumor is concerned with the extent of its growth. The TNM staging system reflects the degree of local extension at the primary tumor site, involvement of local nodes, and presence of metastasis. (Hermanek and Sobin, 1987) (see Chapter 7). Enneking's system also uses histologic and anatomic criteria to define various tumors (Enneking, 1986). Staging helps in planning and standardizing the treatment strategy of these rare lesions.

Treatment. Once identified and staged, decisions about treatment can be considered. Treatment ranges from observation in the case of some benign bone tumors to radical resection in which the entire involved bone and all the tissue compartments adjacent to the tumor are removed. A marginal excision removes the tumor at its border which results in some of the tumor being undisturbed. A wide excision removes some of the normal surrounding tissue leaving none of the tumor (Enneking, 1983). Soft tissue sarcomas often require wide excision to reduce the recurrence rate.

The use of radiation is recommended for some tumors such as Ewing's sarcoma and myeloma, but many malignant tumors are not affected by radiation. For some soft tissue tumors,

TABLE 22-2 DIFFERENTIAL CRITERIA FOR BENIGN LYTIC BONE LESIONS

Mnemonic: "Fegnomashic"

F, Fibrous dysplasia—No periosteal reaction; if in tibia, mention adamantinoma

E, Enchondroma—Must have calcification, except in phalanges; no periostitis

Eosionophilic Granuloma—Must be under age 30 yr

G, Giant cell tumor—(1) Closed epiphyses; (2) epiphyseal and abutting the articular surface; (3) eccentric; (4) well-defined but nonsclerotic border

N, Nonossifying fibroma—Must be under age 30 yr; no periostitis

O, Osteoblastoma—Mentioned whenever A is mentioned, even if over age 30 yr

M, Metastasis and myeloma—Must be over age 40 yr

A, Aneurysmal bone cyst—Must be under age 30 yr; expansible

S, Solitary bone cyst—Must be centrally located; under age 30 yr

H, Hyperparathyroidism (brown tumor)—Must have other evidence of *HAT*

I, Infection—If adjacent to a joint, must involve the joint

C, Chondroblastoma—Must be under age 30 yr; epiphyseal

Chondromyxoid fibroma—Mention when considering nonossifying fibroma

<30 YR OLD	NO PERIOSTITIS OR PAIN	EPIPHYSEAL LOCATION	MULTIPLE SITES
E, G	F	C	F, E, E, M, H, I
A	E	I	F
N	N	G	E, G
C	S	A	E
S	E, G	M, H	I
		A	

Modified from Helms C: Fundamentals of Skeletal Radiology: Benign Cystic Lesions. Philadelphia, WB Saunders, 1989, p 11.

adjunctive radiation is used in an attempt to limit the degree of surgical excision needed. In general, radiation is not recommended for benign conditions.

Chemotherapy is also utilized to help eradicate malignant tumors. When chemotherapy is combined with other modalities such as surgery and radiation, less toxic doses can be used. Chemotherapy has resulted in increased survival rates in clients with Ewing's sarcoma.

Prognosis. The prognosis is based in part on the type of tumor and whether it is benign or malignant. One should not assume that benign means "innocuous." Large fibrous defects in weight bearing bones can cause pathologic fractures. Osteoblastomas in the spine may produce neurologic signs and require resection. Slow-growing tumors should be followed for prolonged periods, to determine the ultimate prognosis. Prognosis can vary from 3- to 5-year survival rates for clients with sarcomas and myeloma, to tumors that are asymptomatic.

Special Implications for the Therapist **22-1**

PRIMARY TUMORS

A therapist's involvement with clients with musculoskeletal neoplasms should begin with increased efforts directed toward early detection and education. Although many musculoskeletal tumors produce symptoms that are also present with more mundane conditions, careful examination and monitoring of a client's response to treatment may lead to earlier detection and treatment. By including the possibility of a primary musculoskeletal tumor in the differential diagnosis of clients who have continued pain despite appropriate rest and treatment, further medical evaluation may be recommended which may help to reveal other pathology.

Therapists are also asked to treat clients who are undergoing treatment for primary musculoskeletal neoplasms. A comprehensive approach should be utilized to ensure that psychosocial aspects, as well as musculoskeletal problems, are addressed. Therapists must understand the pathology of the tumor to understand the entire treatment plan.

Communication within the treatment team among physicians, nurses, and therapists cannot be overemphasized. Communication is essential to coordination and follow-through of the treatment and rehabilitation program. A detailed approach to evaluation and treatment of clients with cancer should be formulated (Pfalzer, 1995).

Specific treatment techniques and goals can be developed with a thorough understanding of the pathology and the medical treatment being undertaken. Surgical procedures will have an effect on multiple organ systems, as will chemotherapy and radiation therapy. A detailed description of pain is always indicated, as described in Chapter 7. There are many other factors to consider before implementing a treatment plan following orthopedic procedures, such as controlling compressive forces and weight bearing, which are discussed under Special Implications for the Therapist: Musculoskeletal Infections in Chapter 21. As discussed, treatment of tumors can result in amputation, prolonged immobilization, resection, or extensive surgical reconstruction, all of which require the involvement of many different types of rehabilitation.

SPECIFIC PRIMARY TUMORS

Bone Island

Overview. Bone islands are oval, usually small, sclerotic lesions of bone. They are one of the most common benign bone lesions. Bone islands are seen in all bones and may present as solitary or multiple lesions. The lesion is well-defined and made up of cortical bone with a well-developed haversian canal system (Fechner and Mills, 1992). The borders blend in with the surrounding bone. The presence of spicules of cortical bone extending from the margins to the surrounding trabeculae is characteristic.

Incidence. A prevalence of 14% has been reported for spinal bone islands (Resnick and Hemcek, 1983).

Clinical Manifestations. Bone islands are always asymptomatic. They are seen on radiographs as incidental findings.

LYTIC PATTERNS

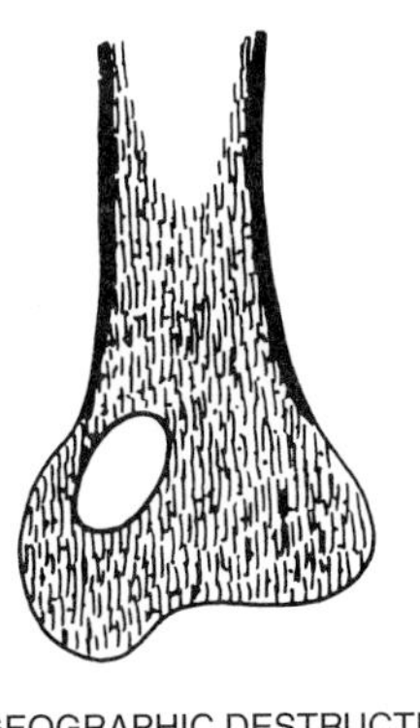

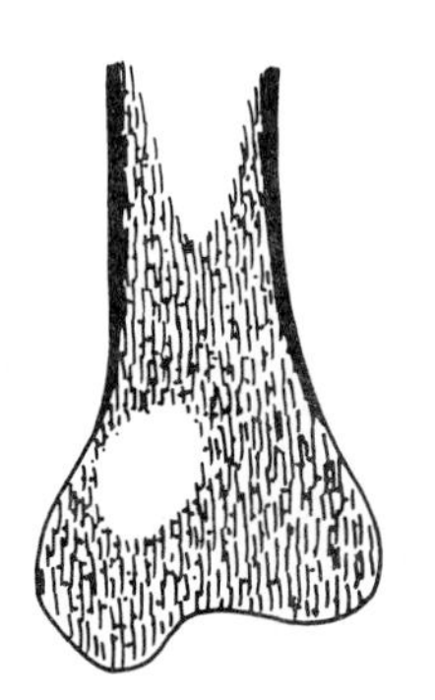

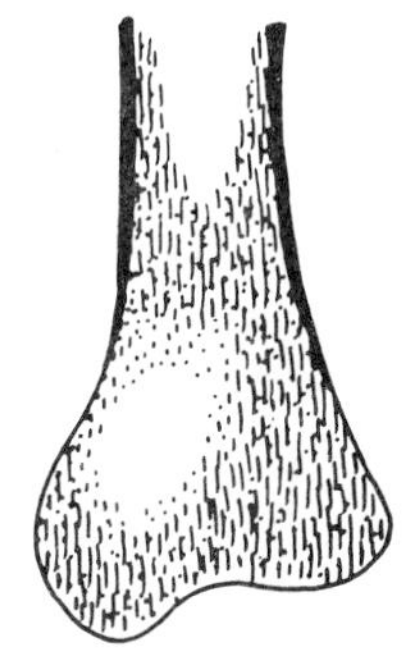

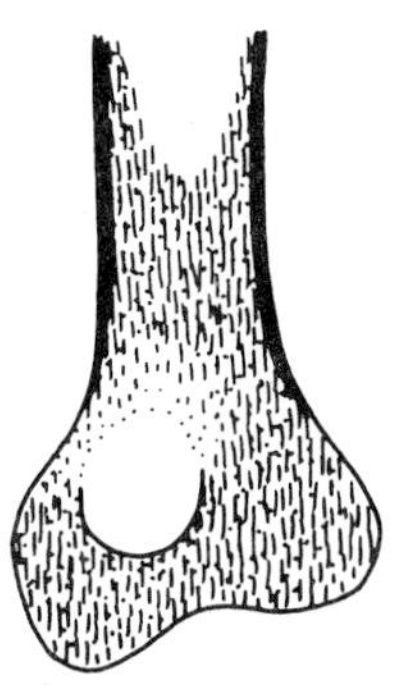

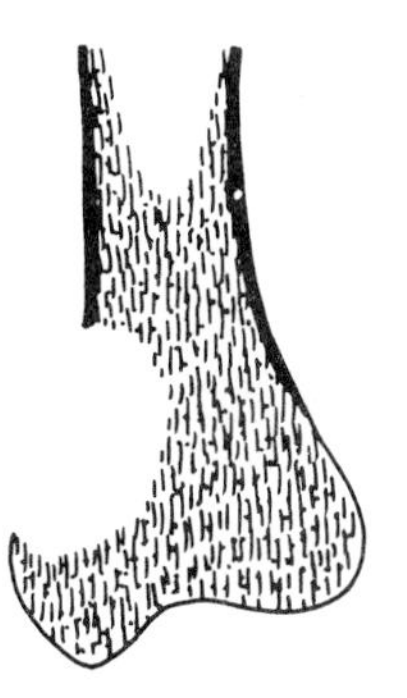

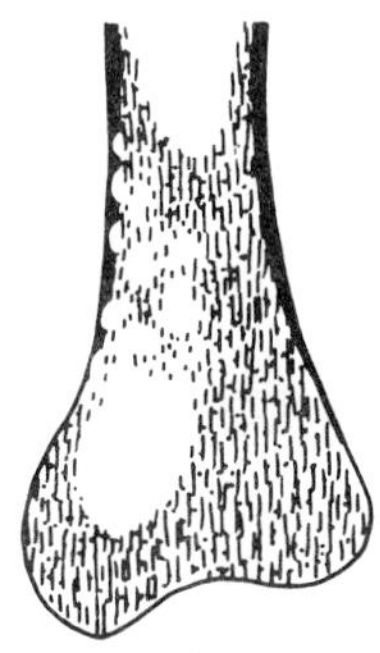

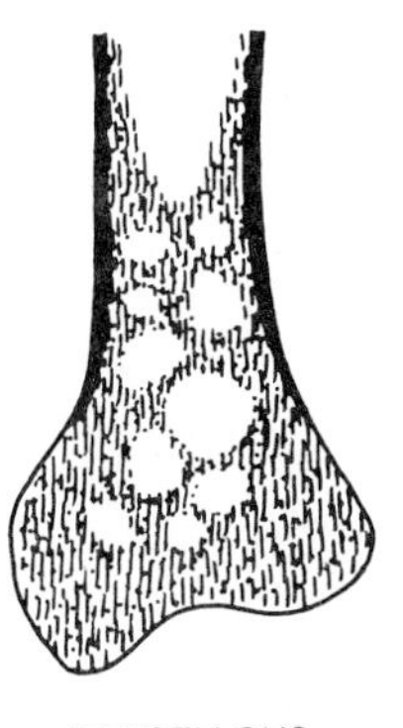

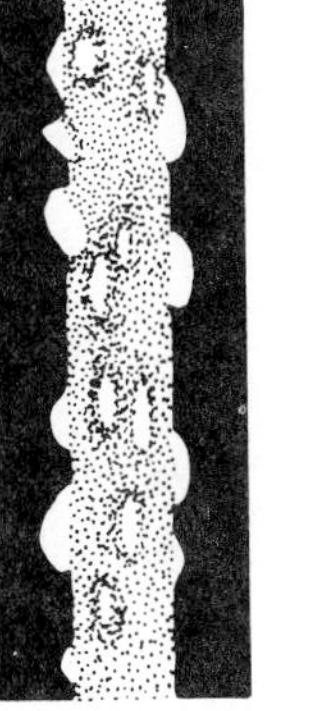

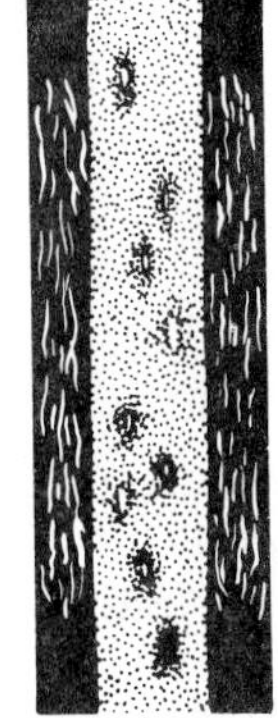

Figure **22–2.** Schematic diagram of patterns of bone destruction (types IA, IB, IC, II, and III) and their margins. *Arrows* indicate the most frequent transitions or combinations of these margins. Transitions imply increased activity and a greater probability of malignancy. (*From Madewell JE, Ragsdale BD, Sweet DE: Radiologic and pathologic analysis of solitary bone lesions: I. Internal margins. Radiol Clin North Am 19:715, 1981.*)

Medical Management

Diagnosis. When the bone islands are small (less than 1 cm), diagnosis with plain radiographs is adequate. They are usually oblong and align themselves with the axis of the bone. A bone scan is usually normal, confirming the absence of malignancy.

Treatment. The emphasis is not on treatment but on the judicious use of diagnostic tools. Biopsies should be avoided. They are usually unnecessary.

Prognosis. Although some bone islands can enlarge they do not transform into malignant lesions.

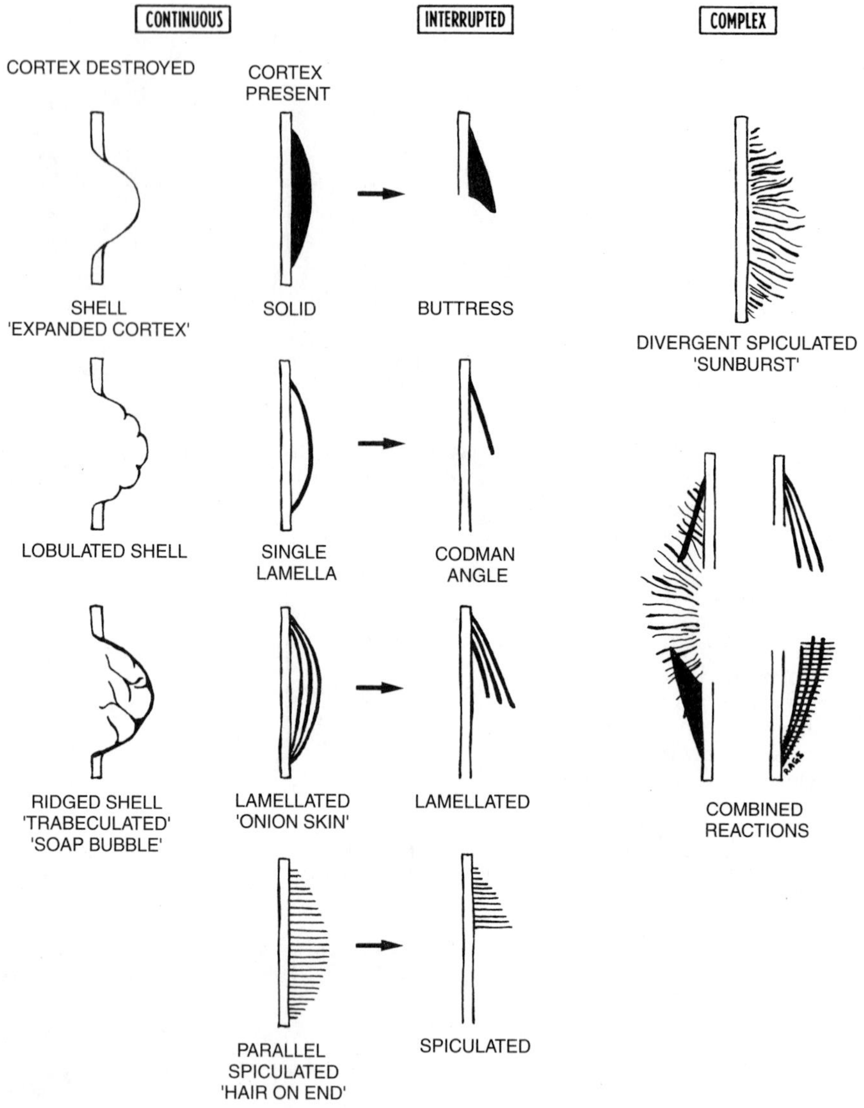

Figure **22–3.** Schematic diagram of periosteal reactions. The *arrows* indicate that the continuous reactions may be interrupted. (*From Ragsdale BD, Madewell JE, Sweet DE: Radiologic and pathologic analysis of solitary bone lesions: II. Periosteal reactions. Radiol Clin North Am 19:749, 1981.*)

Special Implications for the Therapist **22–2**

BONE ISLANDS

Bone islands are seen in radiographs of clients with a variety of musculoskeletal traumas. If clients are aware of these lesions they should be reassured that they pose no significant health concern. Many physicians do not inform patients that bone islands are present. Care must be taken not to alarm the client. The word "tumor" is foreboding and should be used sparingly.

Osteoid Osteoma

Overview. Osteoid osteoma is a benign vascular osteoblastic lesion first described by Jaffe (Jaffe, 1935). It is often found in the cortex of long bones such as the femur, near the end of the diaphysis (Fig. 22–4). Pathologic study shows areas of immature bone surrounded by prominent osteoblasts and osteoclasts. The lesion is vascular but no cartilage is present (Bullough and Vigorita, 1984). The tumor can lead to joint pain and dysfunction which often delay the diagnosis by masquerading as a more common problem such as an overuse syndrome.

Incidence. Osteoid osteoma accounts for about 10% of benign bone tumors. Most of these lesions are found in males under the age of 25.

Clinical Manifestations. Gradually increasing pain, described as a dull ache, is the primary complaint. The pain is often worse at night and can sometimes be relieved by salicylates. Pain relief may be due to the inhibitory effect of aspirin on prostaglandins which are produced by osteoid osteomas. Systemic symptoms are uncommon.

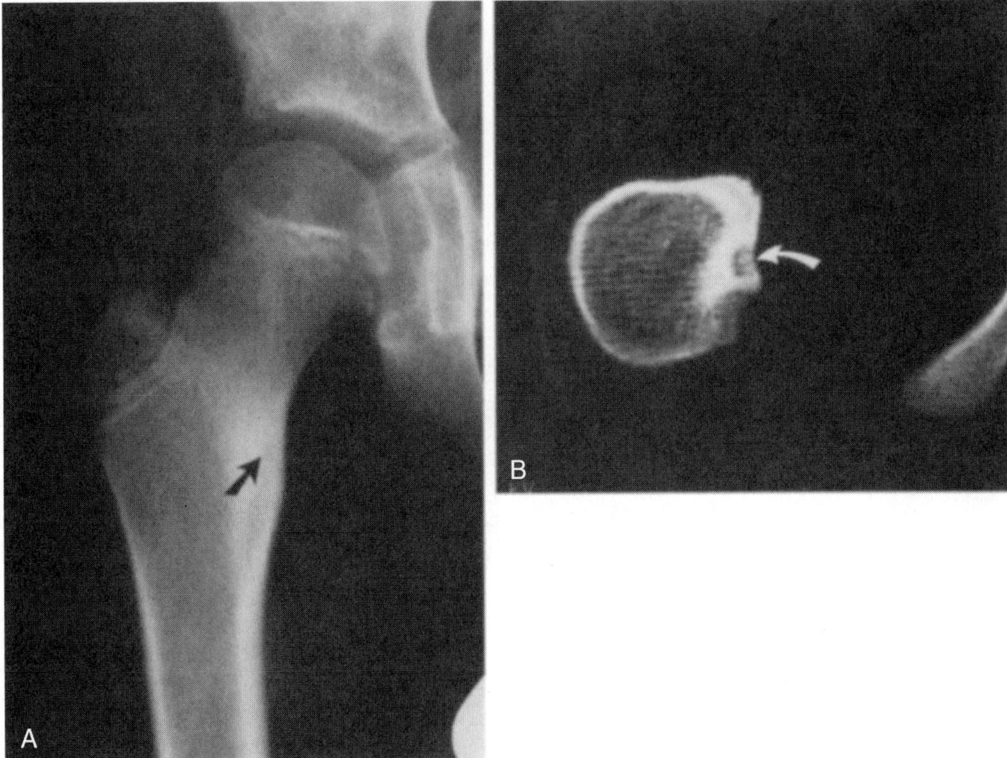

Figure 22–4. Osteoid osteoma. A, Bony sclerosis with cortical thickening is seen in this person with pain in the proximal femur. A faint lucency (*arrow*) can be seen in the area of sclerosis, which is the nidus of an osteoid osteoma. B, A CT scan through the nidus shows it to lie just dorsal to the lesser trochanter (*arrows*). This is a characteristic appearance of an osteoid osteoma with CT. (*From Helms C: Fundamentals of Skeletal Radiology. Benign Cystic Lesions. Philadelphia, WB Saunders, 1989, p 195.*)

Medical Management

Diagnosis. Radiographs can be diagnostic for osteoid osteoma. In some cases the tumor is not easily identified on radiographs and further testing is required, such as a bone scan, which will show a focal uptake of the radiotracer. When the tumor is intra-articular, CT or MRI can be used to accurately locate the nidus when plain films may not be adequate (Fechner and Mills, 1992). Radiographs are normal early in the course. Later, a small (less than 1 cm) translucency or nidus forms which is surrounded by sclerotic bone.

Treatment. In those tumors that are symptomatic, surgical excision of the nidus may be indicated. Since the tumor is small, excision is usually sufficient, although bone grafting may be needed depending on the size and location of the tumor (Gitelis and Schajowicz, 1989).

Prognosis. Recurrence is rare, and a full recovery is common. Differences in the expected rate of recovery may occur depending on the location of the tumor and the extent of excision required.

Special Implications for the Therapist **22–3**

OSTEOID OSTEOMA

The size and extent of the resection may mandate some activity restrictions or weight bearing limitations if the risk of fracture exists. Monitoring bone healing with serial radiographs may help to guide the weight bearing progression. Intra-articular lesions certainly require more extensive rehabilitation for restoration of normal function.

Osteoblastoma

Overview. Osteoblastoma is a benign tumor similar to osteoid osteoma, only larger, with a tendency to expand. Some aggressive forms of osteoblastoma have been recognized (Gitelis and Schajowicz, 1989). Unlike osteoid osteoma, osteoblastomas are often found in the spine. Those found in the long bones are usually in the diaphysis, although as with most tumors they can be seen elsewhere (Fig. 22–5). The histologic makeup of osteoblastoma is very similar to an osteoid osteoma. In fact sometimes it is size alone that differentiates the two, with osteoblastoma being the larger. The lesions are osteolytic and have a sclerotic border.

Incidence. Osteoblastoma occurs most often in males less than 30 years old. Osteoblastomas make up only 1% to 2% of all benign bone tumors.

Clinical Manifestations. When located in the spine, the pedicles are often affected. Pain is the common presentation and may be relieved with aspirin, but usually is not as severe as with osteoid osteoma. Tenderness over the lesion is expected. With a spinal location a functional scoliosis may be observed.

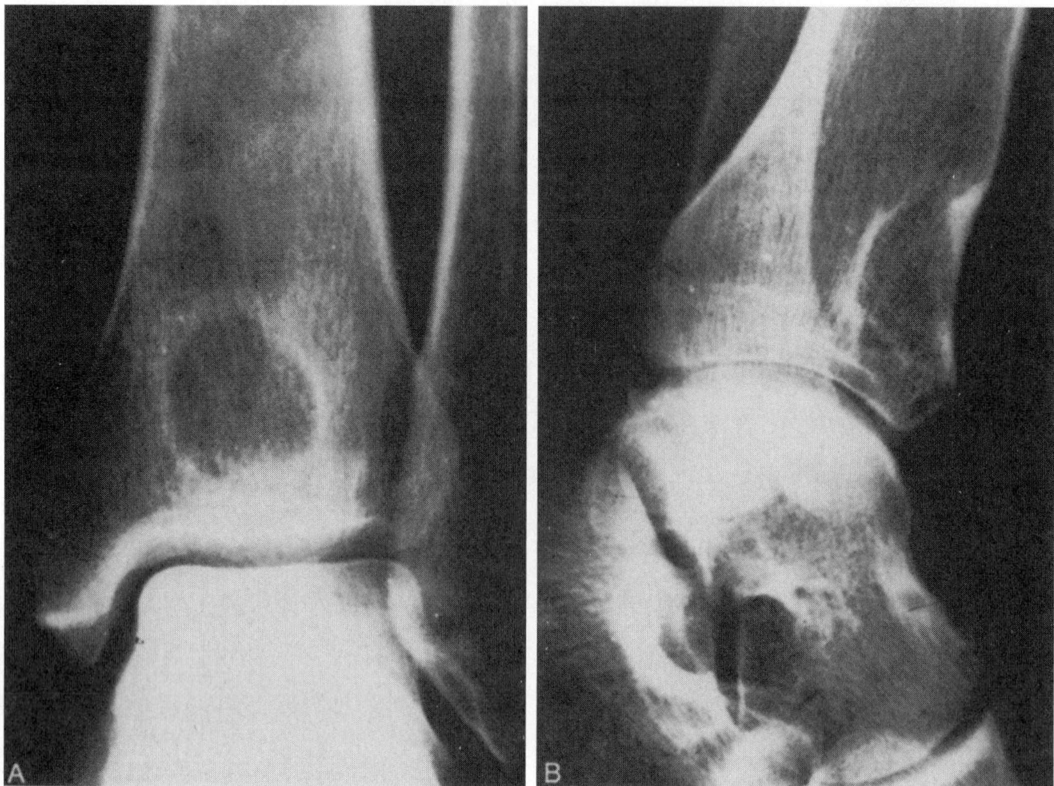

Figure **22–5.** A 24-year-old woman with genuine (conventional) osteoblastoma of the tibia. Anteroposterior (*A*) and lateral (*B*) radiographs show a round radiolucent lesion with slightly sclerotic borders at the lower and anterior aspect of the tibia. (*From Gitelis S, Schajowicz F: Osteoid osteoma and osteoblastoma. Orthop Clin 20:320, 1989.*)

In some cases a neurologic deficit may be present which can mimic other, more common causes of nerve compression.

Medical Management

Diagnosis. Osteoblastoma is seen on plain radiographs but when located in the spine other imaging techniques are also useful. The lesion can have variations in its appearance. Often it looks like a large osteoid osteoma with a well-defined radiolucency in the central portion, with a thin sclerotic border. It can also can be similar to an aneurysmal bone cyst which is expansile, lytic, and has a soap bubble appearance (see Fig. 22–3) (Helms, 1989). CT and MRI are valuable in localizing the tumor and determining the extent of tissue involved. An aggressive lesion can expand beyond the cortex and involve soft tissue.

Treatment. In the long bones, curettage (scraping to remove the contents of the bone cavity) is often adequate. A wider excision is sometimes recommended because of the unpredictable nature of osteoblastoma. This can result in the need to perform reconstructive procedures using autografts or allografts and internal fixation when the tumor is located in the diaphysis of long bones. If the joint is affected, implants may be needed. In the spine, removal of the tumor may lead to instability, which may require fusion and internal fixation (Gitelis and Schajowicz, 1989).

Prognosis. Ninety percent to 95% of osteoblastomas are cured by the initial treatment (Fechner and Mills, 1992). There is a risk of malignant transformation into an osteosarcoma but this can sometimes be determined early and appropriate treatment rendered with adjunctive chemotherapy or radiation. Recurrence of the lesion is reported in 15% of cases (Jackson, 1978).

Special Implications for the Therapist **22–4**

OSTEOBLASTOMA

Surgical excision may be extensive. In the long bones the risk of pathologic fracture is often present. The use of external fixation, allografts, immobilization, and limited weight bearing is common.

Osteosarcoma

Overview. Osteosarcomas are tumors with malignant properties. They are usually destructive lesions with abundant sclerosis both from the tumor itself and from reactive bone formation. A characteristic of osteosarcoma is the production of osteoid by malignant, neoplastic cells. This is seen on photomicrographs and is one of the features used to help differentiate this tumor. Resected specimens usually show that the cortex has been broken by the destructive tumor. Although various types of osteosarcoma exist, including parosteal, periosteal, telangiectatic, and small cell, only the most common, conventional intramedullary osteosarcoma is discussed here.

Incidence. Osteosarcomas account for 15% of all primary bone tumors (Dahlin and Unni, 1986). They occur most often in males under the age of 30. Only myeloma is seen more often. Osteosarcoma can develop in many bones, but is more common in long bones.

Etiology. Osteosarcomas can be primary or secondary. Secondary osteosarcomas are those that develop from other lesions such as Paget's disease, chronic osteomyelitis, osteoblastoma, or giant cell tumor.

Risk Factors. This is one tumor that does appear to have some familial tendencies. A genetic predisposition to primary osteosarcoma, as well as an increased risk of developing secondary osteosarcoma from radiation, is seen in children with retinoblastoma (Fechner and Mills, 1992).

Clinical Manifestations. This tumor seems to appear in bones undergoing an active growth phase. The long bones, such as the femur and tibia, have a relatively more active growth period than other bones, which makes them more vulnerable (Fig. 22–6). Pain is the presenting complaint. The tumor is often located in the metaphysis but does not cross the physis. Even so, joint pain can be present as the lesion penetrates the cortex and invades the joint capsule. Since osteosarcoma can be a rapidly destructive tumor, the pain increases and swelling may develop in just a few weeks.

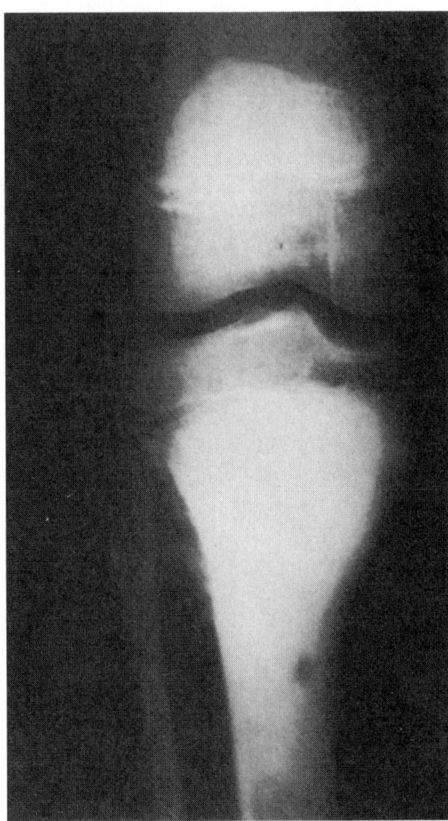

Figure **22–6.** Osteosarcoma. An extremely sclerotic lesion in the proximal tibia of a child is noted, which is characteristic of an osteogenic sarcoma. (*From Helms C: Fundamentals of Skeletal Radiology: Benign Cystic Lesions. Philadelphia, WB Saunders, 1989, p 48.*)

Medical Management

Diagnosis. Plain radiographs often reflect dramatic changes and obvious tumor formation, but important findings can also be subtle. In Figure 22–7 plain films of a pelvis demonstrate minimal changes that could easily be dismissed as insignificant. The CT scan, however, reveals a large osteosarcoma involving the ilium (Helms, 1989). More commonly, radiographs show a rapidly growing lesion with poorly defined margins, and a permeated or moth-eaten appearance in the lytic area.

A biopsy is performed to determine the histologic makeup of the lesion. Serum alkaline phosphatase levels may be elevated, but this is not diagnostic.

Treatment. The current surgical thinking is to use limb-sparing techniques (segmental resection and replacement with bone graft or implant) whenever possible (Fig. 22–8). Many factors, such as age, remaining growth, expected functional outcome, and prognosis, are considered. Chemotherapy and radiation often precede surgery. Chemotherapy is evaluated by its effect on the client as well as on the tumor. Chemotherapy may also help to lessen the chance of "skip lesions," or multiple foci of tumor that can cause recurrence of the tumor after surgery.

Prognosis. Until the 1970s surgery for osteosarcoma consisted of amputation or disarticulation. Even then the survival rate at 5 years was about 20% (Dahlin and Coventry, 1967). The use of radiotherapy and adjunctive chemotherapy results in cure rates of 70% to 80%, whereas surgery alone will probably allow pulmonary metastasis to occur. Even with chemotherapy the outcome is dependent on the ability of the surgeon to achieve a tumor-free margin.

Special Implications for the Therapist **22-5**

OSTEOSARCOMA

Malignant neoplasms usually necessitate aggressive treatment and therefore rehabilitation is more intensive, prolonged, and individualized. Extensive surgery, such as limb-sparing techniques, has provided therapists with an opportunity to assist these clients in maximizing their function (Fig. 22–9).

Since these tumors are treated at regional medical centers, the initial phases of rehabilitation may be implemented by therapists with a great deal of experience working with clients with malignant neoplasms and those who have undergone various reconstructive surgical procedures. When the client returns home a local therapist may be called on to continue the rehabilitation program. Communication with the therapist at the regional medical center to confirm initial treatment, progression, and prognosis is recommended.

Ewing's Sarcoma

Overview. Ewing's sarcoma is a malignant primary bone tumor. Although this type of bone tumor was noted as early as 1866 it was not until 1921 that James Ewing described his experience with the lesion. The pelvis and lower extremity

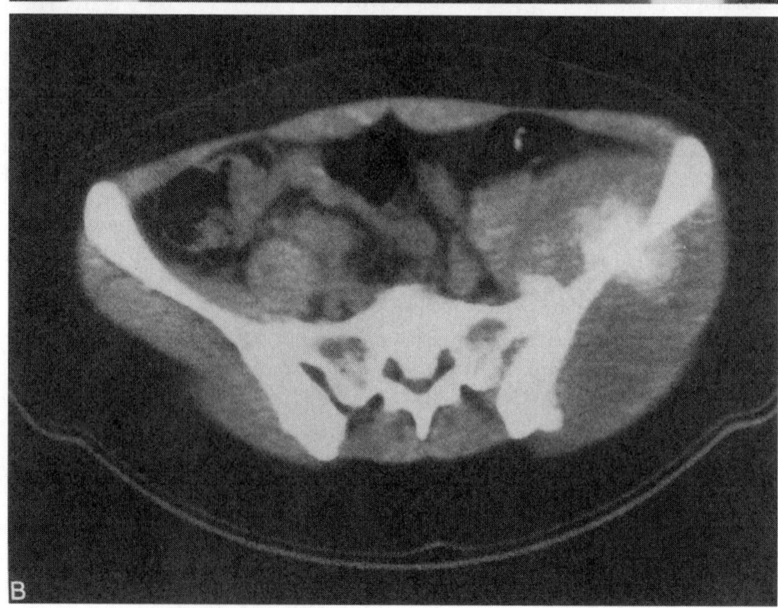

Figure **22–7.** Osteosarcoma. A, A subtle sclerotic lesion is seen in the left ilium adjacent to the sacroiliac joint that was initially diagnosed as osteitis condensans ilii, a benign entity. Because of persistent pain the person returned for a follow-up visit, and a small amount of cortical destruction on the pelvic brim was noted (*arrow*). *B,* A CT scan was performed, which showed a large tissue mass and new bone tumor around the ilium, which is characteristic of an osteogenic sarcoma. (*From Helms, C: Fundamentals of Skeletal Radiology: Benign Cystic Lesions. Philadelphia, WB Saunders, 1989, p 49.*)

are the most common sites. Unlike many tumors there does not appear to be any predilection for a certain part of the bone.

Incidence. This tumor affects young children more than any other primary neoplasm. Most tumors occur in young people under the age of 20 and they have been reported in children as young as 18 months. It makes up about 10% of primary bone tumors.

Pathogenesis. The tumor is soft, sometimes viscous, with hemorrhagic necrosis. The cortical bone is affected via the haversian canals (Eggli et al., 1993). The medullary cavity is affected and infiltration of the bone marrow can progress extensively without radiographic evidence of bone destruction. It is likely that Ewing's sarcoma is the least differentiated of the small cell neoplasms (Fechner and Mills, 1992).

Clinical Manifestations. As with other malignant bone tumors, pain is a common presenting complaint. Swelling may accompany the pain and both are usually progressive. Pathologic fractures occur, but only in 5% of cases. In young children flulike symptoms, including a low-grade fever, may be present.

Medical Management

Diagnosis. Radiographs show an obvious lytic process with a moth-eaten appearance involving a diffuse area of bone (Fig. 22–10). An onion skin formation may be seen which is due to layers of reactive bone. On radiographs the appearance may not differentiate this lesion from osteomyelitis or osteosarcoma. An elevated ESR may be noted but is not diagnostic. CT, MRI, and bone scans can help diagnose the tumor. A biopsy is done to confirm the diagnosis and to help with staging and planning treatment. The biopsy should be performed with the procedure in mind and therefore is best

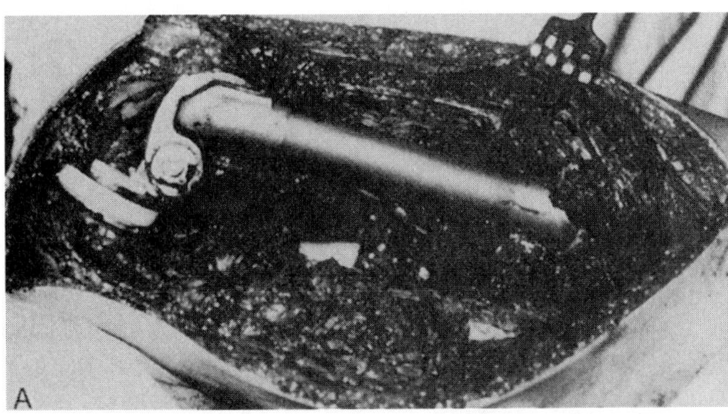

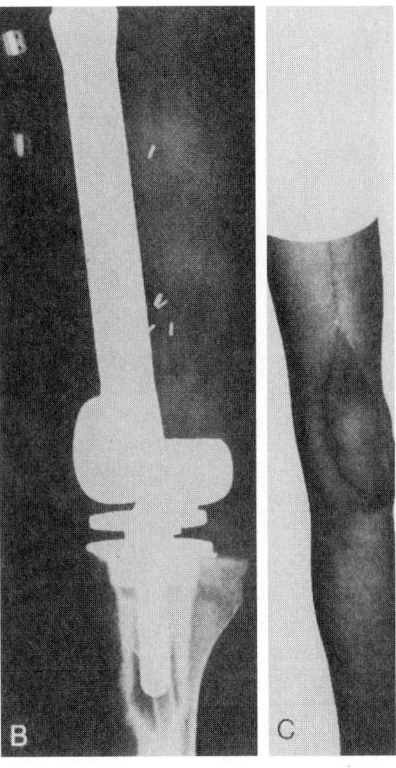

Figure 22–8. A 17-year-old boy with osteosarcoma of the distal femur. A, Intraoperative photograph following resection of the distal femur. B, Postoperative radiograph of custom-made rotating hinge prosthesis. C, Follow-up clinical photograph (3 years after surgery). Soft tissue coverage of the prosthesis by latissimus dorsi myocutaneous free flap with acceptable cosmesis. (*From Klein M, Kenan S, Lenis M: Osteosarcoma: Clinical and pathological considerations. Orthop Clin 20:343, 1989.*)

done by the same surgical team planning to do further resection.

Treatment. Radiation, multiagent chemotherapy, and surgery are used in conjunction to treat Ewing's sarcoma. Surgery can result in amputation, wide resection, or limb-sparing procedures. Radiation therapy is often directed to the primary bone lesion or the entire bone, as well as to both lungs for metastatic disease. Chemotherapy may be beneficial when used before radiation or surgery to minimize exposure.

Prognosis. The prognosis for clients with this tumor is improving steadily. Just a few decades ago only about 15% of clients with Ewing's sarcoma lived longer than 5 years after detection. The 5-year survival rate is now in the 50% to 75% range (O'Connor and Pritchard, 1991). Long-term survival is determined by the presence or absence of metastasis rather than the extent of the local tumor. As many as 35% of clients will have metastatic disease, usually to the lung, at the time of diagnosis (Jaffe, 1989). It is likely that younger children with small, well-defined, distal lesions have the best prognosis.

Special Implications for the Therapist **22-6**
EWING'S SARCOMA

As with osteosarcoma, initial treatment is aggressive, involving extensive surgical resection or even amputation.

Cartilaginous Tumors

Overview. There are many tumors of cartilaginous origin (Table 22–3). Three of the more common tumors of a cartilaginous origin are the enchondroma, osteochondroma, and chondrosarcoma. Determining the aggressiveness of cartilaginous tumors is especially difficult. Even the histologic differentiation is troublesome. Sometimes the presence of pain or the development of pain in a previously diagnosed benign cartilaginous tumor such as enchondroma, is all that raises suspicion of a malignant process or transformation.

Enchondroma

Overview. Enchondroma is a common, benign tumor which arises from residual islands of cartilage in the metaphysis of bones (Fig. 22–11). The hand, femur, and humerus are common sites.

Incidence. Enchondromas account for 10% of benign skeletal tumors. They are seen in persons between the ages of 20 and 40, both men and women.

Pathogenesis. Enchondral ossification is the process by which most bones in the skeleton are formed. A cartilaginous model exists as a precursor to mature bone. A tumor may then develop from cartilage islands displaced from the growth plate during development. This is thought to occur perhaps secondary to trauma or to an abnormality in the growth plate. Histologically, enchondroma consists of hyaline cartilage appearing as lobules rimmed with a narrow band of reactive bone.

Clinical Manifestations. Enchondromas may be asymptomatic. In some cases there may be some swelling. When present in the hands, pain may be a symptom of pathologic stress fracture.

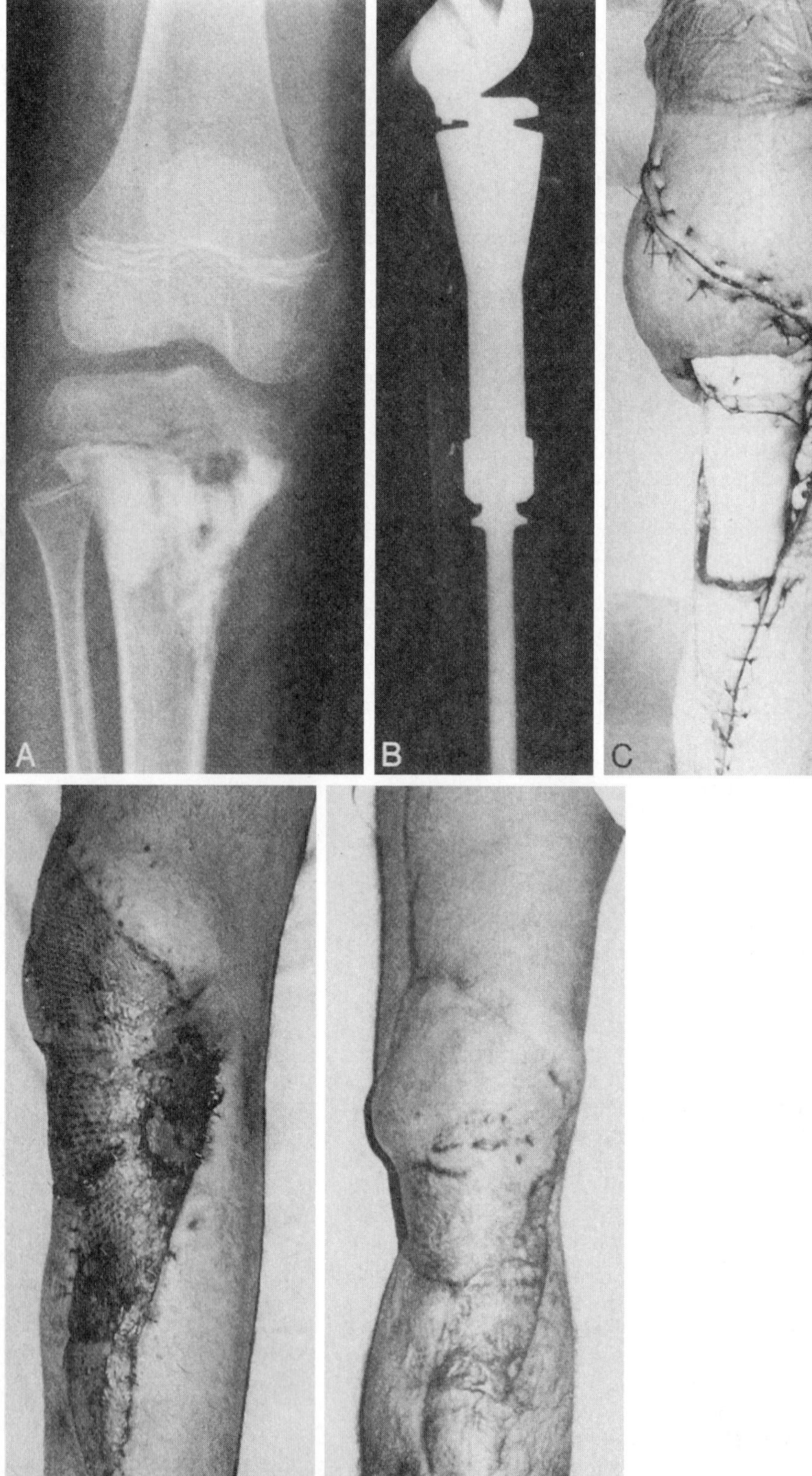

Figure **22–9.** Use of a free muscle transfer to salvage an infected, massive prosthesis. *A*, Preoperative radiograph of a 9-year-old boy with an osteosarcoma. *B*, Following radical resection, an expandable prosthesis was inserted. *C*, When infection occurred, with subsequent breakdown of the wound, the prosthesis was removed, and the area was widely debrided. A spacer of antibiotic-impregnated methacrylate was inserted. *D*, Infection was controlled, and the knee was reconstructed with another prosthesis and a free latissimus transfer. *E*, A satisfactory result was obtained, sparing the leg. (*From Hausman, M: Microvascular applications in limb sparing tumor surgery. Orthop Clin 20:434, 1989.*)

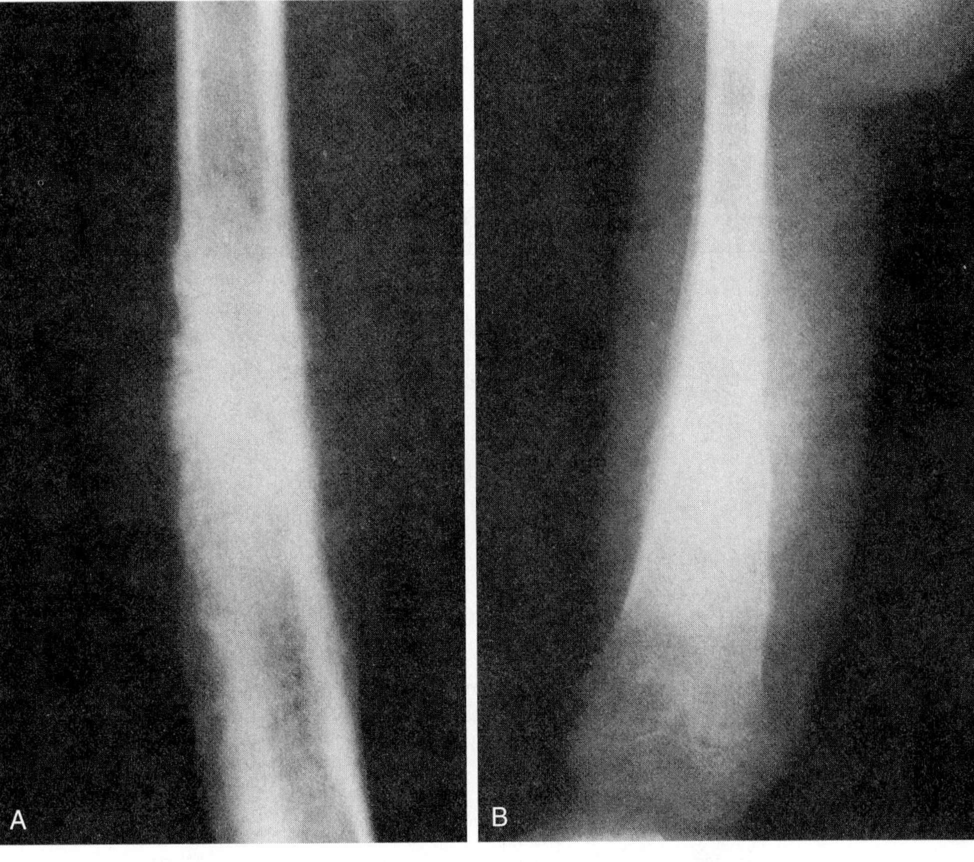

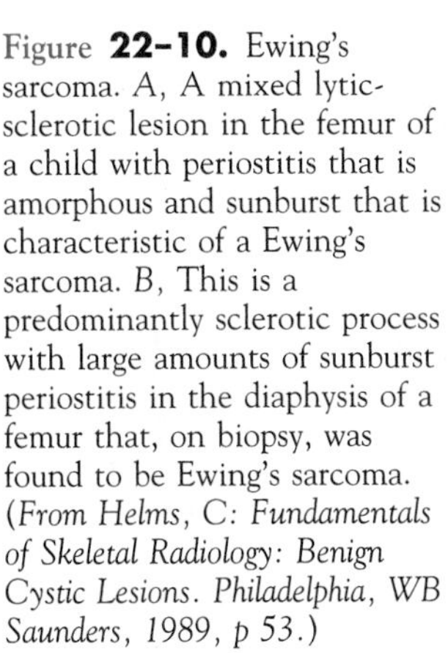
Figure **22-10.** Ewing's sarcoma. *A*, A mixed lytic-sclerotic lesion in the femur of a child with periostitis that is amorphous and sunburst that is characteristic of a Ewing's sarcoma. *B*, This is a predominantly sclerotic process with large amounts of sunburst periostitis in the diaphysis of a femur that, on biopsy, was found to be Ewing's sarcoma. (*From Helms, C: Fundamentals of Skeletal Radiology: Benign Cystic Lesions. Philadelphia, WB Saunders, 1989, p 53.*)

TABLE 22-3 CARTILAGINOUS TUMORS

Benign, fundamentally pure
- Enchondroma
- Ollier's disease
- Maffucci's syndrome
- Parosteal chondroma
- Tenosynovial chondroma
- Soft tissue chondroma

Benign, fundamentally impure
- Osteochondroma
- Osteochondromatosis
- Chondroblastoma
- Chondromyxoid fibroma

Malignant, fundamentally pure
- Primary chondrosarcoma
- Parosteal chondrosarcoma
- Secondary chondrosarcoma

Malignant, fundamentally impure
- Chondrosarcoma with coexistent fibrosarcomatous or osteosarcomatous elements
- Mesenchymal chondrosarcoma
- Secondary chondrosarcoma (transformed from osteochondroma or rarely from chondroblastoma or chondromyxoid fibroma)

Modified from Giudici MA, Moser R, Kransdorf M: Cartilaginous bone tumors. Radiol Clin North Am 31: 238, 1993.

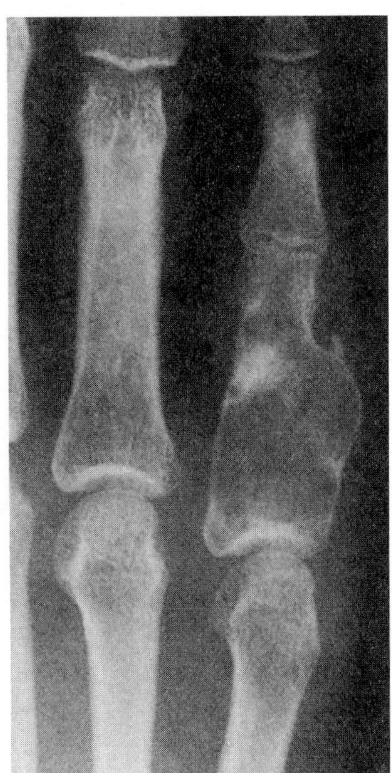
Figure **22-11.** Enchondroma of the proximal phalanx of the small finger in a 27-year-old woman. Note radiolucent, expansile lesion that resulted in attenuation and thinning of the cortex. (*From Greenspan A: Tumors of cartilage origin. Orthop Clin 20:351, 1989.*)

Medical Management

Diagnosis. In those cases where no symptoms are present, plain radiographs or bone scans performed for other reasons reveal the tumor as an incidental finding. Once detected, differentiating the lesion from a chondrosarcoma is crucial. It is not the histologic makeup that is the most informative but rather the radiograph and clinical history. Radiographs of enchondromas do not show cortical destruction. Pain without evidence of a fracture is also suspicious of malignancy rather than enchondroma (Fechner and Mills, 1992).

Treatment. Curettage is a common form of treatment, with or without bone grafting, depending on the size and location of the lesion. Clients with enchondromas in the hand may develop stress fractures that often respond to splinting (Noble and Lamb, 1974).

Prognosis. Malignant transformation can occur, especially in lesions proximal to the wrist and ankle, but is rare (Bogumill and Schwamm, 1984). Recurrence of enchondromas after curettage is less than 5%.

Osteochondroma

Overview. Osteochondroma is the most common primary benign neoplasm of bone. A continuous osseous outgrowth of bone with a cartilaginous cap is characteristic (Fig. 22–12). The outgrowth arises from the metaphysis of long bones and extends away from the nearest epiphysis (Salter, 1970). The metaphysis of long bones, especially the distal femur and proximal tibia, are common sites.

Incidence. The incidence of osteochondroma is unknown. Some reports indicate that males are affected more often but this may be due to the fact that it is often an incidental finding and males may be more likely to have a radiograph taken during the second decade of life when the lesion is usually seen.

Pathogenesis. Osteochondromas are an extension of normal bone and cartilage. The younger the individual, the larger the cartilage cap, which may be up to 3 cm in thickness. The central portion of the lesion is normal medullary bone. The lesion may begin as a displaced fragment of epiphyseal cartilage that penetrates a cortical defect and continues to grow (Milgram, 1983).

Clinical Manifestations. In some persons a mass will be detected. When the tumor is palpable it may, owing to the cartilaginous cap, feel much larger than is apparent on radiographs. (McGuire et al., 1990). Pain may be present if the lesion lies close to tendon, nerve, or bursae. Blood vessels can also be compromised by the tumor (Fig. 22–13). Many tumors are asymptomatic. The lesion has its own growth plate and will usually cease growing when the individual reaches skeletal maturity.

Medical Management

Diagnosis. Plain radiographs may show a slender stalk of bone directed away from the nearest growth plate. This is referred to as a pedunculated osteochondroma. A sessile osteochondroma has a broad base of attachment (Fig. 22–14). In both types the most important feature to note is the continuity of the cortex between the host bone and the tumor.

CT and MRI are not commonly used in the diagnostic

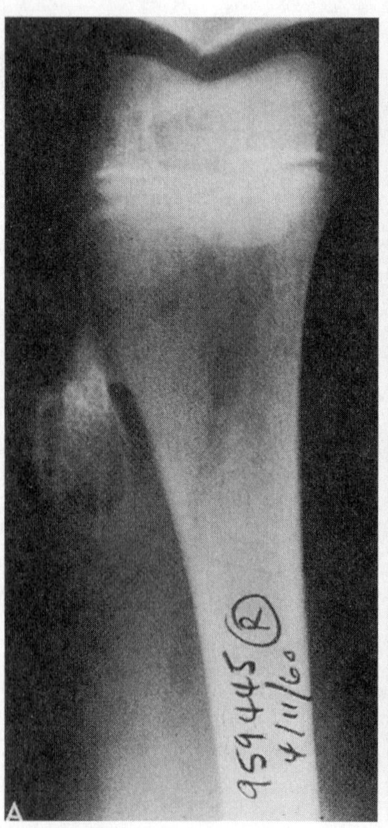

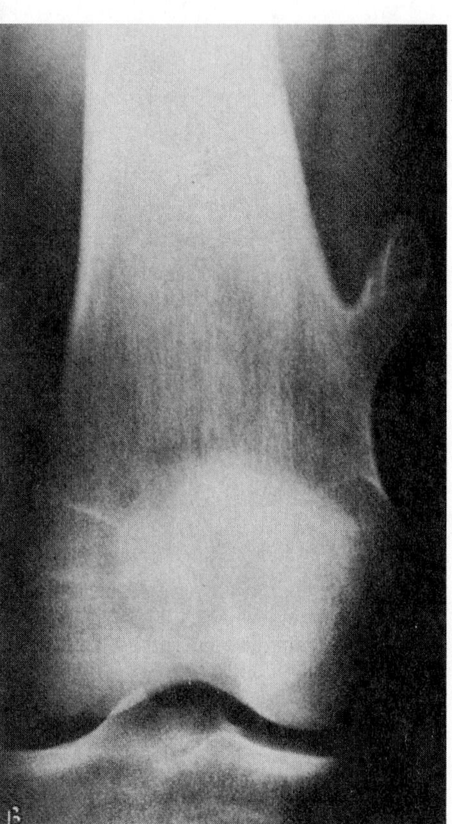

Figure **22–12.** Osteochondroma. Two radiographs (A and B) showing mature osteochondroma: stalked lesion pointing toward the diaphysis and away from the growth plate. (*From Bogumill G, Schwamm H: Orthopaedic Pathology, Philadelphia, WB Saunders, 1984, p 388.*)

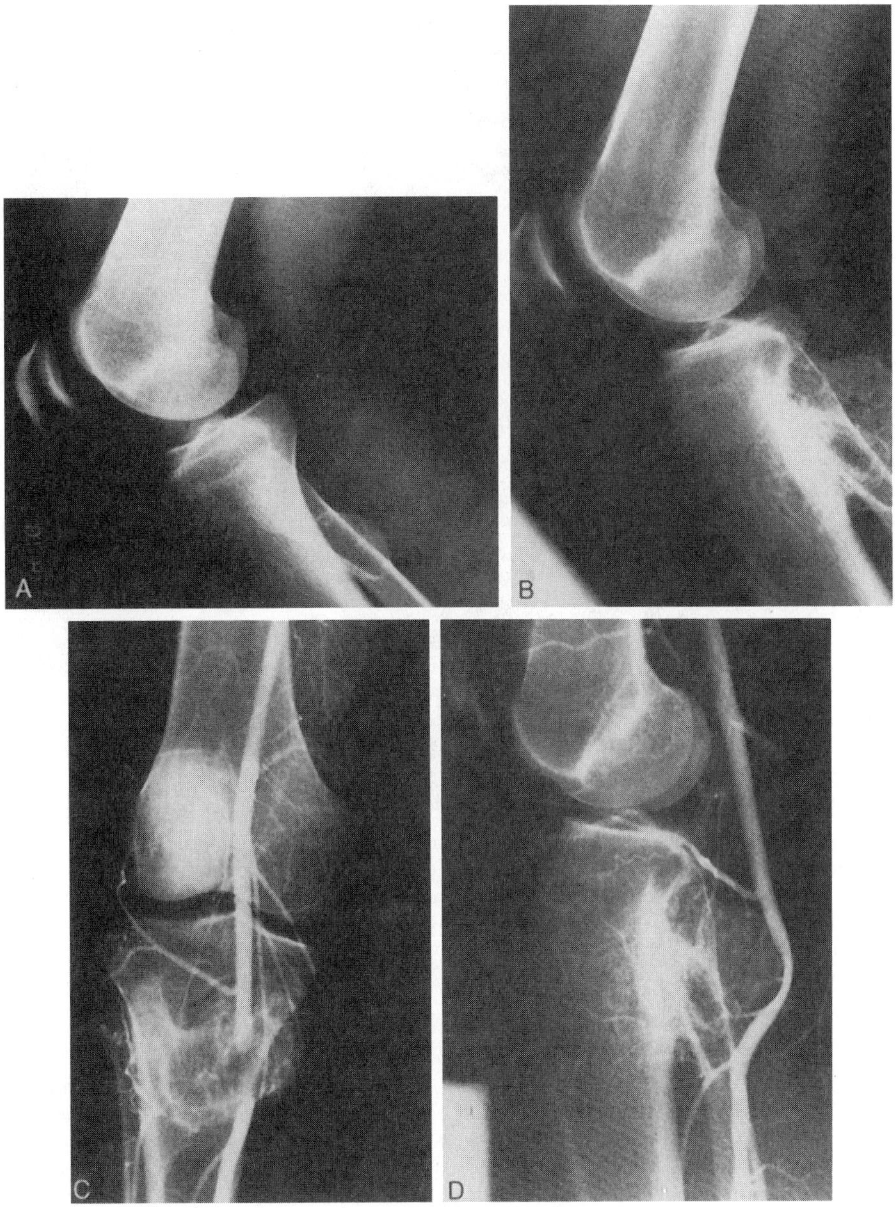

Figure **22–13.** Osteochondroma of the proximal fibula in a young man. *A*, Lateral radiograph of the right knee obtained when the patient was 17 years old demonstrates an exophytic lesion arising from the proximal fibula. *B*, Lateral radiograph obtained 8 years later shows considerable interim growth of the osteochondroma, although a smooth outline is maintained. Anteroposterior (*C*) and lateral (*D*) angiograms demonstrate displacement and marked narrowing of the distal popliteal artery by the tumor. (*From Guidici M, Moser R, Kransdorf M: Cartilaginous bone tumors. Radiol Clin North Am 31:247, 1993.*)

workup of benign lesions, but if there are atypical clinical manifestations or recent changes in the appearance of the lesion on plain radiographs, MRI may be indicated. For example, MRI can demonstrate the continuity of the marrow between the tumor and the host bone, thereby ruling out a periosteal osteosarcoma (Giudici et al., 1993).

Treatment. Since osteochondromas usually cease their growth at skeletal maturity, no treatment is needed unless they are symptomatic. Removal of the lesion is sometimes required when symptoms such as vascular compromise, chronic bursitis, or pain develop secondarily.

Prognosis. Rarely, an osteochondroma can transform into a chondrosarcoma. Those symptomatic lesions that are removed have a very low recurrence rate.

Chondrosarcoma

Overview. Chondrosarcoma is a tumor in which the neoplastic cells produce cartilage rather than the osteoid seen with the osteosarcoma. It can be primary or secondary. Primary chondrosarcomas are more common but their origin is idiopathic. They can be graded based on their microscopic appearance. The presence of a chondroid matrix, extent of necrosis, and type of cells are some of the grading standards used. Secondary tumors are those that arise from previously benign cartilaginous tumors or from a preexisting condition, such as Paget's disease (Klein et al., 1989). Chondrosarcoma is categorized by its location within bone and is called central, peripheral, or periosteal (Fechner and Mills, 1992).

Incidence. Males in their 40s to 60s are those most likely to be affected by primary chondrosarcoma. Of the malignant bone tumors, only myeloma and osteosarcoma are seen more often.

Pathogenesis. The neoplastic cartilaginous cells produce cartilage rather than the osteoid seen with osteosarcoma. Chondrosarcoma is classified by location of the lesion: central,

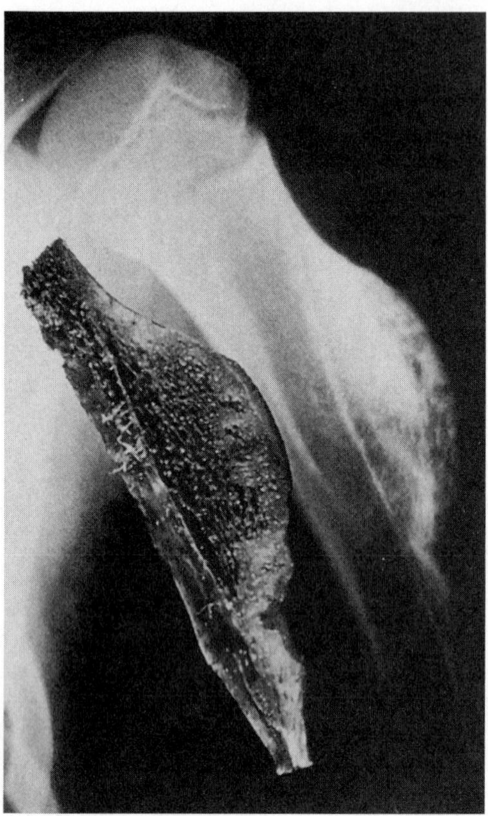

Figure **22–14.** Osteochondroma. Radiograph and gross specimen of the sessile osteochondroma. Note the cartilaginous component causing the radiographic defect in the distal portion. Note also incorporation of hematopoietic tissue into the base of the osteochondroma. (*From: Bogumill G, Schwamm H: Orthopaedic Pathology. Philadelphia, WB Saunders, 1984, p 383.*)

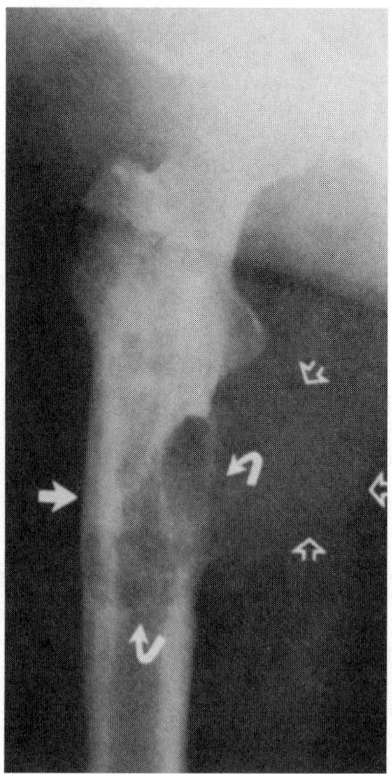

Figure **22–15.** Characteristic radiographic features of chondrosarcoma include thickening of the cortex (*closed arrow*), destruction of the medullary and cortical bone (*curved arrows*), and soft tissue mass (*open arrows*). Note the characteristic punctate calcifications in the proximal part of the tumor. (*From Greenspan A: Tumors of cartilage origin. Orthop Clin 20:359, 1989.*)

peripheral, or juxtacortical. With central chondrosarcoma, the neoplastic tissue is compressed inside the bone and areas of necrosis, cystic change, and hemorrhage are common. Peripheral chondrosarcoma arises outside the bone and then invades the bone. The juxtacortical chondrosarcoma is thought to be periosteal or parosteal in origin.

Clinical Manifestations. Pain is the most common presenting complaint. In some cases the symptoms can exist for years; in others, weeks. The pelvis is a common site of pain, as are the proximal and distal femur and the ribs. The lesion can range from a slow-growing lesion to an aggressive malignancy capable of metastasizing to other organs.

Medical Management

Diagnosis. On radiographs the tumor often shows an expansile lesion in the diaphysis of long bones with cortical thickening and destruction of the medullary bone (Fig. 22–15). The appearance is somewhat variable depending on the rate of growth and the host bone response. Biopsy is important not only for accurate diagnosis but for guiding treatment. Chondrosarcoma can develop on the surface of bone or be multicentric, involving several bones.

Treatment. Treatment of chondrosarcoma is surgical. Curettage is not adequate and recurrence is likely. Wide resections, or limb-sparing procedures are often required.

Prognosis. The prognosis is dependent on the aggressiveness and stage of the lesion. For example a grade 1 lesion is unlikely to metastasize and if it is completely resected a good prognosis follows. A grade 3 lesion is much more likely to metastasize. Those lesions found in the pelvis, or any bone where complete resection is difficult, have a poorer prognosis.

Secondary chondrosarcomas are usually of a low-grade malignancy and have a good prognosis with adequate treatment (Greenspan, 1989).

Special Implications for the Therapist **22–7**

CARTILAGINOUS TUMORS

With *enchondromas,* as with benign neoplasms of bone, limitations on early function may be needed depending on the size and location of the tumor.

Since *osteochondroma* is a benign tumor and will likely require only symptomatic, if any, treatment, the role of the therapist is to educate clients and alleviate any anxiety that may be present.

The special implications of *chondrosarcoma* for the

therapist are similar to those with other malignant neoplasms such as osteosarcoma.

Fibrous Lesions

Overview. Fibrous lesions within bone are a common osseous anomaly. They are usually solitary lesions found in the femur, skull, humerus, and tibia. Adolescents and young adults are affected. These lesions vary from small fibrous cortical defects to larger fibrous dysplasias. While most are benign, fibrosarcoma has many of the features of osteosarcoma. Many children will have defects in the metaphysis, but most will resolve spontaneously. Those that persist are seen in young adult males. The distal femur and tibia are common sites.

Pathogenesis. Although the defect occurs in the metaphysis, during normal bone growth the defect may be "displaced" into the diaphysis. The pathogenesis is unknown.

Clinical Manifestations. Most fibrous defects are asymptomatic. Pathologic fractures may be the initial symptom and occur where there are large lesions. Fibrous defects are usually found as an incidental finding on radiographs.

Medical Management

Diagnosis. Plain radiographs are usually diagnostic. The lesion has an irregular shape with a thin sclerotic border (Figure 22–16).

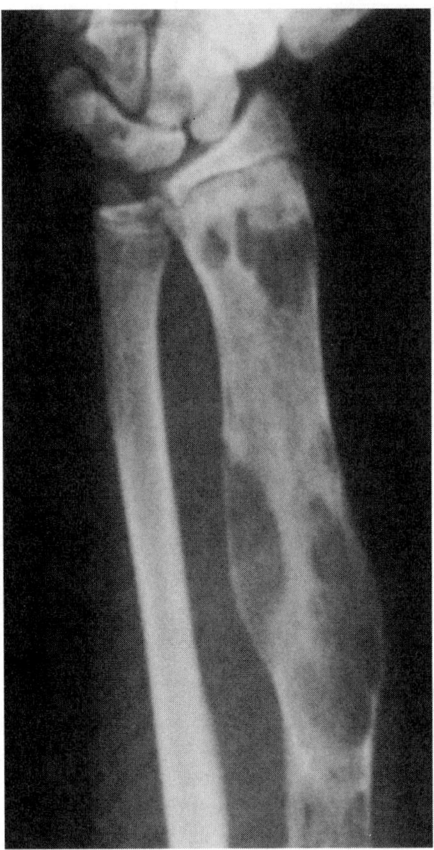

Figure **22–16.** Fibrous dysplasia. A predominantly lytic lesion with some sclerosis and expansion is seen in the distal half of the radius in a child. A long lesion in a long bone typifies fibrous dysplasia. Although parts of this lesion indeed have a ground-glass appearance, most of it does not. Expansion and bone deformity like this is commonly seen in fibrous dysplasia. (*From Helms C: Fundamentals of Skeletal Radiology: Benign Cystic Lesions. Philadelphia, WB Saunders, 1989, p 12.*)

Treatment. Even though this is a benign lesion, treatment sometimes requires surgery. When the dysplasia thins the cortex of a weight bearing bone or occupies more than one half of the diameter of the bone, the risk of pathologic fracture increases. A case reported by Horowitz et al. demonstrated the use of a hip compression screw and fibular allograft strut to restore structural integrity to the femoral neck (Horowitz et al., 1995).

Prognosis. Benign fibrous defects generally have a good prognosis.

Implications for the therapist are similar to those with other benign bone tumors.

Multiple Myeloma

Although multiple myeloma involves bony tissue it is one of a group of disorders called plasma cell dyscrasias (see Chapter 11 for a detailed description of the condition.) Regarding skeletal involvement, the spine, pelvis, and skull are the sites most commonly involved because bone marrow is found in high concentrations in these structures. Deep bone pain is often present clinically and radiographs may demonstrate osteopenia and "punched out" areas of bone with sclerotic borders (in flat bones) (Fig. 22–17). The prognosis is generally poor, with most people dying from the disease within 1 to 3 years after the diagnosis is made.

METASTATIC TUMORS

Overview. Secondary or metastatic neoplasms refer to those lesions that originate in other organs of the body. All malignant tumors have the capability to spread to bone. Although all of the factors that affect the timing and location of metastasis are not known, some patterns do exist. Skeletal metastases are often seen in carcinomas of the lung, prostate, breast, kidney, and thyroid (see Chapter 7).

Incidence and Etiology. Metastatic neoplasms are much more common than primary lesions. In a series of 683 consecutive persons with cancer, 110 had malignant tumors. Over 50% of the metastases involved the spine (Toma et al., 1993). The incidence of skeletal metastasis ranges from 30% to 80% depending on the primary tumor site.

Risk Factors. Primary cancer can metastasize in up to 80% of cases. Risk factors to be aware of are those related to the primary cancer. For some cancers the risk factors are well documented and efforts to educate individuals on health risks should be stressed. Adequate exercise, proper diet, and avoiding tobacco use are the primary preventive measures.

Pathogenesis. The pathophysiology of metastasis is not completely understood (see Chapter 7). Cancer can spread via the bloodstream, lymphatic system, or by direct exten-

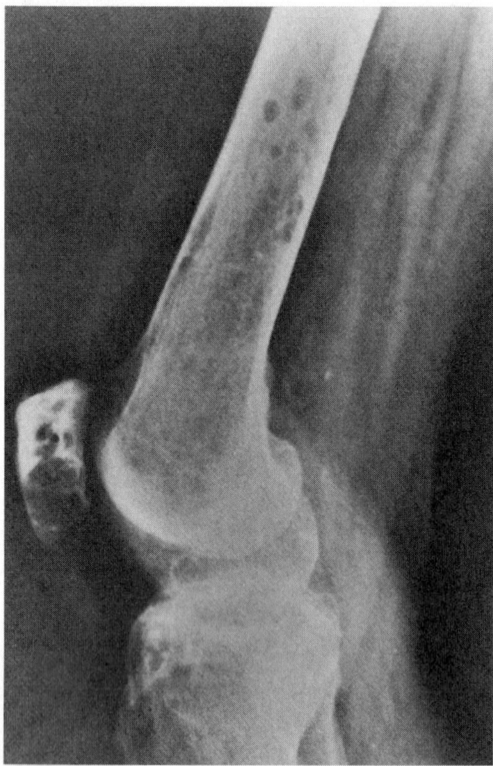

Figure 22–17. Multiple myeloma. Small lucencies in the distal femur, proximal tibia, and patella. (*From Ghelman B: Radiology of bone tumors. Orthop Clin 20:307, 1989.*)

sion into adjacent tissue. Hematogenous spread of the cancer is most common and therefore skeletal metastases are found in areas of bones with a good blood supply. These include the vertebrae, ribs, skull, and proximal femur and humerus. The unique vasculature of the spine contributes to the high rate of spinal involvement in metastatic disease (Batson, 1940).

The development of skeletal metastasis involves a series of events that begins when a tumor cell separates from the primary site, enters the blood system, and then extravasates from the blood vessel to the secondary site (Masayuki, 1995). Separation and clustering of cancerous cells are controlled by adhesion molecules. The presence or absence of certain molecules controls the ability of cells to metastasize. Various types of adhesion molecules have been implicated. Cadherins, integrins, and selectins each have distinct properties which can regulate the propensity for a primary lesion to metastasize to a specific organ (Mundy and Yoneda, 1995).

Metastasis to bone often results in osteolysis. This can occur by systemic changes produced by secretions of humoral factors that stimulate bone resorption or through osteoclastic activation via local mediators (Orr et al., 1995). Osteoblastic activity can also be present, as seen with metastasis from prostate cancer.

Clinical Manifestations. Pain is the most common presenting complaint. However, as many as 50% of persons with breast or prostate metastasis may have no bone pain. Other symptoms, such as swelling, tenderness, or the presence of a mass, are even less likely.

As with primary tumors, pathologic fractures can occur directly from the tumor itself or from the secondary effects of intervention, such as biopsy or prolonged immobilization (osteoporosis). Metabolic changes which increase the risk of fracture can also occur as a result of the disease or treatment.

Medical Management

Diagnosis. Metastases to the skeleton are important to the therapist because the presence of musculoskeletal pain may be the initial symptom of an undetected primary carcinoma elsewhere. A thorough history and a high index of suspicion can lead to the timely identification of a metastatic lesion in the absence of pathognomonic symptoms.

Spinal metastasis may be evident by the loss of the pedicle as seen in the anteroposterior view of a standard spinal radiograph. Another early manifestation is the pathologic fracture of the lesser trochanter (Bertin et al., 1984). Since much of the bone matrix must be destroyed before the lytic process is noted on radiographs, plain films are not sensitive and are not useful in early detection but are more important in staging and treatment assessment. Bone scans are much more sensitive for early detection of skeletal metastasis[3] (Galasko, 1986). Scans are also used to determine the extent of dissemination. CT and MRI also have roles in delineating various types of metastasis and assessing the size and extent of the lesion. Biopsy is sometimes necessary to confirm a diagnosis when the primary source is not known.

Treatment. Treatment of bone metastasis is problematic, costly, and primarily palliative (Houston and Rubens, 1995). Prolonging survival is not always possible, and improving function should be the primary goal. This is becoming more important as treatment for primary cancers improves. Individuals usually die from the primary tumor, not the metastasis. When survival rates and longevity increase, the likelihood of skeletal metastasis increases.

Systemic treatment for skeletal neoplasms includes endocrine therapy (for breast and prostate cancer), chemotherapy, use of radioisotopes, and biophosphonates. These are often combined with other localized treatment such as surgery and radiation therapy.

Pathologic fractures that occur in the femur and humerus often require surgical stabilization. Intramedullary fixation with interlocking devices to limit motion at the fracture site is indicated in many instances. The desire to restore normal anatomy must be weighed against the reality that the individual may have a terminal disease. An estimated life expectancy of at least 6 months is desirable before extensive joint reconstructive procedures are carried out (Harrington, 1995). Where the risk of fracture is great, as when over 50% of the cortex is destroyed, prophylactic nailing of the femur may be indicated (Carnesale, 1992) (Fig. 22–18).

Spinal metastases can cause severe pain, instability, and neurologic compromise. Surgery can take the form of posterior stabilization, excision, and reconstruction or prosthetic replacement. Hosono et al. report on a series of 90 cases where replacement of the vertebrae with a ceramic prosthesis was performed. Dramatic improvements in pain, ambulation, and motor function were noted (Hosono et al., 1995).

[3] Approximately one third of those with skeletal metastatic disease have a positive bone scan yet negative radiograph.

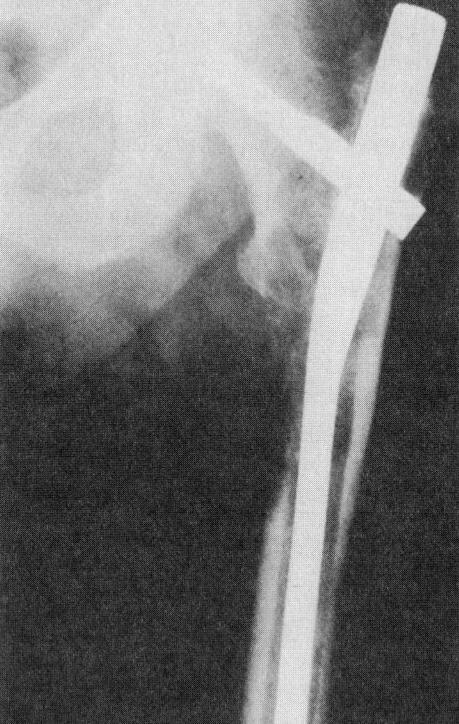

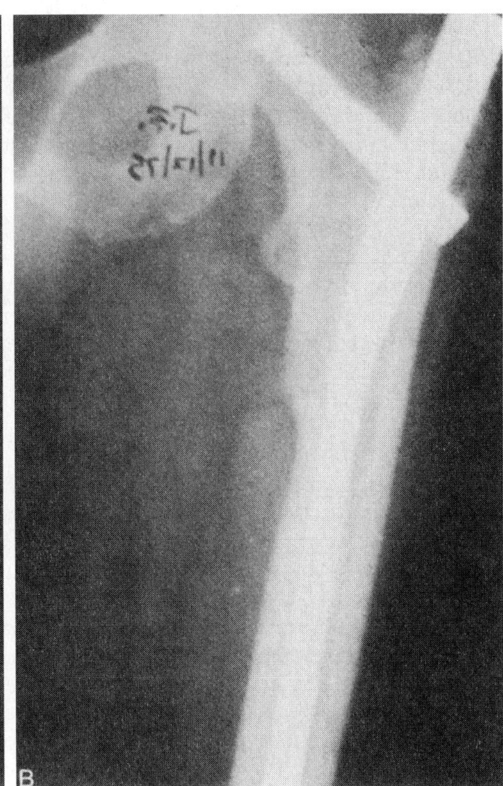

Figure **22-18.** A, Prophylactic fixation in a 63-year-old woman with an impending fracture secondary to breast metastasis treated by Zickel nailing. B, Complete healing of this subtrochanteric lesion 5 months after radiation and chemotherapy. (*From Habermann E, Lopez R: Metastatic disease of bone and treatment of pathologic fracture. Orthop Clin 20:475, 1989.*)

Prognosis. While treatment of the skeletal metastasis may be successful in terms of restoring stability to a pathologic fracture, the prognosis for the primary cancer is still guarded. Only rarely is the skeletal metastasis actually the cause of death. The mean survival time following a pathologic fracture is 19 months, longer for those with prostate or breast cancer, but shorter for those with kidney or lung cancer (Cohen et al., 1990).

Special Implications for the Therapist **22-8**

METASTATIC TUMORS

Early detection is essential for effective treatment. Therapists can play an active role by being aware of the common characteristics of specific tumors whose detection would warrant communication with a physician. In metastatic disease it may be the skeletal lesion that accounts for the initial symptoms. In persons with a history of cancer, the clinician should be vigilant regarding the likelihood and common sites of metastasis. Treatment of clients with metastatic disease is challenging because of the clinical implications of the primary cancer combined with the difficulties associated with the skeletal disease and subsequent medical treatment. Although direct treatment of the malignancy is not within the realm of the physical therapist, clients often need extensive rehabilitation following the medical treatment. Treatment of skeletal metastasis is aimed at improving or restoring function. If the bone has been compromised or fractures have occurred, surgical intervention will attempt to stabilize the defect. Following the surgery, early mobilization, including gait training, bed mobility, and transfers, is essential. Maximizing functional independence is the driving force behind all rehabilitation efforts. Treatment of the primary cancer with chemotherapy and/or radiation therapy often provides additional challenges, such as fatigue and increased risk of infection. For a client with lung cancer, a baseline pulmonary status should be established and proper breathing techniques taught (Gunn et al., 1984).

Primary Cancers Responsible for Bone Metastasis

For discussions of specific primary cancers, see the relevant chapter.

Breast

Carcinoma of the breast is the most likely cancer to metastasize to bone. Common sites include the pelvis, ribs, vertebrae, and proximal femur. See Chapter 17.

Lung

Deaths from lung cancer now outnumber those from breast cancer. Metastasis occurs early in the disease and therefore treatment is often not successful. See Chapter 12.

Kidney

Neoplasms in the kidney metastasize to the vertebrae, pelvis, and proximal femur in about 40% of the cases. See Chapter 15.

Prostate

Most of the new cases are detected in men over the age of 50 (Badalament and Drago, 1990). The prostate is the most common source of skeletal metastases in men. Early detection is important for successful treatment. Therapists should be aware of this possible cause of lumbar spine and hip pain. See Chapter 16.

Thyroid

Cancer of the thyroid is uncommon but does metastasize to bone. Women are affected three times more often than men. Therapists should remember that the development of metastasis may be delayed and may even occur after removal of a cancerous thyroid. See Chapter 9.

Pathologic Fractures

There is a reluctance to ambulate clients who are at risk of pathologic fracture because a measure of risk has not been developed. An active rehabilitation program may not place a client at increased risk of fracture. In fact, in a series of 54 persons with skeletal metastases, six fractures occurred during bed rest, and another eight were "silent" (Bunting et al., 1985). Independent ambulation is such an important factor in maintaining independence that some risk may be warranted. Since many of the people with metastatic disease are elderly, the risk of falling must be considered when planning for ambulation training. Assessment of mental status, balance, strength, range of motion, endurance, vision, ambulation history, and symptoms of dizziness are all significant, and will help to plan ambulation training (Chandler and Duncan, 1993). Even with the most critical analysis of the risks and benefits, therapists who work with individuals who have serious medical conditions such as metastatic lesions and pathologic fractures must be prepared for setbacks and unexpected events to occur when attempting to preserve or maximize function.

Persons who have had a pathologic fracture stabilized are often referred for rehabilitation. Bunting et al. (1992) reported that out of 58 individuals who underwent inpatient rehabilitation 20 (34%) were discharged to their home. Twenty-three could ambulate independently and improvement in their activities of daily living was documented. Of interest was the fact that of the 17 persons who died postoperatively, all had hypercalcemia in the acute or subacute phase (Bunting et al., 1992). Hypercalcemia occurs when bone resorption is greater than new bone formation. The osteolysis that occurs with bone metastasis is one cause of hypercalcemia.

Rehabilitation should begin before any surgical procedures. An understanding of common postoperative impairments will help in treatment planning and prevent or minimize length of hospitalization and foster an early return to independence. Exercise programs directed at strengthening and stretching are often needed. Chemotherapy for some cancers includes the use of steroids which can lead to muscle atrophy, especially of the type II fibers (Levinson, 1993). Isometric exercises may prevent marked atrophy. Radiation therapy can lead to contracture of soft tissues and clients should be taught to stretch susceptible areas before treatment.

References

Badalament RA, Drago JR: Prostate cancer. Postgrad Med J 87:65, 1990.

Batson O: The function of the vertebral veins and their role in the spread of metastases. Arch Surg 112:138–149, 1940.

Bertin KC, Horstman J, Coleman SS: Isolated fracture of the lesser trochanter in adults, an initial manifestation of metastatic disease. J Bone Joint Surg [Am] 66:770–773, 1984.

Bogumill G, Schwamm H: Orthopaedic Pathology. Philadelphia, WB Saunders, 1984.

Bullough P, Vigorita V: Orthopaedic Pathology with Clinical and Radiologic Correlations. New York, Gower, 1984.

Bunting RW, Boublik M, Blevins FT, et al: Functional outcome of pathologic fracture secondary to malignant disease in a rehabilitation hospital. Cancer 69:98–102, 1992.

Bunting R, Lamont-Havers W, Schweon D, Kliman A: Pathologic fracture risk in rehabilitation of patients with bony metastases. Clin Orthop 192:222–227, 1985.

Carnesale P: Malignant tumors of bone. *In* Crenshaw AH (ed): Campbell's Operative Orthopaedics, ed 8. St Louis, Mosby–Year Book, 1992.

Chandler J, Duncan P: Balance and falls in the elderly. *In* Guccione A: Geriatric Physical Therapy. St Louis, Mosby–Year Book, 1993.

Cohen J, Bonfiglio M, Campbell C: Orthopedic Pathophysiology in Diagnosis and Treatment. New York, Churchill Livingstone, 1990.

Dahlin DC, Coventry MB: Osteosarcoma; A study of 600 cases. J Bone Joint Surg [Am] 49:101–110, 1967.

Dahlin DC, Unni KK: Bone tumors: General aspects and data on 8,542 cases, ed 4. Springfield, Ill, Thomas, 1986, pp 269–307.

Deyo R, Rainville J, Kent D: What can the history and physical examination tell us about low back pain? JAMA 268:760–765, 1992.

Eggli KD, Quiogue T, Moser R: Ewing's sarcoma. Radiol Clin North Am 31:325–337, 1993.

Enneking WF: Musculoskeletal Tumor Surgery. Edinburgh, Churchill Livingstone, 1983.

Enneking WF: A system of staging musculoskeletal neoplasms. Clin Orthop 153:106–120, 1986.

Fechner R, Mills S: Tumors of the Bones and Joints. Washington, DC, Armed Forces Institute of Pathology, 1992.

Galasko CSB: Skeletal Metastases. London, Butterworths, 1986.

Giudici M, Moser R, Kransdorf M: Cartilaginous bone tumors. Radiol Clin North Am 31:237–259, 1993.

Gitelis S, Schajowicz F: Osteoid osteoma and osteoblastoma. Orthop Clin 20:313–325, 1989.

Greenspan A: Tumors of cartilage origin. Orthop Clin 20:347–366, 1989.

Gunn AE, Dickison EM, McBride CM: Physical rehabilitation. *In* Gunn AE (ed): Cancer Rehabilitation. New York, Raven Press, 1984, p 23.

Harrington K: Orthopaedic management of extremity and pelvic lesions. Clin Orthop 312:136–147, 1995.

Helms C: Fundamentals of Skeletal Radiology: Benign Cystic Lesions. Philadelphia, WB Saunders, 1989.

Hermanek P, Sobin LH: TNM Classification of Malignant Tumors, ed 4. New York, Springer-Verlag, 1987, pp 7–9.

Horowitz S, Rubin D, Dalinka M, Gannon F: Hip pain in a 24-year-old woman. Clin Orthop 312:271–274, 295–296, 1995.

Hosono N, Yonenobu K, Fuji T, et al: Orthopaedic management of spinal metastases. Clin Orthop 312:148–159, 1995.

Houston SJ, Rubens R: The systemic treatment of bone metastases. Clin Orthop 312:95–104, 1995.

Jackson RP: Recurrent osteoblastoma: A review. Clin Orthop 131:229, 1978.

Jaffe HL: Osteoid osteoma: A benign osteoblastic tumor composed of osteoid and atypical bone. Arch Surg 31:709, 1935.

Jaffe N: Chemotherapy for malignant tumors. Orthop Clin 20:487–503, 1989.

Klein M, Kenan S, Lewis M: Osteosarcoma; Clinical and pathological considerations. Orthop Clin 20:327–345, 1989.

Levinson SF: Rehabilitation of the patient with cancer or human immunodeficiency virus. *In* DeLisa JA: Rehabilitation Medicine: Principles and Practice. Philadelphia, JB Lippincott, 1993, pp 916–930.

Mankin HJ, Lange TA, Spanier SS: The hazards of biopsy in patients with malignant primary bone and soft tissue tumors. J Bone Joint Surg [Am] 64:1121–1127, 1982.

Masayuki M: Cancer metastasis and adhesion molecules. Clin Orthop 312:10–18, 1995.

McGuire MH, Mankin HJ, Schiller AL: Benign cartilage tumors of bone. *In* Evarts C (ed): Surgery of the Musculoskeletal System, ed 2. New York, Churchill Livingstone, 1990, p 4717.

Milgram JW: The origins of osteochondromas and enchondromas. Clin Orthop 174:264–284, 1983.

Mundy G, Yoneda T: Facilitation and suppression of bone metastasis. Clin Orthop 312:33–44, 1995.

Noble J, Lamb DW: Enchondromata of bones of the hand. A review of 40 cases. Hand 6:275–284, 1974.

O'Connor MI, Pritchard DJ: Ewing's sarcoma; Prognostic factors, disease control, and the reemerging role of surgical treatment. Clin Orthop 262:78–87, 1991.

Orr FW, Sanchez O, Kostenuik P, Singh G: Tumor bone interactions in skeletal metastasis. Clin Orthop 312:19–23, 1995.

Parker S, Tong T, Boldlen S, Wingo P: Cancer Statistics, 1996. CA Cancer J Clin 46:5–27, 1996.

Pfalzer L: Oncology: Examination, diagnosis, and treatment. Medical and surgical considerations. *In* Myers RS (ed): Saunders Manual of Physical Therapy Practice. Philadelphia, WB Saunders, 1995, pp 65–417.

Resnick D, Hemcek AA, Haghighi P: Spinal enostoses (bone islands). Radiology 147:373, 1983.

Roach K, Brown M, Ricker E, et al: The use of patient symptoms to screen for serious back problems. J Orthop Sports Phys Ther 21:2–6, 1995.

Salter RB: *In* Textbook of Disorders and Injuries of the Musculoskeletal System. Baltimore, Williams & Wilkins, 1970.

Toma S, Venturino A, Sogno G, et al: Metastatic bone tumors. Clin Orthop 295:246–251, 1993.

SECTION 3

chapter 23

Joint and Muscle Disorders

William G. Boissonnault

People presenting with joint and muscle disorders make up a significant percentage of the therapist's patient population. These conditions are primarily manifested by pain, deformity, and loss of function. Many of the people seen by therapists have joint or muscle conditions secondary to trauma or repetitive overuse. These conditions are generally self-contained or local in terms of involved tissues. Therapists may treat dysfunction in other body regions to reduce the mechanical stresses on the involved joint, but the disorder itself (i.e., degenerative joint disease, bursitis, or tendonitis) does not spread to other body regions. This is in contrast to rheumatic disease, which can be manifested not only by local joint or muscle pain and dysfunction but also by additional complaints associated with other body systems.

Rheumatic disorders are systemic diseases. The pathogenesis and progression of these disorders can affect any and all body systems. The onset of joint pain and loss of function may be accompanied by fever, rash, diarrhea, scleritis, or neuritis. These symptoms are not typically associated with joint or muscle conditions brought on by repetitive overuse or trauma. The presence of these complaints may interfere with the rehabilitation process. Rheumatic disorders are also often marked by periods of exacerbation and remission. During a period of exacerbation the therapist will often need to modify the treatment approach considerably. In addition, aggressive medical treatment (i.e., medications) may need to be initiated to prevent or minimize the tissue destruction that can occur with these disorders. Many of the rheumatic conditions are chronic and progressive, requiring long-term rehabilitation and adjustment of functional goals.

Therapists must be able to differentiate between degenerative joint disease (osteoarthritis) and rheumatic joint conditions. If there is any suspicion of the presence of a rheumatic disorder, immediate referral to a physician is called for. Therapists seeing someone with rheumatoid arthritis must screen for systemic symptoms, and if present or existing complaints worsen, again, immediate communication with a physician is called for. An understanding of the diseases discussed in this chapter will assist the therapist regarding this clinical decision-making process.

OSTEOARTHRITIS

Description. Osteoarthritis, or degenerative joint disease, is a slow, progressive degeneration of joint structures which can lead to loss of mobility, chronic pain, deformity, and loss of function. The most commonly involved joints associated with this disorder are the hip, knee, the lumbar and cervical spine, and the first carpometacarpal and metatarsophalangeal joints. Osteoarthritis is the single most common joint disease and is divided into two classifications: primary and secondary. Primary osteoarthritis is a disorder of unknown cause and the cascade of joint degeneration events associated with it are thought to be related to a defect in the articular cartilage. Secondary osteoarthritis has a known cause, which may be trauma, infection, hemarthrosis, osteonecrosis, and so forth.

Incidence and Risk Factors. The most significant risk factor related to degenerative joint changes is age. It is estimated that 60% to 85% of the population aged 60 years and older have some degree of articular cartilage damage in a number of their joints (Schiller 1994; Mankin and Treadwell, 1986). Interestingly though, only 15% to 25% of these people experience significant symptoms (Davison, 1980). Gender is a factor depending upon which age group is being considered. Males make up the majority of those afflicted with osteoarthritis before the age of 45, whereas females experience this disorder more frequently after the age of 55.

Etiology. The cause of primary osteoarthritis is unknown. Osteoarthritis is termed the wear-and-tear arthritis. The thought is that the articular cartilage breaks down because of an imbalance between the mechanical stresses and the ability of the joint structures to handle the loads (Pigg and Bancroft, 1994). Once articular cartilage breakdown is initiated, a cascade of tissue failure follows.

Pathogenesis. Articular cartilage has an important role in joint physiology. Articular cartilage provides a smooth, relatively friction-free surface between the bony ends making up the joint. In addition, the cartilage attenuates the mechanical load transmitted through the joint. Once the cartilage begins to break down, excessive mechanical stress begins to fall on other joint structures. Eventually, fissuring and eburnation of the cartilage can occur. The joint space narrows as the cartilage thins, and sclerosis of the subchondral bone occurs as new bone is formed in response to the now excessive mechanical load. New bone also forms at the joint margins (osteophytes) (Fig. 23–1).

Immobilization is another factor that can result in articular cartilage degeneration. Secondary to the lack of vascular supply, articular cartilage depends on repetitive mechanical loading and unloading for the nutritional elements to reach the chondrocytes and the cellular waste products to return to the synovial fluid and eventually the bloodstream. The nutritional mechanism of articular cartilage is interrupted by immobilization. The detrimental effects of immobilization are accelerated in the presence of articular surface contact secondary to the immobilization (Pigg and Bancroft, 1994; Salter and Field, 1960). If the nutritional cycle is interrupted long enough, structural changes will occur.

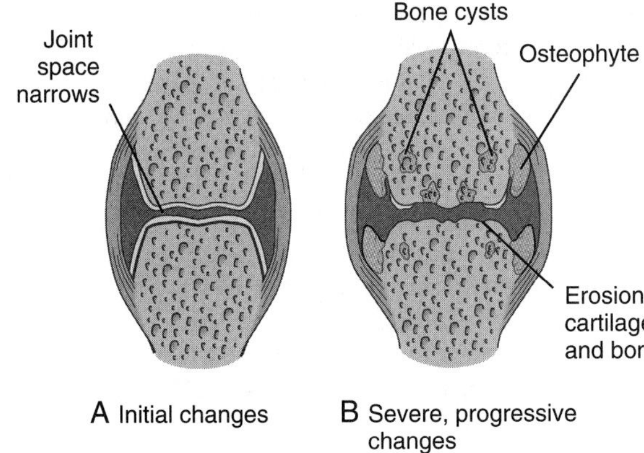

Figure **23-1.** A, Early degenerative changes associated with osteoarthritis include joint space narrowing and articular cartilage erosion. B, Late degenerative changes associated with osteoarthritis include osteophyte formation and articular cartilage fissuring and eburnation.

Clinical Manifestations. The onset of symptoms related to osteoarthritis can occur insidiously or suddenly. For most people, though, the pain complaints progress slowly and gradually. The pain is often described as a deep ache and can occur at rest. Osteoarthritis has also been associated with nocturnal pain (Jonssou and Stromquist, 1993; Foldes et al., 1992). Stiffness of relatively short duration (less than 30 minutes) can occur after periods of inactivity, including sitting and sleeping. Loss of flexibility is usually associated with significant disease and can occur secondary to soft tissue contractures, intra-articular loose bodies, large osteophytes, and loss of joint surface congruity (Schiller, 1994). Crepitus may be noted on physical examination, and enlarged joint surfaces, including osteophytes, may be palpable.

Medical Management

Diagnosis. Osteoarthritis is diagnosed by correlation of history, physical examination, radiologic findings, and laboratory tests, which rule out rheumatic disease. Box 23–1 lists radiographic changes associated with osteoarthritis.

Treatment and Prognosis. Treatment of osteoarthritis is dictated by the extent of the disease and the joints involved. The diseased joints need to be protected from excessive mechanical forces. This may include the use of an assistive ambulatory device, a shock-absorbent shoe insert, or an orthotic device. Educating the client on how to reduce the daily wear and tear on the joint is key. This may include the use of postural supports or a cervical collar or an exercise program to vary the stresses the involved joints are dealing with. Optimizing existing and potential joint function by improving flexibility and strength is important. Medications are administered for pain control. Nonsteroidal anti-inflammatory drugs (NSAIDs) and acetaminophen have been shown to provide pain relief. The advantage of acetaminophen is that it is less toxic than NSAIDs. Surgical intervention is considered when pain and loss of function are severe. Procedures include arthroscopic lavage and debridement, osteotomies or bony resections, and total joint replacement (Pigg and Bancroft, 1994).

BOX **23-1**
Osteoarthritis: Radiographic Findings

Joint space narrowing
Subchondral bone sclerosis
Subchondral bone cysts
Osteophytes

Special Implications for the Therapist **23-1**

OSTEOARTHRITIS

Therapists need to be aware of the potential poor correlation between the extent of radiographic degenerative changes and the presence of symptoms. The assumption that a person with significant, extensive joint degeneration will probably not improve should not be made until a thorough rehabilitation program has been attempted. Conversely, it should not be assumed that someone with minor radiographic degenerative changes cannot be experiencing severe, intense pain. Therapists should rely primarily on the clinical examination findings for direction regarding the development of a treatment program and prognosis.

The medications commonly prescribed for osteoarthritis have significant potential side effects. The NSAIDs have ulcerogenic potential, especially when taken with over-the-counter drugs.* Peptic ulcer disease can be manifested by a multitude of complaints, including indigestion, nausea, vomiting, thoracic pain, melena (black tarry stools), and so forth. The onset of any of these complaints calls for communication with a physician.

People with symptoms associated with osteoarthritis must understand their role in minimizing the mechanical stresses on the involved joint(s). Proper posture, use of supports, avoiding prolonged stressful postures, varying physical activities to vary the stresses (i.e., mix biking with swimming or running), and following through with a flexibility and strengthening exercise program are all components under the patient's control. Educating, motivating, and coaching are important roles the therapist plays to help maximize function and prevent significant recurrence of symptoms.

Lastly, successful management of degenerative joint disease may require evaluating and treating dysfunction of other body regions. For example, someone with osteoarthritis of the knee and pain on ambulation may have significant foot or ankle dysfunction. Treating joint and soft tissue hypomobility, muscle imbalances, and fabricating orthoses may considerably alter the mechanical stresses on the arthritic knee.

* Gastric irritation can result from inhibition of prostaglandin production, which can reduce mucous and bicarbonate production and decrease local blood flow.

DEGENERATIVE INTERVERTEBRAL DISK DISEASE

The degenerative joint process described in the previous section applies to any synovial joint, including the facet joints of the spinal column. Degenerative joint changes are not limited to synovial joints though, and in the spine (particularly the low lumbar segments) they commonly occur at the intervertebral disk articulations (Kraemer, 1995). The intervertebral disk changes include alterations in volume, shape, structure, and composition. Although there is not a 100% correlation between the presence of degenerative disk disease and pain complaints, the structural alterations will decrease motion and alter the mechanical properties of the spine (Buckwalter, 1995).

The intervertebral disk undergoes marked changes with age. The most significant alterations occur in the nucleus pulposus. The number of cells and the concentration of proteoglycans and water decrease. In addition, there is fragmentation of proteoglycans, which contributes to water loss. As the nucleus breaks down, the fibrocartilaginous inner annulus expands. Fissures and clefts may form within the disk, and the height of the disk decreases. This loss of disk height can contribute to the age-related condition of spinal stenosis (Andersson, 1993).

A number of events can contribute to age-related disk degeneration (Box 23–2). The most important appears to be the decreased cellular function and concentration (Urban, 1993; Eyre et al., 1989). The progressive decline in arterial supply to the periphery of the disk and the impairment of nutrient delivery across the cartilaginous end plate contribute to the reduced nutritional supply to the cells, affecting cellular function. In addition, the impaired cartilaginous end plate diffusion results in reduced cellular waste product removal and an increased lactic acid concentration. The resultant decreased pH level compromises cellular metabolism and biosynthesis and can lead to cell death. The reduced biosynthesis can adversely affect the biomechanical properties of the matrix over an extended period of time. Besides the internal events affecting the general health of the intervertebral disk, repetitive external mechanical loading on the structure can lead to fatigue failure of the matrix. Once enough structural breakdown occurs, what once were normal mechanical loads acting upon a normal disk are now excessive loads on a compromised disk. At this point the degenerative process is accelerated (Buckwalter, 1995).

Associated with intervertebral disk degeneration are spinal stenosis and degenerative spondylolisthesis, two common conditions in the elderly. As the intervertebral disk loses height, the annulus may bulge circumferentially and the ligamentum flavum can buckle. Both encroach upon the spinal canal, subarticular (facet) recesses, and the lateral intervertebral foramina. In addition, concurrent osteophyte formation on the vertebral bodies or articular processes may occur, compounding the stenosis.

BOX **23–2**
Events Leading to Disk Degeneration

- Impaired cellular nutrition
- Reduced cellular viability
- Cellular senescence
- Accumulation of degraded matrix macromolecules
- Fatigue failure of the matrix

Degenerative spondylolisthesis is marked by anterior slippage of one vertebra over another with an intact posterior neural arch. The L4–5 spinal segment is the most common site for this to occur (Fig. 23–2). Lytic spondylolisthesis is marked by anterior slippage of one vertebra over another with a defective posterior neural arch (Fig. 23–3). The L5–S1 spinal segment is the most common site for lytic spondylolisthesis to occur. The loss of disk height associated with degeneration allows for a buckling of the annulus and ligamentum flavum, slackening them somewhat. This allows the vertebrae to migrate anteriorly in response to the shear forces inherent to the lumbar lordosis (Herkowitz, 1995). In contrast to the L5–S1 segment, the facet joint orientation at the L4–5 segment tends to be more in the sagittal plane, so there is no structural bar to anterior slippage. The facet joint orientation at L5–S1 tends to be more in the frontal plane, making anterior migration of L5 difficult unless there is a structural defect in the posterior neural arch. Stenosis can be caused by the displacement of one vertebra over another as well as by the concurrent buckling of the annulus and ligamentum flavum.

Special Implications for the Therapist **23–2**

DEGENERATIVE INTERVERTEBRAL DISK DISEASE

See the discussion of osteoarthritis for information related to degenerative disk disease. There are two additional conditions associated with spinal stenosis, cauda equina syndrome and vascular/neurogenic

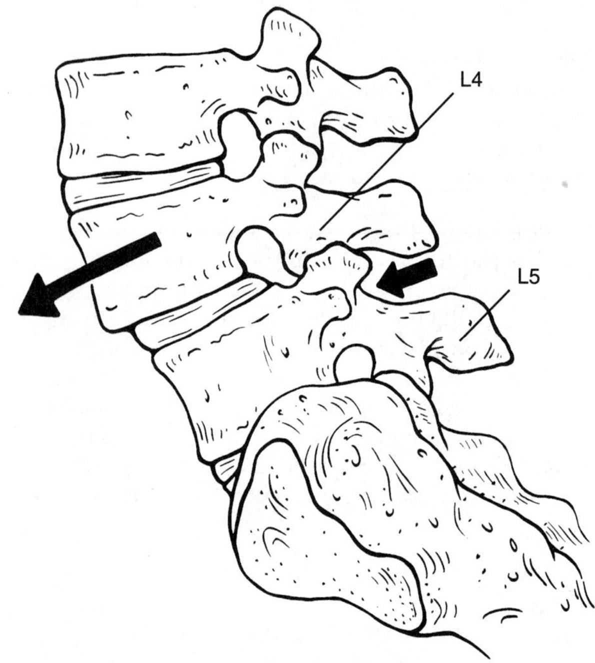

Figure **23–2.** Degenerative spondylolisthesis at L4–5. (*From DeRosa C, Porterfield JA: Lumbar spine and pelvis. In Richardson JK, Iglarsh ZA (eds): Clinical Orthopaedic Physical Therapy. Philadelphia, WB Saunders, 1994, p 144.*)

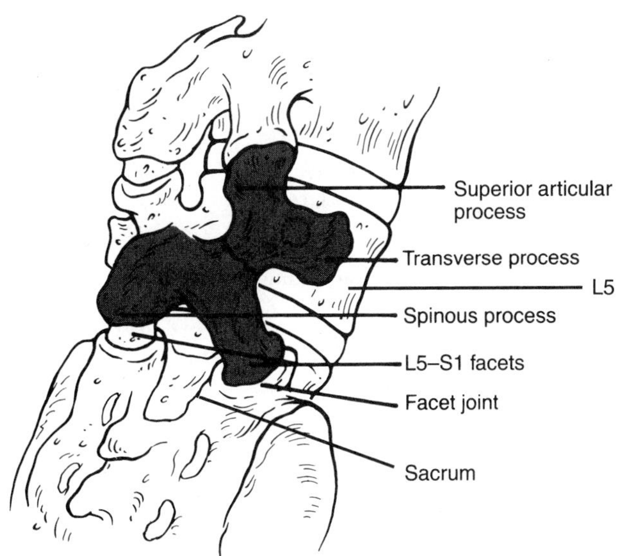

Figure **23-3.** Spondylolysis or posterior arch defect, which can lead to a lytic spondylolisthesis. The "Scottie dog" with a collar, which is visible on the radiograph (posterior oblique view), is outlined. (*From Magee D: Orthopedic Physical Assessment, ed. 2. Philadelphia, WB Saunders, 1992.*)

claudication. Cauda equina syndrome is characterized by pain in the upper sacrum, with paresthesias of the buttocks and genitalia, possibly resulting in bowel and/or bladder incontinence, or sexual dysfunction (difficulty achieving orgasm or inability to achieve or maintain an erection). Numerous conditions may lead to the above manifestations, including spinal canal stenosis. Therapists working with back or neck pain clients should ask about these symptoms and if any are present, immediate communication with a physician is called for (Leonard and Harbst, 1995).

Even with the local degenerative changes in the spine, stenosis may be marked primarily by lower extremity symptoms (neurogenic claudication) as opposed to back pain. The symptoms may include pain, altered sensation, or muscle weakness. The symptoms are typically brought on by walking and are relieved by resting (sitting or lying down) or by flexion of the spine. When a person is upright and walking, the lumbar spine is in a relative backward bent position, which further reduces the size of the foramina and subarticular recesses. When the spine is flexed, the foramina are opened, relieving pressure on the nerves. Similar symptoms are noted with vascular claudication* (see Chapter 10) except that the symptoms are not dependent on the position of the spine (Herkowitz, 1995). Functionally, people with neurogenic claudication lack the backward bending range of motion to tolerate walking. If the therapist can improve overall backward bending range-of-motion by mobilizing the thoracic and upper lumbar regions and by stretching the hip flexors, the patient may be able to assume an upright posture without reaching end range of motion at the involved segments where the nerve compression is occurring. If this can be accomplished, walking tolerance should improve.

* Symptoms and signs associated with tissue ischemia secondary to vascular insufficiency.

RHEUMATOID ARTHRITIS

Description. Rheumatoid arthritis is a chronic, systemic inflammatory disease. A wide range of articular and extra-articular findings are associated with rheumatoid arthritis. Chronic polyarthritis, which perpetuates a gradual destruction of joint tissues, can result in severe deformity and disability. The joints of the cervical spine are commonly involved, potentially leading to atlantoaxial subluxation and spinal cord compression (Oda et al., 1995). The extra-articular changes are varied and widespread, marking the systemic nature of the disease. Systems that may be involved include the cardiovascular, pulmonary, and gastrointestinal systems. Eye lesions, infection, and osteoporosis are other potential extra-articular manifestations (Pigg and Bancroft, 1994).

Incidence. Rheumatoid arthritis has a worldwide distribution and afflicts all races. Approximately 1% to 2% of the adult population has rheumatoid arthritis. Although less common, children can also develop the disorder. Estimates of the incidence in children in the United States range from 60,000 to 200,000 (Schumacher, 1988).

Risk Factors. Age and female gender are the two primary risk factors associated with rheumatoid arthritis. Although the onset of the disorder can occur at any age, the peak onset is usually during the third or fourth decades of life. Women are afflicted two to three times more frequently than men (Schumacher, 1988). Pregnancy and oral contraceptives appear to influence the incidence and severity of the disease. The incidence of rheumatoid arthritis in women who have borne a child is lower, and oral contraceptives diminish the incidence of severe arthritis. A nulliparous woman who does not use oral contraceptives has a fourfold increased risk of developing rheumatoid arthritis (Spector et al., 1990; Hazes et al., 1990).

Etiology. The cause of rheumatoid arthritis is unknown. An immunologic mechanism appears to play an important role.

Pathogenesis. Approximately 80% of people with rheumatoid arthritis are rheumatoid factor–positive (Harris, 1990). Rheumatoid factors are antibodies that react with immunoglobulin antibodies found in the blood. Rheumatoid factor has also been found in the synovial fluid and synovial membranes of those with the disease. It is hypothesized that the interaction between rheumatoid factor and the immunoglobulin triggers events that initiate an inflammatory reaction. As the attracted leukocytes, monocytes, and lymphocytes phagocytose the immune complexes, destructive lysosomal enzymes are released, leading to articular cartilage destruction and synovial hyperplasia. These changes can result in the development of destructive vascular granulation

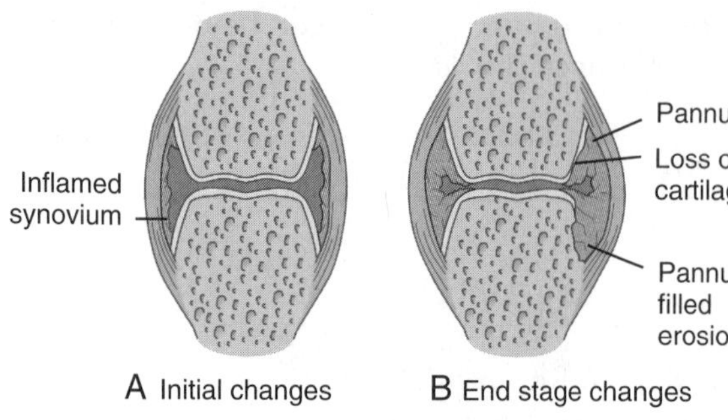

Figure 23–4. *A*, Early synovial changes associated with rheumatoid arthritis. *B*, Late joint changes associated with rheumatoid arthritis, including pannus formation and articular cartilage eburnation.

tissue called pannus. This tissue proliferates, encroaching upon the joint space. The inflammatory cells found within the pannus are destructive, affecting cartilage, bone, and other periarticular tissues (Fig. 23–4). The end result can be joint instability, joint deformity, or ankylosis. These events are irreversible (Pigg and Bancroft, 1994).

The wide range of extra-articular problems are also probably a result of local inflammatory injury induced by the immune complexes traveling through the circulatory system. See Box 23–3 for a list of lesions associated with rheumatoid arthritis.

Clinical Manifestations. Rheumatoid arthritis is typically manifested by both extra-articular and articular complaints (Table 23–1). The symptoms usually begin insidiously and progress slowly. Complaints of fatigue, weight loss, weakness, and general, diffuse musculoskeletal pain are often the initial presentation. The musculoskeletal symptoms gradually localize to specific joints. Multiple joints are usually involved with symmetrical, bilateral presentation. The most frequently involved joints are the wrist, knee, and joints of the fingers, hands, and feet. Involvement of the spinal column is typically limited to the cervical spine, with neck pain reported in 40% to 88% of persons (Boden, 1994). The involved joints can be edematous, warm, painful, and stiff. After periods of rest (prolonged sitting, sleeping, etc.) intense joint pain and stiffness called post-rest gel, may last 30 minutes to several hours

BOX 23–3
Extra-articular Lesions Associated with Rheumatoid Arthritis

- Vasculitis
- Pericarditis
- Interstitial myocarditis
- Coronary arteritis
- Interstitial pneumonia
- Interstitial pulmonary fibrosis
- Pleuritis
- Ocular lesions (scleritis, uveitis)
- Interstitial nephritis
- Felty's syndrome
- Sjögren's syndrome

TABLE 23–1 SYMPTOMS AND SIGNS OF EARLY RHEUMATOID ARTHRITIS (RA)

	SYMPTOMS
Joint stiffness	Found in 98% of clients; most pronounced after inactivity; its duration after arising reflects degree of synovial inflammation; improves with physical activity
Joint pain	Reflects severity of synovitis—may not be a prominent feature at rest
Fatigue	Often pronounced with onset about 4.5 hr after arising; found in 80% of clients; its duration after arising varies inversely with degree of synovitis
Weakness	Nearly universal in RA patients; often out of proportion to degree of muscular atrophy; generally proportional to degree of synovitis
Psychological depression	Common; reflects disease activity, at least in part
	SIGNS
Swelling	Fusiform soft tissue enlargement of small joints and tendon sheaths in hands, wrists, and forefeet most commonly, but can affect any synovial structure in body
Palmar erythema	Very common over palmar and thenar eminences; identical to changes found in liver disease and pregnancy; persists even in remission
Cool moist skin	Over hands and feet; suggests excessive sympathetic tone; true Raynaud's phenomenon is extremely rare
Muscular atrophy	Over hands and feet; suggests excessive sympathetic tone; true Raynaud's phenomenon is extremely rare
Muscular atrophy	Occurs rapidly in severe disease
Contracture of joints	Extension of involved joints is often limited
Nodules	Occur at sites of pressure in about 20% of clients; over olecranon and proximal ulna, over extensor surfaces of fingers, over Achilles tendon ("pump bumps") most commonly, but can occur in tendon substance, bone, sclerae, over pinna of ear, and in visceral organs, especially lung
Synovial hernias	Occur through defects in capsule caused by synovitis; in hands, often mistaken for nodules
Weight loss	May occur rarely, especially with vasculitis; may be a sign of a poor prognosis

Modified from McCarty OJ: Clinical picture of rheumatoid arthritis. *In* McCarty DJ, Koopman WJ (eds): Arthritis and Allied Conditions, ed 12. Philadelphia, Lea & Febiger, 1993, p 788.

as activity is initiated (Pigg and Bancroft, 1994; Schiller, 1994).

As the disease progresses, joint deformity can occur, including subluxation. Deformities in the fingers are common, including ulnar deviation, swan-neck deformity, and boutonnière deformity. The ulnar deviation occurs as the extensor tendons slip to the ulnar aspect of the metacarpal head.

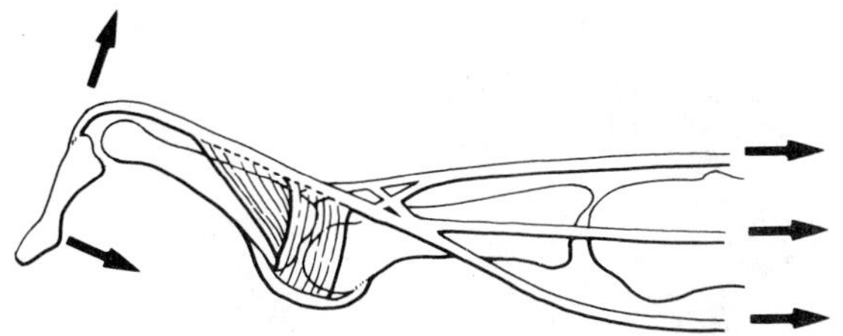

Figure 23-5. Swan-neck deformity. (*From Jacobs JL: Hand and wrist. In Richardson JK, Iglarsh ZA (eds): Clinical Orthopaedic Physical Therapy. Philadelphia, WB Saunders, 1994, p 309.*)

Hyperextension of the proximal interphalangeal joint and partial flexion of the distal interphalangeal joint make up the swan-neck deformity (Fig. 23–5). The boutonnière deformity is marked by flexion of the proximal interphalangeal joint and hyperextension of the distal interphalangeal joint (Fig. 23–6).

The extra-articular manifestations are numerous (see Box 23–3). Many of these manifestations are disabling and some are life-threatening. They could easily hamper rehabilitation efforts, delaying or preventing progress. See Chapters 10 and 12 for a description of the cardiovascular and pulmonary manifestations respectively. Sjögren's syndrome is marked by lymphocytic and plasma cell infiltration of the lacrimal and parotid glands. This can result in diminished salivary and lacrimal secretions. Felty's syndrome is marked by splenomegaly and leukopenia.

Another common manifestation is rheumatoid nodules. These granulomatous lesions usually occur in areas of pressure such as over the extensor surface of the elbow, the Achilles tendon, and extensor surface of the fingers, but they can also occur in the heart, lungs, and gastrointestinal tract. Nodules in these organs can cause serious problems such as heart arrhythmias and respiratory failure (Schiller, 1994).

Medical Management

Diagnosis. In the early stages of rheumatoid arthritis the diagnosis can be difficult because of the gradual, subtle onset of the complaints. The symptoms may wax and wane, delaying the visit to a physician's office. The diagnosis is ultimately based on a combination of history, physical examination,

TABLE 23-2 PROPOSED AMERICAN RHEUMATISM ASSOCIATION CRITERIA FOR RHEUMATOID ARTHRITIS

Four or more of the following conditions must be present to establish a diagnosis of rheumatoid arthritis:

1. Morning stiffness for at least 1 hr and present for at least 6 wk
2. Swelling of three or more joints for at least 6 wk
3. Swelling of wrist, metacarpophalangeal, or proximal interphalangeal joints for 6 or more wk
4. Radiographic evidence of symmetrical joint swelling
5. Hand changes typical of rheumatoid arthritis that must include erosions or unequivocal bony decalcification
6. Rheumatoid nodules
7. Serum rheumatoid factor found present by a method that is positive in less than 5% of normals

Modified from Schumacher HR (ed): Primer on the Rheumatic Diseases, ed. 9. Atlanta, Arthritis Foundation, 1988.

and laboratory tests. Table 23–2 lists the diagnostic criteria proposed by the American Rheumatism Association. The presence of serum rheumatoid factor is supportive of the diagnosis, but can also be found in healthy persons. Synovial fluid analysis will reveal an elevated white blood cell count and protein content. Also, a decrease in synovial fluid volume and viscosity and an increased turbidity may be noted (Schiller, 1994). Lastly, radiographic changes associated with rheumatoid arthritis include joint space narrowing, displacement of subcutaneous fat lines, and osteoporosis of subchrondral bone (Fig. 23–7). As the disease progresses, bony erosion is noted radiographically.

Treatment and Prognosis. The treatment goals for someone with rheumatoid arthritis are to reduce pain, maintain mobility, and minimize stiffness, edema, and joint destruction. Owing to the chronic nature of the disease, patient education and continual adherence to the treatment program are vital. Since the inflammatory process results in progressive joint destruction, controlling inflammation is a primary goal. Medications, rest, ambulatory assistive devices, orthoses, and ice can be used during the acute phase. Salicylates are typically the choice of medication initially. Other NSAIDs may be used if aspirin is not tolerated or is not effective. Medications such as gold compounds, hydroxychloroquine, penicillamine,

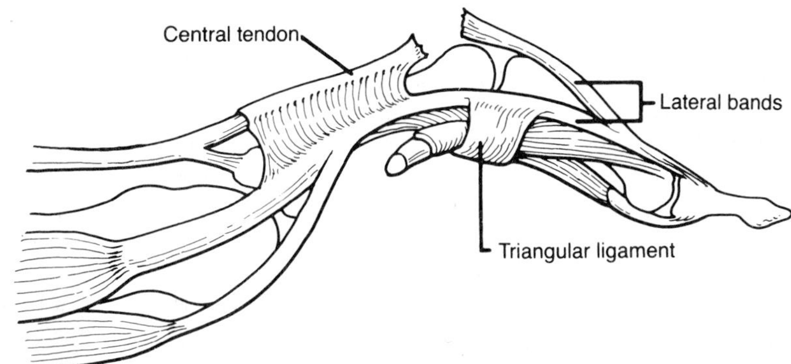

Figure 23-6. Boutonnière deformity. (*From Jacobs JL: Hand and wrist. In Richardson JK, Iglarsh ZA (eds): Clinical Orthopaedic Physical Therapy. Philadelphia, WB Saunders, 1994, p 664.*)

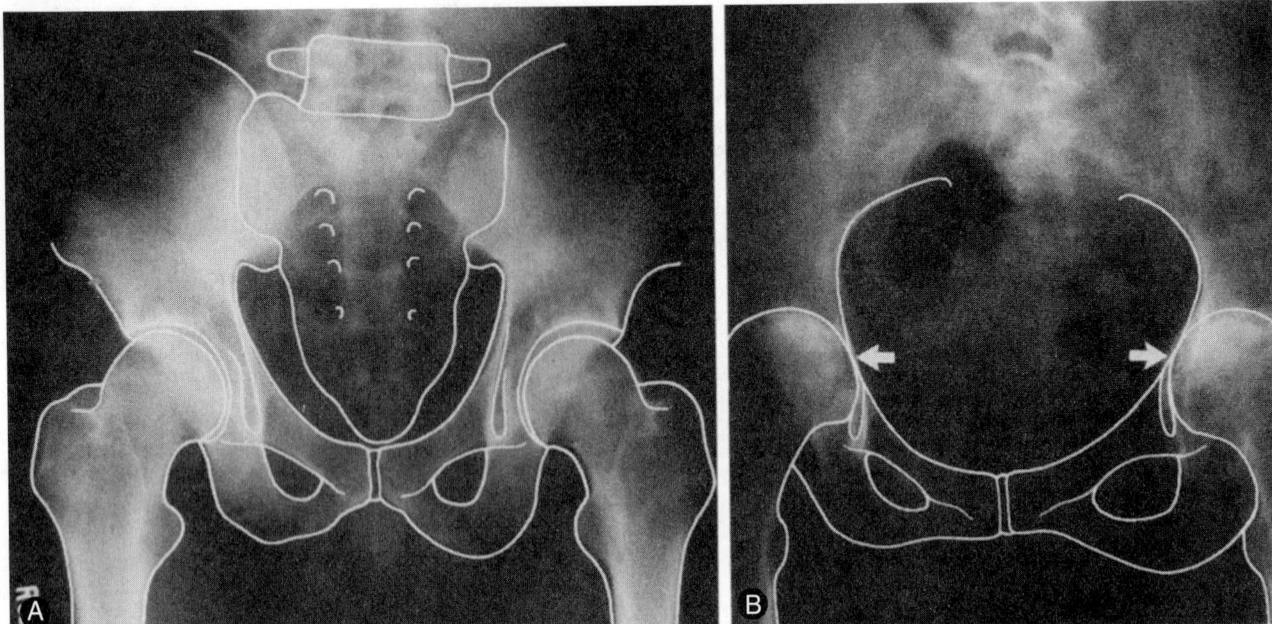

Figure **23-7.** A, Radiograph of normal hips and pelvis. B, Radiograph of rheumatoid arthritis of the hips. Note the narrowed joint space (loss of articular cartilage) and periarticular bone density changes. (*From McKinnis LN: Fundamentals of radiology for physical therapists. In Richardson JK, Iglarsh ZA (eds): Clinical Orthopaedic Physical Therapy. Philadelphia, WB Saunders, 1994, p 673.*)

methotrexate, azathioprine, and sulfasalazine may help induce remission of the disease.[1] Corticosteroids may be used to relieve pain and in clients with unremitting disease with extra-articular manifestations. Intra-articular injections can provide relief of acute inflammation (Pigg and Bancroft, 1994). Administration of these drugs for periods of 3 to 6 months is often necessary for benefit to be noted.

Complete bed rest is rarely indicated and is saved for those with severe, uncontrolled inflammation (McCarty, 1993; Mills et al., 1971). For many people a rest period of up to 2 hours during the day is important for dealing with general body fatigue and protection of involved joints. Splints can be applied to rest involved joints, prevent excessive movement, and reduce mechanical stresses. Crutches, canes, or walkers can be used to reduce weightbearing stresses and enhance balance. Adaptations may be necessary, for example, platform crutches, due to upper extremity involvement.

A balance must be attained between rest and activity. Exercises to prevent contractures, improve strength and flexibility, and enhance aerobic conditioning are an important component of the rehabilitation program (Newcomer and Jurisson, 1994; Harkon et al., 1986).

Surgery may be indicated if conservative care is insufficient regarding pain control and level of function. Synovectomy to reduce pain and joint damage is the primary operation for the wrist. Total joint replacement procedures are performed at the shoulder, knee, and hip. The most common soft tissue procedure is tenosynovectomy of the hand.

[1] Potential side effects of medications include the following; (1) gold—dermatitis, proteinuria, thrombocytopenia, leukopenia, pancytopenia; (2) penicillamine—proteinuria, aplastic anemia, leukopenia, thrombocytopenia; (3) methotrexate—cirrhosis, liver fibrosis.

The natural history of rheumatoid arthritis varies considerably. Approximately one half of those afflicted are only slightly functionally impaired and the other half suffer progressive and disabling joint disease. Death from complications associated with rheumatoid arthritis and its treatment is not rare. These complications include subluxation of the upper cervical spine, infections, gastrointestinal hemorrhage and perforation, and heart and lung disease (Schiller, 1994).

Special Implications for the Therapist **23-3**

RHEUMATOID ARTHRITIS

Therapists see many people with joint pain. Most of these people have joint pain secondary to degenerative osteoarthritis as opposed to rheumatic joint disease, but the therapist must be aware of the symptoms and signs associated with the latter. Quick, aggressive medical treatment is necessary to minimize joint destruction. Joint pain accompanied by systemic complaints, no matter how mild, should raise concern on the therapist's part. Also, insidious onset of polyarthritis should raise suspicion regarding the nature of the pain complaints.

Instability at any joint, particularly at the atlantoaxial segment, requires caution on the therapist's part. Such a joint may present with a marked reduction in range of motion, such as the shoulder or neck feeling "stuck or caught" with a certain movement. A history of periods of significant loss of range of motion alternating with full range of motion suggests joint hypermobility. Restoration of mobility is an important goal, but choosing techniques that are more gentle, or applying traction while stretching, is necessary.

The extra-articular problems may affect the rehabilitation program. For example, if fatigue is present, the therapist may have to allow periods of rest during the treatment session. During periods of symptom exacerbation there is a fine line between overextending the client and maximizing activity. There are times when active exercise may have to be curtailed, but passive stretching remains important to prevent contractures. Aquatic therapy may be beneficial for conditioning, strengthening, and flexibility, while reducing mechanical stress on the joints. Splenomegaly may account for tenderness on palpation and "fullness" or increased resistance of the left upper abdominal quadrant. Deep soft tissue techniques are contraindicated in this area. Percussion techniques may help the therapist delineate the caudal boundaries of the spleen.

Because of the chronic nature of rheumatoid arthritis, treatment is usually an ongoing process. Aspirin and NSAIDs are potentially ulcerogenic, and prolonged use of corticosteroids can lead to osteoporosis. The analgesics and slow-acting antirheumatic drugs such as gold and penicillamine can impair renal function (Bacon, 1993). Periodic screening of each of the body systems is imperative when working with this population.

JUVENILE RHEUMATOID ARTHRITIS

Juvenile rheumatoid arthritis is a chronic inflammatory disease which can range from a mild illness to a severe, destructive arthropathy with significant extra-articular manifestations. A few or multiple joints can be involved. Still's disease, a form of juvenile rheumatoid arthritis, may affect any number of joints, but is characterized chiefly by systemic manifestations (Ostrov, 1995). As with adult rheumatoid arthritis, the cause of this disorder is unknown.

Still's disease is marked by fever and a rash. The fever pattern is marked by spikes reaching 103° to 104° F, and periods between the spikes during which the child feels much better. Lymphadenopathy, myalgias, and hepatosplenomegaly are also often present. The rash typically appears on the trunk and extremities, leaving the palms and soles unaffected. Inflammatory arthritis typically develops at some point and 95% of the children have joint complaints within a year of the initial presenting symptoms. Box 23–4 lists clinical manifestations associated with Still's disease.

BOX 23-4
Clinical Manifestations Associated with Still's Disease

- Fever
- Rash
- Polyarthritis
- Myalgia
- Tenosynovitis
- Skeletal growth disturbances
- Pericarditis
- Pleuritis
- Peptic ulcer disease
- Hepatitis
- Anemia

Medications, including NSAIDs, are administered to control the systemic and articular complaints. Corticosteroids are indicated if severe anemia, unrelenting fever, or vasculitis is present. Physical and occupational therapy are utilized for pain control, maintenance of mobility, and function. By the time these children become adults, only 20% of them have moderate to severe limitations (Ostrov, 1995; Pigg and Bancroft, 1994).

SPONDYLOARTHROPATHIES

Spondyloarthropathies, a group of disorders formerly considered variants of rheumatoid arthritis, are in fact distinct entities with similar features (Box 23–5). The spondyloarthropathies discussed here are ankylosing spondylitis, Reiter's syndrome, and psoriatic arthritis.

Ankylosing Spondylitis

Description. Ankylosing spondylitis is an inflammatory arthropathy of the axial skeleton including the sacroiliac joints, apophyseal joints, costovertebral joints, and the intervertebral disk articulations. Approximately a third of those with ankylosing spondylitis have asymmetrical involvement of the large peripheral joints, including the hip, knee, and shoulder (Pigg and Bancroft, 1994; Schiller, 1994). Figure 23–8 shows the most commonly involved joints. The disorder can ultimately lead to fibrosis, calcification, and ossification of the involved joints. The pain, resultant postural deformities, and complications associated with this disease can be disabling.

Incidence. Ankylosing spondylitis affects approximately 1% to 2% of the population. Nearly 2 million people in the United States have this condition, making it almost as common as rheumatoid arthritis (Ramanujan and Schumacher, 1992).

Etiology. Although the cause of ankylosing spondylitis is unknown, evidence points to a genetic or environmental link. Approximately 90% of those with ankylosing spondylitis are HLA-B27–positive, but of all of the people with this antigen only 2% develop ankylosing spondylitis. However, approximately 20% of people who develop ankylosing spondylitis have a first-degree relative who is HLA-B27–positive (van der Linden et al., 1983).

BOX 23-5
Common Features of the Spondyloarthropathies

- Partiality for involvement of the axial skeleton
- Asymmetrical involvement of a small number of peripheral joints
- Young males most commonly afflicted
- Inflammation at sites of ligament, tendon, and fascial insertion into bone
- Seronegativity for rheumatoid factor, but an association with histocompatibility antigens, including HLA-B27.
- Involvement of visceral systems, including carditis, aortitis, and uveitis

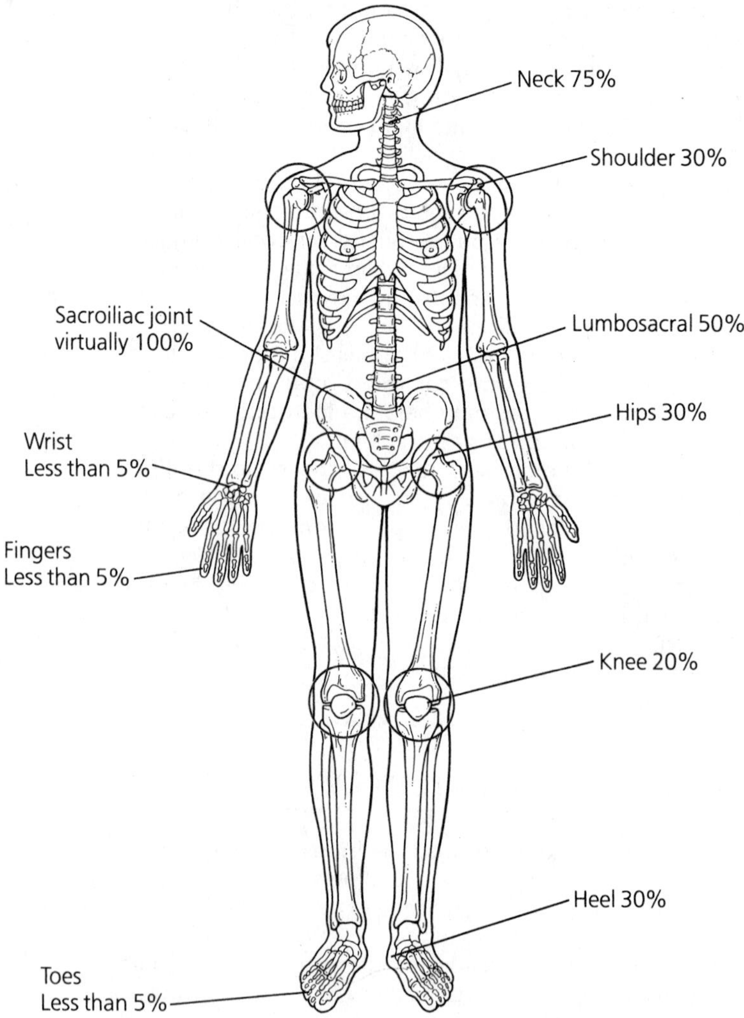

Figure **23-8.** Joints most commonly involved in ankylosing spondylitis and incidence of involvement. (*From Ramanujan T, Schumacher HR: Ankylosing spondylitis: Early recognition and management. J Musculoskel Med 1(1):75–91, 1992.*)

Risk Factors. Gender, age, race, and family history are all important factors regarding the risk of developing ankylosing spondylitis. Although it is more prevalent in males, there is significantly less disparity in incidence between the sexes than was once thought. The belief is that the disorder has been grossly underdiagnosed in women because the disease tends to be milder and peripheral joint involvement is more common, confusing the clinical picture (Arnett et al., 1989; Kidd et al., 1988). The onset of the disease typically occurs between the ages of 20 and 40 years and, as noted under Etiology, the HLA-B27 antigen is associated with the disease. Lastly, ankylosing spondylitis is found more commonly in whites and Native Americans compared with the incidence in blacks and Asians (Arnett, 1987).

Pathologic Manifestations and Complications. Ankylosing spondylitis is marked by a chronic nongranulomatous inflammation. Disruption of the ligamentous-osseous junction results, and reactive bone formation occurs as part of the repair process. Cartilage of the sacroiliac joints may also be involved. The replacement of inflamed cartilaginous structures by bone contributes to progressive ossification which can lead to a fused or bamboo spine, characteristic of end-stage disease.

Longstanding disease is associated with multiple complications. Skeletal complications include osteoporosis, fracture, atlantoaxial subluxation, and spinal stenosis. The stiff and osteoporotic spinal column is prone to fracture from even a minor insult. The lower cervical spine is the most common site of fracture in ankylosing spondylitis (Ramanujan and Schumacher, 1992). The atlantoaxial segment is among the last areas of the axial skeleton to fuse. Because of the inherent mobility of C1–2 and the immobility of the remainder of the cervical spine secondary to the disease, attempts to move the head could result in subluxation. Spinal stenosis can result from the proliferation of bony tissue from the spinal ligaments and facet joints. Stenosis may cause neurogenic claudication and cauda equina syndrome.

Extra-articular complications associated with ankylosing spondylitis are numerous. Uveitis,[2] conjunctivitis, or iritis occurs in approximately 25% of clients (Calin, 1988). Cardiomegaly, pericarditis, aortic regurgitation, amyloidosis, and pulmonary complications may occur. Pulmonary problems include upper lobe fibrosis and decreased total lung capacity and vital capacity.

[2] Inflammation of the uveal tract, including iritis, cyclitis, and choroiditis.

Clinical Manifestations. Insidious onset of back pain and stiffness are often the initial presenting complaints. The pain is usually described as an ache, but can be intermittently sharp. Significant morning stiffness, possibly lasting more than an hour, is often present. In general, symptoms improve with activity and worsen with rest. As the disease progresses it becomes increasingly difficult for the person to tolerate recumbent positions. Progressive disease is marked by new onset of symptoms involving the chest wall and upper thoracic and cervical spine (Ramanujan and Schumacher, 1992; Ball, 1993; Pigg and Bancroft, 1994).

In some cases the initial complaints may occur in areas other than the trunk. One study revealed that 38 of 100 subjects had initial symptoms in the extremities. Twenty-nine of the 38 subjects had pain in the hips or knees. Back symptoms in these 38 people appeared on average 3 years after onset of the peripheral complaints (Maltz et al., 1969).

Besides the symptoms associated with the complications noted previously, other systemic complaints may include weight loss, fever, and fatigue. These are not symptoms typically associated with mechanical causes of back pain and if present should raise concern on the therapist's part regarding the underlying cause of the complaints.

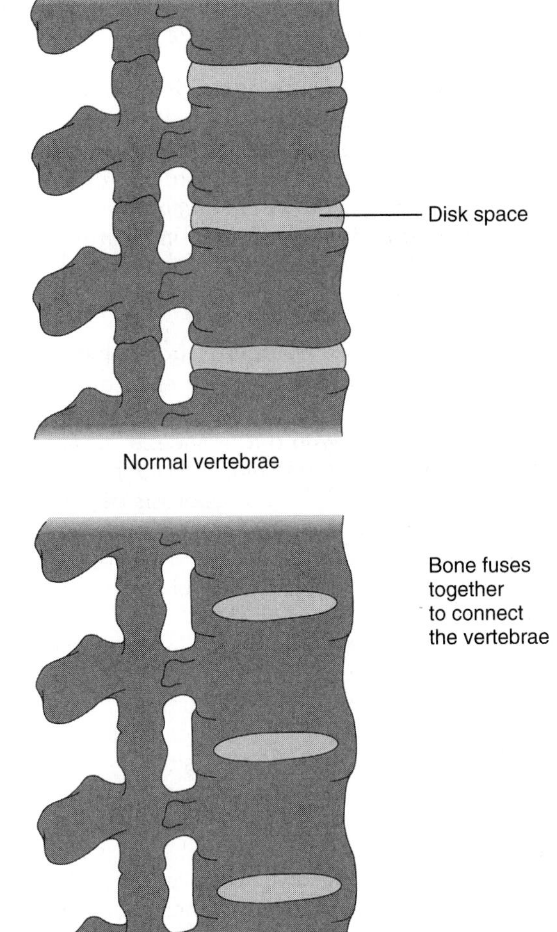

Figure **23–9.** The bony overgrowth associated with ankylosing spondylitis gives the vertebrae a square-shaped appearance.

Medical Management

Diagnosis. In addition to the history, the physical examination, radiography, and laboratory tests are used in the diagnosis. In the physical examination, range-of-motion tests provide important information. Loss of spine mobility in all planes of motion typically occurs. Loss of chest wall excursion is also an indicator of decreased axial skeleton mobility. Circumferential measurements taken at the fourth intercostal space before and at the end of inspiration should reveal an excursion of 4 to 5 cm. In ankylosing spondylitis excursion is less than 4 cm (Bell, 1993; Pigg and Bancroft, 1994). As the disease progresses, a loss of the lumbar lordosis may occur accompanied by increased kyphosis of the thoracic spine. The above findings alone are not diagnostic, but if present, along with the history and radiographic findings, they become significant for the diagnosis.

Radiographs may be negative in the early stages of the disease, but certain findings suggest the presence of ankylosing spondylitis. Findings of sacroiliitis, including blurring of joint margins, juxta-articular sclerosis, erosions, and joint space narrowing, are associated with ankylosing spondylitis. The replacement of ligamentous tissue by bone at the site where the annulus fibrosus of the intervertebral disk inserts into the vertebral body results in a characteristic square-shaped vertebral body (Fig. 23–9). In addition, as bony tissue bridges the vertebral bodies and posterior arches, the thoracic and lumbar spine takes on the appearance of a bamboo spine on radiographs.

Laboratory tests assist primarily by ruling out other diseases. The presence of the HLA-B27 antigen is a useful adjunct to the diagnosis, but is not diagnostic itself, since so many people with other causes of back pain also are HLA-B27–positive. An elevated erythrocyte sedimentation rate and the presence of C-reactive protein may be found, but these findings are not diagnostic (Ramanujan and Schumacher, 1992).

Treatment and Prognosis. The extent of disability in persons with ankylosing spondylitis varies considerably. Periods of exacerbation and remission are common during the course of the disease. The severity of symptoms during the first decade indicates the long-term severity and disabling nature of the disorder. Severe disease is usually marked by peripheral joint and extra-articular manifestations (Pigg and Bancroft, 1994).

The primary focus of treatment is pain relief while maintaining mobility and proper postural alignment of the spine. NSAIDs are commonly administered to control pain and inflammation. Heat is used to relieve stiffness. To avoid long-term complications associated with severe postural deformities, a lifetime commitment to exercise is important. Trunk range-of-motion and strengthening exercises to minimize thoracic kyphosis is essential. The more severe the kyphosis, the more hindered pulmonary function will be and the more pronounced the compensatory forward head posture. Besides their potential for cervical pain and headaches, postural deformities may also affect balance (Pigg and Bancroft, 1994). Avoiding obesity is recommended to reduce stress on weight-bearing joints and the cardiopulmonary system. Lastly, smoking should be discouraged because of its adverse affects on the cardiopulmonary system.

Special Implications for the Therapist **23-4**

ANKYLOSING SPONDYLITIS

Therapists may be treating people with back or hip pain who have yet to be diagnosed with ankylosing spondylitis. If these people begin complaining of new onset of joint pain in the absence of trauma or overuse, low-grade fever, fatigue, or visual complaints, the therapist must consider conditions other than mechanical dysfunction as the root of the problem. Communication with a physician is warranted with this scenario.

Treating a client with a diagnosis of ankylosing spondylitis requires that the therapist entertain different considerations. If the client complains of an onset of sharp pain associated with a fall, sneeze, or lifting a moderately heavy object, one must consider the possibility of a fracture. With osteoporosis being a potential complication, technique modification is warranted. See Special Implications for the Therapist 20–1, Osteoporosis, in Chapter 20 for further discussion.

Therapists play an important role in the rehabilitation of this population (Hicks, 1989; Ball, 1993). Aggressive stretching to address the areas of hypomobility and the muscle imbalances can help maintain as optimal a posture as possible. Strengthening of the trunk extensors is also important. The therapist must be vigilant for an exacerbation of the inflammatory process. Aggressive stretching must be avoided during these phases, and patient communication with the physician is necessary for the development of a proper medication regimen.

Reiter's Syndrome

Description. Reiter's syndrome is one of the most common examples of reactive arthritis. *Reactive arthritis* is defined as a sterile inflammatory arthropathy distant in time and place from the initial inciting infective process (Pigg and Bancroft, 1994). Reiter's syndrome usually follows venereal disease or an episode of bacillary dysentery and is associated with typical extra-articular manifestations.

Incidence. The prevalence and incidence of Reiter's syndrome are difficult to establish because of (1) the lack of consensus regarding diagnostic criteria; (2) the nomadic nature of the young target population; (3) the underreporting of venereal disease; and (4) the asymptomatic or milder course in affected women (Cush and Lipsky, 1993).

Etiology. The most common microbial pathogens are *Shigella*, *Salmonella*, *Yersinia*, *Campylobacter*, and *Chlamydia* species (Cush and Lipsky, 1993; Keat, 1983; Phillips, 1988).

Risk Factors. Age, gender, and medical history are important risk factors associated with Reiter's syndrome. The peak onset of this disorder occurs during the third decade of life. However, children and the elderly can also develop this disease. Males are more commonly affected than females, but not to the extent once thought. The incidence in women is potentially underestimated because their clinical manifestations are less severe than men's and women are more prone to occult genitourinary disease leading to misdiagnosis (Aho et al., 1985; Keat, 1983). A history of infection, especially venereal or dysenteric, is associated with increased risk of developing this condition.

Pathology. Reiter's syndrome is primarily marked by inflammatory synovitis and inflammatory erosion at the insertion sites of ligaments and tendons (enthesitis). Heterotopic bone formation can occur at these sites. Synovial findings include edema, cellular invasion (lymphocytes, neutrophils, and plasma cells) and vascular changes. Extensive pannus formation is rare, unlike in rheumatoid arthritis.

Clinical Manifestations. The triad of symptoms classically associated with Reiter's syndrome are urethritis, conjunctivitis, and arthritis. The urethritis and conjunctivitis often occur early on in the disease. Other ocular manifestations include uveitis and keratitis.[3] The arthritis is usually asymmetrical, often acute, and typically involves joints of the lower extremity, including the knees, ankles, and first metatarsophalangeal joint (Hellman 1995; Pigg, and Bancroft, 1994; Cush and Lipsky, 1993). While most of the symptoms and signs disappear within days or weeks, the arthritis may last for months or years (Hellman, 1995). The digits, especially the toes, can become swollen and distended (dactylitis). Potential mucocutaneous manifestations include mouth ulcers, skin rashes, and balanitis (inflammation of the glans penis or clitoris). The skin lesions may be indistinguishable from those of psoriasis. Low back pain is also a common complaint. The arthritis can progress and spread to the spine and even to the upper extremities.

Medical Management

Diagnosis. Diagnosis of Reiter's syndrome require months to make because the various manifestations may occur at different times. The combination of peripheral arthritis with urethritis lasting longer than 1 month is necessary before the diagnosis can be made (Berkow and Fletcher, 1992). Laboratory tests typically reveal an aggressive inflammatory process. Elevated erythrocyte sedimentation rate and C-reactive protein are detected, and thrombocytosis and leukocytosis are common findings. Up to 70% of those with established Reiter's syndrome may have radiographic abnormalities (Cush and Lipsky, 1993). These abnormalities may include (1) asymmetrical involvement of the lower extremity diarthroses, amphiarthroses, symphyses, and entheses; (2) ill-defined bony erosions with adjacent bony proliferation; and (3) paravertebral ossification.

Treatment and Prognosis. Although Reiter's syndrome is precipitated by an infection, there is no evidence that antibiotic therapy changes the course of the disorder. Treatment in general is largely symptomatic, with NSAIDs being the primary intervention. If the arthritis persists, joint protection and maintenance of function become important. Immobilization and inactivity is usually discouraged, while range-of-motion and stretching exercises are emphasized. Severe disability occurs in less than 15% of those afflicted (Pigg and Bancroft, 1994; Cush and Lipsky, 1993).

---

[3] Keratitis is a fungal infection of the cornea.

Special Implications for the Therapist **23-5**

REITER'S SYNDROME

Questions related to the presence and treatment of infection, current and past, should be asked during the history taking. Also inquire into the person's general health, both current and prior to the onset of the presenting pain complaints. Typically, the onset of joint pain associated with concurrent systemic complaints would raise suspicion. Reiter's syndrome is one condition in which past medical history and general health status may provide the most important information.

Psoriatic Arthritis

Description. Psoriatic arthritis is a seronegative inflammatory joint disease afflicting a small percentage of people who have psoriasis. This joint disorder is associated with radiographic evidence of periarticular bone erosions and occasional significant joint destruction (Bennett, 1993). Psoriatic arthritis tends to progress slowly, and for most of those afflicted it is more a nuisance than a disabling condition (Coulton et al., 1989).

Incidence and Risk Factors. Approximately 1% of the population of the United States has psoriasis. Psoriatic arthritis occurs in 5% to 7% of persons with psoriasis and more often in those with severe psoriasis (Pigg and Bancroft, 1994; Schiller, 1994). Uncomplicated psoriasis typically presents during the second and third decades of life, with the onset of the arthritis occurring up to 20 years later. The disease can occur in children, with onset typically between the ages of 9 and 12 years (Southwood et al., 1989; Shore and Ansell, 1982). Psoriatic arthritis does not appear to have a strong predilection for one sex.

A strong familial association has been noted with this disease. There is approximately an 80% to 90% chance of contracting psoriatic arthritis if one has a first-degree relative with the disorder. This suggests a genetic predisposition (Moll and Wright, 1973a and b; Stern, 1985).

Etiology. Although specific marker genes have not been discovered, there is general agreement that a genetic predisposition exists for psoriatic arthritis.

Pathogenesis. An inflammatory synovitis results in the joint changes associated with psoriatic arthritis. A lymphocyte infiltration into the synovium occurs. Initially the synovium is pale, with edematous granulation tissue extending along the contiguous bone. The synovium later becomes thickened with villous hypertrophy. Eroded articular margins begin to appear at this time. In severe cases the joint space tends to be filled in with dense fibrous tissue (Bennett, 1993).

Clinical Manifestations. The arthritis can be oligoarticular or polyarticular. There is a predilection for the distal interphalangeal joints of the hands. Other joints of the digits may be involved. The joint changes may lead to significant hand deformities, including claw deformity. The digital joint changes and associated flexor tenosynovitis can result in an edematous, thickened digit. Pitting of the nails is also commonly associated with psoriatic arthritis.

Joints of the axial skeleton can also be affected, but typically become involved several years after the onset of the peripheral joint disease. The sacroiliitis is usually unilateral, unlike that with ankylosing spondylitis (Moll and Wright 1973a,b; Gladman et al., 1987). Sacroiliitis can occur in 20% to 40% of clients (Lambert and Wright, 1977).

Although not as common as in rheumatoid arthritis or Reiter's syndrome, extra-articular manifestations can occur with psoriatic arthritis. Inflammatory eye disease, including conjunctivitis and iritis; renal disease; mitral valve prolapse; and aortic regurgitation have been associated with this disorder.

There are some differences in the manifestations of this disease between children and adults. A slight predilection for females is noted in children. In addition, the arthritis may appear before the skin manifestations in a number of children (Sills, 1980). Compared with adults, the onset of the arthritis tends to be more acute in children, with the involvement of multiple asymmetrical joints. The hip joint is much more commonly involved in children (Bennett, 1993).

Medical Management

Diagnosis. The diagnosis of psoriatic arthritis is usually easily made because of the onset of inflammatory arthritis in the presence of obvious psoriasis. Differential diagnosis can be difficult, though, if the psoriasis is absent or equivocal. Laboratory tests do not help except to rule out rheumatoid arthritis. See Box 23–6 lists common radiographic findings in psoriatic arthritis.

Treatment and Prognosis. There is currently no cure for psoriasis or psoriatic arthritis. People with mild arthritis are treated symptomatically with NSAIDs. If there is an acute flare of only one or two joints, local corticosteroid injections may help. Because of the association between severe skin involvement and severe arthritis, treatment of the psoriasis is emphasized with the hope of reducing the arthritis. Multiple medications have been utilized in an attempt to control progressive psoriatic arthritis, but with equivocal results. As noted earlier, for most persons with psoriatic arthritis, the disease is mild, not destructive.

Special Implications for the Therapist **23-6**

PSORIATIC ARTHRITIS

If a flare of the skin condition is noted, encourage the patient to see her or his physician. If the joint inflammation worsens, prompt communication with the

BOX **23-6**
Radiographic Features of Psoriatic Arthritis

- Asymmetrical oligoarticular distribution of disease
- Relative absence of osteopenia
- Involvement of distal interphalangeal joints
- Involvement of sacroiliac joint (unilateral)

physician should occur so the client can be placed on an appropriate medication regimen.

GOUT

Description. Gout represents a heterogeneous group of metabolic disorders marked by an elevated level of serum uric acid and the deposition of urate crystals in the joints, soft tissues, and kidneys. Primary and secondary forms of gout are classified according to the cause of the hyperuricemia. Primary gout refers to hyperuricemia in the absence of other disease while secondary gout refers to hyperuricemia resulting from an antecedent disease (Schiller, 1994). Gout can be manifested by acute or chronic arthritis. Crystals other than uric acid crystals can also form inside joints. An example is calcium pyrophosphate dihydrate crystals which, when present, mark a condition called pseudogout.

Incidence and Risk Factors. Primary gout is predominantly associated with men, as less than 10% of the cases occur in women. Most of the women afflicted with gout are postmenopausal (Levinson and Becker, 1993). Gout is rare in children and the peak incidence occurs during the fifth decade of life. A family history of gout increases the risk of developing the disorder.

Secondary hyperuricemia (gout) can be a result of urate overproduction or decreased urinary excretion of uric acid. People at risk for urate overproduction are those with a history of leukemia, lymphoma, psoriasis, and hemolytic disorders and those receiving chemotherapy for cancer. Alcohol consumption, chronic renal failure, hypertension, hypothyroidism, and hyperparathyroidism can all lead to decreased excretion of uric acid.

Etiology. In many cases of primary gout the specific biochemical defect responsible for the hyperuricemia is unknown. A majority of cases probably result from an unexplained impairment in uric acid excretion by the kidneys (Schiller, 1994). This impairment could result from decreased renal filtration, increased reabsorption, or decreased urate excretion by the renal tubules.

Pathogenesis. Sodium urate crystals precipitate from supersaturated body fluids. These crystals frequently collect on articular cartilage, epiphyseal bone, and periarticular structures. The crystal aggregates result in local tissue necrosis and a proliferation of fibrous tissue secondary to an inflammatory foreign body reaction (Levinson and Becker, 1993).

Clinical Manifestations. An acute attack of gout is manifested by exquisite joint pain, commonly occurring at night. Although the first metatarsophalangeal joint is a common site of pain, the ankle, instep, knee, wrist, elbow (olecranon bursa), and fingers can all be the site of the initial attack. Besides local pain of quick onset, erythema, warmth, and extreme tenderness and hypersensitivity are typically present. Chills and fever may accompany the joint complaints. After recovering from the initial episode the person enters an asymptomatic phase called the intercritical period. This period can last months or years. As the gouty attacks return, the frequency and severity of the episodes tend to increase. These attacks may be precipitated by trauma, surgery, alcohol consumption, or overindulgence in foods with high purine content. The arthritis can become chronic with functional loss and disability (Hellman, 1995; Levinson and Becker, 1993).

Medical Management

Diagnosis. A definitive diagnosis of gout is made when monosodium urate crystals (tophi) are found in synovial fluid, connective tissue, or articular cartilage.

Treatment and Prognosis. The goals of treatment are twofold: (1) to end and prevent acute attacks and (2) to correct the hyperuricemia. NSAIDs are effective in treating the acute attack. Colchicine is another medication given during the acute phase. Involved joints should also be rested, elevated, and protected (crutches, foot cradle, etc.).

Once the acute attack has been relieved, the hyperuricemia must be treated. This requires lifelong management, and compliance is absolutely necessary. Dietary changes, weight loss, and moderation of alcohol intake are all important. Medications such as allopurinol are utilized to reduce the hyperuricemia (Pigg and Bancroft, 1994). Controlling the hyperuricemia is the key to preventing this disease from becoming chronic and disabling (Levinson and Becker, 1993; Ellman, 1992).

Special Implications for the Therapist **23-7**

GOUT

An onset of severe joint pain with a swollen, hot joint should always concern the therapist. Gout, infection, and hemarthrosis are all possible conditions which could account for this clinical scenario. Quick diagnosis and initiation of treatment is necessary to control or prevent damage to the joint structures.

OSTEONECROSIS

Description. The term *osteonecrosis* refers to the death of bone and bone marrow cellular components in the absence of infection. Avascular necrosis and aseptic necrosis are synonyms for this condition. The femoral head is the most common site of this disorder.

Etiology. Osteocytic necrosis results from tissue ischemia. A minimum of 2 hours of complete ischemia and anoxia is necessary for permanent loss of bone tissue (James and Steijn-Myagkaya, 1986). The bony ischemia may be secondary to trauma disrupting the arterial supply or to thrombosis disrupting the microcirculation.

Risk Factors. Box 23–7 lists conditions associated with osteonecrosis. A number of these conditions are linked to osteonecrosis by the development of fat emboli in the vascular tree of the involved bone. The conditions associated with

BOX **23-7**
Conditions Associated with Osteonecrosis

Trauma (e.g., fall)
Systemic lupus erythematosus
Pancreatitis
Diabetes mellitus
Cushing's disease
Gout
Sickle cell disease
Alcoholism
Obesity
Pregnancy
Use of oral contraceptives
Long-term corticosteroid use

the development of fat emboli include alcoholism, obesity, pregnancy, pancreatitis, use of oral contraceptives, and unrelated fractures (Jones, 1993).

Pathogenesis. Certain bones are more vulnerable to osteonecrosis than others. These bones are covered extensively by cartilage, have few vascular foramina, and have limited collateral circulation. The femoral head is a prime example of a bone at risk. The superior-lateral two thirds of the femoral head receives its blood supply almost entirely from the lateral epiphyseal branches of the medial femoral circumflex artery. The only other source of blood for the femoral head is the medial epiphyseal artery (contained within the ligamentum teres) which has limited anastomoses with the lateral epiphyseal vessels (Jones, 1993). Hip dislocation or fracture of the neck of the femur can compromise the precarious vascular supply to the head of the femur. The talus, scaphoid, and proximal humerus are also susceptible to osteonecrosis.

Clinical Manifestations. Pain is the initial presenting complaint. If the femur is involved, the pain may be noted in the groin, thigh, or medial knee area. The pain may be mild and intermittent initially, but will progress, especially during weightbearing activities. An antalgic gait is noted and pain provocation occurs with hip range-of-motion exercises, especially internal rotation and flexion and adduction.

Medical Management

Diagnosis. Plain films may be normal initially in lieu of trauma. Bone scan, magnetic resonance imaging (MRI) and computed tomography (CT) scans are much more sensitive procedures and detect subtle bony changes.

Treatment and Prognosis. The choice between conservative vs. surgical intervention depends on the size of the lesion and whether bony collapse has occurred. If surgery is not indicated, protected weightbearing is essential to prevent collapse of the lesion. Surgical intervention may be hemiarthroplasty or total joint replacement. An osteotomy may be performed to shift the site to where maximal weightbearing occurs on a particular joint surface. The prognosis depends on the extent of damage that has occurred prior to diagnosis in the case of nontraumatic disease.

Special Implications for the Therapist **23-8**

OSTEONECROSIS

When treating people at risk for osteonecrosis, therapists must consider the possibility of fracture if there is a sudden worsening of pain complaints followed by a sudden, dramatic loss in range of motion. Once the diagnosis is made, close communication with the physician is important for safe progression of weightbearing and exercise. Also, an awareness that hip joint pathology may be manifested primarily or completely by knee pain is important. In anyone presenting with knee pain, the lumbar and hip regions should be screened.

LEGG-CALVÉ-PERTHES DISEASE

Legg-Calvé-Perthes disease is epiphysial aseptic necrosis of the proximal end of the femur. This condition occurs in approximately 1 in 1200 children, primarily those between the ages of 3 and 12 years. Legg-Calvé-Perthes disease occurs more frequently in whites than in blacks. The cause is unknown and the clinical manifestations usually begin insidiously. The chief complaint is usually pain noted in the groin, thigh, or knee, with walking or running difficulties.

The disease process consists of four stages: (1) the synovitis stage; (2) the avascular stage, in which the ossification center becomes necrotic and damage to the femoral head occurs; (3) the regeneration stage, in which resorption of necrotic tissue occurs; and (4) the healed or residual stage, in which the newly formed immature bone is replaced by mature bone tissue. The goal of treatment is to limit deformity and preserve the integrity of the femoral head. Conservative care may include minimizing weightbearing forces during ambulation and placement of a hip spica cast or abduction brace to maintain the femoral head in the proper position relative to the acetabulum. Therapists may be involved in gait training, swimming pool therapy, and range-of-motion exercises during this period. Surgery may be performed to contain the femoral head in the acetabulum, especially in children older than 6 years with serious involvement of the femoral head (Gunta, 1994).

CONNECTIVE TISSUE DISEASE

Overview and Incidence. Sometimes people have features of more than one rheumatic disease. This has been called the overlap syndrome or mixed connective tissue disease (MCTD). It includes people who have overlapping features of systemic lupus erythematosus (SLE), scleroderma, or polymyositis. The incidence of this disease is unknown but adults, particularly women, are predominantly affected.

Initially MCTD was considered a distinct entity defined by a specific autoantibody to ribonuclear protein (RNP). More recent studies, have shown, however, that this concept of MCTD is flawed, since with time, in many of the affected people, the manifestations evolve to one predominant disease, and since many people with autoantibodies to RNP have clear-cut SLE. Therefore the designation "overlap connective tissue disease" (OCTD) is becoming the preferred name for people having features of different rheumatic diseases[4] (Hellman, 1995).

Etiology and Pathogenesis. The cause of this disorder is unknown. Persons with this condition often have hypergammaglobulinemia and a positive rheumatoid factor suggesting an immune injury. There is also a high titer of antibody to ribonucleoprotein (anti-RNP), but as previously mentioned this feature is also present in SLE. The cause for the formation and maintenance of the high titer of anti-RNP antibody is unclear. There is no direct evidence that these antibodies induce the characteristic involvement of the various organ systems (Rubin and Farber, 1994).

Clinical Manifestations. OCTD/MCTD combines features of SLE (rash, Raynaud's phenomenon, arthritis, arthralgias), scleroderma (swollen hands, esophageal hypomotility, pulmonary interstitial disease), polymyositis (inflammatory myositis), and in most people, polyarthralgias. Seventy-five percent have rheumatoid arthritis (Merck p. 1288). Proximal muscle weakness with or without tenderness is common.

Pulmonary, cardiac, and renal involvement, as well as such findings as Sjögren's syndrome, Hashimoto's thyroiditis, fever, lymphadenopathy, splenomegaly, hepatomegaly, intestinal involvement, and persistent hoarseness, may occur. Neurologic abnormalities, including organic mental syndrome, aseptic meningitis, seizures, multiple peripheral neuropathies, and cerebral infarction or hemorrhage, occur in about 10% of people affected by this disorder. A trigeminal sensory neuropathy appears to be seen much more frequently in MCTD/OCTD than in other rheumatic diseases (Berkow and Fletcher, 1992).

Medical Management

Diagnosis, Treatment, and Prognosis. Diagnosis is considered when additional overlapping features are present in persons appearing to have SLE, scleroderma, polymyositis, rheumatoid arthritis, juvenile rheumatoid arthritis, Sjögren's syndrome, vasculitis, idiopathic thrombocytopenic purpura, or lymphoma. High titers of antibody to RNP are a characteristic serologic finding, much more often with OCTD/MCTD than with any other rheumatic disease.

General medical management and drug therapy are similar to the approach used in SLE. Most persons are responsive to corticosteroids, especially if administered early in the course of the disease. Mild disease often is controlled by salicylates, other NSAIDs, antimalarials, or very low doses of corticosteroids. High doses of steroids may be used in combination with cytotoxic drugs when the disease is progressive and widespread.

The overall mortality has been reported as 13% with the mean disease duration varying from 6 to 12 years. Causes of death vary without discernible patterns. Sustained remissions for several years on little or no maintenance corticosteroid therapy have been observed in some people.

[4] There is also a condition called undifferentiated connective tissue syndrome (UCTS) in which the systemic rheumatic diseases present have several properties shared to a variable extent by rheumatoid arthritis, SLE, polymyositis, dermatomyositis, and Sjögren's syndrome that make a specific diagnosis for a recognizable connective tissue disease difficult (Reichlin, 1993).

POLYMYALGIA RHEUMATICA

Description. Polymyalgia rheumatica is a disorder marked by diffuse pain and stiffness that primarily affects the shoulder and pelvic girdle musculature. This condition is significant in that diagnosis is difficult and often delayed; severe disability can occur unless proper treatment is initiated; and an association with giant cell arteritis exists. The initial symptoms associated with polymyalgia rheumatica are often subtle and of gradual onset, resulting in a delay of the person seeking care. The complaints also may be localized to one shoulder, leading to an initial diagnosis of bursitis (Healy, 1993). As the disease progresses, carrying out activities of daily living becomes increasingly difficult. Bed mobility and sit-to-stand transfers are among the functional activities affected. Lastly, a significant number (15% to 20%) of those with polymyalgia rheumatica also develop giant cell arteritis. The risk related to the arteritis is blindness secondary to obstruction of the ciliary and ophthalmic arteries (Hellman, 1995).

Incidence and Risk Factors. Female gender, age, and race are the three primary risk factors associated with polymyalgia rheumatica. Women are involved twice as often as men and the disease is rare before the age of 50. White women are more commonly affected than are women of other races. The overall incidence of the disorder is estimated to be 0.5% of the population over the age of 50 (Healy, 1993).

Etiology. The cause of polymyalgia rheumatica is unknown.

Pathology. Despite complaints of pain and stiffness in the muscles, polymyalgia rheumatica is not associated with any histologic abnormalities. Serum creatinine kinase levels, electromyograms, and muscle biopsies are negative in this population.

Clinical Manifestations. Even though the initial muscle pain and stiffness may occur unilaterally, the symptoms are often bilateral and symmetrical. Despite the complaints of difficulties with bed mobility and sit-to-stand maneuvers, muscle weakness is not the problem. Pain and stiffness are the primary issues. Local tenderness of the involved muscles is noted with palpation. In addition, fever, malaise, and unexplained weight loss may occur.

Medical Management

Diagnosis. The diagnosis of polymyalgia rheumatica is often based on the presence of a constellation of findings and the person's rapid response to a trial of prednisone. Besides the complaints noted under Clinical Manifestations, the person may be anemic and present with an elevated sedimentation rate. The lack of rheumatoid factor, the presence of antinuclear antibodies, and histologic changes in the muscles contribute to the diagnosis by excluding other conditions (Healy, 1993; Hellman, 1995).

Treatment and Prognosis. The response of this condition to prednisone is dramatic. In fact, if dramatic improvement is not noted within a week of starting the prednisone, the diagnosis of polymyalgia rheumatica is questionable. Most people require a maintenance dosage of prednisone that is gradually tapered to 5.0 to 7.5 mg/day. The disease is self-limiting in many people within a period of 1½ to 2 years, but recurrence can be as high as 30% in people who received treatment for 1 to 2 years (Healy 1993).

Special Implications for the Therapist **23-9**

POLYMYALGIA RHEUMATICA

When treating someone with a history of polymyalgia rheumatica the therapist must be aware of the potential risk of giant cell or temporal arteritis. An elderly patient with sudden onset of temporal headaches, exquisite tenderness over the temporal artery, scalp sensitivity, or visual complaints should be seen by his or her physician immediately. Also, increased complaints of muscle pain and stiffness should direct the therapist to ask if the client is still taking the prednisone as directed. Owing to the dramatic relief obtained with prednisone, clients may quit taking it prematurely. Careful monitoring of the dosage level is necessary for proper tapering of the medication (Pigg and Bancroft, 1994). Communication with the primary physician is warranted in the presence of the above scenario.

MYOFASCIAL PAIN DYSFUNCTION

Description. Myofascial pain dysfunction is a condition marked by the presence of a clinical entity, myofascial trigger points. These hyperirritable foci located in skeletal muscle or its fascial component were first described in 1952 (Travell and Rinzler, 1952). Upon palpation of these local foci, a characteristic pattern of referred pain is provoked. Pain may be provoked at quite a distance from the points of local tenderness. These trigger points may be a part of a larger syndrome associated with fibromyalgia, but can occur independently of any systemic complaints. The focus of this section is on such conditions. The syndrome associated with myofascial pain dysfunction has also been called fibrositis.

Incidence. Some clinicians believe myofascial trigger points are an extremely common source of back pain (Simons and Travell, 1983). One study reported that 85% of 233 consecutive patients admitted to one comprehensive pain center were diagnosed with myofascial pain syndrome (Fishbain et al., 1986).

Etiology and Risk Factors. The cause of myofascial pain dysfunction is thought to be related to either a sudden overload or overstretching of a muscle or to chronic repetitive or sustained muscle activity (Simons and Travell, 1983). Therefore, people involved in occupations or recreation marked by repetitive or sustained activities or postures are at increased risk of developing this condition. Structural abnormalities could also place a chronic strain on certain muscle groups. Such abnormalities include significant leg length discrepancy, small hemipelvis, short upper arms in relation to torso height, and a foot with a relatively long second metatarsal compared to the first metatarsal (Simons and Travell, 1983). Lastly, other predisposing factors associated with this condition include fatigue, chronic infection, and psychogenic stress (Travell and Rinzler, 1952).

Pathology. To date, the trigger point is viewed as more of a clinical entity than a pathologic entity. Routine laboratory tests and electromyographic examination reveal no abnormalities. Tissue biopsy of a trigger point suggests possible muscle cell metabolic disturbances and impaired local circulation, but gross tissue abnormalities are absent (Travell and Simons, 1983).

Clinically, a trigger point is described as a palpable band within a muscle. An *active trigger point* is defined as a palpable band, which, when palpated, causes local tenderness and referred pain. A *latent trigger point* is defined as a palpable band that is not painful but may cause restriction of movement and muscle weakness. A latent trigger point may become active in the presence of an acute, sudden overload of the muscle or a more chronic strain as described under Etiology. Once present, the trigger points are self-sustained and self-perpetuating hyperirritable foci.

Clinical Manifestations. A taut, palpable myofascial band that is exquisitely tender on palpation with a characteristic and reproducible referred pain pattern (with sustained palpable pressure) is the hallmark of myofascial pain dysfunction. The muscle groups most commonly involved are the postural muscles of the neck, shoulder, and pelvic girdles and the muscles of mastication. The two-volume work by Janet Travell and David Simons describes the pain referral patterns associated with trigger points (Travell and Simons, 1983, 1992). Besides the pain, myofascial pain dysfunction is manifested by a reduced range of motion of joints under the control of the involved muscle, and muscle weakness (Simons and Travell, 1983).

Medical Management

Diagnosis. Because myofascial pain dysfunction is more of a clinical entity, the diagnosis is made solely by clinical examination. Besides the information provided under Clinical Manifestations, Simons and Travell (1983) describe a local twitch response and a jump sign associated with this condition. The local twitch response is a brief contraction of the palpable mass in response to a brisk rolling or snapping palpation of the band. The jump sign is the patient's movement and vocalization in response to pressure exerted on the trigger point.

Treatment. Many techniques aimed at desensitizing trigger points have been employed. These techniques are followed by stretch of the involved muscle. Injections and sustained manual pressure to the trigger point are among the techniques recommended to desensitize the band (Simons and Travell, 1983). Flouromethane spray is also utilized before the stretching procedures to facilitate pain relief and return of function (Travell, 1952).

Special Implications for the Therapist **23-10**

MYOFASCIAL PAIN DYSFUNCTION

This condition is marked by pain patterns often attributed to other conditions such as herniated nucleus pulposus or facet joint disease. Assessment of muscle as the source of pain is an important component of the examination process. Studies done prior to Travell's earlier works demonstrated that muscle irritation could result in referral of pain (Kellgren, 1938). If the therapist notes the clinical manifestations described earlier but in multiple locations, plus other systemic complaints such as fatigue, sleep difficulties, and so on, other conditions (e.g., fibromyalgia) need to be considered. Lastly, client compliance regarding the stretching of the involved muscle is paramount to lasting success of treatment. The client can also apply sustained deep pressure over a trigger point using a tennis ball or some other hard object.

References

Aho K, Leirsal-Repo M, Repo H: Reactive arthritis. Clin Rheum Dis 11:25–40, 1985.

Andersson GBJ: Intervertebral disk: Clinical aspects. *In* Buckwalter JA, Goldberg VM, Woo SL-Y (eds): Musculoskeletal soft tissue aging: Impact on mobility. Rosemont, Ill, American Academy of Orthopaedic Surgeons, 1993, pp 331–347.

Arnett FC: Seronegative spondyloarthropathies. Bull Rheum Dis 37:1–12, 1987.

Arnett FC, Khan MA, Wilkins RF: A new look at ankylosing spondylitis. Patient Care 23:82–101, 1989.

Bacon PA: Extra-articular rheumatoid arthritis. *In* McCarty DJ, Koopman WJ (eds): Arthritis and Allied Conditions, ed 12. Philadelphia, Lea & Febiger, 1993, pp 811–840.

Ball GV: Ankylosing spondylitis. *In* McCarty DJ, Koopman WJ (eds): Arthritis and Allied Conditions, ed 12. Philadelphia, Lea & Febiger, 1993, pp 1051–1060.

Bennett RM: Psoriatic arthritis. *In* McCarty DJ, Koopman WJ (eds): Arthritis and Allied Conditions, ed 12. Philadelphia, Lea & Febiger, 1993, pp 1079–1094.

Berkow R, Fletcher AJ: The Merck Manual of Diagnosis and Therapy, ed 16. Rahway, NJ, Merck, 1992, pp 1337–1338.

Boden S: Rheumatoid arthritis of the cervical spine. Spine 19:2275–2280, 1994.

Buckwalter JA: Spine update-aging and degeneration of the human intervertebral disc. Spine 20(11):1307–1314, 1995.

Calin A: Ankylosing spondylitis. *In* Katz AW (ed): Diagnosis and Management of Rheumatic Diseases, ed 2. Philadelphia, JB Lippincott, 1988, pp 4423–4431.

Coulton BL, Thomson K, Symmons DP, Popert AJ: Outcome in patients hospitalized for psoriatic arthritis. Clin Rheumatol 8:261–265, 1989.

Cush JJ, Lipsky PE: Reiter's syndrome and reactive arthritis. *In* McCarty DJ, Koopman WJ (eds): Arthritis and Allied Conditions, ed 12. Philadelphia, Lea & Febiger, 1993, pp 1061–1078.

Davison S: Rheumatic disease in the elderly. Mt Sinai J Med 47:175–178, 1980.

Ellman MH: Treating acute gouty arthritis. J Musculoskel Med 9:71–77, 1992.

Eyre D, Benya P, Buckwalter J, et al: The intervertebral disk: Basic science perspectives. *In* Frymoyer JW, Gordon SL (eds): New Perspectives on Low Back Pain. Park Ridge, Ill, American Academy of Orthopaedic Surgeons, 1989, pp 147–207.

Fishbain AA, Goldberg M, Meagher BR, et al: Male and female chronic pain patients categorized by DSM-III psychiatric diagnostic criteria. Pain 26:181, 1986.

Foldes K, Balint P, Gaal M, et al: Nocturnal pain correlates with effusion in diseased hips. J Rheumatol 19:1756–1758, 1992.

Gladman DD, Shuckett R, Russell ML, et al: Psoriatic arthritis (PSA)—An analysis of 220 patients. QJ Med 62:127–141, 1987.

Gunta K: Alterations in skeletal function: Congenital disorders, metabolic bone disease and neoplasm. *In* Mattson-Porth C (ed): Pathophysiology (Concepts of Altered Health States), ed 4. Philadelphia, JB Lippincott, 1994, pp 1219–1244.

Harkom TM, Lampman RM, Banwell BF, Castor CW: Therapeutic value of graded aerobic exercise training in rheumatoid arthritis. Arthritis Rheuma 28:32–39, 1985.

Harris E: Rheumatoid arthritis: Pathophysiology and implications for therapy. N Engl J Med 322:1277–1289, 1990.

Hazes JMW, Dijkmans BAC, Vandenbroucke JP, et al: Pregnancy and the risk of developing rheumatoid arthritis. Arthritis Rheum 33:1770–1775, 1990.

Healy LA: Polymalgia rheumatica and giant cell arteritis. *In* McCarty DJ, Koopman WJ (eds): Arthritis and Allied Conditions, ed 12. Philadelphia, Lea & Febiger. 1993, pp 1377–1380.

Hellman DB: Arthritis and musculoskeletal disorders. *In* Tierney LM, McPhee SJ, Papadakis MA (eds): Current Medical Diagnosis and Treatment, ed 34. Norwalk, Conn, Appleton & Lange, 1995, pp 726–732.

Herkowitz, HN: Spine update: Degenerative lumbar spondylolisthesis. Spine 20:1084–1090, 1995.

Hicks JE: Exercise for patients with inflammatory arthritis. J Musculoskel Med 6(10):40–56, 1989.

James J, Steijn-Myagkaya GL: Death of osteocytes. Electron microscopy after in vitro ischemia. J Bone Joint Surg [Br] 68:620–624, 1986.

Johnson KJ, Chensue SW, Kunkel SL, Ward PA: Immunopathology. *In* Rubin E, Farber JL (eds): Pathology, 2nd ed. Philadelphia, JB Lippincott, 1994, pp 140–141.

Jones JP: Osteonecrosis. *In* McCarthy DJ, Koopman WJ (eds): Arthritis and Allied Conditions, ed 12. Philadelphia, Lea & Febiger, 1993, pp 1677–1696.

Jonsson B, Stromquist B: Symptoms and signs in degeneration of the lumbar spine. J Bone Joint Surg [Br] 75:381–385, 1993.

Keat A: Reiter's syndrome and reactive arthritis in perspective. N Engl J Med 309:1606–1615, 1983.

Kellgren JH: Observations of referred pain arising from muscle. Clin Sci 3:175, 1938.

Kidd B, Mullee M, Frank A, et al: Disease expression of ankylosing spondylitis in males and females. J Rheumatol 15:1407–1409, 1988.

Kraemer J: Natural course and prognosis of intervertebral disc diseases. Spine 20:635–639, 1995.

Lambert JR, Wright V: Psoriatic spondylitis: A clinical and radiological description of the spine in psoriatic arthritis. QJ Med 46:411–425, 1977.

Leonard J, Harbst T: Medical emergencies in physical therapy. *In* Boissonnault WG (ed): Examination in Physical Therapy Practice: Screening for Medical Disease, ed 2. New York, Churchill Livingstone, 1995, pp 354–355.

Levinson DJ, Becker MA: Clinical gout and the pathogenesis of hyperuricemia. *In* McCarty DJ, Koopman WJ (eds): Arthritis and Allied Conditions, ed 12. Philadelphia, Lea & Febiger, 1993, pp 1773–1805.

Maltz BA, Sussman P, Calabro JJ: Peripheral arthritis as an initial manifestation of ankylosing spondylitis (abstract). Arthritis Rheum 12:680–681, 1969.

Mankin HJ, Treadwell BV: Osteoarthritis: A 1987 update. Bull Rheum Dis 16:1–10, 1986.

McCarty DJ: Treatment of rheumatoid arthritis. *In* McCarty DJ, Koopman WJ (eds): Arthritis and Allied Conditions, ed 12. Philadelphia, Lea & Febiger, 1993, pp 877–886.

Mills JA, Pinals RS, Ropes MW, et al.: Value of bedrest in patients with rheumatoid arthritis. N Engl J Med 284:453–458, 1971.

Moll JM, Wright V: Psoriatic arthritis. Semin Arthritis Rheum 3:55–78, 1973b.

Moll JM, Wright V: Familial occurrence of psoriatic arthritis. Ann Rheum Dis 32:181–201, 1973a.

Newcomer K, Jurrison ML: Rheumatoid arthritis: The role of physical therapy. J Musculoskel Med 11:14–26, 1994.

Oda T, Fujiwara K, Yonenobu K, et al.: Natural course of cervical spine lesions in rheumatoid arthritis. Spine 20:1128–1135, 1995.

Ostrov BE: Variability complicates systemic-onset juvenile rheumatoid arthritis. J Musculoskel Med 4:26–36, 1995.

Phillips PE: The role of infectious agents in the spondyloarthropathies. Scand J Rheumatol 17:435–443, 1988.

Pigg JS, Bancroft DA: Alterations in skeletal function: rheumatic disorders. *In* Mattson-Porth C (ed): Pathophysiology, ed 4. Philadelphia, JB Lippincott, 1994, pp 1267–1268.

Ramanujan R, Schumacher HR: Ankylosing spondylitis: Early recognition and management. J Musculoskel Med 1(1):75–91, 1992.

Reichlin S: Neuroendocrine-immune interactions. N Engl J Med 329:1246–1253, 1993.

Salter RB, Field P: The effects of continous compression on living articular cartilage. J Bone Joint Surg [Am] 42:31–49, 1960.
Schiller AL: Bones and joints. *In* Rubin E, Farber JL (eds): Pathology, ed 2. Philadelphia, JB Lippincott, 1994, pp 1273–1347.
Schumacher HR (ed): Primer on the Rheumatic Diseases, ed 9. Atlanta, Arthritis Foundation, 1988.
Shore A, Ansell BM: Juvenile psoriatic arthritis—An analysis of 60 cases. J Pediatr 100:529–535, 1982.
Sills EM: Psoriatic arthritis in childhood. Johns Hopkins Med J 146:49–53, 1980.
Simons DG, Travell JG: Myofascial origins of low back pain. Postgrad Med 73:66–108, 1983.
Southwood TR, Petty RE, Malleson PN, et al: Psoriatic arthritis in children. Arthritis Rheum 32:1007–1013, 1989.
Spector TD, Roman E, Silman AJ: The pill, parity and rheumatoid arthritis. Arthritis Rheum 33:782–789, 1990.
Stern RS: The epidemiology of joint complaints in patients with psoriasis. J Rheumatol 12:315–320, 1985.
Travell J and Rinzler SH: The myofascial genesis of pain. Postgrad Med 11:425–431, 1952.
Travell JG, Simons DG: Myofascial Pain and Dysfunction, vol 1. Baltimore, Williams & Wilkins, 1983, pp 5–44.
Travell JG, Simons DG: Myofascial Pain and Dysfunction, vol 2. Baltimore, Williams & Wilkins, 1992.
Urban JPG: The effect of physical factors on disc cell metabolism. *In* Buckwalter JA, Goldberg VM, Wou SL-Y (eds): Musculoskeletal Soft Tissue Aging: Impact on Mobility. Rosemont, Ill, American Academy of Orthopaedic Surgeons, 1993, pp 391–412.
Van der Linden S, Valkenburg H, Cats A: The risk of developing ankylosing spondylitis in HLA-B27 positive individuals: A family and population study. Br J Rheumatol 22(suppl 2):18–19, 1983.

section 4

Pathology of the Nervous System

SECTION 4

chapter 24

Introduction to Central Nervous System Disorders

Kenda S. Fuller

The central nervous system (CNS) controls and regulates all mental and physical functions. It is composed of a network of neural tissue that includes both receptors and transmitters. There is a complex interaction between the areas that control different functions. There is a variety of types of neurons which provide transmission of specific information throughout the nervous system. Disease or trauma of the CNS may affect the nervous system through damage to several types of tissues in a local area, as happens in stroke, or it may cause dysfunction in one type of tissue throughout many areas of the CNS, as in multiple sclerosis.

To understand the pathology of the CNS, an understanding of the general processes involved is necessary, and a review of neurophysiology should be undertaken. It is beyond the scope of this book to provide a comprehensive review, but a brief review of major systems is included here. For the therapist treating a client with a neurologic disorder, it may be necessary to evaluate many aspects of neurologic function.

The history of the onset and nature of the symptoms is critical to establish the diagnosis related to the neurologic disorder. In many cases, based on the history and symptoms, the clinician is able to generate a hypothesis regarding the site in the nervous system that has been affected and the nature of the lesion. A complete history of the nature of the symptoms is also critical to determining which diagnostic tools will provide the most accurate differential diagnosis and best determine the cause. The diagnosis of neurologic disorders remains a clinical specialty, although the use of sophisticated imaging and measurement of neural function have provided insight into the pathology of the nervous system.

The examination of the client with neurologic dysfunction often begins with mental status changes. Alterations of consciousness and disturbances of higher brain function give the clinician clues about the nature of the disease process and the location of damage within the brain. Motor and sensory changes will also reflect the type, level, and extent of damage to the system in the case of both disease and trauma.

Treatment is based on an understanding of the level and type of neuronal dysfunction. Damage or disease of the nervous system often results in changes in the production and uptake of neurotransmitters. The control of neuron damage is sometimes achieved by control of these neurotransmitters. A brief discussion of the chemistry of neurotransmission and of therapeutic drugs acting at the synaptic cleft is included here.

Disability resulting from neurologic disease and trauma can be extensive and care of these clients often requires use of limited resources, namely time and money. With the tremendous advances made in the emergent medical care of trauma victims and people with significant neurologic disease, the number of people living with neurologic sequelae is rising steadily. Theories regarding the most efficient method of reducing the disability resulting from neurologic impairments are created based on our current knowledge of pathogenesis and recovery of neural elements.

SIGNS AND SYMPTOMS OF CENTRAL NERVOUS SYSTEM DISORDERS

Alterations of Consciousness and Disorders of Arousal

Alteration of consciousness is not considered an independent disease entity but a reflection of some underlying disease or abnormal state of brain function. Metabolic or systemic disorders generally cause depressed consciousness without focal neurologic findings. CNS disorders may or may not have concomitant focal signs[1] (Topel and Lewis, 1995). Table 24–1 compares metabolic and drug-induced coma with coma caused by space-occupying lesions.

Disturbances of arousal and attention can range from coma after brainstem injury to confusional states caused by drug intoxication. The human brain possesses a mechanism that allows a waking and sleeping state (arousal) as well as a separate ability to focus awareness on relevant environmental stimuli (attention). Arousal refers to the phenomenon of wakefulness or alertness (Filley, 1995).

To achieve a state of consciousness the cerebral cortex must be activated by the reticular formation, specifically, the ascending reticular activating system (ARAS) in the brainstem. The fibers run from the thalamus to the medulla. The thalamus projects fibers to the cortex. The upper part of this system acts as an on/off switch for consciousness and controls the sleep-wake cycle. The lower part controls respiration (Fig. 24–1).

Clinical disorders of arousal may result in hyperaroused states, and can appear as restlessness, agitation, or delirium. This is presumably due to loss of hemispheric inhibition of brainstem function. Hypoarousal can be described on a spectrum ranging from drowsiness to stupor and coma. Stupor is a state of unresponsiveness that requires vigorous stimulation to bring about arousal. Coma is a state of unarousable unre-

[1] A focal sign represents damage to a distinct area of the nervous system such as hemiplegia vs. a global disturbance such as a change in mental status.

TABLE 24-1 CHARACTERISTICS OF COMAS

MANIFESTATIONS	METABOLIC AND DRUG-INDUCED	FROM SPACE-OCCUPYING LESIONS
Onset	Behavioral changes, decreased attention, arousal	Usually severe headache, focal seizures
Pain response	Present and equal	May be different on each side
Reflexes	Intact deep tendon reflexes, equal responses	Deep tendon reflexes may be unequal; positive Babinski's sign (UMN lesion)
Pupillary reaction	Bilateral normal response	May be unequal
Size of pupil	May be at midpoint with anticholinergics; pinpoint from opiates; dilated from anoxia	Midbrain lesion—midpoint Pons lesion—pinpoint Herniation to brainstem—large
Corneal reflex	Bilateral, intact	Unequal, may be absent
Eye movement	Spontaneous movement without intention; no reaction to VOR	May have paresis of lateral gaze with CN III compression
Decorticate or decerebrate posturing	Absent; movement is normal	Posturing may be present depending on level of lesion
Extremity movement	Equal movement on both sides	Paresis may be unilateral

UMN, upper motor neuron; CN III, third cranial (oculomotor) nerve; VOR, vestibulo-ocular reflex.

sponsiveness. Small and restricted lesions of the brainstem can result in stupor and coma. Massive bilateral hemispheric lesions are necessary to cause coma.

Damage to the cerebral cortex can be caused by loss of blood flow, subarachnoid hemorrhage, anesthetic toxicity, hypoglycemia, hypothermia, or status epilepticus (see Chapter 31). If the link to the reticular formation is destroyed, the person will remain in a persistent vegetative state (PVS). Although the person may make random movements and the eyes may open, mentation remains absent. Akinetic mutism, similar to PVS, reflects damage to the mediofrontal lobe and results in lack of motivation to perform any motor or mental activity (abulia). In the *locked-in syndrome*, there is damage to the pons resulting most often from thrombosis of the basilar artery. This is a remarkable impairment, involving no mental deficit at all, but results in inability to move anything but the eyes.

Supratentorial[2] lesions that cause increased pressure, such as hemorrhage, cerebral edema, or neoplasm, can cause coma by producing tentorial herniation and subsequent compression of the brainstem. There is usually a hemiparesis with a dilated pupil on the side of the lesion due to central compression involving the third cranial nerve by the herniation.

Direct lesions of the brainstem can be related to drugs, hemorrhage, infarction, or compression from the posterior fossa. Disruption of ocular movements is an early sign of brainstem involvement. There is loss of the pupillary reaction to light while the corneal reflex remains intact.[3]

Brainstem death is destruction of both the upper and lower parts of the reticular formation, which will eventually lead to death. There may remain preservation of cortical electrical activity and spinal reflexes, but these are of no consequence as they are unable to be harnessed.

Attention Deficits

Attention is more difficult to relate to brain structure than arousal. However, the acute confusional state is one of the most common neurologic disorders encountered. Although there is not a clear understanding of the mechanism of attention from a neuroanatomic perspective, there appears to be a major role played by the parietal and frontal lobes. Frontal and prefrontal areas of the brain appear to be responsible for mental control, concentration, vigilance, and performance of meaningful activity. Cognition and emotional control are established by extensive white matter connections between the frontal lobes and the remainder of the cerebrum. Diseases that affect the white matter, such as multiple sclerosis (MS), can affect the level of attention without decreasing arousal. Psychiatric disease has an effect on both arousal and attention.

Attention deficits, or the acute confusional state, may be due to a number of causes. Intoxicants, metabolic disorders, infections, epilepsy, blood flow disorders, traumatic injuries, and neoplasms can all be responsible for the change in orientation or attention.

Disturbances of Higher Brain Function

(Filley, 1995; Bach-y-Rita, 1992)

Disturbances of neurologic function can result in behavioral disturbances that mimic disturbances of mental function in psychiatric disorders. *Delusions*, or fixed false beliefs, have been reported in a great variety of neurologic conditions and appear to be associated with the limbic system. Paranoid delusions are common in disorders of the medial temporal or a combination of the frontal and right parietal lobes. *Hallucinations* are sensory experiences without external stimulation.

[2] The tentorium is an invagination of the dura that separates the cerebrum from the cerebellum. Structures above the tentorium are referred to as supratentorial, and structures below the tentorium are referred to as infratentorial. When the supratentorial structures are enlarged, pressure through the tentorium can cause infratentorial damage.

[3] The pupillary light reflex results in constriction of the pupil in response to light; normally there is constriction in both eyes when only one eye is stimulated. A lesion of the optic nerve pathway, which in this case is usually associated with damage to the pretectum, an area between the midbrain and the thalamus, can cause loss of the reflex. The corneal reflex requires an interaction between cranial nerves V and VII via the associated nuclei and therefore can remain intact despite damage to the brainstem, midbrain, or thalamus (Waxman and deGroot, 1995).

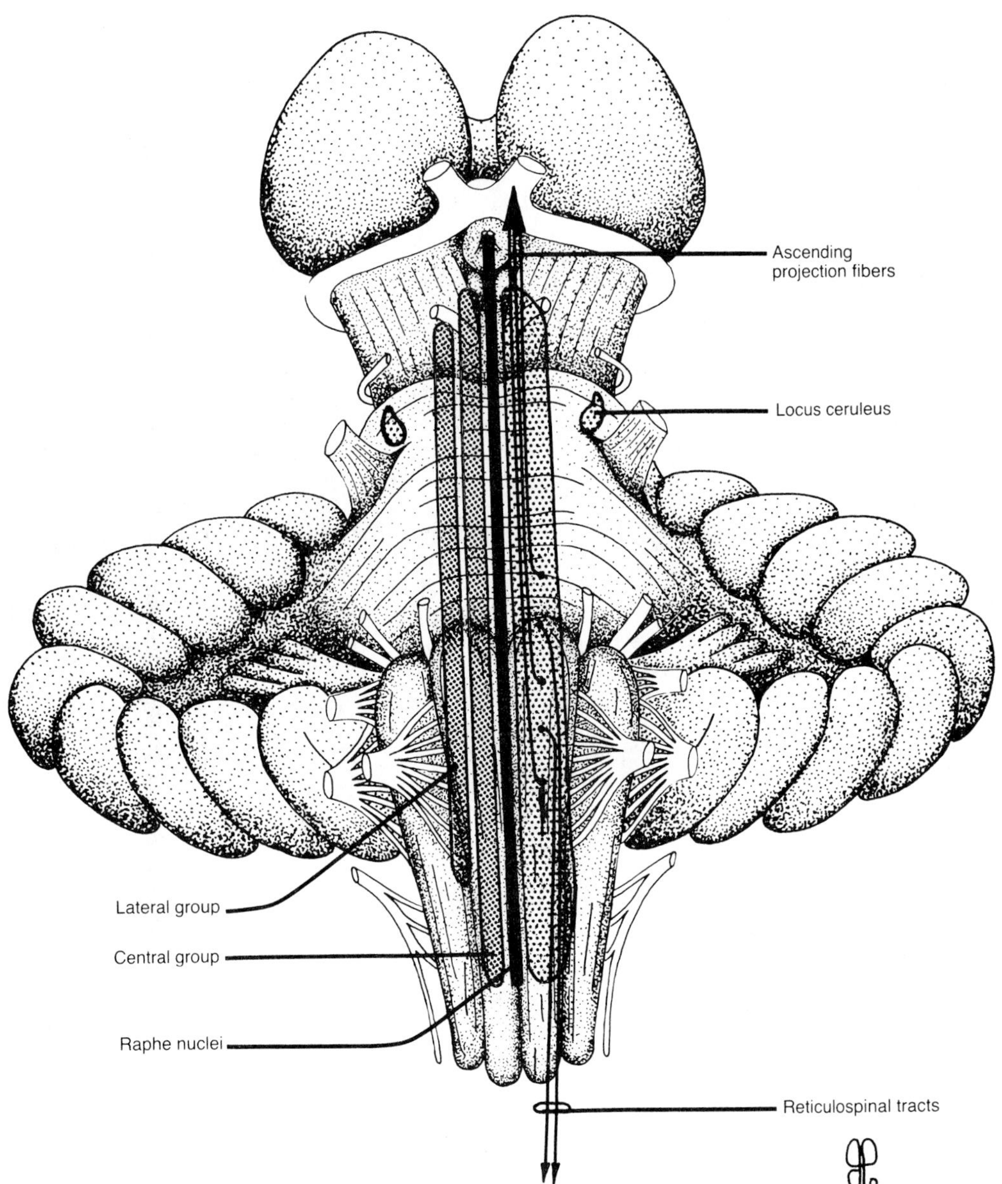

Figure **24–1.** The brainstem (containing the reticular activating system) in relationship to the cerebellum and diencephalon (containing the thalamus and connections to the cortex). Note also its connection to the spinal cord through the reticulospinal tracts. (*From Hendelman WJ: Student's Atlas of Neuroanatomy. Philadelphia, WB Saunders, 1994.*)

Visual hallucinations generally suggest neurologic involvement; auditory hallucinations imply psychiatric disease. Midbrain lesions in the cerebral peduncles can cause hallucinations involving animals. Temporal lesions can cause recurrent auditory experiences.

Memory is controlled by various areas of the brain and a particular area may be responsible for different aspects of memory. *Working memory*, the ability to hold information in short-term storage while permitting other cognitive operations to take place, appears to depend on the prefrontal cortex. Disorders of recent memory, known as amnesia, is a significant neurobehaviorial phenomenon. *Anterograde amnesia*, failure of new learning, and *retrograde amnesia*, failure to consolidate recently formed memories, are common in persons after traumatic brain injury. The inability to acquire new learning is often accompanied by *confabulation*, the fabrication of information in response to questioning. *Declarative memory* is retention of experience or the memory of what has occurred. *Procedural memory* describes the learning of skills and habits, or how something is done.

The hippocampal formation, or hippocampus, contained in the temporal lobe; the thalamus; and the basal forebrain are critical to the performance of recent memory. Sensory information is processed in the amygdala and it is here that the determination of the value of the information is made and stimuli of value are then further processed by the central structures of the diencephalon. The anatomic relationship of these structures is shown in Figure 24–2. Damage to the

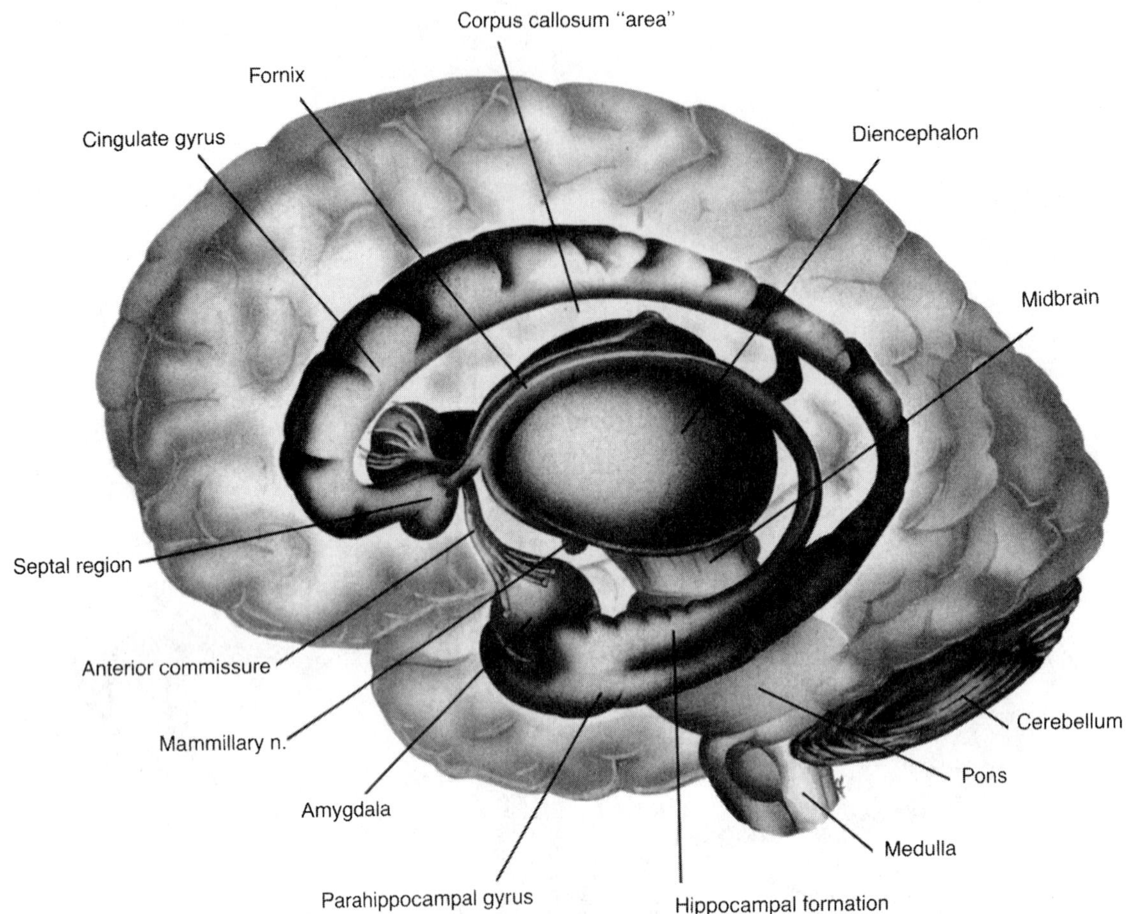

Figure **24–2.** The limbic lobe is the name given to the structures surrounding the diencephalon (containing the thalamus) and midbrain. These structures include the cingulate gyrus, the parahippocampal gyrus, and the hippocampus. Because there is such a close relationship to the prefrontal cortex, some nuclei of the thalamus, the hypothalamus, and the midbrain, the combined elements are referred to as the limbic system. Note the close anatomic relationship to the temporal region of the cortex. (*From Hendelman WJ: Student's Atlas of Neuroanatomy. Philadelphia, WB Saunders, 1994.*)

central structures of the brain can be through direct means such as a tumor, blood flow disorder, or traumatic brain injury and can result in disturbances of memory. Disease processes or toxicity causing a decrease in the flow of nutrients or oxygen to the brain can also lead to memory deficits by affecting this area. Alzheimer's disease appears to result in a loss of cholinergic cells in the forebrain (see Chapter 27).

Language is one of the higher functions of the brain that is affected in many disorders of the CNS. Speech is a more elementary capacity than language and refers to the mechanical act of uttering words using the neuromuscular structures responsible for articulation. *Dysarthria*, a disturbance in articulation, and *anarthria*, lack of ability to produce speech, are disorders of speech, not language. One common language disorder is *expressive aphasia*, a deficit in speech production or language output, accompanied by a deficit in communication, in which speech comes out as garbled or inappropriate words.

Localization of speech production in the left frontal lobe and impaired language comprehension in the temporal lobe demonstrate how higher functions can be related to brain regions. However, language control may be in different areas for different persons and therefore damage to the same area of the brain may produce aphasia in some individuals while others may be spared. Left hand–dominant people may have right hemisphere dominance for language.

Alexia is another symptom of higher brain dysfunction. It is the acquired inability to read. Alexia is typically due to lesions in the left occipital lobe and the splenium of the corpus callosum that prevent incoming visual information from reaching the angular gyrus for linguistic interpretation. When the alexia is combined with *agraphia*, or the inability to write, the inferior parietal and posterolateral temporal region of the left hemisphere is implicated, specifically the angular gyrus, which is responsible for the associations between visual and auditory systems by which one learns to read.

Agraphia can be caused by lesions anywhere in the cerebrum. Because writing is a motor skill, lesions of the corticospinal tract, basal ganglia, and cerebellum; myopathies; and peripheral nerve injuries can all cause abnormal or clumsy writing. These disorders may be seen in addition to neurobehavioral syndromes. Typically the features of agraphia tend to parallel the characteristics of aphasia.

Apraxia is an acquired disorder of skilled purposeful movement which is not a result of paresis, akinesia, ataxia, sensory loss, or comprehension. *Ideomotor apraxia* is the most common and represents the inability to carry out a motor act on verbal command. Ideomotor apraxia appears to be due to a lesion in the arcuate fasciculus. The anterior connection from the left parietal lobe may be disrupted, preventing the motor system from receiving the command to act. A lesion in the left premotor area can cause apraxia by directly interrupting the motor act. Damage to the anterior corpus callosum can lead to apraxia that is evident in the left hand only. *Ideational apraxia* is failure to perform a sequential act, even though each part of the act can be performed individually. The lesion causing ideational apraxia appears to be in the left parietal lobe (as in hemiparesis) or the frontal lobe (Alzheimer's disease), and the syndrome is seen as well with diffuse cortical damage (degenerative dementia).

Agnosia is inability to recognize an object; the previously acquired meaning is no longer attached to it. It is associated with lesions of the sensory cortices involved with seeing, hearing, and feeling. Agnosia is associated with the loss of one sensory modality. It is difficult to assess because the person is often easily able to compensate. When the ability to recognize an object by vision is lost, the ability to recognize that same object by hearing or feeling is retained.

Lobar Disorders

Lesions of the hemispheres or lobes may cause the loss of the functions that each hemisphere controls. Because diseases and damage due to trauma will often affect one area of the brain, the associated syndromes for the main areas of the brain are described. The lobes and the structures contained within each lobe are illustrated in Figure 24–3. These are general descriptions of the syndromes; the specific type of disease or trauma will determine the extent of the syndrome manifested (Filley, 1995; Kandel, 1985; Lindsay et al., 1986; Panter and Faden, 1992).

The *right hemisphere syndrome* represents the inability to orient the body within external space and generate the appropriate motor responses. *Hemineglect* is one of the most common deficits seen with right hemisphere lesions. The individual does not respond to sensory stimuli on the left side of the body and does not respond to the environment surrounding the left side. This results in neglect of the involved extremities and trunk during mobility and self-care activities. The ability to draw in two and three dimensions is lost along with other drawing skills such as perspective and accurate copying. *Spatial disorientation* can result, with the person losing familiarity with the environment and becoming lost in areas which should be familiar. Inability to read and follow a map are clues to right hemisphere deficit.

Disorders of emotional adjustment often follow a lesion in the right hemisphere. These disorders are primarily in the affective domain: interpersonal relationships and socialization. Cortical control of the limbic system is believed to be responsible, but the exact mechanism of control of more complex emotional behavior is not completely understood at this time. There appears to be hemispheric lateralization of emotions with suggestions that the right hemisphere is the dominant hemisphere in controlling emotions.

Temporal and *limbic lobe syndromes* involve the primary emotions, those associated with pain, pleasure, anger, and fear. The limbic system, sometimes referred to as the limbic lobe, is found just above the brainstem.

The limbic system comprises the hippocampus, amygdala, and cingulate gyrus. The hippocampus plays a major role in memory, and the amygdala and cingulate gyrus are involved in emotion. The patterns of emotional memories are formed here and this may be the area that establishes the anxiety and panic that is unconsciously related to an emotional experience that may or may not be remembered. It is thought that the processing of the limbic system is responsible for the fact that emotionally charged experiences will be more easily remembered than those with less emotional stimulation. In lower animals, the limbic system is concerned primarily with the sense of smell, and it is a common observation that smells can trigger a strong emotional response in humans (see Fig. 24–2).

The *frontal lobe* is the largest single area of the brain, constituting nearly one third of the brain's cortical surface. It is phylogenetically the youngest area of the brain and has major connections with all other areas of the brain. The frontal lobe is responsible for the highest levels of cognitive processing, control of emotion, and behavior. An individual's personality is established as a frontal lobe function and one of the most disturbing deficits seen with lesions affecting the frontal lobe is the change from the premorbid personality. A person's character and temperament are changed by damage to the frontal lobe. Slow processing of information, lack of judgment based on known consequences, withdrawal, and irritability are often seen as a result of an insult to the frontal lobe. Disinhibition and apathy are common clinical dysfunctions of the frontal lobe. The person with a frontal lobe disorder may lack insight into the deficits and therefore behavior can be difficult to control.

Cerebellar Disorders

The cerebellum is involved in the coordination of all skeletal movement, and disorders affecting the cerebellum result in discoordinated movement. While there is good understanding of the role the cerebellum plays in movement, and the neuronal substrates have been well identified, movement disorders resulting from cerebellar lesions remain difficult to treat (Urbscheit and Oremland, 1995). The therapist should be able to identify the movement disorders that reflect involvement of the cerebellum.

Through both its ascending and descending projections the medial region of the cerebellum controls the cortical and brainstem components of the medial descending systems. This region of the cerebellum controls axial and proximal musculature. The cerebellum has influence on movement through the vestibulospinal and reticulospinal tracts.[4] Figure 24–4 is a schematic representation of the cerebellum and its connections.

Hypotonicity, or decreased muscle tone, can occur on the side of the lesion or bilaterally if the lesion is central, and is seen primarily in the proximal muscle groups. The person with

[4] The vermis of the cerebellum sends fibers to the brainstem reticular formation and the lateral vestibular nuclei which give rise to fibers that descend to the spinal cord.

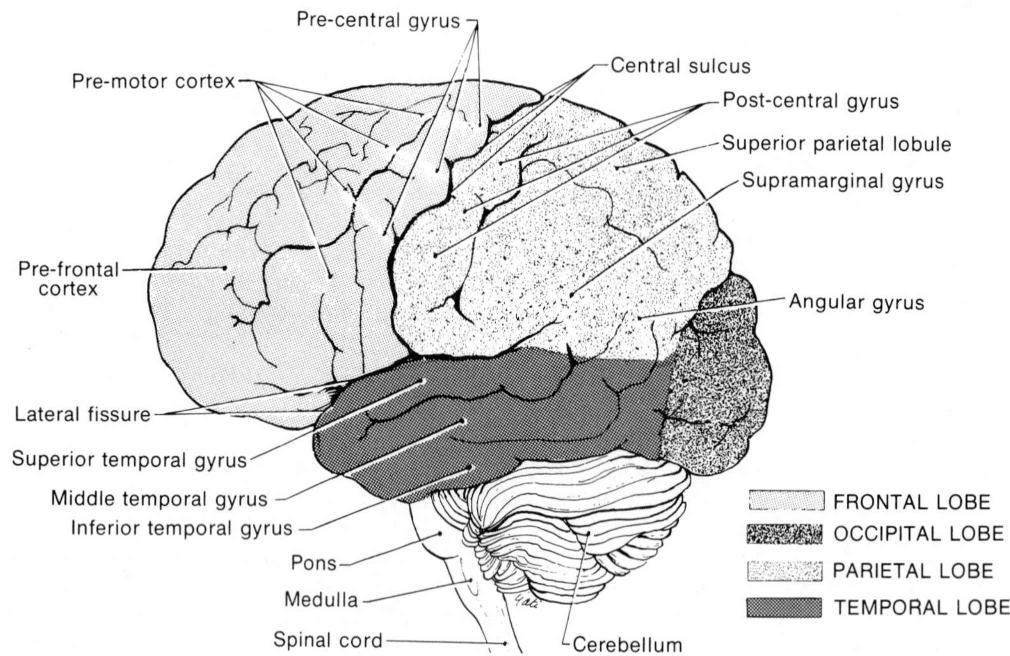

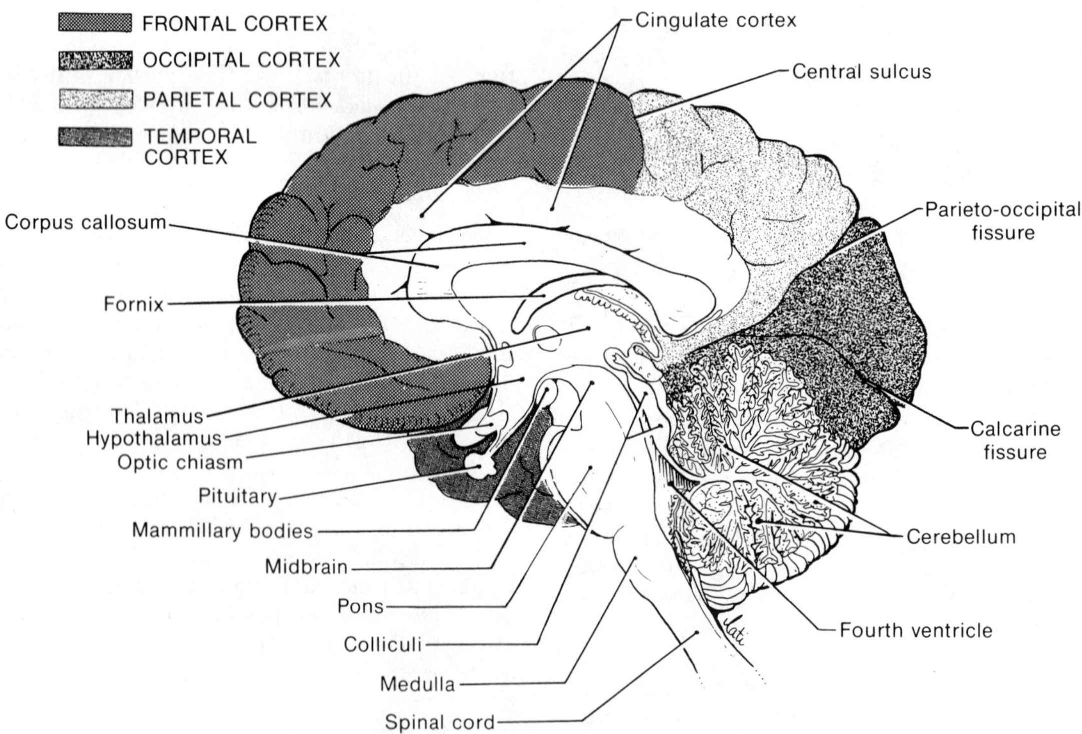

Figure **24–3.** The lobes of the cortex and their relationship to the cerebellum, midbrain, and brainstem. (*From Farber SD: Neurorehabilitation: A Multisensory Approach. Philadelphia, WB Saunders, 1982.*)

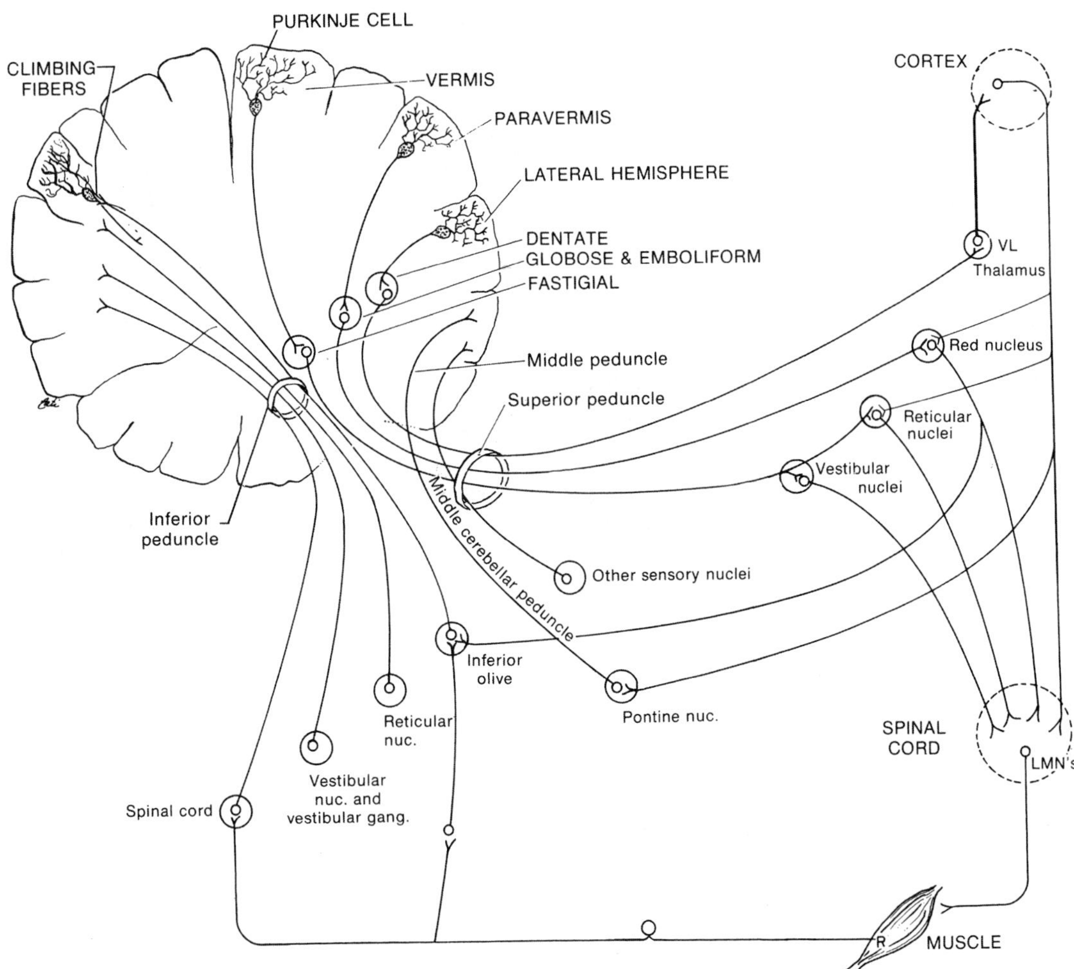

Figure **24–4.** Schematic representation of the cerebellum and its relationship to the cortex and spinal cord through interconnections at nuclei in the thalamus, midbrain, brainstem, and spinal cord. (*From Farber SD: Neurorehabilitation: A Multisensory Approach. Philadelphia, WB Saunders, 1982.*)

hypotonicity is unable to fixate the limb posturally leading to incoordination with movement. *Asthenia*, or generalized weakness, is sometimes seen in the person with cerebellar lesions. Hypotonicity and asthenia, however, do not always occur together. It is believed that both disorders represent loss of input from the cerebellum to the cerebral cortex, but they may represent loss of input to different areas of the cortex.

Cerebellar *ataxia*, or incoordination of movement, is a cardinal sign of cerebellar lesions, and can have different manifestations.

Postural tremor is present when the limbs or trunk is kept in a certain position. It is seen in about 10% of persons with cerebellar dysfunction.

Dysmetria, the underestimation or overestimation of a necessary movement toward a target, is commonly seen with cerebellar disorders. There is an error in the production of force necessary to perform an intended movement. The initiation of movement is prolonged compared to normal and the ability to change directions rapidly is impaired. The resulting overshoot and undershoot during movement is known as an *intention tremor*. *Dysdiadochokinesis*, inability to perform rapidly alternating movements, is also common in cerebellar disorders. The movement is slow, without rhythm or consistency.

Scanning speech is a component of cerebellar dysfunction representing the complexity of the motor activity. Word selection is not affected, but the words are pronounced slowly, and without melody, tone, or rhythm. This reflects the incoordination or hypotonicity of the muscles of the larynx in controlling the voice.

Eye movements are disrupted in the person with cerebellar dysfunction, in both a static head and eye position and with movement of the head. There is *gaze evoked nystagmus*, or inability of the cerebellum to hold the gaze on an object. Vestibulo-ocular function is disrupted. See Chapter 33 for an explanation of the cerebellar association with eye movement.

Decomposition of movement is seen in persons with cerebellar dysfunction. Instead of performing a movement in one smooth motion, the person will move in distinct sequences to accomplish the motion.

Gait disturbance is another disorder related to cerebellar dysfunction. The gait becomes wide-based and staggering. The anterior lobe of the cerebellum is implicated in disorders of gait with loss of balance noted in stance. Proprioception may give inaccurate cues because the cerebellar relays become disrupted. Long loop reflexes lose adaptability and are unable to trigger appropriate responses in the lower leg to maintain balance when the body sways or the surface is moving.

In some persons there is a surprising ability to avoid a fall, although the standing balance is abnormal. When the person is able to perform compensatory movements of the upper body and limbs, falls can be avoided.

Sensory Disturbances

The skin, muscles, and joints contain a variety of receptors that create electrical activity as a result of stimulation (Singer and Weiner, 1994; Burt, 1993). The electrical input is carried to the CNS through the *afferent axons*. The cell bodies rest in the ganglion of the dorsal root that lies adjacent to the spinal cord. The afferent fibers are combined somatotopically in the spinal column and ascend to the brainstem and the cortex. A characteristic of the fibers that run in the dorsal column of the spinal cord is that they synapse at the level of the brainstem nuclei where they cross over to the contralateral (opposite) hemisphere of the brain. When there is a disorder of the brain that affects the afferent system above the level of the brainstem, symptoms occur on the side contralateral to the lesion (Kandel, 1985). For an anatomic view of the ascending fibers from the spinal cord to the cortex, see Figure 24–5.

Disorders of the afferent nerve, dorsal colums of the spinal cord, and brainstem result in changes in the sensory input available. This can manifest as lack of tactile or cutaneous sensation, numbness, tingling, paresthesias, or dysesthesias in the distribution of the nerves affected. When the lesion affects the midbrain areas that modulate and interpret sensory input, the result can cause exaggeration of sensory stimuli. Sensory input from the joints and muscles is known as *somatosensation* or *proprioception*. When this sensory function is lost or disturbed, the person will have difficulty maintaining the body in the appropriate position for the voluntary and involuntary movements necessary for most functional activities, especially those required for postural control.

Disruption of the sensory input provided by the optic nerve is evident in some disorders of the brain, and will result in blindness in some or all of a field of view. Visual-field cuts are common with stroke. Visual hallucinations can also be part of a CNS disorder when the optic radiations or occipital lobe is disrupted, which may also be due to stroke or a degenerative disease such as MS.

Movement Disorders

Motor control is accomplished by the cooperative effort of many brain structures (Shumway-Cook and Woollacott, 1995; Kandel, 1985; Burt, 1993). A hierarchical organization exists that can be described as the interaction of the lower motor neurons with the interneurons that regulate activity initiated in the cerebral cortex. In this structure, plans and strategies for movement are established by the higher centers (cortex); the lower centers (brainstem and spinal cord) are responsible for the execution of the task, making the modifications necessitated by environmental constraints. A schematic view of the tracts as they course through the CNS is shown in Figure 24–6. In addition, the same signal may be processed simultaneously by many different brain structures, though for different purposes, showing parallel distributed processing. In this structure, various areas of the brain, such as the cerebellum and basal ganglia, interact to establish a motor program that modifies the hierarchical information going from the cortex to the spinal cord.

Abnormal movement patterns in neurologic disorders can result from lesions of the CNS at many levels. The parietal and premotor areas of the cerebral cortex are involved in identifying targets in space, determining a course of action, and creating the motor program. The diencephalon contains the thalamus which integrates information from direct connections to the spinal cord, brainstem, and cerebellum and sends it to the cortex. The brainstem contains nuclei that receive the information contributing to postural control and locomotion. In the brainstem is the reticular formation, which regulates arousal and awareness. The spinal cord, or the *final common pathway*, is the last processing level before the motor task is executed by muscle activation. Lesions of the CNS that result in movement disorders are most commonly due to vascular disease, tumor, trauma, or a myriad of degenerative diseases that disrupt the pathways responsible for movement.

Cranial Nerve Involvement

The cranial nerves are peripheral nerves relating to sensation and motor control of the head and neck. Disorders of the CNS often reflect both sensory and motor impairments as the nuclei for the nerves lie within the brainstem and midbrain. An anatomic view of the cranial nerves and the relationship of the nuclei to central structures is provided in Figure 24–7. The sensory and motor functions of the cranial nerves are outlined in Table 24–2.

AGING AND THE CENTRAL NERVOUS SYSTEM

Age-related reduction in adult brain weight represents loss of brain tissue (Fretwell, 1993; Craik, 1993; Lewis and Jordan, 1985; Poirier and Finch, 1990). Neurons are postmitotic and do not duplicate themselves, and therefore, when lost, are not replaced. Glial cells can continue to proliferate but there is an overall decrease in the excitatory neurons. There is highly selective atrophy of brain tissue in the aging CNS. Cell loss is more general in the cerebral cortex and hippocampus, with less damage seen in the brainstem and cerebellum.

The inner structure of the nerve cell changes with aging. The presence of *lipofuscin*, a pigmented lipid found in the cytoplasm, may interfere with normal cell function via pressure on the cell nucleus. The mechanism and relationship to dysfunction is still not clearly understood. Neuritic, or senile, plaques are found outside the neuron filled with degenerating axons, dendrites, astrocytes, and amyloid. The neuritic plaques are thought to occur most often in the cortex and hippocampus and have been associated with dementia. *Neurofibrillary tangles*, abnormal neurofibers which displace and distort the cell body, are found in higher concentrations in the older brain. Neurofibrillary tangles and amyloid are also found in higher concentrations in people with Alzheimer's disease (see Chapter 27).

The blood supply diminishes as well, with a net reduction of 10% to 15%. The relationship of cerebral blood flow, the resultant decrease in the glucose supply to the brain, and

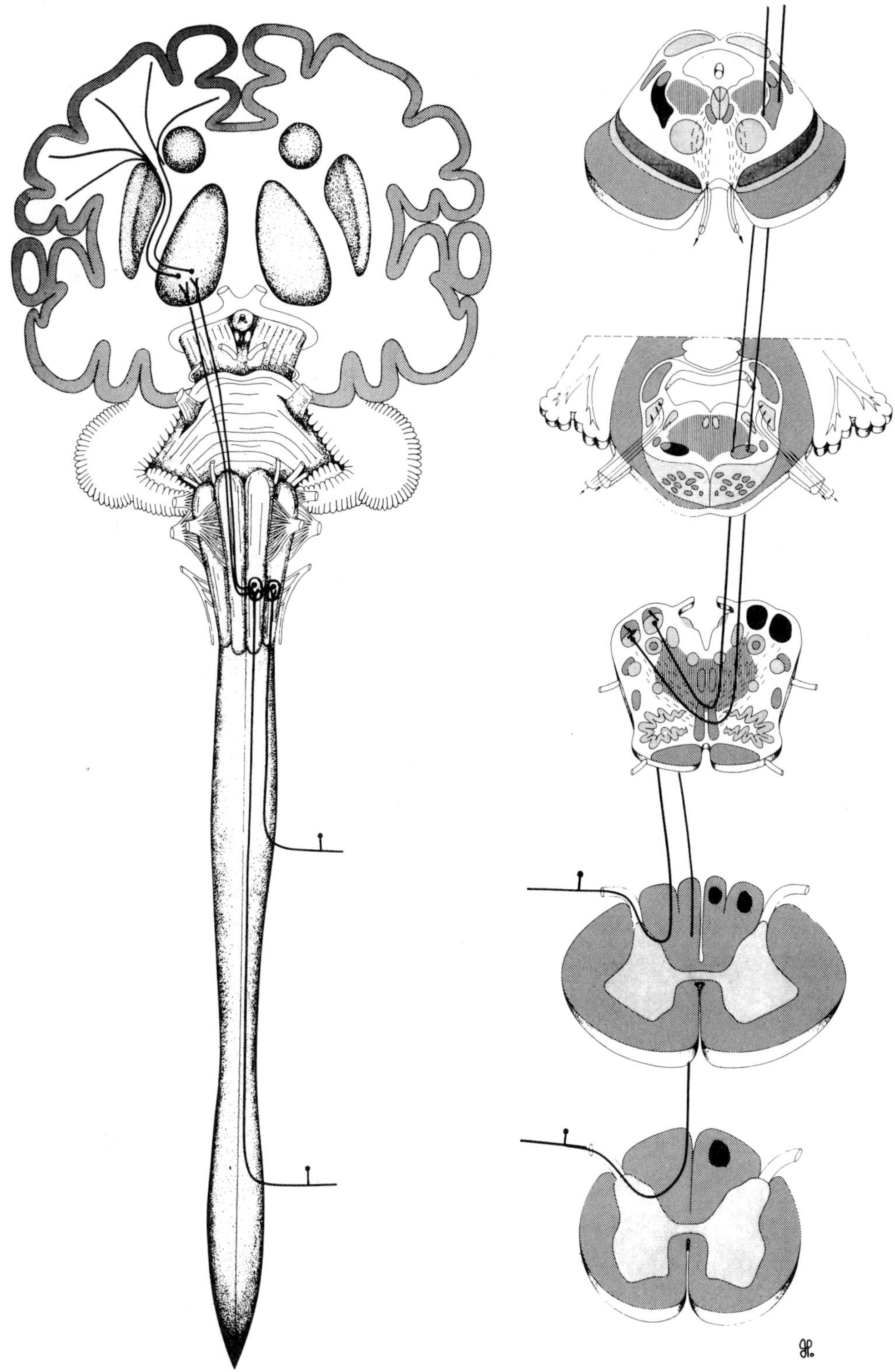

Figure **24–5.** Ascending (sensory) tracts. The dorsal column is represented from the lumbar to the cervical levels of the spinal cord, the pons, and midbrain. The tracts then synapse in the thalamus and travel through the internal capsule to the cortex. (*From Hendelman WJ: Student's Atlas of Neuroanatomy. Philadelphia, WB Saunders, 1994.*)

decreased metabolism are not well established as to cause and effect. All three are noted in the aging brain.

Morphologic changes in the aging brain are accompanied by neurochemical changes. Changes in neurotransmitter activity are seen with aging and are an area of great interest at this time. There is a decrease in the number of some of the receptors as well as decreases in synthesis of some of the neurotransmitters. The neurotransmitters that appear to show the most changes in levels are dopamine, norepinephrine, and epinephrine. Changes in these neurotransmitters may be

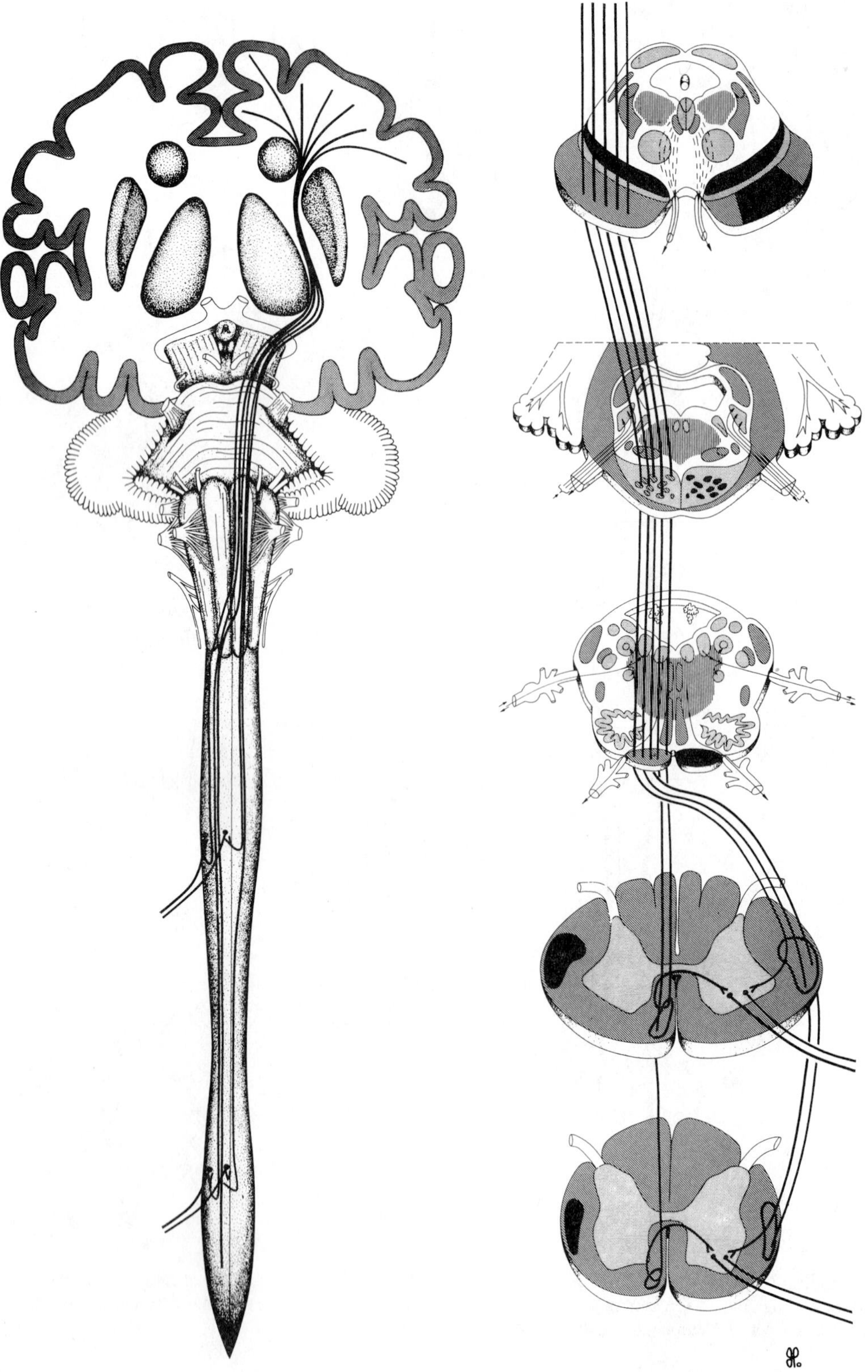

Figure **24–6.** Descending (motor) tracts. The corticospinal tract is represented here, showing the cortical initiation of the neural pathway descending through the midbrain, pons, medulla, and spine. Disruption of the descending tracts results in loss of motor control and abnormal reflexes. (*From Hendelman WJ: Student's Atlas of Neuroanatomy. Philadelphia, WB Saunders, 1994.*)

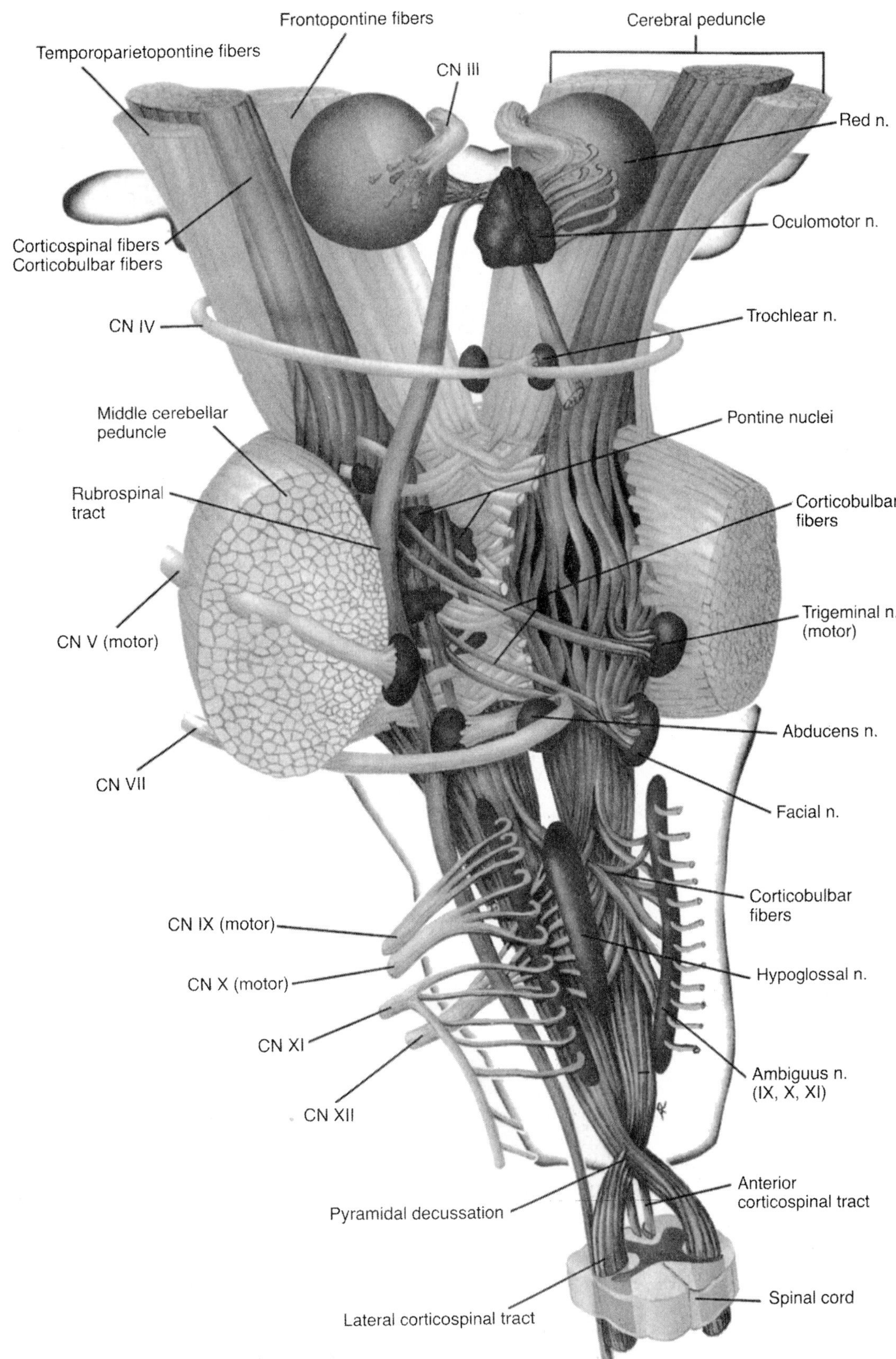

Figure **24-7.** The relationship of the cranial nerves to the structures of the central nervous system, including the nuclei at various levels of the midbrain and brainstem. (*From Hendelman WJ: Student's Atlas of Neuroanatomy. Philadelphia, WB Saunders, 1994.*)

TABLE 24-2 THE CRANIAL NERVES AND THEIR FUNCTIONS

Cranial Nerve	Component	Function
I—Olfactory	S	Olfaction
II—Optic	S	Vision
III—Oculomotor	M	Innervation of inferior oblique muscle, and medial, inferior, and superior rectus muscles of eye
	A	Innervation of ciliary ganglion, which regulates pupillary constriction (pupillary constrictor muscle) and accommodation to near vision (ciliary muscle)
IV—Trochlear	M	Innervation of superior oblique muscle of eye
V—Trigeminal	S	Sensation (epicritic and protopathic) from face, nose, mouth, nasal and oral mucosa, anterior two thirds of the tongue, and meningeal sensation, through all three divisions (ophthalmic, maxillary, mandibular)
	M	Innervation of muscles of mastication and the tensor tympani muscle (through the mandibular division only)
VI—Abducens	M	Innervation of lateral rectus muscle of eye
VII—Facial	S	Taste from anterior two thirds of the tongue
	M	Innervation of muscles of facial expression and stapedius muscle
	A	Innervation of pterygopalatine ganglion, which innervates lacrimal and nasal mucosal glands, and submandibular ganglion, which innervates submandibular and sublingual salivary glands
VIII—Vestibulocochlear	S	Hearing (cochlear division); linear and angular acceleration, or head position in space (vestibular division)
IX—Glossopharyngeal	S	Taste and general sensation from posterior third of the tongue; sensation (epicritic and protopathic) from pharynx, soft palate, and tonsils; chemoreception from carotid body and baroreception from carotid sinus (unconscious reflex sensory information)
	M	Innervation of pharyngeal muscles
	A	Innervation of otic ganglion, which supplies parotid gland
X—Vagus	S	Visceral sensation (excluding pain) from heart, bronchi, trachea, larynx, pharynx, and gastrointestinal (GI) tract to level of descending colon; general sensation of external ear; taste from epiglottis
	M	Innervation of pharyngeal and laryngeal muscles, and muscles at base of tongue
	A	Innervation of local visceral ganglia, which supply smooth muscles in respiratory, cardiovascular, and GI tract to level of descending colon
XI—Spinal accessory	M	Innervation of trapezius and sternocleidomastoid muscles
XII—Hypoglossal	M	Innervation of muscles of tongue

S, sensory; M, motor; A, autonomic nervous system.
From Felten DL, Felten SY: A regional and systemic overview of functional neuroanatomy. *In* Farber SD: Neurorehabilitation: A Multisensory Approach. Philadelphia, WB Saunders, 1982, pp 53–54.

reflected in decreased control over visceral functions, emotions, and attention. Serotonin, involved in central regulatory activities of respiration, thermoregulation, sleep, and memory, appears to be reduced in the aging brain. Depression in the older adult may be related to increased production of monoamine oxidase (MAO), which breaks down catecholamines, which support catechol function related to feeling of well-being. Other changes in the brain related to neurotransmission, such as Parkinson's and Alzheimer's diseases, are described in the chapters that follow.

Nerve conduction velocity decreases with age in both the motor and sensory systems. By the eighth decade there is an average loss of 15% of the velocity in the myelinated fibers.

Neurologic disease is more prevalent in the older person, as is the risk of neurologic sequelae, as a result of intracranial hemorrhage, subdural hematoma, and neoplasms. Awareness of the signs and symptoms of these disorders is essential. The therapist is at times the person who identifies a disease or the potential for a disorder that may manifest during a treatment session.

CELLULAR DYSFUNCTION

As the brain perceives the environment, issues motor commands for coordinated movement, and establishes cognitive strategies, there is a complex organization of the firing of nerve cells (Kandel, 1985). The function of each nerve cell can be described based on the signals received and produced. The cell body, which contains the nucleus, is the metabolic center of the neuron. The cell body receives input from other nerves through synaptic activity directly or on its dendrites.

The cell body generates electrical activity and conducts it through its axon. Axons have branching terminal fibers which end in presynaptic terminals. By means of its terminals, one neuron contacts and transmits information to the receptive surface of another neuron. The point of contact is known as a *synapse*.

In the CNS, a specificity of these connections make up the organized structure of the brain and spinal cord. The size and structure of the neuron reflects its function within the nervous system. Neurons with long axons carry information from one brain region to another; neurons with short axons are interneurons, which are found in the nuclei and reflex pathways.

Another important cell type in the CNS is the *glial cell*. The glial cells provide support and structure for the CNS and play the role that connective tissue performs in other parts of the body. The glial cells are active in the system but are not involved in signaling information.

The oligodendrocyte, one type of glial cell, is responsible for the production of the myelin sheath, which surrounds the axon. Demyelinating disorders are often the result of disrupted function of the oligodendrocyte (Asbury et al., 1986) (see discussion of multiple sclerosis in Chapter 27).

Astroglial changes are widely recognized to be one of the earliest and most remarkable cellular responses to CNS injury. Astrocytes, another type of glial cell, surround the axons of the nerves in the white matter and the cell bodies in the gray matter. Astrocytes are the most numerous cellular element in the brain. In addition to their support function, they appear to serve a nutritive function, as they connect to the capillary wall and to the nerve cell. Astrocytes help to remove neuronal debris after injury and seal off damaged brain tissue. Excessive neurotransmitter substances and potassium in the synaptic cleft are removed by astrocytes. Figure 24–8 shows the oligodendrocyte and astrocyte and their relationship to the neuron and capillary.

Astrocyte swelling is a common pathologic finding and is often seen at the interface with the vascular system. The swelling may be a factor in gliosis, a reaction of the glial cells that produces tissue that is laid down in a scarlike manner (known as the glial scar) (Norenberg, 1994). Glial cells are often implicated in the disease process that affects brain tissue. The glial cell can be the site of neoplastic disorders that disrupt nerve cell function by compressing the nervous tissue (see Chapter 26).

Virtually all communication between neurons occurs via chemical neurotransmitters. A single neuron can release several different neurotransmitter substances and a single neuron can be selectively receptive to different types of neurotransmitters (Fig. 24–9). Neurotransmitters are synthesized within each neuron, stored in presynaptic vehicles, and released from depolarized nerve terminals. They bind specifically to presynaptic or postsynaptic receptors, which recognize the neurotransmitter's chemical conformation. There is a wide range of substances that make up the neurotransmitter substances used by the nervous system. The nervous system makes use of two main classes of chemical substances in signaling, small molecule transmitters and neuroactive peptides. The small molecule transmitters are formed in short biosynthetic pathways. The controlling enzymes are specific to the neuron and determine the properties cholinergic, norepinephrinergic, dopaminergic, etc.

The neuroactive peptides derive from the processing of secretory proteins that are formed in the cell body. The study of neuroactive peptides is important because certain peptides have been implicated in modulating sensibility and emotions. Those that are included here are listed in Table 24–3.

Activation of a receptor by a neurotransmitter can cause changes in a variety of effector molecules. These include alterations in ion channel permeability, stimulation of second messenger synthesis, and regulation of DNA transcription. These biochemical actions alter the electrical activity of the postsynaptic neurons. See the hepatic, pancreatic, and biliary systems in Chapter 14. Many of the pathologic processes described in the following chapters are the result of abnormal neurotransmitter activity.

Neurodegenerative disease results in premature death of neurons in selective brain areas, with other regions and the peripheral nervous system unaffected. The role of the immune system in these diseases has been explored, although there is a long-held belief that the blood-brain barrier[5] protects the CNS from the direct effects of autoimmune responses. Identification of immune system elements is leading researchers toward an understanding of the role of the immune system in diseases such as MS, amyotrophic lateral sclerosis (ALS), Parkinson's disease, and Alzheimer's disease. Molecules in the nerve terminal are converted to neurotransmitters by specific enzymes. Therefore, in some disease processes and response to injury, nerve conduction may be abnormal due to a change in the level of enzyme activity and the resulting neurotransmitter level. Peptide neurotransmitters are synthesized by precursors that are created from direct gene products.

Neurotransmitter pathways can be identified in the CNS. Figure 24–10 shows both inhibitory and excitatory pathways to various parts of the brain.

PHARMACOLOGY OF NEUROTRANSMITTERS

Many important drugs that alter nervous system function act by selective interaction with neurotransmitter receptors (Johnson and Silverstein, 1992; Traub et al., 1992). Drugs that act at synapses either enhance or block the action of these neurotransmitters. Most neurotransmitters with a prominent role in brain function produce very brief receptor-mediated actions at specific groups of synapses. A few of the neurotransmitters are more prolonged and act more widely throughout the extracellular space. The combined action of both a briefly acting and a more enduring neurotransmitter produces a modulation of postsynaptic neuronal activity. Pharmacologic strategies are currently aimed at modulation of neurotransmitter synthesis, release, reuptake, and degradation. These drugs are used in the poststroke, traumatic brain-injured, and spinal cord–injured client to decrease the secondary nerve damage caused by excessive levels of glutamate in the tissue following the initial insult.

The amount of neurotransmitter released in the synaptic cleft is determined by the neuronal firing rate, the quantity of transmitter in the nerve terminal, and the cumulative

[5] The blood-brain barrier is a mechanism opposing the passage of most ions and large-molecular-weight compounds from the blood to the brain.

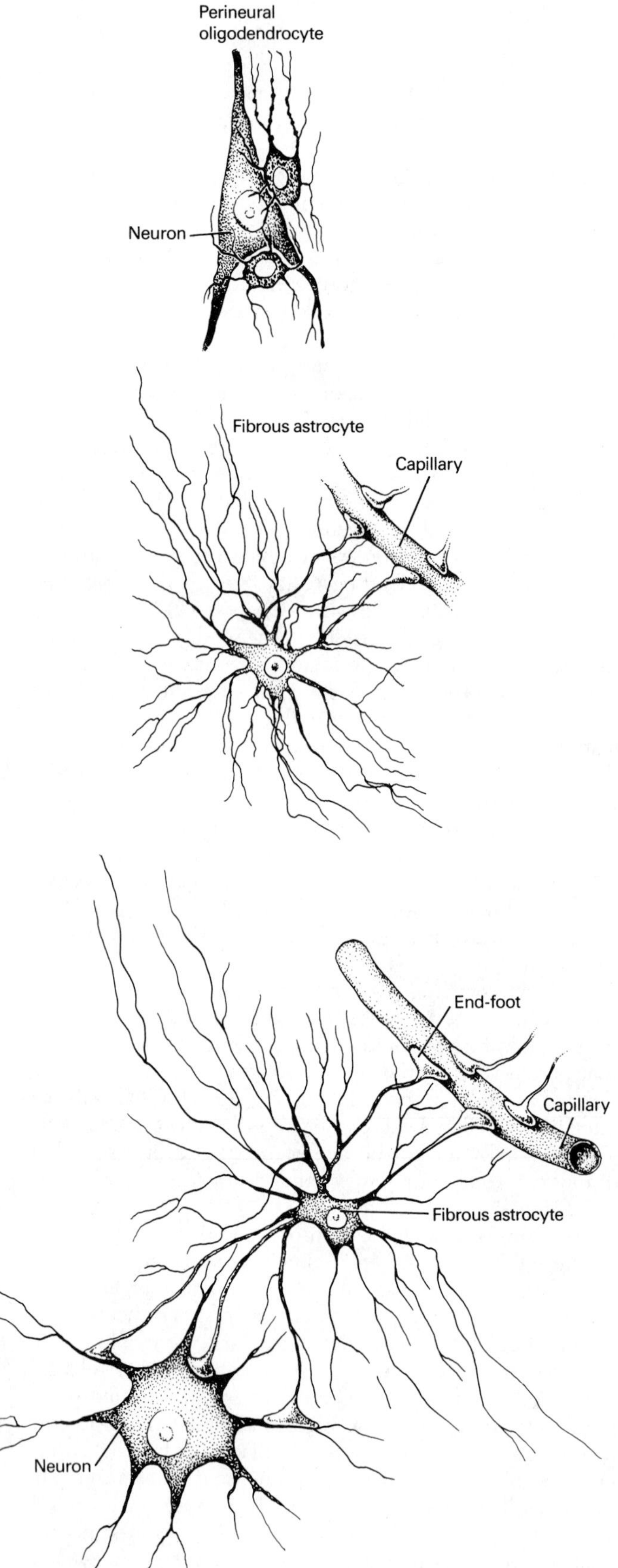

Figure 24–8. The relationship of the glial cells (astrocytes and oligodendrocyte) to the neurons and capillaries. (*From Kandel ER, Schwartz JH: Principles of Neural Science, ed 2. New York, Elsevier, 1985.*)

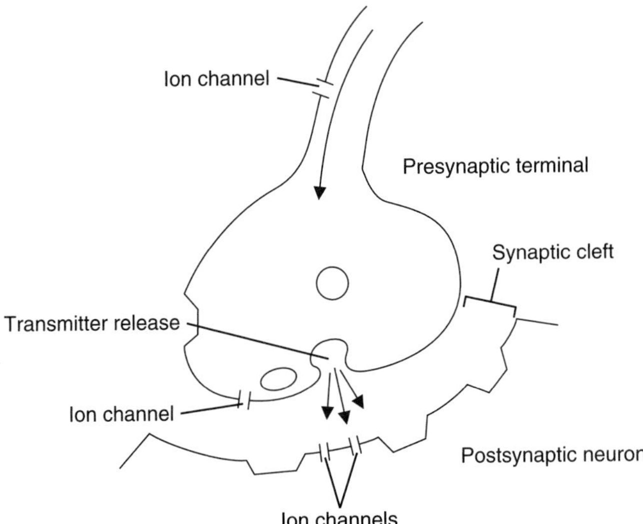

Figure **24-9.** Schematic representation of the postsynaptic neuron and the presynaptic terminal. Transmitter substances are synthesized in presynaptic terminals, released into the synaptic cleft and occupied in the postsynaptic terminal. Modification of the effect of the neurotransmitters at the cleft is the result of the transmitter uptake system, presynaptic receptor sites, and transmitter degradation enzymes released into the cleft. Note the ion channels in both presynaptic and postsynaptic neurons.

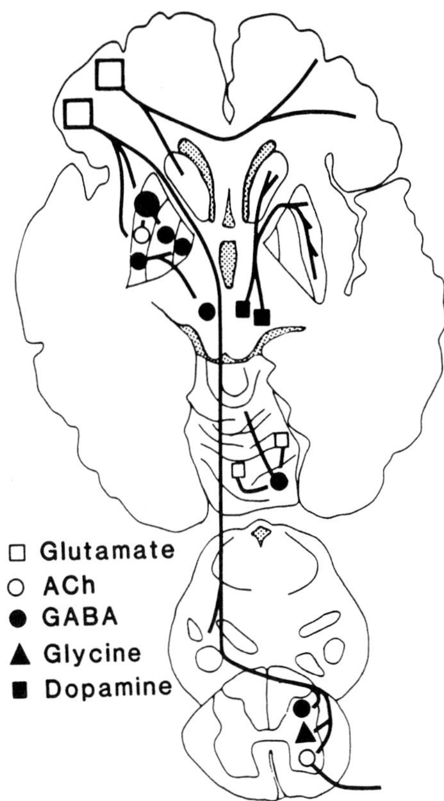

Figure **24-10.** Schematic representation of neurotransmitter pathways involved in motor function. *Black symbols* represent inhibitory pathways and *open symbols* represent excitatory pathways. Schema shows levels of the basal ganglia, cerebellum, pons, and spinal cord. (*From Asbury AK, McKhann GM, McDonald WI (eds): Diseases of the Nervous System: Clinical Neurobiology, vol. 1. Philadelphia, WB Saunders, 1986.*)

regulatory actions of excitatory and inhibitory neurotransmitters. Drugs mediate inhibition of neurotransmitter release by acting at presynaptic receptors. Opiates are one group of drugs that act by the inhibition of neurotransmitter release. Drugs used to control excessive tone in specific muscle groups often work by inhibiting neurotransmitter release.

When the disease process results in decreased neurotransmitter release, as in the neuromuscular junction diseases, drug therapy can stimulate neurotransmitter release. Drugs aimed at maintaining neurotransmitter activity in the synaptic cleft can be useful in these diseases. Another way to regulate the level of neurotransmitters is to influence the rate of chemical degradation. Drugs can inhibit the breakdown of certain elements that may be broken down by natural processes, such as oxidation. One action of these drugs is to prolong the efficacy of released neurotransmitters by inhibiting their degradation.

TABLE 24-3 NEUROTRANSMITTERS

Small molecule transmitter substances
- Acetylcholine
- Dopamine
- Norepinephrine
- Serotonin
- Histamine
- α-Aminobutyric acid (GABA)
- Glycine
- Glutamate

Neuroactive peptides
- Enkephalins
- β-Endorphins
- Glucagon
- Substance P

Trophic factors are essential to maintenance and survival of neurons and their terminals. Nerve growth factor is one such protein that supports the survival of cholinergic neurons. Therapy incorporating trophic factors may be useful in reversing or preventing the degeneration of neuronal terminals in certain neurologic disorders, such as Alzheimer's disease.

Neurotransmitter receptors can be affected by drugs. The receptor is a molecule located on a nerve cell membrane that selectively binds to a particular neurotransmitter. The receptor on the cell membrane is connected to an ion channel or to a second-order enzyme, which can activate or inhibit the nerve's electrical activity. The receptor can be bound to an agonist that activates the neuron, or the neuron can be deactivated by the binding of an antagonist at the receptor site. Identification of the DNA material has led to cloning of the receptor cell in a few neurons.

The excitatory amino acid neurotransmitters constitute 50% of the elements controlling neuronal information flow in the brain. Glutamate is perhaps the most common and most-studied excitatory amino acid. Overactivity of glutamate has excitotoxic effects on neurons. Changes in the target cell can cause abnormal responses to a normal level of glutamate. These include unopposed glutamate transmission, altered receptor function, weakened target cell, and impaired uptake or breakdown in the synaptic cleft. Chronic neurodegenerative disease may be a result of neuronal cell death caused by excessive glutamate or by prolonged glutamate transmission. Loss of cells that inhibit glutamate such as GABAergic neurons (neuroactive γ-aminobutyric acid) result in increased excitation. Overactivity of glutamate is considered a component of epilepsy and the secondary neuronal injury in traumatic brain injury or stroke.

Anesthetic drugs modify the actions of neurotransmitter receptors by changing the membranes of cells on or within which the receptors are located. Other drugs protect the cell membrane in the presence of toxins that act on the membrane. An example is the toxic effects of the free radicals produced in brain tissue after hypoxia, ischemia, and seizures. Damage to the neuron occurs when the free radical is allowed to penetrate the membrane. The best defense is to prevent penetrance.

Many drugs used to treat neurologic disorders influence non-neuronal tissue, including cerebral blood vessels and glia. Cerebral edema is a life-threatening event caused by compression of brain tissue. It can have a vascular component, with increases in permeability of the blood-brain barrier causing an increase in brain water content. Drugs such as mannitol, which controls the edema, or drugs that provide diuresis can help preserve neuronal function. In demyelinating disease, anti-inflammatory and immunosuppressive drugs are used to preserve the function of the glial cells that produce the myelin sheath.

For some of the viruses that invade the CNS there is replication of cells in non-neural tissue. Use of drugs that inhibit RNA or DNA synthesis can prevent viral replication without disrupting neuronal integrity. Acyclovir, used in the treatment of herpes encephalitis, is an example of this type of drug.

The blood-brain barrier is effective at keeping substances in the blood out of the brain, the mechanism being a layer of endothelial cells connected by tight junctions. Use of catheters to deliver the drug directly into the cerebrospinal fluid or brain tissue has enhanced the ability to deliver drugs that act directly on the neuron. Although the catheters have been made more sophisticated and can deliver the drugs in measured doses, complications of administration and uneven levels of absorption continue to be limiting factors. Drugs that bind to natural substances, such as salt or protein, and that penetrate the blood-brain barrier are under investigation.

In infants and children, there is an altered drug metabolism that should be considered whenever administering drugs that act on the nervous system. Intercurrent illness and fever will further alter drug metabolism. An immature blood-brain barrier can also affect the absorption of drugs into brain tissue. When anticonvulsants are administered, close monitoring of blood levels is necessary.

PHYSIOLOGIC BASIS FOR THE RECOVERY OF FUNCTION

Inherent in the recovery of function that has been lost secondary to a neurologic insult is the process of motor relearning, which can be defined as the process of acquisition or modification of movement (Craik, 1992; Shumway-Cook and Woollacott, 1995). Physiologic studies suggest that motor relearning and recovery of function are accomplished through the same neural mechanisms. Neural modifiability may be seen as a change in the organization of connections among neurons and is often referred to as plasticity. Some of the mechanisms for recovery from neurologic insult follow.

Neuronal shock occurs when there is injury to a nerve, and disruption of the neural pathway that extends a distance from the site of injury. When the neurons distal to the injury regain function, which may be soon after the injury, partial function may return.

Injury may be secondary to either swelling of the axon or edema in the surrounding tissue which may block *synaptic activity* in the injured neurons as well as that in the surrounding area. With reduction of the edema, function may return. This is the reason that medications that reduce edema are often given in the context of diffuse brain swelling.

When there is a loss of presynaptic function in one area, the postsynaptic target cells for that area may become more sensitive to neurotransmitters that are now produced in lower concentrations. The compensatory mechanism is known as *denervation supersensitivity*.

Regenerative synaptogenesis occurs when injured axons begin sprouting. *Collateral sprouting* is the process of neighboring axons sprouting to connect with sites that were previously innervated by the injured axon.

Special Implications for the Therapist **24-1**

MOTOR LEARNING STRATEGIES

The recovery of function following nerve injury involves the reacquisition of complex tasks. Clients who have a neurologic deficit must reexplore their own body and its relationship to the environment in order to learn appropriate strategies to move through that environment. Learning involves storage of memory, and can occur in all parts of the brain with both parallel and hierarchical processing. Learning alters our capability to perform the appropriate motor act by changing both the effectiveness of the neural pathways used and the anatomic connections.

The interaction between the client with neurologic sequelae and the therapist is critical for optimal motor learning to take place. Theories underlying the relationship of motor learning and recovery of function are varied, and research continues toward increasing our understanding of that relationship (Schmidt, 1988; Shumway-Cook and Woollacott, 1995). Current theories as the basis for treatment include the following:

Classical conditioning is a form of learning in which a neutral stimulus (the conditioned stimulus) produces a greater response by association with a strong stimulus (the unconditioned stimulus) evoking the response on subsequent trials. This is a result of the conditioned stimulus stimulating the neurons immediately before the unconditioned stimulus through the presynaptic release of calcium ions, which activate specific modulatory transmitters, eliciting the increased response in question.

In *operant conditioning,* a target response, conditioned to occur, is given a reinforcer reward. With repetition, the frequency of the targeted response is increased. Biofeedback is a form of operant conditioning.

Procedural learning results from the repetition of performance of a movement. The rules of the movement, or the efficiencies of control, are thus learned and can be performed repeatedly in the same manner. In a treatment environment, there is emphasis on procedural learning in a variety of environments so that the rules of the task can be demonstrated with more than one set of constraints. This is demonstrated by the client learning the movement strategies to perform a transfer in one environment through repetition or practice, and then learning the movement in another context and environment.

Declarative learning requires knowledge that can be consciously recalled. It involves describing or thinking of the components of a movement prior to execution and then performing the task. This is demonstrated by the client thinking about all the movements required for a transfer before beginning the task.

Other considerations in motor relearning are the methods in which feedback is given regarding the performance of the task. When a task is performed, the individual performing the task has the information available to repeat the motion required to perform that motor task again. The information includes the initial movement conditions, the generalized motor program used, knowledge of the results of the movement, and the sensory consequences of the movement. Motor learning, or the precision of movement, takes place as the client determines the optimal strategy of movement to perform a motor task.

The stages of motor learning involved in learning a skill have been identified. The *cognitive stage* is the first stage and requires a great deal of thought, experimentation, and intervention. Performance is variable, as is seen in the first attempts to walk after brain injury. The second stage of skill acquisition is the *associative stage,* represented by refining of the skill. Fewer errors of performance are experienced, and the motor programs elicited are more consistent and efficient. The final stage is the *autonomous stage* wherein the movement is efficient, and the need for attention to the activity is decreased. The need for feedback during each stage is different. The therapist can enhance treatment by providing the correct amount of feedback for the client attempting to perform a task.

The learning treatment model goes beyond the performance treatment model with a transition from the cognitive stage to the associative stage. In the cognitive stage, the environment is highly structured to allow clients to think and focus on a task. Problem solving is focused on the movement strategies necessary to complete the task. The task may be broken down at this time to work on component parts of the total movement, and practiced with repetition. This is known as blocked or serial practice and can progress from parts of the movement to the whole movement done with repetition and continuous feedback. Transition to the associative stage is necessary at this point or task performance rather than skill acquisition will be developed. For a skill to be acquired, learning principles that promote associative and automatic phases need to be incorporated in the intervention.

References

Asbury AK, McKhann GM, McDonald WI (eds): Diseases of the Nervous System: Clinical Neurobiology. Philadelphia, WB Saunders, 1986, pp 1–3.

Bach-y-Rita P: Applications of principles of brain plasticity and training to restore function. *In* Young RR, Delwaide PJ (eds): Principles and Practice of Restorative Neurology. Oxford, UK, Butterworth-Heinemann, 1992, pp 54–65.

Burt AM: Textbook of Neuroanatomy. Philadelphia, WB Saunders, 1993.

Craik RL: Recovery processes: Maximizing function. *In* Contemporary Management of Motor Control Problems. Proceedings of the II Step Conference. Alexandria, Va, American Physical Therapy Association, 1992, pp 165–173.

Craik RL: Sensorimotor changes and adaptation in the older adult. *In* Guccione AA: Geriatric Physical Therapy. St Louis, Mosby–Year Book, 1993, pp 71–98.

Filley CM: Neurobehavioral Anatomy. Niwot, Colo, University Press of Colorado, 1995.

Fretwell MD: Aging changes in structure and function. *In* Carnevale DL, Patrick M (eds): Nursing Management for the Elderly, ed 3. Philadelphia, JB Lippincott, 1993, pp 113–140.

Johnston MV, Silverstein FS: Fundamentals of drug therapy in neurology. *In* Johnston MV, Macdonald RL, Young AB (eds): Principles of Drug Therapy in Neurology. Philadelphia, FA Davis, 1992, pp 1–43.

Kandel ER: Nerve cells and behavior. *In* Kandel ER, Schwartz JH (eds): Principles of Neural Science, ed 2. New York, Elsevier, 1985, pp 13–24.

Lewis CB, Jordan KS: Clinical implications of neurologic changes with age. *In* Lewis CB (ed): Aging: The Health Care Challenge. Philadelphia, FA Davis, 1985, pp 141–164.

Lindsay KW, Bone I, Callandar R: Neurology and Neurosurgery Illustrated. New York, Churchill Livingstone, 1986.

Norenberg MD: Astrocyte responses to CNS injury. J Neuropathol Exp Neurol 53:213–220, 1994.

Panter SS, Faden AI: Biochemical changes and secondary injury from stroke and trauma. *In* Young RR, Delwaide PJ (eds): Principles and Practice of Restorative Neurology. Oxford, Butterworth-Heinemann, 1992, pp 32–53.

Poirier J, Finch CE: Neurochemistry of the aging human brain. *In* Hazzard WR, Andres R, Bierman EL, Blass JP (eds): Principles of Geriatric Medicine and Gerontology, ed 2. New York, McGraw-Hill, 1990, pp 905–911.

Schmidt RA: Motor Control and Learning: A Behavioral Emphasis, ed 2. Champaign, Ill, Human Kinetics, 1988.

Shumway-Cook A, Woollacott MH: Motor Control: Theory and Function. Baltimore, Williams & Wilkins, 1995.

Singer C, Weiner WJ: The neurologic examination. *In* Weiner WJ, Geoetz CG (eds): Neurology for the Non-Neurologist, ed 3. Philadelphia, JB Lippincott, 1994, pp 1–12.

Topel JL, Lewis SL: Examination of the comatose patient. *In* Weiner WJ, Geoetz CG (eds): Neurology for the Non-Neurologist, ed 3. Philadelphia, JB Lippincott, 1994, pp 43–52.

Traub M, Haigh JR, Marsden CD: Recent developments in the pharmacotherapy of major neurological dysfunction. *In* Young RR, Delwaide PJ (eds): Principles and Practice of Restorative Neurology. Oxford, Butterworth-Heinemann, 1992, pp 66–82.

Urbscheit NL, Oremland BS: Cerebellar dysfunction. *In* Umphred DA (ed): Neurological Rehabilitation, ed 3. St Louis, Mosby–Year Book, 1995, pp 657–679.

Waxman SG, deGroot J: Correlative Neuroanatomy. East Norwalk, Conn, Appleton and Lange, 1995.

SECTION 4

chapter 25

Infectious Disorders of the Central Nervous System

Kenda S. Fuller

Infection of the central nervous system is rare in that there are many protective responses that limit the access of organisms to the nervous tissue. Bacteria and viruses are removed from the blood by the reticuloendothelial system. Immune responses destroy organisms at the site of the infection and in the blood. Most important, there is a mechanism known as the blood-brain barrier that prevents entry of infectious organisms into the brain or cerebral spinal fluid (CSF).[1] The organisms that do enter the brain or CSF may be able to do so when the endothelial cells of the cerebral blood vessels become infected.

Once an infection has reached the brain tissue or CSF, there is less immune protection than in the rest of the body. The CSF has about 1/200 the amount of antibody as blood, and the number of white blood cells is very low compared to the blood. The brain lacks a lymphatic system to fight infection (Davis, 1994)

The signs and symptoms of a central nervous system (CNS) infection depend on the site of the infection and not on the organism. The type of organism determines primarily the length of time it will take the infection to run its course, and the prognosis for neurologic sequelae.

MENINGITIS *(Davis, 1994; Gilroy and Holliday, 1982)*

Definition, Etiology, and Pathogenesis. In meningitis, the meninges of the brain and spinal cord become inflamed. The three layers of the meningeal membranes, the dura mater, the arachnoid, and the pia mater, can be involved. Meningitis is almost always a complication of another infection. Meningitis can be caused by a wide variety of organisms, some of which cross the blood-brain barrier and the blood-CSF barrier. The pia mater and arachnoid become congested and opaque. The relationship of the meninges to the brain tissue is shown in Figure 25–1. The inflammation extends into the first and second layers of the cortex and spinal cord, and can produce thrombosis of the cortical veins. There is an increased chance of infarction, and the scar tissue can restrict flow of CSF, especially around the base of the brain. The block of CSF can result in hydrocephalus or a subarachnoid cyst. The CSF can also become contaminated by a wound that penetrates the meninges as a result of trauma or a neurosurgical procedure (Porter, 1995).

[1] The blood-brain barrier is a mechanism that selectively inhibits certain substances from entering the interstitial spaces of the brain or CSF. It is believed that the astrocytes and the tight junctions between the endothelial cells of the brain capillaries create this barrier. The barrier opposes passage of most ions and high-molecular-weight compounds.

Clinical Manifestations *(Davis, 1994).* Early features of meningitis include fever and headache. The cardinal signs of meningitis include a stiff and painful neck. There is often pain in the lumbar area and the posterior aspects of the thigh. Kernig's sign, pain with combined hip flexion and knee flexion, is positive. As the inflammation progresses, flexion of the neck will produce flexion of the hips and knees. This is known as a positive Brudzinski's sign. The positions for Kernig's and Brudzinski's tests are shown in Figure 25–2. If the infection remains undetected or untreated, the individual may experience seizures and coma, and there will be focal neurologic signs, including cranial nerve palsies and deafness.

Medical Management

Diagnosis, Treatment, and Prognosis. Lumbar puncture is the only absolute means of substantiating a diagnosis of meningitis (see Laboratory Values, Chapter 35). Radiographs are taken to rule out fracture, sinusitis, and mastoiditis. A computed tomography (CT) scan will reveal evidence of brain abscess or infarction which may be responsible for the symptoms.

The time course after onset of the disease is indicative of the type of organism involved. Viral meningitis is hyperacute, with symptoms developing within hours. Acute pyogenic bacterial meningitis can develop in 4 to 24 hours. Individuals with fungal meningitis or tuberculous meningitis develop symptoms over days to weeks.

The viruses causing *viral meningitis* can be isolated in CSF; enteroviruses, including *Enterovirus* coxsackie B, and the causative agent of lymphocytic choriomeningitis (an arenavirus) are common, and herpes simplex virus and mumps virus are a less common cause. Human immunodeficiency virus (HIV) is another virus that can trigger viral meningitis (Baringer, 1992).

Lumbar puncture reveals the following: mononuclear cells in the hundreds, a normal glucose level, a mild increase in protein, and absence of bacterial organisms.

The usual treatment for viral meningitis is symptomatic. Medication is given for the headache and nausea. The prognosis in viral meningitis is excellent, and most clients recover within 1 to 2 weeks.

Acute pyogenic bacterial meningitis primarily affects the immunosuppressed and the young and old. Infections of the neonate are usually produced by *Escherichia coli*. *Haemophilus influenzae* is prominent in children and the immunosuppressed and is a part of the normal flora of the nose and throat that may gain entry to the CSF during an upper respiratory tract infection. Prompt diagnosis is critical in this population as

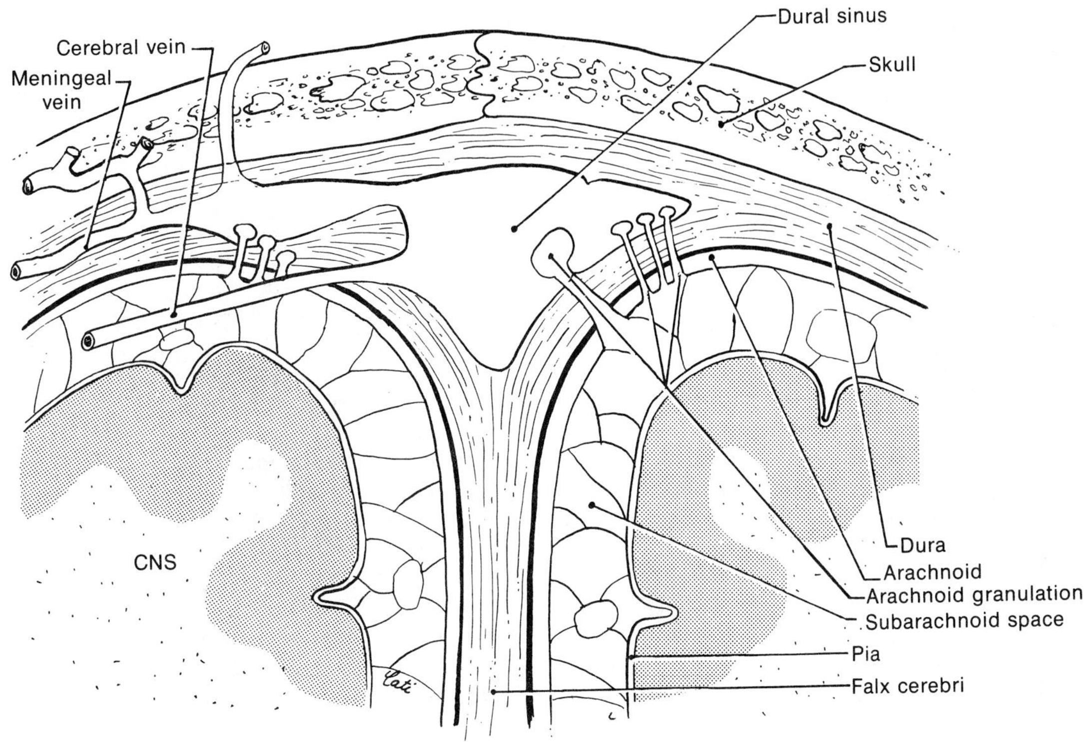

Figure **25-1.** The meninges, showing the relationship of the dura, arachnoid, subarachnoid space, pia, and brain tissue. (*From Felten MD, Felten SY: A regional and systemic overview of functional neuroanatomy. In Farber SD (ed): Neurorehabilitation: A Multisensory Approach. Philadelphia, WB Saunders, 1982, p 6.*)

death can occur without antibiotic treatment. Lumbar puncture is positive for bacterial organisms; the glucose level is less than 50% of the blood serum level. There are thousands of polymorphonuclear cells in the early stages and protein is elevated.

Bacterial meningitis is best treated by the immediate administration of broad-spectrum antibiotics. The appropriate antibiotic is critical because the CNS can sustain long-term damage if the infection is not stopped. The antibiotic must be able to cross the blood-brain barrier and achieve sufficient CSF concentrations to kill the bacteria.

Treatment requires that the individual remain in isolation for at least 3 days until antibiotic treatment is instituted. Bed rest is suggested in the acute phase. Fluid balance and electrolytes are monitored. Antibiotics are administered according to the organisms identified. If there is evidence of cerebral edema or herniation, corticosteroids are given. Seizures can be controlled with diazepam (Valium) or phenytoin (Dilantin). As the infection is controlled, the seizures are resolved, so a short course is all that is usually necessary.

When there is suspected bacterial meningitis in a child or infant it is considered a medical emergency and isolation

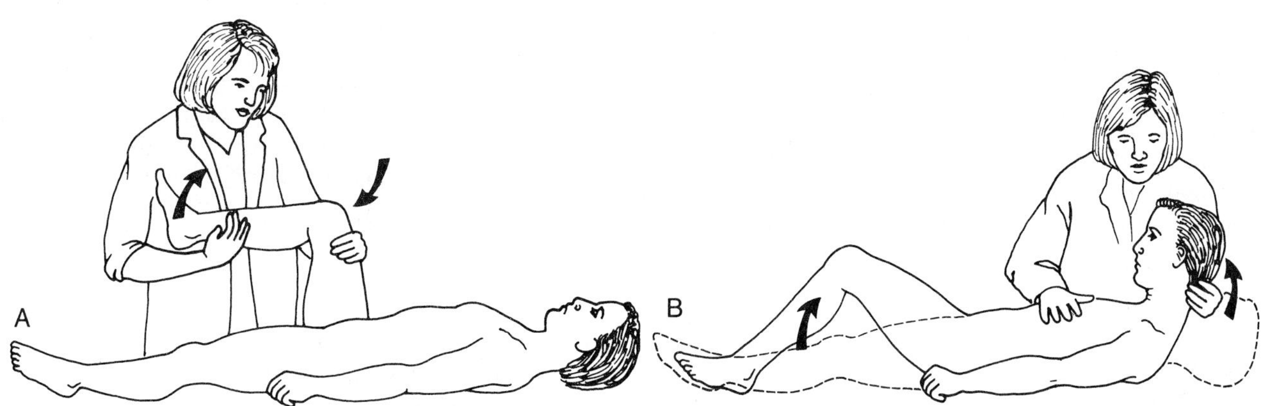

Figure **25-2.** Assessing a client with meningeal irritation. A, Kernig's sign. B, Brudzinski's sign. (*From Schnell SS: Nursing care of clients with cerebral disorders. In Black JM, Matassarin-Jacobs E (eds): Luckmann and Sorensen's Medical-Surgical Nursing, ed. 4. Philadelphia, WB Saunders, 1993, p 763.*)

is the first step taken. The age of the child and the type of organism is reflected in the symptoms. The general picture involves fever, poor feeding, vomiting, a bulging fontanel (in infants), seizures, and a high-pitched cry. Management of the disorder involves antimicrobial therapy, hydration, ventilatory support if needed, maintenance of a stable intracranial pressure, control of seizures and treatment of complications. Mortality ranges from 5% to 25% depending on the infecting bacteria and the health and age of the person infected. Neurologic sequelae remain in approximately 30% of persons with bacterial meningitis.

Tuberculous meningitis is an infection of the leptomeninges (arachnoid and pia mater) by *Mycobacterium tuberculosis*, which enters the body by inhalation. The presence of active tuberculosis elsewhere and CSF examination are usually sufficient to establish the diagnosis. There is a predominance of mononuclear cells, the glucose level is decreased, and protein is increased. It is difficult to identify the tuberculosis bacterium, so clinical signs are important to follow.

Treatment follows the standard for tuberculosis, with antituberculosis drugs given. If there is evidence of spinal arachnoiditis, hydrocortisone is administered. Mortality rates range from 20% to 50%, and survivors may be left with neurologic sequelae similar to those seen in acute bacterial meningitis.

ENCEPHALITIS

Definition. Encephalitis is an acute inflammatory disease of the brain caused by direct viral invasion or hypersensitivity initiated by a virus. The mosquito- or tick-borne virus is responsible for most transmission, but drinking infected goat's milk and other means of contact with the virus can occur. After World War I there was an outbreak of encephalitis that caused lethargy as its primary symptom, and the disease was known as "sleeping sickness." This term for encephalitis, although outdated, persists in nonmedical descriptions of the disease (Baringer, 1992).

Etiology, Risk Factors, and Pathogenesis. The cause cannot be identified in almost two thirds of cases of viral encephalitis. Viral infection may cause encephalitis as a primary manifestation or as a secondary complication. Viruses carried by mosquitoes or ticks are responsible for most of the worldwide known causes. The *herpes simplex virus*, which is a latent infection in most persons, can be responsible, and is the most common cause in the United States. The remainder are caused by bacteria (Davis, 1994).

Encephalitis is characterized by inflammation of, and damage to, the gray matter of the CNS. Neuronal death can result in cerebral edema. There can be damage to the vascular system and inflammation of the arachnoid and pia mater. Herpes simplex virus produces an inflammatory response in the temporal lobe.

Clinical Manifestations. Signs and symptoms of encephalitis depend on the etiologic agent, but in general headache, nausea, and vomiting are followed by alteration of consciousness. Depending on the area of the brain involved, there may be focal neurologic signs, with hemiparesis, aphasia, ataxia, or disorders of limb movement. With herpes simplex encephalitis, there can be repeated seizure activity, hallucinations, and disturbance of memory, reflecting involvement of the temporal lobe.

There can be symptoms of meningeal irritation with stiffness of the back and neck. If the person becomes comatose, the coma may persist for days or weeks.

Medical Management

Diagnosis. The electroencephalogram (EEG) is always abnormal, occasionally showing seizure activity. Lumbar puncture is abnormal with increased protein. The glucose level, however, may be normal and no bacteria grow on culture. Vascular studies and CT scan and magnetic resonance imaging (MRI) show cerebral edema and vascular damage. Brain biopsy is necessary to diagnose herpes simplex.

Treatment. Treatment varies with the infectious agent. No antiviral treatment is available for encephalitis except for that caused by the herpes simplex virus. Acylovir appears to improve the outcome in herpes simplex encephalitis. Close monitoring of the symptoms is critical, especially with the complication of cerebral edema, which may require surgical decompression, hyperventilation, or administration of mannitol. The use of corticosteroids is controversial, owing to the potential suppression of antibody protection within the CNS.

Prognosis. The prognosis depends on the infectious agent. The rate of recovery can range from 10% to 50%, even in individuals may who have been desperately ill at the onset. Individuals with mumps meningoencephalitis, and Venezuelan equine encephalitis have an excellent prognosis. Other encephalitides, such as western equine, St. Louis, and California encephalitis, have a moderate to good rate of survival. Although with the use of medication, herpes simplex encephalitis has a moderately good outcome (20% mortality), neurologic sequelae are common in 50% of persons.

Permanent cerebral sequelae are more likely to occur in infants. Young children will take longer to recover than adults with similar infections.

BRAIN ABSCESS

Definition. Brain abscesses occur when microorganisms reach the brain and cause a local infection. There may be only one area of abscess, or there may be many areas infected, spread by blood-borne pathogens. While the site and size of the abscess influence the initial symptoms, evidence of increased intracranial pressure is common. In persons with a compromised immune system receiving steroids, immunosuppressants, or cytotoxic chemotherapy, or with a systemic illness such as HIV infection, there is an increased risk of developing a brain abscess (Porter, 1995).

Etiology, Risk Factors, and Pathogenesis. While viruses tend to cause diffuse brain infections, most bacteria, fungi, and other parasites cause localized brain disease. Brain abscesses may develop from other infections in the cranium, such as sinusitis or mastoiditis. If the infection is carried in the blood from another site in the body, the abscess will usually develop at the junction of the gray and white matter. Anaerobic bacteria are found in over one half of brain abscesses. The infection usually begins as a localized encephalitis with necrosis and inflammation of the neurons and glial cells. As the process continues, a capsule wall is formed by the proliferation of fibroblasts. There is usually an area of cerebral edema around the abscess. Bacterial and fungal abscesses will continue to grow until they become lethal. Abscesses caused by other parasites are usually self-limiting.

Clinical Manifestations. The person with a developing brain abscess will present with fever, chills, headache, and focal neurologic signs that progress with time. The onset of symptoms may be slow, acting like a slow-growing neoplasm, or it may be rapid and progress to possible herniation and brainstem compression causing death. Seizures are not uncommon. Lethargy and confusion progress with the increased intracranial pressure present with the growing mass. Focal signs reflect the area of the brain that is affected, with paresis resulting from frontal and parietal lesions and visual disturbances noted with occipital lobe dysfunction.

Medical Management

Diagnosis and Treatment. A history of infection or immunosuppression will lead to suspicion of abscess vs. neoplasm. CT and MRI will support the diagnosis based on the different configurations of tumor and abscess. Although the early signs are similar to meningitis, the focal signs of compression in one area of the brain distinguish the abscess over time. The EEG is often abnormal.

Treatment involves the appropriate antibiotic and surgical drainage to reduce the mass effect. Careful clinical observation is necessary with multiple abscesses and CT scans should be repeated often to determine if the abscess continues to expand. Initially, corticosteroids may be used to control the cerebral edema caused by the abscess, but these are used for a short time only because of their interference with capsule formation and immunosuppressive action in the brain.

Prognosis. Mortality from brain abscess can be lowered from 65% to 30% with control of the infection with antibiotics and surgery. Nearly half of the clients are left with some neurologic sequelae, which may include focal signs and seizure activity.

Special Implications for the Therapist **25–1**

INFECTIOUS DISORDER OF THE CNS

The therapist must understand and observe all isolation procedures. Often the treatment of these clients begins in the intensive care unit. Monitoring of vital signs throughout the treatment session may be necessary when the client is in the acute stage.

The client may demonstrate symptoms that are similar to many noninfectious brain disorders. The clinical picture may represent the diffuse disorders typical of brain trauma or there may be only focal neurologic sequelae.

Initially, when the inflammatory response is greatest, there may be a profound alteration of consciousness. Familiarity with the scales used to monitor levels of consciousness, such as the Glasgow Coma Scale (see Table 29–1, Chapter 29) is helpful. The client may be agitated with difficulty in processing sensory input. Increased sensitivity to sound and light is not uncommon. Cognitive and perceptual disorders with memory deficits probably represent the involvement of the brain in the area of the ventricles. It is essential that the therapist understand the behavioral changes that accompany diffuse brain disorders. See Chapter 29 for further details; see also Porter (1995).

Sensory dysfunction should be thoroughly evaluated. If the client has a history of instability of heart rate, blood pressure, or respiration, these should be monitored during the evaluation of sensation, as sensory input may aggravate responses in some individuals. Cutaneous sensation may be affected in different distributions depending on whether the damage is diffuse or deep in one area of the brain. Distorted or absent sensory input can affect mobility and functional status in a dramatic way. For further description of sensory and motor deficits related to specific areas of damage, see Chapter 28.

Movement disorders also reflect the nature and depth of the insult to the brain. Abnormal posturing of the client in the acute phase may be noted and there may be abnormal postural reflexes present. Decorticate and decerebrate posturing are often seen in the early stages of these brain disorders.*

Positioning, and range-of-motion exercises are critical in the early phases as the stiffness of the back and neck can exacerbate the pain. Often, maintaining a darkened environment during treatment will decrease the complaints of headache.

When interacting with the client and family, it is important to be familiar with the acute, subacute, and chronic prognoses related to the type of infection causing the brain injury. When the course of the disease indicates good recovery, the client and family should be given reassurance during the acute and devastating phase of the disease. If the neurologic deficit appears to be more permanent, the client should be referred to a rehabilitation program when medically stable.

* The *decorticate state* is characterized by flexor rigidity of the upper limbs and extension of the lower limbs. The degree of rigidity is associated with tonic neck reflexes, so that when the head is rotated to the right, flexor rigidity is expressed in the left arm. *Decerebrate rigidity* involves extension of both arms and legs; the trunk is arched back with the head flexed. In general, the decerebrate state represents damage at a higher level in the CNS compared to the decorticate state (Carew, 1985).

References

Baringer JR: Viral Infections, *In* Asbury AK, McKhann GM, McDonald WI, (eds): Diseases of the Nervous System: Clinical Neurobiology, vol. 2. Philadelphia, WB Saunders, 1992.

Carew TJ: Posture and locomotion. *In* Kandal ER, Schwartz JH (eds): Principles of Neural Science, ed 2. New York, Elsevier 1985, pp 479–486.

Davis LE: Central nervous system infections. *In* Weiner WJ, Goetz CG (eds.): Neurology for the Non-Neurologist, ed 3. Philadelphia, JB Lippincott, 1994, pp 349–357.

Gilroy J, Holliday PL: Basic Neurology. New York, Macmillan, 1982.

Porter RE: Therapeutic management of the client with inflammatory and infectious disorders of the brain. *In* Umphred DA (ed): Neurological Rehabilitation, ed 3. St Louis, Mosby–Year Book, 1995, pp 335–355.

Schnell SS: Nursing care of clients with cerebral disorders. *In* Black JM, Matassarin-Jacobs E (eds): Luckman and Sorensen's Medical-Surgical Nursing, ed 4. Philadelphia, WB Saunders, 1993, pp 705–772.

SECTION 4

chapter 26

Central Nervous System Neoplasms

Sharon M. Konecne

There are several categories of neoplasia that affect the central nervous system (CNS). *Primary* tumors may develop in the brain, spinal cord, or surrounding structures; secondary, or *metastatic*, tumors may spread to the CNS from another site; or cancer elsewhere in the body may remotely or indirectly affect the CNS, a phenomenon known as *paraneoplastic syndrome*. Additionally, a condition in which carcinoma may spread throughout the CNS with multiple metastatic lesions to the brain or meninges is known as *leptomeningeal carcinomatosis*.

The presence of any CNS tumor is cause for concern. CNS tumors cause early effects mechanically through displacement of brain or spinal cord tissue or by causing a mild block in cerebrospinal fluid (CSF) circulation. They may also compress or destroy local brain or nerve tissue resulting in specific neurologic deficits. Symptoms of brain tumors may vary from headache to the more serious seizures, to blindness, paralysis, and cognitive impairment. Symptoms of spinal cord tumors may include pain, sensory impairments, weakness, and eventually paralysis. Primary CNS tumors do not typically metastasize as do other neoplasms because of the lack of a lymphatic system in the CNS through which cancer cells may be carried to the rest of the body. Cancer cells may infrequently travel through the CSF to the spinal cord. Most primary CNS tumors, however, are locally invasive and because of the critical areas and confined space in the CNS they cause significant morbidity and mortality in every age group.

The diagnosis of a CNS tumor with its threat of significant loss of neurologic and cognitive function is devastating to the client and family. It robs people of independence and dignity, and is viewed as a humiliating and inextricably fatal process. The emotional implications for the affected individual and family can be significant, bringing difficult decisions about treatment options and quality-of-life issues. With both brain and spinal cord tumors, caregiving and financial struggles are frequently encountered.

Despite the inescapable realities of these issues, the situation is improving, with dramatic new advances in radiologic imaging, neurosurgery, and adjuvant therapy. At present, approximately 50% of patients with CNS tumors can be successfully treated and have an excellent long-term prognosis (Thapar and Laws, 1995). A broad knowledge and awareness of current treatment advances provide the health professional with the information and skills to care for the client and family in a sensitive, compassionate, and hopeful but realistic manner.

INCIDENCE

Tumors of the CNS are not uncommon. Accurate estimates are difficult as the incidence is increasing, but primary tumors of the CNS are diagnosed in over 17,000 Americans each year and metastatic tumors are diagnosed in another 17,000 (Hickey, 1992). Although this is a small percentage of the approximately 1.38 million new cases of cancer each year, brain tumors kill more Americans each year than multiple sclerosis and Hodgkin's disease (Snodgrass, 1994). Approximately 8500 deaths each year in the United States are due to primary brain tumors and many more are caused by cerebral metastasis. Primary brain tumors are the second most common form of cancer in children (Weiss, 1995) and primary CNS tumors are the second leading cause of death from cancer in children.

Eighty percent of all CNS tumors are primary, and 20% are metastatic (Gilroy, 1990). The incidence of both primary and metastatic brain tumors is increasing in all age groups in the United States; in people 75 years old and older, primary brain tumors in particular are increasing (Ransohoff et al., 1991).

The incidence of metastatic CNS tumors is on the rise as a result of improved life expectancies from advances in cancer treatment, allowing micrometastases time to develop in the spinal cord and brain and find a safe haven behind the blood-brain barrier through which most chemotherapeutic agents cannot pass. The blood-brain barrier prevents passage of high-molecular-weight compounds through its tight capillary endothelial junctions. More than 60% of tumors in adults are supratentorial, or located in the cerebral hemispheres, whereas the majority of pediatric tumors are infratentorial, involving primarily the cerebellum and brainstem (Chase, 1991).

CLASSIFICATION

The major purpose of tumor classification is to facilitate communication about tumor behavior and treatment, and to design studies to learn more about the tumors (Yates, 1992). A classification system has not been standardized for CNS tumors, but various suggested systems exist, based on a number of distinguishing criteria: neuroembryonal origin, primary vs. secondary, benign vs. malignant, histologic grade, anatomic location, and childhood vs. adult tumors. The World Health Organization (WHO) system of classifying CNS tumors is based on neuroembryonal origin, that is, naming a tumor by the most likely cell of origin, and then adding qualifying phrases to describe the behavior of the tumor (Yates, 1992).

Primary brain tumors originate from the various cells and structures normally found within the brain. Secondary or metastatic brain tumors originate from structures outside the brain, most often from primary tumors of the lungs, breast, gastrointestinal tract, and genitourinary tract (Hickey, 1992).

Primary CNS tumors may also be subdivided into so-called benign tumors, such as meningiomas, neurinomas, and hemangioblastomas, and malignant tumors, such as glioblastomas. A histologically benign tumor has a slow growth rate and is relatively noninvasive. However, because of space-occupying properties in very vital tissue with a resultant high threat of functional limitation, the use of the term "benign" is somewhat misleading. Some authors insist that because of their locations even very slow-growing CNS tumors should be considered basically malignant (Ransohoff et al., 1991). The histologically "benign" tumor may be surgically inaccessible, or located in a vital area, such as the pons or medulla, and will continue to grow, thereby causing an increase in intracranial pressure (ICP), neurologic deficits, herniation syndromes, and finally, death. Malignant tumors typically have a high growth rate and are invasive and infiltrative.

Anatomic location refers to the location of the lesion in reference to the tentorium or cerebral tissue. Table 26–1 gives a classification system based on the anatomic location of the most common CNS tumors.

There are other typically recognized subdivisions. In the brain are two groups of primary tumors: *gliomas*, the most common type, which includes astrocytomas and glioblastomas; and *non-gliomas*, which includes such tumors as meningiomas and pituitary adenomas. Examples of primary tumors in the spinal cord include the more common neurinomas (schwannomas or neurilemomas), and the less frequent gliomas and meningiomas. Some further subgroups of gliomas have been established based on cellular atypism, the presence of mitotic figures, the incidence of endothelial hyperplasia, and the presence of necrotic areas. It is hoped that newer techniques of molecular biology, such as the ability to identify growth factors and inhibitors necessary for cell growth and differentiation, may lead to a more sophisticated subclassification.

Because the clinical presentation, treatment, and prognosis are heavily dependent on the location of involvement and whether the tumor is primary or metastatic, this discussion is divided into three parts: (1) primary brain tumors, (2) primary intraspinal tumors, and (3) metastatic tumors.

TABLE 26–1 CLASSIFICATION OF THE MOST COMMON TUMORS OF THE CENTRAL NERVOUS SYSTEM

Supratentorial tumors
- Cerebral hemispheres
  - Metastases
  - Meningiomas
  - Gliomas (malignant gliomas: anaplastic astrocytoma and glioblastoma multiforme, astrocytoma, oligodendroglioma)
- Midline tumors
  - Pituitary adenomas
  - Pineal tumors
  - Craniopharyngiomas

Infratentorial tumors
- Adults
  - Acoustic schwannomas (neurinomas, neurilemomas)
  - Metastases
  - Meningiomas
  - Hemangioblastomas
- Children
  - Cerebellar astrocytomas
  - Medulloblastomas
  - Ependymomas
  - Brainstem gliomas

Spinal cord tumors
- Extradural
  - Metastases
- Intradural
  - Extramedullary
    - Meningiomas
    - Schwannomas, neurofibromas
  - Intramedullary
    - Ependymomas
    - Astrocytomas

Adapted from Weiss HD: Neoplasms. *In* Samuels MA (ed): Manual of Neurologic Therapeutics, ed 5. Boston, Little, Brown, 1995, p 225.

PRIMARY BRAIN TUMORS

Certain tumor types have a predilection for specific areas of the brain, although they may arise elsewhere in the brain. Topologic distribution and preferred sites of primary CNS tumors are illustrated in Figure 26–1.

Pathogenesis

Brain tumors affect the brain through compression of cerebral tissue, including brain substance and cranial nerves, invasion or infiltration of cerebral tissue, and sometimes, erosion of bone (Hickey, 1992). These mechanisms precipitate pathophysiologic changes such as cerebral edema and increased ICP.

In most brain tumors, vasogenic edema develops in the surrounding tissue of the tumor because of compression. At the cellular level, the increased permeability of the capillary endothelial cells of the cerebral white matter results in seepage of plasma into the extracellular space and between the layers of the myelin sheath. This impairs cellular activity and causes electrochemical instability. Cerebral edema can also develop rapidly from alterations in the blood-brain barrier.

Initially the brain has a surprising tolerance to the compressive and infiltrative effects of brain tumors, and there may be few early symptoms. Compensatory mechanisms to respond to edema and maintain normal ICP include decreasing (1) the volume of brain tissue, (2) CSF, and (3) cerebral blood volume. When the brain can no longer compensate, the resultant increase in ICP leads to more evident signs and symptoms.

Clinical Manifestations

The particular clinical presentation of a brain tumor depends on the compression or infiltration of specific cerebral tissue,

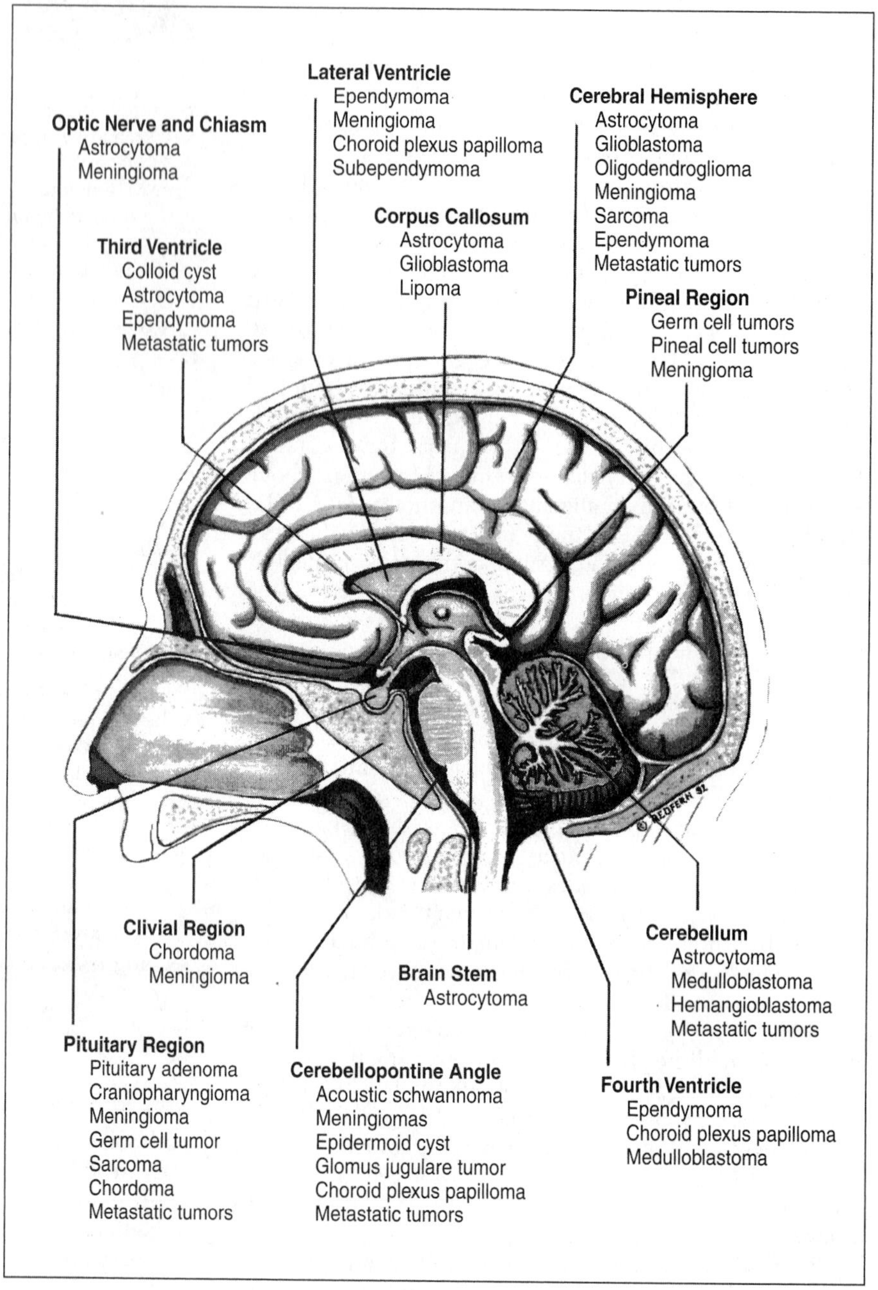

Lateral Ventricle
Ependymoma
Meningioma
Choroid plexus papilloma
Subependymoma

Optic Nerve and Chiasm
Astrocytoma
Meningioma

Cerebral Hemisphere
Astrocytoma
Glioblastoma
Oligodendroglioma
Meningioma
Sarcoma
Ependymoma
Metastatic tumors

Corpus Callosum
Astrocytoma
Glioblastoma
Lipoma

Third Ventricle
Colloid cyst
Astrocytoma
Ependymoma
Metastatic tumors

Pineal Region
Germ cell tumors
Pineal cell tumors
Meningioma

Clivial Region
Chordoma
Meningioma

Brain Stem
Astrocytoma

Cerebellum
Astrocytoma
Medulloblastoma
Hemangioblastoma
Metastatic tumors

Pituitary Region
Pituitary adenoma
Craniopharyngioma
Meningioma
Germ cell tumor
Sarcoma
Chordoma
Metastatic tumors

Cerebellopontine Angle
Acoustic schwannoma
Meningiomas
Epidermoid cyst
Glomus jugulare tumor
Choroid plexus papilloma
Metastatic tumors

Fourth Ventricle
Ependymoma
Choroid plexus papilloma
Medulloblastoma

Figure 26–1. Topologic distribution and preferred sites of primary central nervous system tumors. (*Adapted from Burger PC, Schneithauer BW, Vogel FS: Surgical Pathology of the Nervous System and its Coverings, ed 3. New York, Churchill Livingstone, 1991.*)

the related cerebral edema, and the development of increased ICP (Hickey, 1992). Box 26–1 lists signs and symptoms of brain tumors.

The initial clinical signs of an intracranial tumor are related to the generalized effect of an increase in ICP. Headache is commonly present (in one third of cases), is typically generalized or retro-orbital, and is typically worse in the morning and better later in the day. The headache is intensified or precipitated by any activity that tends to raise the ICP such as stooping, straining, or exercising (see Chapter 13, Box 13–1). Irritation, compression, or traction of pain-sensitive structures such as the dura mater and blood vessels cause the headache. The sixth cranial nerve (abducens), because of its long intracranial path, is highly susceptible to elevated ICP, causing weakness in the lateral rectus muscle and diplopia (Thapar and Laws, 1995). Nausea and vomiting are common.

Other common initial signs are mental clouding, lethargy, alterations in consciousness and cognition, and easy fatigability. With an increase in intracranial CSF pressure, the increase in perioptic pressure impedes venous drainage from the optic head area and retina, causing papilledema (Chusid, 1985). Papilledema, edema of the optic disc, is associated with visual changes, such as decreased visual acuity, and an enlarged blind spot, diplopia, and deficits in the visual fields.

About 20% to 50% of adults with brain tumors develop seizure activity. Seizures may be the first presenting sign of a tumor. The cerebral edema causes hyperactive cells, which produce abnormal, paroxysmal discharges or seizure activity

BOX 26–1
Signs and Symptoms of Brain Tumors

- Headache
- Visual changes
- Nausea
- Vomiting
- Mental changes–impairment of memory, judgment, personality
- Lethargy
- Behavioral changes
- Seizures
- Hemiparesis, hemiplegia
- Sensory impairments
- Cranial nerve palsies
- Language and speech deficits
- Facial numbness
- Hearing disturbances
- Anosmia
- Swallowing difficulties
- Paralysis of outward gaze (6th cranial nerve)
- Papilledema
- Incoordination
- Ataxia
- In children, diastases of cranial sutures and enlarging head size

(Hickey, 1992). As the tumor grows, causing progressive destruction or dysfunction of tissue, locally referable signs may occur (hemiparesis, specific cranial nerve dysfunction, aphasia, visual symptoms, ataxia) which may help to localize the tumor site. Table 26–2 provides a list of signs associated with localized lesions.

Specific Primary Brain Tumors

There are several specific types of primary brain tumors, with similarities in medical management and implications for physical therapy. Therefore, the specific tumors are first presented individually, followed by a discussion of diagnosis, medical management, and therapy implications for all primary brain tumors. Table 26–3 lists the types of primary brain tumors and their percentage distribution.

Gliomas

Gliomas, the most prevalent of primary brain tumors, are tumors of the glial cells, the group of cells that support, insulate, and metabolically assist the neurons. Glial cells are derived from glioblasts. It is of interest to note that neurons, despite their prevalence in the CNS (100 billion in the adult brain, according to some authors), are rarely the cellular basis of neoplastic transformation.

Glial cells, which numerically exceed the number of neurons, are subdivided into astrocytes (star-shaped cells), which provide nutrition for neurons; oligodendrocytes (glial cells with few processes), which produce the myelin sheath of the axonal projections of neurons; and ependymal cells, which line the ventricles (Hickey, 1992). Gliomas are subdivided into *astrocytomas*, *oligodendrogliomas*, and *ependymomas*, named for the cell of origin of the tumor. *Medulloblastomas* are tumors of the vermis of the cerebellum and are classified by some authors as gliomas.

Astrocytomas are given histologic grades of I through IV to indicate the rate of cell division and the degree of differentiation from the original cell type (McGarvey and Walton, 1990). Grade I tumors are the slowest-growing, and grades II, III, and IV are progressively faster-growing with higher rates of mitosis (Pfeifer and Wick, 1995). Astrocytomas are capable at any time of converting to a higher grade. (See further discussion of grading of tumors in Chapter 7.)

Incidence. Gliomas are the most common of the primary brain tumors, accounting for 45% to 50% of all brain tumors, with men more frequently affected than women in a 3:2 ratio. Gliomas are divided into *benign gliomas*, which include low-grade astrocytomas (grades I and II), and *malignant gliomas*, which include anaplastic astrocytomas (grade III), glioblastoma multiforme (GBM) (grade IV), oligodendrogliomas, ependymomas, and medulloblastomas. Low-grade astrocytomas account for 10% to 15% of primary brain tumors (Weiss, 1995) and are the most common type of intracranial tumor in children. Malignant astrocytomas (anaplastic astrocytoma and GBM) are much more common in adults than low-grade astrocytomas, making up 20% to 30% of primary brain tumors. Oligodendrogliomas and ependymomas make up another 1% to 7%. Medulloblastomas make up 3% to 5% of primary brain tumors. Approximately 5000 new cases of malignant gliomas occur each year. The age of peak incidence is 45 to 55 years.

Etiology and Risk Factors. Relatively little is known about the cause of gliomas. They are characterized by a significant genetic heterogeneity, which makes the basic biology of glial neoplasms difficult to understand. It is thought there is a relationship with chromosome abnormalities.

Advances in the fields of molecular biology have allowed identification of mutated genes which increase the cell's susceptibility to the development of certain cancers. These mutated genes that lead to the development of cancer are known as oncogenes. (For further discussion of oncogenes, see Chapter 7.) Another type of chromosome abnormality leads to deletion of the cell's defense mechanism or its normal tumor-suppressing activity. A tumor-suppressing gene is known as an antioncogene. The presence of an oncogene and the absence of a tumor-suppressing gene may be only one step toward tumor formation. Tumorigenesis is thought to be a multistep process with other contributing factors in addition to chromosome abnormalities.

Certain chromosome abnormalities have been linked to specific brain tumor types (Snodgrass, 1994). The oncogene *c-sis* has been identified with GBM. The oncogene *C-erb*B has been identified in 30% of malignant gliomas and is associated with the transforming growth factor receptor. Chromosome 17 abnormalities have been demonstrated to be present in all grades of astrocytomas (Snodgrass, 1994). Oncogenes may have some bearing on other genetic disorders that are associated with brain tumors. Neurofibromatosis, or von Recklinghausen's disease (a familial condition involving the nervous system, muscles, bones, and skin and characterized by multiple soft tumors over the entire body associated with areas of pigmentation) is associated with spinal neuromas, acoustic neuromas, meningiomas, and gliomas. Tuberous sclerosis is associated with astrocytomas. Von Hippel-Lindau disease, a hereditary condition characterized by angiomatosis of the retina and cerebellum is associated with hemangioblastomas (Weiss, 1995). The best-described tumor-suppressor

TABLE 26–2 Signs Associated with Localized Lesions

Location of Lesion	Associated Signs
Prefrontal area	Loss of judgment, failure of memory, inappropriate behavior, apathy, poor attention span, easily distracted, release phenomena
Frontal eye fields	Failure to sustain gaze to opposite side, saccadic eye movements, impersistence, seizures with forced deviation of the eyes to the opposite side
Precentral gyrus	Partial motor seizures, jacksonian seizures, generalized seizures, hemiparesis
Superficial parietal lobe	Partial sensory seizures, loss of cortical sensation including two-point discrimination, tactile localization, stereognosis and graphism
Angular gyrus	Agraphia, acalculia, finger agnosia, allochiria (right-left confusion) (Gerstmann's syndrome)
Broca's area	Motor dysphasia
Superior temporal gyrus	Receptive dysphasia
Midbrain	Early hydrocephalus; loss of upward gaze; pupillary abnormalities; 3rd nerve involvement—ptosis, external strabismus, diplopia; ipsilateral cerebellar signs; contralateral hemiparesis; parkinsonism; akinetic mutism
Cerebellar hemisphere	Ipsilateral cerebellar ataxia with hypotonia, dysmetria, intention tremor, nystagmus to side of lesion
Pons	Sixth nerve involvement—diplopia, internal strabismus; 7th nerve involvement—ipsilateral facial paralysis; contralateral hemiparesis; contralateral hemisensory loss; ipsilateral cerebellar ataxia; locked-in syndrome
Medial surface of frontal lobe	Apraxia of gait, urinary incontinence
Corpus callosum	Left-hand apraxia and agraphia, generalized tonic-clonic seizures
Thalamus	Contralateral "thalamic pain," contralateral hemisensory loss
Temporal lobe	Partial complex seizures, contralateral homonymous upper quadrantanopsia
Paracentral lobule	Progressive spastic paraparesis, urgency of micturition, incontinence
Deep parietal lobe	Autotopagnosia, anosognosia, contralateral homonymous lower quadrantanopsia
Third ventricle	Paroxysmal headache, hydrocephalus
Fourth ventricle	Hydrocephalus, progressive cerebellar ataxia, progressive spastic hemiparesis or quadriparesis
Cerebellopontine angle	Hearing loss, tinnitus, cerebellar ataxia, facial pain, facial weakness, dysphagia, dysarthria
Olfactory groove	Ipsilateral anosmia, ipsilateral optic atrophy, contralateral papilledema (Foster-Kennedy syndrome)
Optic chiasm	Incongruous bitemporal field defects, bitemporal hemianopsia, optic atrophy
Orbital surface frontal lobe	Partial complex seizures, paroxysmal atrial tachycardia
Optic nerve	Visual failure of one eye, optic atrophy
Uncus	Partial complex seizures with olfactory hallucinations (uncinate fits)
Basal ganglia	Contralateral choreoathetosis, contralateral dystonia
Internal capsule	Contralateral hemiplegia, hemisensory loss, and homonymous hemianopsia
Pineal gland	Loss of upward gaze (Parinaud's syndrome), early hydrocephalus, lid retraction, pupillary abnormalities
Occipital lobe	Partial seizures with elementary visual phenomena, homonymous hemianopsia with macular sparing
Hypothalamus, pituitary	Precocious puberty (children), impotence, amenorrhea, galactorrhea, hypothyroidism, hypopituitarism, diabetes insipidus, cachexia, diencephalic autonomic seizures

From Gilroy J: Basic Neurology, ed 2. Elmsford, NY, Pergamon Press, 1990, pp 228–229.

genes are Rb and p53, associated with retinoblastoma and the Li-Fraumeni syndrome, a familial breast cancer associated with soft tissue sarcomas and other tumors.

No risk factors have been identified for the development of brain tumors. The effects of carcinogenic viruses or agents are unclear. There are interesting associations of viruses and brain tumors, such as the Epstein-Barr virus and primary CNS lymphoma, but they are insufficient to constitute direct cause-and-effect relationships. Sustained exposure to certain pesticides, vinyl chloride, nitrosoureas, and polycyclic hydrocarbons has been implicated in astrocytic tumors, but epidemiologic surveys of workers in the farming, petrochemical, and rubber industries have been conflicting (Thapar and Laws, 1995). Infection, trauma, immunosuppression, and radiation are other suspected triggers. It is known that radiation treatment for scalp ringworm in children is associated with an increased rate of developing brain tumors late in life (Gilroy, 1990).

Low-Grade Astrocytoma

Pathogenesis. A low-grade astrocytoma is a benign neoplasm that grows slowly and often becomes cystic. It is composed of astrocytes with densely staining nuclei and scanty cytoplasm and is usually relatively acellular. Cerebral astrocytoma presents as a solid, gray mass with indistinct boundaries (Fig. 26–2). There is a spectrum of differentiation from well-differentiated (grade I) tumors to more anaplastic (grade II) tumors (Gilroy, 1990). Astrocytomas in the cerebellum are often cystic and well circumscribed.

Clinical Manifestations. In adults, astrocytoma typically occurs in the third and fourth decades of life, is usually located in the cerebrum, most commonly in the frontal lobes, but may also be found in the temporal lobes, parietal lobes, basal ganglia, and occipital lobes. Astrocytoma usually appears in the cerebellum in children.

In adults initial symptoms typically are unilateral or focal

TABLE 26-3 PRIMARY BRAIN TUMORS

	PERCENTAGE OF ALL BRAIN TUMORS
Glioma	40–50
Astrocytoma grade I	5–10
Astrocytoma grade II	2–5
Astrocytoma grades III and IV (Glioblastoma multiforme)	20–30
Oligodendroglioma	1–4
Ependymoma (all grades)	1–3
Meningioma	12–20
Pituitary tumor	5–15
Neurinomas (primarily cranial nerve VIII)	3–10
Medulloblastoma	3–5

Adapted from Spencer D, Chyatte D, Collins WF, et al: Neurologic surgery. *In* Schwartz SI (ed): Principles of Surgery, ed 5. New York, McGraw-Hill, 1989, pp 1848.

headaches that become generalized as ICP increases. Frontal lobe tumors may produce personality disorders with changes in behavior and emotional state. Parietal and temporal lobe tumors may cause seizures on one side of the body. Occipital lobe tumors produce visual changes. Refer to Table 26–2 for more details of signs associated with tumor location. In time, astrocytomas, like other gliomas, tend to become more malignant.

In children, cerebellar astrocytomas lead to symptoms of unilateral cerebellar ataxia involving the limbs and trunk followed by signs of increased ICP.

Prognosis. Low-grade astrocytomas treated optimally have 5- to 10-year survival rates of 100% for completely excised lesions, and a 60% 5-year survival and 35% 10-year survival for partially excised lesions with radiation therapy. Untreated low-grade astrocytomas have a 5-year survival rate of 32% and a 10-year survival rate of 11% (Thapar and Laws, 1995). Despite the benign categorization, it must be understood that astrocytomas are nearly always infiltrative lesions, and generally progressive.

Anaplastic Astrocytoma and Glioblastoma Multiforme

Pathogeneis. Anaplastic astrocytoma, which includes grade III and IV astrocytomas, is a rapidly growing, aggressive, infiltrative tumor that is apt to invade both cerebral hemispheres via the corpus callosum. It is a pinkish-gray or multicolored, well-demarcated mass with scattered areas of grossly visible hemorrhage. The blood vessels show endothelial proliferation. There may be areas of cystic degeneration and a central area of creamy necrosis. The histologic distinction of an anaplastic astrocytoma from a glioblastoma is based largely on the absence or presence of tumor necrosis (Weiss, 1995). Microscopically, the tumor is pleomorphic (having various distinct forms) and hypercellular and the cells show hyperchromatic nuclei. There are many mitoses (cells in a state of division), giant cells, and young glial forms.

Clinical Manifestations. Glioblastoma multiforme most frequently arises in the frontal and temporal lobes, with the cerebellum, brainstem, and spinal cord being rare sites for adults. It most frequently occurs in the fifth and sixth decades of life. There is typically a rapid progression of signs and symptoms, with grade IV GBM being particularly aggressive. The presentation may be of unilateral headache that is followed by generalized headache, indicating an increase in ICP. The development of seizures is not unusual.

Prognosis. All malignant astrocytomas will eventually recur. With optimal treatment (excision, radiation therapy) clients with anaplastic astrocytoma (grade III) have a 70% 1-year survival, a 40% 2-year survival, and a 10% to 20% 5-year survival. GBM (grade IV) has a grimmer prognosis with

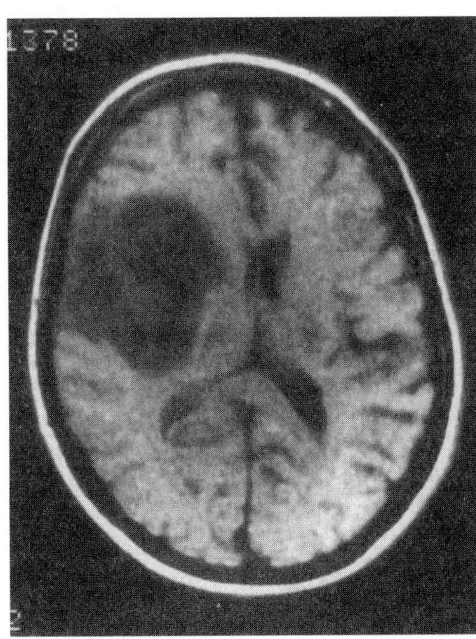

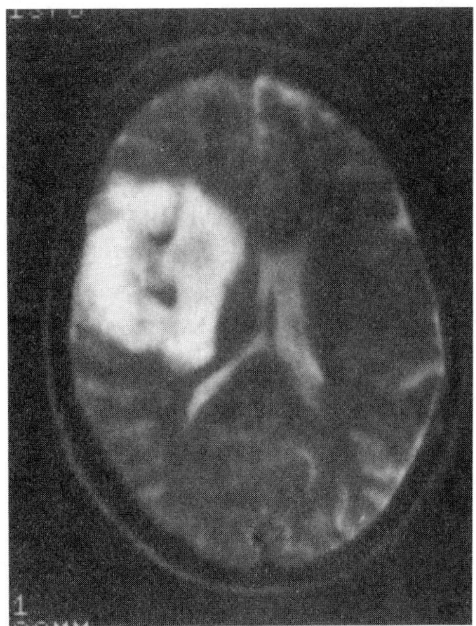

Figure **26–2.** Magnetic resonance T1-weighted image (*A*) and T2-weighted image (*B*) showing an abnormality in the right cerebral hemisphere, compatible with a low-grade astrocytoma or an oligodendroglioma. The individual has been asymptomatic for many years apart from occasional left-sided focal seizure activity. (*From Gilroy J: Basic Neurology, ed 2. Elmsford, NY, Pergamon Press, 1990.*)

a 50% 1-year survival, a less than 15% two-year survival, and rare long-term survival (Thapar and Laws, 1995).

Oligodendroglioma

Pathogenesis. Oligodendroglioma is a slow-growing, solid, calcified tumor arising from oligodendrocytes, the myelin-producing cells of the CNS, and stains for myelin basic protein. It is a gray-pink to red cystic area in the brain and has a honeycomb appearance at low microscopic power due to the presence of a fibrovascular stroma. On higher power the cells have a uniform appearance with a central nucleus surrounded by a clear cytoplasm, or a "fried egg" appearance. Mitotic figures are infrequent. Approximately 70% of these tumors show some evidence of calcification.

Clinical Manifestations. Oligodendrogliomas usually occur in adults and are located predominantly in the cerebral hemispheres, often in the frontal lobes. They expand toward the cortex and may spread through it and eventually attach to the dura (Gilroy, 1990). A history of partial or generalized seizures, usually of long duration, and sometimes with chronic headache, is the typical presentation pattern of oligodendrogliomas. They tend to bleed spontaneously and may present with a strokelike syndrome (Snodgrass, 1994). The hallmark of this tumor radiologically is calcification, which can be identified in the vast majority of people by computed tomography (CT).

Prognosis. With optimal treatment, 5- and 10-year survival rates are 83% to 100% and 45% to 55% respectively. Although post-treatment there may be a long interval of quiescence, oligodendrogliomas will eventually recur, often as a more aggressive tumor with progressing symptoms (Thapar and Laws, 1995).

Ependymoma

Pathogenesis. An ependymoma is a neoplasm derived from the ependymal cell lining of the ventricular system and the central canal of the spinal cord. It is usually reddish, lobulated, and well circumscribed, resembling a cauliflower in shape. Pseudorosette formation, in which the cells are arranged about a clear space or a blood vessel, may occur, and blepharoplasts (small round or rod-shaped intracytoplasmic bodies) may be seen.

Clinical Manifestations. Ependymoma is more common in the fourth ventricle, and is likely to be detected early because of the signs and symptoms of increased ICP in the posterior fossa (e.g., headache, nausea, vomiting, and papilledema). However, supratentorial ependymomas often grow large before detection. Ependymoma is much more prevalent in children than adults, and is the third most frequent posterior fossa neoplasm of children.

Prognosis. The prognosis for ependymomas is improving. Five-year survival rates exceed 80%. Ten-year survival rates are 40% to 60% (Thapar and Laws, 1995).

Medulloblastoma

Pathogenesis. Medulloblastoma is a rapidly growing malignant tumor. The cell of origin is unknown, but it is presumed to arise from the embryonal external granular layer of the cerebellum. It is considered to belong to a group of tumors known as *primitive neuroectodermal tumors* (PNETs). It characteristically metastasizes to the surface of the remaining CNS via the subarachnoid spaces. Grossly it is red and soft and is composed of many closely packed cells, with oval nuclei and many mitoses. Pseudorosette formations are common (Chusid, 1985). It is highly vascular, containing numerous small blood vessels.

Clinical Manifestations. Medulloblastoma is the most common malignant primary CNS tumor in children and the second most common posterior fossa tumor in children. It often develops in the cerebellar vermis and is very aggressive in younger children. Because of its proximity to the fourth ventricle, early development of hydrocephalus is common, along with other signs of cerebellar dysfunction, such as ataxia. Medulloblastomas tend to metastasize through CSF pathways, more predominantly into the spine but also into the supratentorial compartment.

Prognosis. Early in the century medulloblastomas were uniformly fatal tumors. Improvement in therapeutic strategies during the past 30 years has dramatically improved the prognosis. Favorable prognostic factors include age greater than 2 years, undisseminated local disease, and greater than 75% tumor resection. In these clients, the 5-year disease-free survival rate exceeds 60% to 70% in most studies (Thapar and Laws, 1995). In poorer-risk cases, the 5-year disease-free survival rate is about 45% (Thapar and Laws, 1995).

Nongliomas

Meningioma

Meningiomas are slow-growing, usually benign lesions. They occur most commonly along the dural folds and cerebral convexities, though they may occur in the spinal cord as well. Cytogenetic analysis has demonstrated multiple deletions on chromosome 22 in most people with meningioma.

Incidence. Meningiomas represent 12% to 20% of all intracranial neoplasms, and are the second most common primary intracranial tumor in adults and the most common of benign brain neoplasms. They are increased in neurofibromatosis. They are also increased in breast cancer clients. It is important prognostically and for treatment to differentiate a benign meningioma from a metastatic brain lesion originating from a breast cancer.

Pathogenesis. Meningiomas originate in the arachnoid layer of the meninges, and are believed to be derived from the cells and vascular elements of the meninges. They are well-circumscribed globular masses. They may infiltrate the dura, the dural sinuses, or bone, but generally do not invade the underlying brain parenchyma (Fig. 26–3). Meningiomas, because of their proximity to, or invasion of, the bone, are known to provoke a local osteoblastic response termed *hyperostosis*. This may cause a profuse local thickening of the skull.

Most meningiomas grow as well-encapsulated tumors, but others develop in relatively thin sheets along the dura.

Clinical Manifestations and Prognosis. Meningiomas are more common in the later years of life, and are more frequent

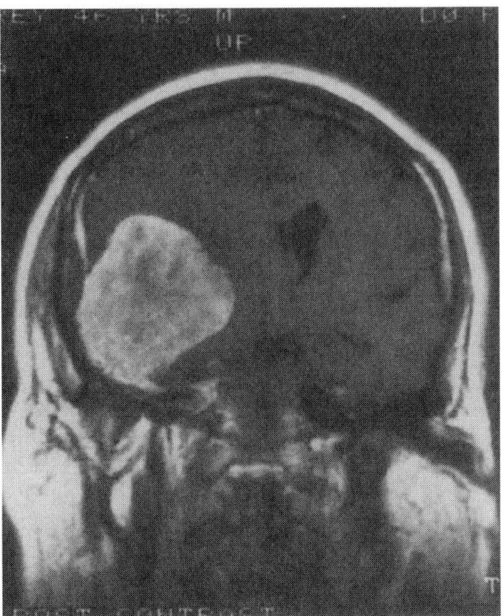

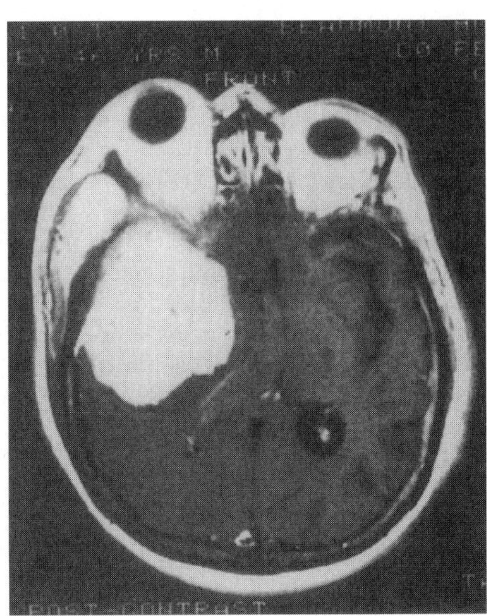

Figure **26–3.** A and B, CT scan showing a meningioma in the right middle cranial fossa with pressure on the right temporal lobe. There is a marked right-to-left shift of the ventricular system. (*From Gilroy J: Basic Neurology, ed 2. Elmsford, NY, Pergamon Press, 1990.*)

in women. Since they are slow-growing, abnormal signs and symptoms may evolve over a period of many years. When located in silent brain areas, some meningiomas can become very large before causing clinical symptoms. Also, they can be discovered incidentally as masses that show little or no growth over time. Neurologic abnormalities depend on the location of the tumor; seizures are a common finding in skull-based lesions.

Meningiomas, when completely resected (surgical accessibility determines excision capabilities), have excellent prospects of long-term cure. Ten-year survival rates for completely excised lesions are 80% to 90%. Partially resected meningiomas have a 50% to 70% 10-year progression-free survival. Malignant meningiomas, about 1% to 10% of meningiomas, have a shorter disease-free interval (Thapar and Laws, 1995).

Pituitary Adenomas

Pituitary adenomas are benign tumors derived from cells of the anterior portion of the pituitary gland. Although pituitary adenomas are the most common of the pituitary tumors, infrequently other types of pituitary tumors may occur in the location of the pituitary gland, or sella turcica (a saddle-shaped transverse depression on the superior surface of the body of the sphenoid bone), and may be primary or metastatic. See also Pituitary Gland, Chapter 9.

Incidence. Pituitary adenomas are common lesions, accounting for about 5% to 15% of all intracranial tumors. They are usually found in middle-aged or older people.

Pathogenesis. Small lesions of the pituitary gland are called microadenomas, are less than 10 mm in diameter, and may be asymptomatic. Larger tumors, or macroadenomas, compress the adjacent normal pituitary gland. Extension of the tumor above the sella turcica will compress the optic chiasm. Figure 26–4 gives the anatomic relations of the pituitary gland, optic chiasm, and surrounding parasellar structures.

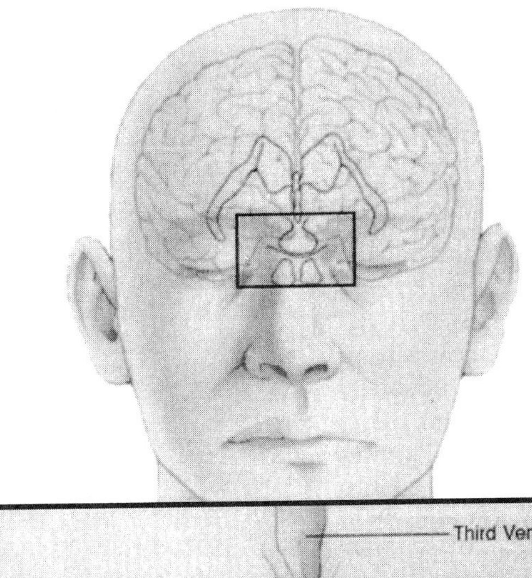

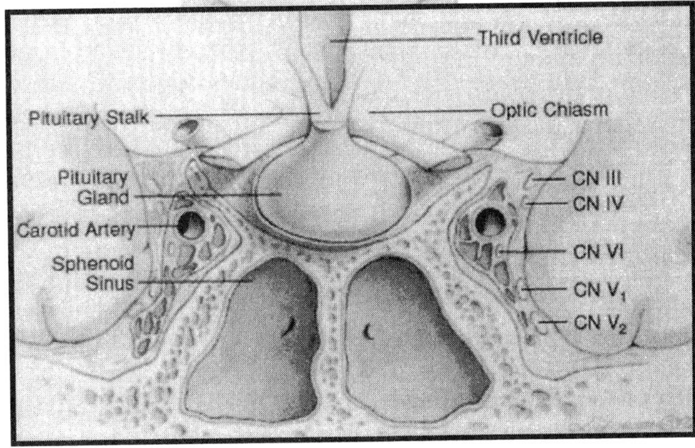

Figure **26–4.** Anatomic relations of pituitary gland and surrounding parasellar structures. (*From Thapar K, Laws ER: Tumors of the pituitary gland. In Murphy GP, Lawrence W, Lenhard RE (eds): American Cancer Society Textbook of Clinical Oncology, ed 2. Atlanta, American Cancer Society, 1995.*)

Clinical Manifestations and Prognosis. In the majority of pituitary tumors, the release of excess pituitary hormones or pituitary insufficiency results in dramatic and unique clinical syndromes. Galactorrhea and amenorrhea, gigantism and acromegaly, and the symptoms of Cushing's disease (hypertension, facial and truncal obesity, osteoporosis, muscle weakness, menstrual abnormalities, and female hirsutism) are among the hormonal symptoms. Pituitary insufficiency, or hypopituitarism, can lead to symptoms such as fatigue, weakness, hypogonadism. A second pattern of presentation consists of regression of secondary sexual characteristics and hypothyroidism. The third pattern of presentation is one of neurologic findings, including headache, bitemporal visual loss, and ocular palsy.

Tumors of the pituitary have become very treatable, with the majority of people enjoying long-term survival or cure. Because visual compromise is a complicating feature of many pituitary tumors, serially recorded visual field deficits can document disease progression as well as responses to treatment.

Neurinomas

Neurinomas are slow-growing, benign tumors originating from Schwann cells. In the brain they most commonly develop on the vestibular component of the eighth cranial nerve, and are called acoustic neurinomas or schwannomas. Acoustic neurinomas account for 3% to 10% of all brain tumors. They occur mainly in the fourth to sixth decades of life. About 5% occur in the context of neurofibromatosis. Neurinomas may also be found attached to other cranial nerves.

Pathogenesis. Acoustic neurinomas typically originate in the internal auditory canal in the transition zone of the oligodendroglial cells and peripheral nervous system Schwann cells. The tumor grows into the cerebellopontine angle, eventually compressing the facial nerve, and encroaches on the brainstem. Some lesions may remain relatively quiescent for long periods of time, but the majority are slow-growing progressive lesions. The tumor is thickly encapsulated, often highly vascular, and microscopically consists of spindle-shaped cells with rod-shaped nuclei often lying in parallel rows.

Clinical Manifestations and Prognosis. Acoustic neurinomas typically present with progressive unilateral sensorineural hearing loss. Other symptoms include tinnitus, vertigo, and unsteadiness. Facial numbness and difficulty swallowing may occur, and weakness of the facial muscles is generally a late feature. Deformity and obstruction of the fourth ventricle leads to hydrocephalus with headache, vomiting, and other symptoms of increased ICP.

In the majority of cases cure is achieved with surgical resection. As acoustic neurinomas are slow-growing, and surgery often accelerates hearing loss, the decision to delay surgery until necessary may be made. However, because the likelihood of hearing retention is greatest when the tumor is small, surgery may be done as soon as possible.

Choroid Plexus Papilloma

This is a low-grade neoplasm of the choroid plexus, the vascular coat along the ventricles carrying blood vessels within the pia mater to each ventricle. It is relatively rare, and is usually found in children. It is often associated with overproduction of CSF and hydrocephalus. Complete removal of the tumor usually results in an excellent prognosis, and resolution of the hydrocephalus. The prognosis for choroid plexus carcinoma, another variation of a choroid plexus tumor, is dismal.

Pinealoma

Pineal region tumors are rare (1% of all intracranial tumors), more common in children, and more common in males than females. These are a heterogeneous group of tumors. Germ cell pinealomas have an embryonal basis and although some are very radiosensitive, others are aggressive, highly malignant, and generally incurable. Pineal parenchymal tumors have a tendency to craniospinal dissemination. Pineal region tumors typically result in obstructive hydrocephalus because of the proximity of the pineal gland to the ventricular system. Ocular abnormalities may also occur.

Management is by shunting the hydrocephalus, if present; radiation therapy; and/or surgical excision. Responsive tumors have a 5-year survival of 70% (Thapar and Laws, 1995). Nonresponsive pineal region tumors have a 1-year survival of only 33%.

Craniopharyngioma

Craniopharyngiomas are histologically benign congenital tumors, and occur most commonly in the suprasellar region in children and adults. They account for 2% to 3% of all intracranial tumors. Based on the location, craniopharyngiomas can compromise a number of important intracranial structures and produce multiple signs and symptoms which include ICP, visual disorders, neuroendocrine disorders, hypothalamus involvement, cranial nerve palsies, hydrocephalus, and progressive dementia. Optimal treatment is controversial, but radiation and/or surgical resection are used. With complete resections or resections followed by radiation therapy, 10-year survival rates of 78% have been reported.

Epidermoid and Dermoid Tumors (Cysts)

These rare benign tumors arise from imperfect embryogenesis of the CNS and account for 2% of intracranial tumors. They are composed of desquamated epidermal cellular debris, keratin, and cholesterol. They grow in basal regions of the brain and tend to enlarge along CSF pathways. The dermoid tumor has the epidermal cellular debris, but mixed with additional dermal elements such as hair, hair follicles, sweat glands, and sebaceous glands. These tumors present with seizures and increased ICP. Complete surgical excision of the tumor capsule and contents is curative (Thapar and Laws, 1995).

Hemangioblastomas

These tumors typically arise in the posterior fossa, primarily in the cerebellar vermis or pons, as solitary lesions with an uncertain origin. Hemangioblastomas are a vascular conglomerate of endothelial cells, pericytes (peculiar elongated cells with the power of contraction, found wrapped about precapillary arterioles), and stromal cells. They make up 2% of all intracranial tumors, are the most common adult intra-axial tumor of the posterior fossa, and occur more commonly in males. These highly vascular tumors attached to the wall of a surrounding cyst are often associated with von Hippel-Lindau syndrome. Hemangioblastomas are considered benign, and complete surgical excision for tumors arising in the cerebellum is curative.

Chordomas

Chordomas rarely arise in the brain and represent less than 1% of all intracranial neoplasms. They are much more typical in the axial skeleton, preferring the clivus (in the posterior cranial fossa), sacrum, and nonsacral spine. They are tumors of bone, presumed to arise from the embryonal notochord remnants. They are considered histologically benign, but have a locally destructive nature, progressive course, and metastatic behavior (Thapar and Laws, 1995). Cranial chordomas typically involve the skull base with a destructive process that invades rostrally into the optic chiasm, into the brainstem, or ventrally into the sinuses. Because of surgical inaccessibility, curative resections are difficult if not impossible. Median survival ranges from 4.2 to 5.2 years, with recurrences likely (Thapar and Laws, 1995).

Primary Central Nervous System Lymphoma

Primary CNS lymphoma (PCNSL) is a non-Hodgkin's lymphoma, and occurs in the absence of systemic lymphoma. This tumor was formerly quite rare, but in the past 15 years has tripled in frequency in the immunodeficient population, that is, clients with acquired immunodeficiency syndrome (AIDS) and collagen vascular disorders, and the congenitally immunodeficient (Weiss, 1995) (see Chapter 10, Box 10–13). It currently accounts for 15% of all primary brain tumors (Thapar and Laws, 1995).

The pathophysiologic basis for development of these tumors is unclear. A large percentage begin as solitary cerebral lesions, but eventually develop into multiple lesions. They typically assume a periventricular pattern, involving the deep white matter, basal ganglia, corpus callosum, and thalamus.

Symptoms and signs generally evolve over several months, including increased ICP (headaches, nausea and vomiting, and generalized seizures). Focal neurologic signs may occur. The appearance on magnetic resonance imaging (MRI) or CT of multiple deep cerebral and periventricular lesions, along with an immunodeficient state, contributes to the diagnosis.

The prognosis is generally poor, with median survival of 10 to 14 months, although adding systemic chemotherapy (methotrexate and cytosine arabinoside) to radiation has improved median survival to 42 months (Thapar and Laws, 1995).

Diagnosis of Primary Brain Tumors

When a brain tumor is suspected on clinical evaluation, a thorough neurologic examination and brain imaging studies are done to confirm its presence and exact location.

MRI has evolved as the most informative brain imaging study due to its superior imaging capabilities and lack of artifact from the temporal bones. With the addition of the gadolinium contrast agent enhancement, which distinguishes tumor from surrounding edema, MRI detects tumors even a few millimeters in size. MRI also defines critical anatomic relationships between the tumor and surrounding neurovascular structures. The multiplanar capability of MRI allows optimal visualization of the anatomy. However, in intraventricular masses, although MRI has many advantages over CT, there are only a few instances when MRI will significantly alter the differential diagnosis (McConachie et al., 1994).

The CT scan is effective in revealing most brain tumors and is widely accessible and convenient. Although its brain imaging capabilities are inferior to MRI, it can identify cerebral edema, midline shift, and ventricular compression of obstructive hydrocephalus. In intraventricular masses, CT is highly sensitive in detecting calcification. Intravenous contrast greatly increases the sensitivity of CT scan for brain tumors.

Although MRI or CT scanning usually provides sufficient information on which to base treatment, occasionally additional tests may be indicated to further delineate the tumor and identify possible surgical hazards. These additional tests include cerebral angiography, which delineates the vascularity within the brain and can help to determine the best surgical approach; visual field and funduscopic examination to identify visual defects that are specific to a particular area; audiometric studies to determine hearing loss; chest films to rule out lung cancer with metastatic lesions to the brain; other studies to rule out a primary lesion outside the brain when a metastatic lesion is suspected; and endocrine studies when a pituitary adenoma or craniopharyngioma is suspected (Hickey, 1992).

Medical Management of Primary Brain Tumors

Surgery, radiation therapy, chemotherapy, and immunotherapy are the treatment options for brain tumors. Management of symptoms and side effects is a major component of medical management.

Treatment

Surgery

Surgical excision is the most important form of initial therapy as it provides histologic confirmation of the tumor and a basis for determining the treatment and prognosis. Surgery reduces tumor load and quickly relieves the ICP and mass effect, thereby improving neurologic function. This cytoreduction may reduce symptoms and enhance the effectiveness of adjuvant therapy (e.g., radiation therapy). The technological and conceptual advances in neurosurgery (intraoperative magnification, ultrasonic aspirators, microinstrumentation, computer-based stereotactic resection procedures, and so on) have allowed safer and more finite approaches to previously inaccessible tumors (Thapar and Laws, 1995).

The goal of surgery is total excision, while minimizing trauma to vital neural structures. For the infiltrative intra-axial lesions, where total excision is not possible, the goal is to provide a measure of temporary control by reducing mass effect and ICP. If the preoperative neurologic deficit is due to destruction of brain tissue by tumor, surgical resection will not improve the situation. But if the deficit is compression-related from the tumor, excision may relieve the compression and allow the deficit to improve. In the case of many benign extra-axial tumors (e.g., meningiomas, schwannomas, pituitary adenomas), cure can be achieved.

Operative complications include hemorrhage, infection, seizures, hydrocephalus due to an impairment of CSF absorption, and neuroendocrine disturbances, especially if surgery is in the region of the pituitary. Brain edema, usually present before surgery, may be severely aggravated during surgery.

Corticosteroids are usually given for several days prior to craniotomy to reduce preoperative edema. Improved surgical techniques have reduced the complications of hemorrhage, infection, and permanent neurologic injury to less than 10% of cases (Thapar and Laws, 1995).

Specific operative techniques include craniotomy and stereotactic biopsy. *Craniotomy* is the resection of the skull overlying the tumor, removal of the tumor, and replacement of the bone flap (Fig. 26–5). *Stereotactic biopsy* of the lesion without craniotomy is used when deep mass lesions are surgically unresectable or when the risk of craniotomy outweighs the benefits. Stereotactic procedures involve creating a burr hole in the brain at an exact location using a computer, radiologic equipment, and a special head-fixation device.

Radiation Therapy

Radiation therapy following surgical resection is of proven effectiveness for most malignant brain tumors. Various brain tumors have different susceptibilities to radiation therapy, but the survival advantage is unquestionable. Unresectable or incompletely resected tumors are especially candidates for radiation therapy. Established radiation doses that avoid exceeding thresholds of CNS tolerance are in the range of 40 to 60 Gy (4000–6000 rad).

Radiation is delivered to a localized area of the brain to minimize the volume of tissue irradiated. Acute reactions to radiation are a result of acute brain swelling, occur during or immediately after radiation, and manifest as an increase in neurologic deficit or increased ICP. Steroid therapy is given to reduce this effect during radiation therapy. A similar delayed postirradiation syndrome 1 to 3 months after radiation can also be controlled by steroids. A third brain reaction known as radiation necrosis may occur months to years after irradiation, and is severe and irreversible. It is presumed to be the result of direct toxic effects on the brain and its microvasculature. There is progressive deterioration, dementia, and focal neurologic signs.

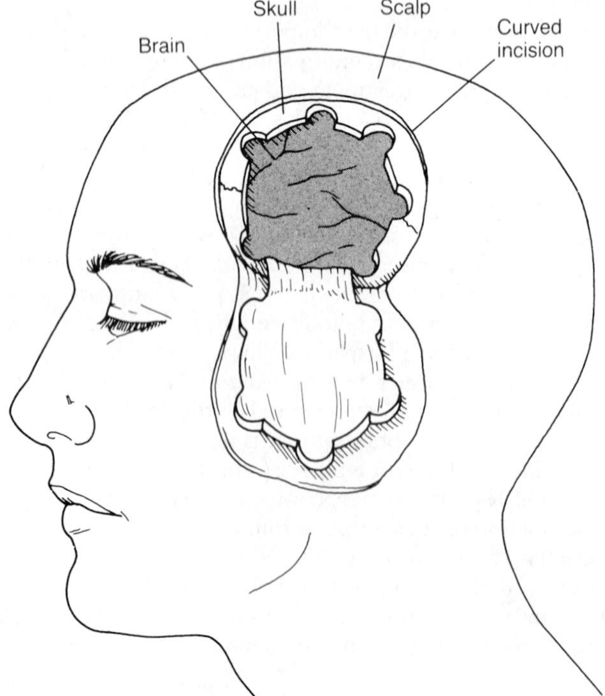

Figure 26–5. Craniotomy with osteoplastic bone flap. (*From Schnell SS: Nursing care of clients with cerebral disorders.* In *Black JM, Matassarin-Jacobs E (eds): Luckmann and Sorensen's Medical-Surgical Nursing, ed 4. Philadelphia, WB Saunders, 1993, p 734.*)

As survival time increases, other long-term complications of irradiation are of concern. Hypopituitarism, radiation-induced occlusive disease of cerebral vessels, and radiation-induced oncogenesis, as well as myelopathies from spinal axis irradiation are included in these complications. White matter injuries have been shown to correlate significantly with radiation dose in long-term survivors (greater than 18 months). These changes correlate with functional neurologic status (Corn et al., 1994), including altered mental status, speech impairments, motor deficit, cranial nerve deficit, personality changes, and other neurologic signs.

Advances in radiation have led to newer methods of radiation delivery. Interstitial radiation therapy, or brachytherapy, involves the placing of the radiation source, such as radium seeds, within the tumor for a period of several days. Brachytherapy has shown promise with GBM and other primary brain tumors. Stereotactic radiosurgery is a technique to deliver a large single fraction of highly focal radiation to a brain tumor. It was originally used to treat functional disorders (e.g., pain and movement disorders), but has recently been used in the treatment of primary and metastatic brain tumors (Loeffler et al., 1995).

The advantages of radiosurgery over surgery are that it avoids risk of hemorrhage, infection, and tumor seeding; links treatment directly to three-dimensional visualization, which reduces the chances of a marginal miss; and requires minimal hospitalization (Loeffler et al., 1995). There are three methods: (1) the gamma knife uses high-energy photon beams from cobalt 201 sources, each directed at a specific isocenter; (2) the linear accelerator-based systems, which are more widely available, deliver high-energy photon beams using converging arcs which intersect at the target site; and (3) the synchrocyclotron proton beam therapy delivers heavy charged particle beams through a small number of portals in the skull (Thapar and Laws, 1995).

Although the gamma knife and the proton beam therapy equipment are of limited availability and expensive, the use of these modalities is rapidly increasing and data on their effectiveness and neurotoxicity are becoming available (Shaw et al., 1995). Radiotherapy may prove increasingly to be a beneficial modality of client care (Schwade and Wolf, 1995) as it becomes more available and easier to deliver, and cooperation between radiation oncologists and neurosurgeons increases. In time, technological modifications will allow treatment at other sites, such as the spine.

Chemotherapy

Chemotherapy has been extensively studied in brain tumors, but has yet to make a dramatic difference in the management of brain tumors, except for certain pediatric neoplasms such as medulloblastoma (Thapar and Laws, 1995).

The blood-brain barrier restricts access to most antitumor agents. A small number of agents are able to transit the blood-brain barrier, including the nitrosoureas (carmustine or BCNU), hydroxyureas, and diaziquone.

BCNU is currently the most effective cytotoxic agent against malignant glioma (Weiss, 1995). Other agents, such as procarbazine, oral lomustine (CCNU), and streptozocin are effective as well.

To bypass the blood-brain barrier, intrathecal (through an Ommaya reservoir surgically placed in the scalp with its tube inserted into the lateral ventricle) or intra-arterial (intracarotid) delivery of other agents, such as methotrexate, vincristine, or cisplatin, can be accomplished. Addition of chemotherapy to surgery and irradiation for malignant gliomas does provide some increases in survival—24-month survival up to 23.4% from 15.9% (Thapar and Laws, 1995).

Immunotherapy

Immunotherapy or biotherapy is the most infrequently used and least proven therapy for brain tumors. Immunotherapy, originally the use of donor serum containing preformed antibodies, now includes the use of interferons and interleukin-2 (see Chapter 4) to boost immune function (Hickey, 1992). The depressed immunocompetence of clients with malignant glioma gives at least a theoretical basis for the potential roles of biologic response modifiers in the treatment of these tumors. Preliminary studies have shown some promise (Thapar and Laws, 1995).

Symptom Management

Brain tumors lead to edema of tissue surrounding the tumor and brain swelling can be massive and extend the neurologic deficits caused by the tumor alone. Antiinflammatory drugs (corticosteroids, such as dexamethasone [Decadron], prednisone, hydrocortisone) are used to provide prompt and effective reduction in peritumoral edema. Improvement in symptoms of ICP and in focal neurologic signs begins within 24 to 48 hours after steroid initiation, and by the fourth and fifth day the maximum degree of improvement is obtained (Weiss, 1995).

Corticosteroids are generally used perioperatively, and are gradually tapered following tumor resection because long-term high-dose corticosteroids precipitate undesirable side effects. Corticosteroids may also be used peri-irradiation, as radiation also precipitates edema. Upon tumor recurrence or progression, corticosteroids may again be instituted to temporarily maximize residual neurologic function.

It is possible for a brain tumor to cause an acute increase in ICP that may be life-threatening because of imminent cerebral herniation. Quick-acting agents are needed to lower the pressure. Mannitol is used as a temporary agent to quickly reduce brain water and relieve the pressure. Steroids are used in conjunction with mannitol to decrease edema.

Anticonvulsants may also be needed to prevent or control seizure activity. These drugs are also used before and after surgery to control symptoms, and are continued as long as they are indicated (Chase, 1991).

Brain tumors also cause a variety of motor, speech, hearing, visual, and other neurologic signs and symptoms. While control of the tumor and edema through medical management is the first priority, residual neurologic problems can significantly lower the quality of life. Timely referral to rehabilitation specialists for management of these functional deficits is important. Splinting, bracing, motor and balance evaluation and training, incontinence training, home adaptation, activities of daily living (ADL) retraining, speech therapy, hearing adaptations, auditory retraining, and vision programs are available to improve and alleviate these functional deficits.

Other specialists are also part of the rehabilitation team. Enterostomal therapists provide help with ostomies; pharmacists provide assistance with pain management; the oncology nurse provides symptom management, psychosocial support, and education; the nutritionist provides diet and nutrition counseling; the social worker assists with community resources and placement in settings for necessary further care; and clergy provide assistance in personal and religious issues.

The psychosocial implications of brain tumors are enormous. Referral to psycho-oncological specialists for alleviation of psychological distress and family disruption, and promotion of role reorganization and adaptation are often of great value. Support groups, psychotropic medications, oncology educational classes for the client and family, and enrollment in one-on-one support programs can be very helpful.

Special Implications for the Therapist 26-1

PRIMARY BRAIN TUMORS

Rehabilitation Referrals

Therapists will undoubtedly encounter clients with brain tumors in their practice. Because clients with brain neoplasms often have mobility and neuromuscular problems such as paresis and balance difficulties, as well as loss of self-care skills, referrals to physical therapy are common. Therapists are likely to see people with brain tumors in all practice settings—acute and subacute care, pediatrics, geriatrics, neurologic practice, skilled nursing facilities, home health, and nursing homes. The person with a brain tumor may also be found in unrelated practice settings when, for example, the presenting problem is cervical pain complicated by a history of a brain tumor, or when the signs and symptoms of a yet undiagnosed brain tumor bring the person to therapy (e.g., unsteady gait and poor balance).

Knowledge Needed for Rehabilitation

A general knowledge of primary brain tumors and their treatment is imperative to provide the therapist with skills for evaluation, treatment planning, and goal setting for this population. Knowledge of malignant vs. benign status, disease progression expectations, complications, precautions, and prognosis are needed to plan treatment and establish goals. The therapist should also be aware of expected focal symptoms in relation to tumor location to anticipate functional changes that may require treatment modifications. It is important to have a working knowledge of the more prevalent brain tumor types, and to be able to differentiate, for example, between a meningioma (a benign, potentially curable tumor) and a malignant glioma (a rapidly growing fatal tumor). Goal setting with the client and family and the appropriate treatment approach to the functional problems may be significantly different when cure is possible compared to when rapid decline is anticipated.

Acute Postoperative Management

When a referral is received for acute postoperative rehabilitation therapy, awareness of general postoperative complications, including atelectasis, pneumonia, cardiac irregularities, fluid and electrolyte imbalances, and renal and gastrointestinal disorders, is important. Observing the client closely during therapy intervention for any significant signs and symptoms, and making appropriate adaptations during therapy, are part of the role of the therapist (Schnell, 1993).

Postoperative Complications of Intracranial Surgery

Potential complications of intracranial surgery may be very serious, even fatal, because of the significant functions performed by the structures involved. Some postoperative complications may improve; others may be permanent.

Increased ICP (due to cerebral edema or bleeding) is the major complication of intracranial surgery. Findings may include decreased level of consciousness with headaches, visual and speech disturbances, muscle weakness or paralysis, pupil changes, seizures, vomiting, and respiratory changes.

Because of increased ICP, further surgical intervention may be needed to release excess fluid. A catheter may be inserted to drain excess fluid from a ventricle or other fluid-filled space, or a Jackson-Pratt suction drain may be needed. CSF leaks postoperatively are evidenced by saturation of the surgical head dressing, or leaking of a clear, thin fluid from the ear or nose that dries in concentric circles.

Management of the postoperative client with increased ICP typically includes, among other things, elevation of the head. A position with the client's head elevated about 20 degrees is often prescribed. The client should be protected from any position that allows stasis of the CSF drainage and should be taught to observe the drainage and to be aware of signs of infection. The client should also be instructed against coughing, sneezing, or blowing the nose.

An erratic body temperature may occur after intracranial surgery. Either hypothermia or hyperthermia may be present. The therapist should check with the nursing staff before beginning therapy if there is a concern about abnormal temperature.

Seizures may also occur, and precautions should be taken during therapy. Meningitis may also occur, caused by irritation of the meninges by infection or blood in the subarachnoid space. If it develops, meningitis typically appears 2 or 3 days after surgery. Chills, fever, nuchal rigidity, headache, irritability, decreased level of consciousness, and increased sensitivity to light are signs of meningitis. It is essential that all care providers practice infection prevention measures such as thorough handwashing when caring for clients that have had intracranial surgery.

Awareness of other signs, such as ecchymosis, periorbital edema, stress ulcer, swallowing and aspiration concerns, and impaired airway protection, is important. Respiratory changes should be monitored carefully. An abnormal respiratory rate and depth may indicate rising ICP. By carefully observing the client during therapy, protecting the client from harm, and alerting nursing staff and physicians to any seizure activity or other adverse signs and symptoms, the therapist can provide a valuable adjunct to postoperative care.

Positioning in the Acute Postoperative Phase

If there is any question about positioning of a client during therapy, check with the nursing staff. Incorrect positioning may have serious, possibly fatal, consequences. The client should not be positioned on the operative side if there is no bone flap. Guidelines for head position include the following: (1) After surgery above the tentorium in the acute phase, do not lower the client's head without the neurosurgeon's direction. (2) If the neurosurgeon orders the client's head to remain flat after supratentorial surgery to remove a chronic subdural hematoma, avoid any activity that would elevate the head until cleared by the neurosurgeon. (3) After surgery below the tentorium, the client may be kept flat and turned every 2 hours. Do not turn client on his or her back, as it could result in serious life-threatening pressure on vital brainstem structures. (4) For posterior fossa surgery, the client is typically positioned on the side with a pillow under the head. This protects the operative site from pressure and minimizes tension on the suture line.

If a bone flap was removed for decompression, place the client only on the side not operated on or the back. This facilitates brain expansion. The client should be turned from the back to the side not operated on if a bone flap is not present.

If a client is neurologically unstable, and with ICP in a critical range (more than 20 mm Hg), avoid therapy procedures that require a flat position (e.g., lowering the head of the bed for range-of-motion [ROM] exercises). Use a pillow under the client's head to facilitate good venous outflow. When the client is side-lying, protect the hips from sharp flexion, which increases ICP.

Treatment Preparation

Before treatment, review the medical chart; the surgical, radiology, and pathology reports; laboratory values; nursing and other reports; and, if needed, call physicians for pertinent information. Hematologic values may be of critical importance for exercise training plans.

Familiarity with cancer terminology aids communication with others on the team. For example, a knowledge of the terminology of tumor staging and grading, of the presence of an Ommaya reservoir, and of the various types of central lines, facilitates interdisciplinary care planning and intervention. The Karnofsky scale (Table 26–4), a functional performance scale, is used in oncology to indicate the client's activity level in the hospital, home, or community, for example, a client's candidacy for home discharge with home health assistance, or need for more supervised care.

Initial outcomes expected for clients with brain surgery include full ROM, active where possible, of all

TABLE 26-4 Karnofsky Performance Status Scale

Condition	Percentage	Comments
Able to carry on normal activity and to work. No special care is needed.	100	Normal; no complaints; no evidence of disease
	90	Able to carry on normal activity; minor signs or symptoms of disease
	80	Normal activity with effort; some signs or symptoms of disease
Unable to work. Able to live at home, care for most of personal needs. A varying degree of assistance is needed.	70	Cares for self; unable to carry on normal activity or to do active work
	60	Requires occasional assistance but is able to care for most needs
	50	Requires considerable assistance and frequent medical care
Unable to care for self. Requires equivalent of institutional or hospital care. Disease may be progressing rapidly.	40	Disabled; requires special care and assistance
	30	Severely disabled; hospitalization is indicated, although death is not imminent
	20	Hospitalization is necessary; very sick; active supportive treatment necessary
	10	Moribund; fatal processes progressing rapidly
	1	Unconscious
	0	Dead

From Baird SB, McCorkle R, Grant M: Cancer Nursing: A Comprehensive Textbook. Philadelphia: WB Saunders, 1991.

extremities, and optimal functioning of respiratory, cardiovascular, and other systems within the precautions indicated. When the client is stable, functional outcomes include independent bed mobility and transfers, ambulation, and self-care skills (ADLs).

Rehabilitation Evaluation for Postoperative Care

During the acute postoperative phase, a thorough evaluation within the constraints of the precautions, including strength, joint ROM, sensory and perceptual status, neurologic signs, pain patterns, and mobility, helps to identify treatable impairments that affect function. During evaluation and treatment, avoidance of any Valsalva maneuver that would increase intrathoracic pressure, thus increasing ICP, is imperative. The therapist should avoid jarring the client's bed or causing sudden movements that would increase pain.

Rehabilitation Intervention

After intracranial surgery, observe the bed rest precautions, usually for 24 hours. If the client is stable, passive ROM exercises may begin. Position changes are important, and use of the draw sheet and adequate help ensure that the patient will not strain with position change and increase ICP. When movement to the bedside chair is safe, lift the client to a reclining chair by a draw sheet with the help of several caregivers, and gradually raise the client's back and head to protect him or her from straining. Bedside sit-and-dangling exercises may also be requested. Blood pressure checks for postural hypotension, close assessment for dizziness and faintness, and monitoring of respiratory and heart rates during activities are essential.

Subacute and Ambulatory Rehabilitation

As the patient becomes more stable and is moved into lower levels of acuity of care, including ambulatory care, further evaluation and progression of the treatment may now be possible. Continued monitoring of vital signs, of any neurologic change, and of any adverse indications such as seizures is important.

Reviewing diagnostic information, laboratory reports, and medical treatment continues to be important as the patient moves into new phases of care. Medical treatment modalities and side effects have a pronounced effect on the client's participation in therapy. Chemotherapeutic and radiation side effects, such as myelosuppression, nausea, and fatigue, may temporarily lower energy levels, requiring adjustment of the therapy program for fatigue. Irradiated areas should be protected against skin injury. No heat or cold or topical agents should be used in the irradiated area during the treatment series or for several weeks after the treatment series until the skin damage has cleared. If there is persistent trophic change in the skin with obvious circulatory impairment, heat or cold should not be applied over the site because of poor dissipation effects.

Steroid Effects

Awareness of steroid effects is important. A person currently receiving radiation to the brain may be placed on dexamethasone during the radiation series, and may demonstrate improved hemiparesis, for example, as a result. However, when radiation therapy is completed and steroid therapy is discontinued, the hemiparesis may worsen. The therapist's approach to the client and family should address any mobility planning issues in view of these possible changes. Likewise, edema fluctuations from the tumor effect itself may cause a puzzling improvement and regression in neurologic status. It is important to approach these cases without creating false hope when there is improved status from edema reduction, or expressing inappropriate negative attitudes when the edema flares.

Long-term management may include family training and education, and more advanced treatment toward self-care and safety. Throughout the rehabilitation process, it is important to avoid activities that increase ICP such as vigorous resistive exercises or isometrics.

Psychosocial Impact

The impact of the diagnosis may be difficult for the client to comprehend. The client who does comprehend may demonstrate extreme behavioral responses or a profound sense of hopelessness. The client should be encouraged to ask questions and express his or her feelings about the situation. The caregiver's support, realistic reassurance, and inclusion of the client and family in the decision-making process will have a positive impact on the quality of life (Hickey, 1992).

Because the diagnosis of a brain tumor is so devastating to the client and family, creating fear and uncertainty, the therapist must have sufficient maturity and psychosocial skills to act in a supportive and understanding way. The challenge is not to provide solutions to these psychosocial problems, but to provide support and validation, and to facilitate referrals to appropriate professionals while addressing the physical problem for which the person was referred.

The Rehabilitation Team

The therapist involved in rehabilitation of the person with a brain tumor is part of a rehabilitation team of professionals that also may be involved in the care. The team may include representatives from nursing, nutrition, respiratory therapy, speech therapy, social work, the chaplain's office, and the physician office staff. An interdisciplinary approach allows access to needed resources.

The therapist must understand that the term "cancer rehabilitation" is used by many other specialists and community programs that provide services for the person with cancer. The American Cancer Society has a rehabilitation program that includes support groups and services. Oncology nurses have become increasingly supportive of cancer rehabilitation and an interdisciplinary approach (Mayer and O'Conner, 1989). Many local groups, such as church and synagogue support groups, provide another aspect of rehabilitation.

In some acute care and outpatient settings, the therapist may be fortunate enough to be part of a more formalized cancer rehabilitation program. The advantages for the client with access to such a program include early and appropriate referrals to skilled professionals and resources, coordination of care and information, and a smooth transition across the continuum of care. Other advantages include enhancement of program development due to collaboration of professionals, outcome studies that will improve the quality of care, and the potential for rehabilitation research.

PRIMARY INTRASPINAL TUMORS

Primary spinal cord tumors are about one sixth as common as primary brain tumors. The histologic types of tumor cells in the spinal cord are the same as those found in the brain, although the prevalence of certain types may differ. The most common tumor in the spinal cord is the schwannoma or neurinoma followed by the meningioma and glioma.

A convenient anatomic classification system of spinal cord tumors is based on the relationship of the tumor to the spinal cord and dura. Figure 26–6 diagrams the location and relative incidence of spinal tumors. Intradural-intramedullary tumors arise within the spinal cord substance. Intradural-extramedullary tumors arise outside the spinal cord but within the dura. Extradural spinal cord tumors arise outside the spinal cord and the dura.

The specific spinal cord tumor types and incidence are discussed first followed by the clinical presentation and medical management.

Intradural-Intramedullary Tumors

Intradural-intramedullary tumors are the least common type of primary intraspinal tumors in adults, but the most common type in children. These tumors account for 5% to 10% of intraspinal tumors. The dominant tumor types are astrocytomas and ependymomas.

Because they are located within the cord itself, intradural-intramedullary tumors are generally derived from the cellular substrate of the spinal cord, such as the astrocytes and ependymal cells, or from the primitive embryonal cells. Astrocytomas may occur anywhere along the spinal cord, and may span several cord segments longitudinally. In children they may run the entire length of the cord.

Although all astrocytomas are infiltrative, most are low-grade and slow-growing in the spinal cord. Ependymomas are generally slow-growing as well, and less infiltrative, and therefore more amenable to surgical excision. Other less frequent types of intradural-intramedullary tumors are hemangiomas, epidermoid and dermoid cysts, teratomas, lipomas, and neuroenteric cysts. Of interest to therapists is chemical meningitis with its significant chronic pain that can occur when epidermoid or dermoid cysts leak debris into the CSF.

Intradural-Extramedullary Tumors

Intradural-extramedullary tumors are the most common type of primary intraspinal tumor in the adult, and account for about 45% of all spinal tumors. Schwannomas and meningiomas are the dominant tumors in this group. Meningiomas are 10 times more common in women than men, and occur in middle age.

Intradural-extramedullary tumors are primary derived from the supporting elements of the CNS, including the meninges and nerve sheath. Occasionally tumors in this compartment are carried down by the CSF from malignant brain tumors (medulloblastomas, ependymomas). Intradural-extramedullary tumors cause compression of the spinal cord, rather than invasion of the cord. Schwannomas are soft, globular masses that arise at the sensory or dorsal nerve root. Occasionally they may straddle the intervertebral foramen and extend outside the foramen, forming the so-called dumbbell configuration. Spinal meningiomas are benign, slow-growing globular tumors that often grow in the thoracic, cervical, and foramen magnum regions. They may be present for many years before symptoms occur.

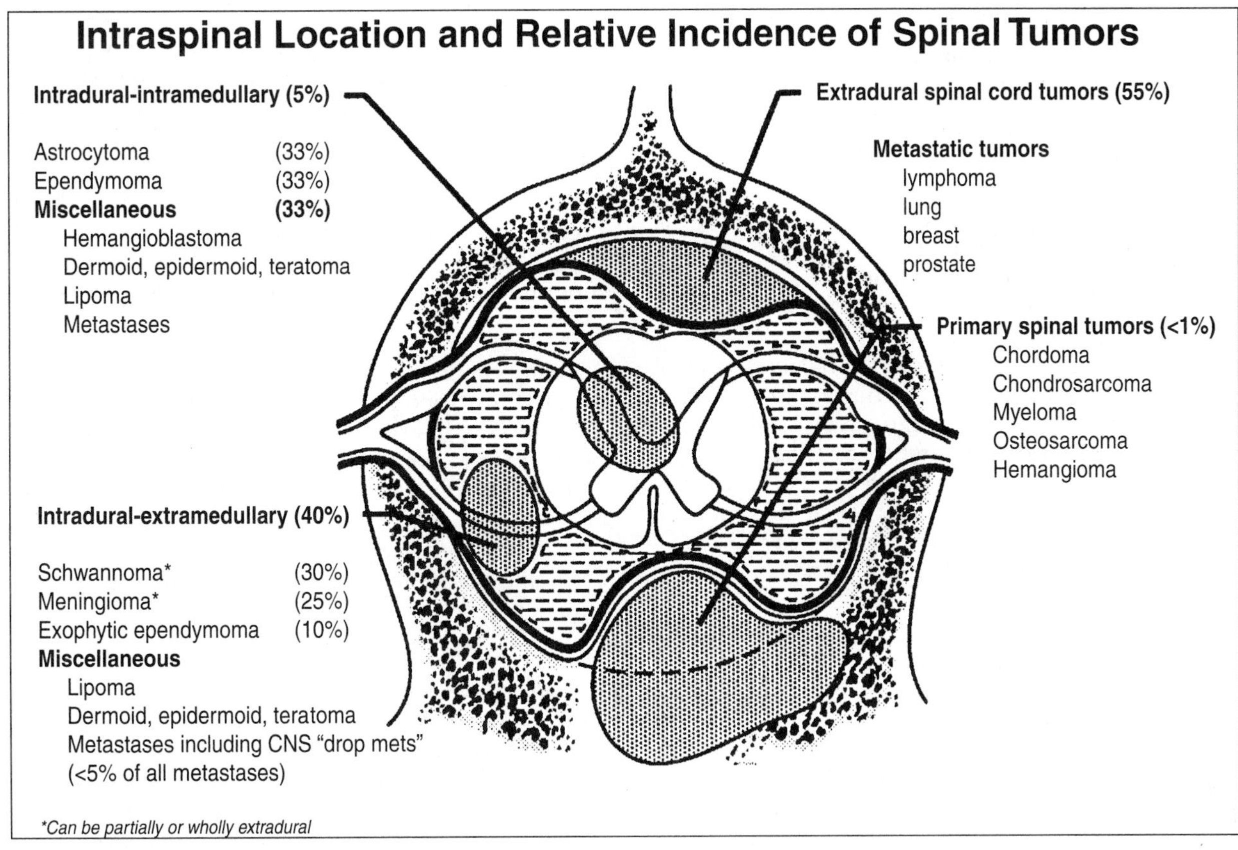

Figure **26-6.** Primary and metastatic tumors of the spine and spinal cord. (*Adapted from Poirier J, Gray F, Escourelle R: Manual of Basic Neuropathology, ed 2. Philadelphia, WB Saunders, 1990.*)

Extradural-Extramedullary Tumors

Extradural-extramedullary tumors are most often metastatic tumors and are addressed under metastatic tumors. There may be an occasional meningioma or schwannoma that arises extradurally, or a spinal chordoma. Spinal chordomas represent less than 1% of spinal cord tumors.

Spinal chordomas are primary tumors that arise from the vertebral bodies, usually in the cervical or sacral regions of the axial skeleton. They are prone to metastasize outside the spinal column. Lesions are characterized by expansive destruction of the bone, for example, the sacrum, or by varying degrees of vertebral collapse.

Clinical Manifestation of Primary Intraspinal Tumors

Spontaneous pain caused by nerve root irritation is a common clinical feature of primary intraspinal tumors and is usually worse at night. Intramedullary tumors have a poorly localized deep burning type of pain in the spine region. Extramedullary tumors have a knifelike radicular type of pain typically radiating to the periphery of the nerve, often aggravated by coughing, sneezing, or straining. The association of asymmetry of reflexes with nerve root pain and an insidious onset is strongly suggestive of spinal cord tumor.

Nerve root pain may be followed by motor weakness and wasting of muscle supplied by the nerve. The motor changes of intramedullary tumors include lower motor neuron changes at the level of the lesion, and may also include upper motor neuron changes at lower levels. The motor changes of extramedullary lesions begin with segmental weakness at the lesion site, and progress to damage to half of the spinal cord (Brown-Séquard's syndrome), and later to a transverse cord syndrome (Thapar and Laws, 1995). This weakness is characterized by upper motor neuron signs, including spasticity. Sphincter weakness, increasing urinary frequency, and urgency may develop. In men, the development of sphincter disturbances is frequently followed by impotence.

Sensory changes in extramedullary tumors usually are along the distribution of the involved nerve roots. Intramedullary tumors result in dissociated sensory disturbances in the limbs below the level of the lesion due to their growth pattern of crossing fibers of the spinothalamic tract. People will often report a feeling of temperature change, particularly a feeling of cold below the level of the lesion. Pain and temperature are compromised, but proprioception and light touch are preserved.

Syringomyelia-like symptoms of loss of pain and temperature sensation below the level of the lesion on one or both sides of the body may occur from damage to the decussating lateral spinothalamic fibers. This is often accompanied by progressive spastic paraparesis caused by pressure on the descending corticospinal tracts. Anterior growth of the tumor produces anterior horn signs, such as muscle weakness, wasting, and fasciculations in the muscles supplied by the anterior horn cells.

Other symptoms of intramedullary cord tumors are papilledema, hydrocephalus, and elevations in ICP. The reason for development of papilledema is unclear, but it is more common with tumors of the thoracic and lumbosacral regions. Box 26–2 lists signs and symptoms of spinal cord tumors.

Medical Management

Diagnosis, Treatment, and Prognosis

After a history and neurologic examination, MRI is the method of choice for the identification of spinal cord tumors. Occasionally plain films may be helpful in treatment planning. Lumbar puncture and CSF examination are no longer used as diagnostic tools.

Surgery is the principal treatment of all primary intraspinal tumors. Complete and curative resection is the objective. Extramedullary tumors can be cured in most cases. Radiation therapy is not required in completely excised lesions. Intraspinal astrocytomas have a lower rate of cure, although surgery and radiation may prolong the disease-free survival. Childhood astrocytomas, however, have a more favorable prognosis, with a 5-year survival rate of 90%.

Special Implications for the Therapist **26-2**

PRIMARY INTRASPINAL TUMORS

Alertness to Signs and Symptoms

As specialists in motor function, therapists may be involved even initially in observing and identifying the signs of spinal cord tumors. Clients referred to physical therapy because of back pain symptoms who have signs of intractable pain, worsening with recumbency, and not relieved by physical therapy should be suspect. Progressive neurologic signs should alert the therapist to the need for medical referral. A thorough initial evaluation of any person with back pain, including symptoms, pain patterns, strength assessment, and other neurologic signs such as impaired bowel and bladder function, changes in deep tendon reflexes, and signs of spasticity, should be the standard of practice to rule out tumors and other systemic disorders.

Rehabilitation Referrals

Neurologic deficits from primary spinal cord tumors resulting in impairments such as weakness in the extremities and trunk, and disabilities such as difficulties with transfers in and out of bed, with ambulation, and with self-care often require rehabilitation therapy. Because of a favorable prognosis with completely excised primary tumors, the approach of the therapist should be toward achieving maximal function and support of the client and family toward long-term goals.

Knowledge Needed for Rehabilitation

As with primary brain tumors, therapists should know the medical management plan, the prognostic expectations, the side effects of treatment, and precautions to prepare for the rehabilitative approach to a client with an intraspinal tumor. Knowledge of the most common intraspinal tumors, their patterns of growth, and neurologic changes assists the therapist in assessing the patient accurately and providing treatment.

Rehabilitation Evaluation

A thorough evaluation of the neurologic and musculoskeletal systems is very important to identify impairments that affect function. For example, an anterior tibialis weakness, or a lower extremity paraparesis may be the impairment that limits mobility and transfers, and may be amenable to therapy. Medical records, laboratory and radiology reports, and other studies should be reviewed by the therapist. If the treatment is provided on an ambulatory basis, blood value determinations should be requested to assist the therapist in planning exercise programs.

Communication with the oncologist and surgeon, keeping abreast of imaging reports and other diagnostic tests, and being alert to other medical management, such as the effect of steroids and chemotherapy, allow the therapist to be more effective in treatment. Postoperative precautions may include protection from spinal torsion, and use of an external support. Protection of irradiated skin follows the same guidelines as given under Primary Brain Tumors.

BOX **26-2**

Signs and Symptoms of Spinal Cord Tumors

- Pain
- Weakness
- Sensory changes
- Urinary frequency
- Urinary urgency
- Sphincter disturbances
- Syringomyelia-like symptoms
- Brown-Séquard–like symptoms
- Hydrocephalus
- Increased intracranial pressure
- Papilledema
- Atrophy
- Hyporeflexia
- Spasticity
- Hyperreflexia
- Gait disturbances
- Sexual dysfunction

METASTATIC TUMORS

The extended survival in all types of cancer has allowed time for metastasis to occur from primary tumors elsewhere in the body. Metastatic complications are an escalating problem. Metastases to the brain and spinal cord are among the most common and most serious complications of metastatic cancer (Thapar and Laws, 1995).

Incidence

Metastasis to the CNS accounts for 20% of all intracranial tumors and 55% of all spinal tumors, a steadily rising figure. The brain is a metastatic site in about 20% of people with primary cancer elsewhere, and the spinal cord is a metastatic site for 10% of primary cancers (Thapar and Laws, 1995).

Pathogenesis

Metastatic tumors reach the brain generally through the arterial blood system. A smaller number arise by direct extension from extracranial sites such as the neck or paranasal sinuses. Most metastatic tumors arise in the distribution area of the middle cerebral artery to the cerebral hemispheres, with most lesions located in the parietal or frontal lobes. About 20% are found in the posterior fossa, primarily the cerebellum. In about half of all cases there are multiple metastatic lesions in the brain (Fig. 26–7).

Metastatic tumors reach the spine and spinal cord through direct arterial dissemination to the vertebral body, by retrograde spread via the vertebral venous plexus as it perforates into the epidural space and vertebral bodies, or by direct invasion from a paravertebral tumor to the epidural space via the intervertebral foramen. The majority of spinal metastases are extradural-extramedullary, although in less than 5% of cases the location is intramedullary. The thoracic spine is the most frequent site of metastasis (70%), followed by the lumbosacral spine (20%) and the cervical area (10%) (Thapar and Laws, 1995).

The most common cancers resulting in brain metastases are lung cancers, especially small cell carcinoma; cancers of the breast, kidney, and gastrointestinal tract; and melanoma. The most common cancers metastasizing to the spinal column are lung, breast, prostate, and kidney cancers and lymphomas. In about 10% of cases, the primary tumor is never found.

Clinical Manifestations of Brain Metastasis

Metastatic brain tumors present with headache, seizures, elevated ICP, and similar signs of primary tumors. However, there may be a much more rapid progression of symptoms, often in days to weeks, as a result of the significant edema that accompanies a metastasis. Cerebellar metastases may cause obstructive hydrocephalus and abrupt deterioration.

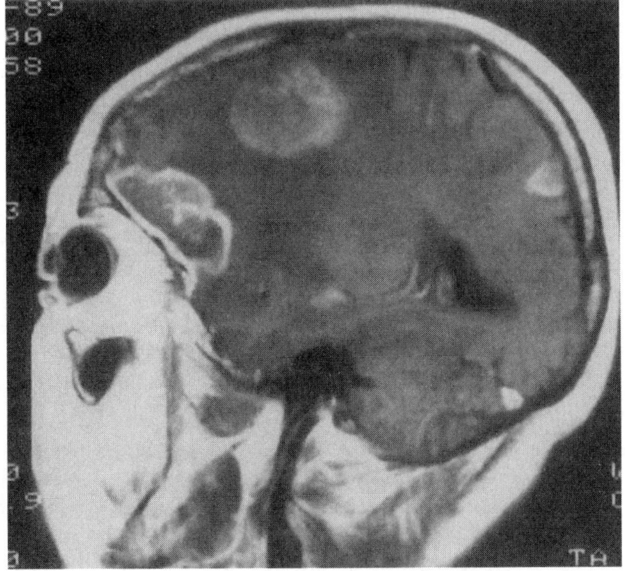

Figure **26–7.** Magnetic resonance scan with gadolinium enhancement showing multiple tumors. (*From Gilroy J: Basic Neurology, ed 2. Elmsford, NY, Pergamon Press, 1990.*)

Medical Management of Brain Metastasis

Diagnosis, Treatment, and Prognosis

MRI is the diagnostic procedure of choice because it is the most sensitive in revealing multiple small lesions. A review of the chest film is often enough to give a presumptive diagnosis of lung cancer. With a history of cancer elsewhere in the body, a solitary brain lesion has about a 90% certainty of being a metastatic deposit (Thapar and Laws, 1995). Because meningiomas have a high prevalence in people with breast cancer, metastatic breast lesions need to be differentiated pathologically from meningiomas for optimal treatment.

Medical management includes corticosteroids, surgical excision when solitary or small numbers of metastases are accessible, and irradiation in almost all cases. Steroids have a dramatic effect in relieving symptoms caused by the significant peritumoral swelling. Radiotherapy provides adequate palliation for many people, as death will occur from the primary cancer, not the brain metastasis.

The prognosis for people with brain metastasis is poor, as the metastasis indicates the primary site has already escaped control.

Clinical Manifestation of Spinal Metastasis

Back pain is the most common and prominent symptom of metastasis to the spinal column and cord, and is present in 95% of cases. Anyone with a known cancer history who presents with new-onset back pain of unknown etiology should be considered to have spinal metastasis until proved otherwise (Thapar and Laws, 1995). Pain is due to stretching of the periosteum, tension or traction on the spinal nerve roots and cord, or compression of the cord and meninges. It is usually a dull ache, worse at night in the recumbent position, and may be local in the spine, or may be a radicular pain.

Without treatment, pain progresses in weeks or months (sometimes days) to weakness, sensory loss, and bowel and bladder sphincter disturbance. These tumors characteristically progress quickly after onset of weakness to cause paraplegia and permanent loss of sphincter control. It is imperative to diagnose and treat the client early, as people treated while still ambulatory will likely remain so, but those who have reached paraplegia and sphincter loss will not typically regain function.

Medical Management of Spinal Metastasis

Diagnosis

A careful neurologic examination, followed by plain films of the spine, are an important first approach, and give the diagnosis in the majority of cases. The most common findings are pedicular erosion, vertebral collapse, pathologic fracture-dislocation, and a soft tissue shadow suggestive of a paraspinal mass (Thapar and Laws, 1995). Bone scans are the next test of choice. If any of these tests are positive, MRI or CT is then done for more definitive imaging of the lesion.

Treatment

Radiotherapy is the treatment of choice of spinal metastasis, to reduce pain, reduce tumor compression, and restore neurologic function. Radiotherapy is also helpful in preserving spinal stability. Surgery is reserved for people with a worsening neurologic deficit during radiation, for those with a spinal instability causing cord compression, for tumors known to be radioresistant, and for those who already have received the maximum radiation.

It should be noted that past attempts at surgical decompression with laminectomy have proved to be disappointing, with neurologic improvement occurring in only 30% of cases (Thapar and Laws, 1995). Surgical access via laminectomy to the typically anterior tumors compressing the cord from a ventral direction is technically difficult. There is evidence that very high doses of corticosteroids relieve local spinal edema. Current practice is to begin very large doses of corticosteroids as soon as a spinal cord compression from metastatic tumor is diagnosed. This dose is continued for several days, then reduced, allowing time for decisions to be made for radiation or surgery (Weiss, 1995).

Prognosis

Prognosis of return of neurologic function is based on the degree of loss before radiotherapy. With radiotherapy, 80% of clients who were ambulatory at the time of treatment remain so, and 30% who were nonambulatory regain gait (Thapar and Laws, 1995). Pain and neurologic function improve in a large percentage of people. Because the metastasis indicates loss of containment of the primary tumor, cure is beyond expectation. However, early diagnosis and treatment lead to the optimal result, the prevention of paraplegia.

Radiation to the spinal cord may cause complications of myelopathy. Although there are no acute effects from radiation to the cord, an early delayed radiation myelopathy after irradiation of the neck is common. Lhermitte's sign (a sudden electric shock sensation brought on by neck flexion), the hallmark of this radiation myelopathy, is present for several months, and then abates. It is not a predictor of late delayed radiation spinal cord injury (Delattre and Posner, 1995). A late effect of radiation to the cord, occurring between 6 and 36 months after radiation, is a chronic progressive myelopathy which begins as a Brown-Séquard syndrome, and progresses over weeks or months to a spastic paresis. There is no effective treatment, but the therapist can provide mobility management for these clients.

Special Implications for the Therapist **26-3**

METASTATIC TUMORS TO THE CNS

Rehabilitation Referrals

Neurologic deficits resulting from metastatic CNS tumors often require physical and occupational therapy. The neurologic impairments from either intracranial or intraspinal tumors may include weakness, paralysis, decreased sensation, and pain leading to loss of mobility and self-care skills. Paraplegia from spinal metastasis requires much rehabilitative intervention.

Alertness to Signs and Symptoms

Since therapists are often in a position to observe the mobility and neurologic status of clients before a diagnosis of a CNS metastasis is made, being alert to abnormal neurologic signs in anyone with a cancer history is vital, particularly in the case of intraspinal metastasis. Spinal cord compression can progress in a matter of hours or days to paraplegia, and a therapist alert to progressive strength and sensory changes can facilitate referral of that person to the physician in time to prevent irreversible paraplegia and sphincter loss. Any signs of intracranial metastasis, such as visual symptoms, or mental status changes in someone with a cancer history, should also be reported immediately to the physician.

Knowledge Needed for Rehabilitation

As with primary CNS tumors, therapists need to know the medical management plan, the prognostic expectations, and the hematologic guidelines for exercise. Goal setting needs to be realistic for noncurable disease, yet not without hope for good management. Families and caregivers may need to have an even greater role in goal setting and training. As with primary brain tumors, the psychosocial implications have a profound impact on the client and family, and the therapist can provide support and even be a sounding board for decision making.

Rehabilitation Precautions

As with primary CNS tumors, there needs to be an awareness of the side effects of the various treatment modalities. Postoperative acute care precautions are discussed under Primary Brain Tumors. A general knowledge of metastatic spread and behavior is helpful. Myelosuppression, fatigue, nausea, and precautions need to be understood. Avoiding modalities such as heat or cold or any topical agents over skin being irradiated is important for skin protection because poor circulation inhibits normal heat and cold dissipation. Once the irradiation sessions are completed and the skin has healed, and depending on skin integrity and adequate circulation, modalities such as heat or cold or transcutaneous nerve stimulation (TNS) may be used. Although ultrasound is not recommended for pain management because of concerns about tumor spread, there may be situations when palliation for pain in endstage disease may allow its use.

Rehabilitation of Metastatic Intraspinal Tumors

It is also helpful to realize that in some cases, a paraplegia from a metastatic spinal cord tumor may respond to irradiation, and improve enough for some return of function, such as limited ambulation. The physical therapist needs to be alert to any neurologic improvement, and adapt the treatment program accordingly.

PARANEOPLASTIC SYNDROMES

Cancer may cause effects on the nervous system not directly related to the primary tumor mass or a metastasis. These so-called remote effects, or paraneoplastic syndromes (see Chapter 7), include such problems as paraneoplastic cerebellar degeneration, brainstem encephalitis, myelitis of the spinal cord, and motor neuron disease. The cause of most paraneoplastic syndromes is unknown, although an immune mechanism is the most likely hypothesis (Posner, 1995). It is postulated that the response of the immune system to the antigen is misdirected and causes neurologic dysfunction.

Paraneoplastic syndromes may be the first sign that there is a cancer present.

Although paraneoplastic syndromes involving the CNS are rare, they are often severe, often associated with an inflammatory CSF, and leave the person with severe neurologic disability. Treatment has not been shown to be successful. Some syndromes are associated with particular tumors, such as paraneoplastic cerebellar degeneration with lung cancer. In this syndrome, the early symptoms are a slight incoordination in walking, with progressive gait ataxia; incoordination of arms, legs, and trunk; dysarthria; and often nystagmus. After a few months the illness reaches its peak and stabilizes. By this time, most clients must have assistance to walk, handwriting is impossible, many cannot sit unsupported, and speech is with great effort.

It is not within the scope of this chapter to elaborate on CNS paraneoplastic syndromes. However, it is helpful for the therapist to have an acquaintance with these syndromes, as they will appear in the practice of caring for people with CNS neoplasms.

LEPTOMENINGEAL CARCINOMATOSIS

Infiltration of the meninges and CSF pathways of the CNS by neoplastic cells is a less common complication of cancer and is known as leptomeningeal carcinomatosis. This metastatic seeding of the meninges is widespread and multifocal, and causes neurologic signs such as radicular pain and weakness, headache, change in mental status, or seizures. Cancers of the breast and lung, non-Hodgkin's lymphoma, melanomas, and adult acute leukemias are the most common primary tumors responsible for carcinomatosis. Diagnosis is by CSF studies, which show malignant cells. Current therapy includes radiotherapy to symptomatic sites, with concurrent intrathecal chemotherapy (Thapar and Laws, 1995). Median survival is about 6 months with treatment.

PEDIATRIC TUMORS

In infants and young children, intracranial tumors are the second most common form of cancer, after leukemia (Thapar and Laws, 1995). The peak incidence of these tumors occurs between birth and age 6 years. Brain tumors are the second leading cause of cancer-related deaths in children below the age of 15.

The most frequently encountered intracranial tumors in children are the astrocytoma, medulloblastoma, ependymoma, and the brainstem glioma (Gilroy, 1990). Brain tumors in children are typically located infratentorially, primarily in the cerebellum and brainstem.

Astrocytomas are the most common type of pediatric intracranial tumor, accounting for about 47% of all brain tumors in children. They are usually well-differentiated grade I tumors. About half of them occur supratentorially, most commonly in the frontal lobes, but also in the temporal and parietal lobes. The cerebellum is the most common infratentorial site of the astrocytoma in children. Cerebellar astrocytoma is more common in males, and usually occurs in the first two decades of life with the median incidence at age 18. In grade I astrocytomas, children have a 10-year postoperative survival rate of 85% (Gilroy, 1990). There are infrequent high-grade astrocytomas with a poorer prognosis.

Medulloblastomas account for 20% to 25% of childhood brain tumors, and are the most common malignant tumor in children. These aggressive tumors are most common in males, and have a peak incidence at age 5 years in children. Evolution of therapeutic strategies to include multimodal chemotherapy followed by surgery has dramatically improved the outlook for children with medulloblastomas (Thapar and Laws, 1990). Medulloblastomas belong to the group of tumors known as primitive neuroectodermal tumors, and arise in the fourth ventricle. Medulloblastomas have a predilection for meningeal seeding. The 5-year survival is about 50%.

Ependymomas usually arise in children from the floor of the fourth ventricle and make up 9% to 20% of childhood tumors. The 5-year survival is 85% when complete resection is possible, and about 45% overall.

Brainstem gliomas may be of several tumor types, including the most common astrocytoma, but also may be glioblastomas or ependymomas. The overall prognosis for brainstem tumors is relatively poor, but occasionally gratifying results are obtained (Thapar and Laws, 1995).

Clinical Manifestations

Clinical manifestations of CNS neoplasms in children are more difficult to evaluate because children are less able to relate and report symptoms. Parents, teachers, and caretakers may notice problems before the child is aware of change (Baird, 1991). Most supratentorial astrocytomas present initially with seizures. Cerebellar astrocytomas produce typical cerebellar findings such as ataxia, and many produce symptoms of increased ICP. Tumors of the cerebral aqueduct or the fourth ventricle, such as an ependymoma or medulloblastoma, typically present at an early stage with headache, nausea, and cranial nerve palsies, but may also produce long-tract signs such as hemiparesis. Hydrocephalus is a complication in patients with ependymoma and medulloblastoma, and a late manifestation of brainstem gliomas (Gilroy, 1990).

Diagnosis and Treatment

Diagnosis is by MRI or CT scan, although the CT scan may not be adequate to detect the early stages of brainstem or fourth ventricle tumors. Early treatment includes high-dose dexamethasone, emergency ventricular drainage in the case of hydrocephalus, and surgical resection. Radiation is the principal form of treatment for brainstem gliomas. Postoperative radiation is indicated for medulloblastomas, and may be helpful in ependymomas and gliomas. Chemotherapy, although generally not beneficial, has been helpful in medulloblastomas.

The risks of brain radiation therapy in children are of great concern. These may include learning disabilities, hypopituitarism, occlusive disease of cerebral vessels, and radiation-induced secondary tumors. Because myelinization of the CNS is not generally complete until 2 to 3 years of age, radiation therapy prior to this age can be especially devastating and is not usually done (Thapar and Laws, 1995).

Spinal cord tumors rarely occur in children. Spinal ependymoma is the most prominent primary intraspinal tumor and has a predilection for the lumbosacral spine. It is treated with resection and radiation therapy. The risks of radiation in children include myelopathy and spinal deformities.

Metastatic spinal cord tumors in children most commonly arise from sarcomas, and less often from neuroblastomas, lymphomas, and leukemias. Metastatic tumors in children occur principally by direct extension from an adjacent primary cancer (Thapar and Laws, 1995), and can be the presenting feature of the primary cancer. This is in contrast to adult spinal tumors where access is by a vascular route and usually occurs in the setting of an advanced malignancy.

Because pediatric metastatic spinal cord tumors are not usually associated with extensive vertebral column destruction, they generally can be removed through a simple laminectomy. An aggressive approach to metastatic spinal tumors in children results in a more favorable outcome in children than in adults (Thapar and Laws, 1995). Ninety-six percent of children have improvement or stabilization of neurologic deficits, and 60% of nonambulatory children regain the ability to walk after treatment.

References

Baird SB, McCorkle R, Grant M: Cancer Nursing: A Comprehensive Textbook. Philadelphia, WB Saunders, 1991.

Chase M: Cancers of the central nervous system. *In* Baird SB (ed): A Cancer Source Book for Nurses, ed 6. Atlanta, American Cancer Society, 1991, pp 253–258.

Chusid JG: Correlative Neuroanatomy and Functional Neurology, ed 19. Los Altos, Calif, Lange, 1985, p 386.

Corn BW, Yousem DM, Scott CB, et al: White matter changes are correlated significantly with radiation dose. Cancer 74:2828–2835, 1994.

Delattre JY, Posner JB: Neurological complications of chemotherapy and radiation therapy. *In* Aminoff MJ (ed): Neurology and General Medicine, ed 2. New York, Churchill Livingstone, 1995, p 437.

Gilroy J: Basic Neurology, ed 2. Elmsford, NY, Pergamon Press, 1990, pp 223–250.

Hickey JV: Neurological and Neurosurgical Nursing, ed 3. Philadelphia, JB Lippincott, 1992, pp 481–504.

Loeffler JS, Shrieve DC, Wen PY, et al: Radiosurgery for intracranial malignancies. Semin Radiat Oncol 5(3):225, 1995.

Mayer D, O'Conner L: Rehabilitation of persons with cancer: An ONS position statement. Oncol Nurs Forum 16:433, 1989.

McConachie NS, Worthington BS, Cornford EJ, et al: Review article: Computed tomography and magnetic resonance in the diagnosis of intraventricular cerebral masses. Br J Radiol 67:240, 1994.

McGarvey CL, Walton JF: Oncology: Principles and management. *In* McGarvey CL (ed): Physical Therapy for the Cancer Patient. New York, Churchill Livingstone, 1990, p 11.

Pfeifer JD, Wick MR: The pathologic evaluation of neoplastic diseases. *In* Murphy GP, Lawrence W, Lenhard RE (eds): American Cancer Society Textbook of Clinical Oncology, ed. 2. Atlanta, American Cancer Society, 1995, pp 79–80.

Posner JB: Paraneoplastic syndromes involving the nervous system. *In* Aminoff MJ (ed): Neurology and General Medicine, ed 2. New York, Churchill Livingstone, 1995, pp 401–406.

Ransohoff J, Kislow M, Cooper PR: Cancer of the central nervous system and pituitary. *In* Holleb AI, Fink DJ, Murphy GP (eds): American Cancer Society Textbook of Clinical Oncology. Atlanta, American Cancer Society, 1991, p 329.

Schnell S: Nursing care of clients with cerebral disorders. *In* Black JM, Matassarin-Jacobs E (eds): Luckmann and Sorensen's Medical-Surgical Nursing, ed 4. Philadelphia, WB Saunders, 1993, pp 705–772.

Schwade JG, Wolf AL: Future trends in radiosurgery. Semin Radiat Oncol 5:246–249, 1995.

Shaw EG, Coffey RJ, Dinapoli RP: Neurotoxicity of radiosurgery. Semin Radiat Oncol 5(3):235, 1995.

Snodgrass SM: Neurologic aspects of cancer. *In* Weiner WJ, Goetz CG (eds): Neurology for the Non-Neurologist, ed 3. Philadelphia, JB Lippincott, 1994, pp 259–267.

Thapar K, Laws ER: Tumors of the central nervous system. *In* Murphy GP, Lawrence W, Lenhard RE (eds): American Cancer Society Textbook of Clinical Oncology, ed 2. Atlanta, American Cancer Society, 1995, pp 378–413.

Weiss HD: Neoplasms. *In* Samuels MA (ed): Manual of Neurologic Therapeutics, ed 5. Boston, Little, Brown, 1995, pp 224–249.

Yates AJ: An overview of principles for classifying brain tumors. Mol Chem Neuropathol 17:106–110, 1992.

chapter 27

Degenerative Diseases of the Central Nervous System

Kenda S. Fuller

Degenerative diseases of the CNS can affect gray matter, white matter, or both. The involvement is often diffuse but usually affects one area or system more than another. In most cases the cause is questionable or unknown. Often the disorder begins in one area of the brain and progresses to other areas causing signs and symptoms which mimic other neurologic disorders. Diagnosis is often made by observing the progression of the neurologic changes and identifying a general pattern consistent with the known disease process. The most common factor in this group of diseases is the slow deterioration of bodily functions controlled by the brain and spinal cord.

In degenerative gray matter diseases the predominent disorder is dementia. The majority of the degenerative diseases that affect the basal ganglia are associated with involuntary movements. Disruption of smooth coordination of muscles can be seen with disease affecting the cerebellum and brainstem.

Disease causing lesions of the white matter affect movement either by increasing the excitabilty of the muscles, resulting in spasticity, or by decreasing the neuronal input with weakness of the muscles. Sensory changes resulting from involvement of white matter are a significant cause for concern. The ability to perform activities of daily living are often restricted when sensation is lost or decreased.

Medical management of degenerative neurologic diseases requires a broad base of practitioners The prognosis in this group of disorders is one of steady decline in function because there is no cure for many of them. Prevention of secondary complications becomes the goal of medical management until medications are found that will change the course of the disease or arrest it.

Therapeutic intervention is intermittent depending on the client's medical or functional status. Treatment, on a one-to-one basis or in groups, focuses on overall conditioning to maintain musculoskeletal and cardiopulmonary fitness at as high a level as possible; to provide recommendations for mobility and functional aids in home and community; and to maintain the ability to communicate as effectively as possible. The cost of care for people with degenerative neurologic disease is significant owing to the protracted time of disability before death and the extent of the disability as a CNS disorder.

Although medical science has made tremendous progress in the past few years, degenerative disorders continue to be a challenge to health-care providers and a scourge to modern society. Many of the disorders appear later in life, and mimic the normal deterioration of the nervous system that comes with aging.

Advances in the field of neuroscience have identified the changes in cell biology that take place in many of these diseases; the understanding of immunohistochemistry has provided insight into possible causes; and manipulation of neurotransmitters and receptors hold promise for future treatment.

The diseases discussed in this chapter are representative of the scope of the neurodegenerative diseases that confront us in our lives and in our practice.

AMYOTROPHIC LATERAL SCLEROSIS

Overview and Definition. Amyotrophic lateral sclerosis (ALS) is the most common form of adult-onset progressive motor neuron disease. It is the most physically devastating of the neurodegenerative diseases. It is a progressive disease of unknown cause, characterized by degeneration and scarring of the motor neurons in the lateral aspect of the spinal cord, brainstem, and cerebral cortex, giving rise to the terms *lateral* and *sclerosis* in identifying the disease. Peripheral nerve changes result in muscle fiber atrophy or *amyotrophy*. The resulting weakness causes profound limitation of movement.

Incidence. The prevalence of ALS around the globe ranges from 4 to 6 per 100,000. ALS is more common in males than in females (Brown, 1994). There is an increased incidence in the Pacific Islands and studies have been done to try to identify a possible environmental cause of increases on the island of Guam. The cycad bean, used as food and medicine, has been implicated. A mechanism to explain this relationship is not at hand (Kurland et al., 1994).

Etiology and Risk Factors. Familial ALS is an inherited autosomal trait. Family linkage studies with DNA probes suggest that there is more than one gene for autosomal dominant ALS; one gene is on chromosome 21. There is also a recessive form of hereditary ALS which has been genetically mapped on the long arm of chromosome 2. This type begins in childhood and is characterized by a prolonged survival. Approximately 90% of ALS occurs sporadically and the cause is unknown. Chronic intoxication with heavy metals such as lead or mercury has been suggested as an etiologic agent. A separate and still unsettled question is whether some cases of ALS represent infection with the poliovirus. Several reports indicate an increased incidence of cancer in patients with motor neuron disease (Brown, 1994).

Pathogenesis. ALS affects the upper motor neurons of the cerebral cortex descending via the corticospinal and corticobulbar tracts to synapse with the lower motor neurons, or interneurons. It can also directly affect the lower motor neuron with disease of the anterior horn cells in the spinal cord and brainstem. The affected cells undergo shrinkage, often with some excessive accumulation of the pigmented lipid (lipofuscin) which normally does not develop until advanced age (Brown, 1994). The production of free radicals may be responsible for the changes in the lipid molecules, eventually causing cell death. There is some evidence that there is a link with an immunoreaction to neuronal gangliosides. Inflammatory cells are present in the spinal cord in ALS, but studies are not conclusive regarding the exact nature of the antiganglioside antibodies. Endogenous excitotoxins, such as the neurotransmitter glutamate, may be an important component of the destruction of neurons in ALS. Although there is evidence that excitatory amino acid (glutamate) levels are altered in ALS, it is unclear whether it is a primary or a secondary finding (Braak and Braak, 1994; Rothstein et al., 1993).

The death of the peripheral motor neuron in the brainstem and spinal cord leads to denervation and consequent atrophy of the corresponding muscle fibers. There is evidence that in the early phases of the illness, denervated muscle may be reinnervated by sprouting of preserved nearby distal motor axon terminals, although reinnervation in this disease is less extensive than in other chronic neurologic disorders.

There is remarkable selectivity of neuronal cell death, involving motor neurons of the brainstem and spinal cord, with relative sparing of the oculomotor nuclei. There is eventual spread into the prefrontal, parietal, and temporal areas, as well as into the subthalamic nuclei and reticular formation. In persons kept breathing with ventilatory support there may be sensory system changes. The areas of the brain controlling coordinated movement (cerebellum) and cognition (frontal cortex) are not affected by ALS.

Clinical Manifestations. The manifestations of ALS are variable depending on whether upper or lower motor neurons are those predominantly involved. With lower motor neuron cell death and early denervation, the first evidence of the disease typically is insidiously developing asymmetrical weakness, usually of the distal aspect of one limb. Cramping with volitional movement in early morning is often reported with complaints of stiffness. Weakness caused by denervation is associated with progressive wasting and atrophy of muscles. Early in the disease there are *fasciculations*, or spontaneous twitching of muscle fibers. Extensor muscles become weaker than flexor muscles, especially in the hands. It is characteristic of ALS that, regardless of whether the initial disease involves upper or lower motor neurons, both categories are eventually implicated. In most persons with ALS, Babinski's and Hoffmann's signs are present or the tendon jerks are disproportionately active (Rowland, 1994). Throughout the course of the disease, eye movements and sensory, bowel, and bladder functions are preserved.

There are four categories of symptoms (Gilroy and Holliday, 1982; Leigh, 1994). The symptoms reflect the area of the CNS that is affected. Figure 27–1 shows the levels of dysfunction associated with the terms that describe them.

1. *Pseudobulbar palsy* reflects damage in the corticobulbar tract.
2. *Progressive bulbar palsy* is a result of cranial nerve nuclei involvement. There is weakness of the muscles involved with swallowing, chewing, and facial gestures. Fasciculations of the tongue are usually prominent. With early bulbar involvement, there can be difficulty with respiration prior to weakness of the limbs. Dysarthria and exaggeration of the expression of emotion, or pseudobulbar affect, indicate involvement of the corticobulbar tract. The oculomotor system is usually not involved and eye movement remains normal.
3. *Primary lateral sclerosis* results in neuronal loss in the cortex. Signs of corticospinal tract involvement include hyperactivity of tendon reflexes with spasticity causing difficulty with active movement. Weakness and spasticity of specific muscles represent the level and progression of the disease along the corticospinal tracts. There is no muscle atrophy and fasciculations are not present. This form of ALS is rare.
4. In *progressive spinal muscular atrophy* there is progressive loss of motor neurons in the anterior horns of the spinal cord, often beginning in the cervical area. There is progressive weakness, wasting, and fasciculations involving the small muscles of the hands. Other levels of the spinal cord can be the site of the initial disease process with symptoms reflecting the level involved. These areas of weakness can be present without evidence of higher-level corticospinal involvement such as spasticity.

ALS with probable upper motor neuron signs reflects a condition where there are no overt upper motor neuron signs, but involvement of the corticospinal tracts is indicated by the incongruous presence of active tendon reflexes in limbs with weak, wasted, and twitching muscles. Upper and lower limbs are usually affected first with progression to facial symptoms and respiratory failure.

Medical Management

Diagnosis. Diagnosis is predominantly made by the clinical presentation and electromyogram (EMG). EMG criteria for the diagnosis of ALS include the presence of fibrillations, positive waveforms, fasciculations, and motor unit potential changes in multiple nerve root distribution in at least three limbs and the paraspinal muscles. These changes occur without change in sensory response (Gilroy and Holliday, 1982; Mitsumoto et al., 1988). Box 27–1 lists the findings in ALS.

There are several disorders that resemble ALS that are treatable. It is critical that the correct diagnosis be made as early as possible. Lymphoma and Lyme disease can cause diffuse lower motor axonal neuropathy. Spinal cord compression can demonstrate similar signs and symptoms due to pressure on the same structures as those affected in ALS. Heavy metal poisoning and inherited disorders as a potential cause of the symptoms can be uncovered by a thorough patient history. Involvement of the sensory system or conduction block with evoked potential testing may indicate other neurodegenerative disease processes (Brown, 1994).

Treatment. There is no known method of arresting the course of ALS. There is, however, much that can be done in the form of symptomatic therapy. The intellect of the client is not affected and health-care providers should emphasize the value of maintaining the highest level of function throughout the course of the disease, educating and supporting the client and family for the rapid decline in function. Symptomatic

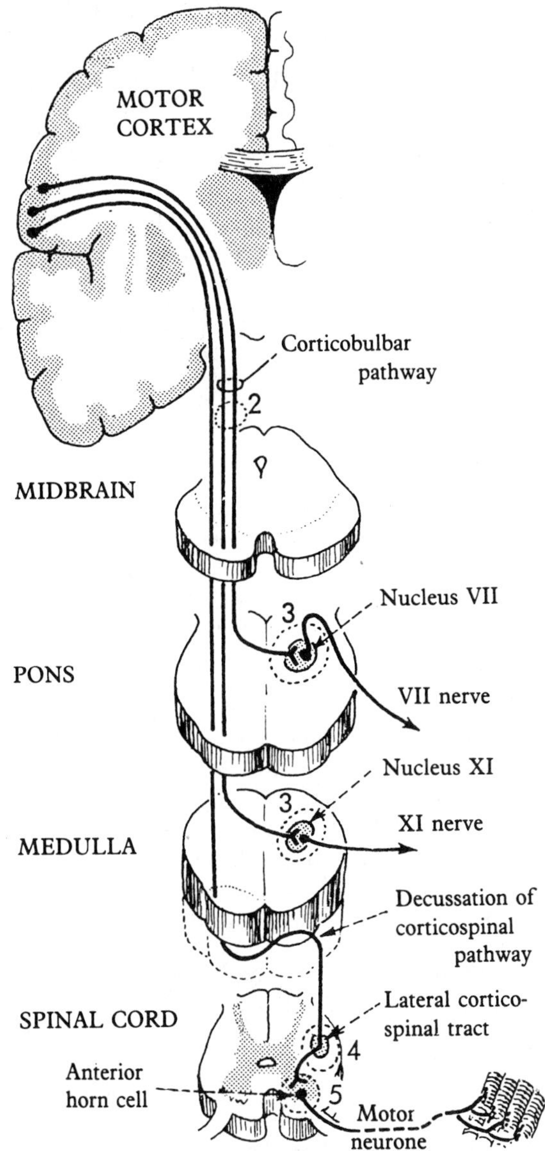

1. The motor cortex.
2. The corticobulbar pathway:
   PSEUDOBULBAR PALSY.
3. The cranial nerve nuclei:
   PROGRESSIVE BULBAR PALSY.
4. The corticospinal tract:
   PRIMARY LATERAL SCLEROSIS.
5. The anterior horn cell:
   PROGRESSIVE MUSCULAR ATROPHY.

The clinical picture is always a mixture of the above.

When 4 and 5 predominate, the term AMYOTROPHIC LATERAL SCLEROSIS is used.

Figure **27–1.** Areas of damage in the central and peripheral nervous system as a result of amyotrophic lateral sclerosis. (*From Lindsay KW, Bone I, Callander R: Neurology and Neurosurgery Illustrated. New York, Churchill Livingstone, 1986.*)

measures may include the use of anticholinergic drugs to control drooling, and baclofen or diazepam to control spasticity.

Maintenance of nutrition is a significant problem, with difficulty chewing and swallowing. Weakness of jaw movement, loss of tongue mobility, and difficulty in lip closure, in addition to impairment of the swallowing reflex, are common. This may lead to respiratory complications from aspiration.

BOX **27–1**

Abnormal Diagnostic Findings in Amyotrophic Lateral Sclerosis

Electromyography shows the presence of fibrillations and fasciculations
Muscle biopsy shows denervation atrophy
Muscle enzymes such as creatine phosphokinase are elevated
Cerebrospinal fluid is normal
There are no changes on myelogram

By modifying the consistency and texture of food and fluids, the risk of aspiration is reduced (Appel and Appel, 1994).

From the earliest stages of care of the client with ALS, there should be emphasis on prevention of respiratory complications. Early evidence of respiratory involvement may be shortness of breath, poor cough reflex, and headache. Use of incentive respirometry, suction, intermittent positive pressure breathing, and postural drainage appear to be useful in maintaining bronchial hygiene.

Respiratory failure and inability to eat are part of the final stages of ALS. Nasogastric tube feeding and use of a respirator may be options to prolong the life of the client. Individual and family wishes concerning these procedures should be discussed as early as possible in the course of the disease, as some clients may experience a rapid decline in function at any time (Brown, 1994).

Prognosis. The course of ALS is relentlessly progressive. Death from the adult-onset sporadic type usually occurs within 2 to 5 years, resulting mainly from pneumonia due to respiratory compromise.

Special Implications for the Therapist: **27-1**

AMYOTROPHIC LATERAL SCLEROSIS

Muscle strength declines in an overall linear progression throughout the course of the disease. The rate of loss is stable within a broad range after the first year, but during the first year there is fluctuation of strength which may be due to the potential for adaptation within the CNS. At this point, the goal of therapy is to maintain general physical activity and muscular tone. Regular exercise in moderation can help alleviate fatigue and have a beneficial effect on the client's general well-being (Bohannon, 1983). Spasticity contributes to complaints of weakness; consistent slow stretching that decreases tone may be of benefit. Cramps, which can be a source of pain, also respond to a daily stretching routine.

Changes in gait are significant and gait analysis is necessary to assess the need for assistive devices. Severe falls caused by weakness are a major problem. Ankle dorsiflexion is lost before loss of strength in plantar flexion. Hamstring strength appears to correlate with walking and the decrease is parallel with the loss of walking ability. The change in isometric muscle strength as a percentage of normal shows a dramatic decrease late in the course of the disease when fewer muscle fibers are available. This is when the greatest functional losses are noted. A surprisingly small amount of muscle activity is necessary across the joints to allow normal function of a joint. Some movement and joint stability are maintained until the degeneration causes atrophy of muscle activity to less than 20% of normal. The weakness and wasting often produce painful subluxation of the scapulohumeral joint and the arm should be supported by external means (Aminoff, 1994). Contractures should be routinely stretched taking care to support the joints as there is minimal control of muscle activity in the late stages. Complaints of pain may begin when the client is unable to shift weight in bed or in sitting. Changing the reclining angle of the bed or wheelchair or the postion of the legs will give some relief. Caregivers need to be educated in this aspect of care.

Braces, other assistive devices, and motorized scooters or wheelchairs help to maintain mobility and freedom. Some clients can be taught to use their abdominal muscles to increase inspiration and expiration when the muscles of the diaphragm and intercostal muscles become weak. In the terminal stages, the comfort of the patient is the therapeutic goal. Table 27–1 describes interventions associated with the various stages of the disease.

ALZHEIMER'S DISEASE

Overview and Definition. Alzheimer's disease (AD) is a progressive dementia, characterized by a slow decline in memory, language, visuospatial skills, personality, and cognition (Miller et al., 1994).

Incidence, Etiology, and Risk Factors. There are approximately 4 million people with AD in the United States. The prevalence is 6% in people over 65 years old, 20% in people over 80, and over 95% in those 95 years old. The cause is unknown, but there appears to be a relationship between genetic predisposition, the abnormal processing of a normal cellular substance, amyloid, and advanced age.

The prevalence of AD rises with each decade. There appears to be a genetic component to AD. There may be an abnormality on chromosome 21. This abnormality shows up in approximately 2% of adults studied, mostly members of families that have a predilection for early-onset AD, that is, onset before age 65. Other chromosomes are being studied with some linkages found with chromosomes 19 and 14 (Miller et al., 1994; Lavretsky and Jarvik, 1994).

Pathogenesis. The first structure to show pathologic changes is the cerebral cortex. Cell death and atrophy are noted, but, because the disease is prevalent in old age, atrophy is not the single response to the disease. There is progressive accumulation of insoluble fibrous material known as *amyloid* that normally does not occur in the human nervous system. Amyloid deposits are the core of "senile plaques" that are believed to take decades to develop. The amyloid core is surrounded by fragmented axons, altered glial cells, and cellular debris. The amyloid deposition appears to have a relationship to β-amyloid protein, a natural substance that is required to maintain fibroblasts and hippocampal cells.[1] "Neurofibrillary tangles" develop among the pyramidal neurons and lead to cell death and atrophy of brain tissue. It is believed that there may be destabilization of microtubules, structural components present in all cells, causing decreases in cell division, and axonal transport of neurotransmitters.

Cholinergic neurons have decreased activity in persons with AD. There is still some question whether this plays a primary role in the disease, or if it is a secondary reaction. Although the cholinergic system is related to memory and cognition, treatment oriented toward cholinergic dysfunction has not been successful in controlling symptoms.

Abnormalitites have been reported in fibroblasts, red and white blood cells, and platelets. Alterations in blood proteins have been observed. The role of these peripheral changes is not clear (Lavretsky and Jarvik, 1994).

Neuropathology is greatest in brain regions just posterior to Wernicke's area, and sensory aphasia often develops. Impairment of judgment is considered to be caused by the disease process in the parietal and frontal lobes. Injury to the parietal and limbic regions may contribute to the psychiatric syndromes. Changes in motor behavior are related to the abnormal processing of information in the hypothalamus and ascending catecholaminergic, serotonergic, and cholinergic cortical projection systems.

Clinical Manifestations. Disorders of higher function are manifest in AD due to cortical lobe dysfunction (Miller et al., 1994) (see Chapter 24). Subtle personality changes occur in AD, such as indifference, egocentricity, impulsivity, and irritability. Often the first symptom is loss of the ability to learn new information. Eventually all learning is lost. Both

[1] The hippocampus is a part of the limbic system and provides memory function.

TABLE 27-1 Exercise and Rehabilitation Programs for Clients with Amyotrophic Lateral Sclerosis

Stage	Treatment
Phase I (Independent)	
Stage I	
Patient characteristics Mild weakness Clumsiness Ambulatory Independent in ADL	Continue normal activities or increase activities if sedentary to prevent disuse atrophy Begin program of ROM exercises (stretching, yoga, tai chi) Add strengthening program of gentle resistance exercises to all musculature with caution not to cause overwork fatigue Provide psychological support as needed
Stage II	
Patient characteristics Moderate, selective weakness Slightly decreased independence in ADL Difficulty climbing stairs Difficulty raising arms Difficulty buttoning clothing Ambulatory	Continue stretching to avoid contractures Continue cautious strengthening of muscles with MMT grades above F+ (3+); monitor for overwork fatigue Consider orthotic support (i.e., AFOs, wrist, thumb splints) Use adaptive equipment to facilitate ADL
Stage III	
Patient characteristics Severe selective weakness in ankles, wrists, and hands Moderately decreased independence in ADL Easily fatigued with long-distance ambulation Ambulatory Slightly increased respiratory effort	Continue stage II program as tolerated; caution not to fatigue to point of decreasing patient's ADL independence Keep patient physically independent as long as possible through pleasurable activities, walking Encourage deep-breathing exercises, chest stretching, postural drainage if needed Prescribe standard or motorized wheelchair with modifications to allow eventual reclining back with head rest, elevating legs
Phase II (Partially Independent)	
Stage IV	
Patient characteristics Hanging-arm syndrome with shoulder pain and sometimes edema in the hand Wheelchair-dependent Severe lower extremity weakness (± spasticity) Able to perform ADL but fatigues easily	Heat, massage as indicated to control spasm Preventive antiedema measures Active assisted passive ROM exercises to the weakly supported joints—caution to support, rotate shoulder during abduction and joint accessory motions Encourage isometric contractions of all musculature to tolerance Try arm slings, overhead slings, or wheelchair arm supports Motorized chair if patient wants to be independently mobile; adapt controls as needed
Stage V	
Patient characteristics Severe lower extremity weakness Moderate to severe upper extremity weakness Wheelchair-dependent Increasingly dependent in ADL Possible skin breakdown secondary to poor mobility	Encourage family to learn proper transfer, positioning principles, and turning techniques Encourage modifications at home to aid patient's mobility and independence Electric hospital bed with antipressure mattress If patient elects HMV, adapt chair to hold respirator unit
Phase III (Dependent)	
Stage VI	
Patient characteristics Bedridden Completely dependent in ADL	For dysphagia: soft diet, long spoons, tube feeding, percutaneous gastrostomy To decrease flow of accumulated saliva: medication, suction, surgery For dysarthria: palatal lifts, electronic speech amplification, eye pointing For breathing difficulty: clear airway, tracheostomy, respirator if HMV elected Medications to decrease impact of dyspnea

ADL, activities of daily living; ROM, range of motion; AFOs, ankle-foot orthoses; HMV, home mechanical ventilation; MMT, manual muscle test.
Adapted from Sinaki M: Exercise and rehabilitation measures in amyotrophic lateral sclerosis. *In* Yase Y, Tsubaki T: *Amytrophic Lateral Sclerosis: Recent Advances in Research and Treatment*. Amsterdam, Elsevier, 1988.

storage and retrieval are impaired. Unlike memory problems associated with frontal or subcortical injury, clues do not help the person with AD to remember. AD causes loss of older memories and recall of events from early life disappears. Language declines in a characteristic progression. Word-finding difficulty is first, followed by inability to remember names (anomia), and finally diminished comprehension.

Visuospatial deficits are an early clinical finding. Navigating the environment, cooking, and fixing or manipulating mechanical objects in the home are all visuospatial tasks that often are impaired in the first stages of AD. Drawing is abnormal; the ability to draw a three-dimensional object is often lost.

The loss of ability to solve mathematical problems and handle money is typical in the early stages of AD. Judgment is impaired and safety in driving is diminished.

Major depression is uncommon but many persons with AD have periods of depressed mood associated with a feeling of inadequacy and hopelessness. AD-associated depression is often more modifiable by environmental manipulation than depressions not associated with AD. As AD progresses, delusions, agitation, and even violence may occur.

Disorders of sleep, eating, and sexual behavior are common. The electroencephalogram (EEG) shows more awake time in bed, longer latencies to rapid eye movement sleep, and losses in slow-wave sleep.

Medical Management

Diagnosis. Use of neuroimaging can be of benefit in the diagnosis of AD. Both magnetic resonance imaging (MRI) and computed tomography (CT) can identify the changes in brain size that are associated with AD. In AD the generalized cerebral atrophy is, however, also present in normal aging and other neurodegenerative diseases (Miller et al., 1994).

Clinical screening tests such as the Mini-Mental State Examination (MMSE) and the Blessed Information Memory Concentration Test can be helpful in determining cognitive function.

Ruling out a partially or completely reversible dementia by performing a blood count, chest film, and general neurologic examination is critical in the diagnostic evaluation of a person with suspected AD.

Treatment. The dementia of AD remains untreatable. Use of anticholinesterases can cause moderate improvement in memory deficits. Treating superimposed medical conditions can be difficult owing to the cognitive deficits. The person with advanced disease and little or no language cannot communicate and small problems can become serious complications. Drug therapies for AD-associated symptoms are often efficacious but can have substantial side effects.

Targeting the role of amyloid precursor protein (APP) may lead to drugs that stop amyloid deposition. Modulation of neurotransmitter substances is currently being studied in hopes it may improve symptoms of cognitive impairment in the early stages of disease. (Whyte et al., 1994).

Manipulation of the environment can be effective. It is difficult to manage aggressive behavior in the home. Long-term care in a facility with a special Alzheimer's unit is often the most appropriate place for that client. Counsel with the family is critical to determine the best long-term environment.

Prognosis. AD is the fourth leading cause of death in adults. The period from onset to death typically takes 7 to 11 years. The rate of decline is variable. Initially, deficits in higher cortical function are the most noticeable. During the middle stages of the disease, the client often develops behavioral and motor problems. Finally, the client becomes mute and unable to comprehend. Death is often secondary to dehydration or infection.

Special Implications for the Therapist **27-2**

ALZHEIMER'S DISEASE

The client with AD has generalized weakness and abnormality of movement. Movements become more stereotyped and rigid. Postural reflexes are diminished and the incidence of falls increases. Falls occur in approximately 30% of clients with AD, which may be attributable to their lack of perception of where their body is in space, and their inability to move adequately around objects. Having the client move in a space that has few obstacles appears to decrease the number of falls.

The therapist often sees a client with AD in a structured living environment, as many people become difficult to maintain at home. Movement and exercise can provide the client with an activity that he or she can succeed in, as well as maintain mobility, good breathing patterns, and endurance. Restlessness and wandering are typical of the client with AD, and a structured exercise program appears to decrease restlessness. Daytime exercise can also help control nighttime pacing and the resulting daytime drowsiness.

Group therapy with simple exercises that use images rather than commands are most effective. Storytelling integrated into the exercise program helps to stimulate thinking as well as movement. Clients need to be able to attend to an activity for at least 5 minutes and the group therapy session must not provide more stimulation than clients are able to tolerate. Exercises should be short and simple and done in the same order each day. The exercise program should include group interaction with physical touching such as holding hands or working in pairs (Bowlby, 1993).

The therapist should be familiar with the warning signs of AD. Because the disease mimics dementia of old age, the symptoms may go unaddressed. It is often the spouse who asks questions regarding the possibility of the client developing AD. Information regarding the types of symptoms related to the disease can be helpful to the family in deciding whether more evaluation is needed. The Alzheimer's Association's 10 warning signs of AD are listed in Box 27–2.

DYSTONIA

Definition. Dystonia is a neurologic syndrome dominated by sustained muscle contractions frequently causing twisting and repetitive movements or abnormal postures often exacerbated by active voluntary movements. Dystonia is both a

BOX 27–2
Ten Warning Signs of Alzheimer's Disease (AD)

1. Recent memory loss that affects job performance. People with AD will forget things often, and may repeat the same question, forgetting the earlier answer.
2. Difficulty performing familiar tasks. The person may make a meal, and then forget to serve it, forgetting even that he or she made it.
3. Problems with simple language: forgetting simple words or using them inappropriately.
4. Disorientation. The person with AD may get lost on his or her own block.
5. Decreased judgment: sometimes forgetting that he or she is responsible for a child's care.
6. Abstract thinking difficulties, for example, forgetting what numbers are for when balancing a checkbook.
7. Misplacing things, such as putting an iron in the freezer.
8. Changes in mood or behavior: getting angry easily, and crying often.
9. Personality changes: becoming irritable, suspicious, or fearful.
10. Loss of initiative: not wanting to get involved in activities he or she previously enjoyed.

From Alzheimer's Association, 919 N. Michigan Ave., Suite 100, Chicago, IL 60611–1676.

symptom and the name for a collection of neurologic disorders characterized by these movements and postures.

Overview. Previously, dystonia was classified according to type, including primary (idiopathic or of unknown cause) or secondary dystonia, occurring as a result of injury or other brain illness. These classifications are still reported in the literature but the current classification scheme for dystonia now describes each person according to three separate categories[2]: age of onset, distribution of symptoms (types of dystonia), and etiology (cause or origin).

The age-of-onset classification includes four subgroups: infantile (under 2 years old), childhood (2 to 12 years), juvenile (12 to 20), and adult-onset (older than 20 years). The distribution of symptoms based on body part affected may be *focal* (affecting a single anatomic area), *segmental* (spreads to one or more adjacent body parts), or *generalized* (one or both legs and another body part are affected).

Focal dystonias are described as *blepharospasm* (uncontrolled blinking or closure of eyelids for seconds to hours), *cervical dystonia*[3] (neck muscles contract, turning the head to one side or pulling it forward or backward), *oromandibular dystonia*[4] (face and jaw muscles contract, causing grimaces or facial distortions), *dysphonia* (affecting speech muscles of the throat, causing strained, forced, or breathy speech), and *writer's cramp* or *occupational cramp* (muscles contract in the hands and forearms).

BOX 27–3
Causes of Secondary or Symptomatic Dystonia

Drugs, including neuroleptics, dopamine agonists, anticonvulsants, and antimalarial drugs
Post hemiplegia, often a delayed reaction to stroke
Focal brain lesions: vascular malformation, tumor, abscess, and demyelination
Traumatic brain injury
Encephalitis
Environmental toxins: manganese, carbon monoxide, and methanol
Hypoparathyroidism
Degenerative disease: Parkinson's disease, Huntington's disease, Wilson's disease, progressive supranuclear palsy, multiple system atrophy
Cerebral palsy

Incidence. An estimated 250,000 persons are afflicted with dystonia in North America. This figure is probably an underestimate because the condition is frequently misunderstood and often misdiagnosed because of its complexity. Focal dystonia is estimated to be six times more common than other well-known neuromuscular disorders such as muscular dystrophy, Huntington's disease, and ALS.

The average age of onset of generalized dystonia is 8 years old. For focal dystonias, the age of onset is between 30 and 50 years. Idiopathic cervical dystonia has its usual onset between 25 and 60 years. Crual dystonia is a gait disorder characterized by plantar flexion of the foot and is seen most often with onset between 6 and 12 years.

Etiology. Several theories have been proposed regarding the cause and pathophysiology of dystonia, including an underlying mental disorder, postinfectious condition, and altered basal ganglia and brainstem function.

Primary (idiopathic) dystonia is the most common diagnosis, accounting for two thirds to three fourths of all cases. A genetic basis is suspected with at least six different genes involved (e.g., persons with generalized dystonia carry a different gene than those with focal dystonias) (Edwards et al., 1995; Third International Dystonia Symposium Proceedings, 1996). Recent advances have been made in the understanding of other inherited dystonias such as dopa-responsive dystonia, sometimes called Segawa's dystonia.

In secondary dystonia, the condition is caused by small areas of brain damage or scarring to the CNS. Box 27–3 lists the major causes of secondary dystonia. Sometimes there are personal or familial extrapyramidal antecedents such as

[2] Theses classifications were presented at the Third International Dystonia Symposium in 1996. A new scheme is being proposed to encompass recent discoveries in the genetics of dystonia. Further information can be obtained about this disorder from the Dystonia Medical Research Foundation (DMRF), 1 E. Wacker Drive, Suite 2340, Chicago, IL 60601-1905, (312)-755-0198, or e-mail: dysfndt@aol.com.

[3] There has been some confusion in the literature regarding the name *cervical dystonia*. This neurologically based movement disorder affecting the head and neck is a separate entity from spasmodic torticollis. Torticollis is a musculoskeletal phenomenon treated as an orthopedic condition (see discussion of torticollis in Chapter 19).

[4] Blepharospasm and oromandibular dystonia combined is called Meige's disease.

tremor, or neck or head trauma.[5] Intramedullary lesions of the cervical cord or focal cerebral lesions as a result of vascular malformation, tumor, or abscess can also result in dystonia. Paroxysmal dystonias, called tonic spasms, can be caused by demyelinating lesions as occur with movement disorders (e.g., multiple sclerosis) (Tranchant et al., 1995).

Dystonias involving hand function are particularly common among certain occupational groups such as keyboard operators and musicians. Focal dystonia related to occupational cramps may be a result of abnormal biomechanics related to the person's inability to move the hand or arm in the range and with the speed necessary to perform the task. In these cases, it may be that there is an aberrant outcome of normal motor learning mimicking neuropathologically based dystonia (Wilson et al., 1993). Focal dystonia involving the hand may also occur as part of a peripheral nerve disorder.

Drug-induced extrapyramidal symptoms may include dystonia as a common side effect associated with antipsychotic drugs (neuroleptics). The fact that β-blocking agents are effective in these cases points to the possibility that neuroleptic drugs increase the activity of β-adrenergic transmitters resulting in various acute and chronic manifestations of neuroleptic-induced dystonia (e.g., blepharospasm, difficulty in opening the eyelids, torticollis, retrocollis, or involuntary extension of the neck) (Inada and Yagi, 1996).

Pathogenesis. Descending pathways involving reciprocal inhibition of motor neurons has been identified as a possible site of pathogenesis in primary (idiopathic) dystonia. Nerve conduction velocity studies have shown that there is a failure of neural activities preparing for a phasic movement. Defective retrieval or retaining of specific motor programs or subroutines in response to sensory stimuli results in co-contraction of agonists and antagonists (Uncini et al., 1994; Rothwell, 1995).

The cause of secondary dystonia is thought to be the result of chemical dysfunction within the putamen, basal ganglia, and related structures of the brain. Messages to initiate the correct muscle contractions required for specific movements are thought to originate in this region. A defect in the body's ability to process inhibitory neurotransmitters such as γ-aminobutyric acid (GABA), dopamine, acetylcholine, or norepinephrine and serotonin may result in poor inhibition of motor control.

Inherited dystonia mapped to chromosome 9 is probably the result of a protein which affects the function of certain nerve cells. The exact malfunction (e.g., whether that protein is missing or produced in excess) remains unknown.

Clinical Manifestations. Since dystonia is a neurologic movement disorder it can take many forms, but it is usually characterized by involuntary, uncontrollable muscular contractions which force certain parts of the body into abnormal movements or positions. Blepharospasm results in uncontrolled blinking or forcing the eyes to keep closed involuntarily. In some cases, only one eye is affected initially but with time both eyes close. The spasms may become sufficiently frequent to result in visual impairment although the eyes and vision are normal.

Other manifestations in the face are involuntary opening and closing of the jaw, puckering of the lips, and repetitive contractions of the platysma muscle. Pharyngeal dystonia is associated with distorted speech so that the person whispers or produces words haltingly and with great effort. Repetitive protrusion of the tongue may occur with speaking or eating.

Involvement of the respiratory muscles has been considered unusual but may in fact be underestimated either because it is not conspicuous or because it is improperly attributed to another cause. Clinical manifestations of respiratory involvement may include involuntary deep and loud inspirations combined with spasms of axial dystonia, breathing arrests, or broken speech caused by deep inspirations when speaking or reading aloud (Lagueny et al., 1995).

Cervical dystonia is the most common focal dystonia and is characterized by rotation of the neck, lateral flexion, and flexion and extension occurring in various combinations. The condition is usually painful, disruptive to functional activity, and leads to osteoarthritis and hypertrophy of the sternocleidomastoid muscle if remission does not occur. Dystonia-induced cervical fracture has been reported (Adler et al., 1996).

Dystonia usually is present continually throughout the day whenever the affected body part is in use. In more severe cases, the dystonia can appear at rest. The symptoms may begin in one area only with a particular movement. For example, it may be apparent when walking forward but not when walking backward, or the foot may turn under after walking or other exercise causing the person to walk on the lateral border of the foot.

Writer's or occupational cramp is a form of dystonia that can be particularly disabling resulting in deterioration in handwriting or in fine motor control. The fingers and wrist flex excessively causing the hand to grasp a pen tightly and press unnecessarily hard on the paper. Another type of cramp that occurs results in extension of the fingers making it difficult to hold a pen. Tremor or myoclonic jerks may occur while writing or trying to play a musical instrument.

Medical Management

Diagnosis. There is no definitive test for dystonia and the diagnosis of primary (idiopathic) dystonia is often delayed a year or more. The clinical presentation of dystonic movements such as head deviation or neck pain (e.g., cervical dystonia) may be the first diagnostic sign. The person will have had a normal perinatal and developmental history. EMG studies show sustained simultaneous contractions of agonists and antagonists (see Pathogenesis for explanation). Determining that there is no evidence for secondary dystonia is essential in the diagnosis of primary dystonia. There should be no precipitating illness or exposure to drugs known to cause dystonia and no evidence of intellectual, pyramidal, cerebellar, or sensory causes.

Treatment. Without a true understanding of the cause of this disorder, treatment remains symptomatic and includes

[5] Dystonia is a rare consequence of head trauma with variable delay between the head trauma and the onset of dystonia. On brain imaging studies (CT or MRI), the most frequent lesion site is the contralateral basal ganglia or thalamus but cases of normal brain scans have been reported. Dysfunction of the lenticulothalamic neuronal circuit seems to be related to the development of dystonia following head trauma (Lee et al., 1994).

drug therapy,[6] including botulinum toxin injections, physical and occupational therapy, and sometimes surgery.

Botulinum toxin type A (Botox), injected intramuscularly, has emerged as a safe and effective symptomatic treatment for a number of conditions associated with excessive muscle activity, particularly focal dystonias involving a limited number of muscles. These injections are effective in improving postural deviation and pain in about 80% of people with cervical dystonias. Injection directly into the actively contracting muscle(s) blocks the neuromuscular junction by acting presynaptically to reduce the release of acetylcholine, producing a chemical denervation.

Decrease of muscle spasm is often accompanied by reduced voluntary movement, and muscle weakness results from this treatment; protocols are being developed to reduce excessive muscle activity without producing significant functional weakness. Response occurs in 3 to 7 days and lasts 3 to 4 months. Dysphagia is the most serious side effect but can be decreased in incidence and severity by injecting lower doses, particularly into the sternocleidomastoid. The need to continue indefinitely with repeat injections approximately every 3 months is a major drawback.

Surgery may be considered only when other treatments are no longer effective, although surgical intervention may also lose its effect over time providing only temporary symptomatic relief. Surgery to interrupt the pathways responsible for the abnormal movements includes thalamotomy (destruction of a portion of the thalamus), pallidotomy (a destructive operation on the globus pallidus), muscle resection, rhizotomy (surgical resection of the anterior cervical spinal nerve roots), and selective peripheral denervation (removal of the nerves at the point they enter the contracting muscles).

Prognosis. Age of onset is the best predictor of prognosis. If dystonia starts in childhood and affects other members of the family, it tends to get progressively worse over the years. If the condition starts in childhood and is secondary to cerebral palsy or other brain injury close to the time of birth, the dystonia tends to remain static for many years. In one third of adult-onset focal dystonia there is progression to segmental dystonia, although there is less than a 20% chance that the disease will progress to generalized dystonia.

Spontaneous remission occurs in 30% of cases within the first year but the majority of clients show steady progression of their focal dystonia with maximal disability occurring after 5 years. Neck pain, occurring in 70% to 80% of clients, contributes significantly to disability. Cervical dystonia has important psychosocial consequences as many people with this condition withdraw from their jobs and social activities (Van Zandijcke, 1995).

[6] Anticholinergics have been the most widely used medications to decrease acetylcholine and correct a cholinergic imbalance in the basal ganglia. Side effects of these drugs vary, with blurred vision, dry mouth, confusion, voiding and sleeping difficulties, and personality changes observed. Use of other drugs such as baclofen (muscle relaxant), carbamazepine (anticonvulsant), and benzodiazepines (regulate GABA systems in the brain) have given mixed results. The combination of carbidopa and levodopa (Sinemet) and bromocriptine increase dopamine transmission and are effective in dopa-responsive dystonia. In some cases, just the opposite—decreasing the brain's capacity to store dopamine, using dopamine antagonists (e.g., tetrabenazine)—may be helpful.

Special Implications for the Therapist **27-3**

DYSTONIA

Treatment Issues

When dystonia originates in the CNS, physical therapy such as massage or electrical stimulation provides only temporary relief from symptoms and does not affect the underlying movement disorder. Likewise, focal dystonia does not respond to facilitatory or inhibitory techniques used for modulating spasticity.

Aggressive treatment may increase the symptoms of dystonia; any treatment should be carried out within the client's tolerance and without increasing the manifestations of the dystonia. A program of therapeutic exercise focusing on improving muscle imbalances and flexibility while providing proprioceptive input is recommended.

Movement should never be forced and all exercises should be performed in a slow, smooth, and controlled manner. Exercise should be stopped if the client experiences pain. Swimming pool therapy is especially helpful in reducing discomfort and facilitating movement. Stretching exercises are helpful in maintaining muscle length and preventing loss of mobility in the joints. Strengthening exercises may be considered for weak muscles opposing the affected dystonic muscles. This is especially important in maintaining good posture and reducing fatigue.

Some degree of the movement associated with dystonia can be controlled with proprioceptive or tactile input. Many people with dystonia use sensory tricks to decrease the severity of the dystonic movements. Resting the head against a high-backed chair, holding the back of the neck, or lightly touching the cheek or chin may return the head to the normal position. No single position should be maintained for long as static positions can aggravate symptoms.

The use of a cervical collar has been tried by some with good results but it is suspected that the sensory information to the skin accounts for this success rather than the mechanical support provided. If the collar minimizes pain or provides a more functional midline position there may be some merit in its use. Otherwise, if it only works as a sensory trick, a piece of cloth wrapped around the neck may accomplish the same effect. The person who uses a cervical collar should be taught to do exercises outside the collar to minimize weakness in the noninvolved muscles.

When the jaw, tongue, or lips are involved, gentle pressure on the lips or teeth may lessen spasm. For example, exerting slight pressure against the jaw on the side to which the head is rotated may decrease or inhibit muscle spasm although this is an immediate and short-term reaction.

The therapist should address all aspects of functional ability with the client who has been affected by dystonia, including stress management, energy conservation, adaptive equipment, mobility, and splinting. In the case of generalized dystonia, splinting has been effective for some people in improving function. In the case of the foot or feet turning in, insoles

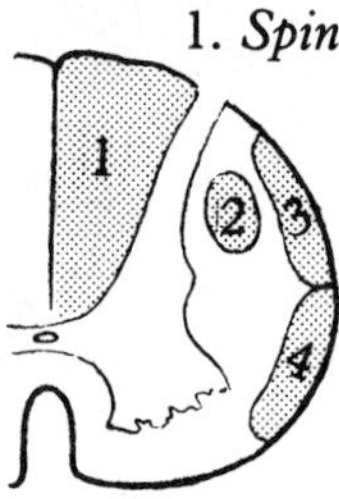

1. *Spinal:* The spinal cord is shrunken, especially in the thoracic region.
   There is degeneration and gliosis of:
   1. Posterior columns.
   2. Corticospinal tracts.
   3. Dorsal spinocerebellar tracts.
   4. Ventral spinocerebellar tracts.

   Dorsal roots and peripheral nerves are also shrunken when cases are advanced.
2. *Cerebellar:* Changes in the cerebellum are less marked. There is Purkinje cell loss and atrophy of the dentate nucleus.

The corticobulbar tract and cerebrum are spared.

Figure **27–2.** Degeneration of the specific area of the central nervous system seen in Friedreich's ataxia. (*From Lindsay KW, Bone I, Callander R: Neurology and Neurosurgery Illustrated. New York, Churchill Livingstone, 1986.*)

placed in the shoes to build up the outer border of the foot may help to put the foot in a neutral position and produce a more normal gait pattern. Guidelines for chewing and swallowing may be helpful for the client with oromandibular dystonia.

There may be further implications for therapy as the relationship of biomechanics, motor programming, and occupational cramps becomes better understood.

Post Botulinum Injection

Once the muscle spasm is reduced following botulinum injection, more normal movement may be possible. The therapist may employ biofeedback to reeducate normal muscle function by increasing awareness of how the muscle is working. This information can be used to grade the activity with the goal of restoring normal movement.

When relief of spasm allows the client to assume a more normal or correct posture, underlying tight soft tissues may benefit from short-term use of physical therapy modalities and soft tissue mobilization to restore full range of motion. The use of palliative treatments such as heat and massage do not provide an objective benefit and are not recommended.

FRIEDREICH'S ATAXIA

Overview and Definition *(Harding, 1993).* Friedreich's ataxia (FA, spinocerebellar degeneration) is the most common of the early-onset ataxias. It is characterized by degeneration of the ascending and descending fibers of the spinal cord, including the spinocerebellar tracts.

Incidence, Etiology, and Risk Factors. FA is a hereditary disease with a prevalence of between 1 and 2 in 100,000. Disease onset before the age of 20 or 25 is typical, the disease usually manifesting between the ages of 8 and 15. It is inherited as an autosomal recessive trait, and is linked to the long arm of chromosome 9. Late-onset FA is less common and is transmitted as an autosomal dominant inheritance.

As only 25% of the offspring of affected parents develop the disorder, there are few cases of siblings with the disorder. The recurrence rate of siblings is 1 in 4, and often the disease is not detected before other siblings are born. Early detection would allow for prudent preconception decisions within the family.

Pathogenesis. The principal changes are cell loss in the dorsal root ganglia and secondary degeneration in the posterior columns and spinocerebellar tracts, most severe in the cervical region. There is loss of the larger cells in the dorsal root ganglia. In addition, there is a loss of large myelinated axons in peripheral nerves. This is seen in very young people and increases with age and disease duration. Degeneration of the corticospinal tracts is evident in many cases, with sparing of the corticobulbar tracts. Figure 27–2 shows some of the spinal cord changes seen as the disease progresses. The cerebellum can be affected to varying degrees, with loss of Purkinje cells in the most advanced cases.

In addition to these neuropathologic changes, there are cardiomyopathic changes resulting in muscle fiber loss and fibrosis in approximately 60% of persons.

Clinical Manifestations. FA is primarily a disorder of movement with ataxic gait the most common presenting symptom. The person begins to stagger and lurch; often a wide-based gait results. Early in the course of the disease, particularly in children, there may be motor restlessness that may look like chorea. Clumsiness, ataxia, and tremor appear in the limbs. Muscle tone is normal at rest, although flexor spasm is common. The plantar reflexes are flexor at the onset but develop to become extensor through the course of the disease. Typically there is an unusual combination or total absence of tendon reflexes with increased extensor reflex activity, or a positive Babinski's sign.[7] Weakness of the limbs follows a progressive course.

Dysarthria and scanning speech are symptoms of loss of normal speech rhythm. Nystagmus is seen in about 20% of clients. Extraocular movements are nearly always abnormal, with broken-up pursuit, dysmetric saccades, and failure of fixation suppression of the vestibulo-ocular reflex (see Chapter 33).

There is loss of vibration and position sense in the extremi-

[7] Babinski's sign reflects upper motor neuron dysfunction. When the plantar surface of the foot is stroked, usually at the metatarsal heads, the great toe extends in response.

ties. Sensation of pain, temperature, and light touch may be diminished in a distal and symmetrical distribution.

Musculoskeletal deformities are a secondary complication of FA. Scoliosis is common, may even be severe if onset is early, and is associated with cardiopulmonary morbidity. Pes cavus, a foreshortening of the foot with cocking of the toes, appears in approximately 50% of clients. This is due to atrophy and contractures of the muscles of the feet at a time when the bones of the feet are malleable. Figure 27–3 shows the common deformities related to FA.

Mentation is usually preserved, although in some instances there is dementia and decrease in intelligence during the course of the disease. Diabetes mellitus occurs in 10% of clients, and a further 20% have impaired glucose tolerance.

Medical Management

Diagnosis. The diagnosis of FA is essentially clinical. For the diagnosis of FA a number of clinical criteria have to be met, which include onset of ataxia before age 25, progressive course, and loss of tendon reflexes.

The condition is most frequently confused with demyelinating forms of hereditary and sensory neuropathies. The differential diagnosis is made by performing an upper limb motor nerve conduction test. The conduction velocity is always above 40 m/sec in FA and slower in the other hereditary neuropathies.

Electrophysiologic studies demonstrate delayed, dispersed somatosensory evoked potentials recorded at the sensory cortex, and abnormal central motor conduction.

CT scans and MRI are either normal or show atrophy in the cerebellum or spinal cord.

Treatment. The results of treating ataxia in FA have largely been disappointing. Treatment of secondary musculoskeletal deformities may be beneficial. Cardiac failure and arrhythmias are treated conventionally.

Prognosis. The prognosis of FA is variable. Over 95% of clients are using wheelchairs for mobility by the age of 45 years, and on average they lose the ability to walk 15 years after onset of symptoms. Reported mean ages of death have been in the mid-30s, but survival into the 50s and 60s can occur, particularly if there is no heart disease or diabetes.

Special Implications for the Therapist **27-4**

FRIEDREICH'S ATAXIA

Education of the family is important. Proper fit of wheelchair and mobility aids should be monitored as the disease progresses.

Clients with FA exhibit multidirectional sway that is complicated by the proprioceptive deficit. These clients then become dependent on visual cues to maintain balance and have more difficulty when the visual environment does not allow for fixation of gaze or is absent.

HUNTINGTON'S DISEASE

Overview and Definition. Huntington's disease (HD) is a progressive hereditary disorder characterized by abnormalities of movement, personality disturbances, and dementia. Known also as Huntington's chorea, it is most often associated with *choreic* movement which is brief, purposeless, involuntary, and random. However, the disease course involves more than just a movement disorder, and hence the name Huntington's disease. HD is a disorder of the CNS and is classified as a neurologic disorder, but as a condition with effects that are complex, management requires a multidisciplinary approach (Harper and Morris, 1991; Wojcieszek and Lang, 1994).

Incidence and Risk Factors. The prevalence of HD in North America ranges from 4 to 8 per 100,000. It is estimated that there are 25,000 cases in the United States. HD may begin at any time after infancy but usually starts in middle age. Twenty-five percent of persons with HD have disease of late onset, which is defined as onset of motor symptoms after age 50. There is almost always a history of an affected parent.

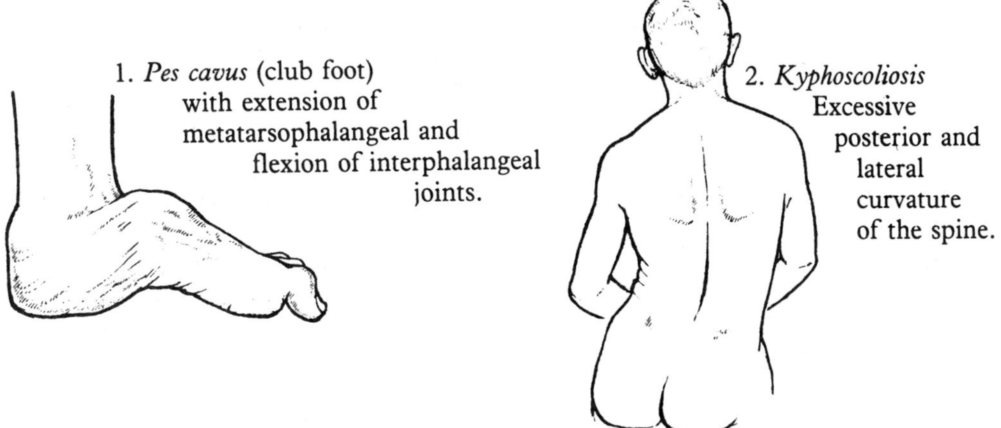

Figure **27-3.** Deformities commonly seen in Friedreich's ataxia. (*From Lindsay KW, Bone I, Callander R: Neurology and Neurosurgery Illustrated. New York, Churchill Livingstone, 1986.*)

There is a 50% risk in each child of an affected adult (Beal et al., 1994). Transmission of the juvenile form of HD (onset before age 20) appears to be primarily from the paternal parent. With adult onset there is more equal transmission from the parents (Harper and Morris, 1991).

HD is an autosomal dominant disease. The genetic marker has been found on the tip of chromosome 4, and is linked to the HD gene. This allows accurate information about the risk to an individual as long as there is a sufficient number of family members with whom to compare the DNA. All of the people who inherit the gene will develop symptoms of the disease if they do not die prematurely. As there is no cure for HD, there is, then, an ethical dilemma associated with testing. Studies are underway to determine the psychiatric and social problems that may result from the knowledge that one will suffer and die from HD (Folstein, 1989).

Pathogenesis *(Beal et al., 1994; Quarrell, 1991; Wojcieszek and Lang, 1994).* While the cause remains unknown, the pathology shows a consistent pattern of tissue changes in the brain The ventricles are enlarged as a result of atrophy of the adjacent basal ganglia, specifically the caudate nucleus and putamen (collectively the *striatum*). This is due to extensive loss of small and medium-sized neurons. The volume of the brain can be decreased by as much as 20%. The dementia of HD has been ascribed to the dysfunction in the striatum. Other subtle changes occur in the cortex and cerebellum, including both loss of neurons and production of glial cells which inhibit neural transmission (Fig. 27–4).

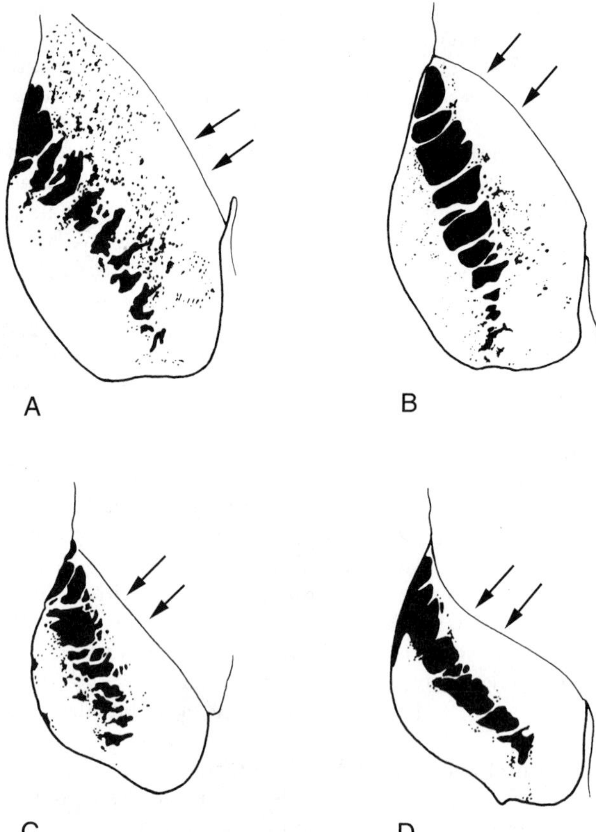

Figure **27–4.** Atrophy seen in the caudate and putamen in a person with Huntington's disease. As the disease progresses (represented by *A* through *D*), there is a change in the caudate at the interface with the ventricle (*arrows*). The outline becomes more and more concave representing the progressive atrophy. (*From Quarrell O: The neurobiology of Huntington's disease. In Harper PS (ed): Huntington's Disease. Philadelphia, WB Saunders, 1991, pp 81–109.*)

As with other progressive diseases there is selective vulnerability of neurons in a particular region with preservation of others. In the early and middle stages of HD neurons projecting from the striatum to the substantia nigra are depleted. This reduces the amount of neurotransmitters, including GABA, acetylcholine, and metenkephalin. This leaves relatively higher concentrations of other neurotransmitters, such as dopamine and norepinephrine. The normal balance of inhibition and excitation responses in the complex organization of the basal ganglia and thalamus that allows for smooth controlled movement is disrupted. The result is an excess of dopamine and excessive excitation of the thalamocortical pathway. This may explain the excessive abnormal involuntary movements described as chorea.

In the later stages of HD, there is a loss of the direct inhibitory substance which causes more inhibition of the thalamocortical output with resultant rigidity and *bradykinesia,* or slowness of movement. By the late stages of HD, virtually all of the caudate nucleus projection neurons are affected. The mechanism of neuronal loss is not known. One hypothesis is that an excitotoxin causes the cell death noted in the basal ganglia.

Clinical Manifestations

Movement Disorders *(Beal et al., 1994; Quarrell and Harper, 1991).* Many patients with suspected early HD will show almost no neurologic abnormality on routine examination other than minor choreic movements. The movements may be suppressed during the examination as they can often be integrated into a purposeful movement such as raising the hand to the head as if to smooth the hair. Early in the course the involuntary movements may appear to be no more than an exaggeration of normal restlessness, usually involving the upper limbs and face. The chorea is increased by mental concentration, emotional stimuli, performance of complex motor tasks, and walking. Problems with voluntary movement may be detected by asking for rapid tongue movements, finger-to-thumb tapping, or testing for *dysdiadochokinesia,* the inability to make rapid alternating movements. There can be early refractoriness of motor tasks such as inability to maintain tongue protrusion or handgrip.

Assessment of muscle strength will usually be normal in early cases but may be affected by any significant bradykinesia or general motor disturbance. Tone will usually be normal initially, but rigidity will become part of the clinical picture in many cases as the disease progresses. The tendon reflexes are usually normal. The "hung-up" knee jerk sometimes seen is produced by interposition of a choreiform contraction of knee extensors upon the normal course of the reflex.

Abnormalities in eye movement are common in HD. Saccades, the ability to move the eyes rapidly from one target to another in order to move the visual focus rapidly to different objects, is disturbed. There is often a decrease in velocity of movement, an undershooting of the target, or a latency in initiation of movement. *Gaze fixation* abnormalities have been noted, that is, inability to fix on a light source without the intrusion of small saccadic movements. *Smooth pursuit*, or tracking of the eye to follow a moving object, is interrupted by the same small jerky saccadic movements. There is often an inability to suppress reflex saccades to a visual stimulus, which leads to visual distractibility.

The term *chorea* is derived from the Greek word for dance, and gait abnormalities are common in HD. When chorea is a predominant sign, persons walk with a wide-based staggering gait. Those persons with bradykinesia and hypertonicity may walk with a slow, stiff, unsteady gait.

Dysarthria, reflected as a decrease in the rate and rhythm of speech, may be mild in the early course with an increase to the point that speech may be unintelligible. In addition to the mechanical problems, neuron loss disrupts linguistic abilities, resulting in reduced vocabulary and syntactic errors. Some persons become mute at a stage before motor disability is severe.

Abnormalities of swallowing, or *dysphagia*, can cause choking and asphyxia. Dysphagia may involve multiple abnormalities of ingestion, including inappropriate food choices, abnormal rate of eating, poor bolus formation, and inadequate respiratory control.

Cachexia, or the wasting of muscle with weight loss, is found despite an adequate diet. This appears to be independent of the hyperkinesia, and is found in persons with rigidity as well.

Sleep disorders become a progressive problem throughout the course of HD. An increased latent period before sleep and increased periods of wakefulness are common in moderately affected persons. Sleep reversal—daytime somnolence and nighttime restlessness—is seen in severely affected persons and is probably related to the dementia. Choreic movements are reduced during the deepest part of sleep.

Urinary incontinence is often a problem. This could be related to dementia, depression, decreased mobility, or hyperreflexia of the muscles that control urine output. There can be a concomitant increase in the incidence of urinary tract infections.

Neuropsychological and Psychiatric Disorders. Early mental disturbances in persons with HD include personality and behavioral changes such as irritability, apathy, depression, decreased work performance, violence, impulsivity, and emotional lability (Morris, 1991; Wojcieszek and Lang, 1994). Intellectual decline usually follows the personality changes. The neuropsychological profile characteristically includes a type of memory disturbance that suggests an impairment of information retrieval. Patients often have difficulty recalling information on command, but are able to give the correct answer in a multiple-choice format. There is difficulty with organization, planning, and sequencing, even when all the information is provided. Other prominent abnormalities include visuospatial deficits, impaired judgment, and *ideomotor apraxia*, the inability to perform previously learned tasks despite intact elementary motor function.

More than one third of persons with HD will develop an affective disorder. Depression is the most common psychiatric condition and does not appear to be simply a reaction to a fatal illness. Evidence for this is the fact that mood disorders are not randomly distributed but occur in subsets of families with HD (Folstein, 1989).

Medical Management

Diagnosis *(Beal et al., 1994; Wojcieszek and Lang, 1994)*. The clinical diagnosis of HD is dependent upon recognition of patterns of symptoms given in the client's history and clinical signs, and the family history. Difficulties in diagnosis arise when the family history appears negative. Some families deny the presence of cognitive or psychiatric disease. Understanding of the clinical signs must take into account the fact that signs change during the course of the illness and that different patterns may be observed depending on the age of onset (Harper and Morris, 1991).

MRI demonstrates atrophy of the striatum which is most easily appreciated as enlargement of the frontal horn of the lateral ventricles. Figure 27–5 shows this change in brain structure. This is not of great diagnostic value unless it is very pronounced, given the normal reduction in brain mass with age and the occurrence of atrophy in other disorders that might be confused with HD. A positron emission tomography (PET) scan will also show atrophy but its value as a diagnostic tool has the same limitations as MRI.

In addition to genetic linkage analysis, which requires testing of family members, it is now possible to evaluate the DNA of an individual to identify specific components that are diagnostic of HD. This eliminates the need to compare DNA of affected family members, but there are still problems with this method because there is a small percentage of affected individuals who do not display the characteristics on the specific gene and there are nonaffected individuals who carry the gene.

Recognition of HD in the elderly person is critical to establish the genetic link for future generations. Often the diagnosis is overlooked in favor of the label of "senile chorea" because there are minimal changes in behavior and cognition. The differential diagnosis of HD in the elderly includes various degenerative, systemic, and drug-related conditions. A patient treated with neuroleptics for a psychiatric presentation of HD, for example, may go on to develop movement disorders and these may be confused with the typical side effects of the medication (Morris and Tyler, 1991).

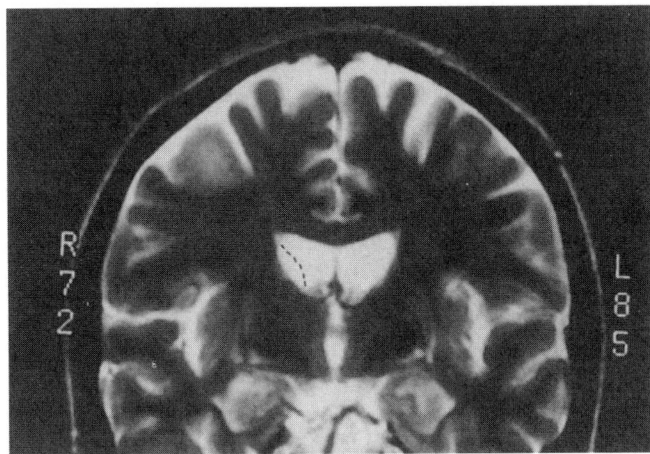

Figure **27–5.** Magnetic resonance scan showing the degeneration of the caudate in a person with Huntington's disease (HD). The *dotted lines* show where the tissue would be in a person not suffering from HD. (*From Ramsey R: Neuroradiology. Philadelphia, WB Saunders, 1994.*)

Treatment. Management of HD requires a team approach including medical and social services (Morris and Tyler, 1991). Education of clients and their families about the implications of the disease is important. Genetic, psychological, and social counseling are required. Organizations designed to help families with HD are often of great help.

Medical treatment is symptomatic. The most useful drugs for the symptomatic relief of chorea are anticonvulsants or antipsychotic agents that block dopamine neurotransmission. They can also help with the emotional outbursts, paranoia, psychosis, and irritability seen in HD. Drug therapy for chorea should be held in reserve if the abnormal movements are slight. There is a high incidence of side effects with the drugs, including acute dystonias, pseudoparkinsonism, and *akathisia*, which is characterized by uncontrollable physical restlessness. The most serious effect is chronic tardive dyskinesia resulting in involuntary movement of the face, tongue, and lips. Another adverse reaction is neuroleptic malignant hyperpyrexic syndrome, characterized by fever and rigidity.

Surgical procedures to remove the medial globus pallidus thought to be overexcited by neuronal loss in the striatum have been tried with mixed results. Implantation of adrenal medullary grafts have not been encouraging; the improvement appears to be transient.

Prognosis. It is characteristic of the disease that younger people, with onset of symptoms at age 15 to 40 years, will suffer a more severe form of the disease than older people, with onset in their 50s and 60s. The advance of the disease is slow, with death occurring on average 15 to 20 years after onset. Survival into the 80s is not uncommon and persons living to over 90 years old have been recorded. Age at onset and death frequently show a familial correlation (Beal et al., 1994; Wojcieszek and Lang, 1994).

Increasing disability from involuntary movements and mental changes often results in death from intercurrent infection. Suicide accounts for approximately 6% of deaths and 25% of persons with HD attempt suicide at least once.

Special Implications for the Therapist **27-5**

HUNTINGTON'S DISEASE

Education of the client and family about movement disorders, including gait and safety in mobility, is the basis for therapeutic intervention. Clients with HD do fall, but it is surprising that mobility is maintained despite the seemingly precarious arrangements of the limbs and trunk. As the disease progresses, postural stability becomes impaired and axial chorea may throw the client off balance. In clients whose bradykinesia is predominant, there is a propensity to "freeze," especially in confined spaces, and this may precipitate falls.

Apraxia, the inability to perform skilled or purposeful movements, may become severe. This impairment may lead to significant disability in performance of activities of daily living. The client may lose the ability to dress, and do self-care activities such as grooming regardless of cues provided by caregivers.

Positioning to prevent soft tissue deformities and safety in transfers should be taught according to the current movement disorder identified. Both the therapist and the family should understand that these techniques may need to be changed as the movement disorder progresses. The therapist should be aware that chorea and bradykinesia can be manifested in the patient at the same time owing to the progressive neuronal loss in the basal ganglia described earlier.

The ability to intervene with neurotherapeutic techniques, including motor learning, may be limited in the face of the concomitant decline in mental function as the motor system impairments progress.

MULTIPLE SCLEROSIS

Overview and Definition. Multiple sclerosis (MS) is typically a disease of young adults that begins acutely or subacutely with an attack of neurologic dysfunction. This disorder affects the CNS, while sparing the peripheral nerves. It is primarily the white matter that is damaged, but lesions of the gray matter have also been found. Characterized by local inflammation, edema, and demyelination, the disease causes a significant decrease in the conduction rate of the axon. This conduction block may account for the fluctuations in function that vary from hour to hour and from day to day and for the worsening of function that follows elevation in core body temperature (Hauser, 1994).

Although it is generally considered a major cause of disability in early to middle adulthood, the course of MS is highly variable. Complications of MS may affect multiple body systems and may require profound adjustments in lifestyle and goals for clients and their families; therefore, a multidisciplinary approach is necessary to optimize clinical care.

Incidence. The incidence of MS in females is twice that in males. MS is uncommon before adolescence, rises steadily in incidence from the teens to age 35, and declines gradually thereafter. There is a slightly later age of onset in men than in women. MS occurring as early as age 2 or as late as age 74 years is rare, but has been documented (Hauser, 1994).

Marked differences in the prevalence of MS exist between different populations and ethnic groups. The highest known prevalence occurs in the Orkney Islands, off Scotland. MS is also common in Scandinavia and elsewhere in northern Europe. In the United States, the incidence is estimated as 30 to 80 per 100,000, or 250,000 to 350,000 people affected. Whites have significantly higher rates of the disease than other racial groups. MS is extremely rare in Japan and virtually unknown in black Africa, but Japanese-Americans and black Americans show an increased prevalence (Rodriguez et al., 1994).

Etiology. It has been established that there is an abnormal autoimmune reaction in the brain tissue in MS, but, the trigger of that reaction is not clearly understood. There appears to be a genetic susceptibility to exposure to a virus. Pedigree study of families multiply affected tends to support the hypothesis that multiple unlinked genes confer susceptibility. The major histocompatibility complex (MHC) on chromosome 6 has been identified as one genetic determinant for MS, but this contributes only a small fraction to the genetic basis of MS (Hauser, 1994). The search for genetic links is ongoing.

Risk Factors. Viral infection can precipitate attacks of MS. In fact, it is the only natural event that has been shown unequivocally to increase the risk of a new attack. Approximately one third of exacerbations are preceded by infection, but only 8% of infections are followed by exacerbations. The role of interferon-γ (increased during infection) and its antagonist interferon-β (dampens antigen recognition) have been shown to affect progression of the disease. In addition, in MS there is an increased susceptibility to infections of the respiratory, digestive, and urinary tracts.

The role of stress and trauma have been studied to determine a link with the appearance of the initial symptoms or to exacerbations of the symptoms, but the mechanism is not yet clearly understood. Research in the area of autoimmune disease and stress is ongoing.

MS is in general a disease of temperate climates. In both hemispheres, its prevalence decreases with lowering of latitude. Migration data in well-defined ethnic populations also indicate an effect of environment on risk. Figure 27–6 reflects the areas that are most prone to an increased incidence of MS. Children born to parents who have migrated from a high-risk to a low-risk area have a lower lifetime risk than their parents. Conversely, migration from a low-risk to a high-risk area confers an increased risk for the children. Limited studies suggest that there is a critical period before the age of 15 that is significant for environmental exposure (Hauser, 1994)

Pathogenesis. MS is believed to be a virus-induced autoimmune disease mediated by lymphocytes and macrophages, the cells of the immune system which trigger the response to changes. Lymphocytes are divided into (1) T cells, which are further divided into suppressor/cytotoxic and helper/inducer cells, and (2) B cells, which produce antibodies (see Immunology, Chapter 5). The role of T cells in MS is not clearly understood, but it is believed that they may be cytotoxic and directly attack and destroy myelin, or that they may be responsible for the secretion of lymphokines that are cytotoxic (Utz and McFarland, 1994) Macrophages are cells that take up and digest cellular and myelin debris and bacteria. The T cells and macrophages infiltrate the tissue and cause the loss of myelin. The area of tissue infiltration is known as a plaque and is easily distinguished from the surrounding white matter.

MS derives its name from the multiple plaques found throughout the brain and spinal cord. The blood-brain barrier becomes more permeable, allowing antibodies and immune cells easier penetration in the area of the plaques. Helper and cytotoxic T cells, B cells, and macrophages are all present in acute plaques. The result is destruction of the myelin sheath, and to varying degrees, the oligodendrocytes, the myelin-producing cells which lie directly beneath the sheath (Herndon, 1994).

Important differences characterize the pathology of acute and chronic forms of the disease. Different neuropathologic manifestations are present in early bouts of chronic MS compared with late stages of disease, particularly with respect to the impairment of oligodendrocytes.[8] In the early stages of MS, a significant number of oligodendrocytes may survive the immunologic insult and be prepared to produce rapid and complete remyelination. In late stages of the disease virtually no oligodendrocytes are preserved, and remyelination, if it occurs at all, occurs only at the peripheral borders of the plaques. In chronic MS the myelin sheath is ultimately replaced by fibrous scarring known as *gliosis*, which inhibits the transmission of nerve impulses. Gliosis is more severe in MS lesions than in most other neuropathologic conditions. In chronic MS lesions, complete or nearly complete demyelination, dense gliosis, and loss of oligodendroglia are present. The edema associated with active disease can cause a mass effect and the plaque can simulate a neoplasm (Hauser, 1994).

Serial MRI studies have shown that new lesions frequently appear at sites of previous activity or within or at the edges of previously stable lesions. New lesions can form within or overlap shadow plaques (areas of thin remyelination) and may contribute to failed remyelination or the conversion of shadow plaques into classic demyelinated plaques (Prineas et al., 1993).

Clinical Manifestations. Sensory changes are most often the initial complaint. This is often a paresthesia or dysesthesia noted in one extremity or in the head and face. Visual blurring or diplopia may be the first sign. Often these symptoms are transient and not even reported. Clients often report a temporary weakness that resolves or moves to another body segment over time. It is usually when there is a pattern or the symptoms are unchanging that the person seeks medical attention. Although MS is a chronic progressive disease, the disease may take a variety of courses. Listed in order of severity, the following courses have been identified (O'Sullivan, 1994a; Weinshenker et al., 1988).

A *benign* course affects approximately 20% of patients and is characterized by an abrupt onset with one or a few exacerbations and complete or nearly complete remissions. These persons experience little or no permanent disability and remain relatively symptom-free.

An *exacerbating-remitting* or *relapsing* course will affect approximately 20% to 30%. The course is similar to a benign course but the symptoms will reoccur between long stable periods and the disease may not progress to increasing levels of disability.

A *remitting* or *relapsing-progressive* course affects 30% to 40%. These persons have acute relapses, but subsequently develop a stepwise or progressive worsening of impairments and disability between attacks.

A *primary chronic* or *progressive* course is found in 20% of persons with MS. The most common clinical presentation of primary progressive MS is myelopathy, a gradual progressive weakening and wasting of muscles, and is typically seen in persons with onset beginning over the age of 40 years. Primary progressive MS may present in other ways, including a progressive cerebellar disorder or dementia.

[8] The oligodendrocyte is a non-neural component of the CNS which is directly related to the cell body or axon. The oligodendrocyte produces the myelin which wraps around the axon of the nerve cell. The myelin sheath increases the speed of the action potential and is critical for smooth and rapid movement.

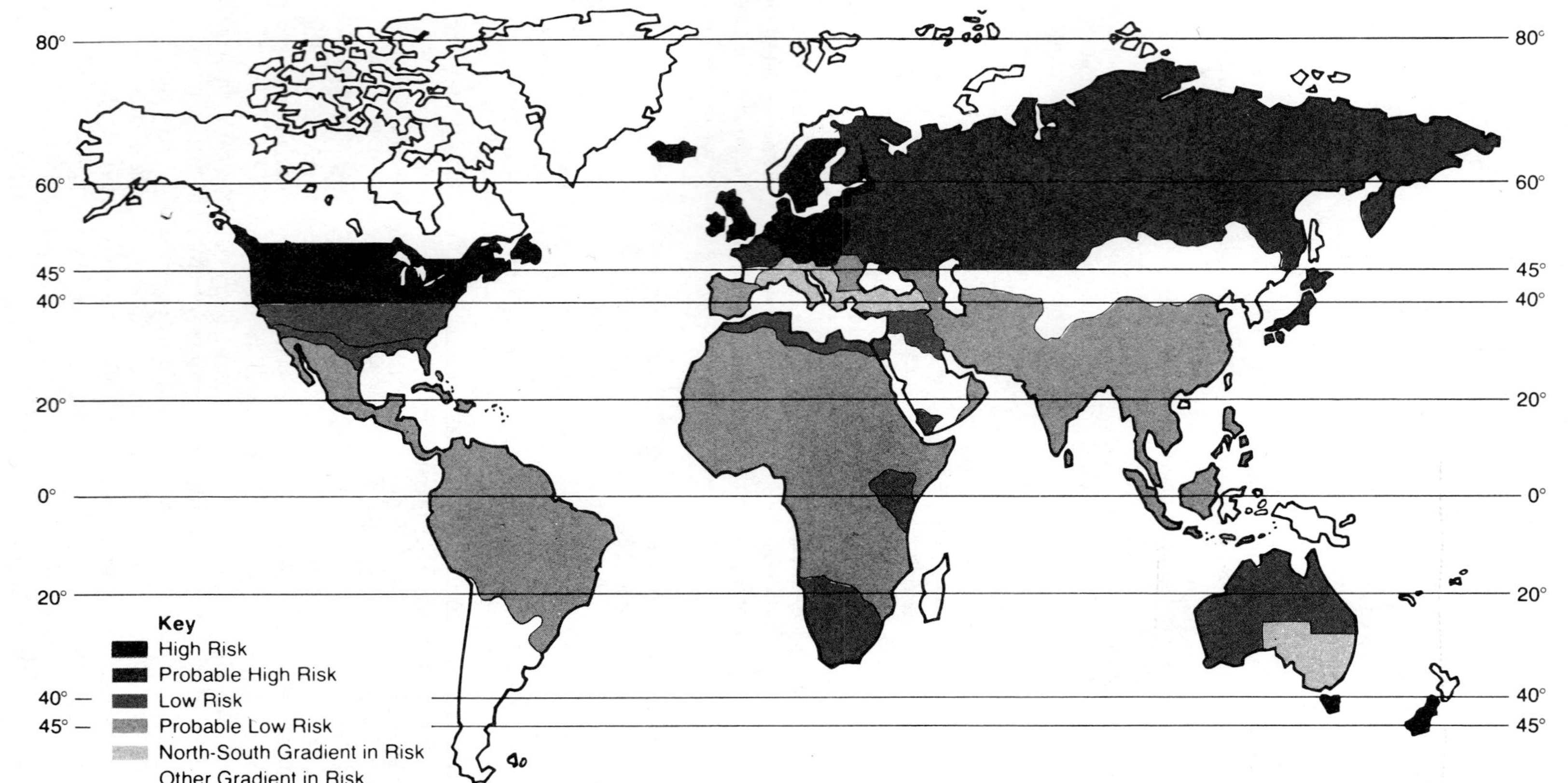

Figure **27–6.** World map showing the relative incidence of multiple sclerosis. Areas of greatest risk are in the northern latitudes. (*From Frankel D: Multiple sclerosis.* In *Umphred DA: Neurological Rehabilitation. St Louis, Mosby–Year Book, 1995.*)

The average frequency of attacks of MS is approximately one a year. The attacks vary in severity; therefore, close surveillence is required to reliably tabulate the attack frequency. Attacks tend to be most common in the early years of MS and become less frequent in later years, regardless of the disability. The risk for rapid development of moderate disability may be greater in persons in whom the frequency of attacks is higher than average. Frequent attacks are less cause for concern than the development of progressive MS, however (Weinshenker et al., 1988).

Signs and Symptoms. Each individual's brain appears to have a different threshold for producing symptoms and signs reflecting the affected regions of the CNS. This threshold, or the capacity of the individual's brain to adapt to the lesions, will determine the severity of the clinical manifestations.

Usually persons with early MS predominantly have one of the initial syndromes which can be categorized as corticospinal, brainstem, cerebellar, or cerebral. The following symptoms can occur in isolation or in combination. More than one syndrome may be found in some individuals (McCance and Heuther, 1994; Hauser, 1994).

Corticospinal Syndrome. The corticospinal syndrome is the most common, involving the corticospinal tracts and dorsal column. Stiffness, slowness, and weakness are components of corticospinal tract impairments. Spasticity is an extremely common problem in patients with MS, occurring in 90% of all cases. Associated signs of upper motor neuron syndrome may include clonus, spontaneous spasm, positive Babinski's sign, and loss of precise autonomic control. Signs of muscle weakness secondary to damage of the motor cortex and tracts reflect the loss of orderly recruitment and rate modulation of motor neurons. Muscle activation patterns and agonist-antagonist relationships are disturbed.

Dorsal column symptoms, which include *paresthesias* (tingling, pricking) or *hypoesthesia* (diminished sensitivity) may begin in one foot, typically in the great toe, and ascend over hours or several days to include the rest of the leg, the perineum, lower trunk, and perhaps the other leg. Other sensory complaints include a feeling of swelling, wetness, or that the body part is tightly wrapped. Involvement of a "cord level" is diagnostically helpful in distinguishing this attack from a peripheral neuropathologic incident. Other positive dorsal column signs are loss of vibration, position, and two-point discrimination. Sensory complaints are often not substantiated by objective findings. For example, the feeling of numbness may not result in a loss of response to pinprick.

Bladder and bowel symptoms occur when the spinal cord is involved. Urgency and hesitancy generally precede incontinence. Residual urine after emptying is a problem for 50% of persons with MS, requiring the use of *Credé's method* (manual pressure on the bladder to express urine) (Betts et al., 1993). Neurogenic disorders may also impair bowel function, resulting in incontinence or constipation. Sexual intercourse can be affected by loss of sensation in the female and impotence in the male. These disturbances have tremendous functional and social implications for the patient. A woman with MS can remain fertile and the fetus is unaffected.

Brainstem Syndrome. The brainstem syndrome reflects lesions of cranial nerves III through XII at the root, nuclear, or bulbar level. Common brainstem symptoms are *gaze palsies*, the loss of active control of eye movement; *nystagmus*, involuntary rhythmic tremor of the eye; and *dysarthria*, abnormal speech resulting from poor control of the muscles of speech.

Intranuclear ophthalmoplegia (INO) is the most common gaze palsy resulting in lateral gaze paralysis and is caused by demyelination of the pontine medial longitudinal fasciculus (MLF), an area of the brain's white matter involved in control of eye movement. Lesions in the MLF and reticular formation can cause other palsies resulting in difficulty with conjugate gaze and ipsilateral gaze palsy. Idiopathic nystagmus that improves over time can be due to lesions in the vestibular nuclei or cerebellum.

Other abnormalities of ocular mobility such as instability of fixation or inability to suppress the vestibulo-ocular response are related to lesions involving brainstem nuclei and tracts. *Vertigo*, the sensation of spinning, may appear suddenly and in dramatic fashion with gait unsteadiness and vomiting. In MS this reflects a brainstem rather than end-organ vestibular disorder; a careful look at associated brainstem symptoms will help to distinguish the cause (see Chapter 33). Trigeminal neuralgia of brainstem origin, resulting in a shocklike pain in the face, while not a common finding, may be an indicator of MS in a young person, especially in the presence of sensory loss. Interruption of brainstem-mediated motor innervation can cause symptoms similar to *Bell's palsy*, twitching of facial muscles, or facial hemispasm.

Cerebellar Syndrome. Cerebellar syndrome deficits are usually symmetrical with all four limbs involved. Manifestations of cerebellar lesions are ataxia hypotonia, and truncal weakness causing postural and movement disorders. Dysarthria of cerebellar origin (scanning speech, producing a prolonged, monotone sound) is common.

Cerebral Syndrome. The cerebral syndrome is characterized by optic neuritis, the manifestation of demyelination of the optic nerve. The optic nerve is an extension of the cerebral cortex, virtually a tract of the CNS, and therefore subject to the effects of demyelination. Optic neuritis typically presents as a painful loss of vision. It is commonly associated with visual field defects, decreased color vision, and reduced clarity of vision. Although not as common as other symptoms, it is highly indicative of MS.

Life-table analysis of patients with a monosymptomatic attack of optic neuritis indicated that approximately 75% of the women and 35% of the men eventually developed MS (Francis et al., 1987). The average time it takes to develop MS after the first attack of optic neuritis is typically 5 to 7 years. Patients with optic neuritis must be carefully evaluated for an ocular mobility abnormality to determine the possibility of a second anatomically distinct lesion (Kaufman and Fratkin, 1992).

Depression and cognitive changes can occur as a direct result of the MS plaques or as a reaction to the diagnosis or disability. Depression may lead to greater disability than that caused by the level of neurologic impairment. Cognitive decline is of significance in about 20% of persons with MS (Shapiro and Laven, 1994). Memory loss is the most common cognitive change. Impaired judgment and euphoria may be present, as well as uncontrollable laughter or crying triggered by emotional stimuli.

Other Clinical Symptoms. Other clinical symptoms are *Lhermitte's sign*, a momentary electric-like sensation evoked by neck flexion or cough, and heat sensitivity, which can cause temporary increase in symptoms after exercise or exposure to heat. Fatigue is present in up to 88% of persons with MS. Fatigue is typically present in midafternoon and may take the form of increased motor weakness with effort, mental fatigue, and sleepiness. Skin breakdown following sensory loss and immobility is a common problem which can be controlled by appropriate skin care and positioning (Hauser, 1994).

Medical Management

Diagnosis. The diagnosis of MS remains a clinical judgment and is based on observation over time. It is established by documenting two separate neurologic lesions in the CNS that are temporally and spatially distinct. Other presentations which may cause diagnostic uncertainty include symptoms with a rapid onset, suggesting a cerebrovascular accident, progressive brainstem syndrome, glioma, or myelopathy. No clinical sign or diagnostic test is unique to MS. It is important to first exclude other potentially treatable causes of the presenting symptoms before making a diagnosis of MS (Hauser, 1994).

Compared with many other chronic illnesses, a considerable period of time may elapse between the onset of the symptoms and the diagnosis of MS, often as long as 5 years. From the patient's perspective, the apparent discrepancies of judgment about the seriousness of the problem often cause frustration and distressing and protracted uncertainty. The patient often undertakes a vigorous and active campaign to obtain more plausible explanations (Miller, 1990).

MRI is the most useful imaging technique for MS. Abnormal scans are present in greater than 90% of persons with MS. Typically seen are ventricular enlargement, low-density periventricular abnormalities, or focal regions of enhancement following injection of a contrast agent. Figure 27–7 shows the plaques seen on MRI. The lesions do not always correlate with the clinical signs and there can be evidence of focal lesions in the absence of disease. However, there is a correlation between periods of clinical worsening of the disease and increases in the total number of lesions, the number of new lesions, and the total area of enhancement on MRI (Smith et al., 1994).

CT can identify large active plaques but is not as sensitive to smaller lesions. It is often used in the search for other neurologic disease.

Cerebrospinal fluid (CSF) analysis often shows increased mononuclear cell pleocytosis, an elevation in total immunoglobulins, and the presence of oligoclonal immunoglobulin, which indicates an inflammatory, viral, or bacterial response. While these values are abnormal in 75% to 90% of persons with MS, abnormal values do not assure that the diagnosis is MS. Metabolites from the breakdown of myelin may also be detected in CSF. Measurement of these myelin basic proteins in CFS is more useful as a predictor of response to steroids used during acute exacerbations than as a diagnostic tool.

Evoked potential response testing may detect slowed or abnormal conduction in visual, auditory, somatosensory, or motor pathways. These tests employ computer averaging techniques to record the electrical response evoked in the nervous system following repetitive sensory or motor stimuli. One or more evoked responses are abnormal in 80% or 90% of persons with MS. Testing is of greatest value when it provides evidence of a second lesion in a patient with a single clinically apparent lesion or when it demonstrates an objective abnormality in a patient with subjective complaints and a normal examination (Hauser, 1994).

Myelography is used to investigate signs of spinal cord involvement. A myelogram may be used to rule out other causes of spinal dysfunction. Demyelinating plaques are not evident with this test (O'Sullivan, 1994a).

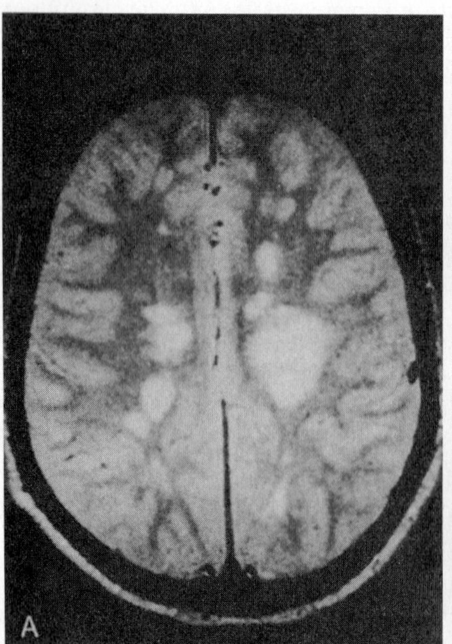

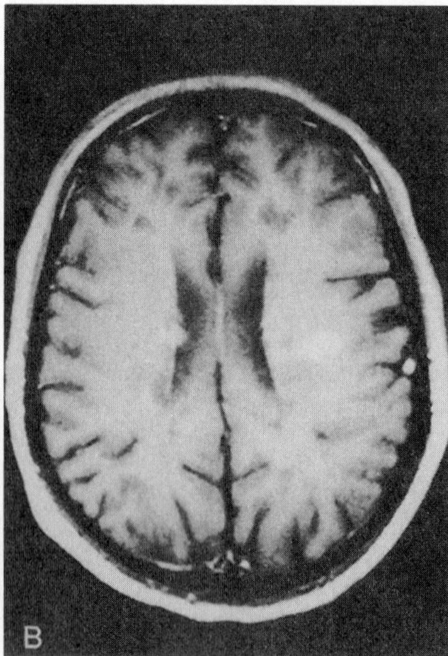

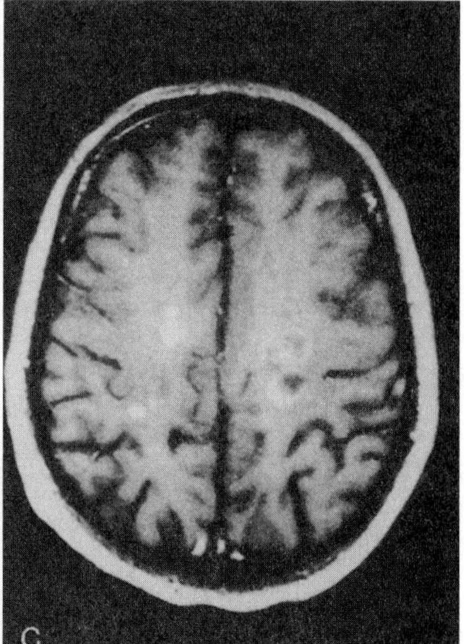

Figure 27–7. A, Typical scattered, variably sized plaques in the brain associated with the diagnosis of multiple sclerosis (MS). B, Contrast-enhanced magnetic resonance imaging reveals scattered area of solid and ring-shaped enhancement. C, Note the atrophy, greater than would be expected for the person's age, a common finding in MS. (*From Ramsey R: Neuroradiology. Philadelphia, WB Saunders, 1994.*)

Treatment. There is no cure or any immunization against MS. Medical management is directed toward the immune system dysfunction, the inflammatory responses, and in controlling symptoms.

Megadose corticosteroids are used in the treatment of MS. Both corticosteroids (prednisone, cortisone, methylprednisolone) and ACTH (adrenocorticotropic hormone) are well known to shorten the recovery period after an acute MS attack. Corticosteroids can alter almost every aspect of the immune system. Corticosteroid restoration of the blood-brain barrier, which becomes less effective during active demyelination or plaque formation, has an antiedema benefit and may prevent circulating toxins, viruses, or immunoactive cells from entering the CNS. There is a change in the activity of the macrophages and lymphocytes resulting in less damage to the myelin in response to steroid therapy (Kupersmith et al., 1994).

The use of interferon beta-1b as a treatment shows promise in controlling the immune system response to MS. The immune response has its own built-in checks to turn off any kind of immune response that is activated, and interferon-β seems to act along a certain number of those pathways. Interferon beta-1b inhibits macrophage-induced, antigen-specific T cell proliferation; it inhibits tumor necrosis factor and it restores some suppressor T cell activity. Treatment with interferon-β has been shown to result in a four- to sixfold reduction in the number of new lesions seen on MRI serial scans compared with those observed in persons given placebo and in persons with the relapsing form of MS (Johnson, 1994). Because the lesions seen on MRI do not correlate with the symptoms, the changes in symptoms must also be less if this drug is to be considered effective.

Drugs with similar properties, such as copolymer 1, cyclophosphamide, and monoclonal antibodies also show promise in the control of the relapsing form of MS. These drugs are being studied to determine if their effectiveness can be increased by combining them (Johnson, 1994).

Cladribine has been shown to improve or at least slow the demyelination activity in chronic progressive MS. Cladribine is a potent lympholytic agent that is also used as an anticancer drug (Sipe et al., 1994).

Drugs that enhance CNS remyelination known as protein growth factors are being studied as a method to restore the loss of oligodendrocytes in MS. Study is underway to determine possibilities of controlling the levels of cytokines such as interleukin-1 and tumor necrosis factor which inhibit regeneration in MS plaques (Pleasure, 1994).

Clinical studies are underway for a computer-designed, synthetic peptide that will target and inhibit the effects of T cells without leaving the person immunodeficient.

Gene therapy also holds promise in the treatment of neurologic diseases such as MS. Use of somatic cell gene therapy to treat cells directly in the brain or spinal cord holds the greatest potential for treatment of such diseases. By means of retroviruses in conjunction with helper viruses, somatic cell gene therapy can correct deficiences in a DNA sequence without producing virus particles and thus can prevent a syndrome from being expressed.

Improvement in the ability to control symptoms through medications has improved the quality of life of the patient with MS. Judicious use of medication can control spasticity, cerebellar incoordination, urinary frequency, pain, and depression. All the current medications available to control these symptoms have potential side effects and therefore must be used judiciously. Careful monitoring of systems affected by MS is essential to medical management.

Prognosis. Life expectancy is not altered to a major extent by MS. According to data from the Mayo Clinic, the mortality rate has not changed in the last nine decades. The risk of dying of MS is strongly associated with severe disability. The death rate in persons who are unable to stand or walk is more than four times that in persons the same age without MS. In mildy disabled patients, the death rate is approximately one and one-half times that of the age-matched population.

There are significant differences in survival curves of disability between persons with a high or low number of attacks within the first 2 years following onset, the time between attacks, and the time it takes to develop moderate disability. Persons with more frequent initial episodes with rapidly developing disability have a poorer long-term outcome (Weinshenker et al., 1988).

Although life expectancy is not significantly changed by the course of MS, lifestyle changes are frequently necessary. Movement impairment is frequently associated with MS and difficulty in walking is a major disability. A majority of people with MS will develop difficulty climbing stairs and close to half will require assistive devices, orthoses, or a wheelchair for locomotion. About one fourth of persons with MS will require human assistance for activities of daily living (Rodriguez, 1994).

The ability to carry on normal life roles is only moderately affected despite the disabilities. Most persons with MS are able to work full time and maintain their usual financial standard of life. Less than one third will require hand controls to drive. Few people require community services (Rodriguez, 1994).

Special Implications for the Therapist **27-6**

MULTIPLE SCLEROSIS

People with MS are advised to be as active as possible in all ways of life. If activity is carried out in accordance with individual strength and abilities, avoiding exhaustion, it will help to prevent complications. Walking becomes difficult because of weakness, spasticity, and tremor. Balance disorders in the absence of weakness are seen that reflect the lesion site in cortical, cerebellar, or brainstem areas (Shapiro and Laven, 1994).

Fatigue and weakness are the complaints most often taken to a therapist. In establishing a training program for endurance and strengthening, careful consideration of the neurologic changes is critical. Clients demonstrating increased reflex activity with exertion will need a longer period of time to recover after fatigue and may notice increased extensor tone and difficulty with flexion. Repetitive submaximal strength training appears to be of benefit to most people, with an increase in both peak torque generated and a decrease in the reported perception of fatigue (Svensson et al., 1994). Changes in strength and endurance are probably due to the normal physiologic changes that are associated with this type of training (Miller, 1990).

Not all people with MS respond with increases in strength and endurance with this type of training. The difference may be due to the level of scarring present in the CNS causing some people to exhibit less adaptability of the system as a whole. Regardless of physiologic changes there is a general increase in well-being associated with training in clients with neurologic disorders, including MS.

Understanding of movement disorders common to lesions in specific areas of the brain and spinal column is essential for the therapist. Analysis of movement is the first critical skill necessary to facilitate the integration of sensory and motor input to maintain postural control. The therapist must be able to identify the impairments to determine the appropriate stretching and strengthening exercises and the need for mobility aids. A successful exercise program is dependent on a number of factors essential to motor learning, including practice, adequate feedback, and knowledge of the results. The client with MS is often restricted in practice by neurologic fatigue and by impairments that disrupt sensory feedback, attention, memory, and motivation. The therapist will need to carefully identify the client's resources and abilities and capitalize on them to minimize the level of disability (O'Sullivan, 1994a).

A common disability scale used by rehabilitation professionals and researchers working with patients with MS is the Kurtzke Expanded Disability Status Scale, (EDSS) (Box 27–4). It is used to monitor changes in disability levels and has value in determining prognosis. Therapists working with this patient population should become adept at using this tool (Mertin and Paeth, 1994).

The day-to-day variation in MS makes determination of the appropriate training program challenging. Use of both impairment and disability scales will assist in monitoring changes. The scales show the relative improvement after intervention, or overall decline regardless of intervention. The scales are useful in tracking the disease process for both the client and the health-care provider. Therapists making decisions regarding the need for adaptive equipment can use the scales to establish trends in the course of the disease.

BOX **27–4**
Kurtzke Expanded Disability Status Scale

0.0 Normal neurologic examination
1.0 No disability, minimal symptoms
1.5 No disability, minimal signs in more than one functional level
2.0 Slightly greater disability in one functional system
2.5 Slightly greater disability in two functional systems
3.0 Moderate disability in one functional system; fully ambulatory
3.5 Fully ambulatory but with moderate disability in one functional system and more than minimal disability in several others
4.0 Fully ambulatory without aid, self-sufficient, up and about some 12 hr/day despite relatively severe disability; able to walk without aid or rest for some 500 m
4.5 Fully ambulatory without aid, up and about much of the day, able to work a full day; may otherwise have some limitation of full activity or require minimal assistance; characterized by relatively severe disability; able to walk without aid or rest for some 300 m
5.0 Ambulatory without aid or rest for about 200 m; disability severe enough to impair full daily activities (e.g., to work a full day without special provisions)
5.5 Ambulatory without aid or rest for about 100 m; disability severe enough to preclude full daily activities
6.0 Intermittent or unilateral constant assistance (cane, crutch, brace) required to walk about 100 m with or without resting
6.5 Constant bilateral assistance (canes, crutches, braces) required to walk about 20 m without resting
7.0 Unable to walk beyond approximately 5 m with aid; essentially restricted to a wheelchair; wheels self in standard wheelchair and transfers alone; up and about in wheelchair for some 12 hr/day
7.5 Unable to take more than a few steps; restricted to wheelchair; may need aid in transfer; wheels self but cannot carry on in standard wheelchair a full day; may require motorized wheelchair
8.0 Essentially restricted to bed or chair or perambulated in wheelchair, but may be out of bed itself much of the day; retains many self-care functions; generally has effective use of arms
8.5 Essentially restricted to bed much of the day; has some effective use of arm(s); retains some self-care functions
9.0 Helpless bed patient; can communicate and eat
9.5 Totally helpless bed patient; unable to communicate effectively or eat or swallow
10.0 Death due to MS

Modified from Kurtzke J: Rating neurological impairment in multiple sclerosis: An expanded disability status scale (EDSS). Neurology 33:1444, 1983.

PARKINSON'S DISEASE

Overview and Definition. Parkinson's disease (PD), or *idiopathic parkinsonism*, is a chronic progressive disease of the motor component of the CNS, characterized by rigidity, tremor, and bradykinesia. Similar movement disorders that arise from abnormalities of the brain in the area of the basal ganglia are referred to as parkinsonism.

Incidence. The prevalence of PD varies between 60 and 120 per 100,000 (Gilroy and Holliday, 1982). PD occurs in about 1% of the population older than 55 years of age and becomes increasingly common with advancing age, reaching 2.6% by age 85. The majority of cases begin between the ages of 50 and 79. As many as 10% will develop initial symptoms before the age of 40. These persons usually have a more benign long-term course. There is no difference in incidence between the sexes (O'Sullivan, 1994b).

Etiology and Risk Factors. The most common form of parkinsonism is idiopathic, implying that the cause is unknown. Parkinsonian symptoms are seen as sequelae in some survivors of encephalitis. Some toxic agents (carbon monoxide, manganese, cyanide, methanol) can damage the basal ganglia and produce parkinsonian symptoms. A rapidly developing parkinson-like disease has been linked to the use of MPTP (1-methyl-4-phenyl-1,2,3,6-tetrahydropyridine), a synthetic narcotic related to heroin. Some neuroleptics can produce a parkinsonian syndrome. In drug-induced parkinsonism, the symptoms can usually be reversed by withdrawal of the drug.

Atrophy of the brain leading to degeneration of neurons in the basal ganglia can be caused by a variety of disorders that are not well understood. These include striatonigral degeneration (SND), Shy-Drager syndrome, progressive supranuclear palsy (PSP), olivopontocerebellar atrophy (OPCA), cortico-basal ganglionic degeneration, and diffuse Lewy body disease. Parkinsonian features can be manifested as a part of other diseases affecting the CNS such as atherosclerosis, ALS, and HD (O'Sullivan, 1994b; Waxman and deGroot, 1995).

Pathogenesis. The signs and symptoms of parkinsonism are neurochemical in origin. The substantia nigra, a nucleus that is part of the basal ganglia, loses its ability to produce dopamine, a neurotransmitter necessary to normal function of basal ganglia neurons. A depletion of 70% to 80% of the dopamine is estimated to occur before clinical signs of the disease are noted. There may also be decreased use of dopamine in the basal ganglia by the neurons normally triggered by the neurotransmitter. The failure of the dopaminergic synapses results in an imbalance in the basal ganglia's mutually antagonistic systems. The cholinergic system, which is triggered by the neurotransmitter acetylcholine, allows the interneurons in the basal ganglia to be activated. The dopaminergic system provides inhibition of the interneurons. When dopamine is decreased and acetylcholine increased, the excessive excitatory output results in a generalized activation of skeletal motor and fusimotor systems. The ultimate effect of the release of cholinergic activity in the basal ganglia is felt at the level of the final common pathway of the motor system, the anterior horn cell. There, there are two basic effects: increased inhibition of the gamma motor neuron and increased alpha motor neuron activity. Both effects cause an increase in muscle activity on both sides of a joint resulting in the cardinal symptoms of rigidity and slowness of movement (Gilroy and Holliday, 1982; O'Sullivan, 1994b).

The function of the basal ganglia is essentially a feedforward/feedback system which is intimately related to the cerebral cortex. Input to the basal ganglia, mostly from the cerebral cortex, comes into the striatum. There nuclei project to the globus pallidus, the major output structure of the basal ganglia. Neurons from the globus pallidus project to different regions of the thalamus, which in turn sends axons back to the cerebral cortex. Figure 27–8 shows this loop. The basal ganglia–cerebral interactions are disrupted by the abnormal function of the basal ganglia. The motor loop, which is thought to serve a direct role in the initiation and scaling of motor activity, derives its input from the premotor, motor, and somatosensory cortices. The complex loop is thought to be involved in motivation and in planning global aspects of behavior. The input is believed to be from the limbic system and prefrontal cortex. The basal ganglia, in association with the frontal lobe, appear to play an important role in the integration of sensory information.

Physiologic studies have shown the basal ganglia to be actively involved in almost all types of movement, including postural responses, alternating movements, and spontaneously occurring movements. Lesions do not produce paralysis or weakness, but rather change the character of movement, leading to loss of adaptive control, slowing of movement, and poor coordination.

In addition to changes in the production of neurochemicals, there appear to be other changes in the brain. Sections of the midbrain show marked diminution of melanin in the area of the substantia nigra. There is diffuse neuronal loss involving the whole of the brain and brainstem with particular involvement of the cerebral cortex, basal ganglia, thalamus, and selected cranial nerves. This may explain the clinical features such as dysphagia, cognitive defects, and postural instability. Falling continues to be a problem, despite control of other symptoms with levodopa, leading to the conclusion that nondopaminergic systems are involved (Fearnley and Lees, 1994).

There is new evidence leading to a theory of either mitochondrial impairment or excess free radical formation as the underlying cause of PD.

Clinical Manifestations. The tremor of PD is the most common initial manifestation, often appears unilaterally, and may be confined to one upper limb for months or even years (Gilroy and Holliday, 1982). It is first seen in the fingers and thumb, referred to as the pill-rolling tremor. Eventually the tremor may spread to all four limbs and the head, neck, and facial muscles. Tension or exertion will cause the tremor to increase and it will disappear during sleep. The tremor is probably initiated by rhythmic discharges of the alpha motor neurons, an activity that is normally suppressed by the action of the gamma motor neuron circuit, the fusimotor system.

Rigidity is an increased response to muscle stretch that appears in both antagonist and agonist muscle groups. Rigidity, like tremor, usually appears unilaterally and proximally in an upper limb, and then spreads to the other extremities and trunk. One of the earliest signs of rigidity is the loss of associated movements of the arms when walking.

Bradykinesia, the slowness of movement seen in PD, is not related to rigidity and is probably the result of a different biochemical dysfunction in the basal ganglia. Akinesia is a disorder of movement initiation and is seen in parkinsonism as a paucity of natural and automatic movements such as crossing the legs or folding the arms. Small gestures associated with expression are reduced. The face is masklike with infrequent blinking and lack of expression. There is a greasy appearance to the skin of the face and occasional drooling due to loss of the swallowing movements that normally dispose of saliva. The slowing of lip and tongue movements during talking causes a garbled speech pattern. There is loss of fine motor skills with the gradual development of small cramped writing or micrographia.

The posture in PD is characterized by flexion of the neck, trunk, hips, and knees (Fig. 27–9). In gait there is a loss of heel strike, reduced toe elevation, reduced movement at the knee joints, loss of dynamic vertical force, reversal of ankle flexion-extension movement, and loss of backward directed shear force (Rajput, 1994).

Most people with PD experience weakness and fatigue once the disease becomes generalized. The person has difficulty in sustaining activity and experiences increasing weak-

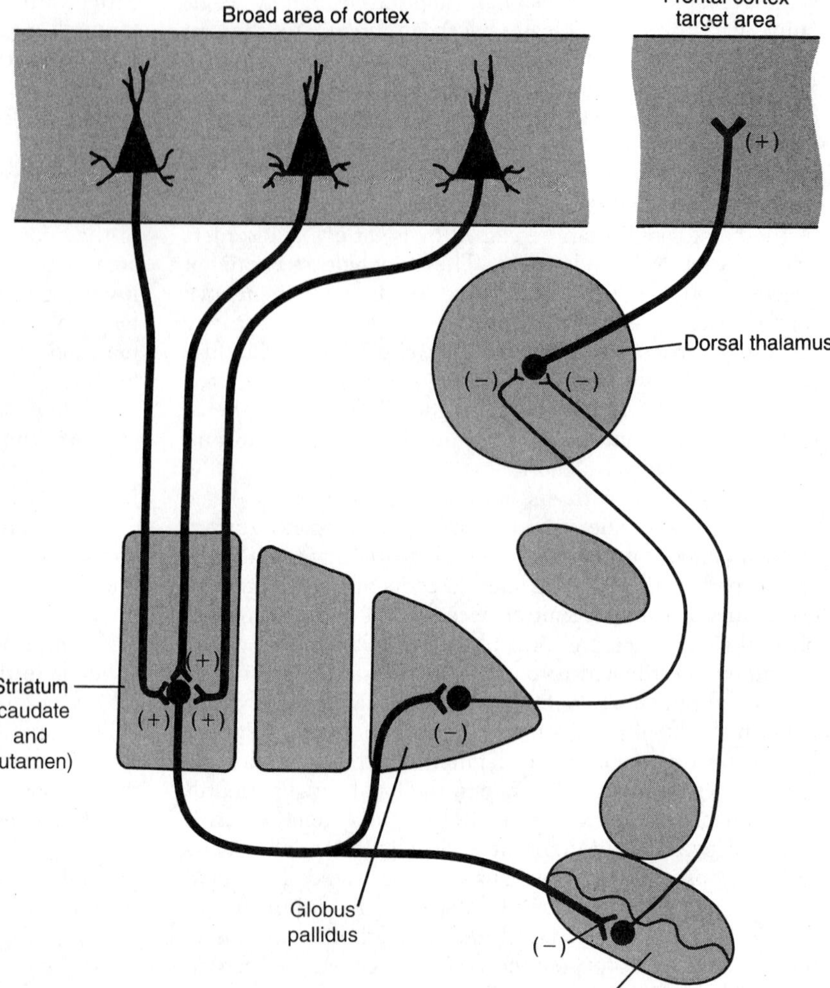

Figure **27–8.** Pathway showing feedback loop of neurons in the basal ganglia, thalamus, and cortex. In Parkinson's disease, this pathway is disrupted. (*From Burt A: Textbook of Anatomy. Philadelphia, WB Saunders, 1993.*)

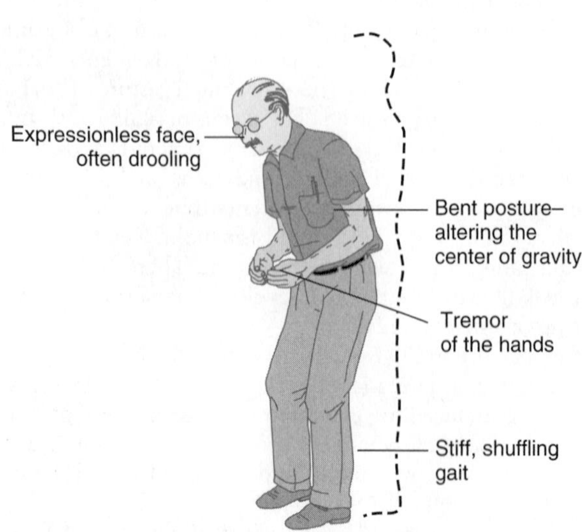

Figure **27–9.** Typical posture that results from Parkinson's disease.

ness and lethargy as the day progresses. Repetitive motor acts may start out strong but decrease in strength as the activity progresses. This compounds bradykinesia and increases immobility.

Many persons with PD experience pain that is poorly localized but that is generally described as cramping in the axial muscles or the limbs. Paresthesias are reported by many persons, including numbness, tingling, and abnormal temperature sensation.

Loss of neurons in the sympathetic ganglia may cause autonomic dysfunction. This results in excessive sweating, excessive salivation, incontinence, and disabling orthostatic hypotension.

Dementia and intellectual changes occur in almost 50% of persons with PD. This is a result of the neurochemical imbalance in the basal ganglia. Bradyphrenia, a slowing of thought processes, with lack of concentration and attention may also occur. Coexisting Alzheimer's disease, organic brain disease, and vascular compromise may also contribute to the dementia.

Depression is common and there is some evidence suggesting that the depression starts before the onset of PD and that it may be related to the dopamine depletion. Behavioral changes such as apathy, lack of ambition, and passivity are common and may be related to the depression. These behaviors may also represent the sensory deprivation secondary to paucity of movement.

Spatial organization is often disturbed resulting in difficulty with orientation to the environment. The inability to distinguish self-movement from movement in the environment can contribute to abnormal balance reactions. Persons with PD show a high dependence on visual information for motor control. There appears to be an inability to choose a balance strategy based on vestibular information even when the visual system is in apparent disagreement (Bronstein et al., 1990).

Medical Management

Diagnosis. Clinical diagnosis of the well-developed syndrome is usually simple because the clinical findings are usually readily visible. Diagnostic problems may occur in mild cases. Depression, with its associated expressionless face, poorly modulated voice, and reduction in voluntary activity, may be difficult to distinguish from mild parkinsonism.

HD presenting with rigidity and bradykinesia may be mistaken for PD unless the family history and accompanying dementia are recognized.

Supranuclear palsy bradykinesia and rigidity are accompanied by a disorder of eye movement, pseudobulbar palsy, and axial dystonia. Essential tremor presents with a tremor of a different character, and there is a lack of other neurologic signs.

Treatment. Drug therapy should be adapted to the person's needs, which may vary with the stage of the disease and the predominant manifestations (Aminoff, 1994). When mobility becomes affected to the degree that walking and self-care activities become difficult, there are medications which can improve the control of movement.

Persons with mild symptoms but no disability may be helped by amantadine. This drug improves all of the clinical features of parkinsonism, but its mode of action is unclear. It is proposed that it increases the synthesis and release of dopamine, and may also reduce reuptake.

Anticholinergic drugs, which reduce cholinergic (excitatory) transmission in the striatum and therefore tend to restore the inhibitory/excitatory balance in the basal ganglia, are more helpful in alleviating the tremor and rigidity than the bradykinesia. They are used in newly diagnosed persons who do not require powerful symptomatic therapy. Anticholinergic drugs are contraindicated in patients with obstructive gastrointestinal disease and are often tolerated poorly by the elderly.

Levodopa, which is taken up by remaining dopaminergic neurons in the basal ganglia and converted to dopamine, improves most of the major features of parkinsonism, including bradykinesia. Levodopa can cause dyskinesias which produce chorea, athetosis, dystonia, tics, and myoclonus. Predictable fluctuations include a wearing-off effect and early-morning akinesia. The duration of each dose becomes shorter.

Carbidopa inhibits the breakdown of levodopa and is often used in conjunction with levodopa. Carbidopa reduces the amount of levodopa required daily for beneficial effects, and is often combined with levodopa in a single preparation (Sinemet). Levodopa should be avoided in persons with malignant melanoma, and in persons with active peptic ulcers, which may bleed.

Bromocriptine acts directly on dopamine receptors and its use in parkinsonism is associated with a lower incidence of response fluctuations. It is often given in combination with levodopa and carbidopa. It should be avoided in persons with mental illness, recent myocardial infarction, or peptic ulcers.

Other drugs are currently being tested that show promise in controlling symptoms in addition to those controlled by levodopa. MAO B inhibitors are believed to decrease the rate of nigral degeneration in PD. Antioxidants and inhibitors of excitatory amino acids show promise. The use of nerve growth factor may prove to be of use in the control of neuronal death.

Fetal cell transplantation shows promise of improved motor function when performed in persons with advanced PD (Tsui, 1994). Another possibility of enhancing fetal cell transplantation is glia-derived neurite-promoting factor (GdNPF). In early animal studies, GdNPF appears to promote survival of dopamine neurons from fetal cells, which may protect adult dopamine neurons from damage induced by PD.

Stereotactic surgery in the lateral ventral nucleus of the thalamus is performed in persons with dyskinesia and tremor that are not controlled by pharmacologic therapies.

Stimulation of the brain with electrodes implanted in the brain and controlled by a disk placed under the skin, and controlled externally through a magnetic field, shows promise in control of the tremor of PD.

Prognosis. In general, all the clinical manifestations in PD worsen progressively, although not to the same extent. Tremor, after reaching peak severity, may become less pronounced with time. Posture and gait abnormalities are the most difficult to control in advanced cases. Demented persons respond poorly (Tsui, 1994).

PD does not significantly reduce life span in most persons who develop the generalized form in their 50s or 60s. However, since there is progressive neuronal loss despite the response to treatment, deterioration continues until death occurs, often from infection or other conditions associated with debilitation.

Since the onset of disease is typically in the fifth or sixth decade of life, and is progressive despite medication, it becomes difficult to separate the complications from the changes seen with aging.

Lack of mobility, loss of balance reactions, and weakness result in more falls than in age-matched normals. Osteoporosis can result from prolonged inactivity and may be present secondary to advanced age of onset. Falls more often lead to fractures owing to the prevalence of osteoporosis. Fracture healing may be delayed or absent.

Special Implications for the Therapist **27-7**

PARKINSON'S DISEASE

Although reduced activity by itself would not seem to be a functional disorder, many of the small automatic adjustments are important for successfully carrying out functional activities. For example, in attempting to rise from a chair a person may fail to make the small initial adjustments of legs that are crucial to standing up. It

BOX **27-5**

Causes of Balance Impairment in Parkinson's Disease

Loss of postural reflexes
Visuospatial deficits
Retropulsion
Start hesitation
"Freezing"
Festinating gait
Orthostatic hypotension
True vertigo

appears that impairment of the normal mechanisms that scale the output of agonist muscles causes the inability to produce quick movements. The client with PD shows relatively small EMG bursts in agonist muscles, and moves the legs in a series of small steps rather than in a single movement. It has been suggested that this disorder may, at least in part, derive from a need to rely on visual feedback, suggesting that there is a disorder of predictive control.

The loss of postural reflexes is the most common cause of balance disorders. Balance reactions are impaired or absent. Clients with PD demonstrate difficulty in regulating feed-forward adjustments of postural muscles using voluntary movement and this is apparent with the loss of anticipatory postural adjustments. There is an abnormality in the processing of vestibular, visual, and somatosensory information contributing to balance. Other causes of imbalance are listed in Box 27–5.

The gait pattern in parkinsonism is highly stereotyped and characterized by an impoverishment of movement. Range of motion in the joints of the lower extremity is often limited. Trunk and pelvic movement is diminished, resulting in a decreased step length and reciprocal arm swing. The gait is narrow-based and shuffling. Persistent posturing of a forward head and trunk typically creates a shift of the center of gravity forward and this may result in a festinating gait. The person takes many short steps to avoid falling forward and may eventually break into a run. Some persons are able to stop only when they come into contact with an object or a wall. Persons with plantar flexion contractures will toe-walk, and this further narrows the available base of support. Kyphosis extensive flexion of the spine, is the most common postural deformity. Scoliosis, an abnormal lateral curvature of the spine, can result from the unequal distribution of rigidity in posture.

The person with PD typically becomes deconditioned. Rapid heart rate and difficulty breathing are common when initiating increased activity in therapy. Vital capacity is reduced as the kyphosis increases and the intercostal muscles develop rigidity. Respiratory complications, which are the leading cause of death, can be prevented to some extent with an early aggressive aerobic exercise program, followed by regular moderate activity as the disease progresses. Control of breathing can be facilitated using verbal and tactile stimuli and should be integrated into any intervention. The Hoehn and Yahr classification (Table 27–2) is a common scale used to classify the disabilities of PD.

TABLE 27-2 HOEHN AND YAHR CLASSIFICATION OF DISABILITY

STAGE	CHARACTER OF DISABILITY
I	Minimal or absent: unilateral if present
II	Minimal bilateral or midline involvement; balance not impaired
III	Impaired righting reflexes; unsteadiness when turning or rising from chair; some activities are restricted, but patient can live independently and continue some forms of employment
IV	All symptoms are present and severe; standing and walking possible only with assistance
V	Confined to bed or wheelchair

Modified from Hoehn MM, Yahr MD: Parkinsonism: Onset, progression and mortality. Neurology 17:427, 1967.

References

Adler CH, Zimmerman RS, Lyons MK, et al: Perioperative use of botulinum toxin for movement disorder–induced cervical spine disease. Mov Disord 11:79–81, 1996.

Aminoff M. Nervous system. *In* Tierney LM, McPhee SJ, Papadakis MA (eds): Current Medical Diagnosis and Treatment, ed 33. Norwalk, Conn, Appleton & Lange, 1994, pp 799–854.

Appel SH, Appel LV: Treatment of amyotrophic lateral sclerosis. *In* Calne DB (ed): Neurodegenerative Diseases. Philadelphia, WB Saunders, 1994, pp 523–542.

Beal MF, Richardson EP, Martin JB: Alzheimer's disease and other dementias: *In* Isselbacher KJ, Braunwald E, Wilson JD, et al (eds): Harrison's Principles of Internal Medicine, ed 13. New York, McGraw-Hill, 1994, pp 2269–2295.

Betts CD, D'Mellow MT, Fowler CJ: Urinary symptoms and the neurological features of bladder dysfunction in multiple sclerosis. J Neurol Neurosurg Psychiatry 56:245–250, 1993.

Bohannon RW: Results of resistance exercise on a patient with amyotrophic lateral sclerosis: A case report. Phys Ther 63:965–968, 1983.

Bowlby C: Therapeutic Activities with Persons Disabled by Alzheimer's Disease and Related Disorders. Gaithersberg, Md, Aspen, 1993.

Braak H, Braak E: Pathology of Alzheimer's disease. *In* Calne DB (ed): Neurodegenerative Disease. Philadelphia, WB Saunders, 1994.

Brown RH: Motor neuron disease and the progressive ataxias. *In* Isselbacher KJ, Braunwald E, Wilson JD, et al (eds): Harrison's Principles of Internal Medicine, ed 13. New York, McGraw-Hill, 1994 pp 2280–2283.

Bronstein AM, Hood JD, Gresty MA, Panagi C: Visual control of balance in cerebellar and parkinsonian syndromes. Brain 113: 767–779, 1990.

Brück W, Schmied M, Suchanek G, et al: Oligodendrocytes in the early course of multiple sclerosis. Ann Neurol 35:65–73, 1994.

Edwards LL, Normand MM, Wszolek ZK: Cervical dystonia: A review of the role of botulinum toxin. Nebr Med J 80:109–115, 1995.

Fearnley J, Lees A: Pathology of Parkinson's disease. *In* Calne DB (ed): Neurodegenerative Diseases. Philadelphia, WB Saunders, 1994, pp 545–554.

Folstein SE: Huntington's Disease: A Disorder of Families. Baltimore, Johns Hopkins University Press, 1989, pp 37–80.

Francis DA, Compston DAS, Batchcor JR, et al: A reassessment of the risk of multiple sclerosis developing in patients with optic neuritis after extended follow up. J Neurol Neurosurg Psychiatry 50:758–765, 1987.

Gilroy J, Holliday P: Basic Neurology. New York, Macmillan, 1982, pp 177–178.

Harper PS, Morris M: The epidemiology of Huntington's Disease. *In* Harper, PS (ed): Huntington's Disease. Philadelphia, WB Saunders, 1991, pp 1–36.

Hauser SI: Multiple sclerosis and other demyelinating diseases. *In* Isselbacher KJ, Braunwald E, Wilson JD, et al (eds): Harrison's Principles of Internal Medicine, ed 13. New York, McGraw-Hill, 1994 pp 2287–2294.

Herndon RM: Multiple sclerosis: Basic science issues. MS Q Rep 12:3–5, 1994.

Inada T, Yagi G: Current topics in neuroleptic-induced extrapyramidal symptoms in Japan. Keio J Med 45:95–99, 1996.

Johnson, K: MRI studies confirm advantages of interferon beta-1b. Peer Peer 1:3–9, 1994.

Kaufman DI, Fratkin J: Multiple sclerosis and the eye. Ophthalmol Clin North Am 5:513–530, 1992.

Kupersmith MJ, Kaufman D, Paty DW: Megadose corticosteroids in multiple sclerosis. Neurology 44:1–4, 1994.

Kurland L, Kurupath R, Williams DB: Amyotrophic lateral sclerosis-parkinsonism-dementia complex on Guam: Epidemiologic and etiological perspectives. *In* Williams D (ed): Motor Neuron Disease, London, Chapman & Hall, 1994, pp 109–130.

Lagueny A, Burbaud P, Le Masson G, et al: Involvement of respiratory muscles in adult-onset dystonia: A clinical and electrophysiological study. Mov Disord 10:708–713, 1995.

Lavretsky EP, Jarvik LF: Etiology and pathogenesis of Alzheimer's disease: Current concepts. *In* Hamdy RC, Turnbull JM, Clark W, et al (eds): Alzheimer's Disease: A Handbook for Care Givers. St Louis, Mosby–Year Book, 1994, pp 80–92.

Lee MS, Rinne JO, Ceballos-Baumann A, et al: Dystonia after head trauma. Neurology 44:1374–1378, 1994.

Leigh PN: Pathogenic mechanisms in amyotrophic lateral sclerosis and other motor neuron disorders. *In* Calne DB (ed): Neurodegenerative Diseases. Philadelphia, WB Saunders, 1994, pp 473–488.

McCance KL, Heuther SE: Alterations of neurologic function. *In* McCance KL, Heuther SE (eds): Pathophysiology: The Biological Basis for Diseases in Adults and Children, ed 2. St Louis, Mosby–Year Book, 1994, pp 571–575.

Mertin J, Paeth B: Physiotherapy and multiple sclerosis—Application of the Bobath concept. MS Q Rep 1:1, 1994.

Miller AE: Clinical features. *In* Cook SD (ed): Handbook of Multiple Sclerosis. New York, Marcel Dekker, 1990, pp 169–175.

Miller BL, Chang L, Oropilla G, Mena I: Alzheimer's disease and frontal lobe dementias. *In* Coffey CE, Cummings JL (eds): Textbook of Geriatric Neuropsychiatry, Washington, DC, American Psychiatric Press, 1994, pp 390–400.

Miller RG, Green AT, Moussavi RS, et al: Excessive muscular fatigue in patients with spastic paraparesis. Neurology 40:1271–1274, 1990.

Mitsumoto H, Hanson M, Chad D: Amyotrophic lateral sclerosis: Recent advances in pathogenesis and therapeutic trials. Arch Neurol 45:189–202, 1988.

Morris M: Psychiatric aspects of Huntington's disease. *In* Harper P (ed): Huntington's Disease. Philadelphia, WB Saunders, 1991, pp 81–126.

Morris M, Tyler A: Management and therapy. *In* Harper P (ed): Huntington's Disease. Philadelphia, WB Saunders, 1991, pp 205–250.

O'Sullivan SB: Multiple sclerosis. *In* O'Sullivan SB, Schmitz TJ (eds): Physical Rehabilitation: Assessment and Treatment, ed 3. Philadelphia, FA Davis, 1994a, pp 451–467.

O'Sullivan SB: Parkinson's disease. *In* O'Sullivan SB, Schmitz TJ (eds): Physical Rehabilitation: Assessment and Treatment, ed 3. Philadelphia, FA Davis, 1994b, pp 473–490.

Pleasure D: New direction in MS therapy: Protein growth factors may enhance CNS remyelination. Peer Peer 1:12–13, 1994.

Prineas JW, Barnard RO, Kwon EE: Multiple sclerosis: Remyelination of nascent lesions. Ann Neurol 33:137–151, 1993.

Quarrell O: The neurobiology of Huntington's disease. *In* Harper P (ed): Huntington's Disease. Philadelphia, WB Saunders, 1991, pp 81–109.

Quarrell O, Harper P: The clinical neurology of Huntington's disease. *In* Harper P (ed): Huntington's Disease. Philadelphia, WB Saunders, 1991, pp 37–80.

Rajput AH: Clinical features and natural history of Parkinson's disease (special considerations of aging). *In* Calne DB (ed): Neurodegenerative Diseases. Philadelphia, WB Saunders, 1994, pp 555–572.

Rodriguez M, Siva A, Stolp-Smith K: Impairment, disability and handicap in multiple sclerosis: A population-based study in Olmsted County, Minnesota. Neurology 44:28–33, 1994.

Rothstein JD, Jin L, Dykes-Hoberg M: Chronic inhibition of glutamate uptake produces a model of slow neurotoxicity. Proc Natl Acad Sci U S A 90:6591–6595, 1993.

Rothwell JC: Physiological study of cervical dystonia. Task-specific abnormality in contingent negative variation. Brain 118(pt 2):511–522, 1995.

Rowland LP: Natural history and clinical features of amyotrophic lateral sclerosis and related motor neuron diseases. *In* Calne DB (ed): Neurodegenerative Diseases. Philadelphia, WB Saunders, 1994, pp 507–522.

Shapiro RT, Laven L: Multiple sclerosis. *In* Good DC, Couch JR (eds): Handbook of Neurorehabilitation. New York, Marcel Dekker, 1994, pp 551–559.

Sipe JC, Romine JS, Koziol JA: Cladribine in treatment of chronic progressive multiple sclerosis. Lancet, 344:9–13, 1994.

Smith ME, Stone LA, Albert PS: Clinical worsening in MS is associated with increased frequency of area of gado-pentetate dimeglumine enhancing MRI lesions. Ann Neurol 33:480–489, 1994.

Svensson B, Gerdle B, Elert J: Endurance training in patients with multiple sclerosis: Five case studies. Phys Ther 74:1017–1026, 1994.

Third International Dystonia Symposium Proceedings, Miami, October 9–11, 1996.

Tranchant C, Bhatia KP, Marsden CD: Movement disorders in multiple sclerosis. Mov Disord 10:418–423, 1995.

Tsui JC: Treatment of Parkinson's disease. *In* Calne DB (ed): Neurodegenerative Diseases. Philadelphia, WB Saunders, 1994, pp 573–582.

Uncini A, DiMuzio A, Thomas A, et al: Hand dystonia secondary to cervical demyelinating lesion. Acta Neurol Scand 90:51–55, 1994.

Utz U, McFarland HF: The role of T cells in multiple sclerosis: Implications for therapies targeting the T cell receptor. J Neuropathol Exp Neurol 53:351–358, 1994.

Van Zandijcke M: Cervical dystonia: Some aspects of the natural history. Acta Neurol Belg 95:210–215, 1995.

Waxman SG, deGroot J: Correlative Neuroanatomy. Norwalk, Conn, Appleton & Lange, 1995.

Weinshenker BG, Bass B, Rice GP: The natural history of multiple sclerosis: A geographically based study. II: Predictive value of the early clinical course. Brain 112:1419–1428, 1988.

Whyte S, Beyreuther K, Masters C: Rational therapeutic strategies for Alzheimer's disease. *In* Calne DB (ed): Neurodegenerative Diseases. Philadelphia, WB Saunders, 1994, pp 647–664.

Wilson FR, Wagner C, Homberg V: Biomechanical abnormalities in musicians with occupational cramp/focal dystonia. J Hand Ther October-December:298–307, 1993.

Wojcieszek JM, Lang AE: Hyperkinetic movement disorders. *In* Coffey CE, Cummings JL (eds): Textbook of Geriatric Neuropsychiatry. Washington, DC, American Psychiatric Press, 1994, pp 406–415.

SECTION 4

chapter 28

Stroke

Kenda S. Fuller

STROKE

Overview and Definition. Stroke, or cerebrovascular accident, is the most common and lethal neurologic disorder and the number one cause of disability in adults. Coronary artery disease often occurs in well-appearing adults, and it frequently sets the stage for the sudden, devastating vascular event that results in destruction of the brain tissue (Duncan and Badke, 1987); that is, stroke is primarily a consequence of an aging cardiovascular system. Concomitant diseases of aging such as arthritis, diabetes, osteoporosis, musculoskeletal fatigue, and decreased general plasticity of the nervous system work together to make the rehabilitation a challenge.

Cerebrovascular disease is caused by one of several pathologic processes involving the blood vessels of the brain. The process may be intrinsic to the vessel, as in atherosclerosis, lipohyalinosis, inflammation, amyloid deposition, arterial dissection, developmental malformation, aneurysm, or venous thrombosis.[1] The stroke may originate remotely, as when an embolus from the heart or extracranial circulation lodges in an intracranial vessel, or the stroke may result from the rupture of a vessel in the subarachnoid space or intracerebral tissue. Figure 28–1 shows the effects of different types of stroke on brain tissue.

Transient ischemic attack (TIA) resembles stroke in its etiology; however, damage to the brain may be nonexistent, the symptoms are more focal in nature, and the affected individual recovers rapidly without permanent deficit. By definition, complete recovery of neurologic function is accomplished within 24 hours, although the majority of TIAs last from 5 to 20 minutes.

Incidence. The average incidence rate of first strokes is 114 per 100,000 persons. First strokes account for about 75% of acute events, and recurrent strokes account for about 25%. The incidence of stroke doubles with every decade after age 55 years. Black men have a 50% higher chance of having a stroke than do white men. Black women have an incidence of stroke that is 130% that of white women. The recurrence rate is highest in the first year after stroke and is more frequent in individuals suffering a thrombotic event and in men. Men have 30% to 80% higher rates of recurrence than do women (Agency for Health Care Policy and Research, 1995).

Risk Factors. Risk factors for stroke can be divided into those that are potentially modifiable and those that are not (see Table 10–2). Hypertension (blood pressure above 160/95 mm Hg), increased cholesterol level, and adult onset diabetes are the most modifiable risk factors. Cigarette smoking increases the risk of stroke by approximately 50% and the risk is directly related to the number of cigarettes smoked per day. Heavy consumption of alcohol, cocaine use, and obesity have been associated with an increase in the incidence of stroke. Among the nonmodifiable risk factors (age, race, and sex), age constitutes the greatest risk. Seventy-two percent of strokes occur in persons older than 65 (Agency for Health Care Policy and Research, 1995).

Fibrinogen is a coagulation factor that has been demonstrated to be associated with increased stroke risk. Fibrinogen is the primary determinant of blood coagulability and plays a crucial role in platelet aggregation. Platelets initiate thrombosis by attracting fibrin and other clot-forming substances (see further discussion in Chapter 8). Conditions associated with increased fibrin deposition or increased blood viscosity include rheumatic heart disease, endocarditis, atherosclerosis, polycythemia, and thrombocytosis.

Ischemic Stroke

Occlusion of Major Arteries

Thrombosis and embolic occlusion of a major vessel are the most common causes of ischemic stroke. The heart is the most common source of embolic material, as a result of damage to heart tissue from atherothrombotic disease. Atrial fibrillation is believed to cause thrombus formation in the fibrillating atrium. Left ventricular myocardial infarction (MI) can be a source of emboli, especially in the first few weeks following the event, when thrombus formation is most prevalent. Mitral valve prolapse or congenital septal defects are also sources of emboli. Cardiogenic embolism during or following coronary artery surgery or intracardiac surgery is a well-recognized complication.

The proximal internal carotid artery is the most common site of atherosclerosis and atherothrombosis leading to stroke. Artery-to-artery embolism, usually arising from an atherothrombotic lesion in the carotid or vertebrobasilar system, may lead to stroke. The emboli from this lesion may travel along the course of circulation and may cause occlusion in the smaller branches. Other causes may be thrombus in the pulmonary vein, fat emboli in the blood, and tumor emboli from a neoplastic process (Feinberg, 1995).

Lacunar infarcts are small infarcts of the end arteries, found in the basal ganglia, internal capsule and pons (see Fig. 28–6). The lacunar infarcts have the characteristics of ischemic necrosis and the cysts are surrounded by *astrocytic gliosis*, or scarring of the support structures of the brain (Hommel and Gray, 1995). These small, cystic spaces resulting from healed ischemic infarcts are common in individuals with hyperten-

[1] Lipohyalinosis and inflammation can cause weakening of the vessel wall. Amyloid deposition develops with age and disease, and can change the status of the vessel wall. Atherosclerosis can be directly responsible for occluding the blood flow in a vessel. Malformations are addressed in the text.

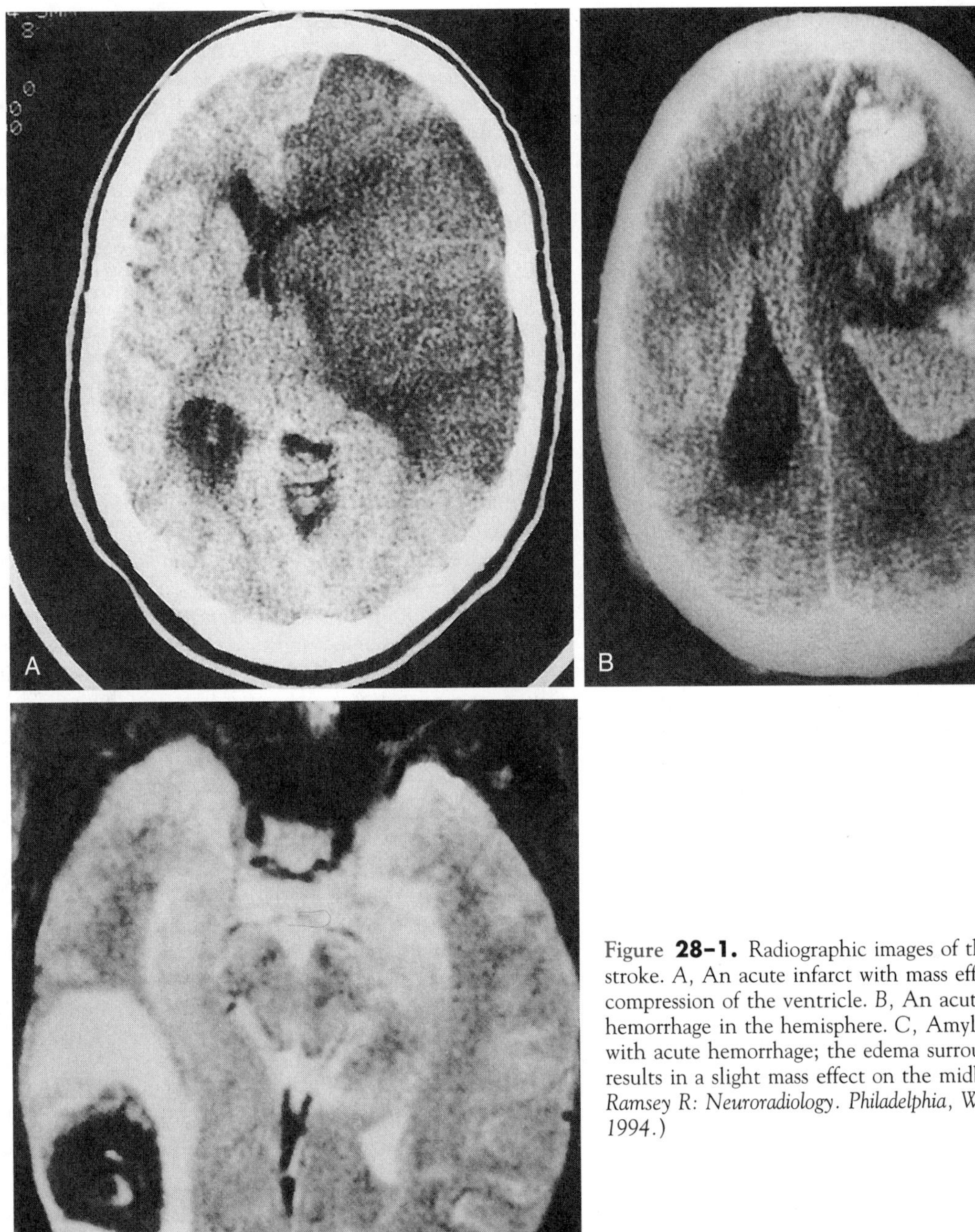

Figure **28–1.** Radiographic images of the brain after stroke. *A*, An acute infarct with mass effect and compression of the ventricle. *B*, An acute intracerebral hemorrhage in the hemisphere. *C*, Amyloid angiopathy with acute hemorrhage; the edema surrounding the area results in a slight mass effect on the midbrain. (*From Ramsey R: Neuroradiology. Philadelphia, WB Saunders, 1994.*)

sion or diabetes. A large majority are asymptomatic, but in about 20% of cases a stroke syndrome occurs with a slowly progressive (over 24 to 36 hours) dysfunction of the cells in the area of the lacune (Pryse-Phillips and Murray, 1992).

Infarction

The tissue of the brain, or the *parenchyma*, is highly vulnerable to an interruption in its blood supply. When the cerebral blood flow falls below 20 mL/100 g of tissue per minute (normal, 50 to 60 mL/100 g of tissue per minute) neuronal functioning is impaired. Infarction causing tissue damage develops when the cerebral blood flow remains below 12 mL/100 g of tissue per minute. Frequently, in an acute infarction, a portion of the affected brain will receive no blood, while a surrounding area will receive sufficient blood from collateral circulation to maintain viability but not to sustain function. This territory has been termed the *ischemic penumbra* (Tuhrim, 1993). Although the major injury to the neurons in the brain is the hypoxia-ischemia related to the occlusion of the artery, causing cell death, further damage to the brain tissue and neurons occurs as a secondary response.

Secondary Vascular Responses

It is postulated that when a cerebral artery is occluded, the formation of thromboemboli begins in the distal vessels of that artery. These presumed microvascular occlusions progressively increase in number and continue to impair blood flow in the brain. Cell death surrounding the area of blocked blood flow may be due to the squeezing effects of microvessels by the swelling of the *astrocyte*, one of the cellular support structures of the nervous system. (See also Cellular Dysfunction in Chapter 24.) Astroglial swelling is one of the earliest cell changes induced by single artery occlusion. The formation of fibrin in the gray matter surrounding the occluded vessel may also contribute to the lack of reperfusion of microvessels. Other factors include parenchymal bleeding, platelet aggregation, endothelial cell swelling (in the walls of the vessels), and vasospasm (Garcia, 1995; O'Brien, 1995).

Secondary Neuronal Damage

After global ischemic injuries to the brain, neuronal groups at locations beyond the immediate site of injury show changes. These neuronal groups, known to be extremely sensitive to ischemia, are traditionally identified as being located in the pyramidal cell layer of the hippocampus and the Purkinje-cell layer of the cerebellar cortex. Neurons at these sites are selectively vulnerable to ischemia, and these neurons may be more susceptible to excitotoxic neurotransmitters, such as glutamate (Choi, 1995).

Changes in the neurotransmitter substances that are normally present in the brain can cause further damage in the hypoxic-ischemic state. In keeping with its widespread role in central excitatory neurotransmission, glutamate is normally present throughout central nervous system (CNS) gray matter. The glutamate is stored in synaptic terminals, and when it is released into the extracellular space, rapid uptake normally occurs, so the resting level of glutamate outside of the synaptic terminal is minimal. After an ischemic event, the cells that normally take up the excess glutamate are compromised, which causes toxic overstimulation of postsynaptic receptors. The ultimate effect of this excessive availability of glutamate is to facilitate the entry of calcium ions into the cells. Excessive numbers of calcium ions begin the process that causes cell death in ischemic necrosis.

Catabolic (destructive) enzymes can be activated by the release of calcium ions and cause further degradation of major neuronal structural proteins. Endothelial cells (in response to changes in perfusion pressure) interact with circulating cells and begin to generate neurotoxic products, such as free radicals. Oxygen free radicals can initiate many destructive processes in the brain tissue.

The overall result of the hypoxic event is a chain of reactions that extend the damage and death of brain tissue beyond the area of vascular supply. Efforts to control the brain damage after stroke focus on changing the natural course of those processes and are discussed in the section on treatment.

Syndromes

Syndromes reflect the dysfunction associated with disruption of blood flow in specific areas of the brain (Kistler et al., 1994). The syndromes are named according to the arteries that feed the specific areas. The syndrome can be partial or complete. When the blockage is in the more proximal component of the artery, the resulting area of hypoxia is greater than if the clot is lodged in a more distal part of the artery. Because of the collateral circulation provided by the circle of Willis, some areas of the brain are supplied by more than one artery. When one artery is blocked, circulation is provided to the tissues through the blood supply of other arteries. In this case, the clinical syndromes are not as extensive. The actual configuration of arteries is different in each individual, so the syndromes described here are not to be considered all-encompassing; this is an overview of the types of symptoms that might be encountered when a particular artery is blocked.

Middle Cerebral Artery Syndrome

If the entire middle cerebral artery is occluded at its stem, blocking both the penetrating and cortical branches, the clinical findings are contralateral *hemiplegia* and *hemianesthesia*, or the loss of movement and sensation on one half of the body. If the dominant hemisphere is affected, *global aphasia*, or the loss of fluency, ability to name objects, comprehend auditory information, and repeat language, is the result. (See discussion of parietal lobe syndromes in Chapter 24.)

Partial syndromes resulting from embolic occlusion of a single branch include *brachial syndrome*, or weakness of the upper extremity, and *frontal opercular syndrome*, or facial weakness with motor aphasia, with or without arm weakness. A combination of sensory disturbance, motor weakness, and motor aphasia suggests that an embolus has occluded the proximal superior division branch and has infarcted large portions of the frontal and parietal cortices.

If Wernicke's aphasia occurs without weakness, the inferior division of the middle cerebral artery supplying the temporal cortex of the dominant hemisphere has been occluded. Jargon speech and an inability to comprehend written and oral language are prominent features. Hemiplegia or spatial agnosia without weakness indicates that the inferior division of the middle cerebral artery in the nondominant hemisphere is involved. Figure 28–2 represents the area of the middle cerebral artery.

Anterior Cerebral Artery Syndrome

Infarction in the territory of the anterior cerebral artery is uncommon and is more often due to embolism than to atherothrombosis. Collateral flow is able to compensate for most occlusion of the artery, so that dysfunction is minimal. If both segments of the artery arise from a single anterior cerebral stem, the occlusion affects both hemispheres. Profound *abulia*, or a delay in verbal and motor response with paraplegia, results. Figure 28–3 represents the area of blood flow of the anterior cerebral artery.

Internal Carotid Artery Syndrome

The clinical picture of internal carotid occlusion varies, depending on whether the cause of ischemia is thrombus, embolus, or low flow. The cortex supplied by the middle cerebral territory is most often affected (for symptoms, see preceding discussion). Occasionally, the origins of both the anterior and middle cerebral arteries are occluded at the top of the

MIDDLE CEREBRAL ARTERY

Anatomy

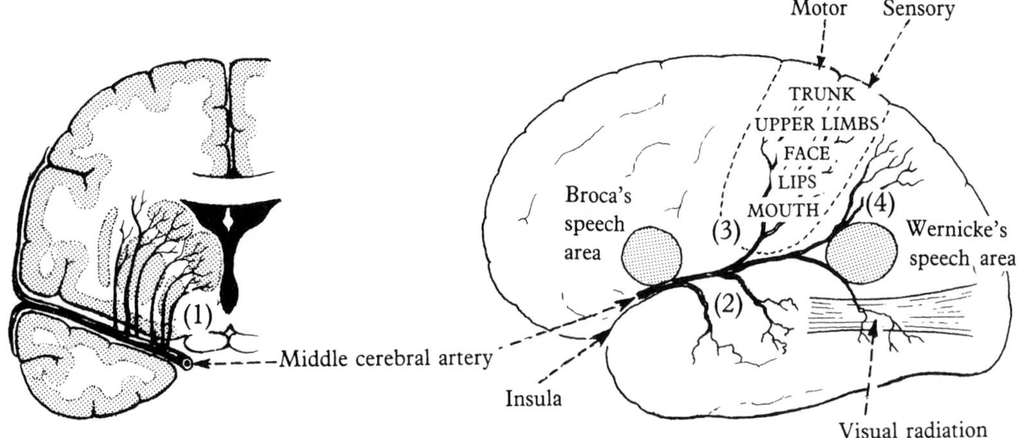

Figure **28-2.** The middle cerebral artery is the largest branch of the internal carotid artery and the most common site of emboli. Its deep branches feed the internal capsule and basal ganglia. On the lateral surface, the branches feed areas of the parietal, frontal, and temporal lobes. (*From Lindsay KW, Bone I, Callander R: Neurology and Neurosurgery Illustrated. New York, Churchill Livingstone, 1986.*)

carotid artery. Symptoms consistent with both syndromes result. With a competent circle of Willis producing adequate collateral circulation, the occlusion can be asymptomatic.

Posterior Cerebral Artery Syndrome

If the proximal posterior cerebral artery is occluded, including penetrating branches, the area of the brain that is affected is the subthalamus, medial thalamus, and ispilateral (same side) cerebral peduncle and midbrain. Signs include thalamic syndrome, including loss of pain and temperature (superficial sensation) and proprioception and touch (deep sensation).

ANTERIOR CEREBRAL ARTERY

Anatomy

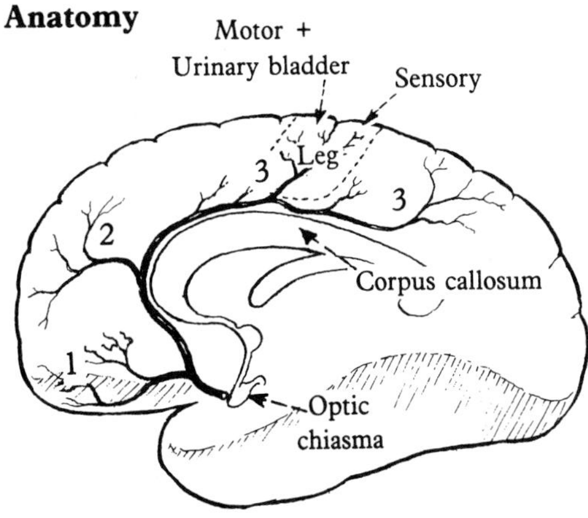

Figure **28-3.** The anterior cerebral artery branches from the internal carotid. Deep branches supply the internal capsule and basal ganglia. Superficial branches supply the frontal and parietal lobes. (*From Lindsay KW, Bone I, Callander R: Neurology and Neurosurgery Illustrated. New York, Churchill Livingstone, 1986.*)

This may develop into intractable, searing pain, which can be incapacitating.

If the posterior cerebral artery is completely occluded at its origin, hemiplegia results from infarction of the cerebral peduncle. Involvement of the red nucleus or dentatorubrothalamic tract can produce contralateral ataxia. When palsy of cranial nerve III occurs with contralateral ataxia, it is known as *Claude's syndrome*, and when third nerve palsy occurs with contralateral hemiplegia, it is known as *Weber's syndrome*. *Hemiballismus*, or the flailing movement of one extremity, usually results from a deep penetrating vessel causing infarct in the contralateral subthalamic nucleus. Paresis of upward gaze, drowsiness, and *abulia*, the lack of interest in movement, can be attributed to occlusion of the artery of Percheron. If the posterior cerebral stem is occluded, causing extensive infarction of the subthalamus, coma and decerebrate rigidity may result.

Peripheral supply of the posterior cerebral artery includes the temporal and occipital lobes. Occlusion of this component of the artery often leads to *homonymous hemianopsia*, in which the visual field defect is on the side opposite to the lesion. *Cortical blindness*, the inability of the brain to record an image although the optic nerve is intact, is one of the visual disturbances that commonly accompanies infarct in this region.

Medial temporal lobe involvement (including the hippocampus) can cause an acute disturbance in memory, particularly if it occurs in the dominant hemisphere. This will resolve because memory has dual representation. Memory is represented on both sides of the brain; if one area is affected the intact side can compensate to a considerable extent. If the dominant hemisphere is affected and the infarct extends to involve the splenium of the corpus callosum, the individual may demonstrate *alexia* without *agraphia*, or impairment of reading without the impairment of writing. *Agnosia*, or difficulty in identification or recognition, affecting the ability to identify faces, objects, mathematical symbols, and colors, may occur. *Anomia,* impaired ability to identify objects by name, and visual hallucinations of brightly colored scenes and objects, can occur with peripheral posterior cerebral infarction. Embolic occlusion of the top of the basilar artery can produce a clinical picture that includes any or all of the central or peripheral territory symptoms. Figure 28–4 represents the area of blood flow of the posterior cerebral artery.

Vertebral and Posterior Inferior Cerebellar Artery Syndrome

Blood supply to the brainstem, medulla, and cerebellum is provided by the vertebral and posterior cerebellar arteries. Collateral circulation is provided by the bilateral component of the vertebral artery—the ascending cervical, thyrocervical, and occipital arteries—so that ischemia is often not manifested in the presence of atherothrombosis.

When infarction ensues, the lateral medulla and the posteroinferior cerebellum are affected, resulting in *Wallenberg's syndrome,* which is characterized by vertigo, nausea, hoarseness, and dysphagia (difficulty swallowing). Other symptoms include ipsilateral ataxia (uncoordinated movement), ptosis (eyelid droop), and impairment of sensation in the ipsilateral portion of the face and contralateral portion of the torso and limbs.

A medial medullary infarction of the pyramid can result in contralateral hemiparesis of the arm and leg, sparing the face. If the medial lemniscus and the hypoglossal nerve fibers are involved, loss of joint position sense and ipsilateral tongue weakness can occur.

The edema associated with cerebellar infarction can cause sudden respiratory arrest due to raised intracranial pressure in the posterior fossa. Gait unsteadiness, dizziness, nausea, and vomiting may be the only early symptoms. Figure 28–5 shows the area of distribution of the superior cerebellar, inferior cerebellar, and anterior inferior cerebellar arteries.

Basilar Artery Syndrome

Atheromatous lesions can occur anywhere along the basilar trunk, but they occur most often in the proximal basilar and distal vertebral area. Ischemia as a result of occlusion of the basilar artery can affect the brainstem, including the corticospinal tracts, corticobulbar tracts, medial and superior cerebellar peduncles, spinothalamic tracts, and cranial nerve nuclei.

If the basilar artery is occluded, the brainstem symptoms are bilateral. When a branch of the basilar artery is occluded, the symptoms are unilateral, involving the sensory and motor aspects of the cranial nerves.

Superior Cerebellar Artery Syndrome

Occlusion of the superior cerebellar artery results in severe ipsilateral cerebellar ataxia, nausea and vomiting, and *dysarthria,* which is a slurring of speech. Loss of pain and temperature in the contralateral extremities, torso, and face occurs. *Dysmetria,* characterized by the inability to place an extremity at a precise point in space, is common, affecting the ipsilateral upper extremity.

Anterior Inferior Cerebellar Artery

Principal symptoms include ipsilateral deafness, facial weakness, vertigo, nausea and vomiting, *nystagmus* (or rhythmic oscillations of the eye), and ataxia. *Horner's syndrome* ptosis, miosis (constriction of the pupil), and loss of sweating over the ipsilateral side of the face, may occur. A paresis of lateral

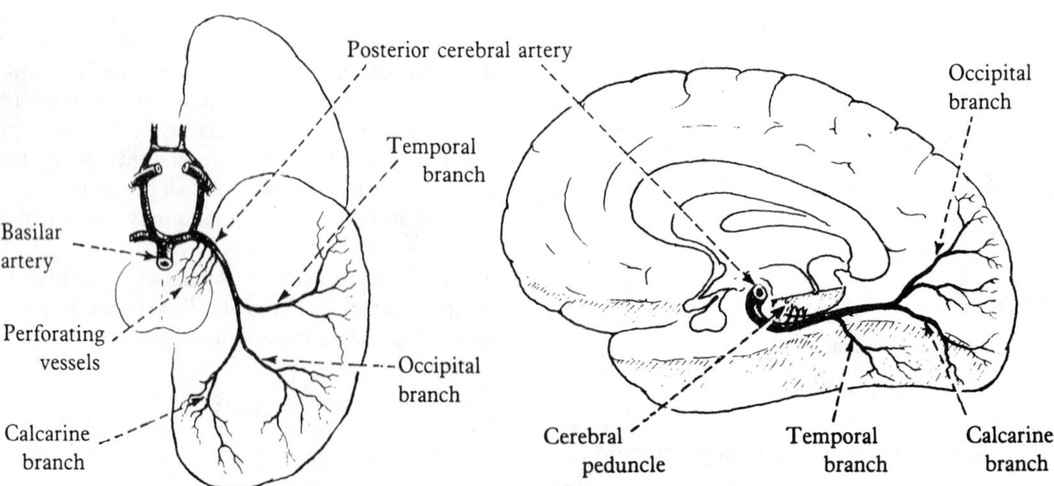

Figure 28–4. The posterior cerebral arteries branch from the basilar artery. The small perforating branches supply the midbrain structures and posterior thalamus. The temporal branch supplies the temporal lobe, and the occipital and calcarine supply the occipital lobe, including the visual cortex. (*From Lindsay KW, Bone I, Callander R: Neurology and Neurosurgery Illustrated. New York, Churchill Livingstone, 1986.*)

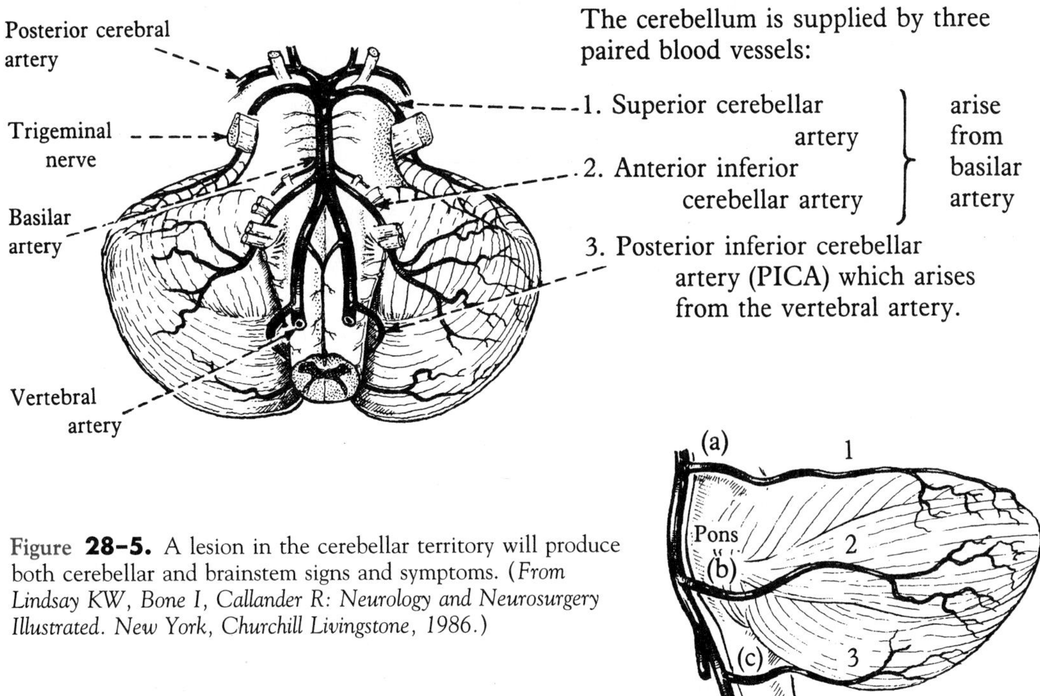

Figure **28–5.** A lesion in the cerebellar territory will produce both cerebellar and brainstem signs and symptoms. (*From Lindsay KW, Bone I, Callander R: Neurology and Neurosurgery Illustrated. New York, Churchill Livingstone, 1986.*)

gaze may be seen. Pain and temperature sensation is lost on the contralateral side of the body.

Lacunar Syndrome

The lacunar syndrome is representative of the area of infarct in which the lacunae are predominant, often in the deep structures of the brain. If the posterior limb of the internal capsule is affected, a pure motor deficit may result; in the anterior limb of the internal capsule, weakness of the face and dysarthria may occur. If the posterolateral thalamus is affected there is a pure sensory stroke. When the lacunae occur predominantly in the pons, ataxia, clumsiness, and weakness may be seen (Fig. 28–6).

Medical Management

Diagnosis. History of the neurologic event should be obtained, including timing, pattern of onset, and course. An embolic stroke occurs rapidly, with no warning. A more progressive and uneven onset is typical with thrombosis. The presenting symptoms will help to determine the location of the lesion. Neuroimaging of the brain has become a standard procedure in the diagnosis of stroke.

Computed tomographic (CT) scans may be normal in the acute stage of an embolic stroke. Bleeding into the brain tissue is seen acutely. Displacement of brain structures, such as the ventricles, by edema can sometimes be seen early in a large infarct. Later CT scans will reveal the area of decreased density. Lacunar infarcts are sometimes visible on CT scans as small, punched-out, hypodense areas (Kistler et al., 1994). The extent of the lesion on CT scan does not directly correlate to the degree of disability for the individual.

Magnetic resonance imaging (MRI) allows for the identification of an ischemic event within 2 to 6 hours of onset. Positron emission tomography (PET) provides information about the local cerebral perfusion and residual cell function. This allows the clinician to determine tissue viability, and it may provide guidance in the medical management of secondary neuron damage with neuroprotective drugs (Baron, 1995). Cerebral angiography can be used in the absence of CT or MRI.

Treatment. Treatment of individuals with ischemic stroke consists of managing the stroke and preventing further embolic strokes. Cerebral perfusion, or the blood flow around the area of the stroke, is the main concern when the cause is embolic. Blood pressure should not be lowered unless it is as high as 180/120 mm Hg. The goal is not to try to normalize the pressure, but to bring it down from dangerously high levels. If the blood pressure is low, raising it is appropriate in the first few hours after the stroke. An excessive rise in blood pressure may cause an increase in edema.

Emboli that lodge in the middle cerebral artery stem can cause enough edema to lead to coma and death if it is uncontrolled. Even a small amount of edema in the cerebellum can cause respiratory arrest from compression of the brainstem. Water restriction and agents that raise the serum osmolarity should be considered with the onset of significant edema.

Anticoagulation

Anticoagulation therapy has played a prominent role in the prevention of acute infarction for several decades, and current research supports use in high-risk individuals. Individuals with atrial fibrillation show increased protection from stroke with the use of anticoagulation therapies.

Warfarin sodium (Coumadin, Panwarfin) appears to be about twice as effective as aspirin in the prevention of stroke

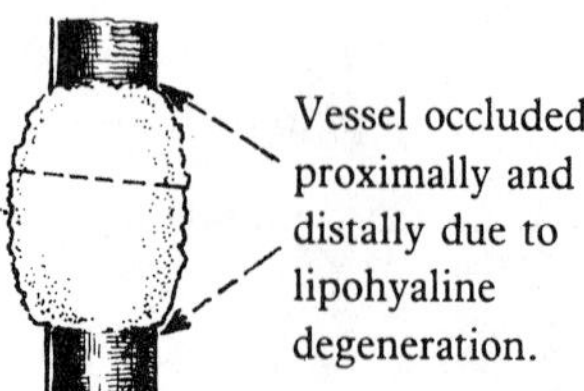

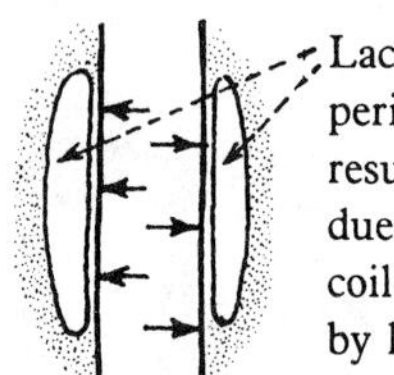

Lacunes are found in hypertensive patients. Their formation is often unassociated with symptoms. However, certain clinical states are recognised:

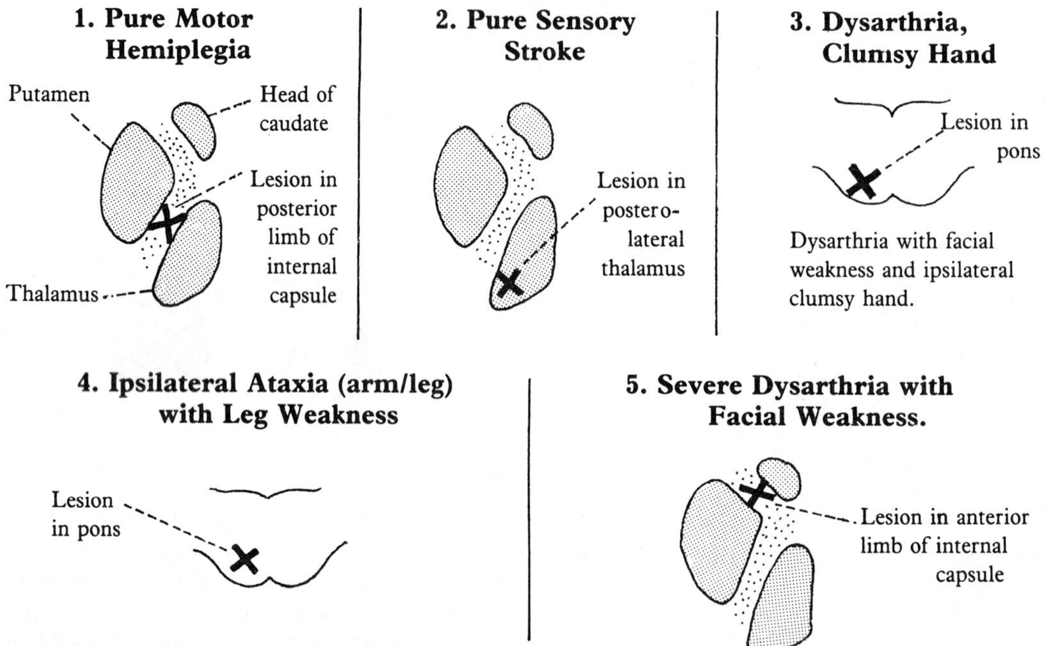

Figure **28–6.** Lacunae are small fluid-filled cavities that surround the small penetrating arteries that are branches of the major cerebral arteries; they are small infarctions produced by occlusions of the small branches. (*From Lindsay KW, Bone I, Callander R: Neurology and Neurosurgery Illustrated. New York, Churchill Livingstone, 1986.*)

in individuals with atrial fibrillation. Persons older than 75 years have the highest risk of stroke and can benefit from anticoagulation; however, risk of bleeding is age related, and the ability to determine the risk-to-benefit ratio is more complex.

Aspirin therapy, however, is considered to be a generally safe, low-cost method of improving protection against stroke. Aspirin is a platelet anti-aggregation agent with moderate side effects. The appropriate duration and dosage of antithrombotic treatment has not been firmly established, and the studies are continuing to look at risk-to-benefit ratios with different dosages and in more complex studies with longer follow-up times (Norrving, 1994).

Thrombolytic therapy remains experimental; however, studies have shown promise. Fibrinolytic agents work by allowing reperfusion of an artery after it has become occluded. Time is of the essence in the use of these drugs, as the ischemic damage worsens with time after occlusion (Zoppo et al., 1994).

Neuroprotection *(Finklestein, 1995; Wahlgren, 1995)*

Medications aimed at creating neuroprotection to decrease the amount of cell death secondary to excitotoxicy are being developed, and clinical studies are under way. Approaches directed at presynaptic reduction of pathologic glutamate release may control the damage caused by excess extracellular glutamate. Reducing the amplification of excitotoxic calcium ion release may also help control cell death. In this category are fibroblastic growth factors, which may improve recovery from calcium overload.

Safety risks exist with these medications, including brain toxic effects, although the side effects are of a short duration, with reversibility after medication is stopped. Time will be of the essence in the administration of these drugs. The window of opportunity may very well be 2 to 6 hours after infarction. Many antiexcitotoxic therapies may be suitable for either hemorrhagic or ischemic stroke and may be given by paramedics before full neurologic evaluation.

Surgical Intervention

Carotid endarterectomy is the treatment of choice for individuals who have had a low-flow or embolic TIA. If stenosis is greater than 70% in a sclerotic lesion at the origin of the internal carotid artery, endarterectomy is indicated. Careful selection of candidates for surgery is essential, as is an experienced team of surgeons and other health-care providers to manage the postoperative course.

Prognosis. The prognosis for survival after cerebral infarction is better than after cerebral or subarachnoid hemorrhage. Loss of consciousness after an ischemic stroke implies a poorer prognosis than otherwise. Individuals with ischemic stroke are at risk for other strokes or myocardial infarctions (Kistler et al., 1994).

Recovery from stroke is the fastest in the first few weeks after onset, with the most measurable neurologic recovery (approximately 90%) in the first 3 months (O'Sullivan, 1994). However, movement patterns can continue to be influenced by intervention with goal-directed activities, and repetition of movement appears to improve the speed and control of the movement in the individual up to 2 to 3 years after stroke.

Intracerebral Hemorrhage

Overview and Definition. Intracerebral hemorrhage (ICH) is bleeding from an arterial source into brain parenchyma (therefore is often referred to as an *intraparenchymal hemorrhage*) and is widely regarded as the most deadly of stroke subtypes. Primary intracerebral hemorrhage describes spontaneous bleeding in the absence of a readily identifiable precipitant and is usually attributable to microvascular disease associated with hypertension or aging. Secondary ICH occurs most often in association with either trauma, impaired coagulation, toxin exposure, or an anatomic lesion.

Supratentorial ICH, so named because it occurs above the cerebellar tentorium, is classified as being *lobar* (i.e., involving the hemispheres of the cerebrum) or *deep* (i.e., implying involvement of structures of the midbrain, such as the thalamus, putamen, or caudate nucleus). *Infratentorial*, below the tentorium, refers to involvement of either the brainstem, usually the pons, or cerebellum (Sacco and Mayer, 1994). Figure 28–7 represents the areas most likely to be involved in ICH.

Incidence. The incidence of ICH is low among persons below the age of 45 years, and it increases dramatically after the age of 65 years. In one study, the incidence of ICH doubled with each advancing decade until age 80 years, after which the incidence became 25 times higher (Sacco and Mayer, 1994). ICH tends to occur more frequently in men. In the United States, blacks are more likely to have an ICH than are whites. Worldwide rates are higher in Asian populations than in Western populations.

Etiology and Risk Factors. Spontaneous ICH in the parenchyma of the brain is usually due to anomaly of the vessel structure or to changes brought on by hypertension (Frank and Biller, 1994). Hypertension represents the single most important modifiable risk factor for ICH. Cerebral amyloid angiopathy (CAA) causing abnormal changes in the vessels of the brain accounts for approximately 10% of ICH. Cerebral amyloid angiopathy is recognized as an important cause of ICH in elderly persons.

Excessive use of alcohol has been associated with massive spontaneous ICH. Alcohol has a number of acute and chronic effects that may contribute to hemorrhagic stroke, including acute and chronic hypertension, impaired coagulation, and direct effects on cerebral vessels.

ICH is the most important adverse effect of thrombolytic therapy. Hemorrhage from fibrinolytic agents can occur within 12 to 24 hours and are typically lobar, occurring in the cortex and subcortical white matter (Sloan, 1994).

Long-term anticoagulant therapy is associated with an increased risk for ICH. Many individuals with anticoagulant-associated ICH are also hypertensive, so that the extent of increased risk is difficult to clearly identify independently (Wilterdink, 1994).

It is possible that use of other medications in conjunction with thrombolytic therapy places individuals at risk for ICH. A number of drugs, such as nonsteroidal anti-inflammatory agents, nitrates, and propranolol may affect platelet function and contribute to bleeding (Sloan, 1994).

Cocaine and amphetamine use is widely acknowledged as an important cause of ICH. Other possible risk factors include liver disease, prior ischemic stroke, and cigarette smoking. Obesity, sickle cell anemia, mitral valve prolapse, patent foramen ovale, and polycythemia all have been identified as possible risk factors. More research in this area is ongoing and will provide more insight into the relationship of chronic disease and lifestyle to ICH.

Pathogenesis. Histopathologic changes in the cerebral microvasculature of hypertensive individuals include processes that affect both the contents and the walls of the blood vessels of the brain. These changes are seen in small cerebral arteries and arterioles where they branch, and they are more severe in the small penetrating vessels in the deep white matter than in cortical vessels of similar size. Changes are more severe distally than proximally. There is a progressive replacement of smooth muscle cells by collagen (hyalinization). Altered permeability of the vessel wall leads to fibrinoid changes in the vessel wall. This results in accumulation of proteinaceous material and fat deposits on the subintimal wall. The vessel wall becomes prone to leakage or rupture (Wilterdink and Feldmann, 1996).

Hypertensives have substantial reduction in the percentage of smooth muscle in the vessel wall. It is believed that this decreased smooth muscle mass represents structural weak-

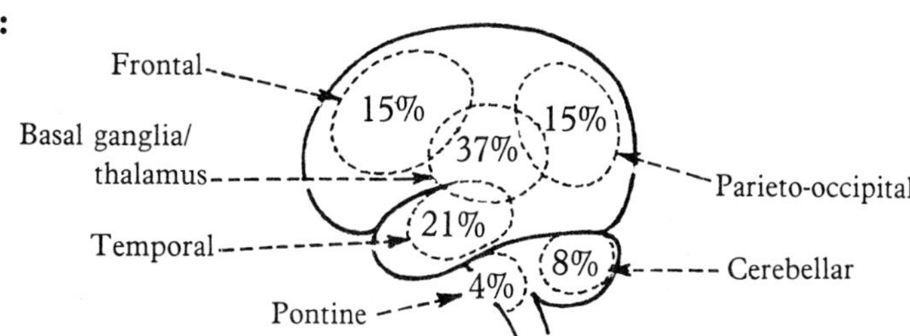

Figure **28–7.** Sites of predilection of intracerebral hemorrhage. (*Adapted from Lindsay KW, Bone I, Callander R: Neurology and Neurosurgery Illustrated. New York, Churchill Livingstone, 1986.*)

ening, resulting in rupture and hemorrhage. Necrosis of the endothelium may be a result of vessel ischemia. The changes in smooth muscle and the thickening of the intimal wall increase the metabolic requirements and impede the flow of oxygen to the outermost part of the vessel wall (Wilterdink, 1994).

CAA is characterized by protein fibrils in the arterioles and small cerebral arteries and is formed by aberrant protein synthesis. Amyloid replaces smooth muscle in the media separating the elastic membranes. Lymphocytic infiltrates, hyaline arteriole degeneration, and fibrinoid necrosis are characteristic changes in the vessel wall. The parenchymal changes seen in CAA reflect the consequences of the vascular pathology and direct deposition of amyloid in the brain tissue. Brains with CAA frequently demonstrate periventricular demyelination, believed to be due to ischemia caused by amyloid deposition in the vessels supplying the deep white matter (Furie and Feldmann, 1994; Harrison, 1995).

In *drug-related ICH*, some underlying vascular pathologic lesion may be present, such as an arteriovenous malformation or chronic vasculitis. The ICH occurs as a result of a sudden increase in blood pressure triggered by the drug. The proposed mechanism for the increased incidence of intracerebral hemorrhage in the individual with increased alcohol ingestion is decreased circulating levels of clotting factors produced by the liver. Thrombocytopenia, which is often associated with alcoholism, may underlie or potentiate hemorrhage (Gorelick and Kelly, 1994).

Hemorrhagic transformation, or conversion of an ischemic cerebral infarction, refers to secondary bleeding believed to occur either with early reperfusion into a damaged vascular bed with impaired autoregulation or as a result of development of collateral circulation into the same vascular bed (Sloan, 1994).

When hemorrhage occurs, it spreads along a path of least resistance, primarily following the fiber tracts of the white matter. Gray matter, with its dense cell structure, is more resistant to the shearing forces of the growing hematoma and is more likely than white matter to be compressed rather than infiltrated by the spreading hematoma. Edema forms in the parenchyma surrounding the hematoma. Blood is reabsorbed by macrophages at the periphery of the hemorrhage, leaving a cavity surrounded by necrotic tissue. This process usually takes weeks or months (Wilterdink, 1994).

Clinical Manifestations. Neurologic symptoms occur gradually, in most cases, representing the expansion of the hematoma. In some cases (approximately 30%) onset is sudden, which is also characteristic of an ischemic stroke. Symptoms worsen due to the bleeding and formation of edema. Once the condition is stabilized, the symptoms improve in parallel with the resorption of the hematoma.

Although headache is an important symptom of ICH, it is present in severe form in only 30% to 40% of cases. Headache is most common as a sign of superficial and large hemorrhages.

The incidence of seizure correlates with the location of the hemorrhage. Cerebral cortex hemorrhage causes the most prevalent seizure activity. Two-thirds of the seizures are generalized and one-third are focal. Focal seizures affect the body on the contralateral side (see Chapter 31). The level of consciousness at onset is unrelated to occurrence of seizure.

Syndromes

Syndromes associated with ICH are representative of the area of bleed and reflect brain activity of the particular site (Wilterdink, 1994; Brass, 1994).

Putamen

Fifty percent to 80% of hemorrhages occur in the putamen. The result is contralateral sensorimotor deficit due to its proximity to the internal capsule. Small putaminal hemorrhages may mimic lacunar syndromes, such as pure motor weakness. A type of aphasia may be present that mimics Broca's aphasia when the lesion is in the mid-putamen. A Wernicke's aphasia is seen with a posterior putaminal lesion. Pupillary abnormalities, visual field loss, and oculomotor deficits are common. Conjugate gaze deviation toward the side of the lesion may be present. Abulia and motor impersistence are seen when the anterior putamen is affected. Headache and vomiting also occur in about 25% of cases.

Thalamus

Sensory loss, or dysesthesias, predominate with thalamic hemorrhage, and some motor deficit occurs secondary to internal capsular involvement. The lateral thalamus abuts the posterior limb of the internal capsule. Oculomotor dysfunction is also seen, the most frequent abnormalities being vertical gaze palsies, often with downward eye deviation and convergence spasm. Constriction (miosis) of the pupil is seen in 50% of cases. In dominant hemisphere thalamic lesions, aphasia, disorientation, and memory disturbances may be seen. With nondominant lesions, *apraxia* (impairment of a learned motor activity) may exist. Midline hematomas are associated with alterations in the level of consciousness during the acute phase followed by prefrontal signs, such as change in character, speaking to oneself, memory disturbance, and impaired learning. Although not as common, the individual may experience symptoms such as headache, nausea, and vomiting in the same degree as with putaminal hemorrhage.

Cerebellum

A hallmark of cerebellar hemorrhages is ataxia. Additional symptoms may be nausea and vomiting, and dizziness with nystagmus and vertigo often is present. The individual may be dysarthric. Brainstem signs, such as facial paresis, can be present with a hemorrhage that extends to the brainstem. The signs of cerebellar hemorrhage should be carefully monitored, as the progression to compression of vital structures in the region of the fourth ventricle and medulla can be rapid and can produce life-threatening changes.

Pons

Brainstem hemorrhages commonly arise in the midline of the pons, leading to coma, quadriparesis, and unreactive pupils with absent horizontal eye movement. Lateral pontine hemorrhage can result in extraocular paresis with deviation away from the side of the lesion. Quick, downward jerks of the eye occur with a slow upward drift. Pupils are small but reactive. Contralateral sensory and motor symptoms and ipsilateral cerebellar signs (see preceding text) are also seen.

Caudate

Caudate hemorrhages can rupture into the ventricles and therefore have a presentation like that of a subarachnoid hemorrhage. Headache, vomiting, and loss of consciousness may occur. The internal capsule may be involved, causing sensorimotor involvement.

Internal Capsule

Internal capsule hemorrhages often result in a pure motor, pure sensory, or sensorimotor stroke with ataxia. The internal capsule is a white matter tract that is situated lateral to the basal ganglia as it connects to the cerebral cortex.

Lobar

Lobar hematomas are centered in the immediate subcortical white matter. Symptoms are lobe-specific (see Clinical Manifestations of Ischemic Stroke, this chapter, and Higher Brain Disorders in Chapter 24). Seizures are more common with lobar hemorrhages than with deeper bleeds.

Medical Management

Diagnosis. The availability of CT allows for prompt diagnosis of ICH. The specific area of damage can be imaged and the amount of blood identified. It has also documented hyperacute clot retraction progression of hypertensive ICH and early hemorrhagic infarction.

MRI can provide multiplanar views and can discriminate subtle tissue changes and rapidly flowing blood. However, it is of limited usefulness in the first 24 hours after ICH. MRI has the capability to detect previous hemorrhage, and it can image the posterior fossa more clearly than can CT.

Prothrombin time, partial thromboplastin time, and platelet count should be performed in all patients to rule out a bleeding disorder. Coagulation factor deficiencies can be detected by evaluation of liver enzymes. Bleeding time, platelet aggregation studies, and fibrinogen assay can also be indicators of disorders related to possible repeat hemorrhage.

A screen for toxic substances in the blood should be performed, especially in the younger population. Acquired immunodeficiency syndrome (AIDS) should be considered as a possible cause of ICH. Biopsy of brain tissue can be diagnostic of cerebral amyloid angiopathy, cerebral vasculitis, and neoplasm. Evaluation of cerebrospinal fluid may indicate levels of toxicity; however, individuals with increased intracranial pressure (ICP) are at risk during the procedure for possible herniation causing compression of the brainstem.

Treatment. The acute reduction of elevated blood pressure is advisable and is most readily accomplished with rapid-acting, potent antihypertensive medication along with effective control of increased ICP, which exacerbates blood pressure elevation (Kelly, 1994). A major issue in the management of ICH is control of edema (see Treatment, Ischemic Stroke, this chapter). Anticonvulsant therapy should be considered with lobar hemorrhage.

The frequency of intracranial hemorrhage may increase with the use of chronic anticoagulation therapy. Treatment with vitamin K is useful to correct an elevated prothrombin time; however, this takes 12 to 24 hours. Fresh-frozen plasma immediately restores diminished clotting factors. Protamine sulfate is the treatment of choice for reversal of the heparin effect. Thrombocytopenia responds to plasma infusion and plasma exchange.

Prognosis. While the overall mortality from ICH is high, functional recovery among survivors is also high. The most important predictor of mortality is hemorrhage size. The individuals who are comatose at onset or who have a wide spectrum of neurologic deficits tend to do poorly compared to those who remain alert and have focal neurologic symptoms. The older the individual, the less complete the expected recovery.

Survival for individuals with hemorrhage in the posterior fossa is more dependent on location of hemorrhage than size. Midline pontine hemorrhage is often fatal, whereas lateral hemorrhages carry a better prognosis (Wilterdink, 1994).

SUBARACHNOID HEMORRHAGE

Overview. Subarachnoid hemorrhage results in frank blood in the subarachnoid space between the arachnoid and the pia, which are contiguous membranes that surround the brain tissue. It can be the result of trauma, developmental defects, neoplasm, or infections that cause rupture into the subarachnoid space. Subarachnoid hemorrhage can be spontaneous and is often seen in normotensive persons. Aneurysm and vascular malformations are responsible for most subarachnoid hemorrhage. About 90% of subarachnoid hemorrhages are due to berry aneurysms. *Berry aneurysm* is a congenital abnormal distention of a local vessel that occurs at a bifurcation, where the medial layer of the vessel is the weakest. Vascular malformations are responsible for approximately 6% of hemorrhages into the subarachnoid space. Included in vascular malformations are venous malformation, arteriovenous malformation (AVM), and cavernous malformation.

Syndromes are associated with the location of the hemorrhage, as they are in ICH (see preceding section for clinical syndromes associated with areas of hemorrhage).

Definite genetic transmission of the tendency to develop berry aneurysm has not been proven; however, a tendency for familial occurrence of aneurysms is apparent. Aneurysms are also more common among individuals with hereditary connective tissue disorders. Individuals with hemorrhage resulting from an aneurysm tend to be younger than those with hemorrhage secondary to hypertension. Aneurysms are associated with a sudden severe headache.

The hematoma caused by an aneurysm can be identified on CT scan and tends to be of a different character than that caused by hypertension. The location of hemorrhage is also a clue to the diagnosis of aneurysm. Primary sites for hematoma due to aneurysms are in the area of the corpus callosum and anterior horns, the frontal lobe, the cavum septum pellucidum, in the area of the frontal horn, or the temporal lobes. Angiography is required to establish that an intracerebral hematoma has been caused by a ruptured aneurysm.

If the resulting hematoma is less than 3 cm, the prognosis is good. Evacuation of hematomas that are larger should include resection of the causative aneurysm. Prompt removal may result in dramatic and early improvement of neurologic function. Repeat hemorrhage is more likely to occur if the hematoma is evacuated without treatment of the ruptured aneurysm (Stern and Agha Kahn, 1994).

Venous malformations are composed entirely of veins, which are usually thickened and hyalinized, with minimal elastic tissue or smooth muscle. The veins converge on a draining vein. Normal brain parenchyma is interspersed among the vessels. Venous malformation is the most common form of vascular malformation, constituting approximately 50% of malformations. The risk of hemorrhage from venous malformation has been estimated at 20% per year. Individuals with a cerebellar malformation have the greatest risk of hemorrhage. Occasionally, seizures may be associated with venous malformations. Headaches and focal neurologic deficits are manifested according to the area of the brain that is disrupted.

In enhanced CT, the venous malformation appears as a linear density, representing the deep draining vein. With significant hemorrhage, the hematoma can appear without use of contrast.

Spontaneous rupture of a venous malformation is not common, and the resulting bleed is often not of great consequence. Surgical resection of the hematoma may be necessary if it is significantly extensive. With evacuation of the hematoma, the malformation is left intact in most cases.

The *arteriovenous malformation* (AVM) is characterized by direct artery-to-vein communication without an intervening capillary bed. The blood vessel contains elastin and smooth muscle cells. Brain parenchyma is found within the AVM, and it is usually gliotic and nonfunctional. AVMs are the result of abnormal fetal development at approximately 3 weeks' gestation. Over 90% of AVMs occur in the cerebral hemispheres. Most AVMs are sporadic, but familial AVMs occur; these appear to have an autosomal dominant inheritance with incomplete penetrance.

The annual risk of bleeding from an AVM is 1% to 4%. AVMs result in a subarachnoid hemorrhage more than 50% of the time. Seizures, headache, or an audible bruit may precede a hemorrhage. Progressive focal neurologic deficits develop in some individuals, and cognitive decline may also precede a hemorrhage. AVM-associated hemorrhages occur predominantly in the third and fourth decades.

Malformations less than 3 cm in diameter are more likely to bleed than are larger AVMs, because arterial pressure is higher in the smaller vessels. A single draining vein, obstructed drainage, or a periventricular or intraventricular location increase the risk of hemorrhage.

Angiography is the definitive diagnostic procedure for an AVM. CT scanning is diagnostic for a dense lesion in the brain. Suspicion of an AVM arises when an area of decreased density is seen around the hematoma and heterogeneous densities appear within the hematoma. MRI is not useful in the diagnosis; however, it can be suspected based on MRI with evidence of intravascular moving blood. An AVM should be suspected as a cause of hemorrhage in persons younger than 40 years, especially if they are normotensive. Figures 28–8 and 28–9 represent the vascular disorder and its appearance on imaging.

Approximately 10% of individuals die from an AVM malformation hemorrhage. In the first year following the hemorrhage, the chance of recurrence is 6%. A concomitant aneurysm increases the chance of recurrent bleeding to 7%.

Neuroradiologic embolization, stereotactic radiotherapy, and surgery are the current treatments for AVM. These techniques are used alone or in combination, depending on the size and site of the lesion.

Cavernous malformations consist of dilated, endothelium-lined, fibrous channels. No smooth muscle or elastin is present in the vascular walls. Neural tissue is present only at the periphery of the lesion. Thrombosis and calcification within the malformation occur, and gliosis (scarring) often surrounds the malformation.

Cavernous malformations represent approximately 10% of vascular malformations. Multiple malformations can occur in the same person. It is believed that cavernous malformations are inherited through autosomal dominance, with close to 100% penetration. Hispanics are at particular risk for the familial disorder. No apparent relationship exists between malformation size and age and the likelihood of hemorrhage. Women tend to be more susceptible to hemorrhage than men. Subclinical bleeding frequently occurs around the malformation.

MRI is the imaging procedure of choice for visualizing cavernous malformations. The malformation appears as a well-defined region with a central area of mixed signal intensity surrounded by a rim of hypointensity.

The majority of individuals recover from a cavernous malformation hemorrhage, and the risk of repeat bleeding is low. Spontaneous rupture of a venous malformation is not

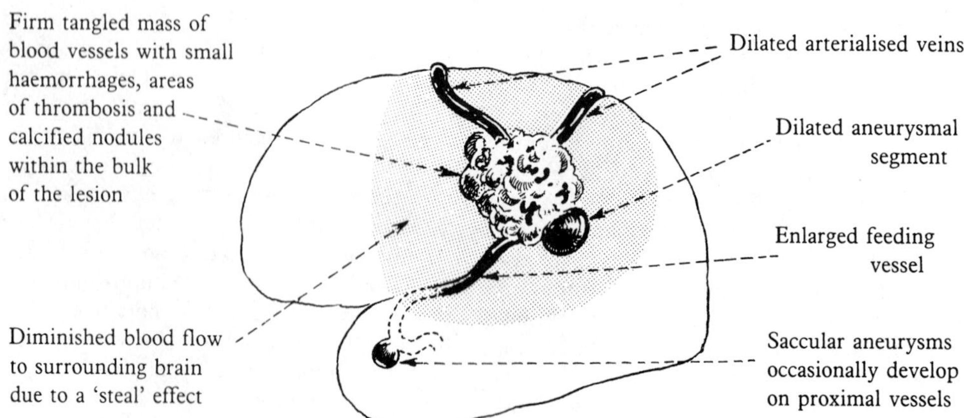

Figure **28–8.** Typical deformation of blood vessels and brain tissue in relationship to an arteriovenous malformation. (*From Lindsay KW, Bone I, Callander R: Neurology and Neurosurgery Illustrated. New York, Churchill Livingstone, 1986.*)

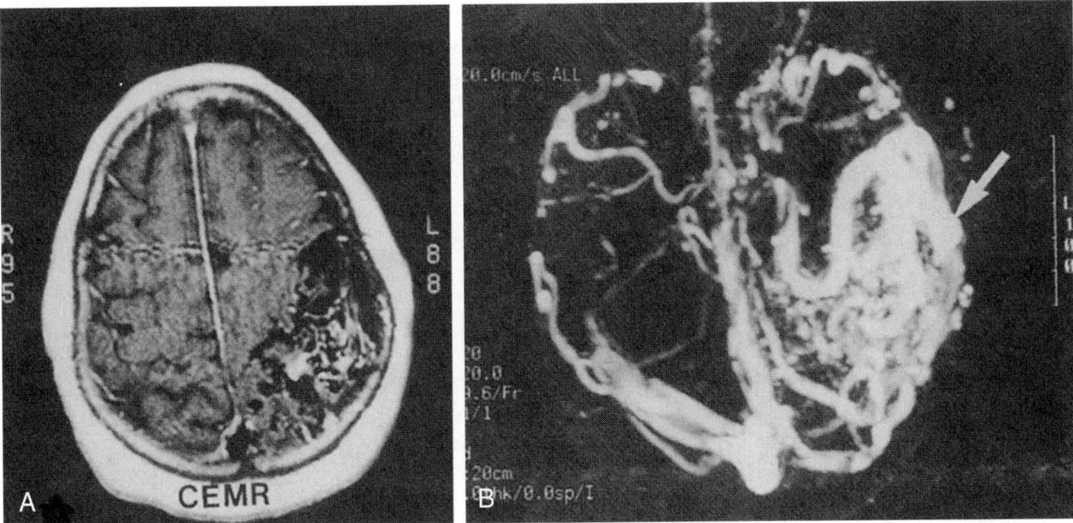

Figure **28–9.** The arteriovenous malformation as seen with (A) MRI and (B) magnetic resonance angiography. *Arrow* points to enlarged vessel in periphery of arteriovenous malformation. (*From Ramsey R: Neuroradiology. Philadelphia, WB Saunders, 1994.*)

common, and the resulting hemorrhage is often not of great consequence.

Surgery is the treatment of choice for malformations that have hemorrhaged and are in an accessible part of the brain. The majority of individuals recover from a cavernous malformation hemorrhage, and the risk of recurrence is low.

SUBDURAL HEMORRHAGE

A subdural hemorrhage is most often the result of tearing of the bridging veins between the brain surface and dural sinus. It results in accumulation of blood in the dural space. If it is a small amount, the body can reabsorb the fluid, if the blood is of great enough volume, as can occur with trauma, it becomes a space-occupying lesion. The lesion is reflected in the area of the hemorrhage and the result can be herniation of the cortex into the adjoining spaces. Compression of the brain tissue can result in both localized lesions and general decrease in the level of consciousness (see Chapter 24). Figure 28–10 represents the pressures on the brain that accompany a subdural hemorrhage.

VASCULAR DISORDERS OF THE SPINAL CORD

Vascular disorders of the spinal cord are rare, and vascular disorders of the brain and spinal cord have many common factors. Due to anatomic differences, some special issues must be considered in vascular disorders of the spinal cord. Infarctions in the spinal cord can be a result of any of the same causes as those in the brain; however, some of the symptoms appear to affect the lower motor neuron at the site of the anterior horn, and the result may be more flaccid extremities and muscle atrophy.

An AVM in the spine can cause pain and burning below the level of the lesion with progressive spastic paraparesis, with or without lower motor neuron lesion. Bowel and bladder dysfunction are seen when the AVM occurs in the lumbar region.

Transverse myelitis, the dysfunction of both halves of the spinal cord in transverse section can be related to vascular disorders. In addition to congenital vascular malformation, transverse myelitis can be caused by viral infection, multiple sclerosis, and degenerative disorders. Necrosis of the spinal cord often occurs at several levels, resulting in sensory and motor loss and pain. The lesion may involve nerve roots or just the central structures. The majority of individuals with transverse myelitis experience some degree of recovery.

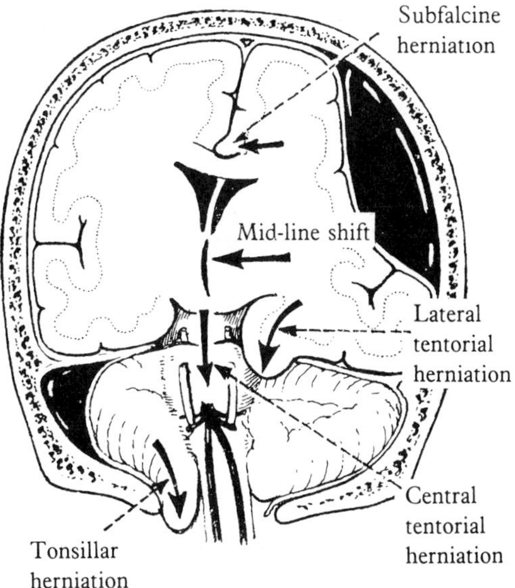

Figure **28–10.** Compression of brain tissue with herniation into adjacent structures produced by the subdural hemorrhage. (*From Lindsay KW, Bone I, Callander R: Neurology and Neurosurgery Illustrated. New York, Churchill Livingstone, 1986.*)

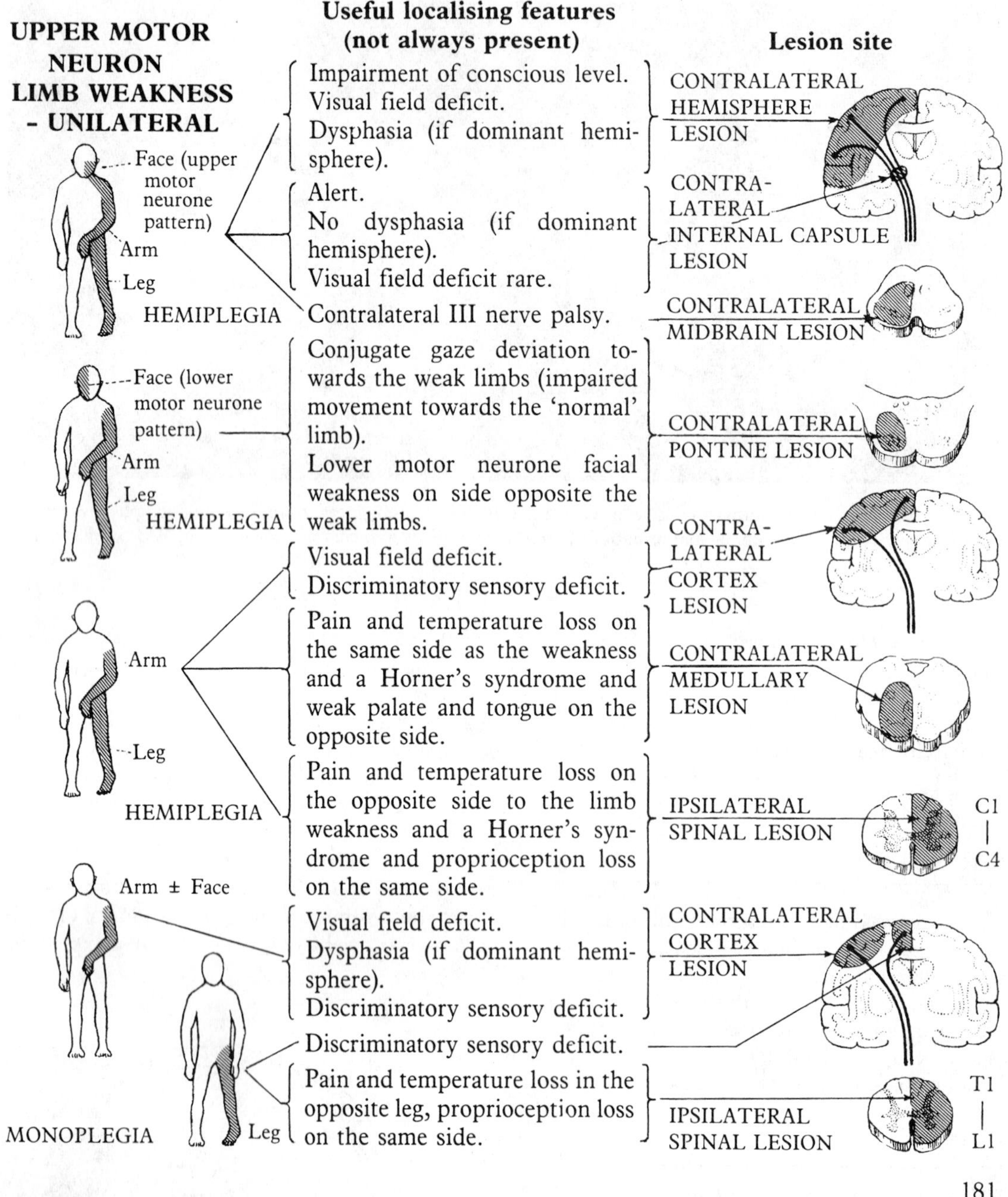

Figure **28-11.** Localizing features of damage to specific areas of the brain and spinal cord. (*From Lindsay KW, Bone I, Callander R: Neurology and Neurosurgery Illustrated. New York, Churchill Livingstone, 1986.*)

Special Implications for the Therapist **28-1**

STROKE REHABILITATION

Loss of sensation and motor control leading to restricted mobility are common after a stroke involving the cerebral hemispheres or the internal capsule. These movement problems may be caused by muscle weakness, abnormal synergistic organization of movement, altered temporal sequencing of muscle contractions, impaired regulation of force control, delayed responses, abnormal muscle tone, loss of range of motion, altered biomechanical alignment, and sensory impairments. Figure 28-11 represents areas of brain damage and associated clinical signs.

Evaluation of the impairments that can lead to an inability to perform functional activities and cause disability is critical. The treatment is then directed at remediation or facilitation to regain lost components, compensation for components that are unlikely to return, and use of motor control relearning (see Chapter 24) (Barton and Sullivan Black, 1993). Box 28-1 describes some of the considerations in treatment.

BOX **28–1**
Interventions Associated with Impairments Related to Stroke

Individuals with some voluntary control but who lack full voluntary control
- Use affected limb in functional tasks (this may include forced use)
- Increase strength
- Improve motor control
- Relearn sensorimotor relationships

Individuals with persistent lack of voluntary control in affected extremity
- Compensatory movements involving nonaffected side may be necessary

Spasticity and contractures
- Antispastic pattern positioning
- Range-of-motion exercise
- Stretching and splinting

Cognitive deficits
- Goal-directed treatment plans

Lack of endurance to exercise
- Cardiovascular training

Clinical Practice Guidelines for Post Stroke Rehabilitation, 1995, includes the following recommendations:

Individuals who have functional deficits and at least some voluntary control over movements of the involved arm or leg should be encouraged to use the limb in functional tasks and should be offered exercise and functional training that are directed at improving strength and motor control, relearning sensorimotor relationships, and improving functional performance.

Individuals with persistent, nonreducible functional deficits should be taught compensatory methods for performing tasks and activities, using the affected limb when possible.

Adaptive devices should be used only if other methods of performing the task are not available or cannot be learned. Their appropriate use should be assessed by a professional, and both stroke survivors and caretakers should be instructed in proper fit and use.

Spasticity and contractures should be treated or prevented by antispastic pattern positioning, range-of-motion exercise, stretching, and splinting. Maintaining soft tissue mobility in the distal extremities is a critical link to the performance of a motor activity.

Cognitive deficits that preclude effective learning are contraindications to rehabilitation. Cognitive and perceptual problems that are not severe enough to preclude rehabilitation require goal-directed treatment plans.

Cardiovascular endurance training is indicated for the stroke survivor; programs incorporating such activities are a part of rehabilitation programs. More research is needed to establish the parameters of cardiovascular training within the limits created by neurologic deficits.

Another important issue it that of sustaining the levels of function achieved during rehabilitation. Failure to maintain functional gains after the course of therapy is a concern for all individuals involved in the management of poststroke rehabilitation. Early and consistent involvement of the family or primary caretakers is paramount, as is the followthrough of a home management program of activity and exercise. The clinician and family should watch for the onset of angina, peripheral vascular disease, and deep vein thrombosis (Agency for Health Care Policy and Research, 1995).

The brain undergoes many natural changes in the months following damage, and it is believed that therapeutic interventions are most helpful in the first 6 to 18 months. Based on the theory of motor learning, the ability to learn a new motor program or a different way of moving does not follow a specific time frame following brain damage.

References

Agency for Health Care Policy and Research: Clinical Practice Guidelines, No. 16. Rockville, Md, US Department of Health and Human Services, 1995.

Baron JC: Positron emission tomography (PET) in acute ischemic stroke: Pathological and clinical implications. *In* Caplan, LR (ed): Brain Ischemia: Basic Concepts and Clinical Relevance. London, Springer-Verlag, 1995, pp 19–28.

Barton LA, Sullivan Black K: Learning treatment strategies applied to stroke rehabilitation. *In* Gordon WA (ed): Advances in Stroke Rehabilitation. Boston, Andover Medical Publishers, 1993, pp 63–78.

Brass LM: Clinical syndromes of intracerebral hemorrhage. *In* Feldman E (ed): Intracerebral Hemorrhage. Armonk, NY, Futura, 1994, pp 223–256.

Choi DW: Excitotoxicity and stroke. *In* Caplan LR (ed): Brain Ischemia: Basic Concepts and Clinical Relevance. London, Springer-Verlag, 1995, pp 29–36.

Duncan PW, Badke MB: Stroke Rehabilitation: The Recovery of Motor Control. Chicago, Year Book Medical Publishers, 1987.

Feinberg WM: Coagulation. *In* Caplan LR (ed): Brain Ischemia: Basic Concepts and Clinical Relevance. London, Springer-Verlag, 1995, pp 85–96.

Finklestein SP: Growth factors in stroke. *In* Caplan LR (ed): Brain Ischemia: Basic Concepts and Clinical Relevance. London, Springer-Verlag, 1995, pp 37–42.

Frank JI, Biller J: Laboratory evaluation of intracerebral hemorrhage. *In* Feldman E (ed): Intracerebral Hemorrhage. Armonk, NY, Futura, 1994, pp 257–290.

Furie K, Feldmann E: Cerebral amyloid angioplasty. *In* Feldman E (ed): Intracerebral Hemorrhage. Armonk, NY, Futura, 1994, pp 49–64.

Garcia JH: Mechanisms of cell death. *In* Caplan LR (ed): Basic Concepts and Clinical Relevance. London, Springer-Verlag, 1995, pp 7–18.

Gilroy J, Holliday PL: Strokes in Children: Basic Neurology. New York, Macmillan, 1982, pp 153–156.

Gorelick PB, Kelly MA: Ethanol. *In* Feldman E (ed): Intracerebral Hemorrhage. Armonk, NY, Futura, 1994, pp 195–208.

Harrison MJ: Neurological complications of hypertension. *In* Aminoff MJ (ed): Neurology and General Medicine, ed 2. New York, Churchill Livingstone, 1995, pp 119–136.

Hommel M, Gray F: Microvascular pathology. *In* Caplan LR (ed): Brain Ischemia: Basic Concepts and Clinical Relevance. London, Springer-Verlag, 1995, pp 215–222.

Kelly RE: Medical therapy, *In* Feldman E (ed): Intracerebral Hemorrhage. Armonk, NY, Futura, 1994, pp 291–302.

Kistler JP, Ropper AH, Martin JB: Cerebrovascular diseases. *In* Isselbacher KJ, Braunwald E, Wilson JD, et al (eds): Harrison's Principles of Internal Medicine, ed 13. New York, McGraw-Hill, 1994, pp 2233–2252.

Lindsay KW, Bone I, Callander R: Neurology and Neurosurgery Illustrated. New York, Churchill Livingstone, 1986.

Norrving B: Medical therapy to prevent stroke. *In* Feldman E (ed): Intracerebral Hemorrhage. Armonk, NY, Futura, 1994.

O'Brien MD: Ischemic cerebral edema. *In* Caplan LR (ed): Brain

Ischemia: Basic Concepts and Clinical Relevance. London, Springer-Verlag, 1995, pp 43–50.
O'Sullivan SB: Stroke. *In* O'Sullivan SB, Schmitz TJ (eds): Physical Rehabilitation: Assessment and Treatment, ed 3. Philadelphia, FA Davis, 1994, pp 327–360.
Pryse-Phillips WE, Murray TJ: Essential Neurology. New York, Medical Examination Publishing Company, 1992.
Ramsey R: Neuroradiology. Philadelphia, WB Saunders, 1994.
Sacco RL, Mayer SA: Epidemiology of intracerebral hemorrhage. *In* Feldman E (ed): Intracerebral Hemorrhage. Armonk, NY, Futura, 1994, pp 3–26.
Sloan MA: Thrombolysis and intracranial hemorrhage. *In* Feldman E (ed): Intracerebral Hemorrhage. Armonk, NY, Futura, 1994, pp 99–150.
Stern BJ, Agha Kahn: Vascular malformations and aneurysms. *In* Feldman E (ed): Intracerebral Hemorrhage. Armonk, NY, Futura, 1994, pp 169–194.
Tuhrim S: Medical therapy of ischemic stroke. *In* Gordon WA (ed): Advances in Stroke Rehabilitation. New York, Andover, 1993, pp 3–18.
Wahlgren NG: Cytoprotective therapy for acute ischemic stroke. *In* Fisher M (ed): Stroke Therapy. Boston, Butterworth-Heinemann, 1995, pp 315–350.
Wilterdink JL: Hypertensive intracerebral hemorrhage. *In* Feldman E (ed): Intracerebral Hemorrhage. Armonk, NY, Futura, 1994, pp 27–48.
Wilterdink JL, Feldmann E: Neuropathology and pathophysiology of intraparenchymal hemorrhage. *In* Gorelick PB (ed): Atlas of Cerebrovascular Disease. Philadelphia, Current Medicine, 1996.
Zoppo GL, Hamann RF, Fitrigde A, et al: Thrombolytic therapy. *In* Feldman E (ed): Intracerebral Hemorrhage. Armonk, NY, Futura, 1994, pp 291–314.

SECTION 4

chapter 29

Traumatic Brain Injury

Kenda S. Fuller

A closed head injury occurs when the soft tissue of the brain is forced into contact with the hard, bony, outer covering of the brain, the skull. Mild closed head injuries can occur after a severe neck injury without the head's actually striking any surface. The symptoms are worse when there is a rotational component to the head injury in addition to the back-and-forth movement. The long-term effects associated with closed head injury vary, depending on the severity of the injury. Differences in recovery are seen in persons who appear to have identical injuries.

A mild head injury occurs when there is no skull fracture or laceration of the brain. Actual loss of consciousness does not always occur, although there is an altered state of consciousness. The person with mild head injury usually has a normal neurologic examination. Often a postconcussive syndrome develops in the person with a mild head injury which can severely limit that person's ability to perform everyday activities (Evans, 1992).

Severe head injuries result from significant bruising and bleeding within the brain. The vast majority of persons with severe head injuries become permanently disabled, spend a significant amount of time in rehabilitation settings, and may be unable to return home (Bernard, 1994).

INCIDENCE AND RISK FACTORS

The National Head Injury Foundation reports the incidence of head injury to be 2 million persons per year. Of those, approximately 90,000 are left with lifelong disabilities that keep them from returning to their preinjury lifestyles.

Males sustain head injury at a rate twice that of females. The incidence of head injury peaks at three different age levels. The first peak occurs in early childhood (1 to 2 years), the second in late adolescence and early adulthood (15 to 24 years), and the third in the elderly (65 years and older).

Of the severely brain-injured, approximately 60% of adults and 92% of children were injured in a motor vehicle accident, either as operator or passenger, as pedestrians, or as bicyclists. The incidence increases with declining income and with rising population density, suggesting that those most at risk for brain trauma are low-income inner-city dwellers (Kraus, 1993).

Alcohol use and abuse is frequently associated with brain trauma. Fifty percent of persons admitted into hospitals with head trauma are intoxicated at the time. Brain injury may be two to four times higher in alcoholics than in the general population (Giles and Clark-Wilson, 1993).

One of the most widespread causes of injury among young people is bicycling. Wearing an appropriate helmet reduces the risk of severe head injury by 88%.[1]

ETIOLOGY

Brain injuries can be open or closed. With an open head injury the meninges have been breached, leaving the brain exposed. Penetrating missile injuries create localized, focal lesions that, when not fatal, cause limited damage to the brain. Figure 29–1 shows the damage from a gunshot wound.

Most non–combat-related head injuries are closed head injuries resulting from falls, assaults, and motor vehicle accidents. Although contusion, or bruising, is the hallmark of traumatic brain injury (TBI), severe or even fatal damage to the brain can occur without contusion (Povlishock and Christman, 1994; Povlishock and Valadka, 1994). With assaults or falls, it is typical to see more focal damage related to the area of primary contact.

Posttraumatic epilepsy (PTE) may emerge months or years following brain trauma and is more common after severe brain injury. Epilepsy occurring within 7 days is often related to severe injury, depressed fracture, or intracranial hemorrhage. Late epilepsy occurs most often as grand mal seizures or temporal lobe seizures (Giles and Clark-Wilson, 1993) (see Chapter 31).

PATHOGENESIS

Motor vehicle accidents often cause complex injury of a diffuse nature. Diffuse brain injury includes axonal injury, hypoxic damage, and diffuse brain swelling. Multiple small hemorrhages may occur and are predictive of a poor outcome.

Primary damage is the result of forces exerted on the brain at the time of injury. Secondary damage refers to changes compromising brain function that result from the brain's reaction to trauma or other system failure. Causes of secondary damage include brain swelling and impaired cerebral perfusion.

Vascular Changes

Focal brain injuries usually result in cerebral contusions. Typically, contusions occur at the poles and on the inferior surfaces of the frontal and temporal lobes. Contusions are usually more severe in persons with skull fracture than in those

[1] Helmets that are certified by the American National Standards Institute provide the greatest protection to the head. Important in the safety issue is proper fit and wearing of the helmet.

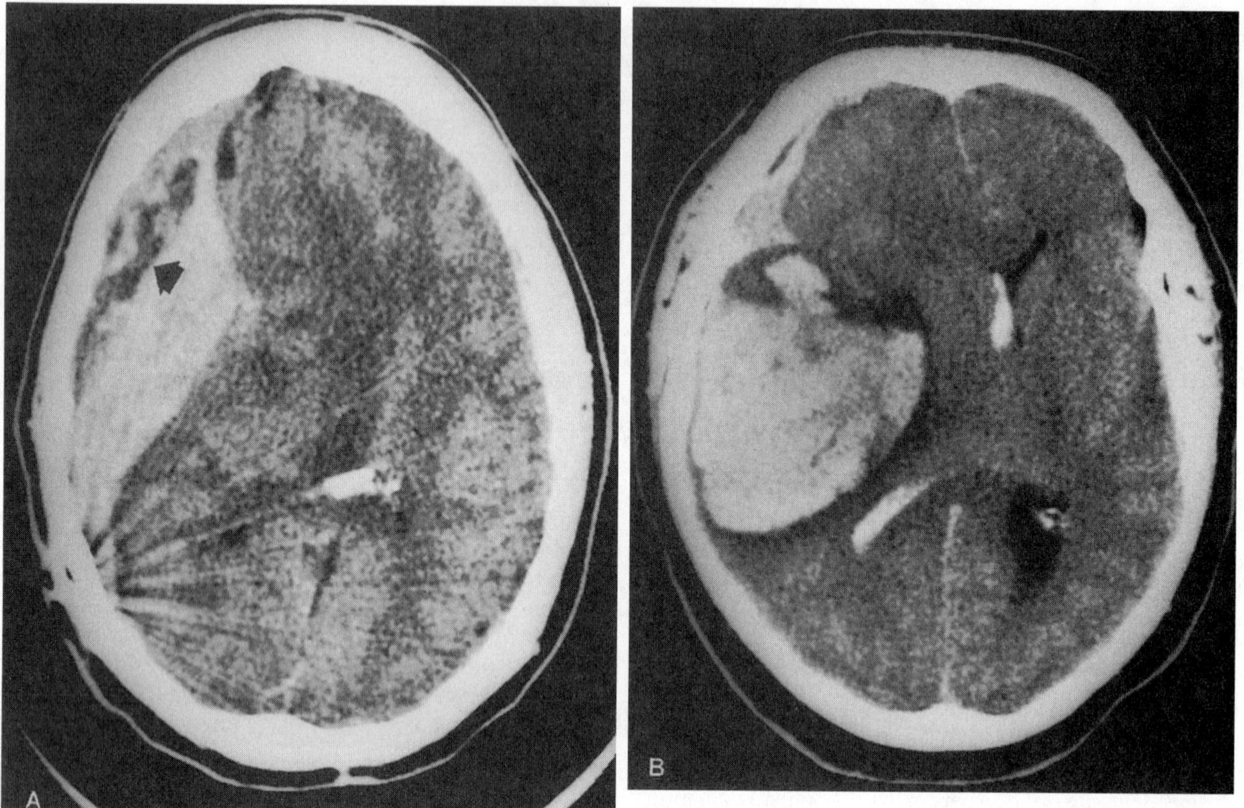

Figure 29–1. Gunshot wound resulting in both intracerebral and epidural hemorrhage. *A*, The bullet is shown on CT scan resting in a midline position with streaking effect of fragments also seen. *Arrow* points to area of decreased density thought to be epidural bleeding. *B*, Large intracerebral hemorrhage is noted with blood present in the ventricle. (*From Ramsey R: Neuroradiology. Philadelphia, WB Saunders, 1994, p 407.*)

without fracture. With fracture of the cranial vault, there may be damage to the superficial epidural vessels and, particularly in the case of falls, rupture of the bridging vessels between hemispheres can occur.

Typically, contusion manifests itself as a wedge-shaped lesion with its apex directed away from the cortical surface. Vascular damage is sustained at the moment of impact and leads to infarction within the cortical gray matter. Glial elements encapsulate the infarction, ultimately creating a residual cystic cavity (Grady and Shapiro, 1995; Domino, 1995).

TBI can be associated with other forms of vascular change. A *gliding contusion*, or hemorrhagic lesions in the parasagittal cortex, may be the result of movement of the cortical gray matter in relation to the underlying white matter, causing shear strains to damage the penetrating vessels found at the gray and white matter interface. Figure 29–2 shows the effects of shearing injury as seen on computed tomography (CT) scan. There can be bleeding into the epidural compartment, creating a mass effect that can displace the brain and increase intracranial pressure (ICP). Figure 29–3 demonstrates the mass effect seen with an epidural lesion, resulting from TBI. The shear and tensile forces of traumatic injury can also create a subdural hematoma by disruption of the bridging veins. Subarachnoid hemorrhage is common due to the rupture of pial vessels within the subarachnoid space. This may trigger vasospasm that can lead to reduced regional blood flow. Injury to the vessels within the white matter can also cause significant neurologic consequences, especially if it is in the area of the basal ganglia.

The impairment of autoregulation of circulation has been described in the presence of moderate to severe head injury. This allows blood flow to the brain to become dependent upon the systemic arterial pressure. Elevated blood pressure can result in hyperemia, with decreased blood pressure causing hypoperfusion. Impaired vascular responsiveness of blood gas changes in head injury results in abnormal arteriolar vasoconstriction in the presence of carbon dioxide.

The overall result of these vascular changes is the decreased ability of the cerebral vessels to maintain necessary homeostasis in the face of changing blood pressure or blood gas composition. Initially, within the first few hours after severe injury, there is decreased cerebral blood flow, both globally and at the impact site, which can induce ischemia. Within 24 hours the blood flow can be at normal or above-normal levels.

There appears to be a change in the endothelium, or walls, of the blood vessels following brain injury. In the normal brain, neurotransmitters such as acetylcholine induce dilation of the vessels through the release of endothelium-derived releasing factor (EDRF), causing relaxation of the smooth muscle in the vessel wall. In the injured brain, this reaction can be missing, resulting in abnormal vasoconstriction.

Additional changes at the level of the endothelium result in disturbed blood-brain barrier in the injured brain. This

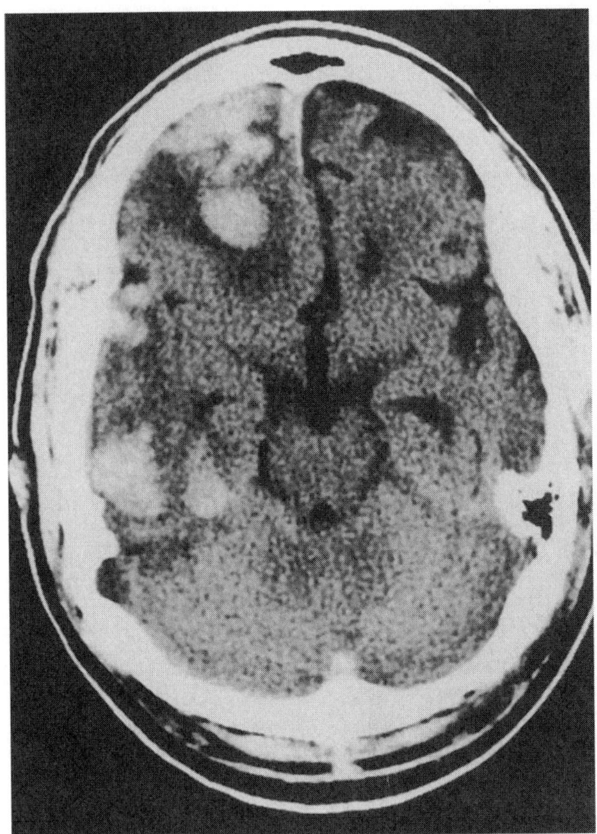

Figure **29–2.** Contusion with shearing injury. CT scan shows multiple rounded areas of blood density with surrounding edema. Many of these areas are at gray–white matter junction consistent with shear injury. (*From Ramsey R: Neuroradiology. Philadelphia, WB Saunders, 1994, p 409.*)

results in leakage of serum proteins and neurotransmitters into the parenchyma, causing edema. The effects of edema in the brain are described in Chapter 24.

Parenchymal Changes

Axonal injury is a consistent feature of the traumatic event. Shear and tensile forces most likely disrupt the axolemma, which impairs transport of proteins from the cell body and causes swelling of the axon (Povlishock and Christman, 1994; Povlishock and Valadka, 1994). The distal axon segment detaches and undergoes *wallerian degeneration*.[2] Reactive axonal swellings (retraction balls), which are full of materials from the axons that are sealed off, develop and can be detected in the injured brain within 12 hours of injury. The myelin sheath pulls away from the axon. The axonal changes are seen throughout the brain regardless of site of impact. The damage is different from that of stroke or tumor, which produces a more complete but local deafferentation.

Typically, with diffuse axonal injury, there remain intact axons interspersed with the damaged axons. Evidence is pointing to the potential for recovery of function based on the possible sprouting of undamaged axons to reoccupy the areas left vacant by degenerating axons.

Study of excitotoxicity related to diffuse brain injury shows that the increase in extracellular neurotransmitters, resulting in increased potassium, causes a massive depolarization of the injured brain. There is a complex interaction of the various amino acids and neurotransmitters which may affect the postsynaptic functions, resulting in secondary dysfunction of the neural mechanisms of the brain. The excitatory neurotransmitter, glutamate, appears to rise to abnormal amounts following brain injury. Glutamate is neurotoxic when concentrations increase. Study of the multiple transmitter systems that are released at the time of injury may reveal further interventions available which may have potential for reducing the amount of neuron damage following brain injury.

During trauma, the brain may shift from its normal symmetrical position, This shift may cause compression of the brainstem, the pituitary, or other delicate brain structures. Since the brainstem controls the body's major visceral functions, brainstem involvement may result in paralysis or death. Because the brain is surrounded by the rigid skull, swelling of the brain pushes tissue through openings in the base of the skull or through the other compartments of the brain a (herniation) (Bernard, 1994). Figure 28–11 (see Chapter 28) demonstrates how compression of the brain tissue leads to herniation.

CLINICAL MANIFESTATIONS

Signs and Symptoms

Levels of Consciousness *(Leahy, 1994; Winkler, 1995)*

Altered level of consciousness is a state that can occur with both diffuse and focal head injuries. Conscious behavior is determined by content and arousal. Content is the sum of cognitive and affective function. Arousal is associated with wakefulness and depends on an intact reticular formation and upper brainstem. Cognition and arousal can be individually impaired or there can be a combination of injury to many degrees.

Coma is regarded as the lowest level of consciousness, and is described as not obeying commands, not uttering words, and not opening the eyes, or a state of unresponsiveness. This indicates advanced brain failure, with bilateral cerebral hemispheric or direct involvement of the brainstem. Coma rarely lasts more than 4 weeks, but some individuals may continue to exhibit a reduced level of consciousness, a condition referred to as *persistent vegetative state*, or postcomatose unawareness. This includes eye opening with sleep-wake cycles, and tracking of the eyes, controlled at a subcortical level. There is no purposeful movement and the individual remains mute.

Other states of consciousness common to closed head injury are *obtundity*, or the slow response to stimulus with disinterest in the environment. *Delirium* is often seen after injury and is characterized by disorientation, fear, and misinterpretation of sensory stimuli.

The Glasgow Coma Scale (GCS) (Table 29–1) is used to assess level of consciousness. Using this scale, three aspects of coma are observed independently: eye opening, best motor response, and verbal response. A score of 8 or less indicates coma.

[2] When there is damage to the axon, each end is sealed off and begins to retract. Wallerian degeneration denotes the distal segment degeneration that results from the loss of axonal transport of proteins to maintain viability.

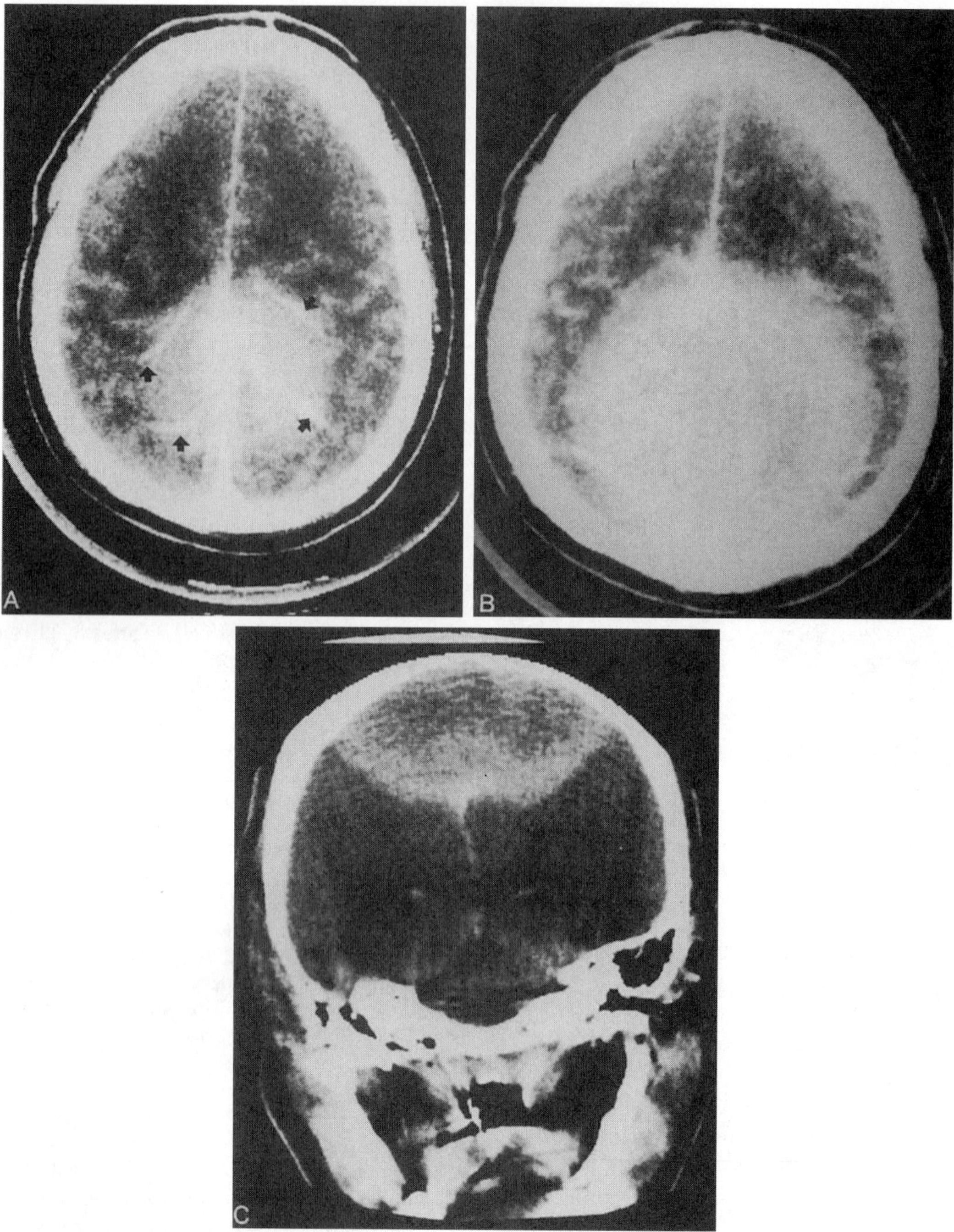

Figure **29–3.** Epidural hemorrhage resulting from a tear in the superior sagittal sinus. A and B, Mass effect of the blood in a rounded configuration. C, Coronal view shows the collection of blood separated by the meninges from the brain tissue. Compression of the brain results in inferior depression of the lateral ventricles. (*From Ramsey R: Neuroradiology. Philadelphia, WB Saunders, 1994, p 406.*)

Cognitive and Behavioral Impairments (*Leahy, 1994; Winkler, 1995*)

Residual cognitive and behavioral deficits most often remain, despite a return to full consciousness. Deficits, including disorders of learning, memory, and complex information processing and loss of abstract thinking and complex problem solving, reflect the frontal lobe pathology associated with TBI. There is often confusion and disorientation, difficulty in problem solving, delayed processing, motor and verbal disinhibition, and lack of initiation. Cognitive deficits are not always directly observable, but the observable behavior gives information regarding ability to integrate cognitive processes. The observable behavior of a brain-injured person is directly related to the integrity of cognitive function. The behaviors often seen—combativeness, agitation, and poor social behaviors—reflect inability to adjust to the environment. Typical behaviors include erratic wandering; motor, sensory, and verbal perseveration; imitation of gestures; restlessness; refusal

TABLE 29–1 Glasgow Coma Scale

Eye Opening	
Spontaneous	E 4
To speech	3
To pain	2
Nil	1
Best Motor Response	
Obeys	M 6
Localizes	5
Withdraws	4
Abnormal flexion	3
Extensor response	2
Nil	1
Verbal Response	
Oriented	V 5
Confused conversation	4
Inappropriate words	3
Incomprehensible sounds	2
Nil	1
Coma score (E + M + V) = 3 to 15	

From Jennett B, Teasdale G: Management of Head Injuries. Philadelphia, FA Davis, 1981, p 78.

BOX 29–1
Cognitive Characteristics and Behavioral Disturbances Associated with Frontal Lobe System Pathology

Cognitive Characteristics
Loss of verbal fluency
Loss of nonverbal or visual design fluency
Decreased modulation of attention; specificity of attention
Increased distractibility and pull toward interfering stimuli
Slowed speed of cognitive processing
Decreased ability to monitor and self-correct performance
General intellectual functions may be within expectations
Mental inflexibility and inability to shift cognitive set (the way a person thinks)
Poor abstract reasoning and complex problem-solving
Inability to apply novel strategies in problem-solving
Loss of concrete thinking

Behavioral Disturbances
Disordered planning and anticipation of events
Disinhibited social behaviors
Psychomotor agitation
Sexual inappropriateness
Euphoria and inappropriate jocularity
Irritability, emotional lability, depression
Abulia, apathy, indifference, flat affect
Paucity of spontaneous movement and gesture
Motor, sensory, verbal perseveration
Dysprosody
Confabulation
Reduplicative paramnesia
Capgras' syndrome
Echopraxis or imitation of gestures
Anosognosia or explicit denial of illness or deficit
Anosodiaphoria or lack of genuine concern about a deficit

Modified from Vomoto JM: Neuropsychological assessment and rehabilitation after brain injury. *In* Berrol S (ed): Physical Medicine and Rehabilitation Clinics of North America. Traumatic Brain Injury. Philadelphia, WB Saunders, 1992, p 303.

to cooperate; and striking out in response to stimulus or in random fashion. Often the individual will attempt to run away from the institution or home. Behavioral changes can be present without cognitive or physical deficits (Sullivan, 1995). Box 29–1 describes some of the typical cognitive characteristics and the resulting behavioral disturbances seen in persons after TBI.

A useful tool to assess behaviors as a function of cognitive recovery is the Rancho Los Amigos Scale (Table 29–2). Table 29–3 lists some of the behavioral disturbances and their manifestations in persons with TBI.

Impairment of memory is common with head injury. *Retrograde amnesia* is the partial or total loss of ability to recall events that have occurred during the period immediately preceding head injury. *Posttraumatic amnesia* is the time lapse between the injury and the point at which functional memory returns. During this time there may be improvement in automatic activities, but there is no carryover of tasks requiring memory or learning. *Anterograde memory* is the ability to form new memory. Loss of anterograde memory is common and manifests as decreased attention or inaccurate perception.

Brainstem Damage

Injury to the brainstem is common in head injury. The area of damage is reflected in the loss of cranial nerve function. The following are signs of specific cranial nerve deficits (Gelber, 1995; Rovit and Murali, 1993).

First Cranial Nerve (Olfactory Nerve). Damage to the olfactory nerve results in anosmia, or the loss of smell. The olfactory nerve is well protected in the cribriform plate, but shearing of the fibers to the extent of damage occurs in about 7% of head injuries. In about 50% of the cases, this is a temporary condition.

Second Cranial Nerve (Optic Nerve). The optic nerve is not a true cranial nerve but rather a direct extension of the brain. The most vulnerable component of the optic nerve in persons with head injury is the portion of the nerve located within the optic canal, damage to which can result in monocular blindness, a dilated pupil with an absent direct pupillary response, and a brisk consensual response to light. Partial visual defects may take the form of scotomata, sector defects, and upper or lower hemianopia.

Third Cranial Nerve (Oculomotor Nerve). This nerve is damaged in less than 3% of persons with head injury. The oculomotor nerve works in conjunction with the trochlear and abducens nerves to move the eyeball in the orbit to maintain gaze stability and scanning. Damage is often due to direct insult to the musculature, but it can also be due to cerebral herniation. Signs of third nerve damage include *strabismus* (squinting), *diplopia* (double vision), and *ptosis* (drop-

TABLE 29-2 RANCHO LOS AMIGOS SCALE FOR LEVELS OF COGNITIVE FUNCTIONING

LEVEL	BEHAVIORS TYPICALLY DEMONSTRATED
I.	No response: Client appears to be in a deep sleep and is completely unresponsive to any stimuli.
II.	Generalized response: Client reacts inconsistently and nonpurposefully to stimuli in a nonspecific manner. Responses are limited and are often the same regardless of stimulus presented. Responses may be physiologic changes, gross body movements, or vocalization.
III.	Localized response: Client reacts specifically but inconsistently to stimuli. Responses are directly related to the type of stimulus presented. May follow simple commands in an inconsistent, delayed manner, such as closing eyes or squeezing hand.
IV.	Confused-agitated: Client is in heightened state of activity. Behavior is bizarre and nonpurposeful relative to immediate environment. Does not discriminate among persons or objects; is unable to cooperate directly with treatment efforts. Verbalizations frequently are incoherent or inappropriate to the environment; confabulation may be present. Gross attention to environment is very brief; selective attention is often nonexistent. Client lacks short-term and long-term recall.
V.	Confused-inappropriate: Client is able to respond to simple commands fairly consistently. However, with increased complexity of commands or lack of any external structure, responses are nonpurposeful, random, or fragmented. Demonstrates gross attention to the environment, but is highly distractible and lacks ability to focus attention on a specific task. With structure, may be able to converse on a social-automatic level for short periods of time. Verbalization is often inappropriate and confabulatory. Memory is severely impaired, often shows inappropriate use of objects; may perform previously learned tasks with structure but is unable to learn new information.
VI.	Confused-appropriate: Client shows goal-directed behavior but is dependent on external input for direction. Follows simple directions consistently and shows carryover for relearned tasks with little or no carryover for new tasks. Responses may be incorrect due to memory problems but appropriate to the situation; past memories show more depth and detail than recent memory.
VII.	Automatic-appropriate: Client appears appropriate and oriented within hospital and home settings; goes through daily routine automatically, but frequently robot-like with minimal-to-absent confusion; has shallow recall of activities. Shows carryover for new learning, but at a decreased rate. With structure is able to initiate social or recreational activities; judgment remains impaired.
VIII.	Purposeful-appropriate: Client is able to recall and integrate past and recent events and is aware of and responsive to environment. Shows carryover for new learning and needs no supervision once activities are learned. May continue to show a decreased ability relative to premorbid abilities, abstract reasoning, tolerance for stress, and judgment in emergencies or unusual circumstances.

From Malkmus D: Integrating cognitive strategies into the physical therapy setting. Phys Ther 63:1958, 1983. Modified from Hagen C, Malkmus D, Durham P: Levels of cognitive functioning. *In* Rehabilitation of the Head Injured Adult: Comprehensive Physical Management. Downey, Calif., Professional Staff Association of Rancho Los Amigos Hospital, 1979, pp 87–88.

ping of the upper eyelid). A dilated pupil and loss of light and accommodation reflexes reflect third nerve palsy. In some cases there is development of misdirection of regeneration resulting in constriction of the pupil when any one of the extraocular muscles supplied by the third nerve is activated. Also, owing to misdirection of the growing axons, the levator muscle of the lid may receive fibers destined for other muscles. When the person affected attempts to look down, instead of the globe moving down, the lid becomes elevated.

Fourth Cranial Nerve (Trochlear Nerve). The fourth cranial nerve is the least frequently injured oculomotor nerve. Damage is usually in the form of contusion or stretching. With severe frontal blows, there can be direct damage to the fourth nerve or hemorrhage of the tentorial incisura. There can be a vertical diplopia mimicking a third nerve palsy. The prognosis for recovery in fourth nerve palsy is poor because the nerve is so slender that it is often avulsed by the trauma.

Fifth Cranial Nerve (Trigeminal Nerve). The most common form of trigeminal nerve injury after head trauma involves the supraorbital and supratrochlear nerves as they emerge from the orbit. Damage results in anesthesia of a portion of the nose, eyebrow, and forehead. Facial trauma may include damage to the fifth nerve, extending the sensory deficits to the cheek, upper lip, gums, teeth, and hard palate. In deep coma the eyelids can be opened easily, and the corneal reflex (indicating fifth nerve palsy) is often absent.

Sixth Cranial Nerve (Abducens Nerve). The abducens nerve is often injured when the head is crushed in an anteroposterior plane with resultant lateral expansion and distortion of the skull. It can also be damaged in fractures of the petrous bone. Vertical movement of the brainstem may severely stretch the sixth nerve as it leaves the pons. There can also be damage in relation to the third and fourth nerves in the orbital fissure. There is failure of the eye to wander outward or abduct when the head is passively turned away from the side of the lesion. Abnormal wandering movements are present in midbrain lesions, and they usually disappear when the person regains consciousness.

Seventh Cranial Nerve (Facial Nerve). Trauma to the facial nerve is common in head injury. With injury to the temporal bone, swelling of the nerve, external compression caused by hematoma symptoms of facial nerve palsy, may occur. Loss of tear production, saliva secretion, and taste in the anterior two thirds of the tongue and loss of stapedius muscle function may be noted.

TABLE 29-3 A TYPOLOGY OF BEHAVIORAL DISTURBANCES AFTER TRAUMATIC BRAIN INJURY

SYMPTOM	DESCRIPTION
Behavioral Excesses	
Inappropriate abrupt physical action	Responds to a situation too quickly without thinking about the adequacy or consequences of the behavior: "doing before thinking." Does not include verbal interruptions.
Tangential verbal output	Expresses one thought after another in disconnected or unrelated sequences: "rambling speech," unable to "get to the point."
Excessive verbal output	Provides too much information; content may be overly detailed or redundant; may be unaware of conversational turn exchange signals or unable to terminate conversation.
Verbal interruptions	Inserts comments that disrupt the flow of conversation or the task at hand; may force other person to relinquish conversational turn before completing the thought.
Inappropriate topic selection	Poor discrimination of appropriate topics for the social context. Revealing statements about personal matters, relationships, feelings that are inappropriate for the social context or level of relationship: "excessive self-disclosure."
Inappropriate word choice	Use of profanity or emotionally charged words that are inappropriate for the social context. Overly explicit descriptions and explanations.
Physical proximity violation	Positions body within a spatial proximity of another person that is inappropriate for the level of relationship or social context: "violating personal space."
Sexual inappropriateness	Acts with intent to develop intimate or sexual contacts or relationships inappropriate for the level of relationship or in violation of social mores (e.g., with adolescent minors); conversation contains sexual innuendos or lewd comments. May misinterpret others' expression of friendship as sexual advances, and responds as above.
Poor social judgment	Unaware of or does not apply rules governing social behavior; does not consider personal safety or safety of others in social context: "rude," "immature," "coarse," "tactless." Violates rules of etiquette.
Irritability	Feelings of annoyance or impatience; may accompany restlessness; easily provoked but generally does not escalate into an anger outburst. Tends to be a constant state, usually neither improving nor worsening by a significant degree.
Lability of affect	Magnitude of affect displayed is disproportionate to the antecedent event or social context and does not necessarily reflect the true nature or extent of feelings.
Anxious affect and rumination	Feelings of worry, tenseness, fearfulness, uncertainty about the future. Complains or verbalizes concern over trivia.
Angry transition—verbal	An escalation of verbal output, where pitch, volume, or speaking rate increases, dysfluency occurs, aggressive content is delivered. Still within the realm of appropriate. A building-up phase before an outburst.
Angry transition—behavioral	Facial flush; posture threatening; personal space may be violated, body positions exaggerated; agitation behavior is evident such as hair pulling, wringing of hands, clutching the fist.
Anger outburst—verbal	Explosive speech, screaming, abusive language, forceful or harmful content, self-deprecating content, or threats toward another person.
Anger outburst—behavioral	Hitting objects, striking out, exaggerated motions, forceful actions.
Behavioral Deficits	
Absence of or decrease in self-directed action	Decrease in spontaneous behaviors, requires prompts for behavioral action.
Depressed mood	Downcast facial expression, tearfulness, verbalizations of sadness, hopelessness, helplessness, low self-esteem; paucity of interest in pleasant events.
Restricted affect	Display of affect less than proportional to the event; face expressionless; voice monotonous; movement fails to reflect stated feelings.

Modified from Vomoto JM: Neuropsychological assessment and rehabilitation after brain injury. In Berrol S (ed): Physical Medicine and Rehabilitation Clinics of North America. Traumatic Brain Injury. Philadelphia, WB Saunders, 1992, p 307.

Eighth Cranial Nerve (Vestibular Nerve). Hearing and vestibular dysfunction occur in head injuries. Transverse fractures of the temporal bone may cause disruption of the auditory and vestibular end organs or transient eighth nerve dysfunction. A blow to the head creates a pressure wave that is transmitted through the petrous bone to the cochlea, resulting in hair cell damage and degeneration of cochlear nerves. For further information on dizziness and vertigo, see Chapter 33.

The Ninth (Glossopharyngeal), Tenth (Vagus), Eleventh (Spinal Accessory), and Twelfth (Hypoglossal) Cranial Nerves. The ninth, tenth, and eleventh cranial nerves pass through the jugular foramen at the base of the skull. The twelfth nerve passes through the hypoglossal foramen nearby. Injury is most often from a missile wound, but fractures of the occipital condyle can also produce lower cranial nerve palsies. Symptoms include cardiac irregularities, excessive salivation, loss of sensation and gag reflex of the palate, loss of taste on the posterior third of the tongue, hoarse voice, dysphagia, and deviation of the tongue to the side of the lesion.

Motor Deficits

Abnormalities of movement include monoplegia, hemiplegia, and abnormal reflexes. Often there is *flaccidity*, absence of motor responses, at the onset, which is gradually replaced by increased tone, spasticity, and rigidity. *Decorticate posturing*, hyperactive flexor reflexes in the upper extremities and hyperactive extensor response in the lower extremities, is common initially and reflects the loss of cortical control. *Decerebrate posturing*, hyperactive extensor reflexes in both the upper and lower extremities, reflects injury at the superior border of the pons resulting in the loss of inhibitory control of the cortex and basal ganglia.

The specific manifestations of hemiparesis may include loss of selective motor control, abnormal balance reactions, and sensory loss. Cerebellar and basal ganglia dysfunction can result in ataxia, dysmetria, and tremor or bradykinesia.[3]

Heterotopic Ossification

Another complication associated with head injury is the formation of *heterotopic ossification* (HO), abnormal bone growth around a joint. The cause and pathogenesis of HO is unknown, but the bone scan shows evidence of increased uptake and there is also elevation of alkaline phosphatase.

The onset of HO is usually 4 to 12 weeks after the head injury, and it is first represented as loss of range of motion. Local tenderness and a palpable mass can be detected, and there can be erythema, swelling, and pain with movement. HO in the hip area can mimic deep vein thrombosis. Peripheral nerve compression will sometimes develop, especially if the HO is in the elbow. HO can also result in vascular compression and possible lymphedema (Varghese, 1992).

MEDICAL MANAGEMENT

Diagnosis

In general, persons who have lost consciousness for 2 minutes or more following head injury should be observed medically. Symptoms of focal neurologic deficits, lethargy, or skull fractures should likewise be monitored. A mental status examination is important in all head-injured persons. Subtle abnormalities may be a guide to significant intracranial injury.

Pupillary examination should document size and reactivity to light. Greater than 1 mm difference in size or asymmetry should be considered abnormal. Once the baseline neurologic status has been determined, repeated evaluations are critical to monitor improvement, provide prognostic data, or detect deterioration, which should be addressed immediately.

Diagnostic imaging can provide significant information, which can guide the intervention and allow a more accurate prognosis to be made.

CT is the primary imaging modality for the initial diagnosis and management of the head-injured person. CT scanning of the head reveals the presence of hemorrhage, swelling, or infarction. An initially normal CT scan, however, is no assurance that hemorrhagic lesions will not occur.

Magnetic resonance imaging (MRI) is complementary to CT and is used in conjunction with, not as a replacement for, CT. The multiplanar capabilities of MRI are important to better demonstrate extra-axial hemorrhage located subfrontally, subtemporally, or along the tentorium. Lesions in the posterior fossa, as well as shear injury, are better demonstrated on MRI than on CT. MRI can also detect small hemorrhages in the corpus callosum, intraventricular hemorrhages, or effacement of basal cisternal structures in the absence of brain shift or mass lesions. This can lead to the diagnosis of increasing ICP, a significant risk in brain injury.

MRI offers a sensitive window of detection for neuropathology from mild TBI. Anatomic distribution of tissue damage and precise indications of the volume of lesions seen on MRI can predict recovery of the brain in the subacute phase. Positron emission tomography (PET) can be used to identify both structural and functional consequences and is especially valuable for mild head injury (Hughes and Cohen, 1993).

Neuropsychological evaluation is valuable in identifying the extent of the cognitive deficits. The evaluation consists of a series of cognitive challenges given to the individual, including assessment of sensorimotor status, attention span, memory, language, sequencing, problem solving, and verbal and spatial integration tasks. Comparisons of normal and brain-injured persons have been well documented, and this remains a good tool to describe deficits, especially for the mildly brain-injured.

Treatment *(Giles and Clark-Wilson, 1993; Grady and Lam, 1995)*

Treatment of TBI requires coordinated care and service from the onset of injury through the person's lifetime. Figure 29–4 represents the levels of care that are utilized in the course of treatment. Note that primary prevention is the first step, and it is only when prevention is not provided that the client must begin the acute medical phase.

Prehospital management of the severely head-injured person includes rapid triage, resuscitation, and efficient transport. Survival and medical management with the goal of stabilization and prevention of secondary complications is the primary medical focus. Hypoxia is a frequent secondary insult; often the upper airway is obstructed and clearing the airway is the first treatment administered. Intubation and ventilation are critical, with positive pressure breathing techniques supplemented by 100% oxygen an early intervention.

Emergency room treatment includes determination of head injury severity, identification of persons at risk of deterioration, and control of hypoxia and hypotension. Prevention of secondary brain damage caused by edema, increased ICP, or bleeding should be addressed. Treatment of the medical complications of the trauma are paramount but will not be discussed here; the focus here is on the control and treatment of neurologic sequelae. Close clinical observation remains the best tool for neurologic monitoring in the early stages of head injury.

Surgical intervention is critical in the presence of hemorrhage to prevent neurologic compromise and can improve both short- and long-term outcomes. Uncal, transtentorial, or ton-

[3] The cerebellum and basal ganglia control the coordination of movement, and diffuse or local damage can cause loss of control of movement in the absence of weakness or tone changes. See Chapter 24 for more information on cerebellar dysfunction. For more information on the manifestations of hemiplegia, see Chapter 28.

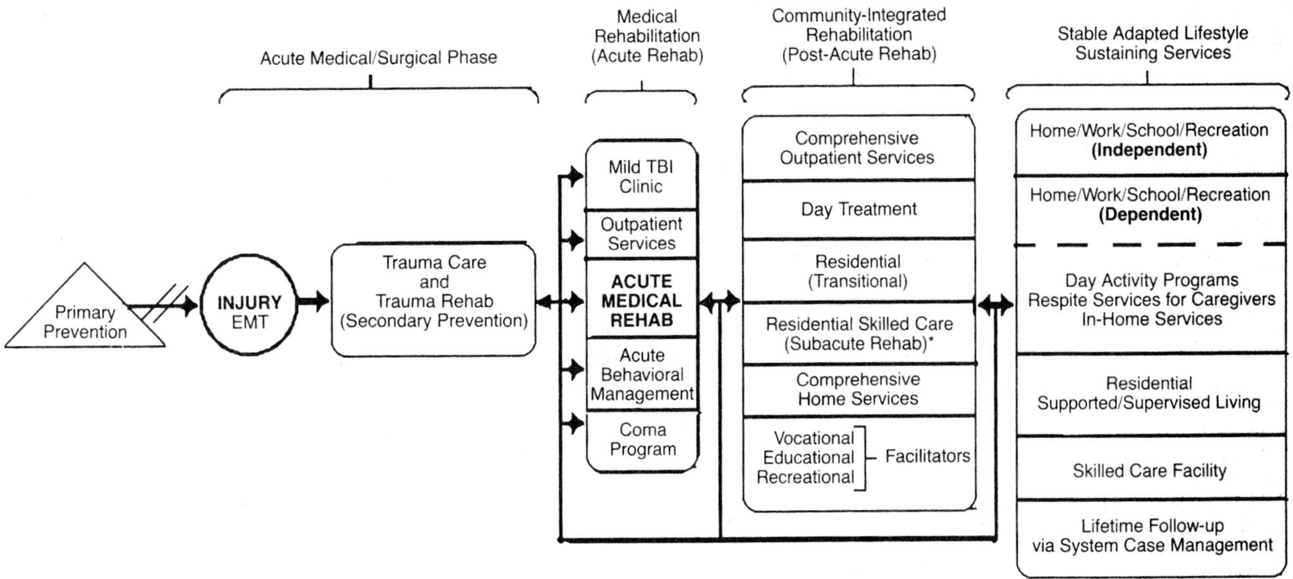

Figure 29–4. System of care for the person with traumatic brain injury, showing the components that should be considered in each phase. (*From Horn LJ: Systems of care for the person with traumatic brain injury. In Berrol S (ed): Physical Medicine and Rehabilitation Clinics of North America. Traumatic Brain Injury. Philadelphia, WB Saunders, 1992, p 479.*)

sillar herniations can occur with hematomas. In some cases, the individual may be lucid after the injury and then, in the presence of undetected hematoma, lapse into coma and die.

Injury to the dural sinus can occur with a depressed fracture over a major sinus and requires evacuation. Decompression of the skull, often using bur holes, is warranted in the presence of significant cerebral edema or subdural hematoma.

Persons with a Glasgow Coma Scale score of less than 8, or persons whose neurologic status cannot be assessed because of administration of sedative drugs or neuromuscular blocking agents, should be monitored for ICP. Monitoring of ICP can be accomplished in a number of ways. The ventriculostomy catheter allows monitoring and drainage of cerebrospinal fluid (CSF), but it is the most invasive method and is associated with risk of infection. The epidural catheter, hollow subarachnoid bolt, and subarachnoid fiberoptic catheter are other options. All must be surgically placed. The noninvasive Doppler waveform can also provide information regarding ICP.

The increase in blood volume is considered to be the most important cause of increased ICP after head trauma. Both hypoxemia and hypercapnia will cause cerebral vasodilation and increase blood volume (see Chapter 4). Hyperventilation is one of the most effective mechanisms for controlling cerebral blood volume. This must be considered a short-term procedure to be used judiciously because of its secondary effect of decreasing cerebral blood flow and causing ischemia.

Cerebral blood volume can also be reduced pharmacologically. Cerebral vasoconstrictive agents such as mannitol, barbiturates, etomidate, and propofol are used to reduce metabolism, blood flow, and blood volume. In clinical studies, the use of mild hypothermia appears to reduce neuronal injury by decreasing the amount of glutamate released. It is important that cerebral venous blood volume be controlled in head injury. Maintaining the head at a 20- to 40-degree tilt will usually provide adequate drainage. However, compression of venous drainage from tracheal ties and collars and extreme neck flexion or extension can occur if precautions are not followed. CSF can also play a role in ICP. This can be controlled by the use of hypertonic saline or mannitol. Removal of CSF can be accomplished by ventriculoscopy.

Because of the intense sympathetic stimulation seen with head injury, hypertension and tachycardia are prevalent. Cushing's phenomenon, a rise in blood pressure in the presence of an acute rise in ICP, most often caused by brainstem compression, may be present. Moderate increases in blood pressure can be tolerated, but extreme hypertension should be treated, as it could lead to increased blood volume.

Abnormal muscle tone can be controlled by nerve and motor point blocks or by the administration of botulinum toxin directly into the muscle belly. Spasticity is controlled by the administration of baclofen, diazepam, or dantrolene.[4]

Rehabilitation of the head-injured person and return to optimal function is the goal once the medical status is stabilized. Highly skilled, specially trained interdisciplinary teams provide an organized approach to the complex deficits encountered after head injury. Rehabilitation management of the patient is dependent on the cognitive and behavioral level of function of the individual. The Rancho Los Amigos Scale (see Table 29–3), which assesses components of cerebral function, is widely used. Treatment protocols are established according to the level at which the individual is functioning.

---

[4] These drugs act at the synaptic junction by presynaptic inhibition, or calcium release. In all cases, there is a decrease in the excitability of the muscle.

Cognitive deficits, as in attention, memory, perception, language, and problem solving, can inhibit the person's ability to cope with a new self. Psychotherapy may help.

Restoration of mobility, self-care, employment, and recreational activities depends on the level of sensorimotor impairment, as well as cognitive status. See Special Implications for the Therapist 29–1: Traumatic Brain Injury.

Prognosis

Injury severity is the main factor determining outcome. The depth of impaired responsiveness and the duration of altered consciousness have been related to outcome. The current gold standard for assessing those mental states in the head-injured person is the Glasgow Outcome Scale (Box 29–2). In addition, the duration of posttraumatic amnesia has been used as a predictor of severity of the head injury.

Other aspects of neurologic functioning are predictive of outcome. Loss of pupillary light reflexes following head injury reflects significant damage to the brainstem and portends a poor prognosis. Oculomotor deficits often signal concomitant cerebral damage resulting in severe cognitive deficits. The degree of hypoxemia and hypotension encountered in the early stages can also have an effect on the long-term prognosis.

CT has increased the ability to predict outcome in the head-injured person with a lesion of the brain parenchyma, intercranial hematoma, subdural hematoma, or massive hemispheric swelling. Acute hemispheric swelling with an extracerebral hematoma is associated with the worst prognosis. Unilateral brain contusion and diffuse axonal injury also carry a poor prognosis. A midline shift of brain structures, absent or compressed basal cisterns (indicating rising ICP), and subarachnoid hemorrhage will increase the the risk of death or remaining in a vegetative state.

BOX **29–2**
Glasgow Outcome Scale

Vegetative State
The client is in a state of nonsentient survival with reduced responsiveness associated with wakefulness. There is no evidence of psychologically meaningful activity, although there may be local motor activity.

Severe Disability
The client is conscious but dependent. There is often spastic paralysis of three or four limbs. Dysphasia that limits communication may be the reason for the dependency, or it may be due to severely restricted mental activity.

Moderate Disability
The client is independent but disabled. The limitations to normal functional levels may be memory deficits and personality changes. Focal brain damage can be evidenced by cranial nerve involvement, posttraumatic epilepsy, hemiparesis, or movement disorders.

Good Recovery
Although there is not restoration of all normal function, the client is able to participate in normal social life and may be able to return to work.

Modified from Jennett B, Teasdale G: Management of Head Injuries. Philadelphia, FA Davis, 1981, pp 304–305.

Special Implications for the Therapist **29–1**

TRAUMATIC BRAIN INJURY

Rehabilitation of the head-injured person involves the therapist at many different levels and in different settings. Understanding the deficits common in acute injury and the natural recovery patterns of the brain dependent on the site and type of injury is paramount for the therapist treating head injury. Approximately 25% of persons with a normal initial CT scan will develop late hemorrhages.

Often the therapist will be involved in a dedicated head injury unit or in a community reentry program. Even in a more general setting, the therapist is often responsible for intervention with persons sustaining head injury, often acutely, or when an individual has been through a rehabilitation setting and is referred for follow-up based on residual deficits. Provision of therapy in the long-term care setting involves care for individuals in persistent vegetative states or with behavioral deficits precluding independent living.

Acute Management *(Gill-Body and Giorgetti, 1995)*

In the acute care setting the therapist is responsible for the evaluation of neurologic function in conjunction with the physicians and nurses. One role may be consistent monitoring of cranial nerve function. In addition, the therapist is involved in monitoring reflexive and voluntary motor behaviors. The treatment plan often includes pulmonary care, positioning, range-of-motion exercises, and relaxation techniques. Movement facilitation begins early in the treatment and continues throughout rehabilitation in many cases. Because treatment starts while the individual is still in the intensive care unit, a discussion of life-sustaining equipment follows.

Chest tubes are common with a pneumothorax or hemothorax. The drainage tube should be kept below the level of the chest at all times. Upper extremity movement should be monitored so as not to interfere with the tube. Nasogastric tube feeding is also common initially, and when a tube is in place, the head of the bed should be placed at 30 degrees to avoid aspiration. Lines such as central venous pressure catheters, pulmonary or arterial lines, and ICP monitors can be compromised during movement, and often the movement will trigger an alarm that can be upsetting for the client and family. Close communication with the nursing staff will give the therapist confidence in moving the person in the intensive care setting.

Pulmonary management is a another critical area. Techniques such as percussion, vibration, and suctioning are used to keep the airway clear but must be done with caution and may be contraindicated in the presence of increased ICP. Monitoring blood gases and oxygen saturation is critical in some clients, as movement may alter these values.[5] Weaning from the ventilator is an individual endeavor. Some clients are able to continue to incorporate activity during weaning, but for others it may mean a decrease in tolerance to movement.

Restoration of normal movement is a major component of the intervention provided by therapists (see Chapter 24). Task-specific training and forced use are interventions which work to prevent the typical compensatory movement strategies common after head injury.

Management of decreased range of motion from overactive musculature or HO is another intervention provided by therapists. Joint contractures are a secondary problem produced by inability of the muscle to return to its normal resting length. Serial casting and dynamic splinting are used to maintain joint motion in the presence of spasticity, rigidity, or HO (Bryan, 1995).

Similar concepts apply to decisions for wheelchair seating and positioning in the nonambulatory individual. Prevention of secondary joint disorders, pain, and disfigurement is facilitated by provision of support in the anatomically proper position. Materials and equipment that are lightweight and provide total contact provide the most comfortable support (Chiu, 1995).

Swallowing deficits and related problems with respiration or coughing occur in approximately one third of persons with head injury. Head, neck, and trunk control affect the ability to swallow. Intervention based on lack of strength and mobility of the perioral structures often starts in the acute phase. Sensation, dentition, tongue control, and laryngeal control are assessed to determine the level of impairment relating to disability of speech and swallowing (Zablotny, 1995).

Cognitive rehabilitation and physical rehabilitation are not aspects of treatment that stand alone. Functional outcomes are limited by the cognitive status, and the understanding of the techniques that foster behavioral modification and learning in the head-injured should be employed by the therapist while motor skill acquisition is being attempted (Sullivan, 1995).

Long-Term Rehabilitation

Community re-entry programs for the head-injured person enhance the transition from rehabilitation unit to independent living. Therapists play a significant role in such programs.

In order to return to a lifestyle that may include work and school, the person with TBI needs to learn how to cope with the multiple demands on his or her attention that are part of that lifestyle. The person with TBI will have difficulty with executive functions such as organizing time and information, self-monitoring, and self-correcting. Self-motivation is often lacking, and structuring is necessary to assure followthrough on assigned activities. Extensive use of checklists and environmental cues are helpful when attempting to reintegrate the client into the community.

TRAUMATIC BRAIN INJURY IN CHILDREN

TBI is one of the leading causes of death and disability in children of all ages (Nelson, 1992). Nonaccidental injury is a common cause of head injury in infants and toddlers and is often the result of the battered-child syndrome. The head injury is often caused by shaking or striking the child.

The pathology of the brain injury in the child reflects damage similar to that in the adult, but, there are differences. Infants typically have tears in the white matter of the temporal and orbitofrontal lobes. The infant will more often sustain a subdural or epidural hemorrhage than an older child but is less likely to have skull fracture because of the pliancy of the skull.

Drowning is the third leading cause of death in children aged 1 to 4 years. Peaks are in 1- to 4 year-olds and in boys in adolescence. Boys are three times more likely to be injured. Rapid resuscitation leads to better outcomes. As in adults, the motor activity return and pupillary light response are prognosticators of outcome (see Chapter 12).

A children's coma scale has been developed for use in children under the age of 3 years (Table 29–4). The highest level of ocular response is eye tracking. The verbal response is rated highest by crying, then by spontaneous respirations, with the lowest score given for apneic breathing. The motor response has a highest score for flexing and extending the extremities.

Early management of the infant or child with TBI follows that of the adult, with some difference in the child's ability to tolerate the medications used. Late seizures are less common with children than with adults, so the need to be maintained on seizure medication is less.

TABLE 29-4 CHILDREN'S COMA SCALE

Ocular response (O)
4 Pursuit
3 Extraocular movement (EOM) intact, reactive pupils
2 Fixed pupils or EOM impaired
1 Fixed pupils and EOM paralyzed

Verbal response (V)
3 Cries
2 Spontaneous respirations
1 Apneic

Motor response (M)
4 Flexes and extends
3 Withdraws from painful stimuli
2 Hypertonic
1 Flaccid

From Raimondi AJ, Hirschauer J: Head injury in the infant and toddler. Childs Nerv Syst 11:12–35, 1984. Infants (younger than 1 year) may have a worse outcome (with scores > 6) than toddlers. A score < 6 relates to a poor outcome for toddlers.

[5] Normal levels of partial pressure of oxygen are between 80 and 100 mm Hg. Normal oxygen saturation is between 95% and 100%. See Table 35–21 and Special Implications 35–9.

Rehabilitation goals for the child are similar to those of the adult, although play is used during therapy. Orthotic and assistive devices are used frequently but for a shorter time than for adults. Agitation is common and is often difficult for the parents and siblings to handle. Aggression, decreased attention span, hyperactivity, and socially inappropriate behavior are seen. These children often require a great deal of behavior modification.

Community reintegration can be as difficult for the child as it is for the adult. Schools are better prepared to handle cognitive delays than abnormal behaviors. Cognitive status may return in one area and remain defective in another. Attention and memory deficits may produce the greatest obstacles to learning.

References

Bernard, PG. Closed Head Injury: A Clinical Source Book. Charlottesville, Va, Michie, 1994.

Bryan VL: Management of residual physical deficits. *In* Ashley MJ, Krych DK (eds): Traumatic Brain Injury Rehabilitation. Salem, Mass, CRC Press, 1995, pp 319–365.

Chiu ML: Wheelchair seating and positioning. *In* Montgomery J (ed): Physical Therapy for Traumatic Brain Injury. New York, Churchill Livingstone, 1995, pp 117–136.

Domino KB: Pathophysiology of head injury: Secondary systemic effects. *In* Lam AM (ed): Anesthetic Management of Acute Head Injury. New York, McGraw-Hill, 1995, pp 25–59.

Evans RW: Mild traumatic brain injury. *In* Berrol S (ed): Physical Medicine and Rehabilitation Clinics of North America. Traumatic Brain Injury. Philadelphia, WB Saunders, 1992, pp 427–437.

Gelber DA: The neurologic examination of the traumatically brain-injured patient. *In* Ashley MJ, Krych DK (eds): Traumatic Brain Injury Rehabilitation. Salem, Mass, CRC Press, 1995, pp 23–42.

Giles GM, Clark-Wilson J: Brain Injury Rehabilitation: A Neurofunctional Approach. San Diego, Singular Publishing Group, 1993.

Gill-Body KM, Giorgetti MM: Acute care and prognostic outcomes. *In* Montgomery J (ed): Physical Therapy for Traumatic Brain Injury. New York, Churchill Livingstone, 1995, pp 1–32.

Grady MS, Lam AM: Management of acute head injury: Initial resuscitation. *In* Lam AM (ed): Anesthetic Management of Acute Head Injury. New York, McGraw-Hill, 1995, pp 87–100.

Grady MS, Shapiro X: Pathophysiology of head injury: Primary central nervous system effects. *In* Lam AM (ed): Anesthetic Management of Acute Head Injury. New York, McGraw-Hill, 1995, pp 11–24.

Hughes M, Cohen WA: Radiographic evaluation. *In* Cooper PR (ed): Head Injury, ed 3. Baltimore, Williams & Wilkins, 1993, pp 65–90.

Kraus JF: Epidemiology of head injury. *In* Cooper PR (ed): Head Injury, ed 3. Baltimore, Williams & Wilkins, 1993, pp 1–26.

Leahy P: Traumatic head injury. *In* O'Sullivan SB, Schmitz TJ (ed): Physical Rehabilitation. Philadelphia, FA Davis, 1994, pp 491–508.

Nelson VS: Pediatric head injury. *In* Berrol S (ed): Physical Medicine and Rehabilitation Clinics of North America. Traumatic Brain Injury. Philadelphia, WB Saunders, 1992, pp 461–474.

Povlishock JT, Christman CW: The pathobiology of traumatic brain injury. *In* Salsman SK, Faden AI (eds): The Neurobiology of Nervous System Trauma. New York, Oxford University Press, 1994, pp 109–130.

Povlishock JT, Valadka A: Pathobiology of traumatic brain injury. *In* Finlayson MA, Garner SH: Brain Injury Rehabilitation: Clinical Considerations. Baltimore, Williams & Wilkins, 1994.

Rovit RL, Murali R: Injuries of the cranial nerves. *In* Cooper PR (ed): Head Injury, ed 3. Baltimore, Williams & Wilkins, 1993, pp 183–202.

Sullivan K: Cognitive rehabilitation. *In* Montgomery J (ed): Physical Therapy for Traumatic Brain Injury. New York, Churchill Livingstone, 1995, pp 33–54.

Varghese G: Heterotopic ossification. *In* Berrol S (ed): Physical Medicine and Rehabilitation Clinics of North America. Traumatic Brain Injury. Philadelphia, WB Saunders, 1992, pp 407–416.

Winkler PA: Head injury. *In* Umphred DA (ed): Neurological Rehabilitation. St Louis, Mosby–Year Book, 1995, pp 421–454.

Zablotny C: Evaluation and management of swallowing dysfunction. *In* Montgomery J (ed): Physical Therapy for Traumatic Brain Injury. New York, Churchill Livingstone, 1995, pp 99–116.

SECTION 4

chapter 30

Traumatic Spinal Cord Injury

Kenda S. Fuller

Spinal cord injury (SCI) can be categorized into traumatic and nontraumatic injuries. Traumatic injury is the most common cause of adult SCI and is the primary emphasis here, although the information is germane to both conditions. SCI is a catastrophic event, of low incidence and high cost. It is most often the highly active persons that incur the types of accidents that cause severe SCI. Within a matter of seconds, the person sustaining a traumatic SCI may become dependent on others or on assistive devices to perform even the most rudimentary activities.

The belief that SCI is irreparable and that there cannot be nerve regeneration in the spinal cord is being replaced by the understanding that there are growth factors available within the cord. Recent advances in medical management, especially in the area of preservation of neurons that typically die as a secondary reaction to trauma, are resulting in fewer complete spinal cord lesions. Transplantation of nerve cells may someday become a reality, as current methods are showing more promise.

Rehabilitation of clients with SCI shows improvement with the availability of more sophisticated muscle stimulation and biofeedback modalities. The painful sequelae of SCI are now better controlled with the use of both medications and electrical stimulation.

INCIDENCE AND RISK FACTORS

Occasionally the spinal cord can be damaged by direct insult from a foreign body such as a bullet or knife, but most often the cord sustains damage as a result of impingement by bony or soft tissue structures, as occurs when vertebrae dislocate or a vertebral body explodes.

Traumatic injury chiefly affects males, with over 80% of all cases occurring in males. It is also an injury of the young, with 50% of the SCI population between the ages of 15 and 30, the median and most common age being 18 years (Buchanan, 1987a,b).

The incidence of traumatic SCI in small children is minor, representing less than 10% of the traumatic SCI population. Most SCI in young children is congenital. The congenital condition predisposes the infant and young child to other central nervous system disorders. Spina bifida, resulting from a defect in closure of the neural tube, causing the contents of the spinal column to protrude, can cause loss of sensory and motor functions in the lower limbs. When there is partial innervation of the spinal cord, orthopedic deformities develop from the imbalance between groups of nerves. Bowel and bladder dysfunction is common, and kidney function is often affected as a result. Brainstem malformation may cause loss of respiratory and bulbar function. Most of these children will develop hydrocephalus, and surgery to correct the spinal defect will include a shunt to maintain flow of cerebrospinal fluid (Schneider and Gabriel, 1990) (see Chapter 20).

DEFINITION AND ETIOLOGY

SCIs are classified as concussion, contusion, or laceration. The spinal cord is often violently displaced or compressed momentarily and the cord appears normal following injury. A *concussion* is an injury caused by a blow or violent shaking and results in temporary loss of function, similar to the cerebral concussion following head injury. *Contusions* are bruises with hemorrhage beneath unbroken skin. Contusions are associated with fractured bone segments striking the spinal cord. *Laceration* (disruption of tissue) of the cord can occur with more severe injuries and, rarely, can result in complete transection of the cord. Extradural hemorrhages are common, although they rarely become large enough to compromise the spinal cord. Subarachnoid hemorrhages, due to contusion and laceration of the cord, are frequent, and can cause further compression of the cord. Secondary neuropathologic changes begin immediately after injury (Kakulas and Taylor, 1992).

Automobile accidents account for over 40% of all SCIs. Falls are the second most common cause and the third most common cause is gunshot wounds. The most preventable cause of SCI is diving, most often in water levels of 4 to 6 ft. Sports accidents resulting in SCI are most prevalent in the contact sports of football and wrestling, high-speed sports such as snow skiing and surfing, and injuries involving a fall from a height such as a trampoline or a horse.

PATHOGENESIS

The mechanism of injury has an influence on the type and degree of the spinal cord lesion. Approximately 50% of injuries come from excessive flexion of the spinal column and are associated with a severe neurologic disorder. Complete spinal cord lesions occur in about one third of flexion injuries. Dislocation in a flexion injury causes a complete lesion 50% of the time. With crush fractures of the vertebrae, there is a 75% chance of a complete spinal cord lesion.

Neuronal Damage

Blunt trauma to the spinal cord results in some primary destruction of neurons at the level of the injury (Fig. 30–1). Neural damage to the spinal cord extends beyond the initial contusion. *Spinal shock,* the loss of sensory, voluntary motor, and automatic control below the level of the lesion, occurs after the trauma. The mechanism is poorly understood, and

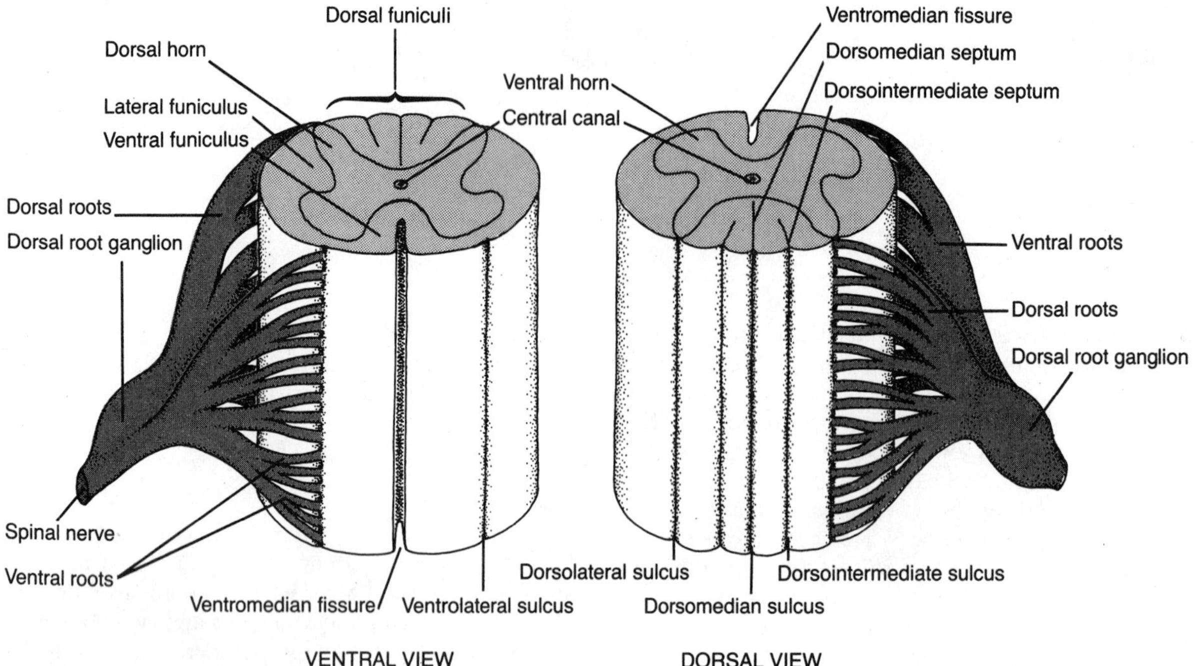

Figure **30–1.** Dorsal and ventral view of a typical spinal segment. Shown are the dorsal and ventral roots as they enter and exit. Shown also are the white matter tracts and the gray matter horns. (*From Burt A: Textbook of Neuroanatomy. Philadelphia, WB Saunders, 1993, p 119.*)

resolves within a few weeks after injury (Waxman and deGroot, 1995).

Demyelination also plays a major role in SCI. The demyelination is probably due to direct trauma to oligodendroglial cells. The myelin sheath becomes thin between the nodes, and this is responsible for a decrease in the peak currents along the axon.

Changes in white matter begin with wallerian degeneration in the ascending posterior columns above the level of the lesion and in the descending corticospinal tracts. There is usually a latent response in the white matter compared to the gray matter, with preservation of the more peripheral white matter tracts (Kakulas and Taylor, 1992).

Discomplete Spinal Cord Lesion

The difference between a complete and incomplete spinal cord lesion may depend on the survival of a small fraction of the axons in the spinal cord. Evidence of axonal conduction across the lesion site has been found in individuals with clinical neurologic diagnoses of complete SCI at that level. This has been termed *discomplete spinal cord lesion*. The surviving axons may be injured and therefore respond subclinically to stimuli. The injured axon conducts slowly and fatigues rapidly. A prolonged refractory period may be responsible for the fatigue (Young, 1991a).[1]

Blood Flow Changes

Changes in blood flow, represented by small petechial hemorrhages, begin soon after the SCI. After several hours there appear to be gross hemorrhages present, preceded by endothelial breakdown and pathologic coagulation products in the blood vessels. Ischemia and necrosis occur primarily in the gray matter, presumably because of the richer blood supply. Macrophages enter the lesion and begin to digest the necrotic debris, converting the complex myelin lipids to neutral fat. Axonal swelling and increased permeability of blood vessels result in a visibly swollen spinal cord (Young, 1991a). Glial cells are activated after about 6 days, and astrocytic fibers form scarlike tissue that lines the cavities created by the necrosis.

Autoregulation of circulation is disabled at the injury site. Systemic pressure changes may be responsible for changes in spinal blood flow, which may cause nervous tissue damage by direct effects. The cause-and-effect relationship between blood flow and spinal injury outcome, however, has not been firmly established. The changes in blood flow may reflect rather than cause secondary injury.

Synaptic Dysfunction

Important changes in the levels of certain ions have been studied recently and appear to have further detrimental effects on the neurons in the spinal cord. Of the many proposed mechanisms of secondary injury, lipid peroxidation has attracted the most attention. SCI causes calcium ions to rush into the cells, disrupting mitochonrial electron transport and activating phospolipases. Injured mitochondria generate oxygen free radicals which break down the membranes and cause lipid peroxides and free arachidonic acid to be released. The free arachidonic acid is converted to prostaglandins and leukotrienes which can cause pathologic and biochemical changes similar to those found in traumatized tissue (Young, 1992b).

Other changes are noted in the spinal cord in the area of

[1] The refractory period is the time following the firing (action potential) of a nerve in which firing cannot be repeated in the same neuron. The refractory period limits the ability of the axon to conduct high-frequency trains of action potentials.

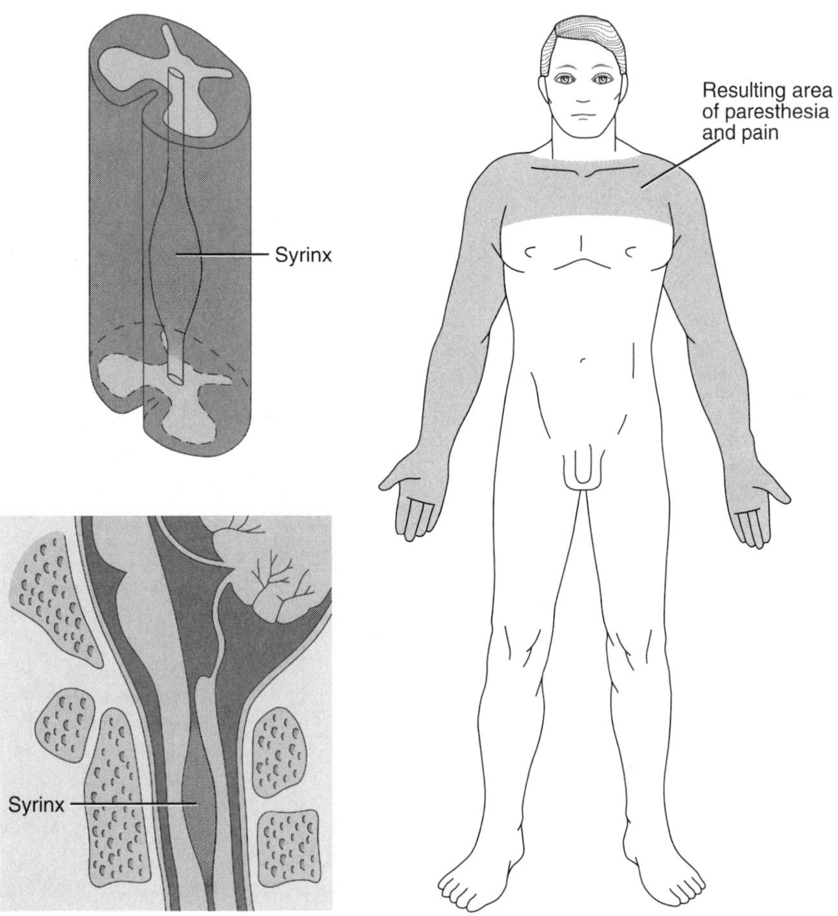

Figure **30–2.** The syrinx formed in the late stages of spinal cord injury as a part of syringomyelia.

injury; levels of high-energy metabolites fall. Ischemia in the area of injury may be due to the presence of norepinephrine, serotonin, histamine, and prostaglandins, all of which cause vasoconstriction. Thrombosis may be another cause of ischemia in acute SCI.

Syringomyelia

Eventually there is nerve root atrophy at the immediate level of injury corresponding to the central gray matter necrosis. The lesion at the level of injury develops the appearance of a cyst, with regeneration of both anterior and posterior nerve roots above and below the area of the lesion.[2]

In the chronic spinal cord lesion, the cysts may continue to develop, become tubular in shape (syrinx), and extend over several spinal levels (Fig. 30–2). This condition is known as *posttraumatic syringomyelia* and may develop up to 30 years after the initial lesion, most commonly within 4 to 9 years after trauma. As the cyst develops, usually below the level of the initial lesion, there can be significant pain as a result of the compromise of the central spinal cord structures such as the substantia gelatinosa and the posterior root entry zone (Williams, 1992)

The thoracic spine is the most common site for the syrinx to develop, with descending and ascending fibers running in the walls of the cavitated lesions. The size and extent of the syrinx is represented by the symptoms, but because of location below the site of the lesion, changes are not easily recognized. The syringomyelia may be responsible for the spasms, phantom sensations, reflex changes, and autonomic visceral phenomena (Kakulas and Taylor, 1992).

CLINICAL MANIFESTATIONS

Level of Injury

SCIs are named according of the level of neurologic impairment (Ragnarsson, 1993; Farcy and Rawlins, 1993). Impairments of sensory and motor systems are used to identify the level. The American Spinal Injury Association (ASIA) has created standards for assessment and classification, which are widely used (Figs. 30–3 and 30–4). The sensory examination consists of testing 28 dermatomes on each side of the body using pinprick and light touch, which are then scored as follows: 0 = absent, 1 = impaired, 2 = normal. Function of the external anal sphincter is tested as a yes or no. The level of inquiry reflects the most caudal level of the spinal cord that exhibits intact sensory and motor functioning.

[2] Nerve root regeneration is similar to a posttraumatic neuroma formation in the peripheral nerves and becomes more and more prominent with time. At present it is conjectural whether Schwann cells associated with nerve root regeneration may supply factors that allow regeneration of central axons in human SCI (Kakulas and Taylor, 1992).

MOTOR

KEY MUSCLES

	R	L	
C2			
C3			
C4			
C5	☐	☐	Elbow flexors
C6	☐	☐	Wrist extensors
C7	☐	☐	Elbow extensors
C8	☐	☐	Finger flexors (distal phalanx of middle finger)
T1	☐	☐	Finger abductors (little finger)
T2			
T3			
T4			
T5			
T6			
T7			
T8			
T9			
T10			
T11			
T12			
L1			
L2	☐	☐	Hip flexors
L3	☐	☐	Knee extensors
L4	☐	☐	Ankle dorsiflexors
L5	☐	☐	Long toe extensors
S1	☐	☐	Ankle plantar flexors
S2			
S3			
S4-5			☐ Voluntary anal contraction (Yes/No)
TOTALS	☐ +	☐ =	☐ **MOTOR SCORE**
(MAXIMUM)	(50)	(50)	(100)

0 = total paralysis
1 = palpable or visible contraction
2 = active movement, gravity eliminated
3 = active movement, against gravity
4 = active movement, against some resistance
5 = active movement, against full resistance
NT= not testable

Figure **30–3.** ASIA motor form. (*Courtesy of American Spinal Injury Association International, Atlanta.*)

Identification of motor impairment is more problematic, given the dual innervation of many of the muscles. The strength of a given muscle is a reflection of the functioning of two or more cord segments. Loss of innervation from a spinal cord level results in weakness of the dual innervated muscle. To determine the level of innervation, the therapist looks for the muscle that has a 3/5 muscle strength and a 4/5 muscle strength in the next most rostral muscle. Volitional contraction of the anal sphincter is also noted.

Differences may exist in the motor vs. sensory levels identified. Asymmetrical damage may result in different levels of neurologic impairment on the left vs. the right side. This is identified by reporting the levels individually, for example, a right C5 and left C6 lesion.

The site of spinal cord damage determines the extent of the physical impairments. Injury of the cord in the cervical region creates quadriplegia (paralysis of all four limbs) or quadriparesis (weakness of all four extremities). In addition to the limbs, the trunk and muscles of respiration are involved. Damage in the thoracic or lumbar region will result in paraplegia or paraparesis involving only the lower extremities and generally the lower trunk.

Lesions are reported as *complete*, or the complete loss of sensory and motor function below the level of the lesion. Complete lesions are caused by a transection, severe compression, or extensive vascular dysfunction.

Incomplete lesions are the partial loss of sensory and motor function below the level of the injury. Incomplete lesions often occur when there is contusion produced by bony fragments, soft tissue, or edema within the spinal canal. The resulting motor or sensory function is called *sparing*. Box 30–1 describes the ASIA method for describing impairment related to SCI.

Spinal Cord Injury Syndromes

Within the category of incomplete spinal cord lesions are the recognizable syndromes that have been identified. Several of the syndromes are illustrated in Figure 30–5.

Brown-Séquard syndrome is characterized by damage to one side of the spinal cord. The most common causes are stab and gunshot wounds. Loss of the entire hemisection of the spinal cord is rare; the natural lesion is always irregular. There is weakness ipsilateral to the lesion. Lateral column damage results in abnormal reflexes, including a positive Babinski sign, and clonus. Often there is ipsilateral spasticity in the muscles innervated below the lesion. As a result of dorsal column damage there is loss of proprioception, kinesthesia, and vibratory sense. On the contralateral (opposite) side, there is pain and temperature loss starting a few levels below the lesion. The lateral spinothalamic tract ascends on the same side for several segments before crossing, giving rise to the discrepancy between the level and contralateral signs.

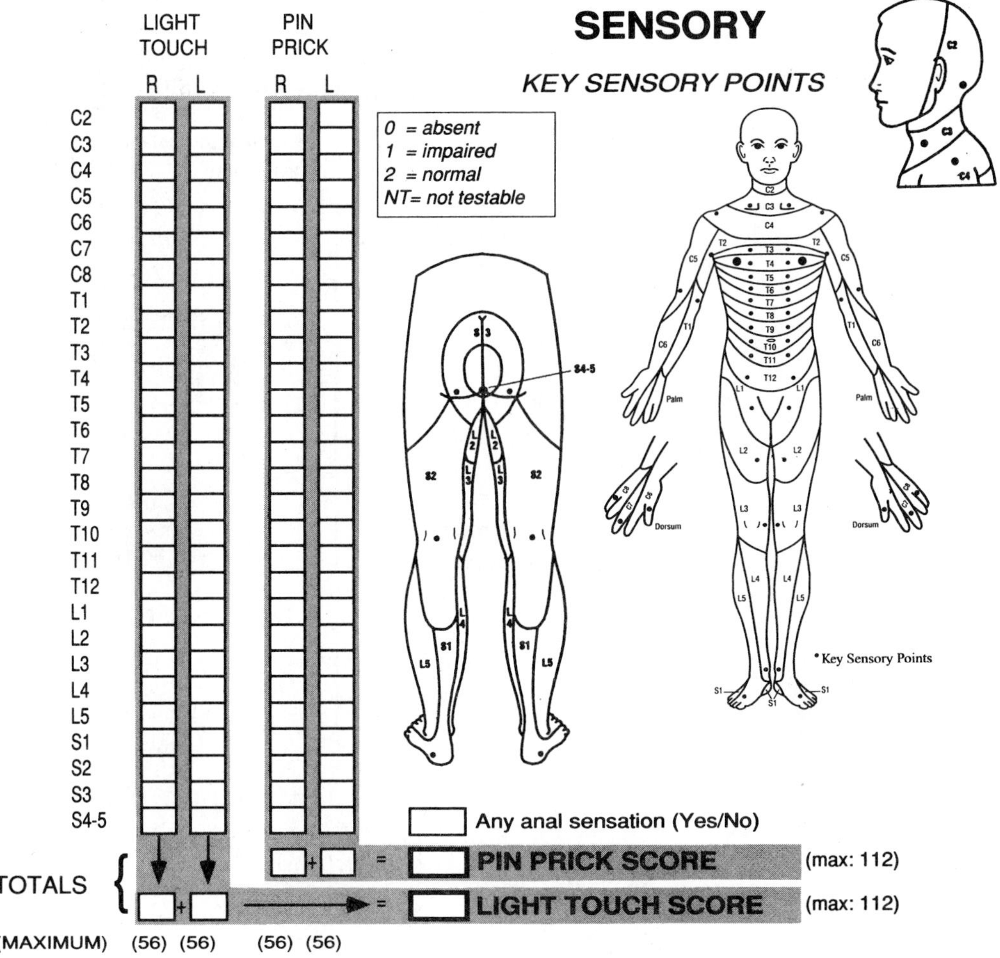

Figure **30–4.** ASIA sensory assessment form. (*Courtesy of American Spinal Injury Association International, Atlanta.*)

Anterior cord syndrome is frequently associated with flexion injuries and is often the result of loss of supply from the anterior spinal artery. Damage to the anterior and anterolateral aspect of the cord results in bilateral loss of motor function and pain and temperature sensation due to interruption of the anterior and lateral spinothalamic tracts and corticospinal tract.

Central cord syndrome is a result of damage to the central aspect of the spinal cord, often caused by hyperextension injuries in the cervical region. There is characteristically more severe neurologic involvement in the upper extremities than in the lower extremities. Peripherally located fibers are not affected and therefore function is retained in the thoracic, lumbar, and sacral regions, including the bowel, bladder, and genitals.

Posterior cord syndrome is extremely rare, with preservation of motor function, pain, and light touch sensation. There is loss of proprioception below the level of the lesion leading to a wide-based steppage gait.

Changes in Muscle Tone

Paralysis of the voluntary musculature is the most obvious effect of SCI. Damage can involve the descending motor tracts, anterior horn cells, or spinal nerves, and it is often seen in combinations of these. When the descending tracts are involved, immediate flaccidity and absent reflexes are present. This is followed by autonomic symptoms, including sweating and reflex incontinence of bladder and rectum. Within weeks there is a gradual increase in the resting tone of the muscles innervated below the lesion, and reflexes appear.

BOX 30–1
American Spinal Injury Association International, Atlanta

American Spinal Injury Association Impairment Scale

A = Complete. No sensory or motor function is preserved in the segment S4–5

B = Incomplete. Sensory but no motor function is preserved below the neurologic level. Sensory function extends through segments S4–5.

C = Incomplete. Motor function is preserved below the neurologic level and the majority of key muscles below the neurologic level have a muscle grade of less than 3.

D = Incomplete. Motor function is preserved below the neurologic level, and the majority of key muscles below the neurologic level have a muscle grade greater than or equal to 3.

E = Normal. Sensory and motor functions are normal.

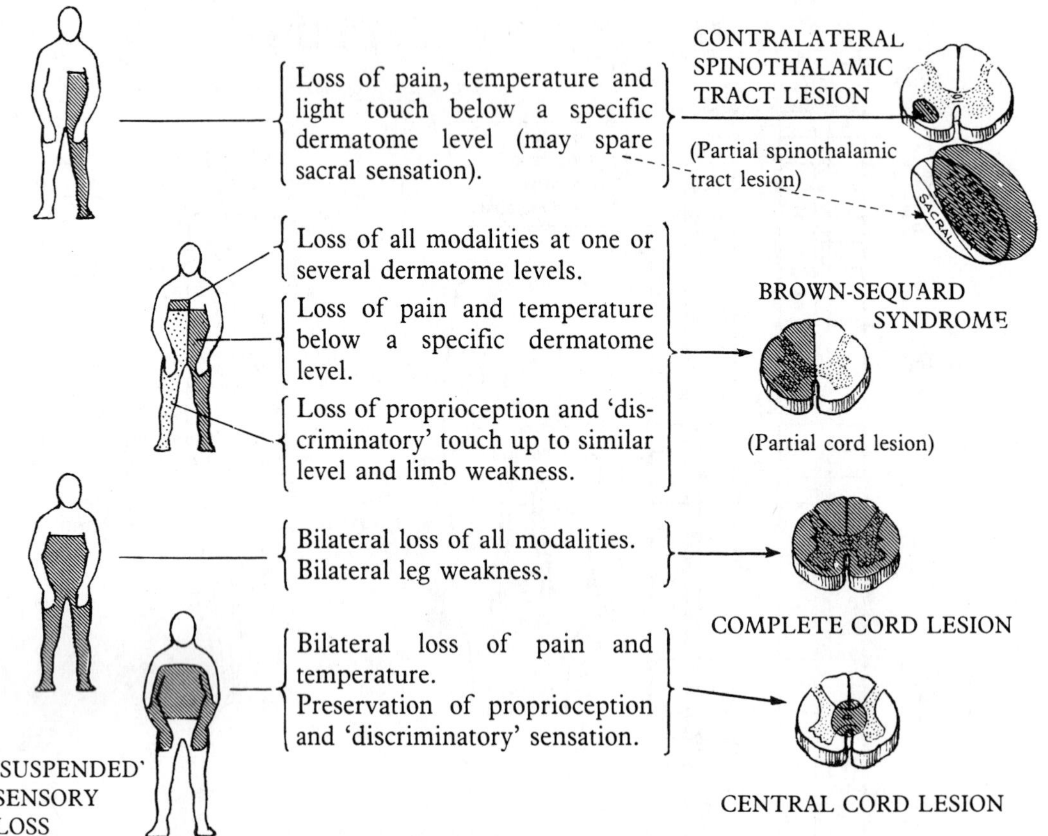

Figure **30–5.** Spinal cord syndromes. Patterns of sensory loss and weakness. (*From Lindsey KW, Bone I, Callander R: Neurology and Neurosurgery Illustrated. New York, Churchill Livingstone, 1986, p 188.*)

Spasticity, an inevitable consequence of spinal cord lesions, manifests itself in many different ways. There is an essential or *basic spasticity*, which may be of some benefit to the individual when emptying the bladder or flexing the hip and knee. Excess spasticity is thought to be due to imposed afferent stimuli. Drug therapy is used to treat the spasticity. Spasticity can be made worse by the presence of constipation, infection, fracture, or a pressure sore below the level of the lesion. In general, a flaccid condition lasts longer, and spasticity comes later in the cervical injury and can be exacerbated by a sudden change in temperature or by physical or emotional stress (Illis, 1992).

Respiratory Complications

Respiratory complications associated with spinal cord lesions can be life-threatening. Lesions above C4 result in paralysis of inspiratory muscles and generally require artificial ventilation due to loss of the phrenic nerve. Pulmonary complications in lesions at C5 through T12 arise due to loss of innervation of the muscles of expiration—the abdominals and intercostals. The position of the diaphragm is compromised and the abdominal musculature is unable to exert pressure during forced expiration. Paralysis of the external oblique muscles also inhibits the person's ability to cough and expel secretions.

An altered breathing pattern develops in conjunction with the loss of the diaphragmatic muscle, the intercostals, and the accessory muscles of inspiration. The upper chest wall flattens and the abdominal wall expands, leading to musculoskeletal changes in the trunk.

Bowel and Bladder Control

The spinal center for urination is the conus medullaris. Primary reflex control originates from the sacral segment. During the stage of spinal shock, the urinary bladder is flaccid. All muscle tone and bladder reflexes are absent. Lesions above the conus medullaris will cause a reflex neurogenic bladder, reflected by spasticity, voiding difficulties, detrusor muscle hypertrophy, and urethral reflux. Lesions at the conus medullaris cause nonreflex bladders, resulting in flaccidity and decreased tone of the perineal muscles and urethral sphincter. Bowel patterns mimic bladder responses in their response to spinal shock; reflex bowel occurs in lesions above the conus medullaris, and nonreflex bowel is caused by damage to the conus and cauda equina.

Sexual Response

Sexual response is directly related to the level and completeness of injury. There are two types of responses, *reflexogenic*, or response to external stimulation seen in persons with upper motor neuron lesions, and *psychogenic*, which occur through cognitive activity such as fantasy, associated with lower motor neuron lesions. Men with higher-level lesions can often achieve a reflexive erection, but typically do not ejaculate. Those with lower lesions can more easily ejaculate, but the ability to achieve an erection is more difficult. With cauda equina lesions, erection and ejaculation are not usually possible.

Menses are typically interrupted for approximately 3 months; fertility and pregnancy are uninterrupted, but the pregnancy must be followed closely, especially in the last trimester. Labor may begin without the woman's knowing it due to loss of sensation, and labor may initiate autonomic dysreflexia (Schneider, 1990).

Autonomic Nervous System Changes

Loss of thermoregulation below the level of the spinal cord lesion is a result of the disruption of the autonomic pathways from the hypothalamus. Vasoconstriction, the ability to shiver, and the ability to sweat are lost. The body temperature then is greatly influenced by the external environment and the sensory feedback from the head and neck must be used to assist in regulating body temperature. The higher the lesion, the more severe the problem.

Autonomic dysreflexia can occur with a lesion above T6. Noxious stimuli (usually visceral) below the level of the lesion trigger a massive uncompensated cardiovascular reaction of the sympathetic division of the autonomic nervous system. Vasoconstriction occurs in the vascular beds of the skin and viscera, causing a rise in blood pressure. Compensatory vasodilation creates flushing of the neck and face. A severe pounding headache follows with sweating and chills without fever. The increase in blood pressure makes the person susceptible to subarachnoid hemorrhage. Autonomic dysreflexia should be handled as a medical emergency (Altrice et al., 1995; Schmitz, 1994).

Musculoskeletal Changes

Joint ankylosis due to *heterotopic ossification*, or ectopic bone formation in the extra-articular soft tissue such as the tendons and connective tissue, can limit range of motion and cause pain. It often develops near the large joints, such as the anterior hip, knee, shoulder, and elbow. It is always found below the level of the lesion, and it develops within the first year after injury. The initial symptoms are soft tissue swelling, pain, redness, and increased temperature in the affected area.

Pain due to irritation of the nerve root is common, especially in cauda equina injury. *Dysesthesia*, impairment of sensation usually perceived as pain, can occur in areas that have no sensation and are often described as "burning," "pins and needles," or "tingling." Disturbances of proprioception are related, and the person feels that a limb is in a different position than it really is in.

Secondary Complications

Secondary complications arise due to loss of motor control and sensation but are not directly related to nervous system disorder. Secondary complications include contractures, deep vein thrombosis, pressure sores, and postural hypotension. Osteoporosis develops below the level of the lesion. In concert with this is the increased concentration of calcium in the urinary system which leads to formation of kidney stones. Musculoskeletal pain can result from faulty posture and overuse of limbs. These disorders are described elsewhere in this book.

MEDICAL ASSESSMENT

Diagnosis

Delayed recognition of SCIs is a significant problem in emergent care of traumatic injuries, occurring in more than 20% of cases (Davis and Rao, 1994; Young, 1991b).

Lateral film studies with plain radiographs are a rapid and effective way of evaluating cervical SCIs with the ability to detect approximately 85% of such injuries (Daffner, 1993). When the open mouth ondontoid view and supine anteroposterior view are added, the accuracy rises to almost 100%. Any area that is inadequately demonstrated in the three-view spinal series is examined by computed tomography (CT). Flexion-extension studies are used primarily to evaluate instability caused by occult ligamentous injury and should not be done if there is any neurologic, bony, or soft tissue injury.

CT demonstrates soft tissue structures and allows visualization of the bony limits of the spinal canal in the axial plane. CT is superior to other diagnostic procedures in demonstrating impingement on the neuronal canal.

Myelography is indicated for optimal visualization of compression of the spinal cord after trauma. Myelography alone is rarely indicated and is used in conjunction with CT. In many cases, magnetic resonance imaging (MRI) has replaced myelography.

MRI in acute SCI is sometimes problematic because of its limited use around ferromagnetic objects such as respirators, oxygen tanks, and traction devices. When these obstacles do not exist, the extent of spinal cord damage and the possibility of disk herniation can be more readily assessed by MRI. The presence of intradural or extradural hematoma can often be demonstrated on MRI. MRI is useful in excluding spinal cord contusion or hemorrhage in persons with neurologic deficits and normal CT and plain films.

In spinal trauma with severe neural malfunction, neurophysiologic studies help in determining which neural elements are involved, which spinal segment is responsible for mechanical or other irritation, and whether the lesion is chronic, acute-progressing, or resolving. Neurophysiologic studies allow intraoperative monitoring and include somatosensory evoked potentials (SEPs); motor evoked potentials (MEPs); neurography; F-wave and H-reflex electromyography (EMG); and sympathetic skin response (SSR). SEPs and MEPs are useful in the investigation of the central nervous system. EMG, neurography, and F-wave and H-reflex studies are used for the evaluation of the peripheral component of spinal injury.

Treatment

Emergent Care

The emergent phase of care is crucial for the person with traumatic SCI (Buchanan, 1987a). It can make the difference between living the rest of one's life with a disability or recovering with only temporary neurologic deficits. An incomplete injury can be significantly worsened by mishandling. Assessment of the likelihood of SCI includes an understanding of the mechanics of the trauma and obtaining vital signs to determine if the individual is in *neurogenic shock*.[3] Movement

---

[3] The sudden disruption of the nervous system results in pooling of blood in the dependent areas of the body. This is reflected by low blood pressure and low heart rate. A person with these symptoms is considered in neurogenic shock, a medical emergency.

of the distal components of the body reflects the intactness of the spinal cord. In the case of a cervical injury, *paradoxical respiration* or abdominal breathing may be present and immediate immobilization should be instituted. Use of a rigid collar and spinal board can help to prevent movement of the spinal column. Oxygen and medication should be given to control the hyperperfusion and swelling of the spinal cord. Transport should be swift, avoiding physical jarring caused by an uneven road surface and sudden stops.

Monitoring in the critical care phase includes cardiac and neurologic status. Orthopedic management may begin at this phase and includes closed and open reduction of the vertebrae and decompression of the spinal cord.

Pharmacologic control of edema, blood flow, and secondary neurologic sequelae shows promise in current studies. Corticosteroids have shown modest results in large doses, but the side effects must be considered and studied further. Lipid peroxidation inhibitors appear to reduce metabolic derangements, protect adenosine triphosphatase (ATPase) activity, and prevent neurofilament loss. Drugs that blockade opiate receptors appear to protect the spinal cord by decreasing endotoxic and hemorrhagic shock. Preservation of spinal cord function can be achieved by modulation of the synthesis and release of neurotransmitters that are produced when there is injury to the nervous system. The dose-response curve remains narrow in most cases.

When considering the appropriate type and dose of medication given to a person with an acute SCI, the degree of SCI must be assessed accurately. A moderate injury may require control of a different set of extracellular substances than that required to control the secondary damage in a severe injury (Young, 1992a).

Experimental studies demonstrate that cooling of the spinal cord within 8 hours following trauma can preserve function. While this has worked well in animal studies, the individual with an SCI often has other complications that preclude immediate surgery. Moreover, the necessary equipment is not available in all institutions and often the injury occurs at night, when the operating room is not fully staffed (Hansebout, 1992).

Management of Complications (Buchanan, 1987b)

Management of complications of SCI is critical. High cervical injuries require immediate placement of ventilation equipment and maintenance of pulmonary hygiene. Therapy consists of intermittent positive pressure breathing (IPPB), bronchodilators, and mucolytics. Prevention of pulmonary infection is critical in SCI.

Electrophrenic respiration is now available. The phrenic nerve is implanted with a single electrode, and the client carries a transmitter to activate the lung. This works well with persons with high cervical lesions and sparing of C3–5 anterior horn cells. This method of respiration more closely mimics normal physiology than does IPPB.

Loss of autonomic nervous system control affects the function of the cardiovascular system. Acute management of blood pressure is critical. The autonomic lesion predisposes persons with high spinal cord lesions to abnormal cardiovascular responses to vasoactive agents. Management of autonomic dysreflexia involves determination of the site and nature of the initiating stimulus and alleviation of the precipitating cause. Drugs may be used to lower the blood pressure and can be chosen based on their site of action.

Treatment of spasticity includes muscle relaxants and spasmolytic agents. Drug management is usually not completely successful, and the side effects must be weighed against the benefits. The client may develop tolerance with prolonged use of one drug. Peripheral nerve blocks provide a temporary reduction of spasticity. If there is long-term severe spasticity, the contractile potential of the muscle can be modified by surgery (Schmitz, 1994).

Fetal Cell Transplants

Transplantation of fetal central nervous system cells shows promise in the treatment of SCI. A transplant of fetal spinal cord tissue may serve as a bridge to permit the regrowth of axons from spinal and supraspinal levels across the site of SCI. At the cellular level, fetal transplants may inhibit formation of glial scar at the site of injury, may inhibit toxic influences at the site of injury, and may provide the mechanism to support axonal growth across the injury site (Bregman and Kunkel-Bagden, 1994).

Pain Management

Management of neurogenic pain in SCI is by systemic or local drug therapy and by neuroaugmentative and neurodestructive intervention. The pharmacologic approach includes nonsteroidal analgesics, opioids, and antidepressants and anticonvulsants (Illis, 1992). Neuroaugmentative procedures include transcutaneous electrical nerve stimulation (TENS), epidural spinal stimulation, and central thalamic stimulation. The last-named has been used primarily in experimental studies to date. Neurodestructive procedures include both chemical and surgical destruction of nervous structures. Procedures may include deafferentation, interruption of ascending pain systems, or destruction of cells in the dorsal horn.

Rehabilitation

Rehabilitation to enhance the function and lifestyle of the SCI client is aimed at the client's achieving the ability to perform most daily tasks. Included are psychosocial adjustment, physical skills, health maintenance, and vocational and avocational adjustments. One goal of rehabilitation is to involve the client in all aspects of his or her rehabilitation, provide the information and environment to foster independence, and to have him or her work as a partner with the clinicians. Rehabilitation involves setting outcome goals, problem solving, and decision making regarding changes in future lifestyle. (See Special Implications for the Therapist 30–1.)

Prognosis

More than 90% of persons admitted to an acute care hospital for treatment of SCI are ultimately discharged home. Morbidity and mortality during the first 4 weeks following SCI are most often related to paralysis of the respiratory muscles. Long-term, urinary tract infection remains the chief cause of death, but control of sepsis has improved markedly since 1970. This is primarily due to improvement in bladder training, antibiotic treatment, control of fluid intake, and surgery of obstruction of the lower urinary tract. The second most common cause of death is respiratory disease, and this is the leading cause of death among high cervical injury clients.

Pneumonia continues at a rate higher than in the general population, with pulmonary edema associated with injuries above T6. Heart disease is common, including myocardial infarction, cardiac arrest, myocarditis, and pulmonary embolism. However, the mortality rate is not much higher than that in the general population and is improving with increased pharmacologic control and improved medical knowledge of the cardiovascular changes accompanying SCI.

Skeletal complications are related to the deformity and degenerative changes. These can lead to pain and further neurologic compromise. Overall, more than half of the spinal cord-injured population will have return of some neurologic function. Compression fractures have the most favorable prognosis for return of function, with crush fractures having the least chance for return of function (Kakulas and Taylor, 1992).

Special Implications for the Therapist **30–1**

TRAUMATIC SPINAL CORD INJURY

Mobilization of the client begins in intensive care. Emphasis here is on respiratory management, positioning and range of motion, the beginning of a strength and endurance program, and education of both the client and family about the process of therapy. The goal of early intervention is to prevent the secondary sequelae, such as pressure sores or contractures that would interfere with the rehabilitation process, and to begin to prepare the musculoskeletal system for a different method of mobility.

It is critical throughout the rehabilitation process that the therapist be cognizant of the systemic and neurologic changes that could be life-threatening, such as orthostatic hypotension and autonomic dysreflexia. Orthotic management of the unstable spinal column is often necessary, and the therapist should be familiar with the types of orthotic devices used. Figure 30–6 illustrates several orthoses used with different levels of spinal cord lesion.

As Box 30–2 demonstrates, the level of the lesion will determine the degree to which independence can be expected in certain activities. The development of wheelchair skills includes transfers, propelling the wheelchair, electric wheelchair propulsion, management of the wheelchair components, and, most important, weight shifts in the chair to prevent skin breakdown. Wheelchair adaptations are necessary for the client with weak upper extremities or poor hand control.

When possible, the client should be taught to maintain range of motion of the extremities independently. Adequate hamstring length is critical for performance of transfers and independent dressing. In determining the training program for an SCI client, there must first be an assessment of physical capabilities and skills. The therapeutic program must work toward developing the necessary range of motion, strength, and skills. Skills needed for mobility without equipment may be different from skills needed for mobility with equipment. In some cases, transfers into and out of bed can only be done with special equipment, such as a transfer board or loop ladder.

Ambulation is a priority concern for many clients with SCI. Research and experience, however, have shown that people with SCIs tend to abandon their ambulation skills after rehabilitation. Often, once the client has experienced walking and knows that it is possible, but at a much greater cost in energy, the speed and ease of the wheelchair make it a better alternative. Walking with an orthosis is not a survival skill.

Functional electrical stimulation is used to augment

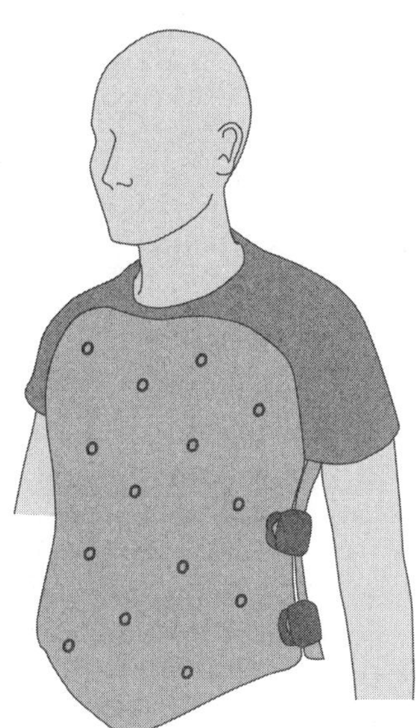

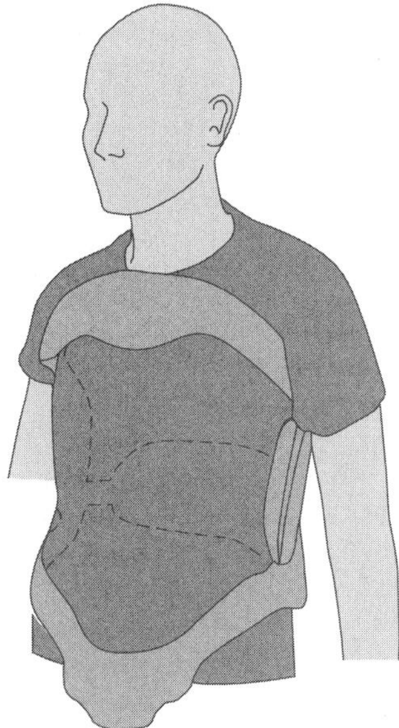

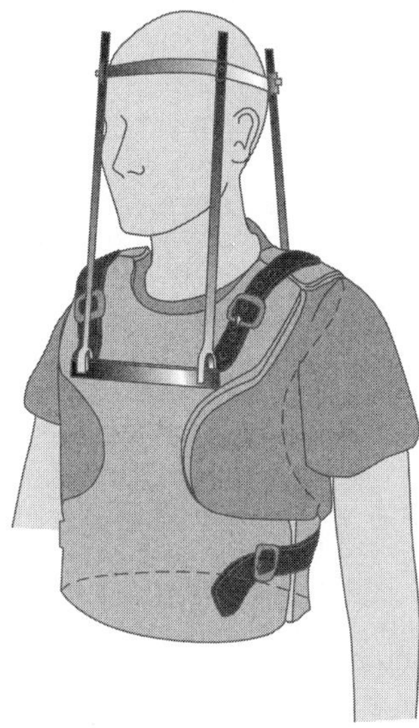

Figure **30–6.** A, Molded thoracolumbosacral orthosis, designed to control extension and rotary movements. B, Hyperextension brace, which restricts flexion in the thoracic area. C, Halo vest, which restricts upper thoracic and cervical motion.

BOX **30-2**
Disabilities Associated with Level of Injury

C1–5 Quadriplegia
Dressing
Dependent in all dressing activities
Bathing
Dependent in all bathing activities
Communication
Independent, with assistive devices for verbal (C1–3), independent verbal (C4–5)
Assistive devices necessary for keyboarding, writing, page turning, and use of telephone

C6–8 Quadriplegia
Dressing
Independent with assistive device in bed (C7) or wheelchair (C8)
Minimal assistance with lower body dressing in bed
Moderate assistance undressing lower body in bed
Clients with C8 lesions are able to dress and undress in wheelchair with assistive devices
Bathing
Minimal assistance for upper body bathing and drying
Moderate assistance for lower body drying (C6)
Independent with assistive devices (C7–8)
Assistive devices (tub chair necessary for tub or shower)
Communication
Independent in verbal communication
Assistive devices necessary for keyboard, writing, and use of telephone
Setup required (C6)

T1 and Below Paraplegia
Dressing
Independent with use of assistive device
Bathing
Independent with use of assistive device with tub bench or cushion on bottom of tub
Communication
Independent

Modified from Altrice MB, et al: Traumatic spinal cord injury. *In* Umphred DA (ed): Neurological Rehabilitation. St. Louis, Mosby–Year Book, 1995, pp 502–506.

ambulation. Several hours of supported standing and limited distances of ambulation can be part of a program to improve respiratory control and loading of the joints with the use of multisite stimulation. For example, stimulation of the common peroneal nerve can facilitate the flexor swing movement, and stimulation of the upper portion of the hamstring and gluteus can facilitate the stance phase. Stimulation of the lower portion of the hamstring and quadriceps can support correction of knee hyperextension (genu recurvatum) (Dimitrijevic and Dimitrijevic, 1992). The use of functional electrical stimulation remains experimental for the most part, but it is gaining more clinical use as the equipment becomes more sophisticated and as understanding of motor control increases.

For further information, see Somers, 1992; Altrice et al., 1995.

References

Altrice MB, Gonter M, Griffin DA, et al: Traumatic spinal cord injury. *In* Umphred DA (ed): Neurological Rehabilitation. St Louis, Mosby–Year Book, 1995, pp 484–529.

Bregman BS, Kunkel-Bagden.: Potential mechanisms underlying transplant mediated recovery of junction after spinal cord injury. *In* Marwah J, Tietelbaum H, Prasad KN (eds): Neural Transplantation, CNS Injury, and Regeneration. Boca Raton, Fla, CRC Press, 1994, pp 81–102.

Buchanan LE: Acute care: Medical/surgical management. *In* Buchanan LE, Nawoczenski DA (eds): Spinal Cord Injury. Baltimore, Williams & Wilkins, 1987a, pp 35–60.

Buchanan LE: Emergency care. *In* Buchanan LE, Nawoczenski DA (eds): Spinal Cord Injury. Baltimore, Williams & Wilkins, 1987b, pp 21–34.

Daffner RH: Imaging of thoracic and lumbar vertebral fractures. *In* Floman YF, Farcy JC, Argenson CA (eds): Thoracolumbar Spine Fractures. New York, Raven Press, 1993, pp 69–98.

Davis P, Rao KC: Spine trauma. *In* Rao KC, Williams JP, Lee BC, et al (eds): MRI and CT of the Spine. Baltimore, Williams & Wilkins, 1994, pp 277–346.

Dimitrijevic MM, Dimitrijevic MR: Clinical practice of functional electrical stimulation. *In* Illis LS (ed): Spinal Cord Dysfunction: Vol 2, Intervention and Treatment. Oxford, Oxford University Press, 1992, pp 168–174.

Farcy JC, Rawlins BA: Physiology and pathophysiology of the neural elements. *In* Floman YF, Farcy JC, Argenson CA (eds): Thoracolumbar Spine Fractures. New York, Raven Press, 1993, pp 35–44.

Hansebout RR: Spinal injury and spinal cord blood-flow: The effect of early treatment and local cooling. *In* Illis LS (ed): Spinal Cord Dysfunction: Vol 2, Intervention and Treatment. Oxford, Oxford University Press, 1992, pp 58–78.

Illis LS: Spasticity: Clinical aspects. *In* Illis LS (ed): Spinal Cord Dysfunction: Vol 2, Intervention and Treatment. Oxford, Oxford University Press, 1992, pp 81–93.

Illis LS: Central pain. *In* Illis LS (ed): Spinal Cord Dysfunction: Vol 2, Intervention and Treatment. Oxford, Oxford University Press, 1992, pp 145–155.

Kakulas BA, Taylor JR: Pathology of injuries of the vertebral column and spinal cord. *In* Vinken PJ, Bruyn GW, Klawans HL (eds): Spinal Cord Trauma. Amsterdam, Elsevier Science Publishers, 1992, pp 21–54.

Lindsey KW, Bone I, Callander R: Neurology and Neurosurgery Illustrated. New York, Churchill Livingstone, 1986, pp 188.

Nawoczenski DA, Rinehart ME, Duncanson P, Brown BE. Physical management. *In* Buchanan LE, Nawoczenski DA (eds): Spinal Cord Injury. Baltimore, Williams & Wilkins, 1987, pp 123–184.

Rägnarsson KT: Rehabilitation principles in the management of thoracolumbar spine fractures. *In* Floman YF, Farcy JC, Argenson CA (eds): Thoracolumbar Spine Fractures. New York, Raven Press, 1993, pp 463–485.

Schmitz TJ: Traumatic spinal cord injury. *In* Schmitz TJ, O'Sullivan SB (eds): Physical Rehabilitation Assessment and Treatment, ed 3. Philadelphia, FA Davis, 1994, pp 533–575.

Schneider FJ: Traumatic spinal cord injury. *In* Umphred DA (ed): Neurological Rehabilitation, ed 2. St Louis, Mosby–Year Book, 1990.

Schneider JW, Gabriel KL: Congenital spinal cord injury. *In* Umphred DA (ed): Neurological Rehabilitation, ed 2. St Louis, Mosby–Year Book, 1990, pp 397–422.

Somers MF: Spinal Cord Injury: Functional Rehabilitation. Norwalk, Conn, Appleton & Lange, 1992.

Waxman SG, deGroot J: Correlative Neuroanatomy, ed 22. Norwalk, Conn, Appleton & Lange, 1995.

Williams B: Post-traumatic syringomyelia (cystic myelopathy). *In* Vinken PJ, Bruyn GW, Klawans HL (eds): Spinal Cord Trauma. Amsterdam, Elsevier, 1992, pp 375–394.

Young W: Clinical trials and experimental therapies of spinal cord injury. *In* Vinken PJ, Bruyn GW, Klawans HL (eds): Spinal Cord Trauma. Amsterdam, Elsevier, 1992a, pp 399–420.

Young W: Neurophysiology of spinal cord injury. *In* Errico TJ, Bauer RD, Waugh T (eds): Spinal Trauma. Philadelphia, JB Lippincott, 1991a, pp 377–414.

Young W: Pharmacologic therapy of acute spinal cord injury. *In* Errico TJ, Bauer RD, Waugh T (eds): Spinal Trauma. Philadelphia, JB Lippincott, 1991b, pp 415–434.

Young W: Therapy for acute spinal cord injury *In* Illis LS (ed): Spinal Cord Dysfunction: Vol 2, Intervention and Treatment. Oxford, Oxford University Press, 1992b, pp 28–58.

chapter 31

Epilepsy

Kenda S. Fuller

There is a fundamental difference between seizure and epilepsy. A *seizure* is a finite event; it has a beginning and an end. *Epilepsy* is defined as a chronic disorder of various causes characterized by recurrent seizures due to excessive discharge of cerebral neurons. Seizures can be induced in any normal human brain with a variety of different electrical or chemical stimuli. The cerebral cortex in particular contains within its anatomic and physiologic structure a mechanism that is inherently unstable and capable of producing a seizure. Seizures are the result of many different underlying physiologic states and therefore there is no single pathognomonic lesion of the brain that causes them. Seizures are commonly divided into two groups, partial and generalized. Some classifications include a third group, partial seizures progressing to generalized seizures. Figure 31–1 shows the seizure types, the typical area of the brain in which the seizure begins, and where it may travel.

DEFINITION

Partial Seizures

Partial seizures have clinical or electroencephalographic (EEG) evidence of a local onset. The abnormal discharge usually arises in a portion of one hemisphere and may spread to other parts of the brain during a seizure. The syndrome is characterized by the locus of onset of the attacks. The seizures are identified as *temporal*, *frontal*, *parietal*, or *occipital*. This group encompasses the most frequent and severe epilepsy problems of adults. Partial seizures can be subdivided into three groups: simple partial seizures, complex partial seizures, and partial seizures which secondarily generalize.

Simple partial seizures are associated with preservation of consciousness and unilateral hemispheric involvement. They may be manifested by focal motor symptoms (jerking) or by somatosensory symptoms (paresthesias or tingling) that spread to different parts of the body. Light flashes, buzzing, or abnormal sensations of taste and smell represent involvement in the areas of the brain that control visual, auditory, or olfactory or gustatory responses. Sometimes there are autonomic or psychotic responses to seizure activity.

Complex partial seizures are associated with alteration or loss of consciousness and bilateral hemispheric involvement. Automatic behaviors, without conscious control, may be manifest.

A *partial seizure secondarily generalized* is a generalized tonic-clonic seizure that develops from either a simple partial seizure or a complex partial seizure.

Generalized Seizures

In a *generalized seizure* there is no evidence of localized onset and the brain shows diffuse EEG abnormalities.

Absence seizures (petit mal) consist of the sudden cessation of ongoing conscious activity with only minor convulsive muscular activity or loss of postural control. Onset and termination of attacks are abrupt. If attacks occur during conversation, the person may miss a few words or may break off in midsentence for a few seconds. The person is unaware of the loss of conscious control. *Atypical absence seizures* are similar to absence seizures but coexist with other forms of generalized seizures.

Myoclonic seizures are sudden, brief, single, or repetitive muscle contractions involving one body part or the entire body. *Atonic seizures* are brief losses of consciousness and postural tone not associated with tonic muscular contractions.

Tonic-clonic (grand mal) seizure is the archetypal seizure, which means total loss of control. The seizure begins with a sudden loss of consciousness, and falls are common. Generalized rigidity (tonic phase) is soon followed by very rapid generalized jerking movements (the clonic stage). In adults there may be incontinence of bowel and bladder. In the tonic phase respiration can cease briefly. Recovery may be swift after a short seizure, but a prolonged seizure may induce a deep sleep. Altered speech and transient paralysis or ataxia may follow, as well as headache, disorientation, or muscle soreness. Another seizure may follow without recovery of consciousness or, after recovery of consciousness, the person may seize again. *Epilepsy with continuous spike waves during slow-wave sleep* is a generalized tonic-clonic seizure which is typical in persons who have an epileptic pattern during slow-wave sleep (Porter and Theodore, 1995).

Epilepsies of Infancy and Childhood *(O'Donohoe, 1994)*

Infantile spasms represent a nonspecific reaction on the part of the brain to a wide variety of insults. It is likely that the condition is more age-specific than disease-specific. It is generally agreed that infants who develop spasms demonstrate a cessation of normal psychological development and frequently show developmental deterioration that relates to the frequency of the spasms.

Severe myoclonic epilepsy of infancy is a syndrome of early normal development followed by treatment-resistant seizures of various types and by psychomotor retardation, usually beginning around 5 to 6 months of age. These attacks are often long and may include status epilepticus. Mental retardation is noted in all cases. *Benign myoclonic epilepsy in infancy* results in bursts of myoclonus in the first or second year of life. There is usually no evidence of prior brain abnormality.

Lennox-Gastaut syndrome usually begins between 1 and 6 years of age. The most common seizures are atonic-akinetic, resulting in loss of postural tone. Violent falls occur suddenly with immediate recovery and resumption of activity, the attack lasting less than 1 second. Injuries to the head and face

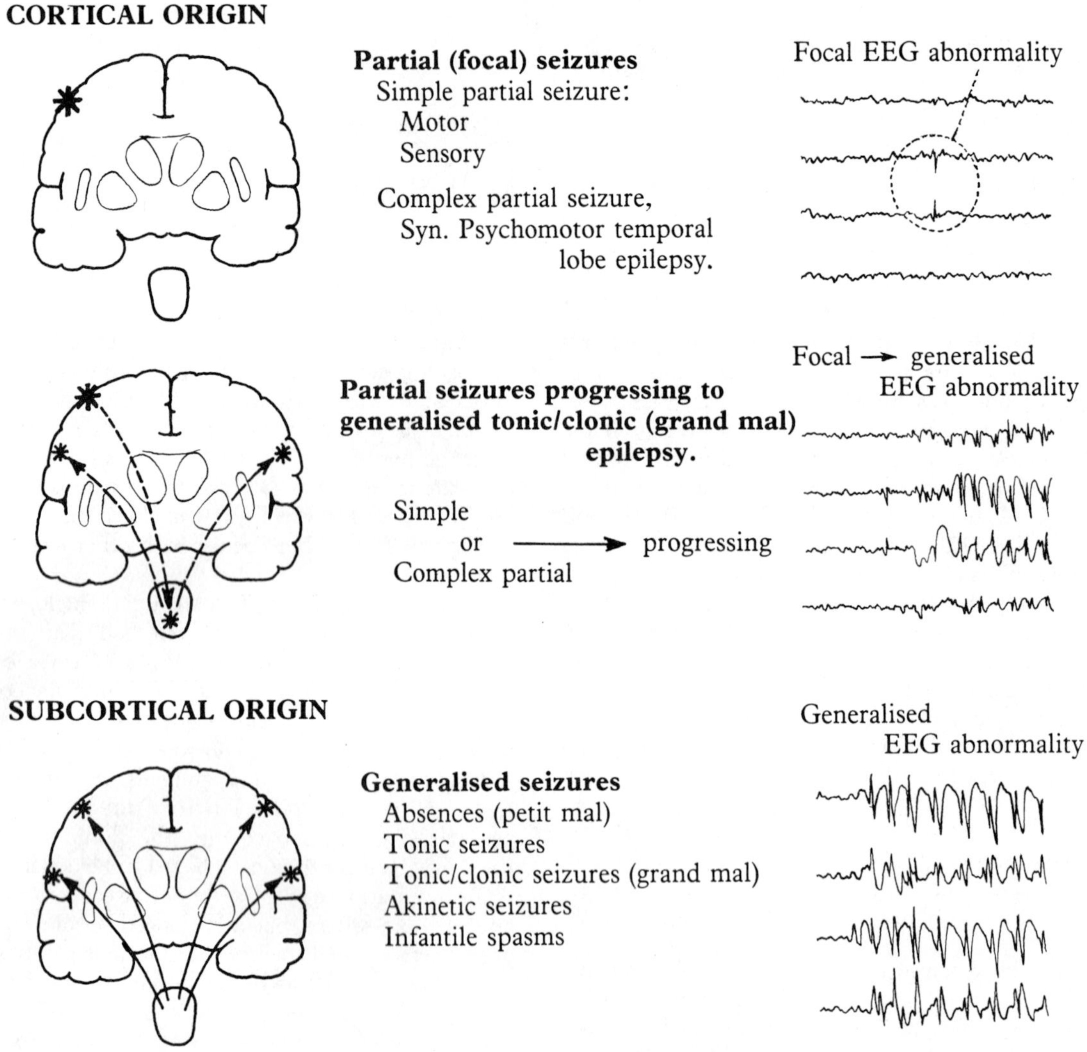

CORTICAL ORIGIN

Partial (focal) seizures
Simple partial seizure:
Motor
Sensory
Complex partial seizure,
Syn. Psychomotor temporal lobe epilepsy.

Focal EEG abnormality

Partial seizures progressing to generalised tonic/clonic (grand mal) epilepsy.

Simple or Complex partial → progressing

Focal → generalised EEG abnormality

SUBCORTICAL ORIGIN

Generalised seizures
Absences (petit mal)
Tonic seizures
Tonic/clonic seizures (grand mal)
Akinetic seizures
Infantile spasms

Generalised EEG abnormality

Figure **31–1.** The nature of the attack is used to classify seizure types. (*From Lindsay KW, Bone I, Callander R: Neurology and Neurosurgery Illustrated. New York, Churchill Livingstone, 1986, p 88.*)

are common. Tonic attacks consist of sudden flexion of the head and trunk. Clusters of attacks are common, followed by automatic behavior. Consciousness is usually clouded rather than completely lost. Neurologic abnormalities such as spasticity are common in the severely affected patients.

Acquired epileptic aphasia (Landau-Kleffner syndrome) is characterized by an acquired aphasia in the absence of other neurologic abnormalities. Often epileptic seizures and psychomotor disturbances develop at the same time or shortly afterward. This disorder often begins between 3 and 9 years of age. The age of onset is critical for the long-term loss of language. It is postulated that recently acquired skills are particularly vulnerable to any disturbance of brain function. Since there appear to be optimal periods of language learning in children, if the formation of intracerebral connections is prevented for any reason, such as by the abnormal neuronal firings of epilepsy, during certain periods of life, then such connections may never become functional and the ability to develop language is lost.

Benign childhood epilepsy with centrotemporal spikes typically occurs between the ages of 3 and 13 and is characterized by brief, simple partial hemifacial motor seizures. *Childhood epilepsy with occipital paroxysms* is a syndrome similar to benign childhood epilepsy with centrotemporal spikes, but it includes visual symptoms at onset and some children have associated migraine headache.

Childhood absence epilepsy begins between 4 and 10 years of age. The attacks may occur many times a day. The attacks were previously described as petit mal, and are characterized by a blank stare with unresponsiveness. The attacks last for between 10 and 45 seconds.

Juvenile myoclonic epilepsy has its onset in early adolescence and begins with early morning jerks of the head, neck, and upper limbs. These may be so violent that objects are thrown to the ground. Consciousness is unimpaired and there is no mental retardation. The attacks occasionally progress to generalized tonic-clonic seizures.

Febrile convulsions, a result of fever, occur in young children who have a susceptibility to convulse in a setting of acute fever. They are rare before 6 months and after 5 years of age. The typical febrile convulsion is brief, generalized, and tonic-clonic in sequence, and the body temperature is high. They occur more frequently when the child is asleep. The convulsion is often the first indication that the child is ill, since 90% of all seizures occur in the first 24 hours of fever. The rise in temperature, which may be due to increased oxygen demands on cerebral oxidative mechanisms, may be the most important factor.

Severe febrile seizures are most often unilateral, and there is a possibility of permanent brain damage, with the development of epilepsy, if the seizure lasts more than 30 minutes.

BOX **31–1**
Causes of Symptomatic Seizure Activity

Head trauma
Intracranial mass
CNS infections
Cerebrovascular disorders
Toxic substances or poisons
Congenital brain defects
Hypoxia
Degenerative brain disorders

INCIDENCE

The prevalence and incidence of epilepsy are difficult to establish because of problems with diagnosis and reporting. The prevalence of active cases is estimated to be between 0.5% and 2.0% (Gumnit, 1995).

Persons presenting with seizures may have almost any disease of the central nervous system (CNS), including some in which imaging studies are normal. Seizures are often the first symptom of an intracranial mass. Head trauma is the most common preventable cause of epilepsy. More than 3000 cases of epilepsy are added every year to the US population because of head injury. Arteriosclerotic cerebrovascular disease is the most common cause of seizures in persons over the age of 50 and often accompanies a stroke (Schnell, 1993).

Although seizure activity in children is rare, at less than 1%, seizures are the most frequent symptoms requiring medical attention in the infant. It has been estimated that 75% of cases of epilepsy have their onset before 20 years of age. Epilepsy in childhood is much more than simply a matter of having seizures. Those affected are vulnerable medically and educationally, and they often face considerable social difficulties as a result of their seizures (O'Donohoe, 1994).

ETIOLOGY AND RISK FACTORS

In a substantial proportion of persons, the cause of the seizures remains undetected. This group of seizures is known as *idiopathic epilepsy*. Genetic factors play a role and seven epilepsy genes have been identified to date. One such gene, for juvenile myoclonic epilepsy, has been located on chromosome 6. This genetic predisposition to seizure activity may explain why one individual with brain damage develops epilepsy while another with similar damage does not develop seizure activity (Porter and Theodore, 1995).

Subclinical infection may be the cause of epilepsy in persons with seizures of unknown origin. With the eventual identification of various agents that can cause disease without overt evidence of inflammation, and with the observation that many viruses are present in latent form in humans, the ability to determine the cause of the seizures may become possible.

The causes of *symptomatic epilepsy* are multiple, and the symptoms may be transient, resolving following treatment of the primary disorder. Box 31–1 describes some of the causes of symptomatic epilepsy. Epilepsy can be caused by virtually any major category of serious disease or disorder of humans. It can result from congenital malformations, infections, tumors, vascular disease, degenerative diseases, or injury. When the seizure is due to a permanent lesion or scar, the seizure activity may persist (Schnell, 1993).

The age-dependent appearance of spontaneous seizures in the primary epilepsies appears to depend on a critical period in cerebral maturation when the genetically determined defect is expressed clinically as a manifest change in behavior. It is believed now that there are changes known as *microdysgenesis* in the brains of these persons. These changes include an increase in cell density, abnormal arrangements of cortical neurons, and an increase in white matter neurons (O'Donohoe, 1994).

Seizures may occur in the neonatal period, within the first 24 to 72 hours, and they are usually of focal cerebral origin. The seizure type relates to the level of development of the brain. The seizures tend to be contralateral, due to the immaturity of the forebrain and corpus callosum, limiting movement from one hemisphere to the other. Seizure activity represents the relative development of the limbic system, diencephalon, and brainstem. Hypoxic-ischemic brain insult is the most common cause of neonatal convulsions and is due to compromise of oxygen to the brain during or prior to delivery. Seizures resulting from cerebral contusion are often a result of prolonged or traumatic labor.

The other important cause of seizures arising in the early neonatal period is hypoglycemia, most often seen in babies who are small for gestational age. The neurologic symptoms of hypoglycemia consist of irritability, drowsiness, hypotonia, and apnea. Approximately half of the babies with hypoglycemia develop neurologic symptoms, and about one fourth of these go on to develop seizures.

Hypocalcemia (serum count below 7 mg/dL) may occur in the first 2 to 3 days of life either in low-birth-weight infants or in association with the complications of birth asphyxia. It may then contribute to seizures but is rarely the primary cause. Hypercalcemia occurring at age 6 to 8 days is usually the primary cause of the clinical features of neonatal tetany, including jitteriness and jaw, knee, and ankle clonus. Hypocalcemia is rare in infants who are breastfed or fed formula created to simulate human milk. Hypernatremia, due to alteration in sodium level, may also lead to neonatal seizures. Hypernatremia is associated with dehydrating illnesses.

PATHOGENESIS

Epileptic seizures result from the sudden, excessive, electrical discharges of large aggregates of neurons. Epilepsy involves variations of the normal physiochemical mechanisms of nerve cells. Epileptogenesis depends on the predisposition of neuronal aggregates of discharge when stimulated and on synchronization of firing of many neurons in a localized area of the brain within the neuronal substrate.

The neuronal membrane potential depends on its selective permeability to different ions. For most synapses the transmitter-receptor complex acts as a gate regulating the permeability of the postsynaptic membrane, with resulting inhibition or excitation (see Chapter 24). It appears that the epileptic discharge is limited to a localized area of the cortex by a ring of inhibition. As the discharges become synchronic and a seizure is initiated, neurons in contiguous and synaptically connected distant areas become part of the seizure.

A common mechanism by which seizures can develop in the brain is decreased inhibition. Another possible explanation of the abnormal potentiation has been linked to a glutamate analogue, *N*-methyl-D-aspartate (NMDA), which is thought to be involved in the excitatory process of epileptogenesis. The NMDA complex is a potential mechanism whereby recurrent epileptic events could induce widespread alterations in neuronal functions (O'Donohoe, 1994).

Another potential explanation of the facilitation of seizures is *kindling*. In the experimental animal model, repeated brain exposures to localized repetitive low-intensity electrical stimuli induce increasingly pathologic responses. This gradual alteration in brain function, once induced, is permanent. While it is not certain that kindling occurs in humans, it remains a possible mechanism for the latent period that exists between the occurrence of a brain insult and the later onset of epilepsy.

Chronic focal epileptogenic lesions can cause distant areas to become capable of generating abnormal electrical discharges and seizures. This focus continues to function independently even after ablation of the primary lesion, a fact which has important implications for the surgical treatment of epilepsy.

CLINICAL MANIFESTATIONS

Signs and Symptoms

In most individuals, seizures occur unpredictably at any time and without any relationship to posture or ongoing activities (Schnell, 1993; Porter and Theodore, 1995). In some individuals, seizures are provoked by specific stimuli such as flashing lights or a flickering television. The presence of focal signs after the seizure suggests that the seizure may have a focal origin. Prodromal symptoms (premonitory symptoms that indicate an impending seizure) may include headache, mood alterations, lethargy, and myoclonic jerking.

In the *tonic phase* of a tonic-clonic seizure, the body becomes rigid and the person is at risk of falling. A cry may be uttered, and the person may become cyanotic. In general the jaw is fixed and the hands are clenched. This phase usually lasts for 30 to 60 seconds. The *clonic phase* begins with rhythmic, jerky contractions and relaxation of all body muscles, especially in the extremities. Figure 31–2 demonstrates the tonic and clonic phases of seizure. Biting of the tongue, lips, or inside of the mouth may occur. Saliva is blown from the mouth, with a froth appearing on the lips.

Minor motor seizures are reflected by involuntary jerking of the major muscles (myoclonic), momentary loss of muscle movement (akinetic), or total loss of muscle tone, which causes the person to fall to the floor (atonic).

Status epilepticus is a condition in which seizures are so prolonged or so repeated that recovery does not occur between attacks. Convulsive status epilepticus occurs when the person has generalized tonic-clonic seizures and there is no return to consciousness between seizures. It is a medical emergency. The molecular events that cause death can occur with the first few seizures. Tonic-clonic status epilepticus is more common in persons whose seizures have a known cause. Often it is the result of tumor, CNS infection, or drug abuse. Febrile seizures are a common cause of status epilepticus in children under the age of 3 years.

Nonconvulsive status epilepticus is difficult to define, but it may be described as a syndrome in which the most fundamental feature is a change in the individual's behavior. There is usually a degree of clouding of mental processes, ranging from drowsiness and confusion to disorientation and dysphagia.

MEDICAL MANAGEMENT

Diagnosis *(O'Donohoe, 1994)*

The history obtained from the client and the observations of bystanders are of importance in establishing a diagnosis and classifying the seizure disorder correctly. To determine seizure type, a series of questions must be answered regarding the location of the seizure activity, the level of consciousness, the level of generalized motor activity, and the preceding level of seizure activity. The state of the client after the episode, including the level of confusion, sleepiness, or headache must be determined.

The EEG has a central role in the diagnosis of epilepsy. The EEG records the integrated electrical activity generated by synaptic potentials in neurons in the superficial layers of a localized area of cortex. In the epileptic focus, neurons in a small area of the cortex are activated for a brief period in a synchronized pattern and then inhibited. Interictal (between seizure) activity on the EEG provides strong presumptive evidence that the event was a seizure. The best way to diagnose the presence of seizures and to classify the seizure is to observe, simultaneously, the seizure and the EEG recording.

Specialized neuropsychological testing is often needed in evaluating clients with seizures. These tests not only help to determine general intelligence and state of brain functioning but also often help to localize lesions.

Metabolic studies are ideally performed at the time of the seizure occurrence, when they are most likely to be abnormal. Glucose level and electrolyte studies, including measurements of calcium and magnesium, are indicated.

A radiographic examination of the brain is indicated to rule out mass effect or vascular disease. Magnetic resonance imaging (MRI) is the method of choice, as the lesions that cause epilepsy are often subtle.

Treatment

Control of seizures is paramount in the treatment of epilepsy, but it is only part of the treatment. Support and education provided by health-care professionals is critical to amelioration of the behavioral, social, and economic consequences of uncontrolled seizures.

Antiepileptic medications are used first in nearly all cases.

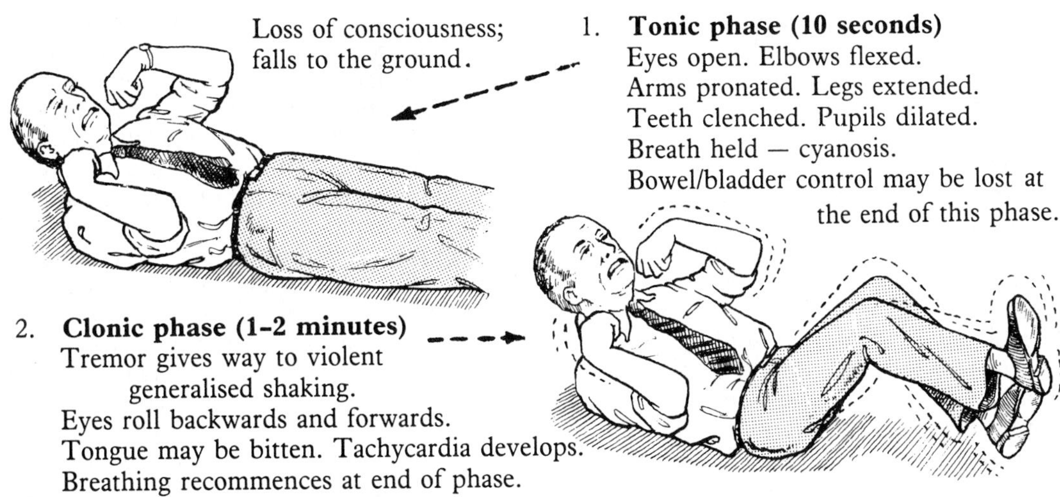

Figure **31–2.** Tonic and clonic phases of seizure activity. (*From Lindsay KW, Bone I, Callander R: Neurology and Neurosurgery Illustrated. New York, Churchill Livingstone, 1986, p 91.*)

The drug of choice is related to the type of seizure. See Box 31–2 for a list of drugs related to seizure type. In most persons with seizures of a single type, satisfactory control can be achieved with a single anticonvulsant drug. Treatment with more than two types of drugs is almost always unsuccessful unless the individual has more than one type of seizure. Monitoring of plasma drug levels has increased the ability to maintain the drug at the maximal tolerated dose. Dose adjustments are carefully monitored, and noncompliance can be identified. In persons who do not comply with the drug regimen, no drug may be better than an inconsistent dosage (Aminoff, 1994).

When drug therapy does not control the seizures or drugs become toxic at effective dosages, then surgical treatment is indicated. Lobectomies, cortical resections, and sectioning of the corpus callosum are the types of surgeries most often performed. *Hemispherectomies*, the removal of one of the hemispheres, can be effective for the severe, uncontrollable seizures usually found in children.

Many persons with epilepsy experience a higher frequency of seizures with large doses of caffeine. Amphetamines and other stimulants should be avoided and some asthma drugs can increase the incidence of seizure activity.

There is some evidence that biofeedback and conditioning techniques are effective in helping to control epilepsy in some persons (Gumnit, 1995).

BOX **31–2**
Anticonvulsant Medications

Generalized Tonic-Clonic or Partial Seizures
Phenytoin (Dilantin)
Carbamazepine (Tegretol)
Valproate (Depakene)
Phenobarbital
Primidone (Mysoline)
Benzodiazepines
  Diazepam (Valium)
  Clonazepam (Klonopin)

Absence Seizures
Ethosuximide (Zarontin)
Valproate (Depakene)
Clonazepam (Klonopin)

Myoclonic Seizures
Valproate (Depakene)
Phenytoin (Dilantin)
Clonazepam (Klonopin)

Prognosis

The danger to life in epilepsy is not great. However, with status epilepticus, 3% of children and 10% of adults die during an attack (Porter and Theodore, 1995).

Death from asphyxia is the greatest concern in instances when the individual has a seizure during eating or when breathing passages are compromised during the seizure or in postepileptic insensibility. Drowning during a seizure has been documented and remains a serious consequence of swimming or bathing alone (Gumnit, 1995).

In persons with epilepsy of no known cause, and a diagnosis made before 10 years of age, there is a 75% remission rate (defined as 5 seizure-free years). A child with epilepsy who has been free of seizures for more than 4 years on antiepileptic drugs has about a 70% chance of remaining in permanent remission when the drugs are withdrawn.

Chronic epilepsy is more likely when there is associated neurologic impairment at birth, when the seizures begin before 2 years of age, and when complex partial seizures are predominant (O'Donohoe, 1994).

Special Implications for the Therapist **31–1**

EPILEPSY

The client who is seizing will normally only need protection from injury in the environment. The therapist should make sure that there are no objects in the immediate area that can be knocked onto the person, and that the individual with seizure activity is lying on a surface that would prevent a fall. Rolling the person onto his or her side may help to keep the airway clear. Observation of physical manifestations, respiratory status, focal or general status, and duration of the seizure are important to the ongoing medical management. When the seizure appears to be generalized, observation of frothing at the mouth, deviation of the eyes, and incontinence will add information for the health practitioners attempting to control the client medically.

If the individual develops status epilepticus, emergency measures must be taken. Irreversible brain damage can result from hypoxia and therefore an airway must be established, possibly through endotracheal intubation. Medication to suppress the CNS given at this point usually includes diazepam or lorazepam, and this is usually effective in controlling the seizure. If the seizure continues, phenobarbital may be administered, and if that is not successful, general anesthesia may be given, and the person may then require ventilatory assistance (Schnell, 1993; Aminoff, 1994).

For the therapist treating a client with epilepsy, it is important to have an understanding of the triggering activities associated with seizure activity. Knowing the type and frequency of seizures will help the therapist to make recommendations regarding activities that can be engaged in safely. If compliance with the medication regimen appears to be a problem, the therapist should give the family information regarding the need to maintain consistent dosages.

If the client is in a work or school setting, the therapist can make specific recommendations to the client's employer or teacher. Side effects of medication can slow cognitive function or alter reaction time. The client sometimes needs to be encouraged to become part of the group activity. Too often, the client has been discouraged from engaging in sports or leisure activities even when the seizures are controlled. When there is a potential safety hazard, the therapist is well suited to recommend adaptations to equipment or the environment to maintain safety. Swimming can even be enjoyed as long as it is supervised directly.

Side effects of medication can produce movement disorders, namely *nystagmus,* rapid movement of the eye; *ataxia,* or inability to control balance in gait; and *dysarthria,* or speech or language disturbance. Lethargy, nausea, irritability, and skin rashes may be due to intolerance to medication. When these symptoms are noted during intervention, the proper health-care worker should be notified. The client and family should have a clear understanding about symptoms related to toxicity or nontherapeutic doses of medication.

Seizures often occur after activity, and so safety measures should be considered even after the activity is finished. Loss of fluids from to sweating during exercise can affect the serum blood levels of medication and increase the metabolism of liver enzymes. Decisions about whether to engage in vigorous activity should be made on the basis of whether seizures are controlled by medication, and only after close monitoring of blood levels of medication after exercise.

References

Aminoff MJ: Nervous system. *In* Tierney LM, McPhee SJ, Papadakis MA: Current Medical Diagnosis and Treatment. Norwalk, Conn, Appleton & Lange, 1994, pp 803–807.

Gumnit RJ: The Epilepsy Handbook: The Practical Management of Seizures, ed 2. New York, Raven Press, 1995.

O'Donohoe NV: Epilepsies of Childhood, ed 3. Oxford: Butterworth-Heinemann, 1994.

Porter RJ, Theodore WH: Epilepsy: 100 elementary principles. Philadelphia, WB Saunders, 1995.

Schnell SS: Nursing care of clients with cerebral disorders. *In* Black JM, Matassarin-Jacobs E (eds): Luckmann and Sorensen's Medical-Surgical Nursing, ed 4. Philadelphia, WB Saunders, 1993, pp 705–771.

SECTION 4

chapter 32

Headache

Kenda S. Fuller

Headache is a common complaint in the history of clients receiving therapy. It is difficult to evaluate; the intensity, quality, and site of pain may provide clues, although there is rarely an underlying structural cause. The duration of the headache and associated neurologic symptoms provide some insight into the origin of the headache. For the therapist, having an understanding of the cause, precipitating factors, and typical course of chronic headache pain is important in order to determine the intervention that will best suit the individual. Although pathologic conditions account for only a few cases of headache pain, it is critical for the therapist to understand what mechanisms may be responsible and when the client may need medical or emergent care. Table 32–1 lists some of the causes of headache that may require immediate medical attention.

A sudden onset of severe headache is usually related to an intracranial disorder such as subarachnoid hemorrhage, brain tumor, or meningitis. These headaches will most often be accompanied by other neurologic signs such as weakness, visual disturbances, and, possibly, altered mental status or coma. A structural lesion is suspected in headaches that disrupt sleep, are triggered by exertion, or cause excessive drowsiness. Headaches can also be associated with systemic illness, fever, and increased blood pressure. Headaches of this kind resolve when the underlying cause is successfully treated.

Chronic headaches of a secondary nature are less likely to be due to a disease or disorder of the brain. These chronic headaches can be a result of cervical joint or soft tissue dysfunction, misalignment of dentures or of the temporomandibular joint, or the result of ocular disorders. Sinusitis and other general medical disorders can have headache as a symptom. Headaches of this nature will be controlled by the management of the underlying cause. Headache with hypertension is rare except with grossly high, episodic hypertension which can give rise to throbbing headache in the occipital region.

Posttraumatic headache is seen often in the clinic as a secondary complaint. This headache is localized to the site of injury, or may be generalized with varying intensity. These headaches are made worse by emotional disturbances, often accompanied by vertigo with change of position, and the client complains of irritability, lack of concentration, and inability to tolerate alcohol. These symptoms are consistent with some of the other chronic headache types but are more difficult to monitor and treat.

The most problematic of headaches are the primary chronic headaches that are episodic and relate to underlying changes in the nervous system that are not clearly understood. The symptoms, once triggered, may be difficult to manage. Included here are the chronic migraine, cluster, and tension headaches. Figure 32–1 illustrates the pain patterns associated with these headache types (Dalessio and Silberstein, 1993).

MIGRAINE

Overview and Definition

Migraine is usually confined to one side of the head, is throbbing, and is episodic. The pain associated with migraine is associated with a change in the vasculature in the brain. Headaches can be classified as *migraine without aura*, sometimes called common migraine, or *migraine with aura*, referred to as classic migraine, reflecting an episode of neurologic changes which appear prior to the onset of the headache.[1] The subset of migraine with aura includes complicated migraine, hemiplegic migraine, basilar migraine, and migraine aura without headache. Ophthalmoplegic migraine is another migraine type, which includes extraocular paralysis (Davidoff, 1995).

Incidence

Migraine is now estimated to afflict 25% of the female population and 8% of the male population, a much higher prevalence than most early studies indicated. It is probable that most cases of migraine are undiagnosed. About 45% of cases of migraine emerge during childhood or adolescence. In the remaining 55% of migraineurs, the first attack generally develops before the age of 40 years. Migraine headaches are estimated to appear earlier in males than in females, and in both sexes migraine with aura is more inclined to develop at an earlier age than migraine without aura (Davidoff, 1995).

Etiology and Risk Factors

Almost all clinical and epidemiologic investigations indicate that adult women are at greater risk for the development of migraine than adult men. For women the frequency of headache is highest during their reproductive years, when the estrogen levels are higher. For men the frequency does not appreciably change between ages 20 and 65 years.

An intrinsic biologic substrate, presumably genetic, predisposes certain people to develop migraine. There is a positive family history of migraine in about 60% of cases, which suggests a hereditary factor. However, the patterns of migraine inheritance are complex, both in the mode of inheritance of migraine and in the role of genetic factors in the pathogenesis.

[1] The headache may be preceded by a short period of depression, irritability, restlessness, or anorexia, and in some persons by flashing lights, visual field defects, and paresthesias. These symptoms may disappear shortly before the headache appears or may merge with it.

TABLE 32-1 PATHOLOGIC CONDITIONS CAUSING HEADACHE

PATHOLOGIC CONDITION	SIGNS AND SYMPTOMS
Subdural hematoma	Mild to severe, intermittent headache; neurologic symptoms include fluctuating consciousness
Subarachnoid hemorrhage	Sudden onset, severe and constant headache, elevated blood pressure; can cause change in consciousness
Increased cranial pressure	Mild to severe headache; neurologic symptoms include hemiparesis, visual changes, and brainstem symptoms, including vomiting, altered consciousness
Meningitis, viral and bacterial	Headache severe with radiation down neck; acutely ill and febrile; positive Kernig's sign
Brain abscess	Mild to severe headache; local or distant infection; may be afebrile; neurologic signs consistent with local site of infection
Central nervous system neoplasm	Localized headache and focal neurologic symptoms; often see cranial nerve symptoms
Toxicity	Generalized headache, pulsating; may show other signs of toxicity
Sinusitis	Frontal or dull headache, usually worse in A.M.; increased pain in cold damp air; nasal discharge
Otitis media, mastoiditis	Feeling of fullness in ear, stabbing pains in head, vertigo, tinnitus, often acutely ill

Twin studies show mixed results. Although there is a higher prevalence of migraine in the maternal line of relatives than in the paternal line, X-linked transmission has been excluded because of the fact of male-to-male transmission. There is evidence that migraine may be inherited as an autosomal dominant trait with partial penetrance or as an autosomal recessive trait. The failure to identify a simple genetic mechanism does not rule out genetic determinants of migraine, but it suggests either that not all migraine syndromes are genetically equivalent or that environmental factors also play a significant role. At one time it was believed that there were personality traits associated with migraine, or a "migraine personality." Migraine appears in all personality types. It may be that a subset of migraineurs have a low pain threshold and seek medical help more often than migraineurs who self-medicate or adjust better to their migraine symptoms.

Attacks may be precipitated by emotional or physical stress, lack of or excess sleep, missed meals, specific foods, and alcohol. Often the headaches are associated with hormonal changes of menstruation and use of oral contraceptives. When the headaches follow a pattern related to hormone changes, pregnancy brings periods of both exacerbation and relief. In the first trimester of pregnancy, there is a rise in the number and severity of migraines. The headaches abate during the second trimester and then increase again in the third trimester. Migraine can be triggered during delivery or may be more prevalent in the weeks and months following childbirth (Dalessio and Silberstein, 1993).

Pathogenesis

The pain of migraine appears to come from a complex inflammatory process of the trigeminal and cervical dorsal nerve roots that innervate the cephalic arteries and venous sinuses. There remains debate in the literature regarding the cause of migraine headache (Lance, 1993; Garcia, 1993).

Vascular and Neuronal Changes

Although migraine has been considered a vascular headache, the role of the vascular changes in the developing headache is not fully understood. Vascular changes occur before and during the migraine headache. In the headache with aura, cerebral blood flow is reduced by about 20% prior to the headache, resulting in cerebral hypoxia. This cerebral hypoxia is thought to be responsible for the neurologic defects that characterize the auras. Blood flow increases during the head-

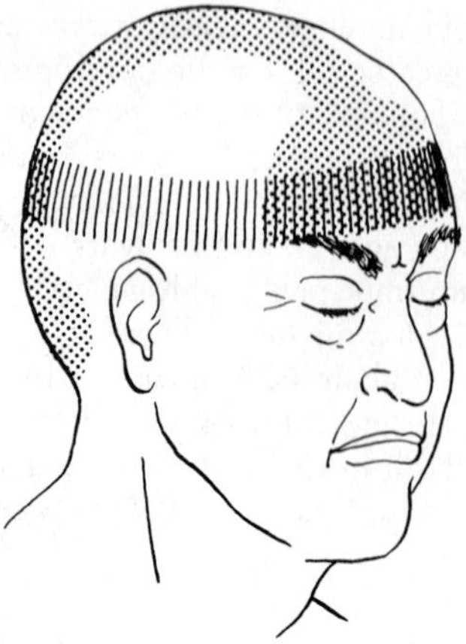

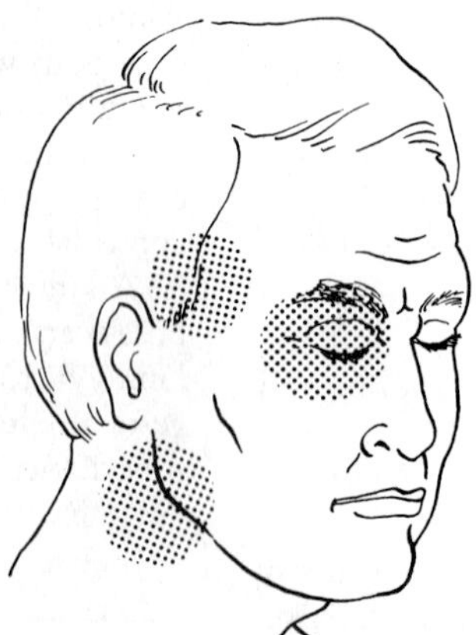

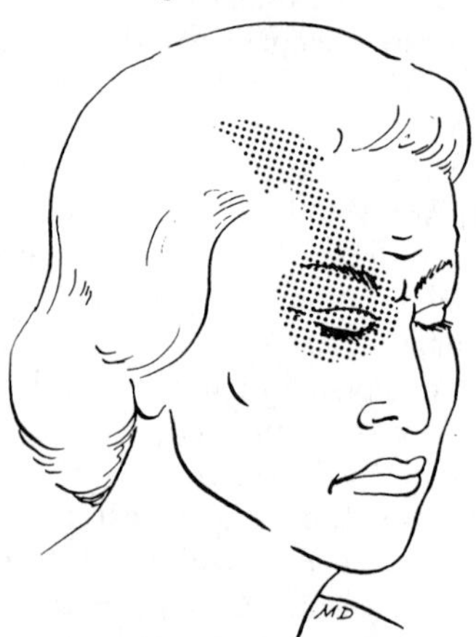

Figure **32-1.** A–C, Types of headache and associated pain patterns. (*From Schnell SS: Nursing care of clients with cerebral disorders. In Black JM, Matassarin-Jacobs E (eds): Luckmann and Sorensen's Medical-Surgical Nursing, ed 4. Philadelphia, WB Saunders, 1993, p 769.*)

ache, although it does not appear to be related to the side of the neurologic symptoms.[2] There appears to be some relationship to the arteries, to referred pain patterns of the veins, and the site of pain.

The brainstem is considered to possibly be implicated in the changes in cerebral blood flow by stimulation of the locus ceruleus or the raphe nuclei.[3] The locus ceruleus receives afferent input from the areas related to internal and external sensory stimuli or to the affective state. It sends projections to the hypothalamus, thalamus, facial nerve nucleus, and the trigeminal nerve. It may be that the trigeminovascular reflex, with excitation of the trigeminal pain pathways and vascular dilation, is a part of the process that results in migraine. The effect of stimulation of the locus ceruleus on target organs is to reduce spontaneous activity and enhance the activity evoked by the sensory systems. The raphe nuclei appear to increase blood flow in the brain. At this time it is not clear whether the two systems work in conjunction or in opposition, but they have a possible influence on blood flow that may be related to migraine headache (Lance, 1993).

The direct relationship of the stimulation of the brainstem and the changes in cerebral blood flow are not fully supported by current knowledge of the connections of the brainstem and cortex. Further research is required to identify those connections. However, there are changes seen in both brain tissue and the vascular system during migraine headache (Davidoff, 1995).

Biochemical Changes

Other possible factors in the pathogenesis of migraine may be secondary to changes in the metabolites and chemical regulators in the brain, the autoregulation of cerebral blood flow, and the neural influences exerted by the release of various types of transmitters from the network of perivascular nerve fibers. In addition, endothelial cells found in the vessel wall synthesize and release substances that produce vasodilation and vasoconstriction of the cerebral vessels. Cerebral blood vessels are very responsive to chemical stimuli such as changes in carbon dioxide tension and oxygen level. Bradykinin, adenosine, and histamine are released by neurons, endothelium, platelets, and mast cells. These substances have been proposed as local regulators of cerebral blood flow (Davidoff, 1995).

The neurotransmitter serotonin has been implicated in the migraine process by the activation of platelet aggregation. Platelets play an important role in the acute inflammatory response. Many persons with migraine show hyperaggregability of platelets when free from headache. Aggregated platelets also release catecholamines which may cause the initial stage of vasoconstriction. Platelet aggregation is increased during the prodromal stage of migraine. This could be due to an increase in epinephrine, thrombin, or arachidonic acid in the circulation in response to anxiety. There appears to be a decrease in aggregation during the actual headache. Platelets contain virtually all of the serotonin present in the blood and release serotonin during aggregation. Reported changes in plasma serotonin may be due to changes in platelet function. Serotonin also excites pain nerve endings and increases the nociceptive (painful) response.

The migraine associated with food with a high tyramine content may occur in persons who have a deficiency of tyramine-*o*-sulfatase. The excess tyramine could be responsible for the release of catecholamines and could initiate the vasoconstrictive stages of migraine. Prostaglandins could also be the cause of the severe systemic upset and the nausea and vomiting that occur. Prostaglandins are also implicated in the bradykinin-induced excitation of nociceptors.

Although it is not clearly understood, there appears to be a relationship between cervical spine dysfunction and a sympathetic nervous system initiation of vascular spasm. Some migraineurs have relief of symptoms when the cervical spine is treated with manipulation or other physical modalities (Edeling, 1994).

Clinical Manifestations

Classic and Common Migraine

A *classic migraine* is preceded by visual symptoms known as an aura. Visual disturbances may consist of field defects, visual hallucinations such as stars, sparks, unformed light flashes (photopsia), geometric patterns, or zigzags of light. A *common migraine* follows some of the same pattern but is frequently bilateral and begins without the aura.[4] Migraine headaches may be dull or throbbing. They usually build up gradually, and may last for several hours or longer. When the headache resolves, there is often a feeling of heaviness and aching in the head, the scalp may be tender, and there may be considerable fatigue. The termination of the headache is often accompanied by a marked diuresis (increased urination).

Focal disturbances of neurologic dysfunction such as aphasia, numbness, tingling, clumsiness, or weakness may precede or accompany the headaches. The basilar artery variant causes transient blindness which is accompanied by dysarthria, disequilibrium, tinnitus, and paresthesia. Sometimes this is followed by loss or impairment of consciousness or by confusion. A headache follows with nausea and vomiting.

Ophthalmoplegic Migraine

Ophthalmoplegic migraine results in pain around the eye and paralysis in the distribution of the third, fourth, or sixth cranial nerve and can produce diplopia or double vision. One of the features of ophthalmoplegic migraine is that the headache always precedes the oculomotor deficit by several hours or days. The paralysis can progress from being transient to lasting several days, and in some persons it becomes permanent. People with ophthalmoplegic migraine typically give a history of many years' duration of common or classic migraine without oculomotor involvement before the development of ophthalmoplegia.

Hemiplegic Migraine

Hemiplegic migraine is an unusual headache. The person experiences symptoms of numbness and weakness preceding

---

[2] If the neurologic symptoms occur contralateral to the decreased flow, it would be consistent that the pain symptoms would occur on the ipsilateral side when the blood flow increases. This has not been shown to always be the case (Lance, 1993).

[3] The locus ceruleus is the origin of the noradrenergic neurons, and the raphe nuclei are the origin of serotonergic neurons, both of which innervate the intracranial vasculature (Davidoff, 1995).

[4] *Classic* and *common* continue to be used to describe migraine types, although the description of migraine with aura and migraine without aura are the newer classifications. Because the terms *classic* and *common* are still used clinically, they are used here.

the onset of the headache. The numbness in the face and arm may spread to involve the whole of one side of the body. The symptoms may be accompanied by dysphasia or aphasia, slow or garbled speech. This type of migraine may alternate with headaches without hemiplegic symptoms. Permanent deficits have been recorded, presumably from the ischemia of the vasoconstriction, but these are extremely rare.

Vertiginous Migraine

Migraine-associated dizziness is a common finding (Cutrer and Baloh, 1992). Nausea, vomiting, hypersensitivity to motion, and postural instability are cardinal signs. Some persons complain of vertigo, a swimming sensation, or imbalance. In others there is a loss of hearing that coincides with the dizziness, but hearing loss alone is rarely associated with migraine (Kayan and Hood, 1984). The vestibulocochlear symptoms occur most often as a part of the headache, although some individuals complain of the dizziness as part of the prodrome. The dizziness is associated with the position of the head in many cases, indicating an association with benign paroxysmal positional vertigo (see Chapter 33). Dizziness does not always accompany the headache but may intermittently coincide with the headache. Changes are sometimes seen on electronystagmography (ENG), indicating a peripheral deficit that is transient.

The mechanisms are still not clearly understood, but it may be that there are neuropeptides released during the migrainous event that could increase the firing of the peripheral vestibular apparatus, or the vestibular nuclei (Parker, 1991). This may result in a transient increase in the firing on one side of the system, causing the subjective sensation of moving. Changes in cerebral blood flow during the migraine may contribute to the dizziness. Prolonged vasoconstriction of vertebral and basilar arteries may be responsible, or it could be the direct mechanical pressure of the dilated vessel during the vasodilating period of the headache.

The diagnosis of vertiginous migraine is made when the episodes of dizziness coincide with a headache, with the aura, or when, in the absence of other migraine symptoms, the dizziness appears in episodes that cannot be attributed to another disease process.

Complicated Migraine

Complicated migraine is the term used when the neurologic manifestations persist beyond the immediate headache period. These symptoms include hemiparesis, hemisensory defects, occlusion of the retinal artery, and ophthalmoplegia. A basilar artery migraine is considered to be in this category and is characterized by loss of vision, dysarthria, ataxia, vertigo, and tinnitus. There is some question as to whether the longer-term deficits are related to actual ischemia during the vasoactive process (Diamond and Dalessio, 1992).

Medical Management

Diagnosis

In most cases the diagnosis of migraine can be established by the history alone. The neurologic examination is normal. Diagnostic procedures are unnecessary and may lead to confusion. An electroencephalogram (EEG) may show focal slowing if taken during an attack of migraine and may create the impression of a space-occupying lesion or infarction.

Treatment

Management of migraines consists of prophylactic treatment, pharmacologic treatment of symptoms, and avoidance of precipitating factors. Rest in a quiet, dark room and taking aspirin or ibuprofen may help (Silberstein and Saper, 1993).

Vasoconstricting drugs such as Cafergot, a combination of ergotamine tartrate and caffeine is often helpful. Caffeine has several properties that may be of benefit in the treatment of migraine. Concurrent oral administration of caffeine with aspirin increases the peak plasma concentration of aspirin. It has mood-altering properties such that the increased mental alertness, lessened fatigue, and feeling of well-being that follow caffeine ingestion counterbalance some of the symptoms of migraine. Caffeine causes cerebral vasoconstriction and may also have anti-inflammatory properties.

Nonsteroidal anti-inflammatory drugs are useful analgesics. Large doses are effective for acute migraine attacks. Sumatriptan is a rapidly effective agent for aborting attacks when given subcutaneously by an autoinjection device. In less severe cases, sumatriptan is given orally.

Prophylactic treatment may be necessary if migraine occurs more than three times a month. The mode of action may involve both an effect on extracerebral vasculature and the stabilization of serotonic neurotransmission. Calcium channel antagonist drugs may reduce the frequency of attacks after an interval of several weeks, but the severity and duration of attacks are not influenced (Aminoff, 1994). Box 32–1 summarizes the acute and prophylactic treatment of migraine.

Prognosis

With menopause and the resultant decrease in estrogen, there is a decrease in the frequency and severity of migraine. However, there have been reports of migraine attacks beginning after the onset of menopause.

There has been some question about the relationship of migraine to increased chance of stroke, but the relationship is not supported in any current study.

BOX **32–1**
Treatment of Migraine

Acute
Rest in dark, quiet room
Nonsteroidal anti-inflammatory drugs
Ergotamine and caffeine
Narcotics
Dihydroergotamine mesylate (intramuscular)
Prochlorperazine (oral, intramuscular, intravenous)
Sumatriptan (subcutaneous, oral)

Prophylactic
β-Blockers
Calcium channel blockers
Carbamazepine
Tricyclic antidepressants
Prednisone

Special Implications for the Therapist **32-1**

MIGRAINE

Biofeedback is the best-known and most widely used nonpharmacologic procedure for the treatment of migraine. Biofeedback allows the client to make intrinsic changes in both the autonomic and somatic nervous systems. The use of biofeedback is not effective for all migraineurs, probably because of the variety of causes of migraine. The mechanism is believed to be a change in the levels of neurotransmitters produced when a person is able to control the stress response. Both thermal biofeedback, the control of temperature in the digits, and electromyographic (EMG) feedback, the control of muscle activity, have been used by therapists in the treatment of migraine.

Treatment of the soft tissues of the neck and occipital structures often will bring some relief to the client with migraine. This may be due to the general relaxation of the skeletal musculature, which reduces stress responses (Edeling, 1994). More research into the sympathetic changes associated with these techniques may bring the therapist further into the treatment of migraine.

CLUSTER HEADACHE

Overview and Definition

Cluster headaches are severe unilateral headaches of relatively short duration (Kudrow, 1993; Sjaastad, 1992). There are two types of cluster headache. The episodic type is the most common, constituting 80% of all cases. Episodic cluster headache is defined by periods of susceptibility to headache, called cluster periods, alternating with periods of remission. They can occur daily or several times a day for a period of several weeks. The headache will then go away for several months and then recur as another series or cluster.

Chronic cluster headache is a term used when remissions have not occurred for at least 12 months and the headaches come at least two times per week. Chronic cluster headache is much rarer than cluster headache.

Incidence

Cluster headaches occur mostly in men between the ages of 20 and 50, predominantly between age 27 and 30 years. Black males appear to have a higher incidence than males of other racial backgrounds.

Pathogenesis

Cluster headaches may be caused by vasodilation in the distribution of one external carotid artery; cerebral blood flow is increased during an attack. Vasodilators such as nitroglycerin will induce cluster attacks. Often, but not always, alcohol induces an acute cluster attack while the person is in an active cluster period. Attacks are commonly induced on awakening from an afternoon nap or from sleep during the night, most commonly 90 minutes after falling asleep. Increased blood flow in cluster headache has been explained as an impairment of autoregulatory responses, reactive hyperemia, or a pain-related activity. The vascular changes may reflect autonomic nervous system dysfunction.

Platelet levels of histamine and serotonin increase during the episode of headache and decrease in the absence of headache. Figure 32–2 shows the relationship among histamine, gastric secretions, and pain. Some evidence supports the theory that there is a decrease in the testosterone level during the period of cluster headache, which suggests a pituitary-hypothalamus involvement. The cluster headache period may be characterized by disturbances in neuroendocrine substances based on the circadian rhythm, which may explain its cyclic nature.

The carotid body may play a major role in the pathogenesis of cluster headaches by its receptor mechanism associated with blood pressure and heart rate. Throughout the course of

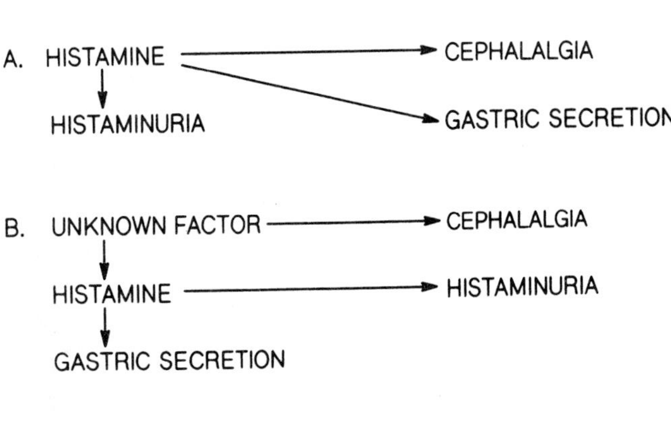

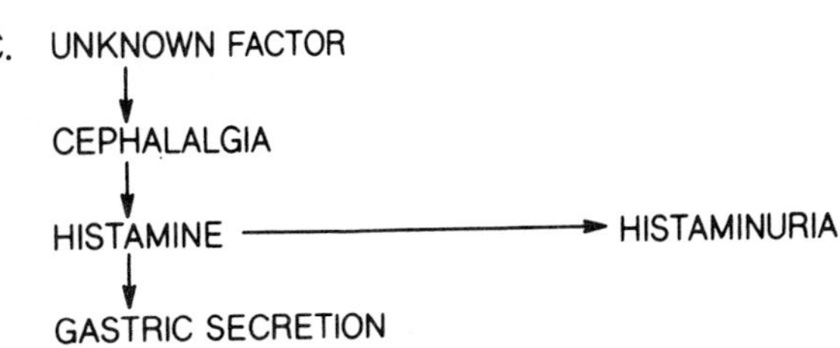

Figure **32–2.** Possible relationship between histamine headache and gastric secretion in cluster headache. A, Histamine as the causative agent. B, Histamine level as an independent phenomenon. C, Increased histamine as a secondary product. (*From Sjaastad O: Cluster Headache Syndrome. London, WB Saunders, 1992, p 150.*)

the cluster period, it may be that the chemoreceptor activity is affected by central control of sympathetic and parasympathetic pathways. The major manifestations would occur during sleep. Sleep apnea and hypoxemia are associated with cluster headaches.

Clinical Manifestations

The onset of cluster headache is sudden, with excruciating pain. In the majority of cluster headache cases, the headache remains on one side of the head throughout life. The headache is usually localized to one eye and the frontotemporal region (see Fig. 32–1). The pain is boring and nonthrobbing. Autonomic symptoms, which are often on the opposite side from the pain, include photophobia or the need to avoid lighted environments, lacrimation or tearing, and nasal congestion. Autonomic changes may be bilateral. Occasionally Horner's syndrome (constricted pupil and droopy eyelid) or forehead sweating will appear on the uninvolved side of the face. Figure 32–3 shows the interrelationship of pain and autonomic symptoms in cluster headache. Persons will occasionally complain of blurred vision on the painful side. Persons with cluster headache generally prefer to assume an erect rather than a reclining posture during attacks.

Persons with cluster headache have some similar physical characteristics, including increased and asymmetrical facial wrinkles and thick "orange peel" skin, giving them the appearance of an alcoholic. Men with cluster headache are on average 3 in. taller than age-matched normals. The typical client with cluster headache smokes cigarettes and drinks alcohol.

Medical Management

Diagnosis

Diagnosis is based on the symptoms and history. Paroxysmal hemicrania, trigeminal neuralgia, and temporal arteritis may have similar symptoms, but they are not episodic.

Treatment

Education should be provided regarding precipitating factors, including alcohol, sleeping patterns that change or involve afternoon naps, negative emotions, and altitudes above 5000 ft. Avoiding these situations may reduce the frequency of cluster headache.

Treatment is similar to that for migraine. Ergotamine-containing drugs are effective vasoconstrictors. Methysergide can be used as a prophylactic. Corticosteroids may be effective in relieving the symptoms.

Upright activities, including walking, appear to be of some relief. Few people choose to lie down during an attack.

Prognosis

In the natural course of this disorder, approximately one third of those who have been subject to cluster headache for 20 years or longer may experience a complete remission. In another one third the attacks may be mild and no longer require medical intervention. The final third continue to have attacks in the same pattern and to the same degree. Cluster headaches do not begin in old age. Most persons have fewer symptoms with progressing age.

Special Implications for the Therapist **32-2**

CLUSTER HEADACHE

It is important for the therapist to be able to recognize the symptoms of cluster headache and to differentiate it from tension headache. A tension headache may be relieved by drinking alcohol; the cluster headache may be triggered by alcohol. Relaxation and stress reduction may be of benefit if the client has a history of episodes triggered by stress response.

Use of thermal and EMG biofeedback may be of benefit (see under Migraine).

MUSCLE TENSION HEADACHE

Overview, Definition, and Incidence

Tension headache associated with muscle contraction is the most common type of headache, occurring primarily as a response to stress (Diamond, 1993) (see Fig. 32–1). The headache is recurrent, lasting for 30 minutes to 7 days, with fewer than 15 headache days per month. The headache is moderate in intensity with no aggravation by physical activity. It is chronic, bilateral, constricting, nonpulsatile, and associated with rigidity or spasm in the neck. Muscle tension

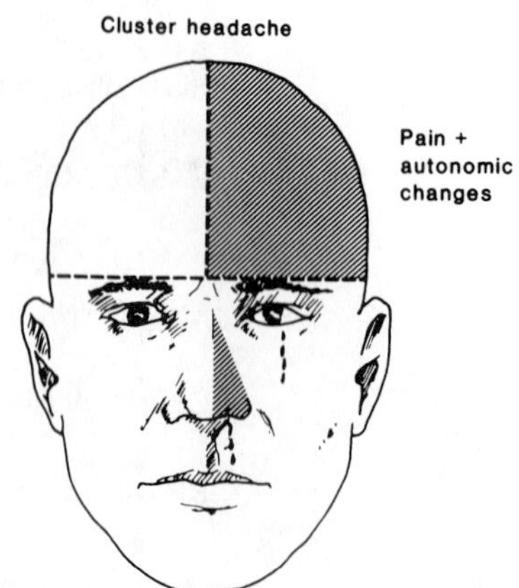

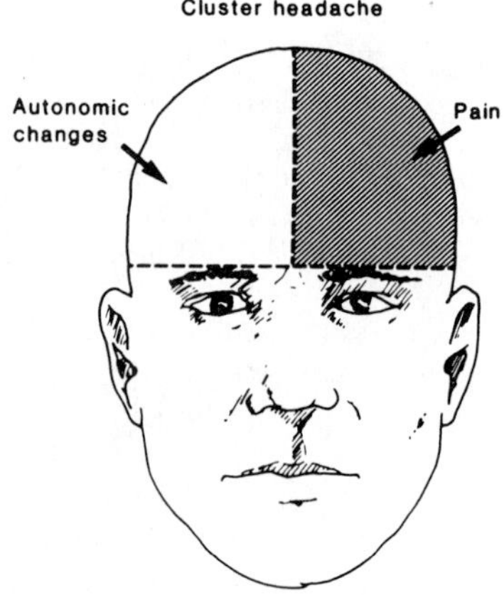

Figure **32-3.** The interrelationship of pain and autonomic symptoms and signs in cluster headache. The usual pattern: pain and autonomic changes on the same side (*left*). Less common pattern: pain on one side, autonomic changes on the opposite side (*right*). (*From Sjaastad O: Cluster Headache Syndrome. London, WB Saunders, 1992, p 49.*)

headache can occur at any age but is more common in adulthood. The lifetime prevalence is 69% of males and 88% of females.

Etiology and Risk Factors

Previous trauma to the neck can precipitate muscle tension headache. The trauma could be a blow, a fall, or a whiplash injury. Because the headaches usually begin a long time after the incident and because the development of the syndrome is insidious, the client does not always relate the two (Edeling, 1994).

Pathogenesis

The headache is often due to anxiety, stress, tension, or psychogenic factors, which may result in disturbance of monoaminergic, serotonergic, and endorphin function, involving the hypothalamus, brainstem, and spinal cord. There may be referral or a central pain phenomenon from the intermingling of major circuits of the brain and spinal cord. Neurotransmitters and brain fluids are known to be abnormal during a bout of tension-type headache. Serotonin content in platelets is decreased and β-endorphin levels are abnormal. Whether this is cause or effect is still being investigated.

Disorders of the cervical spine and atlanto-occipital junction may create localized pain and referred pain to the head. Abnormal posture of the trunk and neck may trigger headache. Alignment of the head in relationship to the cervical spine will affect the length and tension of the muscles and ligaments. When the upper back is rounded, the position of the head is adjusted to maintain the eyes in the vertical position. This often results in shortening of the suboccipital muscles and abnormal positioning of the cervical spine (Edeling, 1994).

Tension-type headaches are common in the geriatric population. Because of arthritic changes in the cervical vertebrae, decrease in general activity, and prolonged sitting, the structures of the atlanto-occipital and cervical region become tight and tender, resulting in prolonged headache.

The role played by emotional factors in the pathogenesis of tension-type headaches has been the subject of much debate. Most investigators concur that pain and psychological factors affect each other. Chronic tension-type headaches may be a manifestation of another medical condition, such as depression.

Clinical Manifestations

Pain in the early stages is infrequent and erratic. Over a period of time the headaches become more regular and more frequent. The once-a-month headache becomes a once- or twice-a-week headache, then a daily headache and finally a constant headache. The headache frequently radiates into the neck and shoulders. The headache can last several days or as long as the tension remains.

Muscle tension headache can cause complaints of poor concentration and other vague, nonspecific symptoms. Visual disturbances are frequently described, as well as tinnitus. Dizziness is reported and clumsiness or disturbed gait is often noted.

The site of the headache varies, with pain frequently occurring on the forehead and temples or at the back of the head and neck. Tenderness of the scalp may accompany the pain.

Medical Management

Diagnosis

The diagnosis of tension headache requires minimal diagnostic tests, as it can be determined by the medical history. A general physical and neurologic examination should be performed to rule out a disease process.

With muscle contraction or tension headache, physiologic movements of the neck often appear to have full range and be pain-free. Restriction of movement at the atlanto-occipital joint can be easily overlooked because it is of small amplitude. However, a restriction here can be the cause of significant headache pain (Edeling, 1994).

Treatment

Simple analgesics are often all that is required. If the client has a high level of anxiety, mild tranquilizers can be effective. If the client is also suffering from depression, a tricyclic antidepressant can help. Often the sleep pattern is disturbed, and the use of tricyclics can improve the sleep pattern; this can lead to a decrease in headache pain.

Prognosis

The headache is closely tied to the level of tension in the muscles of the head and neck. If the underlying reason for the tension is properly addressed, the headaches should subside.

Special Implications for the Therapist **32-3**

MUSCLE TENSION HEADACHE

The chronic headache that arises from the atlanto-occipital and upper cervical joints is a unique syndrome and needs to be differentiated from disorders at other vertebral levels. Description of this syndrome goes beyond the scope of this text. For further information see Magee, 1992; Maitland, 1986. Although this type of headache is responsive to therapy oriented at treating the soft tissue restrictions, the method of examination, assessment, and treatment need to be specific to the neck and occiput (Edeling, 1994).

References

Aminoff MJ: Nervous system. *In* Tierney LM, McPhee SJ, Papadakis MA (eds): Current Medical Diagnosis and Treatment, ed 33. Norwalk, Conn, Appleton & Lange, 1994, pp 799–854.

Cutrer FM, Baloh RW: Migraine associated dizziness. Headache, pp 300–304, 1992.

Dalessio DJ, Silberstein SD: Diagnosis and classification of headache. *In* Dalessio DJ, Silberstein SD (eds): Wolff's Headache and Other Head Pain, ed 6. New York, Oxford University Press, 1993, pp 3–18.

Davidoff RA: Migraine: Manifestations, Pathogenesis, and Management. Philadelphia, FA Davis, 1995.

Diamond S: Tension-type headaches. *In* Dalessio DJ, Silberstein SD (eds): Wolff's Headache and Other Head Pain, ed 6. New York, Oxford University Press, 1993, pp 235–254.

Diamond S, Dalessio DJ: Migraine headache. *In* Diamond S, Dalessio DJ (eds): The Practicing Physician's Approach to Headache, ed 5. Baltimore, Williams & Wilkins, 1992, pp 51–79.

Edeling J: Manual Therapy for Chronic Headache, ed 2. Oxford, Butterworth-Heinemann, 1994.

Garcia JH: Pathology. *In* Olesen J, Tfelt-Hansen P, Welch KM (eds): The Headaches. New York, Raven Press, 1993, pp 175–177.

Kayan A, Hood JD: Neuro-otological manifestations of migraine. Brain 107:1123–1142, 1984.

Kudrow L: Cluster headache: Diagnosis, management, and treatment. *In* Dalessio DJ, Silberstein SD (eds): Wolff's Headache and Other Head Pain, ed 6. New York, Oxford University Press, 1993, pp 171–197.

Lance JW: The pathophysiology of migraine. *In* Dalessio DJ, Silberstein SD (eds): Wolff's Headache and Other Head Pain, ed 6. New York, Oxford University Press, 1993, pp 59–95.

Magee DJ: Orthopedic Physical Assessment, ed 2. Philadelphia, WB Saunders, 1992.

Maitland GD: Vertebral Manipulation, ed 5. Oxford, Butterworth-Heinemann, 1986.

Parker W: Migraine and the vestibular system in adults. Am J Otol 12:25–34, 1991.

Silberstein SD, Saper JR: Migraine: Diagnosis and treatment. *In* Dalessio DJ, Silberstein SD (eds): Wolff's Headache and Other Head Pain, ed 6. New York, Oxford University Press, 1993, pp 96–170.

Sjaastad O: Cluster Headache Syndrome. London, WB Saunders, 1992.

SECTION 4

chapter 33

Vestibular Dysfunction

Kenda S. Fuller

DEFINITION AND NEUROANATOMY

Dizziness is a broad term that describes the sensation that results from the disruption of information from the vestibular, visual, and somatosensory systems. This may be a result of *vertigo*, a false feeling of movement relative to one's environment, a rotational or spinning movement, often associated with nausea. *Lightheadedness* is a common complaint relating to a giddy, faint, dazed feeling. *Disequilibrium* can be described as an unsteady, clumsy, wobbling or swaying.

In order to understand the function of the vestibular system, a general review of the neuroanatomy is necessary (Hain and Hillman 1994; Kelly, 1985; Anson and Donaldson, 1981). The peripheral vestibular system lies within the inner ear, which is bordered laterally by the air-filled middle ear, and medially by the temporal bone. The critical components of the peripheral vestibular system are the three semicircular canals with a center chamber called the ampulla, and the otoliths, which are comprised of the saccule and utricle. Figure 33–1 shows the peripheral vestibular system in relationship to the bony structure and the cochlear system involved in hearing. By virtue of their structure, these organs provide information to the central nervous system regarding angular acceleration, linear acceleration, and static head position.

The semicircular canals are ring-shaped fluid-filled structures oriented three-dimensionally which provide information about angular acceleration. This is accomplished by movement of the fluid (endolymph) in the direction opposite to the head movement. As the endolymph moves, it causes hair cells in the ampulla to deflect away from the direction of movement. The hair cells are attached to the eighth cranial, or vestibular, nerve. The direction of the deflection of the hair cells determines the rate of firing of the vestibular nerve. Figure 33–2 represents the placement of the posterior canal in the head, the relationship of the movement of the head and the endolymph, and the deflection of the ampulla. The vestibular nerve transmits afferent signals from labyrinths along its course through the internal auditory canal and temporal bone to enter the brainstem at the level of the pontomedullary junction. The difference between the rates of firing of the nerves on each side of the head is interpreted by the brain as angular movement of the head.

Both ends of each fluid-filled semicircular duct terminate in the utricle. A portion of the floor of the utricle is thickened and contains hair cells covered with a gelatinous membrane to which calcium carbonate crystals (otoconia) adhere. The orientation of these hair cells is horizontal when the head is horizontal. It is the weight of the otoconia that displaces the hair cells in the utricle during linear acceleration, and gives information about the tilt of the head (the static position of the head with respect to gravity). Figure 33–3 shows how the otoconia sit above the hair cells which lie in the macule. Information from the movement of the hair cell is transmitted to the vestibular nerve.

Hair cells are also found in the saccule. However, in contrast to the utricle, they are oriented vertically when the head is held horizontally. Position of the head is detected, as well as vertically directed linear forces. These components, all working together are responsible for the *vestibulo-ocular reflex*, which maintains gaze on an object while the individual is moving the body or turning the head. Figure 33–4 shows the connection between stimulation of the semicircular canals and eye movement.

The vestibular system is also responsible for motor output through the *vestibulospinal reflexes*. These reflexes are stimulated by the canals and otoliths of the labyrinth and are mediated by the vestibular nuclei, the vestibulospinal tracts, and the spinal cord. These reflexes provide automatic control of the activity of the postural muscles in the trunk and limb. Maintaining equilibrium, or balance, requires a multimodal system integrating vestibular, visual, and somatosensory signals. The integration of these signals in the central nervous system coordinates multiple output responses: eye movement, postural correction, motor skill, and conscious awareness of spatial orientation (Smith, 1993). When the information provided by these systems is incongruent, or when one of the systems is incompetent, the individual will have complaints of dizziness and the ability to maintain balance is compromised.

The vestibular system provides the central nervous system with information about the position and motion of the head in relation to gravity which is critical for sensing and perceiving self-motion. The visual system signals the position and movement of the head with respect to the surrounding objects. The somatosensory system provides information about the position and motion of the body with respect to its support surface and about the position of the body segments with respect to one another (Horak and Shupert, 1994). When functionally useful somatosensory and visual inputs are available, vestibular inputs play a minor role in controlling center-of-gravity position. Somatosensory and visual inputs are more sensitive to body sway than the vestibular system during slow movements, but vestibular input is required for rapid movements. Vestibular input is critical for balance when fast righting reflexes are needed, or when both the somatosensory and visual inputs are misleading or unavailable. (Nashner, 1993c)

Understanding the impairments associated with a balance disorder is critical for the therapist determining intervention. An overview of the special implications for the therapist is included, which encompasses the therapeutic intervention for the disorders described in this chapter.

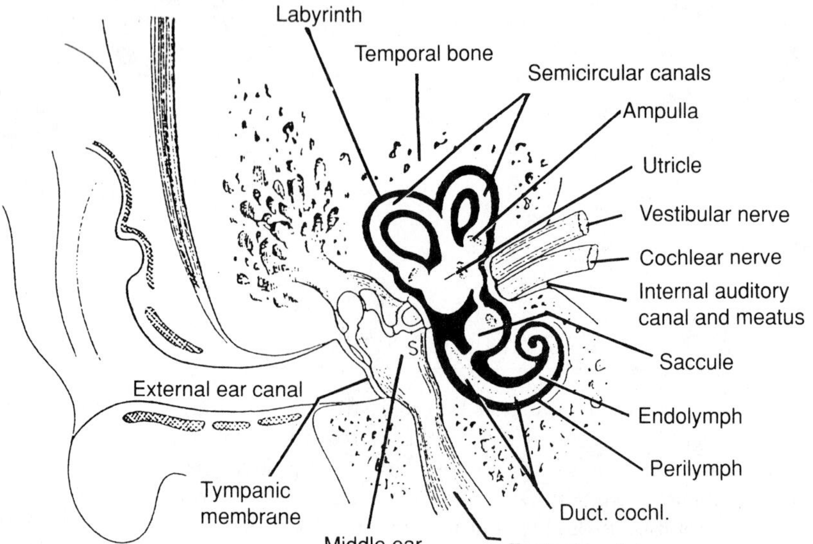

Figure **33–1.** Structures of the inner ear. Note the relationship of the semicircular canals and the cochlear structures. (*From Herdman SJ: Vestibular Rehabilitation. Philadelphia, FA Davis, 1993.*)

SIGNS AND SYMPTOMS OF VESTIBULAR DYSFUNCTION

Dizziness is one of the most common clinical complaints, but the causes are often poorly understood and not clearly documented. The causes of dizziness are multiple. A central deficit is a result of damage to the areas of the brain that process vestibular information. Damage to the peripheral vestibular nerve can be from a nerve pathology, mechanical deformation from a non-neurologic pathology, or trauma to the structures surrounding the nerve. Disorders of the labyrinth can affect the sensory end organs providing input to the vestibular system. In addition to the sensation of dizziness, the main clinical deficit associated with vestibular disorders of central or peripheral origin is loss of balance and inability to walk (Fetter, 1994; Glasscock et al., 1990; Kelly, 1985).

With abnormalities of the vestibular system the *vestibulo-ocular reflex*, which provides automatic control of conjugate eye movement in response to head movement, is disrupted. The lesion can be anywhere from the vestibular end organ, the vestibular nerve, the vestibular nuclei, or the medial longitudinal fasciculus to the ocular motor nuclei. The result is loss of gaze stabilization with head movement. Movement of the head then causes blurring of vision, resulting in dizziness and loss of ability to use visual cues to maintain balance.

Lesions of the vestibular system can result in abnormal

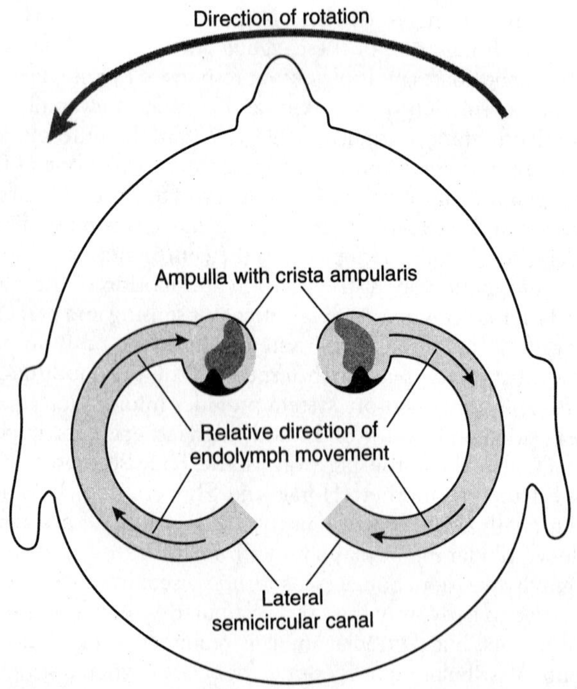

Figure **33–2.** The relative movement of the endolymph with movement of the head in the opposite direction, causing deflection in the structures of the ampulla in the opposite direction to the head. The brain registers this deflection as head movement. (*From Burt AM: Textbook of Neuroanatomy. Philadelphia, WB Saunders, 1993, p 272.*)

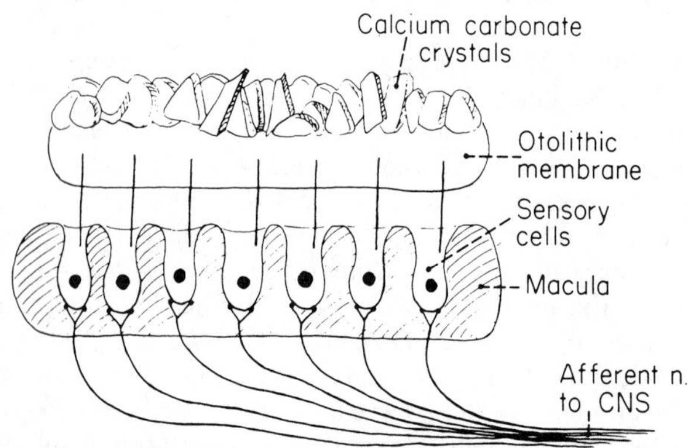

Figure **33–3.** Relationship of the otoconia to the macula and vestibular nerve. (*From Baloh RW, Honrubia V: Clinical Neurophysiology of the Vestibular System, ed 2. Philadelphia, FA Davis, 1990, p 4.*)

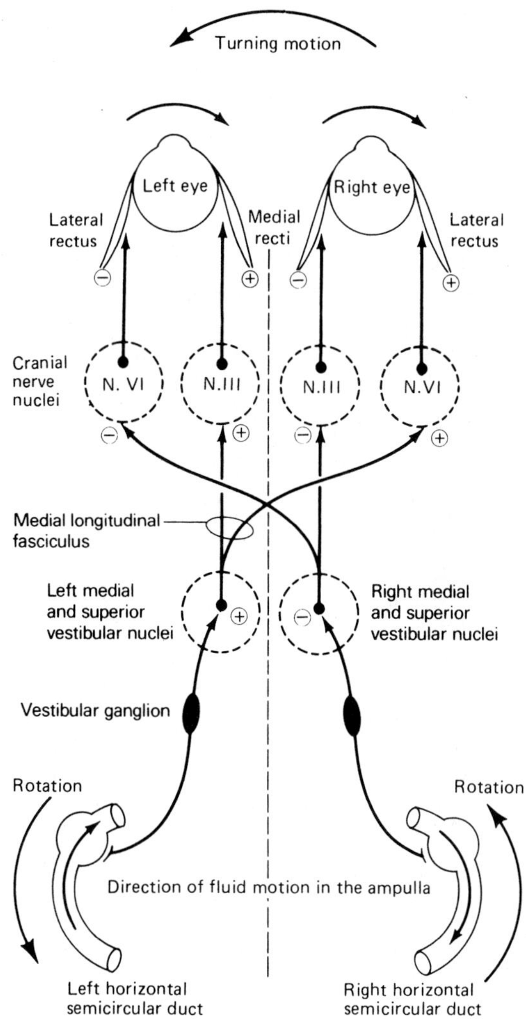

Figure **33-4.** Diagram of the vestibulo-oculomotor reflex showing the relationship of the stimulation of the canals to the movements of the eye. (*From Kelly JP: Vestibular system.* In *Kandel ER, Schwartz JH (eds): Principles of Neural Science, ed 2. New York, Elsevier, 1985, p 594.*)

postural reactions to changes in head and body positions. This results in destabilization when the individual is reliant on vestibular cues for the primary input for balance, as when the lights are low and the ground is soft.

AGING AND THE VESTIBULAR SYSTEM

Vestibular complaints have been recorded in over 50% of elderly people who live alone. Falls in the elderly are a common occurrence, with devastating results including fractures of the hips and pelvis and head injuries (Chandler and Duncan, 1993).

The central mechanisms that are involved in the control of balance do not appear to change excessively with age, but are more likely to be affected by degenerative neurologic diseases such as Parkinson's or Alzheimer's disease. However, there are age-related changes in the peripheral vestibular system. Hair cell receptors begin to decrease at the age of 30 years and by 55 to 60 years there is a loss of the vestibular receptor ganglion cells. The myelinated nerve cells of the vestibular system show up to a 40% loss. There is a reported increase in the incidence of benign paroxysmal positioning vertigo (BPPV) (see later in this chapter) with complaints of dizziness with head movement. This may be due to an increase in the deposits in the posterior semicircular canal. Partial loss of vestibular function in the elderly can lead to complaints of dizziness, with less ability of the nervous system to accommodate the loss compared to a younger person.

In addition to the vestibular losses, there is concomitant loss of other sensory inputs relating to balance, namely, vision and somatosensation. There are longer response latencies and delayed reaction times. Vision changes include loss of acuity, decreased peripheral fields, and loss of depth perception. The loss of input from this combination is slow, with compensation developing through the years. Therefore, compensatory strategy in response to postural instability is not the same as in the person with acute vestibular insufficiency.

There is an overall loss of functional reserve so that the threshold for clinical loss is lowered.[1] This is demonstrated by the increased number of falls in older people with a history of falls compared to an aged-matched group with no history of falls when they are tested with increased challenges to balance. There is an apparent decrease in the ability to integrate the conflicting sensory information to determine appropriate postural responses. Since there are changes as well in motor output, the loss of balance, in addition to lack of sensory organization, may be due to a poor response to vestibulospinal stimulation.[2]

INCIDENCE

Although dizziness is common in all age groups, the frequency of dizziness increases with age. Nearly 7% of people over the age of 45 years visit their physician with this complaint. Dizziness is more often a complaint of women than of men (Draznin and Theriot, 1993).

ETIOLOGY

Lesions of the vestibular system can be broadly categorized into five anatomic sites: (1) the vestibular end organ and vestibular nerve terminals; (2) the vestibular ganglia and nerve within the internal auditory canal; (3) the cerebellopontine angle; (4) the brainstem and cerebellum; and (5) the vestibular projections to the cerebral cortex.

The causes of the lesions are varied and include bacterial infection, viral infection, vascular disease, neoplasia, trauma,

[1] Functional reserve refers to the excess or redundant function that is present in virtually all physiologic systems such that a significant loss of physiologic function can occur before clinical symptoms are seen (Chandler and Duncan, 1993).

[2] While the response patterns are the same in young people and old people, with responses being activated in the stretched ankle muscle and radiating up to the thigh, in some older people, this response is disrupted with the proximal muscles being activated before the distal muscles. In the older person, there appears to be more co-contraction of muscles around the ankle as a result of perturbation (Shumway-Cook and Woollacott, 1995).

metabolic disorders, toxic drugs, and diseases of unknown cause (Britton, 1991; Baloh and Honrubia, 1990).

PATHOGENESIS

Bacterial Infection

The use of antibiotics in general has decreased the incidence of bacterial infections affecting the vestibular system. However, infections still do arise and can be introduced into the vestibular apparatus through the various fluid systems involved or through breakdown of the bony labyrinth.

Persons with bacterial meningitis develop labyrinthitis when bacteria enter the perilymphatic space from the cerebrospinal fluid by way of the cochlear aqueduct or the internal auditory canal. Some bacterial infections result in biochemical irritation of the membranes through a toxic reaction. Both congenital and acquired syphilitic infections produce labyrinthitis as a latent manifestation.

Epithelium from the external canal can develop a cholesteatoma, a slow-growing mass that results from recurrent infection. The cholesteatoma can cause resorption of the adjacent bone by a process of pressure erosion.

Chronic middle ear infections can erode the labyrinths creating a *fistula*, or an opening allowing fluid to pass between the perilymph and the middle ear. Infections of the petrous bone can cause destruction of the bony labyrinth or the eighth cranial nerve in its bony canal.

Malignant external otitis, an infection affecting elderly people with diabetes, begins in the external auditory canal and spreads to the temporal bone, putting pressure on the facial nerve or the surrounding nerves.

The most common intracranial complication of otitic infections is *extradural abscess*, a collection of purulent fluid between the dura mater and bone of the middle or posterior fossa. Spread of the infection across the dura from the epidural space may result in thrombophlebitis of the lateral venous sinus, subdural abscess, meningitis, and brain abscess.

In some cases the damage is temporary, as in serious labyrinthitis, and vestibular and auditory function return to varying degrees. Permanent damage is possible when the infection causes damage to the structures of the labyrinth or the eighth cranial nerve. When the membranous labyrinth becomes permanently damaged, endolymphatic hydrops may result (see Ménière's Disease) and the symptoms can become episodic.

Viral Infection

Viral labyrinthitis is the most common labyrinthitis. Its onset is often preceded by a systemic viral illness such as measles, mumps, or infectious mononucleosis, or it may be an isolated infection of the labyrinth without systemic involvement. Upper respiratory tract illness may also involve the inner ear.

Mononeuritis of the seventh and eighth cranial nerves can be the result of herpes zoster, causing perivascular, perineural, and intraneural infiltration. Other viruses are suspected, but have yet to be positively identified. The cortical vestibular projection fibers can be affected by herpes zoster encephalitis, which has a predilection for the temporal lobe.

Histopathologic studies have suggested involvement of the superior vestibular nerve and vestibular ganglion, often with little or no involvement of the actual end organ. This is true of vestibular neuritis, in which there is no cochlear involvement. However, many viruses do damage throughout the labyrinth and cochlea, Typically, in vestibular neuritis, the end organ is filled with lymphocytes.

Intracytoplasmic particles have been found in the vestibular ganglia. These particles are thought to be dormant forms of a virus, which may produce infection with resultant inner ear disease.

Mycotic Infection

Mycotic infection in the mastoid bone is a major clinical problem. It often occurs in persons with a chronic illness, such as diabetes or a malignancy, who are receiving broad-spectrum antibiotics. The infection enters the middle and inner ear via the nasal sinuses. The infection can spread into the intracranial cavity and create thrombosis of the cerebral arteries. The eighth cranial nerve can be affected along with surrounding cranial nerves in the presence of basilar meningitis.

Perilymph Fistula

Perilymph fistula, an abnormal communication of the inner and middle ear spaces, can cause vertigo. The perilymphatic space is separated from the middle ear by the labyrinthine windows (round and oval), and communicates with the cerebrospinal fluid by way of the cochlear aqueduct and the internal auditory canal. Although most fistulas result from congenital malformations, or prior ear surgery, damage may also be produced by pressure applied via the external ear, the eustachian tube, or by an increase in the pressure of the cerebrospinal fluid, which can result from barotrauma, violent exercise, heavy lifting, or even sneezing (Brandt, 1991). Controversy remains regarding perilymph fistula and its contribution to vertiginous episodes.

Vascular Disease

Vertebrobasilar insufficiency is a common cause of vertigo in persons over the age of 50 years. This is often due to atherosclerosis of the vertebral and basilar arteries. Ischemia confined to the labyrinthine artery distribution results in infarction of the vestibular labyrinth and cochlea. Ischemia can also cause vertigo without hearing loss. A vascular loop compressing the eighth cranial nerve can be a cause of vertigo, tinnitus, and hearing loss. Spontaneous hemorrhage into the inner ear, resulting in vertigo and hearing loss, mainly occurs in persons with underlying bleeding disorders. Leukemia is the most common disorder associated with labyrinthine hemorrhage.

A type of migraine headache which results in symptoms of dizziness is associated with vascular changes in the area of the vestibular apparatus (see Chapter 32).

Neoplasia

Primary carcinoma can directly involve the end organ, the middle ear, or the mastoid. Glomus tumors are the most common tumor of the middle ear, arising from the chemoreceptor system of the 9th through 12th cranial nerves and producing focal symptoms.

Schwann cell tumors arising from the sheath of the vestibular nerve in the internal auditory canal produce symptoms by compressing the nerves. Schwannomas are usually small, firm encapsulated tumors that grow very slowly. Often the term *acoustic neuroma* is used to describe the tumor.

Meningiomas arise from the arachnoid layer in the area of the petrosal and sigmoid sinuses. Displacement of the cranial nerves, brainstem, and cerebellum are common, but they are not invasive.

Gliomas arising from the brainstem grow slowly and progressively disrupt the brainstem centers, invading the vestibular and auditory systems in 50% of cases. Gliomas arising in the cerebellum are relatively silent until there is compression of the brainstem, or obstruction of cerebrospinal fluid. Medulloblastomas, occurring primarily in children and adolescents, are rapidly growing tumors of the vermis and hemispheres of the cerebellum.

Metastatic neoplasms involve the vestibular and auditory function primarily through involvement of the temporal bone. The internal auditory canal is a frequent site of metastatic tumor growth. (See also Chapter 26, Central Nervous System Neoplasms.)

Traumatic Brain Injury

Temporal bone fracture resulting from trauma can lead to tearing of the tympanic membrane or the membranous labyrinth or laceration of the vestibular and cochlear nerve. Labyrinthine concussion in the absence of skull fracture can result in positional vertigo due to canalithiasis (see Benign Paroxysmal Positional Vertigo).

Brainstem injury is usually associated with alteration in the level of consciousness and results in dizziness and disequilibrium with damage to the ascending and descending tracts. Inputs from the visual, vestibular, and somatosensory systems can all become abnormal after blunt trauma to the head. Postconcussion syndrome can result in a nonspecific lightheadedness. Other persistent neurologic symptoms are usually also present.

Metabolic Disorders

When vascular and nerve changes associated with diabetes mellitus occur in the area of the peripheral or central vestibular system, symptoms may develop. Loss of proprioceptive input and visual degeneration will further exacerbate the sense of disequilibrium.

Metabolic disorders affecting the resorption of bone such as *otosclerosis* and *Paget's disease* may develop to the point of causing degeneration of the labyrinths or nerves resulting in vertigo and dizziness.

Toxicity

Aminoglycosides are ototoxic, with streptomycin and gentamicin specifically targeted to the vestibular end organ. Kanamycin and neomycin are toxic to the auditory end organ. Damage to the hair cells in the inner ear can result in complete loss of vestibular function within 2 to 4 weeks after these drugs are given.

Heavy metals such as lead and mercury are known to produce symptoms which may be due to demyelination and axonal damage of the eighth cranial nerve.

Immune Disease

Autoimmune disease can affect the inner ear with resultant vertigo, sensorineural hearing loss, aural fullness, and tinnitus. Symptoms usually progress over weeks or months and there is often a known systemic immune disease such as rheumatoid arthritis.

Allergies

Adverse reactions to foods and chemicals have been recognized as important etiologic agents in allergy. Otolaryngologic allergists have dealt with the clinical aspects of food sensitivity and dizziness after exposure to specific chemicals. There is clinical evidence of the relationship of dizziness to food allergies. The pathophysiology, however, remains unclear (Nonas, 1993).

CLINICAL MANIFESTATIONS

Immediately after the onset of unilateral vestibular dysfunction there is intense disequilibrium. There are profound disturbances of position and motion perception. There is a false sense of angular motion (i.e., rotation). With the eyes closed, the illusion of motion is of the body turning toward the side of the lesion. With the eyes open, the illusion is of spinning of the environment in the opposite direction. There is also a roll-tilt perception around the naso-occipital axis (Baloh and Honrubia, 1990; Goebel, 1993; Halmagyi and Curthoys, 1994; Zee, 1994).

A spontaneous mixed torsional and horizontal nystagmus is often present immediately after unilateral lesions. The slow phases are directed toward the side of the lesion and the quick phases are to the intact side. The nystagmus is often suppressed by gaze fixation.

Any nystagmus that does not decrease with attempted fixation implies abnormal central gaze stabilization. Eyes flickering on and off the target, eyes fluttering around the target, spastic bursts of eye oscillations, any or all of these may be present when there are brainstem or midline cerebellar lesions. *Gaze evoked nystagmus* occurs when the central nervous system is unable to hold the eyes in a lateral position. When looking at a lateral target the eyes drift back toward midline, then immediately back to the target.

Abnormalities of *saccadic eye movement*, the system that generates fast eye movements between two stationary targets, are commonly seen with cerebellar or brainstem lesions. Disconjugate eye movements imply a disruption of the nervous system in the medial longitudinal fasciculus (MLF) which connects the two groups of oculomotor nuclei for conjugate movement.

Smooth pursuit, the ability to track an object across the visual field, can be impaired by lesions in many areas of the brain. Lesions of the brainstem, cerebellum, and occipitoparietal junctional cortex all impair ocular tracking.

In cases of severe unilateral vestibular dysfunction, head shaking will elicit a nystagmus directed toward the intact end organ. This is usually seen in conjunction with other evidence of a peripheral lesion and not in isolation.

Oscillopsia (oscillating vision) is the illusion of environmental movement caused by excessive motion of images of stationary objects on the retina, known as retinal slip. One form of oscillopsia is brought on or accentuated by head movement, and is usually of vestibular origin reflecting an insufficient vestibular occular reflex (VOR). When the vestibular system is unable to keep an image stationary by controlling the movement of the eyes, this slip occurs. Severe or complete bilateral loss of peripheral vestibular system function will result in inability to stabilize vision during head movement and produce oscillopsia. Chronic, uncompensated unilateral lesions can also result in persistent symptoms. Disorders of the central nervous system that change VOR gain or phase, such as lesions of the medial longitudinal fasciculus or an Arnold-Chiari malformation, can also cause oscillopsia.

Nystagmus can cause oscillopsia when the head is stationary. Gaze evoked nystagmus, ocular flutter, and vertical nystagmus can be responsible for the oscillopsia.

Postural Abnormalities

Persons with vestibular disorders often have abnormal perceptions of self-motion (Keshner, 1994). The sensation of spinning, rocking, or that the room is spinning around them is common. Altered postural alignment, sometimes associated with excessive muscle tension and pain, is common with vestibular dysfunction. Sudden loss of vestibular function can result in lateral flexion of the head and an abnormal shift of the center of gravity to the side of the lesion. Vestibular pathology results in an inability to accurately determine one's limits of stability, resulting in maintaining the center of gravity outside of or on the edge of the actual limits of stability, which may cause loss of balance. It is often noted that the person is unable (or unwilling due to fear of falling) to move the center of gravity far enough to perform a functional task such as descending stairs.

MEDICAL MANAGEMENT

Diagnosis

The history of the dizziness should give some indication of the cause of the symptoms (Baloh and Honrubia, 1990). The symptoms may reflect an abnormality in the vestibular system or may be indicative of some other general medical cause leading to a sensation of dizziness. Side effects of medications, anemia, hypoperfusion of the brain from postural hypotension, cardiac arrhythmia, endocrine disorders, or hypoglycemia may mimic a disorder of a vestibular nature.

Electro-oculography (EOG) is a method of measuring eye movement by surrounding the orbit with electrodes. A form of EOG used to evaluate the vestibular system is *electronystagmography* (ENG). ENG is used to measure eye movements caused by activation of the vestibulor-ocular reflex and records spontaneous eye movements caused by alteration of the vestibular discharge rate. The angular velocity, amplitude, and frequency of nystagmus can be quantified using ENG. Recording nystagmus in the dark or with the eyes closed is possible with ENG. Visually controlled eye movements (saccade, smooth pursuit, and optokinetic nystagmus) can be recorded and quantified.

Vestibular nystagmus is most frequently seen in lesions of the labyrinth or the vestibular nerve. Peripheral vestibular nystagmus is usually mixed torsional and horizontal in a fixed direction opposite the side of the lesion. Nystagmus due to a central lesion can be in any direction (vertical, oblique, horizontal, or rotational), may change direction as gaze direction changes, and is not suppressed by fixation of gaze.

Manipulation of endolymphatic flow in the semicircular canals by creating a temperature gradient is known as *bithermal caloric stimulation*. When warm water is infused in the external auditory meatus the skin of the ear canal is heated, resulting in a temperature change which is transmitted to the horizontal semicircular canal. The endolymph closest to the canal wall is heated, causing it to become relatively less dense than the surrounding endolymph. The fluid movement that results from the heating of the endolymph deflects the hair cells in the ampulla, simulating head movement, and the result is a nystagmus with the fast component moving toward the canal that was stimulated. Some direct stimulation of the sensory neurons also occurs. The caloric examination allows the clinician to evaluate each horizontal semicircular canal separately. Figure 33–5 shows how the stimulation results in movement of the endolymph. ENG recordings during this stimulation can indicate abnormalities in different locations of the vestibular system and brain. Table 33–1 gives some interpretations of the results of bithermal caloric testing (Jacobson and Newman, 1993).

Abnormalities of eye movement can be tested by a variety of means. Saccadic eye movements can be induced by using dots or lights at different amplitudes and asking the client to move the focus quickly from target to target. Accuracy can be recorded using ENG, demonstrating the undershooting and overshooting resulting from disorders affecting control of eye movement.

Smooth pursuit, or tracking of the target, is observed by recording the eye movement as the client attempts to follow

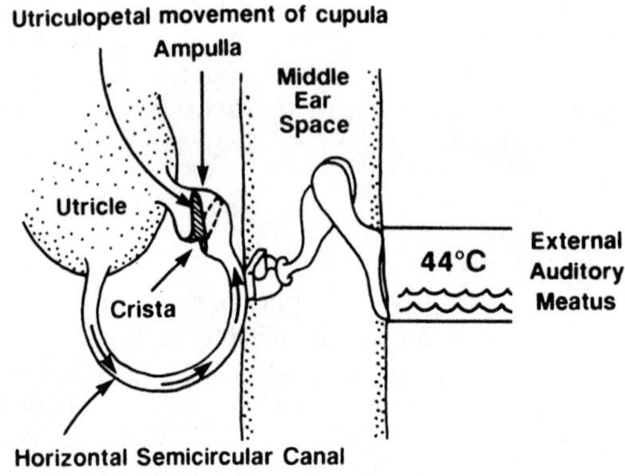

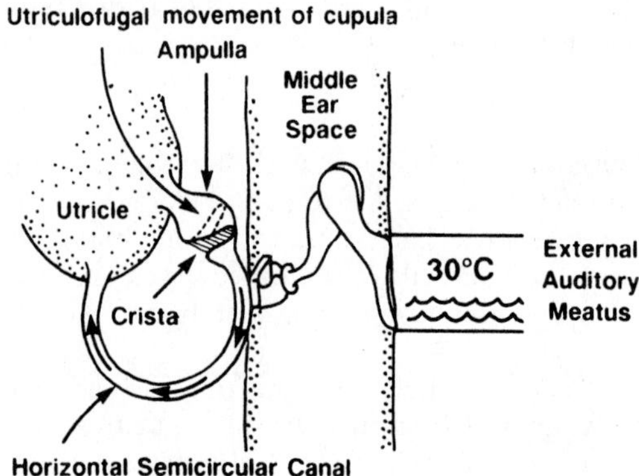

Figure **33–5.** Diagram of the movement of the endolymph in the semicircular canal in response to warm and cold water. (*Adapted from Baloh RW, Honrubia V: Clinical Neurophysiology of the Vestibular System, ed 2. Philadelphia, FA Davis, 1990.*)

TABLE 33–1 Vestibular and Brain Lesions and Their Mechanisms

Impairment	Location of Lesion	Mechanism
Vestibular paresis	Labyrinth, 8th nerve	Decreased peripheral sensitivity
Directional preponderance	Not localizing	Tonic bias in vestibular system
Hyperactive responses	Cerebellum	Loss of inhibitory influence on vestibular nuclei
Dysrhythmia	Cerebellum	Loss of inhibitory influence on pontine nuclei
Impaired fixation suppression	CNS pursuit pathways	Interruption of visual signals on way to oculomotor neurons
Perverted nystagmus	4th ventricular region	Disruption of vestibular commissural fibers

From Baloh RW, Hornrubia V: Clinical Neurophysiology of the Vestibular System, ed 2. Philadelphia, FA Davis, 1990, p 141.

targets at varying velocities. Use of a pendulum or computer-generated movement of lighted targets allows a sinusoidal tracking which can be measured by EOG recording. Two measures are usually applied to the recordings. Pursuit gain compares the velocity of the eye to the velocity of the target. Pursuit phase lag refers to the difference in time between waveforms of the target and the eye movement. A person with normal tracking will predict the target motion and make the precise eye movements necessary to stay on target.

Optokinetic nystagmus (OKN) is the eye movement elicited by tracking of a field instead of a target. The purpose of OKN is to visually stabilize an entire moving visual field. Optokinetic nystagmus is recorded by ENG when a striped drum surrounding the client is moved at a constant velocity. Table 33–2 summarizes the visual ocular control abnormalities produced by focal neurologic lesions.

Rotational testing of the horizontal semicircular canal is provided by use of a motorized rotational chair. Angular acceleration can be controlled and responses to angular acceleration measured. Persons who suddenly lose vestibular function on one side have asymmetrical responses to rotational stimuli. Rotational stimuli are ideally suited for testing persons with bilateral peripheral vestibular lesions because both labyrinths are stimulated simultaneously and the degree of function is accurately quantified. As with lesions of the peripheral vestibular structures, lesions of the central vestibulo-ocular reflex patterns can lead to changes in the gain of rotational-induced nystagmus. Cerebellar dysfunction will result in abnormal amplitudes and dysrhythmia.

Testing of the vestibulospinal reflexes is performed by *posturography*, which evaluates somatosensory and visual influences on posture and equilibrium. The clinical applicability of computerized dynamic posturography (CDP) assessment varies with the chief complaints of the individual. CDP has most clinical value in persons with symptoms of unsteadiness, disorientation, and vertigo in whom the history and physical examination do not suggest an obvious localized cause. In the motor control test (MCT) the individual's postural responses are recorded during displacement of the support surface using electromyogram (EMG) recordings which reflect the activation of the segmental, spinal, and long-loop response pathways. Prolonged MCT latencies are evidence for abnormality in any one or a combination of components comprising the long-loop automatic system and therefore are strong indications for nonvestibular, spinal cord, brainstem, and subcortical involvement.

The *sensory organization test* (SOT), the second component of the CPD, defines six different sensory conditions in which an individual's postural sway is measured. These six conditions vary the amount and accuracy of the sensory information (somatosensation, vision, and vestibular input) available to maintain balance. Vestibular dysfunction patterns are seen in virtually all persons with bilateral peripheral vestibular deficits. These persons are able to maintain balance when the vision or somatosensation is available, but free-fall repeatedly when conditions require dependence primarily on vestibular input. Similar vestibular dysfunction patterns are seen in persons with peripheral vestibular lesions and central nervous system lesions affecting central pathways of the vestibular system. Persons who compensate after a unilateral lesion will have a normal SOT 2 to 4 weeks after the initial insult. An abnormal preference for vision, either alone or in combina-

TABLE 33–2 Visual Ocular Control Abnormalities Produced by Focal Neurologic Lesions

Location of Lesion	Saccades	Smooth Pursuit and Optokinetic Nystagmus Slow Phase
Cerebellopontine angle	Ipsilateral dysmetria*	Progressive ipsilateral impairment
Diffuse cerebellar	Bilateral dysmetria	Bilateral impairment
Intrinsic brainstem	Marked slowing, increased delay time	Ipsilateral or contralateral impairment
Basal ganglia	Mild slowing, hypometria,† increased delay time	Bilateral impairment
Frontoparietal cortex	Difficulty inhibiting reflex saccades	Ipsilateral impairment

* Under and overshoots.
† Undershoots only.
From Baloh RW, Hornrubia V: Clinical Neurophysiology of the Vestibular System, ed 2. Philadelphia, FA Davis, 1990, p 143.

tion with vestibular dysfunction, is most frequently observed in persons with posttraumatic vertigo and unsteadiness. Figure 33–6 shows the sensory conditions during the SOT (Nashner, 1993a,b,c).

Measurement of movement strategies (ankle, hip, and stepping) used to maintain balance is the third component of the CDP. Inappropriate use of ankle movements during large amplitude sway might be an abnormal adaptation used to minimize head movements and associated stimulation of the vestibular system.

When a central cause is suspected based on clinical findings and vestibular testing, magnetic resonance imaging, (MRI) with contrast is indicated. Central brainstem lesions such as stroke, trauma, or multiple sclerosis (MS) can be identified. Neoplasms, including schwannomas, meningioma, and metastasis, can also be identified. Vascular loop or sling can be identified on MRI. Inflammatory lesions can be identified with MRI, including labyrinthitis and inflammatory lesions of the eighth cranial nerve.

There is no reliable single clinical test to establish the diagnosis of Ménière's disease. If the recurrent attacks consist of the typical tinnitus, hearing loss, and vertigo, the diagnosis can be made with some assurance. However, if there are monosymptomatic recurrences, the differential diagnosis is less clear.

Electrocochleography is used to document endolymphatic hydrops. Audiograms are used to measure sensorineural hearing loss. In the early stages of the disease there is a low frequency hearing loss and as the disease progresses the higher frequencies become affected (Arenberg, 1993; Brandt, 1991).

Treatment

When acute vertigo is due to a peripheral vestibular lesion, functional recovery will begin within 2 to 4 weeks. If the symptoms are severe, sedatives may be given, ideally for the first 24 hours only. Vestibular rehabilitation should begin within the first 3 days if possible. (See Special Implications for the Therapist.)

Treatment of recurrent vertigo depends on the nature of the underlying disorder. Persons with migraine-induced vertigo usually can be managed medically. Recurrent vertigo caused by a perilymph fistula usually recovers spontaneously, although some individuals require surgical repair (LaRouere et al., 1993).

When central neurologic conditions result in recurrent vertigo and treatment is unsuccessful in controlling symptoms, vestibular suppression should be considered. Benzodiazepines, antihistamines, or anticholinergic agents are used frequently.

Drug treatment in the suppression of central nystagmus has been of limited value. Optical devices have been used with some measure of success. Persons whose nystagmus is suppressed with convergence may benefit by wearing base-out prisms (Leigh, 1994). In some persons, nystagmus may be less prominent in one gaze angle, and prisms that turn the eyes toward the gaze direction of least nystagmus may be useful.

With the exception of neoplasms, vestibular disorders are chiefly disruptive to lifestyle rather than life-threatening. As described in other sections, surgical intervention is considered for Ménière's disease, BPPV, and vascular disorders when the symptoms are unrelenting. Controversy remains regarding the effectiveness of some of the surgical interventions.

Prognosis

When there is a unilateral lesion in the peripheral vestibular system, and the central nervous system is intact, recovery of function is spontaneous. The recovery is due to the capability of the vestibular system to make long-term changes in the neuronal response to input. The vestibulo-ocular reflex should return to near normal within 2 to 6 weeks so that movement of the head no longer disrupts vision or causes nausea. Recovery, however, is dependent on the stimulus of head movement. Recovery is minimized when the response of the individual experiencing the symptoms is to avoid the provoking motions, and the central nervous system is never given the opportunity to adapt to the asymmetrical firing patterns of the peripheral vestibular system. The vestibulospinal reflexes are slower to return, and the individual may continue to experience insta-

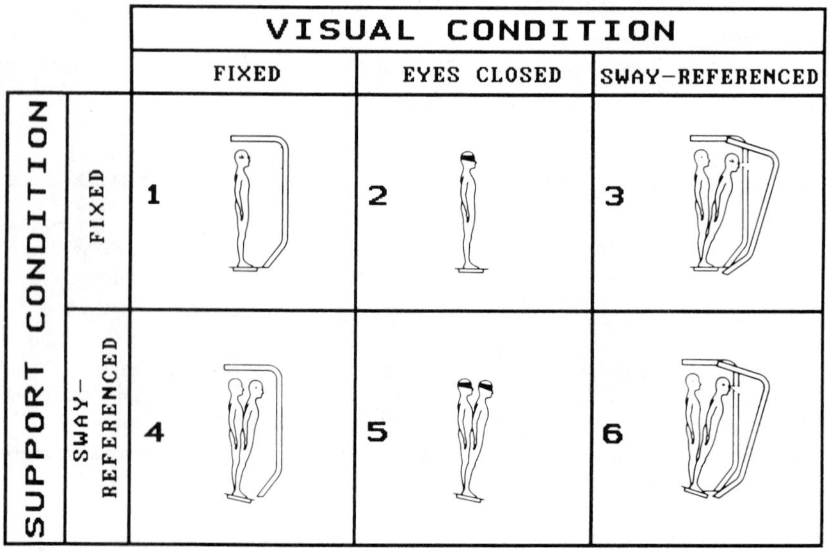

SUPPORT CONDITION	VISUAL CONDITION: FIXED	EYES CLOSED	SWAY-REFERENCED
FIXED	1	2	3
SWAY-REFERENCED	4	5	6

Figure **33-6.** Diagram of the sensory conditions related to the sensory organization test, a component of posturography. (*Courtesy of NeuroCom International, Clackamas, Oregon.*)

bility when turning quickly, or walking on uneven surfaces or in the dark, for weeks after the insult.

Recovery of functional movement can be accomplished by substitution of other sensory mechanisms. Sensory inputs from muscles and joint facets in the neck produce a slow-phase eye movement, known as the *cervico-ocular reflex*, which works in conjunction with the vestibulo-ocular reflex. The use of visual and somatosensory inputs to substitute for loss of vestibular function is possible when the environment provides adequate cues (as in well-lighted environments and firm level surfaces).

Recovery rate in a central vestibular system disorder causing dizziness or disequilibrium is dependent on the nature of the lesion and the concomitant neurologic dysfunction. If it is part of a progressive disease the prognosis is less optimistic than if it is a part of a transient disorder such as a minor vascular incident. A disease such as MS can have episodes of symptoms. When there is a disorder of the central as well as the peripheral vestibular system, as in head injury or in multisensory disorders, the recovery is significantly reduced (Shepard, 1993).

BENIGN PAROXYSMAL POSITIONING VERTIGO

Definition and Risk Factors

Benign paroxysmal positioning vertigo is usually seen in people over the age of 40 years. The otoconia of the utricle begin to loosen and become detached in middle age. Trauma, including direct head blows, whiplash injury, or surgery, can precipitate or accelerate the process and trigger symptoms. Viral neurolabyrinthitis may be responsible for the loosening of particles. Prolonged inactivity of the head can lead to symptoms. Women outnumber men affected by a ratio of 1.6:1. Bilateral involvement is found in 10% of cases. Spontanous remissions are common, but the disorder can recur, and the condition may trouble the individual intermittently for years.

Etiology and Pathology

Densities, known as canaliths, can form in the posterior semicircular canal near the ampulla. It is believed that these densities are formed by the loosening and clumping of the otoconia as described earlier. When the posterior canal is placed in the vertical position (body supine, head extended beyond neutral, and rotated to 45 degrees to the same side) the canaliths begin moving through the endolymph causing drag on the endolymph and creating cupular deflection. This force results in a rotational nystagmus. As the canaliths reach the bottom of the semicircular canal, they slow down and stop moving, and stimulation of the vestibular nerve ceases. Particles can act directly on the cupula. When there is decreased latency of symptoms, or the nystagmus does not fatigue, this may be the mechanism that triggers the symptoms. (Brandt, 1991; Baloh and Honrubia, 1990; Epley, 1993)

Typically, a person with positioning vertigo will complain of brief episodes of vertigo precipitated by rapid head movement in a specific direction. Extension of the neck, often with the head turned to one side, will produce nystagmus. Vertigo can be brought on by looking up to a high shelf, backing out of a car, or most often by lying on one side as one gets into bed or rolling over in bed as one sleeps (Fetter, 1994).

Medical Management

Diagnosis

Diagnostic criteria for BPPV include the following: whirling vertigo induced by a specific head position or movement; a burst of positioning nystagmus that is rotary; latency of symptoms upon placing the head in a provoking position; the nystagmus is *fatigable*, that is, it diminishes with repeated positioning and lasts for less than 30 seconds. Central positional vertigo, which lacks these characteristics, is either induced by head movements that cause a transient ischemia of the pontomedullary brainstem or by a change in head position relative to the gravitational vector (Baloh and Honrubia, 1990; Epley, 1993).

The *Dix-Hallpike maneuver*, passive movement of the head from the upright position to one with the head hanging extended and rotated to 45 degrees, is the standard test performed to establish the diagnosis of BPPV. When the head is in this position, the clinician observes the eyes for evidence of nystagmus. It may take at least 20 seconds for the nystagmus to occur and the nystagmus should fatigue within 60 seconds. The nystagmus occurs when the affected ear is placed down. Figure 33–7 shows the testing positions. Although a positive test is pathognomonic for BPPV, a negative test indicates only that BPPV is not active at that movement. Horizontal canalithiasis can also occur producing symptoms provoked by rolling in the supine position. Nystagmus may occur in both directions, but will be greatest when rolling the head to the involved side (Epley, 1993).

Treatment

Several approaches have been developed to treat persons complaining of BPPV, including maneuvers or positions which attempt to dislodge the provoking substances and move them through the canal system to the common crus. At the conclusion of these procedures, the client is instructed to remain in the upright position for 48 hours, and, in some instances, to avoid the provoking positions for up to 1 week.

Habituation, the repetition of the provoking positions or movements incorporating a wide variety of balance exercises, has been shown to be effective in cases where the individual is unable to tolerate the repositioning procedures, as in a head or whiplash injury. In addition, there is sometimes a vestibular hypofunction accompanying the BPPV that responds to exercises stimulating the vestibular system.

MÉNIÈRE'S DISEASE

Definition, Etiology, and Risk Factors

Ménière's disease is a disorder of inner ear function that can cause devastating hearing and vestibular symptoms. Ménière's disease usually begins in one ear. The attacks increase in frequency in the first years and then decrease. In less than 50% of the cases the late sequelae of the disease is the beginning of involvement in the opposite ear (Brandt, 1991). The disease is equally distributed between the sexes and usually has its onset in the fourth to sixth decade of life. There appears to be a familial connection, with about 15% of persons reporting that blood relatives suffer the same symptoms (Fetter, 1994).

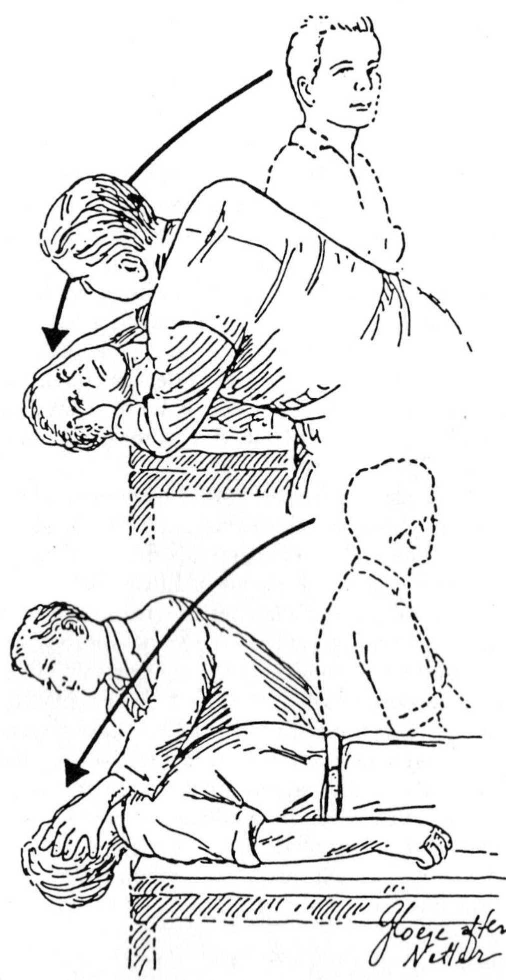

Figure **33-7.** Technique for inducing paroxysmal positional nystagmus, known as the Dix-Hallpike maneuver. (*From Baloh RW, Honrubia V: Clinical Neurophysiology of the Vestibular System, ed 2. Philadelphia, FA Davis, 1990, p 124.*)

Pathogenesis

Ménière's disease is a disorder of the membranous inner ear. Deficits are related to the volume and pressure changes within closed fluid systems. A phenomenon fundamental to the development of Ménière's disease is endolymphatic hydrops. Hydrops, an increase in endolymphatic fluid pressure, is thought to result from endolymphatic sac dysfunction or blockage and affects the ability to resorb the fluid. The increase in the volume of endolymph causes the membranous labyrinth to progressively dilate until the wall makes contact with the stapes footplate and the cochlear duct fills the entire scala vestibuli. Other end-organ pathologies—metabolic, allergic, immunologic, or viral—may be a part of the cause (Arenberg, 1993; Baloh and Honrubia, 1990).

CLINICAL MANIFESTATIONS

The typical attack of Ménière's disease is experienced as an initial sensation of fullness of the ear, a reduction in hearing, and tinnitus. This is usually followed by a rotational vertigo, postural imbalance, nystagmus, and nausea. The vertigo may last from 30 minutes to 24 hours. The symptoms abate over time and the individual regains the ability to maintain balance. However, there may still be some sense of disequilibrium. Hearing slowly returns, but with each attack, there may be a permanent loss of hearing.

MEDICAL MANAGEMENT

Treatment

In Ménière's disease, salt-restricted diets and the use of diuretics help control the fluid balance in the ear, but may not entirely control the vertigo and hearing loss. Vestibular suppressant medication is helpful to control symptoms during acute attacks. Avoiding caffeine, alcohol, and tobacco appears to help.

When medical treatment fails, and the vertigo becomes disabling, surgical treatment is considered. Endolymphatic sac shunting procedures to drain excessive fluid are controversial and may have a placebo effect. Destructive procedures involving portions of the labyrinth, or the vestibular component of the eighth cranial nerve can reduce vertigo without loss of hearing. This is more often done in a young person; ablative surgical procedures in the elderly may have poor results as the central nervous system is unable to compensate for the vestibular loss. Ototoxic drugs can be introduced to selectively damage the vestibular system while preserving auditory functions. This procedure must be carefully monitored for signs of hearing loss. Vestibular nerve section controls vertigo and preserves hearing. (Arenberg, 1993; Brandt, 1991; Fetter, 1994).

Prognosis

Episodes of Ménière's disease occur in an irregular pattern for years, often with long periods of remission. Eventually severe permanent hearing loss develops and the episodic vertigo disappears. Severe symptoms resulting in a sudden fall without warning are referred to as Tumarkin's otolithic crises, which sometimes occur in the late stages of the disease.

Special Implications for the Therapist **33-1**

VESTIBULAR DYSFUNCTION

Clinical evaluation by the therapist of the client with vestibular dysfunction integrates the history with the objective findings of sensory and movement disorders. The therapist is able to look at vestibulo-ocular function as well as vestibulospinal function. Given the history, the therapist makes an attempt to determine whether the lesion is central or peripheral or a combination of both. The nature of the symptoms, and the precipitating, exacerbating, and relieving factors are reviewed.

Testing includes motor control of the visual component, looking for oculomotor control using targets. Gaze stabilization (vestibulo-ocular reflex) is tested by determining the client's ability to maintain visual focus when the head is turning. Evaluating the provoking positions and fatigability of dizziness may help to determine the difference between a canal problem and cerebellar dysfunction. Tests such as the

Fukuda step test may indicate a unilateral peripheral lesion. A careful look at the central nervous system, including cranial nerve function, cerebellum, and brainstem, is critical to determine if there is a central cause or overlay of central on peripheral lesions.

Sensory deficits should be determined. Control of balance in altered sensory conditions which isolate vision, somatosensory, and vestibular inputs is evaluated (see earlier discussion of SOT). When observing upright balance, evaluation of strategy selection is helpful in identifying abnormal reliance on hip or stepping strategy, a common finding in clients with vestibular disorder.*

Musculoskeletal and neuromuscular evaluations are critical to determine compensatory movements based on deficits in these areas that may mimic vestibular dysfunction or detract from recovery. As was mentioned earlier, the correct integration of sensory input is critical for maintaining balance in most situations, and can be responsible for the sensation of dizziness.

Recovery from the dynamic disturbances requires both visual inputs and movement of the body and head. When the client is unable to maintain gaze stabilization and the image moves or slips on the retina, the nervous system will try to adapt and modify the gain of the vestibular system. This is the process of adaptation that is facilitated by the therapist by giving eye-head coordination exercises. Depending on the severity of the symptoms, these exercises may begin in a supine or sitting position in order to decrease the vestibulospinal challenge. The system is progressively challenged by adding activities incorporating movement of the eyes, head, and body, such as bouncing a ball off the wall. During the initial stage, the client may complain of severe vertigo and may be nauseated and vomiting. Exercise will make these symptoms worse. The client should be encouraged to perform the established activities even if it is for brief periods only.

There is an abnormal perception of self-motion in relationship to movement in the environment. Therefore, walking in a crowded environment, riding on an escalator, or walking in a grocery store may create distress for the client. These activities are slowly incorporated into the treatment regimen. For these persons, walking is easier in an empty shopping mall than in a crowded one, and walking with the crowd is less taxing than walking against the crowd.

Adaptation of the vestibular system is context-specific.† Treatment should therefore address the multitude of environments that the person will encounter. Exercises should stress the integration of all the systems involved in balance, synthesizing the visual and somatosensory cues with the vestibular. To stimulate use of somatosensory inputs, environments are designed to disadvantage vision while providing reliable somatosensory inputs (moving the environment while the client is standing on a stable surface). To stimulate the use of visual inputs, environments are designed to disadvantage somatosensation while providing reliable visual cues (looking at a stable visual field with landmarks while standing on foam). The vestibular system is naturally stimulated when visual and somatosensory cues are distorted (standing on foam with rapid head turns, or walking with head turns).

When the balance disorder results in an inability to move the center of gravity through the ranges necessary to perform mobility tasks, the client will benefit from activities directed toward increasing the limits of stability. Center-of-pressure biofeedback has been used successfully in regaining control of center of gravity.

Persons with bilateral peripheral vestibular deficits are unable to see clearly during head movements and are primarily concerned about resulting balance and gait disturbances. Exercises for these clients must be aimed at substitution of visual and somatosensory cues for the lost vestibular function. This is done by having the client perform activities in environments that are manipulated to provide a variety of sensory inputs. Strategies must be developed when the environment provides less than optimal sensory information, such as the use of an assistive device on uneven surfaces, and the use of night lights.

Gaze stability exercise incorporates the vestibulo-ocular reflex, facilitating any possible remaining vestibular function. Head turning with visual fixation also facilitates the *cervico-ocular reflex,* which is effective to a limited degree in facilitating eye movement during head turns.‡ Modifications in saccadic and pursuit eye movements can be used to improve gaze stability with head movement. No mechanism to improve gaze stability will fully compensate for the loss of the VOR, and clients will continue to have difficulty seeing during rapid head movements. Some persons can learn to close their eyes during a turn, and then focus quickly on a stable object to regain stability. This technique increases stability because the disruptive visual input is temporarily eliminated (Foster, 1994).

In clients with chronic complaints of dizziness, effective treatment is often challenging. If the client has self-limited movement of the head and avoided certain changes of position, he or she should be encouraged to reestablish normal movement. Often consistent performance of a gaze stabilization exercise with head movement will decrease dizziness within 4 to 6 weeks in these clients. Practicing activities that increase reliance on existing sensory input can also improve the client's confidence in moving in more complex environments.

For further information see Allison, 1995; Borello-France et al., 1994; and Clendaniel and Helminski, 1993.

---

* An ankle strategy is used when the client is standing on a firm, flat surface. The torque for the motion is controlled at the ankle. A hip strategy is used when the client is standing on a narrow (beam-like) surface, or when the surface is soft. A hip strategy is used on a flat surface when the center of gravity moves beyond the base of support. In a hip strategy, the torque is controlled at the hip. Stepping strategy is used to bring the center of gravity over the base of support when it moves too far to control with an ankle or hip strategy. A suspensory strategy lowers the center of gravity in relation to the base of support.

† Context specificity means that adaptations learned within one sensory context may not work within another. For the vestibulospinal reflexes, this may relate to position of the body, so that if all training is done with the head in an upright position, the client may not be able to maintain balance when the head assumes other postures, such as bending.

‡ The cervico-ocular reflex reflects inputs from the facets and the neck muscles which produce a slow-phase eye movement that is opposite to the direction of the head movement during low frequency, brief head movements.

References

Allison L: Balance disorders. *In* Umphred DA (ed): Neurological Rehabilitation. St Louis, Mosby–Year Book, 1995, pp 802–837.

Arenberg IK: Ménière's disease: Diagnosis and management of vertigo and endolymphatic hydrops. *In* Arenberg IK (ed): Dizziness and Balance Disorders. New York, Kugler, 1993, pp 503–510.

Baloh RW, Honrubia V: Clinical Neurophysiology of the Vestibular System, ed 2. Philadelphia, FA Davis, 1990.

Borello-France DF, Whitney SL, Herdman SJ: Treatment of Vestibular Hypofunction. *In* Herdman SJ (ed): Vestibular Rehabilitation. Philadelphia, FA Davis, 1994, pp 287–313.

Brandt T: Vertigo: Its multisensory syndromes. London, Springer-Verlag, 1991.

Britton BH: Common Problems in Otology. St Louis, Mosby–Year Book, 1991.

Burt AM: Textbook of Neuroanatomy. Philadelphia, WB Saunders, 1993 p 272.

Chandler JM, Duncan PW: Balance and falls in the elderly: Issues in evaluation and treatment. *In* Guccione AA (ed): Geriatric Physical Therapy. St Louis, Mosby–Year Book, 1993, pp 237–252.

Clendaniel RA, Helminski JO: Rehabilitation strategies for patients with vestibular deficits. *In* Arenberg IK (ed): Dizziness and Balance Disorders. New York, Kugler, 1993, pp 663–676.

Draznin E, Theriot KO: Multidisciplinary clinic's model: A comprehensive approach for management of dizziness and balance disorders. *In* Arenberg IK (ed): Dizziness and Balance Disorders. New York, Kugler, 1993, pp 649–654.

Epley JM. Aberrant coupling of otolithic receptors: Manifestations and assessment. *In* Arenberg IK (ed): Dizziness and Balance Disorders. New York, Kugler, 1993, pp 183–202.

Fetter M: Vestibular system disorders. *In* Herdman SJ (ed): Vestibular Rehabilitation. Philadelphia, FA Davis, 1994, pp 80–88.

Foster CA: Vestibular Rehabilitation. Balliere's Clin Neurol 3:577–591, 1994.

Glasscock ME, Cueva RA, Thedinger BA: Handbook of Vertigo. New York, Raven Press, 1990.

Goebel JA: Understanding eye movements in balance disorders. *In* Arenberg IK (ed): Dizziness and Balance Disorders. New York, Kugler, 1993, pp 49–56.

Hain TC, Hillman MA: Anatomy and physiology of the normal vestibular system. *In* Herdman SJ (ed): Vestibular Rehabilitation. Philadelphia, FA Davis, 1994, pp 3–20.

Halmagyi GM, Curthoys IS: Clinical changes in vestibular function over time after lesions: The consequences of unilateral vestibular deafferentation. *In* Herdman SJ (ed): Vestibular Rehabilitation. Philadelphia, FA Davis, 1994, pp 99–107.

Horak FB, Shupert CL: Role of the vestibular system in postural control. *In* Herdman SJ (ed): Vestibular Rehabilitation. Philadelphia, FA Davis, 1994, pp 22–42.

Jacobson GP, Newman CW: Background and technique of caloric testing. *In* Jacobson GP, Newman CW, Kartush JM (eds): Handbook of Balance Function Testing. St Louis, Mosby–Year Book, 1993, pp 156–192.

Kelly JP: Vestibular system. *In* Kandel ER, Schwartz JH (eds): Principles of Neural Science, ed 2. New York, Elsevier, 1985, pp 584–596.

Keshner EA: Postural abnormalities in vestibular disorders. *In* Herdman SJ (ed): Vestibular Rehabilitation. Philadelphia, FA Davis, 1994, pp 47–68.

LaRouere MJ, Seidman MD, Kartush JM: Medical and surgical treatment of vertigo. *In* Jacobson GP, Newman CW, Kartush JM (eds): Handbook of Balance Function Testing, St Louis, Mosby–Year Book, 1993, pp 337–358.

Leigh RJ: Pharmacologic and optical methods of treating vestibular disorders and nystagmus. *In* Herdman SJ (ed): Vestibular Rehabilitation. Philadelphia, FA Davis, 1994, pp 183–192.

Nashner LM: Computerized dynamic posturography. *In* Jacobson GP, Newman CW, Kartush JM (eds): Handbook of Balance Function Testing. St Louis, Mosby–Year Book, 1993a, pp 280–307.

Nashner LM: Computerized dynamic posturography: Clinical applications. *In* Jacobson GP, Newman CW, Kartush JM (eds): Handbook of Balance Function Testing, St Louis, Mosby–Year Book, 1993b, pp 308–334.

Nashner LM: Practical biomechanics and physiology of balance. *In* Jacobson GP, Newman CW, Kartush JM (eds): Handbook of Balance Function Testing. St Louis, Mosby–Year Book, 1993c, pp 261–279.

Nonas NG: Inner ear allergy diathesis and environmental factors: Evaluation and management. *In* Arenberg IK (ed): Dizziness and Balance Disorders. New York, Kugler, 1993, pp 555–562.

Shepard NT, Telian SA, Smith-Wheelock M: Habituation and balance retraining therapy: A retrospective view. *In* Arenberg IK (ed): Dizziness and Balance Disorders. New York, Kugler, 1993.

Shumway-Cook A, Woollacott MH: Motor Control: Theory and Function. Baltimore, Williams & Wilkins, 1995.

Smith DB. Dizziness: The history and physical examination. *In* Arenberg IK (ed): Dizziness and Balance Disorders. New York, Kugler 1993, pp 3–10.

Zee DS: Vestibular adaptation. *In* Herdman SJ (ed): Vestibular Rehabilitation. Philadelphia, FA Davis, 1994, pp 68–78.

SECTION 4

chapter 34

The Peripheral Nervous System

Marcia B. Smith

The peripheral nervous system (PNS) includes all cranial and spinal nerves arising from neurons whose cell bodies are located within the brainstem and spinal cord. Axons extend from the cell bodies to form peripheral nerves. Disorders of the PNS can be broadly divided into neuropathies, in which the pathology is confined to the nerve, and myopathies, in which the pathology occurs in muscle. Disorders of the PNS can be subdivided further according to site of anatomic involvement (Dubowitz, 1978).

Signs and symptoms of PNS involvement relate to the motor and sensory systems. Motor involvement, termed *lower motor neuron (LMN) involvement*, occurs when any of the following sites is affected: the cell body of the alpha motor neuron (anterior horn cell) located within the spinal cord or brainstem; axons arising from these neurons that form spinal and peripheral nerves, and cranial nerves; the motor end plate of the axon; and the muscle fibers innervated by the motor nerve. Similarly, sensory fibers of the PNS will show involvement if a lesion occurs in the dorsal root ganglion where the cell body is located, or peripheral to its location (Fig. 34–1).

STRUCTURE

Nerves in the PNS are supported and covered by connective tissue coverings or tubes: the *endoneurium* surrounds individual axons; the *perineurium* covers groups, or fascicles, of axons; and the *epineurium* surrounds the entire nerve. The surface of an axon is formed by a membrane called the axolemma. Lying between the axolemma and the endoneurium is the Schwann cell (Fig. 34–2). In all but the smallest axons, these Schwann cells form myelin internodes that insulate the axon and allow rapid conduction of an action potential using saltatory conduction. The other fibers are unmyelinated and action potentials are conducted by volume conduction (Table 34–1). Within a peripheral nerve only about 25% of the fibers are myelinated (Gilroy, 1990).

RESPONSE TO INJURY

When either motor or sensory nerves are affected there is a limited response to injury, regardless of the cause. Either the myelin that surrounds the larger nerves can demyelinate or, in more severe involvement, the nerve can degenerate distal to the lesion. *Segmental demyelination* leaves the axon intact as myelin breaks down, while *wallerian degeneration* is the anterograde (distal) degeneration of the axon (Junqueira et al., 1992). Segmental demyelination occurs when nerves are subject to external compression or disease. Wallerian degeneration occurs in any peripheral nerve disorder that directly affects the axon. This includes crush, stretch, or laceration injury, as well as disease.

Diseases that affect the axon or its cell body causing axonal degeneration typically affect the longest nerve fibers first, with signs and symptoms beginning distally and spreading proximally as the disease progresses. Because nerves in the legs are longer, the feet and lower legs are involved long before the fingers and hands. Those conditions that affect only myelin cause segmental demyelination in both sensory and motor fibers. Thus, disruption of the conduction of the action potential from proprioceptors and mechanoreceptors causes sensory changes. In addition, demyelination of motor nerves to muscle and preganglionic fibers of the autonomic nervous system (ANS) create weakness and autonomic involvement.

CLASSIFICATION OF NERVE INJURY

Traumatic injury to peripheral nerves from conditions like compression, ischemia, and stretching can be classified using one of two systems based on the structural and functional changes that occur. Sunderland (1978) classifies nerve injury into one of five degrees indicating the presence or absence of axon and connective tissue, while Seddon (1943) divides nerve injury into one of three categories: neurapraxia, axonotmesis, and neurotmesis (Fig. 34–3A).

Neurapraxia involves segmental demyelination, which slows or blocks conduction of the action potential at the point of demyelination on a myelinated nerve. Neurapraxias often occur following nerve compression that induces mild ischemia in nerve fibers. When segmental demyelination occurs because of disease, the response is often termed a *myelinopathy*. Conduction of the action potential is normal above and below the point of compression and because the axon remains intact muscle does not atrophy. *Axonotmesis* occurs when the axon has been damaged, but the connective tissue coverings that support and protect the nerve remain intact. Prolonged compression that produces an area of infarction and necrosis causes an axonotmesis. In the presence of disease, wallerian degeneration creates an *axonopathy*, which is analogous to an axonotmesis. *Neurotmesis*, the complete severance of nerve fiber and its supporting endoneurium, also produces axonal loss, but in this condition the connective tissue coverings are also disrupted at the site of injury. Neu-

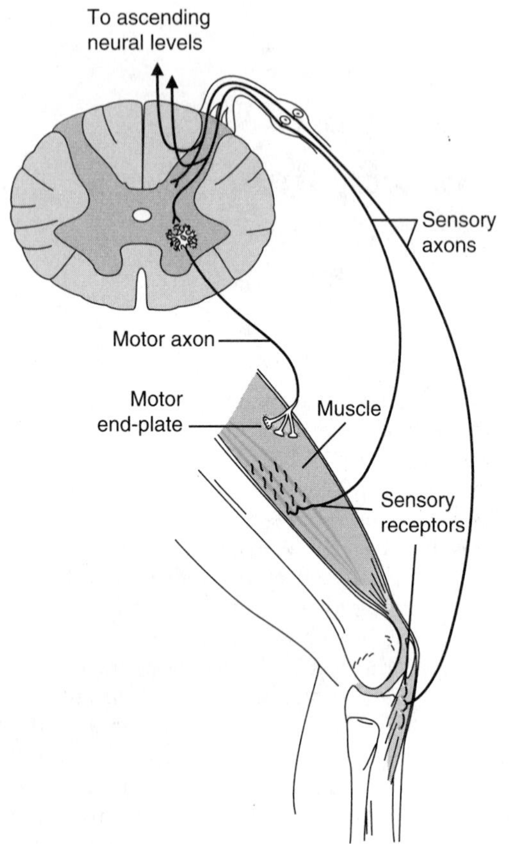

Figure **34–1.** Potential sites of involvement in the peripheral nervous system. Motor: motor neuron cell body, axon, motor end plate, muscle fiber. Sensory: cell body in ganglion, axon, sensory receptor.

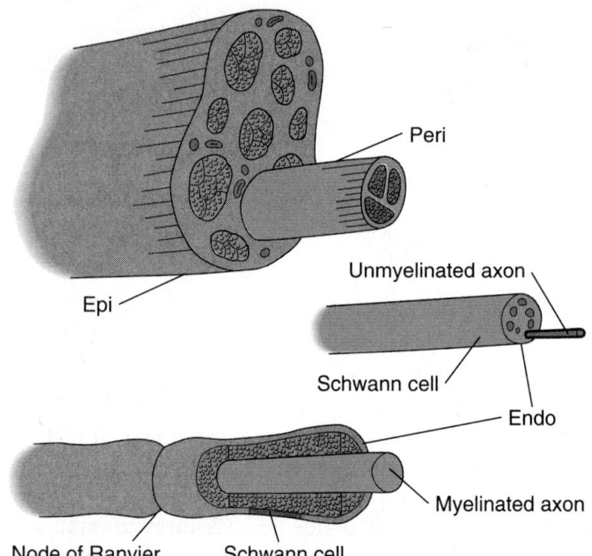

Figure **34–2.** Cross-section of a peripheral nerve showing connective tissue coverings. Externally, the nerve is enveloped by the epineurium (*Epi*); internally, individual axons are surrounded by endoneurium (*Endo*). The perineurium (*Peri*) surrounds groups of axons. Although the majority of the fibers are unmyelinated, they are still associated with supporting Schwann cells. In myelinated fibers, the Schwann cell forms the myelin internode whose borders are formed by the nodes of Ranvier.

rotmesis is caused by gunshot or stab wounds, or avulsion injuries that disrupt a section of the nerve. When axonal continuity is lost (either axonotmesis or neurotmesis), axons distal to the lesion degenerate (*wallerian degeneration*). Because muscle fibers innervated by the axon depend upon the nerve cell body as a source of nourishment or trophic control, when axons degenerate muscle fibers rapidly atrophy (Table 34–2).

If segmental demyelination has occurred, then Schwann cells will mitotically divide and envelope the denuded segment of nerve. Once these cells are in place they will begin to form myelin (Fig. 34–3B). The potential for regeneration after wallerian degeneration is possible as long as the nerve cell body remains viable; new axons can sprout from the proximal end of damaged axons. However, successful functional regeneration requires that the proximal and distal ends of the connective tissue tube align. This occurs relatively easily in an axonotmesis because the connective tissue coverings are intact. In a neurotmesis, without surgical intervention, recovery is less likely because the ends of the endoneurium are not approximated. Without surgery axonal sprouts often enter nearby soft tissue and form a neuroma, or axonal regrowth occurs down the incorrect endoneurial tube (Parry, 1992). Once the axon has established a distal contact either with muscle or sensory receptor, remyelination will begin (Fig. 34–3C).

TABLE 34–1 Relationship of Myelin Thickness, Conduction Velocity, and Sensory and Motor Fibers

Myelin	Conduction Velocity	Sensory Fibers	Motor Fibers
Very thick	Very fast	Proprioception (muscle spindle and Golgi tendon organ)	To skeletal muscle fibers (alpha)
Thick	Fast	Touch, pressure	To muscle spindle (gamma)
Thin	Slower	Touch, temperature	To ANS ganglia
None	Slow	Pain	From ANS ganglia to smooth muscle

ANS, autonomic nervous system.

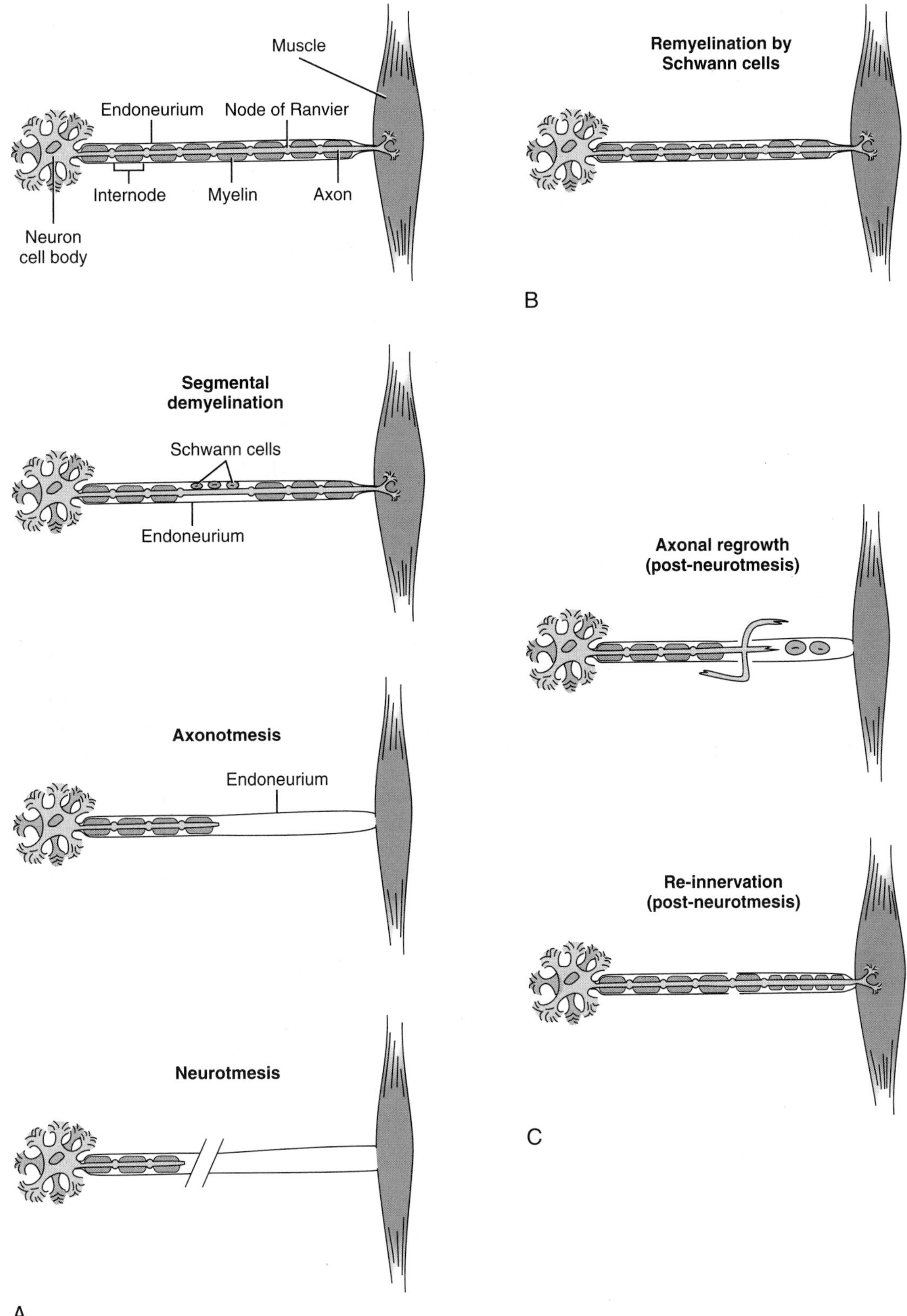

Figure **34–3.** Types of nerve involvement and recovery that occur in peripheral nerves. *A*, Top figure illustrates a normal myelinated nerve. In the picture showing segmental demyelination, one internode of myelin has demyelinated. In the illustration of axonotmesis, the axon and myelin have degenerated, but the connective tissue covering remains intact. In neurotmesis, the connective tissue covering is disrupted at the lesion site. Signs of chromatolysis occur in the cell body following axonotmesis and neurotmesis. Note that muscle atrophies rapidly in the last two conditions because it has lost the trophic influence from the nerve cell body. *B*, The repair process for segmental demyelination occurs rapidly because Schwann cells divide and remyelinate the bare portion of the axon. Shorter internodal distance occurs with remyelination; thus nerve conduction velocity may not return to normal, even though muscle contracts normally. *C*, The repair process for axonotmesis and neurotmesis is more complex. Growth cones from the proximal axon must cross the lesion site and regrow down the connective tissue "channels" and reestablish a motor end plate or sensory connection before remyelination occurs. In neurotmesis the growth cones may enter nearby soft tissue and fail to establish their connections; thus a neuroma is formed.

TABLE 34–2 Relationship of Nerve and Muscle Responses to Disease and Trauma

Level of Severity	Response to Disease	Response to Trauma	Response of Muscle
Mild	Myelinopathy (segmental demyelination)	Neurapraxia (segmental demyelination)	Paresis/paralysis, no atrophy
Severe	Axonopathy (wallerian degeneration)	Axonotmesis (wallerian degeneration)	Paresis/paralysis with atrophy
Severe	—	Neurotmesis (wallerian degeneration)	Paresis/paralysis with atrophy

CLASSIFICATION OF NEUROPATHY

Neuropathies include a wide variety of causes and because of this they can be classified in many ways. They may be classified according to the rate of onset, type and size of nerve fibers involved, distribution pattern, or pathology (Table 34–3). For example, when a single peripheral nerve is affected the result is a *mononeuropathy;* this is commonly a result of trauma. The term *polyneuropathy* indicates involvement of several peripheral nerves. A *radiculoneuropathy* indicates involvement of the nerve root as it emerges from the spinal cord, while *polyradiculitis* indicates involvement of several nerve roots and occurs when infections create an inflammatory response.

In addition to involvement of the peripheral nerve, the motor end plate or muscle itself may be involved in a peripheral disorder. Involvement of muscle, termed *myopathy*, follows a different clinical pattern than nerve. When muscle is involved, the disorder typically is reflected by proximal weakness, wasting, and hypotonia without sensory impairments (Dubowitz, 1978).

SIGNS AND SYMPTOMS OF PERIPHERAL DYSFUNCTION

The presence of signs and symptoms aid in the localization of the level or levels of involvement. Loss of sensory function will follow a peripheral nerve distribution if that is the anatomic region involved, or it will follow a dermatomal pattern when the spinal nerve or dorsal root ganglia (cell body) has been affected (Fig. 34–4).

Similarly, when a peripheral nerve has motor involvement, paresis or paralysis will occur in muscles innervated by that nerve distal to the lesion. When spinal motor nerves are involved, weakness occurs in all the muscles receiving axons from that spinal level (a myotomal pattern). Individuals with only peripheral nerve involvement will have no signs or symptoms of central nervous system (CNS) dysfunction.

Although differences occur in symptom evolution and in progression and severity of a neuropathy, a classic pattern of involvement would occur as follows. Involvement of sensory fibers is reflected by distal sensory deficits with the longest

TABLE 34–3 Causes of Peripheral Neuropathies and Myopathies and Their Effects

Cause	Involvement*					
	Axonal Degeneration	Demyelination	Motor End Plate	Muscle	Motor	Sensory
Charcot-Marie-Tooth disease	X	X			X	X
Mechanical compression/entrapment						
Neurapraxia		X			X	X
Axonotmesis	X				X	X
Neurotmesis	X				X	X
Postpolio syndrome	X				X	
Diabetic mellitus	X	X			X	X
Alcohol	X	X			X	X
Guillain-Barré syndrome	X	X			X	X
Toxins						
Lead	X				X	X
Organophosphate	X	X			X	X
Myasthenia gravis			X		X	
Botulism			X		X	
Muscular dystrophy				X	X	
Inflammatory myopathy				X	X	
Steroid-induced myopathy				X	X	
Overuse myopathy				X	X	
Aging	X	X	X	X	X	X

* The X's indicate the most common types of involvement for each cause.

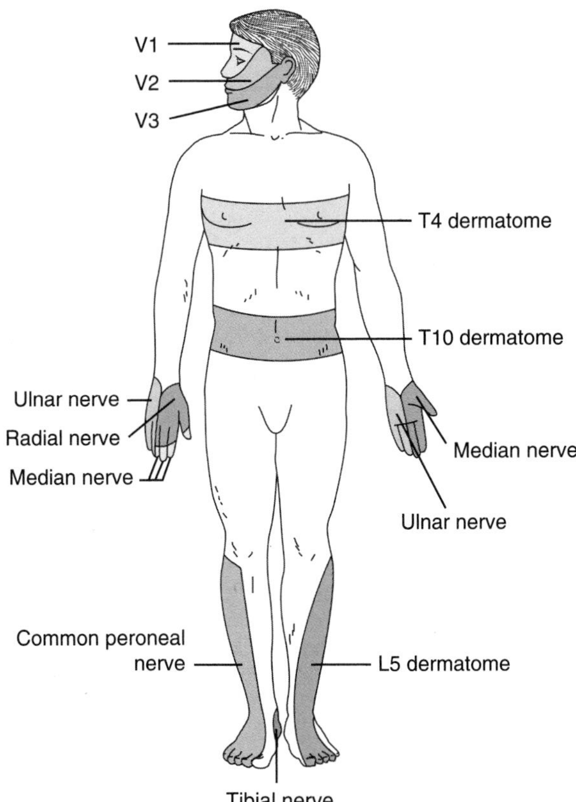

Figure **34-4.** Examples of dermatomal and peripheral nerve patterns. Illustrated are the regions of the skin innervated by the ulnar, median, and radial peripheral nerves in the upper extremity and the common peroneal and tibial nerves in the lower extremity. On the face, trunk, and leg, the dermatomal patterns of sensation are mapped for the trigeminal nerve, T4 (nipples), T10 (umbilicus), and L5, respectively.

nerves in the body involved first. The first noticeable features of neuropathies are often sensory and consist of tingling, prickling, burning, or bandlike *dysesthesias* and *paresthesias* in the feet. When more than one nerve is involved, the sensory loss follows a "glove and stocking" distribution that is attributed to the "dying back" of the longest fibers in all nerves from distal to proximal. (Fig. 34–5).

The most common symptoms of motor nerve involvement include distal weakness and abnormalities of tone (hypotonicity or flaccidity). When clients are asked to walk on their heels, weakness of dorsiflexors becomes obvious. Deep tendon reflexes (DTRs) are diminished or absent. In the presence of axonal degeneration, rapid atrophy occurs, along with electrophysiologic changes (Tables 34–4 and 34–5). Prolonged paralysis gives rise to secondary complications like contractures and edema.

In addition to weakness and hypotonia, a diagnosis of any one of the muscle diseases may be associated with muscle tenderness or cramping. The motor involvement in a myopathy classically is opposite to that of a neuropathy. *In a myopathy the weakness is proximal; in a neuropathy it is distal.*

Finally, because the nerve fibers from the ANS are also located in peripheral nerves, they, too, are subject to the effects of trauma or disease. Preganglionic fibers are myelinated and can be affected by segmental demyelination. In the presence of axonal degeneration, changes will occur in vascular control and sweating. For example, when a person has sustained a laceration of the median nerve in the region of the hand that lacks autonomic innervation, the skin is smooth and does not sweat or wrinkle.

PATHOGENESIS AND DIAGNOSIS OF PERIPHERAL DYSFUNCTION

Trauma, inherited disorders, environmental toxins, and nutritional disorders may affect the myelin (myelinopathy), axon (axonopathy), or cell body of a peripheral nerve. The anatomic region or regions affected determine the severity of the involvement and the amount of function lost (see Table 34–3).

Because the nervous system is the means of signaling from the CNS to the muscle, conduction of the action potential is affected in neuropathies and myopathies. In most disorders electrophysiologic studies are used to determine where and how the nerve or muscle may be affected.

HEREDITARY NEUROPATHIES

Hereditary neuropathies are rare conditions that are genetically determined.

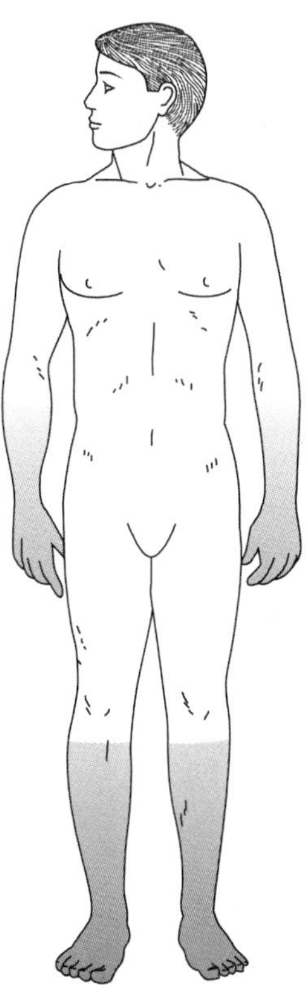

Figure **34-5.** A stocking and glove pattern of sensory loss occurs in polyneuropathy. A gradient of greater distal loss tapering to less proximal involvement is seen.

TABLE 34-4 NORMAL NERVE CONDUCTION VELOCITIES AND DISTAL LATENCIES*

NERVE	MOTOR CONDUCTION VELOCITY (m/sec)	MOTOR DISTAL LATENCY (ms)	SENSORY DISTAL LATENCY (ms)
Ulnar	60 (56–62.7)	2.8 (2.3–3.4)	3.2 (2.9–3.5)
Median	64.3 (59.8–70.4)	3.3 (2.8–4.2)	3.2 (2.9–3.45)
Radial	61.6 (48–75)	2.4 (1.9–2.9)	2.6 (2.0–3.3)
Peroneal	50	5.1	—
Posterior tibial	51.2	2.1–5.6	—

* In general, in the upper extremities, nerve conduction velocity for motor fibers averages about 60 m/sec. Investigators have reported values ranging from 45 to 75 m/sec. In the lower extremity the normal range for motor nerve conduction is in the 40- to 50-m/sec range. Distal latency is a time value, reported in milliseconds, that it takes for an evoked potential to be propagated along the nerve and recorded from either the muscle (motor) or the skin (sensory).

From Goodgold, J, Eberstein A: Electrodiagnosis of Neuromuscular Diseases, ed 2. Baltimore, Williams & Wilkins, 1978, p 109.

Charcot-Marie-Tooth Disease

Charcot-Marie-Tooth disease (CMT), or peroneal muscular atrophy, is an inherited disorder affecting motor and sensory nerves. It was originally described by three neurologists, Jean Martin Charcot, Pierre Marie, and Howard Henry Tooth, in the 1880s. Initially the disorder involves the peroneal nerve and affects muscles in the foot and lower leg. It later progresses to involve muscles of the hands and forearms (Fig. 34–6).

Incidence. Of the neuropathies, CMT is relatively common; it is estimated that 1 in 2500 persons in the United States has some form of CMT. Onset may occur in childhood or adulthood.

Etiology. Most cases of CMT are inherited as an autosomal dominant disorder; however, there are autosomal recessive and X-linked forms. CMT is a genetically heterogeneous polyneuropathy with two forms. In CMT1 chromosome 17 has a tandem DNA duplication, causing segmental demyelination of the peroneal nerve. A less common form, CMT2, is associated with a chromosomal abnormality located on chromosome 1 that causes axonal degeneration. CMT2 has a later onset and less involvement in the small muscles of the hands than CMT1.

Pathology. Extensive demyelination with hypertrophic Schwann cell "onion bulb" formation occurs with CMT1; the hypertrophic Schwann cell creates palpable, enlarged peripheral nerves. Loss of both anterior horn cells in lumbosacral segments of the spinal cord and cell bodies in the dorsal root ganglion lead to axonal degeneration in CMT2.

Clinical Manifestations. In all autosomal dominant disorders there are degrees of genetic dominance. The presence of symptoms are not all-or-none, but are graded. This is termed *variable penetrance*. In CMT1 some members of a family with the genetic mutation may have greater signs of the disorder than others who have only minor involvement (Sheldon, 1992).

CMT is a slowly progressive disorder and though CMT1 begins in childhood, the actual onset may be difficult to determine. Clinical signs of CMT include distally symmetrical muscle weakness, atrophy, and diminished DTRs. The feet have pes cavus deformities (high arch) and hammer toes. Because of the muscles affected, the client will have weakness of the dorsiflexors and evertors and will ambulate with a foot drop (steppage) gait pattern. As CMT progresses, involvement will be seen distally in the upper extremities. Weakness and wasting of the intrinsic muscles of the hand occurs, followed by progressive wasting in the forearms. Because CMT1 demyelinates peripheral nerves, proprioception is lost in the feet and ankles and cutaneous sensation is diminished in the foot and lower legs. Sensory loss is minimal in CMT2.

As muscle atrophy progresses below the knee, the appearance of the client's legs takes on the shape of an inverted champagne bottle because normal muscle bulk is maintained above the knees.

Medical Management

Diagnosis. CMT is diagnosed by history and clinical examination, hereditary picture, electrophysiologic studies, and

TABLE 34-5 RELATIONSHIP OF ELECTROMYOGRAPHIC FINDINGS TO INNERVATION

CONDITION	NORMAL INNERVATION	SEGMENTAL DEMYELINATION	AXONAL/WALLERIAN DEGENERATION	MYOPATHY
Insertion	Normal insertional noise	Normal insertional noise	Increased insertional noise	Increased insertional noise
At rest	Quiet	Quiet	Spontaneous (abnormal) potentials: fibrillation potential, positive sharp wave potential	Quiet, except end stage: fibrillation potentials
Minimal contraction	Normal motor unit potential	Affected fibers: no motor unit potential	Affected fibers: no motor unit potential	Low amplitude, polyphasic potential
Maximal contraction	Complete interference pattern	Nerve partially affected: decreased interference pattern	Nerve partially affected: decreased interference pattern; nerve completely affected: no interference pattern	Low amplitude full interference pattern, accomplished with increased frequency of firing and with moderate effort

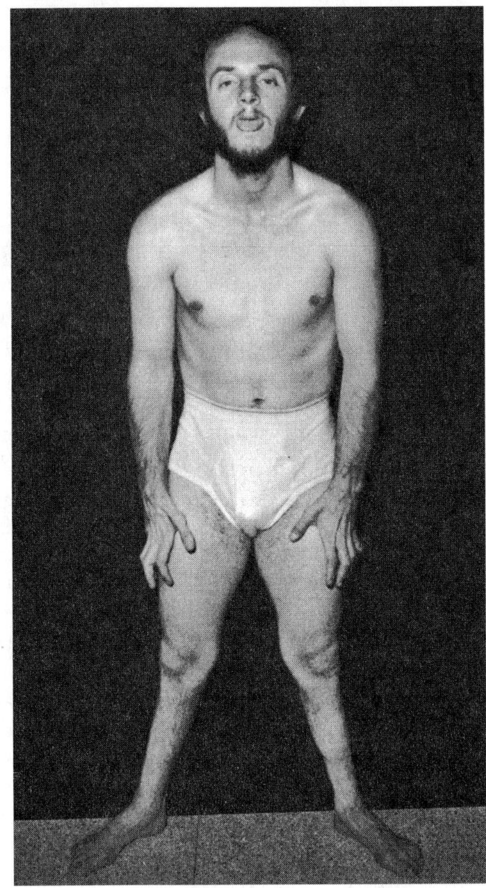

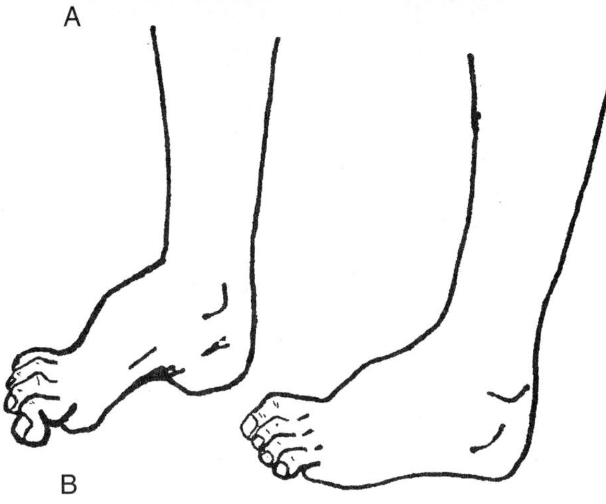

Figure **34-6.** A, A person with Charcot-Marie-Tooth disease. Note the atrophy that occurs distal to the knee, as well as involvement distally in the hands. (*From Ringel S: Clinical presentations in neuromuscular disease. In Vinken PJ, Bruyn GW: Handbook of Clinical Neurology, vol 40. New York, North-Holland, 1979, p 320.*) B, These persons also develop hammer toes and a high-arched pes cavus foot deformity.

nerve biopsy. The nerve biopsy is abnormal and will demonstrate either a demyelinating or axonal degenerative process. Both motor and sensory nerve conduction velocities (NCVs) will be slowed in CMT1, but are normal or only slightly slowed in CMT2.

Treatment. Because CMT is an inherited disorder, there is no specific treatment to alter its course. Treatment is symptomatic to ensure that function is maintained in a safe manner. Footdrop and hand deformities can be helped by orthotic devices. Because the possibility of skin ulceration exists when tactile sensation and proprioception are affected, skin care precautions should be followed when total contact orthoses are used (see Chapter 8). To prevent contractures clients should be instructed in range-of-motion exercises. Whether strengthening exercises can be used to counteract the effects of CMT1 has not been addressed. In CMT2 strengthening exercises will be of little benefit because of the ongoing axonal degeneration.

Prognosis. CMT is a slowly progressive disorder; if unmanaged, contracture formation resulting from weakness will create further gait abnormalities, with clients reporting an increased number of falls. In the upper extremities clients may develop problems with writing and handling objects.

COMPRESSION AND ENTRAPMENT SYNDROMES

The proximity of peripheral nerves to bony, muscular, and vascular structures can cause entrapment or compression syndromes. Clients frequently seek medical attention for the consequences of these disorders.

Carpal Tunnel Syndrome

Carpal tunnel syndrome (CTS) is the most common entrapment neuropathy in the United States. It results from compression of the median nerve within the carpal tunnel at the wrist (Fig. 34–7). CTS is characterized by general signs and symptoms of neuropathies: pain, tingling, numbness, paresthesia and, later, muscular weakness in the distribution of the median nerve.

Incidence. In 1988 the National Center for Health Statistics estimated that 1.89 million workers in the United States were affected with CTS; by 1995 Ellis reported that this figure had increased to over 5 million Americans. The case rate for both men and women peaks between ages 35 and 55 (Palmer and Hanrahan, 1995). Approximately 500,000 surgeries annually are performed for CTS. The incidence of surgery peaks in the 45- to 55-year-old group in women and in the over-65-year-old group in men.

Etiology. Although CTS is associated with occupational activities, any disorder that increases the volume of the contents of the carpal tunnel, or that decreases the volume of the carpal tunnel may impinge upon the median nerve. This includes synovial proliferation in rheumatoid arthritis, edema from local and systemic infections, congestive heart failure, and tumors. Callus formation following fracture, as well as malalignment of fractures, may reduce the volume of the canal. Upton and McComas (1973) reported that a compressive lesion located more proximally on a nerve may predispose it to further injury. Thus, CTS may be present along with thoracic outlet syndrome (TOS) and cervical disk lesions. The increased incidence of CTS has been attributed to both

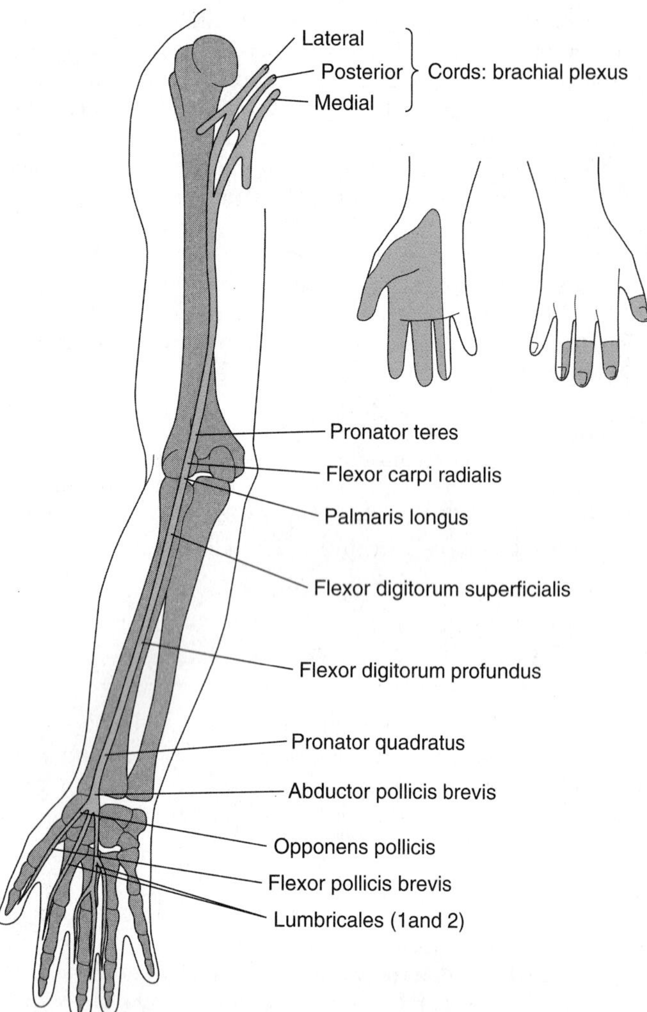

Figure **34–7.** Median nerve innervation with sensory distribution in the hand (dorsal surface, *far right;* volar surface, *near right*).

repetitive single tasks in automated jobs, as well as an increased awareness of CTS as an occupational disorder.

Risk Factors. Exposure to situations that involve repetitive and forceful gripping is a major risk factor for CTS. CTS has been reported in several occupations: meat packers, grocery store and assembly line workers, jackhammer operators, computer operators, grinders, and workers using high-force, highly repetitive manual movements (Hagberg et al., 1992). Also at risk for developing CTS are people with rheumatoid tenosynovitis, edema, pregnancy, and hypothyroidism (Stevens et al., 1992; Table 34–6).

Pathogenesis. In the carpal tunnel where there are 10 structures in a constrained compartment, normal tissue pressures are 7 to 8 mm Hg (Fig. 34–8). In CTS these pressures rise above 30 mm Hg, and go as high as 90 mm Hg when the wrist is flexed. Pressure this great produces ischemia in the nerve. Ischemia accounts for the nocturnal symptoms or those that occur with wrist flexion. Unrelieved compression creates an initial neurapraxia with segmental demyelination of axons. Because the axons have lost their myelin "padding" they are more vulnerable, so that unrelieved compression can create an axonotmesis in which axon continuity is lost and wallerian degeneration occurs.

Clinical Manifestations. Persons with CTS experience sensory symptoms in the median nerve distribution (see Fig. 34–7). Pain may be located distally in the forearm or wrist and radiate into the thumb, index, and middle fingers. It may also radiate into the arm, shoulder, and neck. Nocturnal pain is the hallmark of CTS. Even in the early stages of CTS most people will report being awakened by painful numbness in the middle of the night. Sensory symptoms usually precede motor symptoms. Thenar weakness is seen in advanced cases. In nearly half of all cases, symptoms occur bilaterally. If CTS goes untreated, symptoms escalate into persistent pain with atrophy of the thenar musculature and the person will have a loss of grip strength. The combined loss of grip strength, inability to pinch, and sensory loss causes clumsiness in the hands (Dawson, 1993). Because conditions that impinge nerve fibers in the neck (radiculopathy) or in the thoracic outlet also cause sensory symptoms that are referred to the hand, it is important to ascertain that the symptoms are related to CTS (see Table 34–6).

Medical Management

Diagnosis. The diagnosis of CTS is considered in any person with hand or wrist pain, numbness, and weakness. Diagnosis is determined by history, physical examination, and specialized tests. Provocation tests are used to replicate CTS symptoms. The tethered median nerve stress test has been shown to be a reliable diagnostic indicator of CTS in patients

TABLE 34–6 Causes of Carpal Tunnel Syndrome

Systemic	Neuromusculoskeletal
Arthritis (rheumatoid, gout, polymyalgia rheumatica)	Amyloidosis
Benign tumors (lipoma, hemangioma, ganglia)	Anatomic sequelae of medical or surgical procedures
Endocrine disorders	Cervical disk lesions
Acromegaly	Cervical spondylosis
Diabetes mellitus	Congenital anatomic differences
Hormonal imbalance (menopause, post hysterectomy)	Cumulative trauma disorders
Hyperparathyroidism	Peripheral neuropathy
Hyperthyroidism	Poor posture (may also be associated with thoracic outlet syndrome)
Hypocalcemia	Repetitive strain injuries
Hypothyroidism	Tendinitis
Infectious disease	Tenosynovitis
Atypical mycobacterium	Thoracic outlet syndrome
Histoplasmosis	Wrist trauma (e.g., Colles' fracture)
Rubella	
Sporotrichosis	
Leukemia (tissue infiltration)	
Liver disease	
Multiple myeloma	

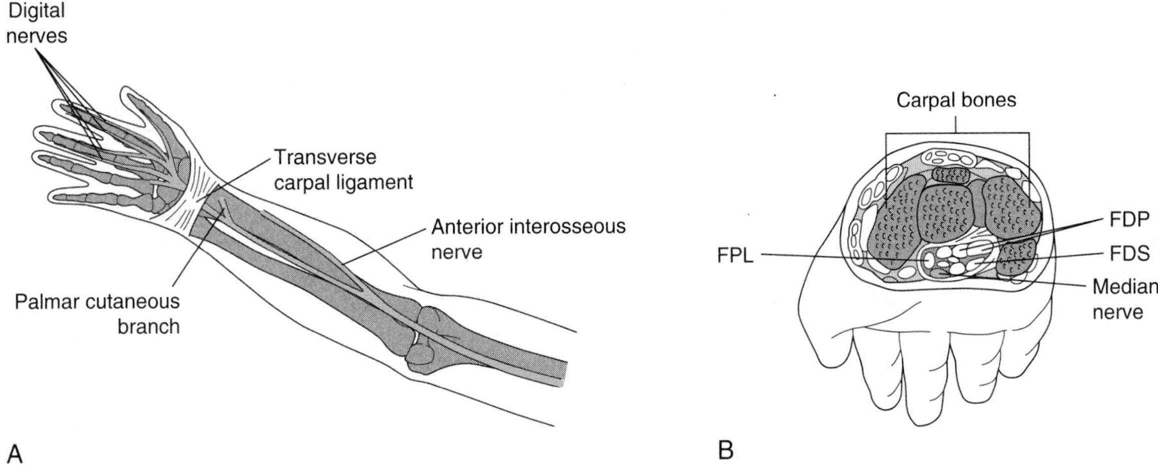

Figure **34–8.** A, Schematic illustration of the route taken by the median nerve as it traverses the volar aspect of the right arm under the transverse carpal ligament. (From Stewart JD: Focal Peripheral Neuropathies, ed 2. New York, Raven Press, 1993, p 158.) B, Cross-section of the carpal tunnel at the wrist. Contents of the tunnel include the tendon of the flexor pollicis longus (FPL), the four tendons of the flexor digitorum profundus (FDP), the four tendons of the flexor digitorum superficialis (FDS), and the median nerve.

with low-grade chronic CTS. The test is administered by hyperextending the index finger with the wrist in a supinated position. The patient with CTS experiences pain as the nerve becomes ischemic from vascular occlusion (LaBan et al., 1989). Phalen's test (wrist flexion to 90 degrees for 1 minute; Fig. 34–9), Tinel's test (wrist percussion over the carpal tunnel; Fig. 34–10), and the carpal compression test (pressure is applied by the examiner by pressing his or her thumbs at the wrist over the flexor retinaculum) are all deemed positive when pain, numbness, and paresthesia are produced. Of these three tests, the carpal compression test is the most reliable (93%), while Tinel's is least reliable (60% to 70%), with Phalen's test reliably reproducing symptoms 90% of the time (Katz, 1994).

Objective tests to confirm the diagnosis include nerve conduction velocity. Changes in the sensory conduction across the wrist are reportedly the most sensitive indicator of CTS (Whitley and McDonnell, 1995). A modified NCV technique, termed "inching," has been shown to provide greater sensitivity and specificity of anatomic involvement for CTS (Imaoka et al., 1992). Although NCV generally provides the benchmark for CTS, a negative NCV study alone does not exclude the possibility of CTS. Finally, magnetic resonance imaging (MRI) has also been found effective in identifying various anomalies, including altered tendon position, altered nerve position, swelling of the median nerve, and thickening of the tendon sheath to aid in establishing the diagnosis of CTS (Middleton et al., 1987). The diagnosis of CTS must be distinguished most often from a cervical radiculopathy or ulnar neuropathy (Dawson, 1993).

Treatment. For patients with mild symptoms, demonstrated by only subjective and objective sensory symptoms, conservative management is generally instituted. Medical management of mild symptoms includes steroid injection into the carpal canal to provide initial relief of symptoms. Early management also addresses ergonomic measures and modification of the client's occupation. Wearing of wrist splints to immobilize the wrist near neutral to minimize carpal tunnel pressures, and patient education are also instituted. With client compliance, this approach is cost-effective compared

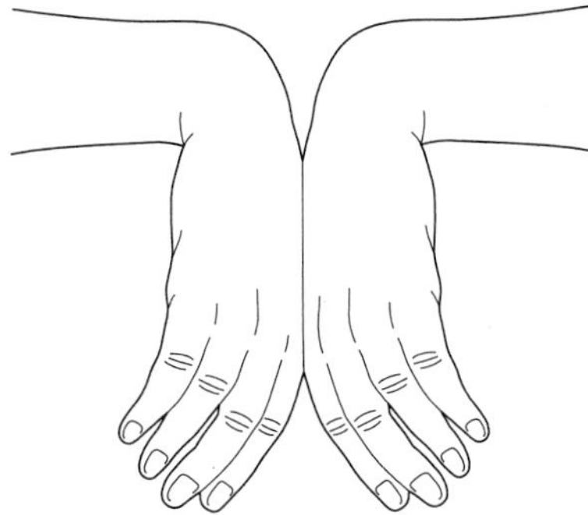

Figure **34–9.** Phalen's test. The volar surfaces of the hands are held together by flexing the wrists to 90 degrees. A positive test will elicit symptoms within 60 seconds.

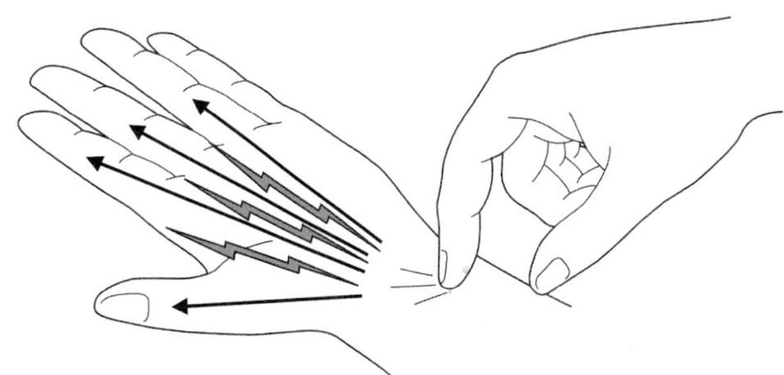

Figure **34–10.** Tinel's test percusses over the carpal tunnel to provoke tingling and burning along the distribution of the median nerve.

to the alternative medical treatment (Siebenaler and McGovern, 1992; Kruger et al., 1991). However, the long-term use of anti-inflammatory medications and immobilization demonstrated a cure rate of only 18%. Relapse was noted within 1 year.

Surgical intervention is advocated for persons without resolution of symptoms following a conservative approach for 2 to 3 months. Surgery is also indicated in untreated persons whose symptoms have lasted longer than 1 year and who demonstrate both motor and sensory NCV involvement, or in persons with denervation as evidenced by fibrillation potentials on electromyography (EMG). Release of the transverse carpal ligament is commonly performed and is usually successful. Complications fall into two categories: errors in diagnosis or surgical technique. Newer surgical techniques (flexor tenosynovectomy with transverse carpal ligament division, endoscopic release of the ligament, and neurolysis of the median nerve) are performed through limited incisions and require less exposure and less manipulation of the nerve than the classic open techniques (Junter, 1995). All have been reported to relieve symptoms. Seventy-six percent of the surgical cases experience return of normal two-point discrimination and up to 70% have normal muscle strength return (Rhoades et al., 1985). Following surgery, nerve and tendon gliding techniques are advocated to reduce scarring, adhesions, and subsequent formation of fibrotic tissue (Totten and Hunter, 1991).

Prognosis. Prognosis relates directly to the severity of the nerve entrapment at diagnosis, clinical cause, and mode of treatment.

Sciatica

Sciatica is a radiculopathy in which the nerve root is affected, most typically by compression. In addition to low back pain, when sensory fibers are affected pain will radiate into one or both legs. One of the reasons the motor and sensory nerves are affected so easily in a radiculopathy is because spinal nerve fibers lack the protection of the same connective tissue coverings that are present in the peripheral nerve (Junqueira et al., 1992). For further information, see Chapter 23.

Bell's Palsy

Incidence. Bell's palsy is a common clinical condition in which the facial nerve is unilaterally affected. Bell's palsy affects 20 of 100,000 people each year. While any age group can be affected, it is most common in persons between the ages of 20 and 40 years.

Etiology and Pathogenesis. The cause of Bell's palsy is uncertain. Days before its onset, the client may recall experiencing severe pain in the area of the mastoid. Pain suggests that this disorder is a product of an inflammatory response. Because the facial nerve lies in the auditory canal, any agent that causes inflammation and swelling creates a compression that initially causes demyelination. However, if the inflammatory response is more fulminating, ischemia will cause an axonal degeneration.

In addition, centrally located structures, such as acoustic neuromas (tumor), can produce unilateral paralysis in the face by impinging on the facial nerve as it emerges from the brainstem.

Risk Factors. People with diabetes mellitus and pregnant women have an increased incidence of Bell's palsy.

Clinical Manifestations. A unilateral facial paralysis develops rapidly, often overnight. Paralysis of the muscles of facial expression on one side creates an asymmetrical facial appearance. The corner of the mouth droops, the nasolabial fold is flattened, and the palpebral fissure is widened because the eyelid does not close. In addition to the motor fibers providing innervation for facial musculature, the facial nerve also innervates the stapedius muscle of the middle ear, and the sensory and autonomic fibers, which innervate for taste, and lacrimation and salivation, respectively. Therefore, involvement of these fibers may produce additional signs and symptoms to those of facial paralysis. If the lesion is proximal to where the fibers of the chorda tympani enter the facial nerve, the client will experience loss of taste on the affected side. In a similar fashion, if the autonomic fibers are involved, the client will experience a dry eye (lack of tearing) and will produce less, but thicker saliva. Some clients report that sounds are louder than normal. This is because the stapes bone of the middle ear is less able to accommodate to sound when the stapedius muscle's innervation is lost.

Medical Management

Diagnosis. Ask the client to wrinkle the forehead, close the eyes tightly, smile, and whistle while you observe for facial asymmetry. In addition to the clinical presentation and history, electrodiagnostic tests can be used to demonstrate whether the lesion is one of demyelination or axonal degeneration. However, EMG as a diagnostic tool is only helpful after the nerve has degenerated; therefore, testing is most accurate after 1 week. Tests of facial nerve excitability will also indicate whether the paralysis is complete.

The LMN involvement of the facial nerve can be differentiated from an upper motor neuron (UMN) involvement to this nerve because with UMN involvement, the client can close the eye and wrinkle the forehead, but cannot smile voluntarily. With LMN involvement, the client is unable to close the eye, wrinkle the forehead, or smile voluntarily.

Treatment. Since the outcome (demyelination or degeneration) is unknown initially, prophylactic administration of high-dose corticosteroids for 5 days, followed by a tapered dose for 5 days, has been advocated. For more severe involvement, this treatment is reported to help prevent permanent damage. Treatment should begin as soon as possible, and no later than 10 days following onset of signs of paralysis.

To protect the cornea, the client should cover the eye with a patch or glasses and use artificial tears. Other palliative treatments, such as gentle massage and gentle heat, may also be used.

Prognosis. For incomplete involvement, typically recovery is complete and occurs over a period of weeks. When involvement is complete, most persons also recover, although the course of recovery is longer. Plastic surgery, using fascial slings to replace active muscle contraction, can help restore facial function when recovery does not occur. Another complication that can occur during recovery is a phenomenon called "crocodile tears." This occurs when motor fibers of the facial nerve cross-innervate the autonomic branch of the greater superficial petrosal nerve. When muscles of the face contract, tears appear (Asbury et al., 1986).

Tardy Ulnar Palsy

Anatomy. The ulnar nerve arises from the lower trunk of the brachial plexus and carries fibers from C8 and T1 nerve roots. At the elbow it passes behind the medial epicondyle and then passes between the two heads of the flexor carpi ulnaris through the forearm to the wrist. The distal portion of the nerve enters the palm by crossing the flexor retinaculum and divides into a superficial and deep branch in the hand (Fig. 34–11).

Etiology. Because of its anatomic location ulnar nerve palsy is a common complication of fractures in the region of the elbow. A late or tardy ulnar palsy may occur years after a fracture and is associated with callus formation or a valgus deformity of the elbow. These produce a gradual stretching of the nerve in the ulnar groove of the medial epicondyle.

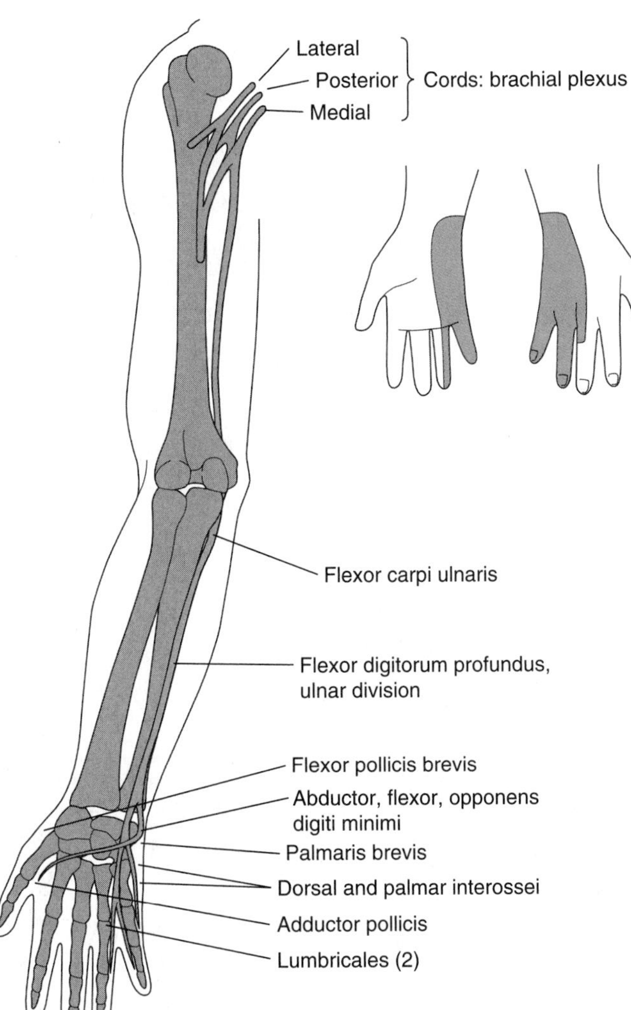

Figure **34–11.** Distribution of the ulnar nerve with sensory distribution to the hand (dorsal surface, *far right;* volar surface, *near right*). A tardy ulnar palsy impinges the ulnar nerve as it passes behind the medial epicondyle of the humerus. (*Adapted from Hollinshead WH, Rosse C: Textbook of Anatomy, ed 4. Philadelphia, Harper & Row, 1985, p 157.*)

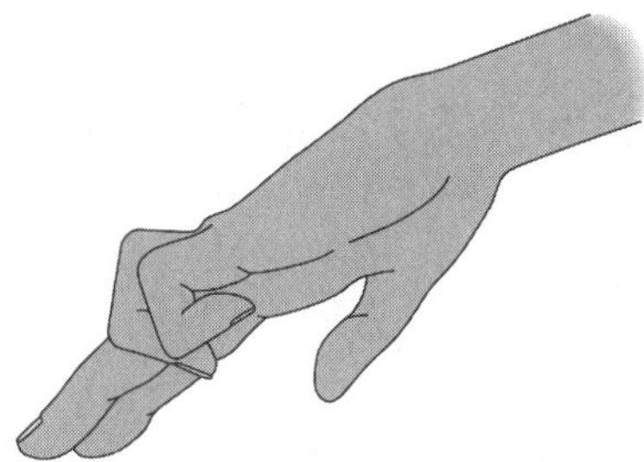

Figure **34–12.** Clawing of the ring and little fingers (hyperextension of the metacarpophalangeal joint and flexion of the interphalangeal joints) due to unopposed action of extensor musculature combined with paralysis of the intrinsic muscles of the hand occurs when there is involvement of the ulnar nerve.

Risk Factors. A similar type of tardy ulnar palsy occurs with repeated trauma for relatively long periods of time in patients with a shallow ulnar groove at the elbow.

Pathogenesis. Compression will initially cause a neurapraxia with demyelination of the nerve; if the pressure goes unrelieved, this will progress to an axonotmesis with denervation occurring below the level of the elbow.

Clinical Manifestations. Expect a clawhand deformity with metacarpophalangeal (MCP) extension and interphalangeal (IP) flexion of the ring and little fingers due to the unopposed action of the extensor muscle group and paralysis of the third and fourth lumbricals which normally flex the MCPs and extend the IPs (Fig. 34–12). Flattening of the hypothenar eminence along with abduction of the little finger coincides with weakness of the palmaris brevis and abductor digiti minimi. Marked atrophy of the interossei on the dorsal surface of the hand with "guttering" between the extensor tendons indicates the presence of denervation. Abduction and adduction movements of the fingers are impaired. Paralysis of the flexor carpi ulnaris (FCU) produces a radial deviation of the hand when wrist flexion is attempted. Sensory loss is variable, but impaired sensation may be expected involving the little finger and the ulnar aspect of the ring finger and along the ulnar aspect of the palm of the hand to the wrist.

Medical Management

Diagnosis. NCV studies are helpful only when sufficient nerve damage has occurred to produce definite strength or sensory changes in the hand. NCVs are slowed through the involved region, but are relatively normal above and below the epicondyle. Payan (1969) reported slowing of sensory or motor NCV across the elbow, prolonged conduction (termed a *latency*) to the FCU, along with changes in amplitude, duration, or shape of the sensory potential across the elbow. Sensory fibers were affected first.

Treatment. To relieve the compression, the nerve is surgically transposed to the anterior aspect of the elbow or a medial epicondylectomy is performed. Symptomatically, the clawhand deformity should be treated with a splint that blocks MCP hyperextension (lumbrical bar) and allows the extensor digitorum to extend the IP joints.

Prognosis. Results of surgery are normally good, with complete restoration of function in the majority of persons (Gilroy and Meyer, 1979). Following nerve transposition, the first sign of return in both sensory and motor fibers was an increase in NCV across the elbow. Significant clinical improvement did not occur until the sensory potential recorded at the wrist had increased in amplitude (Payan, 1970).

Thoracic Outlet Syndrome

Because patients who are diagnosed with TOS have vague symptoms or symptoms that are difficult to interpret, TOS remains a controversial diagnosis. Many patients have been labeled "neurotic."

Definition. This is an entrapment syndrome caused by pressure from structures in the thoracic outlet on fibers of the brachial plexus; in addition, vascular symptoms can occur because of pressure on the subclavian artery (Fig. 34–13).

Etiology. The anatomy of the region of the thoracic outlet is extremely complex. Spinal nerve roots of the brachial plexus interact with surrounding bony ribs, muscles, and tendons (subclavius, anterior and middle scalene, and pectoralis minor) and the vascular supply to the region. In addition to neurologic structures becoming entrapped, arterial and venous structures also may be affected individually or in combination. Thus multiple specialists may be involved in a person's care (Fechter and Kuschner, 1993).

Risk Factors. Postural changes associated with growth and development, trauma to the shoulder girdle, and body composition have all been identified as contributing to the development of TOS. Man's upright posture has contributed to the development of TOS, because gravity pulls on the shoulder girdle creating traction on the structures. Additionally, congenital factors that affect the bony structures, like a cervical rib or fascial bands, also compress the neurovascular bundle.

Pathogenesis. Chronic compression of nerves and arteries between the clavicle and first rib or impinging musculature results in edema and ischemia in the nerves (see Fig. 34–13).

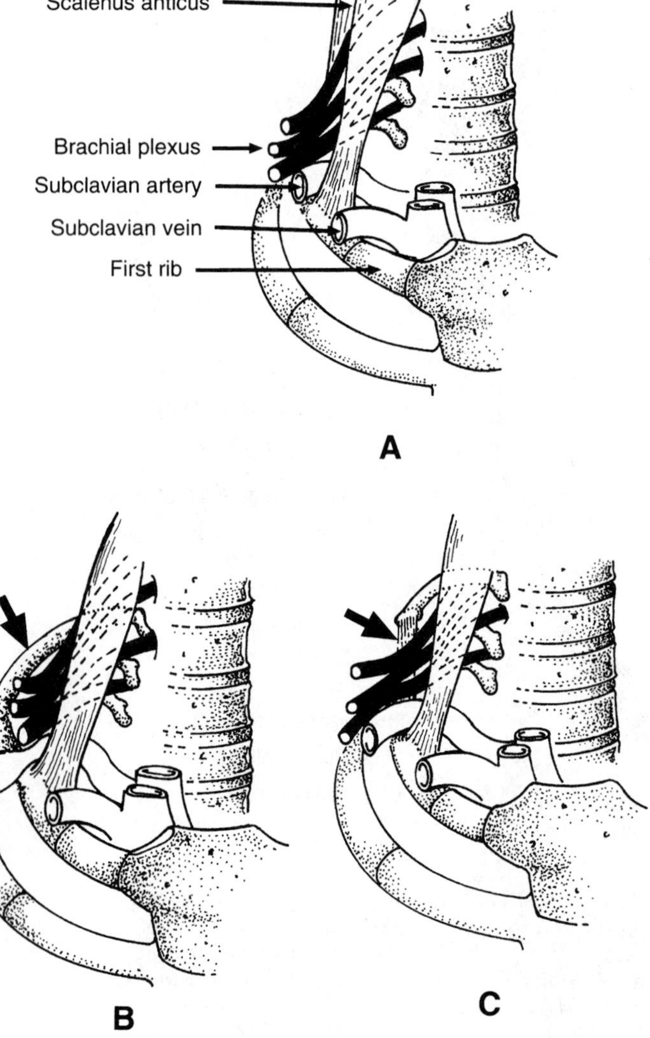

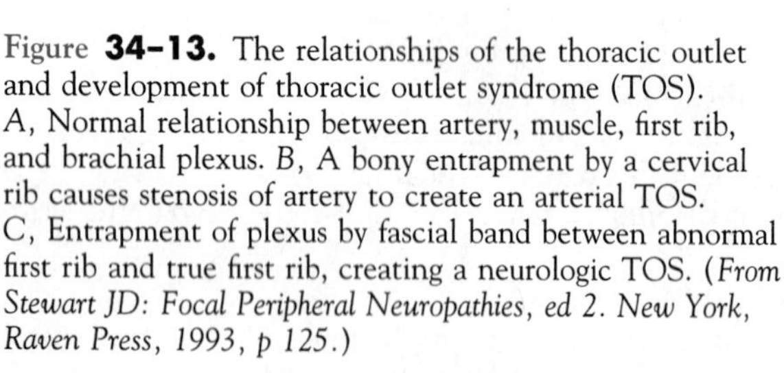

Figure **34–13.** The relationships of the thoracic outlet and development of thoracic outlet syndrome (TOS). A, Normal relationship between artery, muscle, first rib, and brachial plexus. B, A bony entrapment by a cervical rib causes stenosis of artery to create an arterial TOS. C, Entrapment of plexus by fascial band between abnormal first rib and true first rib, creating a neurologic TOS. (*From Stewart JD: Focal Peripheral Neuropathies, ed 2. New York, Raven Press, 1993, p 125.*)

This compression initially creates a neurapraxia in which the axons are preserved, but segmental demyelination occurs. Following loss of myelin the axons are more vulnerable to unrelieved compression. The neurapraxia can progress to an axonotmesis wherein axon continuity is lost and wallerian degeneration occurs.

Clinical Manifestations. Signs and symptoms reflect the structures that have been compressed. When the nerves are compressed, most people report paresthesias in the arm; most often these are nocturnal. Other symptoms may include pain, tingling, coldness, swelling, Raynaud's phenomenon, and paresis. If the upper nerve plexus is involved (C5–7), pain is reported in the neck; this may radiate into the face (sometimes with ear pain) and anterior chest, as well as over the scapulae. Symptoms may also extend over the lateral aspect of the forearm into the hand. If the lower plexus is compromised (C7–T1), pain and numbness occur in the posterior neck and shoulder, medial arm and forearm, and radiate into the ulnarly innervated digits of the hand. Weakness and atrophy may occur in the muscles corresponding to nerve root innervation.

The clinical presentation usually relates to posture and activities that aggravate symptoms. Overhead and lifting activities, along with movements of the head, produce symptoms in the upper plexus.

Medical Management

Diagnosis. Provocative tests are used to elicit symptoms of TOS, but these tests have a high false-positive response. Maneuvers are performed bilaterally and the pulse is monitored to note a change in its quality. The most routine test to demonstrate TOS is *Adson's maneuver* (Fig. 34–14). From the belief that the anterior scalene compresses the neurovascular bundle, the patient is positioned to elicit the symptoms. However, mere obliteration of the peripheral pulse does not necessarily mean that TOS exists as an entrapment problem; sensory symptoms must be reproduced. For persons with a vascular component, blood pressure may differ from side to side.

Several other maneuvers have been found to evoke symptoms: the Allen, Wright, Halstead, costoclavicular, Roos, and provocative elevation tests (Magee, 1992). Each has a positional component where the head, shoulder, or arm, individually or severally, are rotated to compress the vascular and neural structures (Table 34–7).

Radiographic Tests. Radiographic procedures are used to identify bony abnormalities. Presence of a cervical rib may indicate that the nerve has been compressed; however, presence of the rib alone does not necessarily replicate symptoms. Plane films are used to distinguish between a C7–T1 discogenic lesion and TOS.

Electrophysiologic Studies. Because symptoms of TOS are related to neural compression, electrophysiologic studies are valuable in documenting the presence of neuropathy. NCV allows the examiner to pinpoint the lesion, either because of a change in amplitude or a slowing in conduction velocity. Other, more refined electrophysiologic techniques, including somatosensory evoked potentials, and F waves, are used to confirm a diagnosis of nerve root entrapment.

Differential Diagnosis. TOS must be distinguished from other disorders with similar symptoms. These include cervical radiculopathy, reflex sympathetic dystrophy, tumors of the apex of the lung (Pancoast's tumor; see discussion, Chapter 12), and ulnar nerve compression at either elbow or wrist. The sensory pattern of TOS distinguishes it from an ulnar neuropathy, like a tardy ulnar palsy. Because the nerve roots are affected, the sensory changes extend above the hand and wrist into the forearm in TOS and follow a dermatomal

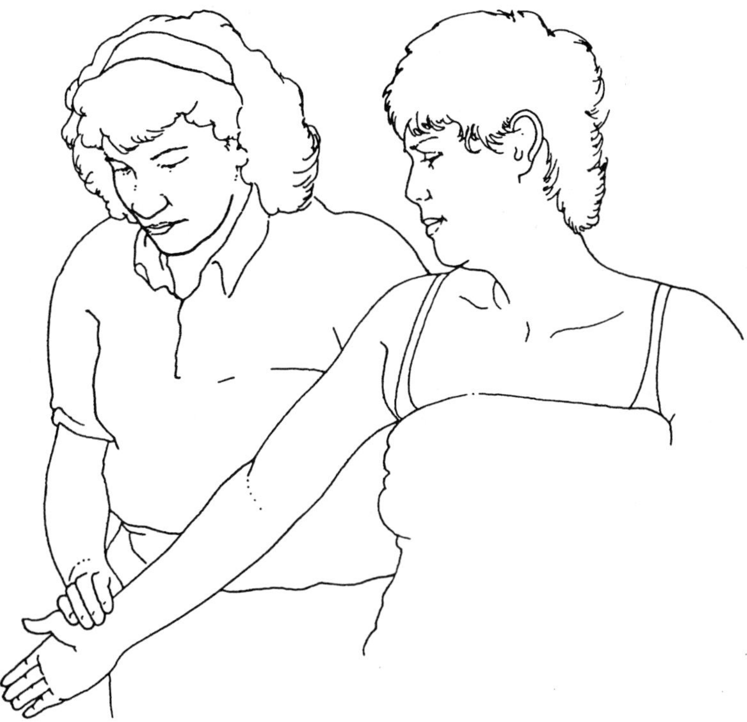

Figure **34–14.** Adson's is one of many diagnostic tests used to examine the upper extremity to determine the presence of thoracic outlet syndrome: arterial or neurologic. The client inhales and holds the breath while extending the neck and turning the chin toward the side that is evaluated. The therapist performing the evaluation palpates the radial pulse to determine the presence of dampening or obliteration. (*From Porterfield JA, DeRosa C: Mechanical Neck Pain. Perspectives in Functional Anatomy. Philadelphia, WB Saunders, 1995, p 151.*)

TABLE 34-7 Special Tests and Patterns of Positive Findings that Characterize Thoracic Outlet Syndrome

	Neural	
Vascular Component	**Upper Plexus**	**Lower Plexus**
Three-minute elevated test	Point tenderness over C5–C6	Pressure above clavicle elicits pain
Adson's sign	Pressure over lateral neck elicits pain or numbness	Ulnar nerve tenderness when palpated under axilla or along inner arm
Swelling (hand, arm)	Pain with head turn or tilted to opposite side	Tinel's test for ulnar nerve in axilla
Discoloration of hand	Weak biceps	Hypoesthesia in ulnar nerve distribution
Costoclavicular test	Weak triceps	Serratus anterior weakness
Hyperabduction test	Weak wrist	Weak handgrip
Upper extremity claudication	Hypoesthesia in radial nerve distribution	
Differences in blood pressure from side to side		
Skin temperature changes		
Cold intolerance		

pattern. Myofascial pain patterns may also mimic TOS symptoms.

Treatment. Management is divided into conservative and surgical approaches. The initial treatment of the person with TOS is conservative when symptoms are mild to moderate in severity. Postural and breathing exercises and gentle stretching are the cornerstone of the initial conservative program. This is followed by strengthening exercises for shoulder girdle musculature, especially the trapezius, levator scapulae, and rhomboids. Initially, overhead exercises should be avoided because they tend to evoke symptoms. Therapists are cautioned against forceful stretching to mobilize the first rib (Leffert, 1992).

Surgical management of TOS is reserved for cases that are refractory to postural and exercise correction and those with vascular compromise (Aligne and Barral, 1992). Once the decision for surgical intervention has been made, the physician must select a procedure and the anatomic approach. There are at least six different surgical procedures and six different anatomic approaches (Table 34–8). In scalenotomy the muscle is detached from the first rib; unfortunately, with this approach a high percentage of people experience recurring symptoms. Scalenectomy, removal of the scalene muscle, is advocated for people who have had recurrence of their symptoms. Clavicle resection is indicated primarily when the clavicle is damaged. The surgical procedure that is most extensively used and reported to provide greatest relief is resection of the first rib using an axillary approach (Roos, 1982).

TABLE 34-8 Surgical Procedures and Approaches for Thoracic Outlet Syndrome

Procedures	Approaches
Scalenotomy	Axillary
Scalenectomy	Supraclavicular
Clavicle resection	Combined axillary and supraclavicular
Pectoralis minor release	Posterior
First rib resection	Subclavicular
Cervical rib resection	Transclavicular

Prognosis. Following surgery 75% of cases have a good or excellent response, while 15% require occasional analgesics, and 10% note no improvement. Complications during surgery include pneumothorax, nerve compression, and transient winging of the scapula because the upper digitations of the serratus are detached.

Special Implications for the Therapist **34-1**

THORACIC OUTLET SYNDROME

Therapists need to consider using an upper quarter screen to rule out cervical radiculopathy or shoulder dysfunction during their evaluation. If this screen is negative, range of motion and posture should be evaluated to identify soft tissue restrictions. The client's response to provocative maneuvers should be assessed along with a sensory evaluation, preferably using Semmes-Weinstein monofilaments. Finally a manual muscle test or other method of evaluating strength should be performed. Treatment is aimed at pain relief along with postural correction (Walsh, 1994).

One of the reasons TOS has been difficult to diagnose relates to the client's subjective report. Frequently the signs and symptoms do not correspond to a single lesion, but to multifocal lesions. For clients who do not respond to treatment, compression at a proximal or distal source might increase the vulnerability of nerves, making them more susceptible to compression at another site. This phenomenon has been termed a "double crush" syndrome and may occur in a few individuals with TOS (Upton and McComas, 1973).

Saturday Night Palsy

Definition and Etiology. This is a radial nerve compression. Damage to the nerve has been associated with compression of the radial nerve at the spiral groove of the humerus in a person who is sleeping off the effects of alcohol. If the radial nerve is compressed in the axilla, the damage is often referred to as a "crutch palsy." See also Chapter 2.

Pathogenesis. Compression of the nerve causes segmental demyelination.

Clinical Manifestations. Symptoms of radial nerve paralysis depends on the level of the lesion. The more proximal the involvement, the more extensive the paralysis. When involvement occurs in the axilla, weakness occurs in elbow extension (triceps), elbow flexion (brachioradialis), and supination (supinator). If the nerve is damaged in the upper arm the triceps is spared. In addition, in both instances there will be paralysis of wrist extensors and the extensors of the fingers and thumb, diminishing grip strength. Sensory loss with radial nerve involvement is variable. If present, it is typically confined to the dorsum of the hand, but may extend to the dorsum of the forearm.

Medical Management

Diagnosis. Diagnosis is by history, clinical examination, and electrophysiologic examination. This type of paralysis is usually classified as a neurapraxia or conduction block, signifying demyelination. There is slowing of nerve conduction in both motor and sensory fibers across the lesion site.

Treatment. Medical management is aimed at asymptomatic management. A cock-up splint is used to maintain the wrist in an extended position until return of function.

Prognosis. If a neurapraxia is reported, normal conduction can be anticipated within a few months because the paralysis is related to a focal demyelination (Goodgold and Eberstein, 1983).

NEUROTMESIS

Definition. A neurotmesis occurs following total loss of axon and connective tissue continuity; the nerve is severed.

Etiology. Neurotmesis occurs following a gunshot wound, stab wound, or avulsion injury.

Pathogenesis. When the axon is lacerated *Wallerian degeneration* occurs distally and, proximally the cell body also responds to the trauma. It swells and undergoes chromatolysis. The ribosomes that normally make protein for the cell disperse throughout the cytoplasm. *Chromatolysis* reflects a change in the metabolic priority of the cell as it switches from daily needs to a repair mode. Distally the axon begins to degenerate and myelin fragments within 12 hours of the lesion. This material is removed by macrophages responding to the inflammatory process (see Fig. 34–3).

As long as the cell body remains viable, a regenerative process begins with sprouting of a growth cone as soon as new cytoplasm is synthesized and transported down the axon from the cell body. As the growth cone grows it releases proteases that dissolve material and permit the axon to enter the tissue more easily. Filopodia, finger-like projections extending from the growth cone, sample the environment searching for chemical and tactile cues to guide the regenerating axon; however, because the tactile cues provided by the endoneurium are absent, many times these fibers become misguided and form a neuroma. The standard used to anticipate return of function is based on a growth rate of 1 mm a day or an inch a month. In reality, this is an average reflecting the delays that occur while the growth cone crosses the repair site and makes connection with sensory end organs or motor end plate. Growth occurs faster nearer the lesion site (3 mm/day) and slower as the length of the axon increases (1 mm/day) (Omer, 1956).

Clinical Manifestations. The degree of involvement relates to the nerve involved and its level of involvement. In any case, an immediate flaccid paralysis occurs in muscles distal to the lesion. Rapid atrophy ensues because of loss of the trophic influences of the nerve that innervated the muscle fibers. Sensory function is also lost below the level of the lesion.

Medical Management

Diagnosis. History and clinical examination are used to diagnose neurotmesis. In addition, electrophysiologic studies may be performed after a week. EMG will demonstrate the presence of fibrillation potentials and positive sharp waves indicating denervation of muscle fiber. EMG can be used to determine whether the lesion is complete or partial.

Treatment. Surgical management is needed to suture the connective tissue bundles together to guide the regenerating growth cone. Various microsurgical techniques are used to try and direct the axon into the appropriate fascicle by restoring connective tissue continuity. Ideally, a primary repair will be carried out; operative delays lead to shrinkage and fibrosis of the distal connective tissue support structures (Holst, 1975).

Other treatments are symptomatic. For the therapist this means splinting to support structures. Use of electrical stimulation to maintain muscle bulk is controversial; recent studies have shown that the chemical signal guiding the nerve (neural cell adhesion molecule, NCAM) disappears when denervated muscle receives electrical stimulation (Sanes and Covault, 1985). However, muscle bulk is maintained for up to 4 weeks. Because denervated skin does not wrinkle after it has been soaked in water, this has been used to evaluate denervation patterns (Phelps and Walker, 1977).

Prognosis. Recovery after neurotmesis is dependent on whether the nerve was repaired and the length of nerve that must be regenerated. Following transection, muscles atrophy rapidly, and after 2 years they have undergone irreversible changes and have become fibrotic. If reinnervation occurs after 1 year, function is poor; with a delay of 18 to 24 months there is no hope for return of function.

METABOLIC NEUROPATHIES

Diabetic Neuropathy

Definition. Diabetic neuropathy is a common complication associated with diabetes mellitus (see Chapter 9). It is defined as a progressive disorder with nerve fiber loss and atrophy, manifested by deteriorating neural function and worsening sensation and motor function. Typically the involvement occurs in a distally, symmetrical pattern, termed a *diabetic polyneuropathy*, although single, focal nerve involvement may be seen. Because diabetes can affect the nervous system differentially, diabetic neuropathy is not a single entity. Instead, it comprises a number of syndromes, each reflecting the type of nerve fiber affected. Currently, there are subclinical and clinical forms. In each, abnormal electrodiagnostic tests are seen. Perhaps the most useful classification is one that differentiates diabetic neuropathy by the commonly occurring pattern of diffuse, symmetrical distal losses to a less common focal and asymmetrical pattern of involvement (Thomas, 1994).

Incidence. Very few studies address the incidence of diabetic neuropathy. The most reliable estimates from clinical studies report that diabetic neuropathy is present in 50% of persons with diabetes longer than 25 years and in 7% of persons within 1 year of diagnosis of diabetes. It can occur in insulin-dependent (IDDM; formerly type I) or non–insulin-dependent (NIDDM; formerly type II) diabetes.

Etiology. This neuropathy is probably caused by the chronic metabolic disturbances that affect nerve cells and Schwann cells in diabetes. A disturbance in sorbitol metabolism results in excess production of sorbitol under conditions of hyperglycemia. This excess sorbitol damages Schwann cells and axons.

Risk Factors. Although hyperglycemia is not directly attributed to damaging nerve fibers causing a diabetic neuropathy, it is a contributing factor. Conversely, some people develop neuropathies when glycemic control is good. A clear relationship does exist between duration of diabetes and development of diabetic neuropathy. After the onset of the neuropathy, control of hyperglycemia is known to enhance the possibility of regeneration of fibers. While studies have confirmed a genetic predisposition to diabetes, they have not confirmed such a predisposition to development of a diabetic neuropathy, nor has a familial tendency been reported. Up to 50% of all people with diabetes never develop symptoms of neuropathy.

Pathogenesis. Many hypotheses exist for the pathogenesis of this disorder. The metabolic effect of hyperglycemia exposes nerves and their associated Schwann cells to glucose. The most prominent change in diabetic neuropathy is loss of both myelinated and unmyelinated axons. Nerves are affected distally more than proximally. Subtle changes have been reported at the nodes of Ranvier in nerves of people with diabetic neuropathies. This is associated with slowing of the NCV (Vinik et al., 1992).

A number of studies suggest that vascular changes affect peripheral nerves in diabetes. Evidence is present demonstrating endoneurial microvascular thickening. In the sural nerve this has resulted in increased numbers of closed capillaries which are believed to cause multifocal regions of ischemia and hypoxia in the nerve, resulting in an axonal degeneration.

Another explanation for the development of diabetic neuropathy proposes that the concentration of nerve growth factor (NGF), which has a structure that is molecularly and physiologically similar to insulin, is reduced. Since NGF acts as a trophic factor, its reduction also reduces nutrition to the nerve.

Clinical Manifestations. The most common form of diabetic neuropathy is one where the nerve has distal and symmetrical involvement. Typically, its onset is insidious, but occasionally signs and symptoms appear acutely. Signs include depression or absence of ankle jerks and loss of vibratory sensation. The lower extremities tend to be the focus of the neuropathy.

Because multiple nerves are affected by diabetes, there is a stocking and glove–like loss of sensation (see Fig. 34–5). However, the stocking is not a single line loss because nerve fibers for each sensory modality will be affected differently. It is as if multiple stockings or gloves are layered into place. No matter the sensation that is lost or impaired, the condition starts distally and proceeds proximally.

When large fibers are affected, loss of position sense and vibration occur as well as touch and ankle reflexes. Clients may report that they feel as if they were walking on cotton or clouds. Small-fiber involvement (nonmyelinated), in contrast, results in loss of pain sensation and loss of thermal awareness. Occasionally, a painful, small-fiber neuropathy will develop manifested by nocturnal pain and paresthesia.

Motor weakness occurs also, distally and symmetrically. Wasting occurs in the musculature of the feet and ankles. In advanced cases the small muscles of the hands are involved.

Medical Management

Diagnosis. The diagnosis is based on the clinical examination, electrodiagnostic studies, quantitative sensory evaluation, and autonomic function testing. Because diabetes is a common disorder and because neuropathies may be related to other causes, mere association of neuropathic signs and symptoms in a person with diabetes is not sufficient to diagnose a diabetic neuropathy. Other causes must be excluded (Harati, 1992). Slowing of NCV is one of the earliest abnormalities present in diabetic neuropathy. Sensory fibers are generally affected first before motor fibers. Autonomic fibers may also be affected.

Treatment. Management is divided into general and specific measures. General measures include control of hyperglycemia and specific measures address the symptomatic management of the disorders (see under Diabetes Mellitus in Chapter 9). Because there is evidence that further complications can be reduced by maintaining control of the diabetes, this is one specific area addressed by health-care professionals. In addition, specific drug therapies are being evaluated. Currently, studies on medications such as aldose reductase inhibitors (ARIs) (Greene et al., 1993) and on gangliosides and NGFs are being conducted and although some show promise, further controlled investigations are needed (Tomlinson et al., 1994).

If the person has a painful diabetic neuropathy an algorithm has been developed that begins with physical modalities to manage pain. This is combined with simple analgesics. Further management may include a trial of capsaicin (topical) or "benign" drugs (Vinik et al., 1992). A common complication of diabetic neuropathy is the development of neuropathic foot ulcers. Institution of foot care procedures is essential (see Table 10–22; and discussion of foot care in diabetes in Special Implication, 9–15. With the development of a footdrop gait, orthotic devices should be considered for the person's safety. The type of orthosis and shoe construction prescribed should be carefully considered based on the sensory picture and the person's ability to demonstrate appropriate foot care.

Prognosis. Diabetic neuropathy is a slowly progressive disorder. Because it is a metabolic disorder, other systems are often affected. Estimates are that over 50% of nontraumatic amputations in the United States are performed in diabetic clients. The presence of autonomic involvement is associated with an increased mortality risk.

Alcoholic Neuropathy

Peripheral neuropathies, typically with distally symmetrical involvement, appear in alcoholics after years of alcohol abuse.

Etiology and Risk Factors. Lesions affecting the peripheral nerves have been attributed to both the toxic effects of alcohol and nutritional deficiencies from poor dietary habits. However, there is more recent evidence that neither age nor nutritional status play a part in development of alcoholic neuropathies. Rather, alcohol-related neuropathies appear to be due to the total lifetime accumulation of ethanol (Estruch et al., 1993).

Pathogenesis. Segmental demyelination progressing to an axonal degeneration has been described in persons with alcoholic polyneuropathy. Changes occur distally at first and become more marked and proximal (Goodgold and Eberstein, 1983).

Clinical Manifestations. Mild forms of alcoholic neuropathy exhibit minor loss of muscle bulk, diminished ankle reflexes, impaired sensation in the feet, and aching in the calves. In addition, vibratory perception is impaired. It begins insidiously and progresses slowly; occasionally the onset may occur acutely. In the most advanced cases symptoms involve all four extremities. Paresthesias of feet and hands may be reported. Bilateral footdrop is observed during gait and a wristdrop contributes to a diminished grip strength because of the client's inability to extend the wrist. Both these features are often combined with varying amounts of peripheral weakness in other muscles.

Medical Management

Diagnosis and Treatment. The diagnosis is made by history, clinical examination, and electrodiagnostic testing. Although diet is no longer implicated as a contributing factor in the development of alcoholic neuropathies, diet to improve nutritional status, along with vitamin supplements and abstinence from alcohol, is the treatment of choice. All other treatment is symptomatic. Orthotic devices, ankle-foot orthoses (AFOs) and cock-up splints, are used to manage weakness and improve function.

Prognosis. If the client abstains from alcohol, mild improvement can be expected, but recovery is slow and incomplete when axonal degeneration has occurred (Palliyath and Schwartz, 1993). Therefore, to anticipate the outcome, review the client's electrophysiologic studies to determine whether demyelination or degeneration is present.

INFECTIONS

Acute Inflammatory Demyelinating Polyradiculoneuropathy (Guillain-Barré Syndrome)

Overview and Definition: Guillain-Barré syndrome (GBS) was originally described by and named for the French neurologists who published case reports describing this syndrome. More recently the syndrome is named according to the pathologic process that occurs: an acute inflammatory demyelinating polyradiculoneuropathy, or AIDP. Since the virtual elimination of poliomyelitis, AIDP is the most common cause of acutely evolving motor and sensory deficits.

Incidence. The annual incidence varies from 1 to 2 cases per 100,000 people. Although AIDP occurs at all ages, peaks in frequency can be seen in young adults and in the fifth through the eighth decades. Occurrence is slightly greater for men than women and for whites more than blacks. Some researchers have noted a seasonal relationship associated with infections.

Etiology and Risk Factors. Evidence supports the view that AIDP is an immune-mediated disorder. Viral and bacterial infections, surgery, and vaccinations have been associated with the development of AIDP. Of the two thirds of persons reporting an acute infection within 2 months preceding onset of AIDP, 90% had illness (e.g., respiratory, gastrointestinal) during the past 30 days. Although a wide range of viruses have been associated with AIDP, they are believed to act as nonspecific triggering agents (Pentland and Donald, 1994).

Pathogenesis. Lesions occur throughout the PNS from the spinal nerve roots to the distal termination of both motor and sensory fibers. The autoimmune theory is the primary theory for the cause of AIDP because evidence exists for antibody-mediated demyelination. Myelin of the Schwann cell is the primary target of attack. Researchers theorize that circulating antibodies penetrate and bind to an antigen (as yet unidentified) on the surface of the myelin and activate either complement or an antibody-dependent macrophage (Murray, 1993). The earliest pathologic changes in the PNS take the form of a generalized inflammatory response. Lymphocytes and macrophages are the inflammatory cells present. Demyelination occurs because macrophages, responding to inflammatory signals, strip myelin from the nerves. After the initial demyelination, the body initiates a repair process. Schwann cells divide and remyelinate nerves, resulting in shorter internodal distances than were present initially.

In addition to the demyelination, there is another process that has longer-lasting effects. Axonal degeneration is believed to occur to some extent in most cases of AIDP. Many believe that the axons are damaged during the inflammatory process, according to what has been called a "bystander effect." Products that are liberated by the macrophages as they strip myelin (e.g., free oxygen radicals and proteases) also damage axons.

Although the autoimmune theory is the main one advanced for this disorder, it may not be the only reason for the development of AIDP. Cases of AIDP have been reported in immunosuppressed patients following renal transplants.

Clinical Manifestations. Various forms of AIDP exist; however, the most common picture is an acute form in which the time from onset to peak impairment is 4 weeks or less. A recurrent form of AIDP is reported in up to 10% of cases. Acute relapses may occur in AIDP, and this may make it difficult to differentiate the acute from the chronic form, called chronic demyelinating polyradiculoneuropathy

(CIDP). Most cases of CIDP progress over a period of months, instead of weeks.

In AIDP, symptoms are characterized by ascending symmetrical motor weakness and distal sensory impairments. The first neurologic symptom is often paresthesia in the toes. This is followed within hours or days by weakness distally in the legs. Weakness spreads to involve arms, trunk, and facial muscles. Flaccid paralysis is accompanied by absence of DTRs. Occasionally, sensory and motor symptoms begin in the hands and arms instead of the feet and legs. Palatal and facial muscles become involved in about half of all cases; even the muscles of mastication may be affected, but nerves to extraocular muscles typically are not involved. Up to 30% of all cases require mechanical ventilation.

Because the preganglionic fibers of the ANS are myelinated, they, too may be subject to demyelination. If this occurs, tachycardia, abnormalities in cardiac rhythm, blood pressure changes, and vasomotor symptoms occur.

In 50% of the cases progression of symptoms generally ceases within 2 weeks and in 90% of the cases progression ends by 4 weeks. After the progression stops, a static phase begins, lasting 2 to 4 weeks before recovery occurs in a proximal to distal progression. This recovery may take months, or even years.

Medical Management

Diagnosis. Careful clinical and neurophysiologic examinations and laboratory tests are needed to diagnosis AIDP. Criteria have been developed by the National Institute of Neurologic and Communicative Disorders and Stroke (NINCDS) (Table 34–9) (Hund et al., 1993).

After symptoms have existed for 1 week, one of the laboratory tests that is important is a lumbar puncture to withdraw cerebrospinal fluid (CSF). Albumin (a protein) is elevated in the CSF with 10 or fewer mononuclear leukocytes present. Electrophysiologic tests will reveal slowed NCVs the entire length of the nerve when demyelination is present, as well as fibrillation potentials when axonal degeneration occurs. In the presence of both, the amplitude of the evoked (NCV) potential will be reduced and the velocity is slowed.

These abnormalities may not be apparent during the first 3 weeks of the illness. In addition, to determine the extent of demyelination of the nerve roots, an F wave electrophysiologic test may be performed. As recovery occurs, the slowed NCVs will persist, even though the person has made a full recovery (Goodgold and Eberstein, 1983).

TABLE 34–9 CRITERIA FOR DIAGNOSIS OF ACUTE INFLAMMATORY DEMYELINATING POLYRADICULONEUROPATHY (AIDP)

Symptoms required for diagnosis
- Progressive weakness in more than one extremity
- Loss of deep tendon reflexes

Symptoms supportive of diagnosis (in order of importance)
- Weakness developing rapidly that ceases to progress by 4 wk
- Symmetrical weakness
- Mild sensory symptoms and signs
- Facial weakness common and symmetrical; oral-bulbar musculature may also be involved
- Recovery usually begins 2–4 wk after AIDP ceases to progress
- Tachycardia, cardiac arrhythmias, and labile blood pressure may occur
- Absence of fever

Cerebrospinal fluid (CSF) features
- CSF protein levels increased after 1 wk; continue to increase on serial examinations
- CSF contains 10 or fewer mononuclear leukocytes/mm^3

Electrodiagnostic features
- Nerve conduction velocity slowed

Adapted from Hund EF, Borel CO, Cornblath DR, et al: Intensive management and treatment of severe Guillain-Barré syndrome. Crit Care Med 21:435, 1993.

Differential Diagnosis. Hysteria is the most common misdiagnosis. Because of the speed of onset, a stroke involving the brainstem will also be considered. Less common causes of acute neuropathies must also be considered, including tick paralysis, and metabolic disorders like porphyria.

Treatment. Because AIDP is believed to be an autoimmune disease, treatment has been aimed at controlling the response. In two major trials plasmapheresis[1] has been shown to significantly improve the impairments in AIDP. Time on respirator and time to independent ambulation (53 days) were both shorter than in the control group (85 days). Plasmapheresis is instituted when respiratory function drops precipitously (to 1.0 to 1.5 L) and the person is placed on a respirator.

High-dose intravenous administration of immunoglobulins (IVIg) has been found safe and effective in the treatment of AIDP (van der Meche and Schmitz, 1992). Results of IVIg using daily infusions of pooled γ-globulin, administered in the first 2 weeks of the disease, suggest that IVIg is as good as plasmapheresis in the treatment of AIDP. It is easy to administer, is readily available, and has fewer risks. Steroids have provided no beneficial effect in the treatment of AIDP (Hund et al., 1993).

Prognosis. The primary methods of managing AIDP have helped to improve mortality rates, which can exceed 5%. Factors that predict a poor outcome include onset at an older age, a protracted time before recovery begins, and the need for artificial respiration. An important objective evaluation finding that predicts a poor outcome is significantly reduced evoked motor potential amplitude, which correlates with the presence of axonal degeneration. Although most persons recover, up to 20% can have remaining neurologic deficits. After 1 year 67% of clients have complete recovery, but 20% remain with significant disability (Feasby, 1992). Even after 2 years 8% have not recovered.

Special Implications for the Therapist **34–2**

ACUTE INFLAMMATORY DEMYELINATING POLYRADICULONEUROPATHY (GUILLAIN-BARRÉ SYNDROME)

Physical therapy is initiated at an early stage in this condition to maintain joint range of motion within the

[1] Plasmapheresis is a technique that removes plasma from circulation and filters it to remove or dilute circulating antibodies. Typically the client will have four to six exchanges of 500 mL per treatment over the period of a week.

client's pain tolerance and to monitor muscle strength until active exercises can be initiated. During the ascending phase when the person is losing function and becoming weaker, he or she can become easily fatigued and overwhelmed. Focus is toward prevention of complications associated with immobilization.

Meticulous skin care is required by all staff members to prevent skin breakdown and contractures. A strict turning schedule is usually established by the nursing staff and should be followed by all other health-care staff as well. After each position change, inspect the skin (especially the sacrum, heels, ankles, shoulders, and greater trochanter). Massage to pressure points stimulates circulation; family or other caregivers can be instructed to perform this on a regular basis.

Care in the intensive care unit requires observation of arterial blood gas measurements. Because the disease results in primary hypoventilation with hypoxemia and hypercapnia, watch for PO_2 below 70 mm Hg, which signals respiratory failure. Report any signs of rising PCO_2 (e.g., confusion, tachypnea). Pulse oximetry may be used to monitor peripheral oxygen saturation (see Chapter 10). Auscultate breath sounds, turn and position the person, and encourage coughing and deep breathing to maintain clear airways and prevent atelectasis. See also Special Implications for the Therapist: Atelectasis, 12–16. The therapist must also follow universal precautions to help prevent any respiratory infection for the client (see Appendix A).

Respiratory support is needed at the first sign of dyspnea (in adults, vital capacity less than 800 mL; in children, less than 12 mL/kg of body weight) or decreasing PO_2.

Ventilation is instituted when pulmonary function is compromised by loss of respiratory skeletal muscle control. Coughing and clearing of tracheal secretions becomes difficult. In addition, weakness of laryngeal and pharyngeal muscles makes swallowing difficult andincreases the risk of aspiration. Early tracheostomy is indicated in people with clinical and EMG evidence of axonal involvement together with respiratory failure.

Clinical indications for weaning from the ventilator include improved forced vital capacity and improved inspiratory force concomitant with improved muscle stretch. Lastly, the chest should be clear of atelectasis. Communication using a communication board or other method is needed during ventilatory support.

Exercise and Guillain-Barré

When the person's condition stabilizes, a therapeutic pool or Hubbard tank can be used to initiate movement in a controlled environment. A major precaution during the early treatment phase is to provide gentle stretching and active or active-assistive exercise at a level consistent with the person's muscle strength. Overstretching and overuse of painful muscles may result in a prolonged recovery period or a lack of recovery. During the descending phase, when the paralysis slowly recedes and physical function returns, neuromuscular facilitation techniques (such as proprioceptive neuromuscular facilitation) may be integrated into the active and resistive exercises.

Deep muscular discomfort or pain in the proximal muscles may be reported by clients. Paresis or paralysis requires positioning and appropriate splinting, which can help alleviate muscle and joint pain. Bed cages may reduce dysesthesias that are present in the feet. Palliative modalities such as hot packs and gentle massage may also bring relief of musculoskeletal pain.

The length of time to maximum impairment (respiratory compromise and motor involvement) has not been found to correlate with outcome. However, the shorter the time it takes for recovery to begin after maximum impairment has been reached, the less likely it is that long-term disability will occur (Ng et al., 1995).

Discharge Planning

When the person is discharged from therapy, recovery may not be complete. Impaired function may require the continued use of assistive devices, and possibly even mobility equipment such as a wheelchair or scooter. The home may require modifications, which should be evaluated and planned for prior to discharge.

Postpolio Syndrome

Overview. Poliomyelitis (polio) virus infection was virtually eradicated in the United States with the advent of the Salk vaccine in the 1950s and the Sabin vaccine in the 1960s. Clinically, the disease was characterized as one of three patterns: (1) an asymptomatic, or (2) nonparalytic infection that produced gastrointestinal, flulike symptoms and muscular pain, or (3) a paralytic infection that also began with flulike symptoms. The paralytic form generally developed within a week following the onset of the symptoms. The virus invaded and damaged motor cell bodies. The extent of the asymmetrical paresis and paralysis that ensued depended on the degree of anterior horn cell involvement. When cell bodies were killed, motor axons underwent wallerian degeneration and muscles rapidly atrophied. Of those persons developing acute paralysis, equal numbers (30%) recovered, had mild residual paralysis, or were left with moderate to severe paralysis. Ten percent died from respiratory involvement. Recovery was attributed to the recovery of some anterior horn cells as well as collateral sprouting from intact peripheral nerves and to hypertrophy of spared muscle fibers (Department of Physical Therapy, 1986).

Polio was a unique neuropathy that created only focal and asymmetrical motor impairments, rather than the typical distal, symmetrical motor and sensory losses associated with other neuropathies. For decades it was considered a static disease; after the initial episode there was no further progression of the disease. The last major epidemics of polio occurred in the early 1950s; thus most of the people who had paralytic polio are at least 40 years old today. Most people had significant recovery of function and went on to live very productive lives.

Definition. Postpolio syndrome (PPS), or postpolio muscular atrophy, refers to new neuromuscular symptoms that occur decades (average postpolio interval is 25 years) after recovery from the acute paralytic episode (Perry and Fleming, 1985).

Incidence and Risk Factors. It is estimated that there are 1.63 million polio survivors in the United States and that one-fourth to one-half of them will develop PPS (Halstead and Rossi, 1985). A previous diagnosis of polio is essential for this diagnosis. As well, the degree of initial motor involvement as measured by weakness in the acute stage is a factor in the development of PPS. These combine with long-term overuse of muscle that places increased demands on joints, ligaments, and muscle (Fredericks and Saladin, 1996).

Etiology. PPS appears to be related to the initial disorder of the motor neuron cell body affected by the poliovirus. Much of the recovery of muscle strength that occurred following the axonal degeneration can be attributed to reinnervation of denervated muscle fibers by collateral spouts from other nearby surviving axons. That is, surviving axons increased the size of their innervation ratio. For example, instead of one axon innervating 3000 muscle fibers in the quadriceps, it then innervated 5000 fibers.

Pathogenesis. Muscle biopsy and EMG both indicate ongoing muscle denervation. PPS seems to be an evolution of the original motor neuron dysfunction that began after the poliovirus affected the alpha motor neuron. PPS is manifested when the compensated reinnervation that occurred cannot maintain that muscle fiber innervation. The nervous system is "pruning back" axonal sprouts that it no longer has the metabolic ability to support; thus new denervation results. Symptoms are related to an attrition of oversprouting motor neurons that can no longer support these axonal spouts (Dalakas, 1995).

Clinical Manifestations. Symptoms vary, but in general muscle strength declines in all people, with periods of stability for 3 to 10 years in muscles that had previously been affected by polio and had fully or partially recovered. Affected persons experience myalgias, joint pain, increased muscle atrophy, and new weakness, as well as excessive fatigue with minimal activity, vasomotor abnormalities, and diminishing endurance. In addition, involvement of respiratory musculature can cause further complications (Jubelt and Drucker, 1993). These all combine to contribute to a loss of function.

Typically, symptoms are related to the individual's activities of daily living: crutch walking, wheelchair propulsion (Fig. 34–15).

Medical Management

Diagnosis. PPS is a clinical diagnosis requiring the exclusion of other medical, neurologic, orthopedic, or psychiatric disorders that could explain the new symptoms. Routine EMG can be used to confirm any new denervation, as can muscle biopsies. Single fiber EMG and spinal fluid studies are rarely needed to establish a diagnosis (Dalakas et al., 1986).

Treatment. Medical management is aimed at symptomatic treatment and modification of lifestyle. Surgery for residual calcaneovalgus deformities at the ankle include triple arthrodesis (Faraj, 1995). Perimalleolar tendon transfers have been performed to compensate for triceps surae insufficiency (DiCesare et al., 1995).

Prognosis. PPS is a slowly progressive disorder with stable periods that last 3 to 10 years.

Special Implications for Therapists **34-3**

POSTPOLIO SYNDROME

Of importance to therapists is the ongoing question of the use of exercise in the management of this disorder. Partially denervated muscle does not have the physiologic capacity to respond to a conventional strengthening program. Instead, programs aimed at nonexhaustive exercise and general body conditioning

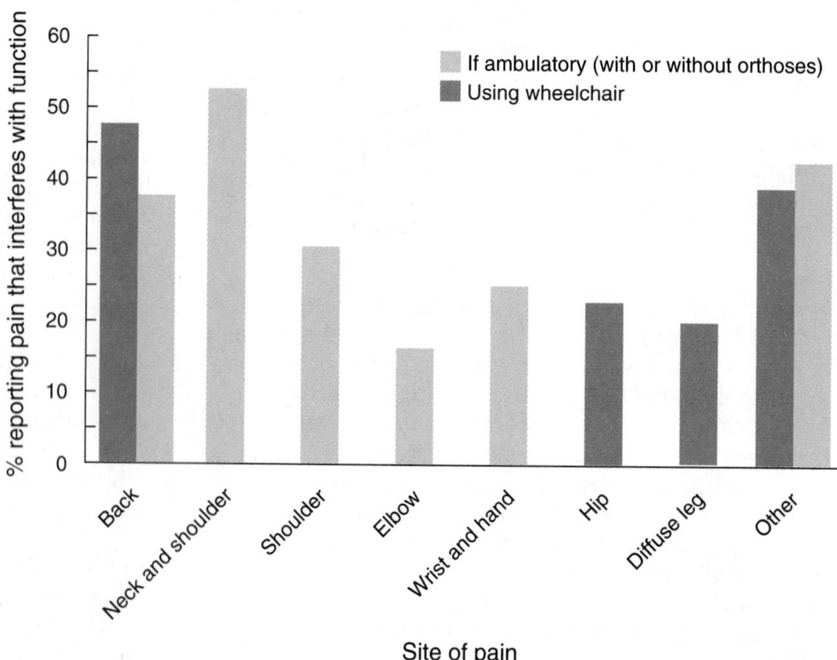

Figure **34–15.** Location of pain reported in ambulatory and wheelchair-bound persons diagnosed with postpolio syndrome. (*Data from Department of Physical Therapy, the Institute for Rehabilitation and Research, Houston: An instructional course on physical therapy management of post-poliomyelitis: New challenges. Presented at the 65th American Physical Therapy Association Annual Conference, Chicago, June, 1986.*)

are preferable (Gross and Schuck, 1989). The client should never exercise to the point of fatigue and vital signs are monitored before and after exercise to assess the client's response to even mild activity. Caution the client to stop if pain persists or weakness increases. Functional exercises of submaximal intensity are stressed with the goal of maintaining and improving endurance and functional capacity. Additionally, clients with PPS may also benefit from lifestyle modifications, including energy conservation techniques. (See Box 7–1.)

Posturally induced mechanical strain and overuse have led to degenerative changes and pain, as well as unstable joints. For these deformities to be reversed, the therapist should explore the use of orthoses, especially for gait. Many clients who have developed PPS are former brace users and may have an aversion to orthoses, but the braces they formerly used were not the cosmetic lightweight braces that can be constructed today.

Herpes Zoster

Varicella-zoster virus (VZV) is a common herpesvirus that affects the nervous system. VZV is the same virus that produces chickenpox in children. Following recovery from that childhood disease, the virus is not eliminated from the body; it lies dormant within sensory ganglia and can become activated later in life to cause herpes zoster (HZ), or shingles.

Incidence. Annually, approximately 1% of the adult population over age 80 years develops HZ each year (Ritchie, 1990).

Pathogenesis. HZ primarily affects the sensory ganglia of the spinal cord or cranial nerves. The virus causes a generalized inflammatory response beginning in the sensory ganglion and spreading along spinal and peripheral nerves to produce demyelination and degeneration.

Clinical Manifestations. The inflammation produces pain and tingling in the involved dermatome with a rash followed by development of vesicles (blisters) that burst and encrust in the same dermatome. The skin lesions last up to 1 month and disappear as the effects of the virus resolve. Thoracic and trigeminal dermatomes are involved most often. Occasionally the inflammation may affect motor neurons and produce LMN signs and symptoms.

Medical Management

Diagnosis and Treatment. The diagnosis is made by clinical presentation. The disorder is treated symptomatically unless there is widespread involvement. Acyclovir, an antiviral medication, is used to control the response. Analgesic drugs may be prescribed to relieve pain.

Prognosis. For immunosuppressed clients, there is a greater risk of developing postherpetic neuralgia and painful dysesthesias as a complication of HZ. Postherpetic pain is very resistant to treatment. Signs of the disorder in immunocompetent persons resolve within a month, but the area that was affected may be partly insensitive. Up to 20% of people who experience HZ will experience a second attack (see Special Implications for the Therapist: Herpes Zoster, 8–4).

Trigeminal Neuralgia

Trigeminal neuralgia (TN), or tic douloureux, is a disorder of the trigeminal (fifth cranial) nerve in which there are intense paroxysms of lancinating pain within the nerve's distribution (see Fig. 34–4).

Incidence. TN is not a common disorder (5 cases per 100,000). It typically occurs in women between the ages of 50 and 70 years.

Etiology. TN arises from many causes: herpes zoster, multiple sclerosis, vascular lesions, or tumors may affect the nerve to produce the painful sensations. Many times it will be referred to as idiopathic because the cause remains undetermined.

Pathogenesis. Researchers hypothesize that the pain is due to ectopic activity generated at the site of involvement. Demyelinated fibers become hyperexcitable. Light mechanical stimulation recruits nearby pain fibers causing them to discharge and create the sensation of intense pain.

Clinical Manifestations. The pain associated with TN has a sudden onset and has been described as sharp, knifelike, lancinating, "like a lightning bolt inside my head" that lasts for seconds to minutes. The sensation is typically restricted to the maxillary (V2) division of the nerve, but it may involve the maxillary and mandibular divisions together. Less likely is involvement of the ophthalmic (V1) division.

The painful sensation often occurs in clusters. Any mechanical stimulation, chewing, smiling, even a breeze, can trigger an attack. Clients avoid stimulating the trigger zone. Remissions occur between attacks, but these remission periods shorten and attacks become more frequent over the course of the disorder. In about 10% of the cases the pain occurs bilaterally.

Medical Management

Diagnosis. Subjective reports of pain in the typical pattern are the basis for the diagnosis. No impairment or loss of sensation or motor control is obvious on evaluation, The person can identify the trigger site. Skull radiographs, computed tomography (CT) scans, and MRI are used to rule out tumors and vascular causes.

Treatment. The preferred treatment of TN is oral carbamazepine (Tegretol, an anticonvulsant). Pain can be controlled with appropriate dosage in about 75% of clients with TN. Side effects of this medication include blurred vision, dizziness, drowsiness, as well as hematologic changes (anemia) and altered liver function. In addition, because carbamazepine has teratogenic effects, it should not be used in the first trimester of pregnancy, nor should it be used by nursing mothers (Gilroy and Meyer, 1979). Other medications, such as phenytoin (Dilantin), are less effective, but should be tried in those who cannot tolerate carbamazepine.

In persons whose pain is refractory to medications, neurosurgical procedures are advised. Radiofrequency rhizotomy is preferred over trigeminal nerve section or alcohol ablation. Microvascular surgery has also been used when small blood vessels have been found to constrict the trigeminal nerve near its root. This procedure provides immediate pain relief; however, it is a major and difficult surgery.

TABLE 34–10 MEDICATIONS TOXIC TO PERIPHERAL NERVES

MEDICATION	USE
Doxorubicin (Adriamycin)	Cancer
Amiodarone	Irregular heartbeat
Chloramphenicol	Antibiotic
Cisplatin	Cancer
Dapsone	Skin diseases
Phenytoin (Dilantin)	Seizures and pain
Disulfiram (Antabuse)	Alcoholism
Ethionamide	Tuberculosis
Metronidazole (Flagyl)	*Trichomonas* infection
Gold	Rheumatoid arthritis
Isoniazid	Tuberculosis
Lithium	Manic depression and headache prevention
Nitrofurantoin (Furadantin)	Urinary tract infection
Nitrous oxide	Anesthetic
Penicillamine	Rheumatoid arthritis
Suramin	Cancer
Paclitaxel (Taxol)	Cancer
Vincristine	Cancer

Adapted from Asbury AK: Disorders of peripheral nerve. *In* Asbury AK, McKhann GM, McDonald WI: Disease of the Nervous System: Clinical Neurobiology. Philadelphia, WB Saunders, 1986, p 326–327.

Prognosis. The efficacy of evaluating treatments for TN is complicated by the fact that the disorder may remit spontaneously. Remissions that occur soon after onset of TN may last for years. For those who do not remit, TN can be managed medically in most cases.

The Trigeminal Neuralgia Association provides information and support for persons with this diagnosis.[2]

TOXINS

In addition to toxic substances in the environment, some medications prescribed to treat medical conditions can be toxic to the PNS (Table 34–10) (Asbury et al., 1986; see also Chapter 3).

Lead Neuropathy

Definition. Toxic substances such as lead affect peripheral myelin or axons.

Etiology and Risk Factors. The leading cause of lead neuropathy is the ingestion of lead from paint by children who live in old homes. However, lead exposure may also occur after inhaling fumes from car batteries, and after drinking contaminated water or moonshine whiskey. Lead neuropathies also occur in workers in industry who use materials containing lead. Most recently the Consumer Product Safety Commission has identified inexpensive plastic miniblinds as a source of lead exposure. As the blind is exposed to sunlight, the plastic disintegrates and sheds dust that is high in lead.

Pathogenesis. Both the CNS and PNS can be affected. In the PNS lead exposure initially causes segmental demyelination, but with prolonged exposure damage to axon cell bodies causes axonal degeneration (Gilroy and Meyer, 1979).

Clinical Manifestations. Unlike most neuropathies, lead neuropathies primarily affect neurons innervating muscles in the upper extremity. After months of exposure, persons with a lead peripheral neuropathy will develop wristdrop.

Medical Management

Diagnosis, Treatment, and Prognosis. Diagnosis is based on the history, clinical examination, and motor NCVs, which will be decreased. If axonal degeneration has occurred, EMG will reveal fibrillation potentials. Other tests to check for concentration of lead in the body are urine evaluation and radiographs to reveal a lead line at the metaphysis in the iliac creases, long bones, and tips of the scapula.

Treatment consists of the removal of the source of the lead toxin along with the introduction of the chelating agent, edetate calcium disodium (EDTA), administered twice daily, to rid the body of lead. Symptomatic management consists of cock-up splints for the wristdrop. Recovery depends on the length of exposure and removal of the toxin.

Pesticides and Organophosphates

Etiology. Insecticides are used extensively worldwide in industry and agriculture. Some compounds have contaminated cooking oils and outbreaks of organophosphate poisoning have been reported following their ingestion. Parathion has been responsible for more accidental poisonings and death than any other organophosphate.

Pathogenesis and Clinical Manifestations. All organophosphate compounds inhibit cholinesterase activity. Organophosphate toxins affect systemic functions throughout the body. Nausea and vomiting, diarrhea, muscle fasciculations, weakness and paralysis, including paralysis of the respiratory musculature, can occur. Death can result from vasomotor collapse that coincides with respiratory paralysis. Symptoms of peripheral nerve involvement appear within days and because they arise quickly, may resemble AIDP. A chronic peripheral neuropathy may persist for months or years.

Medical Management

Diagnosis. Overexposure to organophosphates will reduce cholinesterase activity of erythrocytes to less than 25% of normal. History and clinical evaluation may be accompanied by electrophysiologic studies to indicate the severity of the neuropathy (e.g., segmental demyelination or axonal degeneration or both).

Treatment. Insecticides should be washed from the skin and hair; if toxins have been ingested, emesis or lavage should be carried out. Acutely, atropine is given in doses every 10 minutes until the pupils are dilated, the skin flushed and dry, and the pulse rate rises. Neuromuscular paralysis can be reversed by injection of pralidoxime, a cholinesterase reactivator. Endotracheal intubation and ventilation may be required in the presence of respiratory paralysis. Strictly neuropathic management is aimed at symptomatic management.

[2] Trigeminal Neuralgia Association, PO Box 340, Barnegat Light, NJ 08006.

Prognosis. Recovery is based on removal from the toxin and the degree of involvement. If only segmental demyelination occurs, recovery will occur in weeks to months, but if axonal degeneration is present, recovery will take months to years.

MOTOR END PLATE DISORDERS

Myasthenia Gravis

Overview and Definition. Myasthenia gravis (MG) is the most common of the disorders of neuromuscular transmission. It is characterized by fluctuating weakness and fatigability of skeletal muscles.

Incidence. Estimates from the National Myasthenia Gravis Foundation are that there are over 100,000 clients with MG and an additional 25,000 undiagnosed cases. MG can affect people in any age group, but peak incidences occur in women in their 20s and 30s and in men in their 50s and 60s. Overall, the ratio of women affected compared to men is 3:2.

Etiology. MG is an autoimmune disorder whose action takes place at the site of the neuromuscular junction and motor end plate.

Risk Factors. Disorders associated with an increased incidence of MG are thymic disorders such as hyperthyroidism, thymic tumor, or thyrotoxicosis. There is an association with diabetes and immune disorders, like rheumatoid arthritis or lupus. Exacerbations may occur before the menstrual period or shortly after pregnancy. Chronic infections of any kind can exacerbate MG.

Pathogenesis. In MG, the fundamental defect is at the neuromuscular junction. Receptors at the motor end plate normally receive acetylcholine (ACh) from the motor nerve terminal. An action potential occurs that leads to a muscle contraction. In MG the number of ACh receptors are decreased and those that remain are flattened which results in decreased efficiency of neuromuscular transmission. The neuromuscular junction can normally transmit at high frequencies so that the muscle does not fatigue. Without ACh, the nerve impulses fail to pass across the neuromuscular junction to stimulate muscle contraction. The neuromuscular abnormalities in MG are brought about by an autoimmune response mediated by specific anti–ACh receptor antibodies. The antibodies may block the site that normally binds ACh, or the antibodies may damage the postsynaptic muscle membrane. There may be endocytosis (pinching off of regions of the cell's membrane) of the receptor site.

Although the cause of the autoimmune response in MG is not well understood, the thymus appears to play a role in the disease. Seventy-five percent of persons with MG have abnormalities of the thymus (e.g., thymic hyperplasia or thymoma). Cells within the thymus bear ACh receptors on their surface, and may serve as a source of autoantigen to trigger the autoimmune reaction within the thymus gland (Drach, 1994).

Clinical Manifestations. Although MG encompasses a spectrum of mild to severe, its cardinal features are skeletal muscle weakness and fatigability. Repetition of activity causes fatigue while rest restores activity. Other than weakness, neurologic findings are normal.

The distribution of muscle weakness has a dichotomous pattern affecting only the ocular muscles, or a more variable, generalized pattern occurs. In approximately 85% of persons with MG, the weakness is generalized and affects the limb musculature. This fluctuating weakness is often more noticeable in proximal muscles.

Cranial muscles, particularly the eyelids and the muscles controlling eye movements, are the first to show weakness. Diplopia (double vision) and ptosis (drooping eyelids) are common early signs causing the person to tilt the head back to see (Fig. 34–16). Weak neck muscles may cause head bobbing in this position.

Chewing of meat produces fatigue and the facial expression is one that seems to be "snarling" because the lips do not close. Speech tends to be nasal. Difficulty in swallowing may occur as a result of palatal, pharyngeal, and tongue weakness. Nasal regurgitation or aspiration of food is common.

Medical Management

Diagnosis. History and clinical observation of symptoms of weakness with continued use and improvement with rest are important in diagnosing MG. Several conditions that cause weakness of cranial, or somatic muscles must also be considered. These include drug-induced myasthenia, hyperthyroidism, botulism, intracranial mass lesions, and progressive disorders of the eye. Lambert-Eaton syndrome is a presynaptic disorder of the neuromuscular junction that can cause symptoms similar to those of MG. Lambert-Eaton syndrome is an autoimmune disorder associated with neoplasm, most commonly small cell (oat cell) carcinoma of the lung, which is believed to trigger the autoimmune response.

Three methods are used to diagnose MG: (1) immunologic, (2) pharmacologic, and (3) electrophysiologic testing (Hopkins, 1994). Immunologic testing detects anti–ACh receptor antibodies in the serum. The presence of anti–ACh receptor antibodies is virtually diagnostic of MG, but a negative test does not exclude diagnosis of the disease. There is no correlation between the amount of anti–ACh receptor antibodies and the severity of the disease. However, in a person with MG a treatment-induced fall in the antibody level often correlates with clinical improvement.

The drug edrophonium (Tensilon) is used to demonstrate improvement in the myasthenic muscles by inhibiting acetylcholinesterase (AChE), an enzyme required for ACh uptake. Muscle strength and endurance are measured prior to and following administration of the drug. This test confirms that ACh uptake is part of the pathologic status; however, a control test of saline should also be used for comparison.

Electrophysiologic testing of myasthenic disorders demonstrates a normal EMG at rest. Specialized testing must be employed using repetitive stimulation to demonstrate a rapid decrement in the motor action potential's amplitude. Absence of sensory deficits and retention of tendon reflexes throughout the course of the disease also tend to confirm the diagnosis of MG. Because respiratory impairment is a serious complication of MG, measurements of ventilatory function should be performed (Zulueta and Fanburg, 1994).

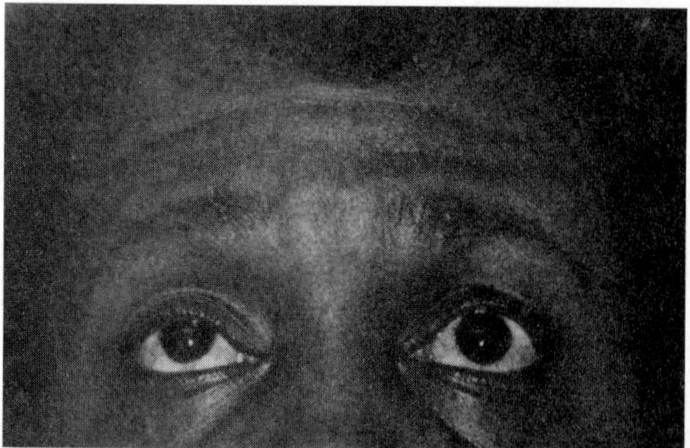

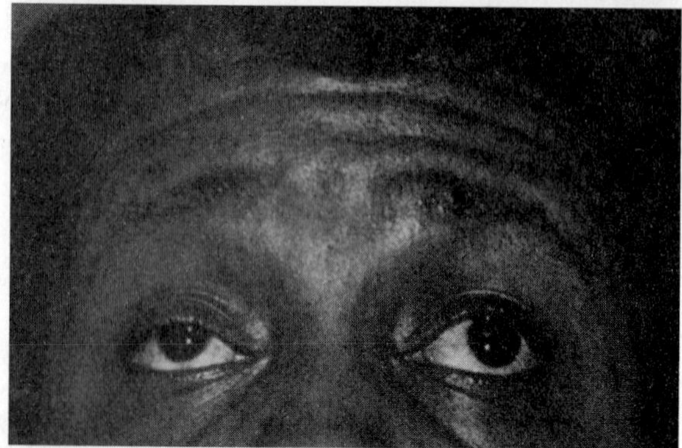

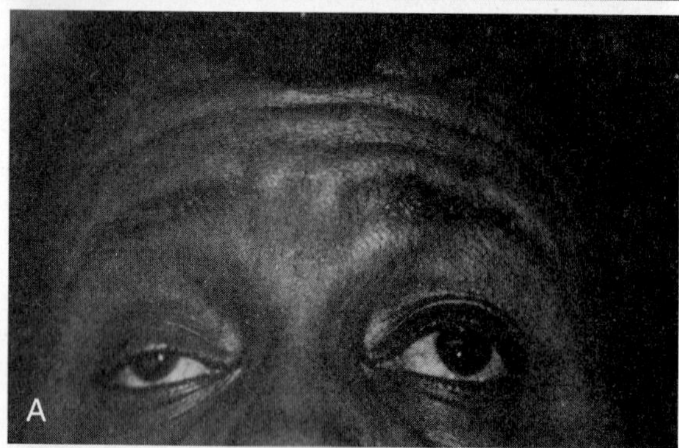

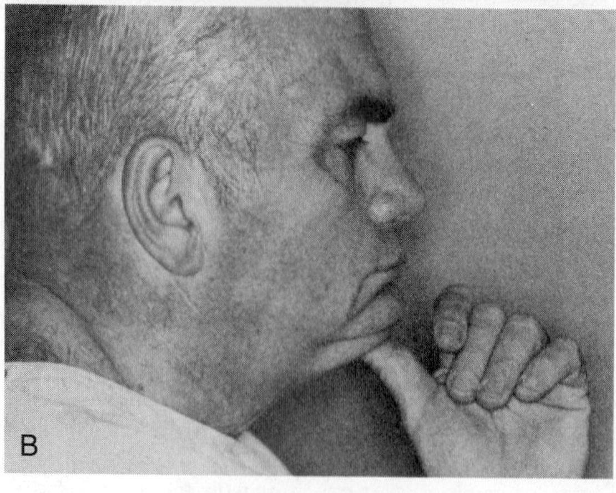

Figure **34-16.** *A*, Weakness of eyelids with sustained upward gaze occurs in myasthenia gravis. *B*, Compensatory movements are adopted to relieve the weakness of the musculature that closes the jaw, that is, passive closure is maintained by the thumb. (*From Hopkins LC: Clinical features of myasthenia gravis. Neurol Clin 12:245, 255, 1994.*)

Treatment. AChE inhibitor medication provides for improvement of weakness, but does not treat the underlying disease. Administration of this medication is tailored to the individual's requirements throughout the day. For example, a person with difficulty chewing and swallowing would take the medication before meals. Side effects of AChE inhibitors include gastrointestinal effects, such as nausea and vomiting, abdominal cramping, and increased bronchial and oral secretions.

Surgical removal of the thymus is successful in 85% of persons with MG. Up to 35% of those undergoing thymectomy achieve a drug-free remission, although this may take years.

Immunosuppression using drugs such as corticosteroids (prednisone) and azathioprine are effective in nearly all persons with MG. Initially, high daily doses are begun; this is followed by alternate-day high doses that are tapered slowly over a period of months. Unfortunately, adverse side effects are associated with high-dose steroids. These include cushingoid appearance, weight gains, hypertension, and osteoporosis (see Chapter 4).

Plasmapheresis is performed to remove substances that affect ACh receptors. However, plasmapheresis produces only short-term reduction in anti-AChE antibodies and is not effective for long-term symptom control.

Prognosis. The course of MG is variable, typified by remissions and exacerbations, especially within the first year after onset. Symptoms often fluctuate in intensity during the day. This daily variability is superimposed on longer-term spontaneous relapses that may last for weeks. Remissions are rarely complete or permanent.

This disorder follows a slowly progressive course. Onset of other systemic disorders and infections may precipitate an exacerbation of the disease, and are the most common cause of a crisis. A myasthenic crisis is a medical emergency requiring attention to life-endangering weakening of the respiratory muscles. A myasthenic crisis requires ventilatory assistance. Treatment of a crisis occurs in the ICU because the client requires careful, immediate control of medications for survival (Chipps, 1991).

When MG begins in children, it is important to establish the form it takes. Ten percent of newborns of mothers with MG develop a myasthenic reaction because AChE antibodies cross the placenta. Newborns with neonatal MG have a weak suck and cry and are hypotonic. Fortunately, this resolves in a few weeks.

Special Implications for Therapists **34-4**

MYASTHENIA GRAVIS

Physical and occupational therapy may be indicated as supportive care to assist the client with MG. In the acute care setting, the therapist must establish an accurate neurologic and respiratory baseline. Tidal volume, vital capacity, and inspiratory force should be monitored regularly during treatment. Deep breathing and coughing should be encouraged. When eating, the person should be instructed to sit upright and to swallow when the chin is tipped slightly downward toward the chest, never with the neck extended because of the risk of aspiration. Finally, the client should never speak with food in the mouth.

The therapist must also be alert to signs of an impending myasthenic crisis (increasing muscle weakness, respiratory distress, difficulty while talking, chewing, or swallowing). Make sure the client recognizes the side effects and signs of toxicity of AChE inhibitor medications. For those receiving a prolonged course of corticosteroids, report adverse side effects to the physician.

Plan therapy and teach the client to plan activities to coincide with periods of maximum energy (see Box 7–1 for Energy Conservation Tips). The home should be arranged to help prevent unnecessary energy expenditure. Frequent rest periods help conserve energy and give muscles a chance to regain strength. The person with MG should avoid strenuous exercise, stress, and excessive exposure to the sun or cold weather. All of these can exacerbate signs and symptoms.

Lohi and colleagues (1993) report that a strength training program eliciting maximal isometric contractions could be instituted in clients with mild to moderate MG. As long as participants were monitored for fatigue during periods of exercise, improvements were noted in all muscles. After 3 months, participants' knee extensor muscles showed the most significant strength gains without adverse reactions.

The Myasthenia Gravis Foundation (800-541-5454) publishes educational materials that can be helpful to the client and family.

Botulism

Definition and Incidence. Botulism is a rare, often fatal condition (20% mortality) caused by ingestion of a potent neurotoxin produced by *Clostridium botulinum* which is found in improperly preserved or canned foods, as well as in contaminated wounds. The Centers for Disease Control and Prevention (CDC) recognizes four categories of botulism: (1) foodborne, (2) wound, (3) infant, and (4) unclassified (Viccellio, 1993). Approximately 10 adult cases and 100 cases of infant botulism are reported each year in the United Sates.

Etiology and Pathogenesis. The anaerobic bacillus releases a protein neurotoxin which is heat-labile; it is destroyed by boiling food for 10 minutes. Therefore, inadequate food preparation allows the neurotoxin to be ingested.

Infant botulism affects babies aged from 3 weeks to 9 months; the most common source of infant botulism arises from the ingestion of honey which is why children of less than 1 year are not allowed to have honey.

Botulism is not always ingested orally. Some cases occur after wounds are contaminated with soil, in chronic drug abusers, after cesarean delivery, and may even occur when antibiotics are administered to prevent wound infection.

When the neurotoxin is ingested, digestive acids and proteolytic enzymes cannot destroy the molecules of the toxin and it is absorbed into the blood from the small intestine. Minute amounts of circulating toxin reach the cholinergic nerve endings at the motor end plate and bind to gangliosides of the presynaptic nerve terminals. Flaccid paralysis is caused by inhibition of ACh released from cholinergic terminals at the motor end plate. Inhibition of ACh release causes a symmetrical paralysis with normal sensory and mental status.

Clinical Manifestations. Onset of symptoms develops 12 to 36 hours following ingestion of food containing the toxin. Signs and symptoms include malaise, weakness, blurred vision and double vision (diplopia), dry mouth, and nausea and vomiting. Progression is variable, but respiratory failure can occur in 6 to 8 hours. People may also report difficulty swallowing (dysphagia), dysarthria (slurred speech), and photophobia. Because the motor end plate is involved, there are no sensory changes. Motor weakness of the face and neck muscles progresses to involve the diaphragm, accessory muscles of respiration, and muscles controlling the extremities. Secondary effects from the flaccid paralysis occur, namely, severe muscle wasting, pressure sores, and aspiration pneumonia.

Medical Management

Diagnosis, Treatment, and Prognosis. A history suggesting a food source and toxin identification made by serum or stool analysis aids in the diagnosis. Electromyographic testing demonstrates a decreasing amplitude and facilitation of muscle action potential following tetanic stimulation. Differential diagnosis includes disorders that also display a rapidly evolving flaccid paralysis, such as Guillain-Barré syndrome, myasthenia gravis, and tick paralysis.

Immediate treatment is directed toward neutralizing the toxin using injectable trivalent ABE serum, an antitoxin. Antitoxin prevents further binding of free botulism toxin to the presynaptic endings. If paralysis occurs because of wound botulism, care should include debridement and antibiotics.

Removal of unabsorbed toxin from the GI tract is accomplished by gastric lavage and induced emesis. Lastly, supportive measures should be instituted in the hospital; intubation and mechanical ventilation are needed when the individual's vital capacity is compromised.

If untreated, this disorder can be fatal within 24 hours of ingestion. Respiratory failure leads to death. In mild to moderate cases, a gradual recovery of muscle strength can take as long as 12 months after onset. After hospitalization, graded rehabilitation is instituted to treat muscle wasting, deconditioning, and orthostatic hypotension.

PERIPHERAL NERVOUS SYSTEM CHANGES WITH AGING

Changes that occur in the PNS may be considered as one segment of a continuum that relates to normal growth and development, or the changes may represent a combination of pathologic processes superimposed on the normal aging process.

Age does not affect the size or number of fascicles, but the perineurium and epineurium do thicken with age and the endoneurium often becomes fibrosed with increased collagen. Even with these changes the cross-sectional area is slightly decreased with age because there is a reduced number of myelinated fibers. Ventral root fibers controlling motion are more affected than dorsal root fibers controlling sensation.

Blood vessels to nerves may become atherosclerotic with aging and occlusion may contribute to loss of fibers. This vascular pathology has been attributed to the reason peripheral neuropathies are seen in older people. When individual myelinated fibers are examined, shorter internodes are seen. This suggests that a demyelinating-remyelinating process occurs with aging.

ANS dysfunction is more common in the elderly. This may be related to the changes seen in the nervous system in the elderly. Cell bodies show chromatolysis, as well as accumulation of lipofuscins, representing diminished ability of the cell to rid itself of toxins. Although a slight loss of cell bodies has been observed in the sympathetic ganglia, there is a greater loss of the unmyelinated fibers in peripheral nerves.

When the motor end plate is examined, age-related changes do occur, but these changes are seen as early as the third decade of life and are not reported in all muscles. When sensory receptors have been evaluated, density and morphology have been found to be altered in the elderly.

NCVs are slowed in the elderly. In addition, the amplitude of the potential is reduced. Shorter internode distances suggest segmental demyelinations and remyelinations, which have been identified in people over age 65 (Jacobs and Love, 1985). EMG studies of elderly people without evidence of neurologic disorders of the PNS show loss of motor units as well as signs of reinnervation. These changes have been observed in people over 60 years of age (McComas et al., 1971).

Healthy elderly, with no evidence of neurologic disease, may provide a clinical history suggestive of peripheral neuropathy. This includes numbness and tingling in the hands and feet along with mild, diffuse weakness—especially in the distal muscles of the hand. Sensory alterations may lead to poor balance and gait instability. On examination, sensory thresholds are increased.

The cause of an aging neuropathy can be attributed to a combination of factors. First, loss of both motor and sensory cell bodies; second, a "dying back" condition, suggesting cells can metabolically support a limited number of fibers or receptors, similar to that seen in other systemic neuropathies. Last, over the course of a lifetime, chronic compression of the peripheral nerves, or repetitive trauma may have damaged the nerves. All these factors, combined with coexisting medical conditions, atherosclerosis, and nutritional deficiencies, may create this neuropathy of aging.

References

Aligne C, Barral X: Rehabilitation of patients with thoracic outlet syndrome. Ann Vasc Surg 6:381–389, 1992.

Asbury AK, McKhann GM, McDonald WI: Disease of the Nervous System: Clinical Neurobiology. Philadelphia, WB Saunders, 1986.

Chipps E: Myasthenia gravis: The patient in crisis. Crit Care Nurs 11:18–26, 1991.

Crutchfield C: Neuromuscular causes. *In* Scully R, Barnes ML (eds): Physical Therapy. Philadelphia, JB Lippincott, 1989.

Dalakas MC: Pathogenetic mechanisms of post-polio syndrome: Morphological, electrophysiological, virological, and immunological correlations. Ann N Y Acad Sci 753:176–185, 1995.

Dalakas MC, Elder G, Mallett M, et al: A long-term follow-up study of patients with post-poliomyelitis neuromuscular symptoms. N Engl J Med 314:959–963, 1986.

Dawson DM: Entrapment neuropathies of the upper extremities. N Engl J Med 329:2013–2018, 1993.

Department of Physical Therapy, Institute for Rehabilitation and Research, Houston: An instructional course on physical therapy management of post-poliomyelitis: New challenges. Presented at the 65th American Physical Therapy Association Annual Conference, Chicago, June 1986.

DiCesare PE, Young S, Perry J, Baumgarten M: Perimalleolar tendon transfer to the os calcis for triceps surae insufficiency in patients with postpolio syndrome. Clin Orthop 310:111–119, 1995.

Drach DB: Myasthenia gravis. N Engl J Med 330:1797–1810, 1994.

Dubowitz V: Muscle Disorders in Children. Philadelphia, WB Saunders, 1978.

Ellis J: Incidence of carpal tunnel syndrome is rising. PT Bull 10:6–9, 1995.

Estruch R, Nicolas JM, Villegos E, et al: Relationship between ethanol-related diseases and nutritional status in chronically alcoholic men. Alcohol 28:543–550, 1993.

Faraj AA: Review of Elmslie's triple arthodesis for postpolio pes calcaneovalgus deformity. J Foot Ankle Surg 34:319–321, 1995.

Feasby TE: Inflammatory-demyelinating polyneuropathies. Neurol Clin 10:651–670, 1992.

Fechter JD, Kuschner SH: The thoracic outlet syndrome. Orthopedics 16:1234–1251, 1993.

Fredericks CM, Saladin LK: Pathophysiology of the Motor Systems: Principles and Clinical Presentations. Philadelphia, FA Davis, 1996.

Gilroy J: Basic Neurology, ed 2. New York, Pergamon Press, 1990.

Gilroy J, Meyer JS: Medical Neurology, ed 3. New York, Macmillan, 1979.

Goodgold J, Eberstein A: Electrodiagnosis of Neuromuscular Diseases, ed 3. Baltimore, Williams & Wilkins, 1983.

Greene DA, Sima AA, Stevens MJ, et al: Aldose reductase inhibitors: An approach to the treatment of diabetic nerve damage. Diabetes Metab 9:189–217, 1993.

Gross MT, Schuck CP: Exercise programs for patients with post polio syndrome: A case report. Phys Ther 69:695–698, 1989.

Hagberg M, Morgenstern H, Kelsh M: Impact of occupations and job tasks on the prevalence of carpal tunnel syndrome. Scand J Work Environ Health 18:337–345, 1992.

Halstead LS, Rossi C: New problem in old polio patients: Results of a survey of 539 polio survivors. Orthopedics 8:845–853, 1985.

Harati Y: Frequently asked questions about diabetic peripheral neuropathies. Neurol Clin 10:783–807, 1992.

Holst HI: Primary peripheral nerve repair in the hand and upper extremity. J Trauma 15:909–911, 1975.

Hopkins LC: Clinical features of myasthenia gravis. Neurol Clin 12:243–261, 1994.

Hund EF, Borel CO, Cornblath DR, et al: Intensive management and treatment of severe Guillain-Barré syndrome. Crit Care Med 21:433–446, 1993.

Imaoka H, Yorifuji S, Takahashi MT, et al: Improved inching method for the diagnosis and prognosis of carpal tunnel syndrome. Muscle Nerve 15:318–324, 1992.

Jacobs JM, Love S: Qualitative and quantitative morphology of human sural nerve at different ages. Brain 108:897–924, 1985.

Jubelt B, Drucker J: Post-polio syndrome: An update. Semin Neurol 13:283–290, 1993.

Junqueira LC, Caneiro J, Kelley RO: Basic Histology. Norwalk, Conn, Appleton & Lange, 1992.

Junter JM (ed): Rehabilitation of the Hand: Surgery and Therapy, ed 4. St Louis, Mosby–Year Book, 1995.

Katz RT: Carpal tunnel syndrome: A practical review. Am Fam Physician 49:1371–1378, 1994.

Kruger VL, Kraft GH, Deitz JC, et al: Carpal tunnel syndrome: Objective measures and splinting. Arch Phys Med Rehabil 72:517–520, 1991.

Kuipers H: Exercise-induced muscle damage. Int J Sports Med 15:132–135, 1994.

LaBan MM, MacKenzie JR, Zemenick GA: Anatomic observations in carpal tunnel syndrome as they relate to the tethered median nerve stress test. Arch Phys Med Rehabil 70:44–46, 1989.

Leffert RD: Thoracic outlet syndrome. Hand Clin 8:285–297, 1992.

Lohi E, Lindberg C, Anderson O: Physical training in myasthenia gravis. Arch Phys Med Rehabil 74:1178–1189, 1993.

Magee DJ: Orthopedic Physical Assessment, ed 2. Philadelphia, WB Saunders, 1992.

McComas AJ, Fawcett PRW, Campbell MJ: Electrophysiological estimation of the number of motor units within a human muscle. J Neurol Neurosurg Psychiatry 34:121–131, 1971.

Middleton WD, Kneeland JB, Kellman GM: MR imaging of the carpal

tunnel: Normal anatomy and preliminary findings in the carpal tunnel syndrome. AJR 148:307–316, 1987.
Murray DP: Impaired mobility: Guillain-Barré syndrome. J Neurosci Nurs 25:100–104, 1993.
Ng KK, Howard RS, Fish DR, et al: Management and outcome of severe Guillain-Barré syndrome. Q J Med 88:243–250, 1995.
Omer GE: Acute management of peripheral nerve injuries. Hand Clin 2:193–205, 1956.
Palliyath S, Schwartz BD: Peripheral nerve functions improve in chronic alcoholic patients on abstinence. J Stud Alcohol 54:684–686, 1993.
Palmer DH, Hanrahan P: Societal and economic costs of carpal tunnel surgery. Instr Course Lect 44:167–172, 1995.
Parry GJ: Electrodiagnostic studies in the evaluation of peripheral nerve and brachial plexus injuries. Neurol Clin 10:921–934, 1992.
Payan J: Anterior transposition of the ulnar nerve: An electrophysiological study. J Neurol Neurosurg Psychiatry 33:157–165, 1970.
Payan J: Electrophysiological localization of ulnar nerve lesions. J Neurol Neurosurg Psychiatry 32:208–220, 1969.
Pentland B, Donald SM: Pain in the Guillain-Barré syndrome: A clinical review. Pain 30:159–164, 1994.
Perry J, Fleming C: Polio: Long-term problems. Orthopedics 8:877–881, 1985.
Phelps PE, Walker E: Comparison of the finger wrinkling test results in peripheral nerve injury. Am J Occup Ther 31:565–572, 1977.
Rhoades CE, Mowery CA, Gelberman RH: Results of the internal neurolysis of the median nerve for severe carpal tunnel syndrome. J Bone Joint Surg [Am] 67:253–256, 1985.
Ritchie AC: Boyd's Textbook of Pathology, ed 9. Philadelphia, Lea & Febiger, 1990.
Roos DB: The place for scalenectomy and first rib resection in thoracic outlet syndrome. Surgery 92:1077–1085, 1982.
Sanes JR, Covault J: Axon guidance during reinnervation of skeletal muscle. Trends Neurosci 43B:121, 1985.
Seddon H: Three types of nerve injury. Brain 66:237, 1943.
Sheldon B: Boyd's Introduction to the Study of Disease. Malvern, Pa, Lea & Febiger, 1992.
Siebenaler MJ, McGovern P: Carpal tunnel syndrome. Priorities for prevention. AAOHN J 40:62–71, 1992.
Stevens JC, Beard CM, O'Fallown WM, Kurland LT: Conditions associated with carpal tunnel syndrome. Mayo Clin Proc 67:541–548, 1992.
Sunderland S: Nerves and Nerve Injuries, ed 2. Edinburgh, Churchill Livingstone, 1978.
Thomas PK: Growth factors and diabetic neuropathy. Diabet Med 11:782–789, 1994.
Tomlinson DR, Stevens EJ, Diemel LT: Aldose reductase inhibitors and their potential for the treatment of diabetic complications. Trends Pharmacol Sci 15:293–297, 1994.
Totten PA, Hunter JM: Therapeutic techniques to enhance nerve gliding in thoracic outlet syndrome and carpal tunnel syndrome. Hand Clin 7:505–519, 1991.
Upton AR, McComas AJ: The double crush in nerve entrapment syndromes. Lancet 2:359–362, 1973.
van der Meche FG, Schmitz PI: A randomized trial comparing intravenous immune globulin and plasma exchange in Guillain-Barré syndrome. Dutch Guillain-Barré study group. N Engl J Med 326:1123–1129, 1992.
Viccellio P (ed): Handbook of Medical Toxicology. Boston, Little, Brown, 1993.
Vinik AT, Holland MT, LeBeau JM, et al: Diabetic neuropathies. Diabet Care 15:1926–1961, 1992.
Walsh MT: Therapist management of thoracic outlet syndrome. J Hand Ther 7:131–144, 1994.
Whitley JM, McDonnell DE: Carpal tunnel syndrome: A guide to prompt intervention. Postgrad Med 97:89–92, 1995.
Zulueta JJ, Fanburg BL: Respiratory dysfunction in myasthenia gravis. Clin Chest Med 15:683–691, 1994.

SECTION 4

chapter 35

Laboratory Tests and Values

Catherine C. Goodman,
William G. Boissonnault,
and Kenda S. Fuller

Many clients entering the health-care delivery system undergo a variety of diagnostic and laboratory tests. These tests provide useful data for the therapist. The therapist needs an understanding of test values, their variations, their interpretations, and their implications for therapy when establishing a plan of care.

With the need for shortened lengths of stay and better client outcomes, therapists in many hospitals are being consulted in the intensive care unit. Advances in medical technology are making it possible for earlier diagnosis, while at the same time improved medical treatment is leading to people with acute medical conditions leading longer lives.

Abnormal test results represent physiologic changes that may contraindicate physical therapy. Neglecting to take these results into consideration before determining goals and designing treatment plans could be harmful and possibly fatal for some clients (Polich and Faynor, 1996).

Only the most common and the most pertinent laboratory tests associated with the three sections of this book (clinical medicine, the musculoskeletal system, and the nervous system) are included in this chapter. For more detailed or more specific procedures, the reader is referred to other texts (Fischbach, 1995; Pagana and Pagana, 1995).

LABORATORY TESTS *(Box 35–1)*

As we have discussed in this book, advances in medicine have resulted in a population who are living longer with a more complex pathologic picture. Orthopedic and neurologic conditions no longer present as singular phenomena but frequently occur in someone who has other medical pathology. We must be cognizant of the ways other conditions and diseases affect the individual's neuromusculoskeletal system and take the necessary steps to treat safely *and* effectively.

For these reasons, many master clinicians within the field of physical therapy are advocating the routine monitoring of vital signs and clinical laboratory data in *all* clients regardless of age, condition, or diagnosis. Other clinicians decide on a case-by-case basis, but even so, these values are being reviewed routinely.

Laboratory values are a useful adjunct to evaluating a client's medical condition and revealing potential precautions for, or contraindications to, therapy, particularly exercise. For example, a low platelet level (e.g., less than 50,000/mm^3)[1] requires careful consideration of the planned treatment program: chest physical therapy is carried out with caution and exercise is restricted (see Table 35–7). Or consider the client with diabetes mellitus who is admitted to the hospital for a myocardial infarction (MI). Cardiac rehabilitation for this person in any setting (i.e., whether or not the facility has a formal cardiac rehabilitation program) requires careful monitoring of glucose levels before, during, and after exercise. However, this same person requiring wound care for a diabetic neuropathic ulcer would not necessarily require blood glucose testing prior to the local application of wound management.

Purpose of Laboratory Tests

Laboratory tests may be utilized by the physician for screening (searching for an occult disease process in an otherwise healthy person), diagnosis (identifying the cause of symptoms), or monitoring (following the progress of a disease) (Polich and Faynor, 1996). A single test may be used differently in different people depending on the need for information. For example, a glucose test may be used diagnostically or as a monitoring test.

Screening tests are used on populations to find high-risk individuals who should be treated differently from the general population. Some of the most common screening tests are carried out on the pediatric population to prevent morbidity and mortality (e.g., hypothyroidism, sickle cell disease, phenylketonuria).

Limitations of Laboratory Tests *(Fischbach, 1995)*

With any laboratory testing procedure there are false-negative or false-positive results. The more tests ordered, the greater the chance that some tests will be false. This phenomenon is purely related to chance because a significant margin of error arises from the arbitrary setting of limits for normal or reference values.[2]

Other factors affecting test results include certain drugs that can produce negative or positive results. Reference ranges vary by laboratory, sex, age, weight, and physiologic status

[1] Abbreviations of conventional units for reporting laboratory test data are listed in Box 35–1.

[2] The range of values for a given test in a so-called healthy person is known as the reference range or expected value, formerly known as the "normal range." The reference range depends on the methods used for the test and must be compared against the reference range specific to that laboratory. It is important to realize that normal ranges of laboratory tests vary from institution to institution; this variability is even more obvious among various laboratory textbooks. The reference ranges provided in this chapter give the therapist a general idea of the values expected for each test, but interpretation of specific individual values must be done using the laboratory reference values (usually provided on most laboratory reports), not these figures.

(e.g., pregnancy). Certain tests have no predictive value such as the electrocardiogram (ECG) which is not sensitive to coronary disease before an MI; a person may have a normal ECG one day and develop an MI the next.

The positive predictive value of a test is dependent on the prevalence of the disease in a population. The less prevalent the disease, the less accurate laboratory results may be. For example, the predictive value of cardiac stress tests in a 40-year-old woman is so poor the test is not recommended. A positive test may be obtained in the absence of cardiac disease; this is an example of how a positive result can occur when the prevalence of (cardiac) disease (in premenopausal women) is low.

TESTS FOR BLOOD COMPOSITION, PRODUCTION, AND FUNCTION

Complete Blood Count

The complete blood count (CBC) is somewhat of a misnomer because this test provides limited data and other blood tests may be required. It is one of the most commonly ordered laboratory tests and is used to assess how the blood cells look (normal or pathologic). The CBC does not test blood cell function; for example, the CBC may indicate a normal number of red blood cells (RBCs) but the fact that the RBCs have decreased hemoglobin content and subsequent poor oxygen transport is not measured.

The CBC is an automated test that determines the actual number of blood elements in relation to volume and quantifies abnormalities. Although it does not test cell function, if the test results are abnormal altered function may be implied and probable cause may be suspected. For example, abnormal white blood cell (WBC) values indicate the functional status of the immune system and the presence of inflammatory processes. This panel of blood tests aids in diagnosing infections, anemias, arthritides, and certain cancers (Tables 35–1 and 35–2).

Red Blood Cell Function

The main function of the RBC (erythrocyte) is to carry oxygen from the lungs to the body tissues and to transfer carbon dioxide from the tissues to the lungs. This process is achieved by means of hemoglobin in the RBCs which combines easily with oxygen and carbon dioxide.

RBC function can be assessed using more than a dozen tests available. Many tests look at the RBCs: their number, size, amount of hemoglobin, rate of production, percent composition of the blood. The RBC count, hematocrit (Hct), and hemoglobin (Hgb) (see Table 35–2) are closely related but provide different ways to look at the adequacy of RBC production (Fischbach, 1995).

White Blood Cell Function

Identifying the specific cells involved in the immune response and observing characteristic abnormalities in the number and percentage of helper T cells, suppressor T cells, and B lymphocytes may provide diagnostic clues to the underlying disease state (Table 35–3) (see also Immunologic Tests). Abnormal levels of blood cell components such as leukocytosis, leukopenia, polycythemia, and anemia are discussed more fully in Chapter 11.

White Blood Cell Differential

A WBC differential estimates the percentage of different types of WBCs (leukocytes) being produced (Box 35–2) and is determined through a peripheral blood smear. A blood smear is a specimen that is prepared by spreading a small quantity of peripheral blood across a glass slide. It is used to show the maturity and morphologic characteristics of blood elements[3] and to determine qualitative abnormalities. When adequately prepared and examined microscopically by an experienced technologist, a smear of peripheral blood is the most informative of all the hematologic tests.

Different disease states produce distinctive patterns of WBCs (Table 35–4). For example, bacterial infections are accompanied by an increase in the number of neutrophils.[4] Close inspection of the nuclei of neutrophils during acute bacterial infection shows the appearance of more immature forms (bands) of neutrophils, indicating that the body is recruiting new neutrophils in response to the infection.

This phenomenon is referred to as a "left shift"[5] and may also occur in response to acute necrosis (e.g., MI) or in response to the immune system forming neutrophils in an autoimmune response. A "shift to the right" occurs when there is an increased percentage of circulating mature neutrophils (e.g., tissue breakdown, as in burns, MI, tumors, gangrene; with allergies; cancer of the liver, gastrointestinal tract, and bone marrow).

The differential count is expressed as a percentage of the total number of WBCs. The absolute number of each type of WBC (there are five types; see Box 35–2) is obtained mathematically by multiplying the percentage of one type

BOX 35–1
Units for Clinical Laboratory Data

g	gram
ng	nanogram
mg	milligram
mL	milliliter
L	liter
dL	deciliter (100 mL)
pg	picogram
mm^3	cubic millimeter
mmol	millimole
U	unit
IU	international unit
mU	milliunit
µg	microgram
µU	microunit
µm	micron
mEq	milliequivalent

[3] All three hematologic lines (RBCs, WBCs, platelets) can be examined on the blood smear. WBCs are examined for quantity, differential count, and degree of maturity. Microscopic examination of the RBCs can reveal variation in size (anisocytosis), shape (poikilocytosis), color, or intracellular content to help classify types and causes of anemia.

[4] Neutrophils are also referred to as segmented neutrophils, polymorphonuclear neutrophils, PMNs, segs, or polys.

[5] The terms "left shift" and "right shift" refer to a previous documenting method by which the number of immature neutrophils (PMNs) usually indicating acute bacterial infection were recorded on the left and the number of lymphocytes (mature neutrophils) were recorded on the right. The term "right shift" is no longer used but the reader will encounter the term "left shift" or "shift to the left."

TABLE 35-1 COMPLETE BLOOD CELL COUNT (CBC)

ABBREVIATION	MEASURE OF
Leukocytes (WBCs)	Number of WBCs
Erythrocytes (RBCs)	Number of RBCs Hematocrit or packed cell volume (PCV) is the percentage of whole blood occupied by RBCs Hemoglobin (Hb) measures the amount (grams) of hemoglobin per 100 mL of blood, to determine the oxygen-carrying capacity of RBCs Mean corpuscular volume (MCV) describes the RBC in terms of size; used to classify anemia Mean corpuscular hemoglobin (MCH) determines average amount of hemoglobin per RBC Mean corpuscular hemoglobin concentration (MCHC) establishes average hemoglobin concentration in 100 mL of packed RBCs
Platelets (thrombocytes)	Responsible for clotting

by the total WBC count. The differential count must be interpreted in relation to the total WBC count. If the percentage of one type of cell is increased it is not known if this reflects an absolute decrease in cells of another type or an actual absolute increase in the number of cells that are relatively increased. If the relative percentage values of the differential are known along with the total leukocyte count, it is possible to calculate absolute values for a more accurate interpretation (Fischbach, 1995).

Plasma

Plasma is evaluated using the erythrocyte sedimentation rate (ESR), electrophoresis of serum proteins (often used to diagnose plasma cell myeloma), and immunoelectrophoresis of serum proteins, which separates and classifies immunoglobulins (serum antibodies).

Sedimentation Rate

The ESR (erythrocyte sedimentation rate) is the rate at which RBCs settle out of unclotted blood plasma in 1 hour, possibly indicating infection or inflammation. This test is based on the fact that inflammatory and necrotic processes cause an alteration in blood proteins, resulting in an aggregation of RBCs, which make them heavier and more likely to fall rapidly when placed in a special vertical test tube. The faster the sedimentation rate or settling of cells, the higher the ESR; a significant increase in the ESR warrants closer investigation (see Table 35–2).

An elevated ESR may be used to monitor the course or response to treatment of certain diseases such as polymyalgia rheumatica, giant cell arteritis, rheumatoid arthritis (RA), systemic lupus erythematosus (SLE), Hodgkin's disease, and tuberculosis; however, the ESR is normal in 5% of all people with RA and SLE.

Although the measurement of ESR is a nonspecific study it is a commonly used index of musculoskeletal dysfunction (e.g., tissue injury or inflammation, bone infections). It provides helpful information when differentiating functional diseases and neuroses from organic diseases.

Hemostasis

Clotting Studies and Bleeding Time

Hemostasis is evaluated using clotting studies and bleeding time. Clotting studies can be used to determine the body's

TABLE 35-2 COMPLETE BLOOD CELL COUNT (CBC) REFERENCE VALUES

AGE	WBCs (Cells/mm³)	RBCs (10⁶/mm³)	ERYTHROCYTE SEDIMENTATION (ESR) (mm/hr)*	HEMATOCRIT (%)	HEMOGLOBIN (g/dL)
Birth	9000–30,000	4.8–7.1	0–2	44–64	14–24
3–6 mo	—	3.1–4.5	Child: up to 10	30–40	10–15
0.5–2.0 yr	6200–17,000	3.7–5.3	—	31–43	11–16
2–6 yr	4500–13,500	3.8–5.5	—	31–43	11–16
6–12 yr	4500–13,500	4.0–5.2	—	35–45	11–16
12–18 yr (male)	4500–11,000	4.5–5.3	—	37–49	13–16
12–18 yr (female)	4500–11,000	4.1–5.1	—	36–46	12–16
Adult male	5000–10,000†	4.7–6.1	Up to 15	42–52	14–18
Adult female	5000–10,000†	4.2–5.4	Up to 20	37–47	12–16

* The ESR or sed rate is not part of the CBC but is rather a separate test. The ESR reference values are included here since the age categories are the same for CBC measurements.

† The reference values for WBCs in adult males and females listed here may be considered high by some. Other reference values may be more inclusive (4300–10,800 cells/mm³).

Data from Pagana KD, Pagana TJ: Mosby's Diagnostic and Laboratory Test Reference, ed 2. St Louis, Mosby–Year Book, 1995, pp 344, 440, 442, 683, 864.

TABLE 35-3 T- AND B-CELL LYMPHOCYTE SURFACE MARKERS

T cells (CD2)	60%–88%
Helper T-cells (CD4)	34%–67%
Suppressor T-cells (CD8)	10%–42%
B cells (CD19)	3%–21%
T helper/suppressor cell ratio	>1.0

Data from Fischbach F: A Manual of Laboratory and Diagnostic Tests, ed 4. Philadelphia, JB Lippincott, 1992, pp 515–516.

ability to initiate the clotting sequence, as well as to diagnose hereditary clotting deficiencies (e.g., hemophilia), and monitor anticoagulant therapy (e.g., Coumadin [warfarin]). Bleeding time is a clotting study that tests the function of platelets (Polich and Faynor, 1996).

Commonly performed studies include the prothrombin time (protime or PT; this test evaluates thrombin production), international normalized ratio (INR; see below), and activated partial thromboplastin time (APTT or PTT; this test assesses plasma clotting factors) (Table 35–5). The PT measures clotting factors V, VII, and X, prothrombin, and fibrinogen. PT results are used to screen for bleeding disorders and to measure the effectiveness of anticoagulation therapy.

In an effort to eliminate laboratory variations in protime tests, the INR has been developed as a way to express PT results.[6] The INR is standardized worldwide and makes results comparable from laboratory to laboratory. The INR is the ratio of the individual's result to the reference range, correcting for variations in PT test materials (Vanscoy and Krause, 1991).

Bone Marrow Aspiration

Bone marrow is located within cancellous bone and in cavities of long bones. A smear is made from a bone marrow aspiration or biopsy to see if the bone marrow is performing its function of manufacturing normal RBCs, WBCs, and platelets. Bone marrow aspiration or biopsy allows evaluation of blood formation (hematopoiesis) by showing blood elements and precursor blood cells, as well as any abnormal or malignant cells. Bone marrow aspiration (BMA) is important in the evaluation of a number of hematologic disorders such as infectious diseases, leukemia or multiple myeloma, and deficiency states (e.g., vitamin B_{12}, folic acid, iron, pyridoxine) (Fischbach, 1995).

Special Implications for the Therapist **35-1**

BLOOD TESTS

Complete Blood Count

Hemoglobin

Decreased hemoglobin may be the result of obvious or occult blood loss, decreased RBC production (e.g., lack of substrate such as iron, vitamin B_{12}, or folate), myeloproliferative processes (i.e., overgrowth of bone marrow caused by cancer), or increased RBC destruction (e.g., disseminated intravascular coagulation or DIC, splenic involvement, or sequestration of sickle cells in sickle cell disease). Increased hemoglobin may be found in cases of dehydration and polycythemia.

Low hemoglobin values (8 to 10 g/dL) typically result in decreased exercise tolerance, increased fatigue, and tachycardia, conditions that may contraindicate aggressive therapeutic measures, including strength and endurance training. Exercise tolerance in anyone with hemoglobin values of less than 8 g/dL is poor and therapeutic intervention is contraindicated (Table 35–6). See also Special Implications for the Therapist: Anemia, 11–3.

White Blood Cell Count

It is important for the therapist to be aware of the client's most recent WBC count prior to and during the course of treatment if that person is immunosuppressed. If the count is low, the client is extremely susceptible to opportunistic infections and severe complications. The importance of good handwashing and hygiene practices cannot be overemphasized when treating these clients. Some centers recommend that people with a WBC count of less than 1000/mm^3 or a neutrophil count of less than 500/mm^3 should wear a protective mask. Therapists should ensure that all equipment is disinfected according to universal precautions (Grant, 1994).

Platelets

Platelets initiate the clotting sequence to plug damaged blood vessels. Where the PT is still being used, generally it is considered therapeutic (i.e., the blood has been sufficiently coagulated in response to blood vessel damage) when the value is 1.5 to 2.5 times the reference range (see Table 35–6). Values 2.5 times the reference range or greater contraindicate physical or occupational therapy intervention because of the increased risk of spontaneous bleeding.

BOX **35-2**
White Blood Cell Differential

The relative proportion of different types of white blood cells including:

Neutrophils (PMNs):
- Segmented or mature neutrophils are white blood cells that constitute the first line of defense against foreign substances (usually bacterial infection)
- Band cells are immature neutrophils that may be called up from the bone marrow to help fight severe (usually bacterial) infections

Lymphocytes: Lymphocytes produce antibodies, fight tumor cells, and respond to viral infection

Monocytes: Monocytes clean up the debris after neutrophils have done their job

Eosinophils: Eosinophils attack parasites and play a role in asthma and allergy

Basophils: Basophils release histamines during allergic reactions

[6] Actual PT test results are currently becoming obsolete. Although the PT value is needed to calculate the INR, eventually only the INR will be recorded, making test results comparable from one laboratory to the next.

TABLE 35-4 Differential White Blood Cell Count Reference Values

Cell	Function	Absolute Count (Cells/mm³)	Differential Count (%)
Neutrophils (PMNs, segs, bands)	Pyogenic infections	1800–7000	50–60
Lymphocytes	Viral infections (measles, rubella, chickenpox, infectious mononucleosis)	1500–4000	30–40
Monocytes	Severe infections	0–800	1–9
Eosinophils	Allergic disorders and parasitic infections	0–450	0–3
Basophils	Parasitic infections, hypersensitivity reactions	0–200	0–1

However, when the INR is recorded (e.g., for most cases of anticoagulant/Coumadin therapy), it is desirable to maintain the INR under 2. A value of 2 to 3 may be considered "therapeutic" for someone being treated with warfarin but when the INR exceeds 2, the therapist should check with the physician to find out whether the client is at increased risk of bleeding. INR values exceeding 3 may place the client at risk of hemarthrosis requiring care during therapy and exercise. Exercise guidelines for the client with reduced platelet counts (thrombocytopenia) or elevated platelet counts (thrombocytosis) (Table 35–7) are discussed in Chapter 11.

Bone Marrow Aspiration

BMA is performed on the sternum, iliac crest, anterior or posterior superior iliac spine (PSIS), and proximal tibia (in children). The preferred site is the PSIS with the client placed prone or lying on the opposite side. Afterward, the client remains on bed rest for 30 to 60 minutes. Some people report tenderness at the puncture site for several days after this procedure and physical therapy should avoid pressure or manual procedures in this area. The application of local heat should be avoided because of the increased risk of bleeding.

SERUM CHEMISTRIES

Iron and Iron Binding

Most of the iron in the body is supplied by the diet, absorbed in the small intestine, and transported to the plasma where it is bound to a globulin protein called transferrin. Transferrin carries the iron to the bone marrow for incorporation into hemoglobin where the majority of iron is located. The serum iron measurement is an indication of the quantity of iron bound to transferrin (normally at 30% to 40% saturation) (see Table 35–15). Iron deficiency results in decreased production of hemoglobin resulting in anemia. Conversely, since iron is necessary for the production of hemoglobin, the measurement of iron is helpful in evaluating anemia (Pagana and Pagana, 1995).

Chronic illnesses such as infections, neoplasm, or cirrhosis are characterized by low transferrin levels, whereas pregnancy is marked by high levels of protein, including transferrin. Because iron requirements are so high late in pregnancy, it is not unusual to find low serum iron levels and a low percentage of transferrin saturation during the third trimester.

Ferritin

Ferritin, the major iron storage protein, is directly proportional to iron storage; the normal adult has approximately 8 mg of stored iron. Ferritin levels in adult men and postmenopausal women are generally significantly higher than in younger adult women. Decreases in ferritin levels are associated with iron deficiency anemia and severe protein depletion (e.g., burns, malnutrition).

Increased levels are seen in the case of iron excess (e.g., hemosiderosis, hemolytic anemia, hemochromatosis) and certain liver disorders. A major limitation to this test is the fact that ferritin levels can be elevated in conditions that do not reflect iron stores such as acute inflammatory diseases, infections, metastatic cancer, and lymphomas.

TABLE 35-5 Platelets

		Coagulation Study		
Age	Platelet Count (Cells/mm³)	International Normalized Ratio (INR)	Prothrombin Time (PT)	Partial Thromboplastin Time (PTT)
Premature infant	100,000–300,000			
Newborn	150,000–300,000			
Infant	200,000–475,000			
Child	150,000–400,000			
Adult, elderly	150,000–400,000	0.9–1.1 (ratio)*	12–15 sec	25–40 sec

* Minimal interlaboratory variability; replaces formerly used prothrombin test (PT).

TABLE 35-6 COMPLETE BLOOD COUNT: EXERCISE GUIDELINES (ADULT)*

White blood cell (WBC) count	<5000/mm³ with fever	No exercise permitted
	>5000/mm³	Light exercise; progress to resistive exercise as tolerated
Hematocrit (Hct)	<25%	No exercise permitted
	>25%	Light exercise permitted
	30%–32%	Add resistive exercise as tolerated
Hemoglobin (Hgb)	<8 g/dL	No exercise permitted
	8–10 g/dL	Light exercise permitted
	>10 g/dL	Resistive exercise permitted
Platelets	<20,000/mm³	No exercise†
Prothrombin time (PT)	Values ≥2.5 times the reference range	Physical and occupational therapy contraindicated
Clients receiving anticoagulant therapy (PT)	INR > 2	Consult with physician (see text)

INR, international normalized ratio.
* These guidelines are only meant as a general recommendation. The therapist must make individual determinations depending on the client's age, general health status, and disease or condition present. For example, someone with an acute episode of urinary tract infection with altered WBC count and fever would be treated differently than someone with a chronic condition such as diabetes mellitus.
† See Table 35–7.
Adapted from Garritan S, Jones P, Kornberg T, Parkin C: Laboratory values in the intensive care unit. Acute Care Perspectives, Newsletter of the Acute Care/Hospital Clinical Practice Section, APTA, winter 1995, p 10.

Vitamin B_{12} and Folate

Vitamin B_{12} is necessary for the production of RBCs. It is obtained from ingesting animal protein and requires intrinsic factor (IF), which is produced by the gastric mucosa, for absorption in the distal part of the ileum. When absorption of vitamin B_{12} is inadequate (e.g., due to a malabsorption syndrome or from lack of IF) pernicious anemia may develop.

Folic acid (folate), one of the B vitamins, is also necessary for normal function of red and white blood cells and for the adequate synthesis of certain purines and pyrimidines which are precursors to deoxyribonucleic acid (DNA). As with vitamin B_{12}, folate depends on normal function of the intestinal mucosa.

Folic acid measurements evaluate hemolytic disorders and detect anemia caused by folic acid deficiency (e.g., dietary deficiency, malabsorption syndrome, pregnancy, anticonvulsant drugs). Elderly persons or those having an inadequate diet are known to develop folate-deficient megaloblastic anemia. The folic acid test may be done in conjunction with tests for vitamin B_{12} levels and is often done to assess the nutritional status of an alcoholic person.

TABLE 35-7 EXERCISE GUIDELINES FOR THROMBOCYTOPENIA*

PLATELET COUNT (Cells/mm³)	EXERCISE
150,000–450,000 (normal range)	Normal activity (unrestricted)
50,000–150,000	Progressive resistive exercise (see below) Swimming Low bench stepping Bicycling (no grade; flat only)
50,000–30,000	Active range-of-motion (AROM) exercise Moderate exercise Stationary bicycling Walking as tolerated Aquatic (pool) therapy
30,000–20,000	Light exercise AROM exercise only Walking as tolerated Aquatic (pool) therapy with physician approval
<20,000	AROM exercise Activity restricted to activities of daily living; walking with physician approval

* These guidelines vary from institution to institution; the therapist should check with each facility for its specific guidelines. Some therapists working in oncology settings report a more liberal exercise guideline. For example, restriction to active range of motion and activities of daily living are indicated only when platelet counts drop below 5000/mm³.

Electrolytes

Electrolytes are chemical substances which when dissolved in water separate into electrically charged particles called *ions*. This process allows the ions in the body fluids to conduct an electric charge transforming ions into *cations*, necessary for metabolic activities and essential to the normal function of all cells. Elevation or depression of electrolytes such as sodium, calcium, potassium, magnesium, chloride, and bicarbonate is diagnostically and clinically significant in a number of metabolic disorders (Table 35–8) (Polich and Faynor, 1996).

Changes in sodium (Na^+) concentration can cause cells to shrink or swell. The brain is most susceptible to these changes. As the brain and other nervous system tissues shrink or swell, mental status changes, intracranial hemorrhage, and coma can result. Potassium (K^+) regulation is critical for neuromuscular function. Abnormal values can cause muscle

TABLE 35–8 Reference Values for Serum Electrolytes

Age	Potassium (mEq/L)	Sodium (mEq/L)	Chloride (mEq/L)	Calcium (mg/dL)	Magnesium (mEq/L)
Newborn	3.9–5.9	134–144	96–106	9.0–10.6	1.4–2.0
Infant	4.1–5.3	134–150	—	—	
Child	3.4–4.7	136–145	90–110	8.8–10.8	
Adult, elderly	3.5–5.0	136–145	90–110	9.0–10.5	1.2–2.0
Critical Values					
Newborn	<2.5 or >8.0				
Adult	<2.5 or >6.5*	<120 or >160	<80 or >115	<6 (tetany) >14 (coma)	<0.5 or >3.0

* These values are related to medical treatment issues; critical value ranges specific to physical and occupational therapy are <3.2 and >5.1 mEq/L. See Special Implications for the Therapist: Electrolytes, below.

Data from Pagana KD, Pagana TJ: Mosby's Diagnostic and Laboratory Test Reference, ed 2. St Louis, Mosby–Year Book, 1995, pp 158, 197, 545, 638, 744.

weakness and irritability. The heart muscle is most susceptible to potassium disturbances.

Chloride (Cl^-) levels tend to follow shifts or losses in salt and water, as occur in dehydration, protracted vomiting, nasogastric suctioning, or diabetes insipidus. Bicarbonate (HCO_3^-) levels reflect acid-base status (Table 35–9). Low values are seen in metabolic acidosis (e.g., diabetic ketoacidosis). The lungs compensate for this condition by "blowing off" carbon dioxide resulting in a decreased bicarbonate concentration. A more detailed discussion of electrolytes is included in Chapter 4. See also Renal Function Tests.

Special Implications for the Therapist **35–2**

ELECTROLYTES

Potassium levels below 3.2 or above 5.1 mEq/L contraindicate physical therapy intervention because of the possibility of arrhythmia and tetany.[7] Exceptions to this guideline are people who are in chronic renal failure and those clients receiving potassium supplementation (e.g., fast-acting oral medication). Usually clients in chronic renal failure can tolerate potassium levels as high as 5.5 mEq/L. Levels less than 2.8 mmol/L or greater than 6.2 mEq/L require immediate medical attention (Kost, 1990).

People receiving potassium supplements may be cleared for treatment with close monitoring of the ECG during activity (see Fig. 4–2). The reader is referred to Chapter 4 and elsewhere (Polich and Fayner, 1996) for a complete discussion of electrolyte imbalances.

Blood Glucose Level

The blood glucose level is the most commonly used indicator of carbohydrate metabolism since glucose is formed from the digestion of carbohydrates and the conversion of glycogen by the liver. The fasting blood sugar (FBS), standard oral glucose tolerance test (OGTT), 2-hour postprandial blood sugar (PPBS), and glycosylated hemoglobin (HbA_{1c}) are various tests used to diagnose hyperglycemia (e.g., diabetes) (Table 35–10).

For the FBS, the client fasts at least 8 hours prior to the collection of blood. An elevated blood glucose level is abnormal in the fasting state but could be within the normal limits if the person has eaten a meal within the last hour. In the OGTT, the person's ability to tolerate a standard oral glucose dose is evaluated by obtaining serum (and urine) specimens for a glucose level baseline before glucose is administered and then at regular intervals after the administration of the glucose. People with an appropriate insulin response are able to tolerate the dose with only a mild rise in serum glucose levels within 1 hour after ingestion of the glucose. Serum glucose levels will be greatly elevated from 1 to 5 hours after this test if there is a deficiency of active insulin or inefficient glucose present.

In the 2-hour PPBS the amount of blood glucose is evaluated 2 hours after a meal (postprandial). For this study, food acts as a glucose challenge to the body's metabolism. In the normal person, insulin is secreted immediately after a meal in response to the elevated blood glucose levels with a return to the premeal range within 2 hours. In hyperglycemia, the glucose level is still elevated after 2 hours.

The glycosylated hemoglobin (GHb) test provides an accurate long-term index of the average blood glucose level. Glycohemoglobin is a minor hemoglobin with A_1 components which are glycosylated (i.e., they have glucose attached to them). The amount of GHb measured in the RBCs depends on the amount of glucose available in the bloodstream over the 120-day life span of the RBC, thereby reflecting the average blood sugar level for the 100- to 120-day period before the test. The more glucose the RBC was exposed to, the greater the GHb percentage. An important advantage of this test is that the sample is not affected by short-term variations such as food intake, exercise, stress, hypoglycemic agents, or compliance.

[7] Table 35–8 lists critical values for potassium levels as less than 2.5 or greater than 6.5 mEq/L. These values apply to medical treatment issues. Therapists must follow a more narrow range of contraindicative values as listed here.

TABLE 35-9 LABORATORY VALUES IN ACID-BASE DISORDERS*

	Arterial Blood			
	pH (7.35–7.45)	PCO_2 (35–45 mm Hg)	HCO_3^- (22–36 mEq/L)	Signs
Metabolic acidosis				
Uncompensated	<7.35	Normal	<22	Headache; fatigue; nausea, vomiting; diarrhea; muscular twitching; convulsions; coma; hyperventilation
Compensated	Normal	<35	<22	
Metabolic alkalosis				
Uncompensated	>7.45	Normal	>26	Nausea, vomiting, diarrhea, confusion, irritability, agitation, muscle twitching, muscle cramping, muscle weakness, paresthesias, convulsions, slow breathing
Compensated	Normal	>45	>26	
Respiratory acidosis				
Uncompensated	<7.35	>45	Normal	Headache, diaphoresis, tachycardia, disorientation, agitation, cyanosis, lethargy, ↓ deep tendon reflex
Compensated	Normal	>45	>26	
Respiratory alkalosis				
Uncompensated	>7.45	<35	Normal	Rapid, deep respirations; lightheadedness; muscle twitching; anxiety and fears; paresthesias; cardiac arrhythmia
Compensated	Normal	<35	<22	

PCO_2, partial carbon dioxide pressure.
* See also Table 4–17.
Adapted from Goodman CC, Snyder TE: Differential Diagnosis in Physical Therapy, ed 2. Philadelphia, WB Saunders, 1995, pp 150, 365.

Special Implications for the Therapist **35-3**

BLOOD GLUCOSE

Although "safe" blood glucose levels are between 100 and 250 mg/dL, the ideal range is between 80 and 120 mg/dL. The therapist should be aware of the goal of medical management for each person. For example, a young person with insulin-dependent diabetes (IDDM) may be working toward tighter control (e.g., 80 to 120 mg/dL), whereas an older adult with non–insulin-dependent diabetes (NIDDM) may be looking for more moderate control (e.g., up to 150 mg/dL). However, in any age group, a blood glucose measurement over 120 mg/dL should be monitored closely. If the blood glucose level is 70 mg/dL or less, a carbohydrate snack should be given and the glucose retested in 15 minutes to ensure an appropriate level.

Insulin therapy can result in hypoglycemia (low blood sugar, also called an insulin reaction). Symptoms can occur when the blood glucose level drops to 70 mg/dL or less. In diabetes, an overdose of insulin, illness, late or skipped meals, or overexertion in exercise may cause hypoglycemic reactions. The clinical picture may vary from a report of headache and weakness, to irritability and lack of muscular coordination (much like someone who is drunk), to apprehension, inability to respond to verbal commands, and psychosis.

It is important to note that clients can exhibit signs and symptoms of hypoglycemia when their elevated blood glucose level drops rapidly but to a level that is still elevated (e.g., 400 to 200 mg/dL). The rapidity of the drop is the stimulus for sympathetic activity–based symptoms; even though a blood glucose level appears elevated, affected persons may still have hypoglycemia (Eaks and Cassmeyer, 1995).

Glucose levels should be monitored before and after exercise (or therapy activities) remembering that the effect of exercise can be felt up to 12 to 24 hours later. Monitoring is not as crucial for the person who has an established pattern of activity or exercise. When a new activity is introduced, as occurs in an exercise or rehabilitation program, monitoring blood glucose levels is recommended until the client's response to the change is known and predictable in maintaining stable blood glucose levels.

The therapist must always be alert for signs of diabetic ketoacidosis (DKA) (e.g., blood glucose levels greater than or equal to 250 mg/dL), a condition that can occur when complications develop from severe insulin deficiency. Observe for symptoms of acetone breath, dehydration, weak and rapid pulse, and Kussmaul's respirations. Most episodes of DKA occur in people with previously diagnosed IDDM. Immediate medical care is essential. If uncertain whether the client is hypoglycemic or hyperglycemic (see Table 9–18), the health-care worker is advised to administer fruit juice or honey. This procedure will not harm the hyperglycemic client but could potentially save the hypoglycemic client. (See also Special Implications for the Therapist: Diabetes Mellitus, 4–15.)

TABLE 35-10 Glucose Tolerance Tests

Fasting Blood Glucose (mg/dL)		Standard Oral Glucose Tolerance Test (mg/dL)		
			Nonpregnant Adult	Pregnant Woman*
Umbilical cord	45–96			
Premature infant	20–60	Fasting	70–115	105
Neonate	30–60	30 min	<200	—
Infant	40–90	1 hr	<200	190
Child <2 yr	60–100	2 hr	<140	165
Child >2 yr	70–120	3 hr	70–115	145
Elderly	Increased range >50 yr	4 hr	70–115	
2-hr Postprandial Blood Glucose (mg/dL)		**Glycosylated Hemoglobin**		
			% of Total	Average Blood Sugar (mg/dL)
0–50 yr	70–140			
50–60 yr	70–150	Child	1.8%–4.0%	
60+ yr	70–160	Adult, elderly	4.0%–8.0%	
		Excellent control	<6.1%	<120
		Good control	6.2%–7.5%	120–165
		Fair control	7.6%–8.9%	165–210
		Poor control	>9.0%	>210

* Two or more must be met and exceeded for a diagnosis of gestational diabetes.
Data from Pagana KD, Pagana TJ: Mosby's Diagnostic and Laboratory Test Reference, ed 2. St Louis, Mosby–Year Book, 1995, pp 414–427.

Renal Function Tests

Renal failure causes metabolic waste products to accumulate in the blood which can be measured to assess renal function. (Polich and Faynor, 1996). The two most commonly measured waste products are serum creatinine and blood urea nitrogen (BUN) (Table 35–11).

Creatinine is a waste product of muscle metabolism. Creatinine levels in serum represent the balance between production by muscle and clearance by the kidneys and is therefore directly proportional to renal (excretory) function. Since muscle mass is relatively constant, changes in creatinine concentration primarily reflect changes in renal function. With aging, there is a decrease in lean body mass (muscle tissue) possibly resulting in decreasing creatinine values. However, serum creatinine may remain normal in an elderly person even with significant declines in creatinine clearance and renal function (White, 1993).

TABLE 35-11 Renal Function Studies

Age	Creatinine (mg/dL)	Blood Urea Nitrogen (mg/dL)
Newborn	0.3–1.2	3–12
Infant	0.2–0.4	5–18
Child	0.3–0.7	5–18
Adolescent	0.5–1.0	—
Adult female	0.5–1.1	10–20
Adult male	0.6–1.2	10–20
Elderly	Decrease in lean body mass may cause decreased values	May be slightly higher than adult values

Data from Pagana KD, Pagana TJ: Mosby's Diagnostic and Laboratory Test Reference, ed 2. St Louis, Mosby–Year Book, 1995, pp 270, 827.

Urea is a waste product of protein metabolism which also is eliminated by the kidney. Renal failure results in elevated serum urea levels expressed as BUN. Other causes of increased BUN include gastrointestinal bleeding and increased protein intake. BUN levels also vary according to the state of hydration (increase with dehydration; decrease with overhydration).

The synthesis of urea also depends on the liver. People with severe primary liver disease will have a decreased BUN. With combined liver and renal disease (as occurs in hepatorenal syndrome), the BUN can be normal, not because renal excretory function is good but rather because poor hepatic functioning resulted in decreased formation of urea (Pagana and Pagana, 1995).

Special Implications for the Therapist **35-4**

RENAL FUNCTION TESTS

Changes in creatinine and BUN levels do not usually contraindicate physical or occupational therapy intervention. However, rising creatinine levels may indicate muscle wasting resulting from an increase in corticosteroid dosage or from exercise beyond the person's physiologic capabilities (Grant, 1994). Additionally, clients with renal disease may have anemia, hypertension, decreased endurance, and general deconditioning (Polich and Faynor, 1996). Any of these conditions can affect physical therapy treatment.

Lipids

The lipids are fat substances associated with arteriosclerotic vascular disease, consisting mainly of cholesterol, triglycer-

TABLE 35-12 LIPID PANEL

LIPID	DESCRIPTION	EXPECTED VALUES (mg/dL)
Cholesterol	Normal constituent of bile; a fat-related compound; the major component of fatty plaques within a blood vessel (atherosclerosis)	<200
High-density lipoprotein (HDL)	HDL is formed in the liver; a source of "good" cholesterol; increased with vigorous exercise, moderate consumption of alcohol, insulin treatment, estrogens	Low risk: >60 Moderate risk: 35–60 High risk: <35
Low-density lipoprotein (LDL)	LDL ("bad" cholesterol); familial predisposition; increased in diabetes mellitus, hypothyroidism, chronic renal failure, pregnancy	High risk: >190
Triglycerides	Triglycerides are compounds containing three fatty acids; they are the principle constituent of body fat (adipose); triglycerides increase in response to a high fat or sugar meal and decrease after exercise (for a 24-hr period)	<150
LDL/HDL ratio	Ratio used to help determine coronary risk	Low risk: 0.5–3.0 Moderate risk: 3.0–6.0 High risk: >6.0
Cholesterol/HDL ratio		Low risk: 3.3–4.4 Average risk: 4.4–7.1 Moderate risk: 7.1–11.0 High risk: >11.0

ides, and lipoproteins, especially high-density (HDL) and low-density lipoprotein (LDL). Body lipids provide energy for metabolism and are necessary for the production of steroids, bile acids, and cellular membranes. A lipid profile will include cholesterol, HDL, LDL, and triglycerides (Table 35–12). Lipid measurements are important in detecting genetically determined disorders of lipid metabolism and in assessing the risk of coronary artery disease.

The liver metabolizes cholesterol to its free form which is then transported in the bloodstream by lipoproteins. HDL, the "good" lipoprotein carries excess cholesterol back to the liver for removal from the body, whereas LDL, the "bad" lipoprotein, carries most of the cholesterol in the body from the liver to other parts of the body (e.g., to the peripheral tissues and blood vessels). Nearly 75% of the cholesterol is bound to LDL and the remaining 25% is bound to HDL.

High levels of free and bound LDL are associated with increased risk for arteriosclerotic vascular disease; high levels of the "protective" HDL are associated with a reduced risk of coronary disease. Although genetic predetermination is the most important factor in lipoprotein levels, smoking, drugs (e.g., oral contraceptives, aspirin, steroids, sulfonamides, estrogens), alcohol, exercise, and diet can alter the ratio of these lipoproteins (see further discussion in Chapter 10).

Triglycerides are a form of fat produced in the liver and stored in adipose tissue as glycerol, fatty acids, and monoglycerides; the liver reconverts these to triglycerides when the body requires an additional source of energy. Triglyceride testing is used to evaluate persons with suspected atherosclerosis and is used as an indication of the body's ability to metabolize fat. Elevated triglycerides along with elevated cholesterol are risk factors for atherosclerotic disease. Because cholesterol and triglycerides can vary independently, measurement of both values is more meaningful than the measurement of either substance alone (Fischbach, 1995).

Serum Enzymes

Enzymes catalyze the chemical reactions that cells need to stay alive, but the enzymes are not destroyed in the reaction and remain in the cell. Normally, these enzymes do not leak into the bloodstream (or leak in small predictable amounts), but when a cell is stressed or damaged it releases its contents (including enzymes) into the bloodstream. Some enzymes are present in almost all cells; others occur mainly in specific organs. The types and amounts of enzymes circulating in the bloodstream (Table 35–13) can indicate which cells (and therefore which organs) are damaged (Owen, 1995).

Cardiac Enzymes *(Polich and Faynor, 1996)*

Cardiac enzymes are monitored following an episode of chest pain or whenever there is suspicion of myocardial infarction. These enzymes change in a predictable pattern in response to a cardiac event when enzymatic contents are released into the bloodstream as a result of myocardial cell injury or death (Table 35–14). In conjunction with these enzyme tests, other common nonlaboratory tests such as ECG, angiography, and stress testing are used to diagnose cardiac disease. See discussion of coronary artery disease in Chapter 10.

Enzyme creatine kinase (CK, formerly CPK) is a very sensitive marker for MI but it is not very specific because any injury to skeletal muscle (e.g., trauma, surgery, muscle disease, heavy exercise, intramuscular injection) can result in an elevated CK level. When both CK and CK-MB[8] levels are elevated, and when the amount of CK-MB exceeds 5% of the CK, the diagnosis of MI is likely. The amount of CK-

[8] CK-MB is an isoenzyme (one of several forms of the CK enzyme) with specificity for the heart. When isoenzymes are separated by electrophoresis, the pattern formed indicates which damaged organ has released the enzymes. CK-MB appears in serum 4 to 6 hours post MI, peaks in 12 to 24 hours (earlier following thrombolysis), and declines over 48 to 72 hours.

TABLE 35-13 Serum Isoenzymes

Isoenzyme	Where Found	Increased In
CK-BB	Brain	Central nervous system surgery, cardiac arrest, Reye's syndrome, cerebral contusion, cerebrovascular accident, malignant hyperthermia, bowel infarction, renal failure
CK-MB	Myocardium	Myocardial infarction (MI), cardiac contusion, cardiac trauma, congestive heart failure without MI, tachyarrhythmias with underlying coronary artery disease, cardiac surgery, myocarditis
CK-MM	Skeletal muscle	Intramuscular injections, skeletal muscle trauma, extreme muscle exertion, tonic-clonic seizures, surgery, excess alcohol (toxic effect on muscle), alcohol withdrawal syndrome, seizures, electric countershock, muscular dystrophy, severe hypokalemia, hypothyroidism, extreme hypothermia or hyperthermia
LDH-1	Heart, kidney, and red blood cells	MI, cardiac contusion or trauma, myocarditis, cardiac surgery; also, renal disease and infarction, hemolysis, hemolytic anemia, hemolysis with prosthetic heart valves, leukemia, pernicious or megaloblastic anemia
LDH-2	Almost all tissues except skeletal muscle	Injury to any tissue except skeletal muscle

CK-BB, -MB, -MM, creatine kinase subunits; LDH, lactate dehydrogenase.
Adapted from Owen A: Tracking the rise and fall of cardiac enzymes. Nursing95 25:35–44, 1995, p 36.

MB correlates with the extent of the MI (i.e., higher levels indicate a larger infarct). Factors that can affect levels of CK-MB include thrombolytic therapy and coronary artery bypass (CABG) (reestablished blood flow through the coronary artery washes out the products of cellular injury).

Lactic acid dehydrogenase (LDH) is an extracellular enzyme widely distributed in the kidney, heart, skeletal muscle, brain, liver, and lungs. Increases in the reported value usually indicate cellular death and leakage of the enzyme from the cell. In the case of an MI, the level of LDH_1 will rise and exceed the normally greater value of LDH_2 in what is referred to as a flipped ratio (see Table 35–14).

Liver Enzymes (*Siconolfi, 1995*)

The liver is one of the first organs exposed to bacteria and toxins in the bloodstream and when the liver is not functioning well these substances may reach the heart and lungs. This is one reason why people with liver failure are at high risk of multiorgan dysfunction syndrome (MODS) (see Chapter 4).

Since no one liver function test can pinpoint the specific liver dysfunction, physicians rely on various tests and measures in conjunction with clinical observations and other diagnostic tests (Table 35–15). There are two different types of tests: those that measure a particular liver function and damage, and those that help to diagnose the cause of liver damage.

Measuring transaminases (enzymes) released into the blood from liver cells when they are damaged provides information about liver function and, in particular, the amount of inflammation in the liver. For example, *alanine aminotransferase* (ALT; formerly SGPT) is an enzyme that serves as a sensitive indicator of hepatocellular damage; most ALT elevations are caused by liver damage. This enzyme is produced predominantly in the liver and to a lesser extent in the heart, kidneys, and skeletal muscle. Another transaminase, *aspartate aminotransferase* (AST; formerly SGOT), may also be elevated in liver disorders but it normally occurs in high concentrations in many organs and is not as specific for liver damage as ALT. Declining serum aminotransferase levels do not necessarily indicate that liver function is improving but

TABLE 35-14 Cardiac Enzymes

Enzyme	Normal Range	Rises In	Peaks In	Returns to Normal In
Creatine kinase* (CK)	15–99 U/L	3–8 hr	10–30 hr	3–4 days
CK-MB isoenzyme	0%–5%	4–8 hr	12–24 hr	2–3 days
Lactate dehydrogenase† (LDH)	48–115 U/L	24–48 hr	72–144 hr	8–14 days
LDH-1 > LDH-2 (flipped ratio)				
LDH-1	17%–28%	8–24 hr	72–144 hr	14 days
LDH-2	30%–36%			

* Creatine kinase is normally higher in males than in females, and in blacks than in whites. Normal values vary according to laboratory.
† Lactate dehydrogenase is normally higher in males than in females.
Adapted from Owen A: Tracking the rise and fall of cardiac enzymes. Nursing95 25:35–44, 1995, p 37.

TABLE 35-15 Laboratory Tests for Liver and Biliary Tract Disease

	Normal Range	Comment
Serum bilirubin		
Direct (conjugated)	0.1–0.3 mg/dL	Increased with obstruction
Indirect (unconjugated)	0.2–0.8 mg/dL	Increased with other problems
Total	0.1–2.0 mg/dL	Increased with cirrhosis, hepatitis, hemolytic anemia, jaundice, transfusion reaction
Urine bilirubin	0	
Serum proteins		
Albumin (A)	3.5–5.5 g/dL	Decreased in liver damage, burns, Crohn's disease, SLE, malnutrition (e.g., anorexia nervosa)
Globulin (G)	2.5–3.5 g/dL	Increased in hepatitis
Total	6–8 g/dL	Decreased in liver damage (synthesis is impaired)
A/G ratio	1.5 : 1–2.5 : 1	Ratio reverses with chronic hepatitis or other chronic liver disease
Transferrin (iron levels)	250–300 μg/dL	Decreased in liver damage; increased in iron deficiency
Alpha-fetoprotein	6–20 ng/mL	Cancer-associated antigen; made by fetus but not by healthy adults; value >1000 ng/mg indicates likely hepatocellular carcinoma
Serum enzymes		
AST	8–20 U/L	Increased in liver damage; released by liver when damage occurs to liver cells; increased with primary muscle diseases (e.g., myopathy)
ALT	5–35 U/L	Same as above
LDH	45–90 U/L	Same as above
GGT	5–38 U/L	Age- and sex-dependent; elevated with significant liver disorder
Alkaline phosphatase	30–85 U/L	Increased in liver tumor, biliary obstruction, rheumatoid arthritis, hyperparathyroidism
Blood ammonia	<75 μg/dL	Great variation in reported values because of methods used; increased in severe liver damage
Coagulation functions		
Prothrombin time	12–15 sec	Prolonged in liver damage, salicylate intoxication, with intake of anticoagulants (warfarin), DIC
INR	0.9–1.1	
Activated partial thromboplastin time	60–70 sec	Prolonged in clotting factor deficiencies (e.g., hemophilia), leukemia, DIC, with administration of heparin
Platelets	150,000–400,000/mm^3	May drop when spleen is enlarged from portal hypertension; decreased in DIC and burns

SLE, systemic lupus erythematosus; AST, aspartate aminotransferase; ALT, alanine aminotransferase; LDH, lactate dehydrogenase; GGT, γ-glutamyltransferase; INR, international normalized ratio; DIC, disseminated intravascular coagulation.
Adapted from Goodman CC, Snyder TE: Differential Diagnosis in Physical Therapy, ed 2. Philadelphia, WB Saunders, 1995, p 291.

may mean that the individual has only a few functional hepatocytes and the liver is dying.

An example of the second kind of testing (i.e., tests that help to diagnose the cause of liver damage) is the test for *γ-glutamyltransferase* (GGT; formerly GGTP). This is a very sensitive enzymatic indicator of hepatobiliary tract disease. It rises rapidly after a small intake of alcohol and can help identify alcohol as a contributing factor to cirrhosis. It also rises in people with hepatitis, hepatic metastases, and obstructive liver disease. Enzymatic tests may be used to follow the progress of individual clients. See discussion of liver in Chapter 14.

Ammonia, a byproduct of protein metabolism, is normally converted into urea by the liver and then excreted by the kidneys. With severe liver dysfunction, or when blood flow to the liver is altered (e.g., in portal hypertension), ammonia cannot be catabolized and the blood levels rise. Any appreciable level of ammonia in the blood affects acid-base balance and brain function.

Special Implications for the Therapist **35-5**

SERUM ENZYMES

Cardiac Enzymes

If the chart notes CPK-MB+, this signifies that an acute MI has occurred. When cardiac enzymes are fluctuating, physical activity is limited and monitoring of oxygenation using pulse oximetry and monitoring vital signs is important. Chest physical therapy treatments should continue according to the individual's tolerance, with frequent rest periods provided throughout the session. Anyone with significant arrhythmia or myocardial dysfunction such as angina, hypotension, congestive heart failure, and so on may be excluded from therapy treatment (Garritan et al., 1995).

Activity may be increased according to the cardiac rehabilitation protocol in use. Always monitor the client for bradycardia or tachycardia, arrhythmias, and associated signs and symptoms of MI (chest pain, unexplained perspiration, nausea, vomiting).

Liver Enzymes

If test results indicate liver dysfunction, monitor the client for signs and symptoms of hepatic disease such as altered behavior or mental status, fluctuating levels of consciousness, edema or ascites, right upper abdominal pain, musculoskeletal pain, and others (see Box 14–1). The client with liver dysfunction is at increased risk of infection requiring careful practice of universal precautions.

The heart tries to compensate for fluid shifts and alterations in vascular status as a result of liver dysfunction necessitating monitoring of vital signs. Heart failure can occur when collateral circulation can no longer support body systems.

When liver dysfunction results in increased serum ammonia and urea levels, peripheral nerve function can also be impaired. Asterixis and numbness or tingling (misinterpreted as carpal or tarsal tunnel syndrome) can occur as a result of this ammonia abnormality causing intrinsic nerve pathology (see further discussion in Chapter 14).

There is also an increased risk of coagulopathy (decreased clotting ability) with liver disease, requiring precautions. Bleeding under the skin and easy bruising in response to slight trauma often occur when the platelet level is abnormally small (thrombocytopenia). This condition necessitates extreme care in the therapy setting, especially any treatment requiring manual therapy or the use of any equipment, including physical therapy modalities and weight training devices (see also Table 35–7 and Special Implications: Thrombocytopenia, 11–11).

Serum Hormones *(Pagana and Pagana, 1995)*

The concentration of hormones in serum can be measured to assess endocrine function in health and disease. Measurement of hormone level is also accomplished by radioimmunoassay, by enzyme-linked immunosorbent assay, and less commonly by bioassay. Measurement of individual hormones does not always permit differentiation between normal and abnormal; sometimes an accurate interpretation of the hormone level requires a knowledge of previous hormone levels (Griffen, 1992).

In the therapy setting, thyroid testing constitutes the majority of serum hormone tests performed, including measurements of thyroxine (T_4), triiodothyronine (T_3), free thyroxine intake (FTI), and thyroid-stimulating hormone (TSH) (Table 35–16). Serum T_4 is a direct measure of the total amount of thyroid function; greater than normal levels of T_4 indicate hyperthyroid states, and subnormal values are seen in hypothyroid states. Newborns are screened by T_4 tests to detect hypothyroidism; mental retardation can be prevented by early diagnosis.

The serum T_3 value is also an accurate measure of thyroid function, although T_3 is less stable than T_4. An elevated T_3 measurement is clinically important in the person with a normal T_4 level in the presence of hyperthyroid symptoms; in this person, the test may identify T_3 thyrotoxicosis. The FTI study measures the amount of free T_4 which is only a fraction of the total T_4 but correlates more closely with the true hormonal status. High FTI calculations suggest hyperthyroidism; low FTI values suggest hypothyroidism.

The TSH concentration aids in differentiating *primary* from *secondary* hypothyroidism. Pituitary TSH secretion is stimulated by hypothalamic thyroid-releasing hormone (TRH). Low levels of T_3 and T_4 are the underlying stimuli for TRH and TSH. Therefore, a compensatory elevation of TRH and TSH occurs in people with primary hypothyroid states, such as surgical or radioactive thyroid ablation, people taking antithyroid medication, or congenital hypothyroidism (cretinism).

In secondary hypothyroidism, the function of the hypothalamus or pituitary gland is faulty because of tumor, trauma, or infarction. Therefore TRH and TSH cannot be secreted and plasma levels of these hormones are near zero despite low T_3 and T_4 levels. The TSH level determination is also used to evaluate and monitor exogenous thyroid replacement and as a screen test in newborns to detect low T_4 levels. TSH and T_4 levels are measured to differentiate pituitary from thyroid dysfunction. A decreased T_4 and normal or elevated TSH level can indicate a thyroid disorder. A decreased T_4 with a decreased TSH level can indicate a pituitary disorder.

Special Implications for the Therapist **35–6**

SERUM HORMONES

Thyroid problems were reported by 7% to 8% of women surveyed in an orthopedic outpatient setting and all of these women were on thyroid replacement medication (Boissonnault and Koopmeiners, 1994). The percentages for the overall therapy population are likely equal or possibly even higher. With adequate replacement therapy, these people will be euthyroid and present no particular problem to the therapist. Replacement needs vary over time, however, and these clients may become hyperthyroid or hypothyroid.

Signs and symptoms of these conditions include myalgia, arthralgia, and numbness (see further discussion in Chapter 9), all symptoms for which the person may seek out a physical or occupational therapist (Boissonnault and Koopmeiners, 1994).

The fact that many women develop carpal tunnel syndrome at or near menopause suggests that the soft tissues about the wrist may be affected in some way by hormones (Grossman et al., 1961; Phalen, 1966). Hormone testing to determine a woman's menopausal status (premenopausal, perimenopausal, postmenopausal) can be done. This information is also helpful when the woman is considering hormonal replacement therapy and can be used by the therapist to facilitate client education regarding prevention of osteoporosis.

IMMUNOLOGIC TESTS

Diagnostic immunology or serodiagnostic testing uses blood tests to aid in the diagnosis of infectious disease, immune

TABLE 35–16 THYROID FUNCTION REFERENCE VALUES

AGE	THYROXINE (T_4) (μg/dL)	TRIIODOTHYRONINE (T_3) (ng/dL)	FREE T_4 INDEX	THYROID-STIMULATING HORMONE (TSH) (μIU/L)
Neonate	10.1–20.0	90–170		3–18 (3–18 mIU/L)
1–4 mo	7.5–16.5			
4–12 mo	5.5–14.5			
1–6 yr	5.6–12.6			
6–10 yr	4.9–11.7	115–190		
>10 yr	4.0–11.0			
Adult, elderly		110–230 1.2–1.5 nmol/L	0.8–2.4 ng/dL (10–31 pmol/L)	2–10 μIU/L (2–10 mIU/L)

Data from Pagana KD, Pagana TJ: Mosby's Diagnostic and Laboratory Test Reference, ed 2. St Louis, Mosby–Year Book, 1995, pp. 788, 795, 797, and 813.

disorders, allergic reactions, neoplastic disease (tumor-related antigens), and in blood grouping and typing (not discussed further here). Blood tests can be used to determine whether particular antigens are present (e.g., bacteria, viruses, parasites, fungi, enzymes).

Immunoglobulins, the general term for antibodies that are produced in response to antigens, are divided into five classes (IgG, IgA, IgM, IgD, and IgE). The globulins in blood serum are separated by an electrophoretic method into the different fractions: α-, β-, and γ-globulin. The different fractions are elevated in specific diseases states. For example, α-globulin is increased in chronic infections and rheumatoid arthritis, and β- and γ-globulins are elevated in multiple myeloma.

Ideally, serum collection is taken at the beginning of the illness during the acute phase and again 3 to 4 weeks later during the convalescent phase. An increase in the quantity (titer) of a specific antibody between these two phases is diagnostically significant. The specific antibody tests for individual antigens are beyond the scope of this chapter. The reader is referred to more comprehensive laboratory and diagnostic manuals (Fischbach, 1995; Pagana and Pagana, 1995).

Rheumatoid Factor

The serum in most people with RA contains an anti–γ-globulin antibody called *rheumatoid factor* (RF). RF is not unique to people with RA but most adults with rheumatoid disease do exhibit it. RF is not usually present in children with juvenile rheumatoid arthritis (JRA) unless the disease has been present for many years.

Antinucleoprotein Antibodies

Total antinucleoprotein antibodies (ANAs) are γ-globulins that react with antigens in all organs of man or animals. These ANAs usually belong to more than one of the five immunoglobulin classes. A positive response is not specific because it is seen in a variety of chronic diseases, but if negative it rules strongly against the diagnosis of systemic lupus erythematosus (SLE) (most people with SLE produce high ANA titers). A negative test does not rule out the diagnosis and a positive test by itself is not diagnostic; it confirms the clinical diagnosis.

Human Leukocyte Antigen

Since the basis of immunity depends on the immune cells' ability to distinguish self from nonself, all cells of the body contain specific cell surface markers or molecules that are as unique to that person as his or her fingerprint. The immune system recognizes these cell markers and tolerates them as self, in other words producing self-tolerance. These cell markers are present on the surface of all body cells and are known as the major histocompatibility complex (MHC) proteins. They were originally discovered on leukocytes and are commonly called human leukocytic antigens (HLA) (see discussion of the major histocompatibility complex in Chapter 5).

HLAs are inherited and can predispose or increase a person's susceptibility to certain diseases (usually autoimmune). Such diseases encompass many that affect the joints, endocrine glands, and skin, including RA, Graves' disease, psoriasis, and many others. Not all persons with a certain HLA pattern will develop the disease, but those that do have a greater probability for its development than the general population. The associations between particular HLA antigens and various disease states are listed in Table 35–17.

TABLE 35–17 DISEASES ASSOCIATED WITH HLA ANTIGENS*

DISEASE	HLA ANTIGEN
Ankylosing spondylitis	HLA-B27 (present in 90% of cases)
Multiple sclerosis	HLA-B27, -Dw2, -A3, -B18
Myasthenia gravis	HLA-B8
Psoriasis	HLA-B13, -B17
Reiter's syndrome	HLA-B27
Juvenile insulin-dependent diabetes	HLA-Bw15, -B8
Graves' disease	HLA-B27
Juvenile rheumatoid arthritis	HLA-B27
Autoimmune chronic active hepatitis	HLA-B8

* HLA testing is used to confirm the diagnosis and is not usually regarded as diagnostic by itself.
Modified from Fischbach F: A Manual of Laboratory and Diagnostic Tests, ed 4. Philadelphia, JB Lippincott, 1992, p 559.

URINALYSIS

Overview

The urine can be examined for a multitude of properties and characteristics such as pH, appearance, color, odor, specific gravity, and the presence of protein, glucose, ketones, and blood. Urinalysis is one of the most useful indicators of health and disease, being especially helpful in the detection of renal or metabolic disorders. Urine is a very complex fluid, composed of 95% water and 5% solids. It is the end product of metabolic processes carried out in the body.

Although urine contains thousands of dissolved substances, the three main components are water, urea, and sodium chloride. Some constituents of the blood (e.g., glucose) have a renal threshold, that is, a certain elevated level must be reached in the blood before showing up in the urine. Almost all substances found in the urine are also found in the blood, although in different concentrations. Urea, for example, is present in the blood, but at a much lower concentration than in the excreted urine (Fischbach, 1995).

Urine Testing *(Fischbach, 1995)*

The reference values and normal findings for a routine urinalysis are listed in Table 35–18. The appearance of a normal urine specimen should be clear, although normal urine may be cloudy due to ingestion of a large amounts of fat, urates, or phosphates. Other causes of cloudy urine may be the presence of pus, RBCs, or bacteria. Urine at 98.6° F may also become cloudy when cooled to room temperature.

Color and Appearance

The color of normal urine is caused by urochrome, a pigment that is present in the diet or formed from the metabolism of bile. Abnormally colored urine may result from a pathologic condition (presence of abnormal pigments) or the ingestion of certain foods (e.g., rhubarb, carrots, beets) or medications (e.g., some laxatives; levodopa for Parkinson's disease; some anticoagulants; chlorzoxazone, a muscle relaxant). Bleeding from the kidney may produce dark-red urine whereas bleeding in the lower urinary tract produces bright-red urine. Dark-brown urine may occur with liver disease or with disseminated intravascular coagulation (DIC).

Specific Gravity and Occult Blood

Specific gravity is a test to measure the kidney's ability to concentrate urine and depends on the state of hydration. A high specific gravity indicates concentrated urine, whereas a low specific gravity indicates dilute urine. Renal dysfunction is suspected when the kidney is unable to concentrate or dilute the urine.

When urine gives a positive result for occult blood, but no RBCs are seen on a microscopic examination, myoglobinuria is suspected. Myoglobinuria is the excretion of myoglobin, a muscle protein, into the urine as a result of traumatic muscle injury (e.g., automobile accident, football injury, electric shock), muscle disorder (e.g., muscular dystrophy, arterial occlusion to a muscle), or certain kinds of poisoning (e.g., carbon monoxide).

Glucose and Ketones

Urine glucose tests are used in screening to detect diabetes, to confirm a diagnosis of diabetes, or to monitor the effectiveness of diabetic control. When the blood glucose level exceeds the reabsorption capacity of the renule tubules, glucose will be spilled into the urine. Sugar may appear in the urine (glucosuria or glycosuria) after a heavy meal is eaten or in conjunction with emotional stress and is not considered pathologic.

Testing for ketone bodies is indicated in anyone showing greater than normal excretion of sugar. Ketone bodies result when carbohydrate metabolism is altered and fat becomes the primary source of energy. The excess production of ketones in the urine (ketonuria) is usually associated with diabetes and provides an early indication of ketoacidosis and diabetic coma.

Electrolytes

Electrolyte balance in the body may be determined by the amount of electrolytes (e.g., sodium, chloride, potassium) excreted in the urine over a 24-hour period. Measuring sodium and potassium is important since these two electrolytes are primary factors in nerve conduction and influence the irritability of the muscles, nerves, and heart. Potassium measurements provide useful information about renal and adrenal disorders and about water and acid-base imbalances. Potassium acts as a part of the body's buffer system regulated by its excretion through the urine.

Drug Screening

The urine may be screened for drugs detectable in urine but not detectable in blood. Such testing may be performed when

TABLE 35–18 ROUTINE URINALYSIS AND RELATED TESTS

General Characteristics and Measurements	Chemical Determinations	Microscopic Examination of Sediment
Color: pale yellow to amber	Glucose: negative	Casts negative: occasional hyaline casts
Turbidity: clear to slightly hazy	Ketones: negative	
Specific gravity (with a normal fluid intake): 1.015–1.025	Blood: negative	Red blood cells: negative or rare
	Bilirubin: negative	Crystals: negative
pH: 4.5–8.0 (average pH: 5–6)	Urobilinogen: 0.1–1.0	White blood cells: negative or rare
	Nitrate for bacteria: negative	Epithelial cells: few
	Leukocyte esterase: negative	

Modified from Fischbach F: A Manual of Laboratory and Diagnostic Tests, ed 4. Philadelphia, JB Lippincott, 1992, p 148.

there is suspected substance abuse, to confirm clinical or postmortem diagnosis, to differentiate drug-induced disease from other causes, or as preemployment testing. Although minor tranquilizers are extensively metabolized and not easily detected in urine (unless an overdose is taken), common urine drug tests look for amphetamines, alcohol, barbiturates, cocaine ("crack"), methamphetamines ("crank"), opiates, marijuana (tetrahydrocannabinol, THC), phencyclidine (PCP), analgesics, sedatives, major tranquilizers, stimulants, and lysergic acid diethylamine (LSD).

MICROBIOLOGIC STUDIES

The pathogenicity of microbiologic organisms is dependent on the number present and the status of the individual's immune system to fight infection. Anaerobic microorganisms considered normal flora are present in the body on the skin, in the mouth, in the vagina, and along the upper respiratory, gastrointestinal, and genitourinary tracts. With air present, anaerobic microorganisms normally do not grow in the upper respiratory tract; the genitourinary tracts are usually a sterile environment preventing growth as well. The gastrointestinal tract is unique in that it normally harbors both aerobic and anaerobic organisms.

Although these organisms are considered normal flora they can be transported to other parts of the body causing severe and often fatal infections, especially when there is a breakdown of the normal defense mechanisms (e.g., immunosuppression, burns). For example, aspiration pneumonia can occur when organisms from the mouth enter the upper airways or infection can develop when *Escherichia coli* from the colon enters the vagina or urethra.

Blood Culture

Blood cultures are obtained to detect the presence of bacteria in the blood. Bacteremia is usually intermittent and transient, except in endocarditis or suppurative thrombophlebitis. Bacteremia is usually accompanied by chills and fever; thus, the blood culture is drawn when the person manifests these signs. Cultures must be performed before antibiotic therapy is initiated; otherwise, the antibiotic may interrupt the organism's growth in the laboratory (Pagana and Pagana, 1995).

Gram Stain

Often the physician will want to begin antibiotic therapy before the blood culture results are reported. In these cases, the specimen can be smeared on a slide and stained for a faster result (less than 10 minutes). All forms of bacteria are grossly classified as *gram-positive* (blue staining) or *gram-negative* (red staining). Knowledge of the organism's shape (e.g., spherical or rod-shaped) also can be very helpful in its identification.

Gram staining can also be used to determine the presence of pathogenic bacteria by culturing the sputum (e.g., pneumonia), pleural fluid (e.g., empyema), throat (e.g., streptococci, meningococci, gonococci), urine (e.g., urinary tract infection), and wounds.

Wound Cultures

Specimens taken from wound cultures may contain a variety of microorganisms that may or may not be pathognomonic; most wound infections are caused by pus-forming organisms. Wound cultures should also be obtained before antibiotic therapy is initiated; otherwise the antibiotic may interrupt the growth of the organism in the laboratory. A Gram stain of the specimen smeared on a slide also can be reported in less than 10 minutes. See further discussion in Chapter 8.

Skin Cultures

The skin of a healthy person may normally contain pathologic organisms such as staphylococci, streptococci, yeasts and other fungi, mycobacteria, *Clostridium* species, and others. When present in low numbers most of these organisms present no problem but when they multiply to excessive quantities a skin infection may develop. Common abnormal skin conditions include pyoderma, folliculitis, furuncles, carbuncles, burns, scabies (and other skin lesions), athlete's foot, and ringworm (see further discussion in Chapter 8).

Special Implications for the Therapist **35-7**

MICROBIOLOGIC STUDIES

Wounds

The physician should be notified of the presence of pus from any deep wound, postoperative incision, or abscess, especially if associated with a foul odor. In the case of suspected gas gangrene tissue, necrotic tissue or debrided material may be cultured. The therapist should be aware that some pathogens are characterized by color and consistency. For example, pus from streptococcal lesions is thin and serous, whereas pus from staphylococcal infections is more gelatinous and pus from *Pseudomonas aeruginosa* infections is blue-green.

The culture should be taken from the suppurative material rather than from the skin edge for a more accurate wound culture.

Skin Lesions

Whenever skin lesions are present the therapist must follow universal precautions carefully both to prevent the spread of infection to the client as well as to prevent self-inoculation and subsequent infection. For a more detailed discussion of skin lesions and their special implications, see Chapter 8.

SPECIAL TEST PROCEDURES

Pulmonary Function Tests *(Pagana and Pagana, 1995)*

Pulmonary function tests are performed to detect abnormalities in respiratory function and to determine the extent of any pulmonary abnormality. These tests are performed most often to differentiate between restrictive and obstructive pulmonary disease,[9] to evaluate the response to bronchodilator

[9] *Restrictive* defects (e.g., pulmonary fibrosis, tumors, chest wall trauma) occur when ventilation is disturbed by a limitation of chest expansion; inspiration is primarily affected. *Obstructive* defects (e.g., emphysema, bronchitis, asthma) occur when ventilation is disturbed by an increase in airway resistance; expiration is primarily affected (Pagana and Pagana, 1995).

therapy, to evaluate the lungs and pulmonary reserve preoperatively (especially for thoracic surgery that will result in loss of functional pulmonary tissue such as a lobectomy or pneumonectomy), and for people with inhalation allergies.

The results of pulmonary function studies may reveal abnormalities in the airways, alveoli, and pulmonary vascular bed early in the course of disease when physical examinations and x-ray studies are still normal. Additionally, the location of an airway abnormality can be determined (i.e., upper airway, large airway, or small airway) (Fischbach, 1995).

Pulmonary function tests routinely determine forced vital capacity (FVC), forced expiratory volume in 1 second (FEV_1), maximal midexpiratory flow (MMEF), and maximal voluntary ventilation (MVV). Additional pulmonary function tests such as arterial blood gases and diffusion capacity[10] may be performed if indicated. More comprehensive studies may also include evaluation of lung volumes and lung capacities including tidal volume, inspiratory reserve volume, expiratory reserve volume, residual volume, functional residual volume, vital capacity, total lung capacity, and dead space (Table 35–19).

Normal findings vary with the person's age, sex, height, and weight. Clients with obstructive and restrictive diseases will have disease-specific changes in lung volumes and capacities. Obstructive lung diseases result in air trapping and associated symptoms. The total lung capacity will be increased with severe disease along with lung hyperinflation (seen on chest radiograph). Restrictive disorders are characterized by decreased total lung capacity, decreased residual volume, and difficulty taking a deep breath (Egloff, 1993). For a detailed description of each of these tests, the reader is referred to a more comprehensive text (Hillegass and Sadowsky, 1994; Watchie, 1995; see also Arterial Blood Gases later in this chapter).

Pulmonary Artery and Pulmonary Capillary Wedge Pressures

To obtain essential information regarding left ventricular function, a balloon-tipped catheter can be introduced into the pulmonary artery to measure the pulmonary artery end-diastolic pressure (PAEDP) and the pulmonary capillary wedge pressure (PCWP) (Table 35–20). PCWP can indicate left ventricular failure coinciding with the onset of pulmonary congestion and pulmonary edema. PCWP can also register insufficient volume and pressure in the left ventricle indicating hypovolemic shock in other conditions.

The balloon is inflated so that it wedges the catheter in a distal branch of the pulmonary artery, occluding the pressure produced by the right side of the heart. The measurement obtained when the balloon is inflated is the PCWP and reflects pressures in the pulmonary capillary bed and left-sided heart function. The balloon must be deflated quickly and should never be left inflated for more than a few seconds so that damage to the pulmonary circulation does not occur (Phipps et al., 1995). The best indicator of left ventricular function is the left ventricular end-diastolic pressure (LVEDP). A direct relationship exists between the three measurements listed in Table 35–20 so that a change in one measurement usually reflects a simultaneous change in the other measurements as well.

Special Implications for the Therapist **35-8**

PULMONARY CAPILLARY WEDGE PRESSURE

With pulmonary artery catheterization, the therapist must know the desirable PCWP level and check the readings; report any significant elevations or changes in waveform that indicate the catheter has become wedged.

Arterial Blood Gases

The blood test used most often to measure the effectiveness of ventilation and oxygen transport is oxygen (O_2) saturation. However, this test only provides an indirect measure of the levels of arterial oxygen and does not provide information about the carbon dioxide level or blood pH. A more comprehensive procedure is the arterial blood gas (ABG) test. ABGs are used to monitor critically ill people (especially anyone on a ventilator), to establish baseline values (e.g., in the perioperative period), to follow up postoperatively, in the detection and treatment of electrolyte imbalances, and in conjunction with pulmonary testing (see previous discussion of pulmonary function tests).

ABG analysis includes information about oxygenation, ventilation, and metabolic function. The test measures the amount of dissolved oxygen and carbon dioxide in arterial blood and indicates acid-base status by measuring the arterial blood pH.[11] The specific measurements include serum pH, partial pressure of CO_2, HCO_3, partial pressure of O_2, and O_2 saturation (Table 35–21). A detailed explanation of these measures and how they interrelate is included in Chapter 4.

Arterial blood is a good way to sample a mixture of blood that has come from various parts of the body and gives the added information of how well the lungs are oxygenating the blood. For example, if the arterial O_2 concentration is normal (indicating that the lungs are functioning normally), but the mixed venous O_2 is low, it can be inferred that the heart and circulation are failing. Arterial samples provide information on the ability of the lungs to regulate acid-base balance through retention or release of CO_2 and the effectiveness of the kidneys in maintaining appropriate HCO_3^- levels (Fischbach, 1995).

Special Implications for the Therapist **35-9**

ARTERIAL BLOOD GASES *(Garritan et al., 1995)*

Whenever the client demonstrates impaired oxygenation status, supplemental oxygen should be continued

[10] This test measures the adequacy of the alveolar membrane and how well oxygen can diffuse from the pulmonary capillaries into the alveolar cells. In some situations (e.g., thickened or scarred alveolar membrane secondary to some cardiac medications or congestive heart failure), blood gets to the alveolar cells but not enough oxygen diffuses across the alveolar membrane.

[11] The pH is inversely proportional to the hydrogen ion concentration in the blood. As the hydrogen ion concentration increases (acidosis), the pH decreases; as the hydrogen ion concentration decreases (alkalosis), the pH increases.

TABLE 35-19 PULMONARY FUNCTION TEST (PFT) COMPONENTS

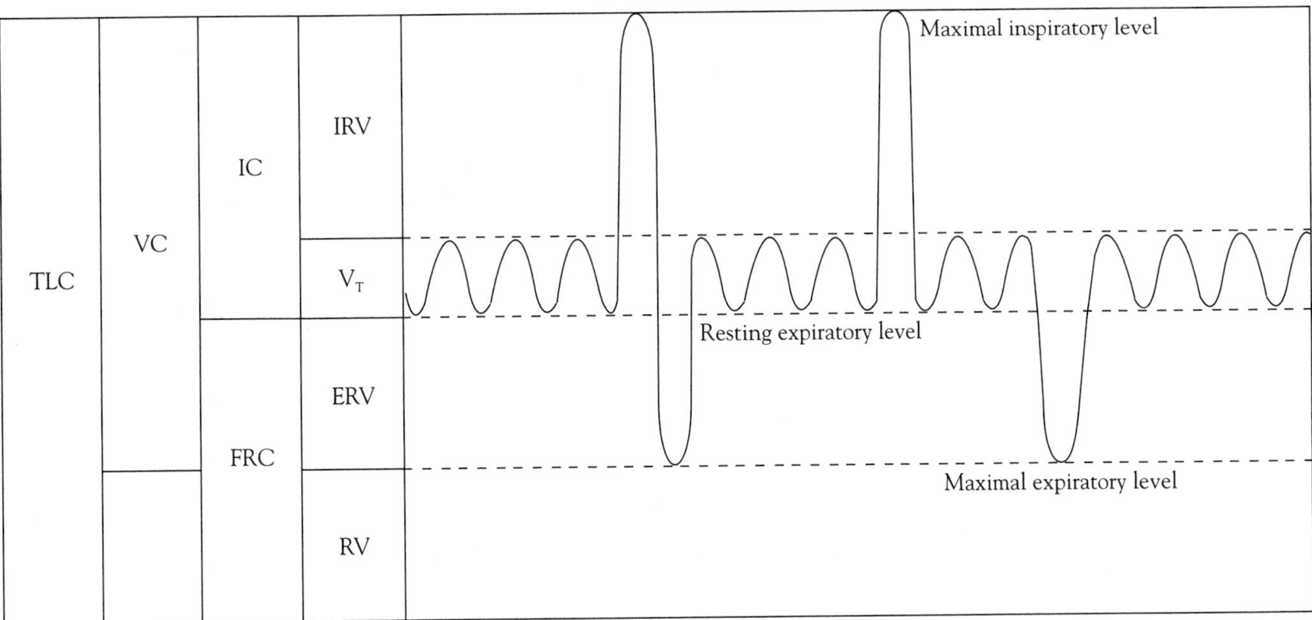

Lung Volumes and Capacities		
VC	Vital capacity	Volume of air that is measured during a slow, maximal expiration after a maximal inspiration; normal range varies with age, sex, and body size
IC	Inspiratory capacity	Largest volume of air that can be inhaled from resting expiratory volume
IRV	Inspiratory reserve volume	The maximal volume of air that can be expired after a normal inspiration
ERV	Expiratory reserve volume	Largest volume of air exhaled from resting end-expiratory level
FRC	Functional residual capacity	Volume of air remaining in lungs at resting end-expiratory level
RV	Residual volume	Volume of air remaining in the lungs at end of maximal expiration
TLC	Total lung capacity	Volume of air contained in the lungs after maximal inspiration
V_T	Tidal volume	Volume of air inhaled or exhaled during each respiratory cycle; normal range is 400–700 ml
f	Respiratory rate	Frequency of breathing is the number of breaths per minute; normal range is 12–22
Lung Mechanics		
FVC	Forced vital capacity	Maximal volume of air that can be forcefully expired after a maximal inspiration to total lung capacity
FEV_t	Forced expiratory volume (in 1 sec)	Volume of air expired during a given time interval (t in seconds) from the beginning of an FVC maneuver
$FEF_{25\%-75\%}$	Forced expiratory $flow_{25\%-75\%}$	Average of flow during the middle half of an FVC maneuver
PEFR	Peak expiratory flow rate	Maximal flow rate attained during an FVC maneuver
MVV	Maximal voluntary ventilation	Largest volume that can be breathed during a 10- to 15-sec interval with voluntary effort
MIP	Maximal inspiratory pressure	Greatest negative or subatmospheric pressure that can be generated during inspiration against an occluded airway
MEP	Maximal expiratory pressure	Highest positive pressure that can be generated during a forceful expiratory effort against an occluded airway

From Black JM, Matassarin-Jacobs E (eds): Luckmann and Sorensen's Medical-Surgical Nursing, ed 4. Philadelphia, WB Saunders, 1993, p 930.

throughout the therapy session. Oxygen saturation should be maintained at 90% or higher[12]. Whenever this is not possible, treatment plans should be modified and the client should not be overexerted, keeping in mind that increased physical activity requires additional oxygen requirements.

Any indication of hyperventilation (e.g., decreased CO_2 level or increased respiratory rate) should be addressed during therapy. Relaxation techniques and breathing exercises such as pursed lip or diaphragmatic breathing can be incorporated into the treatment plan. Hypoventilation as indicated by an increased CO_2 level or shallow breathing may be affected by deep-breathing activities and by positioning (e.g., sitting upright) to improve CO_2 removal and to optimize oxygenation.

[12] Persons with chronic obstructive pulmonary disease (COPD) may retain CO; the use of O_2 is contraindicated in these persons as it can further depress the respiratory drive causing death.

TABLE 35-20 Pulmonary Artery and Capillary Wedge Pressures

Type	Abbreviation	Reference Values (mm Hg)
Left ventricular end-diastolic pressure	LVEDP	12–15
Pulmonary artery end-diastolic pressure	PAEDP	4–12
Pulmonary capillary wedge pressure	PCWP	4–12

From Phipps WJ, Cassmeyer VL, Sands JK, et al: Medical-Surgical Nursing, ed 5. St Louis, Mosby–Year Book, 1995, p 767.

Changes in metabolic components of ABGs (either primary or compensatory) may affect other organ systems and therefore a person's tolerance for physical activity. The therapist must always treat with the client's tolerance in mind and monitor vital signs, observing for associated clinical signs and symptoms.

FLUID ANALYSIS

Cerebrospinal Fluid Studies

Lumbar puncture, using direct percutaneous puncture in the lumbar spine to obtain cerebrospinal fluid (CSF), is used primarily in the diagnosis of central nervous system (CNS) infections, the major indication being the diagnosis of meningitis. Other indications for lumbar puncture are included in Table 35–22. Often it is used as a secondary test to confirm suspicion of disease that may not be fully detectable with neuroimaging, such as with persons with multiple sclerosis.

Contraindications to lumbar puncture include increased intracranial pressure with focal neurologic signs. A computed tomography (CT) scan is done prior to lumbar puncture; evidence of pressure between the infra- and supratentorial structures or evidence of a midline shift as an indication of possible herniation causing pressure on the brainstem is a contraindication to lumbar puncture. Local infection or a bleeding disorder is also a contraindication to lumbar puncture (McConnell and Rillstone, 1994).

The normal composition of CSF is affected by a variety of clinical factors listed in Box 35–3. Testing of CSF involves measurement of a variety of substances and states. Standard pathologic levels of substances found in the CSF are listed in Box 35–4 (Wilder-Smith, 1994). *Appearance* is normally clear; cloudiness is indicative of a disease state, graded from 0 to 4 (indicating progressive levels of cloudiness); 0 denotes a clear fluid and 4 indicates inability to see newsprint through the fluid). Bilirubin, a byproduct of jaundice, can give the CSF a yellow tinge and blood in the fluid will cause it to turn pink.

Cells found in the CSF are usually indicative of an abnormality in the CNS as the CSF is normally virtually free of cells. Cell types found in disease or trauma include WBCs, macrophages, cartilage cells, glial cells, bone marrow, and various tumor cells.

Levels of *inorganic compounds* in the CSF can reflect disorders of the nervous system. Calcium can alter the activation of various neurotransmitters and low levels are implicated in seizure disorders. Low levels of calcium are also associated

TABLE 35-21 Arterial Blood Gas Values

Term	Definition	Reference Value
pH	Measure of blood acidity; ratio of acids to bases	7.35–7.45
Pa_{CO_2} (partial pressure of arterial carbon dioxide)	Pressure or tension exerted by CO_2 dissolved in arterial blood; measures effectiveness of alveolar ventilation (i.e., how well air is exchanging with blood in the lungs)	35–45 mm Hg
HCO_3^- (bicarbonate ion)	Amount of bicarbonate or alkaline substance dissolved in blood; influenced mainly by metabolic changes	22–26 mEq/L
Pa_{O_2} (partial pressure of arterial oxygen)	Pressure exerted by O_2 dissolved in arterial blood in attempting to diffuse through pulmonary membrane	80–100 mm Hg
O_2 saturation	Oxyhemoglobin saturation: percentage of oxygen carried by hemoglobin	95%–100%
Critical Values		
pH	<7.25 or >7.55	
P_{CO_2}	<20 or >60 mm Hg	
HCO_3^-	<15 or >40 mEq/L	
P_{O_2}	<40 mm Hg	
O_2 saturation	<95%*	

* This value varies depending upon the clinical situation. For example, a healthy adult with O_2 saturation levels less than 95% would bear further investigation, whereas in someone who smokes a 95% saturation level would not be suspect.

Adapted from Pagana D, Pagana T: Mosby's Diagnostic and Laboratory Test Reference, ed 2. St Louis, Mosby–Year Book, 1995, p 120; and Garritan S, Jones P, Kornberg T, Parkin C: Laboratory values in the intensive care unit. Acute Care Perspectives, Newsletter of the Acute Care/Hospital Clinical Practice Section, APTA, winter 1995, p 7.

TABLE 35-22 Diagnostic Lumbar Puncture in Adults

Diseases detected with high sensitivity and high specificity
- Bacterial meningitis
- Tuberculous meningitis
- Fungal meningitis

Diseases detected with high sensitivity and moderate specificity
- Viral meningitis
- Subarachnoid hemorrhage
- Multiple sclerosis
- Neurosyphilis
- Infectious polyneuritis
- Paraspinal abscess

Diseases detected with moderate sensitivity and high specificity
- Meningeal malignancy

Diseases detected with moderate sensitivity and moderate specificity
- Intercranial hemorrhage
- Viral encephalitis

Other recognized indications for lumbar puncture
- Toxoplasmosis
- Amebic infections
- Aseptic meningitis
- Inflammatory neuropathies
- Metastatic brain tumors
- Normal pressure hydrocephalus
- Hepatic encephalopathy
- Systemic lupus erythematosus

Adapted from McConnell H: Current and future clinical utility of cerebrospinal fluid in neurology and psychiatry. *In* McConnell H, Bianchine J (eds): Cerebrospinal Fluid in Neurology and Psychiatry. London, Chapman & Hall, 1994, p 232.

with tetany and tumors of the diencephalon. Increased levels of calcium are seen in meningitis. Magnesium levels will drop in the person with meningitis and ischemic brain disorders. Increased levels of magnesium are seen after intracranial hemorrhage. CSF sodium levels normally change as the plasma levels change. Sodium levels can be out of proportion in the CSF in encephalomalacia and tuberculous meningitis. Elevated potassium levels are seen in neonatal hemorrhage, aspiration pneumonia, seizure disorders, and cardiac arrest.

BOX 35-3
Clinical Factors Affecting Cerebrospinal Fluid Composition

- Age
- Sex
- Height and weight
- Activity level, bed rest, hours slept prior to lumbar puncture
- Stress
- Diet
- Drugs
- Disease state
- Genetic, environmental, and experiential conditions

Adapted from Bianchine J, McConnell H: Composition of CSF. *In* McConnell H, Bianchine J (eds): Cerebrospinal Fluid in Neurology and Psychiatry. London, Chapman & Hall, 1994, p 70.

BOX 35-4
Factors Evaluated in Cerebrospinal Fluid

- Appearance
- Cells
- Inorganic compounds
- Acid-base status
- Organic compounds
  - Lactate
  - Glucose
  - Proteins
  - Immunoglobulins
  - Enzymes
  - Amino acids
  - Peptides, neuropeptides

The *acid-base* status of the CSF is an independent variable and does not parallel the acid-base levels present in the blood. Changes in respiration and alterations of cerebral blood flow such as ischemia, subarachnoid hemorrhage, and meningitis will alter the acid-base status of the CSF. In other words, metabolic changes in the CNS associated with brain injury can cause acidosis of the CSF.

Organic compounds are measured in the CSF and abnormal levels indicate pathologic conditions. Lactate plays an important role in regulation of cerebral blood flow. Increased levels in the CSF have been found in seizures, CNS cancers, traumatic brain injury, multiple sclerosis, and CNS infections. Decreased levels are seen in barbiturate coma and poliomyelitis. Any alteration in the glycolytic pathway may result in an increase in the lactate/pyruvate ratio. This response is seen in ischemia, subarachnoid hemorrhage, hypoxia, seizures, and meningitis.

Glucose concentrations in CSF usually parallel plasma levels, but have a 4-hour lag period. Decreased levels are seen as a result of subarachnoid hemorrhage, hypoglycemia, neoplastic or inflammatory infiltration of the meninges, and many forms of meningitis. The CSF normally has a low level of *proteins*, which is increased in a large variety of diseases. Blockage of CSF will result in increased protein levels.

Immunoglobulins, specifically IgG, are found in higher concentrations in multiple sclerosis and other inflammatory conditions. *Enzyme* levels in CSF reflect disease processes. Lactate dehydrogenase (LDH) is increased in meningitis, subarachnoid hemorrhage, leukemia, carcinoma, metastatic CNS cancer, hydrocephalus, epilepsy, and Huntington's disease. A more sensitive breakdown of the type of LDH is used to diagnose different types of meningitis.

Amino acids acting as neurotransmitters in CSF represent an important regulatory mechanism. Levels are increased in meningitis and in CSF blocks, and are decreased in multiple sclerosis. Abnormalities are found in Parkinson's disease and depression.

The CSF plays an important role in the transport of *peptides* to target areas of the brain. *Neuropeptides* (e.g., endorphins) are related to higher brain functions such as learning, memory, posture, and movement, as well as to pain mechanisms. Persons with phantom and neurogenic pain have been found to have low CSF endorphin levels.

Synovial Fluid Analysis

Arthrocentesis, the surgical puncture of a joint cavity for aspiration (withdrawal) of fluid, is performed by inserting a sterile needle into the joint space. Although the knee is the most commonly aspirated joint, arthrocentesis can be done on any major joint (e.g., shoulder, hip, elbow, wrist, ankle).

This test is performed for many different reasons, such as to establish the presence of infection, crystal-induced arthritis, synovitis, or neoplasms. This procedure is also used to identify the cause of joint effusion, to follow the progression of joint disease, and to inject anti-inflammatory medications (usually corticosteroids) into a joint area (Pagana and Pagana, 1995).

Once the fluid sample is obtained, it is examined microscopically and chemically. Normal joint fluid is clear, straw-colored, and viscous because of hyaluronic acid. Viscosity is reduced in people with inflammatory arthritis and the synovial fluid tends to drip like water; fluid of high viscosity forms a "string" several inches long. The *mucin clot* test correlates with the viscosity and is performed by adding acetic acid to joint fluid.

Cell counts are also performed including a WBC count (normal joint fluid contains less than 200/mm^3) and neutrophils (PMNs). A very high percentage of PMNs (greater than 75%) is found in most people with acute bacterial infectious arthritis (Table 35–23). The presence of crystals, which is usually associated with an inflammatory process, can be determined by examining the synovial fluid under polarized light. This test is used to differentiate between gout and pseudogout.

Pleural Fluid Analysis

Thoracentesis is an invasive procedure that requires surgical puncture with a needle (trocar) into the pleural space and drainage of the thoracic cavity. Pleural fluid may be removed as an aid to the diagnosis of inflammatory or neoplastic diseases of the lung or pleura, or it may be used as a therapeutic measure to remove accumulations of fluid from the thoracic cavity. It is performed therapeutically to relieve pain, dyspnea, and other symptoms of pleural pressure.

Pleural fluid is examined for gross appearance; cell counts; levels of protein LDH, glucose, and amylase; Gram stain and bacteriologic culture; and cultures for *Mycobacterium tuberculosis* and fungus. Cytologic study to detect tumor cells is performed with malignant effusions; breast, lung, and lymphoma are the three most common tumors.

Peritoneal Fluid Analysis

Paracentesis is the insertion of a trocar through a small surgical incision into the abdominal cavity for removal of fluid. This procedure may be performed diagnostically to remove and analyze fluid to determine the cause of the peritoneal effusion or therapeutically to remove large amounts of ascitic fluid from the abdominal cavity providing relief from symptoms of dyspnea, distention, and early satiety.

As with pleural fluid, peritoneal fluid is analyzed for gross appearance, RBCs, WBCs, protein, glucose, amylase, ammonia, alkaline phosphatase, LDH, cytology, bacteria, and fungi, as well as other appropriate tests (e.g., urea and creatinine if there is a question of bladder perforation or rupture).

Special Implications for the Therapist **35-10**

FLUID ANALYSIS

Cerebrospinal Fluid

Following lumbar puncture, the client is usually kept in a reclining position for up to 12 hours to avoid the spinal headache that can occur. The client can turn from side to side as long as the head is not lifted. Any report of numbness or tingling in the lower extremities or drainage of blood or CSF at the puncture site must be reported.

Synovial Fluid

After arthrocentesis, the therapist should assess the joint for any pain, fever, or swelling (i.e., indicators of infection). Ice can be applied to reduce pain and swelling and the pressure dressing should be kept on the joint to avoid further joint fluid collection or development of a hematoma. The client should avoid strenuous use of the joint for 48 to 72 hours.

Pleural Fluid

Following thoracentesis, the client is positioned on the unaffected side to rest the site of insertion and allow the puncture site to seal itself. Therapy is not usually performed until the wound has sealed itself; the therapist should check with nursing staff before proceeding with any therapy, especially manual therapy involving the thorax or chest physical therapy (breathing exercises can be initiated sooner than percussion or vibration). If the client has no complaints of dyspnea, normal activity can be resumed approximately 1 hour after the procedure.

Possible aftereffects of the procedure include

TABLE 35-23 CLASSIFICATION OF SYNOVIAL FLUID

	NORMAL	NONINFLAMMATORY	INFLAMMATORY	SEPTIC
Color	Colorless	Straw-colored	Yellow	Variable
Clarity	Transparent	Transparent	Translucent	Opaque
WBCs/mm^3	<200	200–2000	2000–75,000	>75,000
PMNs	<25%	<25%	40%–75%	>75%
Culture	—	—	—	May be +
Crystals	—	—	May be +	—
Examples		Osteoarthritis, trauma, aseptic necrosis, SLE	RA, gout, pseudogout, SLE, seronegative spondyloarthropathies	Bacterial infection, tuberculosis

WBCs, white blood cells; PMNs, neutrophils; RA, rheumatoid arthritis; SLE, systemic lupus erythematosus.
From Koopmeiners MB: Laboratory evaluation for the physical therapist. Presented at Combined Section Meeting, Atlanta, Feb. 15–18, 1996.

pneumothorax, accumulation of air in the tissues of the skin (subcutaneous emphysema), and bacterial infection. Report any signs of dizziness, changes in skin color, and respiratory and heart rate changes. Other signs of complications following thoracentesis include anxiety, fever, restlessness, excessive coughing, blood-tinged sputum, and tightness of the chest. Assess lung sounds for diminished breath sounds, a possible sign of pneumothorax.

Peritoneal Fluid

Following paracentesis, the therapist must watch for signs of hypotension if a large volume of fluid was removed. Vital signs must be monitored for any evidence of hemodynamic changes and any signs of continued drainage, bleeding, or inflammation at the puncture site must be reported. If albumin infusions are ordered after a paracentesis (to compensate for the protein loss—ascitic fluid has a high protein content), the therapist must also monitor for signs of protein and electrolyte (especially sodium) imbalance.

Paracentesis may precipitate hepatic coma in someone with chronic liver disease. The therapist should observe for any indications of shock (e.g., pallor, cyanosis, dizziness), which would constitute an emergency situation.

References

Boissonnault WG, Koopmeiners MB: Medical history profile: Orthopaedic physical therapy outpatients. J Orthop Sports Phys Ther 20:2–10, 1994.

Eaks GA, Cassmeyer V: Management of persons with diabetes mellitus and hypoglycemia. *In* Phipps W, Cassmeyer VL, Sands JK, Lehman MK (eds): Medical-Surgical Nursing: Concepts and Clinical Practice, ed 5. St Louis, Mosby–Year Book, 1995, pp 1281–1354.

Egloff ME: Assessment of clients with respiratory disorders. *In* Black JM, Matassarin-Jacobs E (eds): Luckmann and Sorensen's Medical-Surgical Nursing, ed 4. Philadelphia, WB Saunders, 1993, pp 913–940.

Fischbach F: A Manual of Laboratory and Diagnostic Tests, ed 5. Philadelphia, Lippincott-Raven, 1995.

Garritan S, Jones P, Kornberg T, Parkin C: Laboratory values in the intensive care unit. Acute Care Perspectives, Newsletter of the Acute Care/Hospital Clinical Practice Section, APTA, winter 1995, pp 7–11.

Grant J: Corticosteroid side effects: Implications for PT. PT Magazine 2:56–60, 1994.

Griffen JE: Dynamic tests of endocrine function. *In* Wilson JD, Foster DW (eds): Williams Textbook of Endocrinology, ed 8. Philadelphia, WB Saunders, 1992.

Grossman LA, Kaplan HJ, Ownby FD, Grossman M: Carpal tunnel syndrome—Initial manifestations of systemic disease. JAMA 176:259–261, 1961.

Hillegass E, Sadowsky S: Essentials of Cardiopulmonary Physical Therapy. Philadelphia, WB Saunders, 1994.

Kost GJ: Critical limits for urgent clinician notification at US medical centers. JAMA 263:704–707, 1990.

McConnell H, Rillstone D: Lumbar puncture. *In* McConnell H, Bianchine J (eds): Cerebrospinal Fluid in Neurology and Psychiatry. London, Chapman & Hall, 1994, pp 43–56.

Owen A: Tracking the rise and fall of cardiac enzymes. Nursing95 25:35–44, 1995.

Pagana KD, Pagana TJ: Mosby's Diagnostic and Laboratory Test Reference, ed 2. St Louis, Mosby–Year Book, 1995.

Phalen GS: The carpal tunnel syndrome: Seventeen years' experience in diagnosis and treatment of six hundred and fifty-four hands. J Bone Joint Surg [Am] 48:211–228, 1966.

Phipps WJ, Cassmeyer VL, Sands JK, et al: Medical-Surgical Nursing, ed 5. St Louis, Mosby–Year Book, 1995, p 767.

Polich S, Faynor SM: Interpreting lab test values. PT Magazine 4:76–88, 1996.

Siconolfi LA: Clarifying the complexity of liver function test. Nursing95 25:39–44, 1995.

Vanscoy G, Krause JR: Warfarin and the international normalized ratio: Reducing interlaboratory effects. DICP 25:1190–1192, 1991.

Watchie J: Cardiopulmonary Physical Therapy: A Clinical Guide. Philadelphia, WB Saunders, 1995.

White C: Medications and the elderly. *In* Carnevali DL, Patrick M (eds): Nursing Management for the Elderly, ed 3. Philadelphia, JB Lippincott, 1993, pp 171–191.

Wilder-Smith A: Various factors affecting the composition of CSF. *In* McConnell H, Bianchine J (eds): Cerebrospinal Fluid in Neurology and Psychiatry. London, Chapman & Hall, 1994, pp 57–80.

appendix A

Summary of Universal Precautions*

SOURCES OF POTENTIAL EXPOSURE FOR THE THERAPIST

Universal precautions are intended to prevent occupational transmission of infectious diseases such as tuberculosis, human immunodeficiency virus (HIV), and hepatitis B virus (HBV). Therapists at greatest risk include those who perform electromyographic studies, therapists in direct contact with clients with tuberculosis (see also Table 12–7), and therapists who provide decubitus or pressure ulcer care, treat open wounds, handle bandages and dressings, and assess or treat temporomandibular joint (TMJ) disorder.

Any therapist who assists in toileting or changing diapers (in adults or children) is at increased risk. Other risk factors include human bites, contact with sputum and pleural fluid tinged with blood, or exposure to bloodborne pathogens when working with hospice clients who have acquired immunodeficiency syndrome (AIDS).

MODE OF TRANSMISSION

Although the potential for HBV transmission in the workplace is greater than that for HIV, the modes of transmission for these two viruses are similar. Both have been transmitted in occupational settings *only* by percutaneous inoculation or contact with an open wound; nonintact skin (e.g., cutaneous scratches; chapped, abraded, weeping, burned, or dermatitic skin); or bloody mucous membranes, blood-contaminated body fluids, or concentrated virus. *Blood is the single most important source of HIV and HBV in the workplace.*

In the hospital and other health-care settings, universal precautions should be followed when workers are exposed to blood, certain other body fluids (amniotic fluid, pericardial fluid, peritoneal fluid, pleural fluid, synovial fluid, cerebrospinal fluid, semen, and vaginal secretions), or any body fluid visibly contaminated with blood.[1] These fluids are most likely to transmit HIV. The hepatitis B vaccine substantially reduces the risk of infection and should be available to all employees who have occupational exposure to the virus.

GUIDELINES FOR INFECTED HEALTH-CARE WORKERS

Any health-care worker with HIV or the most virulent form of hepatitis B should not perform "exposure-prone" procedures, in which blood contact might occur. Permission and guidance from special review committees are required before an infected health-care worker can perform such procedures. For the therapist, this would primarily exclude wound care, including debridement and dressing changes. According to guidelines drafted by the Centers for Disease Control and Prevention, at a minimum, the potential client must be informed of the worker's HIV or hepatitis B status.

Barrier Precautions

- All health-care workers should routinely use appropriate barrier precautions to prevent skin and mucous membrane exposure when contact with blood or other body fluids of any person is anticipated.
- Gloves should be worn for touching blood and body fluids, mucous membranes, and nonintact skin of all persons.
- Gloves should be changed and hands washed after contact with each client.
- Apply hand cream after glove removal to prevent skin chapping, which is a potential risk factor for employees. Do not use petroleum-based hand creams or lotions, which can damage latex gloves.
- Masks and protective eyewear or face shields should be worn during procedures that are likely to generate droplets of blood or other body fluids, to prevent exposure of mucous membranes of the mouth, nose, and eyes. See also Guidelines for Therapists for Preventing Transmission of Tuberculosis (Table 12–7) for additional information regarding specific protective masks to wear with the client who has active tuberculosis.
- Fluid-proof gowns or aprons should be worn during procedures that are likely to generate splashes of blood or other body fluids.
- Wash hands before and after client contact, after removing personal protective equipment and gloves, and immediately if hands are grossly contaminated with blood.
- Hands and other skin surfaces should be washed immediately and thoroughly if contaminated with blood or other body fluids. Hands should be washed immediately after gloves are removed. Antiseptic hand cleaner should be used when handwashing facilities are unavailable.
- Sharp instruments, such as scissors or scalpels, should be handled with great care and disposed of in puncture-resistant containers. Needles should never be manipulated, bent, broken, or recapped.
- Pocket masks or mechanical ventilation devices should be available in areas in which cardiopulmonary resuscitation procedures are likely.
- Health-care workers who have exudative lesions or weeping dermatitis should refrain from all direct client care and from handling equipment belonging to the client until the condition resolves.
- Avoid eating, drinking, or smoking in (work) areas in which a potential exists for occupational exposure to hepatitis B virus.

Reference

Kriger JN, Coombs RW, Collier AC, et al: Intermittent shedding of human immunodeficiency virus in semen: Implications for sexual transmission. J Urol 154:1035–1040, 1995.

* Adapted from Centers for Disease Control Guidelines for prevention of HIV and hepatitis B virus transmission to health care and public safety workers. MMWR 38:51–56, 1989.

[1] HBV can be transmitted through infected saliva, but saliva has not been implicated in HIV tranmission except in the dental setting, in which saliva may be contaminated with blood. HBV and HIV transmission has not been documented from exposure to other body fluids, such as nasal secretions, sweat, tears, urine, or vomitus. However, universal precautions still apply whenever handling any body secretions. People who are sexually active should be aware that HIV is intermittently shed in semen (Krieger et al., 1995).

appendix B

Guidelines for Activity and Exercise*

Frequently, older adults with orthopedic dysfunction are inactive, hypertensive, and have multiple risk factors for coronary artery disease. These factors often are not documented and the client is treated as an "orthopedic patient" without regard for the past medical history or current cardiopulmonary condition. For these reasons, the health-care provider must view the effect of other systems on the client's orthopedic condition and rehabilitation outcome. A thorough evaluation may be necessary, and monitoring cardiopulmonary responses to exercise may be required.

Exercise should be specific to the functional and medical needs of each individual. Whenever possible, activity and exercise should be at a level that causes minimal to no symptoms, and progression should be built into the program. For the elderly, physiologic homeostasis may be altered by stress, medications, illness, and exercise. To assist in balancing and maintaining homeostasis, 1 day of rest between each day of exercise is recommended. Common drugs with side effects that may affect an exercise program are listed in Table B–1. Persons who are taking drugs that can cause volume depletion or orthostatic hypotension should have blood pressure and pulse checked in both reclining and standing positions.

Interval training, consisting of short-term periods of ambulation followed by rest, is now recommended (McArdle et al., 1991). Such a program activates the oxygen transport to skeletal and circulatory systems for completion of an ADL activity to develop endurance. Progress slowly by increasing duration to 30 minutes before increasing intensity. Encourage the client to maintain an exercise diary that includes any symptoms that may occur during or after exercise. Review the diary and compare this report to the client's verbal report, as the person may forget or deny important information.

GUIDELINES FOR AQUATIC THERAPY

The hydrostatic pressure of the water may give the body a false impression of increased fluid volume; therefore, individuals will demonstrate lower resting and working heart rates. However, warm pool water temperature combined with the environmental temperature and buildup of body heat through exercise can cause overheating, because the body cannot diffuse the additional heat. In such cases, vital signs may increase. No change should occur in blood pressure in a chest-deep pool when the client's upper extremities remain inactive.

Pool therapy is not recommended for high-risk cardiac clients, for 0 to 6 weeks after myocardial infarction, or in the presence of arrhythmias, especially ventricular fibrillations (the latter requires exercise testing before beginning a pool program; lethal arrhythmias can have serious consequences in a pool setting). Whenever exercise test results are available, compare heart rate in the water to exercise test measures. Work at safe heart rate levels as determined by the exercise testing.

GUIDELINES FOR MONITORING VITAL SIGNS

It is important to know normal responses to movement and activity (including exercise) to be able to identify abnormal responses in the client with a medical diagnosis. Safe and effective exercise can be measured in part by monitoring vital sign responses. Such data can be used as specific outcome measures to substantiate decision making. For example, how quickly the heart rate returns to normal is an outcome measurement of fitness and conditioning.

Anyone with a significant past medical history of cardiovascular or pulmonary disease requires monitoring of vital signs and perceived exertion during exercise. The more coronary risk factors present (see Table 10–2), the greater the need for monitoring. For any client with known coronary artery disease and/or previous history of myocardial infarction, exercise testing should be performed before an exercise program is undertaken. If this testing has not been accomplished and baseline measurements are unavailable for use in planning exercise, the therapist must monitor the client's heart rate and blood pressure and note any accompanying symptoms during exercise. Too rapid a rise in heart rate, respiratory rate, or blood pressure for the workload is a general guideline for modifying the activity or exercise program (see later discussion: Abnormal Heart Rate and Abnormal Respiratory Rate).

Heart Rate (Pulse Rate)

The normal range for the resting pulse rate is 60 to 100 beats/min (BPM). A rate above 100 beats/min indicates *tachycardia;* below 60 beats/min indicates *bradycardia*. Some variations occur with age and training (Table B–2). For example, a well-trained athlete whose heart muscle develops along with the skeletal muscle may have a resting heart rate less than 60 beats/min. The force of the pulse represents the strength of the heart's stroke volume. A "weak, thready" pulse reflects a decreased stroke volume, such as occurs with hemorrhagic shock. A "full, bounding" pulse indicates an increased stroke volume, possibly associated with anxiety, exercise, or some pathologic condition. The pulse force (pulse amplitude) is recorded using a three-point scale as follows (some physicians/nurses use a four-point scale) (Jarvis, 1992):

3+ Full, bounding
2+ Normal
1+ Weak, thready
0 Absent

The pulse should be measured before and during the activity using the same position both times. Count for 6 seconds and add a 0 to that number for a beats-per-minute count or count for 10 seconds and multiply by 6. Heart rate (HR) response should increase gradually with an increase in the workload of the heart. Once a steady state has been achieved, little change should occur in heart rate during sustained endurance activities (e.g., water aerobics, riding a stationary bicycle). Factors affecting heart rate responses are listed in Box B–1.

Heart rate responses are different in the *deconditioned* person because the resting heart rate is higher to begin with. The heart rate increases more rapidly for the same workload when compared to the change in a healthy individual. A rapid heart rate may occur during activity in response to *dehydration*, as the decreased plasma volume results in decreased blood volume and subsequent decreased blood to the heart. A decreased stroke volume (volume ejected per heartbeat) is compensated for by a higher heart rate to match the demands for oxygen by the activity. *Cardiac muscle dysfunction* is the term used when a decreased stroke volume occurs as a result of a diseased cardiac muscle that can no longer contract and pump blood out of the heart normally. Decreased stroke volume results in a more rapid rise in heart rate.

Aging is accompanied by a decreasing maximum heart rate. A guideline for calculating the predicted maximum heart rate (PMHR) is PMHR = 220 − age. For example, for a 70-year-old the PMHR = 220 − 70, or 150 beats/min. For the active, healthy older adult, PMHR = 205 − 1/2 age (Sidney and Shephard, 1977). For example, evaluating the same 70-year-old under these conditions would be 205 − 1/2(70), or 205 − 35, or PMHR = 170.

These formulas cannot be used for the client taking β-blockers for hypertension and angina. β-blockers are medications that block the sympathetic nervous system's input to the β_1-receptors in the heart, therefore affecting heart rate and contractility. The net effect is a decrease in the resting and exercise heart rate (drug-induced bradycardia). Anyone taking these medications may not be able to achieve a target heart rate (THR) above 90 beats/min. A safe rate of exercise will allow the heart rate to return to the resting level 2 minutes after stopping exercise. Avoid increases of more

* Data from Hillegass E, Sadowsky S: Essentials of Cardiovascular Physical Therapy. Philadelphia, WB Saunders, 1994; and Hillegass E: Are You Prescribing Exercise Safely? Activity and Exercise for Patients with Medical Diagnoses. Montana Physical Therapy Association Spring Meeting, May 19–20, 1995.

TABLE B–1 Common Drugs that May Affect an Exercise Program

Drugs	Effects
Tranquilizers	Orthostasis and falls
Antihypertensive agents	Orthostasis and falls Reduced exercise capacity (β-blockers)
Diuretics	Hypokalemia—arrhythmias, muscle cramps Dehydration—orthostasis and falls, thermoregulatory disturbance
Antidepressants	Orthostasis and falls, arrhythmias
Insulin, oral hypoglycemics	Hypoglycemia
β-Adrenergic blockers	Decreased heart rate, fatigue, masking of hypoglycemic symptoms

From Wheat ME, Lowenthal DT: Exercise. *In* Abrams WB, Berkow R (eds): The Merck Manual of Geriatrics. Rahway, NJ, Merck & Co, 1990, p 281.

TABLE B–2 Normal Resting Pulse Rates Across Age Groups

Age	Average Beats/min	Normal Limits (Beats/min)
Newborn	120	70–190
1 yr	120	80–160
2 yr	110	80–130
4 yr	100	80–120
6 yr	100	75–115
8–10 yr	90	70–110
12 yr		
Female	90	70–110
Male	85	65–105
14 yr		
Female	85	65–105
Male	80	60–100
16 yr		
Female	80	60–100
Male	75	55–95
18 yr		
Female	75	55–95
Male	70	50–90
Well-conditioned athlete	May be 50–60	50–100
Adult	—	60–100
Aging	—	60–100

Adapted from Jarvis C: Physical Examination and Assessment. Philadelphia, WB Saunders, 1992, p 202.

BOX B–1
Factors Affecting Heart Rate

- Aging
- Anemia
- Autonomic dysfunction (e.g., diabetes, spinal cord injury)
- Caffeine
- Cardiac muscle dysfunction
- Deconditioned state
- Dehydration (decreased blood volume causes increased heart rate)
- Drugs (e.g., blood pressure medication; asthma inhalants; antihistamines, such as over-the-counter cold medications)
- Emotional or psychological stress
- Fear
- Fever
- Hyperthyroidism
- Infection
- Pain
- Sleep disturbances/sleep deprivation

than 20 beats/min over resting heart rate. (See Exercise and Antihypertensive Medications, Chapter 10.)

Abnormal Heart Rate Response. If the pulse is irregular, count the pulse for a full minute and document the number of beats per minute as well as the number of irregular beats (see next section). Abnormal heart rate responses include a rapid rate of rise in heart rate (judging the activity, age, and training history) or a decreased heart rate with activity (e.g., arrhythmias or pauses in pulse).

A decreased heart rate with activity may occur as a normal response when the person is sympathetically overloaded prior to treatment. For example the person who takes inhalants for asthma just before therapy or who drinks more than 3 cups of coffee within 2 hours of the therapy appointment may have an artificially elevated baseline heart rate response. Over the course of therapy without further stimulation, this person's heart rate may decrease, especially if the therapy session has no exercise component. Factors such as these require individual evaluation of abnormal responses for each person.

Pulse amplitude (weak or bounding quality of the pulse) that fades with inspiration and strengthens with expiration is *paradoxic* and should be reported to the physician (Keene, 1993). A pulse increase of over 20 beats/min lasting for more than 3 minutes after rest or changing position should also be reported.

Heart Rhythm

For the person with an abnormal heart rhythm, palpate the pulse throughout the activity if no electrocardiogram (ECG) or Holter monitor reading is available during exercise. If any abnormal pulse beats are noted (e.g., absent, irregular), count the number of pauses per minute at rest and during activity. There should be no more than 6 abnormal or absent beats per minute. The normal heart rhythm should not change, and individuals with arrhythmias at rest should not show an increase in number of irregular heartbeats with increased activity.

If ischemia occurs as evidenced by angina or (on visual readout) depression of ECG ST-segment (see Fig. 4–2), the person should rest and then return to an activity level below ischemic level. For example, if the ST-segment drops below baseline with activity or the client experiences angina when the heart rate is at 140 beats/min, then reduce the activity level so that the heart rate remains below 140 beats/min.

Respiratory Rate

Normal respiratory rates are presented in Table B–3. The ratio of pulse rate to respiratory rate is fairly constant (4 : 1). The respirations can be counted at the same time that the pulse is counted. If an abnormality is suspected, these measurements should be taken for a full minute. A normal pulmonary response to exercise is an increase in breathing rate and depth based on body type and disease present. Factors that can affect respiratory rate (RR) include the following:

- Altered lung compliance (chronic obstructive pulmonary disease, hyaline membrane disease)

TABLE B-3 NORMAL RESPIRATORY RATES

AGE	BREATHS/MIN
Neonate	30–40
1 yr	20–40
2 yr	25–32
4 yr	23–30
6 yr	21–26
8–10 yr	20–26
12–14 yr	18–22
16 yr	16–20
18 yr	12–20
Adult	10–20

Adapted from Jarvis C: Physical Examination and Health Assessment. Philadelphia, WB Saunders, 1992, p 203.

- Airway resistance (asthma)
- Alterations in lung volumes/lung capacity (smokers, persons with emphysema or occupational lung disease)
- Body position (diaphragm cannot drop down enough to expand the lungs in the fully supine position for the pregnant or obese client)

Abnormal Respiratory Rate Response. An abnormal respiratory rate response is usually characterized by too rapid a rise in respiratory rate for the activity and medical condition of the client. Measuring the respiratory rate may be difficult. Observe how much work is required to breathe, and whenever possible, use a pulse oximeter to measure arterial oxygen saturation noninvasively (Fig. B–1). Using a pulse oximeter with the pulmonary population can provide an outcome measure with exercise for documentation. Normal oxygen saturation is 98%, with no change in this measurement during activity or exercise. Clients with chronic respiratory disease may experience a drop in oxygen saturation that is considered "normal" for them, but this represents a normal response to pathology and is not truly "normal."

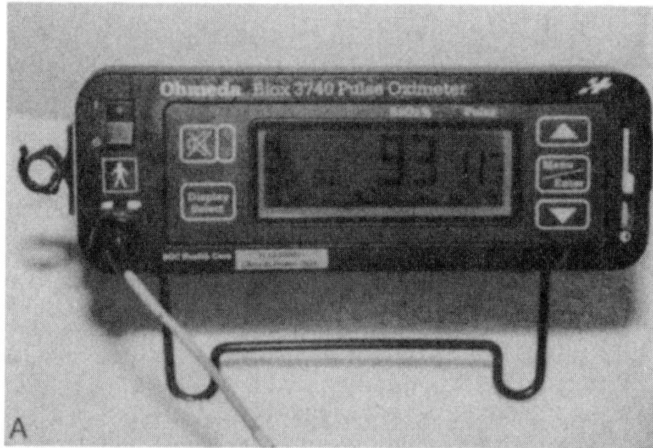

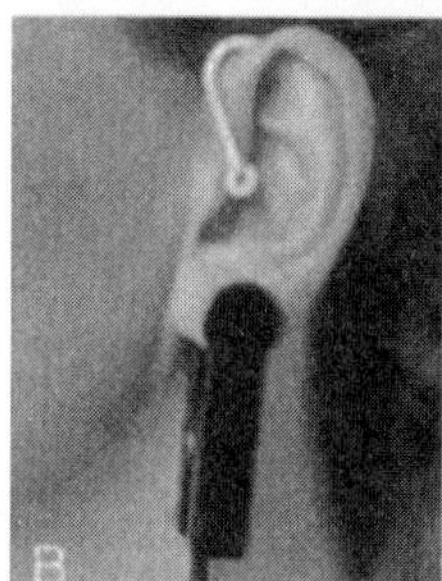

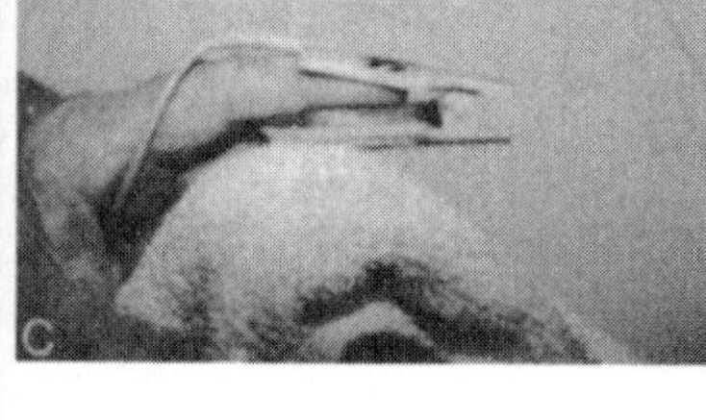

Figure **B–1.** Noninvasive monitoring of oxygen saturation (SaO_2) can be done with a pulse oximeter. This unit (*A*) has an ear probe (*B*) and a finger probe (*C*). The ear probe is used most often to measure oxygen saturation during exercise; the finger probe is used most frequently during stationary activities. (*Courtesy of Ohmeda, Boulder, Colo.*)

Blood Pressure

To monitor effectively, the therapist must be familiar with normal and abnormal blood pressure (BP) responses to exercise and must keep in mind that arterial blood pressure is a general indicator of the function of the heart as a pump and a measure of the peripheral arterial resistance. Systolic pressure measures the force exerted against the arteries during the ejection cycle, and diastolic pressure measures the force exerted against the arteries during rest.

Systolic blood pressure normally rises with increased exertion in proportion to the workload (approximately 7 to 10 mm Hg per MET[1]) with little or no change in diastolic blood pressure (American Heart Association, 1975), and it rises more quickly in males than in females. For example, during endurance activities, the systolic blood pressure gradually increases, but with sustained activity no further change should occur. Exercise involving a small total muscle mass, such as a single extremity, typically elicits minimal incremental changes in systolic blood pressure and greater increases in diastolic blood pressure (Blomquist et al., 1981).

Diastolic blood pressure may increase or decrease a maximum of 10 mm Hg due to adaptive dilatation of peripheral vasculature. A highly trained athlete may exhibit more than a 10 mm Hg drop in diastolic blood pressure as a result of increased vasodilation, but this would be considered an abnormal response in an older or untrained adult. A sustained elevation of the diastolic blood pressure during the recovery phase of activity is also considered abnormal. More specific abnormal responses to activity are discussed in detail elsewhere (Hillegass and Sadowsky, 1994).

If the resting blood pressure is excessively high (systolic blood pressure >200 mm Hg or diastolic blood pressure >105 to 110 mm Hg), physician clearance should be obtained before continuing with evaluation or treatment. Exercise should be terminated if blood pressure becomes excessively high (systolic blood pressure >250 mm Hg or diastolic blood pressure >110 mm Hg) (American College of Sports Medicine, 1991).

Always measure in the same position as the blood pressure can drop quickly with cessation of activity (i.e., do not measure blood pressure while the client is sitting, then ambulate, and recheck blood pressure in the standing position; measure in the standing position, ambulate, and remeasure while standing). In fact, because blood pressure changes can occur within 10 seconds, a truly accurate postexercise blood pressure may be difficult to obtain. Always observe for associated symptoms, such as shortness of breath, dizziness, palpitations, or increase in heart rate.

Abnormal Response. An abnormal blood pressure response may result in hypotension or hypertension as reflected by any of the following responses:

- Too rapid a rise in systolic blood pressure for the workload
- Very little change in systolic blood pressure with excessive workload in an unfit or deconditioned person
- Progressive rise of diastolic blood pressure
- Drop of more than 10 mm Hg in diastolic blood pressure
- Drop in systolic pressure (or both systolic and diastolic pressure) of 10 to 20 mm Hg or more associated with an increase in pulse rate of more than 15 beats/min (depleted intravascular volume)

An *increase* in diastolic blood pressure of 20 mm Hg or more may be a sign that the person has exceeded cardiac reserve capacity and that blood flow to the liver, kidney, and digestive tract has been critically reduced (Amundsen, 1979). A *decrease* in diastolic blood pressure may occur as a result of rapid vasodilation, an effect of training in the athletic individual. A drop in diastolic blood pressure may also indicate normalization in a hypertensive individual as a result of vasodilation and decreased peripheral resistance. For example, this may occur if the hypertensive person experiences a calming effect as a result of participating in a regular routine of exercise

[1] The metabolic equivalent system (METS) provides one way of measuring the amount of oxygen needed to perform an activity: 1 MET = 3.5 mL of oxygen uptake, which a person requires when resting.

BOX B-2
Factors Affecting Blood Pressure

- Age
- Blood vessel size
- Blood viscosity
- Force of heart contraction
- Medications
- Diet
- Time of recent meal (increases systolic pressure)
- Caffeine
- Nicotine
- Alcohol
- Anxiety
- Presence or perceived degree of pain
- Living at higher altitudes
- Distended urinary bladder

after driving in heavy traffic to get to the clinic on time. Other factors that affect blood pressure are listed in Box B–2.

References

American College of Sports Medicine: Guidelines for Graded Exercise Testing and Exercise Prescription, ed 4. Philadelphia, Lea & Febiger, 1991.

American Heart Association Committee on Exercise: Exercise Testing and Training of Individuals with Heart Disease or at High Risk for its Development: A Handbook for Physicians. Dallas, American Heart Association, 1975.

Amundsen LR: Assessing exercise tolerance: A review. Phys Ther 59:534–537, 1979.

Blomquist CG, Lewis SF, Taylor WF, et al: Similarity of the hemodynamic responses to static and dynamic exercise of small muscle groups. Circ Res 48 (suppl):187–190, 1981.

Hillegass E, Sadowsky S: Essentials of Cardiopulmonary Physical Therapy. Philadelphia, WB Saunders, 1994.

Hillegass E: Are You Prescribing Exercise Safely? Activity and Exercise for Patients with Medical Diagnoses. Montana Physical Therapy Association Spring Meeting, Billings, MT May 19–20, 1995.

Jarvis C: Physical Examination and Health Assessment. Philadelphia, WB Saunders, 1992.

Keene A: Physical examination. *In* Black JM, Matassarin-Jacobs E (eds): Luckmann and Sorensen's Medical-Surgical Nursing, ed 4. Philadelphia, WB Saunders, 1993, pp 215–246.

McArdle WD, Katch FI, Katch VL: Exercise Physiology, ed 3. Philadelphia, Lea & Febiger, 1991.

Sidney KH, Shephard RJ: Maximum and submaximum exercise tests in men and women in 7th, 8th, and 9th decades of life. J Appl Physiol 43:280–287, 1977.

index

Note: Page numbers in *italics* indicate figures; page numbers followed by b indicate boxed material; and page numbers followed by t indicate tables.

A

B

C

E

F

G

H

I

J

K

L

M

N

O

R

T

X

ISBN 0-7216-5636-6